Strauss & Mayer's
EMERGENCY DEPARTMENT MANAGEMENT
2nd Edition

Chief Editors

Robert W. Strauss, MD, FACEP
Chief Medical Training Officer, TeamHealth
Knoxville, Tennessee
The Christ Hospital, Dept. of Emergency Medicine
Cincinnati, Ohio
Director, ED Directors Academy
American College of Emergency Physicians
Senior Director, American Board of Emergency Medicine

Thom A. Mayer, MD, FACEP, FAAP, FACHE
Medical Director, NFL Players Association
Founder, BestPractices Inc.
CEO, Survival Skills Solutions
Clinical Professor of Emergency Medicine
George Washington University School of Medicine
Senior Lecturing Fellow
Duke University School of Medicine

Senior Associate Editor

Kirk Jensen, MD, MBA, FACEP
President and CEO, Healthcare Management Strategies LLC
Faculty Member, Institute for Healthcare Improvement (IHI)
Faculty Member, Healthcare Leadership Master's Program, Wake Forest University Graduate School of Arts & Sciences

Associate Editors

James J. Augustine, MD, FACEP
Clinical Professor of Emergency Medicine, Wright State University
Chair, National Clinical Governance Board, US Acute Care Solutions
Vice President of the Emergency Department Benchmarking Alliance

Jean A. Proehl, RN, MN, CEN, CPEN, TCRN, FAEN, FAAN
Emergency Clinical Nurse Specialist, Proehl PRN LLC
Emergency Nurse, Dartmouth-Hitchcock Medical Center
and Gifford Medical Center

Sandra M. Schneider MD, FACEP
Associate Executive Director for Clinical Affairs, American College of Emergency Physicians
Adjunct Professor of Emergency Medicine, University of Pittsburgh
Attending Physician, John Peter Smith Hospital

Section Editors

Sherri-Lynne Almeida, DrPH, MSN, MEd, RN, CEN, FAEN
Nurse Executive Ambulatory Care
Michael E. DeBakey Veterans Affairs Medical Center

Robert A. Bitterman, MD, JD, FACEP
President, Bitterman Health Law Consulting Group

Michael Jay Bresler, MD, FACEP
Clinical Professor of Emergency Medicine
Stanford University School of Medicine

Kathleen J. Clem, MD, FACEP
Professor of Emergency Medicine
Dartmouth Geisel School of Medicine

Jody Crane, MD, MBA, FACEP
Chief Medical Officer, TeamHealth
Faculty, Institute for Healthcare Improvement
Adjunct Professor, University of Tennessee

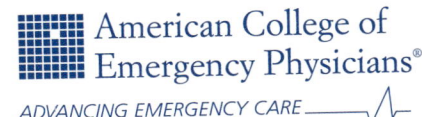

Paula Fessler, RN, BSN, MSN, MS, FNP-BC
Board Member, American Academy of Emergency Nurse Practitioners
Senior Vice President and Chief Nurse Executive
Westchester Medical Center

Michael Gerardi, MD, FAAP, FACEP
Director, Pediatric Emergency Services, Atlantic Health System
Attending Physician, Department of Emergency Medicine, Morristown Medical Center
Associate Clinical Professor of Emergency Medicine, Icahn School of Medicine at Mount Sinai
Past President, American College of Emergency Physicians

Michael A. Granovsky, MD, FACEP
President, LogixHealth
Adjunct Professor of Emergency Medicine
George Washington University

Dan Hanfling, MD
Vice President, Technical Staff, In-Q-Tel
Co-chair, National Academy of Medicine, Forum on Medical and Public Health Preparedness
Clinical Professor of Emergency Medicine, George Washington University
Attending Physician, Inova Fairfax Hospital

Jim Hoelz, MS, MBA, RN, CEN, FAEN
Founder and CEO, Hoelz Healthcare Consulting

Reneé Seminon Holleran, NP-BC, RN-BC, PhD, CEN, CFRN, CTRN (retired), CCRN (alumnus), FAEN
Emergency Medicine, Salt Lake City
Veterans Affairs, Salt Lake City Health Care System
Former Editor, *Journal of Emergency Nursing and Air Medical Journal*
Editorial Board, *Advanced Emergency Nursing Journal*

Gabor D. Kelen, MD, FRCP(C), FACEP, FAAEM
Professor and Director, Department of Emergency Medicine
Director, Center for the Study of Preparedness and Catastrophic Event Response
Director, Critical Event Preparedness and Response
Professor of Anesthesiology and Critical Care Medicine
Johns Hopkins Medicine

Patricia Kunz Howard, PhD, RN, CEN, CPEN, TCRN, NE-BC, FAEN, FAAN
Enterprise Director, Emergency Services
University of Kentucky Healthcare
Past President, Emergency Nurses Association

John McCabe, MD, FACEP
Professor and Chair Emeritus, Department of Emergency Medicine
SUNY Upstate Medical University

Fred Neis, MS, RN, CEN, FACHE, FAEN
Vice President of Strategic Partnerships, Lumeris

Ryan Oglesby, PhD, MHA, RN, CEN, CFRN, NEA-BC
Principal/Global Lead for the Emergency Department and Patient Throughput Assessments
Healthcare Transformation Services, Philips

AnnMarie Papa, DNP, RN, CEN, NE-BC, FAEN, FAAN
Vice President and Chief Nursing Officer
Einstein Medical Center, Montgomery

Randy Pilgrim MD, FACEP, FAAFP
Enterprise Chief Medical Officer
Emergency Medicine Physician
SCP Health

John Proctor, MD, MBA, FACEP, FAAP
Clinical Executive Consultant, Sound Physicians Emergency Medicine
CEO, Enterprise Healthcare Consulting LLC
Clinical Assistant Professor of Emergency Medicine
University of Tennessee Health Science Center

Ali S. Raja, MD, MBA, MPH
Executive Vice Chair, Department of Emergency Medicine
Massachusetts General Hospital
Professor of Emergency Medicine
Harvard Medical School

Nathaniel R. Schlicher, MD, JD, MBA, FACEP
Regional Director of Quality Assurance
TeamHealth Northwest

Steven J. Stack, MD, MBA, FACEP
Adjunct Professor
University of Tennessee Haslam College of Business
Past President of the American Medical Association

Fred "Kip" Wenger, DO, FACOEP, FACEP
Regional Performance Director, TeamHealth

Aaron Wolff, MBA, RN, CEN, PHN
President, Vital Operations Consulting

Publisher's Notice

The American College of Emergency Physicians (ACEP) makes every effort to ensure that contributors and editors of its publication are knowledgeable subject matter experts and that they used their best efforts to ensure accuracy of the content. However, it is the responsibility of each reader to personally evaluate the content and judge its suitability for use in his or her medical practice in the care of a particular patient. Readers are advised that the statements and opinions expressed in this publication are provided as recommendations of the contributors and editors at the time of publication and should not be construed as official College policy. ACEP acknowledges that, as new medical knowledge emerges, best practice recommendations can change faster than published content can be updated. ACEP recognizes the complexity of emergency medicine and makes no representation that this publication serves as an authoritative resource for the prevention, diagnosis, treatment, or intervention for any medical condition, nor should it be used as the basis for the definition of or the standard of care that should be practiced by all health care providers at any particular time or place. To the fullest extent permitted by law, and without limitation, ACEP expressly disclaims all liability for errors or omissions contained within this publication, and for damages of any kind or nature, arising out of use, reference to, reliance on, or performance of such information.

Copyright 2021, American College of Emergency Physicians, Dallas, Texas. All rights reserved. Printed in the United States of America. Except as permitted under the United States Copyright Act of 1976, no part of this publication may be reproduced or distributed in any form or by any means or stored in a database or retrieval system without prior written permission of the publisher. Email us to request permission to reproduce these materials.

To contact ACEP, call 844-381-0911, or 972-550-0911, or write to PO Box 619911, Dallas, TX 75261-9911. Your comments and suggestions are always welcome.

First printing 2014

ISBN 978-1-7366733-0-0

Dedications

To my wonderful wife, Phyllis Bossin, who views life with astonishing clarity and passion and enriches mine every day; to my children, Bo Strauss and Shelby Strauss Demody, for whom I have the utmost love and admiration; to my sisters Susan Stark, my friend and confidant, and Nancy Dale, for always providing insight and perspective; to my late parents Bob and Aileen, for their remarkable intellects and emotional intelligence; and to Aaron and Lauren Bossin Kull, I am grateful that you are part of my family.

Robert W. Strauss

To my brilliant, beautiful, and forever-inspiring wife, Maureen; to our three kind, generous, and thoughtful sons, Greg, Kevin, and Josh; to Josh's wife, Valerie, and their incredible children, Eve, Audra, Clara, and Ryan; to Kevin's fiancée, Nicola, and to the memory of my parents, Bette and "Grandpa Jim" Mayer, and to the memory of Maureen's wonderful parents, Georgette and Dr. John B. Henry.

Thom A. Mayer

Contents

Contributors — xi
Preface — xxiii
Acknowledgments — xxv

VOLUME 1

SECTION 1	**LEADERSHIP PRINCIPLES**	**1**
Chapter 1	Leadership, Management, and Motivation	3
Chapter 2	Vision, Mission, Values, Strategy, and Tactics	21
Chapter 3	Change and Project Management: A Practical Approach	43
Chapter 4	Power vs Influence	59
Chapter 5	Interaction With Hospital Governance	73
Chapter 6	Managing Professionals in Organizations: The Role of Physician and Nurse Leaders	89
Chapter 7	Mentoring and Coaching	103
Chapter 8	Conflict Management	113
Chapter 9	Conducting High-Impact Meetings	133
Chapter 10	Patient Safety: Error Reduction	155
Chapter 11	Defining Patient Experience and Leading Change	173
Chapter 12	The Discipline of Teams and Teamwork	191
Chapter 13	Maintaining Personal and Professional Balance	219
Chapter 14	Ethical Issues in the Emergency Department	237
Chapter 15	Practice Management Leadership: The Role of the Site Medical Director	249
Chapter 16	Women in Emergency Medicine Leadership	267
Chapter 17	Leadership in Times of Crisis	285
SECTION 2	**OPERATIONS: GENERAL**	**301**
Chapter 18	Medical Director Leadership	303
Chapter 19	Nursing Director Leadership	335
Chapter 20	The Medical Director–Nurse Director Relationship	345
Chapter 21	Emergency Department Provider Staffing	359
Chapter 22	Nurse Staffing	373
Chapter 23	Physician and Nurse Productivity Assessments	385

Chapter 24	**Physician Assistants and Nurse Practitioners**	**397**
Chapter 25	**Scribes**	**413**
Chapter 26	**Violence in the Emergency Department**	**433**
Chapter 27	**Emergency Department Facility Design**	**449**
Chapter 28	**Effective Marketing of the Emergency Department**	**473**
Chapter 29	**Multicultural Approach to Emergency Department Patients**	**489**
Chapter 30	**Emergency Department Management Essentials**	**501**
Chapter 31	**The View from the C-Suite**	**517**
Chapter 32	**Emergency Management of Drug and Supply Shortages**	**533**
SECTION 3	**OPERATIONS: FLOW**	**543**
Chapter 33	**Patient Throughput: Why It Matters, How It Is Done**	**545**
Chapter 34	**Patient Flow Principles**	**559**
Chapter 35	**Improving the Front-End Process to Add Value**	**573**
Chapter 36	**Front-Loading Flow**	**585**
Chapter 37	**The Role of Emergency Department Fast Tracks**	**599**
Chapter 38	**Optimizing Patient Throughput**	**613**
Chapter 39	**Role of Observation Units/Rapid Treatment**	**629**
Chapter 40	**Expediting Admissions**	**641**
Chapter 41	**Decision to Discharge: Finishing Strong**	**653**
Chapter 42	**Managing Waits: The Psychology of Waiting**	**669**
Chapter 43	**Hospital-Wide Patient Flow**	**681**
Chapter 44	**Effective Response to Full Capacity**	**699**
Chapter 45	**Defeating Bounce Backs: Managing High-Utilizer Patients**	**707**
Chapter 46	**Innovative Strategies to Enhance Flow**	**721**
SECTION 4	**OPERATIONS: EMERGENCY DEPARTMENT DIVERSIFICATION**	**735**
Chapter 47	**Poison Centers and Medical Toxicology**	**737**
Chapter 48	**Pediatric Emergency Medicine: Improving Quality and Readiness**	**749**
Chapter 49	**Undersea and Hyperbaric Medicine**	**763**
Chapter 50	**Behavioral Health in Emergency Care**	**773**
Chapter 51	**Hospital Medicine**	**785**
Chapter 52	**Disaster Planning and Response**	**805**
Chapter 53	**Military Emergency Medicine**	**823**

Chapter 54	**Freestanding Emergency Departments**	**841**
Chapter 55	**Sports Medicine**	**861**
Chapter 56	**Geriatric Emergency Departments**	**871**
Chapter 57	**Practice Diversification in Emergency Medical Services**	**883**
Chapter 58	**Air Medical Services and Interfacility Ground Transport**	**891**
Chapter 59	**End-of-Life Issues**	**905**
Chapter 60	**Practical Implementation of Opioid-Reduction Initiatives**	**917**
Chapter 61	**Developing and Implementing Emergency Department Ultrasound**	**933**
Chapter 62	**Rural Emergency Departments**	**945**
SECTION 5	**INFORMATICS**	**963**
Chapter 63	**Introduction to Clinical Informatics**	**965**
Chapter 64	**Electronic Health Records**	**969**
Chapter 65	**Electronic Health Record Tracking Systems**	**989**
Chapter 66	**Electronic Health Record Documentation Systems**	**999**
Chapter 67	**Computerized Provider Order Entry and Clinical Decision Support**	**1015**
Chapter 68	**Data Acquisition and Analysis**	**1031**
Chapter 69	**Essential Support Tools and Technologies**	**1049**
Chapter 70	**Social Media in Medicine**	**1059**
Chapter 71	**New Technologies and Applications**	**1065**
Chapter 72	**Telemedicine in Emergency Medicine**	**1077**

VOLUME 2

SECTION 6	**QUALITY AND SERVICE**	**1093**
Chapter 73	**Patient Experience: The Survival Skills Approach**	**1095**
Chapter 74	**Scripts: Using Evidence-Based Language to Improve Service**	**1113**
Chapter 75	**The A-Team Toolkit**	**1129**
Chapter 76	**Complaint Management**	**1143**
Chapter 77	**Effective Medical Staff Relationships: A Case-Based Discussion**	**1175**
Chapter 78	**Improving Performance Through Mutual Accountability**	**1193**
Chapter 79	**Patient Safety and Error Reduction**	**1209**

Chapter 80	Promoting Rational Thinking: An Ethical Imperative	1223
Chapter 81	Debiasing Strategies: Cognitive Pills for Cognitive Ills	1237
Chapter 82	The Revolving Door of Readmissions	1251

SECTION 7 FINANCE 1269

Chapter 83	Developing a Business Plan	1271
Chapter 84	Resource Utilization	1289
Chapter 85	The Financially Successful Emergency Department	1303
Chapter 86	Optimizing Physician Performance Through Incentives	1313
Chapter 87	Optimizing Nursing Performance Through Incentives	1339
Chapter 88	Financially Successful Private Physician Groups	1351
Chapter 89	Financial Success in Academic Emergency Medicine	1361
Chapter 90	Financial Planning for Individuals	1371

SECTION 8 REIMBURSEMENT 1389

Chapter 91	Reimbursement Issues	1391
Chapter 92	Introduction to Coding	1411
Chapter 93	Advanced Billing and Coding	1437
Chapter 94	Facility Revenue Considerations	1461
Chapter 95	Billing and Collecting	1483
Chapter 96	Creating a Culture of Compliance	1499
Chapter 97	Quality and Reporting in the Era of Payment Reform	1517
Chapter 98	Alternative Payment Models	1539

SECTION 9 CONTRACTS 1553

Chapter 99	Negotiation Skills	1555
Chapter 100	Contracts With Physicians	1583
Chapter 101	Contracting With Hospitals	1603
Chapter 102	Employee vs Independent Contractor	1615
Chapter 103	Equity, Parity, and Group Structure	1631

SECTION 10 LEGAL AND REGULATORY ISSUES 1651

Chapter 104	EMTALA for Emergency Department Leaders	1653
Chapter 105	Consent to and Refusal of Medical Treatment	1673
Chapter 106	Emergency Department Documentation	1685
Chapter 107	Reporting Requirements: Confidentiality, Data Breaches, and HIPAA	1697
Chapter 108	Disposition, Discharge, and Follow-Up	1709

SECTION 11 MALPRACTICE — 1733

Chapter 109	Risk Management: Challenges and Opportunities	1735
Chapter 110	Risk Management in Practice	1749
Chapter 111	Medical Malpractice Insurance	1761
Chapter 112	Malpractice: The Personal Toll	1777
Chapter 113	Medical Malpractice	1783
Chapter 114	Anatomy of a Lawsuit	1805
Chapter 115	Being an Expert Witness: Telling the Story of the Case	1815
Chapter 116	Medical Defense Experts: A Defense Attorney's Perspective	1829

SECTION 12 HUMAN RESOURCES — 1835

Chapter 117	Human Resources Management: Basic Principles	1837
Chapter 118	Physician Recruitment, Credentialing, and Orientation	1847
Chapter 119	Physician Retention and Professional Development	1863
Chapter 120	Nurse Recruitment, Orientation, and Credentialing	1881
Chapter 121	Nurse Retention	1897
Chapter 122	Managing Impaired Professionals	1911
Chapter 123	Generational Differences in Emergency Medicine	1927
Chapter 124	Gender Balance	1945
Chapter 125	Burnout: Diagnosis, Treatment, and Prevention	1975
Chapter 126	Compassion Fatigue Resiliency	2001
Chapter 127	Late Career Toolkit	2021

SECTION 13 HEALTH-CARE POLICY — 2031

Chapter 128	Inclusion, Equity, and Diversity	2033
Chapter 129	Health Policy and Advocacy	2047
Chapter 130	Mechanics of Advocacy	2053
Chapter 131	Federal Advocacy	2071
Chapter 132	State Advocacy	2089
Chapter 133	Private Sector Engagement	2105

Contributors

Gallane D. Abraham, MD
Assistant Professor Emergency Medicine
Icahn School of Medicine at Mount Sinai

Paul Allegretti, DO, FACOEP, FACOI
Clinical Professor of Emergency Medicine
Midwestern University/Chicago College of Osteopathic Medicine
Medical Director, Emergency Medicine
Provident Hospital of Cook County

W. Clayton Alexander IV, MBA
Vice President, Geesbreght Group

Andrew Amaranto, MD
Department of Medicine, Division of Cardiology
NewYork-Presbyterian/Columbia University Irving Medical Center
Department of Emergency Medicine
NewYork-Presbyterian Brooklyn Methodist Hospital

Kimberly Anderson, MHA
Performance Integration Director
The Permanente Medical Group, Inc.
Kaiser Permanente South Sacramento Medical Center

Francisco Javier Andrade Jr, MD
Ultrasound Fellow and Clinical Instructor
University of Arizona College of Medicine | Banner Health

Knox Andress, RN, BA, FAEN
Designated Regional Coordinator, Louisiana Region 7 Hospital/Healthcare Coalition
Assistant Director, Louisiana Poison Center
Department of Emergency Medicine
Louisiana State University Health-Shreveport

Louise B. Andrew, MD, JD, FACEP
Former Office and Chair, ACEP Wellness Committee
Senior Member, ACEP Medical-Legal Committee

Jonathan D. Apfelbaum, MD, FACEP, FAAEM
EMS Medical Director, Parker Adventist Hospital
Medical Director, Weber State University Paramedic Program

Tim W. Attebery, DSc, MBA, FACHE
President and CEO, Attebery & Associates
Adjunct Professor
College of Public Health, East Tennessee State University

Andrea Austin, MD, FACEP, FAAEM, CHSE
Associate Physician Diplomate of Emergency Medicine
University of California San Diego

Brooks Babcock, MBA
Senior Vice President, PSR LLC

Stephanie N. Bailey, MD
Emergency Medicine and Primary Care Sports Medicine
Greenville Health Systems
Clinical Assistant Professor
University of South Carolina School of Medicine, Greenville

Erik D. Barton, MD, MS, MBA, FACEP, FAAEM
Chief of Emergency Medicine
Samaritan Pacific Communities Hospital

Denise Bayer, MS, RN, FAEN
Independent Emergency Nursing Consultant
Past President, Emergency Nurses Association

Gigi Baniqued, MHA, MSN, RN, CHC
Director, Supportive Care Services, Continuing Care, and Complex Needs
South Sacramento Service Area
The Permanente Medical Group

Vikhyat S. Bebarta, MD
Director, CU Anschutz Center for COMBAT Research
Director, CU TRIAD Research Colorado
Vice Chair, Strategy and Growth
Professor (tenured), Emergency Medicine and Medical Toxicology, Pharmacology
Department of Emergency Medicine, University of Colorado School of Medicine, Aurora

Kevin H. Beier, MD, FAAEM
Associate Program Director, Emergency Medicine Residency
University of Tennessee

Elijah Berg, MD, FACEP
Chief Executive Officer, LogixHealth

Jeffrey Bettinger, MD, FACEP
Managing Member, BSA Healthcare

Alex Beuning, MD
Emergency Medicine, Mayo Clinic Health Systems

Graham Billingham, MD, FACEP, FAAEM
Chief Medical Officer, MedPro Group and Princeton Insurance Company
Founder, The Center for Emergency Medicine Education

Kevin Biese, MD, MAT, FACEP
Associate Professor, University of North Carolina
Consultant, West Health

Tom Blackwell, MD, FACEP, FAEMS
Assistant Dean, Longitudinal Clinical Education
University of South Carolina School of Medicine, Greenville
Professor of Emergency Medicine, Prisma Health
Executive Director, Greenville County EMS

Kay Bleecher, CRNP
EMS-Nursing Educator, Harrisburg Area Community College
Wellspan Health

Timothy J. Boardman, MD
Assistant Professor and Clinician Educator
Department of Emergency Medicine
Warren Alpert Medical School of Brown University

J. Stephen Bohan, SM, MD
Associate Physician, Brigham and Women's Hospital
Corresponding Member of the Faculty of Emergency Medicine, Harvard Medical School

Ed Boudreau, DO, FACEP, FAAEM, CPPS
CEO, Emergency Physicians Insurance Exchange RRG
Value Stream Managers LLC

Robert M. Bramante, MD, FACEP
Chairman, Department of Emergency Medicine
Catholic Health Mercy Hospital
Progressive Emergency Physicians
Clinical Associate Professor of Emergency Medicine
NYIT College of Osteopathic Medicine
Clinical Assistant Professor of Emergency Medicine
Stony Brook University School of Medicine

Autumn M. Brogan, MD, MPH
Department of Emergency Medicine, Mayo Clinic

John C. Brown, MD, FACEP
Medical Director, San Francisco Emergency Medical Services Agency
Associate Clinical Professor of Emergency Medicine; EMS and Disaster Medicine Associate Followship Director,
University of California San Francisco Medical School
Medical Officer, Disaster Medical Team CA-6

Diane Calello, MD, FAAP, FACMT, FAACT
Executive and Medical Director
New Jersey Poison Information and Education System
Associate Professor of Emergency Medicine
Rutgers-New Jersey Medical School

Janet Carr, MBA
Vice President of Operations, Emergency Medicine
Sound Physicians

L. Anthony Cirillo, MD, FACEP
Board of Directors, American College of Emergency Physicians
Director of Government Affairs, US Acute Care Solutions LLC
Past Chair, Emergency Medicine Policy Institute
Senior Medical Advisor, Graphene Composites - USA
Clinical Adjunct Associate Professor, University of Rhode Island College of Nursing

Mark Collin, MD
Director, Division of Point-of-Care Ultrasound
Director, Emergency Medicine Ultrasound Fellowship
Department of Emergency Medicine
Wellspan York Hospital

Stephen Colucciello, MD, FACEP
Professor and Vice Chair, Department of Emergency Medicine,
Carolinas Medical Center and Atrium Health

Norma Cooney, MD, FACEP, UHM/ABEM
Clinical Assistant Professor of Emergency Medicine
SUNY Upstate University Hospital
Chief Operating Officer, MedSpa Solutions LLC

Michael Corvini, MD, MBA, FACEP, FACP
President, Southeast Group
TeamHealth

Pat Croskerry, BSc, MD, PhD, CCFP, FRCP
Professor of Emergency Medicine, Division of Medical Education
Dalhousie University
Professor
Canadian Patient Safety Institute

Randal L. Dabbs, MD, FACEP, FAAFP
Co-Founder and President, Practice Development
TeamHealth

Keith DellaGrotta, MD, MBA
Assistant Medical Director, Department of Emergency Medicine
West Hills Hospital and Medical Center

Christina Dempsey, DNP, MBA, RN, CNOR, CENP, FAAN
Chief Nursing Officer Emerita, Press Ganey Associates Inc.
Adjunct Faculty
Missouri State University School of Nursing

Colleen Desai, RN
Chief Nurse Officer, Holyoke Medical Center

Joseph P. Dervay, MD, MPH, MMS, FACEP, FAsMA
Flight Surgeon, Space Medicine Operations Division
NASA Johnson Space Center
Clinical Instructor, Division of Emergency Medicine, Dept. of Surgery
Clinical Assistant Professor, Dept. of Preventive Medicine & Community Health
The University of Texas Medical Branch

Taylor T. DesRosiers, MD
Lieutenant, Medical Corps, United States Navy
Naval Medical Center Portsmouth

Jeffrey "Jim" Dietz, MD
Chair, Department of Emergency Medicine (retired)
Coordinator, Vitality Professional Resilience Project (retired)

Sue Dill Calloway, RN, AD, BA, BSN, MSN, JD, CPHRM, CCMSCP
President, Patient Safety and Healthcare Education & Consulting

Valerie Dobiesz, MD, MPH, FACEP
Director of Internal Programs, STRATUS Center for Medical Simulation
Brigham & Women's Hospital
Department of Emergency Medicine, Harvard Medical School

Jeff Druck, MD
Co-Director, Office of Professional Excellence
Assistant Dean for Student Affairs, Office of Student Life
Professor of Emergency Medicine
University of Colorado

Pamela L. Dyne, MD
Professor of Clinical Emergency Medicine
UCLA David Geffen School of Medicine
Designated Institutional Official, Department of Emergency Medicine
Olive View-UCLA Medical Center

Caral Edelberg, CPC, CPMA, CAC, CCS-P, CHC
Honorary Member, American College of Emergency Physicians
Founder and Chairman, Edelberg + Associates

Jim Ellis, MD, FACEP
Emergency Preparedness Consultant, NFL
President, Prisma Health Medical Group-Midlands
Clinical Associate Professor of Emergency Medicine
University of South Carolina School of Medicine-Greenville

Luis F. Eljaiek Jr, MD, FACEP, FAAEM
Medical Director, Physicians Transport Service

Jeffrey Eye, RN, MSN
Vice President, Patient Care Services
Chief Nursing Officer
Murray-Calloway County Hospital

Ugo A. Ezenkwele, MD, MPH, FACEP
Chief, Mount Sinai Queens Emergency Department
Associate Professor of Emergency Medicine
Icahn Mount Sinai School of Medicine

Brian Fengler, MD
Co-Founder and CEO, EvidenceCare

Kathleen Flarity, DNP, PhD, CEN, CFRN, FAEN
Deputy Director, CU Anschutz Center for COMBAT Research
Associate Professor and Research Nurse Scientist, Department of Emergency Medicine
University of Colorado School of Medicine, Aurora
Brigadier General, US Air Force

Cyndy Flores, PA-C
Senior Director, Advanced Providers, Vituity

Edward R. Gaines III, JD, CCP
Chief Compliance Officer, EM Division, Zotec Partners LLC

Gus M. Garmel, MD, FACEP, FAAEM
Clinical Professor (Affiliate) of Emergency Medicine
Stanford University
Senior Staff Emergency Physician, TPMG, Kaiser Santa Clara
Senior Editor, *The Permanente Journal*, KWFCO

Chelsey Geiger, MS
President, CareThrough

Nicholas Genes, MD, PhD, FACEP
Associate CMIO, Mount Sinai Health System
Associate Professor of Emergency Medicine
Icahn School of Medicine at Mount Sinai

J. Eric Gentry, PhD, LMHC, DAAETS, FAAETS
President, FORWARD-FACING INSTITUTE

Aaron George, DO
Chief Medical Officer, Meritus Health

James E. George, MD, FACEP
Co-Founder and Strategic Advisor to the President and CEO, TeamHealth

Michael Gottlieb, MD, RDMS, FAAEM, FACEP
Associate Professor of Emergency Medicine
Director, Emergency Ultrasound Division
Program Director, Clinical Ultrasound Fellowship
Department of Emergency Medicine
Rush University Medical Center

Pawan Goyal, MD, MHA, FAMIA, FHIMSS, FAHIMA
Associate Executive Director, Quality
American College of Emergency Physicians

Louis Graff IV, MD, FACEP, FACP, FACC
Physician Advisor, Hartford Healthcare Corporation
Professor of Surgery and Emergency Medicine, Clinical Professor of Medicine
University of Connecticut School of Medicine

Charles Grassie, MD, JD, FACEP
Retired CEO, Emergency Physicians Medical Group
Emeritus Physician, St. Joseph Mercy Health System

Andrea L. Green, MD, FACEP
Chair, ACEP Diversity, Inclusion, and Health Equity Section
Vituity Healthcare Partner
Department of Emergency Medicine
UMC Medical Center Northeast

Phillip Gruber, MD
Chief Medical Information Officer
LAC+USC Medical Center

Alison Haddock, MD, FACEP
Assistant Professor of Emergency Medicine, Baylor College of Medicine
Vice President, American College of Emergency Physicians

Blaine Hannafin, MD, MBD, RDMS
Chief of Cost Performance, Northern California Clinical Lead for Medi-Cal Operations
Medical Director, Kaiser Geographic Managed Care (Kaiser GMC Medi-Cal)

Gregory L. Henry, MD, FACEP
Clinical Professor of Emergency Medicine
University of Michigan Medical School
Former President, American College of Emergency Physicians
Risk Consultant, Emergency Physicians Medical Group

Judd E. Hollander, MD
Senior Vice President for Healthcare Delivery Innovation, Jefferson Health
Associate Dean for Strategic Health Initiatives, Sidney Kimmel Medical College
Vice Chair for Finance and Healthcare Enterprises, Department of Emergency Medicine
Thomas Jefferson University

Michelle Hoppes, RN, MS, DFASHRM
President/CEO, Michigan Professional Insurance Exchange
Adjunct Faculty, Loyola School of Law

Kenneth V. Iserson, MD, MBA, FACEP, FAAEM, FIFEM
Professor Emeritus, Department of Emergency Medicine
University of Arizona
Visiting Professor, Emergency Medicine Residency
Georgetown Public Hospital, Guyana

Sujit S. Iyer, MD
Director, Pediatric ED Outreach
Associate Fellowship Director
Assistant Medical Director, Pediatric Emergency Medicine
Associate Professor of Pediatrics, UT Austin Dell Medical School
Dell Children's Medical Center of Central Texas

Stephen J. Jameson, MD, FACEP
Chair, ACEP Rural Section
Co-Editor, Emergency Medicine Core Training
Emergency Trauma Center
St. Cloud Hospital

Zachary J. Jarou, MD, MBA
Clinical Associate, Section of Emergency Medicine
Department of Medicine, University of Chicago
Fellow in Administration, Quality, Informatics, and Policy
American College of Emergency Physicians
Immediate Past President, Emergency Medicine Residents' Association

Mark M. Jones, JD, MEd
Retired Partner, Wilson, Elser, Moskowitz, Edelman, and Dicker LLP

Robert Jones, DO, FACEP
Systemwide Clinical Ultrasound Co-Chair, MetroHealth System
Assistant Dean for Clerkship Education
Block 7 Leader, Clinical Ultrasound and Professor of Emergency Medicine
Case Western Reserve University School of Medicine

Thomas Judge
Paramedic/Critical Care
Executive Director, LifeFlight of Maine/ LifeFlight Foundation

Jay Kaplan, MD, FACEP
Medical Director of Care Transformation, LCMC Health
Clinical Associate Professor of Medicine, LSU Health Sciences Center
Attending Physician and Academic Faculty, LSU Emergency Medicine Residency, University Medical Center New Orleans
Past President, American College of Emergency Physicians

Mark Kauffman, BSN, MBA
Director, Strategic Initiatives
Kaiser Permanente South California

Thompson Kehrl, MD, RDMS, FACEP
Chair, Department of Emergency Medicine
WellSpan York Hospital

A. Michael Kelen, CFA, CFP
Director of Financial Services, Sortino Financial Group

Marylou Killian, DNP, RN, FNP-bc, ENP-c, FAEN
Emergency Medicine, TeamHealth

Matthew R. Klein, MD, MPH
Assistant Professor of Emergency Medicine
Northwestern University Feinberg School of Medicine

Kevin M. Klauer, DO, EJD, FACEP, FACOEP
CEO, American Osteopathic Association
Assistant Clinical Professor, Michigan State University College of Osteopathic Medicine
Clinical Assistant Professor, University of Tennessee Health Science Center
Assistant Clinical Professor, Ohio University College of Osteopathic Medicine

Kirk R. Klemme, MD
Addiction Medicine, Aspirus Keweenaw Hospital

Kelly J. Ko, MS, PhD
Director of Clinical Research
West Health Institute, La Jolla, CA

Kathy Kopka, RN, MHSA
Administrative Director Clinical Operations
Skyline Medical Center, HCA TriStar Division, Nashville, TN

Linda Lawrence, MD, CPE, FACEP
Col (ret) USAF, MC
Associate Dean for Clinical Affairs and Clinical Associate Professor of Emergency Medicine
Northeast Ohio Medical University
Adjunct Associate Professor of Military & Emergency Medicine
Uniformed Services University of the Health Sciences

Alexis M. LaPietra, DO, FACEP
Chief, Pain Management and Addiction Medicine
Assistant Professor of Clinical Emergency Medicine
Rowan University School of Osteopathic Medicine

Adriane Lesser, MS
Associate Director, Clinical Research
West Health Institute, La Jolla, CA

Resa E. Lewiss, MD
Director, Point-of-Care Ultrasound
Professor of Emergency Medicine and Radiology
Thomas Jefferson University

Ori Litvak, MBA
Executive Director, Innovation and Process Improvement
LogixHealth

Bernard L. Lopez, MD, MS, CPE, FACEP, FAAEM
Associate Provost for Diversity and Inclusion
Associate Dean for Diversity and Community Engagement
Professor and Executive Vice Chair, Department of Emergency Medicine
Sidney Kimmel Medical College, Thomas Jefferson University

Sujal Mandavia, MD, FRCP(C), FACEP
Clinical Assistant Professor of Emergency Medicine
LAC/USC Medical Center, Keck School of Medicine
Senior Board Examiner, American Board of Emergency Medicine

Nancy Mannion, DNP, RN, CEN, FAEN
President, NMB Global Leadership LLC
Senior Nursing Consultant
Brigham and Women's Hospital

Ricardo Martinez, MD, FACEP
Chief Medical Officer, Adeptus Health
Assistant Professor of Emergency Medicine
Emory School of Medicine

Catherine A. Marco, MD, FACEP
Professor of Emergency Medicine
Wright State University Boonshoft School of Medicine

Donna Mason, RN, BS, MS, CEN, FAEN
Retired Nurse, Emergency Medicine

James C. McClay, MD, MS, FACEP, FAMIA
Chair, Biomedical Informatics Graduate Program
Professor of Emergency Medicine and Informatics
University of Nebraska Medical Center

David A. McKenzie, CAE
Reimbursement Director, American College of Emergency Physicians

Abhi Mehrotra, MD, MBA, FACEP
Vice Chair, Strategic Initiatives & Operations
Professor of Emergency Medicine
University of North Carolina

Sean Michael, MD, MBA, FACEP
Medical Director
Physician Informaticist and Pathways Lead
Department of Emergency Medicine
University of Colorado School of Medicine

Angela M. Mills, MD
J. E. Beaumont Professor and Chair
Department of Emergency Medicine
Columbia University College of Physicians and Surgeons
Chief of Emergency Medicine Services, NewYork-Presbyterian | Columbia

Nicholas M. Mohr, MD
Associate Professor of Emergency Medicine and Anesthesia Critical Care
University of Iowa Carver College of Medicine

William Montei, CPA
Chief Medical Officer, Meglodon Insurance Systems

Michael D. Moon, PhD, MSN, RN, CNS-CC, CEN, FAEN
Former President, Texas Emergency Nurses Association
Professor of Nursing
University of the Incarnate Word
Ila Faye Miller School of Nursing and Health Professions

Lisa A. Moreno-Walton, MD, MS, MSCR, FAAEM, FACEP, FIFEM
President, American Academy of Emergency Medicine
Professor of Emergency Medicine
Director, Latino Health Scholars Program
Louisiana University Health Sciences Center, New Orleans

Rhonda M. Morgan, RN, DNP, CNS, APRN
Professor, King University
Director, Doctor of Nursing Practice Program

Eric J. Morley, MD, MHA, MS
Associate Professor, Vice Chair for Clinical Affairs, and Clinical Director
Department of Emergency Medicine
Deputy CMIO
Renaissance School of Medicine at Stony Brook University

Sergey M. Motov, MD, FAAEM
Research Director, Department of Emergency Medicine
Maimonides Medical Center
Professor of Emergency Medicine
SUNY Downstate Medical College

Karen Murrell, MD, MBA, FACEP
Medical Director, Lodi Memorial Hospital
Performance & Innovation Consultant, TeamHealth
Clinical Consultant, Qventus Inc.

Anthony Nader
Chairman, Inova Health Systems

Joanne Navarroli, MSN, RN, CEN
Chandler Regional Medical Center

Susan Nedza, MD, MBA
Adjunct Assistant Professor of Emergency Medicine
Feinberg School of Medicine
Northwestern University

Lewis S. Nelson, MD
Professor and Chair, Department of Emergency Medicine
Director, Division of Medical Toxicology
Rutgers New Jersey Medical School
Chief of Service, Emergency Department, University Hospital of Newark
Senior Consultant, New Jersey Poison Information & Education System

Diana Nordlund, DO, JD, FACEP
Corporate Compliance Officer, Emergency Care Specialists
Attorney/Partner, Nordlund | Hulverson PLLC
Board of Directors, Michigan College of Emergency Physicians

Marlaina Norris, MD, MBA
Director of Utilization Review and Care Coordination
Vituity Emergency Department
Presence Mercy Medical Center

Charles Noon, PhD, MEng
Professor, Physician Executive MBA Program
Haslam College of Business, University of Tennessee
Faculty, Institute for Healthcare Improvement
Co-Founder/Consultant, X32 Healthcare

Ashley Booth Norse, MD, FACEP
Associate Chair of Operations, Medical Director, and Associate Professor of Emergency Medicine
University of Florida College of Medicine - Jacksonville

Sara Nourazari, PhD
Assistant Professor
California State University - Long Beach

India Owens, MSN, RN, CEN, NE-BC, FAEN
India T Owens Consulting
Adjunct Faculty, Indiana University School of Nursing
Adjunct Faculty, University of Indianapolis

Rebecca Bollinger Parker, MD, FACEP
Chief Coding Officer, Health Care Financial Services of TeamHealth, Knoxville TN
President, Team Parker LLC, Tucson, AZ

Gita Pensa, MD
Clinical Assistant Professor, Department of Emergency Medicine
Warren Alpert School of Medicine of Brown University

Ava E. Pierce, MD, FACEP
Associate Professor and Associate Chair of Diversity and Inclusion
Director of Texas Emergency Medicine Research Associates Program
Department of Emergency Medicine
UT Southwestern Medical Center

Susan B. Promes, MD, FACEP
Professor and Chair of Emergency Medicine
Penn State Milton S. Hershey Medical Center

Ed Racht
Chief Medical Officer, American Medical Response

Mark Reiter, MD, MBA, MAAEM, FAAEM
CEO, Emergency Excellence
Professor and Residency Director, Department of Emergency Medicine
University of Tennessee-Murfreesboro/Nashville
Chair, American Academy of Emergency Medicine Physician Group

Katherine Remick, MD, FAAP, FACEP, FAEMS
Medical Director, San Marcos Hays County EMS System
Executive Lead, National EMS for Children Innovation and Improvement Center
Associate Medical Director, Austin-Travis County EMS System
Assistant Professor of Pediatrics, Dell Medical School at the University of Texas at Austin

Matthew Rice, MD, JD, FACEP
Emergency Medicine Physician
Gig Harbor

Lynne D. Richardson, MD, FACEP
Professor of Emergency Medicine and Health Evidence and Policy
Vice Chair for Academic Research and Community Programs, Department of Emergency Medicine
The Icahn School of Medicine, Mount Sinai

Hammad Rizvi, DO, MBA, CPE, FHM
Senior Vice President, TeamHealth

Kathy Robinson, RN, BSHA, FAEN
Strategic Partnerships Director, National Association of State EMS Officials
Past President, Emergency Nurses Association

Scott W. Rodi, MD, MPH
Inaugural Chair, Department of Emergency Medicine, Dartmouth-Hitchcock Medical Center
Director, Regional Emergency Medicine, Dartmouth-Hitchcock Health
Associate Professor of Emergency Medicine, The Geisel School of Medicine at Dartmouth

Adam Rodos, MD, FACEP
Program Director, Internal Medicine/Emergency Medicine Residency
Director of Quality, Department of Emergency Medicine
Assistant Professor of Clinical Emergency Medicine and Medicine
University of Illinois at Chicago

Marie-Laure Romney, MD, MBA
Vice President of Operations
NewYork-Presbyterian Hospital
Columbia University Irving Medical Center

Mark Rosenberg, DO, MBA, FACEP, FAAHPM
President, American College of Emergency Physicians
Associate Professor and Chairman Emeritus of Emergency Medicine
St Joseph's University Medical Center

Alexander M. Rosenau, DO, CPE, FACEP
Chief, Division of Emergency Medicine, Department of Emergency and Hospital Medicine, Lehigh Valley Health Network
Professor, Morsani College of Medicine, University of South Florida
Former President, American College of Emergency Medicine

William F. Rutherford, MD
Associate Medical Director, IU Health Revenue Cycle Services
Physician Lead, Denial Management

Tracy G. Sanson, MD, FACEP
Founder, TracySansonMD
Emergency Physician, Consultant, Educator

James J. Scheulen, PA, MBA
Chief Administrative Officer, Emergency Medicine and Capacity Management
Johns Hopkins Medicine

Gillian R. Schmitz, MD, FACEP
Associate Professor, Department of Military and Emergency Medicine
Uniformed Services University
Vice Chair of Education
Brooke Army Medical Center

Bill Schueler, MSN, RN, CEN, CPPS, WVTS, FAEN
Patient Safety Specialist, Providence Health - Oregon Region
Owner, WJS Services LLC

Jean Scofi, MD, MBA, MS
Director of Informatics & Analytics
Assistant Director, Healthcare Leadership and Management Fellowship
Assistant Professor of Emergency Medicine
New York Presbyterian Weill-Cornell Medical Center

Aviva Segal, PhD
Faculty, Department of Education, Concordia University
Postdoctoral Fellow, Centre for Research on Children and Families
McGill University, Concordia University

Rahul Sharma, MD, MBA, FACEP
Professor and Chairman, Emergency Physician-in-Chief
New York Presbyterian-Weill Cornell Medicine
Executive Director, Center for Virtual Care
Weill Cornell Medicine

David Singley Jr, MHA
Chief Executive Officer, PSR LLC

Mary Kay Silverman, DNP, RN, CEN, NEA-BC
Director of Pediatric Emergency Services and Pedi/Neo Transport Team
Golisano Children's Hospital of SW Florida

Michael A Silverman, MD, FACEP
Chairman, Department of Emergency Medicine
Virginia Hospital Center

Rebecca Smith-Coggins, MD
Professor (Teaching) of Emergency Medicine
Stanford Hospital and Clinic

Jeff Solheim, MSN, RN, CEN, TCRN, CFRN, FAEN, FAAN,
President, Solheim Enterprises
Past President, Emergency Nurses Association
Past President, Nursing Organizational Alliance

Thomas Spiegel, MD, MBA, MS, FACEP
Assistant Professor of Medicine and Administrative Fellowship Director
Emergency Department Medical Director, Center for Care and Discovery
Section of Emergency Medicine, Department of Medicine, University of Chicago

Donald E. Stader III, MD, FACEP
Emergency Physician, Swedish Medical Center
Founder and President, Stader Opioid Consulting LLC
President, Triage Films LLC

Jennifer L'Hommedieu Stankus, MD, JD, FACEP
Physician, Department of Emergency Medicine
Madigan Army Medical Center
Co-Founder, Comprehensive Medical Legal Consultants LLC

Ryan A. Stanton, MD, FACEP
Central Emergency Physicians
Member, American College of Emergency Physicians Board of Directors
Medical Director, Lexington Fire/EMS
AMR/NASCAR Safety Team

Charles (Chuck) D. Stokes, BSN, MHA, FACHE
Founding Partner, Relia Healthcare Advisors
Former CEO, Memorial Hermann Healthcare System, Houston
Past President, American College of Healthcare Executives

Suzanne Stone-Griffith, RN, MSN, CNAA
Affiliate Faculty, Regis University

Cary J. Stratford, PA-C, DFAAPA
President, Emergency Services of New England Inc.

William Sullivan, DO, JD, FACEP
Emergency Physician, St. Margaret's Hospital
Clinical Assistant Professor of Emergency Medicine
Midwestern University
Law Office of William Sullivan
Co-Founder, BAM Medical Staffing
Senior Editor, *EP Monthly Magazine*

John Sverha, MD
Vice Chair, Department of Emergency Medicine
Virginia Hospital Center
Alteon Health

Abbie G. Tapp-Pearson, RN, MSN, MBA
Director of Clinical Education
Director, TeamHealth Patient Safety Organization

Theresa Tavernero, RN, PhD, MBA
Senior Vice President
Performance & Innovation Consultants

Todd B. Taylor, MD, FACEP
Health Information Technology Consultant
Vice-Chair, ACEP Health Innovation & Technology Committee

Aisha T. Terry, MD, MPH, FACEP
Associate Professor of Emergency Medicine and Health Policy
George Washington University School of Medicine and Hospital
Member, American College of Emergency Physicians Board of Directors

Sarah Todt, RN, CPC, CPMA, CEDC
Senior Director, Revenue Integrity
LogixHealth

Vaishal Tolia, MD, MPH, FACEP
Department of Emergency Medicine
University of California San Diego

Jeremy D. Tucker, DO, FACEP, FACOEP, FACOI
Chief Medical Officer, New Frontier Aerospace
Co-Founder, Drone Delivery Systems Corporation
Chief Medical Officer/Co-Founder, Medssenger
US Acute Care Solutions

Pam Turner, RN, MBA
Independent Healthcare Consultant, Clarksville, TN
Senior Consultant, Quality Matters, Salt Lake City, UT

Joseph Twanmoh, MD, MBA, FACEP, FAAEM
President and Founder, Queue Management LLC

Brad Uren, MD
Associate Professor of Emergency Medicine
University of Michigan

Arjun Venkatesh, MD, MBA, MHS, FACEP
Chief, Section of Administration
Associate Professor, Department of Emergency Medicine
Yale University School of Medicine
Scientist, Center for Outcomes Research & Evaluation
Yale New Haven Hospital

(Asa) Peter Viccellio, MD, FACEP
Professor, Vice Chairman, and Associate Chief Medical Officer
Department of Emergency Medicine
Stony Brook School of Medicine

Barbara Weintraub, RN, MSN, MPH, APN, CEN, CPEN, FAEN
Trauma/EMS Coordinator
Gottlieb Memorial Hospital, Melrose Park, IL

Winnie T. Whitaker, MD, FAAP, FACEP
Assistant Professor of Pediatrics
University of Texas at Austin Dell Medical School
Assistant Medical Director, Pediatric Emergency Medicine
Dell Children's Medical Center of Central Texas
Medical Director, Camp Longhorn

Dennis C. Whitehead, MD, FACEP
Emergency Physician, UP Health System - Portage
Associate Professor of Emergency Medicine
Michigan State University
Past Chair, ACEP Wellness Committee
Past Speaker, ACEP Council

Winnie T. Whitaker, MD
Pediatric Emergency Medicine, Dell Children's Medical Center of Central Texas
Assistant Medical Director and Director of Advance Practice Providers
Clinical Assistant Professor or Emergency Medicine
UT Austin-Dell Medical School

Jennifer Wiler, MD, MBA, FACEP
Chief Quality Officer Denver Metro | UCHealth
Co-Founder CARE Innovation Center | UCHealth
Professor of Emergency Medicine
University of Colorado School of Medicine

Jeannette Wolfe, MD, FACEP
Professor of Emergency Medicine
UMass-Baystate

Christopher M. Ziebell, MD, FACEP
Assistant Professor and Division Chief, Dell Medical School
Emergency Department Medical Director, Dell SETON Medical Center at the University of Texas

Frank Zilm, DArch, FAIA, FACHA emeritus
Chester Dean Director of the Institute for Health-Wellness Design
University of Kansas

Brian J. Zink, MD, FACEP
Senior Associate Dean for Faculty and Faculty Development
Professor of Emergency Medicine
University of Michigan Medical School

Leslie Zun, MD, MBA, FAAEM, FACEP
Professor and Chair, Department of Emergency Medicine
Chicago Medical School
Medical Director, Lake County Health Department and Community Health

Preface

Be not afraid of greatness. Some are born great, some achieve greatness, and others have greatness thrust upon them.

William Shakespeare, *Twelfth Night*

Deep political divides, emerging infectious diseases, inconsistent mandates, recognition of and response to systemic racism, overwhelming burnout and increased risk of suicide, and the safety risks to our team members and families all put inordinate pressure on leaders to get it right.

The health-care sector is undergoing dramatic and disruptive change. National leaders and marketplace pressures are mandating the provision of higher-quality, lower-cost care to an aging population. And so, like the quote from Shakespeare, survival and success during these uncertain times require greatness, strong leadership, and collaboration. Emergency department (ED) leaders must approach these transformative changes with a steady nerve, sustained ingenuity, and a willingness to creatively embrace the ever-shifting landscape.

Approximately, 150 million patients are seen in EDs annually (411,000 patients per day), with 27 million patient admissions from the ED (74,000 patients per day). Furthermore, ED admissions account for 70% of all hospital admissions.[1,2] With such staggering data, it's vital that ED leadership and management continuously assess, adapt, and redesign their approach to patient care. One constant is that EDs continue to be both the critical safety net for their patients, communities, hospitals, and the entire health-care system, *and* a central cog in health-care coordination.

A RAND Corporation research report acknowledged the value of the ED in the health-care system.[3] Though ED care is sometimes referred to pejoratively as "the most expensive care there is," this overly simplistic view "ignores the many roles that EDs fill, and the statutory obligation of hospital EDs to provide care to all in need without regard to their ability to pay." As fewer patients are directly admitted from primary care physician (PCP) practices, PCPs increasingly rely on EDs to perform "complex diagnostic workups and [handle] overflow, after-hours, and weekend demand for care." The report goes on to recognize that the physicians and nurses staffing the EDs "are increasingly serving as the major decision-maker[s] for [the majority of] hospital admissions in the United States."

With approximately one-third of US health-care dollars currently spent on hospital patients, it is no surprise that emergency care providers are under increasing scrutiny.[4-6] On the current growth path, some would argue that health-care costs might "bankrupt America."[7,8] All ED leaders are obligated to actively engage in the health-care debate, and in so doing analyze their services, ensure increasing value, institute evidence-based best practices, provide a caring environment, build transparent and meaningful information systems, and inspire teams of caregivers. Department leaders must go beyond meeting critical metrics; rather, they must create a team that consistently delivers "acts of kindness . . . the highest level of compassion . . . one patient at a time."[9-11]

The purpose of this book is to help leaders respond to the complex and evolving ED environment by organizing the contained information into a unified body of knowledge. The intent is to provide both broad philosophic concepts and granular tools and techniques for delivering best and evidence-based practices. The book is organized into 13 sections, which cover the broad array of ED logistics and operations:

- Leadership Principles
- Operations: General
- Operations: Flow
- Operations: Emergency Department Specialization
- Operations: Informatics
- Quality and Service
- Finance
- Reimbursement
- Contracts
- Legal and Regulatory Issues
- Malpractice
- Human Resources
- Health Care Policy

The mission of this book is to develop and enhance the skills of those leading and managing ED services. It is designed to support the ED and its caregivers—emergency physicians, nurses, department directors, administrators, and other staff members—in the provision of those services. It is our privilege as editors to provide a resource to support that endeavor.

Robert W. Strauss and *Thom A. Mayer*

REFERENCES

1. CDC.gov, "National Center for Health Statistics: Emergency Department Visits." Updated February 21, 2020. Accessed October 31, 2020. https://www.cdc.gov/nchs/fastats/emergency-department.htm
2. Augustine JJ. Latest Data Reveal the ED's Role as Hospital Admission Gatekeeper. Published December 20, 2019. Accessed October 31, 2020. https://www.acepnow.com/article/latest-data-reveal-the-eds-role-as-hospital-admission-gatekeeper/#:~:text=Every%20day%2C%20emergency%20physicians%20in,admitted%20to%20hospitals%-20each%20day.
3. Morganti KG, Bauhoff S, Blanchard JC, et al. The Evolving Role of Emergency Departments in the United States. Santa Monica, CA: Rand Corporation, 2013. http://www.rand.org/pubs/research_reports/RR280.html. Accessed May 23, 2013.
4. Abelson R. "ER's Account for Half of Hospital Admissions, Study Says." http://www.nytimes.com/2013/05/21/business/half-of-hospital-admissions-from- emergency-rooms.html?_r=0. Accessed May 21, 2013.
5. Kavilanz P. "6 Reasons Health Care Costs Keep Going Up." http://money.cnn.com/2012/07/12/news/economy/health-care-costs/index.htm. Accessed July 15, 2012.
6. Gee E. "The High Price of Hospital Care." From Center for American Progress: Healthcare. Published June 26, 2019. Accessed November 22, 2020. https://www.americanprogress.org/issues/healthcare/reports/2019/06/26/471464/high-price-hospital-care/
7. Tikkanen R, Abrams MK. "U.S. Healthcare from a Global Perspective, 2019: Higher Spending, Work Outcomes? Published by The Commonwealth Fund, January 30, 2020. Accessed November 23, 2020. https://www.commonwealthfund.org/publications/issue-briefs/2020/jan/us-health-care-global-perspective-2019?gclid=CjwKCAiAtej9BRAvEiwA0UAWXqXw8XC-a4gihZyf-6PkDhtLhsR8LHsxfGePXrcWu9x31MfgO_jbcxoC7BYQAvD_BwE
8. Brockman K. "The expense nearly half of Americans think can bankrupt them." Published in USA Today, May 31, 2019, Accessed November 21, 2020. https://www.usatoday.com/story/money/2019/05/31/45-american-worried-healthcare-expenses-could-bankrupt-them/1292919001/
9. Feinberg D. CEO UCLA Hospital System in a speech delivered to TEDx uploaded to youtube.com August 2, 2011. http://www.youtube.com/watch?v=cZ5u7p-ZNuE. Accessed November 11, 2011.
10. Michelli JA. *Prescription for Excellence: Leadership Lessons for Creating a World-Class Customer Experience from UCLA Health System*. Co-published by McGraw-Hill Companies and Second River Healthcare Press, Bozeman, MT; 2011.
11. Brenner J, Rosenblatt M. "Transforming Healthcare One Patient at a Time." Published in thehill.com, December 8, 2014. Accessed November 20, 2020. https://thehill.com/blogs/congress-blog/healthcare/226165-transforming-healthcare-one-patient-at-a-time

Acknowledgements

The overwhelmingly positive reaction to the 1st edition of this book was extremely gratifying and deeply appreciated. When the American College of Emergency Physicians approached us about updating the book, we both took several deep breaths but quickly agreed to do so, owing primarily to the dramatic, even cataclysmic changes health care *writ large* and emergency departments, in particular, were undergoing. This meant that leadership and management must adapt and react quickly to those changes while finding innovative and creative ways to change systems and processes. The only reason this work has a chance of being successful is because of the amazing work of our friends, who happen to be among the most talented leaders in the specialty of emergency medicine.

To our senior associate editor, Kirk Jensen, and our associate editors Jim Augustine, Jeanne Proehl, and Sandy Schneider, thank you for your incredible insights, unflagging energy, and pure hard work. The same goes for our section editors, who were the "tactical commanders" responsible for ensuring that the content was consistent, accurate, and timely. Finally, to our authors, all highly respected and busy emergency department leaders: Thank you for your dedication and for sharing your invaluable insights, which will make patient care better and the jobs of those who provide that care easier.

Finally, Linda Sokhor Cooper was our editorial assistant throughout this process, and her contributions to the work permeate every page. Her intelligence is exceeded only by her unflagging positive and proactive spirit, which kept us working when it wasn't always easy to see through to the end. As Shakespeare said of Hermia in *A Midsummer Night's Dream*, "Though she be but little, she is fierce."

DR. MAYER'S ACKNOWLEDGMENTS

Henry Adams once wrote, "A teacher affects eternity. He can never tell where his influence ends." In co-editing this book, I have felt the influence of many teachers who materially contributed to its development, even if they were not explicitly aware of it.

I have had the honor of working with many of the brightest lights of health-care leadership, whose thoughts have deeply influenced my work, including Chuck Stokes, Quint Studer, Dr. Don Berwick, Charles Barnett, Steve Brown, Toni Ardabell, Nicholas Beamon, Candace Saunders, and Drs. Tom Jenike and John Brennan. I am grateful to all of them. My friend Tom Peters is a legend in the field of leadership and management, whose praise for the work I have done is both fulsome and excessive. I simply try to live up to it in large or small ways.

My clinical home at the Inova Health System has exposed me to some of the finest leaders in health care, including its CEO, Dr. Stephen Jones, the chief of clinical enterprise, Dr. Steven Motew, and the president of the Inova Fairfax Medical Campus, Dr. Steve Narang, whose definition of culture as "coming straight from the airway of the organization" is as lyrical and succinct as it is pragmatic. I continue to learn from them and from my emergency medicine colleagues, including Drs. Glenn Druckenbrod, Rick Place, Bob Cates, and Dan Hanfling. Exceeding me in intelligence and wit, they collectively form a leadership brain trust without peer.

While he is mentioned above, Dr. Kirk Jensen has been a sage and gimlet-eyed friend and mentor, whose insights have influenced almost every area of my thinking. The memory of three friends and major contributors to the field of emergency department leadership is always with me: Joan Kyes, Martin Gottlieb, and Dr. Stephen Dresnick.

As the medical director of the NFL Players Association, I have benefited from the wisdom of two executive directors, Gene Upshaw (who gave me the job in 2001) and Demaurice "De" Smith, who is as wise and articulate as he is kind and generous. Sean Sansiveri has been my principal partner in health and safety work, as well as Tom DePaso, Ira Fishman, Dr. Don Davis, Ernie Conwell, Tom Carter, and Mark Verstegen.

Finally, words alone fail to express my respect, esteem, and affection for Dr. Rob Strauss, who has been a friend, mentor, and constant source of wisdom for my entire career. There is no one for whom I have more gratitude, and admiration. He is truly a national treasure to all of those who are fortunate enough to lead emergency departments.

DR. STRAUSS'S ACKNOWLEDGMENTS

I would like to thank several individuals who have helped launch and nurture my professional career. Harvey Meislin introduced me to emergency medicine and helped me discover my professional passion. John Lumpkin, Bob Hockberger, and Frank Baker at the University of Chicago provided both rigorous training and invaluable mentoring. Involvement in emergency medicine organizations has been professionally enriching and has also given me great satisfaction. I am grateful late Hal Jayne for introducing me to the realm of national EM education, both program leadership and teaching. I would like to express my deep gratitude to Greg Henry, both for opening doors that allowed me to attain positions of leadership and for being an inspiration to enhance my skills as an educator.

A special thanks to my friends and colleagues at TeamHealth, who have demonstrated astonishing leadership during good and difficult times. I have the honor to work among people with a steadfast focus on improving health care and supporting the well-being of the clinicians providing that care. Among the exemplary leaders, colleagues, role models, mentors, and friends on this "dream team" are Jody Crane, Lynn Massingale, Michael Wiechart, Leif Murphy, Jim George, Theresa Tavernero, Stan Thompson, Randal Dabbs, David Hogan, Abbie Tapp-Pearson, and John Haeberli.

I am fortunate to have been affiliated with institutions that are deeply committed to providing patient care at the highest levels, including the University of Chicago, which provided my foundation in EM and leadership; St. Francis Hospital in Poughkeepsie, which gave me the opportunity to lead and grow for more than 20 years; and the Christ Hospital in Cincinnati for its consistent commitment to excellence.

And finally, my enormous appreciation to Dr. Thom Mayer, my partner in this endeavor; Thom is brilliant and an inspiration to me and all who have the good fortune to work with him. He has great vision, deep passion, and a profound positive regard for others. Thom is a "level 5 leader" possessing great will and humility. I am one of Thom's innumerable fans, whose life he has indelibly enriched.

LEADERSHIP PRINCIPLES

SECTION 1

CHAPTER 1

LEADERSHIP, MANAGEMENT, AND MOTIVATION

Thom A. Mayer

Give me a lever long enough and I can move the world.

—Archimedes[1]

Management is doing things right; leadership is doing the right things.

—Warren Bennis, *On Becoming a Leader*[2]

People want to be settled; but only insofar as they are unsettled is there any hope for them.

—Ralph Waldo Emerson[3]

Do those served grow as persons? Do they, while being served, become healthier, wiser, freer, more autonomous, more likely themselves to become servants?

—Robert Greenleaf, *Servant Leadership*[4]

For those charged with leading and managing the complexity of daily emergency department (ED) operations, it indeed seems as if they are lifting the weight of the world. Archimedes' wisdom is thus a requisite for lifting that weight and knowing which levers to use, when, and in what circumstances. Fortunately, there is a substantial wealth of scientific, evidence-based wisdom to guide the use of those "levers." The tools of leadership, management, and motivation must all be put to use, to varying degrees, to have a successful ED.

However, all of these knowledge bases have, inherent within them, certain dynamic tensions, comprising elements that may seem contradictory or at odds with the other elements. The great Danish physicist, Neils Bohr, recognized these dynamic tensions when he wisely noted:

> *The opposite of a true statement is a false statement. But the opposite of a profound truth may well be another profound truth.*[5]

Embracing these dynamic tensions is necessary to learn which of the levers will be most effective in any issue facing ED leaders.

Success in the ED requires effective leadership and management to coordinate the multiple processes involved in even the simplest aspects of clinical care. These skills are necessary to enable all members of the ED team to have the training, resources, facilities, staff attributes, and sense of mission required for appropriate clinical care. Leadership and management skills should reside not only with the medical and nursing directors but also with every physician and charge nurse in the ED, since every clinical shift requires onsite leadership to function effectively.

Supreme Court Associate Justice John Potter Stewart once noted:

> *I may not be able to define it, but I know what it is when I see it.*[6]

> **BOX 1.1 ■ DEFINING LEADERSHIP EXERCISE**
>
> **Have you had an excellent leader?**
> - What attributes made that person an excellent leader?
> - How did he or she make you feel as a member of the team?
> - Why did you consider that person an excellent leader?
> - How did he or she motivate you and other members of the team?
> - What results did you and the team attain under that leader?
> - Did you want to be like that leader?
>
> **Have you had a poor leader?**
> - Why did you think that person was a poor leader?
> - What attributes made you feel that person wasn't a good leader?
> - How did he or she make you feel?
> - How did he or she fail to motivate you and the other team members?
> - What results did you and the team attain under that leader?
> - How did that experience change your vision of leadership?

Justice Stewart was talking about a different topic, but his logic is true of leadership as well—it is hard to define, but we know it when we see it. Consider the simple exercise in **Box 1.1**, which can help demonstrate that everyone on the ED team inherently knows what it is like to experience both excellent and poor leadership.

These paradigms of leadership occur in the milieu of cataclysmic change in health care, the most pervasive element of which is the dramatic challenge of *becoming the high-quality, low-cost provider of care*. This is a formidable responsibility that requires us to do more (produce better results) with less (fewer and/or less costly resources). Communicating this imperative to those who lead, manage, and provide bedside clinical care is a distinct challenge that requires a high level of leadership, management, and motivational skills. That is the challenge not only of this chapter but of the entire book.

Having had the privilege of delivering the keynote address on leadership and management to the American College of Emergency Physicians' Emergency Department Directors Academy since its inception, one of my most important messages is this:

> *I don't care how your ED functions when you are there. I know it functions well when you're there. How does it operate when you are not there?*[7]

As harsh as that might sound at first, the point is simple—it is not enough to be a good leader and manager. The test of a leader is the ability to teach, inspire, and act as a catalyst for change. High-functioning leaders train their entire team in effective leadership and management and provide the tools and resources required to achieve those skills.

Prior to the United States entering World War II, Prime Minister Winston Churchill said in a BBC radio address on February 9, 1941:

> *Give us the tools and we will finish the job.*[8]

As leaders, it is our responsibility to give the most effective tools to all our staff, so that these tools are available 24 hours a day, 7 days a week, 365 days per year. One of the central goals of this textbook is to ensure that the principles of ED leadership and management are available to those entrusted with the care of emergency patients. Since its beginnings as a defined specialty in the late 1960s, emergency medicine has depended on a body of knowledge that comprises effective ED management and leadership. This chapter and those that follow seek to provide the best available resources to assist the ED team in delivering the best possible clinical care in environments that are conducive to stellar outcomes and the long-term successful practice of emergency medicine.

WORKING SMARTER, NOT HARDER

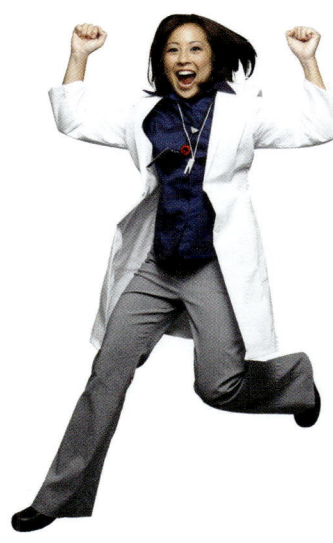

When confronted with the need to improve results, it is common to hear ED staff say, "But we're working so *hard!*" To which the best response is, "Don't work harder, work *smarter!*" Consider the picture at left: Is that you going *in* to work, or going *home?* Because that's the way we should feel going *in* to work every day. The jobs we do in the ED are so fundamentally important and inspiring, if only we can put the right tools in the hands of the team.

The first role of any leader is to equip their team with the tools needed to "work smarter, not harder." One of the core issues of working smarter is understanding what should be changed and what should not. For example, as we will discuss, the core issues of mission, vision, and values should rarely, if ever, change, as they should be constants to which the members of the team are fully committed (see Chapter 2). But the challenges faced in the ED change almost daily, requiring us to work smarter, adapting our approaches to the exigencies and realities of the circumstances. Perhaps the central paradox is that *the path to stability and growth is forever through change and innovation, guided by the wisdom of knowing what to change and what to maintain.*

If we can give the tools of leadership and management to our staff, we can avoid a persistent myth:

Trying to lead physicians/nurses is like trying to lead cats.

That statement is deeply offensive to me . . . because I have cats! Actually, I don't have cats, but the point is clear. Without effective tools, expecting better leadership—and better results—is futile. Without a clearly stated plan that is understood by the entire team, we can't expect effective change. As my colleague Dr. Kirk Jensen and I noted several years ago:

Some is not a number . . .
Soon is not a time . . .
Somehow is not a strategy.[9]

"Some is not a number" emphasizes that we need to define, in an environment where benchmarks matter, what specific metrics are expected to improve. "Soon is not a time" means that improvement must come within specified time frames. And "somehow is not a strategy" emphasizes that there must be a specified plan understood by everyone on the team, delineating what the team will do differently.

This leads to a simple set of principles for leaders to follow when addressing any problem facing the ED team:

- What are the data?
- What is the delta?
- What is the decision?[7]

The "data" are the specifics of an effective metrics-based approach that the team can agree on as a vision for improvement (see the section on Vision below and in Chapter 2). The "delta" is simply the difference between current results and the target. How far are we from our target and why have we failed to achieve it? If we have achieved or exceeded our metrics targets, why and how did that occur? The "decision" is the specific plan for "some, soon, somehow." What will be done differently, how will it be done differently, and why will that result in better performance? This approach simplifies even the most complex problems to actionable, team-based plans. But as simple as this makes improvement efforts, it doesn't change this brilliant insight from Dr. Paul Batalden (adapting the thoughts of Arthur Jones):

Every system is perfectly designed to get precisely the results it gets.[10]

Are your current results (eg, metrics, patient experience scores, safety markers, clinical guideline compliance, etc.) where you want them to be? If so, you have a great system that is "perfectly designed" to get those results. But, for most of us, there is a substantial "delta" between where we are and where we want to be on performance and the strategic deployment of the resources requisite to obtain that performance. If we are in that category, Batalden's fundamental insight is that the *very nature and fabric of the system itself* (not just the components of the system) *must change* if we expect different results.

NAVIGATING THE WHITEWATER OF CHANGE

In the past, change was viewed as dangerous, disruptive, and difficult—not unlike kayaking through class V river rapids. But, previous generations of emergency clinicians could also look forward to calm, placid stretches of "river" where, once change had been weathered, staff could simply operate under newly established processes, free from the threat of change. Unfortunately, the current health-care environment does not afford clinicians with such luxuries. We now live in "perpetual whitewater," where scarcely one change is absorbed before another is upon us.[11]

One of the most important tools for leaders is to become expert change accelerators. The first step in that journey is to realize that resistance to change is not only natural and expected, it fundamentally arises from a fear of the unknown. The more profound the resistance, the deeper the uncertainty for those who will experience the change.

Successfully navigating these "rapids" requires an understanding of Emerson's profound insight that meaningful change requires leaders to become professional unsettlers: people who can provide maximum certainty in the most uncertain of times. ED leaders must understand this dynamic tension between change and providing guidance to those whose lives are being changed. Leaders must become expert change accelerators, capable of providing an environment in which change can flourish and capable of acting as a catalyst for further effective change.

A major part of being an effective change accelerator is understanding that, without resistance, there is no fundamental change, particularly in a complex adaptive system like the ED.[12] An important corollary to this concept is that resistance — an inevitable byproduct of fundamental changes to any system — is a clear sign of uncertainty on the part of those who perceive that their lives are being altered. As a leader, it is your job to deal effectively and proactively with this resistance by providing a reassuring framework for managing the change.

CONNECTING THE GEARS

In his excellent book, *The Fifth Discipline: The Art and Science of Learning Organizations*, Peter Senge emphasized the concept of "shared mental models," defined as "deeply ingrained assumptions, generalizations, or even pictures or images that influence how we understand the world and how we take action."[13] For example, the evidence-based guidelines of the Advanced Trauma Life Support, Advanced Cardiac Life Support, and Pediatric Advanced Life Support courses are shared mental models that create a clear process by which all ED team members will respond, given certain clinical presentations. One of the most important

FIGURE 1.1 ■ Shared Mental Models

Connect the Gears

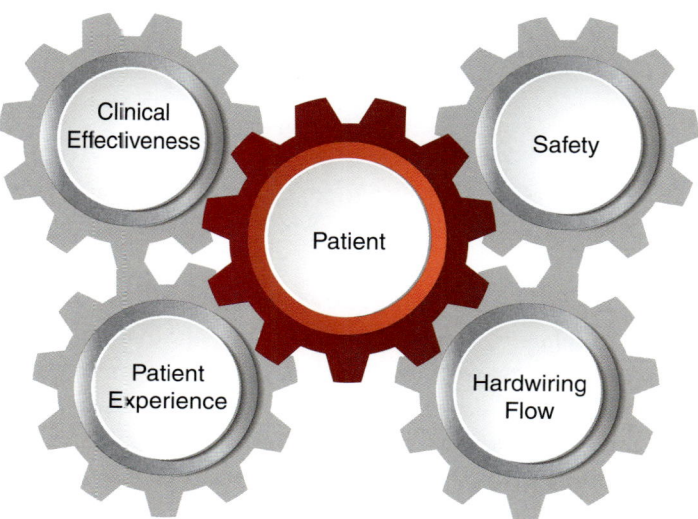

Leaders must be able to "connect the gears" of clinical outcomes, safety, flow, and patient experience, which are connected not only to the patient, but to each other. No gear can be moved without affecting all of the others.

shared mental models for health care leaders and managers is the concept of "connecting the gears" among the requisite components necessary for success (**Figure 1.1**). As discussed above, the patient is at the center of all we do in health care, and all of the "gears" are connected through their relationship to the patient. That much is perhaps intuitive: Each of those disciplines have value only insomuch as they have an impact on the patient.

However, this management approach requires the deeper insight that *moving any one of the gears not only affects the patient, it also affects each of the other disciplines*.[7] For example, adopting a new process of triage bypass (where triage is bypassed when rooms, doctors, nurses, and ED techs are available, thereby allowing the patient to go directly to the room) certainly has an effect on hardwiring flow. But, properly considered, it also has an effect on the patient's experience and safety (by decreasing delays). ("We have a new program that allows you to see the physician and nurse immediately, instead of waiting to be triaged and registered.")

Talented leaders and managers ensure that any new processes not only have a direct effect on the patient but that their essential connections to the other "gears" are considered in detail. This concept is important in every change effort or innovation.

LEADERSHIP AND MANAGEMENT: GENERAL PRINCIPLES

As Harvard Business School Professor John Kotter noted:

> *Leadership and management are two distinctive and complementary systems of action. Each has its own function and characteristic activities. Both are necessary for success in an increasingly complex and volatile environment.* **Most companies today are overmanaged and underled**.[14]

Kotter's insight also applies to hospitals and health care systems, where one of the primary distinguishing features is the *execution* and *agility* of their leaders. In the ED, both

TABLE 1.1 ■ Kotter's Distinctions Between Leadership and Management	
Management	**Leadership**
Planning	Envisioning
Budgeting	Strategies
Organizing	Alignment
Staffing	Empowerment
Controlling	Direction setting

leadership and management skills are required for success. How do these two entities differ? How are they related? Insights from several seminal thinkers on leadership and management assist in answering these questions. The simplest definitions hold that management involves the day-to-day details of an organization, accomplishing its assigned tasks to achieve its desired goals. Management is an activity of maintenance, control, short-range thinking, and bottom-line focus—not unlike progressing persistently along a defined path to a given outcome. Leadership utilizes motivation, vision, empowerment, long-range focus, and the ability to envision new and potentially exciting ways of operating. Not surprisingly, this connotes a more appealing image in which the leader has the view from the bridge and the manager has the view from the trenches.

Kotter summarizes this well:

Leadership is the development of vision and strategies, the alignment of relevant people behind those strategies, and the empowerment of individuals to make a vision happen, despite obstacles. This is in contrast to management, which involves keeping the current system working through planning, operating, organizing, staffing, controlling and problem solving.[15]

Table 1.1 illustrates several important distinctions between leadership and management, two fundamentally different, yet interrelated, concepts (**Figure 1.2**). Much like the dynamic tension that exists between leadership and management, there are similar pressures exerted by *execution*—the ability to produce measurable results despite resistance—and *agility*—the capacity for rapid, responsive change. Execution requires management skills, while agility requires leadership skills. Both are necessary for success.

FIGURE 1.2 ■ The Dynamic Tension of Leadership

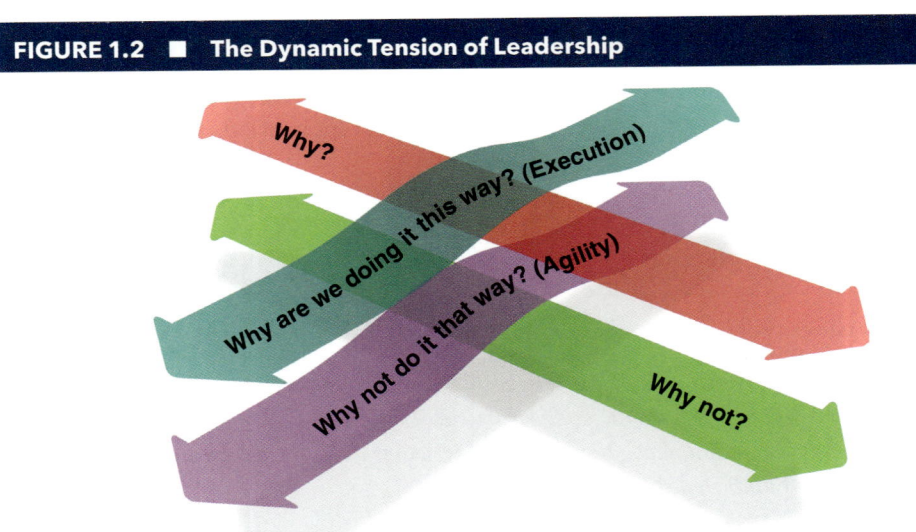

> **BOX 1.2 ■ CASE STUDY ONE**
>
> **The hospital CEO, with whom you have an excellent relationship, tells you in your monthly meeting:**
>
> "It is taking too long to be seen in the ED and our metrics and service scores are suffering. You need to hire more physicians immediately!"
>
> Is this a management issue or a leadership issue?
>
> - The **collection and monitoring** of data are **management** functions.
> - The **interpretation and envisioning** of data are **leadership** functions.
> - Each of these functions must be integrated in order to answer this massive issue intelligently.
> - The key data point (management) with regard to physician staffing is not "*door to doctor*" but rather "*bed to doctor.*"
> - Identifying the key metric is a **leadership** issue.
> - If "door-to-doctor" times are long but "bed-to-doctor" intervals are short, there are likely too few beds or nurses. Leadership may need to change the process by "*frontloading*" care.

Management asks:

Why are we doing it this way? And, how can we execute measurable results that add value to patient care?

Leadership asks:

Why not do it another way, which may be a better and fundamentally different approach to eliminating waste?

The key to the "Why" question is *adding value*; once value is identified, it should be accentuated, and the team needs to be held accountable for performing in predictable ways that support a common goal. The "Why not?" question focuses on ways in which processes can be changed to eliminate waste in order to further the aim of becoming a high-quality, low-cost provider of care. **Boxes 1.2** and **1.3** showcase case studies that illustrate the importance of understanding whether the challenges faced are related to leadership or management and which tools should be used to accomplish the tasks at hand.

Ask your team these "Why" questions:

- Why are we doing this process this way?
- Does it add value? How?
- Is everyone doing it that way if it is truly adding value?
- If not, how can we hold those who are not following the process accountable?

> **BOX 1.3 ■ CASE STUDY TWO**
>
> | **Management** | **Leadership** |
> |---|---|
> | • Collection and monitoring of data | • Interpretation of data's meaning |
> | • Door-to-doctor and bed-to-doctor data collection | • Knowing which data point is key (bed-to-doctor) |
> | **Solution:** more emergency physicians | **Solution:** more ED beds or "frontloading flow" |

> **BOX 1.4 ■ CASE STUDY THREE**
>
> - You have a stable group of ED docs but massive turnover of ED nurses, including the nurse manager position (you have had 6 in 10 years).
> - Your doctors complain that the hospital is hiring ED nurses *"right out of nursing school"* and that there are so many agency nurses that *"we don't even know their names."*
> - The new administrator in charge of the ED (a nurse) says *"Your docs don't understand team work"* and that they *"Complain too much."*
>
> **Conclusion:** The data (management issue) may be correct; the use of agency nurses is a patient safety issue. However, the failure to focus on a team-based solution is a fundamental *leadership* issue.

Now ask these *"Why not?"* questions:

- Why not do this process another way?
- Would that new way add more value, eliminate waste, or both? How?
- What are the obstacles to making this change?
- What will we save by doing things differently?
- How can we be agile enough as a team to successfully make this change?

Bennis, Block, Drucker, Peters, and Kotter, each in a unique way, have contributed to our understanding of these definitions.[15-19] **Box 1.4** summarizes many of these distinctions and is drawn from the works of those authors. It should be referred to during the course of the following discussion. Renowned leadership authority Stephen Covey uses the metaphor of cutting your way through the jungle, which managers do extremely well.[20] But, it takes a leader to climb a tree, survey the landscape, and say, "Wrong jungle!" To which I would add:

Management is about the things we do and how we do them. Leadership is who we are.

Both leadership and management skills are necessary, but it is up to us to determine whether the current challenge we face is primarily a leadership or a management issue.

Leadership Comes at a Price

Uneasy lies the head that wears the crown.

–William Shakespeare,
Henry IV, Part II[21]

Shakespeare's wisdom has held true through the ages and is as accurate now as when it was written in the 17th century. While there are many reasons for that, one of the most important is that people don't typically mind change, but they resent being changed. Being told to do things differently disrupts their lives and forces them into new, unfamiliar processes. And yet, by its very nature, leadership precisely requires us to act as the agent of that disruption. Leaders must be skillful "professional unsettlers," carefully guiding which things to change and which to leave in place. (As noted previously, the decision on what to change and what to leave in place is largely made by whether the process adds value or constitutes waste.) George Bernard Shaw makes the same point in different words:

The reasonable man adapts himself to the world: the unreasonable one persists in trying adapt the world to himself. Therefore, all progress depends on the unreasonable man.[22]

> **BOX 1.5 ■ ATTRIBUTES OF "PROFESSIONAL UNSETTLERS"**
>
> - Passion
> - Patient-first focus
> - Integrity
> - Tenacity
> - Humility

What are the essential attributes of these "unreasonable men" and "professional unsettlers" (**Box 1.5**)? The first is surely *passion*, since only passion for the difficult work of health care leaders can sustain us when times are tough. And, in the current and future health care environment, times will most assuredly always be tough. The second is an unrelenting *commitment to the patient*, which is what drives passion in the first place. In the midst of change, this requires the ability to constantly focus on the questions:

- Is this good for the patient?
- Why is it good for the patient?
- How is it good for the patient?
- Will this benefit one group of patients at the expense of others?

The third is *integrity*, including unalloyed personal honesty in the face of what are inevitably controversial decisions. The crucible of leadership cannot be survived without integrity. The paradox of course is that everyone assumes they have integrity—until it is challenged. The chaos of change always presents challenges requiring integrity.

The fourth is *tenacity*, the ability to persevere while leading from the front by example during the travails of the whitewater of change.

Finally, *humility* is essential, since the terribly difficult times of crisis require an ability to keep this insight at our core: It's never about us, it's about the patients and the people who take care of those patients.

Leadership 1, 2, 3

Parents often tell their children, "You can do this—it is as easy as 1, 2, 3!" The question, of course, is "What are 1, 2, and 3?" On the topic of leadership, three fundamental principles help guide leadership initiatives and help frame a pragmatic understanding of the motivations of others.

1. What is the **"One Myth"** for those involved?
2. What is their **intrinsic motivation?**
3. What is their **self-interest**?

The One Myth

> *There is some One Myth for every man which, if we but knew it,*
> *would tell us all that he did and all that he thought.*
>
> —William Butler Yeats[23]

Yeats's powerful insight is that each person has certain inherent guiding principles that inform and illuminate how they approach issues. The *"One Myth"* is similar to an internal gyroscope or guidance system, a benchmark by which the person can analyze complex issues, particularly through the difficult process of change. Stephen Covey calls this "True North."[23] For Tom Peters it is "Brand You."[24] The "One Myth" is much like a lens through which each of us views our world and our place in it.

> **BOX 1.6 ■ QUESTIONS TO HELP DELINEATE THE "ONE MYTH"**
>
> - *"What excites you most about this?"*
> - *"What concerns you most?"*
> - *"What would success look like to you and your patients?"*
> - *"What role would you like to play as we move forward?"*

Discovering the "One Myth" is complicated by the unfortunate fact that many—perhaps most—people are not fully aware of the "One Myth" that guides their own approach to life. However, as **Box 1.6** illustrates, there are some fundamental questions that can assist the leader in uncovering their own "One Myth" and the "One Myth" held by others.

Within certain medical specialties or subspecialties, there are certain commonalities of the "One Myth." Trauma surgeons, for example, tend to be highly protocol-driven and focused on clear and identifiable processes leading to a defined end point. Internists, while still evidence-based in their approach, face broader, less distinct problems in their practice and focus on details, particularly in how the diagnosis is arrived at. Pediatricians have a common focus on the needs of children, sometimes even to a messianic extent, sometimes assuming that *only they* truly know the needs of children.

We emergency physicians are often called "adrenaline junkies," implying that our "One Myth" is the immediacy of diagnosing and treating life- or limb-threatening problems. We assume the worst—and treat it when it is there—but know that in most cases we will be able to tell patients more about what they "don't have" (ruling out diagnoses) than what they do (ruling in diagnoses).

Simply stated, if you listen carefully and observe astutely, your colleagues will help you discover their "One Myth" as they approach both patient care and the changes needed to deliver that care.

Intrinsic Motivation

Abraham Maslow, Eric Erickson, and many other psychiatrists and psychologists have noted the fundamental role that intrinsic motivation plays in motivating and sustaining change, which is summarized in this insight[25-29]:

All meaningful and lasting change is driven by **intrinsic, not extrinsic** *motivation.*

This insight is particularly important in health care leadership, precisely because of the hierarchical nature of most medical systems, which are often driven primarily, if not exclusively, by extrinsic motivation. Top-down, "Do it because I'm the Boss and I said so," approaches are classic examples of extrinsic motivation.

The word *motivate* is from French and Latin roots that simply refer to "moving" or "movement." This etymological insight is interesting, given the more modern meanings of motivation, which focus on a complex array of factors influencing individuals to act in certain ways. However, an important distinction in motivational theory is that negative, extrinsic motivators simply do not lead to actual motivation but rather to temporary and often begrudging compliance. Herzberg notes that negative, extrinsic motivating factors are at best incomplete, temporary, and unsatisfying.[29] He also

FIGURE 1.3 ■ EXTRINSIC VS NATURAL CHANGE

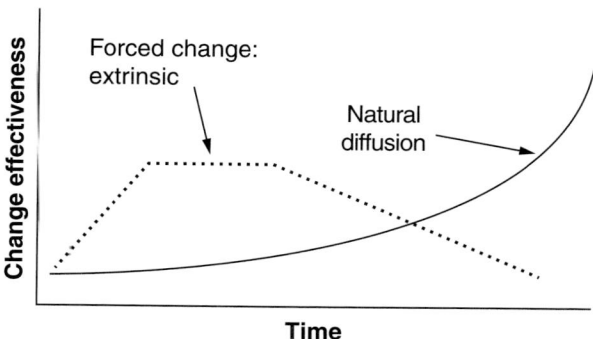

Forced (ie, extrinsic) change can produce early results, but these results quickly plateau before predictably declining. The natural diffusion of ideas requires somewhat longer to produce results, but these changes are often better and more sustainable over time.

makes the important point that what he refers to as positive "KITA" (which he wryly describes as "kick in the... 'pants'") is also a recipe for failure in most settings in which motivation is needed.

The temporary, grudging, and often incomplete compliance resulting from extrinsic motivation produces nonsustainable results. **Figure 1.3** illustrates the insight that forced or extrinsic change does in fact produce rapid results, usually motivated by fear in hierarchical systems. (As Aristotle said. "The prospect of death wonderfully concentrates the mind."[30])

Unfortunately, these results plateau quickly and follow a predictable, steady regression, as shown on the right side of the figure. By contrast, change effectiveness from natural diffusion takes longer to take hold, but these efforts lead to more dramatic, sustainable results over time. However, as **Figure 1.4** shows, change driven by *intrinsic motivation* produces faster results, effectively "shifting" the curve dramatically to the left, making it far more effective, particularly in an environment in which the workforce is comprised of highly trained physicians and nurses, who are accustomed to using data and intrinsic values to guide change.

Intrinsic motivation includes factors such as a sense of personal and professional work, internal recognition for doing a difficult job, personal and professional growth and advancement, and contributing to the overall well-being and health of their patients and the community. Chris Argyris, Peter Senge, Tom Peters, and others have indicated that a principled or value-driven

FIGURE 1.4 ■ EXTRINSIC VS INTRINSIC CHANGE

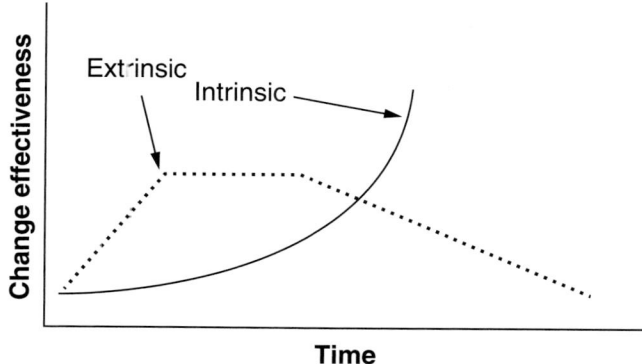

Using intrinsic motivation to drive effective change "shifts the curve to the left" in that it accelerates both the pace of the change and the quality of the results.

> **BOX 1.7 ■ PATIENT-FIRST: MISSION-BASED PRACTICES**
>
> Mission statements that focus on the patient first tap into the intrinsic motivation of emergency personnel, whose inner drive is to assist the ill and injured:
>
> **Rule #1 -** Always do the right thing for the patient
>
> **Rule #2 -** Do the right thing for the people who take care of the patient
>
> **Rule #3 -** Never confuse rule #1 and rule #2.

approach results in professionals and organizations whose goals are clear because they are self-evident.[4,31] Their processes are innovative, they attract high-caliber talent, and they are committed to the patients they serve. As Leonard Berry points out in his study of the Mayo Clinic's success, a "Patient-First" mission always resonates with principled health care providers (**Box 1.7**).[32]

By way of example, improving customer service to patients is one of the most common challenges that ED leaders and managers face. It is not uncommon for hospital executives to take an authoritarian, extrinsic approach to motivation, telling managers, "Get your scores up or I will find someone who can!" However, as illustrated in more detail in Chapter 10, these approaches are rarely successful or sustainable for the long term because they are founded on extrinsic motivation.

Using effective intrinsic motivation requires well-developed communication skills, the most effective of which is *listening*. The ability to listen to an ED staff articulate their vision for providing the best possible patient care is always at the heart of intrinsic motivation in that it helps leaders and managers to understand those with whom they work with and those who provide care to our patients. Simply stated:

The more professionals are involved in the earliest stages of change efforts, the more intrinsic motivation allows for dramatic and successful change.

Self-Interest

Russia is a riddle wrapped in a mystery inside an enigma.

—Winston Churchill[33]

The above quotation is one of Churchill's best known—but, when taken out of context, it is entirely misleading. The conclusions typically drawn from this statement lead the reader 180° off the mark. At first glance, Churchill's words imply that he believed that Russia's behavior was totally unpredictable, but nothing could be further from the truth.

Here is what Churchill did say, in full context, in his BBC radio address on October 1, 1939:

> *I cannot forecast to you the actions of Russia. It is a riddle wrapped in a mystery inside an enigma: but perhaps there is a key.* **That key is Russian natural interest**.[33]

Churchill, far from bemoaning the inability to predict Russia's actions, is telling us that Russia's actions can nearly always be predicted if one can ascertain its national- or self-interest.

Churchill's wisdom leads to a key leadership insight: Always seek to determine, in any endeavor, the self-interest of the stakeholders. If that is understood, success is far more likely. Further, with the intelligence, good grace, and fortune to respect and, to the best extent possible, honor those self-interests, not only will the proximal results of leadership be improved, but the foundation necessary for future success will have been laid.

The obvious question remains: How can others' self-interest be determined? Two key methods are valuable in determining self-interest. The first is simple and straightforward, but often neglected; ask:

What is your self-interest?

For some, this approach is too blunt and direct. If so, the following questions can help determine self-interest in a more oblique way:

- What is the best outcome for your patients?
- What is the best outcome for you and your group?
- How do those outcomes rank against those of other patients and groups in a capacity- and resource-constrained environment?
- What would success look like to you and your patients in this endeavor?
- What does success look like to you and your colleagues?

These questions help determine self-interest. They also help focus on the patient and their needs as the central goals of our efforts. The second way to discover self-interest is a time-honored adage:

The best predictor of future behavior . . . is past behavior.

Thus, observing the actions of others in past situations helps establish a sense of how and why stakeholders have acted in the past, particularly in difficult situations or negotiations. This applies to not just individuals but groups as well. Past observations of change-management efforts and executive committee, department, and quality improvement meetings can help illuminate the self-interests of individuals and the groups they collectively comprise.

SERVANT LEADERSHIP

Robert Greenleaf, a pioneer of organizational learning, is among the most influential people in the field of servant leadership. In a penetrating 1969 essay that dramatically changed the way leaders were viewed, Greenleaf writes:

> *A fresh critical look is being taken at the issues of power and authority, and people are beginning to learn, however haltingly, to relate to one another in less coercive and more creatively supporting ways. A new moral principle is emerging, which holds that the only authority deserving one's allegiance is that which is freely and knowingly granted by the led to the leader in response to, and in proportion to, the clearly evident servant stature of the leader. Those who choose to follow this principle will not casually accept the authority of existing institutions.* **Rather, they will freely respond only to individuals who were chosen as leaders because they were proven and trusted as servants.**[34]

Greenleaf recognized that this new concept would not be welcomed in the existing corridors of power, where too few view themselves as servants and too many have viewed leadership as exerting power and authority over those who are led. The servant leader is always a servant first, then a leader. These are understandably extreme ends of the leadership spectrum, between which, as Greenleaf noted, "are shadings and blends that are part of the infinite variety of human nature."[34]

Servant leadership presents a dynamic tension between the call for service and a legitimate need to exercise accountability. Indeed, the mandate to produce results is built into the performance plan of every leader and manager. This trend in health care is only accelerating.[14] In this environment, how can one emphasize servant leadership?

Consider the following two quotations, which highlight this dynamic tension between servant leadership and accountability. The first answers the question, *"What is the best test of the servant leader?"*

> *Do those served grow as persons? Do they, while being served, become healthier, wiser, freer, more autonomous, more likely themselves to become servants? And, what is the effect on the least privileged in society?*[34]

Greenleaf's focus is clearly on those who are being served, as opposed to those who are leading, and our ability to expand their capabilities. While Greenleaf didn't speak specifically of ED leaders, one can't help being impressed at the applicability of what he says to what emergency physicians and nurse leaders do daily, which is to serve others, to help expand their capabilities, and to consider "the effect on the least privileged in society." Contrast this with these words, which appeared in the same essay, several paragraphs later, speaking to the use of power and accountability among servant leaders.

> *I cannot conceive why anyone would want to be in a position of leadership anywhere unless one is comfortable with getting and using power. The wear and tear on the individual who leads is too great, and nothing, in my judgment, but the satisfaction of using power would compensate for the personal investment.*[34]

As leaders and mangers in the ED, we must be able to create teams capable of serving first, but serving consistently and accountably as well. In the words of political theorist Baruch Spinoza, *"Excellence is what we strive for, but consistency is what we demand."*[35] That requires using power to create teams capable of providing accountable results for the patients as well as for those who take care of the patients. Greenleaf's dynamic tension between servant leaders and their use of power is illustrated in this example. All physician and nurse leaders seek to provide the best patient experience and part of their role is acting as servant leaders to motivate the team to that end. But they are also accountable to "the C-suite" for delivering excellent patient experience scores.

Previously, we noted that extrinsic motivation ("Do it because I say so!" or "Do it or we'll all get fired.") is ineffective. Only intrinsic motivation is likely to motivate professionals. As servant leaders, this distinction is critical. First, by tapping into intrinsic motivation ("Do it because these tools and behaviors *make your job easier*.") servant leaders are far more likely to effectively change behavior, since the team recognizes this is helpful to them as well as the patients. Second, developing and delivering the best service excellence/patient experience tools (with the input of the team) *serves the team* by giving them the needed tools and talents to deliver higher scores. Third, by serving first, leaders can then expect personal and team accountability, precisely because they have provided the requisite skills to perform at a high level.

LIMITS BEGIN WHERE VISION ENDS

Successful leadership does not occur without developing and communicating a clear vision of what constitutes success for the ED team and its patients. Chapter 2 covers vision and mission statements in much greater detail, but an overview is important here. Unless leaders and managers have a clear sense of what is required of them, how can they possibly produce results that patients and those who serve the patients require?

An event occurred on May 6, 1954, which, to the best of human knowledge, had never happened in human history. It transpired at Iffley Road track in Oxford, England, and news of it spread rapidly around the world, even in that far less technologically enhanced world. Many of the most sophisticated medical minds of the time said that the feat was simply impossible—the human body was incapable of attaining it. Others opined that surely a man would die in the attempt.

What happened on May 6, 1954? Roger Bannister, then a medical student at Oxford University studying exercise physiology, ran mankind's first sub-4-minute mile, covering the distance in 3 minutes, 59.6 seconds. In a way that can scarcely be imagined over 60 years later, this event truly stunned the world precisely because so many experts claimed it was impossible (there were admonishments, taken quite seriously at the time, that the heart would burst, the brain would hemorrhage, or the lungs would collapse). This accomplishment was treated, as well it should have been, as a triumph not just of athleticism but of the human spirit.

However, in only 27 months from May 6, 1954, 10 runners had run sub-4-minute miles. In fact, 1 year and 2 weeks later, three men, in the same day, in the **same race**, ran sub-4-minute miles![36] These athletes achieved something for the first time in human history—something that was felt by many to be physiologically unattainable. Yet, once once the *vision* became a reality it became almost commonplace. In fact, by 2012, the 1,000th man had run a sub-4-minute mile.

This is precisely what is meant by "limits begin where vision ends."[37] Tying this insight to the dynamic tension of execution and agility drives our efforts to continuously envision means by which we can drive our ED forward. Unless it can be dreamed, it certainly can't be done. But, once it has been dreamed and then attained, progress is greatly accelerated, like those three runners in the same race. The goal must then be made practical and reproducible, as President Harry S. Truman noted when asked about his philosophy:

The object and its accomplishment is my philosophy![38]

Successful innovation will be the defining attribute of successful health care systems in the quest to provide high-quality, low-cost providers of care.[39] Without a clearly defined and articulated vision, this is simply impossible.

WHAT'S YOUR "ELEVATOR SPEECH"?

Imagine you are headed up to "round" on several patients admitted to the hospital and are waiting for the elevator. The elevator door opens and you see the following people already on the elevator:

- Chief Executive Officer
- Chief Operations Officer
- Chief Medical Officer
- Chief Nursing Officer
- Board Chairman

These administrators will inevitably ask you, "How's it going down in the ED?" You have a journey of five floors to tell the story of your ED. That's your "Elevator Speech." What will you say? It's important that you have the speech ready ahead of time, well thought-out and rehearsed. What should your speech be about? It should always start and end with the patient. Regardless of the issue, the story of the ED should be about the folks we take care of on a daily basis, not just the people who take care of them. For example, if your ED has a serious problem with hospital boarders, you might say:

"We have 12 boarders and only 20 beds. If we don't solve this issue, I can't keep our good doctors."

Or:

"Our nurses have had it with all these boarders. They are leaving in droves because they say they 'didn't sign up to be a floor nurse.'"

Those two statements, while undoubtedly true, focus on the doctors and nurses, not on the patients, who are those who suffer the most. Instead, think about an "Elevator Speech" which focuses first on the patient.

"I'm so glad you asked. We have 12 hospital boarders, some of whom have been waiting over 24 hours for a bed upstairs. Please come with me to the ED and I'll introduce you to them so you can hear what it's been like for them."

Make sure you have your elevator speech ready, and make it about the patient first—every time.

THE POWER OF THE STORY

Our patients come to us for a variety of reasons and clinical presentations, but all need answers to several fundamental questions: Why did their symptoms develop, what do they mean, and how should they be treated? This dynamic requires every emergency clinician to assume the role of "Chief Story Teller," tasked with explaining the reasons for the tests and treatments within the context of each patient's care. This mandate also applies to department leaders, who understand the truth of the great Danish writer, Isak Dinesen (nee Baroness Karen von Blixen), who noted:

All sorrows can be borne if you can put them into a story or tell a story about them.[40]

Leaders at all levels must understand and embrace this insight and put it into work when telling the story of the ED. All great storytellers know, it is not just the story you tell, it's how you tell it. Consider the following examples from history.

Abraham Lincoln did not say:

These dead soldiers inspire us.

But he did say:

That from these honored dead we take increased devotion to that cause for which they gave the last full measure of devotion.

And the world changed . . .
Sir Winston Churchill did not say:

We shall fight as long and wherever we need to.

But he did say:

We shall fight on the beaches, we shall fight on the landing grounds, we shall fight in the fields and the streets, we shall fight in the hills. We shall never surrender.

And the world changed . . .
Dr. Martin Luther King did not say:

I have a negotiating strategy that will accomplish affirmative action.

But he did say:

I have a dream that one day our children will be judged not by the color of their skin but by the content of their character. I have a dream.

And the world changed...

Can a small group of ED team members change the world? Margaret Mead had the answer:

> How can anyone doubt that a small group of dedicated people can change the world. Indeed, it is the only thing that ever has.

As leaders, our words—and the actions they inspire—not only make a difference, they are capable of changing our world for our patients and those who care for those patients.

PUTTING IT ALL TO WORK

How best can these tools be used to make your job easier? The following list can help address any problem leaders and managers may face:

- How would great leaders I have had in the past approach this problem?
- What's the data?
- What's the delta?
- What's the decision?
- Some (what data?), soon (when will it be measured?), somehow (what will be done differently?)
- How can we improve the system itself?
- What's the nature or level of change anticipated?
- How do the "gears" (patient safety, clinical outcomes, hardwiring flow, etc.) connect to the patient and affect the other gears?
- Is this primarily a leadership challenge (agility and change) or a management challenge (execution and accountability)?
- Why are we doing it this way? Why not do it another way?
- How will the leader(s) have to "unsettle" the team to make this change? Which team members will be most "unsettled"?
- What's the "One Myth" for those involved, and how can their intrinsic motivations and self-interests be defined?
- In addressing this issue, how best can we serve the patient and those who serve the patient? Will they more likely become leaders and servants themselves?
- How does this tie into the mission, vision, and values of our ED and health system?
- What's our "Elevator Speech" on this issue?
- How will we tell the story of this issue in a way that helps others understand the challenges we face?

CONCLUSION

Robert Greenleaf said, "Every achievement starts with a goal—but not just any goal and not just anybody saying it. The one who states the goal must enlist trust, especially if it is a high-risk or visionary goal, because those who follow are asked to accept the risking with the leader." Leaders and managers *must* have the ability to tie the passion, energy, and no-harm intent of those they lead in a worthwhile vision, mission, and goals. Again, Greenleaf says it well:

> Not much happens without a dream. And for something great to happen, there must be a great dream. Behind every great achievement is a dreamer of great dreams.

For those who aspire to lead and inspire EDs, perhaps the best advice is the simplest advice: *Dream great dreams!*

REFERENCES

1. Archimedes, quoted by Pappus of Alexandria, *Synagoge*, Book VIII.
2. Bennis W. *On Becoming a Leader*. Reading, Mass: Addison-Wesley; 1989.
3. Emerson RW. Circles. In: Robinson DM, ed. *The Spiritual Emerson Essential Writings*. Boston, Mass: Beacon Press; 2004.
4. Greenleaf RK. *Servant Leadership: A Journey Into the Nature of Legitimate Power and Greatness*. New York, NY: Paulist Press; 1977: 27.
5. Bohr H. My Father. In: *Neils Bohr: His Life and Work*. 1967: 328 New York: Wiley.
6. *Jacobellis v Ohio*, 378 US, 184 (1964) (Stewart JP).
7. Mayer T. *Developing Leadership and Communication Skills*. Dallas, Tex: American College of Emergency Physicians Emergency Department Directors Academy; 2018.
8. Churchill WC. Radio address on BBC, February 9, 1941. In Shapiro FR, ed. *The Yale Book of Quotations*. New Haven, Conn: Yale University Press; 2006.
9. Jensen K, Mayer T. *The Patient Flow Advantage: How Hardwiring Hospital-Wide Flow Drives Competitive Advantage*. Gulf Breeze, Fla: Fire Starter Press; 2016.
10. Batalden P. In a speech at Dartmouth College. 2015. Institute for Healthcare Improvement. Available at: http://www.ihi.org/communities/blogs/_layouts/15/ihi/community/blog/itemview.aspx?List=7d1126ec-8f63-4a3b-9926-c44ea3036813&ID=159. Accessed June 2, 2019.
11. Mayer T. Increasing healthcare's value by reducing waste and clinical variability. Presented at: the American College of Healthcare Executives Senior Executive Program; June 2, 2014; Chicago, Ill.
12. Mayer T, Jensen KJ. *Hardwiring Flow*. Gulf Breeze, Fla: Fire Starter Press; 2010.
13. Senge P. *The Fifth Discipline: The Art and Practice of the Learning Organization*. New York, NY: Doubleday; 1990.
14. Kotter J. What leaders really do. *Harv Bus Rev*. 1990;68(3):103-111.
15. Kotter J. *What Leaders Really Do*. New York, NY: Free Press; 1999.
16. Bennis W. *Still Surprised: A Memoir of a Life in Leadership*. San Francisco, Calif: Jossey-Bass; 2010.
17. Block P. *Stewardship: Choosing Service Over Self Interest*. San Francisco, Calif: Berrett-Kohler Publishers; 1993.
18. Drucker P. The new society of organizations. *Harv Bus Rev*. 1992;70(5):95-104.
19. Peters T. *The Little Big Things: 163 Ways to Pursue Excellence*. New York, NY: Harper Collins; 2010.
20. Covey S. *The 7 Habits of Highly Effective People: Powerful Lessons in Personal Change*. New York, NY: Free Press; 2004.
21. Shakespeare W. *Henry IV, Part II (Folger Shakespeare Library)*. New York, NY: Washington Square Press; 2006.
22. Shaw GB. *Man and Superman, Maxims for Revolutionists*. 1906. London, Penguin Classics, 1957.
23. Yeats WB. *Essays and Introductions*. New York, NY: Macmillan; 1961.
24. Peters T. *The Brand You 50: Fifty Ways to Transform Yourself From an "Employee" Into a Brand That Shouts Distinction, Commitment, and Passion!* New York, NY: Albert Knopf; 1999.
25. Maslow A. *Motivation and Personality*. New York, NY: Harper and Row; 1954.
26. Erikson E. *Childhood and Society*. New York, NY: Norton; 1993.
27. Csikszentmihalyi M. *Flow: The Psychology of Optimal Experience*. New York, NY: Harper and Row; 1990.
28. Kohn A. *Punished by Rewards*. Boston, Mass: Houghton Mifflin; 1999.
29. Herzberg F. One more time: how do you motivate employees? *Harv Bus Rev*. 1968;46(1):53-62.
30. Aristotle. *Poetics*. Ann Arbor, Mich: University of Michigan Press; 1990.
31. Argyris C. *Organizational Traps: Leadership, Culture, and Organizational Design*. Oxford, United Kingdom: Oxford University Press; 2010.
32. Berry LL, Seltman KD. *Management Lessons From May Clinic: Inside One of the World's Most Admired Service Organizations*. New York, NY: McGraw-Hill; 2010.
33. Churchill W. Radio address on BBC, October 1, 1939. In: Shapiro FR, ed. *The Yale Book of Quotations*. New Haven, Conn: Yale University Press; 2006.
34. Greenleaf RK. *Servant Leadership: A Journey Into the Nature of Legitimate Power and Greatness*. New York, NY: Paulist Press; 1977:23.
35. Spinoza B. *Ethics*. London, United Kingdom: Penguin Classics; 1994.
36. Bascomb N. *The Perfect Mile: Three Athletes, One Goal, and Less Than Four Minutes to Achieve It*. Boston, Mass: Houghton-Mifflin; 2004.
37. Jensen K, Mayer TA, Welch SJ, Haraden C. *Leadership for Smooth Patient Flow: Improved Outcomes, Improved Service, Improved Bottom Line*. Chicago, Ill: Health Administration Press; 2007.
38. McCullogh D. Harry S. Truman: 1945-1953. In: Wilson RA, ed. *Character Above All: Ten Presidents From FDR to George Bush*. New York, NY: Simon and Schuster; 1995.
39. von Blixen K. nee Isak Dinesen, in an interview with Mohn B. *The New York Times Book Review*. November 3, 1957.
40. Greenleaf RK. *Servant Leadership: A Journey Into the Nature of Legitimate Power and Greatness*. New York, NY: Paulist Press; 1977:100.

CHAPTER 2

VISION, MISSION, VALUES, STRATEGY, AND TACTICS

Thom A. Mayer, Robert W. Strauss

If a man doesn't know what harbor he is seeking, no wind is the right wind.

—Seneca[1]

The most important questions in life are simultaneously those asked least often.

—Danish philosopher Soren Kierkegaard[2]

Seneca and Kierkegaard's powerful insights are also enigmatic. Without a clear sense of where we are going, it is better to be becalmed than to travel in the wrong direction. Unfortunately, the questions that guide us to where we *should* be going are also the ones least often asked. Patients visit the emergency department (ED) not because they want to but rather because of an unexpected (or postponed) pain, concern, fear, accident, or other perceived life-threatening disruption. They assume they are going to the right place to be cared for by people with the necessary skills and training to address their urgent needs. And they assume they will be treated skillfully and expeditiously by a team dedicated to providing the best clinical care and service.

But has that ED team asked and answered these fundamental questions?

- *What is our Vision*... Why does the ED exist?
- *What is our Mission*... What is the ED attempting to do?
- *What are our Values*... Which core and fundamental beliefs guide the ED?
- *What are our Strategies*... What differentiates this ED from other EDs?
- *What are our Tactics*... How will success be accomplished and measured?

These questions correspond to time-tested and valuable planning tools that guide all successful health-care organizations and their EDs. The definitions in **Figure 2.1** help ED leader(s) guide the direction of their EDs. It is difficult, if not impossible, for health-care professionals to attain and maintain success without a clear sense of direction. Though these concepts are a fundamental activity at the highest level of hospitals and health-care systems, few ED leaders have incorporated their institution's answers to these vital questions into their own guiding principles. It is even rarer for ED leaders to guide their departments through the process of creating or adapting their own vision, mission, values, strategy, and tactics. As a result, it is far too common that the answer to the question asked of an emergency nurse or a physician, "Why are you here and what are you trying to do?" is some variant of (delivered with a look of incredulity), "I'm here to see patients—why do you think I am here?"

This chapter provides practical definitions and frameworks for the development and implementation of the principles of vision, mission, values, strategy, and tactics. Each section uses the experience of the broader business definitions of the terms, while also focusing on the specific application to the health-care and ED environments. Practical examples of each are provided in the text and also in **Appendices 2.1–2.3**.

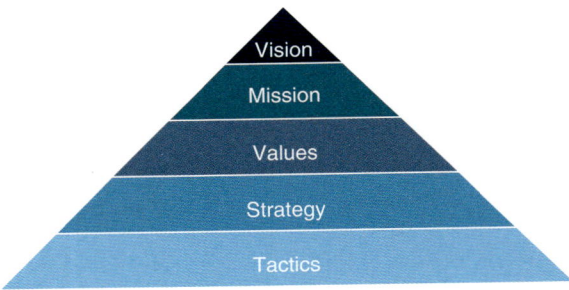

FIGURE 2.1 ■ Vision, Mission, Values, Strategy, and Tactics

1. **Vision:** Why does the ED exist? Why are we here?
2. **Mission:** What is the ED attempting to do?
3. **Values:** Which core and fundamental beliefs guide the ED?
4. **Strategy:** What differentiates this ED from other EDs? Are we making the right choices?
5. **Tactics:** How will this all be accomplished?

VISION: *WHY* DOES THE ORGANIZATION EXIST?

> *He who has a "why" to live can bear almost any "how."*
>
> —Frederick Nietzsche[3]

Failing to provide the *why*, a clear and succinct reason for the organization's existence, is perhaps the most neglected aspect of a health-care organization's development. While mission statements are practically ubiquitous (and often, remarkably similar), it is essential to establish *why* the ED exists prior to defining its mission (*what* the ED, hospital, system is attempting to do).

Effective visions reinforce the core values of the organization while stimulating innovation and encouraging necessary changes. As noted in more detail in Chapters 1 and 3, organizational change requires the wisdom to discern (and celebrate) the fundamentally positive aspects of the team's performance from those that must be transformed. It is challenging to achieve this balance, which accounts for the difficulty of creating effective vision statements in health care.

Building Vision

Collins' and Porras' work on building vision, first published in a *Harvard Business Review* article and later developed more fully in their book *Built to Last: Successful Habits of Visionary Companies*, is an excellent resource to understand the concept of vision and to provide a roadmap to help develop it.[4,5] They note:

> . . .vision has become one of the most overused and least understood words in the language, conjuring up different images for different people: of deeply held values, outstanding achievement, societal bonds, exhilarating goals, motivating forces, or raisons d'etre.[4]

They suggest that effective vision statements must have two components: *core ideology* and *envisioned future*.

Core Ideology

Core ideology asserts what the team stands for—why it exists. It can be further distinguished by its core purpose (the most fundamental reason for being) and its core values (the guiding principles by which it navigates change). The core purpose in health care should always reflect the professional and idealistic motivations for joining this team. This concept is captured by famed management consultant Peter Drucker—the best and most important people in any enterprise are fundamentally volunteers, since they could choose to do the

> **BOX 2.1 ■ EXAMPLES OF HEALTH-CARE CORE IDEOLOGY**
>
> **Mayo Clinic**
> - Patient first
>
> **Saint Mary's Health System**
> - Exceptional care
> - Every patient
> - Every day
>
> **Duke Medicine**
> - Advancing health care together
> - One patient at a time

same work somewhere else or choose to do something else entirely.[6] As a reflection of the *why* of vision, the core purpose is simply an answer to the question, "Why (volunteer) here?" While an understanding of an organization's core purpose is important during successful times, it becomes critical during difficult and evolutionary times like these.

Though often listed separately from the core ideology, core values must be considered in the course of the development and rollout of the vision. Further discussion of core values will be treated in a later section. Examples of core ideology in health care and EDs are listed in **Box 2.1**.

Defining an organization's vision is less about creating a concept or *brand* and more about *discovering* or *uncovering* the organization's *soul* purpose. It is not a "Moses descending from the mountaintop" phenomenon, but rather a search within the organization for its deepest motivations. It cannot be invented or faked. Discovering the vision is not a business strategy about differentiation; it is an essential conversation about what inspires the team.

The Envisioned Future

The envisioned future proclaims what the organization intends to become, the direction in which it will evolve, and the pace required to get there. By definition, these require significant change. Great vision statements envision the future by developing:

- Ambitious plans that inspire change (what Collins and Porras call *big, hairy, audacious goals,* or BHAGs).
- A statement that vividly depicts how the envisioned future will be vibrant, attractive, positive, and meaningful.[5]

Figure 2.2 further illustrates these organizational concepts using the ancient Chinese model of yin (the fundamental unchanging aspects) and yang (the things that must change

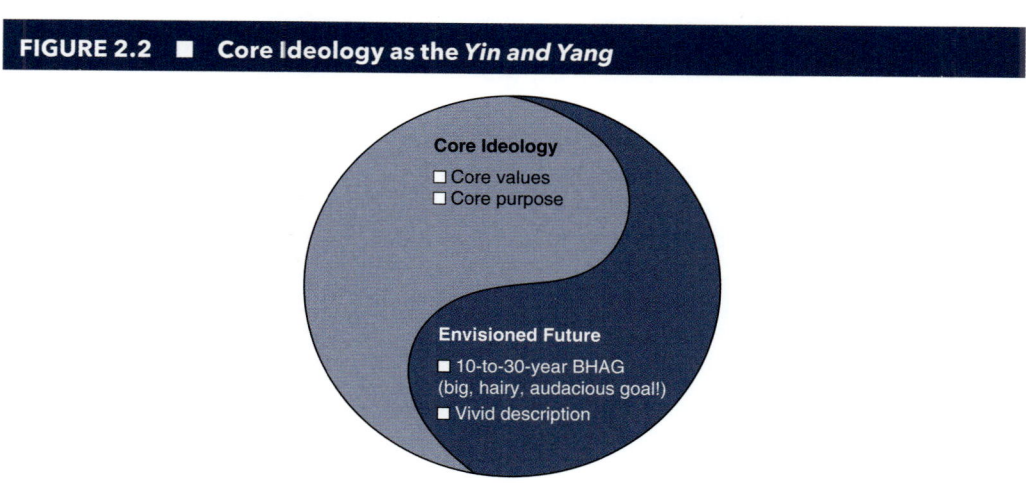

FIGURE 2.2 ■ Core Ideology as the *Yin and Yang*

Adapted with permission from James Collins.

if the team is to *arrive at its destination*). The ED team's BHAGs should not be *sure things*, but rather they should be tangible and not easily attained goals. As Danish physicist Niels Bohr once said to his Nobel Prize-winning protégé, Wolfgang Pauli:

> *We all agree your theory is crazy. The question, which divides us, is whether it is crazy enough.*[7]

As a rule, BHAGs should be attainable about 50% to 70% of the time, clear evidence of their difficulty and the distinct possibility of failure.[5]

Using Vision to Inspire the Team

The language expressing the vision (and the BHAGs driving it) should be chosen carefully for its ability to not only communicate but also inspire current and future team members. Among Winston Churchill's greatest achievements was his ability to use the English language to state great goals and inspire people to achieve them. On May 13, 1940, 3 days after becoming the Prime Minister of Great Britain and facing the Nazi menace, he addressed the House of Commons:

> *You ask: What is our aim? I can answer in one word: Victory! Victory at all costs, victory in spite of all terror, victory however long and hard the road must be.*[8]

On June 18, 1940, again in a speech to the House of Commons, he said:

> *Let us therefore brace ourselves to our duties and so bear ourselves that if the British Empire and its Commonwealth last for a thousand years, men will still say, "This was their finest hour."*[9]

It must be remembered that these words were a form of BHAG. They came at time when the Nazi forces had stormed across Northern Europe and victory was far from certain, even highly unlikely. Indeed, on May 27, 1940, the British Expeditionary Force was desperately evacuated from the beaches at Dunkirk. As American journalist Edward R. Murrow explains:

> *Churchill mobilized the English language and sent it into battle.*[10]

ED vision statements and the BHAGs expressed in them, while not of the world-changing nature of World War II, are critical expressions of the organization's most important aspirations and should have language carefully and skillfully chosen to best express them.

Features of Vision Statements

ED vision statements (and the mission statements addressed in the following section) share these features:

- Developed jointly by the leaders and team members responsible for delivering care
- Integrated with the institution's overall vision
- Focused and concise in nature
- Guides, inspires, and is capable of informing the mission, strategy, tactics, and vision of the organization
- Unique to the organization or the business unit (in this case, the ED)

Developed Jointly

Using the theory, "If they are not with you on the takeoff, they won't be with you on the landing," the first feature ensures involvement of those responsible for providing the service.

As such, it is essential that the leaders charged with directing the service include clinicians when creating the vision. Too often, the leadership team completes these efforts using outside consultants during an offsite meeting or "retreat." The *why* of the ED should describe the reasons talented professionals should want to invest their efforts with this organization as opposed to another ED. This can only occur if both leaders and team members are part of the process.

Integrated

Participation of hospital leadership ensures the vision is integrated with that of the institution. Because EDs are a part of the larger hospital or health-care system, the vision should be closely aligned with the organization's vision. Among the questions that are necessary to ask are:

- How does the ED's vision match the hospital's vision?
- What unique features does the ED have in service of the hospital's vision?

Focused and Concise

Effective vision statements must be succinct. To inspire and motivate staff, vision statements should be expressed in simple, direct language. If it can't be said and repeated back in a few seconds, it won't inspire the staff or even be remembered by them. This language must be carefully crafted if it is to inspire those who:

- Seek to join the team
- Are current members of the team
- Choose to invest their future with the future of *this* ED

Guides and Inspires

The language of a vision statement informs, guides, and inspires not only the team members but also the remaining components of mission, strategy, tactics, and values. Consider this vision statement from the Department of Emergency Medicine at Saint Luke's Hospital (contributed by our colleague Michael Klevins, MD):

> *In everything we do, we believe in putting the patient first. We put the patient first with respect, attention to detail, and a sense of urgency unlike any other emergency department. Our specialty is you.*

A vision statement is not meant to *differentiate* the organization (that is the realm of strategy—addressed later in this chapter). Developing, communicating, and implementing the ED's vision is hard work. It requires convening an already busy team and guiding it through the discovery of its core vision, ideology, and values. Coached effectively through the process, the staff begins to think about the core purpose in deeply meaningful ways. Once completed, the vision statement rarely needs revision, since it is a fundamental and guiding statement, not a trend or leadership style *du jour*. As Collins and Porras note:

> *Once you are clear about the core vision, you should feel free to change absolutely anything that is not part of it.*[4]

Unique

The ability to inspire and inform the mission, values, strategy, and tactics of the team is critical, since the *why* of the vision is the foundation upon which the remainder of the pyramid is based. Finally, the vision statement should reflect the unique *why* of the ED, as opposed to other units or the larger health-care organization as shown in

> **BOX 2.2 ■ EXAMPLES OF ED VISION STATEMENTS**
>
> - "The ED at Inova Fairfax Hospital exists to reinvent emergency care to constantly increase value for our patients and make the team's jobs easier."
> - "The ED of University Hospital exists to provide excellence in clinical care, education of our future physicians, and research to guide that future."
> - "The ED of St. Petersburg General Hospital exists to be the superior choice in emergency health care."

the examples listed in **Box 2.2**. However, the ED's vision should integrate with that of the larger organization.

MISSION: *WHAT* IS THE ORGANIZATION ATTEMPTING TO DO?

Once the vision of the organization is articulated, an equally clear statement must be made of its mission—*what* it is attempting to do. Mission statements, while succinct, are typically longer than vision statements and contain a higher degree of specificity. Like the vision statement, the mission statement should also be capable of motivating the team but with more specific detail. For example, consider the vision and mission statements of Saint Mary's Health System, Duke Medicine, and the Cleveland Clinic (**Table 2.1**).

The vision and mission statements of each institution are laudable, clear, and capable of inspiring those on the team and those seeking to join the team. Each provides excellent descriptions of the *why* and *what* of their respective organizations. However, each organization

TABLE 2.1 ■ Vision and Mission Statements

Organization	Vision	Mission
St. Mary's Health System	Saint Mary's health system will be the leading regional health-care provider.	Saint Mary's Health System provides: • Excellent health care • In a spiritually enriched environment • To improve the health of our community
Duke Medicine	Advancing health together	We will: • Deliver tomorrow's health care today. • Accelerate discovery and its translation. • Create education that is transforming. • Build healthy communities. • Connect with the world to improve health globally.
Cleveland Clinic	Striving to be the world's leader in patient experience, clinical outcomes, research, and education	Provide better care of the sick, investigation into their problems, and further education of those who serve.

differs in geographic scope and aspirational reach, which is to be expected because of the differences inherent among regional, national, and international academic health-care systems. This point deserves emphasis: *vision and mission statements must specifically match the resources and specific challenges of the institution.* Additional examples of effective vision and mission statements are listed in the appendices at the end of this chapter.

CORE VALUES: *WHICH* CORE, FUNDAMENTAL BELIEFS GUIDE THE ORGANIZATION?

Core values are systems of guiding principles that express the timeless character of an organization. They *prescribe* the desired benchmarks that describe the character, behavior, and essential and enduring tenets of those who comprise the team. They should also *proscribe* the pursuit of strategies or tactics that do not reflect or, worse, go against these values. No matter what competitive challenges the organization faces, *values do not change over the course of time.* Values are expressions of the intrinsic nature of the people and the organization and don't, or shouldn't, require extrinsic validation. Ralph S. Larsen, CEO of Johnson & Johnson, expresses this well:

> *The core values expressed in our credo might be a competitive advantage, but that is not why we have them. We have them because they define for us what we stand for and we would hold them even if they became a competitive disadvantage in certain situations.*[4]

Values are the cornerstone to which the team will refer when making decisions about what to do. While values are always important, they are critical in times of crisis, such as those found in our current health-care environment. The only poorly conceived core values are those that do not reflect the true guiding principles of the group or that aren't stated at all. The key is not *what* the core values are but to ensure the values exist and accurately reflect what will guide the team, particularly in times of crisis.

To be effective, there should be no more than four to six "core" values. More are rarely reflective of the core nature of the group and cannot be used to guide decisions. Core values must be so deeply held that they will seldom, if ever, change. If the stated values are subject to market pressures or changes in the leadership team, they are not true core values. As an example, consider the case in **Box 2.3**. One test to ensure that values are deeply held is to ask this question:

> *If the competitive health care market changed and the environment did not reward but punished these values, would those values still be kept or would they be abandoned?*

BOX 2.3 ■ CASE STUDY: CORE VALUES VERSUS ENACTED STRATEGY

An ED physician group has the following core values:

- Equity
- Fairness
- Integrity
- Service to the community
- Patient and family focus

The new hospital leadership team asks the ED group to devise and implement a program to *triage away* patients without health-care insurance when they have nonemergent problems. However, there are few or no community resources to care for uninsured patients. Clearly, there is tension between the stated values of the group and what it is being asked to do. Applying these values to the proposed program will likely cause the group to go against (or change) the hospital's program or their own core values.

TABLE 2.2 ■ Values of Health-Care Organizations	
Organization	Values
Inova Health Systems	• Innovative excellence • Caring about people • Community
Duke Medicine	• Excellence • Safety • Integrity • Diversity • Teamwork
Best Practices	• Integrity • Innovation • Excellence • Execution • Service

Tables 2.2 and **2.3** and **Box 2.4** list examples of value statements of organizations both in health care and in other businesses.

Creating or Revising Core Values

If an organization has a previously stated set of values, any new group should review them to ensure those values are effective in guiding its decisions even in difficult times. The values should be revised if they are inconsistent, ineffective, or, most importantly, do not reflect the core guiding principles and beliefs of the current team.

Alternatively, if the core values of the organization have not been articulated, the ED leaders may assemble the team and identify what is truly central and essential. This process requires the team to develop a consensus. The ED values must incorporate, or at least account for, the values of the overall hospital and health-care system. Several questions are helpful in guiding these conversations.

TABLE 2.3 ■ Values as Core Tenets in Non-Health-Care Organizations	
Organization	Values
Nordstrom	• Service to the customer above all else • Hard work and individual productivity • Never being satisfied • Excellence in reputation
The Walt Disney Company	• Creativity, dreams, imagination • Nurturing "wholesome American values" • Fanatical attention to detail • No cynicism
United States Marine Corps	• Honor • Courage • Commitment

Are these values:

- Intrinsic (from within) or extrinsic (imposed from outside)?
- That team members can describe to their children with pride?
- Deeply held beliefs that will stand the test of time, or merely a product of the times and trends?
- The team will depend on during times of difficulty and crisis?
- That serve to form and sustain the team as they care for patients?

Once completed, the values should provide a reliable benchmark to guide future decisions for the ED team. They should help *prescribe* successful strategies and tactics while *proscribing* decisions that are inconsistent with the core values. The values should be consistent with the mission and vision statements. If not, the deeply held core values should drive a reconsideration of the vision and mission.

BOX 2.4 ■ MAYO CLINIC VALUE STATEMENTS

These values, which guide Mayo Clinic's mission to this day, are an expression of the vision and intent of our founders, the original Mayo physicians and the Sisters of Saint Francis.

- **Respect:** Treat everyone in our diverse community, including patients, their families, and colleagues, with dignity.
- **Compassion:** Provide the best care, treating patients and family members with sensitivity and empathy.
- **Integrity:** Adhere to the highest standards of professionalism, ethics, and personal responsibility worthy of the trust our patients place in us.
- **Healing:** Inspire hope and nurture the well-being of the whole person, respecting physical, emotional, and spiritual needs.
- **Teamwork:** Value the contributions of all, blending the skills of individual staff members in unsurpassed collaboration.
- **Excellence:** Deliver the best outcomes and highest quality service through the dedicated effort of every team member.
- **Innovation:** Infuse and energize the organization, enhancing the lives of those we serve, through the creative ideas and unique talents of each employee.
- **Stewardship:** Sustain and reinvest in our mission and extended communities by wisely managing our human, natural, and material resources.

STRATEGY: *WHAT* DIFFERENTIATES THIS ED FROM OTHER EDs?

The word *strategy* derives from the Greek *strategia*, which means *generalship*. The early literature on strategy was almost exclusively military in nature. There are articles, books, and seminars exploring strategy and strategic planning, with more than a thousand dedicated to health-care strategy. Emergency leaders can choose from numerous definitions of strategy to determine the best approach to this subject.

A Definition of Strategy

We have a strategic plan. It's called "doing _____."

—Herb Kelleher, Founder of Southwest Airlines[11]

For the purpose of this chapter, strategy is defined as the plan, path, or action chosen by health-care leaders to differentiate their organization from others. A fundamental question when developing health-care or ED strategy is:

*Among the many things, which **could** be done in moving forward, what **will** be done to differentiate the organization?*

Health-care systems and EDs increasingly find themselves in capacity-constrained environments. The ability to differentiate an organization is more and more dependent on selecting the most appropriate courses of action. As Michael Porter, a respected voice in strategy, notes:

Strategy is about making choices and trade-offs; it's about deliberately choosing to be different.[12]

While there may be "no bad ideas" in brainstorming sessions that determine vision, mission, and value statements, there are many bad ideas when forming strategies. For instance, if an organizational goal is to maximize return on investment (ROI), the leader must discern and eliminate the bad ideas—those with low ROI and poor capacity to differentiate the ED—from the good ideas—those high-leverage strategies most likely to produce positive and measurable results. Indeed, the capacity to develop and successfully implement strategy becomes a core competitive skill of health-care and ED leaders. Again, Porter's wisdom is helpful:

The best CEOs I know are teachers, and at the core of what they teach is strategy. The chief strategist of an organization has to be its leader – the CEO.[13]

ED medical and nursing directors are the co-CEOs who drive the success of the ED. It is essential for them to successfully discover, implement, and sustain strategies to differentiate their ED. Henry Mintzberg and Tom Peters have framed their work in ways that are particularly helpful for those pursuing strategic objectives in the ED.

Mintzberg on Strategy

Henry Mintzberg was the first to clarify that strategic planning and strategic thinking are not synonymous. In fact, they are in some ways diametrically opposed. He states:

*Strategic planning, as it has been practiced, has really been **strategic programming**, the articulation and elaboration of strategies, or visions, that already exist.*[14]

Strategic thinking is similar to *innovation*, creatively synthesizing varying experiences into a novel approach. Strategic planning may be described as a *calculating* style of management. Strategic thinking is more of a *committing* style of leadership.

The following words from Mintzberg seem as if they were written specifically to address the nature of strategy in health care in general and EDs in particular:

*Real strategists get their hands dirty by digging for ideas, and real strategies are built from the occasional nuggets they uncover. These are not people who abstract themselves from the daily details; they are the ones who immerse themselves in them while being able to abstract the strategic messages from them. **The big picture is painted with little strokes.***[14]

The very nature of the ED hierarchy requires effective nursing and medical directors to be immersed in the details of daily operations. Their insights are essential to meaningful strategic-planning processes. Equally so, the insights and participation of the line nurses and physicians who perform the work of caring for patients are necessary for meaningful strategic planning. There is no "Office of Strategic Planning" in the emergency department! Instead, as Mintzberg's insights point out, both the providers of clinical care and their leaders must be charged with ED strategy development and implementation. In seeking differentiating factors, Mintzberg notes that there are at least four fundamental ways in which strategy may be viewed:

1. Strategy as a **plan**
2. Strategy as a **pattern**
3. Strategy as a **position**
4. Strategy as a **perspective**

Strategy as a Plan

Strategy as a plan means strategy as a guide, a course of action into the future, or a specified path to get from where the organization is to where it seeks to be. Perhaps the largest problem with strategy as a plan used alone is that the world of health care is complex, rapidly changing, and requires substantial commitment of multiple stakeholders. In other words, a plan is not the same as successful execution. For instance, an ED pursuing a *30-Minute Guarantee* as a strategy must utilize multiple resources to accomplish the goal. However, if appropriate processes, staffing changes, intensive oversight, etc., do not support that plan, the strategy (plan) will fail.

Strategy as a Pattern

Strategy can also be viewed as a pattern, a relatively consistent set of behaviors over the course of time. Consider a Level 1 trauma center ED with a strategy focused on providing excellent care to critically injured patients. Excellence requires delivering a consistent pattern of care. However, isolated focus on that pattern of care alone may adversely affect the care to patients with lower acuity problems. The lower acuity patients may experience inattention and long delays and find they are *competing* for the scarce physician, nursing, radiology, and laboratory resources.

Both Minztberg and Greek business theorist Chris Argyris note the importance of distinguishing between an "espoused strategy versus the strategy in action."[15] In an article in *Fortune* magazine, business journalist Walter Kiechel estimates that fewer than 10% of strategies are successfully implemented, a figure Tom Peters instantly described as "wildly inflated."[16,17] Prior to implementation of a strategy, an objective assessment of the current practice patterns can demonstrate the current and anticipated use of resources. For example, the Level I trauma center described previously has demand-capacity mismatches. While a conceptual strategy of pursuing more low-acuity patients may seem attractive, data from the current practice patterns would demonstrate a lack of additional personnel and resource capacity to care for additional patient volume, suggesting that investment in resources and/or flow processes would be needed to enact this strategy.

Strategy as Position

Strategy as position is exemplified by determining which products exist in which markets. As an example, an ED pursues a strategy to attract low-acuity patients through a dedicated fast track. The business plan recognizes significant profitability based on high-volume and low-resource utilization (low utilization of lab and radiology services and use of allied health professionals rather than more expensive physicians). At substantial cost, the fast track is built, providers are hired, processes are changed, and the program is promoted to the community. However, in this market, there is an overabundance of options for low-acuity patients, including a few new community primary care providers and a nearby urgent care center with capacity. In this case, considering the strategic *pattern* of care in the community might have led to a different conclusion about the strategic *position* of this plan.

Strategic positioning seeks to achieve a *sustainable competitive advantage* by identifying, preserving, and amplifying what is distinctive about an ED, either by:

- Performing *different* activities from the competition, that is, developing a dedicated pediatric area with specialists in pediatric emergency medicine, or
- Reliably and safely performing the *same or similar* activities in demonstrably superior ways, that is, adopting a highly evidence-based approach to the most common ED clinical presentations can reliably decrease length of stay, increase reliability, decrease malpractice risk, and increase patient and staff satisfaction.[18]

Strategy as a Perspective

Finally, Mintzberg suggests that strategy may be viewed as perspective, an organization's way of doing things, or as Drucker said, "its concept of the business."[19] This approach may be somewhat less applicable to EDs. As an example, tertiary care EDs in academic medical centers may struggle to define a typical ED strategy when the institution is pursuing national and international strategies.

- The Mayo Clinic has a reputation as a major diagnostic center with clinicians who are well known for their ability to "figure out" complicated medical problems.
- The Cleveland Clinic and Duke Medical Center have enviable reputations as cardiac care centers of international renown, driven by innovation and rapid translation from the bench to bedside.
- UCSF and the Barrow Neurologic Institute are held in high regard for their neurologic centers.

The ED might wish to develop a strategy to serve the local and regional needs of patients within their service areas. However, the EDs of these centers may have difficulty creating strategies that are separate from the broader, more national consultative approach of the health-care system.

Another concept of strategy as perspective is demonstrated by the focus on service throughout the institution.

- The Mayo Clinic describes its "patient-first" focus.[20]
- The Studer Group uses evidence-based leadership principles.[21]
- Many institutions embrace patient experience and patient- and family-focused care.[22,23]

These examples are all ways of pursuing an institutional strategy based on a specific perspective. The associated EDs must participate in the *perspective* and recognize their role within the larger institutional strategy, whether it is a focus on tertiary care, service, or other priorities.

Tom Peters on Strategy

There is one key to excellence. It is called "a bias toward action."

—Tom Peters and Bob Waterman[24]

Since the publication of *In Search of Excellence* in 1982, Peters' voice has been a unique, contrarian, and iconoclastic breath of fresh air in the leadership and management literature. In addition to the call for a "bias towards action" in that seminal work, he has incessantly stressed the importance of the people charged with executing the strategy over the strategy itself:

Get the people and the execution right and the strategy will take care of itself.[25]
Knowing who you are going with tops the list of imperatives in a world of whitewater and knowing that those who you're going with share your passion and determination tops that.[25]

Peters' message is that all service is personal and that health care (emergency medicine in particular) is a personal-service business. Strategies can only rarely create passion in people who have a *job* instead of a *calling* or a *passion for excellence*. Instead, it is the task of the leader to ignite passion in the strategy. In this sense, the leader is in the "talent arbitrage business," leveraging the skills and abilities of the team to drive the strategy.[26] As Collins notes:

First who, then what. First the people, then the direction. Start by getting the right people on the bus.[27]

Putting Strategy to Work in the ED

It is necessary to combine the insights from each of these and other acknowledged visionaries to devise a strategy that differentiates one ED from another. A wide variety of strategies can be pursued, alone or in combination, to achieve effective differentiation.

- *Speed*: Team triage, triage bypass, fast track, 30-minute guarantees, free-standing EDs, etc.
- *Quality*: Trauma, rapid STEMI treatment, and acute care
- *Specialty care*: Pediatrics, geriatrics, sports medicine
- *Service*: Dedication to patient first, caring and curing, call-backs, and rounding
- *Value*: High-quality, low-cost provider of care, best quality per dollar spent
- *Convenience*: Multiple locations throughout a service area
- *Flow*: The ability to add value while eliminating waste in patient care
- *Safety*: Reliably delivering quality care consistently for every patient, every time

This is only a partial list of potentially differentiating strategies. The key to each of these strategies is specifically delineating how the ED will be differentiated from other EDs, either within the service area (to increase market share) or on a national basis (for those hospitals or groups that identify innovation of an entire specialty as one of their goals).

Sentara Health System in Virginia pursues a formula for strategic positioning of its EDs based on the Sentara Vision:

We improve health care every day.

Using its vision as a foundation, each meeting is guided by a strategy that addresses the "four Ms" to make strategic decisions.

- *Mission*: To make the communities we serve healthier places to live, work, and play
- *Market*: To be the number one choice for health care services in the market
- *Medicine*: To set the standard for medical excellence in the community
- *Members of the team*: To be the regional employer of choice

This framework guides ED decision-makers on their strategy decisions and aligns their strategic processes with the broader strategy of the hospital and health-care system. Regardless of the framework utilized or the model of strategy employed, ED medical and nursing leaders should develop an articulated and easily understood strategy to become a fundamental aspect of their department's work.

Other specific examples of ED strategy are listed in **Appendix 2.1**.

TACTICS: *HOW* WILL SUCCESS BE ACCOMPLISHED AND MEASURED?

Strategy refers to the ways in which the ED differentiates itself from other EDs. Tactics refers to the specific ways in which that strategy will be accomplished and measured. Once the vision, mission, values, and strategy of the ED are known and effectively communicated, the specific tactics used to accomplish these become much easier, though they still require substantial attention to detail. In many ways, the remainder of this book is focused on the tactics necessary to accomplish and measure progress toward the strategies identified by the leadership team.

For example, an ED pursues a strategy designed to differentiate itself on speed (door to physician, length of stay [LOS], and ED flow), adding value and eliminating waste at each stage of the process. As a result, the specific tactics to accomplish and measure success toward that strategy are clear, although perhaps not easily executed. The tactics might include front-loading ED flow, development of a results-waiting area, keeping vertical patients vertical and moving, use of scribes to free up physician charting time, and so on.

Another ED may decide to compete on service as a strategy. Tactics could include service-excellence training, effective and timely feedback of results, focused patient satisfaction coaching, service recovery skills, call-back systems, and scripts.

Unlike vision, mission, and values, strategy is not immutable and may occasionally change. Likewise, tactics may be subject to frequent change, as measurements of success or failure will guide modification or replacement of a tactic. The concept of rapid cycle testing (RCT) provides a useful example to understand tactics in health care. RCT recognizes that there are many *potential* solutions to any given problem in the health-care system. It further recognizes that the actual implementation of these solutions is subject to local (and even unit-based) factors.

As a result, to assess whether the proposed "tactic" is going to work, RCT employs focused changes of a limited nature. Thus, tactics may change frequently and according to the demands of the situation. Strategies change far less frequently and only in response to a careful study of the success or failure of the specific tactics, such as RCTs, and the data that arise from them.[28]

Tactics: The Measurement

The data-driven analysis of the proposed tactics is essential in the metrics-driven world of contemporary health care. Every suggested tactic should also contain a measurable data element to judge its success. A simple example involves the strategy of differentiating an ED by efficiency. A tactic to improve ED flow and LOS might include the implementation of a results-waiting area, a place in which patients can wait for their laboratory, and imaging studies without needlessly occupying a bed. Effective measures of this program include:

- Number of "bed turns" in the ED per day (or shift)
- Bed-to-physician times for this group of patients
- Time in bed and time in results-waiting area
- Total LOS for patients using the results-waiting area
- Patient satisfaction
- Employee satisfaction

Appendix 2.1 lists other examples of tactics and strategies.

CONCLUSION

ED professionals cannot be expected to do a good job unless they know:

- Why they are there *(vision)*
- What they are expected to do *(mission)*
- What *values* guide them
- How they are differentiated from other EDs *(strategy)*
- What specific *tactics* will be used to accomplish and measure their progress toward these goals

The development of vision, mission, values, strategy, and tactics statements are an essential leadership function of medical and nursing directors, as well as the ED staff. Accomplishing this is not just a philosophy—it is a *discipline*. Once these principles are understood and effectively applied, patients and those who help those patients are better served. As the president and CEO of one of the most successful health-care systems in the world (Memorial Hermann in Houston) and a leader who has led two different organizations to the Malcom Baldrige Quality Award notes:

> *It is simply impossible to overstate the importance of mission, vision, and values in health care. They must be a part of recruitment, orientation, ongoing education, and, indeed, of the everyday lives of our team and our patients. Otherwise they are sterile words on a wall, not actions in our halls.*[29]

APPENDIX 2.1: STRATEGIES AND TACTICS

Inova Fairfax Medical Campus Department of Emergency Medicine

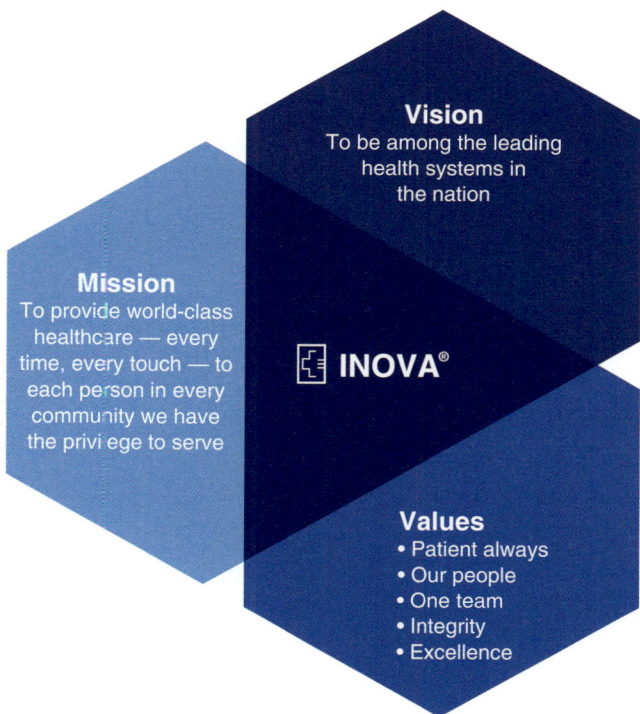

EXAMPLES OF STRATEGIES AND TACTICS

Vision: The ED at Inova Fairfax Hospital (IFH) exists to reinvent emergency care to constantly increase value for our patients.

Strategy: IFH's ED will differentiate itself as the leading ED in the Washington area through excellence and innovation in:

- Trauma and critical care
- Pediatric emergency medicine
- Service excellence
- Patient flow
- Patient safety
- Free-standing emergency department (FSED) care
- Education of emergency medicine (EM) residents and pediatric EM fellows

Trauma and Critical Care Tactics

- Recruitment and retention of emergency physicians with the highest level of skills in trauma and critical care
- Close partnership with trauma surgeons and intensivists
- Close relationship with nursing team
- Provision of Medical Direction for Hospital-Based Helicopter service
- Provision of Medical Direction for Fairfax County and Prince William County electronic medical system
- Provision of Medical Direction for Fairfax County Police Helicopter Unit and Special Operations Command
- Research and education in trauma and critical care

Pediatric Emergency Medicine Tactics

- Recruitment and retention of pediatric emergency physicians who are fellowship-trained in pediatric emergency medicine or residency-trained in emergency medicine and pediatrics
- Strong leadership from the medical director of pediatric emergency medicine
- Close partnership with pediatric nursing director and pediatric nurses
- 24/7/365 coverage of the pediatric ED
- Integration with the general ED physician group
- Integration of pediatric trauma with the trauma service
- Pediatric outreach and telemedicine services
- Community education
- Sustain significant philanthropy

Service Excellence

- Hire right screen for the customer service gene
- Service expectations in the physician contracts
- Service excellence book to all new hires
- Customer service training for all new hires
- All complaints and compliments shared at department meetings—group learning
- Focused patient satisfaction coaching
- Service scores as part of the incentive compensation program
- Mentoring, coaching, and accountability for service

Patient Flow

- Metrics-based accountability
- Hardwiring flow concepts to all physicians
- Flow cascade to add value (direct-to-room, advanced triage and treatment, bedside registration, team triage, etc)
- Lean-based value-added as the core principle
- Team triage 24/7/365 to get the patient and the physician together as rapidly as possible

Patient Safety

- Hire for a commitment to safety and evidence-based protocol participation and adherence
- Require risk-free ED training for all new hires
- Update on risk-free ED every 6 months
- Integration of safety in incentive compensation
- Scribes integrated into the safety culture and programs
- Provide risk-free ED training to all nurses
- Become the recognized leader in the hospital for patient safety

Free-Standing EDs

- Hire for a commitment to FSED concepts
- Accentuate flow, service, and safety
- Exemplary medical leadership
- Grow market share in all FSEDs
- Expand FSED service line
- Pediatric telemedicine
- Onsite ambulance service for "back transports"
- Advertise and exploit "Nation's #1 Free-Standing Emergency Department" status

Education of EM Residents and Pediatric EM Fellows

- Provision of excellent emergency medicine residency, pediatric fellowship, and medical student medical direction
- Hire for educators, not just clinicians
- Faculty appointments for all clinicians
- Evidence-based education
- Conferences, grand rounds, and bedside teaching
- Clinical track and education track options
- Research and publication
- Innovation at the core

APPENDIX 2.2: CROUSE HOSPITAL MISSION, VISION, AND VALUES

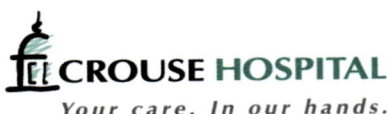

Our Story
(If we can dream it, we can do it.)

As proud members of Crouse Hospital's Emergency Services team, we are at the heart of a Center of Excellence comprised of highly trained and skilled professionals who come together to provide kind, **compassionate**, and **individualized** care to every patient.

We are **mission driven** and our patients recognize and value the care we provide, from the emotional, personal, and clinical experience. Patients know that they are receiving the best care because we listen carefully to them, engage them in their care decisions, and respect them as individuals. The patient experience is confirmed in our satisfaction results, which rate us as a top performer in key areas such as wait times, provider communication, and teamwork.

Our entire team supports, trusts, and respects one another. We stay true to the sentiment of **"family taking care of family,"** as clearly supported by the numerous compliments received from our patients and their families. All team members take the time to recognize the high-quality work of their fellow colleagues. Each member, regardless of his or her role pitches in to ensure our patients receive the best possible care.

Clinical and service excellence is what defines this team. Our experts are frequently recognized, locally and nationally, for their clinical outcomes and creative approaches to improving patient care and the patient experience. Our actions show our strong sense of ownership with our results. We are often invited to present at national conferences to share our expertise with others.

Crouse's Emergency Service team has a **strong partnership** with the EMS community like no other hospital, as evidenced by survey results and feedback. We share our knowledge and support each other at every opportunity. Our partnership is based on respect, value, and trust. We are always engaged collaboratively in quality improvement initiatives with our EMS partners to improve care in the community.

The Emergency Services facility and focus is state of the art. The environment is holistic and **conducive to healing.**

At the end of the day, our patients and their families know they were cared for as if they were one of our own. We are very **passionate and proud** of what we do and how we do it.

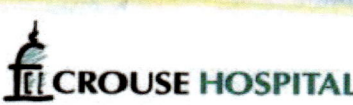

MISSION

To provide the best in patient care and to promote community health.

VISION

To be the leading healthcare provider in Central New York by:

1. being committed to excellence in all areas of our organization by anticipating and exceeding the expectations of those we serve: our patients and their families, physicians, employees, volunteers and other partners;
2. building a dynamic work environment where all are valued, respected and are provided the opportunity for personal and professional growth;
3. developing and building on centers of excellence that support our mission;
4. strengthening relationships with other community providers to enhance the continuum of care for those we serve;
5. operating in a fiscally responsible manner that allows us to provide the best in patient care and technology.

VALUES

C ommunity... working together

R espect... honor, dignity and trust

O pen and honest communication

U ndivided commitment to quality

S ervice to our patients, physicians and ourselves

E xcellence through innovation and creativity

Used with permission from Department of Emergency Medicine, Crouse Hospital.

APPENDIX 2.3: SISTERS OF CHARITY LEAVENSWORTH HEALTH SYSTEM MISSION, VISION, AND VALUES

Our Mission

In the spirit of the Sisters of Charity of St. Augustine, our mission is to extend the healing ministry of Jesus to God's people.

Our Vision

The Sisters of Charity Health System is a beacon of hope devoted to healing and addressing the unmet needs of individuals, families, and communities through a network of innovative services.

Our Values

Compassion: displays a profound sense of interconnectedness by:
- responding to needs, pains oxford, and sufferings of others with concern, empathy, and support
- treating all persons we serve and with whom we co-minister with dignity
- exhibiting an attitude of acceptance and forgiveness
- listening with empathy and attention
- serving as a catalyst for change, especially for the disenfranchised

Courage: dares to take risks that our faith-based demands of us by:
- speaking out on issues that challenge our mission and Catholic identity
- making difficult decisions with integrity and in a timely manner
- promoting economic, political, and social conditions to support the fundamental rights of all individuals that enable them to meet their potential and achieve the common good of society
- addressing institutional problems and issues quickly, objectively, and directly

Respect: values dignity and sacredness of life from conception through death by:
- treating individuals and their families with profound respect and utmost regard
- maintaining an attitude and atmosphere of loving hospitality
- addressing the physical, psychological, social, and spiritual dimensions of the person
- ensuring that diversity exists at all levels
- being trustful and keeping confidences; being truthful, direct, and sincere; apologizing for misunderstandings, inconveniences, or mistakes

Justice: develops right relationships internally and externally by:
- developing or eliminating programs to ensure excellent service and quality
- acting as responsible stewards of all resources
- addressing the needs of the poor and vulnerable
- treating employees justly and respectfully
- advocating to secure the human right to health care

Collaboration: promotes inclusive, compassionate, and collaborative relationships by:
- encouraging interaction internally and externally to empower others for service
- fostering and sharing of gifts and talents within our institution and larger community
- facilitating dialogue and networking with individuals and organizations
- assisting others to realize the importance of their work in contributing to the mission
- promoting a sensitivity to diversity in planning and implementing programs, hiring practices, advertising and other initiatives

Used with permission from SCL Health System.

REFERENCES

1. Seneca LA. *Letters From a Stoic*. London, United Kingdom: Penguin Classics; 1969.
2. Kierkegaard S. *Either/Or: A Fragment of Life*. London, United Kingdom: Penguin; 1992.
3. Nietzsche F. *Beyond Good and Evil*. New York, NY: SoHo; 2008.
4. Collins JC, Porras JI. Building your company's vision. *Harv Bus Rev.* 1996;(74):65-72.
5. Collins JC, Porras JI. *Built to Last: Successful Habits of Visionary Companies*. New York, NY: Harper Collins; 1994.
6. Drucker PF. *The Effective Executive*. New York, NY: Harper Business; 2002.
7. Bohr N. *Symposium on Basic Research*. New York, NY: Columbia University Press; 1958. Quoted by: Wolfie DL.
8. Churchill WS. *Blood, Toil, Tears, and Sweat: The Dire Warning*. New York, NY: Basic Books (Perseus); 2008 (Address to the House of Commons, May 13, 1940, quoted by Lukacs J).
9. Churchill WS. *BBC Archives*. June 18, 1940 (Address to the House of Commons)
10. Murrow ER. Radio broadcast: See It Now. CBS, 1954.
11. Kelleher H. *Nuts: Southwest Airlines' Crazy Recipe for Business and Personal Success*. New York, NY: Bard; 1996. Quoted by Frieberg K.
12. Porter ME. What is strategy? *Harv Bus Rev.* 1996;74:63.
13. Porter M. *Redefining Health Care: Creating Value-Based Competition on Results*. Boston, Mass: Harvard Business School Press; 2006.
14. Mintzberg H. The fall and rise of strategic planning. *Harv Bus Rev.* 1994;72:163.
15. Argyris C. *Knowledge for Action: A Guide to Overcoming Business Barriers in Organizational Change*. San Francisco, Calif: Jossey-Bass; 1996.
16. Kiechel W III. Sniping at strategic planning. *Planning Rev.* 1984:8-11.
17. Peters T. Commentary. *Planning Rev.* 1984:12-13.
18. Mayer T. The pediatric risk free ED. Presented at: *The American College of Emergency Physicians Scientific Assembly*; 2012; Denver, Colo.
19. Drucker PF. *The Drucker Lectures: Essential Lessons on Management, Society, and Economy*. New York, NY: McGraw-Hill; 2010.
20. Berry LL, Seltman KD. *Management Lessons From Mayo Clinic: Inside One of the World's Most Admired Service Organizations*. New York, NY: McGraw-Hill; 2008.
21. Studer Q. *Hardwiring Excellence: Purpose, Worthwhile Work, Making a Difference*. Gulf Breeze, Fla: Fire Starter Press; 2003.
22. Mayer TA, Cates RJ. *Leadership for Great Customer Service: Satisfied Patients, Satisfied Employees*. Chicago, Ill: Health Administration Press; 2004.
23. Mayer T. Putting It All Together: Best Practices in Service Excellence. *Healthc Exec.* 2011;26:56.
24. Peters TJ, Waterman RH. *In Search of Excellence: Lessons from America's Best-Run Companies*. New York, NY: Harper Business; 2004.
25. Peters TJ. *Everything You Need to Know About Strategy: A Baker's Dozen Eternal Verities*. West Tinmouth, Vt: Tom Peters Company; 2001.
26. Daniels P. *The Little Big Things: 163 Ways to Pursue Ways to Pursue Excellence*. New York, NY: Harper Studio; 2011:53. Quoted by Peters TJ.
27. Collins JC. *Good to Great: Why Some Companies Make the Leap and Others Don't*. New York, NY: Harper Business; 2001.
28. Mayer T, Jensen KJ. *Hardwiring Flow: Systems and Processes for Seamless Patient Care*. Gulf Breeze, Fla: Fire Starter Press; 2009.
29. Stokes C. *Remarks to the ACHE Congress*. Chicago, Ill: American College of Healthcare Executives; 2017.

CHAPTER 3

CHANGE AND PROJECT MANAGEMENT: A PRACTICAL APPROACH

Kirk Jensen

And it ought to be remembered that there is nothing more difficult to take in hand, more perilous to conduct, or more uncertain in its success, than to take the lead in the introduction of a new order of things. Because the innovator has for enemies all those who have done well under the old conditions, and lukewarm defenders in those who may do well under the new.

—Nicolo Machiavelli, c.1505 (trans. W. K. Marriott)

The ability to manage projects and facilitate change is a critical skill in any leader's toolkit. A decision to improve the performance of an emergency department (ED) often begins with the realization that current performance and outcomes are inadequate or are not as good as the ED team wishes them to be. In such cases, a common step entails redesigning workflow processes that do not sufficiently meet the needs of patients or staff. Knowing where and how to start can be challenging. Management resources and conferences can provide valuable information and advice based on expert opinion and experience. Networking and site visits can be invaluable. Leveraging the expertise of performance improvement professionals is almost always helpful. The critical element in separating a successful change management effort from an unsuccessful one is seldom the lack of a specific solution. Rather, it is realizing from the outset that the team must not only work to change processes but also to improve behavior, organizational culture and, to some degree, the attitudes of the people who work within it.

While organizational and cultural change is usually necessary to reach the project's goals, obstacles can block the way. This chapter will illuminate how to meet those challenges and overcome those obstacles. As an ED adapts its culture while developing better process and health-care delivery systems, its efficiency, reliability, and effectiveness will increase. Service capability and capacity of the department improve, staff morale and engagement increase, and patient satisfaction scores often rise accordingly.

DEVELOPING GOALS AND DESIGNING PROJECTS

Leading lasting change begins with creating or revisiting the organization's mission, vision, and values statements. (This topic is addressed in more detail in Chapter 2.) Many EDs have never taken the time place to define their goals or their work as a team. If they have, it is common to discover that service goal and delivery statements are gathering dust rather than driving behavior and performance.

Defining a Department's Vision

Successful vision statements inspire and motivate staff while remaining grounded in reality. They document and define principles that serve as a road map to successfully navigate to the department's desired future state. Vision statements are created to embody the organization's core ideology.[1]

When developing mission, vision, and value statements for an ED, it is helpful to understand the questions that are being answered:

- *Mission* is the answer to the question "What is the ED attempting to *do*?"
- *Vision* answers, "Why does the ED exist?"
- *Values* express how the team members will treat each other on the journey to create a new workplace, or "Which core and fundamental beliefs guide the ED?"

The ED's vision statement must describe why the department exists, where it has been historically, and where it intends to go in the future. This written document should be the North Star for the organization, and its elements should guide every decision. Anyone going through this process of organizational change must start with honest questions about what they want. Several specific questions include:

- What are the team members committed to in their respective roles?
- What characteristics would a department have that was effectively and efficiently delivering the desired level of high-quality, safe care?
- What would stand out to patients about their care in such a facility, and what would draw them to it?
- What would stand out to potential recruits about delivering patient care in such a facility, and what would draw them to it?
- What would constitute a satisfactory experience within this high-performing facility?
- What would an ED look like if physicians, nurses, lab technicians, respiratory therapists, and all the other health-care providers worked in concert and left feeling fulfilled at the end of their respective shifts together?
- What is within our capacity and our capabilities?

Pondering these questions with broad input leads a team to develop a vision of a department that delivers on these opportunities. Potentially, pondering these questions will lead to the creation of an ED in which health-care providers are excited to work. It will also create a patient experience that will rival the best any competition could provide. To quote Stephen Covey's landmark book, *The 7 Habits of Highly Successful People*, a redesign team should "begin with the end in mind."[2]

Before a department begins this process of change, it may prove valuable to work through these same questions independently with the physician staffing group. In particular, doctors are trained to be self-sufficient, independent, and critical thinkers. Meaningful process change often involves embracing multidisciplinary teams, consensus building, rapid-cycle testing, and learning through multiple small tests of change and experimentation. The process can test the skill sets, patience, and time commitments of the physician group. The lack of of a consensus between physician and nurse teams can easily torpedo change. In fact, it is often impossible to implement a new process when some doctors and nurses are supporting it while others are undermining it. As a result, it is important and even necessary to review and get advance "buy-in" about the direction of any changes.

The Deming Principle: Reducing Variability

American engineer W. Edwards Deming showed that a critical component in improving quality and efficiency in any process is to reduce or eliminate variability.[3] So a key step is to ensure that there will not be shifts with "A" (committed supporters) doctors and charge nurses and shifts with "B" (noncommitted, nonsupporters) doctors and charge nurses. This initial stage is a good opportunity for the physician and nurse leaders to build their relationship and communication skills (supplemented with formal or semiformal coaching and training of the leaders when necessary). The better the leaders' individual leadership and communication skills, the easier it will be to initiate and sustain change.

The point of reducing variability is to decrease friction and waste in and between the nested and interdependent processes and human interactions that make up the system of care. To be sure, variability may increase value if the processes are changed to meet changing patient care and patient flow needs during the course of the day. For example, direct bedding or "pull until full" is an effective strategy to increase value, but only if ED beds are available, and there is sufficient clinical staff to handle the patient load.

Engaging the Team

Once the ED leaders have a clear idea about where they want to take the department, the other team members must be engaged in developing the vision. People tend to support what they help create. They seldom invest much of themselves in a vision created by someone else and forced on them. If the individual ED members have a meaningful hand in creating the vision, they will "own" it.

An effective approach is to use one of the team members as an objective facilitator, preferably someone who is perceived as capable, fair, experienced, and unbiased. But beware! The vision statement cuts both ways. The organization has to commit leadership and resources to the vision for which the rank and file has publicly declared its support. Both the leadership and the entire ED team must have the same level of enthusiasm and commitment to the vision, the goals, and the processes of change.

John Kotter, a widely recognized authority on leadership, identifies eight principles of leading change in an organization (**Figure 3.1**).[4] Three of these principles deal with the

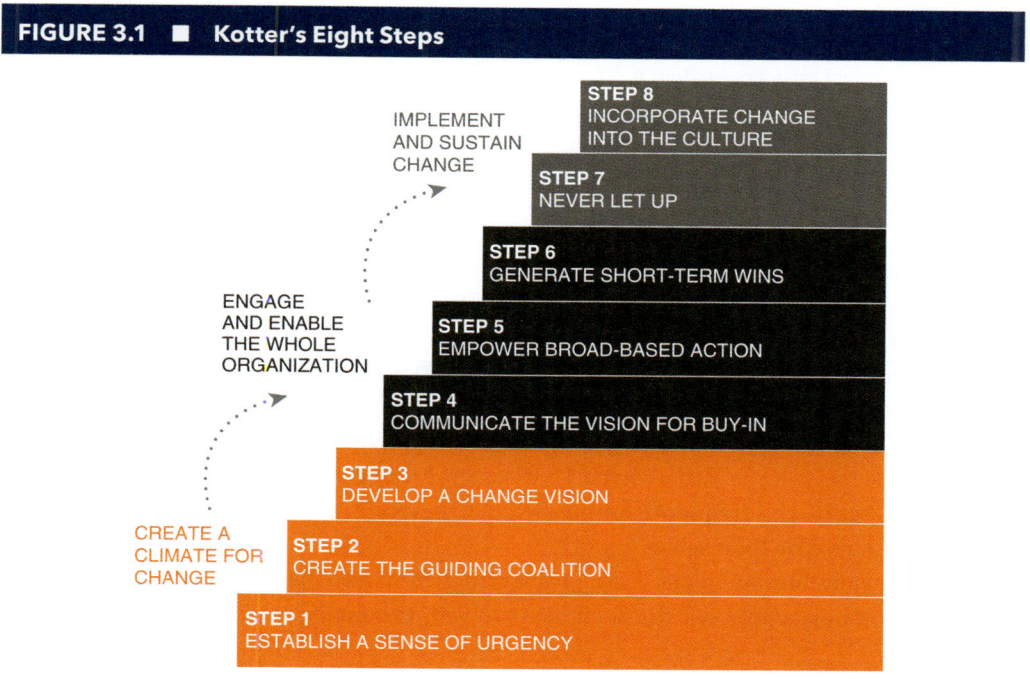

FIGURE 3.1 ■ Kotter's Eight Steps

organization's vision. A key to persuading people to envision the change is to communicate why change is not only necessary but also urgently required. (If it's not necessary, there is no reason to change. If it's not urgent, there is no reason to change now.)

Communication and principled testing and experimentation are as important as creating the vision itself. Everyone on the ED team must understand what the envisioned end point of the project will be—and how achieving the goals will lead them to it. The intent behind principled testing and experimentation along the way is to test ideas and processes and learn while simultaneously engaging the members of the team.

Stephen Beeson has observed that for a vision to have any value, it must guide the daily actions of every member of the health-care team.[5] For that kind of guidance to happen, all members must not only share the vision but also be able to articulate its benefits for each of the key stakeholders. Effective communication has three components:

- *Repetition*: Those leading the effort must communicate the vision regularly, using all available communication channels and resources to do so. Advertisers operate on the premise that consumers must see or hear a commercial multiple times before its message sinks in. The same principle applies to gaining consensus when creating an organization's vision. The organization must repeat the vision over and over until everyone internalizes it.
- *Consistency*: In communicating the vision, the messaging must be consistent. Just as conflicting versions of a commercial would confuse the viewer, offering different messages about the envisioned culture will diminish its impact and create chaos.
- *Accuracy*: The communication and messaging must be accurate in realistically laying out the current state, the future state, and the path for getting there. Trust and clarity are key components in the change management portfolio.

RELATIONSHIP, COMMUNICATION, AND PROJECT MANAGEMENT SKILLS

Before a team creates its vision statement, it is important to analyze both what is and what is not working. In this context, it may be helpful to keep Hoggarth's Law in mind:

> *Attempts to get answers early in a project fail as there are many more wrong questions than right ones. Activity during the early stages should be dedicated to finding the correct questions. Once the correct questions have been identified correct answers will naturally fall out of subsequent work without grief or excitement and there will be understanding of what the project is meant to achieve.*

A corollary is the saying, "Right answers to wrong questions are just as wrong as wrong answers to right questions." In the typical ED, the answer to what is not working well generally falls into two major categories: *human problems* and *system problems*. Attempting to solve system problems when the root cause is human is a recipe for failure. Human issues can include individual idiosyncrasies and personnel problems as well as teamwork-related challenges, problems, or failures. Attempting to solve human problems when the root cause is a systems issue is also a recipe for disaster. Attempting to address human issues is complicated, scary, and frequently unpredictable; therefore, many leaders ignore them and hope they will resolve themselves.

Unfortunately, human issues don't go away; they filter into the departmental gossip pool and evolve into an emotional drain on all involved, producing toxic work environments, low morale, and poor outcomes. Zig Ziglar, the famous motivational speaker, says about employee training:

> What's worse than training your workers and losing them? Not training them and keeping them.[6]

ED Relationship Training

Training ED staff is not like continuing medical education or in-service programs that focus on technical competence. An ED is in the service business, caring for complex people with difficult needs, often under challenging circumstances. How many nurses or physicians were ever given meaningful training in relationship and communication skills? A disappointingly small cohort.

Staff members are expected to come equipped with relationship skill sets to deploy in the workplace, but they may be barely using these skills even at home! Interpersonal and teamwork skills, tools, and techniques are critical for effective, reliable, team-based patient care. However, when directors and managers request interpersonal and team work development training for their staff, the answer from upper management too often takes one of these forms:

- Skepticism about the need and benefits
- Belief that there is no money in the budget for that type of education
- Observation that the organization cannot spare the staff for more than a day

Upper management must be persuaded that excellent team work and interpersonal skills are as important as diagnostic, therapeutic, and technical competence to a smoothly operating, effective ED.

The Motorola Corporation is known worldwide in employee training circles as one of the greatest innovators in human resource management. It was Motorola that launched the Six Sigma–Lean movement, which seeks to lower process defects to the level of 1 in 6 standard deviations from the mean, or 3.4 defects per million. The company is regularly quoted for its assertion that its employee training program yields a 30:1 return on investment.

It is not clear how much the average ED spends on training, but the 2016 American Society of Training and Development Survey found that its benchmark companies averaged 4.3% of revenue spent in this area.[7] A fun exercise is to figure out how much a particular department or hospital invests in this type of training. You might be amazed at how little it is!

Basic Communication Skills

It is often necessary to provide simple ground rules or limited basic training in relationship management and communication before an ED tackles the task of creating a vision statement. Many resources are available for this type of training. A good place to start is "appreciative inquiry"—identifying the thought leaders, informal authority figures, and change agents in the department, enlisting their involvement, and securing their commitment.

Going deeper, it is common in the ED to find that some people feel undervalued or overpowered by others and that their views are ignored or discounted. Many ED team members have seen attempts at change come and go and are resigned to conditions never improving. Some may want to confront chronically disruptive behavior displayed by coworkers but don't know how, are intimidated, or fear retribution. The mission–vision–values exercise is more meaningful and successful if the redesign team can break down some of these barriers at the start and maintain a safe environment that fosters free expression without fear of retribution.

The change initiatives are also more likely to succeed if the team uses a consistent approach toward project management and a common communication convention, particularly for ED leadership. Several excellent resources include *Crucial Conversations, Crucial Confrontations,* and *Healthy Work Environment Initiative*.[8-10] Many local universities also offer programs in project management. However, this type of training is rarely accessed.

Three goals may be accomplished by sending the team offsite for this training: team building, more effective communication, and better working relationships among the group. A retreat site with a strong facilitator is ideal. A successful retreat enables participants to develop a common communication convention and outline a unified approach to project management.

Leadership by Conversation

As already noted, change initiatives are more likely to succeed if management uses a consistent communication convention. One such convention is "leadership by conversation," which is based on recognizing different possible types of conversations and using them to achieve explicit communication.

For example, asking someone to do something entails making a *request*. A request is a specific kind of conversation. To be effective, a request must clearly communicate *what* is being requested and *by when* it is needed. People frequently make a request without taking the time to be clear about what it is they need or specifying a deadline, only to be upset when they don't get the expected results. More explicit communication in the beginning leads to more successful outcomes.

A person who agrees to a request is making a *promise*, which is also a particular kind of conversation. A promise is not an effective promise without an accompanying *by-when*. This closes a loop and enhances the previously mentioned relationship-building skills. The requestor and promisor each make a voluntary *secondary commitment* to the success of the other.

As an example, the requestor makes a note in his or her schedule to call the promisor before the by-when to be sure the promisor either delivers the promise on time or renegotiates the deadline before the due date is missed. Similarly, the promisor makes a note in his or her schedule to call the requestor before the deadline to either reassure the requestor that the request will be met or renegotiate the deadline before it is missed. When an organization consistently uses this convention, a number of things happen throughout its culture:

- People begin to feel good about delivering on their commitments.
- People begin to trust in each other again.
- Resignation (feeling that "nothing is really going to change") fades in the presence of movement, however small.
- People gradually begin to reinvest themselves in the way the department works because there is an avenue for them to be able to contribute to making a difference.

Leadership by communication is just one of a variety of conventions that can be used. It is not important that an ED team uses this particular convention but rather that it uses *an*

> **BOX 3.1 ■ SEVEN BEST PRACTICES IN PROJECT MANAGEMENT**
>
> 1. **Defining the scope and objectives of the project**—know your boundaries from the start.
> 2. **Defining the deliverables**—what tangible items are to be delivered within this project?
> 3. **Project planning**—determine who the project manager will be to lead this effort. The manager will decide what people, resources, and budget are required to complete the project.
> 4. **Communication**—a project plan is worthless if you cannot communicate to the team.
> 5. **Tracking and reporting a project process**—document everything: variations, successes, failures, and discussions.
> 6. **Change management**—managing the changes that occur as the project grows; there will be both human and system issues.
> 7. **Risk management**—risks must be managed to ensure a successful project outcome because they affect the degree to which your project succeeds. Several available methods can help you predict what your risk impact may be; search the Internet or go to your closest library for assistance.

Source: S. Buehring, Project Management Success With the Top Seven Best Practices, at www.projectsmart.co.uk.

effective communication convention and uses it consistently. **Box 3.1** shows approaches for all phases of project management. After these steps, an ED is really ready to take on some change management. But how do the leaders know what to change first?

Strategic Planning

Strategic planning typically starts at the end of the mission–vision–value exercise. Strategy is how the department plans to achieve its goals. Strategy may also encompass what differentiates one's ED and often requires making choices about which direction(s) to pursue.

A "SWOT" analysis is a useful management approach (and acronym) to help everyone define the many elements of the strategic plan. "SWOT" stands for *strengths, weaknesses, opportunities,* and *threats*.

- *Strengths*: An organization should identify and celebrate its existing strengths. In communication convention parlance, a conversation for "acknowledgment" accomplishes that.
- *Weaknesses*: A good facilitator or project lead draws out as many perceived weaknesses as possible in a brainstorming session and lists them on a whiteboard or flip charts. Once this is completed, all present are asked to consider the possibility that some of these problems could be fixed in the next 3 to 12 months and are encouraged to describe which problems seem most important from their perspective. The team can use a type of "multi-voting technique" that allows everyone to vote on which of the problems they would consider to be the top five. (Each person can spread their five votes as they see fit—all five votes on one problem or one each on five problems.) The group should then rank the issues in order.
- *Opportunities*: A conversation for opportunity first asks if each problem is a human problem or a systems problem. Handwashing can prevent illness by preventing the spread of germs. A human-centered problem might be a healthcare worker who does not believe in the need to keep his hands clean. A systems problem might be not having a handwashing station or sanitizer in the work

area. Few human problems lend themselves to a project, whereas most systems problems do. System challenges are often ripe for leadership and team-based projects and solutions (opportunities). Human problems are generally best addressed one-on-one by leadership.

- *Threats:* A conversation for threats asks what elements in the environment external to the group or organization can threaten success. Examples of external threats to the mission of the ED could include competition, an aging workforce, volume overload, or a flu epidemic. To deal with threats, the organization must first define the risk level (low-risk threats may be a low priority), and second delineate the specific responses necessary for high-risk threats. Similar to the multi-voting technique used to identify weaknesses, consider the top five threats. Experience has shown that organizations can take on only so many projects at a time. It is better to accomplish five projects well than to address 10 projects poorly. The exact number of projects a team picks depends on how many (and complex) processes must be addressed when the change initiative begins. In general, shorter, narrower projects succeed more often than longer, broader ones.

IMPLEMENTING CHANGE SUCCESSFULLY

A team must be formed to create and manage the project. Since the team will be implementing changes to the ED, it can be thought of as a "redesign team" (working on a "redesign project"). Three types of participants are key to these initiatives: *project leaders, project team members,* and an *oversight council.*

Project Leaders

Once a team has thoughtfully identified and selected its projects, it must identify the project team leaders. Leadership development and training is a success if some key nurses and physicians (in addition to the nursing manager and the emergency physician director) assume these leadership roles. Over time, project team members often self-identify based upon their interests and expertise, demonstrating their readiness to fulfill the leadership role.

Depending on resource availability and department size, it may be best for team members other than the nurse director or the medical director to assume the position of project team leader. The directors' "real" job often involves coordinating the work of others. They can't do that effectively if their time is consumed leading project teams. The directors' main roles are to ensure resource deployment, enforce accountability and deadlines, and monitor the project's progress.

The project team leader ideally should be someone who is passionate about the issues involved, is committed to finding a solution, and possesses basic project management skills. Once this person is identified, the redesign team can then decide how and when to staff the project and engage key stakeholders. The project leaders must have adequate time to guide implementation of the project. In addition to having a passion for change, the leader should manage the project's progress, that is, keep track of objectives and timelines and ensure that the plan is being implemented day to day in the department.

Project Team Members

Projects may require different levels of expertise and experience. Some will need additional nurses or physicians, and some will need a representative from registration, the lab, radiology, or information technology (IT), and so on. These teams may also include ad hoc members who are necessary only at specific stages of the project. Most experts agree that teams are most effective when they include five to seven permanent team members at most; things often get unwieldy with more than that number. The composition of the team should vary according to the issues to be addressed, and the project team leader should be free to make changes when necessary.

Oversight Council

Individual teams should supervise their own particular projects. Departments embarking on extensive change may benefit by forming an additional supervisory or oversight council to oversee the entire collection of projects. This group should consist of the departmental sponsor from senior administration, the nurse director, the medical director, and all the project team leaders. This group's purpose is to support the project team leaders by removing or negotiating around barriers and, at times, enforcing accountability both within and outside the department. This council must also ensure that project teams have the resources they need to succeed.

Words and Actions

When a project team is ready to start working, it is essential to prepare a written project record. What is not documented, in effect, has not been said or done. To start with, the title of a project itself is important and has two purposes. It should communicate the problem being addressed and the objective metric for evaluating the project's success or failure. For example, "Reducing the Number of Patients Who Leave Without Being Seen by 50%" might be a project title that communicates both the nature of the project and the metric.

There are several reasons to put the intended steps for the project in writing. A written plan:

- Provides a concrete, unambiguous problem definition, project scope, and outline of how the ED wants to proceed
- Creates a map, decreasing the likelihood that team members will stray from the path
- Allows the team to better judge progress; team members have documented clarity about the goals and how they intend to achieve them
- Allows the team to assess how well actions comply with the originally documented intentions

Having the plan in writing also reemphasizes the vision behind this project and allows everyone involved to:

- Know what the goal is and how the team proposes to reach it.
- Know what actions are envisioned and who is to perform them and in what time frame.
- Quickly determine whether progress toward the goal is smooth and what adjustments might have to be made.

Documenting the plan forces the team to be clear and efficient when describing its goals. Involving the team in the writing process allows members to revise the document until everyone agrees that it is a clear reflection of the group's vision. There is a simple way to judge whether the description itself is efficiently written: *The key elements should fit on one page.*

Measuring Progress

Progress is accomplished by action, communication, and follow-through. Action results from acknowledging the requests and promises built on the schedule of "by-whens." While

TABLE 3.1 ■ Reducing the Admission-to-Discharge Interval by 50%.					
Milestone	**Action Step**	**Who**	**By When**	**Status**
Define the best way to determine the admission decision time.	Ask IT if a flag can be added to the ED medical records.	K.J.	October 5	
	If not, can a flag be added to the enterprise system in the nurse's note?	K.J.	October 5	
	Could this time be captured passively using radio-frequency identification technology and at what cost?	T.M.	October 15	

by-whens are always negotiable, it is the project team leader's job to keep the project moving forward. Projects are divided into milestones, or decision points. The project moves from milestone to milestone by a series of action steps.

For example, as demonstrated in **Table 3.1**, the agenda for every meeting of the project team should be accompanied by an action grid that lays out:

- Who has promised to do what task
- When it should be achieved
- Whether the action step is on or behind schedule

A project ends when the milestones are all met. A project is a success if it reaches a valid conclusion.

Using the same example, an ED team determines that reducing the admission decision-to-discharge from the ED time by 50% will only be possible when there are more in-hospital telemetry beds. In this case, the project team has not achieved the goal but has clearly identified the obstacle (what needs to be done to achieve it). The next project might be titled, "How Many New Telemetry Beds are Needed and How Do We Get Them?" The action grid or matrix helps the team regularly assess progress:

- Did the actions the plan calls for occur?
  - ☐ If not, what prevented them?
- Did the actions take place when they were intended to?
  - ☐ If not, what interfered with their achievement?

Metrics are required to gauge how effective the changes are. Evaluation of progress should be based on objective standards of measurement that are consistently used and understood by all the ED staff. Metrics, for example, might involve reductions in turnaround time, unnecessary delays, medication errors, or the number of patients leaving prior to receiving a medical screening examination. Additionally, metrics might relate to patient satisfaction scores and patient complaints and compliments. These metrics should demonstrate progress toward the goals and should also be tied to concrete results specified in advance. A succinct way to express the appropriate metrics is to measure what (if accomplished) will make the project succeed.

Testing Changes

The specific projects identified by the team will show what needs to be done but not necessarily how to do it. It is usually helpful to start small and test often to be sure that any proposed intervention is producing the desired outcome. Testing on a small scale allows for experimentation and learning while improving engagement and buy-in. It often takes

TABLE 3.2 ■ The PDSA Cycle

Phase	Definition	Steps
Plan	Identify the problem that needs fixing to bring about improvement in the process.	• Brainstorming • Pareto analysis • Flowcharting • Cause-and-effect diagrams
Do	Conduct small tests of change.	• Training in small-group leadership skills • Training in conflict resolution • On-the-job training
Study	Determine whether the small tests of change are achieving the results you wish to achieve.	• Data check sheets • Control charts • Key performance indicators • Graphical analysis
Act	Recognize interventions that did not work, and implement the ones that did.	• Process mapping • Process standardization • Formal training for standard processes

a series of small, leveraged successes to overcome inertia. The more an ED can celebrate these gradual improvements in the beginning, the better.[11] Most doctors and nurses have experienced change management programs that did not work well. Achieving incremental successes early in the process lays a foundation of credibility for the current project.

PDSA and Rapid-Cycle Testing

Rapid-cycle testing and PSDA ("plan, do, study, act") are incremental, small-scale approaches to change. Rapid-cycle testing is used in a variety of leadership approaches, including total quality management, kaizen (Japanese for "improvement") groups, and Lean techniques. PDSA is a process also known as the Deming Cycle (**Table 3.2**).[12] (Health care personnel acquainted with the scientific method will find the PDSA process and its iterative cycles very familiar.)

The initial "plan" phase is guided by the team's identification of priority opportunities or problems. Part of determining the best intervention is the "do" phase, which involves testing that intervention on a small scale and building on those results before implementing wholesale transformation. "Study" denotes analyzing the results of the small-scale test and deciding why it worked or didn't. "Act" means one of two things: Recognize that the intervention did work and build on it, or recognize that it didn't work, adjust accordingly, and begin the cycle again (**Figure 3.2**).

FIGURE 3.2 ■ The PDSA Cycle

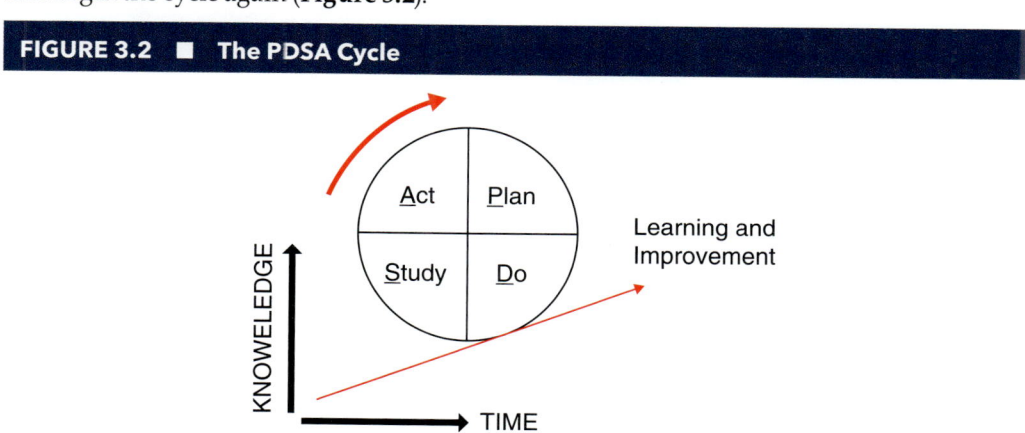

Plan Phase: Everyone involved should understand:

- What the team wants to accomplish
- Who is going to do what by when
- How team members will know if the intended objective improves processes
- How we will know that a change is an improvement

Do Phase: Many ED project teams create implementation processes with a long timelines, such as 1 to 2 years. Just as starting with small changes is usually more effective than starting with broad changes, setting short time frames for components of the project is usually more effective than using a long-term schedule. That is because teams can more easily participate in and manage a project with a focused timeline and limited goals. Senior management, on the other hand, may need or want a project portfolio with a longer time horizon. When two different time frames are necessary, the critical task is to break the big initiatives down into a series of 90-day projects for the implementation teams. Using monthly and weekly milestones focused on specific action steps can help an ED set and achieve realistic goals.

Study Phase: Those running the tests compile written observations for the analysis in the PDSA study phase. The team gathers data throughout the project, since having concrete data is vital for effectively measuring progress. The gathered data should focus on the project goals, the vision statement, and the test of change. It is important to keep the measurement system simple, relevant, and effective.

Act Phase: If the team decides that the intervention was successful, next steps often include ramping up the size and scope of the rapid-cycle testing. An alternative outcome could include selecting some aspects of the proposed change for further improvement—which the team then tests. If the intervention generally did not work, the team reenters the planning phase and, based on the data obtained from the test, designs alternative approaches to accomplish the objective.

When a team recognizes that an intervention did work and implements it broadly, the team is ready to go on to its next project, using the same approach. Culture changes when a successful project (or set of projects) is widely implemented, is recognized by the team as effective, and becomes the new way of operating in the ED. Communication remains important. The team should make sure successes are widely publicized within the system. See **Figure 3.3** for a map of how the PDSA process flows.

For departments that are implementing many changes, the oversight council should regularly review and communicate the overall initiative's progress. This evaluation is important

FIGURE 3.3 ■ The PDSA Cycle Process Flow Map

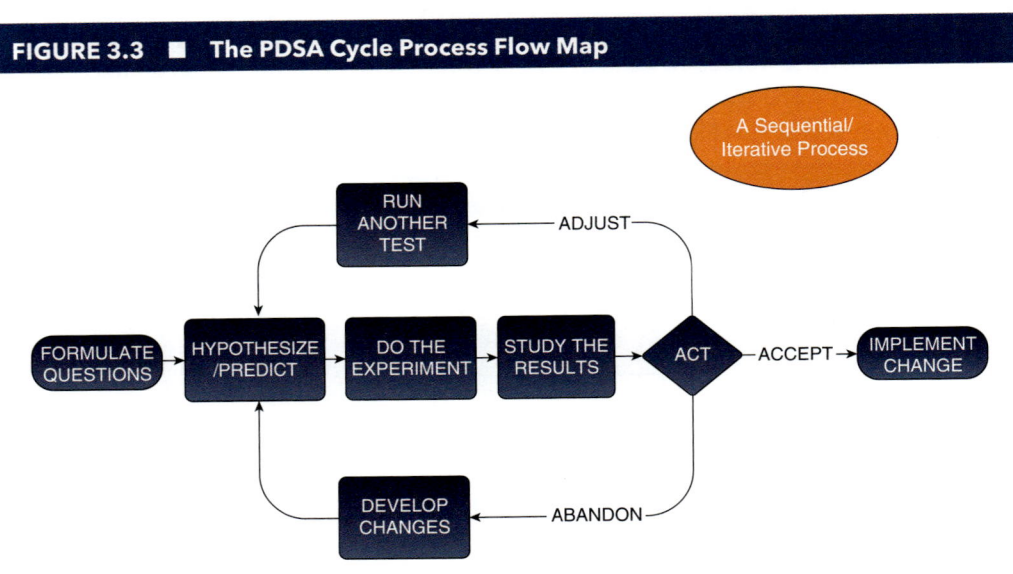

to build a positive culture around change. As noted earlier, most physicians and nurses have experienced change initiatives that started full of promise and then fizzled. By examining the project separately from the day-to-day implementation team, the oversight council helps keep a clear focus on group's overarching goals, resource allocation, and progress.

OPPORTUNITIES FOR SUCCESS

The points discussed in the following sections are important to keep in mind when working through changes in the culture, particularly if they are extensive.

The Right Team

The importance of having the right people on the team cannot be overemphasized. As noted earlier, people should select the projects in which they are most interested and invested. A motivated team goes a long way toward making that project effective. Carrying out training in communication and relationships before a project even begins also makes success more likely. The team should stay focused on working together and working effectively as the project proceeds. Sports teams provide lessons about teams. Talent always plays a role, but a great team is likely one with players who fulfill specific roles that enhance the success of the entire group.

Duke men's basketball coach Mike Krzyzewski uses the analogy of five fingers folded into a fist.[13] A team is more effective than a group of individuals and includes these five elements:

- Communication
- Trust
- Collective responsibility
- Care
- Pride

This principle is important to keep in mind because not every department has a lineup of superstars. "Team" refers to more than just the project team members; it includes everyone working to provide care in the ED. It is important to coach the non-project team ED members in performance improvement skills and mentor individuals one-on-one as projects unfold. Teaching critical relationship skills and coaching through honest evaluation and feedback can help make the individuals in the department the "right people" for any team.

High performance inevitably involves more than just clinical acumen and skills; it involves attitudes. High performers are often called "A-team" members, whose attitudes and aptitudes can greatly enhance team performance.[14] Each project affects people who aren't actually guiding the intervention. The attitude and commitment of the non-team members will also significantly affect how well the intervention is carried out. High performers are engaged and feel responsible for what they and their teammates accomplish. These high performers go about their work with a sense of purpose and passion. Their attitudes are reflected in their behavior.

Empowering the Staff

The secret to motivating clinicians includes emphasizing their desire to serve others and pointing to their healthy self-interest. People typically want to work in a job that is fulfilling. Leaders can inspire their team members by helping them to understand how the planned interventions and improvements enable them to provide better care and make the ED a better place to work. Team members become intrinsically motivated when they begin to understand that the ongoing cycles of change enhance their own self-interests and their ability to serve others. Financial rewards do play a role in motivating health-care workers, as in any other field, but the power of engaging clinicians in worthwhile work and outcomes should not be underestimated.

To discover the driving force that animates particular physicians and nurses on a team, leaders should ask:

- What excites you most about your job?
- What would make the change process succeed?
- What concerns you most about your job?

Conversations around these questions can lead to insights about what will motivate each of the members of the team.

During the design phase of a project, the staff may identify a weakness that hinders their ability to work effectively and efficiently. If an ED project team can improve those processes and align them with staff capability, capacity, and self-interest, the team will empower employees to deliver on the desired outcomes. Team leaders also have to be wary of the impact of perverse incentives. For example, when a staff member is asked why they don't work more diligently and see more patients, that staff member might honestly answer, "If I move patients faster, then I will get more patients, increasing my already heavy workload and perhaps allowing others to sit around and see fewer patients." The team might then work to develop a process that unburdens all staff (e.g., faster admission protocols).

Making Effective Use of Clinicians' Time

Physicians and nurses commonly express dissatisfaction with activities that don't enhance patient care. Requiring doctors and nurses to attend to tasks that should be managed by aides or technicians (or perhaps not be done at all) wastes valuable time. Nurses and physicians should be working in systems that enable them to practice at the top of their licenses. This issue of effective time management also brings to mind what is known as Cohn's Law:

> *The more time you spend in reporting on what you are doing, the less time you have to do anything.*

This insight is salient. Cohn's Law goes on to elaborate on the ultimate effect of this principle wryly:

> *Stability is achieved when you spend all your time doing nothing but reporting on the nothing you are doing.*

A redesign team should ask the staff how process improvements can empower them and make the most effective use of their time. The ED staff will often provide valuable suggestions that can be incorporated into the improvement efforts. Successful adoption of the suggested changes motivates staff while improving the efficiency of patient care.

Potential Pitfalls

Attempts to change organizational culture and performance often fail. The most common reasons for failure are inadequate planning and an inability to successfully execute change over time. Failure is seldom due to a shortage of good ideas.

Failure Factors

Changing a process or a culture is not something someone can do by jumping into it in the middle. In a discussion of other common reasons why such performance improvement initiatives fail, David J. Shulkin notes that laying out too large a scheme on an excessively long timeline is one reason for failure.[15] In addition, he notes other causes of defeat:

- Focusing excessively on processes
- Holding too many meetings
- Trying to micromanage project team leaders (good project managers know when not to manage a project)
- Not having the appropriate incentives or the right people in place

Shulkin's last point is particularly germane in EDs that do not have the luxury of having a full team in place, let alone a team with superstars.

Inspiring Team Members

An effective leader can motivate ordinary people to do extraordinary things. Inspiration begins by building relationships and communication skills. In his book *Conscious Business*, Fred Kofman describes this critical transformation[16]:

> *The exterior of leadership is behaviors. Also, a leader is like the builder or the architect of the ship in developing the social and business systems of the company.... the leader works in a transformational way, touching people's personality and their interiority. As a cultural icon, the leader influences the stories and the shared values and the community.*

By definition, a culture has certain traditional (inertial) ways that people communicate and behave. People generally do not like change and many resist modifying the way they've always operated because it is either working for them or they are comfortable with their abilities within the current cultural framework.[17] We are often tempted to overcome this resistance by providing convincing reasons for change. A better and more realistic approach is articulated by John Shook, chairman of the Lean Enterprise Institute[18]:

> *It's easier to act your way to a new way of thinking than to think your way to a new way of acting. Start by changing what people do rather than how they think.*

Once an ED's behavioral and process changes have been identified and implemented, perhaps the department leaders and the their team can then focus on maintaining the result: *the new status quo*.

CONCLUSION

An effective team begins by assessing the relationship, communication, and performance improvement skills of both the leadership and the rank and file. A team addressing these issues can then focus on projects and outcomes that matter to the entire organization. Training all members of the ED staff in basic relationship and communication skills can be helpful. It is essential that all team members have an understanding of basic performance improvement skills and tools. Finally, the team's chances of achieving meaningful and sustainable change can be greatly improved by establishing the expectation of openness and a safe environment for healthy self-expression.

There can be challenges. One may find some individual ED team members who have become cynical and demoralized because they believe that their opinions go chronically unheard. Some may have developed an abrasive approach to interpersonal relationships, and others have learned to cope with the chronic dysfunction by assuming that conditions will never get better.

Senior management, in partnership with the redesign team, can facilitate the creation of the department's vision statement and project plan. This collaboration begins with the physician and nursing leadership, followed by the project teams, and then the entire staff. Project management training and strategic planning help to identify the high-priority goals and project teams. These teams can outline appropriate interventions and create a written plan with short-term, easily accomplished milestones. Records of team discussions must include the specific tactics and interventions and define the responsible team member and the "by-when." These interventions are evaluated using rapid-cycle testing, which can prompt adjustments and lead to positive change.

Nearly everyone wants to be successful and valued in the organization. The job of a leader is to:

- Inspire the team and its members.
- Show them how to succeed.
- Guide them in their journey toward excellence.
- Celebrate their success.

REFERENCES

1. Cummings TG, Worley CG. *Organization Development and Change*. Mason, Ohio: South-Western; 2005.
2. Covey S. *The 7 Habits of Highly Successful People: Restoring the Character Ethic*. New York, NY: Simon and Schuster; 1989.
3. Deming WE. *The Deming Management Method*. New York, NY: Berkley Publishing Group; 1986.
4. Kotter J. *Leading Change*. Boston, Mass: Harvard Business School Press; 1996.
5. Beeson S. *Engaging Physicians*. Gulf Breeze, Fla: Fire Starter; 2009.
6. Ziglar Z. The Ziglar Weekly Newsletter. WordPress online. Ziglar, Inc.; 2009.
7. American Society of Training and Development. Survey. Available at: http://www.astd.org. 2016. Accessed August 3, 2018.
8. Patterson K. *Crucial Conversations: Tools for Talking When Stakes Are High*. New York, NY: McGraw-Hill; 2002.
9. Patterson K, Grenny J, McMillan R, Switzler A. *Crucial Confrontations*. New York, NY: McGraw-Hill; 2004.
10. AACN. *AACN's Healthy Work Environment Initiative*; 2016 Available at: http://www.aacn.org. Accessed August 3, 2018.
11. Lewin K. *Resolving Social Conflicts: Selected Papers on Group Dynamics*. New York, NY: Harper & Row; 1948.
12. Jensen K, Mayer TA, Welch SJ, Haradan C. *Leadership for Smooth Patient Flow*. ACHE Management Series. Chicago, Ill: Health Administration Press; 2007.
13. Krzyzewski M. *Leading With the Heart: Coach K's Successful Strategies for Basketball, Business, and Life*. New York, NY: Warner Business; 2000.
14. Mayer T, Cates RJ. *Leadership for Great Customer Service: Satisfied Patients, Satisfied Employees*. Chicago, Ill: Health Administration Press; 2004.
15. Shulkin D. Why quality improvement efforts in healthcare fail and what can be done about it. *Am J Med Qual*. 2000;15(2):49-53.
16. Kofman F. *Conscious Business*. Boulder, Colo: Sounds True Press; 2006.
17. Senge, P. *The Fifth Discipline: The Art and Practice of the Learning Organization*. New York, NY: Doubleday; 1990.
18. Shook J. Back to Basics: John Shook on the Role of Questions in Coaching by John Y. Shook, https://www.lean.org/LeanPost/Posting.cfm?LeanPostId=779, The Lean Post, August 29, 2017, originally published February 17, 2009. Accessed August 3, 2018.

ADDITIONAL READINGS

- Berwick D. A primer on leading the improvement of systems. *BMJ*. 1996;312:619-622.
- Berwick DM, Nolan TW. Physicians as leaders in improving healthcare. *Ann Inter Med*. 1998;128(4):289-292.
- Edwards N, Kornacki MJ, Silversin J. Unhappy doctors: what are the causes and what can be done about it? *BMJ*. 2002;324:835-838.
- Fitzsimmons J, Fitzsimmons M. *Service Management: Operations, Strategy, Information Technology*. 5th ed. Boston, Mass: McGraw-Hill; 2006.
- Goldratt E. *The Goal*. Great Barrington, Mass: North River Press; 1986.
- Heifetz R. *Leadership Without Easy Answers*. 1994 Cambridge, Mass. Belknap Press of Harvard University Press, 1994.
- Langley GJ, Nolan KM, Nolan TW. *The Foundation of Improvement*. Silver Spring, MD: API Publishing; 1992
- Langley J, Nolan K, Nolan T, Norman, C, Provost L. *The Improvement Guide*. San Francisco, Calif: Jossey-Bass; 2009.
- Peters T. *The Excellence Dividend: Meeting the Tech Tide With Work That Wows and Jobs That Last*. New York, Vintage Press, Random House, 2018
- Prochaska J, Norcross J, Diclemente C. In Search of How People Change. *Am Psychol*. 1992;47(9):1102-1114.
- Reinertsen J, Pugh M, Bisognano M. Seven Leadership Leverage Points. Innovation Series. 2005. Available at: whitepaper, www.ihi.org.
- Rogers E. *Diffusion of Innovations*. New York, NY: The Free Press; 1995.
- Scott S. *Fierce Conversations: Achieving Success at Work and in Life One Conversation at a Time*. New York, The Berkley Trade Publishing Group; 2002.
- Silversin J, Kornaki MJ. *Leading Physicians Through Change: How to Achieve and Sustain Results*. Chicago, American College of Physician Executives; 2000.
- Sirkin H, Keenan P, Jackson A. The hard side of change management. *Harvard Business Review*. 2005.
- Stone D, Patton B, Heen S, Fisher R. *Difficult Conversations: How to Discuss What Matters Most*. 2010.
- Ury W, Fisher R, Bruce M. *Getting to Yes: Negotiating Agreement Without Giving*. Updated 2011.

CHAPTER 4

POWER VERSUS INFLUENCE

Thom A. Mayer, Robert W. Strauss

Of things that exist, some are in our power and some are not in our power. Those that are in our power are opinion, choice, the things we do like, the things we don't like, and in a word, those things that are of our own doing. Those that are not under our control are our bodies, property, possessions, reputations, positions of authority and in a word things that are not of our own doing. We must remember that those things are externals and are therefore not our concern. Trying to control or to change what we can't only results in torment.

—Greek philosopher Epictetus[1]

DEFINING POWER AND INFLUENCE

Leaders and managers often equate power with influence, two concepts that share a number of common aims, including effecting positive change; producing quality results in a safe, cost-effective system; inspiring staff; and meeting the needs and desires of patients and their families.

Although leadership authority is common to both power and influence, the two approaches are fundamentally different in how they are applied. As Epictetus notes, one individual cannot ever truly persuade or change another. However, effective leaders can influence others to change *themselves*. According to the Greek philosopher, people have power over:

- What they think
- How they feel
- What they say
- What they do

However, an individual has no power over how others react; one can only *influence* others. Far from being a constraint, this frees leaders from illusions of power and helps us understand precisely what is and is not in our control. As Austrian psychiatrist Viktor Frankl notes, "Everything can be taken from a man but one thing: the last of the human freedoms—to choose one's attitude in any given set of circumstances, to choose one's own way."[2]

Power

The word *power* derives from the Latin *posse*, which means "to be able." It is defined as "the ability to produce an effect through the possession of control or authority over others."[3] Power is a zero-sum game—the more that is given away, the less that is maintained. Power typically focuses on short-term results as opposed to long-term relationships because it involves pressuring or even forcing others into action.

If excessively applied, power is fundamentally undemocratic and authoritarian. As classical scholar Friedrich Nietzsche cautions, "Rather perish than hate and fear, and twice

FIGURE 4.1 ■ Three Ways to Influence

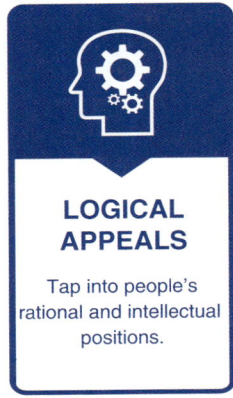
LOGICAL APPEALS
Tap into people's rational and intellectual positions.

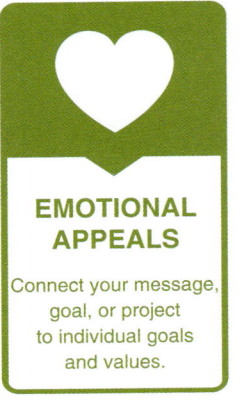
EMOTIONAL APPEALS
Connect your message, goal, or project to individual goals and values.

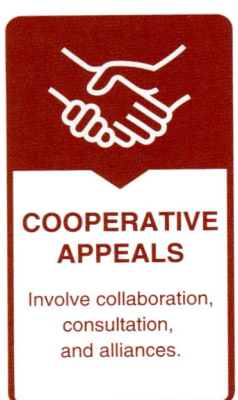
COOPERATIVE APPEALS
Involve collaboration, consultation, and alliances.

rather perish than make oneself hated and feared."[4] If used unwisely, power can cause resentment that leads to turnover among team members.

Influence

The word *influence* is defined as "the capacity to have an effect on something or someone."[3] The word derives from the Latin *influere*, "to flow into"—an apt etymology as we discuss the role of influence in leadership. It raises this question: How can a leader "flow" key elements of teamwork into the team—a common commitment supported by an evidence-based set of skills?

Instead of forcing power on others, influence "invents options for mutual gain" and grows capability.[5] Democratic and interactive, "influence" seeks team input to guide strategies and tactics. If power is a monologue, influence is a conversation. **Figure 4.1** outlines three ways to influence others.

Influence is a fundamentally different approach from power with different consequences for the long-term relationship among team members:

- *Power*: "Managing metrics and mutual accountability are simple realities for the emergency department (ED) team, as we stressed when we recruited you and you accepted our invitation to join the team."
- *Influence*: "How can we work together as a team to discover the best ways to deliver results while making our jobs easier at the same time?"

The Voice of the Patient

ED teams have one true power: *the voice of the patient*. Any and all arguments, negotiations, and decisions should center on this question: "What's the best thing for the patient?"[6] Team members are close to patients at the time of their greatest need, which provides both the opportunity and the necessity for the members of the team to listen to the patients and their families. The most powerful people are those who listen most carefully and astutely. The least powerful are those furthest from patients or those who insist on what they think is best, regardless of the patients' perspectives.

These insights arm the team with the most important knowledge in health care. BestPractices, an emergency physician and hospitalist staffing and management group, applies three essential rules:

Rule #1: *Always* do the right thing for the patient!
Rule #2: Do the right thing for the people who take care of the patient.
Rule #3: *Never* confuse rule #1 and rule #2.[7]

In other words, there is no power greater than the power of the patient. All change efforts should start with a clear understanding of why an action is good for the patient. Consider the following approaches that leaders may use to address the "boarder problem" in the ED:

> **Medical Director to CEO:** *"If this boarder problem can't be solved, the doctors will leave. They didn't sign up for this!"*
>
> **Nursing Director to CNO:** *"The nurses have had it! They came here to be critical care nurses, not 'babysitters' for the floors!"*
>
> **Medical and Nursing Directors (together) at the "C-suite" meeting:** *"Please come to the ED to round and meet the patients and families who have been waiting hours or days for a hospital bed. It's important to understand their experience and hear their voices."*

Of these, the most effective message uses the power of the patient's voice to influence others to action.

Unintended Consequences

Despite the best intentions, detailed plans, elaborate strategies, and excellent tactics, actions almost always result in some unintended consequences. Robert Merton, who coined the term *unintended consequences*, identified one of their sources as "the imperious immediacy of interest . . . instances in which an individual wants the intended consequence of an action so much that he purposefully chooses to ignore any unintended effects."[8] For example, an unintended effect could be the frustration and disengagement of team members responsible for implementing a solution that has been forced on them by someone farther up the chain of command (**Table 4.1**).

TABLE 4.1 ■ Contrasting Power and Influence	
Power	**Influence**
Controls	Convinces
Extrinsic motivation	Intrinsic motivation
Commands and coerces	Convinces and cooperates
Positional	Principled
Power of position	Influence of ideas
Bruises relationships	Builds relationships
Wields power	Exerts and exercises influence
Pushback	**Feedback**
Conscripts	Recruits
Grudging compliance	Gracious assent
Enforced commitment	Voluntary workers
Hurts to fail	Safe spaces to fail
Innovation tough	Innovation easy
Opaque	Transparency
Gives direction	Allows discovery

Power has its own unintended consequences. Organizations that are that are focused on a power approach don't intend to have negative effects that are nevertheless apparent to those within the system, particularly to those who are not in power.

CONTRASTING POWER AND INFLUENCE

None of these statements should be taken as absolutes. Power and influence exist on a spectrum. Very few people are consistently "pure" power leaders or "pure" influence leaders; however, there are times when one or the other approach is necessary. For example, in an ED resuscitation, a power approach may be essential to ensure compliance with protocols. Compliance with evidence-based clinical guidelines is another example in which a power approach can be useful because such protocols are justifiably mandated. Similarly, ensuring that patient safety principles are closely followed requires some level of authority. However, the generation of those evidence-based protocols and patient safety guidelines should be a team effort in which influence is used to convene the members and engage their creativity.

Extrinsic vs Intrinsic Motivation

Extrinsic and intrinsic motivation are diametrically opposed incentives. The phrase "getting people to do what needs to be done" exemplifies a power, or *extrinsic*, approach to motivation. Power and extrinsic motivation are nearly synonymous and typically produce temporary, grudging compliance at best.[9]

By contrast, *intrinsic* motivation ensures compliance because team members realize that a particular action "is the right thing to do." In a word, intrinsic motivation is an attitude. Successful performance through intrinsic motivation creates a sense of satisfaction, internal fulfillment for doing a difficult job, pleasure in growth, as well as desire and grounds for advancement. Intrinsic motivation contributes to the overall well-being and health of both patients and the team.

Whereas extrinsic motivation demands, "Here's what's important for you to do and how to do it," intrinsic motivation asks, "What's important to you and the team and, based on your experience, how can we do it most effectively?" The former is a declarative statement of "You will." The latter is a conversation, recognizing that the people who do the job most likely know how to do it well and will accomplish their goals if given the freedom, resources, and motivation to do so.

Command vs Convince

The very definition of power involves command and control over other people's behaviors by prescriptively defining *what* needs to be done, *how* it will be done, *which* metrics will be used to measure compliance and success, and *when* they will be measured. (Those who have served in the military know that "command and control" has a specific and prescriptive meaning.[10]) A power approach demands specific actions by specific people within a specific timeline. Although it is not the intention of this approach to demoralize the team members, it often does—an unintended consequence of controlling rather than convincing.

Influence relies on framing goals in a way that encourages team members to believe in the importance of the department's mission, vision, and values and work cooperatively to attain these common goals.[11] Consider the process of yearly job evaluations, a tradition typically used to hold people accountable for their agreed-upon responsibilities. In power-focused EDs, those sessions act to reinforce the following notions:

- "You work *for me*, and here's what I think about your work."
- "You need to get *on board* and start doing the following things..."

In EDs focused on influence, job evaluations are far more focused on mutual, rather than individual, accountability:

- "Because we work together, here's what the team tells us went really well, which is deeply appreciated."
- "What areas are you working on to make your job and the team's jobs easier?"
- "Will you help coach and mentor other members of the team with the things you are doing well?"
- "Here are some strategies other team members are using that have gotten great results and made their jobs easier. What are your thoughts on how these might work for you and your patients?"

Because the power approach demands compliance with the desires of "the Boss," it commands and coerces people into specified actions. Paradoxically, in a power culture, it is easy to figure out *what* to do ("Do what I/we say!"), but it is more difficult to figure out *why* it is being done. Hierarchical, pyramidical, authoritarian power cultures have as a central feature the wish for consistency, control, and predictability.

Influence draws on the cooperation, not coercion, of the professionals on the team. The interactive nature of influence still embraces specific goals, but the path forward is wider and more inclusive, resulting in cooperation and, typically, more innovative solutions.

Positional vs Principled

Power is based on the inherent belief that *position* is the guiding force of hierarchical organizations. An entity has one and only one "C-suite" with one and only one "chief." This structure tends to drive toward functional silos, as opposed to cross-functional teams. Research shows that a principled or value-driven approach results in professionals and organizations[5,12-14]:

- Whose goals are clear because they are self-evident
- Whose processes are innovative
- Who attract high-caliber talent to perform in ethical and inspiring ways
- Who will retain that talent in the long term because the focus is on the caregivers

Bruising vs Building

Those who are subjected to controlling, commanding, coercive, positional power cultures resent being constantly told what to do and when to do it. We often hear that people "wield power"—as if power were a weapon to be used against the team. What attitude could be more damaging to individual motivation and team dynamics? Influence seeks not only to produce measurable results but also to build relationships and capabilities for the ongoing success of the team. Instead of wielding power, it is more successful in the long run to exert influence. For ED leaders, relationships matter and must be nurtured to the greatest extent possible.

Conscripts vs Recruits

Wielding power over team members is like conscripting soldiers, enlisting them involuntarily. Influencing team members is like recruiting volunteers. Insisting that people "get on board" is a common management metaphor that has some superficial merit. The metaphor implies that the team is aboard a boat, rowing in the right direction, with everyone pulling smoothly and equally on their respective oars. However, it fails to recognize that not all "oars" are the same; each team member is performing interdependent yet fundamentally different tasks to make "the boat" (presumably the ED) move in the right direction. Although unintentional, the metaphor implies that the leadership has artfully designed the craft and that anyone who is not "on board" is presumably drowning in treacherous waters.

However, a parable by Steven Covey, author of *The Habits of Highly Successful People* and other books, demonstrates a problem with the "power approach." He describes "busy, efficient producers and managers [who might in a demoralizing tone say] 'Shut up! We're making progress!'" in response to team members who question the direction.[15] A power approach can discourage staff from questioning an ineffective process and recommending other ideas.

Working as a team in a multidisciplinary fashion is a necessity in the complex adaptive environment of a busy ED. However, organizational development expert Peter Block refers to onboarding as "soft-core colonialism," with enforced labor devised almost exclusively by the powerful.[16] Demanding compliance with policies and procedures the team has had no voice in developing frequently results in "pushback." Alternatively, seeking feedback on how the system could—and must—be improved to meet the needs of patients and staff results in participation.

A leadership and management system based primarily on a power model creates conscripts instead of recruits. Derived from the military concept of enlisting people by force, power-focused leadership similarly tells the "troops" to toe the line or face the consequences. This is hardly a formula for recruiting the best and brightest professionals. Influence attracts talent by rewarding the unique and important contributions that each individual makes to the team. Influence leaders share and encourage the adoption of a vision. Conscripts are forced to commit to the effort, whereas recruits tap into their passion and dedication.

Beware of the comment, "We all need to get on the same page!" Almost without exception, the true meaning of that statement is, "*You* need to get on *my* page!" This exhortation is a classic power-based statement, although it is disguised as collaborative one. Similarly, when someone demands, "Think outside the box!" they are actually saying, "Think inside *my box!*" Be ready to resist these entreaties, which are rarely based on a broad, consensus-based view.[17]

Building a Voluntary "Army"

Conscripts are forced to commit to the effort. Recruits are chosen for their passion and commitment to the team's mission, vision, and values. They are ready to deliver their total effort, no matter how difficult the task, because their dedication drives them.

Business scholar Peter Drucker understood this well, noting that all knowledge workers are essentially *voluntary* workers.[18] The balance between a power-based and an influence-based system is a calculus in which knowledge workers are willing to do more—*much* more—than what they are paid to do because they understand they are volunteering their heads, hearts, and hands at a level far beyond that for which they are compensated. They deeply believe in and are fundamentally committed to the work. Influence unleashes the power to produce volunteer workers whose potential is virtually unlimited.

Fostering Innovation

Innovation is a distinguishing feature of successful health-care organizations precisely because "the way we're working isn't working."[19] The team knows the system is broken because the processes (and work environment) extract too great a toll on the team members and often result in frustration, failure, and poor patient engagement. It is clear that "the way we're working *is* working" when a passionate, ardent, and enthusiastic team produces sustainable results through processes for which they had some sense of authorship.

In organizations focused on power, innovation may not be welcomed because it questions the way things are currently done and the people who have mandated them.

In a power environment, it takes great courage to point out changes that should be made. Furthermore, innovation failure is poorly tolerated and may lead to humiliation ("Well *that* was a brilliant idea that didn't work! Got any others for us, Einstein?") and self-restraint when suggesting further changes.

Approached correctly, the process of innovation is accompanied by the risk of failure. After all, innovation that works 100% of the time isn't really innovation—it's simply the early adoption of best practices. By enlisting input from the team, influence encourages diversity of opinion when considering potential solutions. The adoption of one approach means others have not been chosen. Influence creates safe spaces to fail and encourages participants to learn from these mistakes. In the authors' experience, a failure rate of about 40% is typical for organizations "out on the edge" of health-care innovation.[20]

For example, Thomas Watson, Sr., the founding CEO of IBM, recalled the story of an employee whose mistake cost the company $1 million. When the contrite employee tendered his resignation, Watson exclaimed, "Fire you? You must be mad—I just spent $1 million *investing* in you!" From that day forward, one of IBM's guiding principles has been "forgive thoughtful mistakes!"[21]

In his book *The Fifth Discipline*, Peter Senge describes the concept of the "no-blame" learning organization. In it, he lists the 11 "Laws of the Fifth Discipline" (**Table 4.2**). These

TABLE 4.2 ■ Senge's 11 "Laws of the Fifth Discipline"

	The Law	Implication
1.	Today's problems come from yesterday's solutions.	Today's problems resulted from previous well-meaning solutions. Engage all the stakeholders.
2.	The harder you push, the harder the system pushes back.	Invite and engage the stakeholders and create a safe milieu in which ideas can grow.
3.	Behavior grows better before it grows worse.	Initial behavior may be supportive, but the team will have to be recruited again and again.
4.	The easy way out usually leads back in.	When challenged, many resort to old habits because they are tried and tested, although not necessarily effective.
5.	The cure can be worse than the disease.	Sometimes leaders lock on a solution (good or bad) and stop looking to improve.
6.	Faster is slower.	Sustainable solutions require time to absorb, revise, achieve nuance, and gain stakeholder acceptance.
7.	Cause and effect are not closely related in time and space.	Impatience is the enemy of successful change. Slower may be faster.
8.	Small changes can produce big results, but the areas of highest leverage are often the least obvious.	A diverse group of empowered stakeholders can collaboratively define the small, focused actions that produce the most impactful solutions.
9.	You can have your cake and eat it too, but not at the same time.	Solutions are not either/or but rather often require collaboration and innovation.
10.	Dividing an elephant in half does not produce two small elephants.	It takes more than one person to solve the problem. Understand the problem, find the solution, unblind your team, and collaborate.
11.	There is no blame.	Lasting solutions rely on recognizing "they" are part of "our" team.

"laws" recognize the necessity of deep stakeholder engagement and the perception that "they" are part of "our" team.[13]

Opacity vs Transparency

Many power-driven organizations have an unspoken (and certainly unwritten) philosophy that those in power should have access to and control over information that is unavailable to others in lower positions. If information and knowledge are power (and they certainly are in health care's "perpetual whitewater of change"), should they be hoarded by those in authority? Limiting the distribution of information puts control in the hands of a few and "blinds" those stakeholders who could use the information to make intrinsically motivated improvements. As illustrated by the parable "The Blind Men and the Elephant"—in which six blind men touching different parts of an elephant give entirely different definitions of the animal—unless knowledge is fully shared, people create their own reality with limited information.

> *A team that regularly says, "I don't understand what's going on . . . why exactly are we doing this?" is mired in the opacity of power.*

Alternatively, information and knowledge should be widely disseminated to support learning. Strong influence-driven organizations choose transparency and broadly share the most reliable information with the people doing the work. Dashboards should be available to show the data that drive decisions on a real-time basis, whenever possible.

> *A team that regularly says, "I just saw yesterday's results; our team is doing a terrific job!" exists in the liberating glow of transparency.*

Direction vs Discovery

An organization focused on power is ultimately directive in nature. It tells the team what to do, how to do it, and when to do it. "Complete these tasks without questioning the reason or method, and when you finish, come back and I'll give you further direction." For example, when attempting to improve core measures compliance, a power leader might say, "Here are the core measure guidelines. Follow them to a 'T' as I've laid them out. Don't deviate from those guidelines, no matter the circumstances. And don't forget to document that you followed them; we don't get 'credit' for compliance unless you do." Aside from being fundamentally disrespectful to the team members, such an approach smothers creativity and innovation.

An influence-driven approach recognizes the importance of core measures, acknowledges that an evidence-based approach is needed to meet them, and emphasizes thorough documentation in all areas requiring compliance. But influence starts by gathering the stakeholders in a discovery meeting to share the importance of the outcomes (the "why"). The influence leader then addresses any questions and encourages the team to discuss options to achieve success. The meeting continues with a discussion of how the evidence-based guidelines can best be tailored to the requirements of the ED. An influence leader might ask, "What obstacles might prevent you from meeting the core measures through evidence-based guidelines? How can we remove those obstacles together to allow the best patient care with the most efficient delivery and documentation of that care?"

Diminish vs Encourage

A common approach to leadership is: "Follow the rules! If something went wrong, somebody is to blame." But how does this approach make team members feel? In a word, diminished. Authoritarian systems claim they are hiring professionals for their creativity but then subject them to a system in which failure to follow the rules or achieve the desired outcomes is punished. As astronaut and physician James Bagian points out, accidents in aviation are approached differently than accidents in health care: "In health care, when something goes wrong, we ask, 'Who messed up?' In aviation accidents, we ask, 'What happened?'"[22] Even though outcome failure is most frequently process based, individuals in power-centered health-care organizations are often blamed.

Errors are inevitable. Blaming individuals is short sighted because only a small percentage of mistakes are the result of an individual's actions; finger-pointing seldom prevents them. In fact, experts who study human error have concluded that mistakes by individuals during operations account for only 15% of those that occur in complex systems. The other 85% arise from flawed processes.[23]

Rules, particularly those based on evidence, are important. However, it is up to people to put these rules into action in a fluid and changing environment. If team members are treated like fungible, interchangeable "FTEs" instead of professionals, they may adhere to the rules strictly, even when the situation requires a nuanced approach. Those who consistently feel diminished and fear humiliation will be afraid to speak up or modify "mandatory" processes even when appropriate.

Influence leaders recognize that, although evidence-based approaches can be "the rule" within a complex adaptive system, the role of individual team members' judgment and critical thinking skills must be allowed to adapt the rules to the circumstances. Members of these teams are encouraged to "break the rules on behalf of the patient," which means using one's common sense and judgement to do whatever is necessary to produce the best outcome. With this approach, patient outcomes will be optimized, and team members will feel encouraged, not diminished or devalued.

Outcomes of Power and Influence

Applying the lessons of power and influence leads to predictable behaviors and outcomes among team members who work in those respective environments.

Complain: If the primary management method is power, the most common outcomes are resistance, obstruction (often passive–aggressive), sabotage, second-guessing, asking for overrule, and/or push back from the shadows. As frustrating as these complaints may be, they should be expected. A few situations require a pure power approach, but they are rare. This approach should be avoided because it results in dissatisfaction.

Comply: When a blend of power and influence is used, the expected outcome is compliance, which may, at times, be grudging. When compliance is the general response, attitudes don't change, only behavior does. The reaction may be temporarily effective, but it is unlikely to be long-lasting or assimilated. Although the team members comply, they aren't necessarily convinced. Compliance won't guide the team members to the team purpose because they haven't been a part of developing the solutions presented. Compliance also can't tap into the team's innovation and creativity.

Commit: When influence is the dominant approach used, the results are predictable:

- Voluntary support
- Less required outside monitoring (more self-monitoring)
- Shared goals that are understood
- Higher sustained effort over time with greater self-motivation and less scrutiny
- Increased interpersonal interaction and commitment

THE PLACE FOR POWER, THE OPPORTUNITY FOR INFLUENCE

Despite all the limitations and unintended consequences of power, there are still circumstances in which the paradigm of power is situationally effective, efficient, and practical.

The most effective use of pure power occurs in situations that are time sensitive, require precision, and have a single answer. For example, when the security of ED team members is at risk, a focused, directive response is required to protect them. When these dangers occur, immediate, forceful action to remove the physical or psychological threat is essential. Crisis situations may also require staff to follow a specified authoritarian sequence, at least until the danger passes. (Some leaders may regard regulatory surveys and investigations [e.g., COBRA investigations or trauma site surveys] as crises, but these issues are best handled proactively so they don't escalate.)

Most other situations call for influence-driven ED leadership. Because it is difficult to change others, leaders can direct their considerable influence by using the "voice of the patient" to help team members develop their own intrinsic motivation. Leaders can describe the nature of the patient's problems, associated parameters, resources available, and the value of success, then invite the team to help devise collaborative solutions.

An Alternative Model

An alternative model integrates influence as the primary mental model for ED leadership but also injects power into the equation when needed. Generally, influence should be the consistent driver to educate, motivate, and inspire professionals who provide care in the complex adaptive system of the ED. With the exceptions listed above, influence is more effective than power. Team members should be recruited, or re-recruited, with a clear statement that a culture of influence, supported only when necessary by power, guides the ED.

However, there are times in the life span of a change effort when immediacy, quick results, and directive leadership may be needed, either to accelerate the pace of change or cement a consistent solution. Using power at the appropriate inflection points of the journey can be highly effective, particularly if it is fully articulated and used for a limited amount of time. Use the tactics of influence to convene and motivate the team, and reserve "power" for when compliance is essential to progress.

Influencers as Mentors

To be effective as an influencer, it is essential to be an effective mentor. Mentoring is an important part of talent development and is best used to influence others to "flow into" patterns of behavior that help the patient and the team. To influence effectively, leaders can adopt the efficient method of terse, staccato mentoring conversations:

- "You did well."
- "Here's how you did well."
- "How can we help others do well?"
- "How will you mentor others to do well?"
- "How can the leadership team support you in these efforts?"

Trust, Humility, and Commitment

> *We learned about gratitude and humility—that so many people had a hand in our success, from the teachers who inspired us to the janitors who kept our school clean... and we were taught to value everyone's contribution and treat everyone with respect.*
>
> Michelle Obama[24]

Unfortunately, some power-driven leaders focus on themselves, their needs, and the continuing reaffirmation of their expertise. This self-aggrandizing approach fails to recognize that the team must understand, contextualize, and believe in the vision in order to deliver inspired, best-practice patient care. Influence-driven leaders do not focus on themselves; instead, they humbly recognize that others are responsible for the department's success.

One of the most trusted and admired leaders in health care is Chuck Stokes, the president and CEO of the Memorial Hermann System in Houston and past president of the American College of Healthcare Executives. One of his insights is that the best leaders are people of profound humility. This deeply humble nature is a foundation on which other leadership characteristics, such as confidence, are built. As the theologian C.S. Lewis notes, "The truly humble man will not be thinking about humility: he will not be thinking of himself at all."[25] Or in the words of Harvey Mackay, businessman and best-selling author:

> *[Humility is becoming a lost art] in an era of self-promotion and making sure you get all the credit you deserve. Humility is not difficult to practice. It doesn't involve downplaying your achievements. It doesn't mean that you won't be recognized for your contributions. It does mean that you realize that others have been involved in your success and you are prepared to be involved in theirs. Anyone who thinks he or she is indispensable should stick their finger in a bowl of water and notice the hole it leaves when they pull it out.*[26]

Humble leaders can recognize and appreciate both their own and other team members' unique contributions. In his moving eulogy for President George Herbert Walker Bush, Senator Alan Simpson noted:

> *Those who travel the high road of humility are not bothered by heavy traffic.*[27]

Although analogies between military combat and the stressful circumstances of the ED must be carefully drawn (and with great respect for those who have defended their country in battle), the military has focused a great deal of attention on "unit cohesion" and the role that trust and leadership play in building that cohesion.[28] Glenn Gray, Paul Fussell, and Karl Marlantes have written eloquently on the fundamental reason soldiers, sailors, airmen, and Marines are willing to place their lives at risk: their dedication to their comrades and resolve to not let them down. As difficult as working in the ED can be, we certainly aren't being shot at; still, we must do our jobs while demonstrating dedication to our team and our patients.

Case History

The ED at Inova Fairfax Medical Campus is a regional level I trauma center that sees more than 120,000 patients annually. Hospital boarding is a daily reality for the doctors and nurses practicing there. In March 2016, patient experience scores as measured by Press Ganey fell below the 10th percentile (**Figure 4.2**).

Nursing and physician leadership jointly delivered a coordinated message, combining power and influence approaches. The power aspect consisted of delivering the message that the "C-suite" and Board of Directors were demanding the implementation of a plan to improve these low scores. But this message was tempered by one seeking to influence the staff by reiterating the idea that a positive patient experience could be attained by focusing on "A-team behaviors," including being proactive and communicating effectively.[32] Equally important was the message that, just as A-team behaviors and habits should be accentuated (through influence), negative B-team behaviors needed to be eliminated (a power message). The focus throughout the rollout was firm yet inclusive, seeking input from the team at each step of the process.

Leaders invested in the team by providing focused patient satisfaction coaching. This influence-driven approach showed that the time, energy, and effort of personalized

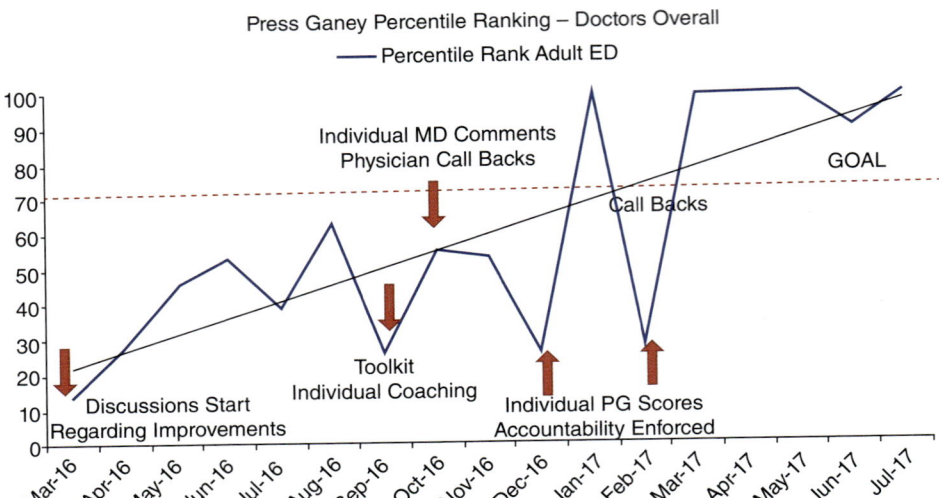

FIGURE 4.2 ■ Inova Fairfax Patient Experience Scores and Interventions

coaching could produce results. Other investments in the staff included individualized patient comments for the doctors and the introduction of a patient-callback system, which some staff initially resisted but later felt was helpful to their practice patterns. (Power was used to ensure compliance with the callback system. However, the widespread adoption of the program was influenced by "champions" who advocated for it by sharing how the program had helped them.)

After several reporting periods demonstrated score increases, a sharp decline occurred 9 to 10 months into the program. A natural response would have been to exert power to ensure compliance. Instead, the leadership team refocused on the role of influence by having individual team members explain how the program helped change their practice and job satisfaction. In addition, "shadow-shifting," in which A-team nurses and doctors observe and coach B-team staff during patient encounters, was initiated. This program became a symbol of the leadership's deep commitment to helping clinicians improve their scores. However, to be clear, "shadow-shifting" was framed as a *choice* with wording such as this:

> We have all agreed as a team that our definition of quality patient care includes service quality and patient experience. We've also committed our entire team to a culture of mutual accountability and coaching and mentoring each other in ways that work. (Examples of using influence.) But your scores continue at the bottom, so you have a choice. You can accept the resource of "shadow shifting," which has clearly worked for others. Or you can find ways of your own to improve. But, either way, improvement is essential, not just desired. It's your choice, but failure to improve is not an option.

Over a one-year period, patient experience scores increased by 600%, an improvement that was sustained for more than two years. Combining messages and techniques of power and influence was necessary for success. The program blended "delivering the results that matter" with a "culture of mutual accountability" and reinforced effective A-team tools. It is important to note that, as **Figure 4.2** shows, improvements are often followed by declines, resulting in a pattern that resembles ventricular tachycardia. But this pattern should be expected, and effective leadership teams should be well prepared to use a culture of influence punctuated by power to achieve sustainable results. Similar examples can be found when taking measures to improve hardwiring flow, patient safety, and clinical protocols.[33-35]

CONCLUSION

Power and influence are related yet different pathways by which common goals can be achieved. In situations that require immediate, specific, directive actions, power can be highly effective. However, in situations involving teams of highly educated professionals working interdependently in a complex, adaptive system (essentially *every* ED), influence should play a significant role in guiding leadership and management. Effective influence strategies generate intrinsic motivation, pride, and sustainable results. An innovative alternative model integrates influence as a primary guiding force and uses power at appropriate inflection points.

REFERENCES

1. Lebell S. *Epictetus: Art of Living. The Classic Manual on Virtue, Happiness, and Effectiveness.* New York, NY: Harper Collins; 1995.
2. Frankl V. *Man's Search for Meaning.* Cutchogue, NY: Buccaneer; 1992.
3. *Merriam-Webster's Collegiate Dictionary.* 11th ed, Versailles, Ky: Printing Quad Graphics; 2014.
4. Nietzsche, F. *The Portable Nietzsche.* New York, NY: Penguin Books; 1976.
5. Fisher R, Ury W, Patton B. *Getting to Yes: Negotiating Agreement without Giving In.* 3rd ed. New York, NY: Penguin Books; 2014.
6. Mayer T. *Developing Leadership and Communication Skills.* Dallas, Tex: American College of Emergency Physicians, Emergency Department Directors Academy; 2019.
7. Best practices. Available at: http://www.best-practices.com/. Accessed January 20, 2019.
8. Merton RK. The unintended consequences of purposive social action. *Am Sociol Rev.* 1936;1(6):894-904.
9. Teresa M, Amabile R. Toward new conceptualizations of intrinsic and extrinsic motivation in the workplace. *Hum Res Manag Rev.* 1993;3(3):185-201.
10. US Department of Defense. Joint Chiefs of Staff. Available at: http://www.jcs.mil/Portals/36/Documents/Doctrine/pubs/dictionary.pdf. Accessed January 20, 2019.
11. Mayer T. *Rewarding the Champions, Corralling the Stragglers.* Dallas, Tex: ACEP, Emergency Department Directors Academy; 2019.
12. Block P. *The Answer to How Is Yes: Acting on What Matters.* San Francisco, Calif: Berrett-Koehler; 2003.
13. Senge P. *The Fifth Discipline: The Art and Science of the Learning Organization.* New York, NY: Doubleday; 2006.
14. Peters T. *The Excellence Dividend: Meeting the Tech Tide with Work that Wows and Jobs That Last.* New York, NY: Viking/Penguin; 2018.
15. Covey S. *The 7 Habits of Highly Effective People.* Salt Lake City, UT: Franklin-Covey; 2004.
16. Block P. *Stewardship: Choosing Service Over Self-Interest.* San Francisco, Calif: Berrett-Koehler; 2014.
17. Mayer T. *The Discipline of Teams and Teamwork.* Chicago, IL: ACEP, EDDA 2; 2019.
18. Drucker P. *The Effective Executive.* New York, NY: Harper Collins; 2006.
19. Allen W. *The Complete Prose of Woody Allen.* New York, NY: Picador Press; 1998.
20. Mayer T. Learning to love the job you have while creating the job you love. The James Mill, Jr. Memorial Lecture. American College of Emergency Physicians Scientific Assembly.
21. MBI Concepts Corporation. On Thoughtful Mistakes. 2019. Available at: https://www.mbiconcepts.com/watson-sr-and-thoughtful-mistakes.html. Accessed January 2, 2020.
22. Bagian J. Interview. Available at: https://psnet.ahrq.gov/perspectives/perspective/211/In-Conversation-With--James-P-Bagian-MD-PE. Accessed June 20, 2019.
23. Weick KE, Sutcliffe KM. *Managing the Unexpected: Assuring High Performance in an Age of Complexity.* San Francisco, CA: Jossey-Bass; 2001.
24. Obama M. Transcript: Michelle Obama's Convention Speech. September 4, 2012. Available at: https://www.npr.org/2012/09/04/160578836/transcript-michelle-obamas-convention-speech. Accessed July 3, 2019.
25. Lewis CS. *Mere Christianity.* New York, NY: Harper One; 1952. Book 3, chap 8.
26. Mackay H. Business success tips: lessons they don't teach you in school. 2013. Available at: https://harveymackay.com/lessons-they-dont-teach-you-in-school/. Accessed January 2, 2019.
27. Simpson A. Eulogy for President George Herbert Walker Bush, delivered at the National Cathedral.
28. United States Marine Corps. Improving Unit Cohesion: The First Step in Improving Marine Corps Infantry Battalion Capability. 2018. Available at: http://www.2ndbn5thmar.com/coh/mcbreen2002.pdf. Accessed January 20, 2019.
29. Gray JG. *The Warriors: Reflections on Men in Battle.* New York, NY: Harcourt Brace; 1996.
30. Fussell P. *The Great War and Modern Memory.* Oxford, United Kingdom: Oxford University Press; 2000.
31. Marlantes K. *What It Is Like to Go To War.* New York, NY: Atlantic Monthly Press; 2011.
32. Mayer T, Cates R. *Leadership for Great Customer Service.* 2nd ed. Chicago, Ill: Health Administration Press; 2014.
33. Mayer T, Jensen K. *Hardwiring Flow.* Gulf Breeze, Fl: Fire Starter Press; 2012.
34. Mayer. Creating the risk-free emergency department. Available at: https://www.envisionphysicianservices.com/campaigns/breakthrough-series/presentation-materials/presentations/dr-kirk-jensen-high-leverage-patient-safety-strate.pdf. Accessed January 3, 2019.
35. Mayer T, Jensen K. *Innovative Strategies for Hardwiring Hospital-Wide Flow.* 2018. *Management in Healthcare.* 2(4):373-387.

CHAPTER 5

EMERGENCY DEPARTMENT INTERACTION WITH HOSPITAL GOVERNANCE

Thom A. Mayer, Robert W. Strauss, Anthony Nader, Rhonda Morgan, Tim Atteberry, Charles Stokes

The hospital is altogether the most complex human organization ever devised.

—Peter Drucker[1]

Health care is in the midst of cataclysmic change, making Peter Drucker's observation even more important than when it was made over 15 years ago. Hospitals and health-care systems are becoming larger and more complex enterprises, with many factors driving change:

- Consolidation of payers and providers is accelerating the need for meaningful economies of scale.
- Economic pressures mean revenue constraints and squeezed margins.
- An increased focus on the entire continuum of care, including hospital integration, physician integration, insurance/risk integration, and managing population health, requires operational change into new territory.
- The definition of quality has evolved from one more narrowly focused on safety to one encompassing all six of the Institute of Medicine's dimensions of quality, captured in the acronym STEEEP (safe, timely, effective, efficient, equitable, and patient centered).[2]

All of these factors exert pressure on board members, who must guide the organization's response to this demand for change. As such, the education of board members will continue to evolve as the health-care system adapts to meet the public's needs.

Governance refers to the structure by which hospitals or health-care systems respond to their stakeholders (or shareholders in for-profit systems). (A stakeholder is anyone who in any way is involved in or affected by an organization.) Health-care boards ultimately bear the responsibility for clinical quality, patient satisfaction, fiscal viability, patient safety, and strategic direction of the organization. To these is added the complex issue of population health, as boards become more and more responsible for care delivered far beyond the hospital's walls. There are over 7,500 health systems and hospital boards in the United States (including subsidiary and joint venture organizations), comprising over 120,000 board members.[5]

Hospital administrators are responsible for the day-to-day operations and strategic direction of their institution. The hospital governance structure is the entity to which the emergency department (ED) administrative leadership reports. Although the specific structure and terminology of boards vary, all health-care organizations have a well-defined process by which medical staff report their collective findings and recommendations to their parent board.

These well-defined processes include medical staff credentialing; quality improvement and patient safety activities; patient satisfaction; mission, vision, and strategy statements; and financial management. A careful reading of any medical organization's bylaws, rules,

> **BOX 5.1 ■ STRATEGIC RELATIONSHIPS FOR ED LEADERS**
>
> - Hospital board memberships
> - Board member relationships
> - Administration liaisons
> - Medical staff
> - Nursing staff
> - Patients

regulations, and administrative policies makes it clear that the ultimate source of governance is the health-care system's board of directors, trustees, or governors.

Despite these well-defined processes, quality is often a lesser priority for boards than financial reporting and oversight. Epstein and Jha reported that "quality performance was on the agenda at every board meeting in 63% of US hospitals, and financial performance was always on the agenda in 93% of hospitals."[4] However, Jha and Epstein found that boards that were engaged in quality and safety oversight had demonstrably better outcomes.

Hospitals vary widely in actual governance structures, depending on their status as not-for-profit versus for-profit and private versus public or academic. However, all health-care institutions share a common requirement to be responsive to their stakeholders through a formal process. The primary duties of the governing board are to set organizational strategies (into which performance and outcomes must be integrated) and recruit, hire, hold accountable, and evaluate the chief executive officer (CEO).

The governing board has oversight for overall organizational performance and is responsible for ensuring that the organization remains true to its mission, values, and goals; revising those principles when needed; and developing and executing a strategic plan.

In summary, the board oversees the accountability for quality and safety, organizational financial performance, and a shared responsibility for community and regional health care. The board ultimately warrants the quality of patient care provided by the organization and the value of the services provided to its customers. In most organizations, as already noted, the board is the entity responsible for ensuring the performance of (hiring, firing, and evaluating) the CEO of the organization. Finally, the board must be self-accountable in selecting competent board members; maintaining a succession plan; incorporating new thought leaders; providing continuing education and training for board members; and cultivating relationships that impact operations, quality, performance, and outcomes.

For ED leaders, six core strategic relationships address key concerns of the hospital board. These are listed in **Box 5.1**.

Nash and colleagues note:

> *Hospitals and healthcare systems continue to experience unprecedented demand for good governance — a demand that extends far beyond traditional notions of financial oversight.*[5]

Patient safety and quality of care are chief among those emerging demands, both of which require substantial board oversight. An understanding of the governance function of the board is a core foundation on which the successful long-term practice of emergency medicine and nursing should be built.

HOSPITAL BOARD COMPOSITION, PURPOSE, GOALS, AND OBJECTIVES

To begin to understand governance structures, it is necessary to ask the "why," "how," "who," and "what" of such organizations. The "why" must be asked, answered, and understood first. In the words of philosopher Friedrich Nietzsche, "He who has a strong enough 'Why' can bear almost any 'How.'"[6]

The "Why" of Hospital Governance

The "why" of governance can be answered from the perspective of the board itself, the health-care system, and the community. From the perspective of the community, it is necessary to have an organization capable of overseeing the extraordinarily large number of resources that any hospital requires to function. Even the smallest of hospitals is responsible for millions of dollars in operating budgets, is entrusted with the well-being of multiple patients on a daily basis, manages multiple teams of staff members—all while answering to the public they serve.

In both large and small communities, hospitals and health-care systems are among the largest employers. Even in most proprietary hospital settings, the board is structured to help ensure that local accountability is addressed.

High Quality, Low Cost

In the increasingly capacity-constrained environment of the health-care system, all institutions find themselves in pursuit of a common goal: to become the high-quality, low-cost provider of health care.[7] While high quality, low cost may seem an oxymoron, there is a constant challenge to raise quality while eliminating excess costs. "Doing more with less" was the mantra of yesterday. Today and tomorrow, health-care systems and providers must "do *better* with less." A great deal of attention will be placed on reducing waste and eliminating futile interventions and treatments to reduce cost and suffering. This approach requires a much broader range of skills than were required in the "cost-plus" system of the past, which resulted in insurers reimbursing unnecessary claims and perpetuated the fee-for-service model.

The current environment requires hospital administrations, medical staffs, and boards to exercise a broader range of skills to accomplish this "why." The principles of Lean management and Six Sigma, intended to add value while eliminating waste, are now widespread in health care.[8,9] Reducing wasteful spending is a path to improving clinical outcomes, not a tool to ration care. In his writing, Atul Gawande eloquently expresses the art of maximizing quality outcomes and patient satisfaction by doing better—not doing more. This concept was poignantly illustrated in Gawande's book, *Being Mortal*.[10] Indeed, the health-care industry is ripe for disruptive innovation and core changes to the system that will usher in a new model, a different market, a set of new values, and alternate methods of delivery. Boards must be equipped with pioneering leaders who possess the skill and mindset to craft workable, accessible, accountable, and affordable health care for the future.

Expanded Responsibilities

Traditionally, hospital boards have been a part of a three-legged table responsible for the operations of health-care institutions:

- *Hospital administration*: Responsible for the overall operations of the facility.
- *Medical staff*: Responsible for providing clinical services.
- *Hospital board*: Responsible for oversight of the medical staff and hospital administration.

Metaphorically, the weight of quality patient care (including all six STEEP elements) rests upon the strength and balance of this three-legged table. In many cases, boards focused on financial oversight and have served largely perfunctory roles in other areas. Community, regulatory, payor, and government oversight has dramatically changed board responsibility and participation in health-care governance. Board members must now assume a substantially greater level of participation and responsibility and, as a result, must

> **BOX 5.2 ■ SHORTELL'S CHARACTERISTICS OF EFFECTIVE BOARDS**
>
> - Manage and lead a diverse group of stakeholders.
> - Involve physicians in the management and governance process.
> - Meet the governance needs required of the changing health-care environment.
> - Embrace the challenges of change in a value-based purchasing environment.
> - Successfully translate strategy formulation and implementation as interdependent and interrelated processes.

have a broader and deeper skill base. Indeed, at least 13 states now require some form of board orientation, including either mandated or voluntary education programs.[11]

From the perspective of the board members themselves, directors generally serve for various reasons including community service (a desire to give something back to the community), professional stimulation, and the enjoyment of participating in the growth of an important local institution. The Greek word *koinonia*, which means a deep and abiding sense of community commitment, might best describe the primary reason that many board members serve.

The "How" of Hospital Governance

The "how" of hospital operating boards relates to their ability to effectively discharge their duties—the "what" listed earlier. Health-care management expert Stephen Shortell notes that effective boards share the characteristics listed in **Box 5.2**.[12] To accomplish these responsibilities, board members are increasingly assuming roles as risk takers, strategic directors, experts, mentors, and evaluators. As Abraham Lincoln noted in his 1862 message to Congress:

> *The dogmas of the quiet past are inadequate to the stormy present. The occasion is piled high with difficulty, and we must rise with the occasion. As our case is new, so we must think anew, and act anew. We must disenthrall ourselves, and then we shall save our country.*[13]

Although the ever-changing health-care environment poses significant challenges, doing things the "old way" will not serve hospital boards in their attempt to create a new and successful future. "Thinking anew" and "acting anew" will surely be necessary, both now and in the future.

The values of the board and administrators define the organizational culture and are essential to "how" hospital governance is achieved. Few things are more nebulous or weighty than an organization's culture. The board sets the culture of the organization. **Box 5.3** summarizes the primary indicators of organizational culture, as characterized by Edgar Schein, an expert on organizational development and culture.[14]

> **BOX 5.3 ■ SCHEIN'S PRIMARY MECHANISMS OF CULTURE**
>
> - What does the board pay attention to?
> - Is finance more important than quality?
> - What measures and benchmarks are used?
> - Does the board see the trees or the forest (ie, the "big picture")?
> - Is continued education valued/required?
> - Does attendance at board meetings matter?
> - How does the board react to critical incidences?
> - How are agendas developed?
> - How does the board allocate rewards and status?
> - How are new board members recruited and oriented?

The Institute for Healthcare Improvement has published resources for board governance arising from a landscape scan of current boards, a review of existing peer-reviewed literature, and expert meeting, comprising communication with health care and governance experts. These resources include the "Framework for Effective Board Governance of Health System Quality" and a "Governance of Quality Assessment Online Tool." Both documents present a perspective on the "how" of hospital governance.

The "Who" of Hospital Governance

The "who" describes the typical composition of a health-care board. In the past, boards often were composed of "pillars of the community," including local leaders and wealthy donors. Over time, potential new members of the board began to be nominated by organizations with substantial, and in some cases vested, interests in the operations of the institution.[15] For example, virtually all hospital boards include physician representation (often the president of the medical staff, members nominated by the county medical society, or, less commonly, members nominated from medical specialty groups). Similarly, community organizations, state and local governments, and citizens' groups have also played a larger role in the nominating process. As governance restructuring attempts to streamline boards by consolidating functions, membership is now more commonly based on qualifications tailored to the specific expertise needed by the board in its deliberations.

Several meaningful trends have emerged in board selection. First, boards generically are becoming smaller in size and fewer in number. Ackerman and Prybil in their study of health-care boards found that larger boards have[15-17]:

- Less accountability
- Less sense of ownership
- Less active discussion and engagement
- Less preparedness for meetings
- Less director satisfaction
- Less ability to react

Modern boards are highly likely to change their composition, with members selected for expertise in:

- Clinical care
- Safety
- Systems integration
- Population health
- Chronic illness care
- Social media
- Branding
- Cybersecurity

Boards are also trending toward diversity of race, gender, age, ethnicity, geography, and even social status. These selections should be driven by the need to reflect the strategic imperatives of the organization.[16]

Another imperative is board selection for risk oversight; specifically, there is growing concern for risks which damage or threaten the "brand" of the institution. Boards are also ultimately responsible for ensuring the system has a clearly delineated crisis management team with a detailed response plan, including risk mitigation. Very few health-care systems will escape the need to deal with crisis management.

In summary, selection of board members is increasingly based on a combination of factors, including diversity of membership, community involvement, trust and expertise in health care, commitment, required areas of expertise, and the ability to articulate the perspective of the organization and its stakeholders. Because of the increasing consolidation of governance structures (see the following discussion), participation on boards represents a substantial time investment, particularly when board meetings, committees, and subcommittees are considered. As a result, it is unusual for boards to retain token membership from a group or an individual who is not able to meaningfully participate on an ongoing basis to bring continuity and objectivity to the proceedings of the governance structure.

The "What" of Hospital Governance

In its simplest terms, the "what" of boards is the responsibility to oversee the operations of the entire health-care facility and the accountability for all of the assets that have been entrusted to that health-care organization. **Box 5.4** lists typical primary functions for which boards are responsible.

Over the past 20 years, evolving health-care reform has significantly impacted the "what" of hospital governance. Increased regulatory requirements have radically impacted reimbursements and the fiscal well-being of health-care organizations. The regulatory changes include the Centers for Medicare and Medicaid Services (CMS) process of care measures and the hospital star rating system, instituted in 2015.[18] Reimbursements from CMS and other payers are further affected by outcomes and performance metrics including, for EDs, timely and effective care measures (**Box 5.5**). In addition to those listed below for ED throughput, other care measures for specific medical diagnoses, such as heart attack and pneumonia, are greatly impacted by ED care and processes. Gone are the days when payers were passive payers of claims; they are now active purchasers of quality. The governing board must oversee processes that ensure that quality standards and benchmarks are met for the benefit of patients, the organization, and the community.

BOX 5.4 ■ PRIMARY BOARD FUNCTIONS

- Setting the strategic direction of the institution
- Formalizing strategic planning activities
- Selecting the CEO and evaluating her or his performance in a metrics-based fashion
- Evaluating financial performance
- Evaluating and setting priorities for capital expenditures
- Ensuring system operational performance
- Setting hospital policies
- Ensuring compliance with regulatory agencies
- Exploring philanthropic opportunities
- Meeting obligations to provide health care to the community
- Developing communication strategies to key stakeholder groups
- Delegating appropriate responsibilities to board subcommittees and management team members
- Evaluating quality improvement, patient satisfaction, patient safety, medical staff satisfaction, and employee satisfaction
- Recruiting new board members
- Developing, where appropriate, clinical research opportunities

> **BOX 5.5 ■ TIMELY AND EFFECTIVE CARE MEASURES**
>
> - ED patient volume
> - Median time from ED arrival to time of departure from the ED for admitted patients
> - Median time from admit decision to time of departure from the ED for patients admitted to inpatient status
> - Median time from ED arrival to ED departure for discharged patients
> - Door to diagnostic evaluation by a qualified medical professional
> - Median time to pain management for long bone fracture
> - Left without being seen
> - CT scan results delivered within 45 minutes for a patient with an acute ischemic or hemorrhagic stroke

It is the job of the board to ask the extraordinarily difficult questions, such as:

- How will scarce resources be deployed in an increasingly cost-constrained and competitive environment?
- How will relationships between hospitals and physicians be structured?
- Where should the organization place its emphasis in helping to devise a reasonable health-care structure that will serve the organization and the community, both now and in the future?

Board Structure and Fiduciary Responsibility

Governance structure encompasses multiple aspects of the board, including overall size, number, and types of committees, relationships to other boards in the system or in multistate hospital systems, rules for member recruitment, retention and rotation off the board, and mechanisms for evaluation. Operating boards have a fiduciary responsibility to wisely and judiciously use the assets of the community (nonprofits) or shareholders (for-profits) for the benefit of the organization's social mission.

This responsibility simultaneously requires board members to address the complex, rapidly changing, and capital-constrained environments in which they find themselves. A *fiduciary* is a person who has the legal duty, created by his or her undertaking, to act primarily for the benefit of others in related matters.[19] This fiduciary duty entails four obligations.

Duty of obedience: The duty of obedience means that the fiduciary person or board has an obligation to be compelled by legal norms to act in ways that support the stated vision, mission, and values articulated in the health-care system's formal statements. Just as the vision, mission, and values vary from organization to organization, so does the specific duty of obedience—but not the primacy of the duty itself. For example, when a board chooses to pursue a new product or service line, it is ultimately the board's responsibility to ensure that it is consistent with the health-care system's mission, vision, and values.

Duty of care: The duty of care ensures that the board (and its members) operates in good faith, exercises the care that a reasonable and prudent person would exercise in like circumstances, and acts in the best interests of the corporation. In exercising the duty of care, the board must consider patient safety and quality in every aspect of its decisions. Board members must diligently inquire about any potential problems that might arise.

Duty of loyalty: The duty of loyalty means that the board members owe their allegiance (in their deliberations and decision-making) to the hospital stakeholders rather than to personal interests or interests of other individuals or organizations. Balancing the desires of the medical staff with those of the hospital is an example of the duty of loyalty.[20]

Duty of disclosure: The duty of disclosure requires that board members inform fellow board members and management about any information known to the board member that is material to corporate decisions.

In addition, boards are covered by two important rules. The Business Judgement Rule protects a disinterested director (informed and on a good faith basis) from personal liability if a decision that the director approved proves to be a mistake. The Confidentiality Rule states that the board member must keep confidential all matters involving the organization that have not been publicly disclosed.

CHANGING NATURE OF BOARDS

Few areas in society are changing as rapidly as health care. As hospitals undergo innovation, regulatory change, financial constraints, political pressures, resource redistribution, and so on, their structures evolve in new, challenging, and exciting directions. Governance is also changing to meet the evolving needs of the organizations and the communities they serve. A recent governance benchmarking study identified several trends among the systems studied, including changes in the areas listed in **Box 5.6**.

The imprimatur of safety and quality is a major challenge for those charged with governance (**Box 5.7**). A hospital board would not be able to effectively govern without the financial data necessary to understand growth and operations. Similarly, the governing board must gather and understand meaningful data about safety and (medical) quality, areas typically outside of the scope of most new board members. Boards therefore need increasing education regarding the development and deployment of sophisticated measurements of complex, adaptive systems, which is precisely what even the smallest hospitals are.

To answer these and other difficult questions, many health-care systems are utilizing "balanced scorecards" to measure progress toward the stated mission, vision, and values (**Table 5.1**). The balanced-scorecard tool, introduced by Harvard Professors Robert Kaplan and David Norton in 1996, helps leaders stay the course and clarifies the resources necessary to achieve the desired vision of the organization.[21] Just as pilots depend on their aircraft instrument panel, the balanced scorecard provides leaders and board members with critical information about performance, results, and the internal and external environment. This strategic tool helps leaders set goals, allocate resources, set priorities, and evaluate progress.

BOX 5.6 ■ TRENDS IN BOARD GOVERNANCE

- Fewer governance layers
- Evolution of smaller boards with composition based on expertise and utility
- Redefined roles and priorities for greater clarity
- Greater use of councils, forums, and management assignments as integrating mechanisms
- Increased physician participation
- Consolidation of committees, clarification of charters
- Focus on strategy, strategic finance, and system oversight
- Increased emphasis on patient safety and quality of care

> **BOX 5.7 ■ BOARD QUALITY AND SAFETY QUESTIONS**
>
> - From a quality and safety perspective, how good is the care delivered in the institution?
> - Is the care provided getting better or worse? If so, by what measures?
> - How can the care provided be improved?
> - What resources will be needed to improve care?
> - In saying "yes" to one area of improvement in a resource-constrained environment, what other areas will need to be told "no"?

Just as the name implies, the scorecard balances critical strategic variables, sets a benchmark, and tracks progress.

Duke University Health System was an early proponent of the use of balanced scorecards.[22] A study of 35 hospitals in Michigan and Tennessee showed that scorecards are being used routinely to present a framework through which quality and safety can be measured and understood.[23] (The outcomes measured in this study were valid for identifying hazards rather than measuring processes in safety and quality themselves.)

TABLE 5.1 ■ Pillar Management (Balanced Scorecard) With Discrete Goals

Service	Quality	People	Finance	Growth	Community
IMPROVE:	**IMPROVE:**	**IMPROVE:**	**IMPROVE:**	**IMPROVE:**	**INCREASE:**
Patient satisfaction	Clinical outcomes	Employee satisfaction	Operating income	ED volume	Philanthropy
Physician satisfaction	Percentage of evidence-based care	Physician satisfaction	Collection	Revenue	
Throughput/ED access metrics		Staff turnover rate	Case mix	Throughput	
			Amount of cash on hand	Physician activity	
			Operating margin	New patient encounters	
				Retail/joint ventures	
REDUCE:	**REDUCE:**	**REDUCE:**	**REDUCE:**	**REDUCE:**	
Claims	Nosocomial infections	Turnovers	Cost per discharge	ED patients who left without treatment	
Legal expenses	Medically unnecessary days and delays	Vacancies	Accounts receivable days	Outpatients No-shows	
Malpractice expenses	30-day readmission rate	Agency costs	Advertising costs	Surgical volume/procedures	
Patient complaints	Medication errors	Overtime	Length of stay		
Post-anesthesia hold hours	Mortality rate	Physicals and cost to orient			
	Patient-harm events	Staff vacancies			
		Time to fill key positions			

> **BOX 5.8 ■ CHARACTERISTICS OF SUCCESSFUL BOARDS**
>
> - Leadership maintains an up-to-date medical staff development plan.
> - Major new clinical programs meet both the stated mission/vision statements and quality and safety performance criteria.
> - Patient satisfaction scores are reviewed (with comparative data) at least quarterly.
> - Physician satisfaction scores are reviewed (with comparative data) at least yearly.
> - A governance self-assessment for patient safety and quality is reviewed annually.
> - Metrics-based accountability for all clinical services is standard and applied across all boundaries.
> - Information technology challenges are an important part of the board's agenda.
> - Philanthropy is integrated into future planning for additional sites and/or clinical services.
> - Hospital-physician alignment is a core operating strategy.
> - Growth is strategically and tactically managed.

Another study of effective hospital governing boards indicated several general trends that are prevalent in most successful hospitals and health-care systems (**Box 5.8**).[24]

ED LEADERS AND GOVERNANCE

In the past, common wisdom held that a physician need only practice good medicine to be successful. Although it is questionable whether that statement was ever accurate, leadership and management skills are now essential to the successful practice of medicine and nursing, particularly in the ED. Principles such as quality improvement, patient safety, hardwiring flow into operations, risk reduction, change management, strategic planning, boundary management, and stakeholder analysis are all necessary components of the day-to-day landscape of emergency care. Because hospital trustees are increasingly fluent in these principles, it is necessary for ED leadership to understand and practice these principles on a day-to-day basis.

Health-care boards have historically relied on articulate, experienced physician leadership to help guide the direction of the organization. This trust is particularly true of those (ED) leaders who are capable of dispassionately discussing appropriate deployment of resources that best meet the needs of the institution and its patients. Unfortunately, some physician attitudes and behavior could be described as narrow-minded at best and self-serving at worst. Increasingly, those physicians have tended to be in the minority, and their fellow physicians have offered to the board a mature, balanced, and articulate perspective. Members of the governance structure look to the medical staff and its physician leadership for assistance in several ways (**Box 5.9**).

> **BOX 5.9 ■ ROLES OF PHYSICIAN LEADERS**
>
> - Visionary leadership
> - Medical expertise
> - Objective presentation of medical data
> - Organizational perspective
> - Consistency and constancy
> - Objective and disciplined debate of issues
> - The voice of the medical staff as customer
> - Administrative leadership

Visionary leadership: First, and most important, board members look to some physicians to become visionary leaders of the medical staff, particularly those who understand the need for change, can effectively communicate that vision to their fellow physicians, and are willing to play a substantial role in the development and implementation of change strategies.

Medical expertise: Second, leadership among physicians is essential because of their medical expertise. This competence is critical in areas such as physician credentialing, acquisition and the use of medical technology, clinical quality review, and medical ethics. For example, some institutions have chosen to delegate decisions on capital budget requests to medical staff committees. Members of those committees can help assess the relative need for certain technologies compared with others in the institution. Such an approach has the advantages of allowing substantial physician input, while establishing leadership on the part of the physicians, who will be tasked with saying "no" to their colleagues when those budget requests are not ranked highly enough.

Objective presentation of medical data: A third important requirement is the ability to present medical information objectively, simply, and concisely, and yet comprehensively enough for nonphysician board members to understand. For example, the physician members or representatives to the board may be asked to explain the proposed substantial capital outlay for the three-dimensional magnetic resonance imaging equipment for tumor localization in a hospital that has a substantial commitment as a cancer center. Similarly, it may be necessary to explain why substantial funding is essential for development of a cardiac short-stay unit with immediate access to cardiac stress testing in an institution with a deep commitment to comprehensive cardiac care. As another example, the board may query its medical members about evidence-based protocols for patient safety.

Organizational perspective: A fourth area needed from physician leaders is a sense of organizational perspective. While the physician's primary duty is always to the patient, clinicians must also respect the broader interests of the organization and those it serves. The increasing presence of accountable care organizations and population health management represents place substantial pressure on physicians to consider the interest of *his or her* practice versus that of the broader organization. Organizational perspective is necessary to ensure that whether in committees, at the executive level or at the board level, physicians keep the best interests of the institution in mind.

For example, in many states, the credentialing of podiatrists and advanced practice providers is a matter of statutory compliance. It is important that a physician who is a member of the credentials committee should respond objectively to the merits of qualified individuals applying in these categories regardless of the physician's personal preference or feelings about the role of such providers.

Consistency and constancy: Foremost among issues of consistency is regular attendance at appropriate functions, particularly for physician members of the board. The hours required of board members is increasing as the complexity of the work increases. Physicians must be responsible members and do the work required to prepare for board meetings. A "part-time" attitude is poorly perceived by other members of the committee who have taken the time and effort from their busy professional lives to ensure that they are available for the operations of the institution. No matter how busy the physician is, he or she must ensure that appropriate time is budgeted for assigned meetings.

As with all commitments, legitimate reasons for absences do arise, in which case physician members must extend the courtesy to the other members of the committee. The absentee physician should inform the group of the impending absence and make arrangements to obtain information on any issues to be addressed.

Objective and disciplined debate: It is important for physician members to debate issues vigorously, appropriately, and professionally. This must occur with objectivity and openness to legitimate expression of differences in perspective or opinion. Once the discussion is completed and an agreement is reached or decisions are made, all members of the group must be able to move forward as a team, while supporting the collective decisions that are reached. Physician leaders (as with all board members) should identify areas in which real or perceived conflicts of interest arise and, when appropriate, recuse themselves from either debate or vote on the issue.

Voice of the medical staff as customer: Another important role of physician leaders is described by the literature as representing the voice of the medical staff customer. As an internal customer of the health-care organization, the physician board member can offer an insightful perspective of this group of important internal customers. He or she can be particularly effective when dispassionately discussing the expectations of diverse physician members with differing points of view. The physician board members can also ensure that appropriate information flows back from the board to the physician medical staff members. This two-way communication ensures that medical staff members are aware of the reasons for board decisions, deployment of resources, assignment of capital, and other board actions.

Administrative leadership: Finally, with increased involvement, there is an expectation of higher levels of management skills among physicians. Hospitals have always relied on articulate and informed physician leadership to support the institution's goals and objectives. More recently, physicians with new talents, skills, and techniques have emerged, allowing them to participate more meaningfully in management decisions and interactions with the board. Increasingly, physicians occupy some of the top levels of institutional management. The use of many of the skills described in this book, including boundary management, negotiation techniques, strategic planning principles, continuous quality improvement, financial and outcomes management, contribute to physicians' understanding of hospital operations.

RELATIONSHIP OF EMERGENCY PHYSICIANS AND NURSES WITH THE BOARD

Without exception, the ED is widely recognized as the hospital's "front door." For many families, the ED is their *only* hospital experience from both a clinical and a branding standpoint. The ED leaders must therefore identify and respond to the needs of the community.

With ED leaders' development of appropriate skills and demonstrated commitment to the institutional vision, the board and hospital management will look to the ED leaders for their expertise beyond the clinical management of patients. Effective leaders with broad perspective are often encouraged to participate in the broader operational management of the organization.

Virtually all quality and high-performance medical institutions have the expectation and assumption that quality and safe medical care are provided. Emergency physicians and nurses who are not good practitioners will have a brief tenure in these organizations. In this regard, the board and management are looking for "Quality Plus," which means demonstration of expertise well beyond meeting the diverse clinical needs of the patients presenting to the ED.

Other expectations from the board include a substantial capacity for change and adaptation. The modern health-care system must be able to partner with its ED leaders to anticipate the direction, magnitude, and pace of change in a multitude of different areas.

Among the many skills required of the emergency physician group, one of the more important is *change management*. A strong corollary to this capacity for change is a deep level of commitment to the institution's clinical leaders. The board expects all contract providers, including emergency physicians, to have goals and objectives that are consonant with those of the overall organization. Although this statement is easy to make, its implications can be far-reaching and yet quite difficult to accomplish.

Metrics-Driven Outcomes

As an example of expectations that, in this era, go beyond quality care, the goals of many health-care institutions now include effective operations, demonstrated accountability, and a strong culture of metrics-based management. In such a culture, ED leadership must embrace the board's vision and successfully address the measure(s) chosen by the board. In contradistinction, resisting or, worse, arguing about the "statistical significance" of the measures is a clear path to failure.[25] The ability to deliver outcome progress across the selected metrics is critical to ongoing success.

Active and Effective Participation

The appropriate interaction between the board and the effective ED leadership team is always cooperative, collegial, and consonant with the objectives of the organization. It is extremely rare for hospital governance to want contract groups to be purely subservient or less than full, active, and respected members of the medical staff. Instead, the proactive modern health-care board looks to its emergency physicians for cooperation and guidance in achieving the organization's stated aims of caring appropriately for the institution's patients and actively participating in the dialogue about the organization's strategic direction.

Board Oversight and Involvement

Board members have a fiduciary duty to the community at large to administer the assets with which they have been entrusted in the most effective, efficient, and responsible manner possible. At times, this may create adverse economic tensions between the hospital or health-care system and individual physicians or groups. Simply stated, the board members' collective duty is to the community and institution it serves and not specifically to physicians' economic interests.

It is unusual for the board to participate actively in the renegotiation of contracts with physicians. However, boards increasingly ensure that contractual performance expectations with specific metrics appear in the contracts with hospital-based physician groups.

ADVICE FOR ED LEADERS

Several aspects of an institution's governance require careful attention and ED leadership.

Role of the Board

First, ED leaders should understand the intended role of their institution's board. Both written descriptions of the role of the board and (usually) the overall strategic plan for the institution are generally available. Familiarity with how the board operates, its composition, and the strategic plan for the institution are all important to the successful practice of emergency medicine and nursing.

Interaction With the Board and Administration

Second, it is important to gain an understanding of how physician leaders can interact with the board and administration to enhance the mission of the organization, accomplish its stated purposes, and participate meaningfully in the organization's endeavors. Participation by members of the ED group in the hospital medical staff committee structure is to demonstrate that all members of the group are committed to the institution.

Familiarity With Board Members

Third, the leadership of the medical staff and the ED should get to know the members of the board. Meetings should be scheduled to accommodate the board member's agenda, and the board members will appreciate having an advanced understanding of the substance of the meeting. Most board members genuinely appreciate the opportunity to express their opinion about how the ED group can best fit the needs and the strategic initiatives of the hospital. Such meetings are an excellent opportunity for leaders of the ED to communicate to board members. These meetings allow the emergency physicians to share the group's commitment to quality patient care and caring, as well as the philosophy of the "safety net" that the department offers to the community at large.

However, it is important that the ED leaders, when meeting with board members, avoid administrative "end-runs." While it is appropriate to discuss organizational strategic initiatives, it is inappropriate to advocate for operational changes and pet projects more related to the administrator's scope of responsibility. It is ineffective and poorly perceived when physician leaders use their relationship with board members to help lobby either for personal financial gain or for development of the physician's "pet projects." Although educating the board to the unique perspective of emergency medicine is appropriate, caution should be undertaken whenever personal, professional, and financial objectives begin to become interwoven into the dialogue. It is necessary to immediately acknowledge clearly and openly when any potential conflict of interest develops.

Board member rounding is an increasingly common practice in health-care facilities. This experience is scheduled and performed with a member of the administrative team. It provides a valuable opportunity for emergency physicians and nurses to get to know board members and for the board members to be visible and to see the health care "work in action." Physician and nurse leaders should round with board members together and carefully choose the time to stress the issues facing the ED. For example, rounding on Saturday night is more likely to demonstrate the difficult issues facing the ED than Tuesday morning.

It is also important to use interactions with members of the board to determine how ED operations can fit into the overall strategic objectives of the institution. The board has a unique perspective on the institution's resources, commitments, and its vision for the future. Interaction with the board and its members can provide invaluable information that can guide the ED team in its endeavors.

Concierge Emergency Medicine

Many primary care physicians have developed "concierge" practices, limiting their panel of patients to a limited number who pay a premium for these services. Of course, this is not an option for emergency medicine. However, emergency physicians should practice "concierge emergency medicine" by giving a card with their home and cell phone number to board members and VIPs, encouraging them to call whenever they need emergency care. Simply calling ahead to the ED or, when possible, meeting them there is a very powerful symbol of the department's commitment to the board. It is also a powerful symbol that the ED operates around the clock and that its leaders share the same commitment to all patients.

CONCLUSION

During meetings with members of the board, it is imperative to establish a relationship of trust, cooperation, communication, and integrity. This positive relationship can be developed by demonstrating an unwavering commitment to the institution and its strategic objectives. Physicians communicating with the board must demonstrate commitment to the strategies of the institution rather than a short-term desire to accomplish more narrow and personal objectives. Speaking with the "voice of the patients" and telling their stories is always the most effective way to communicate with board members.

Finally, when speaking with the board and administration, it is important for emergency physicians to clearly describe the emergency physicians' commitment to the organization and the willingness of the team to adapt, change, and facilitate the transition from the current to the future state of health-care delivery. This capacity to work as team members within the framework of a broader, more overarching goal occurs daily in the clinical delivery of care in the ED. Applying this principle to interactions with the board is a natural step toward the growth and development of the ED as a critical aspect of the institution's future.

Interactions with members of the board can be extraordinarily enriching to a physician, both personally and professionally. Board members' backgrounds represent a diverse and rich resource for any physician who takes the time and effort to engage them in constructive dialogue. The perspective they bring to an understanding of health care's role in the community is truly invaluable and is certainly worth the investment of time, energy, and effort to help ensure development of a strong and positive relationship between the ED and the board.

REFERENCES

1. Drucker, P. *Managing in the Next Society*. New York, NY: St. Martin's Press; 2002:119.
2. Tyler, LJ. Governance and Organizational Structure. American College of Healthcare Executives Board of Governors Examination. Available at: http://www.ache.org/mbership/BOGEXAMOT_V3/slides/1-Governance-and-Organizational-Structure.pdf. Accessed October 25, 2018.
3. Callender AN, Hastings DA, Hemsley MC, Morris L, Peregrine MW. *Corporate Responsibility and Health Care Quality: A Resource for Health Care Boards of Directors*. Washington, DC: US Department of Health and Human Services, Office of the Inspector General; 2007.
4. Nash DB, Murphy SP, Mullaney AD. Governance: current trends in board education, competencies, and qualifications. *Am J Med Qual*. 2011;26(4):278-283.
5. Jha AK, Epstein AM. Hospital governance and the quality of care. *Health Aff (Millwood)*. 2010;29:182-187.
6. Nietzsche F. *Basic Writings of Nietzsche*. Translated by W. Kaufmann. New York, NY: Modern Library; 2000.
7. Mayer T. Leadership for great customer service: getting the "why" right before mastering the "how." *Healthc Exec*. 2010;25(3):66-68.
8. Mayer T, Jensen K. Flow and return on investment in healthcare. *Intl J Six-Sigma Competitive Advantage*. 2008;4(3):192-195.
9. Mayer T, Jensen K. *Hardwiring Flow: Systems and Processes for Seamless Patient Care*. Gulf Breeze, Fla: Fire Starter Press; 2009.
10. Gawande, A. *Being Mortal*. New York, NY: Metropolitan Books; 2014.
11. The Governance Institute. *Governance Structure and Practices: Results, analysis, and evaluation. 2009 Biennial Survey of Hospitals and Healthcare Systems*. San Diego, Calif: The Governance Institute; 2009.
12. Shortell SM. New directions in hospital governance. *Hosp Health Serv Adm*. 1989;34(1):7-23.
13. Lincoln A. 1862 address to Congress.
14. Schein, EH. *Organizational Culture and Leadership*. 5th ed. Hoboken, NJ: John Wiley and Sons; 2017.
15. Prybil LD, Peterson R, Breszinski P, et al. Board oversight of patient care quality in community health systems. *Am J Med Qual*. 2010;25(1):34-41.
16. Ackerman FK, Prybil LD. *The Future of Healthcare Governance: Meeting Board Challenges in Unforgiving Times*. Chicago, Ill: ACHE Congress; 2017.
17. Ackerman FK. The Future of Governance: Healthcare Boards with Challenging Times. *Prescriptions for Excellence in Health Care*. Summer 2013; 20:11.
18. Timely and Effective Care Measures. Medicare.gov. Available at: https://www.medicare.gov/HospitalCompare/data/Data-Updated.html#MG3. Updated July 25, 2018. Accessed October 25, 2018.

19. Murphy S, Peregrine M. Corporate governance: A practical approach to governance for hospital and health systems boards. In: Gosfield AG, ed. *Health Law Handbook*. Eagan, Minn: Thompson Wentworth; 2008:225-253.

20. Goeschel CA, Wachter RM, Provonost PJ. Responsibility for quality and patient safety: hospital board and medical leadership. *Chest*. 2010;138(1):171-178.

21. Kaplan, RS, Norton, DP. *The Balanced Scorecard: Translating Strategy into Action*. Boston, Mass: Harvard Business School Press; 1996.

22. Silow-Carroll SS. Duke University Hospital: Organizational and tactical strategies to enhance patient satisfaction. The Commonwealth Fund. 2008; 5(1206). Available at: http://www.commonwealthfund.org/usr_doc/Silow-Carroll_Duke_case_study_1206.pdf?section=4039. Accessed May 29, 2012.

23. Goeschel CA, Berenholtz RA, Culbertson RA, Pronovost PJ. Board quality scorecards: measuring improvement. *Am J Med Qual*. 2011;26(4):254-260.

24. Valentine ST, Masters GM. *For Board Members Only: 10 Trends That Will Define Healthcare in 2012*. San Diego, Calif: The Governance Institute; 2012.

25. Mayer T. *Leadership and Motivation*. Presented at the American College of Emergency Physicians Emergency Department Director's Academy, Dallas, Tex, November 13, 2018.

CHAPTER 6

MANAGING PROFESSIONALS IN ORGANIZATIONS: THE ROLE OF PHYSICIAN AND NURSE LEADERS

Thom A. Mayer, Robert W. Strauss, Theresa Tavernero, Jay Kaplan

American health care is in the midst of dramatic and sustained change, which necessitates leading and managing across the inherent boundaries within the emergency department (ED). Success requires becoming high-quality, low-cost providers, which requires increased alignment, cooperation, and coordination among physicians, nurses, and health-care organizations.[1] Successfully integrated health-care systems establish highly metrics-driven approaches to management, respond proactively to regulatory and technological demands, adopt evidence-based medicine practices, and, increasingly, address the mandate to "do more with less."

DEFINING OUTCOMES

One characteristic of successful health-care organizations is consistent collaboration among nursing, physician, and administrative leaders in the development of strategies and systems that promote high-quality health care at the lowest possible cost, while making their teams' jobs easier. Quality is more than measurably superior clinical care. Excellence in health care also includes customer service, operational efficiency, hardwiring flow, and patient safety.

Because outcomes depend on clear goals, metrics, and knowledge, traditional boundary management will not suffice. Rather, physician and nursing leadership and management skills are requisite, not merely recommended, for success in health care. This approach is particularly necessary in the ED, where multiple stakeholders are the rule and not the exception.

The core principle of collaboration involves *aligning strategic incentives*, so that all stakeholders and team members develop a common understanding that is articulated clearly and can be demonstrated through tangible actions and behaviors.

The Fundamental Questions

Aligning strategies requires asking and answering the fundamental questions:

- What does success look like in our organization?
- How will that success be measured and when?
- What will we do if we fall short?
- How will we sustain gains when they occur?

Once these questions are asked and the team adopts the answers, Nietzsche's wisdom is helpful in answering "How will we commit to the strategy?"

He who has a strong enough "Why" can tolerate almost any "How."[2]

FIGURE 6.1 ■ The Balanced Scorecard Approach to Health Care Metrics

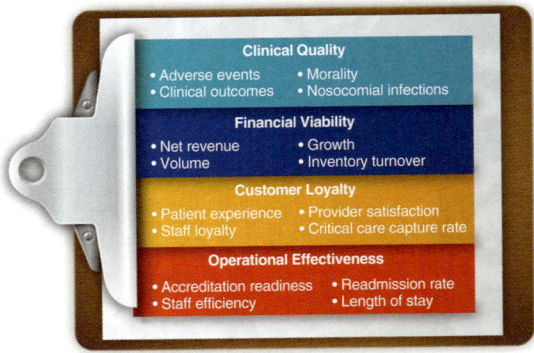

A Direct Relationship to Mission/Vision and Values

Aligned strategic incentives should tie directly to the organization's mission/vision and values (M/V/V). In other words, an ED team that has a clear sense of M/V/V can meet almost any challenge or barrier and develop strategies or tactics needed to overcome them.

Leaders must articulate the department's strategic goals and incentives clearly and consistently in a manner that makes sense to the staff and other stakeholders. Goals must be simple, measurable, achievable, realistic, and time targeted (SMART).[3] Strategic incentives should be consistently conveyed and reinforced using multiple vehicles of communication, such as staff meetings, daily team huddles, e-mails, and memos as well as 1:1 communication as leaders round with staff.

Most organizations now use some form of "balanced scorecard" or "pillar management" system to delineate what the strategic goals are and how they tie to the purpose of the organization (**Figures 6.1** and **6.2**).[4] These goals should be incorporated and hardwired into

FIGURE 6.2 ■ Pillar Reporting Scructures

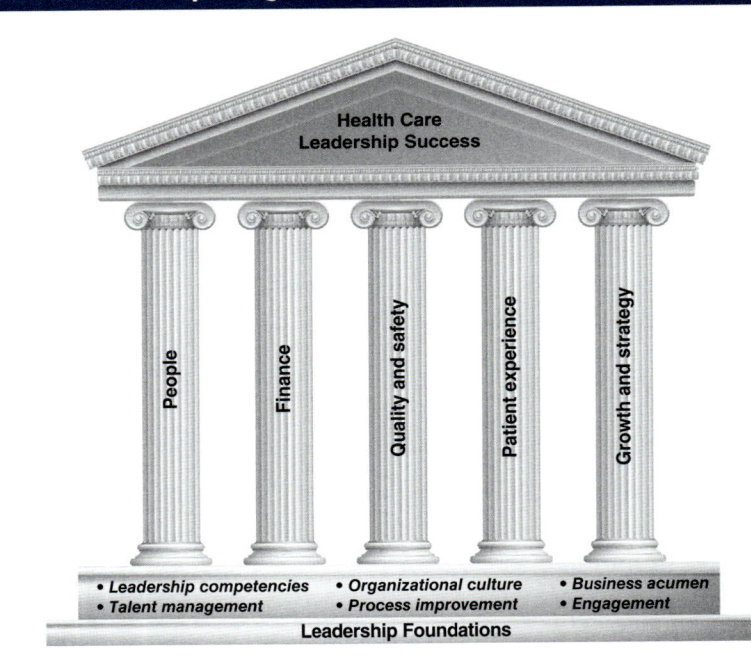

Pillar management reporting structures measure progress across the pillars of *people, finance, quality and safety, patient experience,* and *growth and strategy.* Many not-for-profit hospitals also include *community.*

daily practice and publicly posted so that every single member of the team can be clear about how they contribute.

PHYSICIAN–NURSE TEAMWORK: DYAD LEADERSHIP

To accomplish the organization's and the department's strategic goals as an integrated team, the team must be led by collaborative leaders. In particular, ED leadership is by nature and necessity a "team sport." One of the most significant improvements has been the development of physician and nurse leader teams or "dyads" working as a team. This change has been critical to effectively and collaboratively serving our patients and the professionals who serve these patients. A competent coordinated team is best positioned to create a patient-centric, aligned, and efficient approach (see Chapter 20: ED Physician/Nurse Director Relationship).

Dyad leadership is a partnership in which the respective skills, abilities, and training of the leaders combine to benefit each other, the ED team, and the patients and families they collectively serve.[5]

Origins/Adoption

The dyad concept has its origins in the sociology literature and typically refers to two persons involved in an ongoing relationship focused on a common set of mission, vision, and values. The Mayo Clinic was among the first health-care organizations to develop a model based on the following principles[6]:

- Common core values
- Willingness to work across boundaries toward a common mission and vision
- Clear and transparent communication focused on the needs of the patient
- Mutual respect, embodied in daily action
- Complementary competencies

There is a rich heritage of excellence in leadership and management across medicine and nursing boundaries, including centers such as Duke University Medical Center,[7] Mayo Clinic,[8] Cleveland Clinic, Virginia Mason Medical Center, Kaiser Permanente,[9] and others. The best of these programs have close, collaborative, and collegial partnerships between their physician and nurse leaderships. However, the pace of change and the push for integration in health care have accelerated rapidly and require leaders to simultaneously address physician and nurse shortages as well as a more culturally and generationally diverse workforce. These transformations will continue to drive the need for the presence of excellent physician and nursing leaders armed with new 21st century competencies in all organizations.

Advantages of Dyad Relationship

Traditional physician–nurse leadership models do not achieve their full potential because, while working together, each leader often has different goals, measurements of success, reporting structures, and approaches. Alternatively, dyad models have *joint goals and accountability with a clear division of responsibility*. The dyad model differs from traditional physician-nursing models in the very language used in trying to solve problems (**Table 6.1** and **Figure 6.3**).

The question arises, "How, specifically, does the division of labor occur in such a model?" In fact, shared collaborative responsibility focuses on leveraging strengths without worrying about who has the authority. So, in answer to . . .

TABLE 6.1 ■ Traditional versus Dyad Model

Traditional Model Language	Dyad Model Language
That's not a doctor problem, it's a nurse problem.	It's *our* problem!
Ask the charge nurse.	Time to get a clinical huddle to solve this.
The nurse (our) scores are fine.	It's a problem for the team, let's work together.
We're working two nurses short.	We're down two, but we're not out. Let's change our current process and fix it.

Who is in charge in this model?

. . . collaborative physician and nurse leaders will say, "*We* are!" In a joint accountability model, if a problem is brought to either of the leaders, that leader will accept the challenge of addressing the issue and ensure that his/her dyad teammate is aware and shares in the development and implementation of an effective solution.

Effectively structured and executed, dyad leadership allows a unique perspective that combines the respective strengths of the diverse training and background of medical and nursing leadership. Most important, it recognizes that all EDs are by their very nature *complex adaptive systems*.[1] Such a systems approach is at the heart of dyad leadership, a model that is based on ensuring psychological safety across complex boundaries.[1]

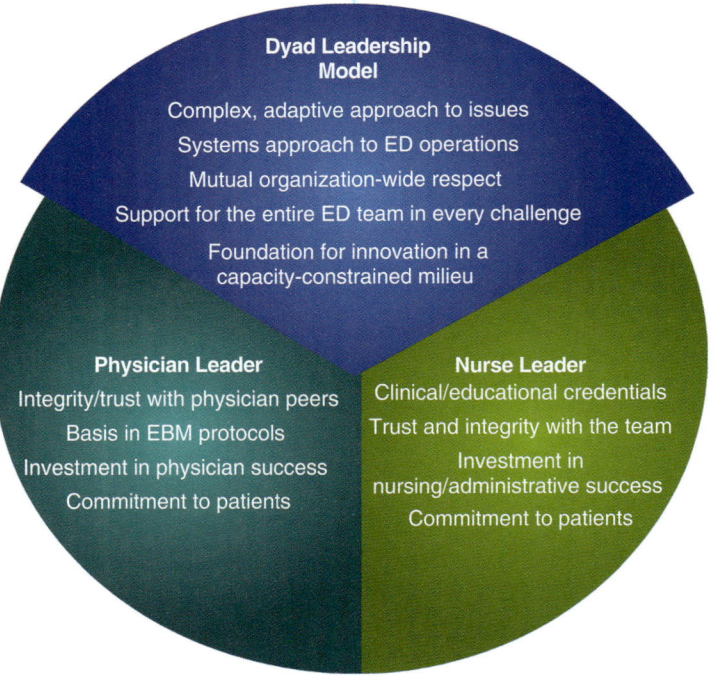

FIGURE 6.3 ■ Advantages of the Dyad Leadership Model

Effective team leadership in a dyad model has some additional characteristics when applied to the ED, including:

- Alignment of strategic incentives
- "No Blame-Game Zone" characterized by mutual support
- Members working to the "top of their licenses"
- Joint accountability for mutually developed metrics
- Eliminating rather than perpetuating functional silos
- Joint recruitment of team members
- Joint celebration of wins
- Jointly developed, specific plans for improvement
- "Boundaryless" EDs[10]

If the relationship between the physician and nurse administrative ED leaders is characterized by these elements, it functions as a dyad. Robert Greenleaf's model of servant leadership serves the dyad leadership model well, particularly his emphasis on the necessity of being "servant first, then leader." The quality of having "a scientist's mind, but a servant's heart" should inform dyad leaders in all their work.[11] The physician/nurse leader pair is critical to the success of any service and organization, especially the ED.

TRAINING DIFFERENCES AMONG DOCTORS AND NURSES

Traditional Approaches

Emergency physicians and nurses have traditionally been trained in distinct and seemingly disparate fashions. Critical thinking, an essential skill possessed by virtually every successful leader, is widely taught in nursing schools and has long been ingrained in the culture of nursing education (**Table 6.2**).[12,13] Unfortunately, this vital problem-solving approach is seldom taught in medical schools and residency programs, where physicians have historically been trained to function as independent, autonomous

TABLE 6.2 ■ Critical Thinking in Emergency Nursing

Skill	Example in Action
Analyzing	Discovering functional relationships
Applying standards	Judging by evidence-based standards
Discriminating	Differences and similarities
Information seeking	Searching for evidence
Logical reasoning	Drawing conclusions from evidence
Predicting	Envisioning a plan and results
Transforming knowledge	Putting the plan to work

TABLE 6.3 ■ Differences in Physician and Nurse Training/Education	
MD	**RN**
Autonomous	Interdependent
Authoritarian	Collaborative
Hierarchical	Team focused
Intense, focused time	Expanded time
Outcomes-driven	Interactive service
Technical expertise	Critical thinking skills
Linear perspective	Circular perspective

decision makers. To bridge this divide (**Table 6.3**), physicians must also understand the basis and theory of critical thinking and its important role in effective department leadership.[14,15]

Today's Multidisciplinary Approach

Working in the complex environment of multidisciplinary teams is now an essential feature for *all* physicians and nurses, not just leaders and managers. In general, this transition has been easier for nurses, as they have always taken an interdisciplinary approach to the care given to their patients.

Specific training in leadership and management skills is essential to effectively address the current health-care environment. The accelerating pace of change now requires a consistent and reliable approach to patient care, a highly metrics-driven focus, and evidence-based leadership.

Even the simplest ED patient interactions require training and development of *all* emergency physicians and nurses in some leadership and management skills—not just those with leadership and management titles. The most effective EDs have adopted a dyad leadership model on every clinical shift. Beyond providing basic medical and operational knowledge as part of the training, more efforts and emphasis are needed on the application, practice, and coaching of leaders (dyads). Simply stated, no ED can function successfully unless it is effectively led by the physician–nurse team guiding it on a day-to-day, hour-to-hour basis.[16]

DIFFERENCES BETWEEN CLINICIANS AND LEADERS-MANAGERS

There is a clear understanding of the importance of leadership among clinicians in the senior administrative ranks and dyad models. As an example, most hospitals and health-care systems have multiple layers of administrative management, including a chief medical officer (CMO) and a chief nursing officer (CNO) roles. This recognition has led to the advent of combined MD/MBA, RN/MBA, and executive MBA and/or MHA programs.

A large body of literature indicates that divisional/departmental physician and nurse leaders have an even larger need for leadership education when compared to other health-care administrators. Emergency department physicians and nurses have received substantial clinical education and skills training; in most cases, they have had little in the way of formal leadership and management training.[17] While physicians and nurses are educated to provide high-quality clinical care to patients, very few have been educated to manage or lead the processes and teams that deliver that care. Even fewer understand how to develop, assess, and improve plans to address human and programmatic barriers to effective care.

Most current physician and nurse leaders rose to management positions because they were so good at their craft that someone said to them, "You are really good at what you do, why don't you become the director of the department?" Without other training, these leaders often find themselves underprepared for the challenges in creating the vision and building an engaged and high-performing team to deliver coordinated care. The recognition of inadequate training is leading to enhanced leadership and collaboration training, as increasingly organizations invest not only in leadership training but also training in dyad models themselves.

The Skills Required of Leaders

Physician and nurse leaders require skills in team building, collaborative decision-making, development of evidence-based approaches to clinical care, analytics, performance coaching, strategic planning, negotiation skills, and development and implementation of service excellence programs. Lemire identified 5 key leadership skills for nurse and physician leaders which are necessary to influence organizational success, including being a(n) visionary, expert achiever, communicator, mentor, and critical thinker.[18]

Implied in these skills is the leader's understanding and application of emotional intelligence, which is defined as an awareness and regulation of one's self and others that can enhance and positively impact the outcome of interactions and relationships.

What are the differences between clinicians and leader-managers? Kurtz used behavior-oriented assessments to help delineate the differences between clinicians and managers, which are listed in **Table 6.4**.[19,20] In their clinical roles, physicians and nurses have been

TABLE 6.4 ■ Differences Between Clinicians and Managers

Clinicians	Managers
Doers	Planners, designers
One-on-one interactions	One-to-many interactions
Reactive personalities	Proactive personalities
Require immediate gratification	Accept delayed gratification
Deciders	Delegators
Value autonomy	Value collaboration
Independent	Participative
Patient advocate	Organization advocate
Identify with profession	Identify with organization

trained as doers, inasmuch as they prefer and are drawn to hands-on involvement in patient care. However, in making the transition to leaders, clinicians must become planners and designers of the clinical services and their interface with the health-care organization. They must also learn to be influencers and coaches developing comfort with working in the "gray areas," holding people accountable for set expectations and being a conduit between administration and staff while advocating for the team and patients.

By nature of their training and philosophy, clinicians are used to one-on-one interactions with their patients and largely judge their success by the outcomes of those interactions. On the contrary, to be successful, leadership and management require numerous interactions with multiple providers and stakeholders, often in diverse and disparate settings. Kurtz found that clinicians tended to be more detached, independent, and self-sufficient and were not "joiners" to the extent that leaders and managers are required to be.

Reactivity versus Proactivity

Provision of clinical services is fundamentally a reactive process, since the clinician waits for the patient or family to request medical care and then responds to the specific needs. The leader is proactive and anticipates the needs. The leader must plan both for the expected and the unexpected. As an example of a clinical rather than leadership perspective, when an ED physician or nurse is asked "Is ED flow predictable?" the clinician's response is predictable, though surprising. "No, we never know what's coming through the door!"

The fact is that the flow, arrival, acuity, and even the clinical presentations of ED patients are highly predictable. **Figure 6.4** shows the classic sinusoidal curve seen in all EDs, with lower patient volumes seen past midnight into the morning hours, followed by a predictable rise through the midmorning to a peak in the afternoon and evening hours. And ask any ED clinician what the busiest day of the week is and they will all answer, "Monday, of course."

Leaders and the most experienced clinicians understand that ED patient flow is in fact highly predictable and take a more proactive approach. They have learned that ED life should not be surprise to us if we are proactive, not reactive. Emergency medicine residents, fellows, and nursing students should be taught the results of predictive data analysis, which

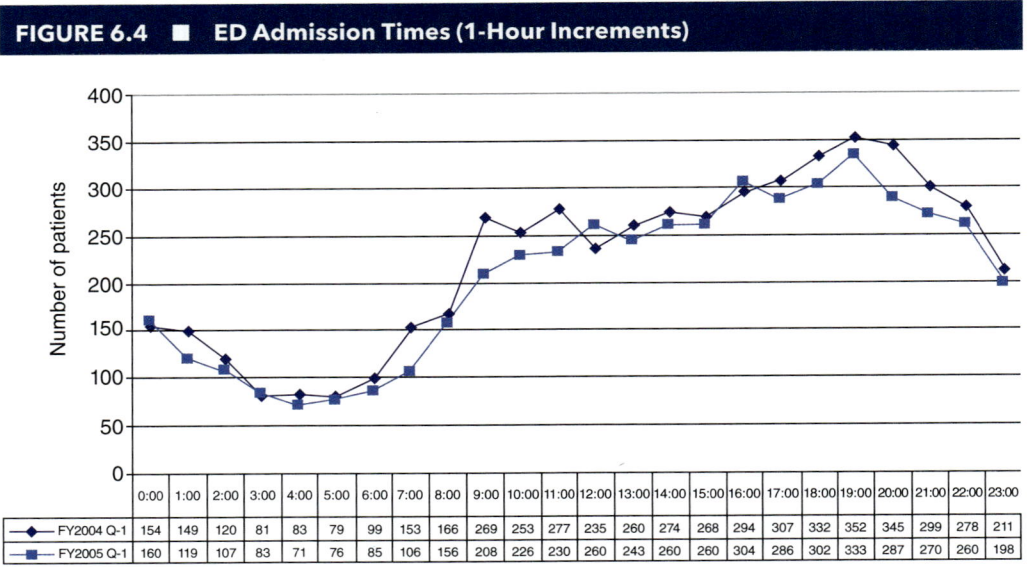

FIGURE 6.4 ■ ED Admission Times (1-Hour Increments)

	0:00	1:00	2:00	3:00	4:00	5:00	6:00	7:00	8:00	9:00	10:00	11:00	12:00	13:00	14:00	15:00	16:00	17:00	18:00	19:00	20:00	21:00	22:00	23:00
FY2004 Q-1	154	149	120	81	83	79	99	153	166	269	253	277	235	260	274	268	294	307	332	352	345	299	278	211
FY2005 Q-1	160	119	107	83	71	76	85	106	156	208	226	230	260	243	260	260	304	286	302	333	287	270	260	198

[Trend-Star Data: Q-1 FY04 & 05]

allows them to predetermine the numbers and types of patients that are likely to arrive. In essence, they can say, "We knew you were coming—we just didn't know your name!"[21]

A noted and somewhat striking difference between ED clinicians and leaders is that clinicians have a greater desire for immediate gratification (or satisfaction) of their professional, psychological, and personal needs. Indeed, this is often why nurses and doctors are drawn to the specialty. In contradistinction, leadership and management require the ability to delay gratification for weeks, months, sometimes even years to see the results of their planning. The clinical strategy for caring for trauma or chest pain patients is clear, immediate, and produces results rapidly; it's a sprint. However, pursuing a strategy of developing an effective protocol, team approach, interdisciplinary management, and effective transitions of the trauma or chest pain patient is a much slower process that requires stamina and patience. However, the result of effective programmatic change has long-term positive effects on all patients, not just one.

Developing a Culture of Collaboration

Changing the culture of a department might take even longer. Consider changing the thinking of the staff from "we're here to care for the sickest patients" to "we're here for anyone who walks through our doors." Changing systems is easier than changing people or culture, but the success of any systems' change depends upon the engagement and buy-in of the people who drive it. It is important to note that the leaders set the tone of the department and help shape culture. The physician and nurse leader, individually and as a leadership team, must model what is expected and desired of the entire staff.

Some physicians are drawn to their specialty because of a perception of autonomy. Physicians have traditionally been viewed as the primary person responsible for directing patient care. The term "doctor's orders" alone speaks to this concept. However, in the ED, physicians and nurses have always worked as a team, seamlessly coordinating their care for the good of the patient. Thus, collaboration, while a trait required of leaders and managers, is essential to every clinician in the ED. Indeed, it is wise to note:

> *The #1 way to assess the health of an emergency department is the working relationship of the doctors and nurses!*[22]

Physician and nursing leaders play a pivotal role in creating an environment that promotes job satisfaction, which in turn is highly correlated with patient satisfaction and quality outcomes.

Kurtz also noted that clinicians often view themselves as independent patient advocates who identify with their profession. Leaders and managers are seen as integrated into a team with the broader needs of multiple and diverse patients as their primary advocacy and therefore identify with the organization. This has been referred to as "The Problem of the Apostrophe" (**Table 6.5**). Clinicians typically say they are responsible for "my patient's needs," while leaders are charged with the responsibility for "our patients' needs," as well as those who care for them. It is telling how moving the apostrophe one letter can dramatically change the nature of the interaction.

TABLE 6.5 ■ The Problem of the Apostrophe[a]	
Physician/Nurse Clinician	**Physician/Nurse Leader**
"My job is to meet my patient's needs."	"Our job is to meet our patients' needs."

[a] Individual physicians and nurses focus on the *individual* patient, while leaders focus on *many* patients. Simply moving the apostrophe one letter makes a huge difference.

> **BOX 6.1 ■ ORGANIZATIONAL OBSTACLES IN THE CLINICIAN TO PHYSICIAN MANAGER ROLE[22]**
>
> 1. Failure to set clear objectives
> 2. Failure to delineate specific responsibilities
> 3. Failure to provide adequate and timely feedback
> 4. Neglecting to provide practical experience to develop managerial skills
> 5. Failure to mentor and/or guide physician in this transition
> 6. Surrounding a physician with incompetent or inadequately trained staff
> 7. Failure to reward or recognize exceptional performance

THE TRANSITION FROM CLINICIAN TO LEADER-MANAGER

McCall and Claire identified seven critical transformations in the transition process from clinician to manager (**Box 6.1**).[23] The skills required and the psychological demands are quite different between the two roles. McCall and Claire's work is based on interviews and delineates the importance of the seven factors during the transition process. They note that several of the clinician's skills can easily be adapted to managerial roles, including:

- Analytical skills of diagnosis
- Self-confidence deriving from mastery of clinical skills
- Comfort with decision-making
- Interpersonal sensitivity that comes from dealing with patients and families in difficult situations

However, their study clarified that these skills and abilities alone were insufficient for a successful transition from clinician to manager. They identified six specific types of transitions that are critical to the shift, including three psychological adjustments and three specific new skills or abilities (**Table 6.6**).

The Three Psychological Adjustments

Adjustment 1

The first psychological adjustment requires moving from hard-earned independence and autonomy as a clinician to a much more dependent role as a manager. Clinicians are able to independently adapt and individualize care. In contrast, nurse and physician leaders cannot simply rely on their own initiative to modify practices but rather are significantly more dependent on collaborating with others to create a group approach.

TABLE 6.6 ■ McCall and Claire's Psychological Adjustments and New Skills[22]

Adjustment 1. From independence/autonomy to (inter-) dependence
Adjustment 2. From a clinician focused on a patient's care to a leader focused on successful systems
Adjustment 3. From organizational naiveté to organizational reality awareness
Skill ability 1. From demand and control to persuasion, ambiguity, and communication skills
Skill ability 2. From comfortable colleague friendships to authority-based relationships
Skill ability 3. From perceived clinical competence to recognized management/leadership competence

For example, the medical and nursing directors of the department may develop a series of strategies designed to enhance patient flow, including triage by-pass, standing orders at triage, and team triage. However, implementation of these programs requires dependence on multiple staff members adapting their current functions and following the newly devised processes for the good of the patients. It can be particularly difficult for clinicians to adopt new processes when they have competently and pridefully performed the old function (triage) with success. Wise leaders and managers involve multiple staff members in the design of these processed changes, which allows the clinicians to both guide the program changes and create more nuanced and adoptable programs.

The best leaders and managers do not insist that all the questions are answered by them. Rather, they ask questions to foster an empowered staff and a supportive environment. A team comprising staff and leadership will usually find better solutions than will either alone. Further, it is more difficult to adopt a solution in which one has not participated. There are two related aphorisms:

Leaders know they have done a good job when they work themselves out of a job.

An ED's success can be measured not by how it operates when the leaders are present, but rather how it functions when they are not present.[21]

Adjustment 2

Second, the leader–manager must make the transition from a clinician focused on individual patient care to a manager focused on the system needs of the entire ED (as well as the entire health-care system's goals and objectives). McCall and Claire note that, traditionally, "physicians are fiercely independent, pursuing personal or professional agendas rather than department agendas."[22] Physician and nurse leaders must ensure that the focus is on the needs and programs of the entire ED team.

For example, common clinical and managerial issues should be decided in a team forum, perhaps at a monthly ED meeting. Collaboration and engagement of nurses, physicians, clerical staff, and all team members driving "bottom-up" solutions are essential. Successful EDs incorporate team governance models that utilize an evidence-based and highly collaborative approach to finding negotiated solutions to arrive at the best processes and policies.

"We agree to disagree" is not an acceptable outcome of a process or policy discussion. Instead, successful ED leaders promote consistent team adoption of group determined solutions.

Adjustment 3

The third psychological adjustment involves a transition from relative "naiveté" about organizational dynamics to acceptance of organizational realities and priorities. Change may seem particularly slow to the new leader, who ruminates, "This is a good idea, why can't we simply make the change now." New leaders may find it difficult to realize true and lasting change requires collaboration, compromise, and perseverance. Further, they must learn specific organizational dynamics skills and abilities, including conflict resolution and negotiation skills. McCall and Claire note:

The rationality of the clinic is based on fact, logic, and linearity. The rationality of the organization is very different—it rests in getting people to accept and act on a decision. Facts don't always triumph, people don't always rally around logic, and power, position, and different perspectives effect outcome.

The Three New Skills/Abilities

In addition to these psychological adjustments affecting the transition from clinician to manager, the authors also noted that three new skills or abilities were also requisite. The new skills/abilities can be quantified and taught. They are somewhat different from those required for success in the clinical setting.

New Skill/Ability 1

The first involves a transition from demand and control in the clinical setting to persuasion, ambiguity, and communication skills in the setting of the leader and manager. In fact, over the last decade, the expectations of patients and their families have changed to now include effective communication skills.

Since the early 2000s, communication skills and professionalism have been listed in the Accreditation Council for Graduate Medical Education residency program requirements as core competencies (IV.A.5.d).(1), "Residents are expected to: communicate effectively with patients, families, and the public, as appropriate, across a broad range of socioeconomic and cultural backgrounds."[24]

New Skill/Ability 2

The second of the new skills or abilities requires a transition from comfortable, established relationships with professional colleagues to authority-based, boss-subordinate relationships. It is difficult to transition from the relationship of a colleague (friend) to that of a supervising clinician leader. Yet, success requires the new leader to lead. On the other hand, the new leader is not required to be a strict autocrat. Many successful health-care systems have moved away from authoritarian, hierarchical approaches to team governance, but authority-based relationships still commonly exist and development of this skill must be considered.

New Skill/Ability 3

The third skill requires shifting from hard-won competence in medicine to competence in management – a skill that can be equally challenging but is seldom as well respected. Emergency physicians, in particular, have long valued the "pit doc" capable of rapidly managing multiple complex patients. They have rarely, however, held the role of medical director in the same high esteem. In fact, some smaller emergency physician groups still insist that medical directors work full-time clinically with little nonclinical compensation.

Regardless of how good a clinician is or how strong his or her communication skills are, it is also essential to develop the leader's abilities related to organizational learning, negotiation, strategic planning, service excellence, change management, and patient safety. These skills and abilities are all distinct, quantifiable, and crucial to the success of the organization and the department in particular.

Taken together, competence in these six areas can lead to what Peter Senge refers to as *personal mastery*.[25] This requires an intentional change in one's personal identity, learning competencies, demonstrating skill mastery, and earning esteem.

Overcoming Barriers and Developing a Dyad Relationship

Successful transitions from the role of clinician to the role of leader and manager are most likely to occur when potential personal and organizational obstacles are addressed in advance. Personal barriers may include defense mechanisms (especially denial), errors in leader (candidate) selection, and an inability to build effective support systems.

The common organizational impediment involves poor preparation. This often includes a lack of groundwork in considering the people and processes affected by the change, particularly if the leader is moved into a newly created role. The institution's insufficient consideration and inadequate planning often leads to poor understanding and adoption of the new role/person. There are multiple examples of failure, or delayed acceptance, because of a poorly thought-out implementation strategy.

Returning to the dyad concept, effective transitions of nurse and/or physician clinicians to collaborative leadership roles necessitate respectful relationships between the departmental leaders. In many institutions, this primary relationship is made difficult because physician and nurse leaders report to different hierarchies with conflicting goals.

For instance, the nurse leader may report to the hospital CNO, while the physician leader may report to his/her group and the hospital CMO. Further, the dyad leaders usually find themselves in arranged relationships, sometimes working with noncollaborative counterparts. The psychological adjustment needed in this working relationship requires recognizing the relationship of a primary dyad, setting unified goals, and clarifying mutual expectations. It takes time and effort, but the dyad must develop processes to ensure clarity of roles and shared goals. Specifically, dyad members must communicate regularly and commit to including each other in planning, problem-solving, and departmental communications. This commitment entails defining frequent regular meetings to review and work on priorities. Nurse and physician leaders must support one another and back one another up. This is what high-performing leadership teams do to ensure that they optimize their relationships and lead their teams.

CONCLUSION

Although the transition from clinician to leader-manager can be daunting, the process is significantly facilitated by leaders availing themselves of the rich literature on the core competencies of leadership.

Leadership Competencies

The radical changes in American health-care point to the need for articulate, passionate, and committed leaders to successfully shepherd those changes. The requirements of effective ED nurse and physician leaders create the foundation for success in this complex environment. Indeed, many CMOs, CNOs, COOs, and even CEOs are former emergency physicians or nurses, whose skills, talents, and successes were recognized by the organizations they serve. As these roles evolve, organizations have invested in integrated training for their nurse and physician leaders. To become institutional leaders, clinicians must additionally develop competence (executive skills) in[26]:

- Strategic business planning, analytics, and financial management
- Empowerment, developing appropriate reward systems, staff development
- Mission/vision development and articulation
- Change management skills
- Negotiation and conflict resolution
- Stakeholder analysis, boundary management, and service excellence skills

Reaching Our Potential

All of these competencies are addressed in this text, because we must develop these skills to help our EDs—and the professionals and staff comprising them—reach their fullest and most enlightened potential as centers of excellence for the patients we ultimately serve. We are the front lines of health care and the safety net for our society's health-care needs. We can only be successful if we recognize that our clinicians must *all* be leaders if we are to succeed.

One of the leader's most important goals is to recognize that professionals in health-care organizations require a unique set of skills and abilities, and it is our responsibility to help develop them. While it is not an easy work, it is perhaps our best hope for further developing both the clinical and leadership practice of emergency medicine upon which all our success depends. We must collaborate with our dyad leadership to lead and manage across the inherent boundaries of the complex adaptive system comprising the ED. This effort requires more than a philosophical and cultural commitment; it requires the use of specific tools, processes, and behaviors to have the team pull together to "connect the gears" for the good of the patient and the team providing care.

REFERENCES

1. Mayer T. *How to Lead a Team*. Dallas, Tex: American College of Emergency Physicians' Emergency Department Directors Academy; 2018.
2. Nietzsche F. *The Twilight of the Idols*. Oxford, UK: Oxford University Press; 1998.
3. Doran GT. There's a S.M.A.R.T. way to write management's goals and objectives. *Manag Rev*. 1981;70(11):35-36.
4. Inamdar N, Kaplan RS, Bower M. Applying the balanced scorecard in healthcare provider organizations. *J Healthc Manag*. 2002;47(3): 179-196.
5. The Advisory Board. Dyad leadership. https://www.advisory.com/research/physician-executive-council/prescription-for-change/2015/03/dyad-leadership-slides. Accessed March 30, 2018.
6. Cortese DA, Smoldt RK. 5 success factors for physician-administrator partnerships. https://www.mgma.com/resources/resources/business-strategy/5-success-factors-for-physician-administrator-part. Accessed March 30, 2018.
7. Stead EA Jr. *What This Patient Needs is a Doctor*. Wagner GS, Cebe B, Rozear MP, eds. Durham, England: Duke University Press; 1990.
8. Berry LL, Seltman KD. *Management Lessons from Mayo Clinic: Inside One of the World's Most Admired Service Organizations*. New York, NY: McGraw-Hill; 2008.
9. Lawrence DM. *Best Care, Best Future: A Guide for Healthcare Leaders*. Bozeman, Mont: Second River Healthcare; 2014.
10. Hirschhorn L, Gilmore T. The new boundaries of the "boundaryless" company. *Harv Bus Rev*. 1992;70(3):104-115.
11. Mayer T. Leadership, management and motivation, In: Strauss RW, Mayer T, eds. *Emergency Department Management*. 2nd ed. Dallas, Tex: American College of Emergency Physicians Press; 2019.
12. Turner P. Critical thinking in nursing education as defined in the literature. *Nurs Ed Perspect*. 2005;26(5):272-277.
13. Zori S, Morrison B. Critical thinking in nurse managers. *Nurs Econ*. 2009;27(2):75-79.
14. Reinertsen JL. An interview with James L. Reinertsen. Interview by Penny Carver. *Jt Comm J Qual Patient Saf*. 2011;37(5):196-200.
15. Contino DS. Leadership competencies: knowledge, skills, and aptitudes nurses need to lead effectively. *Crit Care Nurse*. 2004;24(3):52-64.
16. Mayer T. *Developing Leadership and Communication Skills*. Dallas, Tex: American College of Emergency Physicians Emergency Department Directors Academy; 2018.
17. Porter ME, Teisberg EO. *Redefining Health Care: Creating Value-Based Competition on Results*. Boston, Mass: Harvard Business School Press; 2006.
18. Lemire JA. Redesigning financial management education for the nursing administration graduate student. *J Nurs Adm*. 2000; 30(4):199-205.
19. Kurtz ME. The dual dilemma. In: Curry W, ed. *The Physician Executive*. Tampa, Fla: American College of Physician Executives; 2002.
20. Adapted from Kurtz ME. The dual role dilemma. In: Curry W, ed. *The Physician Executive*. Tampa, Fla: American College of Physicians Executives; 1988.
21. Mayer T. *Leadership for Great Customer Service*. Dallas, Tex: American College of Emergency Physicians' Emergency Department Directors Academy; 2018.
22. Mayer T, Tavernero T, Strauss RW, Jensen K. The discipline of teams and teamwork in emergency medicine. In: Strauss RW, Mayer T, eds. *Emergency Department Management*. 2nd ed. Dallas, Tex: ACEP Press; 2019.
23. McCall MW Jr, Claire JA. *In Transit: From Physician to Manager*. Philadelphia, Pa: Wharton Center for Applied Research; 1990.
24. ACGME Common Program Requirements—Educational Program-IV.5.d)(1). http://www.acgme.org/Portals/0/PFAssets/ProgramRequirements/CPRs_2017-07-01.pdf. Accessed April 18, 2018.
25. Senge P. *The Fifth Discipline: The Art and Practice of the Learning Organization*. New York, NY: Doubleday; 2006.
26. Mayer T. *The Business Case for Flow*. Dallas, Tex: American College of Emergency Physicians Emergency Department Directors Academy; 2018.

CHAPTER 7

MENTORING AND COACHING

Brian J. Zink

I am always ready to learn, although I do not always like to be taught.

—Winston S. Churchill

Professional success and satisfaction in the world of medicine are related to many factors, one of the most important being the influence of mentors and coaches. This principle has been borne out in studies of career development and in the narratives of those who have risen to leadership positions. Many different definitions and understandings exist on what constitutes mentorship and coaching.

From the education literature comes a definition of mentoring that has been adopted and used in medicine: "a dynamic, reciprocal relationship in a work environment between two individuals where, often but not always, one is an advanced career incumbent and the other is a less-experienced person. The relationship is aimed at fostering the development of the less-experienced person."[1] In most effective mentoring relationships, the skills of both parties advance.

DEFINING MENTORING AND COACHING

A mentoring relationship is a one-on-one, supportive relationship between a more senior person and more junior person, while a coaching relationship usually involves an individual who is teaching one or more individuals, even a whole team, a particular skill. The definitions blur somewhat depending on the individuals involved and the nature of the relationship. For example, the concept of peer-to-peer mentoring does not utilize a more senior mentor. Rather, the wisdom gained by one or more people who are at the same level is shared to collectively advance those individuals. The meaning of "coaching" can also be more expansive—for example, faculty physicians who are called "coaches" work one-on-one in a confidential manner with individual medical students in at least one medical school.[2] Some would view this type of interaction more as a mentor relationship than coaching. Executive coaches, usually supported and funded by health systems, are utilized by many physician, nurse, and administrative leaders when they start in new leadership roles.[3]

Other terms for a mentor/coach include advisor, role model, confidante, advocate, and supporter. An extension of the traditional mentoring role is described in the newer term "sponsor," which arose from efforts to advance women in their professions. Sponsorship involves a more active role in promoting the career of the mentored person through advocacy and connections. (Coaching, including Focused Coaching™ and "shadow shifting," are addressed in detail in Chapters 12 and 78.)

Whether the title of a person who helps another advance is mentor, advisor, coach, sponsor, or some other term, the key concept is that no one can achieve true leadership success in emergency medicine without having strong relationships with other people who show them the way, teach them skills, help prevent and learn from mistakes, and offer opinions and support as career opportunities arise.

The Evidence for Mentoring and Coaching

The data for the value of mentoring are compelling. In the education realm, it has been repeatedly shown that students who have mentors, particularly those who are disadvantaged, are much more likely to enroll in college and eventually become leaders than those without a mentor.[4] In academic medicine, a large systematic review found that effective mentorship was associated with increased productivity of faculty members and that mentored faculty were promoted more quickly and were less likely to leave their medical schools.[5] Perhaps the best way to reinforce the value of mentorship is to ask those who are successful and admired in medicine if they benefited from strong mentor relationships—the answer is almost universally "yes."[6-9]

MENTORSHIP

Setting Goals and Expectations

The mentoring or coaching relationship should be defined and structured, and responsibilities agreed to before it commences. In emergency departments with established mentorship programs, this relationship should be discussed in the recruitment process so the goals, expectations, and responsibilities are clear. Both the mentor and the mentee should benefit from the relationship. Because most mentor–mentee relationships have a power discrepancy, the potential for conscious or unconscious exploitation of the mentee exists and must be guarded against. A mentor/mentee agreement may not go so far as to generate a written contract, but it is advisable to have a written understanding, or at least an email exchange, that defines the goals and expectations of the relationship. Some components to include when setting up the agreement for a mentoring relationship are summarized in **Table 7.1**.

Mentor and Mentee: A Two-Way Relationship

While a classic view of mentorship and coaching is that a gray-haired sage takes a bright-eyed, naive student under his or her wing and selflessly provides wise guidance and advice, the reality is that mentorship and effective coaching only works if there is active engagement from both sides. As noted above, the relationship should be reciprocal. To borrow from ecological terms, this is known as mutualism—both organisms benefit. The "win–win" of mentoring can occur in many different ways. For most mentees, the knowledge, skills,

TABLE 7.1 ■ Questions to Address Before Establishing a Mentoring Relationship
Will the mentor function as a primary mentor, secondary mentor, or one of a group of mentors?
What specific goals does the mentee have for his/her development?
How often will meetings and communication occur?
How will the mentoring and communications occur?
If there is scholarly output from the relationship, how will authorship and presentation work?
Are there any conflicts of interest on behalf of the mentor in serving in this role for the mentee?
Is there a defined time period for the mentoring relationship?

experience, and advice provided by the mentor or coach are a valuable "win." On the other side of the equation, the satisfaction of seeing a more junior person advance and contribute is enough of a reward to make the mentoring effort worth it. This "giving back" to the profession to ensure a positive future in health care is the most virtuous form of mentorship.[5-10]

On the practical side, the mentee can provide value to the mentor by doing basic work that, while building skills and knowledge, helps the mentor's team accomplish their goals. For example, a mentee can organize, review, and analyze data from a study or project and provide that to the mentor for use in the next steps of the project. A mentee may write drafts of policies, articles, chapters, or scientific papers for mentor review and critique. The mentor benefits as the draft helps to advance the writing project, and the mentee receives instruction and critique on his or her writing skills. As mentees become more developed, they may be asked to step in for the mentor in some situations (e.g., attending a hospital committee meeting in place of the mentor).

A study of mentoring relationships for academic physicians across two large medical centers found that success depended on the relationship having reciprocity, mutual respect, clear expectations, personal relationships, and shared values. On the other hand, failed mentor relationships were noted to have poor communication, lack of commitment, personality differences, and perceived or real competition between mentor and mentee.[8]

While a solid two-way commitment and working relationship is necessary for effective mentoring and coaching, mentors are often very busy people. Mentees are important to mentors, but they may not always be the highest priority in a given week. Therefore, the activity and degree of engagement of the mentee is crucial to make the relationship work. As mentorship expert Dario Sambunjak notes, "Mentees should take the initiative for cultivating the relationship with their mentors (taking the driver's seat). It is important that mentees have commitment to the success of the mentoring relationship and passion to succeed in their career."[6] The terms "managing up" or "leading up" describe how the mentee can foster the relationship by initiating communications, preparing agendas for mentoring meetings, and focusing the mentor on the key needs at that point in the relationship. A passive approach where the mentee waits for the mentor to initiate the next communication is unlikely to work.

Characteristics of an Effective Mentor

An effective mentor or coach must have the time, experience, and willingness to engage in the role. Common features of high-quality mentors, some of which are innate but many of which can be learned or practiced, are summarized in **Table 7.2**.

TABLE 7.2 ■ Characteristics of an Effective Mentor
Altruism: puts the interests and needs of the mentee first
Credibility: has knowledge, skills, reputation, and experience that can benefit the mentee
Accessibility: is able to communicate and meet regularly and reliably
Patience: has an understanding approach with those who are inexperienced
Good listener: fully hears and comprehends what the mentee is relating by using active listening
Gives excellent feedback: can offer constructive, honest, reliable assessment and advice
Trustworthy: keeps information confidential
Connector: introduces mentee to other influencers and helps build new relationships
Motivator: provides a positive outlook and a push forward for the mentee when needed

FIGURE 7.1 ■ Challenge Support Grid for Mentorships[9,11]

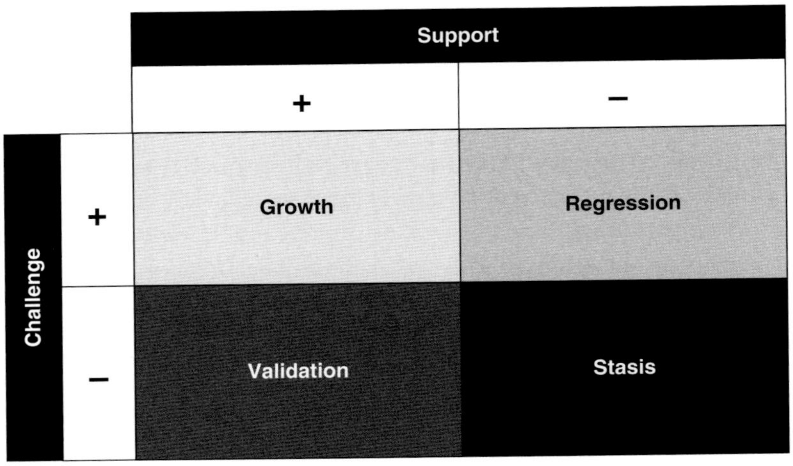

	Support +	Support −
Challenge +	Growth	Regression
Challenge −	Validation	Stasis

Adapted from original by Daioz (1956) and updated by Ramani et al (2006).

Some individuals naturally become excellent mentors and coaches as they progress in their careers. However, as not everyone is innately a highly skilled teacher, most people can benefit from specific training in how to be an effective mentor or coach. Institutional courses or sessions may be offered, and many national medical organizations offer workshops on mentoring and coaching. Since having an adequate number of mentors or coaches is a common problem in medicine, training up mid-career physicians, nurses, and administrators to become available mentors and coaches is essential.

One quandary is that potential mentees become very aware of who are the best mentors, and requests for mentoring can saturate these mentors. If this is the case, it is important for the mentor to have a list of other qualified mentors to provide to the requesting mentee. As a mentee learns about the characteristics of a potential mentor, a certain amount of flexibility and tolerance is required, as not all mentors possess all the positive characteristics. For example, a mentor may have outstanding content knowledge but may not be the best communicator. For these reasons, it is important to have multiple mentors, as described below, who can fill various needs.[9-10]

The best mentors both challenge and support the mentee. Consequences of the challenge/support dynamic are summarized in **Figure 7.1**. Mentees will grow and thrive if the mentor provides positive support and a real challenge to develop. They will regress or not progress if support is not adequate and will be validated but will not grow if there is support but no real challenge. If a mentor is too busy to truly engage the mentee, the most common result is stasis: the mentee does not learn or contribute in the mentor's realm. In this case, the mentor should recognize that the relationship is not working and take steps to correct it or refer the mentee to someone who can provide better mentorship or coaching. Finally, there is often a need to "mentor the mentors" to ensure there is a consistently high level of interaction with demonstrably improved results and relationships, as opposed to simply assuming that the mentorship program is producing good results.

Characteristics of an Effective Mentee

Just as certain qualities contribute to the competence of a mentor, there are key characteristics and skills for mentees that lead to productive mentoring relationships. A basic quality is being "coachable": open and receptive to the guidance and instruction

TABLE 7.3 ■ Characteristics of an Effective Mentee
Prepared: reads in advance, develops agenda or talking points, formulates questions
Team player: willing to pitch in and help, even if not directly his/her assignment
Reliable: punctual, shows up, meets deadlines, delivers high-quality work
Creative: brings interesting and fresh perspectives to the mentor's world
Communicative: keeps everyone informed, verbally or electronically
Feedback: able to both receive evaluation from mentor and provide feedback to the mentor

of the mentor or coach and willing to work to improve knowledge and skills. Beyond that openness to mentoring or coaching, other characteristics that lead to successful relationships are summarized in **Table 7.3**.

The Mentorship Network

While the image of a Yoda-like figure who provides solitary mentorship to a developing hero is appealing, it is also more fantasy than reality. Almost all successful leaders and managers in health care will list at least several mentors or coaches who they have utilized over the course of their careers. Mentees should have a stable of mentors, each providing a different component to the overall mentoring experience. Just as a horseman might choose a draft horse for one task, a pleasure horse for another, and race horse for another, a health care mentee might utilize one mentor to learn a specific clinical skill, another for career advice, and another to make key connections at a national meeting. In addition, if only one mentor is used, that mentor had better know everything, which is highly unlikely in any setting. Having multiple formal or informal mentors to acquire multiple skills is a sound strategy (**Figure 7.2**).

The mentor milieu naturally changes over time. The importance and engagement of mentors fluctuates, with some becoming former or occasional mentors as new mentors enter the team. The value of having multiple mentors for academic researchers was demonstrated in a qualitative study of National Institutes of Health K grant awardees, which showed

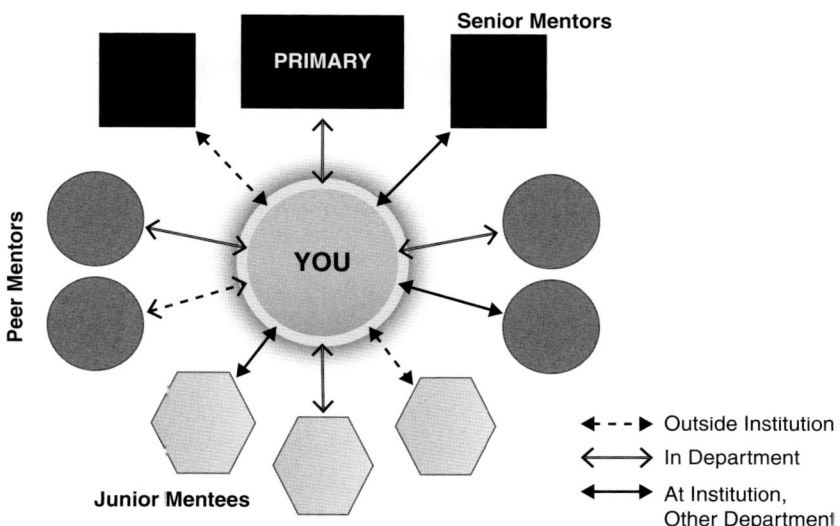

FIGURE 7.2 ■ Mentorship Network Map

this "polyga-mentoring" approach to be widespread and viewed very favorably.[12] Peer-to-peer mentoring, also known as horizontal mentoring, is common and viewed as valuable because individuals can practice mentoring others at their level before they become senior mentors. Peer mentoring does not take the place of having more experienced mentors.[10,13]

One way of defining the group of mentors that contribute to a developing person's success is to construct a mentorship network or map. This process schematically lays out the collection of mentors, with some being senior, some being peers, some internal to the institution, and some external. The diagram also includes the mentees of the individual, painting the whole scope of mentor/mentee involvement. It should be viewed as a living diagram, updated with mentors and mentees written into the bubbles as they enter and exit the person's life. An example of a how a mentor network map can be constructed is provided in **Figure 7.2**.

Finding and Choosing Mentors and Coaches

Some mentors or coaches are organically found as a person enters a new stage of life. It may be a respected professor or teacher, a new manager, or a senior coworker. Institutions may have a program that assigns a mentor or coach to a more junior employee. However, in most cases, mentors or coaches must be sought. As new employees survey their landscape, they will identify those in leadership positions who might function as mentors: those who are slightly ahead in rank and respected by peers. One or more people from each category can be approached as possible mentors. As noted, an explicit request ("Can you serve as a mentor for me?") and the ability to set expectations in advance are key. Depending on the reach and exposure of the individual, mentors or coaches external to the institution or those who have been important in the past should be included. The eye of an external mentor or coach in helping a mentee can give fresh perspectives and ideas for how to deal with local issues and problems.[4-8]

It is the responsibility of leaders in emergency care to ensure that their employees have good mentoring and coaching. The benefits of creating strong mentor/coach relationships are clearly worth the time and money invested in doing so. The methods used vary, but one way to start is by helping new employees find a primary mentor and beginning a mentor network in their first year of employment. Some institutions assign a mentor or coach for a new employee or trainee. This may be beneficial, but since the mentee has not chosen the individual, the fit in personality and style may or may not lead to a productive relationship.

Another approach, which may work better over time, is to make sure the new employee or trainee is receiving basic guidance from managers in their first few weeks or months. Afterward, meet with them to discuss who they have identified as potential mentors/coaches and how to move forward with establishing the reciprocal relationships that they choose. A launch program that includes attention to developing a mentor network can be very effective in the onboarding process for new employees. The annual review is a great time for the leader or manager to go over the employee or trainee's mentor network diagram (**Figure 7.2**) to determine if there is an adequate level of mentoring and coaching.

MYTHS AND MISCONCEPTIONS

Misconceptions are common and arise out of the common frustrations and challenges in a process that is often unstructured. These misconceptions sometimes impair the development of strong relationships, and mentors must recognize when they are circulating in the minds of mentees. Some of these are listed below.

Communication skills, both verbal and nonverbal, play a major role in the development or resolution of conflict. Poorly developed skills often heighten discord and dissent, especially in an environment prone to high stress and miscommunication.

Personal Response to Stress and Conflict

Individuals respond to stress and conflict by habit, that is, learned patterns of behavior. In general, habits are advantageous because they allow people to perform activities and tasks without thinking. People perform thousands of minor tasks every day without conscious effort. For example, when driving a car, habits allow the driver to accelerate, turn the steering wheel, watch the scenery, and listen to the radio at the same time.

In a calm environment, individuals exhibit routine behavior patterns. However, when under substantial stress, a person typically responds with a consistent and individualized pattern of behavior known as a "crisis pattern." Some people confront stressful predicaments with maladaptive behavior patterns—provocation, accusation, anger, withdrawal, or disdain—that exacerbate the situation. These behaviors may be particularly ineffective (and often disruptive) in an environment that requires decisive, collaborative, and articulate communication and responses, such as the ED.[23,24]

Implicit Bias

Discrimination, although sometimes subtle, exists in all areas of the hospital, especially the ED. This creates further inequities and conflict. Because waiting times and level of caring by practitioners are key factors in patient satisfaction, biases that prolong waiting and decrease practitioner compassion seem particularly unfair and inappropriate. Biases that exist among staff members may further undermine care. Common types of inherent bias include gender, generational, ethnic, financial, and educational. In health-care settings, "presenting complaint" bias can also influence perception and compassion.

- *Gender bias*[25-28]: It is well-documented that female patients presenting with cardiac illnesses are approached, evaluated, and treated less aggressively than male patients with similar complaints. Women presenting with abdominal pain or chronic pain syndromes experience a similar type of bias. Another form of gender bias occurs when patients request that the evaluating practitioner be of the same gender.
- *Ethnic and cultural bias*[29,30]: Patients of non-white ethnicities are more likely to perceive and report caregiver bias than their white counterparts. Differing ways of responding to pain and language barriers may frustrate staff members and lead to ethnic bias.
- *Financial or socioeconomic bias*: Emergency providers may exhibit bias against uninsured or homeless patients who have few options for urgent or ongoing care. Conversely, emergency staff may treat patients who are well dressed or appear to have financial means with greater courtesy and respect.
- *Educational bias*: Closely associated with financial and socioeconomic bias, providers may demonstrate bias against patients with less education. These individuals may be less articulate and less able to understand or follow written or verbal instructions in accordance with the health-care provider's intent. Furthermore, health-care workers may react negatively to patients who use "street" grammar, slang, or idioms because they may be perceived as indicators of educational status.
- *Presenting-complaint bias*: Most practitioners prefer straightforward presenting complaints, and they may avoid patients who present with vague or confusing complaints that are difficult to assess, choosing to see "easier" cases first. Typical presentations that lead to presenting-complaint bias include chronic back pain, fibromyalgia, constipation, generalized weakness, confusion, and behavioral issues.[31] Presenting-complaint bias may lead to caregivers forming opinions about the patient prior to evaluation.

Myth 1: My Mentor/Coach Should Be Like Me

Although an exact match of mentor/mentee gender, ethnicity, personal style, and so on, may be desirable and comfortable for the mentee, such pairings are not always possible. If the mentee only seeks someone like himself or herself, it may drastically limit the number of potential mentors. Further, it can simply reinforce common beliefs and skills instead of developing broader perspectives. Many successful mentoring and coaching relationships thrive on differences, as each person learns more about the other's perspectives, culture, or approach. This is especially true for those who are underrepresented in medicine (URiM). Because the number of URiM mentors or coaches is limited, not every URiM mentee may be able to find a mentor in their realm who matches their race, ethnicity, or gender identity. The URiM mentors often become saturated with mentees. In this case, the mentor can identify non-URiM mentors who have served as strong advocates for URiM mentees and may be able to direct them to URiM mentors who are outside their realm. Women in medicine may have difficulty finding female mentors and may have to look beyond their immediate job group for a female mentor while utilizing male mentors who have shown that they can successfully mentor women. Many national organizations have subgroups that address common issues for professional women and foster mentoring relationships.

Myth 2: The Best Mentor(s) Will Be Experts in My Focus Area

Not every mentee can find a great local mentor in their area of focus, especially if it is a narrow field. While it is desirable to have a mentor or coach who is well-versed in the mentees' subject area, some of the best mentors may come from an associated realm or even a totally different field. As mentors become more experienced, they can apply their wisdom and provide different perspectives than someone who is closely matched to the mentee's focus area. Many instances exist where a mentor from another field provides a creative, innovative suggestion that helps the mentee advance in their area.

Myth 3: I Need to Have a Close, Personal Relationship With My Mentor or Coach

While the most fulfilling mentor/mentee relationships may evolve to become close, enduring personal relationships that extend beyond the workplace, this dynamic is unnecessary and is more likely to be the exception. As noted above, a professional mentor/mentee relationship with defined expectations and goals can be highly successful and beneficial for both parties without becoming a close personal relationship.

Myth 4: I Need to Spend a Lot of Time With My Mentor or Coach

The quality of interactions is far more important than the quantity. Many mentor/mentee and coaching relationships in medicine are not like a traditional apprentice role, where there is daily direct contact and supervision. Whether interactions are weekly, monthly, or even less frequent should be determined by the needs of the relationship and may change over time. If the mentee can utilize a mentor network, it may be that some mentors are only utilized a couple times per year, and the communications may be electronic rather than face-to-face. On the other hand, mentors should be available when needed, and the mentee should feel comfortable in contacting mentors "off schedule" for pressing, time-dependent matters.

Myth 5: I Am Stuck With a Mentor, Even if I Don't Like Them

Some mentoring relationships do not work out. Whether it is a lack of commitment or availability from the mentor, personality conflicts, or inappropriate behaviors, the relationship can be terminated. If a mentee is dissatisfied, it is likely that the mentor also feels this way. When issues arise, it is important to refer back to the initial agreement for the mentoring relationship and note where expectations are not being met. If there are irreconcilable issues, a professional agreement to end the relationship through a face-to-face meeting is necessary. Because of the power dynamic, a mentee may be tempted to slink away and let a poor mentor relationship dissolve, but this could result in negative feelings from the mentor that could impact the mentee's career path. Mentor–mentee relationships typically evolve with distinct phases: initiation, a positive mentoring phase, a less frequent interaction phase, and finally, a termination of the relationship as a true mentoring relationship. This evolution will happen naturally, and the phases may not be clearly evident or declared during the relationship but should be expected. Issues may arise if the mentee or mentor does not appreciate that the relationship is evolving, and the terms of the relationship may need explicit discussion.[6]

Myth 6: Only Physicians Need Mentoring

While mentoring programs are extremely important to the development of physicians, all members of the emergency department team can benefit from these programs, including nurses, advanced practice providers, and even ED technicians, unit secretaries, and essential services personnel (imaging and laboratory technicians). Many large volume, high-acuity EDs have developed nursing fellowship programs, the best of which assign mentors to new nurses.

CONCLUSION

While few would dispute that having strong mentoring or coaching relationships is crucial for the career development of individuals and the success of organizations, far too many people in the early and middle stages of their careers in health care lack adequate mentorship and coaching. The tendency is to focus on the day-to-day activities of a busy unit like the emergency department and to not step back and look at how employees are progressing.

It is the responsibility of the manager or leader to make sure that mentoring and coaching relationships are developing for each employee. This takes conscious effort, meetings with the employee to assess mentoring, and advice on how to best achieve strong mentoring. Mentors and coaches also need training in order to be effective. The investment of time will be rewarded, as study after study has shown that people who have strong mentoring and coaching relationships perform better and have higher job and career satisfaction than those who do not.

On the mentee side, a deliberate approach is also necessary. Actively seeking mentors or coaches, defining relationships, setting expectations, and taking the time to fully utilize mentors and coaches will be worth the effort.

The future of emergency patient care will be brighter if both mentors and mentees seek each other out and build the relationships and networks that produce happy, productive, empowered emergency care providers and staff.

REFERENCES

1. Healy CC, Welchert AJ. Mentoring relations: a definition to advance research and practice. *Educ Res*. 1990;19(9):17-21.
2. University of Michigan Medical School website. Available at: https://medicine.umich.edu/medschool/education/md-program/m-home. Accessed July 4, 2019.
3. McAlearney AS. Executive leadership development in U.S. health systems. *J Healthc Manag*. 2010;55(3):206-222.
4. The National Mentoring Partnership website. https://www.mentoring.org/why-mentoring/mentoring-impact/. Accessed June 16, 2019.
5. Sambunjak D, Straus SE, Marusic A. Mentoring in academic medicine: a systematic review. *JAMA*. 2006;296(9):1103-1115.
6. Sambunjak D, Straus SE, Marusic A. Systematic review of qualitative research on the meaning and characteristics of mentoring in academic medicine. *J Gen Intern Med*. 2010;25(1):72-78.
7. Carey EC, Weissman DE. Understanding and finding mentorship: a review for junior faculty. *J Palliat Med*. 2010;13(11):1373-1379.
8. Straus SE, Johnson MO, Marquez C, Feldman MD. Characteristics of successful and failed mentoring relationships: a qualitative study across two academic health centers. *Acad Med*. 2013;88(1):82-89.
9. Ramani S, Gruppen L, Kachur EK. Twelve tips for developing effective mentors. *Med Teach*. 2006;28(5):404-408
10. Balmer DF, Darden A, Chandran L, D'Alessandro D, Gusic M. How mentor identity evolves: findings from a 10-year follow-up study of a national professional development program. *Acad Med*. 2018;93(7):1085-1090.
11. Daloz LA. *Effective Teaching and Mentorship: Realizing the Transformational Power of Adult Learning Experiences*. San Francisco, CA: Jossey-Bass; 1986:209-235.
12. Ripley E, Markowitz M, Nichols-Casebolt A, Williams L, Macrina F. Training NIH K Award recipients: the role of the mentor. *Clin Transl Sci*. 2012;5(5):386-393.
13. DeCastro R, Sambuco D, Ubel PA, Stewart A, Jagsi R. Mentor networks in academic medicine: moving beyond a dyadic conception of mentoring for junior faculty researchers. *Acad Med*. 2013;88(4):488-496.

CHAPTER 8

CONFLICT MANAGEMENT

Robert W. Strauss, Gus M. Garmel

> *Peace is not the absence of conflict but the presence of creative alternatives for responding to conflict—alternatives to passive or aggressive responses, alternatives to violence.*
>
> —Dorothy Thompson, journalist (1894-1961)

Wherever people coexist, conflict exists. Frequently, a difference exists between what people desire and their current conditions. This discrepancy is especially true in a crisis-oriented environment like the emergency department (ED), where rapid and high-pressure interactions occur among individuals. In the ED, conflict is intensified as a natural consequence of urgency, the pursuit of incompatible objectives, individuals under stress, and unmet expectations.[1,2]

CONFLICT IS INEVITABLE

Examples of conflict in the ED include the following:

- An emergency medical technician (EMT) arrives in the ED with a patient and expects that staff will immediately attend to the new patient respectfully. Instead, the EMT finds an overwhelmed and somewhat agitated health-care worker who angrily responds, "Can't you see we're busy?"
- A patient with chronic back pain expects immediate treatment and dramatic relief. The busy, perhaps overwhelmed health-care worker arrives 30 minutes later to assess the patient and finds a sarcastic and disdainful patient who claims, "I thought you forgot about me."
- A cardiologist arrives in the ED after leaving his busy office, demanding that a nurse attend to his needs immediately.
- An emergency physician becomes increasingly frustrated because it seems that nothing is getting done and patients are languishing. He loudly calls out to a nurse who just picked up a phone call, "That's great! You're on the phone while patients are sick and waiting!"
- The mother of a crying child walks up to the triage nurse after waiting for more than an hour and is told, "Ma'am, we have sicker patients than your child . . . you'll just have to go back to your seat and wait!"
- An emergency nurse refuses to give a physician-ordered treatment because the nurse believes it may be inappropriate.

Benefits of Conflict

Although the foregoing examples demonstrate negative aspects of conflict, conflict is often beneficial. High-functioning organizations are not conflict-free; rather, they recognize conflict as an opportunity to address unresolved issues and make improvements. The benefits of conflict include the following[3]:

- ***Improved solutions:*** A disagreement voiced and examined allows a deeper investigation into the problem, perhaps incorporating a perspective not yet considered. Attention to alternative views may create more nuanced solutions addressing several perspectives.

- ***Improved efficiency:*** A poorly introduced process change may lead to resistance, delayed implementation, and perhaps failure. Effective leaders recognize that change is fluid and requires "after-action reviews" and "tweaking." Reviewing what worked and what did not opens the process to fine-tuning by those responsible for and affected by its implementation. Identifying conflict and encouraging feedback on process changes fosters buy-in and early adoption.
- ***Enhanced morale:*** Poorly managed or ignored conflicts may lead to brooding and unwillingness to participate in current and future solutions. Addressing concerns or conflicts early decreases resistance to new ideas, programs, and processes and is more likely to result in the successful implementation of those new ideas. Individuals recognize they are respected and their ideas can contribute to the solutions of complex problems. Addressing the issues of people within the group strengthens relationships and enhances morale.

When a patient, family member, or colleague's dissatisfaction is acknowledged, caregivers have an opportunity to make a change to better meet the needs of those they serve. Quality service can only be sustained in organizations that care about the people delivering those services and those to whom the services are delivered.

Costs of Conflict

Although conflict in the ED is unavoidable—and can have benefits, as previously noted—it is vital to understand its associated costs (especially when conflict is not handled early and productively).[4] Unresolved conflict interferes with patient satisfaction, throughput, quality of care, and patient safety. Staff morale and pride are likely to decline with high levels of conflict, resulting in greater turnover from dissatisfaction with the work environment.[5] In high-conflict EDs, leaders will likely spend more time hiring for open staff positions and addressing an increasing number of complaints from patients, medical staff members, and other hospital units.

In the ED, a stressful, noxious work environment negatively affects the staff. In a toxic work environment, poor communication is more likely, which directly affects patient care through increased errors. Some staff members may avoid work by calling in sick, leaving the department understaffed. Repeated conflict and professional dissatisfaction may lead to frustration, anger, family strife, substance abuse, and chemical dependency in staff members. Furthermore, patients can recognize conflict among staff members, which may reduce their satisfaction.

ORIGINS OF STRESS AND CONFLICT IN THE ED

Stress is widespread in EDs for practitioners, patients, and their family members. Clinicians confront numerous situations for which there are few or no positive solutions. Many patients waiting to be seen believe their problems are emergent in nature and require immediate attention; most of them are anxious and in pain. They or their family members may be standing in the hallway or waiting area with arms folded, glaring at the staff while waiting for attention. Overwhelmed staff who are too busy to adequately respond to meet their patients' expectations may avoid these individuals, creating even more conflict.

The Health-Care Setting

Keeping up with the changing health-care setting and expanding numbers of regulatory mandates generates ongoing stress among ED leaders and staff. Health-care reform brings with it pressures to provide nearly perfect care, eliminate pain, address patients' service needs in a timely manner, and ensure quality. Managed care organizations, insurance providers, hospitals, and accountable-care organizations critically review resource use in the ED and advocate limiting the battery of tests and procedures performed. Conversely, specialty training, peer-review organizations, patients and their families, and malpractice fears create pressure to leave no stone unturned when providing emergency care to the public. Furthermore, the lack of historical clinical perspective that exists in an established patient relationship often results in emergency caregivers using additional resources.

Organizational Climate

The hierarchical structure of the ED creates additional tension. Significant inequality of status and pay exists among physicians, nurses, technicians, and clerical staff. Physicians outrank each other in terms of seniority, partnership, leadership, training, or skill set, and they outrank the nursing staff. Some nurses outrank other nurses. Technicians and secretaries are often (incorrectly) considered less significant than clinical staff members. Intensifying this stress is the traditionally held "captain of the ship" mentality—the belief that one person must be in charge of all patient care decisions. When a speaker has power over the listener and the situation is stressful, the potential for conflict is far greater.

Limited resources place further pressure on ED staff. Downsized staffs (in both the ED and the hospital), limited budgets for facility and equipment upgrades, and prolonged "holding" of patients waiting for disposition contribute to suboptimal service.[6] The limited resources severely challenge staff members as they strive to meet patients' needs and provide quality service.

Unhealthy Work Environment

The stresses of delivering emergency care can create symptoms of post-traumatic stress disorder (PTSD)—depression, anxiety, stress, and anger—in many health-care staff. Emergency physicians are more than twice as likely to suffer from PTSD than those in the general public.[7,8] One 2005 study described seven emergency medicine residents who "reported sufficient symptoms to meet the *DSM-V* criteria for PTSD."[9] Those who develop PTSD-like symptoms work in environments with these characteristics:

- *Intensive*: The work is exhausting.
- *Dangerous*: Emergency care is often a matter of life and death. The margin for error is slim and mistakes, which are inevitable, must be kept to a minimum. Contagious diseases and increasing violence in the ED environment also carry personal risk to health-care providers.
- *Litigious*: The fear of malpractice is pervasive among most emergency practitioners.
- *Unpredictable*: There is always a pending sense of the unknown. One moment the ED may be empty; an hour later, it may be overwhelmed by injured and critically ill patients.
- *Unmet expectations*: When the patient or private attending arrives, the ED staff member's complete and immediate attention is required.
- *Uncontrollable*: There is often a sense of crisis and inability to address urgent demands.[10]

In addition to the effects of environmental stress, ED staff have little opportunity to recover or rest. Shifts are often without breaks; meals are always rushed and often missed. Sleep patterns are irregular because of shift work and 24-hour coverage mandates, despite an increasing body of knowledge that describes the biologic and physiologic stresses of changing sleep habits.[11-13]

In describing stress and burnout among emergency care providers, emergency physician Debra Roberts Slapper notes that "individuals prone to burnout are high achievers who have intense schedules, do more than their share on every project, and don't admit their limitations. As we age, our bodies tolerate the physical stresses less well. Twelve-hour shifts, eating on the run, no time for breaks, and sleep disturbances make us feel 70 when we are only 35."[14,15] Given the lack of control over patient volume, job insecurity, challenges with professional and patient relations, the mountain of knowledge and skill that must be maintained (often at one's fingertips), and the emotional roller coaster of "routine" practice, it is understandable that many emergency providers struggle with full-time clinical practice.[16,17]

The Four Cs

Patients arrive at the ED with certain expectations about the attention they will receive. These expectations are numerous, sometimes unrealistic, and often difficult to achieve.[18-20] **Box 8.1** lists the Four Cs, or general expectations, of patient satisfaction.

Convenience (expeditious care): Convenience and time are crucial to most patients seeking emergency care. Longer wait times are associated with lower patient satisfaction.[21] When patients have a choice about emergency care, they generally choose the place that will see them immediately and get them out most quickly. Patients place time-pressure on ED providers, particularly when they have (or think they have) a true emergency. After all, rapid assessment is the *sine qua non* of emergency care.

Caring (concern and kindness): Of equal or greater importance to many patients is provider caring. Rapport and trust must be established rapidly. Initially, patients judge the staff and their experiences not by the level of care, but by the level of *caring*. The responsibilities of ED caregivers are to take care of the patients' needs, both physical and emotional.[13] Caring goes beyond providing a high standard of care. Most patients prefer a warm, friendly, and concerned health-care provider who delivers "good" care to an unfriendly and distant provider practicing on the cutting edge.

Care (quality): Because the actual quality of care is quite difficult for the patient to assess, this expectation is generally considered only when there is no improvement or something goes wrong. Patients take for granted that emergency care is exceptional.

Cost (acceptable or not): Patients who are treated expeditiously with caring and quality tend to be somewhat less concerned about the cost of their care. This is especially true when the outcome of their care is favorable, and they feel better (or relieved) after their experience. Conversely, cost may be an issue for patients who experience provider-in-triage models during which patients may be evaluated, treated, and released quickly yet receive a large bill. Furthermore, cost is more likely to become an issue when a patient perceives that any aspect of care is absent, substandard, inadequate, or does not meet their expectations.

BOX 8.1 ■ THE FOUR Cs OF PATIENT SATISFACTION

- Convenience
- Caring
- Care
- Cost

> **BOX 8.2 ■ MEHRABIAN'S COMPONENTS OF PERSUASION**
>
> | Component | Weight |
> |---|---|
> | Verbal content | 7% |
> | Vocal expression | 38% |
> | Visual cues | 55% |
> | **Total** | **100%** |

PROVIDER COMMUNICATION: SKILLS, BIASES, AND RESPONSE TO STRESS

To be successful, ED personnel must move rapidly from situation to situation, communicating effectively in each. For example, a provider may be required to resuscitate a critically ill patient, admit a patient to a reluctant staff member, and put a fearful child at ease, with each situation requiring a different skill set with respect to conflict management. Regardless of the situation, skillful communicators recognize the importance of words, tone, and body language when trying to persuade others and manage conflict.

Components of Communication

The three classic components of communication are verbal content (words), vocal expression (tone), and visual cues (body language). Some may be surprised to learn that verbal content plays a relatively small role in persuasion. In fact, in some situations, less than 10% of persuasion may be the result of the actual words used.[22] Success in swaying one's perception or opinion is often the result of other forms of communication—the tone, posture, expression, and movement of the communicator.

Albert Mehrabian, one of the foremost communication experts of his time, performed experiments to demonstrate the importance of verbal and nonverbal communication (**Box 8.2**).[22] He examined the contribution of verbal content, vocal expression, and visual cues to persuasion and believability when trying to convince others of something they did not currently believe. Mehrabian found that only a small percentage of communication in that setting relates to the words used; instead, persuasion relies heavily on vocal expression and visual cues. However, in a pressured environment, it is typical to communicate with attention to the words only, ignoring other aspects of communication. This focus on words only may result in verbal incongruence, which Mehrabian described as incongruity between the spoken words and the manner in which they are delivered (vocal tone and body language).

The following examples illustrate verbal incongruence:

- A parent with tight lips, tense body, and threatening posture attempts to verbally reassure a child, "I'm not angry with you!"
- An ataxic patient staggers into the ED with a strong odor of alcohol on his breath and slurs, "I only had a coupla beers."
- On learning of his wife's death, a grieving husband begins shaking uncontrollably with tears streaming down his cheeks. When a caring health-care provider offers solace, he continues to say, "I'm fine! Really, I'm just fine!"

Implicit biases may lead to health-care disparities by affecting clinical judgment and decision-making. As such, it is incumbent on ED personnel to recognize and thoughtfully reflect on how these stereotypes and prejudices may affect their patient care.

CONFLICT MANAGEMENT: GENERAL PRINCIPLES AND FRAMEWORKS

Several conceptual frameworks are useful in managing conflict. These include shared governance, leadership choices, and taking personal responsibility for behavior change.

Shared Governance

Instituting shared governance programs (SGPs) is an excellent method of reducing intradepartmental conflict. Unlike traditional quality processes that emphasize blaming outliers, SGPs emphasize collaborative improvement of processes by generating broad participation. Staff members are encouraged to give input, requesting their feedback acknowledges their expertise in and direct responsibility for system efficiency. Shared governance programs decrease departmental stress and increase accountability, both of which are critical elements in creating a team approach to problem-solving and, ultimately, decreasing conflict.

Leadership Choices

In an organization committed to SGPs, leaders may choose to regularly meet one-on-one with employees (i.e., Studer's "rounding for outcomes") to identify evolving problems.[32,33] Judgments about who is right or wrong are de-emphasized; instead, staff members are empowered to work with leaders to initiate solutions in a timely manner. Creating an open environment, seeking critical feedback, and avoiding blame all decrease stress and may prevent conflict before it occurs.

Personal Responsibility for Behavior Change

The first step in behavior change requires individuals to recognize they have no control over anyone's behavior but their own. Some individuals think, "It sure seems like there are a lot of difficult people out there. I don't do anything to provoke them." However, the most difficult people often don't realize they're triggering stressful interactions. A person who regularly becomes frustrated during times of stress may significantly contribute to the frustration of others, further increasing conflict. That person's conduct and communication skills merit review and self-reflection (i.e., "What is my role in this?").

Behavior patterns are extremely difficult to change. People frequently repeat previous behaviors whether successful or not; they don't always learn from their mistakes. If we extrapolate from the experiments of the psychologist Guthrie, responses to stimuli tend to become habitual.[34] Thus, it is likely that if a person has an ineffective response to a stressful situation, that same response will recur when that person is confronted with similar circumstances. In fact, in times of crisis, most people tend to repeat an individualized, consistent pattern of behavior they developed in childhood. Reflecting on one's own response to stress can lead to adaptation and more appropriate responses. Consider the admonition, "When angry, count to ten before you speak." While a somewhat simple intervention, it is an example of placing "time and space" between the stimulus and the response.

> *Human freedom involves our capacity to pause between stimulus and response and, in that pause, to choose the one response toward which we wish to throw our weight.*
>
> —Rollo May[35]

> **BOX 8.3 ■ CONCEPTUAL MODELS OF CONFLICT**
>
> - Thomas-Kilmann conflict mode
> - DISC personality profile
> - Meyers-Briggs
> - *Getting to Yes* by Fisher and Ury

MODELS FOR ASSESSING AND RESPONDING TO CONFLICT

By adopting a conflict management framework, leaders can take a broader view of conflict, thus facilitating resolution. There are several ways to view conflict; four methods are listed in **Box 8.3**.

Thomas-Kilmann Conflict Mode

Thomas and Kilmann defined a matrix illustrating five distinct styles of negotiation (that is, responses to conflict) that fall along two axes (**Figure 8.1**).[36] One axis, assertiveness, describes the extent to which individuals attempt to satisfy their own concerns. The other axis, cooperativeness, identifies the extent to which an individual attempts to satisfy another person's concerns.

The five styles of negotiation are:

- *Competing*: assertive, uncooperative
- *Avoiding*: unassertive, uncooperative
- *Accommodating*: unassertive, cooperative
- *Compromising*: intermediate assertiveness, cooperativeness
- *Collaborating*: assertive, cooperative[37]

Each style may be useful in a particular situation; for example, competing may be best when the outcome is more important than the relationship. Simultaneously, certain styles

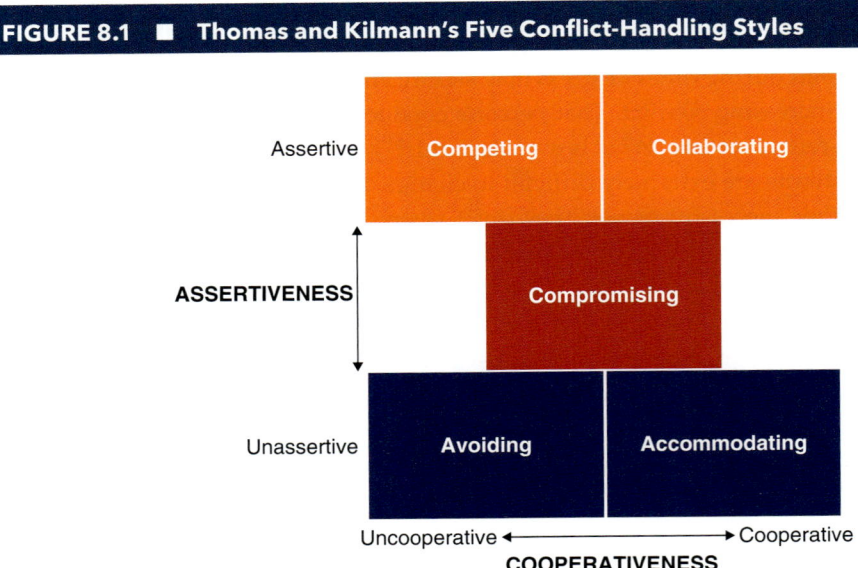

FIGURE 8.1 ■ Thomas and Kilmann's Five Conflict-Handling Styles

TABLE 8.1 ■ Negotiation Response Styles

Response	Assertiveness Level	Cooperation Level	Use When	Avoid When
Avoiding	Low	Low	Relationship and outcome are unimportant	Relationship or outcome are important
Accommodating	Low	High	Relationship is more important than outcome	Outcome is important
Competing	High	Low	Outcome is more important than relationship	Relationship is important
Compromising	Moderate	Moderate	Outcome and relationship are somewhat important	
Collaborating	High	High	Outcome and relationship are very important	Relationship or outcome is unimportant

should be avoided when the goals or outcomes are important; for example, the avoiding style should not be used when the outcome is important (**Table 8.1**).

The collaborating style is the most complex style of conflict resolution; yet, it is the best method to adopt when the relationship is long term and the outcome is important to both parties. The style has a "win-win" goal—both parties achieve desired, acceptable outcomes. Collaboration is characterized by high assertiveness and high cooperativeness; it integrates perspectives. Exploring the issues in depth and confronting differences are integral components of this strategy. This style often results in increased commitments and improved relationships among parties.

DISC Personality Profile

The DISC personality profile is a model based on observable behaviors. First introduced by William Marston in 1926, DISC describes four distinct traits of behavior: dominance (or drive), influence, steadiness, and compliance.[38] The intent of the profile is to help individuals understand their own and others' traits so they can avoid, reduce, or manage conflict while working with others (**Table 8.2**).

TABLE 8.2 ■ DISC Traits

Trait	Description
Dominance	Achievers and self-starters. They are direct, decisive, driven, and push themselves and others.
Influence	Enjoy people and attention, life of the party. They are motivators, fun, and persuasive.
Steadiness	Understanding, supportive, and good listeners. They are loyal and steady.
Compliance	Neat and organized. They are analytical, systematic, detailed, and accurate.

The DISC model identifies an individual's primary trait, although people may display additional traits or styles when interacting in different roles (e.g., department chair, clinician, spouse, parent, etc.). DISC profile tests are available online, providing immediate results that offer detailed personality assessments. With the newer "Everything DISC" profiling system, the test-taker responds to several phrases using a Likert scale to identify the degree to which the phrase describes the individual.

The profile may be used to help an individual work more effectively with others; many businesses use it to enhance teamwork, improve relations, and decrease work conflict.[39] Residency training programs have had success using this tool with residents and residency administrators.

Myers-Briggs Type Indicator

The Myers–Briggs type indicator (MBTI) is adapted from Jungian theory of personality types.[40,41] Although initially created to help individuals determine the job best suited for their personality type, the MBTI is currently the most widely used personality assessment tool. The MBTI categorizes people by attitudes, functions, and lifestyles (**Table 8.3**). The Myers–Briggs test is intended to help people understand how they perceive the world and make decisions. Its advantages include its widespread use and depth of evaluation. However, its interpretation is complicated and difficult to apply in daily activities.

Getting to Yes by Fisher and Ury

Getting to Yes is a popular book written by the cofounders of the Harvard Negotiation Project, Roger Fisher and William Ury. It advocates the concept of principled conflict resolution that

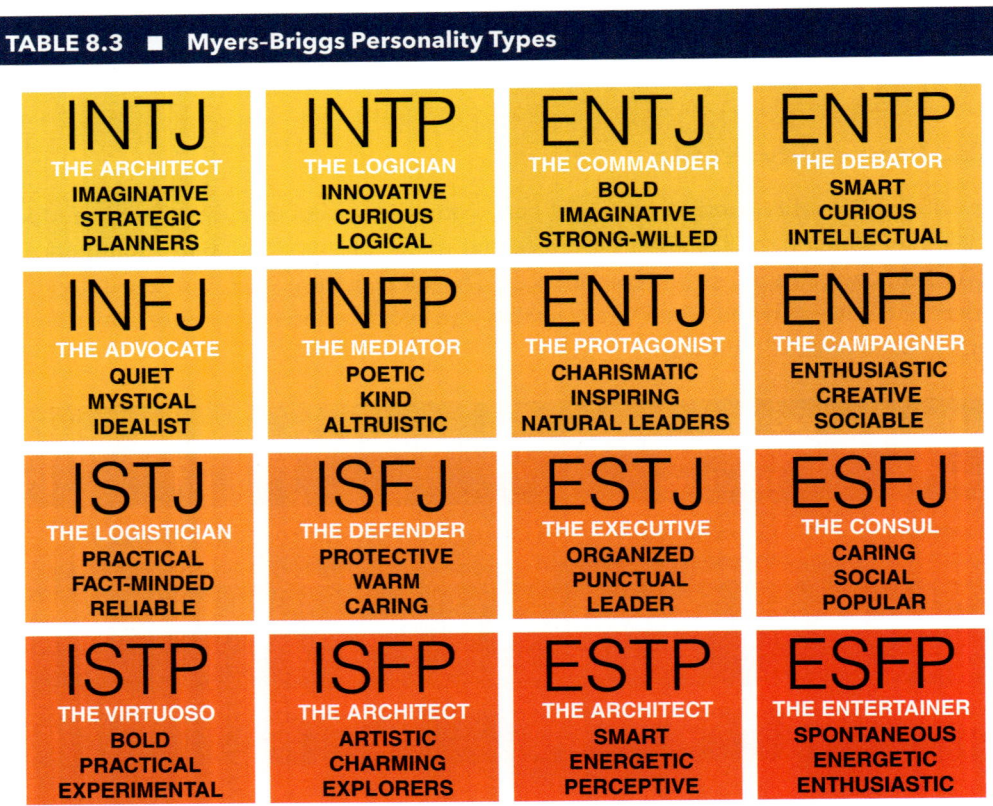

TABLE 8.3 ■ Myers-Briggs Personality Types

> **BOX 8.4 ■ FISHER AND URY'S *GETTING TO YES* SOLUTIONS**
>
> - Separate people from the problem.
> - Focus on interests, not positions.
> - Generate options for mutual gain.
> - Insist on objective criteria.

seeks "win-win" solutions similar to Thomas–Kilmann's collaborating style.[42] By being "hard" on concepts and "soft" on people, principled conflict resolution clarifies problems, validates emotions, discusses and explores interests, and develops objective criteria for solutions. Advantages of the approaches described in this book include their universal appeal, applicability of concepts, and utility for multiple situations (**Box 8.4**).

CONFLICT MANAGEMENT: SPECIFIC SKILLS

When used properly, many techniques can help manage and resolve conflict. However, even correct strategies may exacerbate disagreements when applied inappropriately. Conflict management begins with creating trust and listening effectively.

Creating Trust

It is difficult to negotiate where neither will trust.

—Samuel Johnson[43]

Effective communication occurs most easily in an environment of trust and respect. Supervisors who live in their offices except when criticizing staff or mandating new programs create an environment of apprehension and distrust. Leaders must get close to the people providing the services so they can understand the issues and conflicts first hand. Criticism of the night or weekend staff by ED leaders who never work nights or weekends often falls on deaf ears.

Alternatively, workers are more likely to listen to compassionate leaders with whom they identify. Leaders who listen to and acknowledge team members' issues are more likely to be perceived as understanding and more likely to be heard by the other side. The Mazda Way, for example, demonstrates a corporate-wide approach that hinges on a commitment to seven basic principles: integrity, flawless execution, continuous "Kaizen," challenger spirit, self-initiative, "Tomoiku," and "One Mazda." Each principle recognizes that *people* are the company's most important asset (**Figure 8.2**).[44]

Effective Listening

Although effective ED care requires rapid identification of problems and immediate response, staff members may move too quickly in some situations. Some health-care providers interrogate patients and staff in hurried and impatient tones, interrupting responses to their questions with further questions. When rushed, people may gloss over subtleties. Obtaining nuanced information depends on building trust and rapport. When people believe the other person is not listening, they may become frustrated, reserved, and vague, resulting in a breakdown in communication and withholding of sensitive information. Effective listening, a first step toward resolving the problem, is critical to improving trust, patient satisfaction, and outcomes. It is also one of the key qualities that minimizes litigation and conflict.

FIGURE 8.2 ■ The Mazda Way

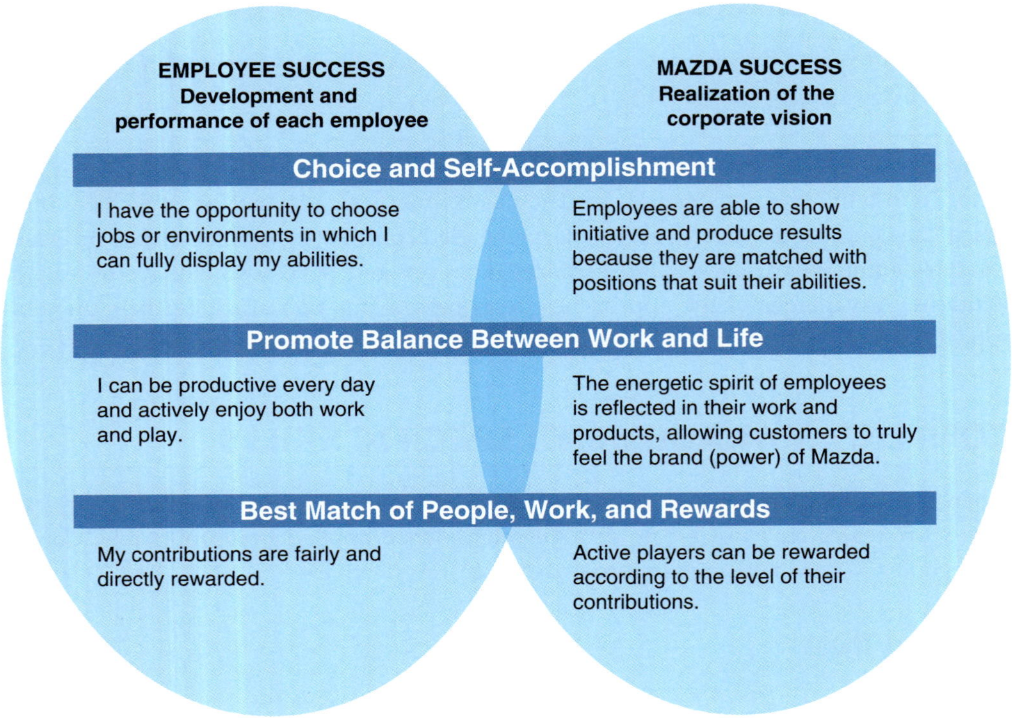

EMPLOYEE SUCCESS
Development and performance of each employee

MAZDA SUCCESS
Realization of the corporate vision

Choice and Self-Accomplishment

I have the opportunity to choose jobs or environments in which I can fully display my abilities.

Employees are able to show initiative and produce results because they are matched with positions that suit their abilities.

Promote Balance Between Work and Life

I can be productive every day and actively enjoy both work and play.

The energetic spirit of employees is reflected in their work and products, allowing customers to truly feel the brand (power) of Mazda.

Best Match of People, Work, and Rewards

My contributions are fairly and directly rewarded.

Active players can be rewarded according to the level of their contributions.

Many effective listening styles and techniques have been described in the literature.[45,46] In general, effective responses are neutral, without criticism or judgment, and often validating. Accepting the speaker's concerns creates the opportunity for clarification and further exploration (see **Box 8.5** for listening styles).

Consider the responses to the following comment by a staff member: "I just can't stop thinking about the child from the accident."

Impatient response: "You're overreacting, and you're getting too emotional about it. I would just put it out of my mind if I were you."

Although perhaps well meaning, this advice ignores the feelings of the staff member. This response inadvertently communicates criticism, dismissal, and lack of concern for the staff member's distress.

Passive response: "Hmmm."

Passive listening requires the listener to be quietly attentive. This behavior may encourage the speaker to continue discussing the issue and possibly get to the crux of the problem. Difficult issues take time to divulge and, like onions, may require peeling away layers before getting to

BOX 8.5 ■ LISTENING STYLES

- Passive
- Reflective
- Empathetic
- Validating

the center. A passive type of response can also help defuse angry reactions. To feel comfortable revealing a problem, people often need time and, at the very least, a safe environment.

Reflective response: "It seems like it's difficult to get him out of your thoughts."

Reflective listening involves providing objective feedback to the person expressing a concern. In its most rudimentary form, this response involves repeating the words back. This technique encourages the speaker to elaborate.

Empathetic response: "It sounds like you're worried about him."

This listener has decided to try to understand the speaker to get on the same side of the table. The listener has suspended a personal frame of reference and attempted to rephrase content and reflect feeling. This type of nonjudgmental and concerned listening allows speakers to address their feelings about the problem.

Sympathetic response: "I understand what you're going through. The same thing happened to me."

Sympathizing should be used with caution. Insincere sympathy may seem patronizing. Furthermore, the recipient of the "sympathetic" response may not believe that the person offering the sympathy really understands.

Acknowledging and validating response: "Yes, it is difficult to see a child suffer. Would you like to talk about it?"

When done correctly, acknowledging and validating responses allow the speaker to know the listener has heard and is substantiating the concern. Frequently, the speaker confirms the response by saying something like, "Yes, that's it exactly," or nodding in affirmation.

Eye Communication

Skilled communicators maintain good eye contact when listening to and speaking with others.[47] The pattern of eye contact (minimal, intermittent, or continuous) used by one person in a conversation will generally be copied unconsciously by the other person. Looking into another's eyes while listening (and speaking) demonstrates interest and attentiveness. Conversely, avoiding eye contact may be interpreted as a lack of interest. The listener can create an even greater sense of apparent interest by facing the other person and giving occasional nods of affirmation, a form of acknowledgment.

Focus on Interests, Not Positions

Positions are generally driven by underlying interests. As an example, consider two chefs who both insist on using the one remaining orange to create a dessert.[48] Positional bargaining would lead to an argument and perhaps one winner and one loser. However, once the underlying interests were understood (Chef A needed the rind, while Chef B needed the juice), both could be satisfied. Some of the most difficult people exhibit positional bargaining, as shown in the following example:

Admitting resident: "That's the third sick patient you've asked me to admit in the last hour. I won't do it." The position is "NO!"

Responding to the position is "taking the bait" and getting hooked into a win-lose situation. *A positional response might be:* "Oh, yeah? Well, you have to—and now! If you don't, I'll call your attending!"

> **BOX 8.6 ■ DISCREPANCY BETWEEN WORDS AND INTENT**
>
> | The actual words spoken: | The thoughts underlying the words: |
> |---|---|
> | A: Did you discharge the patient yet? | I have some free time, so if it isn't done yet, I can do it. |
> | B: I told you I would do it when I get the chance, and I will! Don't keep bugging me about it! | I have been incredibly busy doing more important things, and now you're criticizing me for taking five minutes for myself to get a cup of coffee. |
> | A: Well, never mind! | That is what I get for offering to help. |

Positional bargaining may, in fact, get the desired result. However, it generally creates a winner and a (resentful) loser. Furthermore, if these two parties work with each other again, the loser typically remembers and may try to get even.

The effectiveness of interest-based rather than position-based bargaining is evident in successful conflict management, negotiation, and complaint management. Continuing to concentrate on the interests of both parties often mitigates difficult situations. By focusing on the interest of the admitting resident, a solution may become clear immediately. A good interest-based listener will interpret the underlying message from the admitting resident as:

I'm tired, overwhelmed, and feeling out of control. I don't think I can handle another patient right now.

Responding to the message rather than the words would lead to a more effective reply:

Yes, your night has been difficult. I can hold the patient here for another 45 minutes until 3 A.M., while you catch up. Can you commit to being here by 3 A.M.?

Avoiding a direct response to the resident's position and instead responding to the resident's interests and needs may require minor compromise, but it allows both sides and the patient to get their needs met—everybody wins.

Separating the People From the Problem

Everyone has irritating behaviors. Although most people seek mutually satisfying and trusting relationships, they may quickly become suspicious and angry when someone is offended. In a stressful and hurried environment such as the ED, communication is often truncated and may inadvertently aggravate a situation. Under duress, stressed health-care professionals may not take the time to be polite ("Please . . ." or "When you get a chance, could you . . ."). Instead, they use verbal shortcuts ("Get the . . . now!"). Such communication may result in or increase conflict, especially between individuals without a history of positive exchanges. Successfully separating the person from the problem requires recognizing that people generally try to satisfy their own needs and obligations. To successfully resolve conflict, it may be necessary to discern the other person's underlying intent. Note how differently the scenario in **Box 8.6** would conclude if the underlying intent were recognized.[49]

When someone perceives a person's intentions as dishonorable, future actions tend to be interpreted in that same light. To avoid a conflict, a participant must examine the other person's motivations in a sincere and noncritical way. This may be accomplished by simply asking, "What was your reason for asking me if I had discharged the patient yet?" Or, "Why did you react negatively when I asked if you had discharged the patient yet?" Eventually, by continuing to explore each other's intentions, a positive outcome can be achieved, and miscommunication can be averted.

Responding to Emotion

Emotional actions breed emotional reactions. When one person is behaving obnoxiously, it is tempting to reciprocate with anger or respond emotionally by yelling, crying, door-slamming, or stomping. An emotional response may provide a momentary feeling of relief; however, this type of response will almost always make resolution and subsequent interactions more difficult or impossible. Silence is a powerful alternative response to difficult emotional interpersonal conflicts because escalation is less likely when one party avoids emotional engagement. Furthermore, those who can maintain composure and continue to focus on the interests of the other party (or parties) are more likely to enhance the resolution process.

THE MANDATE FOR BEHAVIORAL FEEDBACK

In the stressful ED environment, leaders may find it necessary to provide feedback to individual staff members. To encourage change, leaders should provide feedback. Behavioral feedback is mandated in Accreditation Council for Graduate Medical Education training programs, which evaluate behavior using the competencies of "professionalism" and "interpersonal and communication skills."[50]

Because inappropriate behavior can undermine the culture of safety, The Joint Commission mandates that "[institutional] leaders create and implement a process for managing disruptive and inappropriate behaviors."[51]

Structuring Feedback

Although feedback may be mandated or a consistent part of a program, behavioral commentary is often met with resistance unless structured in a manner that encourages receptivity. Feedback is accepted most readily when it is presented with positive, instructive, or constructive language and without blame, criticism, or judgment. The best environments for process improvement are those in which bidirectional feedback is encouraged, establishing a culture of feedback.

The "I" Message

The word "criticism" connotes judgment and disapproval; it should be avoided when commenting on behavior. Terms such as "input" or "feedback" are more readily accepted because they connote more objective and helpful consideration. Additionally, feedback is received more favorably when it is internally focused (on the person giving the feedback) rather than externally focused (on the person receiving the feedback) because it allows the feedback recipient to maintain self-esteem. Finally, labeling, personal attacks, and generalizations should be avoided. For example, the following comment voiced in an attempt to create positive behavior change is likely to be rejected:

"You are always too argumentative!"

> **BOX 8.7 ■ THE THOMAS GORDON MODEL**
>
> - When we/you . . .
> - I feel . . .
> - Because . . .

When giving feedback, emphasizing a point by using terms such as "always" and "never" will be poorly accepted because the recipient will likely perceive the comment as an unwelcome exaggeration. Furthermore, the term "argumentative" is a label describing a personal trait; it is unlikely to lead to a helpful insight or resolution. Conflict resolution expert Thomas Gordon suggests a more effective alternative for providing behavioral feedback: using "I" statements.[52] He advocates structuring feedback in three parts, with a clear description of the behavior and how it affects the person offering the feedback (**Box 8.7**).

- *When I/we*: The "when" statement should be specific, concrete, and observable. Simply and objectively recount the occurrence with a statement such as "When we argue. . . ." Avoid attacks and labeling, such as, "When you argue with me." Specific and objective words will be more easily accepted. For example, avoid a statement such as, "When you act the way you do . . .," which is too vague, or "When you behave like a jerk . . .," which attacks the person receiving feedback by labeling them.
- *I feel*: The "I feel" statement should express a sincere feeling that is consistent with the situation, such as "I feel angry (frustrated, upset, embarrassed)." Avoid phrases that are blaming or do not describe a feeling, such as "I feel like a child," (how does a child feel?) or "I feel like you don't care" (accusatory).
- *Because*: The "because" statement provides an opportunity to share motives and the desired outcome. A good example is, "I feel frustrated because it seems my ideas are not considered." Again, blaming should be avoided. Speakers should focus on the way the behavior affects them and their perception.

Effective "I" Statements

Using the Gordon model, the person providing feedback can effectively share the concern without blaming the other person, labeling, or exaggerating. In **Box 8.8**, the examples in the first column will probably be ineffective because the recipient of the feedback is likely to perceive blame and disapproval. The "I" statements in the second column are more likely

> **BOX 8.8 ■ EXAMPLES OF EFFECTIVE "I" STATEMENTS**
>
> | Blaming | Constructive |
> |---|---|
> | You are always too argumentative! | When we argue, **I feel frustrated** because it seems my ideas are not respected. |
> | I am furious with you because you always ignore me! | When I am ignored, **I feel upset** because my ideas aren't considered. |
> | You are so disrespectful; I can never count on you! | **I feel frustrated and resentful** when you arrive late for a shift because it disrupts my plans and I do not know whether to take care of waiting patients. |

to be met with receptivity, resulting in an effort to further examine and resolve the issue. Constructive feedback clarifies the problem, describes the resulting feeling, and defines the underlying issue to address. When done well, there is no blaming. This technique allows both parties to objectively examine ways to resolve the problem.

CPR: Content, Pattern, Relationship

In *Crucial Accountability* and *Crucial Conversations*, Patterson et al. promote the mnemonic CPR—content, pattern, relationship—as a way to appropriately respond during a confrontation without avoidance or aggression.[53,54] First, the leader identifies the *content*, or problem, in the current situation and then relates the present situation to a history of similar events, the *pattern*. Finally, the leader addresses their continuing interactions and trust of the parties, that is, the *relationship*. The CPR approach may be used to move toward a fair solution for all parties, and it is particularly valuable when a habitual pattern is noted. For example:

Content: A practitioner might say to a colleague who takes multiple long breaks, "Janet, I've noticed that you have taken five or six long breaks during the shift today."

Pattern: "I've noticed the same pattern when we've worked together recently."

Relationship: "Janet, I must be able to rely on you when we are working together. This pattern leads me to question whether or not I can."

While it appears simple, CPR can be difficult to put into practice when there is strong emotional content. With practice, CPR helps transition conflict from confrontation to resolution by avoiding blame or emotional finger pointing and, instead, objectively describing what has happened and what the speaker would like to see happen.

Averting Public Ridicule

Occasionally, an angry person may verbally abuse another person in a public space. This behavior makes most observers uncomfortable, and the unfortunate recipient of the ridicule will likely feel humiliated by this exposure. The person expressing discontent may not even recognize the inappropriateness of their behavior.

If a patient, coworker, or medical staff member is publicly expressing emotion in a loud or disruptive manner, the dysfunctional communication should be interrupted. The following process may help resolve the situation. The intervening person can:

1. Walk up to and stand in front of the speaker.
2. Gain the person's attention, and establish eye contact.
3. Quietly and firmly say, "I see you're upset. I'd like to talk with you about this issue over here."
4. Move to a more private space.
5. Address the issue.

Most angry people will go with the person who has offered to address the problem. Physically moving will itself begin to decompress the situation. (Note: This technique should not be used if there is any potential danger.)

Responding to a Complainer

In a busy ED, patients' expectations often go unmet. The two most common complaints from patients are "It's taking too long!" and "Nobody cares!" People who wait for a prolonged period and are treated rudely may be particularly vocal or hostile when expressing their discontent.

Habitual blamers tend to be angry and believe they should get their way; anything less may feel unacceptable. They may even believe they have not gotten what they deserve because people are insensitive and purposefully obstinate. Blamers often use personal pronouns, generalizations, and extreme language to make their point. They tend to be dramatic in both tone and gesture. Blamers may shake their finger, pound their fist, and be verbally threatening. The blamer, in essence, tries to place the responsibility for his or her problem on someone else. For example, a blaming patient who is tired of waiting might exclaim, "Why is it that every time I come here, I always have to sit around and wait for hours and hours? Don't any of you people care about anyone? Can't you see that I'm in agony?" But what the patient means is, "I want to be taken care of now!"

A placating patient is, in many ways, like a blaming patient.[55] The placater acts as if he or she or the system is personally responsible for the problem. The placater, like the blamer, uses many personal pronouns, generalizes, and places emphatic stress on words. However, instead of aggressively placing the responsibility for the problem on others, a placater is apologetic and appears to assume responsibility. A placater who is frustrated because of a prolonged wait might say, "I don't know why it is that I always seem to come when it is so busy. I don't like to complain, and I know that you doctors and nurses are so busy and my problem is so insignificant," when what they really mean is, "I want to be taken care of now!"

There are many ways to respond to complainers. Before choosing a response, recognize that a verbal assault is not necessarily directed at the unfortunate recipient. Although tempting, one should avoid taking the bait. An opportunity is created to address concerns when a complaining person confronts or blames someone.[54,55] An effective response may lead to immediate resolution, whereas an ineffective or defensive response may exacerbate the problem. Blaming the blamer will likely exacerbate the conflict, whereas placating, offering a blameless apology, or acknowledging and validating the patient's concerns might help resolve the issue.

Blaming a Blamer

If the health-care professional takes complaints personally, a blaming professional might blame the blamer and respond by saying, "Can't you see that we're busy? We're working as fast as we can! Your constant interruptions are delaying our getting to you. If you will just sit quietly and wait, we'll take care of you when it is your turn. There are people here who are really sick!"

Blaming a blamer puts the responsibility back on the original blamer. Joining this mudslinging contest gets everyone dirty; there are no winners. Inevitably, blaming back leads to escalation of the conflict. When the opportunity arises, the blamer will take his or her frustrations to the next level, with a letter to the CEO or an editorial to the local newspaper.

Placating

Professionals in a service industry such as health care commonly placate to resolve conflict. The placating professional apologizes and either assumes personal responsibility or apologizes for the inadequacy of others, such as, "I'm very sorry, I wish I could have been here sooner. You must be upset. It's been so busy and one of the x-ray machines is broken. I'm very sorry." What they really mean is, "It's not my fault."

Placating in response to conflict works—to some degree. Generally, it avoids escalation and allows the other side to blame the obliging apologizer. This behavior, however, causes the placater to feel inept and impotent. Furthermore, it does not substantially improve the situation.

Blameless Apology

An effective alternative to placating is the blameless apology: "I am sorry you've had to wait so long." This approach is reassuring and expresses concern for the perceived issue without assuming responsibility for the problem. It demonstrates that the provider cares and is listening.

Acknowledge and Validate

A particularly effective way of responding is to acknowledge and validate the expressed complaint. Ideally, the provider addresses the underlying concern. This approach eliminates blame, deals directly with and validates the patient's concern, and provides the complainer with what she really wants—attention, empathy, and responsiveness. This technique avoids "biting the hook" by assuming responsibility or blaming others. For example, "Yes, it's frustrating to wait when you're in pain. I'm here to take care of you now."

Objectively repeating the complaint from the complainer's perspective demonstrates an understanding of the issue. When possible and appropriate, the provider should immediately offer complainers the care and caring they want. If unable to provide a solution now, then it is appropriate to let the complainer know when to expect one

CONCLUSION

Conflict is inevitable and it has both benefits and costs. To effectively manage conflict, the parties must treat each other respectfully, recognizing that the other participants have real interests and needs that are important. Active listening and empathy may be the most important skills necessary to achieve satisfactory resolution. The other parties should not be considered adversaries to be overcome because winning at the expense of others does not bode well for future collaboration.

The process of developing collaborative solutions—satisfying their needs while achieving your goals—takes time and skill. The focus should be on creating an environment of mutual respect. Even when a conflict must be addressed immediately and unilaterally, such as in the emergent management of a critically ill patient, real-time input should be encouraged and respected.

When dealing with conflict, consider and respect the needs of others without neglecting your own. A culture of collaboration is essential to achieve the goal of providing high-quality care and caring in an ED environment.

With appreciation to Mary Kaye Halterman for contributions to a previous version of this chapter.

REFERENCES

1. Garmel GM. Conflict resolution in emergency medicine. In: Adams JG, Barton ED, Collings JL, et al., eds. *Emergency Medicine: Clinical Essentials*. 2nd ed. Philadelphia, Pa: Elsevier/Saunders; 2013.

2. Strauss RW, Garmel GM, Halterman MK. Conflict management. In: Strauss RW, Mayer T, eds. *Strauss and Mayer's Emergency Department Management*. Philadelphia, Pa: McGraw-Hill; 2013.

3. Tjosvold D. *Learning to Manage Conflict: Getting People to Work Together Productively*. New York, NY: Lexington Books; 2000.

4. Knaus WA, Draper EA, Wagner DP, Zimmerman JE. An evaluation of outcome from intensive care in major medical centers. *Ann Intern Med*. 1986;104(3):410-418.

5. Azoulay E, Timsit JF, Sprung CL, et al. Prevalence and factors of intensive care unit conflicts: the conflicus study. *Am J Respir Crit Care Med*. 2009;180(9):853-860.

6. Aiken LH, Clarke SP, Sloane DM, Sochalski J, Silber JH. Hospital nurse staffing and patient mortality, nurse burnout, and job dissatisfaction. *JAMA*. 2002;288(16):1987-1993.

7. Delucia J. Rate of post-traumatic stress disorder in emergency medicine physicians. Presented at: Society for Academic Emergency Medicine Meeting; May 10-13, 2016; New Orleans, La.

8. Vanyo L, Sorge R, Chen A, Lakoff D. Posttraumatic stress disorder in emergency medicine residents. *Ann Emerg Med*. 2017;70(6):898-903.

9. Mills LD, Mills TJ. Symptoms of post-traumatic stress disorder among emergency medicine residents. *J Emerg Med*. 2005;28(1):1-4.

10. Adriaenssens J, De Gucht V, Maes S. Determinants and prevalence of burnout in emergency nurses: A systematic review of 25 years of research. *Int J Nurs Stud*. 2015;52(2):649-661.

11. Puttonen S, Härmä M, Hublin C. Shift work and cardiovascular disease—pathways from circadian stress to morbidity. *Scand J Work Environ Health*. 2010;36(2) 96-108.

12. Coffey LC, Skipper JK, Jung FD. Nurses and shift work: effects on job performance and job-related stress. *J Adv Nurs*. 1988;13(2):245-254.

13. Perry SJ, Wears RL, Croskerry P, et al. Process improvement and patient safety. In Marx, JA, Hockberger RS, Walls RM, et al. *Rosen's Emergency Medicine: Concepts and Clinical Practice*. 7th ed. Philadelphia, Pa: Mosby; 2010:2547-2553.
14. Slapper DR. Emergency medicine is here to stay. What about emergency physicians? *American College of Emergency Physicians News*. 1991;10:7.
15. Lowry F. Emergency department staff not immune to PTSD. *Medscape*. March 5, 2015. Available at: https://www.medscape.com/viewarticle/840980. Accessed July 14, 2018.
16. Whitehead DC, Thomas H, Slapper DR. A rational approach to shift work in emergency medicine. *Ann Emerg Med*. 1992;21(10):1250-1258.
17. Kuhn G, Goldberg R, Compton S. Tolerance for uncertainty, burnout, and satisfaction with the career of emergency medicine. *Ann Emerg Med*. 2009;54(1):106-113.
18. Cooke T, Watt D, Wertzler W, Quan H. Patient expectations of emergency department care: phase II—a cross-sectional survey. *CJEM*. 2006;8(3):148-157.
19. Thompson DA, Yarnold PR, Williams DR, Adams SL. Effects of actual waiting time, perceived waiting time, information delivery, and expressive quality on patient satisfaction in the emergency department. *Ann Emerg Med*. 1996;28(6):657-665.
20. Toma G, Triner W, McNutt LA. Patient satisfaction as a function of emergency department previsit expectations. *Ann Emerg Med*. 2009:54(3):360-367.
21. Anderson RT, Camacho FT, Balkrishan R. Willing to wait?: The influence of patient wait time on satisfaction with primary care. *BMC Health Ser Res*. 2007. Available at: https://bmchealthservres.biomedcentral.com/articles/10.1186/1472-6963-7-31. Accessed July 11, 2018.
22. Mehrabian A. *Non-Verbal Communication*. Chicago, Ill: Aldine-Atherton; 1972.
23. Leape LL, Fromson JA. Problem doctors: is there a system-level solution? *Ann Intern Med*. 2006;144(2):107-115. doi:10.7326/0003-4819-144-2-200601170-00008.
24. McDonald O. American College of Physician Executives. Disruptive physician behavior. QuantiaMD. 2011. Available at: http://www.quantiamd.com/q-qcp/Disruptive_Physician_Behavior.pdf. Accessed July 19, 2018.
25. Kaul P. Differences in admission rates and outcomes between men and women presenting to emergency departments with coronary syndromes. *Can Med Assoc J*. 2007;177(10):1193-1199.
26. Katz JD. Gender bias in diagnosing fibromyalgia. *Gend Med*. 2010;7(1):19-27.
27. Chen EH. Gender disparity in analgesic treatment of emergency department patients with acute abdominal pain. *Acad Emerg Med*. 2008;15(5):414-418.
28. Safdar P. Impact of physician and patient gender on pain management in the emergency department—a multicenter study. *Pain Med*. 2009;10(2):364-372.
29. 29. Stepanikova I. Effects of poverty and lack of insurance on perceptions of racial and ethnic bias in health care. *Health Serv Res*. 2008;43(3):915-930.
30. Cabana MD, Lara M, Shannon J. Racial and ethnic disparities in the quality of asthma care. *Chest*. 2007:1329(5)810S-817S.
31. Dutch MJ, Taylor D, Dent AW. Triage presenting complaint descriptions bias emergency department waiting times. *Acad Emerg Med*. 2008:15(8):731-735.
32. Studer Q. *Hardwiring Excellence*. Pensacola, Fla: Fire Starter Publishing; 2003.
33. Thomsen S. 5 Questions to ask when leadership rounding on the front lines. Huron. 2015. Available at: http://www.myrounding.com/blog/5-questions-to-ask-when-leadership-rounding-on-front-lines. Accessed July 2, 2018.
34. Hill WF. *Learning: A Survey of Psychological Interpretations*. New York, NY: Harper & Row; 1990.
35. May R. *The Courage to Create*. New York, NY: Norton Paperback, 1975.
36. Thomas-Kilmann conflict mode instrument. Available at: http://kilmanndiagnostics.com/Library/_notes/TKI_Sample_Report.pdf. Published 1974. Accessed April 2011.
37. Wikipedia, Thomas-Kilmann Conflict Mode Instrument. Available at: https://en.m.wikipedia.org/wiki/Thomas%E2%80%93Kilmann_Conflict_Mode_Instrument. Accessed December 15, 2019.
38. Marston WM. *Emotions of Normal People*. New York, NY: Harcourt, Brace and Co; 1928.
39. Center for Internal Change, How to Determine. DISC Profile. 2019. Available at: http://www.onlinediscprofile.com/. Accessed December 15, 2019.
40. The Myers-Briggs Foundation, The Myers-Briggs Type Indicator. 2019. Available at: http://www.myersbriggs.org/. Accessed December 15, 2019.
41. Wikipedia, Myers'-Briggs Type Indicator. 2011. Available at: http://en.wikipedia.org/wiki/Myers-Briggs_Type_Indicator. Accessed February 2011.
42. Fisher R, Ury W, Patton B. *Getting to Yes: Negotiating Agreement Without Giving In*. London, England: Penguin Books; 2011.
43. Johnson S. *Rasselas, Prince of Abyssinina*. Chapter 37. London, United Kingdom: Cassell and Company; 1889. Available at: http://www.gutenberg.org/files/652/652-h/652-h.htm. Accessed June 30, 2018.
44. Three pillars of Tobiuo, Mazda Sustainability Report. 2017:93. Available at: http://www.mazda.com/globalassets/en/assets/csr/pdf/pdf_employee.pdf. Accessed June 24, 2018.
45. Burley-Allen M. *Listening: The Forgotten Skill*. New York, NY: John Wiley and Sons, Inc; 1995.
46. Nichols MP. *The Lost Art of Listening: How Learning to Listen Can Improve Relationships*. New York, NY: The Guilford Press; 2009.
47. Argyle M. *Bodily Communication*. New York, NY: International Universities Press; 1988.
48. MIT, Interests vs. Positions. Available at: http://web.mit.edu/negotiation/www/NBivsp.html. Accessed December 15, 2019.
49. Tannen D. *You Just Don't Understand: Women and Men in Conversation*. New York, NY: William Morrow Paperbacks; 2007.
50. Common Program Requirements. Competencies. 2019. Available at: acgme.org/What-We-Do/Accreditation/Common-Program-Requirements/articleid/3845. Accessed December 12, 2019.
51. Behaviors that undermine a culture of safety, Sentinel Event Alert. 2008. 40. The Joint Commission. Available at: http://www.jointcommission.org/assets/1/18/SEA_40.PDF. Accessed July 14, 2018.
52. Gordon T. *Teacher Effectiveness Training: The Program Proven to Help Teachers Bring Out the Best in Students of All Ages*. New York, NY: Bantam Books; 2003.
53. Patterson K, Grenny J, Maxfield D, et al. *Crucial Accountability*. New York, NY: McGraw-Hill; 2013.
54. Patterson K, Grenny J, McMillan R, et al. *Crucial Conversations*. New York, NY: McGraw-Hill; 2012.
55. Haden-Elgin S. *The Gentle Art of Verbal Self Defense* (Revised and Updated). New York, NY: Fall River Press Edition; 2009.

CONDUCTING HIGH-IMPACT MEETINGS

CHAPTER 9

Robert W. Strauss

Every meeting generates a host of little follow-up meetings—some formal, some informal, but both stretching out for hours. Meetings, therefore, need to be purposefully directed. An undirected meeting is not just a nuisance; it is a danger. But above all, meetings have to be the exception rather than the rule. An organization in which everybody meets all the time is an organization in which no one gets anything done. Wherever a time log shows the fatty degeneration of meetings—whenever, for instance, people in an organization find themselves in meetings a quarter of their time or more—there is time-wasting malorganization.

—Peter Drucker[1]

When professionals achieve greater success in organizations, they tend to spend more time in meetings, considering strategic options, developing plans, solving problems, and sharing critical information. Some managers spend more than 50% of their average work week in meetings, in addition to the time spent preparing for and performing tasks assigned in a meeting.[2-4] An endless stream of meetings can leave little time for other work.

Hofstra University and Harrison Consulting Services determined that three-fourths of business leaders spend more time in meetings now than they did a few years ago and expect to spend even more time in meetings in the future.[4] This time expenditure would be acceptable if meetings were valuable, yet people often state that meetings actually interfere with accomplishing their objectives. A poll of 471 management leaders conducted by Communispond reported that 70% of the participants found meetings "a waste of time," and a study of 38,000 Microsoft employees determined that 70% found meetings unproductive.[3,5] Accountemps determined that an average executive spends 2 months each year in unnecessary meetings.[6]

WHY MEETINGS FAIL

Meetings are indispensable when you don't want to do anything.
—John Kenneth Galbraith, economist (1903-2006)

Meetings usually fail for one or more reasons[7-10]:

Poor leadership: The chair is disorganized, does not establish order or exert the discipline necessary to control input. Meeting leaders may be overly talkative, perhaps insisting on their own point of view; conversely, they may be too reserved to provide meaningful input. These chairs may not establish or follow an agenda and have little regard for the time or input of the participants, blocking effective communication.

Poor participation: The participating members are disinterested (information is not relevant to them), routinely unprepared or late (are not held accountable), or participating in other endeavors (side conversations, catching up on other responsibilities, or texting) during the meeting.

Poor time management: Meetings that neither begin nor end on time are discouraging to participants who are unable to rely on an efficient process. Consider those participants who show up on time only to find that the meeting begins late or the leader has not yet shown up. Even more frustrating are meetings that go beyond the predefined ending time, interfering with other appointments.

Poor organization: These meetings lack a clear purpose or agenda, and they may begin late or run overtime. The members may speak anytime without being recognized, and there is one digression after another. Emotional responses may be directed at another person. The room is too hot, and members cannot see visual aids.

Poor meetings waste time that could have been devoted to more valuable efforts. So why have meetings? Because effective, well-organized, and well-led meetings are a center of creative and effective communication. To be effective, meetings require thoughtful preparation, sensitive and purposeful leadership, and a strong focus on meeting the group's objectives.

THE VALUE OF MEETINGS

Reasons to Avoid a Meeting

First, determine whether the meeting is necessary (**Box 9.1**).[11] Meetings that occur out of habit (e.g., "because we always meet") should be reconsidered and possibly eliminated. If the organizer cannot develop a meaningful agenda, then find an alternative method for accomplishing the goal. Unfortunately, some ritualistic meetings, like Linus's blanket, are not easily abandoned. An example might be meetings held at the same time each month about the same topics.

If there are no decisions to be made or you are unsure what will be accomplished, skip the meeting. A meeting is unnecessary when there is no important information to share, no question to be asked, no problem to be solved, or the answer is already known and the leader does not need permission or buy-in to accomplish the goal. Avoid meetings when greater involvement will only confuse the issue.

Reasons to Have a Meeting

Most meetings have one of two purposes: information transmission or problem-solving. Meetings may be an efficient way to communicate to a large group or the most effective way to make certain decisions (**Box 9.2**).[12,13]

Information transmission: This type of meeting provides a forum for the simultaneous dissemination of information and creates a pool of consistent knowledge. Typical examples include defining and promoting a group's mission, educational seminars, training sessions, project reports, and program updates.

BOX 9.1 ■ REASONS TO AVOID A MEETING

- No decisions to be made
- No meaningful information to share
- Information easily shared by memo, newsletter, or e-mail

> **BOX 9.2 ■ REASONS TO HAVE A MEETING**
>
> **Can you answer YES to all these questions?**
>
> 1. Do I know what problem I want to solve?
> 2. Do I need help or input?
> 3. Does help or input require simultaneous involvement of others?
> 4. Must the meeting be in person?

If the presentation is long or the group is large, audiovisual aids can enhance engagement and interest by helping the participants focus on the major points. During or after this type of presentation, the speaker should check for understanding and reactions and provide any necessary clarifications.

Problem-solving: Problem-solving meetings are generally held to identify and address issues, develop solutions, make determinations, and identify implementation steps (**Box 9.3**). The premise of a problem-solving meeting is that that an issue exists that the members of the group have an interest in and can help solve. A group is generally more creative and better at decision-making than an equivalent number of individuals working alone.[3]

An additional advantage of group decision-making is that participation creates awareness of and commitment to the solution, which results in more effective and complete implementation. Jim Whitehurst, CEO of Red Hat, states that if those affected are involved from the start, change occurs more easily.[14] If the problem is solvable by a single person and commitment to the decision is unnecessary, a problem-solving meeting may be unnecessary.

Hospital staff and administration carry out their business by committee. Emergency department (ED) team members are uniquely positioned to be valuable contributors to these meetings because they interact with the entire medical staff, every inpatient unit, all hospital-based programs, thousands of community members, and large portions of the community's support and service programs.

By working toward the common good of the institution, ED clinicians can be instrumental in designing and implementing the institution's programs. The ED team can have a meaningful voice and presence that foster their recognition as peers and leaders. Over time, active participation will provide a broader perspective on the ED and its issues, so members of the ED should have representation on all key committees (**Table 9.1**).[15,16]

Telemeetings: the Alternative to In-Person Meetings

Virtual or online meetings are an excellent alternative to in-person meetings, particularly when necessary members are not near the hospital. The requirements are minimal: a computer, an Internet connection, and conferencing software. There are both advantages and disadvantages to choosing telemeetings over in-person meetings as well as rules and protocols to make telemeetings effective.

> **BOX 9.3 ■ VALUE OF PROBLEM-SOLVING MEETINGS**
>
> - Identify issues.
> - Analyze situations.
> - Clarify goals.
> - Develop solutions.

TABLE 9.1 ■ Critical ED Committees

Committee	MD	RN	Advantage of active membership
Executive	✓		• Ensures ED's perspective is represented • Allows venue for discussion of ED strategic initiatives • Permits simultaneous dialogue with most medical staff and administrative leaders • Limits or prevents backstabbing complaints about the ED
Disaster	✓	✓	• Uses ED practitioners' unique knowledge of and expertise in EMS, triage, resource use, emergency intervention, communications, etc • Creates hospital and community leadership opportunity • Ensures best use of ED resources in a disaster
Credentials	✓		• Ensures ED's perspective is represented • Promotes fair evaluation of emergency physician candidates • Permits deep insight into medical staff members' interests and issues • (May) advance ED interests related to medical staff responsibilities
ED steering or governance	✓	✓	• Advances shared ED governance, responsibility, and accountability • Broadens representation • Creates a forum for consensus development, strategic planning, and team building
Performance improvement	✓	✓	• Reviews and provides perspective on high-visibility cases • Integrates ED quality programs in hospital-wide programs • Develops performance improvement strategies
Safety	✓	✓	• Aligns and integrates hospital safety standards • Analyzes hospital and ED safety issues • Develops plans to refine hospital and ED safety plans • Interacts with hospital leaders and board members

Advantages

- *Ease of attendance*: The most common reasons for scheduling online meetings are increasing attendance, improving productivity, and decreasing the time, burden, and expense of travel. Participants attend by simply turning on a computer and connecting to the meeting. When a member is hundreds of miles away, participation might only be possible online.
- *Informal*: Members can participate in a relaxed setting without the need to dress in formal attire.
- *Fewer documents*: Digital attachments significantly reduce the number of paper documents typically provided to support onsite presentations.

Disadvantages

- *Distractions*: Because their inattention may not be noticed, online members may be tempted to multitask, especially when the topic is of limited interest to the participant. Loss of focus limits the potential of the discussion.
- *Personal connection*: Because so much communication and interpersonal feedback is related to body language, a presenter will not have the ability to observe and respond to the reception of the distant members, particularly with voice-only participation.

- *Sensitive discussions*: Meetings intended to address difficult issues or those requiring particularly nuanced decisions are best managed in person.
- *Technical issues*: There are several technical problems that can delay or disrupt an online meeting. Generally, all participants must have the same conference software loaded and running. The push of a (wrong) button might disconnect everyone. Inadequate Internet connections hamper communication.

Of note, video conferencing addresses many of the disadvantages of voice-only meetings. Video conferencing participation is enhanced when the entire group (not just the person speaking) is visible. With generally available software, presentation materials can be reviewed in real time, participants can see each other's reactions, and attention is substantially improved.

Telemeeting Rules

Participation protocols for telemeetings can and should be discussed and agreed on in advance. Ground rules are particularly valuable when there is no access to video, and it is difficult to know who is present, when to speak, or the reactions of others to the discussion. Some basic considerations include the following[17]:

- *Announce your arrival.* If late, do not interrupt, but rather wait for a pause in the discussion.
- *Limit background noise.* Keep your phone on mute when not speaking. Ensure there is no musical or promotional background when on hold.
- *Know the agenda.* Familiarize yourself with the meeting schedule and materials ahead of time.
- *When speaking, introduce yourself each time.* "This is Rob, I'd like to consider . . ." Be brief, be courteous, and avoid interrupting.

MEETING PREPARATION

Good meetings are well-orchestrated events. The first critical element of successful meetings is *planning*; organizing the meeting in advance allows the group to most efficiently accomplish its objectives (**Box 9.4**).[18] Preparing for a meeting includes developing objectives, creating an agenda, inviting the appropriate people, and preparing the room logistics. Less time is spent in meetings when more time is spent preparing for them.

Determine the Purpose

All too often, meetings seem to exist without purpose. A poorly clarified set of goals and objectives for the meeting confuses participants and wastes their time. When preparing for a

---

BOX 9.4 ■ MEETING PREPARATION

- Determine the purpose.
- Develop an agenda.
- Select participants.
- Set the scene.
- Seat for success.

meeting, leaders should determine its intended purpose in order to share its importance and specific goals. Thoughtful preparation and distribution of clearly stated objectives improves the likelihood of accomplishing them. If several objectives are listed on the agenda, they should be prioritized to ensure that the most important issues receive appropriate attention. Once the objectives are clear, the meeting leaders should create a plan to accomplish those objectives and to figuratively "write the minutes before the meeting."

Effective leaders do not necessarily define the outcome of the meeting, but they *do* determine how to achieve to an outcome. In other words, they create an essential agenda that addresses several critical questions:

- What will be discussed?
- Who needs to be present?
- How long will it take?
- What outcomes address the meeting's purpose?

Develop an Agenda

The agenda is the most important document required for a successful meeting.[3,7] An agenda is a road map, timetable, overview, advertisement, and goal-setter (**Box 9.5**). It cues the presiding officer, enlists the attention of members, and keeps participants moving in the same direction at the same time. More time spent preparing an agenda will mean less time in the meeting. The agenda should be complete but accomplishable. If the time runs out before the meeting does, participants will be left with the impression of disorganization and poor prioritization. The agenda should be circulated in advance to allow members to plan for their participation.

State goals and objectives. The statement at the beginning of the agenda communicates the chair's overall vision for the meeting.

List discussion topics. Participants prefer to know in advance what will happen and what is expected of them. An agenda that is divided into its component parts will help organize and focus the discussion, allowing the chair to redirect a wandering group. It may be helpful to mark items for information, discussion, or decision-making to cue members to expectations. When developing the agenda, leadership consultant Roger Schwarz recommends seeking input from the participants on specific agenda items that are of particular interest to them.[19]

Sequence topics. Provide an orderly framework for the meeting's topics by placing them in a logical sequence. When discussion flows from one topic to another, it becomes easier to develop support for the issue and the meeting is more manageable. A well-organized approach will facilitate work on key concepts. Some leaders suggest beginning with topics that require creativity, which allows adequate time to be spent on the most complex issues. Others recommend an orderly progression of topics beginning with easier, less taxing topics, and proceeding to more difficult and complex issues.

BOX 9.5 ■ MEETING AGENDA ITEMS

1. Title of meeting
2. Date, start and end times
3. Location
4. List of invited individuals
5. Meeting goals and objectives
6. List of topics:
   a. Use action verbs to describe the objective.
   b. Provide a brief summary (optional).
7. Supporting documents

Distribute in advance. Circulating the agenda in advance enables members to come to the meeting prepared. This practice also allows the group members to confirm the time of the meeting and review the topics for discussion. The chair must consider each topic and come prepared. Advance circulation eliminates the most common cause of confusion at the beginning of a meeting, the question of what is being discussed, and shows consideration for participants.

Provide supporting documents. Supporting documents should be attached and sent in advance with the agenda, so that members may become familiar with the information before the meeting, unless the documents contain confidential information that must be protected.

List action items. Most agenda items require specific action by members of the group.[20,21] The group members will accomplish more when the agenda specifically defines what is to be done with a topic. When creating an agenda, it may be helpful to review *Bloom's Taxonomy Action Verbs*, including the following examples[22]:

- Review the available options to . . .
- Determine the best approach to . . .
- Establish guidelines for . . .
- Develop education program for . . .
- Identify potential contributors to . . .

Select Appropriate Participants

The planner must decide who should attend the meeting, avoiding these common but irrelevant reasons[23,24]:

- *"They've always been at the meeting" (a ritual).* Inviting individuals who will not meaningfully contribute to the discussion is a waste of time and can disrupt the meeting.
- *"Let's get agreeable members for quick and easy decisions" (a rubber stamp).* Homogeneity (choosing those with a similar perspective) leads to quick decisions that have worked in the past. Few alternatives or creative options will be considered, and leadership challenges will be rare. A homogeneous group falls prey to "groupthink" and tends to exhibit stereotypic behavior and superficial decisions.[25]
- *"Let's include everyone" (a public relations event).* Large groups (more than 12-15) tend to be ineffective at decision-making.

Relevant considerations for membership include the following[23,26]:

- ***Topic expertise:*** the knowledge and potential to contribute
- ***Authority:*** the power to make a decision
- ***Responsibility:*** the ability to implement a decision
- ***Stakeholder or end user:*** those directly affected by the decision

A diverse group produces the most innovative thinking because they bring more information, alternatives, opinions, and creativity. Decisions made by a diverse group will occur more slowly, but these decisions are generally more nuanced, complex, and lasting. The group will be less complacent and will drive for innovative solutions.

Set the Scene

Although the perfect meeting environment will not guarantee a success, an uncomfortable room that is hot, stuffy, noisy, or overly dark will certainly increase the likelihood of failure. When planning the room setting, consider the following physical characteristics:

Room size: Choose a room that corresponds to the group's size. A small group in a very large room will create distance between individuals that hinders communication, undermining attention, and group cohesiveness.[2,13,23] A small room may quickly get hot, stuffy, and oppressive, squelching meaningful discussion. People seated too closely together may be uncomfortable and become agitated.

Room aesthetics: Dissention is more likely to occur when people are crowded into an unattractive room for a prolonged period. Poor aesthetics can produce monotony, irritability, fatigue, and hostility. A red room quickly becomes unpleasant. Lighter shades of blue, green, or beige are the most relaxing and conducive to successful group communication and "relaxed concentration."[2,24]

Environment: The environment is rarely considered by meeting attendees unless there is a problem. The room should be attractive, clean, well ventilated, and well lit and allow an unobstructed view of the presenters and audiovisuals. Acoustics should be adequate and the temperature comfortable. Refreshments may be appropriate because "breaking bread" creates a more cohesive group; the meeting should make everybody feel nourished.

Seating arrangement to enhance success: Seating configuration should be specifically designed to accomplish the meeting's objective. A formal classroom or theater-style configuration limits interaction, which is ideal for an information transmission meeting such as a lecture or training seminar (**Figure 9.1**).[2,8,24]

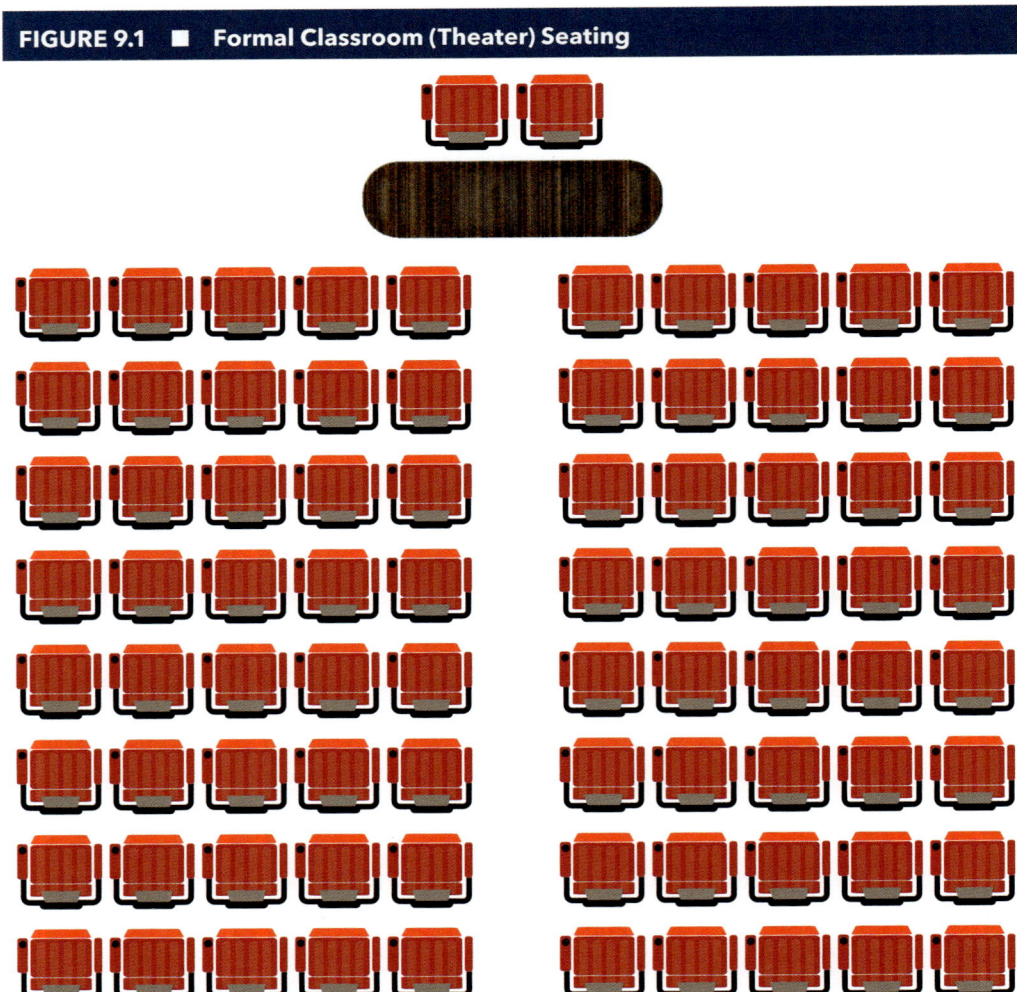

FIGURE 9.1 ■ Formal Classroom (Theater) Seating

FIGURE 9.2 ■ Circular Seating

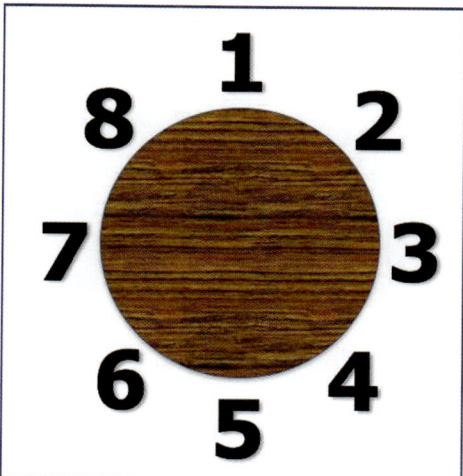

Circular seating limits the authority of any individual and encourages all members to participate.

A decentralized or circular arrangement (**Figure 9.2**) encourages the exchange of ideas and is more appropriate for a smaller group when the goal is problem-solving or decision-making. These configurations enhance group interaction and are particularly suitable for meetings addressing complex issues requiring careful deliberation.

A circular arrangement maximizes interaction and participation but removes the leader from the position of power, which may lead to more disagreements. However, because satisfaction with decisions is generally based on participation, members will tend to be more satisfied with and confident about the solutions when they contribute. The solutions from an engaged group will tend to be more detailed and contain fewer errors.

Positions of Power and Weakness

The positions of the group members in a noncircular seating arrangement will significantly influence their participation and control of the meeting.

Positions of dominance: The head of the table is the most dominant position.[2,27] Leaders tend to sit at the head of the table; therefore, the people who sit at the head of the table tend to emerge as leaders (**Figure 9.3**). Attention is focused at the head of a table: it is easy to hear and be heard, to see and be seen.

FIGURE 9.3 ■ Dominant Seating Positions

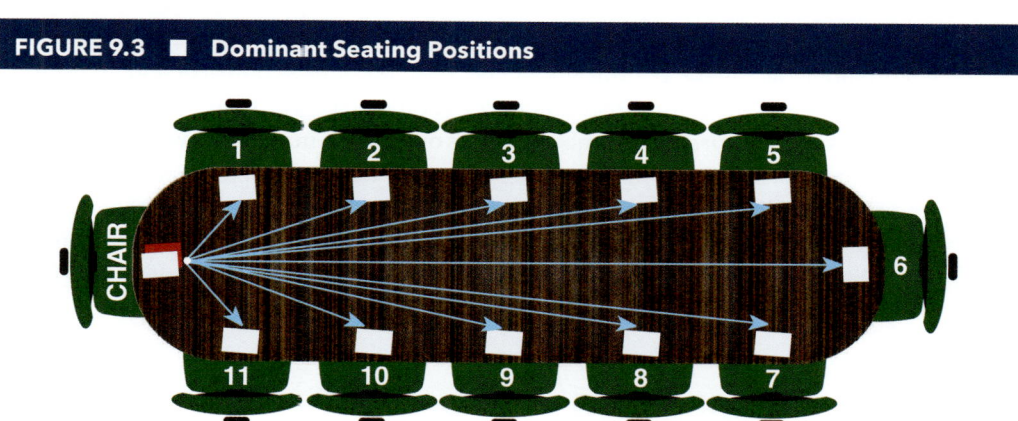

Positions around the table significantly influence the participation of the members. leaders sitting at the head of the table simultaneously have visual access to and influence over all members.

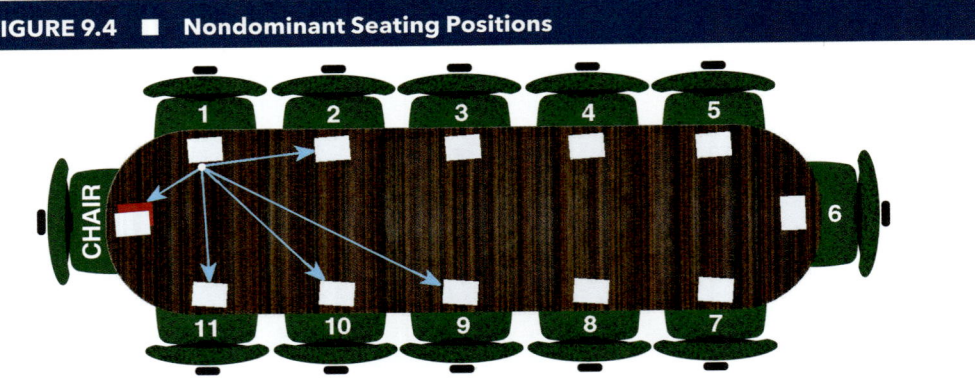

FIGURE 9.4 ■ Nondominant Seating Positions

Corner sitters have the least visual access to and influence over most members, other than the chair.

Positions of nondominance: Corner and middle seats are nondominant positions. Corner sitters tend to be the least active (**Figure 9.4**), but they can potentially influence the chair during a sidebar conversation. A leader who sits in a nondominant position may have to struggle for attention and control. Sitting in the middle of the long side of a table will limit visibility and communication, particularly with those facing the same direction. A chair who sits in the corner is in the weakest position with the least visual access to other participants.

Strategic placement of group members: It may be possible to place members of the group to create the most favorable interaction.[2,21] Any manipulation of seating must occur before the meeting begins. Methods include setting place cards, inviting a member to sit next to you, or having allies invite someone to sit next to them. Specific placement strategies include the following:

- ***Distracters***: Overly talkative members may be placed in a corner (i.e., positions 1, 5, 7, or 11) to minimize their interactions and influence.
- ***Shy members***: Reticent group members may be placed at the other end (head) of the table (i.e., position 6). This placement encourages participation, and the withdrawn member may emerge as more of a leader.
- ***Squabblers and socializers***: Argumentative and overly social members should be placed apart but facing the same direction (e.g., positions 1 and 5). This placement limits direct interaction and conflict by limiting proximity and visual confrontation.
- ***Opponents of the chair***: A pontificator or powerful opponent should be encouraged to sit next to the chair (i.e., positions 1 or 11), separated from his or her support system. Given the choice, adversaries tend to sit across from each other and surround themselves with their supporters. This arrangement occurs frequently during a negotiation. Placing the pontificator next to the chair limits control of and access to others and gives the chair direct influence over the possibly disruptive member.
- ***Inner versus outer circle***: A member who sits outside the inner circle will generally feel excluded; a member who sits in the inner circle will tend to participate more actively in the discussion. When attending lectures, many choose the front of the room because it encourages a sense of involvement and allows direct access to the speaker. Sitting in the back of a room discourages involvement and allows the attendee to focus attention on other issues.

RUNNING THE MEETING

A poorly run meeting is like a poorly run resuscitation: No one is in charge and everyone feels that things are out of control. Whether or not the desired outcome is achieved, everyone involved will believe the process could have been better.

Why are meetings so bad—why do they fall short? A study of business managers reveals that 78% have no formal training in running meetings; this percentage is much higher for health-care workers.[3,28] As much as half of a director's nonclinical time is spent attending, doing the work assigned from, or preparing for meetings led by people who have little or no formal training.

Setting the Tone

The conduct of the chair determines the extent to which the meeting will reach its potential. The leader must set the tone. The chair begins to establish credibility by arriving early and sitting at the head of the table. The posture, confidence, and enthusiasm of the leader influence the perceptions of the group members. If the chair is businesslike, committed, and task-oriented, the group members are more likely to meaningfully participate. If the chair is confused, lackadaisical, or unfocused, the result may be aimless discourse. If the chair tells too many jokes or grandstands, others will do the same.

Skillful guidance: Leadership is the ability to exert interpersonal influence. The chair should be like a stage director, bringing the issue and associated information onto the stage, directing and rallying the forces, channeling opinions and ideas into meaningful conclusions, and moving the issue offstage by thoughtfully and deliberately transitioning to the next issue.

Chair participation depends on the type of meeting. If the purpose of the meeting is to disseminate information and the chair is the person with the greatest expertise, the chair may take a substantial role in the discussion. However, if the meeting is intended to be a problem-solving meeting, the participation of the chair may be limited. During a problem-solving meeting, the chair may become more of a facilitator, encouraging the expression of all the opinions and generally refraining from advocating any particular viewpoint.

Chair's opinion: Generally, the chair's responsibility is to ascertain the group's resolve rather than to impose his or her own.[3] Achieving this goal requires effective listening and keen attention.

Rule: The role of the chair is not to accomplish his or her goals but to encourage the group or committee to recognize common goals and implement them. Accomplishing the group's goals (not the leader's) should be the focus.

A chair should avoid strongly advocating for his or her own opinion before carefully listening to the opinions of others. The "listen first" strategy allows other viewpoints to be heard and relevant concepts to be incorporated into the chair's view. A chair who strongly believes one solution is best loses objectivity and cannot effectively facilitate discussion.

On occasion, the chair may believe that a particular decision of great importance may have only one satisfactory solution. In this case, the issue should be resolved by premeeting "jawboning." This process entails the chair or others speaking individually with committee members in advance of the more public discussion. It may be wise to determine the answer to a controversial issue before, rather than during, the meeting. In fact, if committee members cannot be convinced of a particular solution before the meeting, the chair is unlikely to convince them in the meeting. In other words, the chair should solve difficult and disruptive issues before the meeting and take a stand on an issue only when the outcome is assured.

Beginning the Discussion

As stated earlier, poorly articulated agendas and goals create confusion. Effective leaders establish a clear direction and stick to it.

Describe a clear purpose. Effective leaders begin with a brief review of the agenda and start each topic with a concise presentation of the decision to be made (i.e., an orientation to the goals). This is the time to pronounce the importance of the discussion that will occur, its value to the people, organization, patients, community, and/or participants. The leader may describe the method to achieve the goal, with an impartial review of the alternatives. Describing and following an intended order of discussion will help members stay on track and discourage digression.

Create ground rules. Members of a new group will arrive with expectations based on their individual experience. Formulating expectations or ground rules during the formative phase of a group can help the team function most effectively.[23] The ground rules can be divided into process, decision-making, and after meeting. In the following section, types of ground rules are listed for consideration by the group.

Establishing Ground Rules

- *Agendas*:
  - ☐ Distributed at or before meeting
  - ☐ Followed in an orderly fashion during the meeting
  - ☐ When nonagenda items will be discussed (at the beginning or end of the meeting, or placed on a future agenda)

- *Attendance*: standards set by group
- *Promptness*:
  - ☐ Expectation of timeliness
  - ☐ Notification of late arrival or nonattendance
  - ☐ Begin and end on time

- *Participation*:
  - ☐ Are all members encouraged to speak?
  - ☐ Must members be recognized by the chair before speaking?
  - ☐ Limit sidebar conversations.
  - ☐ Limit back-and-forth conversations between two people.

- *Respect*:
  - ☐ One speaker at a time
  - ☐ Cell phone and texting rules

- *Roles*:
  - ☐ Taking notes
  - ☐ Facilitation

- *Conflict management*: for example, disagreement is acceptable, but personal attacks are unacceptable.

Decision-Making Ground Rules

- *Agreement*: Contrary views are encouraged; silence equates to agreement.
- *Chair's opinion*: As facilitator, the chair should remain neutral when possible.
- *Complex decision techniques*: Encourage brainstorming and use of the nominal group technique (see below).
- *Conclusion*: Move toward a conclusion, limit nonpertinent discussions, and request a vote or consensus.
- *Commitment to decision*: All should be in support of the group's decisions (e.g., 70% rule).

> **BOX 9.6 ■ MANAGING AIRTIME**
>
> - Allocate ample time.
> - Limit the time spent on a topic.
> - Sequence discussants.
> - Limit two-way debates.
> - Intermittently summarize the discussion.
> - Avoid speaking too much.
> - Resolve issues in advance.

After-Meeting Ground Rules

- *Next meeting*: Schedule the next meeting before the current one ends.
- *Task completion*: Review assignments before adjourning, and define member expectations.
- *Sharing materials*: Create and distribute the meeting minutes and assignments, and formulate a management action plan (see "Distribute the Minutes" below).

Managing Airtime

The chair should guide discussion to a meaningful conclusion. This responsibility often requires actively sequencing the speakers and determining when and for how long each person speaks. There are many methods to control the discussion on a topic (**Box 9.6**).

Allocate ample time. A well-conducted meeting starts and ends on time. The chair should stress promptness because late members distract on-time participants from the discussion. Further, topics or background information that have been presented and perhaps resolved may require time-wasting reexamination to bring the late arriving members up to speed.

Participants generally appreciate meetings that end early because they get unexpected time for other activities. Conversely, participants may become frustrated by meetings that end late and infringe on other priorities. Additionally, the chair who allows meetings to run over time will be viewed as disorganized at best and disrespectful at worst.

Limit time on the topic. Time limits set in advance help govern the discussion and discourage rambling. Within reason, the chair should adhere to those limits. If a topic requires more time than originally planned, the chair may seek group agreement to extend the time on the current topic by reducing time on another topic. Time limits for individual members may be necessary when there are many people eager to speak, the topic is controversial, or there are domineering members of the group.

Sequence discussants to provide order. It may be expedient for the chair to exercise control over who will speak next. It is frustrating to politely raise one's hand to be recognized, especially when others interrupt the discussion.

A chair may provide order by:

- asking members to raise a hand to be recognized,
- scanning the room to recognize when others wish to speak,
- acknowledging (perhaps with a head nod) that a speaker's turn will come in order,
- creating a list of speakers in the order they raised their hands,
- calling on speakers according to the list, or
- discouraging members from interrupting and talking out of turn.

To emphasize this procedure, the chair can intermittently state the sequence of speakers, which will let all members know that they will get a chance to speak. Members can then focus on the discussion rather than worry about working their way into it.

Limit back-and-forth dialogue. Back-and-forth debate frustrates other members of the group who may wish to have their opinions heard. The chair may simply state that others would like an opportunity to discuss the topic and describe the order of the next speakers. This process reminds the members that the chair will control the discussion.

Intermittently summarize the discussion. Summarizing the discussion helps all participants understand the status of an issue, and acknowledging the points of view may help difficult participants who believe that they are not being heard and continue to repeat the same position.

Avoid speaking too much. Some meeting leaders may be tempted to speak at length on every topic, believing that they know more and are responsible for driving the discussion. This approach may have a chilling effect on others and limit discussion by those who are uncomfortable venturing an opinion. In his book, *How to Run a Meeting Without Talking Too Much*, Art Markman suggests that meeting leaders[29]:

- determine in advance when they will speak,
- avoid speaking on every topic,
- prepare and then further condense remarks, and
- encourage input and let others know that their participation is anticipated.

Issues that do not require discussion in the meeting should be resolved in advance. Limit circulation of handouts during the meeting. Meeting attendees will complain if materials that could have been digested before the meeting are instead reviewed or, worse, read at the meeting because their time is being wasted. Alternatively, the chair can assign a member to summarize background materials or list possible solutions to a problem that does not require the group's deliberation in the meeting.

Facilitating the Discussion

Digression is the soul of wit. Take the philosophic asides away from Dante, Milton, or Hamlet's father's ghost and what stays is dry bones.

—Ray Douglas Bradbury, writer of fantasy and science fiction novels

Although digressions in artistic works may add context and flavor, in meetings they create confusion. Wandering discussion is a common problem in meetings; participants do not believe it is their responsibility to direct the discussion, and some leaders wish to avoid appearing overbearing. The result is a tortuous, and sometimes *torturous*, discussion. The chair should carefully monitor discussion and focus the group's attention on the issue. Periodically, the chair can refocus the discussion by summarizing its main points and reflecting on its relationship to the agenda item. Effective chairs continually ask themselves the following questions:

- What is being discussed now?
- Is it relevant?
- Will this discussion move us toward resolution?
- If not, how can I refocus the discussion without stepping on the speaker?

The chair is a type of gatekeeper, encouraging pertinent discussion and curbing unnecessary input. Groups require and appreciate guidance to an end—a decision. When the discussion is poorly focused, the chair must adhere to an orderly process to clarify the discussion and concentrate on the issue at hand. When ideas are widely scattered and disjointed, it may be helpful to use specific problem-solving steps (see "Problem-Solving Techniques").

Digressions occur for several reasons, including disinterest in the current discussion, a "hot-button" issue that has been triggered, or the group leader's loss of focus. Managing off-topic discussions requires a balance of discipline and sensitivity. Once recognized, a digression may be dealt with by one of these methods:

On topic, out of order (i.e., subsequent agenda items): Issues that are slated for later discussion may be noted with a commitment to address the issue later, "Yes, this is an important topic that we will address in a few minutes when we get to . . . Now I'd like to focus on . . . ." If the issue needs to be addressed out of order, the leaders should note the change in agenda order and commit to come back to the slated item.

Off-topic (unrelated) items: Off-topic discussions, although important, may not be part of the meeting's purpose. If the item does not need to be dealt with immediately, then the new issue should be recognized as important but not for the day's agenda. The chair may additionally agree to address the topic at the end of the meeting, if time permits; discuss it privately after the meeting; or save the matter for a subsequent agenda.

Closing the Discussion

Seasoned leaders effectively close discussion. Conversely, inexperienced chairs may allow a discussion to continue beyond its useful time to avoid being perceived as heavy-handed. The chair is responsible for determining when the discussion has gone on long enough, such as when no new concepts are being presented or when the group appears to have reached consensus. Common closure misconceptions include the following:

- *Everybody must speak.* The discussion must go on until everybody has said as much as he or she wants to on the topic. Although group input is critical to resolving issues, it is unnecessary for each and every member to participate without limits.
- *Everyone must agree.* Although it is preferable that the group comes to consensus, it may not be possible. When the chair recognizes that the sentiments of the individual members are established, it may be the time to conclude the discussion. The chair should then summarize the information and ask for consensus or a vote. Decisions made by consensus are preferable to those made by vote because it encourages the support of members who may be responsible for implementation.
- *We must decide all the details now.* Determining the fine points may unnecessarily prolong a meeting. Instead, an individual or subcommittee may be assigned to develop the implementation process.

When a stated goal of the agenda has been met, it is helpful to conclude the segment with a summary of any decisions, assignments, and implementation plans that have been made—and then move on.

PROBLEM-SOLVING TECHNIQUES

When you come to a fork in the road, take it.

—Yogi Berra, MLB Hall of Famer and three-time MVP

Group decisions have several advantages over decisions made by an individual. Groups working together to resolve important issues are generally more satisfied with the

> **BOX 9.7 ■ GROUP PROBLEM-SOLVING METHODS**
>
> - Identify the problem.
> - Describe the facts.
> - Determine alternative solutions.
> - Choose the best solution.
> - Determine an implementation method.

outcome, have a greater sense of unity, create more nuanced decisions, and develop greater commitment to the decision. Various problem-solving methods incorporate the advantages of group participation in the decision-making process. Most problem-solving techniques involve an orderly sequence of steps (**Box 9.7**).

Brainstorming

Brainstorming is a simple, effective, easy-to-use method of problem-solving that has broad application.[30] Brainstorming is valuable because it encourages group creativity and reduces personal bias. The five steps of brainstorming are:

- *State the problem.* The specific issue or problem to be resolved is presented, and ideally the group commits to solving the problem. The leader describes the technique, time limit, and ground rules.
- *Generate solutions.* Ideas, suggestions, and recommendations from the participants are called for. During this stage, judgment should be suspended to allow members to suggest imaginative ideas without the fear of criticism or ridicule. The chair may state that "there are no bad ideas" to encourage participation. Another way to think about this is that innovative and nontraditional ideas should be encouraged because the current approach has not worked, and a nonthreatening environment engenders the greatest creativity. Alex Faickney Osborn, an advertising executive who popularized the term "brainstorming," suggested that "quantity breeds quality."[30] In other words, the more ideas that are considered, the greater the likelihood of finding an effective solution. All ideas should be listed on a visible medium such as a whiteboard to allow structured exploration.
- *Develop criteria.* This step provides a bridge between generation and selection of solutions. The group examines individual and group values and agrees on the standards against which the solutions will be judged. This step may be difficult and require thorough examination. The criteria should be listed near the possible solutions. Once the group agrees on acceptable criteria, selecting a solution is simplified.
- *Compare solutions to criteria.* Each option is discussed in relation to the developed criteria, and solutions that do not meet the most important criteria should be eliminated or receive a low ranking. Over time, consensus begins to emerge.
- *Reach consensus.* When the group has reached consensus, the facilitator should review the group's decision, test understanding and agreement, ask for commitment, and develop the implementation steps.

Nominal Group Technique

The nominal group technique is another popular method of quickly solving complex and controversial issues.[31] This technique ensures the involvement of each participant and maintains confidentiality in decision-making. Once the group is gathered, the facilitator poses the question and leads the members through the following six steps:

- *Develop individual answers.* Each member of the group develops solutions to the problem.
- *Compile group's solutions.* The facilitator asks each individual to contribute one idea at a time with a brief explanation. Each suggestion is recorded on a visible medium such as a flip chart or video screen. This process continues until all ideas are presented.
- *Clarify each idea.* Each idea is reviewed with details described. The facilitator and members of the group ask for explanations and clarifications. Similar or duplicative ideas are combined.
- *Take preliminary vote.* Each person individually prioritizes and ranks the listed solutions. An anonymous vote is taken to determine which alternatives the group considers the best.
- *Discuss differences of opinion.* The initial ranking compiled by the group vote is discussed. Major differences are examined to ensure each member clearly understands the information.
- *Select preferred solution.* After the discussion is completed, members again prioritize their solutions. A final anonymous vote is taken, and a solution is chosen.

NAVIGATING IMPASSES

Problem-solving meetings depend simultaneously on controlled flow of the discussion by the leader and active participation of the members. However, some members may be too active, dominating the discussion, whereas others may be reticent to participate. Although leaders are responsible for facilitating the discussion, they are not totally responsible for the success of the meeting.

Successful leaders have highly evolved interpersonal skills: they can balance the human desire to participate with the need to control direction and input. Judgment should be withheld to avoid stifling participation and creativity. Simultaneously, the leader must limit and guide the discussion to move it to conclusion.

Dealing With Difficult People and Emotions

A lively meeting discussion with important consequences can rouse participants' emotions and bring out participants' individual personality traits. Good leaders are able to validate the concerns and emotions of the participants while continuing to refocus on the issues.

Emotional responses: Great meetings accomplish results of importance to those involved. The significance of these issues naturally evokes strong feelings from the participants. Some group leaders may discourage the expression of feeling because they fear the exposure of too much emotion. They may be concerned that emotional expressions will damage relationships and distract from the problem-solving process, or they may believe that a meeting is successful only if everybody is affable, preferring positive "public relations" to meaningful decision-making.

Emotional responses to issues should be accepted rather than avoided. In fact, the chair would be well advised to express gratitude for the display of concern about such an important issue. However, personalized (ad hominem) attacks toward an individual should not be tolerated. The leader should immediately restore order, perhaps saying, "This is not the forum for this type of discussion. We will remain objectively focused on the issue." The chair could use this awkward moment as an opportunity to refocus the discussion by providing an objective summary of the issue and the decisions yet to be made.

Dominator: The dominator tends to monopolize the discussion and exclude other participants.[32] There are several types of dominators: talkative people, self-appointed experts, and angry members with an ax to grind. Their common characteristic is a desire to talk without listening; many want to run the meeting. The person who does the most talking usually feels as though the most was accomplished.

The chair should not allow a single member to inhibit group creativity. Doing nothing in response to a dominator may allow the meeting to spiral out of control. Conversely, a head-to-head confrontation may create an intolerable, although entertaining, conflict. At best, the meeting becomes a spectacle; at worst, the chair will lose. In either case, many good ideas may be stifled, and everyone present will be uncomfortable. Dominators can be valuable participants, however, and should not be totally silenced. There are many more subtle and successful methods for dealing with the dominator:

- *Arrange seating.* Chairs may (just prior to the beginning of the meeting) ask a dominator to sit next to them in the less powerful corner position. Placing the dominator next to the chair allows the chair to influence the dominator, and the corner position decreases the visibility and influence of the dominator on the rest of the group.
- *Limit discussion in advance.* Impose structure by setting ground rules with the group. For example, "In order to ensure that everyone has input into this important discussion, we'll limit each person to 2 to 3 minutes and allow everyone who wishes to speak to do so before a second round of comments."
- *Control the discussion.* Considering the comments of the early speakers, the chair may then carefully direct the discussion toward reticent participants by asking what they think.
- *Avoid dialogues.* The leader should take responsibility for recognizing each speaker prior to speaking and ensure that the dominator does not control the discussion.

Body language may also be successful when managing the dominator. Looking at the dominator, holding up the index finger, or even an open palm out to signal "stop" will usually quiet the speaker. Standing will draw attention directly to the chair and away from the dominator. If it is still difficult to control the dominator, take a brief recess and use the time to talk directly to the dominator. Explain the value of the group process and of allowing other, quieter participants to speak.

Silent members: Even in meetings with significant group participation, one or more members may not be actively engaged in the discussion. This may occur because the members are shy or feel inhibited by more dominant members. To gain the greatest value from the group process, the leader should sensitively recognize the reticent members and encourage their input.

Avoid calling attention to silence as a means of changing it or making a joke at the expense of a quieter member. Although perhaps well meaning, these techniques will further discourage participation and potentially create enmity. To encourage silent members, seat them in a power position such as the end of the table. Bring the reticent member forward by asking a simple, direct question such as, "John, have you had experience with this situation?" Allow the quiet member early and easy success by responding supportively and integrating his or her reply into the discussion.

Handling Difficult Situations

In moderation, emotion, disagreement, and conflict may result in the most creative, well-thought-out decisions. However, when tempers rise and anger threatens to derail the meeting, the chair must take decisive action without becoming embroiled in the conflict. The only thing worse than watching meetings deteriorate is participating in the destruction. The worst response is anger. It may relieve the tension of the chair, but it will add to everyone else's.

Focus on interests. Frequently, the disagreeing members will have adopted different positions on the same issue. To defend their position, the members may become contentious. This situation can usually be resolved simply by refocusing the discussion on the interests of the parties.[33]

Intervene with process checks. When the discussion wanders or the meeting falls off track, the chair may use several methods to bring the meeting back into focus:

- Ask a particularly rational member, "How do you think we should address this?" This technique will usually direct the group's attention to the new speaker and allow the chair the opportunity to regain focus and control.
- Make a general statement such as, "We are clearly off track and moving in different directions. Does anybody have an idea of how to get back on track?" This question usually works because the members concentrate their attention toward reestablishing an orderly discussion.
- Suggest taking a break. During the recess, the chair has an opportunity to gain composure, establish control over dominators, discuss methods of moving forward, and enlist support from group members.

CLOSING THE MEETING

Ending the meeting well is as important as beginning it and running it (**Box 9.8**). The meeting should end when the anticipated decisions are made, there is no new information, or a subcommittee can better deal with the remaining issues.

End on time. Leaders should make every effort to end meetings on time. Participants perceive leaders as disrespectful when they allow meetings to run longer than scheduled. Conversely, meetings that end early are particularly pleasing to the participants. If there are a few minutes left, it may be helpful to offer the participants an opportunity to briefly voice critical issues that were unaddressed during the meeting. Few will speak, but for those who do, this opportunity may make the difference between leaving the meeting satisfied or frustrated. Rarely, an issue of significance may be raised and cannot be resolved in the remaining time. These issues can usually be addressed after adjournment or at the next meeting.

Summarize accomplishments. The chair may wish to allot specific time on the agenda to summarize the meeting's accomplishments and to review important decisions in

---

BOX 9.8 ■ CHECKLIST FOR CLOSING A MEETING

- End on time.
- Summarize accomplishments.
- Assign or clarify tasks.
- Schedule the next meeting.
- Assess the meeting.
- Distribute the meeting minutes (after).

relation to the meeting's intended goals. Praising the group will help end the meeting on a positive note.

Clarify responsibilities and deadlines. It is appropriate during the closing for the chair to clarify what is to be done, by whom, and by when. This review ensures that participants understand, acknowledge, and commit to their responsibilities between meetings. Each participant should leave with a clear understanding of his or her obligations. Some enthusiastic participants may accept unrealistic deadlines because they are focused on the goal of the moment without considering their other commitments. As such, the chair should rein in unrealistic deadlines and set more credible time frames for task completion.

Schedule the next meeting. If a follow-up meeting (not already scheduled) is necessary, it may be appropriate to schedule it before adjourning. Defining the best time may be easier when many or all the essential members are already in the room. This strategy will assist members to develop a commitment to the deadlines. However, when specific deadlines cannot be determined in advance, then a general time frame and a mechanism for contacting members should be established.

Assess the meeting. Although meeting leaders often believe that their meetings were successful, others may not agree. A meeting's success should be determined by asking its participants, either directly at the end of the meeting or perhaps with an anonymous questionnaire sent after. Many evaluation tools are accessible online. Generally, all assessments attempt to answer four questions[34]:

1. *Effectiveness*: Were the meeting goals clear, and did the meeting accomplish those goals?
2. *Time and organization*: Were the planning and execution (logistics) effective?
3. *Leadership*: Did the group and leader ensure appropriate tone and participation?
4. *Next steps*: Did the participants clearly understand follow-up actions and specific responsibilities?

Distribute the minutes. Minutes are created to record what has occurred and to remind participants of what needs to be done; they should be quickly distributed after the conclusion of the meeting. The chair is responsible for creating minutes that accurately reflect the essential elements of the meeting. Simple management action plan templates are useful for documenting most meetings (**Table 9.2**), but more sophisticated and detailed project management tools may be necessary for long-term processes involving multiple stakeholders (**Table 9.3**). The minutes should detail the agreed-upon actions, deadlines, and individuals

TABLE 9.2 ■ Simple Management Action Plan				
Topic	**Issue and Approach**	**By Whom**	**By When**	**Current Status**
	Develop plan to achieve 75%	J. Jones, RN; F. Smith, MD	Next meeting	Data reviewed
Improve bed-to-doctor time	Current: 19 minutes Goal: 15 minutes	All providers	3 months	1. Data reviewed 2. Developing alert system 3. Assess individual providers

TABLE 9.3 ■ Comprehensive Management Action Plan

Topic	Action Step/Expected Outcome	Measurable Objective	Person Responsible	Start Date	Target Date	Completion Date	P: Progress, B: Barrier, S: Solution
Customer satisfaction	Train staff in AIDET	Checklist	All staff	02/01	03/01	03/01	P–Training complete
	Implement AIDET	Survey	All staff	03/01	05/01	Pending	B–Resistant staff S–Directors to counsel individuals
	Inform patients 54%→90%	Survey	All staff	03/01	06/01	Pending	P–Trained P–90th percentile S–Counsel low performers
	Address pain 37%→75%	EDPECS chart review	Physicians and APCs	04/01	07/01	Pending	P–Protocol adopted B–Inconsistent Rx S–Review individual performance S–Provide feedback

responsible for completion of the actions. The chair may occasionally communicate with the meeting members to check on their progress.

CONCLUSION

Meetings are conducted by, attended by, and intended for *people*. A good meeting:

- is in a comfortable environment,
- values and appreciates its members,
- provides an orderly approach to issues (agenda),
- uses time efficiently, and
- accomplishes its tasks during and after the meeting.

By addressing the needs of the participants, leaders can conduct efficient and effective meetings.

REFERENCES

1. Doyle M, Straus D. *How to Make Meetings Work*. New York, NY: Jove Publications/The Berkley Publishing Group; 1982.
2. Woods RH, Berger R. Making meetings work. *Cornell Hotel Restaur Adm Q*. 1988;29:100-106.
3. Tobia PM, Becker MC. Making the most of meeting time. *Train Dev J*. 1990;44:34-38.
4. Thomas K. *The Firefly Effect: Build Teams That Capture Creativity and Catapult Results*. Hoboken, NJ: Wiley; 2009.
5. Wakin E. Make meetings meaningful. *Today's Off*. 1991;25:68-69.
6. Ashenbrenner G. Planning effective meetings. *Buss Cred*. 1988;90:43-46.
7. Bailey J. The fine art of leading a meeting. *Work Wom*. 1987;12:68-70, 103.
8. Blanchard K. Meetings that work. *Today's Off*. 1987;22:9-11.
9. Drucker P. *The Effective Executive: The Definitive Guide to Getting the Right Things Done*. New York, NY, Harper Collins Publishers; 2006.
10. Surveys by Thom Mayer MD of >3,500 attendees at ACEP's Emergency Department Directors Academy 2004–2018.
11. Sanders EG. *Do You Really Need to Hold That Meeting, HBR Guide to Making Every Meeting Matter*. Boston, Mass: Harvard Business Review Press; 2016.
12. Kirkpatrick DL. *How to Conduct Productive Meetings: Strategies, Tips, and Tools to Ensure Your Next Meeting is Well Planned and Effective*. Alexandria, Va: ASTD Press; 2006.
13. Michaels EA. Business meetings. *Small Buss Rep*. 1989;14:82-88.
14. Stevenson A. Decisions are better made as a group. http://www.spring.st/libby-vanderploeg. Accessed May 18, 2018.
15. Strauss R, DeHart D. Administrative responsibilities. In: Strauss R, ed. *Contracts: A Practical Guide to Emergency Physicians*. Dallas, Tex: ACEP; 1990.
16. Strauss R, DeHart D. Medical staff interrelationships and clinical responsibilities. In: Strauss R, ed. *Contracts: A Practical Guide to Emergency Physicians*. Dallas, Tex: ACEP; 1990.
17. iToolkit.com. How to lead conference calls for optimum participation and results. https://www.ittoolkit.com/articles/lead-conference-calls. Accessed May 21, 2018.
18. Streibel BJ. *Plan and Conduct Effective Meetings: 24 Steps to Generate Meaningful Results*. New York, NY: McGraw-Hill; 2007.
19. Schwarz R. *How to Design an Agenda for an Effective Meeting, in HBR Guide to Making Every Meeting Matter*. Boston, Mass: Harvard Business Review Press; 2016.
20. Cathcart J. How to plan a meeting. *Market Commun*. 1987;12:82-83.
21. Linkemer B. *How to Run a Meeting*. New York, NY: AMACOM; 1987.
22. Wikipedia, "Bloom's taxonomy." https://en.wikipedia.org/wiki/Bloom%27s_taxonomy. Accessed May 18, 2018.
23. Streibel BJ. *Manager's Guide to Effective Team Meetings*. New York, NY: McGraw-Hill; 2003.
24. Frank MO. *How to Run a Successful Meeting in Half the Time*. New York, NY: Pocket Books; 1989.
25. Janis I. *Groupthink: Psychological Studies of Policy Decisions and Fiascoes*. London, England: Wadsworth Publishing; 1982.
26. Jewett M, 3M Meeting Management Team. *How to Run Better Business Meetings: A Reference Guide for Managers*. New York, NY: McGraw-Hill; 1991.
27. Zaremba A. Meetings and frustration. *Supervision*. 1989;49:7-9.
28. Sigband N. Meeting with success. *Personnel J*. 1985;19:48-55.
29. Markman A. How to run a meeting without talking too much. *Harvard Business Review*. May 3, 2018. Accessed May 19, 2018.
30. Osborn AF. *Applied Imagination: Principles and Procedures of Creative Problem-Solving*. New York, NY: Scribner;1979.
31. Delbecq AL, VandeVen AH. A group process model for problem identification and program planning. *J Applied Beh Sci VII*. 1971;466:91.
32. Bean GJ. Don't let a dominator spoil the meeting for everyone. *Marketing Commun*. 1989;22:6.
33. Fisher R, Ury W, Patton B. *Getting to Yes: Negotiating Agreement Without Giving In*. New York, NY: Penguin Books; 2011.
34. iToolkit.com. The meeting is over. Now it's time to evaluate and improve! https://www.ittoolkit.com/articles/post-meeting-assessment, Accessed May 21, 2018.

CHAPTER 10

PATIENT SAFETY: ERROR REDUCTION

Kirk Jensen, Robert W. Strauss

One definition of insanity is doing the same thing, over and over again, but expecting different results.

—Rita Mae Brown, *Sudden Death*, 1983

Patient safety is a fundamental priority. All participants in health care want a safe and error-free environment for patients who maximize quality patient care outcomes. This desire has always been critically important to physicians and nurses; recent decades have witnessed even greater emphasis on safety by hospitals, regulatory organizations, and health-care professionals. Through extensive research in various fields, health-care professionals have come to realize that keeping patients safe is a complex endeavor that affects not only the quality of the care provided but also the satisfaction of patients and the morale of the people who work in the emergency department (ED).

Achieving a safe and reliable ED requires leaders to *intentionally* create a culture of safety. Establishing this culture requires organizational leadership to determine how and why errors occur and focus on what can be done to prevent them (see also Chapter 79). A 10-year study of ED cases that led to malpractice suits concluded that 80% of the mistakes were preventable.[1] These findings suggest the possibility of (and an opportunity for) substantially reducing errors in the ED.

DEVELOPING GOALS AND MEASURING PROGRESS

Creating a Culture of Safety

The key to developing a culture of safety is to focus on processes, people, places, and performances that ensure a "high-reliability department"—an essential prerequisite for a safe environment. When operational reliability is attained, the number of errors and near misses are reduced (many are prevented from occurring), and the effects of errors that do happen can be mitigated. EDs that focus on optimizing their patients' experiences and outcomes continuously emphasize the reliability of their processes. Reliability science dictates a focus on developing and maintaining consistent, evidence-based, and best-in-class processes that are linked to clinical, operational, and service outcomes. Successful, reliable, quality EDs do not wait for problems to occur but rather focus proactively on both what goes right and what could go wrong.

Social psychologists Karl Weick and Kathleen Sutcliffe have identified five characteristics of high-reliability organizations that guide the thinking and actions of the people in them

> **BOX 10.1 ■ WEICK AND SUTCLIFFE'S FIVE CHARACTERISTICS OF HIGH-RELIABILITY ORGANIZATIONS**
>
> - Preoccupation with failure
> - Reluctance to simplify interpretations
> - Sensitivity to operations
> - Commitment to resilience
> - Deference to expertise

(**Box 10.1**).[2] A healthy preoccupation with failure allows leaders to design processes that both minimize the possibility of mistakes and mitigate the harm that may occur when errors do happen. Emergency physician James A. Espinosa and statistician Thomas W. Nolan describe a three-pronged approach to the design of safe and reliable systems: prevent identify, and mitigate (**Box 10.2**).[3] Several methods, such as an analysis of data and trends, daily or weekly flash reports, and rounding on errors can dramatically increase the awareness of mistakes and "near misses."

Measuring Improvement

Emergency departments should continuously track the incidence of both errors and near misses. Documentation of fewer and less serious mistakes will demonstrate the result of improvement efforts. Fewer errors and near misses mean better care. However, the opportunity and the potential impact are even greater because addressing an error reliably often has a ripple effect.

Examining error rates from a mathematical and probabilistic perspective provides several eye-opening facts (**Table 10.1**). Consider the following example. Assume a doctor or nurse has a 95% pretreatment probability of "getting it right" (i.e., not making any errors) when treating an individual patient. In other words, this caregiver has only a 5% chance of making an error, or "getting it wrong." However, if that doctor or nurse cares for 25 patients—not unrealistic in a typical ED shift—then the chances of treating *all* 25 patients without making *any* mistakes drops to 30%. (In other words, these clinicians have a 70% chance of getting it wrong on at least one of these cases.) After four shifts (having seen 100 patients), the clinician only has a 0.6% chance of delivering error-free care!

When the probability of getting it right (performing perfectly) on any one case increases to 99%, the chances of not making any mistakes in the management of all 25 patients rises

> **BOX 10.2 ■ ESPINOSA AND NOLAN'S APPROACH TO SAFE AND RELIABLE SYSTEMS**
>
> 1. **Prevent:** Design the system to prevent failure.
> 2. **Identify:** Design procedures and relationships to make failures visible when they do occur so that they may be intercepted before causing harm.
> 3. **Mitigate:** Design procedures and build capabilities for fixing failures when they are identified or mitigating.

TABLE 10.1 ■ Probability of Performing Perfectly	
Number of Elements	**Probability of Performing Perfectly**
1	.95
25	.28
50	.08
100	.006

to 78%. Therefore, reducing the rate of errors does improve performance, but the error rate is not reduced to zero. As the math demonstrates, increasing the probability of getting it right has a substantially positive impact on outcomes, but it still leaves a significant element of risk in the equation.

Reporting errors is a measurable metric. ED leaders can and should track this statistic in order to improve safety—leaders cannot anticipate what *might* go wrong if they do not know what *did and does* go wrong. Keeping track of mistakes is a necessary part of creating a culture of safety. Paradoxically, increasing the observation and reporting of errors will usually lead to an initial increase in the identification of reported errors, even as actual error rates (the actual commission of errors) decline. However, encouraging awareness and open reporting, acting on the results, and monitoring progress will lead to improved performance and outcomes.

ACHIEVING HIGH RELIABILITY

- Everyone makes mistakes.
- No one makes a mistake on purpose.
- Not all mistakes lead to harm.

Health-care professionals should constantly consider these concepts when addressing errors, misses, and near misses. Doctors, nurses, and hospitals have traditionally approached mistakes with the "sharp end of the stick," routinely assigning blame when mistakes occur. Blaming creates an underground culture in which caregivers bury and avoid sharing mistakes. Creating a culture of safety requires moving away from a "blame, shame, and train" culture. Embracing an "every defect a treasure" philosophy and focusing on learning, rather than blaming, should be the approach of the ED leadership—expose errors and near misses and "put them to work." The need for an active, nonpunitive review process is critical to encourage active reporting of errors.

There are several environmental or structural components within the ED that can contribute to adverse events. EDs that are overcrowded and overwhelmed are more likely to experience adverse events. Even the most competent and conscientious staff members are more likely to make mistakes or errors in judgment when stressed and overtaxed. Improvement requires:

- Accepting that clinicians will make mistakes, particularly when stressed and overwhelmed
- Avoiding blaming the staff for the errors (unless willful or intentional)
- Designing processes and implementing solutions that reduce the likelihood of such mistakes and lessen their impact when they do occur

Errors in Complex Systems

The implication of the probability principle delineated earlier is that increasing the number of elements (e.g., decisions or steps) involved in an action or process increases the likelihood of errors and near misses. This was clear in the example where the number of patients treated increased from 1 to 25 and the likelihood of errorless performance plummeted. This implication has even more relevance in complex systems, such as health-care delivery, where multiple decisions are made in the diagnosis and treatment of each patient. Each additional decision and decision-maker introduced into a process or system increases the likelihood that more errors will occur.

As Jensen and Kirkpatrick note, "Errors are an intrinsic performance characteristic of complex systems."[4] This point illustrates why errors are inevitable and why blaming individuals will seldom help prevent them. Experts who study human error, in fact, have concluded that mistakes by individuals during operations cause only 15% of the errors that occur in complex systems. The other 85% arise from *flawed processes*.[2]

Catastrophic errors can occur in a variety of fields, such as the operation of nuclear power plants, manufacture of chemicals for industrial use, and on the flight deck of an aircraft carrier. Researchers in these fields have responded by designing safety into their processes. As a result, these organizations have extraordinarily low error rates and excellent records of avoiding catastrophic consequences. In addition to highly reliable processes, they maintain a safety culture that avoids blame and encourages the reporting of errors and near misses to allow process review, study, and modification.

The traditional assessment of and approach to safety overemphasizes the performance of the individual. It is important to highlight that health-care delivery in emergency medicine is team based and *process oriented*; an ED cannot optimize its outcomes by focusing on physician and nurse performance alone.

Learn From Mistakes

Errors should be viewed as opportunities to review, study, and modify. ED leaders can and should learn from errors by exposing mistake-prone weaknesses that are built into their department's processes. Errors that almost happen but are averted—"near misses"—are particularly good opportunities to learn because no harm occurred and there is a lesser propensity to deny or cover up the event. When department leaders know the strengths and weaknesses of their ED, they can adjust their processes to reduce the potential for mistakes. This illustrates why a blame-avoidant or "just culture" encourages staff members to report errors and champion systemic improvements.

A punitive organization stokes employee fear and a "code of silence." In an environment characterized by the fear of blame, reprisal, and censure, people and their mistakes are driven underground. Conversely, when the doctors, nurses, and other members of the department realize that reporting errors will not bring censure but will instead be considered valuable and appreciated input, they will respond by sharing more information and insights. As a corollary, the ED should have an effective system for analyzing and providing feedback to the clinicians about errors and near misses.

Design and Redesign the System

Effective approaches to reducing errors include appreciative inquiry (identifying what works well), focusing on possible errors (thinking about what could go wrong), and responding to identified errors (finding root causes and changing processes to avoid future occurrences).

Appreciative Inquiry

Appreciative inquiry should play a central role in efforts to improve. "What's working well?" and "What's good about what you are currently doing?" can effectively promote improvement.[5] Additional questions are:

- What works well?
- Why does it work well?
- Who works well?
- Can these processes and outcomes be replicated and spread?

Focus on Possible Errors

A counterintuitive paradox is that one of the better ways to succeed is to concentrate on failure. Thinking about what *could* go wrong is a key starting point in process design or process redesign. The focus should be not only on the end point—obvious mistakes that might occur—but also on the potential trail of decisions, actions, and communications that create the end points. Consider these questions:

- What circumstances could lead to situations that create mistakes?
- What set of small errors or near misses can have a cumulative effect. For example:
  - ☐ The doctor misses a vital element in the patient's history.
  - ☐ The doctor overlooks a relevant observation in the nursing notes.
  - ☐ The nurse forgets to perform and act on repeat vital signs.
  - ☐ A simple key lab test result is missed.

The cumulative effect of small mistakes can grow into a major error that has a profound effect on a patient's outcome. Projecting how such a series of errors might accumulate can be valuable in redesigning processes so as to prevent them.

Response to Identified Errors

When errors do occur and staff members report them, managers should examine "root cause" processes, step by step. For instance, they should ask what it is about these processes/handoffs that might have caused this error and what changes to the processes would make it less likely to happen. They should then incorporate those changes into a modified process, perhaps encouraging some redundancy—not too much but just enough—to build in a margin of safety. Encouraging the frontline staff to continually seek ways to improve process and performance contributes significantly to an effort to improve quality and safety. The frontline staff are knowledgeable and should be empowered to promote a culture of safety.

An Ongoing Process

This approach entails an ongoing process. ED leaders and their staff should continually:

- Adjust their processes.
- Monitor their results.
- Consider the possibilities for failure (and error proofing) that exist in the redesigned processes.
- Seek error reports.
- Examine what caused the new errors.
- Once again, redesign.

Relentless pursuit of this strategy will steadily decrease the rate of error and near misses in an ED. As previously noted, despite a department's best efforts to anticipate mistakes and design and adjust the system to prevent them, some mistakes will happen. Thus, mitigating the effects of errors that do happen is also a crucial element of an effective system. Leaders

> **BOX 10.3 ■ MITIGATING HARM FROM ERRORS**
>
> Dr. Casey is an excellent emergency physician at the Pixley Medical Center. He reads imaging studies correctly 99% of the time. On a particular day, the number and acuity of patients entering the department was unusually high. As a result, Dr. Casey was somewhat overwhelmed and distracted, and he misread Ms. Buchanan's study. He prescribed an incorrect medication based on his reading.
>
> Fortunately, the Pixley ED management anticipated this possibility, however unlikely, and created a prevent-identify-mitigate set of processes to address the potential error. Dr. Jones, the radiologist, reads over all ED images as a matter of course. She recognizes Dr. Casey's mistake and notifies him. Dr. Casey calls Ms. Buchanan and tells her that upon further evaluation by the radiological staff, the images do not show what his initial reading indicated and that she should not use the prescribed medication. His phone call is timely, and Ms. Buchanan does not take any of the medication.
>
> **Conclusion:** An *error* has occurred, but the ED's processes have been *designed* to *identify* this type of error, *prevent* the (highly trained) emergency physician from *compounding the problem*, and *mitigate* its effects to *prevent harm*.

must oversee an ongoing effort to examine processes, identify mistakes, and learn from them. In other words, they should ask what steps they can take once an error occurs to prevent its impact from compounding and causing harm (**Box 10.3**).

Manage High-Risk Situations

Being able to predict likely errors and error-prone situations has important implications for high-risk and problem-prone situations. This knowledge allows ED leaders to more easily manage those potential problems by developing processes and fail-safe procedures in advance. "Scenario planning" is a highly useful tool in the patient safety toolbox that allows leaders to assess and plan for high-risk, high-volume, or problem-prone scenarios. Examples of such scenarios include patient handoffs, seasonal illness surges, and situations that trigger malpractice claims.

Patient Handoffs

Patient handoffs provide one illustration of analysis and scenario planning. Review and analysis of potential problems that can arise from handoffs, followed by refinement of handoff methods, perhaps with the aid of a standardized approach or checklist, enables the design of an improved process that minimizes risk.

Seasonal Illness Surges

Surges such as an influenza epidemic are another high-risk situation. Hospitals know these surges may bring large numbers of patients to the ED in the fall and winter. Scenario planning—considering what, when, and how many—enables effective preparation. Using the "threat model," EDs can:

- Implement processes and procedures to manage larger than usual numbers of patients (volume pressures or threats).
- Create alerts for patients who are prone to severe complications from influenza ("needle in the haystack" pressures or threats).
- Develop processes that prevent patients from infecting other patients (contagion threats).
- Address potential clinician illness (staffing threats).

> **BOX 10.4 ■ THE 10 MOST PREVALENT MALPRACTICE CASES IN EMERGENCY MEDICINE**[6]
>
> 1. Acute myocardial infarction
> 2. Chest pain, not further defined
> 3. Symptoms involving abdomen and pelvis
> 4. Injury to multiple parts of the body
> 5. Appendicitis
> 6. Fracture of vertebral column
> 7. Fracture of the radius or ulna
> 8. Aortic aneurysm
> 9. Open wound to fingers
> 10. Fracture of the tibia or fibula
> 11. Others

Common Malpractice Cases

Common malpractice incidents are a third high-risk situation that can often be addressed in advance. Several studies, some privately held, others publicly accessible, have dissected this issue. **Box 10.4** outlines potential high-risk or problem-prone situations. **Box 10.5** highlights the results of another analysis that looked at 98 malpractice claims and stratified the primary body system or disease process involved.[6,7]

Identifying and studying the most frequent types of malpractice risks faced by ED staffs enables the development of standard and hardwired patient care plans. It is critical that these "hardwired" approaches—best practices coupled with a reliable set of processes—are known and understood by all staff. This scenario planning helps to eliminate potentially serious errors. Having trigger awareness, processes, and people in place to handle these scenarios helps prevent undesired outcomes that occur when departments are unprepared for predictable high-risk or problem-prone situations.

Emphasize Situational Awareness

Often, individual ED doctors and nurses provide excellent care to individual patients and yet are unaware of problems developing in the department and with other patients around them. "Situational awareness" occurs when members of the staff are focused not only on their patients but also on the department as a whole and are ready to act in support of the team when necessary. It also means that the staff member managing a patient knows how to assess and communicate the patient's needs and the resources necessary to meet those needs.

> **BOX 10.5 ■ PRIMARY BODY SYSTEMS/DISEASES LEADING TO MALPRACTICE CLAIMS**[7]
>
> - Neurologic, 28 (28.6%)
> - Gastrointestinal, 15 (15.3%)
> - Cardiovascular, 9 (9.18%)
> - Obstetrics and gynecology, 9 (9.18%)
> - Orthopedics, 8 (8.16%)
> - Respiratory, 8 (8.16%)
> - Other, 21 (21.4%)

Promoting situational awareness is another ED leadership tool that builds a culture of safety. When encouraging team situational awareness, leaders should continually emphasize safety as a central concern for the whole department. Awareness *and* communication are key aspects of effective situational awareness. When designing safety processes, managers should strive to ensure that staff adopt common language to communicate assessments in the same manner.

Emphasize Teamwork

Situational awareness decreases errors by emphasizing teamwork, common language, and consistent communication. As an example of situational awareness embodied in action, nurses or other staff are encouraged to ask if their colleagues need help and provide support when the answer is yes. Clear communication of the "why," goals, and methods of error reduction is critical to team buy-in. Education, training, coaching, and mentoring of staff are therefore key attributes of a high-performing team and department.

Several approaches to effective teamwork have evolved from crew resource management (CRM), a set of training procedures aimed at improving safety by reducing human error. Similar programs and techniques that can enhance coordinated work as an ED team include MedTeams, TeamSTEPPS, callouts and check backs, and the two-challenge rule.

MedTeams and TeamSTEPPS: One widely used "team" method in emergency medicine is MedTeams, an ED-specific application of techniques developed in CRM. TeamSTEPPS is a nearly identical teamwork system developed jointly by the Department of Defense and the Agency for Healthcare Research and Quality.[8,9]

Callouts and Check Backs: An example of CRM practice for effective communication is the combination of callouts and check backs:

- Callouts—The doctor or nurse examining or treating a patient declares *out loud* what he or she is doing and what needs to be done for the patient.
- Check backs—Other staff members *repeat back* the intention or instruction, so the doctor or nurse is sure it has been understood and will likely be carried out.

The Two-Challenge Rule: The two-challenge rule is another important tool. All staff members are encouraged to professionally challenge the attending physician's orders and staff intentions if they are unclear or seem likely to cause an error.

OPPORTUNITIES TO ELIMINATE ERRORS

A number of ways to help eliminate errors are discussed in the next sections.

Make Errors Visible

As emphasized earlier, leaders should encourage doctors, nurses, and all those who interact with the department to identify and report errors. Implementing this transparent process helps all team members learn from specific, concrete examples. One method of creating visibility is to:

TABLE 10.2 ■ An Example of an Error-Reporting Chart

Record Number	Incident Description	Category	Results of Review	Recommended Improvements	Time Frame	Responsible Person/Group

- Prepare an easy-to-use error-reporting tool and summary chart (**Table 10.2**).
- Ensure that the tool is available throughout the ED (computerize it).
- Promote the system so that all staff members:
    - ☐ Know about it
    - ☐ Are confident they won't face punishment for reporting errors
    - ☐ Recognize that they are improving the team's care of patients

Implementation Time Frame

Time frame development steps:

- Create a time frame for the initiation of the error identification program, perhaps 30 or 90 days.
- Teach the staff how to identify and report mistakes, near-misses, and other concerns.
- Compile and review cases, looking for patterns. Once patterns have been identified, management and staff can consider adjusting or redesigning relevant processes.
- Repeat the process. Safety requires an ongoing review of processes to look for new patterns. This, in turn, enables the ED to further refine its approach. As noted earlier, it is healthy to anticipate the presence or possibility of failure in order to reduce its likelihood.

After-Action Review

While the ED staff is tracking errors, leaders, staff, and safety committee (if established) should actively address them. An "after-action review" is an effective way to rapidly address change. This concept has its origin in the military[10]:

> The United States Army and Marine Corps use after-action reviews in war-gaming exercises and combat situations to hone both strategy and day-to-day tactics. Units preparing to go to war conduct an exercise against a force stationed in the United States. The attacking force—the force headed overseas—is always better equipped, has ten times the number of men, and has daily access to the plans of the defending force. Nine times out of ten, however, the defending force wins. It wins because after-action reviews after every engagement, every day. The unit command of the defending force collates the lessons learned each day and then gets those lessons out to the commanders in the field so they can implement the "lessons learned" the next day.

After-action reviews in EDs allow staff members to review cases either in real time or shortly after. A department should use these reviews for both successfully managed cases and ones that lead to concerns. Reviewing well-managed cases allows the staff to look at what worked well and what might have gone wrong but did not. The ED staff can define the processes that led to success, replicate them, and anticipate what could have gone wrong to

> **BOX 10.6 ■ THE PROCEDURE FOR AFTER-ACTION REVIEWS**
>
> 1. What results did we intend to achieve in this case?
> 2. What measures can we use to assess the results?
> 3. What challenges might we have expected beforehand that we might face in future cases?
> 4. What lessons do we learn from our actions and their consequences in this case?
> 5. How can we succeed in similar cases in the future?
> 6. How can we implement what we have learned into our processes?

prevent future failure. **Box 10.6** demonstrates this procedure for examining cases. This is a procedure that can be conducted at the bedside as well as in a conference room. It is too valuable a tool to not be used by the health-care team.

Decrease Complexity

In the earlier example in which a doctor or nurse treating one patient has a 95% chance of avoiding errors, that doctor or nurse has only a 28% cumulative chance of having gotten it all right after seeing the 25th patient. As noted in **Table 10.1**, increasing the chances of success from 95% to 99% would lead to a considerably higher probability of getting it right on all 25 patients (78% but still not 100%). This mathematical analysis has a useful implication for emergency medicine.

Reduce Elements of Care

Reducing the complexity (number of elements, steps, or decisions) in a set of processes increases the chances of providing care (succeeding) without mistakes. This principle can be applied broadly. For example, there may be many steps, people, and handoffs necessary to treat a single patient. When staff members examine the ED's process flow analysis for complex patients, they may discover ways to decrease the number of steps, handoffs, and decisions—complexity. Reducing the number of elements will not only decrease the error rate but also increase efficiency within the department's operations.

Work as a Team

Reducing the complexity embedded within the elements and processes of care can significantly reduce the risk of error. Working as a coordinated, communicating team (rather than as a group of independent individuals) is critical to success. A useful definition of an effective team is a coordinated group with a/an[11]:

- Clear and inspired common sense of purpose with a commitment to excellence and improvement, ideally a purpose the team members have helped shape
- Deep and abiding respect among the team members for the unique roles and talents each brings to the endeavor
- System of value-added processes designed to accomplish clearly defined goals
- Process for providing real-time communication and feedback
- Culture that celebrates team success while coaching members through a system of mutual accountability

Simplification reduces complexity and, therefore, the potential for errors. As such, leaders should also look for ways to standardize patient care delivery approaches for specific diagnoses and streamline their ED procedures, handoffs, and reporting (automation can help standardize this).

Emphasize Communication

A common theme running throughout this discussion is *the importance of teamwork and communication*. When effective teamwork is present in an ED, so is effective communication. When errors, near-misses, or patient safety concerns occur, openly communicating about them leads to knowledge and redesign that prevents recurrences. Predicting and planning for high-risk situations requires clear communication of the relevant changes in operational protocols for successful implementation. Several additional communication processes add value to a department striving to implement a culture of safety.

Conduct Patient Safety Rounds

Managers and clinical leaders can make regular patient safety rounds, speaking with patients and staff about concerns, workload, communication, teamwork, near-misses, patient safety threats, and other staff insights. This permits leaders to engage employees and patients and ascertain their experiences, perceptions, and concerns. These observations can be applied to process analysis and redesign.

Establish Patient Communication Standards

Clear communication with patients by physicians, nurses, technicians, and others in the department leads to better and safer care and more satisfied patients.[12] The implications are significant, as nearly three-fourths of patients who sue for malpractice have experienced a poor interaction with staff and cite it as a major driver behind their legal action.

Share Process Information

When managing patients, clinicians can emphasize their commitment to safety by explaining the reason behind a particular action. This information simultaneously reassures patients and increases their engagement. For example, it may be helpful to specify why the clinician is checking their armband (to ensure they're receiving the right treatment) or shutting the door (to protect their privacy).

Educate Staff on Safety Issues

Education is another component of creating a culture of safety and harm reduction. For example, it is essential to educate doctors, nurses, mid-level providers, and other staff members about techniques for fostering effective teamwork, protocols for managing high-risk situations, and standard ED processes. A safety culture calls for staff who share a common and consistent purpose and speak a common professional language. The ED leaders need to communicate a serious, ongoing commitment and a deliberate educational approach to the program. New employees should undergo early training in the ED's safety protocols.

Utilize SBAR

The SBAR method (**S**ituation, **B**ackground, **A**ssessment, and **R**ecommendation) is a widely used communication model.[13] When managing a patient, the **S**ituation might entail describing the patient's complaint and associated information, such as blood pressure and temperature. **B**ackground might include the patient's general medical history, current medications, and pertinent lab or radiology results. **A**ssessment might be the caregiver's appraisal of the medical problem and the patient's current condition. **R**ecommendation involves next steps or actions, perhaps asking the physician to see the patient immediately or recommending consideration of certain tests or treatments.

An additional benefit of communication techniques or models like SBAR is that the technique often becomes a standard method of communication in interactions among caregivers. When a refined communication model becomes pervasive, all employees are more likely to communicate effectively, enhancing the implementation of standards for best practices in patient care.

Build Reliability Into the ED

Everything must be made as simple as possible. But no simpler.

—Albert Einstein

Employees and team members should be able to clearly and effectively articulate the department's standard procedures and processes for patient care. This goes beyond understanding relevant patient care pathways. Staff need a deep appreciation for roles, responsibilities, and timelines and must be able to articulate "who does what by when." For instance, if they cannot clearly articulate the standard processes for chest pain management, even the relatively simple process of obtaining an immediate electrocardiogram will be unreliable. The people engaged in implementing the processes must be able to clearly articulate the roles they play as well as the "why." Building reliability into processes reduces the risk of error.

One reliability technique is to design prompts based on triggers. For instance, when a caregiver recognizes that a patient might have pneumonia, there could be a trigger for the implementation of standardized physician orders. The trigger could even be an electronic alert from the diagnostic imaging department that indicates the pneumonia pathway should be started when an infiltrate is identified by the radiologist.

A high-reliability process is more likely in place when *all* involved employees understand:

- The standard best practices for specific high-risk situations
- Their role in the delivery of those best practices
- The "why" of the best practice in relation to medical outcomes and patient safety

If every clinician in the ED knows how to apply standard best practices, the odds of providing errorless, harm-free care increases dramatically. The use of focused training exercises, staff interviews, patient safety walk-rounds, and even exit interviews can be valuable and effective ways to ascertain if all staff understand and are prepared to act on these best practices.

Standardizing processes does not always reduce the aggregate number of steps. While achieving high reliability may reduce the number of process elements or decisions, it might also add prompts or alerts to build an appropriate level of system redundancy (*just enough and no more*) to reduce risk. For instance, if mistakes are more likely to occur at certain points in processes, then designing a standard practice to back up (make redundant) the primary interaction can introduce increased reliability. Over-reading of radiology images is an example of redundancy built into the delivery process to increase reliability and reduce errors and harm.

Another way to enhance reliability is to *think as little as possible*. This may seem like a strange and counterintuitive goal, but true thinking is hard and complex work. Just consider

> **BOX 10.7 ■ SOURCES OF POTENTIAL ERROR IN A BUSY ED[14]**
>
> - High level of uncertainty for diagnosis
> - High number of decisions made in typical shift
> - High cognitive load in processing large amounts of data
> - Short time frames for assessing patients
> - Multiple transitions for many patients
> - Multiple interruptions for doctors and nurses

the number of actions, communications, protocols, and procedures that physicians and nurses must perform for each and all patient encounters during a shift (**Box 10.7**).[14]

Thinking is hard work. Physician and Harvard professor Lucian Leape has observed that the more expertise someone has, the less they are required to actually think.[15] To demonstrate this, imagine a recognized authority talking about his or her subject of expertise. The expert is likely to speak quickly and succinctly, pointing out important considerations. The concise, discerning, and focused discussion does not occur because the expert is thinking hard; rather, it is because the expert has a deep well of knowledge from which they can draw. Rather than spending a significant portion of their time "thinking hard," the goal of every ED staff should be to become experts at pattern recognition. *Hardwiring* these patterns is an excellent safety practice in the ED.

Think About Thinking

To interpret how errors occur and can be prevented, cognitive psychologists assert that it is necessary to understand the different ways in which people think. Leape cites the work of James Reason, who identifies two primary kinds of thinking:[16]

- Automatic (unconscious) thinking, which people use in many of their daily activities
- Conscious (controlled) thinking, which they use to solve problems

Other experts have identified three additional types of thinking: skill based, rule based, and knowledge based.[17]

Automatic (skill-based) thinking: This type of thinking uses the pattern recognition mentioned previously and is similar to what Leape calls "schemata." Schemata are a group of small patterns within a larger action that a person has done over and over and can be accomplished without thinking about them (i.e., unconscious thinking). Errors associated with automatic thinking often occur when an individual's concentration is broken by distractions and interruptions. Another kind of error in this category occurs when a familiar pattern deviates from the expected (e.g., the hoof beats are from a zebra and not a horse). If the deviation goes unrecognized, the provider might continue to respond as if the more familiar original pattern existed—possibly leading to a mistake.

Conscious thinking: Unlike automatic thinking, conscious thinking is slow and requires the person to consciously consider the consecutive steps necessary to solve a problem.

Knowledge-based thinking: This is similar to conscious thinking. Knowledge-based thinking requires people to address problems that may not entirely resemble situations they have encountered before. Mistakes in knowledge-based thinking, as the name implies, indicate that the provider does not have adequate knowledge or misinterprets the problem.

Rule-based thinking: This somewhat blends two types of thinking. People typically use rule-based thinking when encountering situations they cannot handle automatically but fall into categories with which they have considerable experience. As a result, they follow a programmed sequence for a that kind of problem; if x, then y, as Leape expresses it. Mistakes in rule-based thinking generally occur when providers choose the wrong rule as a result of perceiving the situation incorrectly or when they misapply the rule in what Leape calls "misapplied expertise."

Resulting Errors

Understanding the types of thinking enables people to more easily grasp the kinds of errors that result from them. When applying these insights to the ED, experts theorize that healthcare professionals use:[14,18]

- Pattern recognition when symptoms clearly indicate a specific course of treatment
- Rule-based thinking in high-stress emergencies
- Conscious, knowledge-based thinking when symptoms are vague and could indicate one of a wide range of potential diagnoses

Errors are most likely to occur in the third type of thinking (knowledge based), particularly when judging a patient's condition prematurely without waiting for confirming evidence.

Incorrect diagnoses are the leading cause of serious errors in emergency medicine. Some researchers surmise that "dual-process thinking" may be the most effective approach to problem solving in the ED.[14] The first of the two processes, as described by critical-thinking expert Pat Croskerry, uses pattern recognition for familiar symptoms and results in rapid treatment; the second process uses knowledge-based thinking, which is slower but necessary when symptoms do not lead to an obvious diagnosis. Glatter, et al assert:

The key to effective emergency medicine [is to combine the two types of thinking into] a balanced blend that adjusts to contingencies of clinical circumstances.

PITFALLS FOR PATIENT SAFETY

All humans err frequently—systems that rely on error-free performance are doomed to fail.

–Lucien Leape[15]

Traditional medical training has indoctrinated the idea that doctors and nurses should aim for a mistake-free performance, and hospitals and professional boards often hold their clinicians to that lofty standard. Research into complex systems, however, demonstrates that perfection is an unrealistic goal that fails to appreciate that many errors are intrinsic to the system itself. ED leaders who reflexively single out, blame, and punish their clinicians for their mistakes are doomed to fail. In fact, they may paradoxically ensure that process-based errors (85%) continue unabated.

In an environment of blame, management is reactive to mistakes. Reactively focusing only on the *results* of failure rather than the *potential* for failure and the *processes* involved in failure ensures that failure will continue to occur. Alternatively, organizations with a high-reliability mindset continually focus on the potential for failure and on "what *might* go wrong." Examining weak and vulnerable processes allows safety-conscious organizations to predict and potentially modify the patterns that lead to mistakes.

Multitasking and Interruptions

In 2009, Clifford Nass—a Stanford professor and an expert on communication, organizational theory, and multitasking—decided to study how serious multitaskers perform.[19] Impressed with their skills, he hoped to improve his own. To his complete surprise, he discovered that serious multitaskers were not effective at accomplishing their tasks. When he studied their outcomes, he observed that they did not achieve quality results. Those who multitasked the most actually performed the worst. The appearance of continuous activity and effective multitasking masked the poor outcomes. And yet, the multitaskers remained convinced they were great at accomplishing their tasks and able to do even more.

One Carnegie Mellon study demonstrated that doing several things at once reduces the mental attention a person can devote to each individual task. One lesson for emergency medicine is that the more doctors, APPs, and nurses attend to multiple tasks at the same time, the greater the likelihood they will fail at some of them. The probability of failure at any one of those tasks increases. Thus, examining processes that demonstrate the focus (and distractions) of a healthcare provider's attention may illuminate where failure is more likely to occur.

Interruptions similarly reduce productivity. A study in the archives of surgery found that surgery residents committed 8 times more errors when there were common disruptions in the operating room than when there were not any interruptions or distractions.[20] Residents committed major surgical errors in 8 of 18 simulated procedures that involved disruptions. In comparison, they committed a major surgical error in only 1 of the 18 procedures that did not involve any disruptions. In emergency medicine, doctors average over 10 task interruptions every hour.[21,22] After nearly 20% of the interruptions, the physicians never returned to the original task!

Some interruptions cannot be avoided. However, observing patient care delivery processes to identify when interruptions are most likely to occur and for what purpose may demonstrate opportunities for improvements.

Failures in Communication

According to the Joint Commission, poor communication is the leading cause of sentinel events in the ED. Misunderstandings can occur when clinicians approach conversations using different mental models, language, and communication protocols. Different communication styles, particularly between nurses and physicians (often due to differences in their training), can cause errors, which are more likely to occur during patient handoffs.[11] This risk can be reduced and the probability of success increased by ensuring that staff members use clear, standard communication practices that are capable of crossing authority gradients and boundaries. Analysis, the development of common language protocols, education, and role-modeling are good starting points for improving communication and decreasing the potential failure rate.

CONCLUSION

To create a culture of safety, the ED staff and its leadership must aspire and work to achieve a highly reliable organization that continually strives to optimize performance, reduce the rate of errors, and mitigate harm when errors occur. High-reliability EDs occur when effective communication and teamwork are regular features of the department and when clearly understood standard protocols and processes are put in place. Always working toward optimizing patient safety and reducing errors means appreciating and encouraging positive performance, while simultaneously:

- Focusing on potential failures
- Looking for weaknesses in the processes
- Ensuring open review of errors that do happen
- Learning from those mistakes
- Adjusting and then readjusting those processes for continuous improvement

Safety and error prevention strategies, tools, and techniques provide effective ways to achieve these goals. As an ED staff builds and hardwires a culture of safety, the team members find that the care provided to patients is both safer and of higher quality. Inevitably, the patients and the people providing care to those patients will be more engaged and gratified.

REFERENCES

1. Risser DT, Rice MM, Salisbury ML, Simon R, Jay GD, Berns SD. The potential for improved teamwork to reduce medical errors in the emergency department. *Ann Emerg Med*. 1999;34(3):373-383.
2. Weick KE, Sutcliffe KM. *Managing the Unexpected: Assuring High Performance in an Age of Complexity*. San Francisco, Calif: Jossey-Bass; 2001.
3. Espinosa JA, Nolan TW. Reducing errors made by emergency physicians in interpreting radiographs. *BMJ*. 2000;320(7237):737-740.
4. Jensen K, Kirkpatrick DG. *The Hospital Executive's Guide to Emergency Department Management*. Marblehead, Mass: HCPro; 2010.
5. Eaton SE. Appreciative inquiry. an overview. http://www.scribd.com/doc/56010589/ Appreciative-Inquiry-An-Overview. Accessed August 7, 2013.
6. Brown TW, McCarthy ML, Kelen GD, and Levy F. An epidemiologic study of closed emergency department malpractice claims in a national database of physician malpractice insurers. *Acad Emerg Med*. 2010;17(5):553-560. www.aemj.org.
7. Carlson JN, Foster KM, Pines JM, et al. Provider and practice factors associated with emergency physicians' being named in a malpractice claim. *Ann Emerg Med*. 2018;71(2):157-164.e4.
8. Morey JC, Simon R, Jay GD, et al. Error reduction and performance improvement in the emergency department through formal teamwork training: evaluation results of the MedTeams project. *Health Serv Res*. 2002;37(6):1553-1581.
9. Agency for Healthcare Research and Quality. TeamSTEPPS. https://www.ahrq.gov/teamstepps/index.html. Accessed December 2, 2019.
10. US Army. A Leader's Guide to After-Action Reviews. Training Circular 25-20. Washington, DC. http://www.au.af.mil/au/awc/awcgate/army/tc_25-20/table.htm. Accessed August 7, 2013.
11. Mayer T, Tavernero T, Jensen K, Strauss R. The discipline of teams and teamwork in emergency medicine. In: Strauss RW, Mayer TA, eds. *Strauss and Mayer's Emergency Department Leadership*. New York, NY: McGraw-Hill; 2013.
12. Beckman HB, Markakis KM, Suchman AL, Frankel RM. The doctor-patient relationship and malpractice. Lessons from plaintiff depositions. *Arch Intern Med*. 1994;154(12):1365-1370.
13. Haig KM, Sutton S, Whittington J. SBAR: a shared mental model for improving communication between clinicians. *Jt Comm J Qual Patient Saf*. 2006;32(3):167-175.
14. Glatter RD, Martin RE, Lex J. How emergency physicians think: highlights of the Fourth Mediterranean Emergency Medicine Congress (MEMC IV). http://www.medscape.com/viewarticle/57539. 2008. Accessed December 2, 2019.
15. Leape LL. Error in medicine. *JAMA*. 1994;272(23):1851-1857.
16. Reason J. *Human Error*. Cambridge, England: Cambridge University Press; 1990.
17. Rasmussen J, Jensen A. Mental procedures in real-life tasks: a case study of electronic troubleshooting. *Ergonomics*. 1974;17(3):293-307.
18. Croskerry P, Cosby KS, Schenkel SM, Wears RL, eds. *Patient Safety in Emergency Medicine*. Philadelphia, Pa: Lippincott Williams and Wilkins; 2009.
19. Ophir E, Nass C, Wagner AD. Cognitive control in media multitaskers. *Proc Natl Acad Sci U S A*. 2009;106(37):15583-15587.
20. Carnegie Mellon University. Carnegie Mellon study provides conclusive evidence that cell phones distract drivers. *ScienceDaily*. www.sciencedaily.com/releases/2001/07/010727094311.htm. Accessed 27 July 2001.
21. Feuerbacher RL, Funk KH, Spight DH, Diggs BS, Hunter JG. Realistic distractions and interruptions that impair simulated surgical performance by novice surgeons. *Arch Surg*. 2012;147(11):1026-1030. doi:10.1001/archsurg.2012.1480.
22. Chisholm CD, Collison EK, Nelson DR, Cordell WH. Emergency department workplace interruptions: are emergency physicians "interrupt-driven" and "multitasking"? *Acad Emerg Med*. 2000;7(11):1239-1243.

ADDITIONAL READINGS

- ACEP. Patient safety in emergency medicine, August 18, 2008, by Pat Croskerry, MD, ed, Karen S. Cosby, MD, FACEP, ed, Stephen M. Schenkel, MD, MPP, ed, Robert L. Wears, MD, MS, ed.
- ACEP Patient Safety Task Force. Patient safety in the emergency department. Dallas, Tex: American College of Emergency Physicians; 2001.
- Aiken L, Clarke S, Sloane D. Hospital nurse staffing and patient mortality, nurse burnout, and job dissatisfaction. *JAMA*. 2002;288(16):1987-1993.
- Bogner M. *Human Error in Medicine*. Hillsdale, NJ: Lawrence Erlbaum Associates; 1994.
- Bosk C. Forgive and remember managing medical failure. Chicago, Ill: University of Chicago Press; 1984.
- Brennan TA, Leape LL, Laird NM, et al. Incidence of adverse events and negligence in hospitalized patients. *N Engl J Med*. 1991;324:370-376.
- Croskerry P. Critical thinking and decision making avoiding the perils of thin-slicing. *Ann Emerg Med*. 2006;48:720-722.
- Dynamics Outcomes Management (website), A Short History of CRM.
- Green LV, Soares J, Giglio JF, et al. Using queuing theory to increase the effectiveness of emergency department provider staffing. *Acad Emerg Med*. 2006;13(1):61-68.
- Haig KM, Sutton S, Whittington J. SBAR: a shared mental model for improving communication between clinicians. *Jt Comm J Qual Patient Saf*. 2006;32(3):167-175.

- Helmreich R. On error management: lessons from aviation. *BMJ*. 2000;320:781-785.
- Institute of Medicine. *To Err Is Human*. Washington DC: National Academy Press; 1999.
- Kachalia A, Gandhi TK, Puopolo AL, et al. Missed and delayed diagnoses in the emergency department: a study of closed malpractice claims from 4 liability insurers. *Ann Emerg Med*. 2007;49:196-205.
- Kohn LT, Corrigan JM, Donaldson MS, eds. *To Err Is Human: Building a Safer Health System*. Washington, DC: National Academy Press; 1999.
- Lardner R. Effective shift handover: a literature review. Health and Safety Executive. 1996. http://www.npsf.org/download/Focus2004Vol7No2.pdf.
- Leape L. Error in medicine. *JAMA*. 1994;272:1851-1857.
- Morey JC, Simon R, Jay GD, et al. Error reduction and performance improvement in the emergency department through formal teamwork training: evaluation results of the MedTeams Project. Health Services Research [December 2002 publication]. In Press.
- Reason J. *Managing the Risks of Organizational Accidents*. Burlington, VT: Ashgate Publishing; 1997.
- Risser DT, Rice MM, Salisbury ML, Simon R, Jay GD, Berns SD. The potential for improved teamwork to reduce medical errors in the emergency department. The MedTeams Research Consortium. *Ann Emerg Med*. 1999;34:373-383.
- Sexton JB, Thomas EJ, Helmreich RL, et al. Error, stress, and teamwork in medicine and aviation: cross sectional surveys. *BMJ*. 2000;320:745-749.
- Spear SJ, Schmidhofer M. Ambiguity and workarounds as contributors to medical error. *Ann Intern Med*. 2005;142(8):627-630.
- Spear SJ. Fixing healthcare from the inside, today. *Harvard Business Review*. September 2005.
- Uhlig P, Haan C, Nason A. Improving patient care by the application of theory and practice from the Aviation Safety Community. Presented at: the 11th annual Ohio State Symposium Aviation Psychology, Columbus, Ohio, March 6, 2001.
- Wears RL, Perry SJ, et al. Shift changes among emergency physicians: best of times, worst of times. *Proceedings of the Human Factors and Ergonomics Society 47th Annual Meeting*; October 13-17, 2003; Denver, Colo.
- Wears R, Leape L. Human error in emergency medicine. *Ann Emerg Med*. 1999;34:370-372.
- Weick K, Sutcliffe K. *Managing the Unexpected: Assuring High Performance in an Age of Complexity*. San Francisco, CA: Jossey-Bass; 2001.

CHAPTER 11

DEFINING PATIENT EXPERIENCE AND LEADING CHANGE

Thom A. Mayer

Every system is perfectly designed to get precisely the results it gets.

—Paul Batalden, MD[1]

Emergency nurses and physicians have often expressed concerns, and even complained, about the best way to measure patient satisfaction. With the introduction of the Emergency Department Consumer Assessment of Healthcare Providers and Systems (ED CAHPS) survey, emergency departments (EDs) are moving into a new era in which patient experience is center stage. These changes define the experience of care, imply how to improve the delivery of that care, and affect provider compensation.[2]

The foundation for success in patient experience requires it to be an *evidence-based discipline*. It is guided by careful study of what works (and what does not) for providing quality care to ED patients, from both a clinical and service perspective.

DEFINING PATIENT EXPERIENCE

While there are many definitions of patient experience, perhaps one of the most widely acknowledged is from the Beryl Institute (**Figure 11.1**).[3] It is important to note that patient satisfaction surveys simply require the patients to rate their satisfaction with specific aspects of their care. The delivery and assessment of patient *experience*, however, provides a richer, deeper tapestry than patient satisfaction. The concept of "experience" offers a

FIGURE 11.1 ■ Beryl Institute Definition of Patient Satisfaction

The sum of all interactions, shaped by an organization's culture, that influence patient perceptions across the continuum of care

— The Beryl Institute

wonderful opportunity to design evidence-based approaches to provide better service and get better results. It provides a more complex palette from which to paint, since it provides a more nuanced understanding of care.[4]

Moving From Patient Satisfaction to Patient Experience

Until recently, patient satisfaction has been one of the critical parameters by which ED care has been measured. But that simple concept has matured into a broader, more sophisticated, richer, and more actionable view of the entire patient experience, not just the degree to which the patient was satisfied. While this may initially seem a subtle distinction, a fuller understanding of patient experience reveals how it allows implementation of a far more effective set of tools to address patient satisfaction.

Patient satisfaction surveys merely ask patients a series of questions about the people and processes they encountered during their visit. Using Likert scales to rank responses to ordinal data, patients simply state how satisfied they were.[5,6] The most widely used survey tool uses only four questions concerning physicians and five concerning nurses in the ED. While many providers and administrators may feel they are judged (and "live or die") by those scores, patient satisfaction provides only a very rough approximation of what actually transpired during a visit. Further, the limited information provided by the scores generates, at best, only very crude tools for improving the actual care provided.[4-6]

In addition, some of the information is nonactionable, making it difficult to take the patients' experience of care into account to make clear and meaningful improvements.[7] Excellent coaching has guided teams in the "satisfaction era." Now, however, organizations must prepare for a huge leap forward if the culture, tools, and strategies outlined here are implemented. Patient experience and patient engagement are, or should be, welcomed because they will allow exponential expansions of the previous constructs and permit ED leaders to significantly enhance the patients' and staff's experience (**Figure 11.2**).

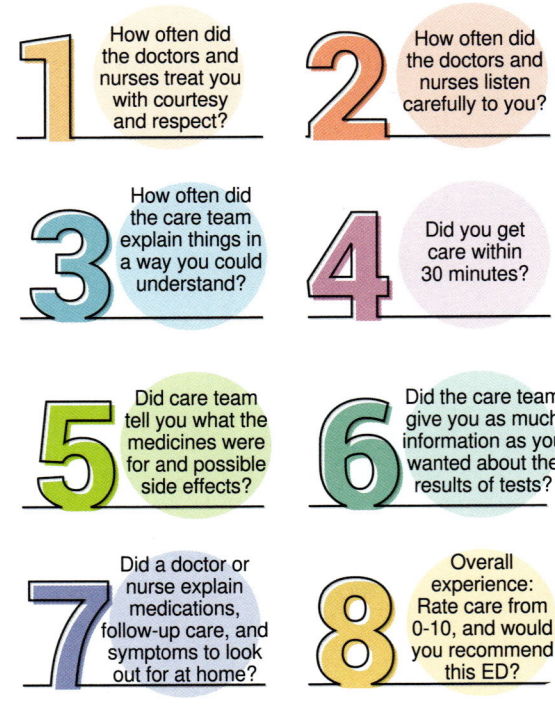

FIGURE 11.2 ■ Core ED CAHPS Survey Categories

1. How often did the doctors and nurses treat you with courtesy and respect?
2. How often did the doctors and nurses listen carefully to you?
3. How often did the care team explain things in a way you could understand?
4. Did you get care within 30 minutes?
5. Did care team tell you what the medicines were for and possible side effects?
6. Did the care team give you as much information as you wanted about the results of tests?
7. Did a doctor or nurse explain medications, follow-up care, and symptoms to look out for at home?
8. Overall experience: Rate care from 0-10, and would you recommend this ED?

The best definition of patient experience is the difference or "delta" between what the patient *expected* and what the patient *experienced*. Thus, patient experience, far from being an abstract concept, is the simple calculus of how patients compare their expectations entering the ED with the reality of what they saw, heard, felt, and thought through the course of their ED journey.[8] The questions that arise are:

- What does the ED look like through *their* eyes?
- How can ED team members in a capacity-constrained environment deliver care in a way that allows them professional enjoyment?

A critical question then is, "How can ED team members discover the expectations of the patients and families?" It's very simple. Ask them:

What are your expectations for this emergency department visit?

This simple, direct question allows patients to express their expectations in the earliest phase of their care and delivers a common understanding of why they came to the ED.

Expectation Packets

Discovering expectations at the beginning of every visit is essential to understanding patient experience. From the most acutely ill or severely injured ED patient to those with coughs, colds, and sore throats, the patients and their families bring a set of expectations to the encounter. Consider them *expectation packets*, which describe the anticipated mental model of what they expect over the course of their ED visit. These packets must be unpacked. While the expectations can be accurate or inaccurate, they must never be ignored. In theology, the process of unpacking (making a critical interpretation of) expectations is referred to as *exegesis*.[9]

A health-care service problem exists when many providers and staff believe it is their job to simply provide *adequate* care and meet the patients' expectations—no more and no less. But if the health-care system does no more than meet expectations, the encounter went as expected and the patient is "merely satisfied." People content with merely meeting expectations are "just-enoughers," similar to the staff who are doing "just enough" to meet organizational expectations and thus keep their jobs. These team members do not have poor character; they simply have not been inspired to strive for *excellence over adequacy*. If the ED leaders only want to meet expectations, it will be difficult to attain success in the "always" era of ED CAHPS.

In the current, highly competitive, and capacity-constrained health-care market, is "just good enough" enough? To consistently meet and exceed the targets, ED teams must do more. Besides, no one wants to lead a team of people who wake up in the morning thinking:

I can't wait to get out there and perform at an average level!

If the person lying on the stretcher were a member of an ED team member's family, would anyone consider average percentile performance "good enough?" Hospital boards and leadership teams can no longer accept the mean—they seek excellence. If patient satisfaction is low (e.g., the 15th percentile), moving to the 50th percentile is on the path to the top—but it should just be a temporary stop on that journey.

The Source of Patient Complaints

When their expectations are not met, patients are dissatisfied and often complain (see Chapter 76). The difference between patient expectations and the care delivered dictates the

FIGURE 11.3 ■ Understanding Expectations is the Key

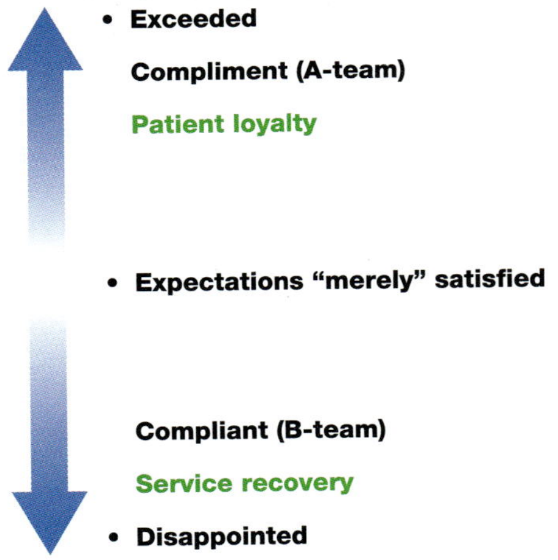

- Exceeded

  Compliment (A-team)

  Patient loyalty

- Expectations "merely" satisfied

  Compliant (B-team)

  Service recovery

- Disappointed

focus of the resulting complaint (**Figure 11.3**).[10] Occasionally, ED staff members believe that patients' or their family's expectations were unreasonable; these clinicians ignore the critical importance and responsibility of negotiating expectations, a bedrock skill for everyone in the ED.

Emergency department team members should relate to patient expectations by considering their own service experiences. Dirty trays and seats and observable broken items on an airline lead passengers to wonder how well the maintenance crews are servicing the rest of the plane or how attentive the ground crews are at getting luggage to the right destination. Patients are equally attentive and readily extrapolate from dirty linens and unkempt rooms that they are receiving sloppy, poor clinical care. These are "quality surrogates." They are not, strictly speaking, markers that indicate quality, but they are elements that patients, families, and even staff view as evidence of the organization's commitment to excellence.[11]

Emergency providers are generally focused on a patient's clinical diagnosis so they can "fix it." In fact, that's why most of them gravitated to the ED in the first place—the lure of immediate gratification and the excitement of addressing urgent needs. This is consistent with the colloquial ED phrase, "treat 'em and street 'em," meaning to take care of the patients and discharge them in a quick manner. This approach, of course, assumes that the patient only wants an answer and to be told what to do. Beyond that, however, patients want an answer to the broader, rarely asked question:

What matters to you?

Understanding this primary patient need drives all the other inflection points, including moving from:

- A provider-centered to a patient-centered focus
- Viewing care as episodic to viewing the patient's continuum of care
- Passive patient involvement to including patients as full participants in their own care—the most important of these points

Creating Patient Loyalty

Caregivers in the ED can go well beyond addressing expectations. The key is *exceeding* expectations, a dynamic that produces loyal patients. The "delta" between what was expected by the patient and the patient's actual experience can be:

- *Negative*—Expectations that exceed experience create disappointed patients who, if they voice their dissatisfaction, become "complainers."
- *Positive*—An experience that exceeds expectations creates loyal patients who not only received outstanding care, but also perceived that excellence.

Most health-care personnel readily recall a grateful patient who went out of his or her way to express gratitude to the provider whose care and caring went above and beyond. Often, these interactions are the fuel that keeps those health-care workers going. For emergency physicians, that fuel is embodied in this concept:

The six most treasured words an emergency physician can hear from a patient are . . .

"Do you have a private practice?"

Those words mean that not only have they exceeded the patient's expectations, they have demonstrated the skills that the patient would want in their personal physician. Just as failing to deliver on expectations largely stems from behaviors, language, processes, and perceived delays, similarly, exceeding expectations and creating loyal patients derives from positive behaviors, evidence-based language, and hardwiring flow into the equation.

Precision Patient Care

Discover what is important to the patient by simply asking them:

What's the most important thing we can do to make this an <u>excellent</u> emergency department experience for you?

It is then appropriate to individualize and "precision guide" care (use Precision Patient Care [PPC]) by tailoring management to the individual patient's needs.[12] Most patients have never been asked this simple question; yet, it allows the team, and the emergency nurse and physician specifically, to be guided by the patient's personal desires and expectations.

While based on the presentation, there will be consistent responses and variations (below), which will help focus the care. Rather than assuming what the patient/family wants, using PPC helps to ensure the patient participates in driving the team's approach and guiding the care toward the "most important thing" that they have identified:

Patient Complaint	Most Important Thing
Abdominal pain	"Make sure it isn't cancer/appendicitis."
Chest pain	"Make sure it isn't a heart attack."
Pediatric fever	"Is it meningitis?"
Extremity trauma	"Is it a fracture or a sprain?"
Pediatric facial laceration	"Will there be a scar?"
End-stage cancer	"Keep me comfortable, no mechanical devices."

The following personal story (from author Thom Mayer) is an example of what can happen if PPC is not used and assumptions are made regarding what is most important to the patient:

One evening, I saw a 15-year-old lacrosse player with an inversion injury to the ankle with lateral pain and swelling. I performed a careful evaluation, during which I explained everything that I was doing, described the anatomy of the ankle in detail, and discussed first-, second-, and third-degree sprains. Although a fracture seemed unlikely, I described why we were obtaining an ankle film. I even "predischarged" her, explaining she would be on crutches for several days and in a posterior splint while using rest, ice, compression, and elevation therapy.

When the radiograph was completed, I pulled the computer into the room and demonstrated to the athlete and her family that the images confirmed my clinical diagnosis and we would be discharging her soon. I asked what questions she had, and I thought she might be overreacting when she burst into tears.

It was then that I realized I had forgotten to use PPC and had not asked, "What's the *most important thing to you* that would make this a great ED visit?" She told me she was a recruited athlete, the state championship was in four days, and several college coaches were going to be there to scout her. Playing in that game was the most important thing to her. I felt foolish. While I had made the correct clinical diagnosis, I had failed her by not considering what this injury meant to her.

I learned late, but not too late, what was important to the patient and was able to arrange aggressive cold compression treatments, physical therapy sessions with the local experts, and ankle strapping by an athletic trainer. She was able to play in the final in front of numerous women's college lacrosse coaches—and me! (She ended up with an excellent college placement.)

The story illustrates that making the clinical diagnosis is only one part of the obligation to the patient. Precision Patient Care allows the clinician to determine what the clinical diagnosis means for the *person with the diagnosis*.

> *It is better to know what kind of person has the disease than what kind of disease the person has.*
>
> —Sir William Osler[13]

GETTING THE "WHY" RIGHT BEFORE THE "HOW"

Highly trained and motivated members of the ED team always want to know, "*How* do we provide a great experience for all of our patients?" That question misses the point: it is essential to discover the "why" that motivates professionals before the details of the evidence-based "hows" can effectively be put into action.

Very few clinicians would claim that EDs are optimally designed, staffed, funded, resourced, supported, and maintained. Further, the processes by which care is provided are often flawed, as virtually all EDs operate in a significantly capacity-constrained environment.[14] Indeed, the status quo is producing burnout in physicians, nurses, and other staff at unprecedented and unacceptable rates (see Chapters 13 and 125).[15] Emergency department teams and their leaders must not only change the culture but also the means by which care is delivered. These changes require an evidence-based approach matched directly to an assessment, such as a survey tool.

Improving the ED patient experience also requires improving the staff experience. Highly effective evidence-based solutions exist, and these approaches make it easier for both patients and those who care for them.[16]

Making the Job Easier

Health care is an art, a science, and, at its core, a personal service business. Successful execution of a service excellence/patient experience strategy requires that ED team members understand the importance of and embrace service excellence, and ensure that it is delivered consistently. Many team members feel that a significant cause of failure is that service excellence is only "embraced" to improve scores and build market share. (Try telling nurses in a busy ED that the reward for great patient experience is more patients!) Prior to asking others to master the "how-to," it is necessary for them to comprehend the "why."

This question can be answered by asking the ED staff to finish this sentence:

The No. 1 reason to get patient experience right in health care is . . .

Among the answers, staff will state it is good for the patient, the family, patient safety, risk reduction, market share, and customer service scores. These are all correct; however, leaders must emphasize that, although giving good care to patients is the primary motivation, there is another reason why the staff will want to strive for service excellence:

It makes their job easier.

Health-care workers, like most people, do not change easily. The most compelling, effective, and sustainable reason to change is that it makes the job easier for those providing the clinical care and service. Improving the patient experience makes the job of the health-care worker easier for a multitude of direct and indirect reasons, including:

- Satisfied patients are, by definition, happier with the care provided and with those who provided it. As a result, these patients and their families are more likely to express gratitude at the time of care and on subsequent surveys.
- Clinicians who have been sincerely praised feel good about the care they've provided and often consider what led to the praise in an attempt to reproduce that behavior.
- Satisfied patients are much more likely than dissatisfied patients to trust the clinicians and follow their instructions, resulting in improved health.
- Members of a dedicated team feel good when they work harmoniously to efficiently provide care and effectively communicate with each other and the patient.

Providing quality clinical care at the bedside is a difficult job that seems to get more challenging every day. It should not be a surprise that team members push back when leaders say, "Oh, and by the way, get your patient experience scores up, too." For too many care providers, patient experience is just one more mandate among an already overwhelming list of "musts." To demonstrate this concept, simply ask members of the staff the simple question:

Do you offer good customer service?

Some will say "yes" and some will say "no," but the vast majority will say "sometimes" or "it depends." To determine the specific cause of this variability, consider asking the staff the following:

Are there days when you come to work, see the people you are working with, and say to yourself, "Bring it on! Whatever we've got to do today, these folks can make it happen!"?

The answer will be "yes." When asked to describe what they call those staff members, they will answer: the "A-Team" (**Box 11.1**). Interestingly, when A-Team members are

---

BOX 11.1 ■ HOW OTHERS PERCEIVE A-TEAM MEMBERS

- Positive
- Proactive
- Confident
- Compassionate
- Competent

- Good communicators
- Team players
- Trustworthy
- Does whatever it takes
- Have a sense of humor

> **BOX 11.2 ■ HOW A-TEAM MEMBERS PERCEIVE THEMSELVES**
>
> - Things can improve, and so can I.
> - I am committed to my team and the success of each member.
> - I'm a professional and, as such:
>   - I can learn more and be better at what I do.
>   - I want honest feedback so I can grow.

asked how they think about themselves, they will somewhat consistently describe a set of characteristics similar to those listed in **Box 11.2**, clarifying that they are striving to improve. Also, ask the ED team:

> *Are there also days when you go to work, see who you're working with, and think, "Oh, no! I can't work with them — I worked with them yesterday. Who in the world makes the schedule around here, anyway?"*

That team is known as the B-Team (**Box 11.3**). Everyone on the staff can name these low-performing members except, of course, the B-Team members themselves. As the reader might expect, the B-Team member's self-perception is entirely inconsistent with the perception of their team members. Most B-Team members have an inflated view of their own capacity and leadership skills. If they are asked about their own characteristics, they might provide a list similar to the one in **Box 11.4**.

Finally, ask the staff:

> *How many B-Team members does it take to destroy an entire shift?*

They will respond in unison and emphatically, "Just one." One person can spoil, or at least lower, the morale of an entire busy clinical unit. It happens every day. Regardless of how it is described, these insights point to ways to use the performance gap to drive intrinsic instead of extrinsic change.

> **BOX 11.3 ■ HOW OTHERS PERCEIVE B-TEAM MEMBERS**
>
> - Negative
> - Overreactive and hypersensitive
> - Confused about the team goals
> - Negative, backstabbing communicators
> - Lazy, shifting responsibility
> - Frequently arrive late to work
> - Always have an excuse about why they didn't . . .
> - Constant complainers with a victim mentality

> **BOX 11.4 ■ HOW B-TEAM MEMBERS PERCEIVE THEMSELVES**
>
> - We tried that before.
> - I've been disappointed.
> - Suggestions involve too much risk.
> - They have different values; I'm better.
> - It's just a job; I can't wait to retire.
> - I'm really good just the way I am.

The "Why" in Practice

Once the A-Team and B-Team dichotomy has been explained, demonstrated, and addressed, there is an opportunity to make two important points:

- The "why" of patient experience programs is that they make the staff members' jobs easier. If not, it is not really customer service but rather something masquerading as service. Illustrate the point by employing the A-Team and B-Team exercises described above. The A-Team attributes are evidence-based customer service behaviors; B-Team attributes are customer disservice behaviors, and these actions make the jobs of the rest of the team harder. All staff want to work with A-Team members.
- The "why" of patient experience also gives everyone hope that—finally—the B-Team members will be held accountable for their actions, which affect our patients and their families and destroy our morale. Without this intervention, staff members are left to wonder when, if ever, accountability will be enforced.

Therefore, the role of the leader is to identify, accentuate, train for, and reward A-Team behaviors while simultaneously searching for, confronting, and eliminating B-Team behaviors, which should not be tolerated (see Chapter 78). Leaders who accept the responsibility of ensuring patient focus and team collaboration and accountability tap into the wisdom of people like psychologists Abraham Maslow and Erik Erikson and psychiatrist Viktor Frankl.[17-20] All, in their own way, recognized this sage insight:

All meaningful and lasting change is intrinsically, not extrinsically, motivated.

Helping ED team members understand that the leadership team is dedicated to making their jobs easier not only communicates the "why" of patient experience, it also demonstrates that the leaders will be ready to bear almost any "how." The result of combined leader and staff buy-in is that patient experience scores will rise and stay elevated because the "servant hearts" of the team will become intrinsically motivated to make their own jobs easier and make others' jobs easier, as well.

Then, and only then, is it appropriate to move on to the question of "how," as Peter Block indicates in the title of his provocative book *The Answer to How is Yes: Acting on What Matters*.[20] Leaders are more successful when they focus less on the scores and instead focus on the "why," asking:

What have I done today that makes life easier for my staff?

In doing so, a powerful and sustainable force in your organization will be unleashed—intrinsic motivation for staff to *always* be members of the A-Team.

Maslow's Hierarchy and Intrinsic Motivation

There are important parallels between Abraham Maslow's work on the hierarchy of needs and best practices in health care (**Figure 11.4**).[17] Maslow notes the hierarchy of human needs ranges from the most basic physiological needs (food, water, and warmth) to attainment of the most self-actualized needs (talent, creativity, and fulfillment). However, Maslow had two additional insights, which are often overlooked:

1. The first is that one cannot move to the next (higher) level until *all* the needs of the lower level are met.

2. The second is that, even if a person has risen to the highest levels of self-actualization, if *any* of the needs of a lower level are suddenly lacking, that person slides back to the lowest level of unmet needs.[17]

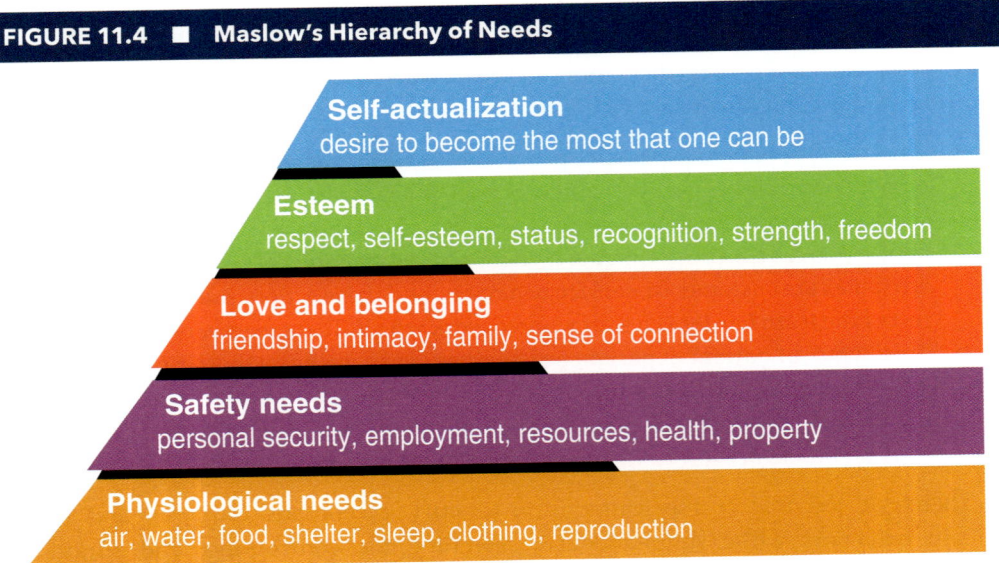

FIGURE 11.4 ■ Maslow's Hierarchy of Needs

Similar to Maslow's hierarchy of human needs, health-care organizations have a parallel set of needs, ranging from the physiological needs of basic staffing (right people, right number, right mix) to the most elevated, that of a best practice, best-in-class learning organization. Like Maslow's two additional insights, an ED can't achieve or sustain a fully developed culture of patient experience (best practices) unless and until it has met *all* the needs of the lower level, including staffing, effective leadership, teams and teamwork, flow, workforce, and patient satisfaction. Attaining the highest level is dependent on successfully achieving all of the needs of the lower levels.[21]

The second of Maslow's overlooked insights is equally germane, since even those teams that have fully met lower-level needs and become a best practices learning organization may "slide down the pyramid" if a lower-level need is no longer addressed. For example, assume an ED has achieved excellence in patient experience. Today, however, there are 10 hospital boarders and the nursing staff has three unreplaced "call-in" staff members. At least for that day, there is a high likelihood that the team may fall to the lowest levels of unmet organizational needs.[17] These critical leadership and management challenges must be regularly assessed and addressed to sustain best practices.

The Power of One

The importance of the "why" before the "how" is illustrated by the concept of "the power of one" (**Figure 11.5**). There are certainly some jobs in which people wonder if their efforts make a difference. This is not a concern in the ED, where "the power of one" simply recognizes that one doctor, one nurse, one team, one patient, one family all make a difference. The question is:

What will that difference be?

Use Patient Experience Surveys as a Tool, Not a Club

The dogmas that have guided ED caregivers in the past do not adequately address the current tasks. Leaders and team members must think anew and act anew to successfully move forward.[22] They must confront the reality of patient experience, the new means of assessing ED care in positive, creative, and proactive ways, starting with this insight:

Don't use the ED CAHPS survey as a club! Use it as a tool!

FIGURE 11.5 ■ The Power of One

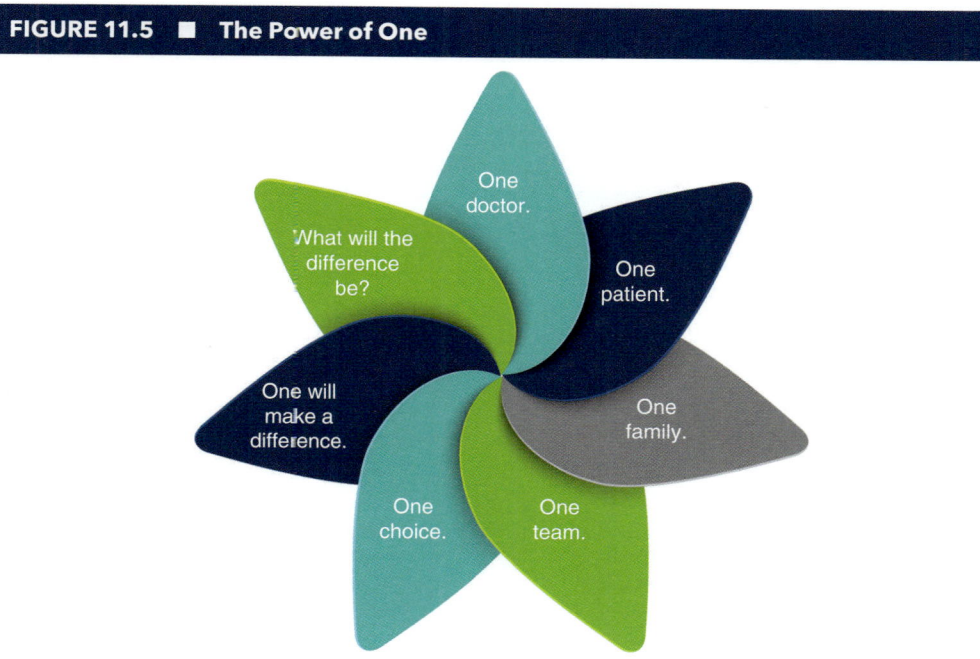

In the past, surveys were too often used as a club to beat people into submission to get their scores higher (often without any coaching or mentoring on how to do so). Instead, the survey should be used as a tool, a creative way to improve the language, transitions, and processes of clinical care as well as the entire experience for patients and their families.

Paul Batalden's insight that health-care systems are perfectly designed to produce precisely the results they get mandates action to change the system. Improved results require new and modified processes. Poor outcomes are the result of poor systems, ineffective leadership strategies, and a culture hardwired to deliver ineffective daily actions.

Fortunately, patient experience surveys, properly viewed and utilized, provide detailed and actionable information. Practices can be improved by identifying how they are experienced by the patient and how they can be used to make our jobs easier. **Figures 11.6** and **Table 11.1** summarize the details of ED CAHPS, which show:

- How the ED team is perceived
- What can be done to improve how the care is experienced
- How the ED CAHPS and other feedback can be used as tools, not clubs

Making Commitments... Ensuring Success

The core of all ED missions is commitment to the patient. Organizations like the Mayo Clinic ("The needs of the patient come first."), Cleveland Clinic ("Patient first"), Duke University ("Caring for our patients, their loved ones, and each other"), and other health-care systems have, each in their different voices, made the same bedrock commitment to keep the patient at the center of their efforts.[23-25] These commitments, while essential to success, are not enough to ensure success in the current complex health-care environment.[26]

Chris Argyris noted that there is a fundamental difference between the espoused theory (the theory promoted by leadership and management) and the theory in action (which reflects how the organization actually operates).[27] Every ED should carefully examine how closely its espoused theory matches that theory in action. For instance, if the espoused theory is "patient-centered care," it is appropriate to ask: Is the patient

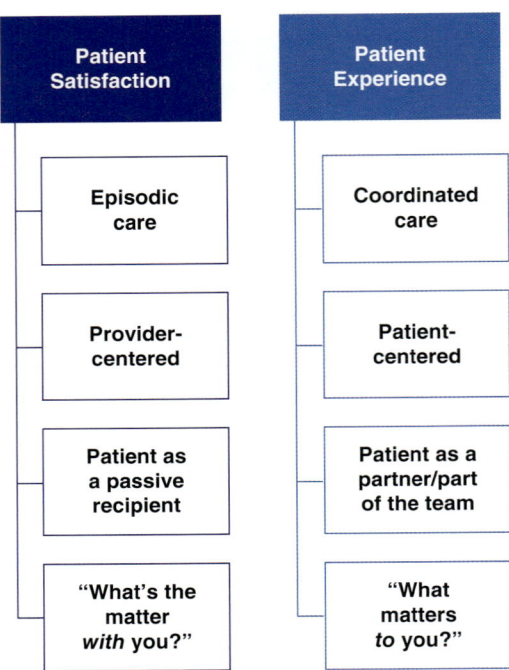

FIGURE 11.6 ■ Moving from Patient Satisfaction to Patient Experience

really at the center of everyone's actions, or is it simply a popular idea to which the organization gives lip service? What *actions* are actually occurring with each patient? Stated another way, pay attention to the "happenings in the halls" instead of the "words on the walls."[28]

Shared Mental Models

Whether tacitly or explicitly, the elements of patient experience are held together by the commitment to the patient through *shared mental models*. As Peter Senge notes in his seminal work, *The Fifth Discipline: The Art and Practice of the Learning Organization*, every organization has its shared mental models, which he defines as:

> . . . deeply held internal images of how the world works, images that limit us to familiar ways of thinking and acting. Very often, we are not completely aware of our mental models or the effects they have on our behavior.[29]

TABLE 11.1 ■ Satisfaction Surveys vs ED CAHPS

Satisfaction ratings reflect...	Patient experience ratings reflect...
Superficial evaluations	More detailed evaluations
Simple perception of care	The depth of the interaction
Board areas evaluated	Involvement and participation in treatment
General evaluation	Actionable concerns
Evaluation of what accured	What actually accured
Evaluation of staff/services	The quality of the experience
Less clarity on how to improve	More detail on what and how to improve
No input from admitted patients	Admitted patients included

The Reputational Calculus of Exceeding Expectations

Emergency departments represent a phenomenal marketing and branding opportunity for the entire health-care system. Data from the Emergency Department Benchmarking Alliance indicated that current ED usage comprises nearly 475 annual visits per 1,000 people, an increase from 350 a decade ago.[30] This staggering figure underscores the power of the community to affect the reputation of an ED. Good reputations, both in life and in the ED, are hard-won but can be lost in an instant.

Previously, reputations traveled at the speed of sound, meaning one person would share details of their ED visit at home, at school, at work, at the grocery store, or at the place of worship. These days, reputations move at the speed of light because people are transmitting their experiences on social media and e-mail. Indeed, these "reputation electrons" are even being sent from the waiting room and the treatment areas; some patients are not even waiting until they leave the premises to share their stories!

Emergency department team members believe it is unfair that satisfied patients only occasionally share their experiences, while dissatisfied patients seem to extensively broadcast their complaints. Many physicians and nurses believe that unhappy patients tell everyone about their experience, and happy patients tell no one. The real data on the topic, however, are more complex.

One of the first insightful voices on the concept of customer loyalty is Frederick Reichheld of Bain & Company.[31] His work is credited with providing a clear lens through which to view the role of exceeding expectations in service industries. Unhappy customers tell an average of 15 to 20 people about their bad experience. "Crusaders," who are on a mission to spread the bad news about their care, tell 24 to 30 people.

As **Figure 11.7** shows, patient complaints are a form of the "iceberg phenomenon," where there is much more under the surface than appears. (These data originally came from the Technical Assistance Research Project and reflect non-health-care experience, but this finding has been replicated in health care.[32]) The impact on the staff—and some

FIGURE 11.7 ■ The "Iceberg" Effect

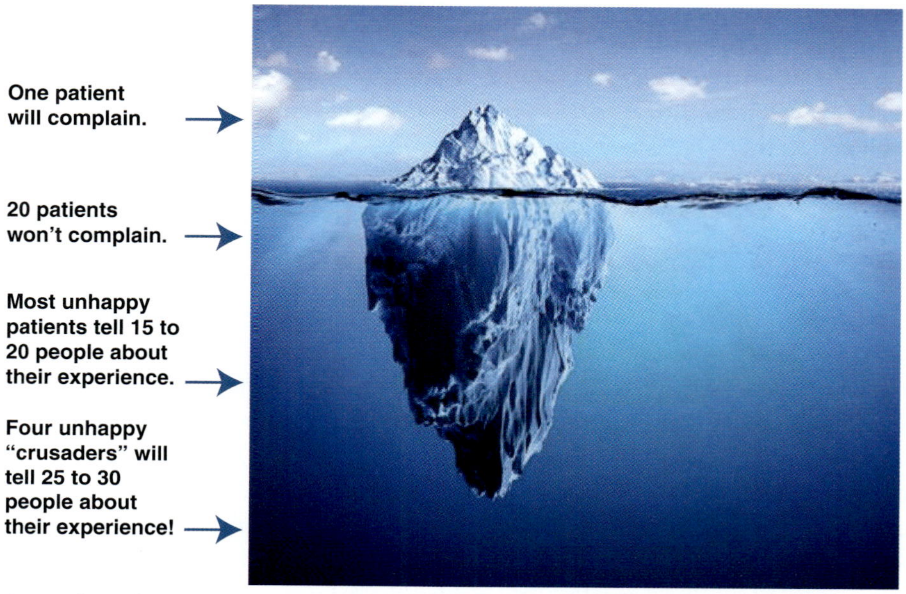

- One patient will complain.
- 20 patients won't complain.
- Most unhappy patients tell 15 to 20 people about their experience.
- Four unhappy "crusaders" will tell 25 to 30 people about their experience!

Approximately 70% of these patients will become loyal customers if their complaint is properly resolved. That number rises to 96% if the complaint is resolved *quickly*!

FIGURE 11.8 ■ The "Mt. Everest" Phenomenon

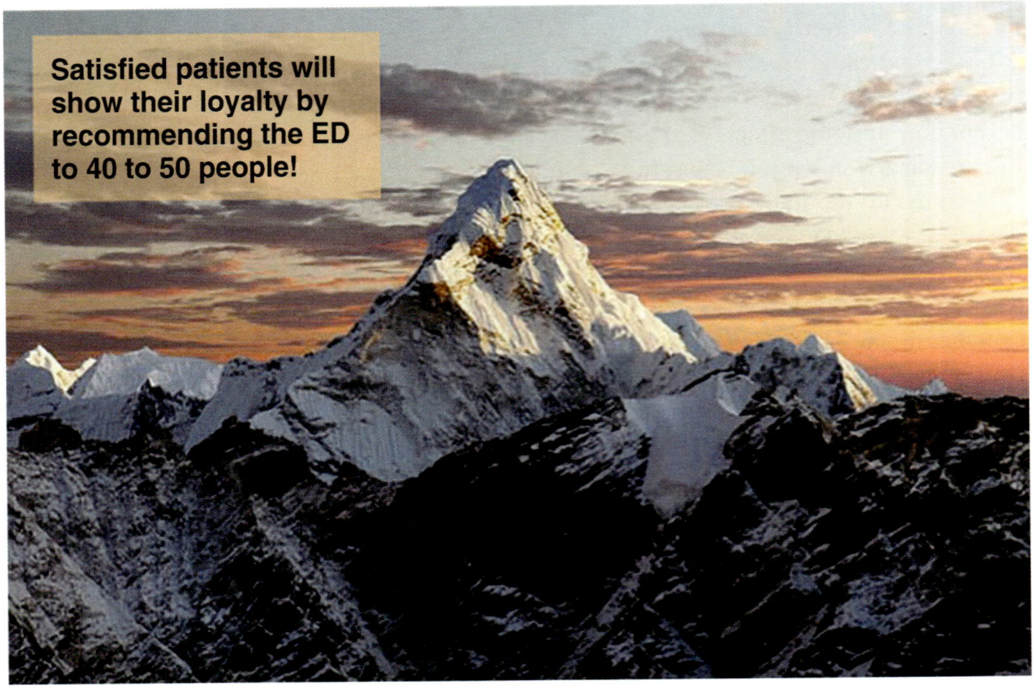

Satisfied patients will show their loyalty by recommending the ED to 40 to 50 people!

managers—may be a type of hopelessness: "What can you do? We can't win with odds like that." However, an astounding statistic discovered in ED research holds promise.[33]

Studies show that patients whose expectations have been exceeded tell an average of 40 to 50 people how happy they were with their experience. Therefore, it is critically important for leaders to understand, promote, and advance the concept of patient loyalty. Extrapolating from the "iceberg" metaphor of patient complaints, there is also a "Mt. Everest phenomenon" of patient satisfaction, which can be recognized and achieved by most ED staff (**Figure 11.8**).

Strengthening patient loyalty requires a systematic approach to understanding and exceeding expectations. Loyal patients are satisfied and recognize, tacitly if not explicitly, that their expectations have been exceeded; whereas each unsatisfied, nonloyal patient has their own strongly felt issue.

Moving Into the "Always" Era of Health Care

There are many important distinctions between previous patient satisfaction surveys and ED CAHPS surveys. However, the most important difference by far is that EDPECS, like all other Consumer Assessment of Healthcare Providers and Systems (ED CAHPS) surveys (the results of which are used by Medicare to determine hospital payments), includes "always" as a top score for many of its questions.

Several organizations only give credit for "top-box scores." In terms of ED CAHPS, the top box is the highest score: "always." These health-care organizations and hospitals define success by the percentage of patients who answer "always" on the core questions; any other score, including "usually," is considered a failure. In the final version of the ED

CAHPS survey, the total number of "always" questions is now down to six, three each for the physicians and nurses in these areas:

- Doctor/nurse showed courtesy and respect
- Doctor/nurse took the time to listen carefully
- Doctor/nurse explained things in a way you could understand

Health-care workers in a system that measures "top box" results do not get partial credit. It's "always" or "nothing!" The same is true for net promoter score surveys (NPS) and loyalty questions.[34] On a scale from 1 to 10, credit is given only for scores of 9 and 10. In fact, the NPS system considers scores 7 and 8 as "neutral" and 6 and below as "detractors." To determine the NPS, the total number of detractors are subtracted from the total number of promotors (**Figures 11.9**).

Clinicians, particularly those working in EDs, may initially resist moving into the "always" era of measurement. As a way of illustrating this, when coaching the staff, consider asking this question:

Have you "always" been a good ...

- *Mother/daughter?*
- *Father/son?*
- *Husband/wife?*
- *Boss/employee?*

"Always" seems to be a pretty tough standard to meet when put that way. But consider asking this follow-up question:

What if that were your mother/father, son/daughter, sister/brother, grandmother/grandfather on the ED stretcher, wouldn't you want "always" for them?

The answer will be a resounding "YES!" It's helpful to remember that just because it may be difficult to always provide excellence, it doesn't mean that "always" isn't worth striving for. The key for leaders is to help their staff understand that in the "always" era, there are evidence-based disciplines that *must be used on every patient, every time, all the time!*

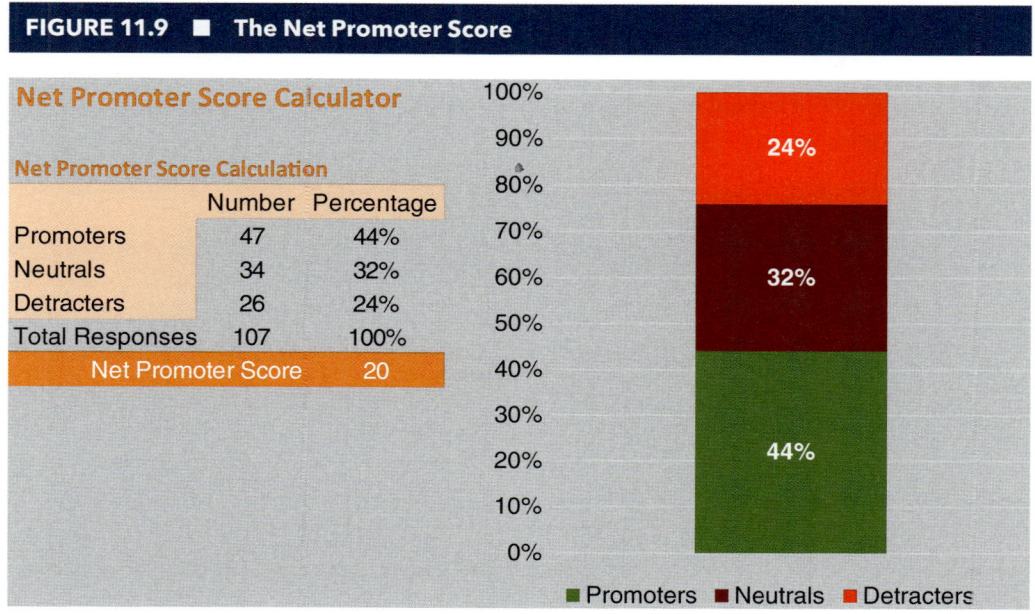

FIGURE 11.9 ■ The Net Promoter Score

In his wonderful reflections on the meaning of having lived through the Holocaust, Austrian neurologist Viktor Frankl makes this critical point:

> *Everything can be taken from a man but one thing: the last of human freedoms — the ability to choose one's attitude in any given set of circumstances — the ability to choose one's own way.*[25]

While "always" surveys may be offered by the Centers for Medicare and Medicaid Services, in every circumstance, ED team members retain the choice of how to react by choosing their attitude. It is "the power of one" simply stated in a different way. It is choosing to use the survey as a tool instead of a club, to treat the survey as an open-book test, (see Chapters 3 and 74) and to use all the evidence-based resources available to make the job easier in pursuit of "always."

There is only one way this can happen, and that is to apply the available evidence on what works (and what doesn't) in a highly disciplined fashion and freely choose to make it better for those we serve, noting that success makes the job easier. Add to this the fact that pushing back against "always" will *always* be a waste of time, energy, effort, focus, heart, soul, mind, and purpose.

CONCLUSION

Patient experience differs from patient satisfaction in important ways and offers a more nuanced and actionable way to make the job easier, which is the primary "why" of an evidence-based approach to ED leadership. Patient experience is defined as the "delta" between the patient's expectations and the patient's experience. If the experience falls below expectations, the patient is unhappy and complains, telling 20 people. But if a patient's expectations are *exceeded*, they demonstrate their loyalty by telling 40 to 50 people about how pleased they were.

Getting the "why" right before the "how" is a key to success. A primary "why" is that it makes the job easier. All meaningful and lasting change is intrinsically, not extrinsically, motivated. This essential concept requires health-care providers to change the underlying key question from "What's the matter *with* you?" to "What matters *to* you?" Making the patient part of the team and using PPC are the two most important tools in this transition. The survey is a tool for guiding improvement rather than a club to harass staff, and each and every team member makes a difference each time they care for a patient ("the power of one"). In the "always" era of patient experience, these evidence-based tools are essential to helping the team choose to always achieve excellence.

REFERENCES

1. Batalden P. Available at: www.ihi.org/communities/blogs/origins-of-every-system-is-perfectly-designed-quote. Accessed December 27, 2019.
2. Mayer T. EDPECS is Coming! Preparing for the New Patient Experience Reality of Emergency Medicine. Presented at: ACEP Scientific Assembly 2019; October 29, 2019; Denver, Colorado.
3. The Beryl Institute. Available at: https://www.theberylinstitute.org/page/About. Accessed December 27, 2019.
4. Mayer T. Leadership for great patient experience: the survival skills approach. In: Strauss R, Mayer T, eds.) *Emergency Department Management.* 2nd ed. Dallas, Tex: American College of Emergency Physicians; 2020.
5. Press Ganey Associates. Patient experience: build the patient-consumer relationship throughout the healthcare journey. Available at: https://www.pressganey.com/solutions/patient-experience. Accessed December 27, 2019.
6. Urden L. Patient satisfaction measurement: current issues and implications. 2002. Lippincott's Case Management. 7(5):194-200.
7. Mayer T. Creating a culture of customer service. Making employees' jobs easier is the key to success. *Healthc Exec.* 2015;30(3):58, 60-61.
8. Mayer T. Patient experience in emergency medicine. 2020. Delivered to the ACEP Emergency Department Directors Academy, Dallas, Tex, February 5, 2020.

9. Gerber A, Lungen M, Lauterbach KC. Evidence-based medicine is based in Protestant exegesis. *Med Hypotheses*. 2005;64:1034-1038.

10. Mayer T. Beyond customer service: a guide to delivering on patient experience. 2020. Presented to the ACEP Emergency Department Directors Academy, Dallas, Tex. April 16, 2020.

11. Pelligrino ED. *For the Patients' Good: The Restoration of Beneficence in Health Care*. New York, NY: Oxford University Press; 1998.

12. Mayer T. Precision Patient Care™ moving forward. Presented at: the Institute for Healthcare Improvement Open School, December 6, 2019.

13. Osler W. *Aequanimitas*. Philadelphia, Pa: HK Lewis Publishers; 1904.

14. Jensen K, Mayer T. *The Patient Flow Advantage*. Gulf Breeze, FL, Fire Starter Press; 2014.

15. Mayer T. Getting back to the job you love: reconnecting with passion to battle burnout. *Healthc Exec*. 2020.

16. Mayer T, Cates RJ. *Leadership for Great Customer Service: Satisfied Employees, Satisfied Patients*. Chicago, Ill: Health Administration Press; 2004.

17. Maslow A. A theory of human motivation. *Psychol Rev*. 1943;504 (4):370-396.

18. Eriksen E. *The Life Cycle Completed*. New York, NY: Norton Books; 1997.

19. Frankl V. *Man's Search for Meaning*. Boston, Mass: Beacon Press; 2006.

20. Block P. *The Answer to How is Yes: Acting on What Matters*. San Francisco, Calif: Berrett-Koehler; 2003.

21. Mayer T, Jensen K. *Hardwiring Flow: Systems and Processes for Smooth Patient Flow*. Gulf Breeze, Fla, Fire Starter Press; 2004.

22. Lincoln A. Annual Message to Congress. December 1, 1862. Available at; http://www.abrahamlincolnonline.org/lincoln/speeches/congress.htm. Accessed December 27, 2019.

23. Berry LL, Seltman KD. *Management Lessons From Mayo Clinic*. New York, NY, McGraw-Hill; 2008.

24. Lee TH, Cosgrove T. Engaging doctors in the healthcare revolution. *Harvard Business Review*. May-June 2014.

25. Duke Health. Available at: https://corporate.dukehealth.org/who-we-are/mission-vision. Accessed December 29, 2019.

26. Stanford Encyclopedia of Philosophy. Necessary and sufficient conditions. Available at: https //plato.stanford.edu/entries/necessary-sufficient/. Accessed December 29, 2019.

27. Argyris C. *Organizational Traps: Leadership, Culture, and Organizational Design*. Oxford, United Kingdom: Oxford University Press; 2010.

28. Mayer T. Rewarding the champions and corralling the stragglers. In: Strauss R, Mayer T, eds. *Strauss and Mayer's Emergency Department Management*. 2nd ed. Dallas, Tex: American College of Emergency Physicians; 2020.

29. Senge P. *The Fifth Discipline: The Art and Science of the Learning Organization*. New York, NY: Doubleday; 2006.

30. Emergency Department Benchmarking Alliance. EDBA Annual Report 2018. Available at: www.edbenchmarking.org. Accessed December 28, 2019.

31. Reichheld F. *The Loyalty Effect: The Hidden Force Behind Growth, Profits, and Lasting Value*. Boston, Mass: Harvard Business School Press; 1996.

32. Zimkowski R. The effect of loyal patients in healthcare. *Healthc Financ Manage*. 2004.

33. Mayer T. Putting it all together: best practices in service excellence. *Healthc Exec*. 2011.

34. Reichheld FF, The one number you need to grow. *Harvard Business Review*. 2003. Available at: https://hbr.org/2003/12/the-one-number-you-need-to-grow. Accessed December 28, 2019.

CHAPTER 12
THE DISCIPLINE OF TEAMS AND TEAMWORK

Thom A. Mayer, Robert W. Strauss, Theresa Tavernero, Mary Kay Silverman, Kirk Jensen

Alone we can do so little. Together we can do so much.

—Helen Keller[1]

Emergency departments (EDs) can be exciting, stimulating, and rewarding places to work, particularly for those drawn to a wide range of patients with varying acuity. Emergency physicians and nurses are typically extremely intelligent, highly motivated professionals who work with an impressive group of support personnel. Thus, we know that we have a "team of experts." But that is quite different from being certain that we have "an expert team." Do those smart people work together in smart ways? Are they taught the fundamentals of teamwork as a part of their orientation to the ED team, or are teamwork skills simply assumed?

Successful ED leaders recognize that certain evidence- and experience-based principles are requisite for teams to interact successfully. A "high-performance team" has been defined as "a group of people with specific roles and complimentary talents and skills, aligned with and committed to a common purpose, who consistently show high levels of collaboration and innovation, produce superior results."[2]

IT TAKES A TEAM

Emergency department care is a "team sport" by its very nature. Nurses, physicians, and essential services personnel (e.g., laboratory, radiology, ED technicians, unit secretaries, registration, inpatient admissions, housekeeping, and others) must function as a team in order to deliver quality patient care in a predictable, reliable, and sustainable fashion. Effective patient care can only be provided with coordination and collaboration among diverse—and sometimes disparate—groups of people. Beyond the technical training, patient care requires multiple interdependent processes carried out by individual team members of different levels. Physicians, nurses, technicians, clerical staff, and other personnel working together as a team can create high-performance EDs that set themselves apart from the ones that struggle to merely survive. Teamwork is also key to effective recruitment and retention of team members. Without teamwork, burnout is almost inevitable in the ED (see Chapter 125).

Each team member brings their own unique talents, skills, abilities, background, and motivation for a shared common purpose. While members of high-performance ED teams may not contribute equally, all contribute uniquely—and to the best of their abilities—for a single, clear, measurable common purpose: to benefit the patients and families whose care is entrusted to the team. The care of those patients and their families is the *raison d'être* of emergency medicine.

The difficult work of patient care is exponentially easier if teamwork is a fundamental part of the mission, vision, values, and culture of the ED. The staff's ability to consistently deliver clinical and service excellence to patients is substantially enhanced in a work environment characterized by teamwork, which itself becomes a source of ongoing professional satisfaction.

Danish philosopher Søren Kierkegaard once noted that it is a fundamental paradox of the human condition that the most important questions are simultaneously those asked least often.[3] "Are you a team?" is an extremely important question. Too often, we assume that the people assembled in the ED are a team, yet the principles outlined in this chapter are not a fundamental part of their daily work. To help guide answering this question, consider these additional questions:

- What are you most proud of as a team?
- What are the best things you do as a team?
- What are you least proud of as a team?
- What are the things you need to work on as a team?
- Does the rest of the team agree with you?
- If not, why?

Then move on to these questions:

- What's the strongest aspect of your team?
- What's the weakest aspect of your team?
- What are you doing to ensure your strongest asset is consistent?
- What are you doing to ensure you eliminate your weakest asset?

This exercise helps team members better understand their interactions, as well as areas that work well and those that need improvement.

Seams of the Teams

The "seams of the teams" are the multiple ways in which team members interact.[4] ED processes are filled with service transitions and repeated handoffs from one team member to another during even the simplest of cases. Focus first on what you are doing well, the things you are most proud of in caring for patients. Then ask, "Do we do those things 100% of the time with every patient?" Don't be surprised if a sheepish, "Well . . . no," is the response. Begin by ensuring that the positive team elements are accentuated with every staff member. These are the "A-Team" behaviors we are doing, but we're just not doing them all day, every day, with every patient.

Now focus on the things you are *least* proud of. Begin discussions on how those areas can be made to work more smoothly and consistently—and don't be surprised when the very process of doing this exercise helps improve teamwork.

Making the Patient a Part of the Team

The fundamental question is this: "Is the patient a *recipient* of care, or are they a *participant* in their care?" Unfortunately, when we ask this question in our work with teams, the most common response is a somewhat blank, quizzical look, followed by, "Actually, I've never thought about that." As we move from patient satisfaction to patient experience, making the patient a clear part of the team will be of paramount importance to ED success (see Chapter 11). These are the questions the team must ask and answer:

- Are we making the patient part of the team?
- How, specifically, are we doing that?

- Is everyone on the team doing that consistently with every patient?
- If we asked the other team members (teams and seams) these questions, would we get the same answers?
- If we asked the patient, would they agree?

Too often, patients end up being simply a recipient of care—at least from their perspective. Teaching the team to use scripts or evidence-based language is an important start, for example:

> *Mr. Jones, we have a team of dedicated professionals who are here to serve you, but you are the most important member of our team. We want to keep you fully informed of every aspect of your care, so please let us know if you have any questions at any time.*

Experience working with hundreds of ED teams demonstrates this concept of making the patient a part of the team can be one of the most helpful and transformational of the teamwork tools.

Just as the patient needs to be proactively made a part of the team, the family/caregivers also need to be enlisted actively in discussions about the diagnosis, treatment, and follow-up care. This is particularly true with pediatric and geriatric patients. (Of course, for patients who are of the age of consent, their permission is required before discussing elements of their care.)

Hire Right for Teams

Recruiting new members onto the team is one of the most important decisions ED leaders make. If you believe teamwork is an essential value for success, what are you doing to "hire right" for teamwork?[5] Too often, leaders simply assume that the people they are recruiting have effective teamwork skills. Here are several ways to build teamwork into the hiring process:

- **Ask their previous employer/training program.**
    - ☐ "Tell me about this person's teamwork skills."
    - ☐ "Please give me some examples of how they exhibit teamwork."
- **Build teamwork questions into the interview process.**
    - ☐ "How important is teamwork to you in your daily work?"
    - ☐ "Give me an example of how you went above and beyond for your team."
    - ☐ "Have you ever thought about the patient being a part of the ED team?"

If teamwork is an important value for your ED, make sure it is a part of your hiring process as well as the orientation and coaching/mentoring process, discussed later in this chapter. Physician and nurse leaders should consider themselves the "chief talent officers" responsible for recruiting the best talent to the team, and teamwork must be cultivated as a part of this process.

DEFINING TEAMS AND TEAMWORK

The words team and teamwork are so widely used that most people tacitly believe they know what they mean. Actually, most teams have never explicitly taken the time to come to a common definition of the terms, as the insightful quote from Jon Katzenbach and Douglas Smith clearly shows:

> *The word* team *gets bandied about so loosely that many managers are oblivious to its real meaning — or its true potential. With a run-of-the-mill working group, performance is a function of what the members do as individuals. A team's performance, by contrast, calls for both individual and mutual accountability.*[6]

> **BOX 12.1 ■ THE ELEMENTS OF HIGH-PERFORMING TEAMS[5]**
>
> - Deep sense of purpose
> - Clear performance goals
> - Specific processes to accomplish the goals
> - A common mission and individual responsibility
> - Complimentary and sometimes interchangeable skill sets

A clear definition with measurable and actionable elements is essential for understanding teamwork in health care. Without such a pragmatic definition, it is likely that the words of the late Peter Drucker, one of the world's great thinkers on leadership and management, will be as applicable to health care as they were to business: "Team building has become a buzzword in American business. The results are not overly impressive. Teams are tools. Teamwork is neither 'good' nor 'desirable'—it is a fact. Whenever people work together or play together, they do so as a team."[7]

A team is defined as two or more people who share a common goal and work interdependently to accomplish that goal.[8] A group differs from a team in that members of the group may share a common goal but may not work together to accomplish it. This is a subtle but crucial point, as it is possible to assemble a group of health-care providers in the ED who share the common goal of quality patient care but who cannot achieve this goal because they do not function as a high-performance team. While there are many formulations and definitions of effective teams (**Box 12.1**, **Figure 12.1**), the most necessary elements are as follows:

- A clear, inspired, and common sense of purpose with a commitment to excellence and improvement at the forefront that the team members have helped shape.
- Deep and abiding respect among team members for the unique roles and talents each brings to the endeavor, as well as a genuine appreciation for the contributions of others.
- A system of processes designed to accomplish clearly defined goals, which are capable of revision and improvement over time.
- A culture which celebrates team success, while coaching members whose performance needs improvement through a system of mutual accountability.

To understand this definition of teams in health care, an exegesis of each element is necessary.

Common Sense of Purpose

Health care can be quite confusing, even to those involved in its daily work. The best way to prevent such confusion is to ensure that each member of the team has a clear, succinct understanding of the purpose for which the team exists. While it may seem obvious that excellence in patient care is the primary purpose, team members often get distracted by process details and extraneous task-related issues. Thus, it is necessary to constantly refocus on the common purpose.

Daily Reinforcement: Ritz-Carlton

How often should that common sense of purpose be reinforced? In world-class organizations, the answer is "every day!" The Ritz-Carlton hotels have a well-earned reputation for excellence in the hospitality industry, but how exactly they got that reputation is lesser known. In this context, two critical concepts are worth emphasis.

FIGURE 12.1 ■ John Wooden's Pyramid of Successful Teams

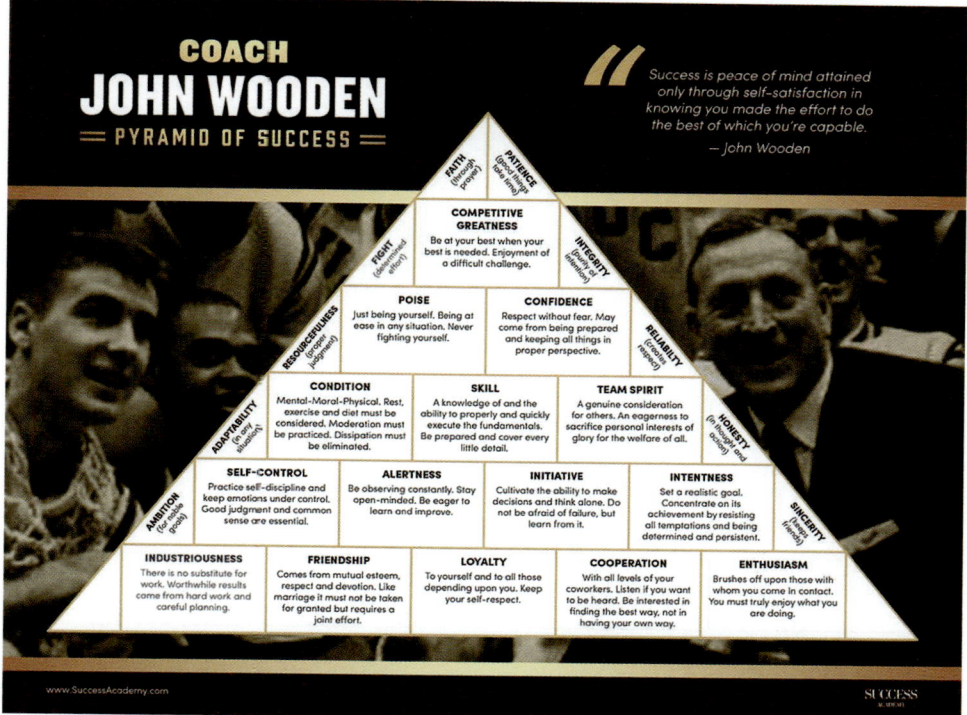

The first concept is the importance of having a clear vision for their staff, which succinctly states their purpose, known as the credo.[9] Some health-care organizations have used this concept to help focus their staff on mission, vision, and values (**Figure 12.2**). The credo in health care is an excellent idea, but it must be backed by a system that can be practically applied by the staff.

This leads to the second concept: a practical method to regularly deliver this common purpose in the patient care setting. For that reason, Ritz-Carlton and many highly successful hospitals and health-care systems have adopted a "daily huddle." The purpose of the huddle is to have a focused daily gathering across all units and departments that emphasizes a particular aspect of the credo, any safety concerns the team may have, or a common sense of purpose for that day or shift.

Daily Huddle: Bon Secours Richmond

At Bon Secours Health System Richmond, the use of daily huddles has had dramatic results. As an example, one huddle focuses on anticipation: knowing what patients and families want before they ask for it. This is one of many reasons that Bon Secours is considered a world-class health provider. The huddle goes on to emphasize the importance of observing patient and family body language and using active listening as keys to building loyal, engaged relationships. Each huddle ends precisely the same way for this faith-based system, with the three questions and answers included in **Box 12.2**.

Creating a Meaningful Vision

Each organization must discover or uncover its own deep sense of purpose and give that purpose its own unique voice. Successful teams share a sense of purpose that includes not only a commitment to excellence but also an understanding that the rapid pace of change

FIGURE 12.2 ■ Ritz-Carlton Credo Card

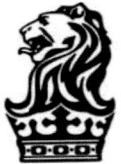

THE RITZ-CARLTON®

THE CREDO

"WE ARE LADIES AND GENTLEMEN SERVING LADIES AND GENTLEMEN"

The Ritz-Carlton is a place where the genuine care and comfort of our guests is our highest mission.

We pledge to provide the finest personal service and facilities for our guests, who will always enjoy a warm, relaxed, yet refined ambience.

The Ritz-Carlton experience enlivens the senses, instills well-being, and fulfills even the unexpressed wishes and needs of our guests.

Three steps of service are (1) A warm and sincere greeting. Use the guest's name, if and when possible. (2) Anticipation and compliance with guest needs. (3) Fond farewell. Give them a warm goodbye and use their names, if and when possible.

THE RITZ-CARLTON BASICS

1. The Credo will be known, owned, and energized by all employees.
2. We are Ladies and Gentlemen serving Ladies and Gentlemen.
3. The three steps of service shall be practiced by all employees.
4. Smile — "We are on stage." Always maintain positive eye contact.
5. Use the proper vocabulary with our guests (eliminate "hi," "folks," etc).
6. Uncompromising levels of cleanliness are the responsibility of every employee.
7. Create a positive work environment. Practice teamwork.
8. Be an ambassador of your hotel in and outside of the work place. Always talk positively.
9. Any employee who receives a guest complaint "owns" the complaint.
10. Instant guest pacification will be ensured by all. Respond to guest wishes within ten minutes of the request. Follow up with a telephone call within twenty minutes to ensure their satisfaction.
11. Use guest incident action forms to communicate guest problems to fellow employees and managers. This will help ensure that out guests are never forgotten.
12. Escort guests, rather than pointing out directions to another area of the hotel.
13. Be knowledgeable of hotel information to answer guest questions.
14. Use proper telephone etiquette. Answer within three rings and, with a "smile," ask permission to put a caller on hold. Do not screen calls. Eliminate call transfers when possible.
15. Always recommend the hotel's food and beverage outlets prior to outside facilities.
16. Uniforms are to be immaculate. Wear proper footwear and your correct nametag.
17. Ensure all employees know their roles during emergency situations and are aware of procedures.
18. Notify your supervisor immediately of hazards, injuries, or assistance needs you have.
19. Practice energy conservation and proper maintenance of hotel property.
20. Protecting the assets of a Ritz-Carlton Hotel is the responsibility of every employee.

requires a constant spirit of innovation. "We've always done it that way" is a recipe for disaster.

Finally, and perhaps most importantly, if the team is to have a passionate commitment to the common sense of purpose, the team members themselves must actively help shape and articulate the sense of purpose. The phrase "if they are not with you on the takeoff, they won't be with you on the landing" certainly applies here.[10] As team members change and new team members are onboarded, each should be oriented to the common sense of purpose and given the opportunity to discuss and improve it. The team's statement of purpose should reflect the organization's mission, vision, and values (see Chapter 2).

> **BOX 12.2 ■ BON SECOURS HUDDLE QUESTIONS**
>
> - **Where are we?** We are on holy ground.
> - **Why are we here?** We are here to serve.
> - **What are we?** We are world class.

Critical Thinking Skills

Part of assuring a common sense of purpose is developing a common understanding of the reasoning process by which decisions are made. It is important to understand that modern emergency nursing leaders appropriately place a premium on the value of critical thinking skills, which is concept not often taught in medical schools, residency, or orientation of physicians. Critical thinking is the ability to be in control of one's thinking while in the process of thinking. It includes the ability to consciously examine the elements of one's reasoning, or that of another, and evaluate that reasoning against universal intellectual standards, including:

- Clarity
- Accuracy
- Precision
- Relevance
- Depth
- Breadth
- Logic

All sources of information must be examined for their applicability and reliability in the clinical setting. Critical thinking integrates the intellectual traits of humility, autonomy, integrity, courage, perseverance, confidence, empathy, and fair-mindedness.[11] When emergency physicians and nurses understand the critical thinking skills concept, it facilitates developing a common sense of purpose shaped by team members.

Deep Respect

High-performance teams require a common sense of purpose and a recognition of individual roles. The care of each patient in the ED requires multiple service handoffs among many different people from highly variable educational backgrounds and training, ranging from high school graduates to nurses and physicians with many years of professional training. And yet, there is a common sense of purpose. Team members must be well prepared to accomplish their own responsibilities and to work adaptively with other team members who have different roles.

High-performance teams ensure that service transitions are handled in a positive and proactive manner. Using effective scripts to manage that transition is extremely helpful. For example, a triage nurse stating, "Janice will be your primary nurse—she's one of our best!" primes the patient and family to feel that they will be well cared for in a professional fashion. These types of verbal skills assure patients and families that the service transition has been anticipated and handled well. Quint Studer refers to this as "managing up."[12] **Box 12.3** shows other examples of this technique.

> **BOX 12.3 ■ LEADING UP-MANAGING EXPECTATIONS**
>
> Teams can dramatically assist in service handoffs by "managing up" with these verbal approaches, which ensure that the patient and their family approach the next team member with a positive attitude.
>
> - "Janet is your nurse today, and she's the best we have."
> - "Let me introduce you to my partner Dr. Smith, who will be taking over your care. I have briefed him on your care, and he is an excellent physician."
> - "Unfortunately, the bone is broken. The good news is that Dr. Theiss is on call, and he is a great physician."
> - "You will need to be admitted. I spoke to your doc, and he want our specialist in Hospital Medicine to care for you. Dr. Rodriquez will be taking care of you, and he is excellent."

Contrast the triage nurse's comment above with a different greeting: "Have a seat. Someone will call you." The first message communicates, "I care, and we are prepared to treat you with excellence." The second message communicates, "I/we don't care."

A critical responsibility of ED leaders is to ensure that all team members know the roles and responsibilities of others and that a culture of mutual trust and appreciation exists. This knowledge and trust accelerate and accentuate the team's effectiveness. Perhaps Rudyard Kipling said it best: "For the strength of the pack is the wolf, and the strength of the wolf is the pack."[13]

A Pertinent Example

James Adams, chair of the Department of Emergency Medicine at Northwestern University, shares the following vignette about the dramatic value of teamwork:

> *A patient presented to triage when no beds were available. Per protocol, an electrocardiogram (ECG) was performed at triage by an ED technician, whose responsibility it was to take the ECG to an emergency physician in the acute care area. The quiet and unassuming ED technician expected the worst when he took the ECG to a particularly acerbic, gruff emergency physician. The emergency physician snatched the ECG tracing out of the tech's hands, quickly read it, and diagnosed an acute anterior myocardial infarction. The patient was quickly rushed into the treatment area and then onto the cardiac catheterization lab. But not before the emergency physician sought out the ED tech and said, "You just saved that guy's life."*

Not only did that tech feel incredible and, in that moment, recognize his unique sense of purpose, but also the story became a part of the lore of the ED. That's the power of teamwork and the way in which it strengthens "the pack."

Dyad Leadership

One of the most important developments that assures deep respect among team members is the concept of dyad leadership, a partnership where physician and nurse leaders work as a team to use their respective skills and training for the good of the ED team and the patients for whom they care (see Chapter 6). It recognizes that all EDs, by their very nature and the processes that guide them, are complex adaptive systems that require a team approach to function effectively. It is this systems-based approach that is at the heart of dyad leadership, based on psychological and practical safety across complex boundaries, leading to adaptive and cooperative leadership. When someone asks, "Who is in charge of the ED?" dyad leaders proudly answer, *"We* are!"

A System of Value-Added Processes

Good teams rarely make it up as they go along. Excellent, high-performing teams never do. Instead, they develop clearly delineated processes that all team members know and that are designed to produce measurable results.

The Indianapolis Colts 2006 Super Bowl-winning NFL team ran the "no-huddle" offense to near perfection. Quarterback Peyton Manning and center Jeff Saturday, along with the entire team, were able to set the offensive formation, snap count, and specific play, all of which were designed to maximize the chance of success against the defensive set they encountered on that specific down and distance. A complex set of hand signals, verbal calls, and last-minute adjustments and audibles were used to choreograph maximum productivity out of the offense. (The verbal signals have been described as so complex that some claim, inaccurately, that they are in the Celtic language.)

Among the highest performing sports teams, there is variability of performance from play to play, series to series, and game to game. The same is true of high-performance ED teams, in which the system is extremely well known to the team members and is designed to deliver specific, measurable results. Sometimes, changing even a single—albeit critical—team member can dramatically change team results. Similarly, the high-performance ED team carefully designs processes intended to add value (to the patient, family, and providers of care) while predictably and reliably producing measurable results in diverse areas (clinical, service, financial, patient safety, etc.). The processes all combine for the good of the patient and for those who care for the patient.

Consider the cascade of processes used at triage, which vary according to the specific circumstances and demand–capacity constraints at the time of service. In the traditional triage model, each patient presenting via ambulance was triaged at the entry point, after which only the high-acuity patients were sent directly to the treatment area. Far more commonly, patients were sequentially sent to the waiting room following triage, then to registration in a cubicle, then to the waiting room again, and then after being called by the primary care nurse, finally placed in a room. The wait continued as the patient was subjected to "secondary triage" until the emergency physician arrived to begin the evaluation and treatment.

ED teams began to evaluate these processes from the patients' perspectives and to implement the critical concepts of adding value and eliminating unnecessary waste. It became abundantly apparent that a cascade of more innovative processes could be put in place for the good of the patient and for the good of those taking care of the patient. Bedside registration, triage bypass (also known as "pull until full" and direct bedding), advanced triage orders and treatment, and team triage are all examples of variable processes used according to demand–capacity circumstances, which are mutually conceived, widely understood, and put to use for the good of the patient.

Prepare and Adapt

As the play call varies for a sports team, the specific process used by the high-performance ED team may vary according to the specific circumstances the team faces and the resources available at the time. Triage bypass is an excellent process when there are ED beds available. When all of the ED beds are full, standing medical orders for advanced triage and treatment become the preferred process or "play call." When all ED and hospital beds are full and there are hospital boarders occupying ED beds for extended periods of time, team triage is a high-performance adaptive process that can be used to alleviate the bottleneck. Team triage consists of placing an emergency physician and nurse, often along with registration personnel and a medical scribe, in the triage area to manage patients until beds become available in the treatment area. Well-prepared and effectively coached teams, whether in sports or in the ED, have prepared in detail (and together) to address these types of challenges.

Execution and Agility

Execution encompasses much more than efficiency. It is the ability to consistently, reliably, and efficiently produce desired results with the minimal amount of waste, despite obstacles. The more long-term and ultimately more satisfying benefit is the creation of *agility*: the talent and capability to change and adapt systems, processes, disciplines, and behaviors in ways that allow the team to create a new and more sustainable future. High-performance teams that execute with agility improve the system and its processes to benefit the patient and staff. Any ED team that has designed new processes, such as the triage cascade mentioned previously, has felt this effect.

Creating a Culture of Success

Peter Drucker wrote that "culture eats strategy for breakfast." That is certainly true in health care. Further, culture is not governed by the leaders; both the leaders and the followers determine culture. Chris Argyris wisely noted the difference between the espoused theory versus the theory in use.[14] The former is typically a piece of paper or a poster, while the latter is the way leaders and their teams actually perform their day-to-day duties.

To be effective, leaders must continually share the vision describing their intended culture prior to creating a plan of action. With an understanding and commitment to the vision, even in the face of adversity, a team can reach great heights.

What is the culture of the ED, and do the leaders and members of the team embody that culture in their every action? Culture lives in the hearts and minds of those who provide the service to the patients. It must be exemplified from both a top-down and bottom-up perspective. If the culture is not defined and effectively articulated in an inspirational vision, and if leaders at every level do not embrace and consistently embody that culture in their every action, there is little chance of having a high-performing, highly reliable organization.

The Words on the Walls vs the Happenings in the Halls

Unfortunately, many organizations, including EDs, have one culture on paper and quite another when you view the actions and decisions of those who provide the actual care for the patient. The "words on the walls" may proclaim a commitment to quality, safe patient care in a friendly environment, but do the "happenings in the halls" belie a different reality?[15] Observe the daily interactions among team members to see if these match. If they do, compliment the team members publicly. If the "words" and the "happenings" reveal a mismatch, leaders should find ways to have private discussions about why the culture isn't embodied in daily action, starting with your own leadership.

Celebrating Success

High-performance team cultures seek and celebrate team success, not just success for the individual members. Sports team analogies abound in this regard. A quarterback or running back may have a great game from a statistical standpoint, but that counts for nothing if the team loses. Hall of Fame and six-time NBA champion Bill Russell repeatedly said that his numbers counted for nothing if his team did not win the championship.[16] John Wooden, whose teams won more NCAA Division I men's basketball titles than any coach in history, never

> **BOX 12.4 ■ "NONTEAM" STATEMENTS**
>
> - "That's not a 'doctor' problem, it's a 'nurse' problem."
> - "That's not a 'nurse' problem, it's a 'doctor' problem."
> - "That's not our problem, it's a radiology (or lab, registration, inpatient, etc.) problem."
> - "Our patient satisfaction scores are fine. It's the doctors (or nurses, lab, etc.) who are pulling us down."
> - "That's not in my job description!"
> - "Nobody told me . . . this is the first I've heard about it!"

asked any of his players to "win"—but he asked every one of them to perform to the very best of their ability.[17]

Poor Team Approaches

Similarly, ED teams should be focused on team results and team success, not just on parameters affecting individuals or subgroups of the team. For example, statements like those in **Box 12.4** are evidence individuals are not functioning as a team. These statements are evidence that teamwork has broken down and individuals or groups of individuals have failed to embrace the interests of the team and the patients the team serves. High-performance team leaders are sensitive to the early signs that the team structure and morale are breaking down and are prepared to deal with it.

Recognizing Conflict

The inability to deal with conflict constructively is another sign of an ineffective team. Negative methods of handling conflict involve making conflict personal or assuming areas of conflict are resolved when they have simply been described but, in reality, were ignored.

An effective team-building approach involves raising and discussing an area of concern or conflict. Each team member is asked to take copious notes during these deliberations, particularly regarding the decisions and resolutions discussed. At the end of the meeting, the team leaders(s) collect the notes and confidentially review the conclusions of the team members. Even in high-functioning teams, there is often discrepancy among what is recorded in the notes. In poorly functioning teams, there may be minimal overlap in the notes, reflecting the inability of the team to share a common vision or recognize common deviations from that vision. This discrepancy may be particularly pronounced on a team with members driven by individual success rather than team success.

Coaching and Mentoring

It is the nature of a team that individual team members have variable levels of talent, ability, motivation, and results. Team members may be motivated by a steadfast love for the team and the work it does, but they will have varying abilities. Effective team leaders create a culture in which coaching and mentoring are part of the fabric of the organization. There will always be an A-Team and a B-Team, as well as some C-Team members in the mix. Does the team have both the culture and the wherewithal to provide a path for low performers to raise their performance?

Coaching and mentoring are essential for individual and team accountability. If a culture of accountability does not exist, there is no need for coaching and mentoring. Individual accountability is a precursor of team accountability. This concept of individual accountability may seem paradoxical, since the focus is on the team. However, the actions of the individual team members comprise, collectively, the performance of the team. If

> **BOX 12.5 ■ COACHING AND MENTORING TIPS**
>
> - Ensure that the culture of performance, as well as the concept of coaching and mentoring, are well known and widely accepted by the team.
> - Make performance about metrics, not opinions.
> - Make team-based performance and the associated metrics the rule, not the exception.
> - Ensure accountability is a function of both the members and leaders of the team.
> - Identify mentors (see discussion) who are willing and able to assist in the process.
> - Pair B-Team members with A-Team mentors over the course of several shifts.
> - During the coaching and mentoring effort, point out specifically what the A-Team members are doing that makes them so widely admired.
> - And if all else fails, act on behalf of the team to remove low performers who will not change.

individual team members cannot be depended upon to do their jobs consistently well, the team can never perform at the high levels demanded of EDs. Delivering consistently high levels of performance over time requires mutual accountability.

There is a wealth of literature on coaching and mentoring, and **Box 12.5** lists several simple concepts that are particularly pertinent.[18-20]

QUALITIES OF HIGH-PERFORMANCE TEAMS

The ED is a dynamic, episodic, and complex high-risk environment. Effective patient care requires teams to work under pressure and time constraints as they deal with rapidly evolving, ambiguous situations. When considering the characteristics of the best ED teams, it is important to determine what qualities these teams possess that make them so effective, that is, what these teams do differently that sets them apart from the rest of the ED teams. When studying high-performance teams, the key elements that contribute to their effectiveness are listed in **Box 12.6**.

Leadership

Every great team requires effective leaders. There are several levels of leadership involved in an ED. Effective and collaborative medical directors and nursing leaders partner together to build a solid foundation for the ED team by establishing the ground rules, setting the goals, and communicating the vision. The department leaders shape, reinforce, and maintain the ED culture. Their attitudes, values, and examples dramatically influence how team members work together and treat one another, which sets the stage

> **BOX 12.6 ■ KEY ELEMENTS OF EFFECTIVE TEAMS**
>
> - Leadership
> - Team structure
> - Shared goals
> - Planning and problem solving
> - Communication
> - Conflict management
> - Balanced workload
> - Process improvement

in the development of the culture. The style of leadership (i.e., dictatorial, participative, or servant leadership) colors the personality of the department. Effective leaders show respect, demonstrate consistency, empower the staff, and hold them accountable. Prior to implementing teamwork initiatives, ED leaders should honestly assess their own teamwork competencies.

Medical Directors/Nursing Leaders

Most commonly, ED leaders are thrown together into an arranged partnership, not one of their choosing. Initially, the ED medical and nursing leaders must work on the marriage of leadership goals, looking honestly at their respective strengths and weaknesses and using the dyad leadership approach discussed earlier. Like all strong marriages, this assessment requires an honest dialogue to clarify each other's needs, priorities, and hot buttons. It is necessary to establish personal communication ground rules, such as the frequency of meetings, types of issues, and methods of communication (email, phone, in person).

Effective leaders understand and commit to each other, even when they do not fully agree on an issue. This commitment and understanding occurs through a disciplined approach that includes regular meetings during which goals are established, metrics are reviewed, and issues are identified and discussed. Effective leaders confront issues and address conflict constructively, always with the goal of enhancing collaboration. Because medical and nursing leaders frequently work independently (in silos) and answer to different senior administrators, it is imperative that critical strategic goals like throughput and patient satisfaction are approached in an aligned manner. This medical and nursing leader alignment has to be genuine, transparent, and cohesive. As this dyad develops, it becomes apparent to the team that it functions as a unified model. The culture of "us versus them" dissipates as it becomes apparent that it is a one-team culture. The reward for this forward-thinking and unified relationship is improved quality and safety through strategies based on collaboration and mutual commitment.

Charge Nurses/Flow Coordinators

Charge nurses are critical members of the leadership team who influence teamwork and impact ED operations. They are the frontline floor leaders who manage the ED operations and influence teamwork 24 hours a day, 7 days a week, 365 days a year. Charge nurses serve as extensions of the medical directors and nursing leaders and work on a moment-to-moment basis to ensure that processes flow in a coordinated and effective fashion. The clinical responsibility of the charge nurses should be limited to allow them to maintain global awareness of the ED so that they can help solve problems, serve as resources and experts, and ensure that the teamwork is balanced.

A common reason for team ineffectiveness is the lack of ability and skill of the charge nurse. Not every nurse is suited to be a charge nurse. In addition to core clinical knowledge and skills, the qualities and skills of effective charge nurses are listed in **Box 12.7**.

In some organizations, charge nurses are often placed in their role based on seniority, experience, or department necessity rather than demonstrated possession of the critical skills required of the role. These improperly prepared nurses are often thrown into the role without training or mentoring, and the competencies needed to be successful are often insufficiently developed. High-performance teams recognize the importance of this role for the success of the team and invest in proper selection, training, and practice. Success needs to be clearly defined, and charge nurses require coaching and feedback to improve their skills. The charge nurses' roles and duties should be clear and standardized as much

> **BOX 12.7 ■ QUALITIES OF AN EFFECTIVE CHARGE NURSE**
>
> - Highly organized
> - Communicates effectively
> - Manages conflict well
> - Works well under stress
> - Maintains credibility and respect of staff

as possible to prevent variation from one shift to another. Forward-thinking EDs include physician and staff input into the evaluation of charge nurses' performance; similarly, progressive physician groups routinely include feedback from their nursing colleagues in evaluating their staff. The Center for Creative Leadership refers to this as "360-degree feedback."[21]

Team Structure

An effective team structure promotes patient-centered positions, care, and flow within a geographical pod that focuses care for a specific segment of patients (i.e., acute, fast track). The team members within this structure might comprise a physician and/or mid-level provider, nurse(s), ED tech, unit secretary, and possibly, a physician scribe. A team leader who is responsible for coordinating care and for continually clarifying each team member's role and expectation is designated.

Some team leaders may create clarity through assignments of specific rooms, while others may accomplish this through assignment of functions and tasks. Some best practice EDs employ a process in which the physician and nurse greet and conduct a joint intake assessment, reducing the number of times patients are asked questions and preventing potential in answers. One of these models designates a nurse to carry out the physician orders and discharge patients. A clear structure enhances the team's situational awareness and encourages the physician to communicate the plan of care to the entire team in the presence of the patient. Coordinating care through a team approach has a very positive impact on patient satisfaction.

Routinely, teams are organized hierarchically with staff members having specialized roles and responsibilities. Effective team members communicate and use adaptive mechanisms as they perform tasks and share information. This requires teamwork skills—competencies that enable people to contribute effectively—as well as task-work skills—those abilities that relate to specific job performance.

Shared Goals

Typically, asking the frontline staff member about the goals for the ED will lead to several different responses, demonstrating an inconsistent vision and absence of a team concept. Some may believe the goal is simply to survive the shift. Others may honestly state that they have no idea.

The SMART Principle

The consistent articulation of goals by members of the team requires thoughtful and consistent leadership communication, ideally following the SMART principle. To simply tell the staff that the goal is to improve patient satisfaction is too vague and leads to an unreliable understanding of what is expected. The strategies to accomplish goals should be specific and define both the "what" and examples of "how." For instance, it is effective to specifically state that the team goal is to improve patient satisfaction by having all staff members introduce themselves by name, describe their roles, and inform the patient about their care and delays. This approach is clear and sets achievable, simple, measurable strategies to accomplish the goal.

To improve the patient satisfaction score for teamwork, some EDs employ the strategy of frequently using the keyword "team" when speaking to the patient. When patients are then asked in a survey whether the ED worked as a team, they recall the word being used and are more likely to respond favorably to the question.

Change Requires the Team to Focus on the Goals

When staff members understand the reasons behind departmental change, they are more likely to adopt the goals—particularly those that add value to the patient and the staff. Establishing baseline measures and comparing results over time help the team to recognize progress, refocus efforts, share in celebrations of success when appropriate, and understand the impact of their efforts.

Behavioral change requires time and coaching. To avoid overwhelming staff with too many changes, effective leaders allow plenty of time for staff to practice and implement a new process before adopting a new and different goal. Unified and consistent SMART goals encourage the team to work interdependently, regardless of the difference in team member's roles. For instance, a team that adopts the goal of ensuring a door-to-doctor time of less than 30 minutes compels each team member to work toward removing any barrier that gets in the way of meeting that team goal.

Balanced Workload

Homeostasis is important to the function of all organisms, including teams. A common reason for team stress and conflict is workload imbalance. The entire team becomes unbalanced when some team members are overburdened with work and others are not assuming their share.

The workload of a team operates much like a stack of spinning plates. With constant attention, the plates can be kept turning with minimal effort. However, as one plate starts to falter, more energy and spin must be applied to that plate to keep it moving. The attention to that plate takes attention away from others, and these begin to wobble, lose momentum, and eventually topple. To keep all the plates spinning simultaneously, workload must be appropriately distributed and balanced.

Effective teams build processes to maintain homeostasis. They adopt a culture that balances effort among the team members and employs a practice of "no one sits until everyone sits." Members of high-performance teams offer help without being asked and ask for help without fear of refusal or derision. They maintain situational awareness and anticipate patient and team member needs. They optimize downtimes by continuing to prepare (i.e., stock rooms, review cases, and practice skills). These team members understand that losing situational awareness results in errors during both low- and high-volume periods.

Process Improvement

The final essential element of high-performance teamwork is process improvement. Highly effective teams employ continuous process improvement to reinforce teamwork. They actively solicit and share feedback to improve the entire team. The team maintains vigilance to avoid errors and hardwires processes that help the team communicate and maintain situational awareness. They keep abreast of best practice strategies and maintain a culture of excellence in which each team member is respected and valued for their unique contribution. New ideas are encouraged, and the team ensures that they have fun in the process.

THE TOOLS OF TEAMWORK

Peter Senge refers to shared mental models, which are "deeply ingrained assumptions, generalizations, or even pictures or images that influence how we understand the world and how we take action."[22] Shared mental models and anticipation help us understand how the team is likely to function in certain situations, as well as how other situations differ and require other skills.

Anticipation

One of the most powerful teamwork tools is anticipation, which is the ability to use observation, experience, and discipline to help guide decision-making in critical situations while remaining open to fresh possibilities. Anticipation allows us to use our considerable past experience in working with others to make reasonable assumptions on how the team will function, particularly in stressful situations, relieving us of the need to make it up as we go. The military services are masters of this teamwork skill, which creates, in their term, unit cohesion. But the ability to see variability as a part of anticipation, as Ferguson noted, is also important.

A simple example of anticipation and a shared mental model is the care of a trauma victim who has blunt force trauma to the chest, resulting in subcutaneous emphysema. Because of the teamwork skills, evidence, and experiential-based care in which we have trained, the entire team knows that the physician will reach for a 36F trocar chest tube for a tube thoracostomy, and the nurse will have it ready. That is anticipation and a shared mental model of clinical care by a highly trained team of people.

Demand-Capacity Leadership

Demand–capacity leadership is a skill closely related to anticipation (see Chapter 46). While often applied to hardwiring flow, the five demand–capacity questions are essential to effective teamwork:

1. Who is coming?
2. When are they coming?
3. What are they going to need?
4. Are we going to have what we need?
5. What will we do if we don't?

Teams must have a common understanding that emergency care is in fact highly predictable if historical data and experience are used in an anticipatory fashion. For example, what is typically the busiest day of the week? Monday, of course, which we know both from experience and from data. The team schedule should be made in anticipation of when the patients arrive, as well as what type of patients will arrive. It is one responsibility of ED leaders to ensure the staffing and scheduling models are supported and benchmarked among other like departments.

The position statement "Staffing and Productivity in the Emergency Department" by the Emergency Nurses Association supports the evaluation of staffing and productivity is based on:

- Patient census and acuity
- Direct and indirect time for care delivery
- Experience and skill mix of the ED staff
- The impact on patient and emergency nurse safety and satisfaction
- The recruitment and retention of qualified nurses[23]

Matching patient demand to capacity is an essential skill of the ED team, led by its leaders but provided at the bedside each day. Routine use of the five demand–capacity questions fosters teamwork.

Eliminating Silos

The term "functional silo" was first coined in 1988 by Phil Ensor, a consultant to the Goodyear Tire and Rubber Company, but it applies to health care as well.[24] A functional silo is a part of an organization or process which, while functioning practically in an inter-related fashion, tends to act as a stand-alone, independent entity. Effective teamwork requires the ability to recognize and eliminate functional silos through prospective, proactive efforts to help individuals and elements of the team fully recognize and embrace the inter-related and essential work each does for the good of the patient and the team.

Empowerment

Effective teamwork is impossible without empowerment, which involves the power, authority, and ability to make decisions at the level at which the care is provided. Never make decisions at a higher level that can and should be made at a lower level.[5] Empowerment requires not just an understanding of teamwork, but the role of trust in the care of the patient and the functioning of the team. Encourage departmental councils that are multidisciplinary, staff facilitated and chaired to create the atmosphere that fosters positive change, higher quality, and safer patient care by those who do the work every day.

Make sure your team has a thin rulebook, not a thick rulebook. Make it easy for them to understand your culture of excellence and teamwork and turn them loose—don't make them look up what they are supposed to do at every step. Give them wide corridors for success. The skill "managing up" mentioned previously is a classic example of empowerment, as is the story by Dr. Adams and the ED tech.

High-Reliability Principles

Karl Weick and Katherine Sutcliffe coined the term "High-Reliability Organizations (HROs)"[25] following their study of high-risk, high-pressure organizations, including nuclear power plants, naval aircraft operations, and . . . EDs. The five principles they delineated for success in these high-performing teams were:

Anticipation: Staying Out of Trouble

1. Preoccupation with failure
2. Sensitivity to operations
3. Reluctance to simplify

Containment: Getting Out of Trouble

4. Commitment to resilience
5. Deference to expertise

These concepts a critical part of developing and maintaining highly functioning teams in stressful situations and should be a part of the teamwork skills used by ED leaders (see Chapter 10).

Reliable and Redundant Communication Skills

As described previously, high-performance team members actively communicate with one another to ensure that each person understands the mental model and plan of care and works to safely provide the care. The physician has the responsibility to communicate what is going on with the patient. All team members share in the responsibility to provide information and carry out the tasks necessary to confirm or challenge the diagnosis. Structured communication ensures team effectiveness by enhancing situational awareness of the patients and their status. Continual communication of information and changes in patient status is vital to teamwork and error avoidance.

Team Huddles

Team huddles are also a key aspect of ensuring that ED operations are performed as a team. The concept of huddles was invented by a football coach for a deaf school to ensure that the other team could not see the signals they were calling by American Sign Language.[26] Huddles are particularly helpful at the start of a shift, at predefined intervals (e.g., every four hours), and when ED conditions, patient load, or patient acuity have changed dramatically. Clinical huddles serve several purposes, including:

- Promoting a trusting and safe clinical environment
- Improving quality of care
- Decreasing and/or eliminating communication gaps
- Creating shared mental models
- Using anticipation and demand–capacity skills
- Identifying bottlenecks
- Identifying opportunities to leverage flow
- Assigning clear responsibilities

The ED nurse and doctor can assemble the team and, within minutes, review the current status of the patients, the clinical team, and the overall ED. Current and anticipated workloads, life- and limb-threatening presentations, and a shared understanding of the operational and clinical situation (a shared mental model) can all be reviewed in a short and productive period of time. Any needed changes in process, performance, or personnel can be implemented to ensure patient safety and team integrity. Communication huddles are also beneficial prior to performing a patient procedure. All team members huddle to plan how the procedure will be conducted. A team leader and other procedural roles are identified, the process is discussed, and potential safety concerns are addressed, including what the patient and family's role is during the procedure. Doing this builds trust among all participating team members and ensures everyone has a clear understanding of the process.

To be effective, huddles should be focused, limited to a few crucial elements, and not exceed more than a few minutes. Team members review specific team goals and operational issues that impact the provision of patient care (i.e., staff call-in, CT down). Time is taken out to appreciate and recognize team members. Team huddles also add value during volume and

FIGURE 12.3 ■ SBAR Technique

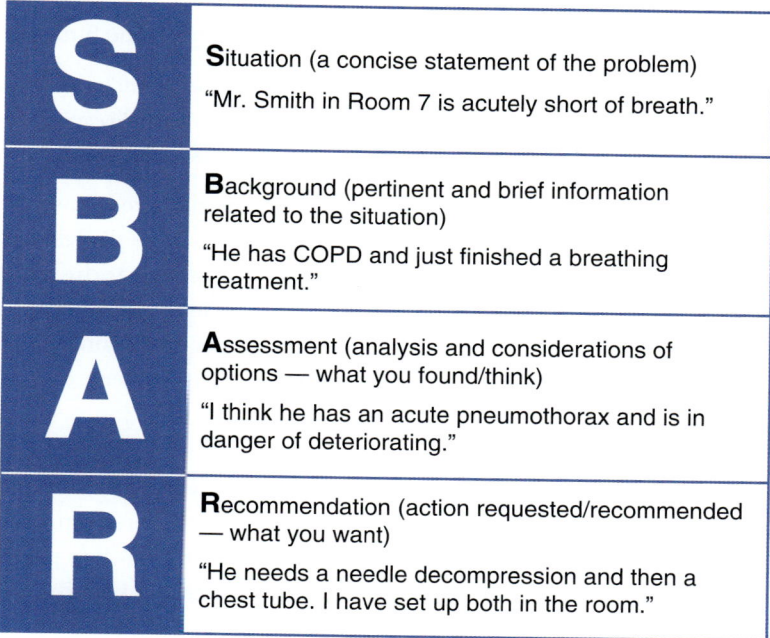

acuity surges, when a team is most vulnerable to losing situational awareness and control. Team huddles can help reduce demand–capacity mismatches leading to gridlock, such as ambulance diversion, as early shared input can both optimize patient flow and recognize the need for additional resources before it is too late. The SBAR technique is an effective communication tool to use during and outside of team huddles (**Figure 12.3**).

Questions for the Team Huddles

For most teams, starting the team huddle concept requires having a set of questions to begin the process, including:

- Where is this patient on their journey through our ED?
- What are the constraints, bottlenecks, and rate-limiting steps in their care?
- Who will eliminate those steps, and how?
- How much more time will be needed to complete their care?
- Are they "vertical" enough to come out of a room into the hallway?
- Are they likely to require admission? If so, can we call for the bed now?

Just as a huddle in football helps ensure the entire team understands the formation and the play, clinical huddles develop the same sense of situational awareness and anticipation.

Resistance to Team Huddles

The biggest source of resistance to team huddles is that it represents something new, which speaks to the need for structure and a common set of questions to decrease this resistance. It does create a team-based understanding of what the physician and nurse are thinking, so in that sense it requires more transparency, which some people find difficult at first. We once heard an emergency physician say the huddles create a "forced intimacy," to which he objected. This statement misses the point of huddles. Huddles force teams to communicate regularly with each other for the benefit of the patients, those who care for the patient, and the institution.

Conflict Management

While conflict is unavoidable, the way in which conflict is addressed and managed differentiates effective teams from dysfunctional ones. Katzenbach and Smith note:

> *When conflict arises in the middle of discussing a complex problem, it is actually considered good for the team process. The conflicting viewpoints are an opportunity to evaluate a problem from different perspectives and then take a decision based on a thorough assessment.*[27]

The inability to effectively deal with conflict is a commonly cited reason for ED team dysfunction. Since conflict management is not a standard part of professional training, it should be included in staff training for the entire ED team. Addressing conflict is uncomfortable for many, and some individuals avoid it fearing that confrontation may risk personal friendships. Because team members are interdependent, conflict between two members may have deleterious effects on the entire team and the patient.

Conflict Resolution Training

Some conflicts can be resolved through establishment of clear goals, expectations, and roles. Regardless of the situation, high-performance team members commit to resolving conflict with the best interest of the patient and team in mind, rather than personal interest or gain. It is helpful for the team to create and commit to a code of conduct, establishing rules of engagement around conflict. Those who cannot or will not commit to the rules do not have the best interest of the team and patient as a priority and should be removed from the team.

Conflict management training requires teaching staff to effectively confront one another in a healthy and professional manner. Training must be followed by practice. Clinical simulation through role playing scenarios and video feedback are powerful adult learning tools. Providing conflict resolution scripts or templates are helpful to produce a positive outcome.

TeamSTEPPS, a teamwork program developed by the Department of Defense (DoD) and described in more detail later, uses the acronym DESCC (**Figure 12.4**) to help frame the conflict conversation.[28] ED team members should be encouraged to address conflict directly rather than hand it off to the team leaders.

Conflict Resolution Techniques

Some EDs use team huddles to rapidly and openly identify and address team issues. The questions posed include:

- What have we done well today as a team?
- What has not gone well today?
- What can we do to improve as a team?

In these huddles, each team member is encouraged to share his/her perspective on problems and conflicts. Hardwiring and regularly practicing this technique make it easier to discuss and handle conflict in this forum. Team members skilled at conflict resolution may be employed to help coach and mentor others who are less comfortable.

Conflict can be used to help team members strengthen teamwork as they learn the importance of addressing differences and collaborating to understand what each can do to help the patient and the entire team. Effective teams appreciate and value conflict while respectfully addressing and managing it.

FIGURE 12.4 ■ DESCC Approach to Conflict Confrontation

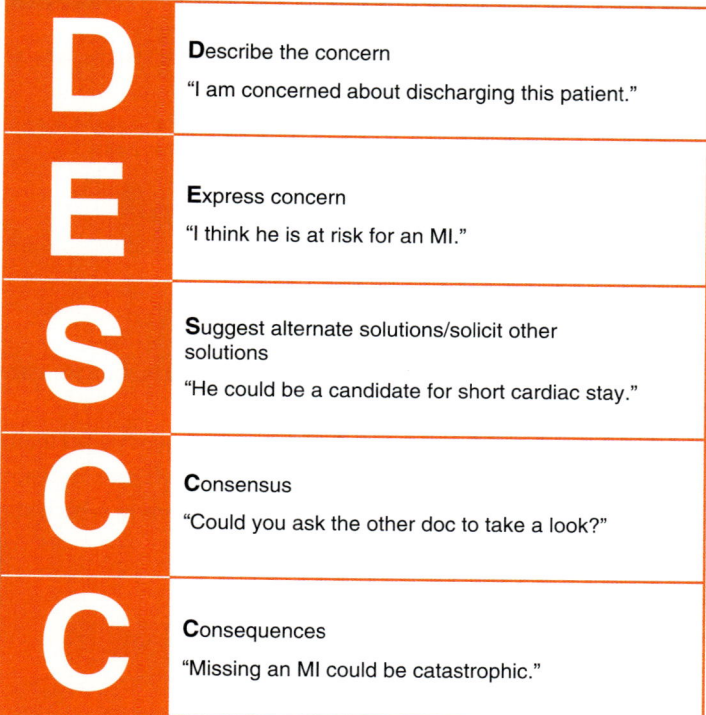

TeamSTEPPS

In 1979, the National Aeronautics and Space Administration convened an expert panel to address the fact that the major source of aviation accidents was human error.[28,29] Its purpose was to develop ways in which human error could be reduced or eliminated, both in commercial and DoD aviation. In addition to developing programs focusing on cognitive, interpersonal, and communications skills in aviation, the program resulted in the development of a program named Crew Resource Management (CRM).[30]

Crew Resource Management

The goal of CRM was to "make optimum use of all available resources—equipment, procedures, and people—to promote safety and enhance the efficiency of flight operations." Soon after its implementation, the CRM program was shown to have dramatically reduced aviation mishaps. Its potential applicability to EDs was recognized as there are similarities between the ED and the airline's team structure and dynamics. Both the pilot and the ED physician serve as the captain of the ship. They both rely on others with different education, roles, skills, and backgrounds in order to successfully fly the plane or treat a patient and prevent a bad outcome. Both environments are stressful, critical to life and death, and involve rapidly changing conditions. To avoid fatal crashes and medical errors, both teams must carefully synchronize their efforts. Recognizing the fundamental team structure of both aviation and ED operations and the communications that drive them were essential to the improvement process. As Frankel and colleagues note, "Currently, we can assure our

> **BOX 12.8 ■ TEAMSTEPPS**
>
> - Anticipate the needs of other team members.
> - Adjust to others' actions and the changing environment.
> - Possess a shared understanding of how processes and plans function and how they are carried to completion.
> - Communicate clearly, concisely, and efficiently.
> - Ensure that the patient is a key part of the team whenever possible.

patients that their care is always provided by a team of experts, but we cannot assure our patients that their care is always provided by expert teams."[31]

As a response to this critical dilemma, the DoD and the Agency for Healthcare Research and Quality adapted and expanded the principles of CRM into a resource for better teamwork practices in health care called TeamSTEPPS, an acronym which stands for:

- **T**eam
- **S**trategies and
- **T**ools to
- **E**nhance
- **P**erformance and
- **P**atient
- **S**afety

Implementing TeamSTEPPS

TeamSTEPPS begins with the insight that effective teamwork absolutely depends on the team's ability to anticipate and respond (**Box 12.8**). The program helps bridge the uncomfortable fact that health-care professionals are rarely trained together, much less in team-based settings. Rather, they are trained not only as individuals, but in a relatively rigid, hierarchical educational structure. TeamSTEPPS' curriculum is centered around four core competencies (**Table 12.1**).[32]

TABLE 12.1 ■ TeamSTEPPS Competencies	
Competency	**Definition**
Team leadership	The ability to direct and coordinate activities of team members, assess team performance, assign tasks, develop team knowledge and skills, motivate team members, plan and organize, and establish a positive team atmosphere.
Situation monitoring and awareness	Mutual performance monitoring is the capacity to encourage and develop a shared understanding of the team environment and performance progress.
Mutual support	Mutual support requires the capacity to anticipate team members' needs and shift workload to maximize efficiency and balance.
Communication	Effective communication ensures accurate, timely, concise, mission-critical exchange of information among all team members to increase reliability and patient safety.

TABLE 12.2 ■ Principles of Effective Communication	
Complete	Communicating all relevant (and no irrelevant) information
Clear	Conveying information that is simple and plainly understood
Brief	Communicating in a clear, concise manner
Timely	Offering and requesting pertinent information, verifying authenticity, and acknowledging receipt

While all the core competencies are important, none is more important than effective communication skills, which is central to the success of the others. The standard for all forms of communication is that they must be complete, clear, brief, and timely (**Table 12.2**).

There are several examples of CRM training programs available. They all share the same basic goals, framework, language, and methodology. TeamSTEPPS is a superb example of a teamwork program tailored to and field-tested in the ED.

CREATING A TEAM CULTURE

As leaders work to create teams and improve teamwork in the ED, there are critical steps that can lead to success. Teamwork is the foundation of effective operations and, as such, team improvement requires digging beneath the surface to ensure that the infrastructure is strong. Medical directors and nursing leaders interested in building or improving their team culture will find it very helpful to review the steps listed next, initiate a dialogue, and develop a plan together.

Build a Powerfully Inclusive Team

- Conduct a team self-assessment. Use the key elements of effective teams that have been discussed in this chapter. Individually assess the team and then compare results and engage in a dialogue.
    - Define weak elements of the team.
        - If several, determine the highest priorities.
    - Define areas of strength and use them as an example to reinforce areas of excellence.
- Conduct leader self-assessment. Honestly appraise the leaders' strengths and weaknesses.
    - Determine the team's assessment of the leaders.
    - Give constructive feedback.
    - Have an honest and open dialogue about priorities, hot buttons, preferences of communication, and the greatest concerns.
    - Establish rules of engagement and commit to supporting one another in public.
    - Be vigilant about (hardwire) regularly meeting and focusing on joint goals.
- Evaluate the team and confront areas of weakness.
    - Determine the clarity of the team members' roles.
    - Evaluate whether the right people are in the right roles.
    - Address the performance of the team members who have been chronic low performers, particularly if they are bringing down the entire team.
    - Review the employment selection criteria.
    - Consider behavioral interview criteria for attitude above skill in hiring interviews. (Skills can be taught, but attitudes are difficult to change.)

- Develop the charge nurses. Train them on key elements of teamwork, communication, and conflict management.
  - ☐ Coach them and give them practice time.
  - ☐ Reduce variation between charge nurses by standardizing required processes, such as team huddles.
- Jointly select teamwork goals.
  - ☐ Apply the SMART principle: are goals simple, measurable, achievable, realistic, and timely?
  - ☐ Develop a process to track positive changes toward teamwork goals to be shared with staff.
- Identify and select a multidisciplinary team comprised of different roles and shifts (charge nurse, staff nurse, ED tech, unit secretary, charge physician).
  - ☐ Train them on key elements of teamwork, communication, and conflict management, and empower them to create strategies to improve teamwork (i.e., code of conduct, reward, and recognition).
  - ☐ Hold this team accountable to develop and implement changes based on the team goals selected.
- Inform the rest of the staff. Communicate the goals, changes, and expectations. Include everyone and encourage team to submit ideas for improvement.
  - ☐ Require team members who criticize to come up with an alternative solution.
- Once the teamwork improvement strategy is implemented, be visible in the department to ensure compliance.
  - ☐ Give feedback, recognize good behavior, and correct bad behavior.
  - ☐ Praise in public, correct in private.
- Ensure data are regularly updated and shared with staff to communicate progress.
- Allow time with the new process. A minimum of 3 months is suggested to ensure staff has had enough time to adopt the change. Do not make changes too quickly or frequently.
- Gather postimplementation data to evaluate impact of improvement strategy.
- Evaluate and make improvements before moving onto a different goal (**Figure 12.5**).

FIGURE 12.5 ■ The Plan-Do-Check-Act (PDCA) Cycle

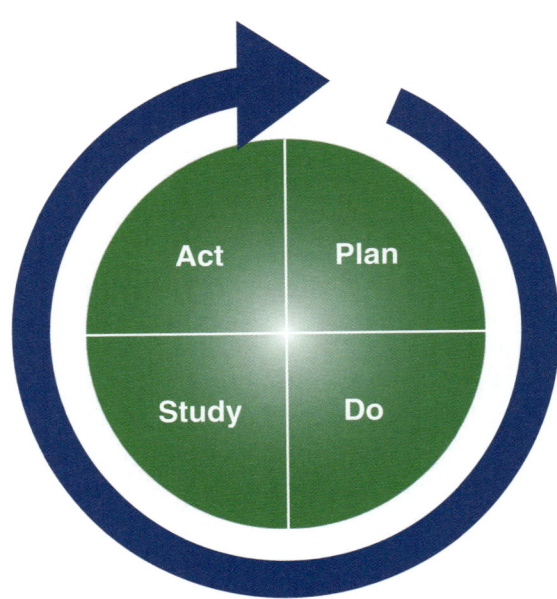

> **BOX 12.9** ■ **"I" IS APPROPRIATE AND USEFUL WHEN ADDRESSING CERTAIN WORK ATTRIBUTES**
>
> - Quality of the individual's contribution to the team effort
> - Personal involvement and collaboration
> - Self-motivation
> - Self-esteem
> - Personal development of individual traits, skills, and habits
> - Technical proficiency
> - Work habits

Is There an "I" in Team?

When discussing teams and teamwork, the use of the personal pronoun "I" is often derided as being disruptive to team building. Nonetheless, every team member brings their own unique blend of talents, skills, abilities, and work/life experience to the job. Taking the "I" completely out of a talented person is neither possible nor desirable. Indeed, for high-performing teams to be effective in producing results, team members must have a sense of both team and individual responsibility. It is only when "I" is overemphasized, overused, or applied at the wrong place or time that it becomes destructive to morale and counterproductive to performance. Every team has—and needs—its top performers to help set the pace.

"I" is appropriate in several different circumstances or situations; for example, when one is assuming personal responsibility for results, or a process is directly dependent on an individual team member. The unique perspective of an individual can be useful in multiple circumstances (**Box 12.9**).

- "I will inform your family of the results of your test."
- "I took your input from my last performance review, and I have made serious efforts to improve."
- "I'll get your pain medication and be back within 10 minutes."

Perhaps most importantly, when leaders recognize and praise the efforts of and results by team members, those team members are far more likely to commit to the team's purpose and goals. Thus, there is always a place for both "I" and "we" in effective teamwork. Katzenbach and Smith have it precisely correct: "'I' represents belief in the self and the quest for accomplishments. 'We' represents commitment and allegiance to the team effort."[33]

What to Do When the Team Breaks Down

If you could get all the people in an organization rowing in the same direction, you could dominate any industry, in any market, against any competition, at any time.

In the *Five Dysfunctions of a Team*, Patrick Lencioni describes the reasons why teams fail to accomplish their objectives. Any experienced provider has participated in groups that share a number of these dysfunctions (**Table 12.3**).[34]

Given the increasingly metrics-driven approach to ED performance, it is relatively easy to tell when a team is in profound trouble—their performance metrics are well below target, usually for prolonged periods. However, waiting until performance metrics deteriorate is a major mistake. The dysfunctions that Lencioni delineates are almost always evident to astute leaders long before a dramatic drop in performance occurs.

The first place to look for team dysfunction is at "the seams" of the team: the areas of interactions or handoffs between team members or subsets of the team. Nurse–physician

TABLE 12.3 ■ Lencioni's Five Dysfunctions of a Team

Dysfunction	Negative Consequences
Absence of trust	Lack of trust leads team members to avoid sharing mistakes and hesitate to ask for or offer help. Meetings avoid open discussion and become boring.
Fear of conflict	In an untrusting environment, controversy and conflict are avoided and honest opinions and perspectives of others are not sought.
Lack of commitment	Team members who are not given the opportunity to have their opinions considered and participate in development and debate do not buy-in to the team goals.
Avoidance of accountability	This dysfunction results from a lack of commitment to the team goals. As a result, team members avoid confronting colleagues who are not goal focused or productive.
Inattention to results	Without accountability, members of the team focus on individual, rather than organizational, advancement.

and physician–nurse handoffs are, not surprisingly, the most common seams where problems occur, simply because of the sheer volume of their interactions. In addition, look for seams in which communication, rather than technical aspects of care, is at the core of the dysfunction. Classic examples of communication dysfunction include:

- "The emergency physician will be right in to see you."
- "The nurse will be right with you to give you your pain medication."
- "The ED tech will give you crutches and instructions on how to use them, and then you are good to go."

First, functional communication statements personalize the team members by using names whenever possible. Second, effective teams manage the time frames for patients through expectation creation (see Chapter 39).

- "Dr. Smith, our emergency physician on duty today, is with another patient, but will be in to see you as soon as possible. I'll make sure he knows you are here and brief him on the nature of your problem."
- "I know Connie, your nurse, has several patients now, but I'll personally make sure she knows you need the medication I have ordered."

Communication Seams

It may be necessary to find a way to break the norms which have created the problem and develop a bold, swift, and specific method to rectify them. Determine if the problem is poor role clarity, ineffective communication, lack of understanding of service handoffs, poorly led meetings (which devolve into complaint sessions instead of constructive solutions), or misplaced blame. Build on the strengths of the highly performing team members and use them to coach and mentor those who are struggling. Publicly praise B-Team members when they make progress. Be specific: "Great job today with Mrs. Smith. The way you communicated with her and the family decompressed a difficult situation and made things easier for the rest of the team."

Moving to the Other Side

Well-chosen team-building exercises allow team members to open up and interact with each other in a more positive and constructive fashion. One of the most time-honored and effective teambuilding techniques is called "moving to the other side" and involves having team members state the problem—not from their own perspective but that of the other team members. This helps them understand and articulate the problem from a wholly different and often unique perspective. "I've been doing this job for 15 years, but I really never thought of it that way" is a common response in this exercise.

Building team spirit is critical to success. It begins by reaffirming the common purpose and is accentuated when team leaders celebrate success. Turning a team around is one of the most difficult challenges nursing leaders and medical directors face. It is also one of the most gratifying when the difficult work is completed.

MAKING THE "C-SUITE" PART OF THE ED TEAM

The need for establishing teamwork is perhaps obvious, even if difficult to achieve and sustain. Somewhat less obvious is the importance of ensuring that other, outside key stakeholders are included as essential members of the ED team, even though they are often not a part of the direct clinical care of the patient. Each of the following stakeholders are highly influential decision makers for issues that are critical for successful ED operations. All of these "C-Suite" people should be made to feel a part of the team, since they can have a powerful influence on the ED and, in particular, its integration into the hospital and overall health-care system's goals and objectives.

Keep these team members proactively informed both of key issues facing the ED and of the positive results the team generates. Never fail to thank them for their assistance. Keep them informed of patient compliments, improvements in patient satisfaction scores, and other performance metrics. As the specialty of hospital medicine becomes further developed and increasingly critical to department operations (by ensuring patients are admitted from the ED in a timely and efficient fashion), having a positive relationship both with the chief medical officer and the medical director of the hospital medicine (hospitalist) service will be important, and they need to feel a part of the ED team.

All of these people, and many more, must understand that they are a part of the team. Without their understanding of and commitment to the culture of the ED, success is impossible. With them as informed allies, progress is highly likely. Several steps help ensure this success:

- Ensure they know the ED is the "front door" of the hospital.
- Align strategic incentives with the leadership team.
- Note the critical role the ED plays for hospital admissions (over 50% in most).
- Define success through metrics, then meet or exceed them.
- Take them with you to do rounds in the ED.
- Meet frequently—at least monthly, preferably—and do it as a team.
- Copy them on important issues.
- Be the people to come to with any problem, ED-related or not.
- Be responsive and anticipate problems.
- Practice "concierge" emergency medicine: give them your cell phone number and encourage them to use it for family, friends, VIPs, etc.

CONCLUSION

Teamwork is a discipline which requires the requisite skills, abilities, and techniques to bond people of different professional and educational backgrounds over the common purpose of excellence in patient care. Establishing and cultivating teams is a never-ending challenge, but one which is deeply satisfying to both the nursing and physician leaders of the ED and the team members they represent. Using the principles described in this chapter helps teams rise from mediocrity to elite-level performance. Most importantly, it creates an environment where highly talented people want to work in a team environment.

REFERENCES

1. Keller H. *The Story of My Life*. New York, NY: Random House; 2004.
2. Wikipedia. High-performance teams. 2013. Available at: https://en.wikipedia.org/wiki/High-performance_teams. Accessed December 18, 2019.
3. Kierkegaard S. *Either/Or: A Fragment of Life*. London, England: Penguin; 1992.
4. Mayer T. *Teams and Teamwork*. Presented at: American College of Emergency Physicians Emergency Department Directors Academy, Session 2, March 29, 2019; Dallas, Tex.
5. Mayer T, Cates R. *Leadership for Great Customer Service: Satisfied Employees, Satisfied Patients*. 2nd ed. Chicago, Ill: Health Administration Press; 2014.
6. Katzenbach JR, Smith DK. *The Wisdom of Teams: Creating the High Performance Organization*. New York, NY: Harper Collins; 2003.
7. Drucker P. There's more than one kind of team. *WSJ*. 1992. Accessed April 9, 2009.
8. Coutu D. Why teams don't work. *Harv Bus Rev*. 2009;87(5):98-103.
9. Ritz Carlton Credo. https://www.ritzcarlton.com/en/about/gold-standards. Accessed April 9, 2020.
10. Mayer T. *Customer Service in Emergency Departments*. Presented at: American College of Emergency Physicians Emergency Department Directors Academy, Session 1, February 5, 2019; Dallas, Tex.
11. Croskerry P, Mayer T. *Teaching Critical Thinking: An Ethical Imperative*. In: *Strauss and Mayer's Emergency Department Management*. 2nd ed. Dallas, Tex: American College of Emergency Physicians; 2020.
12. Studer Q. *Hardwiring Excellence*. Gulf Breeze, Fla: Fire Starter Press; 2008.
13. Kipling R. The law of the wolves. *The Jungle Book*. Mineola, NY: Macmillan and Co; 2010.
14. Argyris C. *Organizational Traps: Leadership, Culture and Organizational Design*. New York, NY: Oxford University Press; 2010.
15. Mayer T. *Sustaining the Patient Flow Advantage*. Presented at: VA Health System Collaborative on Hardwiring Flow, 2018; Dallas, Tex.
16. Russell B. *Russell Rules: 11 Lessons on Leadership From the 20th Century's Greatest Winner*. New York, NY: New American Library; 2002.
17. Wooden J, Jamison S. *The Essential Wooden: A Lifetime of Lessons on Leaders and Leadership*. New York, NY: McGraw-Hill; 2007.
18. McManus P. *Coaching People*. Boston, Mass: HBR Press; 2009.
19. Baron L, Morin L. The impact of executive coaching on self-efficacy related to management skills. *Leadership Org Dev J*. 2010;31(1):18-38.
20. Coutu D. What coaches can do for you. *Har Bus Rev*. 2009;87:91-97.
21. Van Velsor E, ed. *Center for Creative Leadership Handbook of Leadership Development*. San Francisco, Calif: John Wiley and Sons; 2010.
22. Senge P. *The Fifth Discipline: The Art and Science of the Learning Organization*. New York, NY: Doubleday; 2006.
23. Staffing and productivity in the emergency department. Emergency Nurses Association website. Available at: https://www.ena.org/docs/default-source/resource-library/practice-resources/position-statements/staffingandproductivityemergencydepartment.pdf?sfvrsn=c57dcf13_8. Accessed January 7, 2019.
24. Ensor PS. The functional silo syndrome. Association for Manufacturing Excellence website. Available at: http://www.ame.org/sites/default/files/target_articles/88q1a3.pdf. Accessed January 7, 2019.
25. Weick K, Sutcliffe K. *Managing the Unexpected: Sustained Performance in a Complex World*. 3rd ed. Hoboken, NJ: Doubleday; 2015.
26. Okrent A. The true origin story of the football huddle. *The Week*. 2014. Available at https://theweek.com/articles/451763/true-origin-story-football-huddle. Accessed April 10, 2020.
27. Katzenbach JR, Smith DK. The discipline of teams. *Harvard Business Review*. 1993. Available at https://hbr.org/1993/03/the-discipline-of-teams-2. Accessed April 10, 2020.
28. TeamSTEPPs pocket guide app. Agency for Healthcare Research and Quality website. Available at: https://www.ahrq.gov/teamstepps/instructor/essentials/pocketguideapp.html. Reviewed April 2018.
29. Alonso A, Baker DP, Holtzman A, et al. Reducing medical error in the military health system: how can team training help? *Hum Resour Dev Rev*. 2006;16(3):396-415.
30. Kanki BG, Helmreich RL, Anca J. *Crew Resource Management*. San Diego, Calif: Academic Press; 2010.
31. Frankel AS, Leonard MW, Denham CR. Fair and just culture, team behavior and leadership engagement: the tools to achieve high reliability. *Health Serv Res*. 2006;41:1690-1709.
32. Clancy CM, Tornberg DN. TeamSTEPPS: Integrating teamwork principles in healthcare practice. Patient Safety and Quality Care website. Available at: http://www.psqh.com/novdec06/ahrq.html. Accessed January 7, 2019.
33. Katzenbach JR, Smith DK. Team Building Portal website. Available at: http://www.teambuildingportal.com/articles/effective-teams/i-out-of-team. Accessed November 10, 2011.
34. Lencioni P. *The 5 Dysfunctions of a Team: A Leadership Fable*. San Francisco, Calif: Jossey-Bass; 2002.

CHAPTER 13

MAINTAINING PERSONAL AND PROFESSIONAL BALANCE

Robert W. Strauss, Jay Kaplan, Alex Rosenau, Tiffiny Strever, Thom A. Mayer

Wellness is a state of mental and physical health and well-being that includes a balance between work and personal life. Although the emergency department (ED) workplace environment presents many challenges to achieving wellness, professional stress can negatively affect personal, physical, psychological, spiritual, and mental health.

An intact workforce capable of adequately performing its mission requires competent, healthy, high-functioning professionals who are aware of the implicit stresses and have mechanisms and resources available to address them. ED leaders must first acknowledge the existence of stress. By understanding the causes and effects of long-standing stress, leaders can work to implement the changes necessary to create a more balanced environment. Great leaders demonstrate concern for their colleagues and coach them toward a more balanced lifestyle while exemplifying appropriate wellness behaviors themselves.

The benefits of attaining self- and situational awareness in order to improve work-life balance are substantial and include quality communication, effective teamwork, and enhancing career enjoyment and longevity. Health-care workers in a state of well-being, including good mental health, are better able to provide safe, timely, and quality care to their patients.

Emergency physicians and nurses spend more of their waking time at work than in any other single activity. Yet it is clear how important enjoyment of personal time is to a fulfilled life. As author Rabbi Harold Kushner has wryly observed[1]:

Nobody on their deathbed has ever said 'I wish I had spent more time at the office.

In order to more deeply understand the concept of this vital relationship between work and home life, it is helpful to start with several definitions (**Table 13.1**).

TABLE 13.1 ■ Balance, Health, and Mental Health	
Term	**Definition(s)**
Balance	• Stability produced by an even distribution of weight on each side of the vertical axis • Equipoise between contrasting, opposing, or interacting elements • Equality between the totals of the two sides of one account • An aesthetically pleasing integration of elements
Health	• The condition of being sound in body, mind, and spirit • Freedom from physical disease or pain
Mental Health	"The ability to negotiate the daily challenges and social interactions of life without experiencing undue emotional or behavior incapacity."[1]

Excessive stress and "burnout" are more likely to occur when individual providers fail to develop work-life balance strategies and when the workplace environment does not provide organized resources to address the inherent stresses. (Burnout is addressed in more detail in Chapter 125.) Emergency caregivers are exposed to enormous strain, as they must care for patients who may have life-threatening disorders, demand immediate attention, expect unrealistic outcomes, and who do not expect to be in the ED. It is stressful to provide this unscheduled care on a shift-work basis in high-acuity, time-sensitive situations.

STRESS

Hans Selye, an endocrinologist and Nobel Prize nominee, defined stress in his landmark book, *The Stress of Life*.[2] Acknowledging the contributions of the great physiologists Claude Bernard (who developed the concept of the "milieu intérieur") and Walter Cannon (who described the body's "homeostasis"), Selye writes that stress is a nonspecific physical response to any demand. His work describes stress as potentially positive (eustress) or negative (distress), explaining that stressful experiences lead the body to react through a "general adaptation syndrome" (**Table 13.2**). A person's stress response stems from how they perceive and are able to cope with a particular situation.

Stress and Illness

Psychiatrists Thomas Holmes and Richard Rahe examined the medical records of over 5,000 patients in an attempt to determine whether stressful events resulted in illness.[3] Patients were asked to compile a list of 43 life events based upon a relative score. The researchers classified different life events as having specific "Life Change Units"; for example, the death of a spouse was the highest stressor on their list at 100 units; divorce received a score of 73. Positive events were also counted, with marriage having a score of 50; gaining a new family member generated a score of 39. Their results led to the creation of the "Social Readjustment Rating Scale." Their findings were dramatic and demonstrated the increased likelihood of having a life-threatening illness or injury following a stressful event:

- A person with a total score of 150 in the previous year had a 50% increased likelihood.
- A person with a score of 300 or greater had a 90% increased likelihood.

Post-Traumatic Stress

Post-traumatic stress (PTS) occurs when there is exposure to extreme, dramatic, or persistent mental, physical, psychological, or spiritual stress or trauma. Post-traumatic stress is a

TABLE 13.2 ■ Selye's General Adaptation Syndrome	
Phase	**Explanation**
Alarm	The body recognizes that there is a danger and prepares to respond; this is the fight or flight reaction. Activation of the hypothalamic-pituitary-adrenal axis and sympathetic nervous system occur. Adrenalin/noradrenalin and cortisol are pumped into the bloodstream.
Resistance	With high levels of circulating hormones, the body is primed to respond to the demand. Once the stressor has been removed, the body begins to restore balance. This becomes a time of renewal and restoration (if the stressor has been removed).
Exhaustion	If the stress continues unabated, there is no time for renewal; over time, the body is left with little ability to resist. There is no longer an adaptive reserve, and illness and disease occur.

natural and predictable reaction to extreme stress. Symptoms include an easily triggered startle response, flashbacks to the traumatic event(s), insomnia, emotional distance, and increased or unexplained anger that is out of proportion to the current situation. These symptoms may occur immediately but more commonly occur weeks to months after the event. When PTS is not appropriately addressed, it becomes entrenched. The goal is to recognize and address PTS to prevent the syndrome of impairment, often referred to as PTSD (post-traumatic stress disorder), which is a distinct diagnosis in the *Diagnostic and Statistical Manual* but is rarely made in ED workers who are often exposed to PTS. The Department of Defense has also emphasized that PTS is a normal response and should only be described as a disorder when specific criteria are met.

A less recognized condition is secondary traumatic stress (STS), which occurs when a person not directly experiencing the traumatic event experiences the same symptoms as the one who is involved. This has also been called "bystander syndrome." As an example, a health-care worker can develop STS symptoms by simply listening to someone describe their harrowing trauma; by caring for a patient suffering from the effects of that trauma, such as severe burn or death of a child; or by empathizing with a family who has just unexpectedly lost a loved one. This stress syndrome is likely to be due to the phenomenon of *neural entrainment* in which the brain waves in the auditory, frontal, and parietal lobes "sync" closely between the speaker and the listener, producing a "memory" for the listener, despite never having witnessed the event.[4]

Emergency care workers can develop PTS experiences at work. Most non-health-care workers rarely witness firsthand the death of another person. Yet, emergency clinicians regularly experience the stress of observing death and being involved in efforts to prevent it. It is even more stressful when the victim is a child, young adult, or subject to a prolonged, unsuccessful resuscitation.

Following an unsuccessful resuscitation, there is rarely time to process the complex thoughts and feelings surrounding that death. Instead, the health-care workers must repress their feelings and address the increasing queue of waiting patients, many of whom are acutely ill and have their own unique emotional and clinical needs. After managing patient after patient, these caregivers must complete their documentation, complete transitions of care at the change of shift, and then travel home, carrying all their suppressed emotional stress. With increasing acuity and relentless pressure to perform, ED caregivers increasingly exist in states of chronic low- to mid-level stress, without an opportunity to adequately recover.

Unfortunately, training cannot prepare emergency caregivers for these types of situations. And while critical incident stress debriefing (CISD) has an important role in recovery, it is only in the most severe situations that CISD teams are called to assist.

Burnout

Burnout in health care represents a failure of *adaptive capacity* to balance *job stress* with the *requisite resources* to deal with the stress, resulting in three highly negative, yet completely understandable and predictable, responses[5]:

1. Overwhelming emotional exhaustion
2. Cynicism born of detachment and depersonalization
3. Loss of effectiveness and personal accomplishment

It is likely that burnout occurs along a continuum depending on the duration, constancy, and intensity of a clinician's stress. Adverse patient care events and/or destructive personal life events can occur if the spectrum of symptoms continues unrecognized and unaddressed. Not only is burnout widespread (50+% in some studies), it also has a profoundly deleterious effect on the clinicians themselves and on the care they provide (safety and quality). Burnout manifests itself across six core domains[6]:

1. Mismatch in workload demands and capacity
2. Loss of control
3. Lack of or insufficient rewards and recognition
4. Lack or breakdown of community
5. (Un)fairness
6. Values conflict

Many studies of physicians in training and practice have been published.

- In 2012, Shanafelt et al. found that 45.8% of physicians reported at least one symptom of burnout.[7] Substantial differences in burnout were observed by specialty, with the highest rates among physicians at the frontline of care access (family medicine, general internal medicine, and emergency medicine). Compared with a probability-based sample of 3,442 working US adults, physicians were more likely to have symptoms of burnout (37.9% vs. 27.8%) and to be dissatisfied with work–life balance (40.2% vs 23.2%) ($P < .001$ for both).
- In 2018, a survey published by Medscape reported that 54% of physicians in all specialties reported burnout, depression, or both.[8] Forty-eight percent of emergency physicians reported burnout, depression, or both. The rate of burnout was 10% higher for female physicians than for males.
- In a 2018 paper published in the *Journal of the American Medical Association*, "Association of Clinical Specialty with Symptoms of Burnout and Career Choice Regret Among U.S. Resident Physicians," 45.2% of second-year residents reported burnout (53.8% among emergency medicine residents), while career choice regret was 14.1% (11.4% in emergency medicine).[9]
- In a literature review on burnout in medical students published in 2013, 50% of medical students were felt to experience burnout.[10]

There are now multiple citations that connect physician burnout to poorer clinical outcomes for patients:

- In a study of pediatric residents, 39% reported burnout. Residents with burnout had significantly greater odds ($P < .01$) of reporting suboptimal patient care attitudes and behaviors, including discharging patients to make the service more manageable, not fully discussing treatment options or answering questions, making treatment or medication errors, ignoring the social or personal impact of an illness, and feeling guilty about how a patient was treated.[11]
- In a study of intensive care units, it was shown that patient safety and clinician burnout are dependent on one another. Researchers identified different predictors for the safety outcomes: standardized mortality ratios, length of stay, and clinician-rated safety. Evidence was found that mortality adjusted for severity of disease is higher on units with high emotional exhaustion. Our results led us to the conclusion that clinician psychological health and patient safety could and should be managed harmoniously.[12]
- In their paper, "From Triple to Quadruple Aim; Care of the Patient Requires Care of the Provider," Bodenheimer and Sinsky point out that burnout is associated with lower patient satisfaction and reduced health outcomes, and it may increase costs.[13]

A review of the manifestations of burnout published by the American Association for Physician Leadership (previously American College of Physician Executives) revealed the personal and professional signs of burnout[14]:

Personal Signs of Burnout

- Depersonalization
- Suicide
- Substance abuse
- Failed relationships
- Emotional exhaustion
- Cynicism

Professional Signs of Burnout

- Physician turnover
- Decreased patient adherence
- Increased lawsuits
- Deceased patient satisfaction
- Decreased work productivity
- Increased medical errors
- Decreased quality of care

These findings not only highlight the personal toll of unaddressed stress, they also build a case for managers and leaders to prioritize the prevention and treatment of burnout. Stress should be addressed at the personal, departmental, and business unit level to ensure patient safety and avoid the real financial costs of personnel attrition, the degradation of patient safety, and lost market shares.

THE UNIQUE STRESSES OF THE EMERGENCY CARE WORKER

Although the Social Readjustment Rating Scale is an effective predictor of stress and subsequent injury and illness in the general population, the stresses experienced by emergency health-care workers are unique.

Patient-Related Stressors

Stresses related to ED patient care include the following:

- ED patients arrive any time of the day or night in an unscheduled manner and without the benefit of a medical history previously known by the provider. Yet the large amount of unfiltered and often nonpertinent patient information in today's electronic medical records is expected to be integrated into an individual's care in real time.
- Emergency care workers have little or no control over what they will experience during their day. While arrival patterns are actually predictable over time, the acuity and special case variation impact each hour of each day differently. ED staff can rapidly go from caring for patients at a comfortable relaxed pace to chaos.
- Most ED patients have a sense of urgency that can only be satisfied by the immediate and full attention of the health caregivers.
- There is not a preestablished and trusting patient–physician relationship. Rapport must be created in the first few seconds of the encounter in an often-difficult, impersonal environment. Frustration with many pre-encounter issues like parking, telephone triage, department triage, and registration often increases the challenge of establishing rapport with the patient.

- Patients and their families commonly come to the ED upset, in pain, and in physical and/or emotional crisis.
- The expectations and needs of the patients are varied, and health-care workers must constantly readjust their approach to each unique situation.
- Unlike specialty/subspecialty care providers, emergency clinicians must be able to readily apply a broad foundation of knowledge to a diverse patient population with whom they have no previous relationship.

Additionally, there are substantial physiologic stresses associated with changing shifts, which may affect ED workers by:

- Altering their sleep patterns and circadian rhythms
- Decreasing their ability to cope with the usual demands of daily living, including personal and family needs
- Creating social isolation from friends and family due to significant evening and weekend work obligations
- Limiting the sense of belonging and engagement with the greater hospital community

All emergency care workers are expected to function without error in a culture of patient safety; yet, they practice in uncertain circumstances, with incomplete information, and with constantly changing demands. Most ED personnel describe both emotional and physical exhaustion when practicing in a busy ED environment (see **Box 13.1**).

Personal Stressors

All members of the emergency care team are subject to certain general stressors. Family and personal events, including pregnancy, marital discord and divorce, dysfunctional relationships, financial pressures, and various impairments, can affect each team member's

---

BOX 13.1 ■ TYPICAL STRESSORS AMONG ED PERSONNEL

- Constant pressure to provide unassailable patient care:
  - Outcomes—the patient's well-being
  - Diagnoses—the threat of malpractice litigation
  - Experience—the threat of a patient complaint
- Continuing reappraisals and requirements to demonstrate credentials and skill sets through recurrent observation, testing, hospital, and payor credentialing, peer review, e-learning, and regulatory inspections
- Inadequate assurance of professional security: A physician or nurse's position may be lost with little warning, and one bad outcome could potentially lead to termination.
- Risk of violence directed at staff
- Risk of infectious disease exposure
- Declining physician compensation as Medicare and other reimbursements are reduced
- Pressure to increase productivity with similar or fewer resources
- The practice of boarding admitted patients in the ED requires significant personnel, operational, and space resources further creating stress by:
  - Increasing the queue of waiting patients
  - Decreasing the safety of all patients
  - Creating frustration of ED workers

sense of well-being and performance. Reorganization of departments and service lines, changes in corporate ownership, requirements for involuntary overtime, workforce reductions, and decreases in compensation or benefits can create additional worker strain, uncertainty, and sense of loss. These institutional events can lead to anger and disillusionment.

Finally, beyond these corporate stressors, other associated workplace issues contribute to the emergency care worker's psychological burden:

- Litigation threat and adverse litigation outcomes
- Time pressure
- Limited opportunity to maintain or advance current knowledge base
- Legislatively enacted requirements, such as mandatory continuing medical education for child abuse, opioid stewardship, patient safety, HIV, and so on
- Fatigue from frequent shift changes
- Loss of authority and control
- Threat of workplace violence

Stress-Related Burnout

The concept of burnout, which was first defined in psychological literature in the 1970s, applies to a combination of emotional exhaustion, cynicism, and loss of personal accomplishment.[15,16] These three components are measured with the Maslach Burnout Inventory–Human Services Survey, a 22-question survey that takes 15 to 20 minutes to complete.[17] Burnout may result from situations that are particularly emotionally demanding. Lack of sleep is also a contributor. The occurrence of burnout depends not only on the particular set of circumstances, but also on the attitudes, coping mechanisms, and preparation of the person exposed to the demanding situation.

Prolonged, persistent stress without relief can have long-lasting negative effects on the individual, eventually leading to a state of burnout. In a study of paramedics, high-stress clinical situations led to high cortisol levels with a delayed return to baseline. Prolonged stress and handling patients in immediately life-threatening situations measurably affected the neuroendocrine stress response.[18]

The full syndrome of burnout generally entails a combination of depersonalization, low sense of personal accomplishment, and mental (or emotional) exhaustion. Interestingly, a survey demonstrated that 32% of emergency physicians exhibited emotional exhaustion, one of the three major characteristics of burnout.[19] Uncertainty and anxiety about the potential for bad outcomes was found to be the strongest predictor of career burnout.

Yet, in many cases, these same doctors found satisfaction with their careers. Emergency care providers rarely have a preexisting relationship with their patients. Nevertheless, the exigencies of time-sensitive clinical syndromes, severe pain, and presentations with high levels of uncertainty lead to deep concerns about the outcomes of their patients. This involvement may account for the surprising lack of depersonalization that otherwise might be expected with patient unfamiliarity, demands of shift work, and effects of mental exhaustion.

ADDRESSING WELLNESS

American College of Emergency Medicine

Organized emergency medicine has created committees and interest groups to address wellness. The Wellness Section of the American College of Emergency Physicians (ACEP) is a leader in promulgating and implementing wellness strategies for emergency

TABLE 13.3 ■ Examples of ACEP Wellness Resources

Media	Title
Book	*Wellness Guide Book: Being Well in Emergency Medicine*
Video	• Leadership Resiliency During Times of Constant Change • ZDoggMD Talks to Emergency Physicians About Happiness and Health
Papers	• Health Resource Document For Emergency Physicians • Wellness on Physician Wellness Throughout the Various Stages of Their Life and Career • Resources on PTSD • Litigation Stress: a Primer

physicians. As an example, for many years, a "wellness booth" was operated at ACEP's annual *Scientific Assembly*. More than 50% of the physician visitors to the wellness booth indicated that the testing provided at the conference was their only regular health care, which included multiple test panels to assess the health of emergency medicine professionals (cholesterol, chemistries, complete blood count, prostate-specific antigen testing, immunizations, vital signs, burnout surveys, and other assessment and prevention methodologies).

ACEP currently offers multiple resources designed to address personal wellness. Several of these are listed on its website (**Table 13.3**).[20] An example of a wellness approach is the Wellness Wheel (**Figure 13.1**).[21]

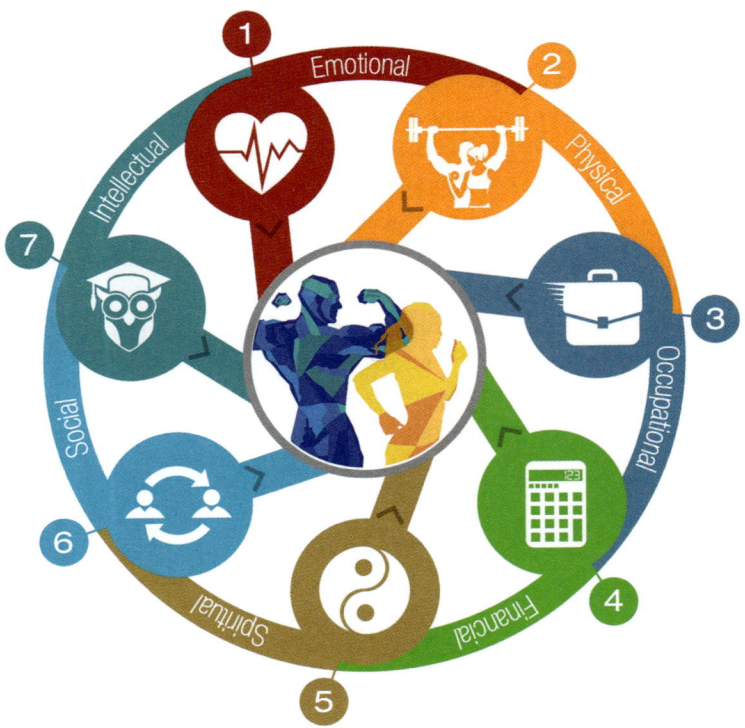

FIGURE 13.1 ■ The Wellness Wheel

Regulatory and Deeming Organizations

Organizations such as the American Board of Medical Specialties, Accreditation Council for Graduate Medical Education, and the Residency Review Committee for Emergency Medicine have continued to develop duty-hour rules for residents to humanize the training experience and improve patient safety.[22] These same rules are influencing providers beyond training as the association between fatigue and errors is becoming clearer. Though controversial, the duty-hour rules for residents continue to evolve to protect the integrity of the educational experience, advance patient safety, and reduce errors caused by clinician exhaustion.

The National Academy of Medicine

Formerly the Institute of Medicine (IOM), the National Academy of Medicine published a landmark series of reports, *Quality of Health Care in America*, which were designed to assess the US health-care system.[23] The report's statistics on preventable mortality shocked the medical community and the nation at large. The first report, "To Err is Human: Building a Safer Health System," was released in November 1999 and focused attention on the specific issue of medical errors in the hospital setting. The report alerted the public to the concept of patient safety and the value of systems optimization to prevent error.

The IOM panel released a second report, "Crossing the Quality Chasm: A New Health System for the 21st Century," in March 2001.[24] This second report recommended a sweeping redesign of the health-care system and provided a framework for improving the quality of care. These reports contain information that is consistent with the concepts of patient safety and physician wellness.

In 2016, The National Academy of Medicine (NAM) initiated an Action Collaborative on Clinician Well-Being and Resilience (**Figure 13.2**). ACEP and the Society for Academic Medicine were sponsoring organizations. Similar to its landmark report in 1999, "To Err is

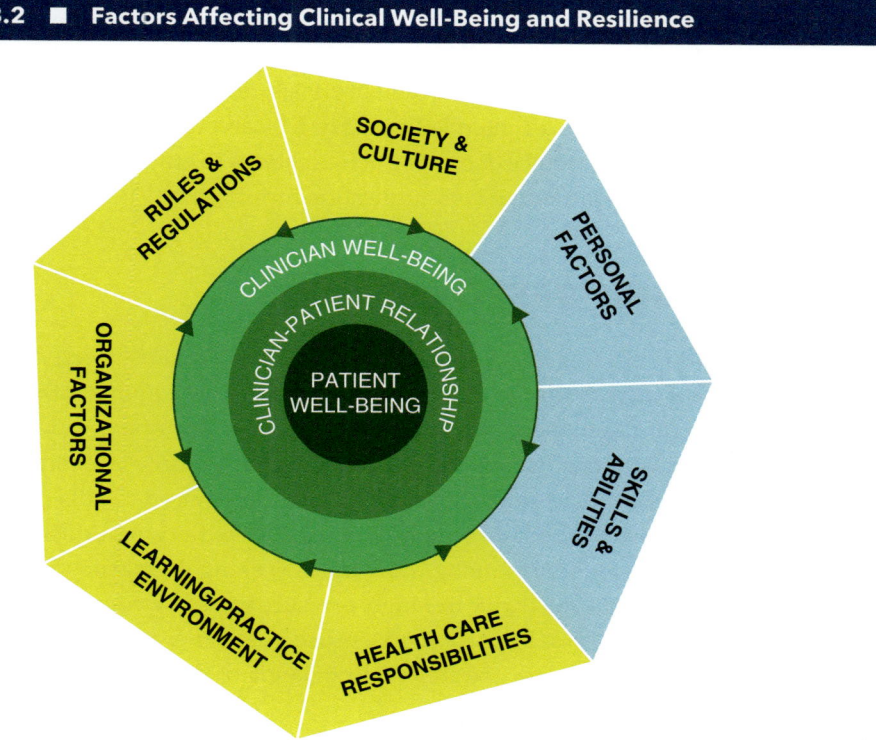

FIGURE 13.2 ■ Factors Affecting Clinical Well-Being and Resilience

Human," NAM has put together a consensus group to report on "To Care is Human." The Action Collaborative has created a new Conceptual Model of Clinician Well-Being. Of note, many of the variables that affect clinician well-being have been identified as external factors rather than intrinsic capabilities of the health-care provider.[25]

American Medical Association STEPS Forward

The American Medical Association (AMA) developed "STEPS Forward," an online program intended to identify, prevent, and treat burnout. The program is comprised of 50 modules focused on patient care, workflow and process, leading change, professional well-being, and technology and finance.

The AMA recommends using the 11-item "Mini-Z" burnout assessment survey, which includes a useful calculator for quantifying the organizational cost of physician burnout and the return on investment for interventions that reduce it (https://stepsforward.org/modlues/joy-in-medicine).

Institute for Healthcare Improvement Joy at Work

In 2017, the Institute for Healthcare Improvement (IHI) released *IHI Framework for Improving Joy in Work*, a white paper that identifies four steps for leaders and a broad framework for improvement[26]:

1. Ask staff, "What matters to you?"
2. Identify unique impediments to joy in work in the local context.
3. Commit to a systems approach to making joy in work a shared responsibility at all levels in the organization.
4. Use improvement science to test approaches to improving joy in work in your organization.

Other organized medical and nursing groups that continue to address wellness include the Emergency Medicine Residents' Association, Society for Academic Emergency Medicine, and Emergency Nurses Association.[27–29]

Patient safety, medical quality improvement efforts, resident work-hour constraints, and benchmark expectations are all intended to make ED careers more manageable. Standout employers realize the importance of making active choices in annual hours worked, lengths of shifts, behavioral standards, and communication scripting.

ED LEADERSHIP RESPONSIBILITY

The proper selection of caregivers is critical. Emergency physicians in one Australian study were found to have Myers-Briggs personality profiles that significantly differed from those of the general population, with ENTJ (extraversion, intuition, thinking, judgment) being the most frequent type for emergency medicine physicians.[30] Generally, people with these characteristics are "natural born leaders . . . career focused . . . dislike mistakes and inefficiencies . . . and hold onto submerged emotions." These findings underscore the degree of self-selection that may occur among individuals seeking emergency medicine careers, since the ability to tolerate and thrive in a high-pressure work environment is a determinant of career satisfaction.[33] It is important to ensure that emergency medicine residency candidates are a good match for the inherent demands of the profession and the specific demands of a particular practice.

Identifying Stress and Burnout

Nursing and medical leaders have an important role to play in identifying stress and burnout among their colleagues, employees, and associates (see Chapter 125). Direct observation, reports from work associates, quality reviews, and compliments and complaints from physicians, staff, and patients should continually inform the department leaders. Certain verbal expressions and nonverbal signs may signal a problem. Clinical problems, decreasing patient satisfaction (as noted by trends in surveys or complaints), tardiness, absenteeism, avoidance by other employees, and changes in behavior and personality are harbingers of burnout.

Medical and patient care nurse directors are not immune to stress. To the contrary, the responsibilities of meeting financial performance, ensuring staffing needs, providing employee oversight, addressing complaints, and successfully accomplishing productivity goals, in addition to clinical obligations, all contribute to significant leadership stress.

Emergency Medicine's Longitudinal Study

Between 1994 and 2008, a longitudinal study examined career satisfaction and burnout among emergency physicians.[32] Approximately two-thirds of respondents reported high career satisfaction, with more than 75% reporting that emergency medicine had met or exceeded their career expectations. Despite these encouraging numbers, nearly one-third of respondents reported that burnout was a significant problem.

This survey noted a high correlation between certain career characteristics and high satisfaction. For example, emergency medicine physicians involved in teaching, consulting, institution leadership roles, or organized medicine leadership roles were twice as likely to report high career satisfaction. Job security and job excitement were also positive correlates.

Conversely, factors associated with low career satisfaction included:

- Insufficient time for their personal lives
- Long shift length
- High census
- Lack of subspecialty support
- Unsupportive hospital administration
- Self-reporting of burnout

Major contributors to burnout included:

- Poor control over the workday environment
- Poor sense of personal reward
- Lack of control over shift length, night shifts, patient acuity
- Lack of resources for patient needs
- Fatigue
- Lack of time to attend educational conferences

The longitudinal study noted that physicians who felt dissatisfied with professional autonomy or compensation were more likely to seek new positions. In fact, dissatisfied physicians were found to be three times as likely to leave the practice of medicine. These studies strongly indicate that emergency medicine providers—and, by extrapolation, *all* ED workers—can benefit from an environment that supports wellness, work–life balance, and career longevity. Such a positive environment supports patient satisfaction and practitioner wellness, long-term employment, and quality care. Responsible leaders identify and ameliorate stressors. While personal resilience is a significant factor in well-being, the underlying nature of the ED environment is highly influenced by hospital, network, and department leadership.

Solutions to Enhance Wellness and Prevent Burnout

Burnout has significant effects on the functioning of an ED. An ED leader who fails to consider and plan to reduce burnout and its causes may find that nurses and physicians deliver lower quality care, have greater absenteeism and worse morale, and experience higher-than-average job turnover.[16] Physician quality measures, 360-degree surveys, and peer satisfaction surveys provide windows into employee functioning. Patients treated by physicians and nurses with low job satisfaction and high stress have lower satisfaction and lower compliance with care instructions.[16]

Schedule Adjustments

Methods of preventing stress and enhancing wellness include schedule adjustments that provide opportunities for physiological sleep, ensure personal time prior to and after shifts, and optimize circadian rhythms. Examples of strategies that are helpful to the entire group of workers include:

- 8- and 9-hour shifts (rather than traditional 12-hour shifts)
- 1-hour shift overlaps (reducing care transition, enhancing contemporaneous chart completion, and confining work to the workplace)
- Scribes (often improve documentation and reduce uncompensated post-shift work)
- Rewards for those who commit to full-time night-shift work (increased hourly rates and/or reduced weekly hour commitments—notably, these commitments are helpful to the entire group)

Note, these strategies also partially address the frequently noted difficulties associated with the aging caregiver.

Critical Incident Stress Debriefing

It is helpful to provide staff support following an unexpected clinical outcome, disaster, death of a young patient, or particularly disturbing emotional trauma. Involving the at-risk staff in a CISD can provide immediate support and help gauge how the physicians, nurses, and other staff members are reacting.

Improving the Environment of Care

Environmental strategies to improve physician wellness are predicated on the belief that there is a direct correlation between the wellness of the workforce and the delivery of patient care. To accomplish this goal, some institutions provide incentive programs that include smoking cessation, a monetary dollar credit for participating in a well-equipped health club/gym with proof of regular usage, weight loss programs, and lifestyle education.

Creating Standards for Effective Communication

The successful ED demands teamwork among a variety of professionals and essential personnel. A healthy practice environment requires workers who effectively communicate, have procedural competency, and are able to focus in the face of frequent interruptions. Language and communication protocols can create an environment that is conducive to wellness, enhance patient safety, and foster a culture of respect and teamwork. Scripted

Table 13.4 ■ ICARE Communication Strategy

I Introduce yourself and **I**nspire confidence (manage up).

C **C**onnect with the patient and make **C**ontact (visual, physcial, emotional).

A **A**cknowledge (listen without interruption) and **A**rticulate your thoughts.

R **R**eview your plan of care; **R**emember to say how long it will take.

E **E**ducate about home care; **E**xit after asking, "What questions do you have?"

methods of communication bring a sense of control to the emergency physician, helping to prevent burnout. Specific examples include:

- *ICARE:* An acronym used to effectively communicate with patients and families. This program has been adopted by EDs to facilitate communication with patients **(Table 13.4)**.
- *SBAR:* Standardizes communication, especially during patient handoff transitions and specialty backup consultation requests. It helps to ensure patient safety. SBAR stands for *situation, background, assessment,* and *recommendation*.[33]
- *The 4 Cs:* Civility, collegiality, collaboration, and community—guide relationships among emergency care providers and their many audiences, including specialists, ancillary departments, and others. The 4 Cs employ relationship rules to build teams and ensure a culture of respect.
- *EI (emotional intelligence):* Effective emotional intelligence depends on self-awareness, managing one's emotions, having social awareness, and ultimately addressing other's emotions.[34]
- *Crucial conversations:* A crucial conversation occurs when people are discussing difficult issues with high stakes, different points of view, and high emotions. The book *Crucial Conversations* describes techniques designed to master communications involving these difficult discussions.[35]

The systems described above emphasize that effective communication is the most important competency required for optimum team interaction. A team that fully understands its common goals and trusts its members is most likely to adequately and safely treat patients, make appropriate disposition decisions, and decrease the stress caused by the clinical and administrative practice of emergency medicine.

Addressing Impairment

In addition to workplace and family stress, emergency care workers are subject to the same types of impairments that affect the general population (see Chapter 122). Department leaders must be familiar with their institution's guidelines (HR/medical staff bylaws) regarding the identification, treatment, and work continuation of addicted or impaired professionals. State licensure and employment credentialing scrutiny are high stressors for impaired clinicians, who may choose to suppress or hide the impairment, ultimately to their own detriment.

Referral to an employee assistance program and, in certain situations, an impaired physician/nurse program at the state level can help an ED worker salvage a career threatened by addiction. Absolute privacy and confidentiality are necessary to protect the employee and avoid legal implications and grievance filing.

PERSONAL GOAL ACHIEVEMENT

There are many reasons why people are drawn to work in the ED, for instance, the excitement and adrenalin, the lifestyle (limited hours and minimal on-call responsibilities) the capacity to make a difference, and the life-saving work. However, because the work is so intense and, at times, so rewarding, it may be necessary to make a concerted effort to avoid becoming too narrowly focused on career at the exclusion of personal fulfillment and a balanced life.

Career longevity and satisfaction often require ED workers to actively seek opportunities for personal and professional balance. This goal is rarely achieved by chance. Caregivers are well advised to continually define personal values/goals and determine the best method to achieve them.

A Personalized Strategic Plan

A simple exercise to create goals requires about 1 hour. By answering the questions listed here, one can begin the process of goal setting:

- What do I want to accomplish professionally?
- What do I want to do personally?
- What do I want in terms of relationships?
- What do I want to have?
- How much money do I want to make?
- Where do I want to go professionally and personally?
- What do I want to give and contribute?
- What do I want to learn?
- What are my dreams?

It is advisable for a person completing this exercise to write down a large number of goals and then assign them to groups:

- 1—critically important
- 2—desirable but less important
- 3—"would be nice" but unimportant

Additionally, it is important to establish target dates for accomplishing these goals, with particular attention to group 1 goals. This type of strategic plan should be reviewed and revised on a regular basis, as goals, opportunities, and circumstances change. It is often helpful to create separate lists for personal and professional goals and then work toward goal integration and balance. Separating these goals permits reflection on the relative number on each list and allows consideration of ongoing realignment to achieve greater balance.

Goal Sharing

Since very few people achieve success entirely by themselves, enlightened leaders work to formalize pathways to support well-being. It may be valuable to share personal and professional goals with trusted professional colleagues (and significant others). If several members of a collaborative group attempt the same exercise, the group can engage in a discussion to review both individual and group goals. The aspirations of some group members may not be consistent with the goals of the group. Recognizing these differences may be particularly valuable when addressing potential conflicts. From these discussions, groups can implement changes that incorporate the needs of the individuals and the group, such as altering the schedule and shift length, hiring additional practitioners, creating productivity plans, permitting more vacation

TABLE 13.5 ■ The Adult Apgar Tool

	Almost Always Score = 2	Some of the Time Score = 1	Hardly Ever Score = 0
1. I am satisfied with the **Access** I have to my emotions—to laugh, to be sad, to feel pleasure or even anger.			
2. I am satisfied that my life's **Priorities** are mine and clearly reflect my values.			
3. I am satisfied with my commitment to personal **Growth**, to initiate and embrace change.			
4. I am satisfied with the way I ask for **Assistance** from others, professionally and personally, when in trouble.			
5. I am satisfied with the **Responsibility** I take for my well-being—physically, emotionally, and spiritually.			
Total Score = 0-10			

time and periodic sabbaticals, encouraging development of entrepreneurial programs, and so on. Goal sharing can be crucial to both individual and group career planning.

Performance Improvement Processes

The individual can utilize the performance improvement phases of the change cycle—plan, develop, change, assess—to achieve personal and professional balance. Once goals are set, specific change methodologies may be implemented to attain goals.

Adult Apgar Score

The Adult Apgar Score (**Table 13.5**) created by emergency physician Shay Bintliff is an instrument that can be used to monitor clinician wellness. Rather than passively accepting a situation like burnout, health-care providers can monitor their own work–life balance and satisfaction and use this information to steadily realign activities to achieve goals. This is a slow and steady process.

> *You cannot change your destination overnight, but you can change your direction overnight.*[36]

Renewal Investment Plan

The acronym "RIP" is used in a new context by Tom Peters, the gifted management consultant and inspiring speaker. He suggests using the abbreviation to represent "renewal investment plan."[37] An active approach to health and wellness is necessary for an emergency caregiver to achieve career longevity. Specific methods can be applied. A formalized RIP may include wellness considerations, including:

- *Rest:* Too little sleep over long periods creates stress and limits recovery. Adequate sleep on a regular basis requires thoughtful planning, particularly for ED workers who shift from days to nights and back. Some people are proponents of setting an alarm as an alert for when it is time to go to sleep. It is particularly important to rest before late evening and night shifts, and it may be necessary to engage family members in the process to ensure undisturbed sleep time.

- *Exercise*: An exercise program usually requires a regular pattern (timing, location, type). For instance, most studies suggest that people who exercise early in the morning are more successful in maintaining an ongoing and regular exercise program. Aerobic exercise builds physical and mental stamina, and it is ideally accompanied by strength training to maintain muscle mass and stretching to maintain flexibility.

Another important consideration is *where* to exercise. Exercising at home may be distracting for some who require the discipline imposed by a gym or workout facility. Alternatively, exercise at home takes significantly less time (travel) and may avoid undesirable social distractions. Some have achieved success by making home exercise a family event; for instance, walking or jogging with children or a significant other reinforces the importance of healthy activities and ensures valuable time together.

- *Family/significant other time*: Amidst busy and sometimes-harrowing work lives, it is necessary to ensure adequate time to connect with loved ones. Thoughtless or even unnecessary time at work and away from a growing family cannot be recovered.
- *Scheduled downtime*: Many in medicine and nursing are overachievers or at least overly busy. It may be helpful to ensure time to just "be" rather than "do." This may be partially accomplished by shutting off the connection to work. Even leaders can occasionally put the smartphone away. The ubiquity of technology handcuffs the unwary, significantly limiting free and family time. To provide balance and limit the infringement of professional interruptions, it may be appropriate to take electronics-free hours at home (and electronics-free days when on vacation). The constant urge to check in or review e-mails and texts is a form of withdrawal from others. Consider what is communicated when one is engaged in a discussion and looks away to respond to a text, Facebook notice, or e-mail: *This alert is more important than continuing our current conversation.*

Traditional approaches to stress management, such as yoga, exercise, meditation, and self-reflection, are other effective methods of reducing existing stress.

- *Spirit*: Derived from the Latin word "spiritus," which means breath, "spirit" is used here to consider what gives a person a sense of meaning and perspective. Whether it takes the form of religion, volunteerism, helping others, and so on, it provides a more selfless view that goes beyond the needs of the individual.

    Some ED caregivers find that volunteer efforts help them to focus their attention toward some of the same motivations that led them into their fields. Examples include working in a local free clinic, an economically disadvantaged region or country, or disaster sites. Individuals may find these activities personally satisfying while simultaneously bringing benefit to all involved.

- *Nutrition*: A nutritional diet is an important component of physical and mental health. The ravages of unhealthy eating habits, such as obesity, diabetes, coronary artery disease, and digestive problems, are self-evident. Typically, emergency care workers have poor diets—perhaps ordering pizza frequently, eating available sweets, and drinking multiple sugar-filled sodas during a shift. To avoid this non-nutritious approach to diet requires thoughtfulness, planning, and effort.

CONCLUSION

Focusing on and achieving personal and professional balance can lead to a long and fulfilling career in emergency medicine. Alternatively, unaddressed stress may lead to burnout, limit career enjoyment, and ultimately reduce the effectiveness of the health-care worker, even to the point of threatening patient safety. ED leaders must help to identify and systematically decrease workplace stressors among their partners, coworkers, and themselves. The promotion of wellness, identification and treatment of stress, and recognition and referral of impairment are all important aspects of mindful leadership, resource stewardship, patient safety, and responsible business practices.

REFERENCES

1. Kushner quote, "My Favorite Quotes." 2017. Available at: https://www.cs.cmu.edu/~roni/quotes.html. Accessed August 2, 2020.
2. Selye H. The general adaptation syndrome and the diseases of adaptation. *J Clin Endocrinol*. 1946;6:117-231.
3. Holmes TH, Rahe RH. The Social Readjustment Rating Scale. *J Psychosom Res*. 1967;11(2):213-218.
4. Liberzon I, Abelson JL. Context processing and the neurobiology of post-traumatic stress disorder. *Neuron*. 2016;92(1):14-30. Available at: https://www.ncbi.nlm.nih.gov/pmc/articles/PMC5113735/. Accessed December 9, 2019.
5. AHRQ. Physician burnout. 2017. Available at: https://www.ahrq.gov/prevention/clinician/ahrq-works/burnout/index.html. Accessed July 29, 2020.
6. Saunders EG. 6 causes of burnout, and how to avoid them. Harvard Business Review. 2019. Available at: https://hbr.org/2019/07/6-causes-of-burnout-and-how-to-avoid-them. Accessed July 5, 2020.
7. Shanafelt.
8. Medscape.
9. Dyrbye LN, Burke SE, Hardeman RR, et al. Association of clinical specialty with symptoms of burnout and career choice regret among US resident physicians. *JAMA*. 2018;320(11):1114-1130. doi:10.1001/jama.2018.12615.
10. Ishak W, Nikravesh R, Lederer S, et al. Burnout in medical students: a systematic review. *Clin Teach*. 2013;10(4):242-245. doi:10.1111/tct.12014.
11. Baer TE, Feraco AM, Tuysuzoglu Sagalowsky S, et al. Pediatric resident burnout and attitudes toward patients. *Pediatrics*. 2017;139(3):pii:e20162163. doi:10.1542/peds.2016-2163.
12. Welp A, Meier LL, Manser T. Emotional exhaustion and workload predict clinician-rated and objective patient safety. *Front Psychol*. 2015;5:1573. doi:10.3389/fpsyg.2014.01573. eCollection 2014.
13. Bodenheimer T, Sinsky C. From triple to quadruple aim: care of the patient requires care of the provider. *Ann Fam Med*. 2014;12(6):573-576.
14. Klevos GA, Ezuddin NS. In Search of the most effective interventions for physician burnout. American Association of Physician Leadership. 2018. Available at: https://www.physicianleaders.org/news/discussion-burning-brightly-burning-out. Accessed December 4, 2018.
15. Felton JS. Burnout as a clinical entity: its importance in health care workers. *Occup Med*. 1998;48(4):237-250.
16. Kuhn G, Goldberg G, Compton S. Tolerance for uncertainty, burnout and satisfaction with the career of emergency medicine. *Ann Emerg Med*. 2009;54(1):106-113.e6.
17. Maslach C, Jackson SE. Maslach Burnout Inventory. 2020. Available at: https://en.wikipedia.org/wiki/Maslach_Burnout_Inventory. Accessed August 3, 2020.
18. Sluiter JK, Van der Beek AJ, Frings-Dresen MHW. Medical staff in emergency situations: severity of patient status predicts stress hormone reactivity and recovery. *Occup Environ Med*. 2003;60(5):373-375.
19. Popa F, Arafat R. Occupational burnout levels in emergency medicine: a two stage nationwide study and analysis. *J Med Life*. 2010;3(4):449-453.
20. American College of Emergency Physicians. Wellness resources. 2020. Available at: https://acep.org/life-as-a-physician/wellness/#sm.00017ymcj87ifcnbscu2qymretd8k. Accessed August 3, 2020.
21. American College of Emergency Physicians. The wellness wheel. 2020. Available at: https://www.acep.org/search/?searchtext=%22wellness%20wheel%22#sm.00017ymcj87ifcnbscu2qymretd8k. Accessed July 24, 2020.
22. ACGME. Improving physician well-being, restoring meaning in medicine. 2020. Available at: https://acgme.org/What-We-Do/Initiatives/Physician-Well-Being. Accessed July 18, 2020.
23. Kohn LT, Corrigan JM, Donaldson MS. *To Err Is Human: Building a Safer Health System*. Washington, DC. Committee on Quality of Health Care in America, Institute of Medicine, National Academy Press; 2020.
24. Institute of Medicine. *Crossing the Quality Chasm: A New Health System for the 21 Century*. Washington, DC The National Academies Press; 2001.
25. Sharing knowledge to combat clinician burnout. 2020. Available at: https://nam.edu/clinicianwellbeing/. Accessed July 19, 2020.
26. IHI. 2017. Available at: https://www.ncha.org/wp-content/uploads/2018/06/IHIWhitePaper_FrameworkForImprovingJoyInWork.pdf. Accessed December 8, 2018.
27. EMRA. Wellness articles 2020. Available at: https://www.emra.org/emresident/articles/categories/topics/wellness. Accessed August 3, 2020.
28. SAEM. Wellness and resilience. 2020. Available at: https://www.saem.org/resources/wellness-and-resilience. Accessed August 3, 2020.

29. ENA 2019. Wellness, Available at: https://www.ena.org/search?indexCatalogue=dev&searchQuery=wellness&wordsMode=AllWords. Accessed July 25, 2020.
30. Available at: https://www.myersbriggs.org/my-mbti-personality-type/mbti-basics/Published 2020, Accessed August 1, 2020.
31. Boyd R, Brown T. 2005. Pilot study of Myers Briggs type indicator personality profiling in emergency department senior medical staff. *Emer Med Australas*. 2005;17(3):200-203.
32. Cydulka R, Korte R. Career satisfaction in emergency medicine: the ABEM longitudinal study of emergency physicians. *Ann Emerg Med*. 2008;51(6):714-722.
33. Available at: http://www.ihi.org/IHI/topics/patientsafety/safetygeneral/tools/SBARTechnique-forCommunicationASituationalBriefingModel.htm.
34. Goleman D, Boyatzis RE, McKee A. *Primal Leadership: Learning to Lead with Emotional Intelligence*. Boston, MA: Harvard Business School Press; 2004.
35. Patterson K, Grenny J, McMillan R, et al 2012. *Crucial Conversations: Tools for Talking When Stakes Are High*. McGraw-Hill.
36. Rohn J. *The Treasury of Quotes*. Southlake, Tex: Jim Rohn International; 2001.
37. Peters T. *The Brand You 50: 50 Ways to Transform Yourself from an 'Employee' into a Brand that Shouts Distinction, Commitment and Passion*. New York, NY: Alfred A. Knopf; 1999.
38. Available at: www.sourcesofinsight.com/ghandi-quotes/. Accessed December 9, 2018.

ADDITIONAL READINGS

- Bintliff S, Jay Kaplan JA, Meredith JM III, eds. *Wellness Book for Emergency Physicians*. 2004.
- Carius M. Avoiding "training toxicity": staying human during residency. *Annals Emerge Med*. 2001;38(5):596-597.
- Chapman D. Burnout in emergency medicine: what are doing to ourselves. *Acad Emerge Med*. 4(4). First published online.
- Chipman C. If the walls could speak. *Annals Emerge Med*. 2002;40(1):120-121.
- Available at: http://www.studergroup.com/newsletter/Vol1_Issue3/vol1_i3_sec7.htm.
- Salluzzo RF, Mayer TA, Strauss RW, et al, eds. *Emergency Department Management, Principles and Applications*. St Louis, Mo: Mosby Year Book Inc; 1997.

CHAPTER 14

ETHICAL ISSUES IN THE EMERGENCY DEPARTMENT

Catherine A. Marco

A variety of ethical dilemmas are commonly encountered in the emergency department (ED), including both organizational and clinical dilemmas. An organized approach to the assessment and management of these ethical dilemmas promotes prompt and consistent resolution to promote patient safety and well-being. This chapter will address basic principles of bioethics and case discussions to illustrate these principles.

CASE STUDIES

Case One

As the chair of the Department of Emergency Medicine, it has come to your attention that a faculty member has posted a patient case, including radiographs, on Facebook. Although there is no disclosure of protected health information, you are concerned about possible ramifications for the patient, faculty member, and your department. How should you address the issue of social media in your department?

Case Two

A 56-year-old man presents to the ED with abdominal pain, in obvious discomfort. Vital signs are stable. A police officer approaches you to mention that the patient is suspected of drug trafficking and requests that you do a body cavity search. How should the emergency practitioner respond? Should departments have a policy about this issue?

Case Three

Your institution wishes to begin advertising ED wait times on a billboard sign. The CEO demands a 20-minute guarantee for patients to be seen by a physician. What are the ramifications of such an approach? What is your role as chair/medical director/nursing director in promoting this approach or refuting it?

Case Four

A 22-year-old man presents to the ED with altered mental status. He is agitated, combative, and refuses to answer questions. He attempts to strike and bite the staff and demands to leave, announcing, "I know my rights! Let me out of here!" Should the patient be allowed to leave the ED?

PRINCIPLES OF ORGANIZATIONAL ETHICS

The practice of ethics is to *understand and examine the moral life*.[1] Code of ethics have guided behavior for centuries. The Hippocratic Oath is recognized as one of the earliest codes of medical ethics, but other examples relevant in emergency medicine include the American Medical Association code of ethics (with its earliest version published in 1847)[2] and the American College of Emergency Physicians (ACEP code of ethics, 1997 through 2017; **Table 14.1**).[3]

Health-care organizations and ED leaders should commit to ethical and legal principles that protect the best interests and safety of patients. Priorities for health-care organizations should include patient care, population health, expertise based on trustworthy standards and self-regulation, accountability for delivering services, and advocacy within society for health values.[4]

The American College of Healthcare Executives has developed a code of ethics that states, "The fundamental objectives of the healthcare management profession are to maintain or enhance the overall quality of life, dignity and well-being of every individual needing health care service and to create an equitable, accessible, effective, and efficient health care system."[5]

Business practices in health care should balance the primary responsibility to patients with the fiduciary duty to stakeholders, since conflicts in these two duties may arise when an action seemingly promotes one duty over the other. In many cases, seeking financial profit may seem self-serving but is actually necessary to provide quality patient-centered care. As the adage states, "No margin, no mission."

TABLE 14.1 ■ ACEP's Principles of Ethics

The basic professional obligation of benevolent service to humanity is expressed in various physicians' oaths and codes of ethics. In addition to this general obligation, emergency physicians accept specific ethical obligations that arise out of the unique features of emergency medical practice. The principles listed below express fundamental moral responsibilities of emergency physicians.

1. Emergency physicians shall embrace patient welfare as their primary professional responsibility.
2. Emergency physicians shall respond promptly and expertly, without prejudice or partiality, to the need for emergency medical care.
3. Emergency physicians shall respect the rights and strive to protect the best interests of their patients, particularly the most vulnerable and those with impaired decision-making capacity.
4. Emergency physicians shall communicate truthfully with patients and secure their informed consent for treatment, unless the urgency of the patient's condition demands an immediate response or another established exception to obtaining informed consent applies.
5. Emergency physicians shall respect patient privacy and disclose confidential information only with consent of the patient or when required by an overriding duty such as the duty to protect others or to obey the law.
6. Emergency physicians shall deal fairly and honestly with colleagues and take appropriate action to protect patients from health-care providers who are impaired or incompetent or who engage in fraud or deception.
7. Emergency physicians shall work cooperatively with others who care for, and about, emergency patients.
8. Emergency physicians shall engage in ongoing study to maintain the knowledge and skills necessary to provide high-quality care for emergency patients.
9. Emergency physicians shall act as responsible stewards of the health-care resources entrusted to them.
10. Emergency physicians shall support societal efforts to improve public health and safety, reduce the effects of injury and illness, and secure access to emergency and other basic health care for all.

PRINCIPLES OF MEDICAL ETHICS

Codes of ethics often include common principles such as *beneficence* (doing good), *nonmaleficence* (*primum non nocere*, or "do no harm"), respect for patient *autonomy*, *confidentiality, honesty, distributive justice,* and *respect for the law.*

Ethical dilemmas commonly arise in clinical medicine when there is a conflict between two principles or values. Ethical dilemmas may be very complex and a single best course of action may be difficult to identify. One approach to resolving ethical dilemmas is the ABCs of medical ethics (**Table 14.2**).[6]

TABLE 14.2 ■ The ABCs of Medical Ethics[7]

A. Assessment: Gather information, communicate with patient and other parties, and *assess* objectives of interventions.

1. Gather information about the case. Obtain information about the background, clinical information, and expected outcomes of various courses of action.
2. Communicate with the patient regarding goals, values, and objectives of medical care in this clinical scenario. Discuss patient preferences.
3. If the patient is unable to communicate, obtain information regarding advance directives, previous conversations, or family opinions regarding patient preferences.
4. Communicate with family and friends regarding their opinions, goals, and values (if the patient consents to this step).
5. Consider the involvement of additional parties, such as pastoral care, social work, or an ethics committee.

B. Bioethical Principles and Values: Identify and prioritize principles of *bioethics* and values relevant to the case.

1. Identify bioethical principles applicable to the case. Principles may include:
   a. Respect for patient autonomy
   b. Beneficence
   c. Nonmaleficence
   d. Justice
2. Identify values applicable to the case. Values may include such concepts as honesty, integrity, altruism, respect for life, justice, freedom, and others.

C. Capacity: Assess *capacity* of the patient to participate in medical decision-making.

1. Assess the decisional capacity of the patient.
2. If the patient does not possess decisional capacity, identify any advance directives or other communications of patient wishes.
3. If necessary, identify a surrogate decision maker to speak on the patient's behalf. This is often defined by state law and may include a hierarchy such as spouse, adult children, parents, and others. If no surrogate can be identified, a court-appointed surrogate may be named.

D. Decision: Make a timely *decision*.

1. Identify possible courses of action.
2. Weigh positive and negative ramifications of each possible course of action.
3. Select the course of action that best adheres to the ethical principles and values of the patient and the physician.
4. Make the decision in a timely fashion to allow for the best possible outcome.

E. Evaluation: *Evaluate* the outcome and ramifications of the decision.

1. Review the clinical outcome.
2. Assess the opinions of the patient, family, and health-care providers.
3. Analyze in retrospect whether other options may have been preferable.

Emergency department providers should begin with a thorough assessment of all relevant facts, apply principles of bioethics, assess patient capacity, make a timely decision, and evaluate the clinical scenario. In some circumstances, caregivers may also seek additional resources, such as hospital administration, legal counsel, an institutional ethics committee, or the judicial system.

ADMINISTRATIVE AND CLINCIAL ETHICAL ISSUES

Many administrative and clinical ethical dilemmas can be resolved by the application of ethical and legal principles. Institutional and departmental policies should guide clinicians in commonly encountered dilemmas based on these ethical and legal principles.

Privacy and Confidentiality

Confidentiality is an important ethical concept that promotes trust in the patient–clinician relationship. Confidentiality has been recognized as an important value for centuries. The Hippocratic Oath describes this duty as: "Whatever I see or hear in the lives of my patients, whether in connection with my professional practice or not, which ought not to be spoken of outside, I will keep secret, as considering all such things to be private."[8]

More recently, federal law delineates this responsibility under the Health Insurance Portability and Accountability Act of 1996 (widely known by its acronym, HIPAA), which includes regulations requiring medical personnel and health-care institutions to protect patient information. Although this requirement can be challenging in the ED environment, confidentiality should be an absolute priority. Access to patient records should be limited to those directly involved in health care with some notable exceptions. These exceptions include disclosure for public health safety, safety of individuals (duty to warn), and judicial proceedings.

Electronic Communications and Social Media

Many providers use electronic means for professional and personal communications. Electronic communications may be useful for patient care (communication with consultants), research (use of databases), and education (patient cases, data, Centers for Disease Control and Prevention, online services, and images). Many health-care providers also use social media for professional networking (LinkedIn, Doximity, blogs, and so on) and for personal or social networking (Facebook, Twitter, SnapChat, Instagram, blogs, and others). The lines that separate professional and social networking often become intertwined through professional groups that use social media (eg., "EMDocs," a private Facebook group).

All electronic communications, both professional and social, should protect patient privacy and confidentiality. Protected health information should be disclosed only on secure networks and when necessary for clinical care. Organizations may have specific policies that delineate appropriate use of electronic communication for patient care through secure electronic means and may limit or prohibit any use of patient data, including radiographs and photographs, on social media or other public communications.[9,10] Guiding principles are listed in **Table 14.3**.[11]

Law Enforcement in the ED

Emergency practitioners frequently interface with law enforcement in the ED. Patients may be in police custody or may be "a person of interest." Significant issues may arise,

TABLE 14.3 ■ Guiding Principles for the Use of Electronic Communication and Social Media by Health-Care Practitioners

1. Understand privacy settings and use them to the fullest extent to safeguard personal information on social networking sites. Consider separating personal and professional content.
2. Routinely monitor personal and professional online presence to ensure that information is accurate, appropriate, and professional.
3. Maintain boundaries of the patient–health-care provider relationship and ensure patient privacy and confidentiality when interacting online.
4. Be forthcoming about employment, credentials, and conflicts of interest.
5. Posted information should be supported by current peer-reviewed literature whenever possible and should clearly indicate whether it is based on studies, consensus, experience, or personal opinion.
6. Posted content may be available to anyone and may be misconstrued. Recognize that online behavior can negatively impact reputation among patients and colleagues, represents one's practice institution(s), and may have permanent consequences for medical careers.

including the appropriate handling of illegal items and patient consent for specimen procurement or questioning. Emergency practitioners should work prospectively with law enforcement to ensure timely and appropriate medical care, with patient welfare as the primary priority.[12,13] Common ethical issues between ED caregivers and law enforcement should be discussed and, where possible, policies and procedures should be put in place.

Conflicts of Interest

Conflicts of interest may arise on an organizational level or on an individual level. A conflict of interest may occur when an organization or individual has a financial, professional, or personal interest or responsibility that may interfere with their primary duties.[14] Organizations and institutions should have policies to delineate the appropriate management of real or perceived conflicts of interest. When conflicts of interest are identified, they should be managed appropriately, which may include disclosure, recusal, or transfer of duties.

Quality Metrics

Quality metrics serve an important function in promoting timely and quality health care.[15] Any metric being instituted in the ED should be evaluated for its reasonableness, application, effect on patient safety, and impact on staff and other patients.

Many quality metrics serve to promote timely access to care. For example, evaluating time-to-physician goals ("door-to-doc time") can improve patient satisfaction and reduce the number of patients who leave without being seen.[15-18] Other examples of metrics designed to promote timely access may include additional triage resources, reducing time to triage, direct-to-bed initiatives with bedside registration and triage, and improved throughput times to increase available treatment beds.[19-23] The institution of any metric should include consideration of potential unintended consequences. For example, a metric to designed to guarantee a short door-to-physician time may interrupt other critical tasks. Interruptions of practitioner tasks may result in deleterious effects such as disrupted workflow, inefficiencies, medical errors, or decreased patient satisfaction.[24-27] Metrics that interfere with clinical judgment about treatment priorities may interrupt or interfere with quality care.

Informed Consent and Informed Refusal of Care

Informed consent is an essential component of emergency medical treatment (See Chapter 105, "Consent to and Refusal of Medical Treatment"). Most patients can provide informed consent for ED treatment. Specific informed consent should also be obtained for emergency medical interventions of significant risk.

Refusal of care also requires an assessment of decisional capacity. Patients have the right to refuse emergency medical treatment at any time during their evaluation and treatment. "Left prior to medical screening examination" refers to patients who leave the ED before being evaluated. "Left without being discharged" refers to patients who "elope" by leaving the ED following some aspect of evaluation but without a conversation regarding refusal of treatment or discharge instructions. Refusal of care or "AMA" (against medical advice) refers to patients who leave the ED before completion of recommended diagnostic studies or treatment and are designated by the provider as having made a decision to refuse medical advice.

Patients leaving AMA provide a significant challenge to emergency providers. It has been estimated that approximately 1% to 3% of patients leave the ED AMA.[28-31] Patients who leave AMA have a higher rate of return ED visits, hospital admissions, and mortality.[32-42] Certain patient factors are associated with a higher incidence of leaving AMA, including male gender, younger age, alcohol use, illicit substance use, weekend treatment, Medicaid insurance, and no medical insurance.[31,43,44]

The assessment of decisional capacity is an essential skill for emergency physicians and nurses to ensure the patient is able to make an informed choice.[45] Assessment of capacity should precede informed consent for treatment or informed refusal of care. There is significant variation in providers' assessment of decisional capacity.[46-48] Capacity includes four essential elements: understanding, appreciation, reasoning, and expression of choice.[49] A patient must be able to understand the information delivered, appreciate how to apply this information to his or her own situation, reason to make an appropriate decision, and communicate that choice (**Table 14.4**).

Capacity is a dynamic, task-specific attribute.[50] Individuals may have impaired capacity from a reversible condition, such as acute intoxication, and may return to full decisional capacity when the condition has resolved. When patients in the ED refuse any component of emergency care (diagnostic tests, treatments, or disposition decisions), there should be an assessment of the patient's decisional capacity. There should also be consideration of the spectrum of potential outcomes as a result of the patient's choice based on the seriousness and severity of the condition.[51] For example, a patient may have decisional capacity to agree to or refuse radiographs for an extremity injury but may lack capacity to weigh the risks and benefits of high-risk emergency surgery.

Multiple clinical conditions may impair capacity. These conditions may include cognitive disorders, neurologic disorders, medication effects, alcohol intoxication, substance abuse, psychosis, pain, anxiety, or any other condition that impairs ability to make an authentic choice.[52-55] An assessment of capacity and its relation to the patient's baseline capacity must be performed prior to refusal of care. It may be helpful to gather additional information from relevant

TABLE 14.4 ■ Elements of Decisional Capacity

1. Understanding (ability to receive information)
2. Appreciation (ability to process information and apply it to one's circumstances)
3. Reasoning (ability to deliberate)
4. Expression of choice (ability to make and articulate a decision)

sources, with the patient's permission. Such sources may include family, friends, primary care provider, or other individuals familiar with the patient's baseline level of functioning.

Assessment tools may be helpful when determining decisional capacity, particularly in high-risk settings. There is no evidence to establish a single tool as a valid gold standard for assessment of capacity, and the use of any of these approaches represents only one part of the clinical assessment of capacity.[56-60] Examples of assessment tools that may be used in the ED include the Mini Mental State Examination; Montreal Cognitive Assessment, MacArthur Competence Assessment Tool for Treatment, Competency Interview Schedule, Structured Interview for Competency and Incompetency Assessment Testing and Ranking Inventory, Hopkins Competency Assessment, Mini-Cog, Aid to Capacity Evaluation, and the Capacity Assessment Tool.[61-69]

For patients who lack decisional capacity, a surrogate decision maker or advance directive may be helpful in clarifying the patient's wishes. State laws vary regarding the identification of surrogates. Some states require a legally appointed surrogate and others designate a hierarchy of surrogates, often including a spouse, adult children, or parents. If no surrogate is available, medical interventions should be performed using the standard of what a reasonable patient would desire under those circumstances.

When a patient refuses care, this creates conflict between the provider, who wishes to provide the best possible medical care, and the patient, who knows his or her goals and values best. Ensuring an optimal physician–patient relationship and developing trust may mitigate this conflict and promote a mutually agreeable resolution.

The appropriate management of a patient who wishes to refuse medical care includes the following elements: determination of decision-making capacity; assessment of the reasons for refusal of care; delivery of information, including the risks and benefits of the proposed therapy; discharge planning, including the best treatment alternative; and documentation. One approach to the AMA patient is the "AIMED" framework (assess, investigate, mitigate, explain, and document).[70] A reasonable course of action can often be negotiated. For example, a patient who is unwilling to be hospitalized for symptoms of chest pain may agree to urgent outpatient cardiology follow-up.

Proper documentation of AMA can confer medicolegal protection in three potential ways.[71] Against medical advice documentation can:

- Define termination of the legal duty to treat the patient.
- Create the defense of "assumption of risk" by the patient.
- Provide evidence of the patient's refusal of treatment.

Documentation of an encounter in which a patient refuses treatment should include several essential elements (**Table 14.5**).[72] Unfortunately, such notes are often suboptimal. In one recent study, only 17 charts (4.1%) met minimal standards that apply to unstable patients, according to the Emergency Medical Treatment and Active Labor Act. Decisional capacity, one component of the AMA, was documented in only 22% of charts.[73]

TABLE 14.5 ■ Documentation of Refusal of Care

1. Assessment of decisional capacity
2. Delivery of information including the proposed intervention and risks of refusal
3. Delivery of information including alternatives to the proposed intervention
4. The patient's understanding of risk and voluntary decision
5. Discharge instructions, including follow-up care
6. Invitation to return for care at any time

End of Life

Patients frequently present to the ED near the end of life. A discussion with the patient (or family, with permission) is important to establish goals of care. Advance directives may be helpful for understanding end-of-life wishes, particularly when managing patients who are unable to speak for themselves. The American College of Emergency Physicians' Policy on Ethical Issues at the End of Life provides guidance (**Table 14.6**).[74] Advance directives can be useful in communicating the patient's wishes, should the patient be unable to do so. Advance directives and code status are especially important in emergency medical decision-making.[75-77] Types of advance directives include:

- *Durable power of attorney*: Durable power of attorney (or health-care proxy) specifies a surrogate decision maker in the event that the patient no longer has the capacity to make medical decisions.
- *Living will*: The living will is a document suitable for terminally ill individuals.
- *Do-not-resuscitate (DNR) orders*: The DNR order specifies specific actions that are not desired by the patient, for example, intubation or cardiopulmonary resuscitation. These orders are recognized in many states.
- *Physician order for life-sustaining therapy (POLST)*: POLSTs are medical orders that specify the patient's treatment wishes.[78] They are increasingly recognized among states and require the signature of a physician or other licensed health-care provider. POLSTs express patient goals and values as medical orders that are easily understood and specific enough to apply to most medical encounters.

TABLE 14.6 ■ Ethical Issues at the End of Life

The American College of Emergency Physicians (ACEP) believes that:

- Emergency physicians play an important role in providing care at the end of life.
- Helping patients and their families achieve greater control over the dying process will improve end-of-life care.
- Advance care planning can help patients formulate and express individual wishes for end-of-life care and communicate those wishes to their health-care providers by means of advance directives (including state-approved advance directives, do-not-attempt resuscitation [DNAR] orders, living wills, and durable powers of attorney for health care).
- To enhance end-of-life care in the ED, ACEP believes that emergency physicians should:
  a. Respect the dying patient's needs for care, comfort, and compassion.
  b. Communicate promptly and appropriately with patients and their families about end-of-life care choices, avoiding medical jargon.
  c. Elicit the patient's goals for care before initiating treatment, recognizing that end-of-life care includes a broad range of therapeutic and palliative options.
  d. Respect the wishes of dying patients, including those expressed in advance directives. Assist surrogates who make care choices for patients who lack decision-making capacity based on the patient's own preferences, values, and goals.
  e. Encourage the presence of family and friends at the patient's bedside near the end of life, if desired by the patient.
  f. Protect the privacy of patients and families near the end of life.
  g. Promote liaisons with individuals and organizations in order to help patients and families honor end-of-life cultural and religious traditions.
  h. Develop skill at communicating sensitive information, including poor prognoses and the death of a loved one.
  i. Comply with institutional policies regarding recovery of organs for transplantation.
  j. Obtain informed consent from surrogates for postmortem procedures.

Despite the important function of advance directives, only a minority of patients have completed one. In addition, few patients who have completed them arrive in the ED with the necessary documentation.[75-77] Some patients present with nonstandard advance directives, such as letters, notes, tattoos, or other unofficial communications. In such situations, explicit communication with the patient and family is essential to establish patient wishes and goals of therapy. If the patient's wishes are uncertain, resuscitative efforts should be undertaken while attempting to verify the patient's wishes.[78]

Allowing family members to be present during resuscitative efforts has proven to be a beneficial practice. Family presence during resuscitation may serve to improve family comprehension, relieve guilt or disappointment, and may be a helpful part of the grieving process.[79-84] When family members are invited to be present, it is helpful to provide a staff liaison to assist with communication and education about medical procedures and other issues.[7]

CASE RESOLUTIONS

Case One

Organizations should have clearly communicated policies that dictate appropriate use of social media. Protected health information should be used only when necessary for clinical care and using secure communications methods. If organizations choose to allow limited social media posts, protocols should dictate the absolute exclusion of any protected health information or derogatory content toward patients or institutions. The faculty member and the other members of the department should be advised of these issues.

Case Two

Departments should have clear policies to guide providers about appropriate interactions with law enforcement. Patient welfare should be the primary responsibility. Procedures should be undertaken only with patient consent unless required by law.

Case Three

Quality metrics can be important in promoting timely quality medical care. The specific departmental environment and staffing should be assessed to determine whether this type of metric will enhance patient care or, perhaps, detract from some aspect of care. Advertising of metrics should be carefully considered, particularly regarding the potential inappropriate prioritization of time over quality of care. Consideration of the appropriate resources necessary to deliver on the "20-minute guarantee" with administration should be a part of the process.

Case Four

Emergency care providers should apply principles of patient autonomy and beneficence to cases in which a patient wishes to refuse medical care. The appropriate actions include assessment of capacity, delivery of information, and documentation. For a patient who does not possess decisional capacity, it is appropriate to ensure the patient's welfare by detaining the patient until he or she regains decisional capacity. Departmental policy may be helpful in delineating actions and documentation to ensure consistent application of these principles.

CONCLUSION

Ethical dilemmas are commonly encountered in the ED. A variety of dilemmas may be seen, including those related to the organization, procedures, policies, and clinical care. An organized approach to the assessment and management of ethical dilemmas promotes prompt and consistent resolutions as well as patient safety and welfare. Emergency department leader involvement in the development of institutional policies may be helpful in promoting the consistent application of bioethical and legal principles in the ED.

REFERENCES

1. Beauchamp TL, Childress JF. *Principles of Biomedical Ethics*. 7th ed. New York, NY: Oxford University Press; 2012.
2. The American Medical Association Code of Ethics. https://www.ama-assn.org/delivering-care/ama-code-medical-ethics. Accessed July 16, 2018.
3. American College of Emergency Physicians. Code of ethics for emergency physicians. *Ann Emerg Med*. 2017;70(1):e7-e15.
4. Ozar D, Berg J, Werhane PH, Emanuel L; for the National Working Group on Health Care Organizational Ethics. *Organizational Ethics in Health Care: Toward a Model for Ethical Decision Making by Provider Organizations*. Chicago, Ill. American Medical Association; 2000.
5. American College of Healthcare Executives. 2017. *ACHE Code of Ethics*. https://www.ache.org/abt_ache/code.cfm. Accessed September 8, 2018.
6. Marco CA, Shriner C. The ABC framework for ethical decision making. *Med Educ*. 2010;44(5):489-526.
7. Morrison LJ, Eby D, Veigas PV, et al. Implementation trial of the basic life support termination of resuscitation rule: reducing the transport of futile out-of-hospital cardiac arrests. *Resuscitation*. 2014;85(4):486-491.
8. Greek Medicine: The Hippocratic Oath. https://www.nlm.nih.gov/hmd/greek/greek_oath.html. Accessed July 27, 2018.
9. Pillow MT, Hopson L, Bond M, et al. Social media guidelines and best practices: recommendations from the council of residency directors social media task force. *Western J Emerg Med*. 2014;15(1):26-30.
10. Farnan JM, Snyder Sulmasy L, Worster BK, et al. Online medical professionalism: patient and public relationships: policy statement from the American College of Physicians and the Federation of State Medical Boards. *Ann Intern Med*. 2013;158(8):620-627.
11. McGrath J, Gorgas DL, Sahlani L. Social media and electronic communications. In: Marco CA, Schears RM, eds. *Ethical Dilemmas in Emergency Medicine*. New York, NY: Cambridge University Press; 2015.
12. Baker EF, Moskop JC, Geiderman JM, et al. Law enforcement and emergency medicine: an ethical analysis. *Ann Emerg Med*. 2016;68(5):599-607.
13. American College of Emergency Physicians Policy Statement: Law Enforcement Information Gathering in the Emergency Department. https://www.acep.org/globalassets/new-pdfs/policy-statements/law.enforcement.information.gathering.in.ed.pdf. Accessed September 8, 2018.
14. American College of Emergency Physicians. Conflicts of Interest. *Ann Emerg Med*. 2017;70(1):118-120.
15. Berg LM, Källberg AS, Göransson KE, et al. Interruptions in emergency department work: an observational and interview study. *BMJ Qual Saf*. 2013;22(8):656-663.
16. Holden RJ. Lean Thinking in emergency departments: a critical review. *Ann Emerg Med*. 2011;57(3):265-278.
17. Slash door-to-doc time, boost patient approval. *Hosp Case Manag*. 2011;19(9):142-143.
18. Lean-driven improvements slash wait times, drive up patient satisfaction scores. *ED Manag*. 2012;24(7):79-81.
19. Fernandes CM, Price A, Christenson JM. Does reduced length of stay decrease the number of emergency department patients who leave without seeing a physician? *J Emerg Med*. 1997;15(3):397-399.
20. Rowe BH, Channan P, Bullard M, et al. Characteristics of patients who leave emergency departments without being seen. *Acad Emerg Med*. 2006;13(8):848-852.
21. Clarey AJ, Cooke MW. Patients who leave emergency departments without being seen: literature review and English data analysis. *Emerg Med J*. 2012;29(8):617-621.
22. Lorch AC, Martinez M, Gardiner M. Analysis of a patient intervention to reduce patients who leave without being seen in an ophthalmology-dedicated emergency room. *J Healthc Qual*. 2018;40(1):e15-e19.
23. Nestler DM, Fratzke AR, Church CJ, et al. Effect of a physician assistant as triage liaison provider on patient throughput in an academic emergency department. *Acad Emerg Med*. 2012;19(11):1235-1241.
24. Blocker RC, Heaton HA, Forsyth KL, et al. Physician, interrupted: workflow interruptions and patient care in the emergency department. *J Emerg Med*. 2017;53(6):798-804.
25. Biron AD, Loiselle CG, Lavoie-Tremblay M. Work interruptions and their contribution to medication administration errors: an evidence review. *Worldviews Evid Based Nurs*. 2009;6(2):70-86.
26. Chisholm CD, Collison EK, Nelson DR, et al. Emergency department workplace interruptions: are emergency physicians "interrupt-driven" and "multitasking"? *Acad Emerg Med*. 2000;7(11):1239-43.
27. Berg LM, Källberg AS, Göransson KE, et al. Interruptions in emergency department work: an observational and interview study. *BMJ Qual Saf*. 2013;22(8):656-663.
28. Centers for Disease Control. National Hospital Ambulatory Medical Care Survey: 2011 Emergency Department Summary Tables. Available at https://www.cdc.gov/nchs/data/ahcd/nhamcs_emergency/2011_ed_web_tables.pdf. Accessed January 22, 2017.
29. Ding R, Jung J, Kirsch T, Levy F, McCarthy M. Uncompleted emergency department care: patients who leave against medical advice. *Acad Emerg Med*. 2007;14(10):870-876.
30. Alfandre D. "I'm going home": discharges against medical advice. *Mayo Clinic Proceedings*. 2009;84(3):255-260.
31. Lee C, Cho J, Choi S, et al. Patients who leave the emergency department against medical advice. *Clin Exp Emerg Med*. 2016;3(2):88-94.
32. Gabayan GZ, Asch SM, Hsia RY, et al. Factors associated with short-term bounce-back admissions after emergency department discharge. *Ann Emerg Med*. 2013;62(2):136-144.e1.

33. Gabayan GZ, Sarkisian CA, Liang LJ, et al. Predictors of admission after emergency department discharge in older adults. *J Amer Ger Soc.* 2015;63(1):39-45.

34. Choi M, Kim H, Qian H, Palepu A. Readmission rates of patients discharged against medical advice: a matched cohort study. *PLoS One.* 2011;6(9):e24459.

35. Southern WN, Nahvi S, Arnsten JH. Increased risk of mortality and readmission among patients discharged against medical advice. *Am J Med.* 2012;125(6):594-602.

36. Glasgow JM, Vaughn-Sarrazin M, Kaboli PJ. Leaving against medical advice (AMA): risk of 30-day mortality and hospital readmission. *J Gen Intern Med.* 2010;25(9):926-929.

37. Yong TY, Fok JS, Hakendorf P, Ben-Tovim D, Thompson CH, Li JY. Characteristics and outcomes of discharges against medical advice among hospitalised patients. *Internal Med J.* 2013;43(7):798-802.

38. Geirsson OP, Gunnarsdottir OS, Baldursson J, Hrafnkelsson B, Rafnsson V. Risk of repeat visits, hospitalisation and death after uncompleted and completed visits to the emergency department: a prospective observation study. *Emerg Med J.* 2013;30:662-668.

39. Jerrard DA, Chasm RM. Patients leaving against medical advice (AMA) from the emergency department—disease prevalence and willingness to return. *J Emerg Med.* 2011;41(4):412-417.

40. Southern WN, Nahvi S, Arnsten JH. Increased risk of mortality and readmission among patients discharged against medical advice. *Am J Med.* 2012;125(6):594-602.

41. Baptist AP, Warrier I, Arora R, Ager J, Massanari RM. Hospitalized patients with asthma who leave against medical advice: characteristics, reasons, and outcomes. *J Allergy Clin Immunol.* 2007;119(4):924-929.

42. Fiscella K, Meldrum S, Barnett S. Hospital discharge against advice after myocardial infarction: deaths and readmissions. *Am J Med.* 2008;120(12):1047-1053.

43. Jeong J, Song KJ, Kim YJ, et al. The association between acute alcohol consumption and discharge against medical advice of injured patients in the ED. *Am J Emerg Med.* 2016;34(3):464-468.

44. Ti L, Ti L. Leaving the hospital against medical advice among people who use illicit drugs: a systematic review. *Am J Public Health.* 2015;105(12):e53-e59.

45. Marco CA, Brenner JM, Krauss CK, McGrath NA, Derse AR; ACEP Ethics Committee. Refusal of emergency medical treatment: case studies and ethical foundations. *Ann Emerg Med.* 2017;70(5):696-703.

46. Marson DC, McInturff B, Hawkins L, Bartolucci A, Harrell LE. Consistency of physician judgments of capacity to consent in mild Alzheimer's disease. *J Amer Geriatr Soc.* 1997;45(4):453-457.

47. Braun M, Gurrera R, Karel M, Armesto J, Moye J. Are clinicians ever biased in their judgments of the capacity of older adults to make medical decisions? *Generations.* 2009;33(1):78-91.

48. Sessums LL, Zembrzuska H, Jackson JL. Does this patient have medical decision-making capacity? *JAMA.* 2011;306(4):420-427.

49. Grisso T, Appelbaum PS. *Assessing Competence to Consent to Treatment: A Guide for Physicians and Other Health Professionals.* New York, NY: Oxford University Press; 1998.

50. Larkin GL, Marco CA, Abbott JT. Emergency determination of decision making capacity: balancing autonomy and beneficence in the emergency department. *Acad Emerg Med.* 2001;8(3):282-284.

51. Appelbaum PS, Grisso T. Assessing patients' capacities to consent to treatment. *N Engl J Med.* 1988;319(25):1635-1638.

52. Boettger S, Bergman M, Jenewein J, et al. Assessment of decisional capacity: prevalence of medical illness and psychiatric comorbidities. *Palliat Support Care.* 2015;13(5):1275-1281.

53. Restifo S. A review of the concepts, terminologies and dilemmas in the assessment of decisional capacity: a focus on alcoholism. *Australas Psychiatry.* 2013;21(6):537-540.

54. Kolva E, Rosenfeld B, Brescia R, Comfort C. Assessing decision-making capacity at end of life. *Gen Hosp Psychiatry.* 2014;36:392-397.

55. Karlawish J, Cary M, Moelter ST, et al. Cognitive impairment and PD patients' capacity to consent to research. *Neurology.* 2013;81(9):801-807.

56. Sturman ED. The capacity to consent to treatment and research: a review of standardized assessment tools. *Clin Psychol Rev.* 2005;25:954-974.

57. Appelbaum PS. Clinical practice. Assessment of patients' competence to consent to treatment. *N Engl J Med.* 2007;357(13):1834-1840.

58. Dunn LB, Nowrangi MA, Palmer BW, Jeste DV, Saks ER. Assessing decisional capacity for clinical research or treatment: a review of instruments. *Am J Psychiatry.* 2006;163(8):1323-1334.

59. Bremault-Phillips SC, Parmar J, Friesen S, et al. An evaluation of the decision-making capacity assessment model. *Can Geriatr J.* 2016;19(3):83-96.

60. Finney GR, Minagar A, Heilman KM. Assessment of mental status. *Neurol Clin.* 2016;34(1):1-16.

61. Palmer BW, Harmell AL. Assessment of healthcare decision-making capacity. *Arch Clin Neuropsychol.* 2016;31:530-540.

62. Folstein MF, Folstein SE, McHugh PR. "Mini-mental state." A practical method for grading the cognitive state of patients for the clinician. *J Psychiatric Res.* 1975;12(3):189-198.

63. Edelstein B. Challenges in the assessment of decision-making capacity. *J Aging Studies.* 2000;14(4):423-437.

64. Nasreddine ZS, Phillips NA, Bedirian V, et al. The Montreal Cognitive Assessment, MoCA: a brief screening tool for mild cognitive impairment. *J Am Geriatr Soc.* 2005;53(4):695-699.

65. Grisso T, Appelbaum PS, Hill-Fotouhi C. The MacCAT-T: a clinical tool to assess patients' capacities to make treatment decisions. *Psychiatr Serv.* 1997;48(11):1415-1419.

66. Bean G, Nishisato S, Rector NA, Glancy G. The psychometric properties of the competency interview schedule. *Can J Psychiatry.* 1994;39(8):368-376.

67. Tomoda A, Yasumiya R, Sumiyama T, et al. Validity and reliability of structured interview for competency incompetency assessment testing and ranking inventory. *J Clin Psychol.* 1997;53(5):443-450.

68. Carney MT, Neugroschl J, Morrison RS, Marin D, Siu AL. The development and piloting of a capacity assessment tool. *J Clin Ethics.* 2001;12(1)17-23.

69. Borson S, Scanlan J, Brush M, Vitaliano P, Dokmak A. The mini-cog: a cognitive 'vital signs' measure for dementia screening in multi-lingual elderly. *Int J Geriatr Psychiatry.* 2000;15(11):1021-1027.

70. Clark MA, Abbott JT, Adyanthaya T. Ethics seminars: a best-practice approach to navigating the against-medical-advice discharge. *Acad Emerg Med.* 2014;21(9):1050-1057.

71. Levy F, Mareiniss DP, Iacovelli C. The importance of a proper against-medical-advice (AMA) discharge: how signing out AMA may create significant liability protection for providers. *J Emerg Med.* 2012;43(3)516-520.

72. Monico EP, Schwartz I. Leaving against medical advice: facing the issue in the emergency department. *J Healthc Risk Manag.* 2009;29(2):6-15.

73. Schaefer MR, Monico EP. Documentation proficiency of patients who leave the emergency department against medical advice. *Conn Med.* 2013;77(8):461-466.

74. American College of Emergency Physicians. Ethical issues at the end of life. *Ann Emerg Med.* 2016;68(1):142.

75. Taylor DM, Ugoni AM, Cameron PA, McNeil JJ. Advance directives and emergency department patients: owners rates and perceptions of use. *Intern Med J*. 2003;33(12):586-592.

76. Llovera I, Ward MF, Ryan JG, et al. Why don't emergency department patients have advance directives? *Acad Emerg Med*. 1999;6(10):1054-1060.

77. Harrison L, O'Connor E, Renner CH, Kluesner N. Assessing the accessibility to the IPOST at admission to the emergency department. *Am J Emerg Med*. 2019;37(1):162-163.

78. Iserson KV. Nonstandard advance directives in emergency medicine: what should we do? *J Emerg Med*. 2018;55(1):141-142.

79. Morrison LJ, Kierzek G, Diekema DS, et al. Part 3: Ethics: 2010 American Heart Association Guidelines for Cardiopulmonary Resuscitation and Emergency Cardiovascular Care. *Circulation*. 2010;122(18 suppl 3):S665-S675.

80. Millin MG, Khandker SR, Malki A. Termination of resuscitation of nontraumatic cardiopulmonary arrest: resource document for the National Association of EMS physicians position statement. *Prehosp Emerg Care*. 2011;15(4):547-554.

81. Critchell CD, Marik PE. Should family members be present during cardiopulmonary resuscitation? A review of the literature. *Am J Hosp Palliat Care*. 2007;24(4):311-317.

82. Mortelmans LJ, Van Broeckhoven V, Van Boxstael S, et al. Patients' and relatives' view on witnessed resuscitation in the emergency department: a prospective study. *Eur J Emerg Med*. 2010;17(4):203-207.

83. Itzhaki M, Bar-Tal Y, Barnoy S. Reactions of staff members and lay people to family presence during resuscitation: the effects of visible bleeding, resuscitation outcome, and gender. *J Adv Nurs*. 2012;68:1967-1977.

84. Jabre P, Belpomme V, Azoulay E, et al. Family presence during cardiopulmonary resuscitation. *N Engl J Med*. 2013;368(11):1008-1018.

CHAPTER 15

PRACTICE MANAGEMENT LEADERSHIP: THE ROLE OF THE SITE MEDICAL DIRECTOR

Michael Silverman

The site medical director (SMD) leads and manages the provider group while serving as a clinical role model. Every day can pose complex new challenges—whether presenting to a board committee, meeting with the chief executive officer (CEO), defending a case during a Centers for Medicare and Medicaid Services (CMS) investigation, or counseling a physician on inappropriate behavior. Depending on the hospital organization chart, the SMD may be called chair, chief, director, or medical director. In most hospitals, the SMD supervises the provider group (physicians and advanced practice clinicians [APCs]) while working collaboratively with the nurse director (or manager) responsible for the nursing aspects of care. Together, the two leaders oversee the performance and metrics of the ED.

SMDs must assume responsibility for provider group staffing, quality of care, and clinical operational efficiency. The SMD is the face of the department, interacting with hospital administration, outside departments, and patients. Whether addressing quality performance measures or responding to a CMS investigation, responsibility for the quality of care also falls to the SMD.

A leader must develop a clear vision and collaborate with others to implement it. Unfortunately, physician training typically encourages independence rather than teamwork. Despite the countless hours of education provided in medical school and residency, emergency physician training does little to address the skills necessary to lead a team. Effective leadership requires the ability to motivate others, delegate responsibility, define metrics, set and modify goals, encourage and give feedback, hold others accountable, and share the accolades that come with success.

THE LEADERSHIP SKILL SET

It is amazing what you can accomplish if you do not care who gets the credit.

—Harry S. Truman

The Healthcare Leadership Alliance (HLA) has identified five broad categories of essential competencies for physician leaders (**Figure 15.1**). Within this overall construct, HLA has defined more than 300 specific competencies for physician leaders.[1]

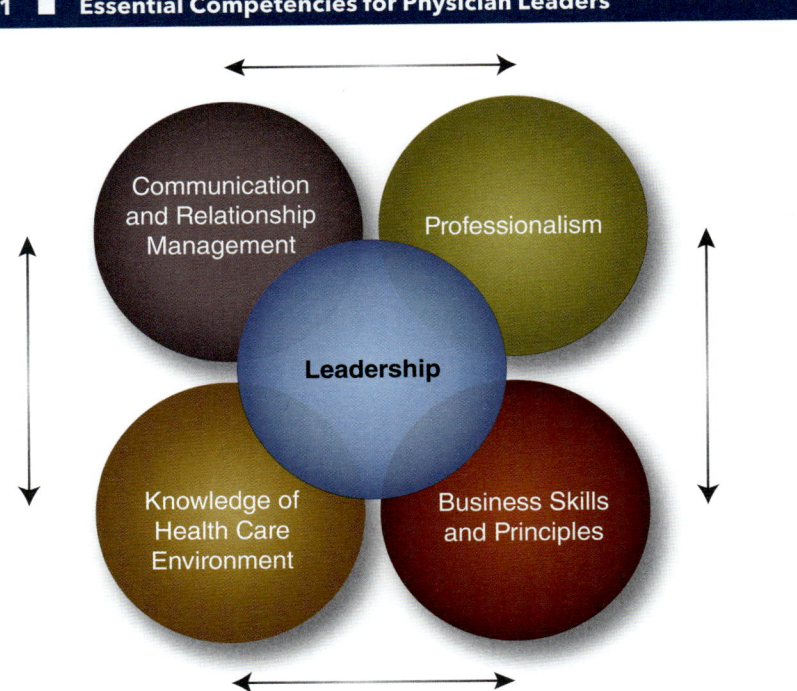

FIGURE 15.1 ■ Essential Competencies for Physician Leaders

For the purposes of this book, we will discuss four essential competencies for physician leaders:

- Core knowledge
- High emotional intelligence (EQ)
- Creative vision
- Organizational altruism

A fifth element is not a competency but a key ingredient in developing the essential competencies:

- Mentorship

Core Knowledge

SMDs must possess an excellent fund of knowledge in medicine as well as in business and human resource (HR) management. For example, the SMD must be able to confidently review and discuss a case with medical accuracy in front of other department chairs. The SMD must also be able to speak the language of the business office, present proposals that resonate with the finance team, and manage a myriad of personnel issues.

High EQ

The second essential competency is high emotional intelligence. High EQ includes effective communication skills. Many leadership mistakes made in communication and poor communication are the root cause of a high percentage of patient complaints. The two primary EQ categories are personal (how we manage ourselves) and social (how we handle our relationships).

In medicine, where physician intelligence generally comes with the territory, EQ may be even more important than IQ. It is how we communicate and work with others that often defines success. There have been thousands of journal articles on EQ since Daniel Goleman's groundbreaking book, *Emotional Intelligence: Why It Can Matter More Than IQ*.[2]

Creative Vision

Leadership is about vision, and the third competency on the broad list of necessary leadership skills is having vision and effective change management skills. In collaboration with the nurse leader, the SMD sets the direction of the department and is responsible for aligning the team's goals to achieve success.

Organizational Altruism

Finally, effective leaders have organizational altruism. This involves broad, systemic rather than personal or parochial thinking. Effective leaders recognize that that they are part of a larger organization and goals must be aligned. Another way of thinking about this is to avoid focus on personal success at the expense of others. Within every organization, all leaders have bosses and, ultimately, one of the leader's jobs is to make their leaders successful.

Mentorship

Fortunately, these critical leadership skills can be taught. Ideally, a potential leader has an early career mentor from whom he or she can learn. Consider the following personal testimony.

> *I was incredibly lucky to have a fantastic mentor early in my career. He brought me to essentially every meeting that he attended. I was exposed to multiple chair-level issues when I was just a couple of years out of residency. As another example, I had a good friend who became president of his company, all while learning the ins and outs from different mentors, taking advantage of behind-the-scenes discussions after meetings.*

More Paths to Leadership Skills

A mentor can dramatically accelerate a young leader's professional growth, not only by providing exposure and opportunities but also by discussing the behind-the-scenes thought processes and issues that arise from challenges outside of the clinical arena. There are often opportunities within the hospital to learn leadership skills. Joining and participating in various committees allows an aspiring leader to watch, listen, and learn invaluable skills. Those who contribute and consistently focus on the broad improvement of the organization, rather than on personal departmental needs, are often rewarded.

Assuming medical staff leadership roles is an excellent way to advance professional skills and become influential. Many medical staffs will pay for formal training outside of the hospital, and some hospitals are part of a larger network that holds leadership seminars. It is increasingly common for physician staffing companies to provide leadership development classes. The American College of Emergency Physicians offers an excellent, tiered set of courses known as the ED Director's Academy.

Additionally, there are multiple resources for self-advancement through online materials, professional seminars, books on critical leadership skills, and self-assessment programs. Some of the greatest lessons come from reading, observing, and learning about extraordinary leaders in fields that have nothing to do with medicine. A discerning student of leadership can learn to communicate effectively and lead a group in critical situations both in and out of the ED.

In many cases, leaders are chosen based on their clinical acumen and apparent leadership potential. Yet, it is often their management skills that create long-term success. Managers define purpose and assign tasks. Managers maximize efficiency by nurturing skills, developing talent, and inspiring results. Supervising a group (often comprising physicians and APCs) requires the ability to influence numerous aspects of ED operations and personnel. Among the most important attributes of a successful ED are the positive morale and mood of valued team members. This leads to employee satisfaction and retention, which impacts overall compliance with the department's goals and objectives. Ultimately, highly motivated and experienced staff who are aligned with the department's and institution's goals are more productive and efficient. Inevitably, their professional satisfaction is manifested in a highly satisfied patient population.

BUILDING THE TEAM

One of the keys to being a successful SMD is to hire the "right" people. After all, if the team "gets it," the ED is sure to face fewer complaints (from patients, nurses, and physicians from other departments), callouts, and bad outcomes. Since there are other chapters in this textbook that deal more extensively with recruiting, onboarding, and retention, these concepts will only be covered briefly here.

Recruiting

Recruiting starts before the interview. Effective leaders carefully evaluate each candidate's CV (*curriculum vitae*: the resumé) for red flags, such as an extended residency, job gaps, frequent job changes, or an overemphasis on non-work life. Once a decision is made to interview an applicant, the leader should be prepared to devote several hours to the process.

The Interview

An effective interview can easily consume two hours; if the candidate is a true superstar, it is appropriate to extend a lunch invitation. Consider also inviting a couple of other members of the ED team so the applicant can get a good feel of what the group is like. At the end of every interview, each candidate should walk out thinking "this is the best job, and I want to join this team." While this may not be realistic, it is certainly the goal. On the flip side, if the desirable candidate instead joins a competitor, it is appropriate to be a gracious loser. People change jobs frequently in emergency medicine, so if they do not join your team on the first round, perhaps they might want to join the team later. Emergency medicine is a very small world, so maintaining healthy relationships is important for everyone.

Learning About the Candidate

During the interview, the SMD should attempt to understand the candidate's personality, goals, and commitment to and excitement about emergency medicine. What is the applicant looking for in a team, and is this candidate a good fit?

Stanford Professor Robert Sutton's book *The No-Asshole Rule—Say No to Jerks*[3] (the title says it all) helps to define what is and is not acceptable on a high-functioning team. By the end of the interview, it is important to clearly establish the expectations of the candidate (schedule, productivity, patient satisfaction, and so on), answer any questions, and sell the benefits of the group/practice. Afterward, a careful and discerning reference check is necessary, as program directors are also trying to "sell" their residents and sometimes give an overly positive review. When they are desperate to fill holes in the physician schedule, it is easy for an SMD to ignore reference-related warnings, only to later regret the decision.

> **BOX 15.1 ■ CASES THAT MAY REQUIRE COMPLEX MANAGEMENT DECISIONS**
>
> - Resuscitation (medical, trauma)
> - Psychiatric patient requiring transfer
> - Patient brought in by the police
> - ST-elevation myocardial infarctions
> - Code stroke
> - Opioid addiction
> - Requiring management or follow-up by an uncovered service

Onboarding

The onboarding process starts early in the recruitment process. Expectations are discussed during the interview and then continue with the occasional e-mail until orientation starts. It is a best practice to send an orientation manual two to three weeks before the first shift. An on-site orientation meeting in the week leading up to the start date should be scheduled to discuss key aspects and priorities of the department. Another best practice is to schedule at least three orientation shifts in which the new practitioner serves as an extra provider and can be assigned to a mentor.

There are several patient types that new providers should manage during orientation so they can get help troubleshooting the expected obstacles. Examples might include patients or conditions listed in **Box 15.1**.

The SMD might wish to work side-by-side during at least one orientation shift with each new provider. Some sites assign a "big brother" or "big sister" to help mentor the new provider, with the intent of also building a bond for the new provider with an experienced clinician and to help answer the questions that arise early in a career or at an institution.

It is essential to check in with new clinicians every few weeks and provide low-stress feedback during the first 6 months. At 6 and 12 months, SMDs should provide more formal feedback. There is tremendous growth in the first years out of residency, and as a manager, we can positively impact this growth and ensure the new providers are assimilated into the department culture while improving their individual performance. Some important areas of feedback are listed in **Box 15.2**.

> **BOX 15.2 ■ COMMON TYPES OF PROVIDER FEEDBACK**
>
> - Productivity
> - 360-degree evaluation
> - Patient experience of care
> - Imaging utilization (computed tomographic scan)
> - Against Medical Advice and Left Prior to Medical Screening Exams
> - Average patient length of stay
> - Documentation quality
> - Complaints/compliments
> - Clinical concerns
> - Coordination of care effectiveness
> - Practice-based learning
> - Professionalism
> - Provider feedback re: practice

Retaining Providers

Retaining physicians is one of the keys to maintaining a high level of performance. The SMD should provide support, coaching, and mentoring to the clinical staff so that each person can reach his or her performance potential. High-performing providers should be kept engaged, making it critical that the leader recognizes when providers want to do more, keeping each member of the group growing professionally. Essentially, every emergency care provider who interviews for a job wants to work in an ED with a team atmosphere—a key for retention. Team building takes place over time.

Not every management decision will be popular. In fact, those decisions that involve change in well-practiced routines are likely to meet resistance. Nonetheless, it is critical to discuss the "why" of change and get fresh ideas and feedback on proposed changes from those who will be responsible for making the change operational. As a personal example:

> *A few years ago, my CEO made it very clear that we needed to reduce our left-without-being-seen (LWBS) rate. When we discussed the causes and options in staff meetings, there were a lot of reasons why the LWBS had climbed but no clear solutions. Ultimately, the decision was made to see patients in the waiting room after triage when necessary (we did not have a provider in triage). The decision to do this was complex and unpopular, but when we discussed the "why" behind it, the team realized it was the right decision for the patient and ultimately led to a reduction in patients who LWBS.*

The team culture is also best achieved when working together with the nursing team. The first step needs to be the nurse and physician leaders presenting a unified front when it comes to how the ED is run. Joint presentations, frequent leadership meetings and discussions, attending the other's staff meetings, and copying each other on e-mails are the starting points. Additionally, physicians can present education topics at nursing meetings; convene nursing and physician leaders (and nonleaders) for retreat-like events to discuss issues and future improvements; and organize social functions.

Protected Time

Most SMDs would like more protected time as their actual administrative hours worked typically exceed their administrative protected time. Some groups rotate the SMD job among the physicians and do not provide any protected time to the SMD. This approach is inconsistent with the recognition that leadership involves a set of skills developed over time that are neither possessed nor enjoyed by all who hold the position; not everyone can be an effective leader. Protected time is necessary to be successful as the group leader. The leader should have adequate time to do the work and attend the meetings that come with the position.

Alternatively, there are some SMDs who believe they should not work clinically at all but rather should be spending all of their time functioning as the leader of the group. This is not an effective leadership strategy as it is important to have the clinical credibility that is earned by being "in the trenches." Intradepartmental staff members may not believe that a nonworking SMD has the nuanced understanding of the department necessary to make recommendations for change. It would be extremely rare to come across the chair of another department (in a community setting) who does not work clinically.[4]

There is always plenty of work to do. With each promotion up the administrative ladder, more time is required in the hospital. The amount of protected time should be based on the average expected work requirement on a week-to-week basis—including, among other tasks, meetings, chart reviews, recruitment, and so on, and other flexible and open time blocks to respond to urgent requests. Additional time is required to "steer the ship." The SMD should have time to think about long-term planning and new projects. Stacking meetings together to create "meeting days" is one trick to allow free days for clinical time. A good rule of thumb for an SMD in a moderate-volume ED would be a 50-50 split between protected time and clinical time. A smaller ED and hospital will likely have fewer meetings, and therefore, the SMD gets less protected time, while a busier and more complex organization may require more administrative time, utilizing an associate SMD, and assigning administrative duties to other members of the provider team. This approach must be balanced with maintaining enough clinical hours, so the SMD can maintain his or her skill set and clinical competence.

Protected time is not typically paid at the clinical rate. Depending on the pay rate, assistant directors or others with smaller amounts of protected time may actually spend more than the expected time on administrative activities. For example, if an assistant director is contracted for 4 hours a week, there may be many weeks that require 8 hours of work and rarely weeks requiring less than 4 hours. This is likely to occur early in a clinician's administrative growth as the new "green" administrator will typically be less efficient. As a physician climbs the administrative ladder to become an experienced SMD, success breeds further opportunity and is the best method of negotiation when looking for more protected time.

MANAGING THE TEAM

The SMD must have or develop expertise in multiple areas, including HR protocols, group finances, and group performance metrics. The world of HR starts with an alphabet soup of initials and acronyms for terms that define regulations and laws that managers must follow. It is beyond the scope of this book to cover all employment legislation, but the following are the laws that most frequently impact SMDs. It is considered standard practice that every SMD should have access to an HR specialist who can assist with HR issues, many of which are listed in **Box 15.3**.

The Fair Labor Standards Act

The Fair Labor Standards Act addresses overtime pay and other related issues. Highly compensated practitioners, such as physicians, are "exempt" from overtime pay regardless of how many hours we work in a week. Alternatively, APCs are generally classified as "exempt" if salaried or "nonexempt" if they are paid hourly or weekly. A nonexempt employee (e.g., an APC paid hourly) is entitled to and must be paid overtime at 1.5 times the

---

BOX 15.3 ■ ED-RELATED EMPLOYMENT LAWS

- The Fair Labor Standards Act
- The Equal Pay Act of 1963
- Civil Rights Act of 1964
- Title VII of the Civil Rights Act of 1964
- The Age Discrimination in Employment Act of 1967
- The Occupational and Safety Health Act
- The Family Medical Leave Act
- The Pregnancy Disability Act
- The Americans with Disabilities Act and Amendment Act of 2008

rate of regular pay for hours worked over 40 per week. Note that the regulation differs for an APC employed on an hourly basis by a group and by the hospital. For example, during a single pay period, an APC works 24 hours for 1 week and 42 hours the second week. The group would have to pay 2 hours of overtime pay (over 40 hours in a week). However, the hospital's overtime payment is calculated based on greater than 80 hours in a 2-week pay period and no overtime payment would be due.

Exempt positions are not entitled to overtime but are paid for the job performed versus the hours worked. This explains why the SMD or nursing director may be present 50 hours in a week and not get overtime pay. Physicians, attorneys, and teachers are examples of professions that are considered exempt.

The Equal Pay Act of 1963 and the Civil Rights Act of 1964

The Equal Pay Act of 1963 and the Civil Rights Act of 1964 were passed to help end discrimination in the workplace. The Equal Pay Act states that an employer must not discriminate on the basis of gender and cannot pay different wages to employees of the opposite gender for equal work performed under similar working conditions.

There are some exceptions to the law, including differences due to a seniority system, merit system, or system that measures earnings by the quantity or quality of production. So, while pay may vary based on experience or productivity, a male and a female hired from residency, starting at the same time and required to perform the same duties, should be getting the same pay.

Title VII of the Civil Rights Act of 1964

Title VII of the Civil Rights Act of 1964 is a federal law that prohibits workplace harassment and discrimination. It covers all private employers, state and local governments, and educational institutions with 15 or more employees and prohibits discrimination against workers based on race, creed, color, national origin, religion, or gender. Workplace harassment can occur at a work-sponsored event, via social media, by sending out an "inappropriate" joke in a group e-mail, or by posting something that someone finds offensive in the physician lounge.

Interactions at work should remain professional at all times and in all situations. What one person considers harmless flirting could make someone else very uncomfortable and could be considered sexual harassment. This can also occur via social media, such as Facebook, where posting racist or sexist posts could make workplace colleagues uncomfortable and even cause them to leave their job.

The Age Discrimination in Employment Act of 1967

The Age Discrimination in Employment Act of 1967 (ADEA) protects individuals who are 40 years of age or older from employment discrimination based on age. The ADEA's protections apply to both employees and job applicants. Under the ADEA, it is unlawful to discriminate against a person because of his or her age with respect to any term, condition, or privilege of employment, including hiring, firing, promotion, layoff, compensation, benefits, job assignments, and training. The ADEA permits employers to favor older workers based on age even when doing so adversely affects a younger worker (less than 40 years old). Here are examples of actions that could result in the practice being sued for age discrimination:

- The SMD hires a younger physician instead of an older physician because the SMD, without evidence, believes that a younger physician will be faster than an older physician, although the older physician meets the essential job requirements. The practice could be sued for age discrimination.
- A scheduler decides that an older physician (older than 40 years) is not fit to work nights because he/she is "old" and takes the older physician off nights against her wishes.

The Occupational and Safety Health Act

The Occupational and Safety Health Act (OSHA) requires employers to provide workers a place of employment free from recognized hazards to safety and health, such as exposure to toxic chemicals, excessive noise levels, mechanical dangers, excessive heat or cold, or unsanitary conditions. This law also includes significant reporting requirements for work-related injuries.

The ED is a risky work environment, and it is important that both the provider and the employer follow the law. Consider this example:

- A provider accidentally experiences a needle stick while caring for a patient. The provider notifies the SMD, who reviews the patient's chart and finds no history of blood-borne illness. As a result, the SMD does not follow the proper reporting channels (notifying the practice or the employee health) and does not recommend prophylactic coverage. The provider eventually develops hepatitis C.

This would be a workmen's compensation and OSHA violation, which could result in a fine to the company. Most workplace safety programs are in place to ensure compliance with OSHA regulations, which translates to employee safety.

The Family Medical Leave Act

The Family Medical Leave Act (FMLA) is a federal law that allows eligible employees to take up to 12 weeks of unpaid leave for personal or family emergencies without job or benefit loss. The employee must be reinstated to the same or similar position with the same or similar pay, benefits, and terms and conditions of employment. The FMLA covers the categories listed in **Box 15.4**.

To qualify for FMLA, the employee must:

- Work a minimum of 1250 hours during the 12 months prior to the start of leave
- Work at a location in which 50 or more employees work at that location or within 75 miles
- Have worked for the employer for 12 months (not required to be consecutive)

BOX 15.4 ■ FMLA CATEGORIES

- Birth
- Adoption
- Foster care placement of child
- Leave for employee's illness
- Care for seriously ill member of employee's immediate family
  - Parent
  - Spouse
  - Child

It is not uncommon for a provider to start maternity leave prior to completing 12 months of work. Officially, FMLA would not apply to this employee, and she could be replaced. However, this might be a short-sighted decision by the SMD since the SMD recently made the decision to hire her. While the provider in this case might be out for 12 weeks while her job is held, technically she would be taking "a leave of absence" rather than "unpaid leave" under FMLA since she did not meet the FMLA requirements.

This is similar to the situation that many people experience who start a new job but miss a lot of work for illness early in their employment and as a result get fired. These new employees are not eligible for job protection under FMLA. To protect members of the military and their families, the original FMLA was later amended to include leave due to the requirements of active duty or the call to active duty status of a spouse, son, daughter, or parent. The FMLA now allows up to 26 weeks of job-protected leave in a single 12-month period to care for a covered service member with a serious injury or illness.

The Pregnancy Disability Act

The Pregnancy Disability Act says an employer cannot treat a woman differently just because she is pregnant. As an example, the SMD cannot use pregnancy as a reason to not hire someone. Further, a pregnant provider cannot have her job responsibilities changed without her consent. The SMD also cannot consider time off related to pregnancy in any performance evaluations.

Examples of violations of this law include:

- Reassigning a pregnant employee to a nonclinical project because the SMD thinks she "should not" be on her feet anymore.
- Mandating that FMLA begins at the 37th week of pregnancy in case the employee delivers early. (The SMD does not want to have to scramble for shift coverage at the last minute.)

The Americans With Disabilities Act and Amendment Act of 2008

The Americans With Disabilities Act and Amendment Act of 2008 is a federal law that protects employees from employment discrimination if they have:

- A physical or mental impairment that substantially limits one or more major life activities, major bodily functions, or physical activities
- A record of such an impairment or are regarded as having such an impairment

Examples of major life activities include the ability to care for oneself, seeing, hearing, eating, sleeping, walking, lifting, and communication. Bodily function disabilities include functions of the immune, digestive, or respiratory system. Physical impairments include conditions that require use of a wheelchair or conditions that may not be readily apparent such as insulin-dependent diabetes. An impairment that is "episodic or in remission" is a disability even when inactive "if it would substantially limit a major life activity when active." Examples may include cancer, epilepsy, and post-traumatic stress disorder.

In order to be covered under this program, the individual must be qualified to perform the essential functions of the job, with or without reasonable accommodation, such as installing a ramp or adjusting a computer desk to accommodate an employee in a wheelchair.

Get HR Help

Many SMDs spend a lot of time on HR issues that may require a significant amount of expertise to safely navigate. It is recommended that SMDs regularly communicate with or get a consult from the institution's HR professional before acting to limit a provider's (or potential provider's) activities or responsibilities.

Often a quick phone call or an e-mail will either confirm the SMD is on the right path or the projected course requires a correction. If a situation seems difficult, there is probably a reason to get help. And every time someone uses one of the big buzz words, such as hostile work environment, harassment, bullying, disability, family medical issues, or pregnancy, get your HR professional involved.

Practical Management Issues

There are practical issues SMDs should address with employees. Most SMDs at some point will encounter a provider who regularly shows up late, performs well below the productivity of the group, does not complete charts in a timely basis, or does not comply with a hospital directive—for instance, transfer all ST-elevation myocardial infarctions to the partner hospital or refer patients only to our approved list of primary care providers. While there are several approaches to correcting this, the first step is to recognize that there is a problem and that you, as the SMD, have responsibility for fixing it.

It is possible to divide corrective actions into four phases, ranging from a group communication to putting an employee on a performance improvement plan (PIP) with noncompliance leading to termination. An infraction like admitting the patient to the wrong physician or forgetting to call the house officer for an admission could result in a dual response, such as a general e-mail reminder to the group and a direct conversation with the provider to ensure that the issue is well understood.

Cup-of-Coffee Conversation

This somewhat casual, and generally brief, conversation with the involved provider might be considered a "cup-of-coffee conversation." The conversation could cover the "why" of proper communication and its importance as it relates to patient care. It should be explained that by not properly communicating and "closing the loop," in addition to causing frustration for our inpatient colleagues, there can be delays in orders and delays in patient care that can lead to poorer outcomes as well as increased patient discomfort and pain.

This "coffee talk" is designed to be less formal and intimidating than meeting with someone in the SMD's office while still giving the time needed to discuss the issue. For example, the conversation could address a repeat mistake or a minor behavioral issue leading to a nursing complaint. None of these first examples necessarily requires a note in a provider's HR file.

More Serious Issues

As the significance of these issues increases or the provider's response is determined to be inadequate, the formality and tone of the meeting must escalate.

The SMD should hold these meetings in his or her office and send a request to meet to the provider, such as "I want to meet with you regarding . . ." or providing the clinician with a specific date and time to meet. If the latter, it typically occurs on a nonclinical day to avoid having the provider start a shift after receiving negative feedback that could impact the provider's job performance.

For these types of meetings, documentation in the HR file is appropriate. That documentation should be consistent with the institution's quality process in a way that limits discoverability. It should be sent to the HR person and include:

- Date and time of the meeting
- Subject(s) discussed in detail
- Any action and follow-up plans

Performance Improvement Plans

Placing a physician on a PIP in many systems can be the final warning with a clear message that recurrence or a failure to improve will result in job termination. A PIP is a written document that outlines the following:

- Performance issues at hand
- Specific corrective actions that are required
- Target end points needed to be successful
- Time frame (which may range from immediate to several months)
- Specific description that failure to achieve described thresholds will result in a consequence (typically termination)

Termination

Terminating a physician "for-cause" requires data-bank notification. As a result, for-cause terminations are uncommon. If the provider reaches the PIP time limit without improvement, and if termination seems inevitable, a conversation can be held with the employee to recommend resigning rather than initiating a "for-cause" termination that may make getting credentialed at another site difficult. The National Practitioner Data Bank (NPDB), managed by the US Department of Health and Human Services, is a web-based repository of information that collects, stores, and distributes information regarding malpractice payments, credentialing and privileging issues, and terminations. Hospitals have reporting regulations to follow and rely on the NPDB as part of the credentialing process.

Case example 1: Untimely completion of charts: It is common to find a provider who regularly falls behind on completion of charting. This deficiency impacts the billing and the revenue cycle of both the group and the hospital. Electronic medical record (EMR) data management generally generates reports (available to directors) that show which providers have issues with chart completion.

This problem typically reaches the attention of the SMD when they start getting e-mails from the hospital medical records department, the Chief Financial Officer, or the Chief Information Officer. The first step may be a phone call to the provider requesting his or her urgent attention to the matter, but because of the potential consequences to the hospital as well as the group finances, the SMD must hold the provider accountable. If the provider continues to fall behind, the next step may require a PIP mandating that the provider meet a defined standard, such as 98% chart completion within 1 week of patient management.

Case example 2: Referral to a nonpartner hospital: Hospital systems benefit from referrals from other hospitals in the system. The system CEO is usually aware of every patient being transferred to system and nonsystem hospitals. As a result, hospital leadership will generally react negatively to inappropriate transfers to an outside-the-system hospital, occurring when a practitioner does not follow the hospital rules. While one mistake may be explainable, multiple transfer errors will be perceived as a provider who does not align goals with those of the institution.

This problem, once recognized, requires an urgent meeting with clinician explaining why the hospital wants patients to stay within the system. There are numerous examples in which providers perceived to demonstrate misalignment with the institution's appropriate goals have been removed from the ED staff, and contracts have been lost over this issue. This problem requires aggressive action.

Case example 3: Recurring arguments with hospitalists: ED providers and hospitalists disagree from time to time. However, when a single provider in the group is constantly battling with the hospitalists and telling the SMD about another fight he or she had, the SMD will likely have to address a clinician issue.

This behavioral issue requires provider feedback and may be a great opportunity to discuss more productive communications. While receptive providers may respond to a cup of coffee conversation, often this communication requires mentoring, coaching, and case reviews over a period of time.

Nursing Collaboration

SMD collaboration with nursing is an essential component of ED team effectiveness. To address the challenges of the ED, the SMD must be able to work with the ED nursing leader in a mutually respectful way. If their goals are aligned, a plan can be implemented enabling the physician and nursing leaders can achieve their goals.

Physicians and nurses rely on each other in the clinical area and in the administrative world as well. Like any relationship, the relationship between the SMD and nursing director develops over time and relies on trust and communication. The SMD and nursing director will usually have regular meetings (often weekly) and then touch base throughout the day and week as needed.

Many SMDs will sit with their nursing directors for at least a few minutes a day and additionally text and talk throughout the day, filling each other in on issues and other meetings. The more formal weekly meetings are used for more in-depth discussions and big picture planning.

The SMD and nursing leader should jointly create targets and priorities for the department that are aligned with institutional goals. By working together on this list, the 2 leaders can strategize about how each team (physician and nursing) can collaborate to help each other accomplish their objectives. It is important to present a unified front to the executive suite and to the staff. While disagreements may occur in private, they should never be voiced in public. This is accomplished through having shared priorities and similar messaging. Both the hospital executive team and the staff will feel better knowing their ED leadership team is working together. A best practice could include the physician and nurse directors together preparing for a meeting with any of the C-suite members—CEO, Chief Nursing Officer (CNO), Chief Medical Officer (CMO), and so on—and then debriefing after the meeting.

Trust is critical when discussing issues related to individual and groups of physicians and nurses. Each leader may become aware of problems related to the other leader's team. The relationship must allow for direct and honest discussion, and the two leaders need to trust each other to deal with the problems brought to them about their respective employees.

Many SMDs have been fortunate to have had excellent relationships with their nursing directors. Others have been unable to establish an effective and trusting partner relationship with their counterparts, resulting in a dysfunctional ED and often ending with one of the leaders being replaced.

Governance

There are several employment and governance models used by ED groups. There are several variations based on who employs or engages the providers:

- Hospital employs providers
- Hospital contracts a group that employs providers
- Hospital contracts group that engages providers as independent contractors (ICs)

In addition to the method of engagement, the group's governance may range in decision-making by utilizing a democratic approach, single owner group (autocratic), or decision-making by a board or leadership team.

Employee Versus Independent Contractor

Employees are typically contracted to a set number of hours within a given time period (usually monthly, quarterly, or annually) and receive a variety of benefits. Working over the hourly commitment may result in overtime pay rates (despite being an exempt employee) or additional vacation (paid time off [PTO]).

Independent contractors (ICs) usually agree to work a fixed number of hours for a time period, getting paid a higher hourly rate in return for having to purchase their own benefits except malpractice coverage (usually purchased by the group). The IC model typically offers flexibility to both the practitioner and the staffing group.

Because the tax implications differ between the two, it is wise to consult a tax professional. Most who have worked in both models have been equally content.

Decision-Making

The most important governance issue for most providers relates to how decisions are made. For example, financial decisions such as paying a stipend for nights, adding extra coverage, or changing the benefits package may be made by the owner, partners, local group, or regional leadership. All of these decisions have financial implications to the bottom line. Ultimately, regardless of the employment model, the SMD will be intimately involved in weighing the pros and cons of the impact on the providers, patients, flow, and finances. Often, the SMD must be the voice of reason and speak up against a hospital administration, a democratic group, or a CMO, that may be too focused on the bottom line. On the other hand, the SMD must be able to recognize that an added expense may not improve ED performance or provider satisfaction.

Managing the Finances

The sophisticated SMD understands that medicine is a business and that businesses accrue revenues and expenses.

Revenue and Expenses

Each patient visit will ultimately result in a bill to the patient. Depending on the ED patient acuity and payer mix (percentage of patients self-pay versus insured, and the type of insurance they may have), reimbursement for services will be defined by the contracted rate with the insurance companies plus the patient co-pay or totally from the patient (if uninsured). While physician charges to the patient may be in the $400 to $600 range, the typical collection will average between $100 and $200 per patient. The total collections plus any stipends define the revenue.

Profit then is achieved by deducting expenses from total revenues. Expenses include:

- Provider payroll (including salaries, benefits, such as insurance, CME, PTO for physicians and APCs)
- Coding and billing costs
- Malpractice insurance
- Administrative overhead and support (scribes, office space, chart coordinators, and so on)
- Administrative salaries (including the SMD and other stipends within the group)
- Legal and accounting costs
- Recruiting expenses
- Other expenses

Other expenses, such as a provider in triage, may not generate revenue but be advantageous by making the other providers more efficient. Increased efficiency may lead to higher productivity for the provider.

When profit (revenue greater than expenses) is realized, it can be:

- Distributed among partners in a privately held group
- Spread across to other physician specialties or the hospital's bottom line if a hospital employee
- Invested back into the company or group to fund a new position
- Used to repay a start-up loan

Unprofitable EDs and Subsidies

Some EDs are not profitable due to poor payer mix, low volume, or operational inefficiency. In these circumstances, it might be advisable for the physician group to negotiate a subsidy from the hospital to help balance the books. A subsidy may be a fixed financial arrangement between the hospital and the provider's contracting company to ensure that the company can provide the required ED services. Alternatively, the subsidy might have a flexible stipend with increased payments for achieving specific metrics (for patient experience, operational efficiency, productivity, and others.).

The hospital might consider paying a subsidy if the:

- Is unable to manage the ED without the services of the contracted group
- Recognizes the benefits the ED management group will bring
- Understands that volume and patient acuity (payer mix) are low and generate inadequate revenues to pay market salaries

Subsidies have become less common over the years as hospitals have increasingly shifted the ED financial responsibility to management companies. Additionally, contracts are frequently written with decreasing subsidies over time. As mentioned, subsidies are also attached to achieved metrics.

Hospitals have also recognized that many ED practices are quite profitable while the hospitalist program usually requires a significant subsidy. As more contracted groups provide hospitalist services, hospitals have bundled the ED and hospitalist contracts together, forcing the ED management group to subsidize the hospitalist program with its own profits rather than hospital monies.

Administrative Salaries

An important component of the overall financial budget is how the administrative salaries are paid. This may include the salaries of the SMD, assistant directors, and other paid positions (e.g., emergency medical services, stroke and education directors, physician scheduler, and so on). Stipends are often used in an effort to retain talent, provide professional growth opportunities, and get providers involved. All administrative stipends are expenses against revenues that may otherwise get distributed to the physicians in salary increases or bonuses. There is not a single approach to subsidies, salaries, and positions since the specific needs of the group and hospital will vary based on size and complexity.

However, there is a general market rate so that an SMD or assistant SMD may have a sense of what their responsibilities (clinical and administrative) and associated annual income should be. The SMD and other ED leadership team members must have appropriate time and financial incentive to be available, successful at the job, and interested in continuing to contribute to the ED (rather than looking for their next job).

Managing the Metrics

There is hardly a click that occurs in the EMR that does not have an associated time stamp. Add to this both the dramatic rise in publicly reportable metrics and the increased focus on payments for demonstrated outcomes, and it becomes clear that the pressure to manage the metrics is only growing. The SMDs may be challenged to balance their focus on the regularly changing publicly reportable metrics as well as the key metrics that allow them to review operational efficiency.

Sophisticated SMDs know that one of the keys to their success is to make their boss, the CEO, look good. The SMDs do that by achieving success in the areas that matter most to him or her. Executive teams typically use a red-yellow-green dashboard to show at a glance the key metrics throughout the hospital. While green is at or better than goal, yellow might be near goal, and red is clearly not achieving the goal. The SMD can feel a lot better about his or her department and job stability when the ED dashboard is all (or mostly) green at the Medical Executive Committee meeting or meeting with the CEO. The CEO will usually have goals established by the hospital board and hold the SMD accountable for those goals related to the ED. It is typical for the CEO to ask the SMD to achieve several goals. However, there are usually several processes, or components, that must be addressed by the SMD (along with the nursing director) to accomplish each of the goals.

For example, the CEO may want a particular length-of-stay goal for patients who are discharged from the ED. To address that metric, the SMD and operations improvement team will have to understand each step of, and bottlenecks related to, the care processes, including:

- The front end (comprising all door-to-provider processes: door-to-triage, triage-to-bed, bed-to-provider)
- Provider evaluation to disposition decision (all evaluation and management processes)
- Back-end process (disposition decision to actual movement out the door, including patients admitted)

Furthermore, because metrics are based on 24/7 data, the SMD may need to review metrics by hour of the day and by day of the week. Operational adjustments based on the data will be different for each phase of patient care and, perhaps, different for various shifts and days of the week.

Managing the metrics also requires providing regular and specific feedback to the providers. Sharing key performance indicators (KPIs) in a daily dashboard or table format is a great way to keep providers (and nursing staff) aware of the ED's focus areas. The dashboard can be e-mailed out daily or posted in a high traffic staff area. It is important for everyone to understand the goals and current progress toward achieving them.

Many SMDs have a portion of their compensation tied to performance, often ranging from 10% to 25% of their total compensation. Selecting several categories that align the SMD job responsibilities with the institution's KPIs is an effective way to develop bonus criteria. As examples:

- Recruitment and retention of providers (e.g., 90% staffing with full-time providers)
- Left Prior to Medical Screening Exam with a number, perhaps 50% of the current percentage
- Door-to-provider time
- Provider-related Patient Experience of Care survey percentile

Bonuses can be further divided into tiers of achievement that include partial payment for a lower level of achievement, increased payment for moderate improvement, and a full bonus for reaching the goal.

It is common for leaders to focus on what they are incentivized to achieve, so while SMDs may not be able to accomplish "everything," human nature may lead to SMDs choosing to focus on the goals with the biggest potential for payout.

Having described "human nature," it is important to remember that it is not all about the money. A CEO once said, "My decisions always put the patient and hospital first even if it was not in the best interest of my bonus."

This concept should resonate with all SMDs because occasionally there is a conflict between the right decision for the department (patients and staff) and our own personal financial opportunity. As an example, a medical director might be incentivized to reduce staffing while simultaneously recognizing that such a cut might create unsafe clinical conditions.

Managing the Future

Leadership development and succession planning are key responsibilities of the SMD in order to address the potential for future leadership changes. For all groups, the contractual relationship is at high risk when there is a change in the SMD position. While this risk is high when the SMD is retiring, the risk may be particularly acute if the hospital leadership is asking for a change in the ED leadership.

Another time of uncertainty and possible contract loss occurs when there is a change in the hospital leadership team (most notably the CEO, CMO, or CNO). It has long been recognized in business that developing leaders to seamlessly replace those who leave is essential. In health care, this "obvious" contingency planning is often overlooked. It is a best practice for EDs to develop leaders and create a succession plan with the next leader in mind. The current SMD should plan for a future in which he or she is no longer present. A fruitful succession plan requires leaders to provide growth opportunities, delegate responsibility, offer mentorship, ensure accountability, and publicly praise success.

CONCLUSION

Successful leadership requires a skill set that is not acquired during medical school or residency. However, it can be learned through a purposeful process of observation, reading and self-study, class work, on-the-job-training, and, most important, mentored opportunity. The role of an SMD can be challenging, rewarding, and frustrating, sometimes all in the same day. The most effective leaders rely on communication, teamwork, and collaboration.

REFERENCES

1. Stefl ME. Common competencies for all healthcare managers: the Healthcare Leadership Alliance model. *J Healthc Manag.* 2008;53(6);360-373.
2. Goleman, D. *Emotional Intelligence: Why It Can Matter More Than IQ.* New York, NY: Bantam Publishing; 1995.
3. Sutton RI. *The No Asshole Rule.* New York, NY: Business Plus; 2007.
4. Silverman MA. *Director's Corner: Lessons in Emergency Medicine Leadership and Management.* Galesville, Md: Plaster Publishing; 2014.

CHAPTER 16

WOMEN IN EMERGENCY MEDICINE LEADERSHIP

Andrea Austin, Valerie Dobiesz, Resa E. Lewiss, Rebecca Bollinger Parker, Tracy Sanson, Aisha T. Terry

Each time a woman stands up for herself, without knowing it possibly, without claiming it, she stands up for all women.

—Maya Angelou

Despite widespread conversation about inequity, there continues to be a pronounced leadership gap for women in emergency medicine. Many of the challenges faced by emergency departments (EDs), such as pay inequity and sexual harassment, might be more readily addressed if women were better represented in positions of leadership. Supporting and developing women in their careers improves the working environment for all. Interviews, chapters, articles, and focus and working groups by and about women in medicine describe how they've felt tokenized, abused, and discriminated against. It is time to take immediate, concrete action to address obstacles facing women emergency physicians.

BARRIERS AND MICROAGGRESSIONS

There are a multitude of reasons women lag in senior leadership positions and have not kept pace with the number of women entering medicine. Fundamentally, it is thought to be due to the overarching issues related to a "glass ceiling" as well as a " leaky pipeline."[1]

Barriers

The glass ceiling refers to a multitude of invisible barriers women face related to institutional culture as well as deeply embedded unconscious gender-based biases, stereotypes, and accompanying assumptions that impede career advancement.[1,2] The leaky pipeline refers to the loss of women faculty along the advancement pathway from challenges with work–life integration to a lack of leadership development and sponsorship for women among other factors.

Both the glass ceiling and leaky pipeline act as barriers to advancement and are integral in understanding the current paucity of women in leadership roles. Efforts to address these obstacles must include efforts to address institutional, structural, and individual frameworks that act as impediments to advancement. These barriers are often subtle and unintentional but are nonetheless pervasive, insidious, and cumulative in constraining women from advancing in leadership within medicine.

Research has also documented subtle but significant gender differences in the evaluations of male and female medical students and residents in written evaluations at important career stages. Stereotype-based cognitive bias may manifest as:

- Overt gender bias, such as the belief that women are less committed to their careers than men

- Implicit bias, which is much more elusive since there is a lack of awareness of its existence and it may be counter to personal beliefs (self-image), yet still influence decisions and perceptions[2]

Other barriers described are that women are "less apt to see themselves as qualified for top positions" despite having the same training and credentials as their male counterparts. Those leaving academia in the leaky pipeline report fewer role models combining careers and parenting, a lack of collaborative work cultures, and a lack of support in building professional networks.[3,4] Several studies have also described high work–family conflict, gender discrimination, lack of mentorship, greater interest in teaching over research, and a failure to advance or be promoted to a leadership role.[5-7] Well-documented gender disparities exist in academic rank and salary in full-time US academic emergency medicine faculty which may also impact retention of female faculty.[7] Women earned less than men when controlled for rank, clinical hours, and level of training.[7]

Microaggressions

The term *microaggression* was originally coined by Chester M. Pierce, a Harvard University psychiatrist, to describe daily insults and dismissals that he witnessed inflicted on African Americans in the 1970s.[8] The conceptual framework of microaggressions was later broadened to other groups and defined as "brief and common verbal, behavioral, or environmental indignities, whether international or unintentional, which communicate hostile, derogatory or negative slights, invalidations, and insults to an individual or group because of their marginalized status in society."[8] These microaggressions can be based on gender, race/ethnicity, sexuality or sexual orientation, intersectionality, among others. Microaggressions are thought to be a major contributing factor to the persistent disparities women, as well as underrepresented in medicine faculty, face in advancing to senior leadership positions in medicine.

There are multiple forms and degrees of microaggressions that women may face including sexual objectification, second class citizenship, sexist language, assumption of inferiority, restrictive gender roles, denial of the reality of sexism, denial of individual sexism, invisibility, sexist humor/jokes, and environmental invalidations (e.g., unequal pay, glass ceiling, media images). Women may also face additional negative impacts with intersectionality with membership in other marginalized groups. Gender-based microaggressions manifest in a multitude of ways not only inequities in pay, promotion, and advancement but can also have negative impacts on physical and mental health. It is well-documented that there are gender disparities for women in medicine in academic rank, wages (salary and bonuses), resource allocation, and leadership positions not explained by differences in productivity or attrition from the workforce.[9-18] Common microaggressions encountered by women emergency physicians were described in a recent commentary as patients asking "When will I see the doctor? "Are you the nurse?" when in the caring for patients.[19] Another example of a microaggression in academic medicine recently reported is that women are less likely to be introduced by their professional titles compared with men at grand rounds.[20]

The sexual harassment of women in academic medicine remains prevalent according to the National Academies of Sciences Engineering and Medicine (NASEM) report in 2018, with half of all medical trainees reporting sexual harassment from faculty or staff.[21] Academic medicine has a prevalence of sexual harassment almost double other science and engineering specialties.[21] What is striking, but not unexpected due to the power dynamics and workplace culture, is that according to the AAMC's 2017 Medical School Graduation Questionnaire, only 21% of medical students who experienced harassment reported the incident citing the following reasons: "I didn't think anything would be done about it" (37%),

"The incident did not seem important enough to report" (57%), "fear of reprisal" (28%), and "I did not know what to do" (9%).[22]

The NASEM report describes sexual harassment as a "chronic debilitating disease" in medicine with a need to address prevention measures. According to NASEM, "the cumulative effect of sexual harassment is a significant and costly loss of talent in academic science, engineering, and medicine, which has consequences for advancing the nation's economic and social well-being and its overall public health."

Microaggressions occurring in medicine may be overt and obvious but more often are more subtle prejudices and unconscious biases that are either not recognized or addressed but nonetheless are present and harmful. These microaggressions may be brief, everyday occurrences that may be unintentional or unnoticed by the perpetrator when they occur. They may seem benign or innocuous to the aggressor, however, to the person from a marginalized group, these behaviors have a powerful cumulative negative effect on stress levels and mental health.[9] Over time these occurrences are perceived as discrimination and can result in decreased motivation, job dissatisfaction, burnout, increased stress, poor performance, decreased self-confidence, and well-being that may contribute to women leaving academia. This attrition of women faculty due to the cumulative effect of microaggressions only serves to exacerbate gender disparities in leadership as talented qualified women leave.

There may be other unintended negative consequences of microaggressions in the workplace on witnesses, who if incidences are left unacknowledged, may perceive these behaviors as institutionally condoned and socially accepted behaviors. Witnesses may recognize these behaviors as microaggressions but may feel pressure due to social norms to refrain from addressing them and learn that these are expected and tolerated behaviors. When microaggressions are allowed to go unchecked, this creates hostile work environment for marginalized groups.

A study involving medical school faculty found six types of workplace gender-based microaggressions were common: encountering sexism, sexually inappropriate comments, pregnancy and childcare bias, having their abilities underestimated, being relegated to mundane tasks, and feeling excluded and marginalized.[9] This study found significant gender differences in perceptions of prevalence of microaggressions, with women reporting workplace microaggressions as highly prevalent whereas men in the same settings found them to be uncommon (**Box 16.1**). This clearly demonstrates that privilege is not apparent to those that have it; however, bias and discrimination are readily apparent to those that experience them.[9]

What can be done in emergency medicine to address microaggressions which may be a key contributing factor in the persistent lack of advancement for women physicians? Fundamentally, there must be individual, interpersonal, institutional, and structural

---

BOX 16.1 ■ EXAMPLE OF UNCONSCIOUS OR IMPLICIT BIAS: MEDICAL STUDENTS AND RECOMMENDATIONS

"In 2017, after a panel discussion on diversity and inclusion, two medical students approached me who were working hard to match into emergency medicine. They had done an away rotation at a prominent academic emergency department in hopes of garnering strong recommendations. Toward the end of their month, one of the senior male faculty members invited all the male students to a social event involving sports and did not invite the female students. They felt very uncomfortable and were concerned that the male students, through the benefits of social interaction, would receive much stronger recommendations. They also felt they did not have the power to attend the event if they were not invited."

targeted changes beginning with an awareness that microaggressions exist and have negative unintended impacts on the advancement of women. The perpetrators of these microaggression may be well intentioned but unaware of the potential impact of their words or behaviors. We must all develop an awareness of our own biases, prejudices, and stereotypes in order to become allies and advocates for change in order to mitigate disparities in medicine and for all faculty to thrive.

Bias-prevention training and coaching targeting individuals and institutions is essential. Creating environments that are collegial and respectful of all physician while enabling anonymous pathways for reporting these behaviors, acting on them expeditiously, and establishing a zero-tolerance policy are needed. Specific sensitivity training is recommended for all physicians at all levels in identifying and addressing microaggressions when they occur real time in the workplace. Fundamentally, an organization must truly value and actively promote a culture of equity, parity, safety, and respect for all physicians in order to mitigate microaggressions that are prevalent in medicine and remain significant barriers to the advancement of women in leadership.

HIRING, RETAINING, AND PROMOTING WOMEN OF COLOR

An underrepresented person is defined as one whose percent representation within a particular group is less than their percentage of the general population. Historically, underrepresented minorities in medicine have consisted of African Americans, Mexican Americans, Native Americans (American Indians, Native Alaskans, and Native Hawaiians), and mainland Puerto Ricans.[23] Following the 2003 Supreme Court case Grutter versus Bollinger which debated the constitutionality of affirmative action, however, many would argue that there was a movement to be mindful of the inaccurate use of the word "minority" in certain contexts given that it is typically relative and sometimes based on self-perception.

The use of "underrepresented" to describe a paucity of diversity is therefore often preferred. The sentiment of such language should be applied to the recruitment and retention of people of color within medicine and health-care leadership. While the objective percentage of people present in a group relative to the general population should be considered, understanding how well or poorly represented their voices are in terms of bringing diversity to and being included in that group should also be made paramount. To that end, while women have surpassed men in terms of medical school applications, overall, women of color still lag behind men of color in terms of active practice of medicine for all underrepresented groups except for African Americans. Further, among younger cohorts (34 years and younger) of physicians, women outnumber men in most racial and ethnic groups yet are underrepresented in leadership roles and faculty promotion.[23]

Given the professional strides that are being made by women, it is especially important that health care administrators within emergency medicine and otherwise understand why recruiting and retaining underrepresented women physicians (URWPs) into leadership must remain a priority. Companies with an increased number of women on boards show a correlation with great ethical standards.[24] Additionally, one solution to persistent racial and socioeconomic disparities in medicine is to recruit more leaders in medicine that reflect the communities they serve. Studies have shown that racial congruence between patients and physicians is associated with longer visits, greater utilization of the health care system, and improved patient satisfaction. Language concordance between patients and physicians has also been associated with greater compliance with the prescribed plan.[25-27]

Further, it is vital that medicine is practiced with utmost competence to ensure the best outcomes and that leaders have excellent skills. There is a growing body of literature that supports that women physicians have equal to even better patient outcomes. Women physicians are more likely to care for patients with complex psychosocial issues and also other women.[28,29] Women patients who suffer a myocardial infarction were more likely to survive with a woman physician,[30,31] and hospital readmissions were lower among patients cared for by women hospitalists.[32] These improved outcomes are likely attributable to better communication and collaboration, both of which are integral to excellent leadership.

To hire, retain, and promote URWPs, ED administrators need a comprehensive and consistent approach. Hiring practices must be intentional about attracting a diverse applicant pool. Pipeline initiatives should reach out to high school students.[33] Additionally, selection committees should also represent a diverse set of demographic characteristics. While it should be mandatory for everyone to have implicit bias training, it is particularly critical for those involved with interviews, hiring, and selection to regularly undergo such training. Additionally, selection committee members must receive training on employment laws and specific site policies to avoid legal or ethical breaches with selections.

Faculty promotion and board-level positions have not significantly increased in the last 20 years. The US population is comprised of approximately 13% of African Americans, while only 4% of US medical school professors and only 5% of active physicians are Black.[23] Similarly, while 16% of the US population identifies as Hispanic, physicians identifying as Hispanic is only 4%.[34] The small numbers of URWPs in the workplace can lead to social isolation. Social isolation in the workplace is a large contributor to burnout and job dissatisfaction for URWPs.[33,35] The contributors to social isolation manifest in a myriad of ways.

Tokenism continues to be an issue, in which some efforts are made to recruit minorities to committees or positions, but there are no systemic changes made to facilitate inclusion and their success. Tokenism in its worse form occurs when organizations attempt to block accusations of discrimination while avoiding the underlying discrimination and biases within workplaces.[33] Underrepresented women physicians also face accusations that they were admitted to medical school or later positions via affirmative action.[33] This belief places a lot of pressure on URWPs to be "twice as good" to counteract the affirmative action myth. When a critical mass of URWPs is present in the workplace, tokenism and affirmative action-related myths are less likely to take hold within departments.

Along with social isolation, URWPs can face their work being devalued (**Box 16.2**).[33,35] It is important that when URWPs express interest or are recruited for diversity initiatives in their

---

BOX 16.2 ■ ADDRESSING UNCONSCIOUS OR IMPLICIT BIAS, ONE SOLUTION: AMPLIFYING COLLEAGUES

"During a formal board meeting, in a board with only 20% women, there was an ongoing discussion and brainstorming session regarding a crucial topic. One of the younger board members, a woman, proposed a very good idea. The group skimmed over it and continued discussions. The second or third comment, made by a male member, proposed the same idea which the board overwhelmingly agreed was a terrific idea. They did not recognize that the young woman physician had just proposed the exact idea. As a senior female leader, I stopped the conversation and pointed out that the original idea had been stated by this female board member. The group paused and, after some thought, agreed this was true. The individual thanked me later and greatly appreciated the support."

workplaces, that their time and efforts are recognized and compensated.[33,35] The expectation to be the subject matter expert for all diversity matters and be on all diversity-related committees, especially without proper compensation, can be a contributor to burnout.[35] Additionally, the type of academic and administrative projects they select may face increased scrutiny and be less valued.[33,35] For instance, a junior professor who is interested in community health outreach initiatives may have her work viewed as less academically rigorous and interesting compared to a colleague who chooses work in a traditionally valued area of study.

It is critical to acknowledge the intersectional experiences of URWPs. Intersectionality refers to the idea each person has a unique experience related to their socioeconomic, race, and gender identities.[36] This translates into URWPs experiencing both racism and sexism that greatly compound workplace dissatisfaction and burnout.

There continues to be extremely high rates of harassment in workplaces, with up to 50% of medical students experiencing sexual harassment.[21] Along with overt acts, microaggressions are equally important for leaders to address within their departments and organizations. Microaggressions are defined as indirect, subtle, or unintentional discrimination against members of a marginalized group.[37] Many that have experienced microaggressions describe it as "death by a thousand paper cuts," the idea that these seemingly small comments, even when unintentional, have a profound cumulative effect on URWPs.

Underrepresented women physicians are more likely to come from diverse socioeconomic backgrounds as well. Irrespective of marital status and earnings, mothers serve as the breadwinner in half of all American households with children under the age of 18. More than four in five (81.1%) Black women are breadwinners in their households, and the majority (60.9%) of Black women are raising their families alone. Approximately 67% of Native American mothers are breadwinners and those who are single double those who are married. Women of color are particularly more likely to find themselves balancing work and childcare alone.[38] Some URWPs may have less family financial resources and thus higher student debt loans and more financial obligations for family members. When debt levels exceeded $200,000, more emotional exhaustion was reported among women physicians, compared to men (60% vs 49.8%).[36] Especially within academic medicine, efforts to increase financial compensation or diversity income opportunities through community hospital partnerships may increase recruitment and retention of URWPs. The unique social and economic realities of women of color must be acknowledged and addressed through workplace regulations such as family and sick leave policies which systemically foster successful careers.

RETAINING AND PROMOTING WOMEN PHYSICIANS

We are optimistic that the disparities for women in medicine can be addressed and rectified. Lewiss et al, in a 2019 article for the *Journal of Women's Health*, outlined concrete steps to increase the retention and promotion of women physicians in academia.[39] Gender equity solutions that come from the top are more effective than those which place responsibility on women to do the work themselves.[40] As an example, The National Institutes of Health director, Francis Collins, states that he would no longer sit on all-male panels or "manels." Behaviors such as these may accelerate a culture shift at scientific and medical society conferences and raise awareness of the invisibility of women and underrepresented groups. Journal editorial boards should also make changes by inviting more women to join their ranks.

Institutional, hospital, and departmental leadership must step up and speak up, serve as allies, sponsor women, and select women to serve as chairpersons and deans. Institutions must critically and humbly review their promotion processes and promote the many qualified women to full professor. There must be a commitment to advancing the careers of women in STEMM by institutions of higher education and research. This scrutiny and intervention in promoting the advancement of women must be an early and continuous appraisal of policies and processes, as aggressions and inequities start in the early career and increase by mid-career.

Diversity, equity, and inclusion (DEI) training for all staff increases knowledge and raises awareness of issues faced by women physicians. There is some evidence to suggest that this training can change culture and may lead to a trend toward hiring more women faculty.[41,42] Prioritizing DEI work can be a first step toward transformative change. Focus groups and discussion spaces allow staff to express concerns and give leadership an opportunity to address questions and begin a dialogue.

The literature suggests that sponsorship rather than mentorship plays a more important role in promoting women to leadership because sponsors are positioned and have the power to advocate for advancement. In this way, men can make a difference in the career advancement of women.[43-45] A 2019 letter to the American College of Surgeons gave specific strategies on what it means to be a male ally. "To be genuine champions for women colleagues by leveraging power and influence to nominate women for leadership positions, awards, and speaking opportunities. One subtle yet important action that male allies can take is to credit women for their work and ideas, even in their absence. To implement meaningful change, male allies must not only be at the table creating policy change that addresses workforce disparities but must also be intentional in inviting women to the table, advocating for women colleagues, and fostering an environment that equitably supports all trainees, physicians, and scientists."[46]

We must also address some of the realities and false narratives that concentrate the power, status, and income primarily among the male physicians. Ely and Padavic, in a 2020 *Harvard Business Review* article, note "*why* women remain so dramatically underrepresented in promotions to positions of senior rank, is an unfortunate but inevitable 'truth'—that goes something like this:

> *High-level jobs require extremely long hours. Women's devotion to family makes it impossible for them to put in those hours, and their careers suffer as a result.*[47]

We call this explanation the work/family narrative, women were held back because, unlike men, they were encouraged to take accommodations, such as going part-time and shifting to internally facing roles, which derailed their careers."[47] The work/family narrative oversimplifies the cause and misses the fact that childless women bear the brunt of derailed careers, as well. This narrative is often echoed by leadership and the women ushered into noncareer advancing roles (**Box 16.3**).[48] It is time to assertively address personal biases about

BOX 16.3 ■ EXAMPLE OF IMPLICIT BIAS: PREGNANCY[48]

Dr. Hala Sabry, in an *ACEPNow* article from September 2016, described how she was overlooked for a leadership position in her department because of a pregnancy. The medical director assumed she would not be interested in the role with a new baby and was confused when she confronted him. In the end, the implicit bias shut down communication. Opening the dialogue also opened up opportunities for Dr. Sabry.

a parents' role at home and work, as well as the long-term career and income impact of parental accommodations. Action items for departmental and institutional leadership:

- Provide education on workforce gender disparities.
- Critically and regularly assess work environments in the ED, hospitals, institutions, business entities, and professional societies.
- Critically and regularly review assignments to ensure opportunities are equally career advancing for all employees.
- Actively include qualified women using data-driven best practices.
- Develop mentorship and sponsorship programs.
- Recruit male allies at all levels of leadership.
- Develop clear metrics and accountability mechanisms at all levels of the institution/business entity.
- Apply an intersectional approach to strategic plans.
- Improve human resources and employee experiences.

It isn't enough for institutions to advertise themselves as "equal opportunity employers." Leadership must be intentional and proactive in analyzing and updating the ED and institutional structures, policies, and practices. Leadership must reevaluate their efforts and share regular, transparent updates on the structures, policies, and practices that impact their employees and their careers. Leadership has the opportunity to evaluate their role in a system that blocks, diminishes, and negatively impacts women's advancement. It is time for leadership to listen, learn, and take action.

POLITICAL AND NATIONAL LEADERSHIP

The US Federal Glass Ceiling Commission defines the *glass ceiling* as "the unseen, yet unbreachable barrier that keeps minorities and women from rising to the upper rungs of the corporate ladder, regardless of their qualifications or achievements." As a complement, the *glass cliff* phenomenon speaks to how women are more likely than men to achieve leadership roles during periods of crisis or downturn, when the chance of failure is highest due to the circumstance of timing. Studies have also shown that women are more likely to occupy precarious leadership positions that are associated with a higher risk of failure, typically due to being appointed to lead during organizational crisis or because they are not provided with the resources and support needed for success.[49,50] The metaphor of the glass cliff refers to a danger which involves exposure to the risk of falling, which is not readily apparent. Evidence of this phenomenon has been documented in the fields of law, business, political science, and others.[51,52]

Historically, the field of medicine has also been affected by the *glass ceiling* and *glass cliff* phenomena. For women, while prudent to recognize the existence of these inconspicuous, potential barriers and hazards, it is also imperative to understand that many have previously managed to break through the *glass ceiling* and fly above the *glass cliff*, avoiding failure. One such woman was Harriot Kezia Hunt (**Figure 16.1**), a physician, who was a leading voice in the women's movement of the mid-19th century. In 1850, she attended the first National Woman's Rights Convention where she championed a woman's right to vote, earn income, and receive medical education in order to practice medicine. Against all odds, Dr. Hunt's tremendous work in part led to the opportunity for women to practice medicine today and be successful leaders.[53,54]

Over two centuries later, women physicians continue to break through *glass ceilings* and safely sojourn *glass cliffs*. In 2018, Dr. Kim Schrier became the first woman physician elected to serve as a voting member of the United States Congress. Dr. Schrier was a Democrat from

FIGURE 16.1 ■ Harriot Kezia Hunt, MD (1805-1875)

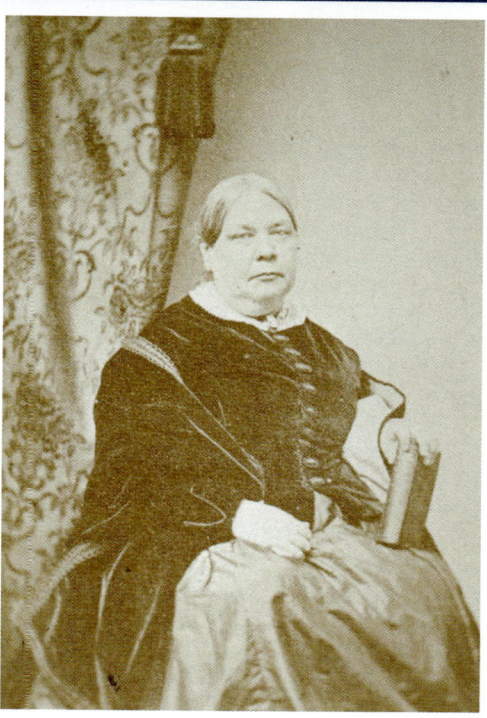

Sammamish who practiced pediatrics at a Virginia Mason Medical Center clinic. Having essentially no prior political experience, she ran in the midterm elections for the state of Washington's 8th Congressional District, a seat which had long been held by a Republican.[55] She went on to win the Democratic nomination and defeated Republican Dino Rossi by a 52.4% to 47.6% margin.

When Representative Schrier was asked why she decided to run for Congress, she responded that "when I saw some of the changes happening under the new administration—threats to the Affordable Care Act and protections for people with preexisting conditions, environmental hazards, threats to nutrition programs, and early childhood education—I just decided that maybe a better role for a person with type 1 diabetes who is also a pediatrician was to step up and represent the real needs of our district."[55] When Representative Schrier was asked about how her perspective as a woman physician differed from that of her male physician colleagues in Congress, she said, "there was a time when there really weren't women doctors. And I think it's made a huge difference for women to have somebody who really firsthand understands they're going to bat for women. I feel exactly the same way about Congress. If you really want a doctor who is going to put the interests of children and women at top of mind, it really helps to have a woman there. We know from the data that when women win, we talk about things like paid family leave and early childhood education and nutrition programs and what's really best for the families in this country. It's not that men don't get it. It's just that women get it on a different level."[55]

Representative Schrier's story of unprecedented leadership illustrates an important lesson; when one has the courage to get off the sidelines and instead be a part of creating the change that one wants to see, the possibilities are limitless, regardless of seen or unseen barriers and hazards.

The US population is about 51% women; approximately 45% of medical school students are women. Further, only 38% of emergency medicine residents are women. Within

> **BOX 16.4 ■ EXAMPLE OF IMPLICIT ORGANIZATIONAL BIAS: BREAKING THE GLASS CEILING**
>
> "I began as a business leader as a woman physician executive at the regional level after running a fantastic large ED, awarded by a prestigious hospital system as 'Emergency Department of the Year.' In my regional role I excelled at client relationships including the C-Suite, contracting, legal issues, managing P&L (profit and loss) and financial spreadsheets, recruiting, starting new businesses; all the parts of the business of medicine that result in a successful practice and highly impact the bottom line. I was complemented, given more responsibility and promoted. As I was promoted, I eventually advanced to duties across the whole enterprise but found myself asked to take on nonbusiness duties, for example, education and communications. When I requested to do more work related to finance and practice management, I was declined and told I was needed more for these other duties. I complied, being a servant leader, and taught others the business skills I knew. However, when president/CEO positions became available I was not fully qualified to apply nor in the position politically to pursue the top job. And when the company took a disastrous financial downturn, my position was the first to be eliminated."

emergency medicine's parent specialty organization, the American College of Emergency Physicians (ACEP), only 25% of active members are women.[56] Only 27% of ACEP's policy-making council is made up of women, and historically, ACEP's Board of Directors has been heavily male. In recent years, the composition of the ACEP board has been more diverse, however. In 2017 to 2018, in fact, five of the 15 ACEP Board members were women, making up one-third of this governing body.

Within emergency medicine, there is a plethora of outstanding groups and organizations such as ACEP's American Association of Women Emergency Physicians, the Society for Academic Emergency Medicine's Academy for Women in Academic Emergency Medicine, and open-access resources like Females Working in Emergency Medicine (FemInEM), which serves as a key facilitator by having created speakers' bureaus, idea exchange, pipeline initiatives, and community. Yet despite these resources and the data that show that women leaders are more than capable of leading with excellence, there is still disparity in female leader representation in the 21st century (**Box 16.4**). A minority of the numerous past presidents of emergency medicine specialty organizations, for example, have been female (**Table 16.1**). How do we close these gaps?

One way to address these issues is through organized initiatives that have systemic effects:

> *When one further considers that our nation has even more religious, cultural, sexual, gender identity, and other forms of diversity — far beyond the obvious visual distinctions — it is apparent that the magnitude of the opportunity for improvement is enormous.*[57]

The preceding quote is from the *Annals of Emergency Medicine* article, "Why Diversity and Inclusion Are Critical to the American College of Emergency Physicians' Future." This article and a 2016 Diversity Summit kicked off then-ACEP President Dr. Rebecca Parker's diversity and inclusion platform. Dr. Aisha Terry (formerly Liferidge) was appointed to lead those efforts, which sought to increase awareness, specify barriers, and identify solutions for enhancing diversity within ACEP and emergency medicine. The task force focused on identifying gaps through data collection, internal organizational reform, and increasing awareness about bias relative to clinical practice and workforce. Several products in perpetuity were born out of this initiative, including the creation of ACEP's Diversity, Inclusion, and Health Equity Section, the development and launch of an online course,

TABLE 16.1 ■ Past Female Presidents of EM Organizations

ACEP

- Nancy Auer (1997-1998)
- Angela Gardner (2006-2007)
- Linda Lawrence (2008-2009)
- Sandra Schneider (2009-2010)
- Rebecca Parker (2016-2017)

Society of Academic Emergency Medicine (SAEM)

- Mary Ann Cooper (1987-1988)
- Sandra Schneider (1999-2000)
- Katherine Heilpern (2008-2009)
- Jill Baren (2009-2010)
- Debra Houry (2011-2012)
- Cherri Hobgood (2012-2013)
- Deborah Diercks (2015-2016)
- Andra Blomkains (2016-2017)

American Academy of Emergency Medicine (AAEM)

- Lisa Moreno-Walton (2020-2022)

Emergency Medicine Residents' Association (EMRA)

- Jennifer Waxler (1993-1994)
- Maryanne W. Lindsay (1994-1995)
- Cherri Hobgood (1997-1998)
- Kristin Harkin (1998-1999)
- Melissa Graber (2000-2001)
- Angela Siler-Fisher (2002-2003)
- Comilla Sasson (2004-2005)
- Aisha Terry (Liferidge) (2006-2007)
- Jordan Celeste (2013-2014)
- Alicia Kurtz (2016-2017)
- Hannah Hughes (2019-2020)

"Implicit Bias in Clinical Practice: Protect Your Patients and Yourself," and the passage of two key resolutions during ACEP's 2019 Council meeting—one favoring pay transparency and another that outlined expectations around diversity and inclusion for emergency physicians and academicians.[58]

Policies such as these will be used to translate hopes for gender equity into concrete action which results in diversification of our workforce and ultimately improves the care we provide. ACEP's Diversity and Inclusion initiative sparked incremental change through organizational leadership, which then influences culture.

Individual leadership can also bring about big change. Big journeys of great impact often start with small, individual steps. Whether through political activism, elected political office, or organized medicine, female physician leaders possess the unique opportunity to use their broad perspective to influence various walks of life and impact the world. Successful leadership as a female physician requires intention, rather than passivity, in all you do:

- **Be intentional ... about everything.**
  - Be intentional about your visibility. This is important in terms of mentoring others because "you can't be what you can't see." It is also important to foster hope for others but showing them what change looks like.
  - Be intentional about getting the recognition you deserve. Humbly accept praise with no apology. Gracefully toot your own horn when deserved and no one else will.
  - Be intentional about forming a coalition. Surround yourself with a cohort of mentors, mentees, and supporters who share your mission and vision.
  - Be intentional about seeking frequent, constructive feedback. We will all forever continue to learn and grow.
  - Be intentional about checking yourself and your own biases. Practice what you preach; if you believe that diverse representation and perspectives yield better solutions, then there have to be more than just women at the table.
  - Be intentional about bringing someone along for the journey, to help them achieve their dreams. Don't break through the *glass ceiling* alone; make sure someone is on your heels as you soar to the top so that they, too, can break through a different section of the ceiling, and others should follow in succession; eventually, the entire ceiling will be obliterated.

Rise to the challenge of striving to make our specialty, our practice, and our world a more equitable place, in order to provide our diverse patient population with the most competent, minimally biased care that they need and deserve.

CONCLUSION

Over the last 50 years, women in medicine made tremendous strides; there is much work left to accomplish. The pipeline of women physicians is stronger than ever. In 1970 in the US women made up only 7.6% of physicians.[59] Starting in the medical school class matriculated in 1992, women made up 40% or more of US medical students in the United States. And for the first time in 2018, women made up the majority of matriculated US medical students.[60]

However, the emergency medicine workforce does not reflect these percentages yet in the attending staff or leadership positions. The most recently published data from the ACEP from 2016 demonstrate only 26% of active (attending) members were women, with the percentage of women in leadership positions decreasing with only 12.5% of national board members being women. As noted above, only five women served as ACEP president in the organization's more than 50-year history. As a result, ACEP instituted and continues to actively pursue diversity, inclusion and cultural sensitivity in its short- and long-term strategic plans and initiatives.[57]

Organizational Considerations

The first step to affect real and lasting change in any organization requires the full commitment of the organization itself and from its senior leaders, from both men and women. The majority, that is., non-Hispanic men, must be fully committed, engaged, and vocal supporters. Additionally, organizations should recognize the process is a multiyear, requiring strategic planning, resources, and intentional actions to advance and secure lasting change.

To prepare for the strategic planning, a good first step for any organization is to perform an environmental survey, gathering as much data as possible. Initially, the organization should turn inward, assessing data points such as the percentage of women physicians within their staff and throughout their leadership tracks. The organization should review common gender gaps such as tenure and promotion, current pay, interview process, succession planning, and policies regarding diversity and inclusion. Externally organizations should query like groups and organizations as well as medical organizations such as the Association of American Medical Colleges (AAMC), ACEP, and nonmedical resources such as the Stanford's Clayman Institute for Gender Studies and the Harvard Business Review for comparison data and best practices. The data and information will then formulate the organization's short-term, midterm, and long-term planning. Organizations should also plan periodical reassessments to confirm the effectiveness of planned programs and either further support or redirect efforts accordingly.

Common Best-Practice Interventions

Implicit bias, and the concepts surrounding its pervasive presence within our society and organization, is an excellent place to begin conversations around culture change within an organization.

Implicit (Unconscious) Bias Training

Common approaches include engaging the formal initiatives from AAMC or ACEP, Harvard Project Implicit program, or external formal education resources.[62] Many organizations invest in formal "train the trainer" programs who can then bring back key concepts for strategic planning and ongoing organizational education.

Understanding and addressing implicit bias then becomes a cornerstone, supporting other key organizational initiatives. Additionally, for clinicians, these concepts can be applied directly to clinical care, thus grounding the understanding and acceptance by physicians and other clinicians. Medicine inherently includes implicit biases that must be recognized and addressed to deliver high-quality care. The latter can also engage the health care system and emphasize the importance of addressing the implicit bias issue.

Hiring, Promotion, and Retention

As a part of their strategic plan, organizations and leaders should review and improve their approach to hiring, promotion, and retention.

Hiring: When filing a position, the job should be posted and clearly available for anyone to apply. Additionally, organizations should purposely look for candidates within their organization to encourage them to apply, including diverse, nontraditional candidates. The job itself should have clear criteria on duties, responsibilities, and qualifications available to applicants, interviewers, and selection committee. Best practice for interviews includes standardized questions and a panel of diverse interviewers who are blinded as much as possible to the gender and other nonrelevant applicant background to minimize bias. Selection should also be blinded as much as possible.

It is clear that gender bias in interviewing and selection exists. One set of studies showed that when interviewers are shown the same CV, one applicant name is male and the other female, all interviewers regardless of gender perceive the male applicant more qualified than the female applicant. This was true of ethnic named applicants as well.[63,64] Another study demonstrated how blind orchestral auditions, which included a visual barrier on stage and the removal of shoes by the auditionee, with interview panels, improved the percentage of female orchestral members from 6% to 21%.[65]

Organizations should also invest in developing a strong pipeline of applicants. Programs for women physician leaders should include typical professional development programs supplemented by programming specifically geared toward women. For example, women succeed more when they have the ability to network, participate in affinity groups and with a sponsorship program. They also succeed more when men participate as well. Examples of these type of programs include conferences focused on gender issues, regular affinity group meetings such as Lean In Circles, and formal sponsorship programs for women physicians.

Promotion: Organizational leaders and all physicians must be thoughtful and proactive on addressing common leadership culture behavior gaps related to gender.[66] For example, as women move up the leadership ladder, they often end up in positions, or performing duties, that do not impact the return on investment (ROI), for example, human resources, marketing, or education. Without a clear ROI, these positions do not prepare them to apply for the most senior levels of leadership such as an executive office or chair/dean position. Matching interest, skills, and pathways of advancement for women should be given careful consideration by leaders, mentors, sponsors, and women physicians themselves. Any role or project assumed should have a clearly described ROI, with numeric values attached when possible.

Additionally, women commonly say "yes" to less desirable projects that may be mission critical to the organization, but not held in high value. Later on, these women are not available for career-advancing opportunities because of prior commitments. Thus, women should carefully consider and prioritize each project based on ROI or the ability to describe the ROI, for the organization, impact on career advancement, or other prioritized reason.

Finally, all organizations should have a thoughtful and intentional succession planning processes, especially for senior leaders. It should be multiyear, with a longitudinal perspective of the needs of the organization and the potential candidates. Succession planning should also intentionally diversify the pool of candidates to ensure the most talented and diverse candidates advance to the next level.

Retention: Organization cultural best practices must include flexibility for women physicians. Women are usually the caretakers of their families carrying a disproportionate caretaker load in their personal lives. Additionally, those who have or adopt children have specific needs during that time of their life. Considerations include maternity leave, lactation support including at work, flexibility in schedule, and career path. Some organizations include a period of years of part-time leadership positions, so the woman physician has flexibility without exiting the leadership track. These factors should be considered for all physicians, as human beings, and plays heavily in increasing wellness and resiliency for physicians on the whole.

Leaders and colleagues should carefully monitor and address organizational cultural issues known to occur disproportionately to women. Examples include interruptions during meeting discourse, addressing women by their first name rather than professional names in formal settings, and not being recognized for contributed ideas. Simple approaches such as stopping interruptions, addressing all physicians the same, to processes such as amplification where members within the group acknowledge, vocally reinforce, and recognize a woman colleagues' idea, are great ways to start.[67]

Pay Gap

As outlined earlier in the chapter, a pay gap continues to exist for women physicians. In the referenced 2016 *JAMA* article, the investigators found that, after controlling for specialty, age, faculty rank, and metrics of clinical and research productivity, male physicians earned nearly $20,000 yearly more than female physicians. As female physicians advance in their careers, this pay discrepancy continues. Many theories have emerged regarding the reasons why such as negotiation skill, personal ambition choices, or implicit or explicit bias regarding women as people and professionals.[68]

Negotiation skills, the negative perception of woman negotiation styles, and employer approaches to negotiation are crucial. Clearly, a fair first negotiated salary is a cornerstone for the woman physician and her potential employer. Not only does it set the monetary stage for years to come, but also it establishes the ongoing relationship. For the woman applicant, common best practices include surveying the market for current salaries, asking for what you want, combating the imposter syndrome, and have a Plan B to fall back on to embolden negotiation skills are all effective.[69,70] Employers should recognize the negative perception people have when women negotiate for higher pay. Best practice for employers includes stop asking what applicants previously earned, set salaries based on the job itself and not the individual applicant, and consider sharing the salary range explaining final salary will be determined by the applicant's skills and experience.[71] Additionally, organizations should conduct internal reviews of salaries and benefits at regular intervals and make any corrections in identified discrepancies.

Post-COVID Considerations

At the time of this writing, the United States was immersed in the COVID pandemic, changing society forever. Shelter in place laws, working from home, and virtual meetings exacerbated many gender issues. For those women who are mothers, children at home and attempting homeschooling exacerbated the so-called "motherhood penalty." Employers should understand this impact and loss of social support for women and recognizing how this effect may promote implicit biases about women being inherently less competent or valuable. Decreasing the pressure and recognizing this delicate balance which women disproportionately carry is crucial as well. Be careful regarding virtual meetings and run them equitably, with inclusive intent. Leaders should broaden their virtual screens beyond their inner circle, to be sure to engage all team members. Be careful during virtual meetings to limit side conversations and private chats and invite each participant to contribute and participate. Be sure any teambuilding or social events include the entire team to foster connectivity and inclusiveness.[72]

Diversity and inclusion is a focus in the United States in medicine and business. The population of the United States is diversifying more than ever, with current minority groups expected to become the majority of the US population by 2044.[73] AAMC includes diversity, inclusion, and health equity as one of its four missions. ACEP and other specialties have included the topic in its short- and long-term strategic plans. Focusing on women in diversity and inclusion initiatives is a first common approach, allowing for other diverse groups to be included immediately, while setting a foundation to expand to other diverse groups in the future. In the end, all organizations want to recruit, retain, and promote the highest quality physicians. Diversity and Inclusion should be a cornerstone to any great organization, and especially to medicine and emergency medicine whose mission impacts the most diverse group of all: our patients.

REFERENCES

1. Surawicz CM, Women in leadership: why so few and what to do about it. *J Am Coll Radiol.* 2016;13(12 pt A):1433–1437.

2. Carnes M, Bartels CM, Kaatz A, et al. Why is John more likely to become department chair than Jennifer. *Trans Am Clin Climatol Assoc.* 2015;126:197–214.

3. Guptill M, Reibling ET, Clem K. Deciding to lead: a qualitative study of women leaders in emergency medicine. *Int J Emerg Med.* 2018;11:47.

4. Bickel J, Wara D, Atkinson B, et al. Increasing women's leadership in academic medicine: report of the AAMC Project Implementation Committee. *Acad Med.* 2002;77(10):1043–1061.

5. Westring A, McDonald JM, Carr P, et al. An integrated framework for gender equity in academic medicine. *Acad Med.* 2016;91:1041–1044.

6. Edmunds LD, Ovseiko PV, Shepperd S, et al. Why do women choose or reject careers in academic medicine? A narrative review of empirical evidence. *Lancet.* 2016;388(10062):2948–2958.

7. Madsen T, Linden J, Rounds K, et al. Current status of gender and racial/ethnic disparities among academic emergency medicine physicians. *Acad Emerg Med.* 2017;24(10):1182–1192.

8. Sue DW. *Microaggressions in Everyday Life: Race, Gender, and Sexual Orientation.* Wiley; 2010: xvi. ISBN 978-0-470-49140-9.

9. Periyakoil VJ, Chaudron L, Hill E, et al. Common types of gender-based microaggressions in medicine. *Acad Med.* 2020;3(95):450–457.

10. Tesch BJ, Wood HM, Helwig AL, et al. Promotion of women physicians in academic medicine. Glass ceiling or sticky floor? *JAMA.* 1995;273(13):1022–1025.

11. Sege R, Nykiel-Bub L, Selk S. Sex differences in institutional support for junior biomedical researchers. *JAMA.* 2015;314(11):1175–1177.

12. Blumenthal DM, Olenski AR, Yeh RW, et al. Sex differences in faculty rank among academic cardiologists in the United States. *Circulation.* 2017;135(6):506–517.

13. Jena AB, Khullar D, Ho O, et al. Sex differences in academic rank in US medical schools in 2014. *JAMA.* 2015;314(11):1149–1158.

14. Reed DA, Enders F, Lindor R, et al. Gender differences in academic productivity and leadership appointments of physicians throughout academic careers. *Acad Med.* 2011;86(1):43–47.

15. Jagsi R, Griffith KA, Stewart A, et al. Gender differences in the salaries of physician researchers. *JAMA.* 2012;307(22):2410–2417.

16. Jagsi R, Griffith KA, Stewart A, et al. Gender differences in salary in a recent cohort of early-career physician-researchers. *Acad Med.* 2013;88(11):1689–1699.

17. Carnes M, Bland C. Viewpoint: A challenge to academic health centers and the National Institutes of Health to prevent unintended gender bias in the selection of clinical and translational science award leaders. *Acad Med.* 2007;82(2):202–206.

18. Carr PL, Raj A, Kaplan SE, et al. Gender differences in academic medicine: retention, rank, and leadership comparisons from the National Faculty Survey. *Acad Med.* 2018;93(11):1694–1699.

19. Mannix R, Lee L. Doctoring while woman. *Acad Emer Med.* 2020;27(5):434–436.

20. Files JA, Mayer AP, Ko MG, et al. Speaker introductions at internal medicine grand rounds: forms of address reveal gender bias. *J Women's Health.* 2017;26(5):413–419.

21. The National Academies of Sciences Engineering Medicine Consensus Report. *Sexual Harassment of Women. Climate, Culture, and Consequences in Academic Sciences, Engineering, and Medicine.* Washington, DC: National Academies Press; 2018. Available at: https://www.nap.edu/catalog/24994/sexual-harassment-of-women-climate-culture-and-consequences-in-academic. Accessed August 8, 2020.

22. AAMC. 2017 Medical School Graduation Questionnaire. 2017. Available at: https://www.aamc.org/media/8746/download. Accessed August 8, 2020.

23. American Association of Medical Colleges. Available at: https://www.aamc.org/data-reports/workforce/interactive-data/figure-20-percentage-physicians-sex-and-race/ethnicity-2018. Accessed August 6, 2020.

24. Bernardi R, Bosco S, Columb V. Does female representation on boards of directors associate with the 'most ethical companies' list? *Corp Reput Rev.* 2009;12(3).

25. Oguz T. Is patient-provider racial concordance associated with Hispanics' satisfaction with health care? *Int J Environ Res Public Health.* 2018;16(1):31.

26. LaVeist TA, Nuru-Jeter A, Jones KE. The association of doctor-patient race concordance with health services utilization. *J Public Health Policy.* 2003;24(3-4):312–323.

27. Strumpf EC. Racial/ethnic disparities in primary care: the role of physician-patient concordance. *Med Care.* 2011;49(5):496–503.

28. McMurray JE, Linzer M, Konrad TR, et al. The work lives of women physicians results from the physician work life study: the SGIM Career Satisfaction Study Group. *J Gen Intern Med.* 2000;15(6):372–380.

29. Guarín-Nieto E, Krugman SD. Gender disparity in women's health training at a family medicine residency program. *Fam Med.* 2010;42(2):100–104.

30. Greenwood BN, Carnahan S, Huang L. Patient-physician gender concordance and increased mortality among female heart attack patients. *Proc Natl Acad Sci USA.* 2018;115(34):8569-8574.22.

31. Centers for Disease Control and Prevention. LowerYour Risk for the Number 1 Killer of Women. CDC Features. 2018. Available at: www.cdc.gov/features/wearred/index.html. Accessed January June 23, 2019.

32. Tsugawa Y, Jena AB, Figueroa JF, et al. Comparison of hospital mortality and readmission rates for Medicare patients treated by male vs female physicians. *JAMA Intern Med.* 2017;177(2):206–213.

33. Albert MA. #Me_Who anatomy of scholastic, leadership, and social isolation of underrepresented minority women in academic medicine. *Circulation.* 2018;138(5):451–454.

34. American Association of Medical Colleges, ed. Diversity in medical education: facts and figures 2016. 2016. Available at: http://www.aamcdiversityfactsandfigures2016.org/. Accessed August 2, 2017.

35. Blackstock U. Why Black doctors like me are leaving faculty positions in academic medical centers. Available at: https://www.statnews.com/2020/01/16/black-doctors-leaving-faculty-positions-academic-medical-centers-comment-page-3/. Accessed March 22, 2020.

36. Silver JK, Bean AC, Slocum C, et al. Physician workforce disparities and patient care: a narrative review. *Health Equity.* 2019;3(1):360–377.

37. Sue DW, Alsaidi S, Awad MN, et al. Disarming racial microaggressions: microintervention strategies for targets, White allies, and bystanders. *Am Psychol.* 2019;74(1):128–142.

38. Institute for Women's Policy Research. Quick Facts. 2016. Available at: https://iwpr.org/wp-content/uploads/wpallimport/files/iwpr-export/publications/Q054.pdf. Accessed August 5, 2020.

39. Lewiss RE, Silver JE, Bernstein CA, et al. Is academic medicine making mid-career women physicians invisible? *J Women's Health.* 2019;00(00).

40. Laver KE, Prichard IJ, Cations M, et al. A systematic review of interventions to support the careers of women in academic medicine and other disciplines. *BMJ Open.* 2018;8:e020380.

41. Carnes M, Devine PG, Baier Manwell L, et al. The effect of an intervention to break the gender bias habit for faculty at one institution: a cluster randomized, controlled trial. *Acad Med.* 2015;90(2):221–230.

42. Devine PG, Forscher PS, Cox WTL, et al. A gender bias habit-breaking intervention led to increased hiring of female faculty in STEMM departments. *J Exp Soc Psychol*. 2017;73:211–215.
43. Ibarra H, Carter NM, Silva C. Why men still get more promotions than women. *Harvard Business Review*. 2010. Available at: https://hbr.org/2010/09/why-men-still-get-more-promotions-than-women. Accessed July 01, 2020.
44. Travis EL, Doty L, Helitzer DL. Sponsorship: a path to the academic medicine C-suite for women faculty? *Acad Med*. 2013;88(10):1414–1417.
45. Ayyala MS, Skarupski K, Bodurtha JN, et al. Mentorship is not enough: exploring sponsorship and its role in career advancement in academic medicine. *Acad Med*. 2019;94(1):94–100.
46. Jain S, Madani K, Flint L, et al. What does it mean to be a male ally? Implementing meaningful change in gender representation in medicine. *J Am Coll Surg*. 2020;230(3):355–356.
47. Ely RJ, Padavic I. What's really holding women back? *Harvard Business Review*. 2020. Available at: https://hbr.org/2020/03/whats-really-holding-women-back. Accessed July 01, 2020.
48. Sabry H. Better communication with medical leadership brings more opportunities for emergency physician mother. *ACEP Now*. American College of Emergency Physicians. 2016. Available at: https://www.acepnow.com/article/better-communication-medical-leadership-brings-opportunities-emergency-physician-mother/2/. Accessed August 1, 2020.
49. Ryan MK, Haslam SA. The glass cliff: evidence that women are over-represented in precarious leadership positions. *Br J Manage*. 2005;16(2):81–90.
50. Ryan MK, Haslam SA. Introducing the Glass Cliff. *BBC News*. 2004. Available at: http://news.bbc.co.uk/2/hi/uk_news/magazine/3755031.stm. Accessed July 31, 2020.
51. Ashby JS, Haslam SA, Ryan MK. Legal work and the glass cliff: evidence that women are preferentially selected to lead problematic cases. *William Mary J Women Law*. 2007;13(3).
52. Ryan MK, Haslam SA, Kulich C. Politics and the glass cliff: evidence that women are preferentially selected to contest hard-to-win seats. *Psychol Women Quart*. 2010; 34(1):56–64.
53. Mansky J. SmithsonianMag.com. 2017. Available at: https://www.smithsonianmag.com/science-nature/woman-who-paved-way-female-physicians-america-180967104/. Accessed August 8, 2020.
54. Wikipedia. Harriot Kezia Hurt. Available at: Https://en.wikipedia.org/wiki/Harriot_Kezia_Hunt. Updated July 19, 2020. Accessed August 8, 2020.
55. Rubin R. Dr Schrier goes to congress as second woman physician. *JAMA*. 2019;321(15):1443–1445. Available at: https://jamanetwork.com/journals/jama/fullarticle/2729714. Accessed August 8, 2020.
56. *ACEP Diversity and Inclusion Survey*. AAMC Partner. 2018. Available at: https://www.emra.org/emresident/article/implicit-bias/. Accessed August 8, 2020.
57. Parker et al. Why diversity and inclusion are critical to the American College of Emergency Physicians' future success. *Ann Emerg Med*. 2017;69(6):714–717.
58. ACEP eCME. Unconscious bias in clinical practice. Available at: http://ecme.acep.org/diweb/catalog/item? id=2215016. Updated 2020. Accessed August 8, 2020.
59. Freedman J. Women in medicine: are we "there yet"? 2010. Available at: http://www.medscape.com/viewarticle/732197. Accessed June 14, 2016.
60. American Association of Medical Colleges. AAMC data warehouse. 2020. Available at: https://www.aamc.org/media/37706/download. Accessed May 6, 2020.
61. Stanford. The Clayman Institute for Gender Research. Available at: https://gender.stanford.edu/about/mission. Updated 2020. Accessed August 8, 2020.
62. Harvard IAT. Project Implicit®. Available at: https://implicit.harvard.edu/implicit/takeatest.html. Updated 2020. Accessed July 2, 2020.
63. Moss-Racusin CA, Dovidio JF, Brescoll VL, et al. Science faculty's subtle gender biases favor male students. *Proceedings of the National Academy of Sciences*. 2012. Available at: https://www.pnas.org/content/109/41/16474. Accessed August 8, 2020.
64. Eaton AA, Saunders JF, Jacobson RK, et al. How gender and race stereotypes impact the advancement of scholars in STEM: professors' biased evaluations of physics and biology post-doctoral candidates. *Sex Roles*. 2020;82:127–141.
65. Goldin C, Rouse C. Orchestrating impartiality: the impact of "Blind" auditions on female musicians. *Am Econ Rev*. 2000;90(4): 715–741.
66. Furmans V. Where are all the women CEOs? 2020. Available at: https://www.wsj.com/articles/why-so-few-ceos-are-women-you-can-have-a-seat-at-the-table-and-not-be-a-player-11581003276. Accessed May 15, 2020.
67. The Amazing Tool that Women in the White House Used to Fight Gender Bias. 2016. Available at: https://www.vox.com/2016/9/14/12914370/white-house-obama-women-gender-bias-amplification. Accessed May 15, 2020.
68. Arora VM. It is time for equal pay for equal work for physicians—Paging Dr Ledbetter. *JAMA Intern Med*. 2016;176(9):1305–1306. Accessed August 8, 2020.
69. Mohr TS. Why women don't apply for jobs unless they're 100% qualified. 2014. Available at: https://hbr.org/2014/08/why-women-dont-apply-for-jobs-unless-theyre-100-qualified. Accessed May 15, 2020.
70. Parker RB. Negotiating the best deal: advice from an expert. 2015. Available at: https://feminem.org/2015/09/20/negotiating-the-best-deal-advice-from-an-expert/. Accessed August 8, 2020.
71. Frank L. Why banning questions about salary history may not improve pay equity. 2017. Available at: https://hbr.org/2017/09/why-banning-questions-about-salary-history-may-not-improve-pay-equity. Accessed May 15, 2020.
72. Ammerman C, Groysberg B. Why the crisis is putting companies at risk of losing female talent. 2020. Available at: https://hbr.org/2020/05/why-the-crisis-is-putting-companies-at-risk-of-losing-female-talent? fbclid=IwAR29tq_ZWwchFgOfsM3YDAo00Fzmb3Cz25UknAdNXVwXVPKth_ZEjYIQp5g. Accessed May 15, 2020.
73. Colby SL, Ortman JM. *Projections of the Size and Composition of the US Population: 2014 to 2060, Current Population Reports, P25-1143*. Washington, DC: US Census Bureau; 2015

CHAPTER 17
LEADERSHIP IN TIMES OF CRISIS
Thom A. Mayer

*When we are no longer able to change a situation,
we are challenged to change ourselves.*

—Viktor Frankl, MD, *Man's Search for Meaning*[1]

*You have been stationed in a key post, not some lowly
place, and not for a short time but for life.*

—Epictetus, *Discourses, 3.24.31–36*[2]

The first section of this book has focused on leadership principles in "normal" times, although life in the emergency department (ED) can seem anything but normal given the often-surreal environment in which we work. Chapter 52 eloquently discusses ED disaster planning and response, but here the focus is on crisis leadership principles, through a personal lens. It has been my privilege to have led organizations through many disasters throughout my career, having served as a command physician for the Pentagon rescue and recovery operation on September 11, 2001, incident commander for the inhalational anthrax crisis in Washington, DC, and medical director for the National Football League (NFL) Players Association.[3]

Leadership in normal times is what we *can* do . . . but leadership in times of crisis is what we *must* do; after all, failed leadership worsens the crisis and its consequences. Crisis leadership is not simply a mindset or attitude, it is also a *discipline*, guided in part by those who have been there previously. While hope is not a plan, neither is despair. In a crisis, leaders must be able to use strategic optimism to illuminate a path forward, demonstrating the potential for success where others see only possibilities for failure.

A Crisis is Nonnegotiable

Although negotiation skills are an essential part of leadership (see Chapter 99), you cannot negotiate with a crisis. For example, the coronavirus (COVID-19) is immune to negotiation; it is a blunt reality with which we are forced to deal. Crisis leadership is nonnegotiable; it must occur as the crisis continues to expand. We must fit our lives and our systems into the disaster for as long as it lasts, not the other way around. To be clear, negotiation skills are critical in stakeholder analysis, boundary management, and leading teams in a crisis, but the nature of the crisis itself is nonnegotiable.

HARDWIRING, TRAINING, AND DISCIPLINE

Emergency department leaders are seemingly perfect for crisis management by virtue of their training and constant exposure to ambiguity. When normal people hear a loud bang or witness a catastrophic accident, they do what tens of thousands of years of evolution have taught them—run away! It is simply a matter of self-preservation. Military personnel, law enforcement officers, fire and emergency medical service professionals, and emergency team members do the opposite—they run into the fire, toward the chaos. Nearly every crisis facing health care in the past 20 years has first manifested itself in the interface between ED leaders and the community. What goes against nature in others is a part of our nature, which makes ED nurses and physicians inclined to be great crisis leaders. At times when others would be most distressed, emergency clinicians become almost preternaturally calm. That calmness comes from a combination of factors, each of which are deeply interrelated.

Evidence-Based Discipline

Emergency medicine is based on a foundation of evidence-based and evidence-influenced approaches to our daily challenges, both clinical and administrative. During the COVID-19 pandemic, I found my words published as the *New York Times* quote of the week: "We will go anywhere the science takes us and nowhere the science doesn't."[4] While I was speaking of the NFL Players Association's (NFLPA's) values, my words could just as easily have applied to emergency teams in times of crisis.

Preparation

Emergency department leaders are always deeply involved in (and often lead) disaster preparedness efforts in their communities; yet, these plans and drills are designed to merely approximate crises. They cannot duplicate them. Excellent leaders recognize this and prepare for the unexpected, which accounts in part for the calmness they exhibit in the face of disaster.

Deep Empathy

It is virtually impossible to practice emergency medicine without a profound commitment to the needs of the patient. Underlying all clinical care should be the deep and sustained inclination to empathy, which is the capacity to feel and understand the perspective of others *from their frame of reference*. Practicing empathy is a part of daily life in the ED. Our ability to understand issues from the patients' and families' perspectives is also an essential component of crisis leadership.[5]

DEFINING A CRISIS

Although there are many definitions of a crisis, all share the essential features shown in **Figure 17.1**.[6]

Undesirable

Crises by their very nature are are unwanted, unwelcome intrusions into our lives. If they were desirable, they would be called opportunities. The ancient Chinese definition of crisis is said to combine the symbols for danger *and* opportunity (**Figure 17.2**). The very fact that the event is undesirable often galvanizes people to reach across boundaries and come to common solutions.

FIGURE 17.1 ■ Essential Components of a Crisis

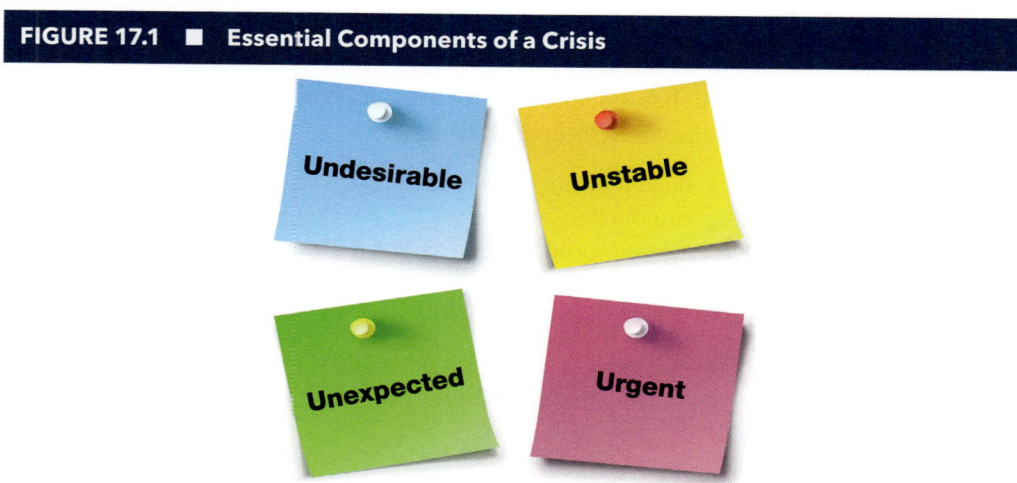

Unstable

Every crisis is at least initially unstable, as the facts on the ground continue to evolve. This instability drives the need for the leader to deal with ambiguity, even while seeking time-sensitive clarity. The tenuous nature of any crisis calls into question the validity of associated decisions, which are difficult to make with precision during times of change.

Unexpected

While most health-care systems have a defined disaster plan, each event is unique and never completely follows the expected course. As my great friend and one of the world's premier authorities on global preparedness Dan Hanfling says, "These pesky disasters don't seem to be able to read our disaster plans!" This does not mean that disaster planning and preparedness are unimportant. Rather, it means that it is impossible to predict precisely what form a new challenge will take, which accentuates the need for a disciplined response. To quote former Secretary of State Henry Kissinger, "There can't possibly be a crisis next week—my schedule is already full."[7]

Urgent

Once the crisis occurs, the response must be urgent, time sensitive, and cognizant of potential spread or deterioration (absent strong, decisive, and effective leadership). A crisis

FIGURE 17.2 ■ Chinese Symbol for Crisis: Danger + Opportunity

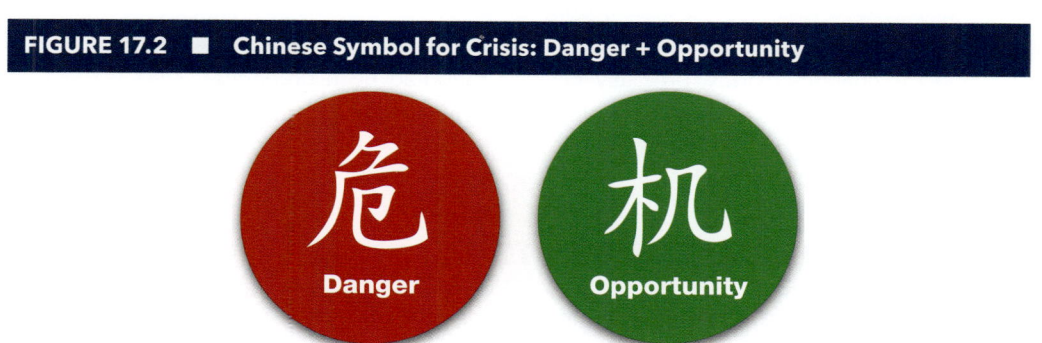

does not initially permit sustained periods of reflection (although as the event continues, leaders should build time for reflection into their day). Action is essential.

The COVID-19 pandemic has put medical leaders under intense, sometimes unfair scrutiny. These sorts of questions have been common in the ED:

- "Come on, Doc—what do you mean you don't know?"
- "It's a virus—how bad could it be?"
- "Surely there is *something* that could be done to stop the spread?"
- "How can doctors transplant hearts and lungs and yet you can't stop a simple virus?"

When an ED leader is in the midst of a crisis, it is important to weave the undesirable, unstable, unexpected, and urgent elements of the situation into the story—for the sake of the crisis team and broader public.

The Transitional Nature of a Crisis

An essential feature of a crisis is that it is *transitional*. In the midst of a disaster, people are forced to move from one set of facts and assumptions to a new, often fundamentally different set. The work of the great sociologist Kurt Lewin is particularly helpful in understanding this transitional nature. Lewin's work on change management stressed, among other things, the importance of[8]:

- *Unfreezing*: Normal operations are insufficient for the new and emerging reality, so systems, processes, and attitudes must be adaptive.
- *Moving*: Resiliency is fundamentally the capacity to move quickly, efficiently, and effectively in response to the crisis, seeking the input of team members at each step and building a powerful guiding coalition. This also means moving in the right direction, so the situation is made better, not worse.
- *Refreezing*: Once resiliency/adaptive capacity and teamwork have created a new normal, systems and processes must be communicated to the team members, who will hold themselves mutually accountable for them.

Depending upon the length of the crisis, this cycle may need to be repeated many times. For example, during the COVID-19 pandemic, viral testing strategies have changed dramatically as sensitivity and specificity have continued to improve, and nasopharyngeal swabs (relatively invasive and uncomfortable) have given way to point-of-care saliva testing. In informing the parties involved in the negotiations to open NFL facilities to players, coaches, and the team staffs, SARS CoV-2 was continuously described as a novel and emerging infectious disease, meaning many facts about the virus were initially unknown.

When changes to protocols transpired, as they inevitably would in a pandemic, NFL players accepted the changes readily, precisely because they had been prepared. Crisis leadership requires an understanding that our explorations are necessarily transitional and sometimes seemingly unending.

CRISIS LEADERSHIP ESSENTIALS

In reflecting on a career of crisis leadership, several essential tenets emerge, many of which are not a part of the traditional crisis leadership literature.

A Discipline, Not a Motto

The discipline required to effectively plan is essential during times of crisis. Two of the greatest World War II commanders were General Dwight D. Eisenhower, Supreme Commander of the Allied Expeditionary Force, and General George S. Patton, Commanding General of the US Third Army in Europe, close friends who had differing perspectives on planning. Patton once said, "A good plan violently executed now is better than a perfect plan executed next week."[9] He also noted that even the best of plans fall apart with the first contact of battle, as several other military giants have described over the centuries. Eisenhower, who began his WWII duty as the director of the War Plans Division in Washington, explained, "In war, planning is everything, but plans are nothing."[10] The discipline of preparing for ambiguous eventualities is a core essential for crisis leadership.

Mission, Vision, and Values

When the stakes are high—and the stakes are never higher than when leading a crisis—the best compass is your own personal mission, vision, and values and those of your organization. You will likely find some mention of honesty, humility, tenacity, and integrity—core values that make excellent guideposts for navigating a disaster. A crisis is the wrong time to be developing core ideals. You must own and embody the values of your organization and yourself *before* the crisis occurs.

In representing the health and safety needs of the 2,500 active players in the NFL, the most powerful sports organization on earth, I am often asked where the courage came from to confront them. After all, the NFLPA represents the interests of the players, but the NFL represents those of the owners. The answer is simple: Every decision I made was guided by the NFLPA's Core Health and Safety Values:

1. Health and safety are nonnegotiable.
2. We will go anywhere the science takes us and nowhere the science does not.
3. Whole player, whole life, whole family.

As long as my words and actions reflected those core values, I simply could not go wrong.

The Speed of Trust

Chief among your core values should be trust; effective leadership simply cannot be done without it. Hopefully, the arc of your career will have embodied building trust with your colleagues, which is a well to which you will return throughout your career. Trust earned and "banked" will be your most valuable asset. Hall of Fame basketball player Grant Hill describes how Duke University men's basketball coach Mike Krzyzewski told his 1991 team that they would win the National Championship, after which he asked Grant, "Do you believe it?" Grant replied, "Coach, I believe it because you said it!" That's trust.

Trust *yourself*; you are made of strong stuff, or you would not have been asked to lead. Open your heart and then follow it. Take the time to pause, reflect, and reconsider the challenges facing you and your team. You will have to forgive others in your role as a crisis leader, but that starts with forgiving yourself. Mistakes will be made. There is neither time nor energy for recriminations. Each day when you arrive at the scene for crisis leadership, pause and throw your guilt about previous decisions or words in the trunk. Guilt will not fuel you in a crisis; it will merely distract you. Keep these thoughts in mind:

- Trust yourself.
- Trust your teammates.
- Be the teammate you would want others to be.
- Bring out the best in others, and they will bring out the best in you.
- Remember there are always ways in which things could have been done better—leave your guilt in the trunk of your car—don't bring it into the crisis.

Systems and the Crisis

Every system is perfectly designed to get precisely the results it gets.

—Paul Batalden, MD[11]

Health-care improvement expert Paul Batalden's insights are widely quoted but often poorly understood. It is the system that has indirectly allowed the crisis to occur, and the system itself fuels the lurking crisis. Our systems are designed to work in "normal" situations, not necessarily in times of disaster. To keep the system functioning during periods of great stress, the following steps are important:

- Understand the system in as much detail as possible, preferably proactively, but immediately during crises.
- Get educated—quickly yet effectively—on those elements of the system with which you are less familiar.
- Make it clear that you will need the team to continuously update you on the system.
- Remove "blame from the game" by assuring the team that whatever part(s) of the system failed, those who designed them are to be consulted, not blamed.

Ask and answer the following questions:

- What elements of the system failed?
- Why did they fail?
- How does the system need to be adapted to meet the demands of the crisis?
- How will the team ensure accurate and timely information to make these decisions?
- Which stakeholders will need to be enlisted to make these changes in the system?

What You Control and What You Don't

There is a natural tendency for those charged with leading in a crisis to assume control. However, it is wise to recall the wisdom of the Stoic philosophers, who cautioned that much less of our lives are under our control than we think. As Epictetus writes:

Happiness and freedom begin with a clear understanding of one principle: some things are within our control and some things are not. It is only after you have faced up to this fundamental truth and learned to distinguish what you can and can't control that inner tranquility and outer effectiveness become possible.[12]

Leading in a crisis requires the inner peace that comes from understanding this wisdom. The concept that we cannot control what happens to us but we can always control how we feel and what we do about it is best summarized by Victor Frankl, "Everything can be taken from a man but one thing: the last of human freedoms—to choose one's attitude in any given set of circumstances, to choose one's own way."[1]

FIGURE 17.3 ■ Leading in Times of Crisis

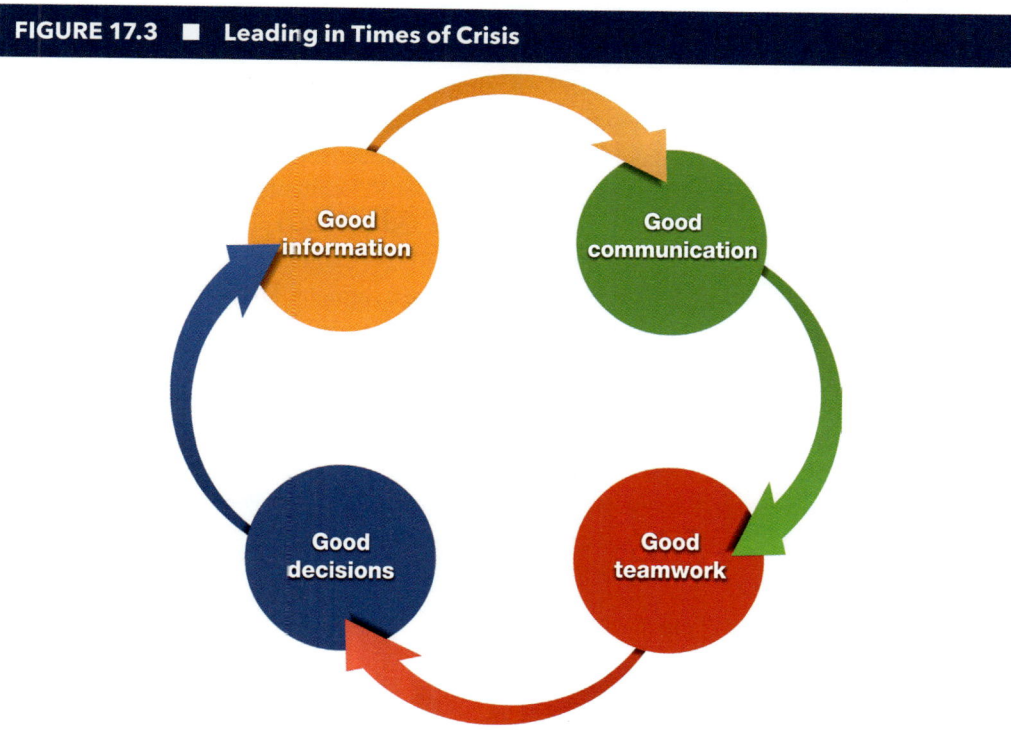

Crisis Recognition and Redundant Communication

I've discovered that reliable information is central to recognizing and circumscribing any crisis. Without good information, there cannot be good communication, which drives the good teamwork needed to make good decisions (**Figure 17.3**). While the need for reliable facts may seem obvious, information in the midst of a crisis is fluid and subject to numerous inaccuracies, largely because it is so difficult for people to say, "I don't know." Very few of us want to seem uninformed during times of upheaval. Will Rogers understood this well, saying, "It ain't what you don't know that will hurt you—it's what you think you know that ain't so."[13]

As a crisis leader, it is important to ensure that the team understands the premium of accurate information and insist, whenever possible, on receiving redundant sources of information. Despite the best plans and discipline, communications in a crisis are often the weakest links in the chain. In physical disasters, a reliance on ordinary means of communication can lead to failure. For example, the Pentagon Rescue and Recovery Operation on September 11, 2001, relied on cellular phone communication while most of the network was down. All emergency plans should rely upon redundant communications networks as well as concepts like call-backs and call-downs used in crew resource management (see Chapter 12).

To determine if the information relayed during a crisis is timely and accurate, ask the following questions:

- Do I have all the facts?
- Are there two or more sources to confirm these facts?
- Which facts don't I have that I wish I did?
- Who can help me get these facts?
- How will we, as a team, judge their accuracy?
- What questions haven't I asked that I should have asked?
- What else should I know and why should I know it?

The Leader as Chief Storyteller and Chief Sensemaker

The story of the crisis must fundamentally be a human story of the heart to be fully understood and interpreted. There is no greater way to lead through the crisis than to control the narrative by accepting the dual roles of chief storyteller and chief sensemaker.[14] These roles require a largely innate talent that arises from the daily care of ED patients, whose days have been disrupted by pain, injury, or other symptoms. Doctors and nurses explain the possible reasons for patients' symptoms and explain how the team will use diagnostic tools to determine the etiology of their complaints and devise the most effective treatment. The same approach applies to crisis management, in which the leader's role is to tell the story of the event in terms the team and the public will understand and even embrace.

To tell the story of an unfolding event, emergency clinicians must rely on their education and experience, particularly their knowledge of history and literature. For example, one of the questions I am asked most often is, "What was the Pentagon like on September 11?" People still want to hear the *story* of that crisis. When I arrived at the Pentagon, the south wall was literally blown apart, and flames and smoke were billowing high into the clear blue sky (**Figure 17.4**). Dante's opening lines of *The Inferno* immediately came to mind:

In the middle of the road of my life
I awoke in a Dark Wood
Where the True Way was wholly lost.
Death could scarce be more bitter
But if I would show the good that came from it
I must talk about things other than the good.[15]

The power of the story and the path it illustrates have tremendous importance in these troubled times. On the dark night of September 11, 2001, I saw several young Marines rigging a makeshift flag, which they taped to a small fire engine at the Pentagon heliport. The scene,

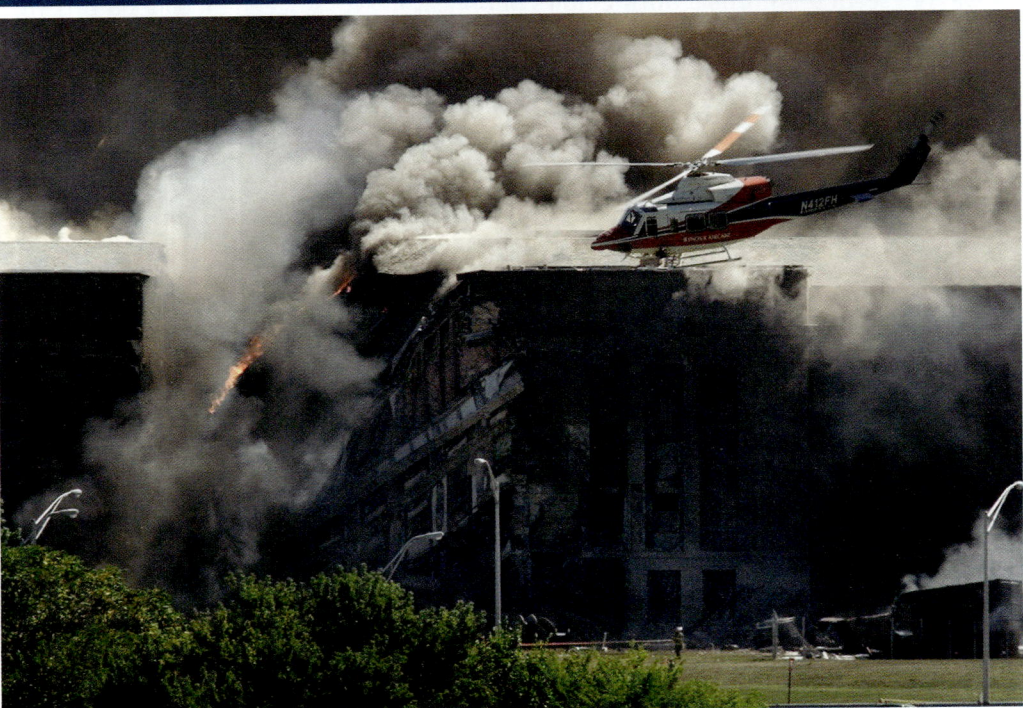

FIGURE 17.4 ■ Inova Rescue Helicopter Arrives at the South Wall of the Pentagon on September 11, 2001

which was near the impact zone of American Airlines Flight 77, was evocative of the great Joe Rosenthal photograph of the flag-raising at Iwo Jima, and I intuitively knew what needed to be done. I radioed the US Army major in charge of logistic operations and asked him to get the biggest flag he could find and put up on the wall of the Pentagon. I believed that a symbol of the triumph of the American spirit needed to be next to the horrible charred breach in the Pentagon wall, where it would be an unmistakable symbol of resistance to the tyranny of terrorism.

When President George W. Bush and Secretary of Defense Donald Rumsfeld arrived the next day, a massive flag was unfurled on the Pentagon's wall precisely as I was shaking hands with the President. That flag, which flew there for weeks, communicated to the world: You can burn our buildings, you can kill our people, but you can never kill the American spirit. It was unfurled again on the first, second, and tenth anniversaries of the September 11 attacks. Let me be clear—I claim no great leadership role at the Pentagon. Indeed, I am in awe of the leadership provided by those with whom I served there. Nonetheless, vision can often be communicated in stories and symbols that assume deeper meanings than we initially intended. Indeed, images of the Pentagon flag and the flag raised by three New York City firefighters at the World Trade Center are the two most frequently downloaded photographs from 9/11. (**Figure 17.5**).[16]

In addition to telling the story of the crisis, ED leaders must also act as chief sensemakers. The chief storyteller role entails blending the aspects of the crisis into a meaningful story, but the chief sensemaker role, while deeply related, integrates the *big story* into the *big picture*.

FIGURE 17.5 ■ Pentagon Flag Unfurled on September 12, 2001

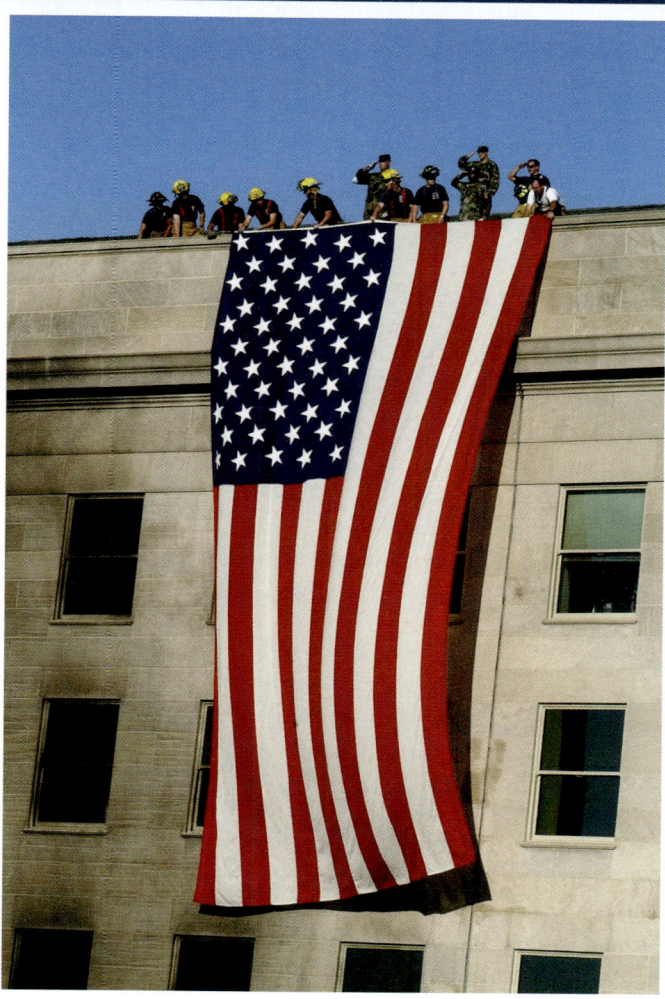

When our middle son, Kevin, was 9 years old, I came home from work one evening to find him deep into his literature homework. He asked if I could help him, so I read the passage carefully, thought for a minute, and simply told him what it said. His responded, "Dad, I know what it *says*—what does it *mean*?"

In order for the medical team and public to know what a crisis *means*, we must incorporate sensemaking into our storytelling. The chief storyteller provides the narrative detail of what the crisis entails, the best approaches to address these possibilities, and the framework and time frame in which these steps will occur. The chief sensemaker role is layered over this and provides the context of meaning. Sensemaking means navigating the crisis with a compass instead of a map. (And it is wise to recall Count Korzybski's cautionary words: "The map is not the territory."[17]) Organizational theorist Karl Weick explains it well, "To lead in the future is to be less in thrall of decision-making and more in thrall of sensemaking."[18] Storytelling and sensemaking should be embraced and respected; we make a difference in people's lives, in part by appropriately exercising control on behalf of our patients.

Building a Powerful Guiding Coalition

If crisis leadership is not for the faint-hearted, neither is it for a lone individual. The efforts should also include a team—a powerful guiding coalition of trusted key people. One person cannot sustain crisis leadership efforts alone. The Biblical example of the Battle of Refidim between the Israelites and the Amalekites described in the Book of Exodus illustrates this well. As Joshua led the battle for Israel, Moses watched from a hill and noticed a strange thing: "And it came to pass, when Moses held up his hands, that Israel prevailed: and when he let down his hands, Amalek prevailed."

It seems simple enough: Keep your hands up and Israel will prevail. However, the battle raged on for hours, and Moses' arms tired and fell to his sides. Solution? Moses' brother Aaron and a trusted colleague named Hur stood on each side of Moses, each holding up an arm. You will need a similar support system during times of crisis. You simply cannot sustain the effort alone. Choose members of that powerful guiding coalition carefully, and the best litmus test is *trust*.

Learning to Suck Down in a World Full of Suck-Ups

When the mantle of crisis leadership is thrust upon you, there will always be those who choose to *suck up* to the person in charge. There is no time for sucking up in a crisis, but there is a role for *sucking down*. Let's explore that idea.

Defining Sucking Up

All of us have clear memories of the suck-ups that we have known in life. When they are successful at ascending the leadership ladder, we shake our heads in amazement and disbelief. As executive leadership coach Marshall Goldsmith notes:

> *If leaders say they discourage sucking up, why does it happen so often? Here's a straightforward answer: Without meaning to, we all tend to create an environment where people learn to reward others with accolades that aren't really warranted. We can see this very clearly in others. We just can't see it in ourselves.*[19]

While on the surface, sucking up may seem a matter of degree—overdoing flattery in an overbearing way; however, at its essence, sucking up reveals the fundamental belief that success, advancement, and the answers to our questions are somehow *above us* in the organization. In this sense, sucking up is a matter of substance. We do it because we somehow cannot trust that the answers we seek are within us. Thus, even if the right questions are being asked, we are looking in the wrong place.

Defining Sucking Down

Sucking down consists of a fundamental and deeply held belief that the locus of power, knowledge, and meaning in a crisis lies within the organization. This includes actively seeking answers from those supposedly below us. It is important to note that sucking down does not preclude looking above in the organization, only in doing so exclusively. Sucking down thus includes perspectives from throughout the organization, while sucking up places its focus above.

Sucking down is effective for leaders because it puts them in touch with those who actually do the work. When I found myself wearing the Command Physician vest at the Pentagon on what became one of the defining days of our generation, the lessons I learned came not from listening to the generals, cabinet secretaries, and other potentates but rather from listening below—to the firefighters, paramedics, physicians, nurses, and law enforcement officers. For days, it seemed that most of my sentences began:

I need your help with this . . .
Help me understand this . . .
What's your take on this?
Help me understand how this works . . .
I've got a tough decision; I need your input on . . .
How would you handle this problem?

Gearing up in self-contained breathing apparatus to go into the still-burning Pentagon on September 11 required a certain amount of courage, especially when you are as claustrophobic as I am. But sucking-down listening also requires effort and courage. Effort is required not only because such downward-reaching conversations are counterintuitive but also because they seek out those who may have the answers when it seems we should have such answers ourselves. Any such courage is born from humility—the ability to say, "I don't know, but I would like to learn. Will you help me?"

Sucking-down leaders have a distinct advantage in environments filled with uncertainty precisely because they are more adaptable and resilient. They detect problems earlier and act on them. Organizations with sucking-down leaders are therefore more flexible; problems are discussed regularly, freely, and without fear of criticism for having pointed out the crisis team's frailties.

An example of the power of listening down comes from the bioterrorism crisis of 2001. Scarcely a month after the September 11 attacks, anthrax-laced letters were sent to the Philip A. Hart Senate office building in Washington, DC. Within days, hundreds of patients (many of them postal workers) came to our ED desperately concerned that they might have been poisoned. At that time, we did what most people would do; we listened to recognized authorities with demonstrated expertise; in this case, that was the Centers for Disease Control and Prevention (CDC). In other words, we practiced sucking-up listening. What we heard were reassurances that, unless you were on the fifth and sixth floors of the southeast wing of the Hart building between 9:00 am and 7:00 pm on October 15, 2001, there was absolutely nothing to be concerned about.[20] Based on what was thought to be good science, the CDC declared that it was impossible to have contracted anthrax unless you had been in that specific building on those specific floors at the time the letter was opened.

Several days later, however, a postal worker named Leroy Richmond from the Brentwood neighborhood of Washington DC came to our ED, where he told his emergency physician, Dr. Cecele Murphy, "I think I have anthrax." Listening upward—consulting the expert authorities—would have led Dr. Murphy to tell this patient, "Don't worry—the experts say you're okay." Fortunately, she instead did what all great physicians do—she listened to the patient, who told her, "My chest feels very strange. I know my body and something just doesn't feel right."

Dr. Murphy recognized Osler's wisdom that it is more important to know what sort of patient has the disease than what sort of disease the patient has. Because she listened *down* to the patient and not *up* to the experts, Dr. Murphy obtained a chest x-ray and then a more detailed computed tomography (CT) examination of Mr. Richmond's chest, which revealed dramatic evidence of potentially fatal inhalational anthrax. Quite simply, even though he did not appear acutely ill, the patient's chest was literally dissolving—and he was getting worse by the hour. (Even today, looking at the chest CT gives me cold chills.) Following Dr. Murphy's diagnosis, Mr. Richmond was treated aggressively and survived his terrible illness. Sucking-down listening has its rewards.

About a week later, I stood in Mr. Richmond's hospital room where, in spite of the seriousness of his disease, he was doing extremely well, sitting up and conversing with his family while CNN droned in the background. Suddenly there was a news conference from Washington, DC, where an official announced, "The Inova Fairfax Hospital patient is gravely ill and facing." Complete silence fell upon the room. Holding a piece of fruit in his hand, Mr. Richmond turned to me and said, "Doc, is there something you're not telling me?"

In the midst of disaster, when communications need to be at their best, they are often misinformed. Strategic listening works because it is omnidirectional and involves listening within and throughout the organization. It produces *listening redundancy*, ensuring that we hear information from multiple sources, in a variety of voices, all of which must be interpreted and unified.

Strategic listening requires listening in nontraditional ways to nonevident sources, uncovering surprising and sometimes even shocking insights into how things work and how people interact, all by connecting the web of conversation. Dr. Murphy certainly understood the advice of the CDC, but she listened more closely to her patient, even though his presentation did not fit the textbook description of anthrax.

Listening strategically allows us to build strength, adaptability, and the capacity for change by helping those we serve discern the fundamental interdependency of the system in which we operate. Because people feel free to communicate problems (or the potential thereof), they are able to anticipate difficulties far earlier and more effectively.

In addition to possessing a servant's heart, those who suck down have a clear and guiding sense of their own limitations, particularly when they are charged with crisis leadership. This requires the realization that we are in less control than many people would like to think. Far from being masters of our own—and other's—destinies, leaders who suck down are effective because their mission to serve is matched by a realistic sense of their own place in life.

Sucking-up leaders often think, "Thank goodness for *me*—if *I* weren't here, this would be a real mess!" Sucking-down leaders, on the other hand, embrace their responsibilities but understand their limitations. The sucking-down leader's focus is not on what they bring to the organization but on what they can help others accomplish.

Strategic Optimism in a Crisis

Are you an optimist or a pessimist (or a realist . . .)? When you see a partially filled glass of water, do you consider it half-empty or half-full? That test is often used to guide assessments of optimism versus pessimism. (Shortly before he passed away, I asked my father that same question. He thought for a moment, smiled, and answered, "It depends upon whether you're pouring . . . or drinking." It's all about perspective . . .)

Several years ago, I developed a concept known as *strategic optimism*.[21] It starts with the principle that life's greatest asset is our capacity to assess a situation with the most positive practical possibility. (There are many other definitions, but that is mine.) Since strategic optimism is an asset, we are duty bound to maximize its return on investment (ROI) to increase our wealth. None of us have unlimited energy and optimism, so we must use these qualities wisely.

Before their respective deaths, I had the rare honor of interviewing both Admiral James B. Stockdale and Senator John S. McCain III, both of whom had been guests of the "Hanoi Hilton, the most brutal, torture-ridden prisoner of war camp during the Vietnam War."[22] Each man told me separately that those who died first in that brutal environment were blind optimists, meaning they were divorced from reality and constantly felt they would be liberated "quickly, soon, or even the next day." These individuals had squandered their optimism on an unreasonable belief. Stockdale called on what he described as "brutal optimism":

> *I never lost faith in the end of the story. I never doubted not only that I would get out, but also that I would prevail in the end and turn the experience into the defining event of my life. This is a very important lesson. You must never confuse the faith that you will prevail in the end with the discipline to confront the most brutal facts of your current reality.*[22]

To lead in a crisis, start with brutal optimism—a realistic assessment of the situation. Write those facts down, in all their starkness. Be prepared to feel slightly demoralized. Now turn to the faith that you will prevail in the end, and invest your optimism to maximize your ROI. This is the *strategic optimism* concept; since your optimism has boundaries and limits, use it to your strategic advantage by placing your energy in the right places at the right times.

As you assess the harsh reality of the crisis, where will you strategically invest your optimism? Will you invest it wisely, or will you squander it on false hopes and unreasonable expectations? Just remember, the more wisely you invest, the greater your return.

DEALING WITH THE PRESS

Dealing with the press is simply a necessary and unavoidable aspect of leading through a crisis. Preparation and teamwork allow your message to be delivered effectively and succinctly. An ED leader's responsibility entails communicating the story and meaning of the crisis in a light that best reflects the organization's efforts toward finding a solution

Most hospitals have proactively established relationships with the press as well as a template for crisis management, so it is critical to work closely with institution leaders throughout this process. The director of communications will be your key partner during the crisis. These invaluable professionals often have existing relationships with journalists and are experts at developing appropriate media messaging. Whenever possible, speak with the director of communications prior to holding a press conference to discuss these questions:

- What is the information we want to communicate to the press and public?
- What is the best "sound bite" for communicating this message?
- What are the toughest questions we will be asked, and who is likely to ask them?
- How will we answer those difficult questions?

Using the Sound Bite Wisely

It is wise to remember former Secretary of State Henry Kissinger's opening question during a large press conference: "Do any of you have questions for my answers?"[23] It is essential to work with the crisis leadership team to think through the best sound bites for

> **BOX 17.1 ■ NFLPA SOUND BITES**
>
> - "This is a novel virus and an emerging infectious disease. We have to discover the facts about it over time, which we will communicate to you as we learn them."
> - "We will go anywhere the science takes us and nowhere it does not."
> - "This is a contact disease in a contact sport, so this is a risk-mitigation effort not a risk-elimination equation."
> - "We cannot fit the virus into football—we must fit football into the virus."
> - "This virus has one natural enemy and one only, and that is transmission. If you kill transmission, you kill the virus."

communicating the desired central message. During the NFL response to the COVID-19 pandemic, the NFLPA's message stressed several essential sound bites (**Box 17.1**), which served the organization well and were widely quoted by journalists. In each crisis, think through the simplest, most effective way to communicate your message.

In general, journalists genuinely want to tell a compelling story and approach the situation from the following perspective:

- Holding true to their core value of "the public's right to know"
- Reporting all sides of the story
- Getting information that no one else has
- Speaking to credible, on-scene witnesses (including you and members of your team)
- Obtaining memorable sound bites

Additional suggestions for communicating with the press include:

- Use the journalist's name when possible: "Andrea, that is an excellent question."
- When asked a yes-or-no question to which there is not a single-word answer: "That's an interesting and complex question, and it deserves a full response" or "I find when that question is asked, people want to know these details . . . ."
- Praise the team: "I can't emphasize enough the incredible job this team has done in managing this crisis."
- When asked a repeat question: "I'm sorry if I wasn't clear, but here are the facts as we know them now . . ."

What You Know and What You Don't

First, state clearly that you do *not* know all the facts. Second, state the facts that you *do* know. While you may not have all the answers, you can at least provide hope and create trust by offering reassurance that facts will be revealed as they become clear. During the Beltway sniper attacks in 2002, the only female fatality occurred in Fairfax County, Virginia, where I serve as the operational medical director of Tactical and Special Operations, including the police helicopter unit. Police Chief Colonel Tom Manger was interviewed on the night of the shooting, and his responses to the reporters need no improvement. In precise, staccato language, he clearly identified the known facts of the case.[24] Over the course of the next 10 days, clues from this shooting led to the arrest and successful prosecution of the two men who committed the nine murders.

Finally, be prepared to learn from each interaction, ask for feedback on what you could have done differently, and participate in ongoing after-action reviews (see the next section). To the best extent possible, develop a positive relationship with journalists; there is a very good chance you will see them again in the next crisis.

LEARNING FROM THE CRISIS

As the crisis begins to wind down—a process that may take days, weeks, or even months—make sure the team takes time to reflect on and learn from the event. The best way to do so is to use a format developed jointly by the United States Marine Corps (USMC) and the US Army: after-action reviews (AARs). The concept of AARs arose from a military approach known as "red teaming," a time-honored concept of employing a dedicated unit to act as an opposing force in training operations. This method helps prepare other units with battle strategies and tactics prior to deployment to war zones.[25]

After-action reviews follow a specific set of questions that are designed to improve future operations. They should be treated as verbs (something you do) not nouns (a thing or box that must be checked). In crisis leadership, AARs should be a part of the daily debriefing but also used as the crisis winds down. **Box 17.2** further defines AARs.

Once the Crisis Is Over

Take the time at the end of the crisis to celebrate the team's work, both formally and informally. You will find that bonds form in a crisis that endure for years. As the great writer Sebastian Junger notes in *Tribe: On Homecoming and Belonging,* the challenges of a crisis "thrust people back into a more ancient, organic way of relating."[26] It is wise to celebrate and accentuate those bonds, often with a celebratory event, but always with public thanks and praise. It is also wise for crisis leaders to send a written message to the members of the team, praising their integrity, courage, and performance when their community needed them most.

The Sisyphean Nature of Crisis Leadership

The nature of a crisis inevitably calls to mind the ancient Greek myth of Sisyphus, who was condemned by the gods to ceaselessly roll a massive stone to the top of a mountain, only to have it roll back to the bottom, where the process would begin again without end. Yet despite Sisyphus' eternal punishment, Homer called him the wisest and most prudent of mortals.[27] During the COVID-19 pandemic, the Sisyphean nature of health-care providers and their leaders was pointed out.[45] The constant effort, often against seemingly insurmountable odds, may be an apt metaphor. However, it should not be considered a sad one. Perhaps the best-known iteration of the tale is in the philosopher Albert Camus' essay *Myth of Sisyphus*. It is an excellent exegesis, well worth reading and rereading by those charged with crisis leadership, for it ends with these telling words, "One must imagine Sisyphus happy."[28]

BOX 17.2 ■ AFTER-ACTION REVIEWS

After-action reviews are NOT:
- Meetings
- Reports
- "M & M" sessions without structure
- A "box to be checked"

After-action reviews ARE:
- An opportunity to learn "how to think," not just "what to do" during a crisis
- A chance to accentuate the positive while learning what not to change in the future
- An opportunity to create organizational learning
- A way to connect recent past experience with positive future action[42]

Those who are privileged to lead in a crisis must also be imagined happy because it is worthwhile to be of service to others during the most challenging and difficult of times. It is where our deep joy intersects the world's deep needs.

CONCLUSION

Leadership in health care is never more necessary than in the midst of a crisis, which is an undesirable, unstable, unexpected, and urgent challenge requiring decisive and definitive action. In a crisis, the leader must act as chief storyteller by explaining what is happening and chief sensemaker by explaining what it all means. Since all crises are complex, adaptive situations, a systems approach must be used. Leaders must have a powerful guiding coalition of people, who are chosen based on trust rather than hierarchy. Leaders are encouraged to invest their optimism wisely to gain the maximum ROI, and deal with the press in a positive, thoughtful, and proactive fashion, crafting the message carefully. After-action reviews are an effective tool for continuously improving a department's crisis response. While the work of crisis leadership is taxing, the rewards of a job well done are immense.

REFERENCES

1. Frankl V. *Man's Search for Meaning*. Boston, Mass: Beacon Press; 2006.
2. Epictetus. *Discourses-3.24: 31–36*. London: Penguin Classics; 2008
3. Beaton A. The doctor and the 'badasses' keeping NFL players safe from the coronavirus. *Wall Street Journal*. May 27, 2020. Available at: https://www.wsj.com/articles/the-doctor-and-the-badasses-keeping-nfl-players-safe-from-the-coronavirus-11590580800. Accessed June 19, 2020.
4. Mayer T. *New York Times Quote of the Day*. April 26, 2020.
5. Mayer T, Cates R. *Leadership for Great Customer Service: Satisfied Employees, Satisfied Customers*. 2nd ed. Chicago, Ill: Health Administration Press; 2014.
6. Mayer T. Crisis Management or Crisis Leadership: Lessons from 9/11, the Anthrax Crisis, and Duke Lacrosse: The Colin Rorrie, Jr. Lecture. Presented at: American College of Emergency Physicians Scientific Assembly, 2002, Chicago, Ill.
7. Kissinger H. *World Order*. New York, NY: Penguin; 2014.
8. Lewin K. *A Dynamic Theory of Personality: Selected Papers*. London: Read Books; 2014.
9. Patton GS. *War As I Knew It*. New York, NY: Houghton Mifflin; 1995.
10. Eisenhower DD. Quoted in Ambrose SE. In: Ambrose SE, ed. *The Supreme Commander: The War Years of Dwight D. Eisenhower*. New York, NY: Anchor Books; 1970.
11. Batalden P. *Like Magic (Every system is perfectly designed…)*. Institute for Healthcare Improvement; 2015. Available at: http://www.ihi.org/communities/blogs/origin-of-every-system-is-perfectly-designed-quote. Accessed June 19, 2020.
12. Frankl V. *Man's Search for Meaning*. Boston, Mass: Beacon Press; 2006.
13. Rogers W. *Never Met a Man I Didn't Like: The Life and Writings of Will Rogers*. New York, NY: Avon Books; 1991.
14. Mayer T. *Battling Healthcare Burnout: Learning to Love the Job You Have while Creating the Job You Love*. San Francisco, Calif: Berrett-Koehler; 2021.
15. Alighieri D. *The Inferno*. New York, NY: New American Library; 2003.
16. Little B, Howard BC, Handwerk B. *Remembering 9/11 in Pictures*. National Geographic. Available at: https://www.nationalgeographic.com/news/2016/09/september-11-pictures-remembrance/. Accessed June 19, 2020.
17. Korzybski A. *Science and Sanity: An Introduction to Non-Aristotelian Systems and General Semantics*. New York, NY: The International Non-Aristotelian Library; 1933.
18. Karl E. Weick . Reprinted from The Collapse of Sensemaking in Organizations: The Mann Gulch Disaster by Karl E. Weick published in Administrative Science Quarterly Volume 38 (1993): 628–652 by permission of Administrative Science Quarterly. © 1993 by Cornell University 0001-8392/93/3804-0628.
19. Goldsmith M. Are you encouraging suck ups? *Huffington Post*. July 2009. Available at: https://www.marshallgoldsmith.com/articles/are-you-encouraging-suck-ups/. Accessed June 19, 2020.
20. Centers for Disease Control and Prevention. Investigation of bioterrorism-related anthrax and interim guidelines for exposure management and antimicrobial therapy. *MMWR Morb Mortal Wkly Rep*. 2001;50:909–919.
21. Mayer T. *Creating Great Patient Experience*. Presented at: American College of Emergency Physicians Emergency Department Directors Academy, February 5, 2020, Dallas, Tex.
22. Stockdale J. *A Vietnam Experience: Ten Years of Reflection*. Palo Alto, Calif: Hoover Press; 1984.
23. Kissinger H. Available at: https://www.nytimes.com/1978/04/16/archives/what-will-henry-do-for-an-encore-kissinger-kissinger.html. Accessed June 19, 2020.
24. Manger T. Available at: https://www.upi.com/Archives/2002/10/15/Ninth-death-tied-to-Washington-area-sniper/7531034654400/. Accessed June 19, 2020.
25. Darling M, Parry C, Moore J. Learning in the thick of it. *Harvard Business Review*. 2019, Special Issue:102–111.
26. Junger S. *Tribe: On Homecoming and Belonging*. New York, NY: Hachette; 2016.
27. Homer. *The Iliad*. Translated by Fagles R. New York, NY: Penguin; 1990.
28. Camus A. *The Myth of Sisyphus*. New York, NY: Alfred Knopf; 1990.

OPERATIONS: GENERAL

SECTION 2

CHAPTER 18

MEDICAL DIRECTOR LEADERSHIP

Thom A. Mayer, Robert W. Strauss, AnnMarie Papa

Uneasy lies the head that wears the crown.

—William Shakespeare, *Henry IV*[1]

The emergency department (ED) medical director role is among the most sought after and least understood in all of medicine because people assume it is stimulating, rewarding, and gratifying. However, many who have held the position found it to be difficult, thankless, demanding, and even demeaning. The job of coordinating multidisciplinary services provided by a diverse group of clinicians in a capacity-constrained environment requires talent, energy, and enthusiasm. By nature, EDs are complex adaptive systems that require their leaders to adopt a systems approach.[2] Successful directors are:

- *Leaders* who collaborate, share compelling visions, provide guidance and mentoring, support organizational alignment, delegate authority, act as role models, and mentor the team
- *Managers* who accomplish critical tasks, develop and implement improvement strategies, provide clinical expertise, set standards, ensure compliance, obtain and provide feedback, conduct meetings, handle complaints, provide a framework to attain metrics goals, and recruit, orient, hire, and fire employees
- *Innovators* who challenge the status quo, generate new ideas, problem-solve creatively, and courageously go where other physicians may not care to venture

Although challenging, successfully guiding the development of a high-performing ED can result in gratifying improvements in patient care, effective development and growth of staff, and personal and professional development of the director. Regardless of the size, sophistication, and level of service provided in the ED, effective physician and nursing leadership is necessary for success. In the current health-care environment, sound leadership and management skills are required to provide the appropriate training, resources, facilities, and staff to deliver quality patient care and caring. The ED medical director must work collaboratively with other leaders and managers, including the nursing leader, to achieve at least two goals:

1. Develop systems and processes that consistently provide good outcomes for ED patients. These must work in the absence of senior or middle management and function effectively 24 hours a day, 7 days a week.
2. Design systems and processes that consider and incorporate both the interests of clinical patient care and the needs of the providers responsible for that care. Stress and burnout can in part be attributed to failure to address the needs of the providers and staff.

More succinctly stated, the two goals are to *make our patients' lives better and make our jobs easier.* Superficially, the ED medical director appears to be a position of power, control, and authority. Nothing could be farther from reality. In fact, the critical competencies necessary for success in this rapidly changing health-care environment are collaboration, cooperation, empowerment, alignment of incentives, and stewardship.[3]

Robert Greenleaf, an authority on the concept of servant leadership, noted that effective leaders of multidisciplinary teams must be "influencers" who are capable of helping guide, rather than control, others' behavior.[4] *When faced with the choice of power or influence, always choose influence.* In emergency medicine, we can influence others by using the "voice of the patient"; those who use it well will effectively influence others.

THE TRANSITION FROM PHYSICIAN-PROVIDER TO PHYSICIAN-LEADER

The difficult and daunting job of the ED medical director requires an effective transition from a clinical care provider to a physician-leader. Physician-managers must possess the talents, skills, and techniques needed to both provide and coordinate clinical and administrative services.

Management is doing things right; leadership is doing the right things.

—Warren Bennis[5]

Multiple Interdependent Processes

The transition from a skilled clinician to a talented leader is difficult. Consider these differences:

- The skilled clinician provides excellent care to *one patient at a time* and effectively navigates through the multiple, cross-functional processes involved in even the simplest of patient encounters.[6]
- The talented leader affects *all ED patients* and staff and improves patient care by collaborating with others, establishing goals, empowering staff, measuring processes, creating rapid cycle corrective actions, providing feedback, rewarding excellence, addressing deficiencies (people and processes), communicating progress, and performing (as the small print says) "other duties as assigned!"

The specific interdependent tasks and processes that clinicians and leaders must address include prehospital care, triage, registration, resource allocation, diagnostic evaluation (including ancillary services), therapeutic interventions, patient and family education, discharge processing, consultation, and admission to the hospital (**Box 18.1**).[7,8] If any critical step in this multitude of processes is performed incompletely or ineffectively, the patient or family may not care how well the other functions were performed.

In the ED environment, designing a system that allows 999 of 1,000 processes to function correctly is a recipe for failure, not success. It is not surprising that multitasking and process improvement are taught to leaders outside health care in a game known as "Friday night at the ER."[9] This game teaches systems thinking through a series of practical choices. The participants "learn to collaborate and innovate while considering the effects of their actions on the larger system." In particular, the game teaches the critical leaderships skills of:

- Applied systems thinking
- Collaboration across boundaries
- Smart innovation
- Data-driven decision-making
- Designing structures for desired behavior

> **BOX 18.1 ■ AMERICAN BOARD OF EMERGENCY MEDICINE LIST OF TASKS**
>
> **Emergency physicians simultaneously consider multiple factors that may alter the direction of patient management.**[6]
>
> - Prehospital care
> - Emergency stabilization
> - Performance of focused history and physical examination
> - Modifying factors
> - Professional issues
> - Diagnostic studies
> - Diagnosis
> - Therapeutic interventions
> - Pharmacotherapy
> - Observation and reassessment
> - Consultation
> - Transitions of care
> - Prevention and education
> - Documentation
> - Multiple patient care
> - Team management
> - Mass casualty and disaster management
> - Patient-centered communication skills
> - Prognosis

By nature, health care is prone to "functional siloing," a term first coined by Phillip Ensor to describe potentially divergent goals and processes within an organizational unit.[10] The complex interrelationships between the various elements and providers may go unrecognized, resulting in ineffective service transitions during the multiple clinical encounters. Emergency departments are organized across at least four distinct yet interrelated functions, which usually report through different vertical structures (**Table 18.1**). Within these core functions are other essential providers, including unit secretaries, ED technicians, housekeeping, security personnel, volunteers, and social workers. Although ED operations consist of vertical silos, the patient moves through the clinical encounter in a horizontal, process-oriented fashion. Managing the clinical

TABLE 18.1 ■ Traditional ED Organization

The goal of all members of the interdisciplinary team is efficient, quality patient care. However, each type of provider reports to a different hospital administrator, and each of the administrative leaders may have different goals.

ED Staff Provider	Function	Direct Report	Admin Leader
Emergency physician	Provide clinical care and coordination of medical resources	ED medical director	Chief Medical Officer
Emergency nurse	Perform triage and primary nursing functions, implement physician orders, apply critical thinking skills, and coordinate nursing resources	ED nursing director	Chief Nursing Officer
Essential services personnel	Provide laboratory, imaging, and other essential services	Imaging, lab director	Chief Operations Officer
Registration personnel	Obtain demographic and financial information, manage hospital admissions and bed control	ED registration director	Chief Financial Officer

FIGURE 18.1 ■ FUNCTIONAL SILOS

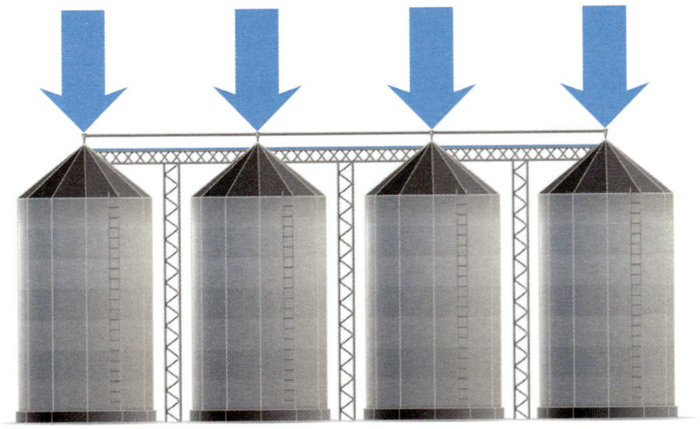

Patients often assume that the components of the ED (e.g., nursing, physician, registration, lab, radiology) exist as separately functioning silos. To avoid this misperception, the medical and nursing directors must make sure their multiple service transitions are filled by "A-team processes" in which these changes are anticipated and effectively managed.

encounter across these cross-functional processes is at the heart of the ED medical and nursing directors' roles.

The leader should ensure the functional silos are filled with "A-team processes" (**Figure 18.1**). These processes include handoffs from nursing (triage) to registration to nursing (assessment) to the physician (evaluation and treatment) to nursing (treatment) to essential services (imaging, lab, respiratory therapy, etc.) and then back to nursing (treatment and reevaluation) to the physician (reassessment and disposition) to nursing (disposition). Because each handoff relies on complex interactions, efficient care requires each transition to operate in a seamless, "boundaryless" manner (**Figure 18.2**). In other words, highly organized, well-designed systems fill the functional silos with "A-team processes."[11]

Medical Directors Must Lead

An essential competency of an ED medical director is the ability to work in a collegial and cooperative fashion with other leaders, both within and outside the department. Although the importance of the physician director–nurse director relationship is discussed in detail in other sections of this book, it must be emphasized that this critical relationship is the most

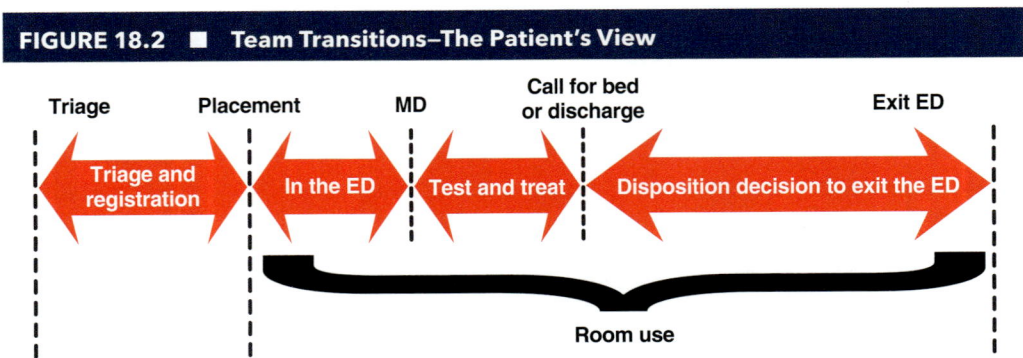

FIGURE 18.2 ■ Team Transitions–The Patient's View

important partnership in the entire ED. Continually cultivating this relationship requires a substantial commitment of time, effort, and energy to ensure communication, collaboration, integrity, and mutual accord.

The physician and nurse directors should strive to develop a common:

- Mission, vision, and values for the ED
- Philosophy of leadership and management
- Understanding of the working relationship among team members

The medical and nursing leaders should meet frequently and formally (preferably weekly) to discuss departmental operations, problems, and future directions. Beyond the formal meetings, each must commit to inform the other of any issues or problems that may affect the ED, its patients, and providers. These communications should occur on a timely basis and can occur by means of telephone, voicemail, e-mail, memos, texts, or informal face-to-face meetings. The relationship between the two leaders should be highly supportive both during private discussions concerning ED operations and in related communications to other team members. Similarly, the ED medical director must work cooperatively with leaders and managers in other departments, so interdepartmental services and processes can be coordinated smoothly and proactively.

QUALIFICATIONS

The medical director's qualifications may vary based on the size and type of ED. For example, the specific qualifications required to lead a 100-bed ED in an academic teaching institution with 120,000 annual visits are different from those required to lead a 15-bed ED in a 250-bed community hospital with 25,000 annual visits. Nonetheless, several essential characteristics should be sought in every ED medical director (**Box 18.2**).

Clinical Skills

The ED medical director should be board certified in emergency medicine. Although the supply of board-certified emergency physicians is lower than the demand, even small hospitals in rural settings should seek a board-certified physician to oversee and lead the ED. For children's hospitals, the ED director should be board certified (Certificate of Added Qualifications, or CAQ) in pediatric emergency medicine, an examination jointly administered by the American Board of Pediatrics and the American Board of Emergency Medicine (ABEM).

BOX 18.2 ■ MEDICAL DIRECTOR QUALIFICATIONS

Clinical Qualifications

- Demonstrated clinical excellence
- American Board of Emergency Medicine certification or eligibility
- Ability to deliver performance metrics
- Use of clinical guidelines
- Commitment to personal education and professional growth

Personal Qualifications

- Leadership skills and experience
- Ability to build teams
- Communication skills
  - Written
  - Verbal
  - Listening
- Integrity and intellectual honesty

Board certification in emergency medicine or pediatric emergency medicine ensures baseline clinical competence and indicates the director has completed stringent training and peer review that addresses the multiple problems faced as a director. Although the medical director should be a respected and experienced clinician, the director does not need to be the best clinician in the group. In fact, mature physician-leaders often surround themselves with highly qualified clinicians, any one of whom may be able to outshine the director in a given clinical area.

Completion of various protocol-oriented courses as a qualification can be a source of contention for emergency physicians. Some hospitals and health-care systems consider certification in Advanced Trauma Life Support, Advanced Cardiac Life Support, and Advanced Pediatric Life Support courses essential for emergency physicians. Conversely, ABEM has a standing "Policy on Third Party Standards" that affirms:

> *ABEM unequivocally states that ABEM certification and ABEM MOC supersedes any perceived need for credentials that are established by third party standards. Specifically, it is unnecessary for an ABEM-certified physician who is actively participating in ABEM MOC to also acquire and maintain credentialing by third parties through short courses such as Advanced Pediatric Life Support (APLS), Advanced Cardiac Life Support (ACLS), or Advanced Trauma Life Support (ATLS), in addition to a specific number of CME hours in a specified content area of Emergency Medicine.*[12]

In fact, in May 2018, the American College of Surgeons agreed:

> *The American College of Surgeons Committee on Trauma (ACS-COT) recently revised the criteria for trauma CME for trauma centers. Effective immediately, certified physicians from any ABMS Member Board with an MOC program that includes sufficient trauma content will not need to acquire trauma CME credits. ABEM and every major EM organization submitted the trauma content of ABEM's MOC Program and it was found to meet this standard, so ABEM-certified physicians participating in MOC no longer need to fulfill the ACS-COT trauma center verification trauma-related CME requirement.*[13]

Nonetheless, hospital policy and regulatory requirements (e.g., Level I Trauma Center verification) guide certification in these courses. Regardless of certification requirements in such courses, knowledge of their precepts and protocols may help guide the medical director's departmental education programs. Further, some ED leaders may seek to attain instructor-level status because it can be beneficial to the department's public relations, perceptions among the medical staff, and educational functions.

Leadership Skills and Experience

The successful medical director effectively addresses problems by:

- Actively seeking out potential problems
- Thoroughly investigating, critically analyzing, and accurately describing factors constituting those problems
- Clearly and effectively communicating the causes of the problems
- Objectively and sensitively recommending appropriate solutions
- Assiduously following through on recommendations for continuous improvement and innovation

Attaining skills through previous experience as a medical director can be helpful, although it is not a requirement. However, developing the mind-set of a physician-manager is essential. This approach entails learning, collaboration, empowerment, and motivation.

Management training itself can be attained through a variety of programs, including masters' programs, readings in the management literature, and courses offered by the American Association for Physician Leadership, the American College of Emergency Physicians Emergency Department Directors Academy, and business schools, some of which offer programs designed specifically for physician executives, for example, executive MBA programs.

Clear Communication

The medical director must have excellent written, verbal, and listening communication skills.

Written Skills

The director should be an effective, concise writer, capable of reducing issues to a single page that outlines the problem, addresses its components, and suggests potential solutions in a focused fashion. Good editing skills, brevity, and clarity of thought are requirements for effective leadership. Physician managers should also be aware of both the positive and negative "power of the carbon copy."

- *Positive*: Issues that cross departmental (divisional) boundaries should be copied to representatives of the affected departments to ensure the awareness of those who need to know. Written records of any important verbal conversations should be maintained. Whether the conversation has been in person, by e-mail, or via telephone, a brief communication summarizing the issue and its resolution creates a paper (or e-mail) trail documenting the manner in which issues are being addressed.
- *Negative*: A negatively interpreted comment sent by e-mail or text, written memo, or left as a phone message and received by or forwarded to the "wrong" person can create significant unintended consequences. Once delivered, the sender has no control over the message. For this reason, thoughtful and careful editing of all communications should ensure there are no personal attacks, blaming, or harmful or injurious comments that could be negatively perceived as an ad hominem attack. When addressing areas of deficiency, failed service, or other performance issues, the facts can usually be presented in a way that speaks to the issue and remains factual, nonblaming, and dispassionate. *Attacks on a problem, properly framed and communicated, can be helpful. Attacks on people seldom are.*

Verbal Skills

The verbal abilities of the medical director can be determined by the manner in which the physician handles both bedside communication with patients and their families and communication with care providers.

Verbal communication should always be imbued with a profound respect for the person's value. For example, consider what messages the speaker delivers to the listener and how the listener may perceive the speaker with these different statements:

- "Mrs. Smith in bed 3 with abdominal pain" versus "The belly pain in . . ."
- "Mr. Jones with chronic pain syndrome in room 15" versus "The chronic drug abuser in . . ."

To some, this level of communication may seem unimportant; however, patients, their families, and ED staff readily notice such thoughtful verbal communication.

TABLE 18.2 ■ Active Listening

Active listening increases the listener's retention from 25% to over 80% and is substantially more likely to get to the speaker's true intent. One tool to accomplish this is to repeat the last words or phrase you heard, which may encourage the speaker to expand on what was said.

Repeat the last word or phrase said to you.	**Patient:** "And the worst thing is that I was in so much pain." **You:** "Pain?"
Then listen more.	**Patient:** "Yes, it was unbearable, no one seemed to care!" **You:** "No one cared?" **Patient:** "They didn't, and that was what offended me most."

Additionally, staff members who begin to depersonalize patients stop seeing them as people with problems who have sought care and expertise from the providers. Rather, they begin to see the patients as obligations that make the provider's day more difficult. These negative perceptions occur slowly, but they inexorably lead to frustration and burnout.[14] The medical director therefore should both have and insist on the utmost professionalism in all verbal communications, whether in clinical or management settings.

Listening Skills

Many managers believe they are expected to have all the answers; in fact, most people would prefer someone who can listen intently and in an open fashion. In many cases, the listener should repeat what has been heard to ensure that effective communication of the issues has occurred.

Effective listening requires *active* listening (**Tables 18.2** and **18.3**). When a speaker has a one-sided conversation with another person, the listener is passively listening. Multiple studies indicate that passive listening results in less than 25% retention of what is said. However, if the listener actively listens, retention rises to nearly 80%.[15]

TABLE 18.3 ■ The Five Whys

Patient	Service Recovery Leader
"I was very unhappy with my ED visit."	"Why?"
"The quality of care was horrible!"	"Why?"
"Communication was poor."	"Why do you say that?"
"They didn't contact the right doctor."	"Why was that an issue for you?"
"I wanted them to call the Kaiser doctor."	"Why?"
"My insurance won't pay for this on-call doctor." (An apparent quality issue now appears to be a payment issue.)	

For example, consider the perceptions, understanding, and retention of patients and family members when the ED staff member provides the following discharge instructions:

A. *"This is what you should do when you leave . . ."*

B. *"Discharge instructions are very important. We want to be sure that you understand what you should do when you leave . . ."*

C. *"Discharge instructions are very important. We want to be sure that you understand what you should do when you leave . . . Because these instructions are important to your continuing improvement, I would like you to repeat the instructions back to me just to be sure that you understand."*

With scenario A, the patient may not focus closely on or realize the importance of the instructions. With scenario B, the patient may pay more attention, but the clinician does not know if the patient understands the instructions. By repeating the instructions in scenario C, the patient will demonstrate their understanding and the clinician can be certain that the patient has listened if they repeat the instructions correctly. Instruction C is the best tool to ensure the patient is listening and to assure the patient that *you* are listening.

Another tool of active listening is the "Five Whys" first promoted by Sakichi Toyoda, the founder of Toyota.[16] As **Table 18.3** demonstrates, continuing to ask "why" helps the listener drill down to the root cause of the problem in a way that simply asking "why" once cannot accomplish.

Patients may get a patient satisfaction survey, which may include questions such as:

- *"Were you given discharge instructions?"*
- *"Did the staff care about you as a person?"*

If the staff consistently uses "A," the patients might answer both questions as "No." If the staff consistently uses "B," the patient would likely say "Yes," they were given "discharge instructions." However, the patients might not understand their instructions. If the staff consistently uses "C," the patients are involved in active, not passive, listening and they are far more likely to understand and retain that understanding. With C, the patients will probably answer both survey questions with a "Yes" and give high scores.

Integrity

Although qualifications are specific and quantifiable, perhaps the most important characteristics possessed by a medical director (as with most leaders) are integrity and intellectual honesty. Medical directors must often make difficult judgments, astutely assess complex interpersonal relationships, and acknowledge and address existing deficiencies of the ED staff and operational processes. Confidentiality, trust, and maturity are the attributes that personnel respect most, and yet these characteristics cannot be easily measured. The medical director should have a strong sense of personal worth, decency, and integrity to deal successfully with the problems inherent to the job.

Intellectual honesty is another critically important attribute. To defend the ED, its practitioners, or its processes, some leaders find fault with or lay blame on others outside the department. The intellectually honest leader recognizes that some problems do belong with the physician group, an individual physician, a faulty internal process, or the medical director. The effective medical director starts with an open mind, seeks out and investigates problems, and, when appropriate, accepts responsibility for problems that originate in the ED. Under such circumstances, having the integrity to acknowledge and address the issue will gain respect throughout the institution.

Charles Stokes, the CEO of Memorial Hermann Health System, believes that personal integrity is the most important asset for a leader at any level of health care. The ability to integrate the "passion of the heart with the intellect of the head" will always be valued by those driven to succeed in health care.[17]

Specific Roles

An ED medical director must share responsibility and collaborate with nursing and other leaders to ensure that the ED:

- Is committed to excellence
- Has a fair and reasonable management structure
- Focuses on constant improvement
- Continues to be responsive to the needs of its patients and their care providers

To accomplish these critical elements, the ED's leadership must achieve four primary goals:

- Establish and manage the boundaries of the organization.
- Provide a constant commitment to excellence and quality.
- Ensure superb customer service.
- Develop the providers and staff (hold clinicians accountable for quality, defined in highly specific and measurable ways).

MANAGING THE BOUNDARIES OF THE ORGANIZATION

The ED medical director must begin by assessing the core purposes, functions, and processes of the ED, as well as its vision, mission, and values (see Chapter 2). For instance, the director must ask if the primary purpose of the ED is to be a:

- Community hospital resource for convenience care?
- Level I trauma center?
- Pediatric emergency regional resource?
- Gatekeeper for primary care physicians and managed care organizations for after-hours care?
- Regional tertiary care resource?
- All or combinations of the above?

These and many other questions must be asked and answered collaboratively to ensure that leaders, managers, and providers of clinical care have a clear understanding of the boundaries and purpose of the ED.

These boundaries create both constraints and opportunities to achieve excellence and therefore must be discussed with the administration, medical staff, and hospital governance structure. Ensuring consistency in the vision of the ED's function aligns goals, encourages development of a strategic plan, and permits discussion about the resources necessary to achieve those goals (see Chapter 5). Virtually all EDs are undergoing constant change; therefore, the boundaries of the organization are subject to iterative revision.

In addition to establishing departmental boundaries, the ED medical director also must have a clear sense of the boundaries of his or her specific job. These boundaries are largely defined by two important sources: hospital administration and the emergency physician group.

Current Assessment

Establishing boundaries must always begin with an accurate assessment of the current state of the organization and the intended goals of the ED medical director and department leadership. This assessment requires a clear understanding of the core businesses of the ED. Substantial data must be obtained, including a statistical analysis of acuity of care, percentage of patients admitted to the hospital, financial pay or mix, effect of managed care, and so on, to understand how the department's revenue is generated.

Once data are gathered, it is important to determine the financial, physical, and human resources required to provide the intended services. Examples of resources include the physical plant, nursing resources, technicians, ED physicians, core secretaries, registration personnel, equipment and supplies, the operational budget, and other essential services (e.g., radiology, lab).

Gap Analysis

The gap analysis clarifies the adequacy of current resources when matched against the identified core business goals, that is, the organizational boundaries established by the administration, medical staff, and ED leadership. For example, if prompt ED care is a stated goal (core business), but the resources are insufficient to deliver this goal (i.e., inadequate space and staff), this resource–goal mismatch (gap) requires an objective, open, and honest discussion of the problem.

Short-Term Goals

To address recognized gaps, ED leaders must establish initial goals of the ED. Succinctly stated, "What needs to be done now?" Defining immediate goals requires support from the ED's internal and external stakeholders. Once short-term goals are determined, the ED medical director must ask the difficult question, "What magnitude of change is required to complete these goals?" Change of any magnitude requires a clear understanding of change management and its principles (see Chapter 3).

When involving the stakeholders, the leader should determine the current culture of the organization by asking the following questions:

- What are the primary mind-sets and decision-making processes of the organization's leaders?
- Are the organization's imperatives derived from quality improvement and management-by-objective concepts of learning organizations, lean engineering, and so on?

After completing the current assessment and designing a plan for initial changes, a wise leader chooses conservative, attainable goals. Leaders who try to accomplish too much too quickly are destined for frustration and failure. It may have taken years to establish the current processes and habits and the leader must understand the "why" of the current approach. Otherwise, an enthusiastic yet injudicious medical director will likely encounter many unforeseen hurdles and face many failures.

Selecting smaller, easier changes that improve the caregivers' ability to provide care—and makes their jobs easier—builds a foundation for success and enthusiasm for future changes. Leaders should involve those who are responsible for implementing change early in the process: "If they are not with you on the takeoff, they won't be with you on the landing."[18] The success of a change process depends far less on the energy, enthusiasm, and skills of the leader, who is only one person, than on that leader's ability to empower, motivate, and steward the staff to deliver effective and meaningful change.

Stakeholder Analysis and Boundary Management

Stakeholder analysis and boundary management are two closely related tools that can help the ED medical director define the boundaries of the organization. Boundary management may be further differentiated by boundary types.

Stakeholder Analysis

This analysis simply identifies the key stakeholders, delineates their "stake" or interests in an issue, seeks their input, and enlists their support for the necessary process changes. This tool requires a clear understanding of the process, its component parts, and recognition of organizational dynamics (including resistance to change).

Boundary Management

Older style or "traditional" boundaries of organizations are structured along areas of function, hierarchy, and geography. These "hard-wired" boundaries create rigid structures and limit innovation. This inflexible organizational approach has one advantage: Managers and employees within the structure usually have roles that are simple, clear, and relatively stable, even if they are not particularly functional.

Eliminating boundaries can enhance programs. In the 1990 General Electric Corporation Annual Report, CEO Jack Welch described his vision of "A boundaryless company where we knock down the walls that separate us from each other on the inside and from our key constituencies on the outside."[19] Welch recognized the need for an organization where vertical hierarchies are replaced with horizontal, functional networks and in which cross-functional teams participated with suppliers and customers to improve services.

"Seamless" and "boundaryless" operations have emerged, and new types of functional boundaries replaced older, traditional, less functional boundaries. Business consultants Larry Hirschhorn and Thomas Gilmore define these new boundaries as *authority, task, identity* (sentient), and *political* (**Table 18.4**).[20]

TABLE 18.4 ■ Key Boundaries and Their Implications

Boundary	Key Issues	Sharing Factors	Skills
Authority	Control, accountability	• Number of levels • Culture of "direct talk" • Delegation practices	• Setting and accepting limits • Letting go • Challenging colleagues and leaders • Absorbing risk and uncertainty
Task	Productivity, effectiveness	• Division of labor • Work design • Organization design • Customer requirements	• Linking data to performance • Balancing integration and specialization
Sentient	Loyalty, identity	• Professional groupings • Cultural identities • Regional ties • Group identifications	• Promoting identification, avoiding groupthink • Understanding stereotyping
Political	Rewards, equity, and security	• Differing interests • Power distribution	• Negotiating differences • Linking conflict to collaboration • Understanding the dynamics of bargaining, gaming

Authority Boundary

The authority boundary seeks to determine "Who is in charge of what? What am I authorized to do?" In traditional organizations, those in authority, "the bosses," were easy to identify. They issued the orders that the workers followed. Even though those closest to the product or service could often ascertain a better way, they were not usually given the opportunity to share the improvement and, in fact, were discouraged from doing so. More flexible organizational leaders understand that the individual with formal authority is not necessarily the one closest to the delivery of the service and often does not have the most up-to-date information about a given patient or customer need.

This authority boundary can be seen in the relationship between the ED nurse and physician. The nurse spends substantially more time with the patient and often knows more about how the patient feels, what the response has been to therapy, and the concerns of and interactions with the family. The physician, who has more authority over the management of the patient, does not possess all the nurse's information. The care givers' approach to the authority boundary largely determines the interaction between ED physicians and nurses and may limit or enhance the communication of critical information.

When examining the authority boundary, several questions must be addressed:

- Where does the individual, process, or organization get its authority to do its work?
- How does each provider within the process or organization hold others accountable, particularly in areas of cross-functional dependency?
- Are individuals encouraged to cross "traditional" authority boundaries to communicate important information?
- Who is responsible for what aspect of patient care?
- Are these responsibilities cross-trained or are they solely delineated to specific individuals or job descriptions?

The last two questions have significant overlap with the task boundary.

Task Boundary

The fundamental question of the task boundary is "Who does what?" In the complex setting of the ED, every patient encounter requires multiple providers to complete multiple tasks under changing conditions.

In traditional EDs, the specialized and job-specific tasks performed by various staff and providers interferes with the critical need for shared communication and purpose required of the team approach—the heart of a well-functioning department. Consider a technician who responds to a request to perform an ECG by saying, "I'm not assigned to those beds." Staff and providers should coordinate their separate efforts by using known effective teamwork methodologies to overcome traditional task boundaries. High-functioning ED teams eliminate silos and create a shared understanding of purpose by adopting proven communication tools, frequent huddles, cross-training, quality improvement, and reengineering methods.

Identity Boundary

The identity boundary asks the following questions:

- Who is and isn't one of us?
- Who are the members of the ED team and what are the criteria for membership?
- What loyalties do the ED team members feel toward each other, and how strong are those loyalties?
- How clearly are the identities of the team members aligned with their purpose?

Strong identity boundaries cause individuals to trust "insiders" and become wary of "outsiders." A renewed focus on purpose increases recognition of identity boundaries, leading staff to drop this identity barrier and become more inclusive, energized, and motivated. "Team spirit" grows when identity boundaries expand. However, simply expanding who is and who is not "one of us" while maintaining a sharply defined identity boundary still risks poor relationships between the ED and "other" areas of the hospital.

Political Boundary

The fundamental question of the political boundary is "What is in it for us?" This boundary provides the context in which the ED fits with other stakeholders in the health-care system and clarifies how power is negotiated among the different stakeholder groups. Properly framed, the ED's political boundary is powerful because it is founded on patient care, interaction with the community, and interrelationships with the entire health-care organization. Although the concept of health-care politics is a negative term to some, it grows out of the interaction of the multiple internal and external stakeholders. When operating at the political boundary, staff face the challenge of defending their patients' interests and those of their department without undermining the effectiveness and coherence of the organization.

Table 18.4 summarizes the skills required to manage effectively across the authority, task, political, and identity boundaries. Emergency department leaders can effectively use boundary management and stakeholder analysis skills to accomplish the following tasks:

- Implement specific strategies.
- Address changes needed within the ED.
- Align the ED's and the organization's goals.
- Identify dysfunctional relationships.

Because of the highly cross-functional nature of ED operations, "managing across the seams" is an important ED leadership strategy.

COMMITMENT TO QUALITY

The ED leader must demonstrate a consistent, passionate, and unwavering commitment to excellence in the clinical care of patients. Although the term "quality" is perhaps overused, it essentially means "to enhance the value of the services (provided to the patient)."[21] This "lean" definition of quality is derived from a value-added, waste-eliminated perspective. Experts have defined "value" as a ratio of benefits received to the burdens endured in each phase or aspect of health care (**Box 18.3**).[22] Thus, value can be added by increasing the

---

BOX 18.3 ■ THE VALUE-ADDED EQUATION

Value in health care is often described as a ratio of quality to cost. However, for the bedside clinician, quality is assumed and cost is unknown. A more practical definition views value as a ratio of benefits received to burdens endured to receive those benefits.

- **What are the benefits received?**
    - If obvious, reaffirm them.
    - If not obvious, inform them.

- **What are the burdens endured?**
    - If necessary, explain them.
    - If unnecessary, eliminate them.

- **Would you tolerate this ratio?**

benefits, decreasing the burden, or some combination of both. The more value added, the higher the quality of the service.

Perhaps a clearer standard than "quality" is a commitment to excellence, which implies the product or service has been carefully constructed, regularly reviewed, and appropriately revised to meet the highest possible standards. However, assessing clinical excellence and quality in the ED requires substantially more effort because of the broad diversity of emergency functions performed and each department's commitment to a specific purpose. For example, an ED may be excellent at providing general medical care for undifferentiated emergencies. However, that same ED may not provide the highest standard for patients with a major traumatic injury or an ST-elevation myocardial infarction requiring emergent placement of a cardiac stent. An assessment of the existing state of clinical excellence requires, among other things, a comprehensive clinical review of charts, outcomes, staff knowledge and competence, and patient and staff satisfaction.

Resource Management in Value-Based Health Care

Effective ED medical and nursing directors manage the financial and nonfinancial resources of the department. These leaders must be capable of taking a global view of the resources required to provide excellent patient care. As our health-care system continues its journey from "volume-based" to "value-based" reimbursement, these skills will increase dramatically in importance. Population-health initiatives are also an important factor to consider in resource management in our increasingly capacity-constrained environment.[23]

For example, an ED is charged with developing a "fast-track" alternative to normal operational flow. The additional resources required to implement this program should be carefully considered. The ED medical director (along with his or her management colleagues) must ensure there is a clear vision and set of goals for the service. For instance, are the goals of the program:

- More rapid care?
- More cost-competitive care?
- After-hours gatekeeper for minor illnesses?
- A competitive alternative to urgent care centers?
- A means of "decompressing" the main ED?
- A new "profit center?"

The answers to these questions will guide the systems and processes to best deliver the service. Additionally, the leadership must determine if additional staff and space should be provided to develop such a program? If not, simply expanding the use of existing resources (both staff and space) could unintentionally lengthen turnaround times for all patients, and both "fast-tracked" patients who are not acutely ill and "non-fast-tracked" patients who are managed in the main department would have fewer resources and longer lengths of stay.

The effectiveness of resource management will determine the success or failure of the program over time. Other resource-related questions include:

- Are the system, space, and policies designed with patient input to ensure the program addresses customers' needs?
- What information systems will be put in place to track progress of the product line?
- What are the timeframes for evaluation and reassessment?

SERVICE EXCELLENCE

Patient experience and service excellence in health care have become critical goals for EDs, and they are often the most difficult to achieve and maintain. The ED medical director must ensure the staff is focused on providing efficient, compassionate, team-based care; this model works best for both patients and their caregivers.[24] Included in this group of caregivers are physicians, nurses, housekeepers, technicians, registration personnel, unit secretaries, security guards, EMS personnel, medical staff members, administrators, essential services providers, and so on. This approach expands the identity boundary. Only by working collaboratively to ensure a patient-focused service can all team members enjoyably, efficiently, and effectively take care of patients.

Service to the Patient and Family

The raison d'être of any ED is the patient (**Box 18.4**). This principle should be a part of every ED's mission statement. When designing the ED's commitment to excellence and quality, the leaders should account for the patient's interests, well-being, hopes, and expectations. Service to the patient should imbue all levels of the organization from the ED physicians and nurses to the housekeepers and security guards. Customer satisfaction leads to employee satisfaction, and aggressive customer service programs can benefit both the patient and the provider.[25]

The medical director should encourage emergency physicians to visit patients they have admitted to the hospital. These visits provide great customer service and an opportunity to monitor the patient's progress. The visit often leads to positive, collegial discussions with medical staff members, who may for the first time realize that emergency physicians care about the progress of patients and their outcome. Additionally, emergency physicians may have business cards printed, which can be shared appropriately with patients.

Service to the Administration

As financial and nonfinancial incentives become more aligned between hospitals and physicians, hospital administrators increasingly look to all hospital-based physicians to work closely and cooperatively with the needs of the institution. Most hospital administrators look to the ED medical director to ensure that operations and clinical competence in the ED are provided seamlessly. Alignment of strategic incentives is a core guiding principle in these efforts.

BOX 18.4 ■ PATIENT-FIRST PRACTICES

The mission of the ED should always start with the patient, not with those who take care of the patient.

Rule #1 - Always do the right thing for the patient.

Rule #2 - Always do the right thing for those who take care of the patient.

Rule #3 - Never confuse rule #1 with rule #2.

Administrative Liaisons

The ED medical director should meet frequently (both formally and informally) with the appropriate administrator(s) to ensure a common vision for the ED and a clear understanding of day-to-day operations. The content and timing of these meetings should be planned rather than being spontaneous. The ED medical director should consider providing a written agenda before the meeting to ensure the administrator(s) is(are) aware of the relevant issues. Stakeholder analysis and boundary management skills should be used to keep appropriate administrators informed of issues that affect their departments.

For example, in many hospitals, the administrator who is responsible for essential services (imaging, laboratory tests, bed board, and so on) plays a different role than the emergency services administrator. Because many of these interdepartmental responsibilities overlap, ED leaders are encouraged to develop collaborative relationships with non-emergency personnel. The administrator overseeing the ED should be:

- An insider (identity boundary) who perceives a strong alignment with the ED
- Included in all significant discussions
- Aware of day-to-day activities and metrics

Anything less than a feeling of being one of "us" is counterproductive and creates unnecessary barriers. To accomplish this, the administrator should be invited to selected ED staff meetings, physician group meetings, and social functions.

Whenever possible, the medical director should attend appropriate management team meetings to ensure the medical director's and the ED's perspectives are integrated into the overall operations of the hospital. Further, it provides the director with exposure to and perspective on the organization's philosophy and operational structure. As actor Woody Allen wryly noted,

80% of success is showing up!

"Rounding" with administrators includes them as part of the team and helps them understand patients' and team members' perspectives. I (Thom Mayer) had the privilege of working with a hospital CEO (Steve Brown) who was truly a "roll your sleeves up and get out and see the patient" leader. On many occasions when I was scheduled to meet in his office, I would instead call up and say, "Time for a walkie-talkie," which meant we would walk the ED and talk with the patients and staff. That gave him—and by extension the entire administrative team—a perspective that would otherwise have been impossible to obtain. Additionally, it changed the perception of the ED from an "uncaring upper-floor administration" to "an administration that seeks to understand us."

Establishing and Maintaining Credibility

The ED leader can establish leadership and management credibility by applying sound business principles to clinical practice. Whenever possible, enlisting the administrator's guidance to access management information, courses, or advice can help develop a personal and professional relationship. Medical directors should emphasize their willingness to learn additional management and administrative skills and techniques.

In times of change, learners inherit the earth, while the learned find themselves beautifully equipped to deal with a world that no longer exists.

—Eric Hoffer[25]

The medical director should encourage the other emergency physicians to spend time in common medical staff meeting areas, such as the physician lounge or lunchroom, discussing common issues and/or problems with medical staff members. Presence and discussion outside the ED allow emergency physicians to address any questions about the department and be perceived as an ordinary member of the staff. When possible, a legible copy of the ED medical record should be forwarded to the patient's private physician. This information:

- Alerts the physicians about the ED visit so they are not blindsided by a patient who believes the primary care provider should have known
- Familiarizes the physicians with the specific presentation and care delivered to their patients in the ED, including changes in management and medications
- Increases the respect for the diagnostic and therapeutic interventions provided by the emergency physicians
- Enhances the perception of the emergency physician as a consultant

Similarly, the emergency physicians should be encouraged to routinely review discharge summaries on admitted patients and copies of office notes from attending physicians.

Service to the Medical Staff

A number of factors are involved in serving the medical staff, including addressing complaints, concerns, and conflicts; recognizing boundaries, and fostering good relationships between the ED physicians and other medical staff.

Complaint Management

When complaints or concerns arise from the medical staff, the medical director must handle them immediately and objectively (see Chapter 76). Whenever possible, the attending physician and emergency physician should meet face-to-face to resolve any issues, questions, or concerns about clinical care. When broader conflicts arise between individual physicians and/or departments, the medical director must assess stakeholder issues related to the problem before confronting the complaining physician or chair. This assessment includes speaking to all parties involved and determining the facts before the discussion. Whenever possible, these quality problems should be resolved in private rather than during a large meeting, when some physicians may "grandstand" in front of an audience. The medical director should have sufficient moral character to apologize freely for mistakes made in the ED, while at the same time defending staff who may have been criticized unfairly.

Stakeholder Analysis and Boundary Management

The tools of stakeholder analysis and boundary management are effective when dealing with the medical staff. The medical director should respect and appropriately address the boundaries between and within departments. The medical director should be aware of and develop potent allies within the medical staff who can be of assistance when negotiating solutions. In particular, "premeeting jawboning" may help resolve important issues that will be subject to close votes in committee. Communication with and development of support from medical staff members before the meeting creates more nuanced and effective solutions (**Table 18.5**). The ED medical director can use these boundary management processes to develop a reputation for honesty, fairness, and common sense that is earned through positive interactions with the medical staff.

TABLE 18.5 ■ SBAR: Standardized Communication Technique to Concisely Organize Discussion on Critical Issues[26]

S	Situation	A concise statement of the issue
B	Background	A concise statement of what led to the occurrence, that is, how it happened
A	Assessment	A critical appraisal
R	Recommendation	A description of the actions that should be taken to achieve resolution

Addressing Conflicts

Despite attention to all these issues, conflicts still arise. When general conflicts occur, particularly those discussed "off the record in back hallways," remember that some medical staff members retain the dated concept of emergency physicians as hospital-based physicians who are pawns of the administration. These physicians may assume the medical director will automatically side with the hospital administration. Although the ED medical director and the physician group should be aligned strategically with the objectives of the hospital, medical directors must honestly express their opinions, even when they conflict with those of the administration, and focus on what is best for the patient and the clinical staff. The successful medical director seeks to resolve disputes in private, not in public, particularly when the ED is going to win on a given issue, to avoid subjecting the "loser" to what might be perceived as the "humiliation of defeat."

As with complaint management, areas of known staff conflict should be addressed preemptively and solved in person. Medical directors should keep hospital administrators informed about any substantial conflicts between the ED group and members of the medical staff. Although most hospital administrators understand the "patient first, caregiver second" concept, these conflicts should still be discussed with them (in advance, if possible). The administrator's advice and/or perspective can be extremely helpful in resolving difficult issues.

Checklist for Medical Staff Success

The medical director must actively manage the relationship between the ED physician group and the medical staff. Among the ways to establish a common dialogue are to:

- Identify the needs of the attending physician prospectively.
- Recognize there is a tendency to blame the ED.
- Attend executive committee, medical staff department, and hospital section or operations meetings.
- Socialize with the attending physicians.
- Respond rapidly to issues and complaints.
- Resist the temptation to immediately justify and instead commit to investigating complaints.
- Consistently treat medical staff members as respected colleagues.
- Pay close attention to stakeholder analysis and boundary management.
- Actively participate in the medical staff structure and in the county or state medical society, demonstrating a commitment to the needs of the medical community.

Service to Our Team and Ourselves

Finally, we should always remember we owe an extremely high level of service to ourselves and our team. We can show respect and service to our fellow team members in the following ways:

- Show up on time (or early), every time.
- Show up ready to work.
- Work at an acceptable pace, rising to the occasion when volume, acuity, stress, and/or complexity increases.
- Ask for input from the team members.
- Respect your nursing colleagues and other staff members in the department.
- Thank your colleagues at the end of every shift and several times during the shift.
- Do sign-out rounds at the bedside.

And we should never neglect to recognize our good fortune for having the privilege of working as an emergency physician, engaged as a leader of a team of dedicated, highly trained professionals who have the honor of caring for our patients.

Service to Emergency Nurses

As important as the other elements of service are, the single most important service is to our emergency nursing teammates with whom we have both a sacred bond—caring for patients—and a unique relationship.

INTERACTION BETWEEN EMERGENCY PHYSICIANS AND EMERGENCY NURSES

The interaction between emergency physicians and nurses is among the most complicated, confusing, and compelling in all of medicine. Only in the ED do physicians and nurses work so closely for long periods every day under varied conditions. For 8 to 12 hours at a time, teams of doctors and nurses work side by side to meet the needs of patients, their families, and the other customers of ED processes. To a significant extent, the culture, growth, and success of an ED can be gauged by the quality of the relationship between the emergency physicians and emergency nurses. Despite the significance of this working relationship, typically little explicit thought and effort are expended to understand and address how to

TABLE 18.6 ■ Differences in Physician and Nurse Perspectives

Physicians and nurses are educated and trained in fundamentally different ways, despite the common focus on patient care. The medical and nursing directors should be aware of these differences and ensure the bond between the emergency nurses and physicians is strong.

Physician Perspective	Nurse Perspective
Autonomous	Team dependent
Authoritarian	Collaborative
Hierarchical	Communicative
Intense, focused time	Expanded time
Outcomes driven	Process driven
Technical expertise	Interactive, service
Problem solver, evidence-based	Critical-thinking skills
Linear perspective	Circular perspective

work collaboratively with our ED partners to ensure the very best patient care. The Institute for Healthcare Improvement has recommended the S-B-A-R tool as an effective tool to communicate among care givers.[26]

As shown in **Table 18.6**, there are fundamental and deeply rooted differences in the ways physicians and nurses are educated. As a result, the ED medical director and nursing director must work together very closely to:

- Develop trust in each other.
- Ensure consistent values and attitudes.
- Communicate effectively with each other.
- Speak in one voice when communicating with others.
- Create a safe, complementary relationship.
- Develop integrated quality and operational programs and metrics.
- Participate in common education and training programs.
- Manage complaints and professional issues together.
- Inspire the next generation of ED leaders.

The Origins of Physician and Nursing Education and Training

American medical education has been based on an authoritarian, hierarchical educational model with relatively strict progression of the student, resident, and junior physician through the stages of education and development. Medical schools and residences have reinforced classic concepts of doling out information, procedures, and prestige based on the level of training of the student or physician. The titles themselves reflect this authoritarian structure: junior student, senior student, intern, junior resident, senior resident, chief resident, and fellow. Such hierarchic structures are also maintained during the initial phases of clinical practice, with the use of titles such as "provisional" and "active" staff members and "junior" and "senior" partner.

Physician education is highly "ends driven": The primary, driving goal is to make a specific diagnosis and offer appropriate treatment. In an increasingly technological environment, physicians have developed a near obsession to use all available technology and resources to ensure the most accurate diagnosis and provide the best available treatment. Although the means of attaining the diagnosis and treatment are important, the primary focus is on the result.

Nursing education is far less authoritarian and hierarchical in nature. Beginning in nursing school and continuing through nursing practice, the educational process is more collaborative than medical education and practice. Nursing practice is highly process driven, not ends driven, with a primary focus on the manner in which interventions are undertaken. The policies and procedure manuals of most EDs demonstrate this contrast.

- Nursing policies and procedures tend to be highly process driven, reflected in the delineation of purposes and objectives.
- Physician protocols are more algorithmic, reflecting some process orientation but almost always driven toward specific ends.

Approaches to Patient Care

Care given by emergency physicians and emergency nurses differs in the amount of time spent with the patient. Emergency physicians are usually limited to discrete, intermittent interactions with patients and their families; these interactions are always outcome- or ends focused. The questions a physician asks involve time, intensity, duration, and quality of symptoms. This staccato litany of questions uses a linear approach and includes the review of systems, past medical history, family history, and social history. These questions are often read off a specific form to ensure documentation for both medical and billing purposes.

Nursing interactions are more holistic in nature and consider the patient's clinical presentation, social problems, and family interaction. In the best of EDs, mechanisms are in

> **BOX 18.5 ■ ELEMENTS OF AN EFFECTIVE ED TEAM**
>
> - **Proactive approach:** Understand the boundaries and interactions between nurses and physicians to identify and eliminate fragmentation. Avoid divisiveness and recognize that if a problem exists in the ED, "It's *our* problem."
> - **Clear communication of desired outcomes:** Leaders should recognize interdependency and continually promote "team" collaboration and celebrate individual and group successes.
> - **Open communication lines:** In particular, emergency physicians must seek input and insight from bedside emergency nurses who generally have significant information about the patient. This process emphasizes "double-loop learning," a concept of continual feedback and information sharing described by Argyris.[29]
> - **Recognition of organizational boundaries:** Work collaboratively with nursing colleagues to develop and implement "nurse-driven, physician-approved protocols." This process respects differences, decreases boundaries, and ensures multidisciplinary input.
> - **Empowerment and stewardship:** Leaders can define the desired approach, but the ED team members must accept responsibility for "real-time" implementation. Success only occurs in a respectful, encouraging, collaborative culture.

place to ensure that communication between emergency physicians and nurses routinely reflect these interactions. Although their approaches are different, establishing shared and open communication between nurses and physicians ensures accurate and complete transmission of information and the most appropriate treatment (effective "authority boundary" management).

Creating a Patient Care Team

How can the medical and nursing directors most effectively cooperate to ensure optimal ED operations? Mutual accountability is essential.[27] The seminal work of Katzenbach and Smith provides an instructive, terse, and accurate definition: "A team is a small number of people with complementary skills who are committed to a common purpose, performance goals, and approach for which they hold themselves mutually accountable."[28]

The charge nurse and charge physician must have clearly delineated roles and responsibilities (**Boxes 18.5** and **18.6**) that establish close cooperation and ensure the

> **BOX 18.6 ■ MEDICAL DIRECTOR "UNDER FIRE"**
>
> When the medical director is facing criticism, regardless of the source, a disciplined approach to the situation must be undertaken to maximize the chances of success.
>
> - Don't take it personally: Remove the "I" from the problem.
> - Focus on the issues and interests.
>   - Listen, don't defend.
>   - Define the problem area(s).
>   - Determine the underlying cause(s).
>   - After listening, objectively restate the issue.
> - Set priorities, action plans, and timeframes.
>   - Create timeframes.
>   - Define measurements to show progress.
> - Use available resources.
> - Focus on the issues and interests.
>   - Recruit supportive stakeholders
> - Focus and follow-up.
>   - Document and share progress.
>   - Demonstrate ED leadership's role.
> - Approach problems with ferocity, equanimity, and class.

department is effectively managed on a shift-to-shift basis. Equally important, as already discussed, is a strong, supportive, and cooperative relationship between the medical and nursing directors. These two professionals must not only be role models for the staff, their collaboration should itself provide a model for the rest of the staff to follow. The trust and mutual respect built into their relationship are the essential building blocks for a strong ED.

Team-Building Strategies

What can the ED medical director and nursing director do from a practical standpoint to ensure a team approach to the physician–nurse interaction?

Proactive approach: There should be a clear understanding of the boundaries and a collaborative interaction between nurses and physicians, both at the management level and at the bedside. Leaders must invest substantial efforts to identify and eliminate fragmentation of ED operations and processes. The nonproductive language, "that's a nursing problem" or "it's a doctor problem," creates a destructive, all-too-common "zero sum mentality" form of communication.

Instead, the department should proactively establish the concept of a team of professionals working collaboratively to address the needs of both the patient and the providers. Service failures do occur. Instead of creating divisiveness, they should act to strengthen the bounds between team members, as well as the processes by which they function.

Clear communication of desired outcomes: The medical director and nursing director should clearly and concisely communicate the desired results of the team. These goals often include not only patient care but also the working relationship and interdependency of team members. Identifying and celebrating "small victories," such as complimentary letters from patients, encourage cooperative and collaborative behaviors. Medical directors should develop those who exhibit these desirable behaviors as role models for the department.

Open communication lines: Directors should encourage open communication, particularly at the bedside. Emergency nurses spend substantially more time with patients than do emergency physicians, and mature emergency physicians listen carefully to their insights, judgments, and evaluations. The ED nurses can provide critical information about a patient's clinical presentation, signs and symptoms, perceptions, response to therapy, and family situation.

From a theoretical standpoint, modern learning theory emphasizes the concept of double-loop learning, as presented by Argyris.[29] This involves continual feedback loops of information during the course of the learning process. The concept of double-loop learning lends itself to the interaction between ED nurses and physicians, that is, multiple providers obtain information from diverse sources. A double-loop learning environment helps providers to assimilate that information.

> *Example: In the course of care of a patient with congestive heart failure, the emergency physician and nurse obtain multiple inputs of information from diverse sources, including EMS providers, the patient, the family, medical records, and attending physicians. Technologic information such as the electrocardiogram, chest radiograph, pulse oximetry, BNP, and other laboratory studies are added to the baseline information. This information is shared and assimilated into the patient's ED evaluation and treatment. During the ED evaluation and therapy, both the physician and nurse constantly reassess these data points. They participate in the patient's care from similar yet different vantage points. With double-loop learning (collaboration and sharing of multiple information inputs from different sources with diverse points of view), it is possible to provide the most effective patient care in a complex environment.*

Recognition of organizational boundaries: Leaders must recognize authority, task, political, and identity boundaries (addressed previously) while focusing on outcomes, not on "who's the boss here?" The nature of the protocol-oriented approach in emergency medicine, including concepts such as advanced triage and advanced interventions, attests to the degree to which most EDs cooperate in managing boundaries on an ongoing basis. Although these protocol-oriented approaches to care are often "nurse driven," they must be "physician approved." For that reason, many organizations have titled these "physician-approved, nurse-driven protocols." This name respects and values the clinical and organizational boundaries of all involved.

While breaking down the traditional boundaries, effective ED leaders seek input from team members when redesigning processes that affect them. High-functioning EDs have a long history of enlisting input from providers to assist in process-management and quality-improvement issues.

Empowerment and stewardship: The medical and nursing directors should cooperate to create a sense of empowerment and stewardship within the ED. Although the leadership can help define the collaborative nature of the desired approach, providers must accept responsibility for managing such relationships in the midst of an ED with multiple organizational boundaries. When areas of objection or concern occur, leaders should address them immediately and in private (never at the bedside or within earshot or view of patients or family). When necessary, team members can meet with their respective nursing and physician colleagues to help resolve areas of substance.

PROVIDER DEVELOPMENT

The effective ED medical director creates an environment in which the staff can continue to grow and develop both as individuals and professionals. This leadership role requires a clear understanding of a combination of disciplines, including the principles of administrative management, departmental operations, and human-resource management.

The development of the ED providers may be the medical director's most difficult role. It requires a clear understanding of a fundamental, basic truth—personal and professional development requires a spirit of continuous improvement, which can only occur in an organization and culture that values professional growth and learning. These principles include:

- Selecting the right staff
- Orienting that staff appropriately
- Developing appropriate performance reviews
- Ensuring that retention and development programs are in place
- Providing appropriate team-building activities

Selecting and Orienting ED Team Members

If I had to pick one single attribute that is most important to whatever modest success I have been fortunate enough to attain, it would be this—I always hired people, any one of whom could outperform me in their given area of interest or expertise.

–Thom Mayer, MD[30]

The ED is a complex, process-rich environment. Working effectively to provide excellent care within that environment requires several personal and professional proficiencies, including clinical, interpersonal, and management skills. For that reason, a careful and prospective approach to the selection of the ED staff is essential for success. Several steps are required.

Clarifying Expectations

Emergency department leaders should clearly articulate expectations to all the staff. Among those expectations are the adoption of and commitment to the vision, mission, goals, and objectives of the ED. Prior to hiring any staff, these expectations (and accountabilities) should be made clear, as should elements of clinical, interpersonal, personal, and professional commitment. Concepts such as effective problem-resolution and the methods by which patient complaints are handled should be clarified. In other words, all potential ED staff should understand what the organization does, how it does it, and how it adapts to change, improvements, complaints, and adversity.

Developing Broad Support

Leaders should cultivate institutional investment and participation in the hiring process with "buy in" from stakeholder groups. Colleagues from nursing, the medical staff, and administration should interview candidates applying for more senior positions with broader or supervisory responsibilities. A candidate chosen through this process will likely have the early support of key stakeholders who are invested in the success of the individual.

From the candidate's perspective, inclusion of high-level institutional stakeholders in the interview process is a symbol of institutional commitment and a demonstration of the importance of the position. For example, if the president of the medical staff, chief executive officer of the hospital, and appropriate community members do not interview an ED medical director candidate, a clear message that the ED is not a high priority for the institution is communicated.

Interview Process

A thoroughly planned and executed interview explores important issues such as approaches to problems, leadership and governance, philosophy of care, and cultural fit with the institution. For example, a candidate who has a high degree of authoritarian, hierarchical need for control will likely fail in an institution that believes in a highly participatory, shared accountability model of operations. In most cases, the interviews should be summarized, preferably in writing, to allow those responsible for selecting the ED staff members to have input and communicate their own reasons for favoring one candidate over another.

In the long-term, the "fit" of the candidate will be in large part dependent on the match of the candidate's aspirations/desire for growth and the opportunities the organization offers that individual. Often the interview process can help the medical and nursing directors to identify areas in which growth and development of an individual might be necessary. A particularly helpful question that can be used when selecting ED staff (after an initial bond exists) is: "What is the worst thing I am going to hear about you, and from whom will I hear it?" The thoughtfulness and reflection inherent in the answer can be helpful in the selection of the "right" personnel.

It's also important to ask, "What's the nurses' facial expression when they see *your name* on the schedule?" That not only tells the candidate that interactions with nurses are critical to success in your ED, it also implies that you will be asking that question when you call their former place of employment or residency program.

Orientation

Orientation should be handled with a great deal of prospective thought and guided by clearly established policies. New providers should work one to two shifts with another provider to learn practical approaches to operational processes in the ED, including its flow and staffing patterns, relationship to the medical staff, use of essential services (imaging and lab), interaction with EMS, back-up plans, EMR, IT support, and so on.

Performance Review

After the initial integration of new staff into the department, leaders can conduct performance reviews that provide the practitioner with feedback about progress and impressions. These should occur at least at 1-, 3-, 6-, and 12-month intervals.

The concept of performance reviews has undergone considerable revision over the last several years. The Joint Commission requires physicians to undergo Ongoing Professional Practice Evaluation as part of the re-credentialing process. "Traditional" performance reviews assess the practitioner's compliance with pre-established standards laid out by the organization. These types of reviews use clearly defined categories by which the individual is evaluated. However, experts have questioned the utility of such traditional performance reviews and their potentially negative outcomes on organizations and the individuals evaluated by them.[31] Such performance reviews are controlling, confining, and ineffective. Organizational consultant Peter Block suggests, "We need a reward system that gives preference to service over self-interest."[3]

He recommends three essential elements to help develop a performance-review system that emphasizes stewardship over power and control. The performance review should:

- *Affirm the purposes of the organization,* including its commitment to excellence, the boundaries of the organization, and the development of the providers with whom the individual works.
- *"Share the wealth" of the organization.* In many cases, pay increases themselves depend on the results of the performance review. However, such reviews are increasingly structured to help individuals expand their personal and professional horizons, and to maintain or increase financial compensation. To further align the individual with the organizational goals, some organizations have incorporated gain sharing, cross-training compensation, and equity options.
- *Drop the cloak of secrecy.* Secrecy about performance reviews may be a manifestation of structural inequities. Performance reviews should be regularly shared with staff members and daily feedback should be provided to the staff to reaffirm the overall purposes of the organization. Performance reviews should simply confirm or summarize the period under review, with specific attention given to prospective goals and objectives for the individual, team, department, and institution.

Provider Retention and Development

Effectively managed EDs seek providers who are responsible, innovative, and motivated by commitment to and satisfaction from providing daily ED care to patients. The cost of turnover is extremely high among professionals and is estimated to be at least 1.5 to 2 times the actual salary of the practitioner. Emergency provider groups will benefit by ensuring the right staff members are selected and a provider retention and development program is in place. The provider group should establish long-range goals that facilitate interchange among individuals to address several different areas, including the following:

- Daily work demands and stresses
- Job security
- Wages
- Benefits
- Provision of adequate leadership
- Equity and parity in participation
- Professional status
- Support for professionals and their families
- Personal and professional development

The ED medical director should have a formal individualized provider retention and development structure. Individualized retention programs recognize and incorporate the specific needs of each member on the ED team. For example, a physician might wish to maximize short-term earnings to address burdensome loans, whereas another physician might have more interest in maximizing long-term earning to create wealth, ensure job security, and plan for retirement or children's education. The provider retention and development program must be adapted over time to meet the changing needs of the group members.

Counseling, Discipline, and Dismissal

Building an excellent team of clinicians requires creating a learning organization, selecting the right staff, orienting them appropriately, and helping them coalesce as a team. However, counseling, discipline, and even dismissal of staff are sometimes necessary. Counseling and discipline of ED providers must be handled in a professional, fair, and equitable manner. All related discussions should be held in private to ensure confidentiality.

Minor differences among staff may often be settled quickly and without significant leadership involvement. For example, if a practice habit causes annoyance or dismay to particular doctors or nurses, those professionals should be encouraged to resolve those issues directly and at the time they occur, rather than involving leadership and dealing with it later. "Keeping small problems small" is an important strategy in the ED environment.

More significant problems, such as the enforcement of counseling or disciplinary procedures, must be handled impartially and in a consistent manner. Otherwise, the staff may conclude that discipline is being used in a punitive fashion only against specific members of the staff. A perception of an unfair and biased disciplinary process has a deleterious effect on ED operations and morale. If "favorites" of the medical or nursing director are perceived to "get away with" behaviors for which others are disciplined, those "unfairly" treated may seek employment elsewhere.

Complaints and concerns: Each complaint should be addressed objectively and directly with the individual at or near the time it occurs, and always within a few days of being informed. When managers do not inform an individual about complaints until they are a certain number or severity, the staff member may correctly state: "You never told me about this and I could have dealt with it right away."

While some ED leaders believe they are doing the staff member a favor by not sharing minor complaints, most staff members believe the leaders are withholding important information. Consider the points of view of a staff member when confronted by the director who makes one of the following statements:

- "I just received a complaint about the interaction that you had with... Let's discuss it and figure out a way to address it." (Message: "My director is trying to help... she's on my side.")
- "I've gotten six complaints about your care and patient interactions over the last few months. Most of them relate to your attitude... the most complaints in the group... this issue must be addressed." (Message: "My director didn't tell me before this became so serious... he's not really on my side.")

Written documentation describing the nature and type of complaint or concern should be provided to the professional. Individual staff members should get timely information about the complaints, their type and frequency, and group comparison data.

Counseling and disciplinary procedures: Considerable thought must be given to the counseling and disciplinary procedures. In most hospitals, a clearly defined Human Resources policy governs the disciplinary process for employees but may be less clear for independent contractors or employees of a contracted group. If the institution's policies do not fully address the emergency providers, then the group should develop their own. All such policies typically progress along specified steps:

1. Verbal warning
2. Written warning
3. Counseling and corrective actions
4. Termination

Although it may not be necessary for the physician group to have precisely the same approach as the hospital, some sense of parity should exist between the physician and nursing structures, particularly regarding process and severity.

When contract termination or reassignment of a provider is necessary, several specific steps should be followed closely:

1. Obtain appropriate legal advice whenever considering contract termination. Attorneys can help ensure the appropriate process is followed, documentation is in place, and thought has been given to other alternatives.
2. Document the events leading up to the decision. Contract law in the appropriate jurisdiction should be researched to ensure substantial compliance.
3. Think the process through carefully yet quickly. Questions medical directors should ask themselves include the following:
    - Am I being fair?
    - Is this in the best interest of:
        - ☐ patient care?
        - ☐ the physician group?
        - ☐ the hospital?
        - ☐ the individual physician?
    - Are there any other alternatives to contract termination that would definitively resolve the issue?

Termination: When contract termination is necessary, the medical director should provide advance notice to key stakeholders, such as the administrator, chief of staff, and ED nursing director, and ensure absolute confidentiality outside of the "need to know" circle. The information must not reach the physician before the medical director directly informs him or her. Once the decision to terminate is made, it is usually best to move quickly yet judiciously with considerable prospective thought regarding the following:

- With whom will I review the situation and the approach to termination?
- How will the information be communicated to the provider?
- What is going to occur?
- What alternatives are available?
- What effect will the contract termination have on the corporation, the team, and the individual?

Such news should be delivered in person with a witness present, particularly if the information is unexpected or the situation inflammatory. When the actual meeting occurs, sharing the information about the reasons for termination may depend on the type of termination. If the termination is "without cause," a minimalist approach is often best; that is, "Unfortunately this is not a good fit and we are exercising our right to 'terminate without cause' as described in paragraph 7C of our contract with you . . ."

If the termination is "for cause," then it may be appropriate to briefly lay the appropriate groundwork but move to the termination itself in a rapid fashion. When explaining the "for cause" reasons for the termination, address the behavior, documented clinical deficits, or the problem, not the person. The medical director should be firm in his or her decision, unless the individual presents serious reasons for reconsideration.

Reconsideration is unusual because a contract is terminated generally only when all other alternatives have been exhausted. The medical director should outline the plan for completion of duties or activities and assist the practitioner, to a "reasonable" extent, in the transition to a new position. A concise and direct written letter should summarize the meeting, including a description of how the contractual relationship will end and any agreed-on transition period.

Once the contract-termination meeting has occurred, the medical director must be aware of the potential reactions of other staff members. It may be appropriate to let others know of the separation while protecting the confidentiality of the physician terminated. Hearing from the director may be helpful because contract terminations generally cause substantial concern or turmoil among other team members who may be approached for support by the terminated individual. The medical and nursing director should work carefully on any staff termination to help address such boundary-management issues.

Personal Development

The medical director is responsible for establishing a program for the personal development of the ED team. For instance, the Inova Fairfax Hospital ED management developed the Emergency Department Survival Skills course to meet this need. This and other similar courses recognize that emergency medicine requires a specific set of abilities beyond clinical competence to provide high-quality clinical and customer care and ensure the long-term viability of the providers.

Effective training teaches customer service, stress recognition and management, conflict resolution, time management, communication skills, and team building. Although these skills are primarily directed at the ED professional environment, they often help guide individuals in their personal lives as well. A successful program reduces patient complaints, improves customer satisfaction, and enhances employee satisfaction and retention.

Whether or not a formal professional and personal training approach is in effect, the ED medical director, in collaboration with the ED nursing director, should make every effort to foster the personal development of the members of their team. Appropriate guidance, leadership, coaching, and support should be given to team members whenever they ask or are in need. These conversations require a private and professional approach, strictly respecting the boundaries established by each individual.

Handling Criticism

Regardless of the time, effort, and attention focused on leadership and management issues, the ED medical director may occasionally come under substantial criticism for the manner in which the department is functioning. When such the circumstances arise, objectively and methodically address the issue(s) (**Box 18.6**).

Although it is tempting to take all criticism personally, the first step is to remove the "I" from the equation. Although the criticism seems (and in some cases is) personal, the medical director should not react as if it is. Although this approach avoids defensiveness and the temptation to blame others, it requires substantial integrity and self-control.

Developing an Action Plan

Listen carefully to the substance of the criticism and the interest of the person bringing the criticism. Without this understanding, it is unlikely the required improvements can be accurately recognized or implemented. Listen, do not defend the ED or its providers, and do not blame. Occasionally, the person presenting the complaint is the cause of the problem. However, "blaming the blamer" is ineffective and leads to conflict escalation.

Emergency physicians learn early to be "fix-it" doctors. They have a natural tendency to approach administrative problems with an immediate solution. It is tempting to respond with an immediate "fix" that does not consider, examine, or address the underlying "root cause." However, many problems are complex and require "peeling" (like an onion) to get to the core issue. At this discovery stage, the ED director should listen carefully to what is being said, reserving comments or rebuttals for a more appropriate time. After listening to the substance of the criticisms, the issue may be restated to ensure the area of concern is understood.

The director should describe potential qualifications and/or inaccuracies in the original statement of the problem *only of these are clear*. However, a detailed response to the criticism should be reserved until the director has performed an appropriate investigation and thoughtfully considered the issue and its resolution.

Set specific priorities and action plans to address the areas of criticism. The director may set specific timeframes during which the problem will be analyzed and solutions presented. This approach ensures a brief "breathing period" while the problem is dissected. A specific timeframe also establishes an appropriate sense of urgency among team members. The director (and team) should work collaboratively to develop a mutually acceptable means to measure progress. This ensures subsequent agreement when considering whether progress and resolution have occurred. It further permits consideration of the components of a problem's resolution, allowing focus on possible barriers.

Too often, problems are addressed by "patchwork" or Band-Aid solutions that only resolve the symptom and not the root cause. To develop a thoughtful, reasoned, and successful solution, all appropriate resources (e.g., consultants, administrators, task forces), effective tools (e.g., "The Five Whys"), and necessary data (e.g., IT support, benchmarking) should be used. Communicate with supportive stakeholders, perhaps an administrator or medical staff leader, to gather their assistance and, when necessary, advocacy.

To ensure continuing focus on the improvement process, the director must develop mechanisms with appropriate timeframes during which interval successes or failures are evaluated and communicated. The information should be fed back to those who lodged the criticism. This regular communication demonstrates that improvement is a process and emphasizes the leadership role of the medical director.

Whenever the medical director or the ED is "under fire," problems should be approached with tenacity and ferocity. The response to any criticisms raised should be aggressive, responsive, and decisive. When EDs and their leadership are criticized, medical directors should understand that their and the group's practice, standing in the community, livelihood, and career are on the line. However, negative perceptions can be changed. Just as desperately ill patients can be revived to live long and productive lives, an ED practice and its leaders can become reinvigorated and filled with determination to improve poorly performing areas.

CONCLUSION

Navigating the broad array of the ED medical director roles and responsibilities can be difficult, challenging, and at times overwhelming. Yet, the successful director can create satisfying improvements in patient care, develop a high-performing ED, and expand the horizons of the team members who comprise that department. Medical directors can help to ensure the viability of their ED and the patients who rely on it for timely and excellent care. Successful leadership requires committing to excellence, establishing the boundaries of the organization, collaborating with nursing leadership, forming strong partnerships throughout the organization and community, and developing providers and staff.

REFERENCES

1. Shakespeare W. *Henry IV. Part I*. New York, NY: Washington Square Press; 1994.
2. Senge P. *The Fifth Discipline: The Art and Practice of the Learning Organization*. New York, NY: Doubleday; 2006.
3. Block P. *Stewardship: Choosing Service Over Self-Interest*. San Francisco, Calif: Barrett-Koehler; 1993.
4. Greenleaf R. *Servant Leadership: A Journey into the Nature of Legitimate Power and Greatness*. New York, NY: Paulist Press; 2002.
5. Bennis W. *On Becoming a Leader*. New York, NY: Perseus; 2009.
6. American Board of Emergency Medicine: Physician Tasks. Available at: https://www.abem.org/PUB-LIC/portal/alias Rainbow/lang en-US/tabID 4223/DesktopDefault.aspx. Accessed March 15, 2018.
7. Counselman FL, Babu K, Edens MA, et al. The 2016 Model of the Clinical Practice of Emergency Medicine. *J Emerg Med*. 2017:52(6):846-849. Available at: https://www.jem-journal.com/article/S0736-4679(17)30108-7/fulltext. Accessed May 29, 2018.
8. Welch S, Jensen K. The concept of reliability in emergency medicine. *Am J Med Qual*. 2007;22(1):50-58.
9. Kim D. Friday night at the ER. Available at: www.fridaynightattheer.com. Accessed March 15, 2018.
10. Ensor PS. Organizational Renewal—Tearing Down *the Functional Silos*. Target. 1988:16.
11. Mayer TA, Cates R. *Leadership for Great Customer Service: Satisfied Employees, Satisfied Patients*. 2nd ed. Chicago, Ill: Health Administration Press; 2014.
12. ABEM Policy on Third Party Standards. Available at: https://www.abem.org/public/docs/default-source/policies-faqs/policy-on-third-party-standards.pdf? sfvrsn=4. Accessed May 24, 2018.
13. ACS CME Dropped for MOC participants. *ABEM News*. May 14, 2018. Available at: https://www.abem.org/public/news-events/news/2018/05/14/acs-cme-dropped-for-moc-participants. Accessed May 22, 2018.
14. Mayer TA. Active Listening: The 2nd A Team Behavior. Available at: www.best-practices.com. Accessed March 15, 2018.
15. Hoppe MH. *Active Listening: Improve your Ability to Listen and Lead*. Greensboro, NC: Center for Creative Leadership; 2006.
16. Toyoda S. 5 Whys (Defining the Root Cause). Available at: https://en.wikipedia.org/wiki/5_Whys. Accessed June 1, 2018.
17. Stokes C. Presidential Address to the American College of Healthcare Executives. Chicago, Ill, March 24, 2018.
18. Mayer T. *Leadership for Great Patient Experience*. Presented at: the American College of Emergency Physicians' Emergency Department Directors' Academy; Dallas, Tex; February 5, 2018.
19. Welch J. *Annual Report: 1990* General Electric Corporation. Boston, MA.
20. Hirschhorn L, Gilmore T. The new boundaries of the "boundaryless" company. *Harv Bus Rev*. 1992;70(3):104-115.
21. Jensen K, Mayer T. *The Patient Flow Advantage: How Hardwiring Hospital-Wide Flow Drives Competitive Advantage*. Gulf Breeze, Fla: Fire Starter Press; 2014.
22. Maddox KE, Epstein AM, Samson LW, et al. Performance and participation of physicians in year one of Medicare's Value-Based Payment Modifier Program. *Health Aff (Millwood)*. 2017;36(12):2175-2184.
23. Mayer TA, Cates RJ. *Leadership for Great Customer Service*. Chicago, Ill: Health Administration Press; 2007.
24. Studer Q. *Results that Last: Hardwiring Behaviors That Will Take Your Company to the Top*. Hoboken, NJ: John Wiley; 2008.

25. Hoffer E. *The Passionate State of Mind*. New York, NY: Doubleday; 1955.
26. Institute for Healthcare Improvement. "SBAR Tool: Situation-Background-Assessment-Recommendation. Available at: http://www.ihi.org/resources/Pages/Tools/SBARToolkit.aspx. Accessed May 31, 2018.
27. Mayer T. Physician accountability: leading in a world of metrics mania. Presented at: the ED Practice Management Association Annual Meeting; Ft. Lauderdale, Fla; May 1, 2018.
28. Katzenbach J, Smith DK. *The Wisdom of Teams: Creating the High Performance Organization*. Boston, Mass: Harvard Business School Press; 1993.
29. Argyrgis C. Double-loop learning in organizations. *Harv Bus Rev*. 1977;115-125.
30. Mayer T. Remarks to the O.W. "Red" Haven Award 50th Anniversary, Anderson, Ind. May 15, 2018.
31. Kohn A. *Punished by Rewards: The Trouble with Gold Stars, Incentive Plans, A's, Praise and Other Bribes*. Boston, Mass: Houghton-Mifflin; 1999.

This chapter focuses on the ED nurse leader, who may fill the role of nursing director, nurse manager, or shift leader. Regardless of the exact management structure and job titling a particular emergency department (ED) employs, it is clear that those who have nursing and medical leadership roles share important responsibilities for the quality of care the department provides.

TODAY'S ED NURSE LEADER

The ED is often a profitable business unit and a portal into other important clinical and revenue-generating services offered by the organization, such as the surgical, neurosciences, cardiac, and imaging services. The ED is increasingly important in population health management. As community organizations develop plans for tracking and fostering the care of specific populations, the role of emergency services must be included. Additionally, the ED has its own role in reaching out to the broader population; no longer just the front door of the hospital, the EDs have become a gateway to a variety of corridors for the communities they serve.

Let's first consider the nursing leadership role itself. For any leader to be successful, certain elements must be in place, including:

- Well-defined expectations for the role
- Clear goals for success of the department
- A collaborative environment that includes physician partners and organizational departments
- A supportive executive team that provides for the mentoring and growth of its leadership team

The potential nurse leader must choose to be in this difficult role for the right reasons, both personal and professional. Each leader must be able to answer some tough questions, outlined in **Figure 19.1**. Being a leader in today's ED requires skills beyond outstanding clinical abilities. Strategic planning and project management experience, financial savvy, and communication skills are just a few of the many strengths that today's hospital departmental leaders must possess to ensure success. Because they will work closely with a number of stakeholders, including community services, physician leaders, care coordinators, and other hospital and community providers, ED nursing leaders must be able to work in a collaborative, team-based environment.[1]

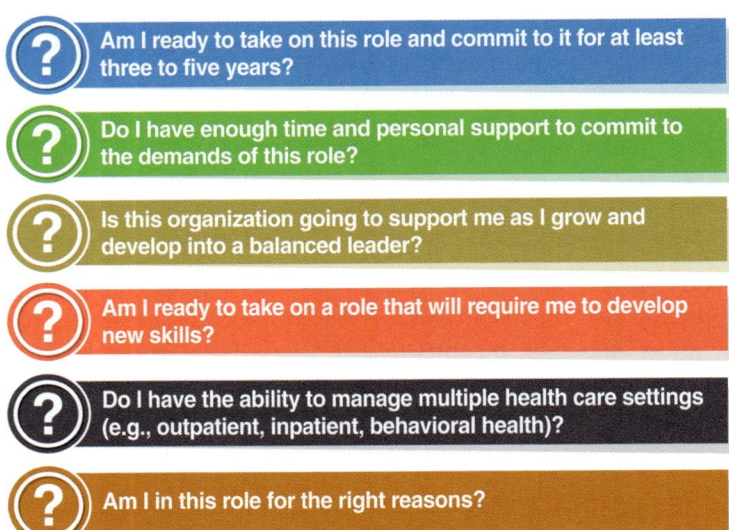

FIGURE 19.1 ■ ED Nurse Leader Questions to Self

- Am I ready to take on this role and commit to it for at least three to five years?
- Do I have enough time and personal support to commit to the demands of this role?
- Is this organization going to support me as I grow and develop into a balanced leader?
- Am I ready to take on a role that will require me to develop new skills?
- Do I have the ability to manage multiple health care settings (e.g., outpatient, inpatient, behavioral health)?
- Am I in this role for the right reasons?

Nursing Leadership in the Modern Health-Care Environment

Historically, "good ED nurses" were those who were organized and always willing to help out; as a result, they were frequently asked to assume the role of the department leader. Training for these positions was often limited and focused primarily on tasks instead of role development. Poorly selected candidates combined with inadequate training and support led to frustration and high turnover in ED nurse leader positions. Instability in these roles or frequent turnover can heighten anxiety and frustration throughout the organization. Demands from ED nurse leaders have prompted organizations to improve how people are prepared for this complex role.

In the 1950s, emergency and accident care was provided in one or two rooms of a facility in which nurses had operational and administrative responsibilities but no formal recognition or authority.[2] Now, ED nurse leaders are crucial in meeting the broad needs of the community and organization. As emergency services have expanded and ED visits have risen, leadership development programs have been initiated to prepare potential nursing leaders for the challenges ahead. These responsibilities may include:

- Leading performance improvement projects
- Developing business plans
- Having responsibility for productivity and fiscal performance
- Developing and delivering presentations to senior and executive members of the organization

The program modules are scheduled at intervals with project assignments for each module. This approach gives the participant the opportunity to develop cohesive working relationships with other departments. The programs often assign a mentor and an executive sponsor during the 6- to 12-month period leading up to placement in a permanent ED leadership role.

The ideal nursing director candidate should have ED clinical and supervisory experience in addition to the appropriate leadership skills and training. The ED nursing director must also be able to articulate the department's vision and inspire the staff to embrace it. To achieve the vision—and to provide high-quality care to a variable patient population—effective and efficient processes must be in place. Each process must take into account the

FIGURE 19.2 ■ Daily Responsibilities of ED Nursing Directors

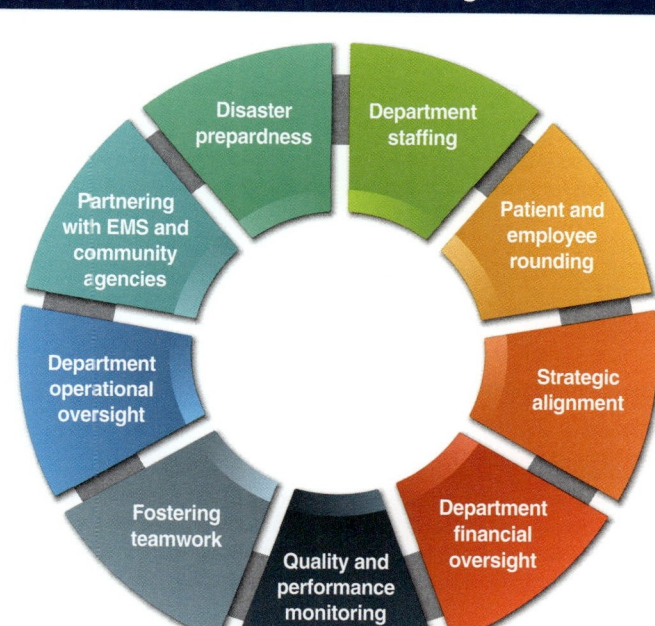

following: patient, employee, and physician satisfaction; quality and regulatory guidelines; and financial impact. Daily responsibilities for the ED nursing director are outlined in **Figure 19.2**.

Ongoing Leadership Growth and Development

A National Center for Healthcare Leadership white paper identifies four qualities that are associated with powerful learning experiences[3]:

- A compelling need for substantial change
- A set of unfamiliar responsibilities
- A greater responsibility or latitude of decision-making
- The need to deal with significant adversity, failure, or both

The ED leader is a visible institutional leader who must work with other nursing and ancillary leaders in the organization; an ED director must focus on the organization in its entirety. Therefore, it is particularly important for senior leaders to invest time, effort, and patience in identifying and developing high-potential future leaders. The Emergency Nurses Association (ENA) has developed professional nurse leader standards, outlined in **Figure 19.3**.

One of the ways health systems can align leadership development programs with the overall mission and goals of the organization is to ensure that these activities are centralized. By centrally coordinating the activities of its component parts, the organization can more easily ensure vertical alignment with high-level strategic objectives.[4]

ED leaders' annual goals should cascade down from their administrative line officer. The goals should be specific, measurable, achievable, relevant, time bound, and related to the organization's mission. ED nurse leaders, in collaboration with their physician partners, will develop several tactics for each goal (see Chapter 18). At a minimum, progress should be evaluated quarterly, and adjustments can be made if necessary. The goals and tactics should be shared broadly with the ED leadership team and staff and with all organizational

FIGURE 19.3 ■ Emergency Nurses Association's Leadership Standards

Emergency nurse leaders uphold a commitment to quality, safety, and cost-effective care using evidence-based practice.

| Emergency nurse leaders support lifelong learning for themselves and others. | Emergency nurse leaders support certifications in emergency nursing practice and model professionalism by joining and participating in their specialty nursing associations. |

↓

Emergency nurse leaders support learning and practice transformational leadership styles.

| Emergency nurse leaders promote an environment that is conducive to professional nursing practice and foster the mentorship of developing nurses. | Emergency nurse leaders who are expected to provide care at the stretcher maintain the same competencies as the staff registered nurses. |

department leaders. The ED nurse leader should work collaboratively with the interdisciplinary team to create and share a vision of how the tactics can be accomplished.

Other professional development resources that can assist in the nurse leader's development include national leadership organizations organizations, many of which have state and local chapters that offer a variety of educational programs (**Figure 19.4**). Professional organizations further benefit their members through networking opportunities, updates on legislative changes, and volunteer opportunities in the community.

Specialty certification demonstrates a commitment to professionalism and advanced learning. A nurse leader's enthusiasm about achieving certification can inspire other frontline staff to obtain and maintain specialty certifications. Specialty and leadership

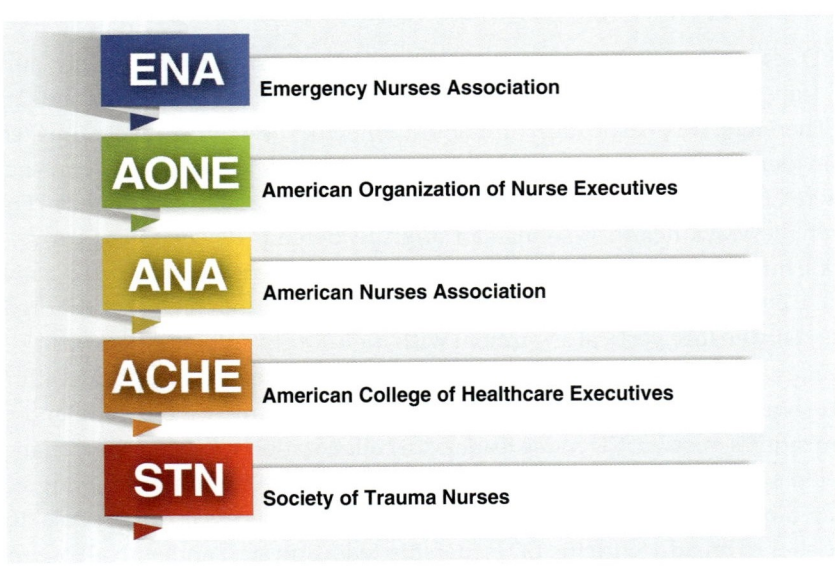

FIGURE 19.4 ■ Professional Nurse Leader Organizations

- **ENA** — Emergency Nurses Association
- **AONE** — American Organization of Nurse Executives
- **ANA** — American Nurses Association
- **ACHE** — American College of Healthcare Executives
- **STN** — Society of Trauma Nurses

conferences provide current information in a rapidly changing health-care arena. Nursing journals also provide up-to-date information on current research, processes, and procedures.

TRADITIONAL ED LEADERSHIP MODELS

Although the broad functions and leadership roles of EDs have undergone—and are undergoing—continuous change, it is helpful to understand the traditional roles and reporting structures from which these new models are emerging.

Traditional Leadership Roles

The traditional ED leadership team consisted of a nurse director and/or nurse manager along with a shift leader (charge nurse, clinical coordinator, or others). In recent years, the roles of directors and managers have often been blurred. Some organizations eliminated one of the positions, whereas others kept both but without clear role delineation. As the ED has emerged as a leading strategic source of growth, models of governance have also changed. Although the director and manager duties vary from institution to institution, we are seeing more distinction in role nomenclature and duties, as depicted in **Figure 19.5**.

The *shift leader* oversees shift operations, such as productivity, assignments, patient flow, and patient experience optimization, and serves as the frontline for dealing with customer concerns.

The *nurse manager* is a middle manager who collaborates with other midlevel department leaders throughout the organization and with some external organizations, such as EMS and

FIGURE 19.5 ■ Traditional ED Nurse Leader Roles

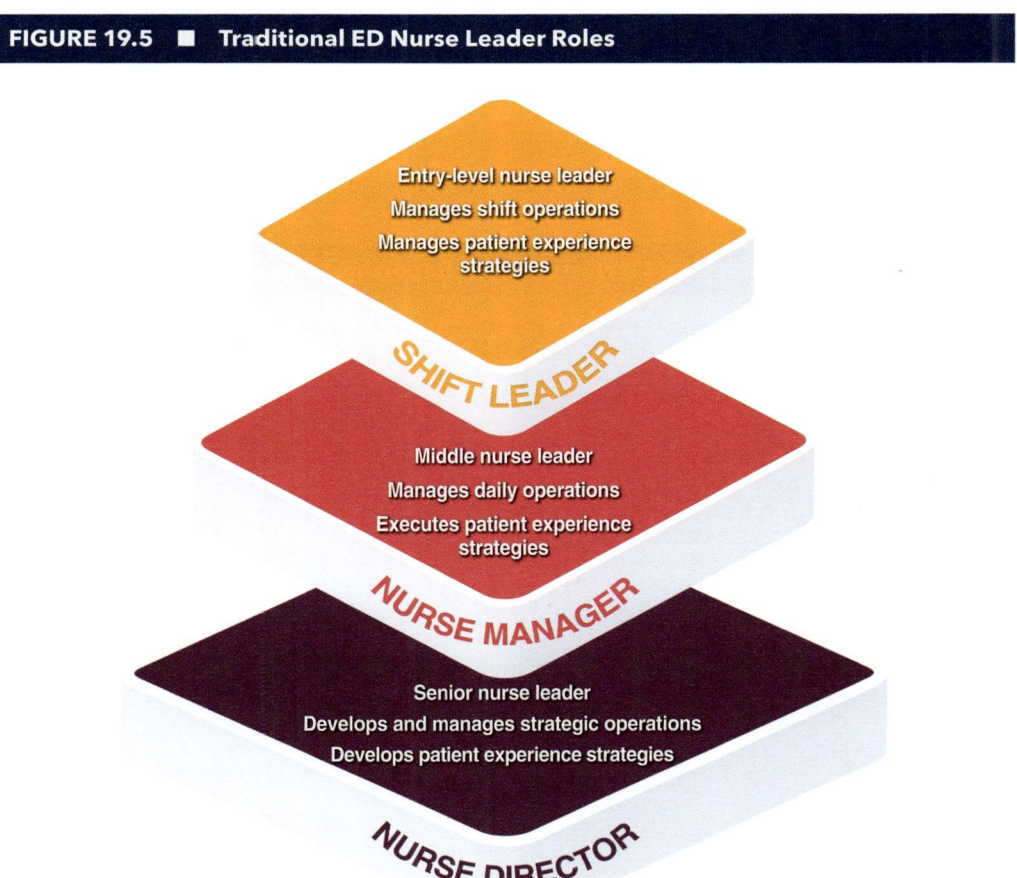

behavioral health institutes. Most nurse managers are more focused on tasks that ensure quality patient care and a healthy working environment for the clinical team.[7] Nurse managers lead by example when mentoring frontline staff and shift leaders. The nurse manager must possess the skills necessary to foster bidirectional communication between the senior department leader and frontline staff. Other responsibilities of the nurse manager include overseeing daily personnel issues, quality programs, professional growth opportunities for charge nurses and frontline staff, and department regulatory compliance.[8]

Depending on the size of the ED and the span of control by the department leader, additional managers may be required. The ED *nursing director* at most health-care organizations is a senior nurse leader who works directly with the executive team to develop operational and strategic plans.[7]

The ED leader uses creative skills to design strategies that meet the needs of the organization and are willingly adopted by the clinical staff. Communication skills include the ability to create a departmental environment that embraces these strategic plans by setting clear expectations in a systematic manner.[8] The ED leader oversees the development and management of the department's operational and staffing budgets and maintains current knowledge of the many regulatory and compliance standards.

ENA promotes the premise that all ED nurse leaders must be transformation leaders who encourage emergency nursing professionally and ensure quality care and a safe environment for all ED patients.[9]

Traditional Reporting Structure

Figure 19.6 illustrates the traditional reporting structure for the ED through the institutions' nursing leadership organization. Many health-care institutions employ a variation of this traditional structure, which may include freestanding EDs, pediatric EDs, and other strategic alignments that fall within the emergency service line. The number of vice president positions that oversee ED service lines has risen. Numerous ED nurse directors or managers might report to the ED vice president, but the traditional reporting model remains

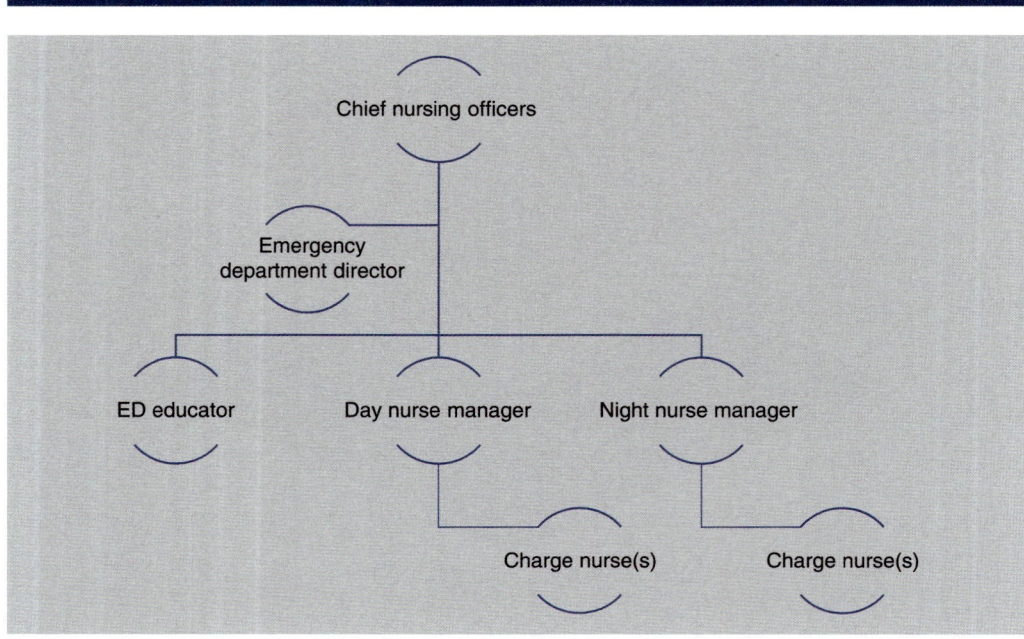

FIGURE 19.6 ■ Traditional ED Nurse Leader Reporting Structure

FIGURE 19.7 ■ ED Dyad Reporting Structure

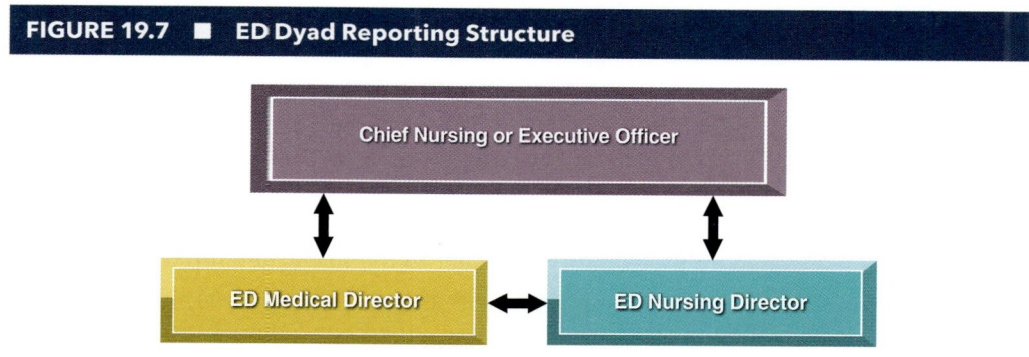

mainly within the nursing structure as the structure that supports all patient care activities. As the complexity of the health-care environment evolves and the strategic importance of the ED increases, leadership structures for emergency services will continue to evolve.

DYAD LEADERSHIP MODEL

Many health-care systems have implemented a dyad leadership model: a team approach in which responsibilities are shared by physician and nurse leaders. This team approach is effective because it mirrors the coordinated approach to successful patient care. ED leadership naturally leans toward the dyad model because it promotes a unified front.[10] According to the Studer Group, a successful dyad model in the ED must share common goals, combine nursing and physician communication into one aligned communication, and recognize the team together.[11] The alignment that occurs from a well-executed dyad model can eliminate the silos that often occur in the traditional ED leadership model.

Dyad Reporting Structure

The organizational chart in **Figure 19.7** illustrates changes to the traditional reporting structure for the ED. In many institutions, the operational importance of the ED has transitioned from the nursing reporting structure to the chief operating officer reporting structure. However, some institutions have kept the ED within the nursing realm to ensure the alignment of all patient care activities. The role of the ED medical director varies within institutions; depending on the physician group, the reporting structure may include additional expectations for the physician group.

FUTURE LEADERSHIP MODELS

The future of health care is unknown to many institutions and regulatory bodies; however, all can agree that the complexity of the ED and its strategic importance within the health-care system will continue to evolve. The traditional and dyad leadership models will also change.

Triad Model

A few health-care organizations have transformed the dyad model into a triad model in which a business or operations leader joins the medical and nursing teams. The reporting structure may evolve in several directions, such as by adding an operating or strategic planning officer who may report to the nursing officer.

Support Structure

The traditional ED leadership support structure consists of a department clerk who performs a variety of duties that allow the nursing leaders to focus on their most important daily tasks. Many midsized and large departments also have the support of a dedicated educator or clinical specialist who develops an education plan for the front-line staff that is specific to the type of patients treated at their institution.[12] Several large facilities have also added a nurse quality manager to the ED leadership team to ensure that the multitudes of quality metrics are met. The quality director also typically ensures that appropriate education is developed to increase the knowledge of the ED care team concerning how to produce quality patient outcomes, reduce the number of poor patient outcomes, and mitigate organizational risks.

THE STRATEGIC IMPACT OF HEALTH-CARE CHANGES

In an era of rapidly developing changes to the way health-care is delivered and monitored—in both the hospital and the wider community—changes to the functions of the ED and its leadership are bound to follow.

Population-Based Health Care

There are expectations for any leader, whether new or seasoned. These expectations include the optimization of performance measures, clinical outcomes, and customer experience. The ED leader will face new challenges, including:

- Addressing the role of the ED in their community's population health
- Ensuring the ED collaborates with other access points to provide health care
- Supporting the capture and navigation of both new and existing patients to ensure the correct care in the correct environment

Collaboration by hospital executive leadership, physicians, and staff will be critical as these health-care changes become the new reality. **Figure 19.8** illustrates the ED's potential role in population health.

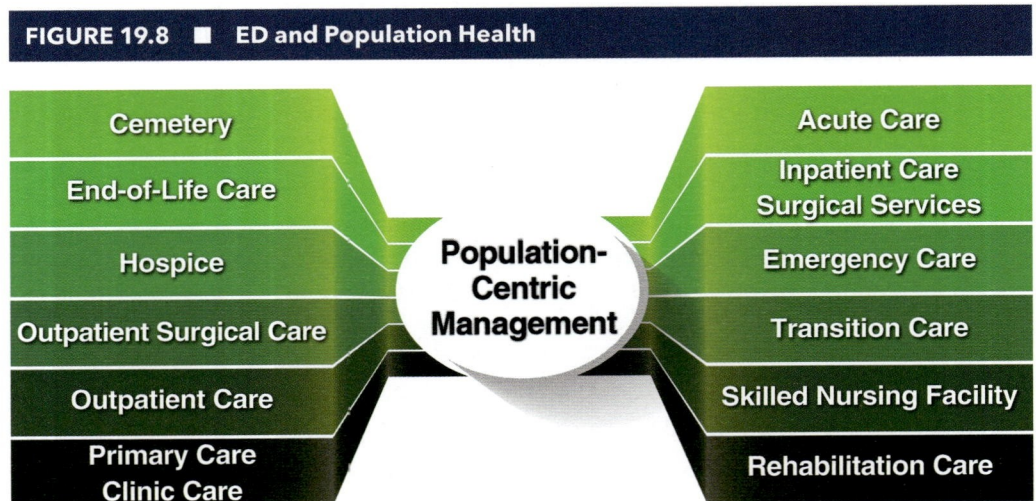

FIGURE 19.8 ■ ED and Population Health

Performance Measures

There are many resources leaders can access to improve their departments. The emergency staff alone cannot effect outcomes. These changes require skills in both collaboration and communication. The ED is a "team sport" that relies on unity in purpose and process with the staff who are employed by or frequently interact with the department. ED leaders, executive leaders, nurse leaders, and physician leaders must all be aligned on the goals, timeline, and requisite cost required to move their metrics. Developing a team-based committee structure to drive these goals forward is not only helpful but also necessary to affect change in such a large and complex department.[13]

A scorecard should be widely shared so that all members of the team can monitor their incremental successes and understand any lapses; scorecards can also be used to educate the ED care team. Scorecards come in many forms: a traditional paper format, a simple white board, or an integrated electronic board that can be updated daily or in real time. Interdisciplinary team training that includes nurses, physicians, and laboratory, imaging, and leadership staff can be used to achieve targets for key operating metrics. To achieve improved quality outcomes, the nurse leader must understand the organization's quality improvement framework and internal resources and, if necessary, petition executive leadership for additional training and support.

Service Excellence

Many organizations already take a programmatic approach to customer experience excellence; some may have even engaged a national company to supply coaching and support. Using internal resources and expertise, some health-care organizations have developed and branded their own programs. All ED leaders must be educated and engaged with the approach being used and should become comfortable with and proficient in both patient and staff rounding. Organizations may have daily and monthly expectations for the ED leadership team (including shift leaders) regarding customer excellence. Typical expectations include:

- A percentage of patients who are rounded on, with staff feedback and correction or recognition
- Shift handoffs that integrate key metrics of performance
- Medical staff minutes to stimulate and engage the clinical staffs
- Stoplight reports
- Individual staff conversations

Managing the department's human capital is a critical skill that is proven to lead to excellence in customer expectations.

CONCLUSION

Health-care and organizational leadership has dramatically changed over the past 20 years and will be faced with many challenges in the future. The ED will continue to be a pivotal department in the evolving medical landscape. Large integrated health-care systems are already exploring alternative access points to manage populations within their service areas. EDs of the future may take on responsibilities that integrate outpatient clinics and urgent care treatment to control access to the ED and the inpatient setting.

Regardless of how the volume-to-value shift in health care occurs, the ED will remain part of the long-term equation; thus, nurse leaders must be educated and conversant with the potential changes ahead. By understanding their health-care organization's strategic direction, nurse leaders can focus on what is most important to their ED patients and staff. Furthermore, staying involved with key nursing organizations can improve professional agility and help prepare nurse leaders for the every-changing role of the ED.

REFERENCES

1. Taplin SH, Foster MK, Shortell SM. Organizational leadership for building effective health care teams. *Ann Fam Med.* 2013;11(3):279-281.

2. ENA Position Statement Nurse Leaders in Emergency Care Settings. Emergency Nurses Association. 2018. Available at: https://www.ena.org/docs/default-source/resource-library/practice-resources/position-statements/nurseleaders.pdf?sfvrsn=316948d8_10. Accessed July 9, 2018.

3. Garman AN, Lemak CH, Developing Healthcare Leaders: What We Have Learned, and What is Next, National Center for Healthcare Leadership White Paper. Published 2011, https://nchl.memberclicks.net/assets/Website/Developing%20Healthcare%20Leaders_What%20we%20have%20learned%20and%20what%20is%20next.pdf, Accessed September 14, 2020

4. Anderson MM, Garman AN, Leadership Development in Healthcare Systems: Toward an Evidence-based Approach, National Center for Healthcare Leadership White Paper, Published 2014, https://static1.squarespace.com/static/59a33ae4f14aa15be9df1f78/t/59e26c8d18b27d395c999e65/1508011150861/NCHL_Leadership_Survey_White_Paper_Final_05.14_updf.pdf, Accessed September 14, 2020

5. Department of Emergency Medicine, School of Medicine, University of Alabama at Birmingham. Available at: https://www.uab.edu/medicine/em/about/mission-vision. Accessed date 9, 2018.

6. Department of Emergency Medicine, Dalhousie University. Available at: https://medicine.dal.ca/departments/department-sites/emergency/about/mission-vision.html. Accessed date July 9, 2018.

7. Eileen Williamson MR. Nurse manager vs. nurse leader: what's the difference? OnCourse Learning. 2017. Available at: https://www.nurse.com/blog/2017/05/23/nurse-manager-vs-nurse-leader-whats-the-difference/. Accessed May 25, 2018.

8. *The Role of the Nurse Manager.* Rockville, MD: Agency for Healthcare Research and Quality. Available at: http://www.ahrq.gov/professionals/education/curriculum-tools/cusptoolkit/modules/nursing/index.html. Accessed July, 2018.

9. Melanie Crowley MR. *Nurse Leaders in Emergency Care Settings* (2. E. Committee, Editor). Emergency Nurses Association. 2017. Available at: https://www.ena.org/docs/default-source/resource-library/practice-resources/position-statements/nurseleaders.pdf?sfvrsn=316948d8. Accessed May 25, 2018.

10. Daniel Meltzer MM. How dyad leadership sets up emergency departments for success. Studer Group Insights. 2016. Available at: https://www.studergroup.com/resources/articles-and-industry-updates/insights/march-2016/how-dyad-leadership-sets-up-emergency-departments. Accessed May 30, 2018.

11. Studer Group. 3 Powerful Ways to Make an Impact in the Emergency Department. Insights Blog. 2018. Available at: https://www.studergroup.com/resources/articles-and-industry-updates/insights/march-2018/3-ways-to-impact-ed. Accessed May 30, 2018.

12. Al-Sawai A. Leadership of healthcare professionals: where do we stand? *Oman Med J.* 2013;28(4):285-287.

13. Agency for Healthcare Research and Quality: TeamSTEPPS: Research/Evidence Base. Available at: https://www.ahrq.gov/teamstepps/evidence-base/emergency-care.html. Accessed December 14, 2019.

The emergency department (ED) is a microcosm of its hospital and its parent health-care system. Both the nursing director and physician medical director are charged with providing optimum medical care to patients while also demonstrating the institution's overarching mission philosophy and achieving its goals. Accomplishing these ends requires more than good "management" and attention to operational details. Inspirational leaders must transform a collection of individuals into a loyal and highly motivated team that is passionately committed to a common vision of excellence. The director team must lead by personal example, attention to morale, creation of an environment of learning, and clearly communicated expectations.

WHY PHYSICIAN-NURSE COLLABORATION MATTERS

Nowhere is the need for effective leadership more evident than in the daily turmoil of a busy ED. The ED leadership structure is unique because the physician and nurse directors work closely together with frontline staff with a degree of visibility and integration not often found in other areas of the hospital. The nurse and physician directors influence and guide the unit in tandem, with overlapping responsibilities. Highly effective nurse–physician leadership teams function as single entities rather than a pair of individuals. Patients, staff, and the hospital and health-care system profoundly benefit from a collaborative approach to leadership.

First and foremost, patients obtain better outcomes and have a better experience when the team strives toward common goals through a shared vision of excellence in all facets of patient care. The ED is unique in the rapid delivery of intensely focused initial care to the entire spectrum of illness and injury while orchestrating multiple handoffs to nursing units, diagnostic areas, surgery, and/or intensive care units—all while appearing, to the untrained observer, to be on the verge of chaos. Such efficiency only occurs when physicians and nurses work collaboratively to rapidly arrive at the correct diagnoses, initiate appropriate treatments, shorten lengths of stay (LOS), improve patient satisfaction, and foster teamwork.

In the truest sense, care in the ED results from the combined efforts of housekeepers, maintenance, secretaries, security, ancillary staff, nurses, and physicians—the entire hospital staff. Job satisfaction and morale increase when the directors are "in sync," reducing burnout and turnover while improving retention of experienced and effective team members. Alternatively, when the nurse director and physician director aren't aligned in collaborative leadership, team members sense the discord, choose sides, have fewer common goals, and often quickly look for new positions.

Nurses who quit often state they love their work but have become frustrated by the *job* (i.e., the work environment and the leader).[1] The *Gallup Business Journal* states that "at least 75% of the reasons for voluntary turnover can be influenced by managers."[2] In other words, people most often leave their managers, not their company. The negative effects of poor leadership are profound; ineffectively led groups are significantly less productive and unhappier in their work.

For the hospital and the health-care system as a whole, ineffective leaders produce inefficient teams that produce poor patient flow—the death knell for an ED. This, in turn, can lead to increased costs. For example, the hospital may see costly new construction as the solution to bottlenecks. However, efficient care may prevent such a futile response when the issue is truly operational inefficiency. Conversely, excellent ED leadership increases staff retention and ameliorates the exorbitant costs of frequent recruiting, hiring, and training of new employees. Finally, efficient teams may decrease legal fees and settlements as satisfied patients are less likely to engage in costly litigation.

Leadership teams that are focused on quality and service decrease institutional expenses and, by improving operational efficiency, increase the revenue necessary to carry out their mission. Patient satisfaction scores, LOS, mortality, and other measures of quality are increasingly available to both consumers and third-party payers. Highly satisfied patients are loyal and advertise by word-of-mouth, resulting in even more patients. Similarly, all of these metrics are used by payers who often mandate where their members receive service. Contract negotiations with those payers can be further influenced by proven efficiency, quality, positive patient outcomes, and patient satisfaction.

KEY FACTORS IN PHYSICIAN–NURSE LEADER COLLABORATION

Trust

Trust is vital for any relationship to flourish and be sustained. Excellent nurse–physician leadership teams are:

- Confident in each other's abilities
- Certain that each will act responsibly
- Assured that each will set good examples while honoring the collaborative nature of the relationship

Trust between the nursing director and the physician director can develop naturally through mutual day-to-day communications, decisions, and respectful actions. However, lives change, people retire, inspirational leaders often advance, and poor leaders may be replaced. When choosing a new coleader, it is imperative that the remaining director is included in the interview and selection process. Without basic compatibility and shared visions, a noncollaborative and ineffective leadership team is the inevitable result. Realistically, there is no guarantee that coleaders will achieve consistent synergy, even with the best intentions. However, mutual trust among the leaders is required to achieve operational efficiency.

Self-Assessment

A wise leader will engage in a period of self-reflection before selecting a new partner or investing time in improving collaboration with a current codirector. Since all leaders have both strengths and weaknesses, simply seeking a clone of the remaining director limits potential growth of the ED. Without insight into one's own personality, leadership style and tendencies, strengths and weaknesses, it is impossible to discern if the leader candidate has the characteristics necessary to build a superior leadership team. A committed leader should use available tools to discern what might have led to the development of their specific leadership tendencies, strengths, and weakness.[3-5] Such tools may provide insight into repetitive and negative behaviors that are not team-oriented. Recognition of personal strengths and weaknesses allows leaders to develop a personal action plan and build a collaborative practice.

In addition to understanding one's own strengths and weaknesses, it is also critical to understand the talents, traits, behaviors, and preferences of one's coleader. For example, an engaging speaker who delights in giving presentations may dislike the "detail work" required to formulate the presentation. An ideal counterpart would be a partner who wishes to avoid the "on-stage" presentation, preferring the behind-the-scenes support work involved in data collection and the creation of graphs and visual aids. Identifying each other's traits, strengths, and weaknesses leads to many opportunities for a synchronized approach and maximizes efforts/success.

Effective Communication

Being conscientious of one's self and others is only part of the collaboration equation. Leaders must openly and honestly communicate their thoughts with one another. Honesty includes sharing differences of opinion, but the setting and manner in which such disagreement is expressed must be respectful and controlled.

Physicians and nurses often approach problems differently, in part because of their diverse training and job descriptions. Nurses may tend toward detail, while physicians may engage more in global thinking. Each leader brings a different perspective to the table that inevitably leads to more nuanced, complete, and well-thought-out programs and processes. The nurse and physician directors must then effectively communicate the result of their collaboration to all stakeholders. Collaborative work results in improved outcomes, efficiency, shared credit, and opportunities to further build trust.

Values

Values are the broad and overarching drivers of our decisions and actions in both our personal lives and at work. Differences in values create conflicts if they are not recognized and addressed, and they can destroy the leadership team's approach to the most basic communications and actions. Aligned values simplify coleadership, but absolute congruity is neither possible nor desirable.

It is imperative that directors discuss how they will achieve alignment when divergent values are discovered. For example, if one leader highly values treating everyone equally while the other believes in a hierarchal system, there is potential for destructive discord. If these differences are publicly displayed, the result may be confusion, frustration, and friction among team members. Public disagreement creates an opportunity for staff to choose sides, contributing to division. Effective leaders define when and how these issues will be handled, optimally in private negotiations and respectful communication.

Attitudes

Attitudes are the outward manifestation of values. Leaders who appreciate and respect all patients, regardless of their "desirability," are more likely to be cheerful, optimistic, and able to motivate their subordinates to treat patients well. These directors are also more likely to be interested and skilled in collaboration.

Communication

Each person has an individual and specific communication style. Recognizing personal styles, triggers, and responses is essential to positive interpersonal negotiations. (Several self-assessment tools, such as the Thomas-Kilmann Conflict Mode Instrument, DISC Personality Profile, and the Meyers Briggs Test and Personality Assessment are readily available to assess one's own communication/negotiation style and easily recognize the style of others).[3,5,6]

Knowing one's own and another's general communication style, triggers, responses to feedback, and successful methods of influence are very useful in situations that are volatile or have the propensity to lead to antagonistic behaviors. For instance, if one leader tends to have a fiery response to challenges from staff, it would be appropriate to rely on a fellow director to express the unified opinion in a composed way, particularly to a potentially contentious issue. It takes practice, discipline, and a trusting relationship to avoid unnecessarily inserting an opinion or statement that will lead to rancor and loss of message.

Assertive communicators are clear in their intent, demonstrate respect for others, and allow little opportunity for confusion. This method yields positive results when used in conversations and negotiations throughout the health-care organization. Other communication styles are less likely to produce successful resolutions. Passive communicators allow others to direct the conversation, making clarity and advocacy difficult to achieve.

Ironically, aggressive communicators often think of themselves simply as assertive and efficient communicators, yet there are essential differences. Aggressive communicators use body language and poor etiquette to dominate the conversation, usually in a way that makes it difficult for others to communicate their position. This style leads to long-term adversarial relationships. Passive-aggressive communicators are generally frustrated and clearly transmit their intended message to others—"I'm not interested in what you have to say." and "I don't intend to collaborate with you." In such a situation, the likelihood of a win-win result is virtually nonexistent.

Body Language

Attitudes are often evident in body language. A significant portion of communication is nonverbal, and volumes may be communicated without a single word. Body language is the most difficult element of communication to change, since the behaviors are largely subconscious. While body language is clearly visible to those who are observing, the "speaker" is frequently unaware of the "message" being delivered—the body language that may drown out his or her spoken words.

Common examples of negative body language include the following habits[7]:

- *Rolling one's eyes*: communicates disdain, contempt, or incredulity.
- *Looking past someone when speaking*: communicates impatience and a lack of desire to engage directly. It further limits the opportunity to obtain visual cues that may be helpful in making the communication more effective.
- *Crossing arms across the chest when listening*: communicates disinterest, nonlistening, defensiveness, or hostility.
- *Making overly dramatic negative facial expressions*: communicates rejection of ideas.

- *Frequently checking the time*: communicates boredom.
- *Stroking the chin*: communicates a decision-making process and may imply, "I'm judging you."
- *Faking a smile*: communicates fraudulent behavior. Genuine smiles involve the whole face and wrinkle at the corners of the eyes. Fake smiles only involve the mouth and lips.

Effective open-minded leaders are willing or even eager to have these negative body language activities pointed out and take action to eliminate them. The effort to improve is a commitment to personal growth that advances communication. For example, making eye contact while speaking demonstrates acknowledgment, conveys interest, and improves communication. Eye contact by the speaker allows that speaker to gauge whether what is being said is understood by observing the facial expressions of the listener.

Emotional Intelligence

Emotional intelligence (EI) is the ability of individuals to perceive and address emotion in themselves and others.[8-10] The ability to recognize and regulate one's emotions to either enhance or suppress *feeling* in communication is a valuable skill. EI may be thought of as a social awareness that guides interactions, such as when to speak, listen, expand a conversation, or close it. Communicators with high EI can successfully harness their emotions. They tend to exhibit positive body language, develop and hone their communication skills, and adapt as the interaction unfolds. Effective communicators can emotionally take a step back from an interaction and correctly identify what the other person is communicating and how they are being perceived by the other person. Communication coaches can help develop these important skills. Trusting partners can rely on each other to develop a system of signals when the interaction requires use of a different approach.

Creating Safety in the Relationship

Partner trust is essential to achieving desired outcomes. Agreeing to "always assume good intent" of the other is a basic tenet of a trusting relationship. Since the discussions between coleaders may involve nuanced and sometimes uncertain areas of planning, human resources, operational changes, complaint management, corrective actions, and so on, it is essential that both leaders have access to a safe, nonjudgmental "neutral zone" when communicating privately. Adhering to these principles allows the relationship to flourish and grow. It allows each partner to develop an understanding that the other will protect the integrity of the relationship by dealing with conflict or differences within the relationship first. If at any time this agreement is violated, the power and absolute necessity of an apology cannot be minimized if trust and an effective partnership are to be regained. It is much easier to maintain a framework of "always assume good intent" when the coleaders know and trust each other. It is important to keep promises and commitments between coleaders, including the commitment to the relationship. Therefore, in new coleader relationships, this tenet should be discussed and agreed to as the basis for establishing a safe relationship.

COMMUNICATING WITH EACH OTHER

There are several methods for successful communication. These include establishing processes, establishing time for consideration, using mediation when necessary, and meeting regularly.

Addressing Concerns

It's been said that integrity is how people act when they think no one else is watching—that actions are consistent with the values and principles one espouses whether or not these actions are known by others. Integrity is vital in the handling of complaints and concerns from patients, coworkers, administration, and regulatory bodies. It also plays a critical role in the relationship between coleaders.

Well-established care pathways are used to treat diseases and to approach medical care situations. Their use ensures consistency and reduces the opportunity for errors and miscommunications. Consistent pathways can also be used to handle intra- and extra-departmental administrative issues and will yield similar results.

As an example, determining the specific responsibilities for managing complaints establishes clear lines of responsibility within the department and with hospital leadership. The complaint management pathway might define that:

- The medical director will handle pure physician issues.
- The nurse director will handle pure nursing issues.
- Both leaders will address interdisciplinary issues.

Even when an issue or complaint is related to a single discipline (medical or nursing), it is appropriate to share the information with the coleader to ensure transparency. This shared information avoids inadvertent "blindsiding" and associated distrust. If an administrator or other leader within the institution finds one of the ED leaders ignorant of a critical issue, that administrator may become concerned about the competence and communication between the ED leaders. Viewing an issue as solely a "nursing problem" or "doctor problem" is overly simplistic and ignores the collaborative approach necessary for strong team leadership.

Ideally, each coleader will trust the judgment of the other, both in terms of handling and communicating issues. Both must understand and believe that simply ignoring issues only leads to perpetuation and perhaps escalation of the problem, much like ignoring hypertension or an abscess. Conversely, working together to address issues and setting clear expectations with accountability are more likely to lead to resolution and nonrecurrence. Leaders may have to overcome the natural tendency to be defensive about their own team members.

Allowing Time for Consideration

Since the first report of an issue or problem is unlikely to be entirely accurate, it is appropriate for both directors to avoid the tendency to immediately react and instead "ponder," insisting on details and performing a more thorough investigation. This approach might result in a mutual decision to further monitor an apparent issue and ensures that both leaders remain vigilant to ongoing indicators of a problem.

Staff may occasionally challenge leadership and inadvertently cause "splitting behavior." When publicly confronted with an unexpected question from staff on a difficult topic, there is a tendency to feel pressured and to give a definitive and immediate answer. Providing an immediate answer may undermine a coleader who may have already answered the question differently or may have a substantively different opinion. When uncertain, it's prudent to defer immediate comment, allowing time for consideration and coleader discussion prior to answering. Leaders should respond without misdirection, stating simply, "I need to get all the facts and discuss that with _____." This has the dual result of de-escalating the issue as well as publicly demonstrating respect for the other leader.

Mediation

There is a time in all relationships when coleaders may reach an impasse and, despite discussion, are unable to resolve a difference of opinion. This situation, as well as recurring and unresolved issues, may require mediation. Leaders with foresight anticipate this possibility and set up a mutually agreed upon mediator and establish parameters for seeking mediation. By establishing a mediation process in advance, an impasse can be readily addressed. Mediation with a known, mutually acceptable, fair, respected, and open-minded professional who understands the ED is likely to lead to an outcome that both parties can accept. In some situations, there may not be a middle ground—one partner may have to abandon their position to the other in the interest of maintaining the relationship and team cohesiveness.

Director Meetings

Regular face-to-face meetings between coleaders are essential. Some ED leaders may prefer recurring formal "appointments" to achieve a collaborative and informed decision-making process. Other leaders may prefer frequent (even daily or more), informal chats. In any case, like any partnership, it is difficult to "row in the same direction" if there isn't frequent, comprehensive, and honest communication. Consistently monitoring and addressing daily operations and staffing ensure maximum communication and minimum surprises.

The standing agenda for formal meetings could include these topics:

- Patient satisfaction and complaints
- Staff satisfaction
- Staff performance
- Key operational metrics
- Administrative issues
- Prioritized improvement projects

As already mentioned, this meeting provides an opportunity to ensure both leaders are aware of all complaints directed at the ED and to discuss priorities and plans of action.

ROLES OF THE DIRECTORS WITHIN THE GROUP

Effective leaders work closely with and involve staff in decision-making. This approach has several advantages. It improves staff satisfaction, creates more nuanced decisions, enhances buy-in, and hardwires practice changes.

Nurse Staff Meetings

Nurse leadership and nursing staff use various meeting formats to achieve participative leadership—shared governance. In these meetings, staff members' opinions are solicited on various issues, and members' opinions are considered during decision-making. Some decisions and action plans are formalized in this group with the guidance of the leader. This dialogue between staff and leadership clarifies goals and objectives for the team.

Including the physician leader in the operations portion of a nursing staff meeting presents the nurse and physician leader as equals and coleaders, and staff observes mutual respect and collaboration in action. Further, by attending these meetings, the medical director can gain a fuller understanding of the perceptions and challenges of frontline, care-delivering staff. Physician participation in nurse staff meetings fosters the nursing staff's perception that the medical director and the staff physicians care about their needs and professional observations.

The directors can use this forum to encourage the staff to share their observations and requests directly and on the spot. The input they solicit can potentially modify their approaches to accomplish the established goals of the department. The availability of immediate input both to and from the medical director and shared decisions by the coleaders can improve efficiency and effectiveness of decision-making and planning.

Provider Meetings

Providers (physicians and sometimes advanced practice providers) also benefit from regular organized meetings. The opportunity to gather to communicate and share ideas is as important to the success of physician groups as it is to nursing staff. The presence of the nurse director at provider meetings sends the powerful message of collaboration and mutual respect that helps to solidify the concept of coleadership and validates the observations and requests of the nursing staff. Including nursing leadership at physician meetings also allows the nurse leader to hear nursing-related concerns from providers.

Combined Communications

Circumstances frequently call for a unified communication to the entire department. Examples include:

- Changes in leadership at any level from the ED itself to the highest corporate levels
- Changes in corporate vision and mission statements
- Messages with fiscal impact on frontline staff
- Public relations issues
- Operational and staffing changes
- Roll out of a major project

Staff trust in leadership is improved with ample communication during crucial times. A cohesive message indicating high-level and combined support for major initiatives or serious problems reassures staff that their leaders are working in tandem toward established goals. Properly constructed messages motivate the team and clearly communicate how the project, resolution of the problem, or major change of any type will help the ED and staff to:

- Achieve agreed upon goals.
- Reestablish why those goals are priorities.
- Modify tactics to achieve those goals.
- Define the expected outcomes—the "Why."

Some leaders prefer to use additional communication tools, such as a newsletter. Ideally, staff participate in, contribute to, and possibly coauthor this form of communication. This type of newsletter might include:

- A welcome to new staff members
- Important information about other staff members
- Progress on projects, patient satisfaction, LOS
- ED social gatherings, holiday parties
- Educational items of interest
- Follow-up or reinforcement of new patient care processes

MISSION, VISION, PLANNING

Simply stated, the primary goal of the ED is to take care of patients (and their families) and to take care of the people who take care of the patients. An effective and collaborative team consistently works toward these ends. To be successful within the global organization, ED staff and leaders must continually participate in the creation, modification, and delivery of the overarching goals of the department. Many EDs will create their own mission and vision statements that align with those of the organization. This helps staff to identify their own philosophy, strategies, and goals of patient and staff caring and integrate them into their daily practice. Collaboration between the physicians and nurses to develop departmental-level mission and vision statements ensures alignment between the two teams (see Chapter 2).

Mission Statement

The mission statement is a clear and concise document that answers three questions:

- What are the needs that we serve to address?
- How do we meet those needs?
- What are the principles we incorporate while doing that work?

An effective mission statement resonates with the group it guides and is developed or modified by representatives of that group. Since the mission of the ED is the same for physicians and nurses, a shared mission statement is in order. The mission statement must be fundamental and relevant to be of value. Slang or jargon should be avoided to ensure the message is clear and understandable to all stakeholders. The mission statement should be dynamic and action oriented. To ensure relevancy and alignment with the corporate mission, the departmental mission statement should be updated every few years.

The physician and nurse leader might wish to collaboratively develop a leadership mission and vision statement around their relationship. This statement would act as a guiding framework. This mission statement should answer the same three questions and might look something like this:

> *The emergency department exists to serve all patients in need. The directors of the emergency department exist to provide clear and consistent leadership and strategic planning to enhance the team's ability to provide the highest quality of care possible. The directors adhere to the tenets of equality, mutual respect, and integrity in the accomplishment of this mission.*

Vision Statement

The vision statement is a long-standing and high-level conception of what the organization wishes to be. The vision statement is the framework for strategic long-term and short-term planning. Similar to the mission statement, the ED directors can develop their own vision statement, an example of which is below:

> *The leadership of the emergency department engages in transformational behaviors and collaborates to ensure outcomes that are in alignment with corporate goals.*

Department vision statements created by staff might incorporate the concepts of delivering high-quality, compassionate care while being fiscally responsible. The department must be aware of and support organizational goals. Integrating the ED leadership's and department's mission and vision statement with corporate goals further enhances organizational alignment.

While the ED statements should be fully aligned with those of the institution, they should not be the same. Rather, the ED team should spend the time to ensure that its statements are specifically relevant to what the department does and wants to accomplish.

The ED statements may be thought of as visible and viable plans that outline what the ED stands for, where it is going, what it delivers, and how it will comport itself while on that journey. These plans are important to keep the team moving in the same direction and are a guide to newcomers of "how we do it here."

Strategic Planning

A gap analysis highlights the difference between where the organization wishes to be—the vision statement—and where the organization actually is. The gap is assessed by asking three simple questions:

- What is the current state?
- What is the desired state?
- What are the steps and resources needed to get to the desired state?

The gap analysis leads to the strategic plan for improvement. The leadership team develops the strategic plan, a formal outline for achieving the vision of the department and the organization. Staff should have the opportunity to participate by sharing their thoughts about the strategic plan through staff and clinical practice meetings. However, it is the role of the ED leaders to discern which suggestions are (and are not) in line with the organization's mission.

Strategic planning takes into consideration both the resources that are available and necessary to get to the desired state and the key "players" or stakeholders of influence necessary to achieve success. This planning concludes with goals and tactics that are specific, measurable, and accomplishable in a timely manner. It is helpful to organize the goals into discreet 90-day action steps, providing a manageable way to communicate and track progress. The strategic planning requires collaboration and agreement between the nursing and medical director.

USING QUALITY-IMPROVEMENT MODELS

Communicating goals using a respected quality improvement model will align leadership and frontline staff and ensure all parties are shooting at the same target. It is common for EDs to use the "Model for Improvement," which incorporates the testing phase of "Plan, Do, Study, Act."[11] The ED leadership team should determine which of the various improvement models will work best for the selected strategies and personnel. The leadership team may wish to employ the improvement model used by the parent organization, which may be more likely to achieve institutional acceptance. An aligned or "common" model uses language that is mutually accepted by all participants and clearly communicates the department's status of change.

Rolling Out Improvement Projects

Once the strategic plan and goals are developed, project development teams may be utilized as the means to roll out the project and achieve the goals.

Staff Involvement

A high level of staff engagement helps in the development and rollout phases. Identifying "champions" from among the frontline staff creates broad buy-in of the staff. Frontline staff involvement also provides the leadership with valuable insights and details about how the work actually is, and should be, done on the unit. The team process ensures that decisions are made based on realistic assessments of current and desired processes and outcomes.

Prior to implementing change, Lean processing can be helpful. ("Lean" is a management philosophy based on stripping away wasteful activities [e.g., ones that waste time and add no value to the process] and keeping or creating activities that add value for the patients, staff, and so on.) Thinking through the project from the "Lean" point of view can help staff members from many disciplines within the department create process maps detailing how work is currently accomplished. Another process map can then be created to detail how work will be accomplished in the future. Process maps visually communicate the expected overall change and the specific points and components of change. The consistent input of staff leads to a workable plan that is supported and avoids "work-arounds" that introduce variability and frustration.

Minimizing Variability

Variability, workarounds, and "one-offs" defeat successful implementation of new processes. Minimizing variability is essential to the successful rollout of a new plan. Efficiency and safety are most likely to occur when the approach is consistent and functions independently of the specific nurses and doctors who are working on any given day. Since the ED is filled with strong-willed people who like to think independently, it is important to hold the staff accountable to following the standard work, which is sometimes the most difficult part of the process.

Any new process or procedure should not be arbitrarily changed for a minimum of 30 days to reduce variability and confusion. This allows the staff to adjust to the new process before modifying it if necessary. However, an exception to the "30-day no-change rule" may be necessary if a member of the team identifies a process that is potentially harmful to a patient. Then, the concern must be immediately communicated to the floor leader (charge nurse or shift coordinator), who may determine that it is necessary to immediately modify or suspend the process.

Communicating the change to all staff can be accomplished by using an immediately recognizable process or form (e.g., a pink form) that describes the algorithm and includes the changes. The staff must know that a posted pink sheet communicates an immediate safety-related change. Other changes or procedural tweaks are deferred until the clinical practice meeting during which the team can discuss the issues and decide if changes are necessary to fine-tune the process.

Goal Evaluation

Goal evaluation should be performed quarterly to ensure continued alignment of unit and organizational needs. Leaders may begin the year by soliciting staff input for unit improvements. One method of collecting this information is an exercise called "What's working/What's not?" This technique may occur during a staff/team meeting. Each participant is given a stack of Post-it notes. On each note, staff members write one thing that is working or not working. (Each separate idea goes on its own note.) The small size of the note leads to concise ideas and avoids rambling complaints.

The leaders can then take the notes and sort them under the headings of Operations, People, Budget, and Quality. Several ideas may be similar, and common themes can be selected as high priorities for action. Coleaders can identify "low-hanging fruit"—ideas that are easily achieved. Rapid fixes encourage staff by demonstrating that their voices are heard. Since nothing breeds success like success, such easy harvesting allows and encourages the incorporation of more ideas into the strategic plan.

Effective leaders celebrate successes, which have a far greater impact when they are delivered jointly and regularly to both nursing and physician staff during "huddles." As more and more goals are achieved, the team and leadership become deeply invested in quality and continual improvement.

Interacting With the C-Suite

Collaborative and effective leaders plan interactions with institutional leadership, including the chief medical officer (CMO), chief executive officer (CEO), chief nursing officer (CNO), chief operating officer (COO), chief quality officer (CQO), and chief financial officer (CFO).

Although medical and nursing coleaders may in many ways be equal, the leaders should thoughtfully consider which of them is most likely to have the greatest influence with a particular institutional leader. For example, the CMO or CNO may be more receptive to hearing an update or a request from the ED medical director or nursing director, respectively. At the same time, hearing a consistent message from both leaders solidifies the perception of alignment and may help garner institutional support. It is critical that the ED leaders specifically agree about the priorities and language used to deliver the messages. Consistent descriptions and language when expressing concerns, requests, and plans demonstrate teamwork and a well-thought-out plan.

It is important to adapt the message to the audience. When considering proposals, the CFO generally prefers financial return on investment statements and cost outlay information. The CNO is interested in patient outcomes, processes, and satisfaction. The CQO has an interest in the impact on quality indicators. The same message, given to different members of the C-suite at different times, should be tailored to the specific listener.

INSPIRING THE NEXT GENERATION OF LEADERS

Forward-thinking leaders identify, develop, and prepare the next generation of leaders. By setting an example, the coleaders can model the philosophy of collaboration. Frequent teaching, observation, feedback, and coaching discussions with emerging leaders help to ensure growth, loyalty, and support on the front lines. Commitment to individual development strengthens the individual, team, and department.

Setting specific expectations, evaluating performance, and creating accountability identify leaders who are and are not meeting expectations. It is important to provide early feedback to potential leaders who are underperforming; if feedback fails to improve the leader's performance within a relatively short time frame, termination from the position should follow. Leaving an underperforming leader in a position lowers morale and is counter to continued momentum.

CONCLUSION

Collaborative leadership in the ED setting is critical to patient care, the ED team, and the hospital. Trust is the foundation on which successful coleadership is built. Understanding one's self and applying the information learned in self-reflection fosters the development of a strong leadership team. Setting a pattern of frequent, open, and honest communication is integral to success. Certain failure will occur when there is lack of communication and frequent unilateral decision-making.

The broader ED and administrative teams quickly recognize poor collaboration between the ED coleaders. Divided coleaders fail to fully achieve the goals of the team and the hospital.

Divergent strategies (like working to accomplish goals separately without the knowledge or support of the coleader) severely limit the potential successes of the ED and can compromise patient care. The hallmark of effective coleadership is that the nurse and medical directors discuss, work through, and agree on departmental and interpersonal strategies. ED leaders who engage in mentoring and personal and professional growth as they continue on their journey of collaborative leadership are the most likely to succeed.

REFERENCES

1. Raup GH. The impact of ED nurse manager leadership style on staff nurse turnover and patient satisfaction in academic health center hospitals. *J Emerg Nurs*. 2008;34(5):403-409.
2. Robison J, Turning Around Employee Turnover, http://businessjournal.gallup.com/content/106912/turning-around-your-turnover-problem.aspx. Published May 8, 2008, Business Journal, Accessed June 10, 2020
3. MBTI, http://www.myersbriggs.org/. Published 2020, The Myers & Briggs Foundation, Accessed May 25, 2020
4. The Keirsey Group, The Four Temperaments, http://www.keirsey.com/. Published 2020, Accessed June 11, 2020
5. Your Life's Path, Thee DISC Profile, http://www.thediscpersonalitytest.com/. Published 2020, Accessed April 5, 2020
6. Kilmann RH, Thomas-Kilmann Assessment Tool, http://www.kilmanndiagnostics.com/. Published 2020, Accessed June 11, 2020
7. Psychology Today, Body Language, http://www.psychologytoday.com/basics/body-language. Published 2020, Psychology Today, Accessed April 3, 2020
8. Mayer JP, Salovey P, Caruso DR. Emotional intelligence: new ability or eclectic traits? *Am Psychol*. 2008;63(6):503-517.
9. Salovey P, Mayer JD. Emotional intelligence. *Imagin Cogn Pers*. 1990;9(3):185-211.
10. Goleman D. *Working With Emotional Intelligence*. New York, NY: Bantam Books; 1998.
11. Institute for Healthcare Improvement. Available at: www.ihi.org. Accessed April 2011.

Physician staffing is one of the most important and fundamental competencies required of emergency medicine and hospital leaders. Not only are providers (physicians and advanced practice providers [APPs]) the costliest resource, but they, along with nursing staff, are among the scarcest resources in the emergency department (ED). Given that quality, flow, and patient satisfaction depend on a timely and engaging initial provider–patient encounter, effectively staffing EDs is one of the most essential tasks we do for our patients.

Understanding key academic principles, defining demand, and understanding variability of demand and subsequent capacity, including all the elements that create these variations, are keys to optimal staffing. This chapter addresses each of these key concepts in detail to provide insight into the best practices for provider staffing.

APPLYING ACADEMIC PRINCIPLES

Effective and efficient staffing requires the application of some important academic principles, including the theories of queuing and constraints. Effective provider workflow can be analyzed and improved with Lean principles (adding value, eliminating waste) and other performance improvement techniques. Time studies, workflow analyses, spaghetti diagramming, human factors analyses, and other techniques provide valuable insight into the causes of and solutions for inferior provider productivity.

Queuing Theory

Queuing theory can help optimize shift design by taking into account the rates of patient arrival and service (and all their variations). Queuing theory asserts there is a definable average arrival rate for every ED for any given hour and that each caregiver has a definable service rate at which they can see patients. Service rates vary by provider according to personal characteristics, system design elements, and environmental factors. The interaction between arrival rates and service rates determines how responsive the system is (i.e., the length of patient wait times) under average operating conditions.[1]

Theory of Constraints

The theory of constraints (TOC) also significantly affects staffing efficiency. A constraint or bottleneck is anything that slows the flow or throughput of patients. The TOC maintains that if the activities in a process and the providers responsible for those activities are clearly defined, the busiest caregiver will often be the greatest constraint to throughput. This basic concept has profound implications for staffing EDs because it sets forth that provider efficiency is inextricably related to the other system resources, such as nurses and beds. The TOC asserts that if providers are the bottleneck, then all efforts must be focused on reducing provider demand or increasing provider capacity. However, if there is another constraint in the system (e.g., nurses or beds), then enhancing provider productivity will not significantly improve overall throughput.

As an example of this TOC concept, consider a four-bed fast track with an average patient arrival rate of three per hour. This fast track area is staffed by one nurse and one doctor. Assume that the doctor can see three patients per hour, performing the history, physical, and any requisite procedures. The nurse spends 30 minutes with each patient on average, taking history and vital signs, performing the nursing physical examination, administering medications, and documenting each of these actions.

Now, calculate the number of patients managed in this scenario in an average hour. The correct response is two patients per hour. In this example, the nurse is the constraining resource at two patients managed per hour (whereas the doctor sees three patients per hour); adding a doctor or additional beds does not increase throughput. The only method to enhance throughput is to offload tasks from the nurse, which can be accomplished by eliminating no-value-added nursing tasks or by transferring value-added work to another provider who is not as busy.

For example, the physician could assume the discharge process or the nurse could defer some of the initial assessment to the doctor's notes. If 10 minutes of work per patient can be eliminated, the nurse's throughput increases to three patients per hour. Interestingly, even if additional arriving patients exceed the average arrival rate, the reduction in nursing tasks will likely drive down length of stay (LOS), improve door-to-doctor times, and reduce the number of patients who leave prior to the medical screening examination.

OPTIMIZING PROVIDER PRODUCTIVITY

The basic approach to optimizing provider staffing involves three steps:

1. Defining **demand** and variation around demand
2. Defining **provider capacity**
3. Optimizing factors that affect **service capacity**: provider, operational, and environmental

This chapter expands on this basic approach to staffing, addressing each of these three steps; but first, we take a look at the benefits of optimizing provider productivity and the common mistakes that interfere with or prevent it.

Benefits

Why should provider productivity and staffing alignment be optimized? Why not continue to staff according to feel and intuition? With the current focus on "doing more with less," healthcare organizations expect providers to manage more patients per hour, and precious resources cannot be wasted. These demands drive up stress levels, upset work–life balance, and contribute to burnout.

Simply put, provider productivity is the sum of staffing efficiency during every hour of the year. Thus, capacity should reflect demand. By using Lean principles, systems can be designed with less waste, greater provider productivity, and increased provider satisfaction. Effective systems provide necessary services, lead to improved patient satisfaction, and create additional revenue for provider compensation.

Common Mistakes

After performing more than 1,000 analyses over nearly two decades, we have identified some common missteps made by medical directors when staffing and scheduling their departments.

Missing the Ramp Up

Many of the EDs evaluated failed to provide sufficient capacity to meet demand early in the day. This mistiming forces providers to manage too many patients, and insufficient front-end effort pushes most of the work later in the patient encounter or shift. This delay creates a situation in which the individual provider has many patients taking up space in the department while awaiting completion of their evaluations and dispositions. The result is bed congestion and batching of admissions at the end of the shift.

As a simple illustration, presume the provider is expected to see 10 patients in the first hour of a shift. Mathematically, this expectation allows a maximum of 6 minutes with each patient and that maximum can only be achieved if patients arrive in exactly 6-minute intervals. However, because of other responsibilities and the time it takes to move from room to room, the provider will likely spend 5 minutes or less with each patient.

Now, assume the provider can manage an average of two patients per hour (30 minutes of work for each patient). In the first hour, the provider has performed 50 minutes of work and generated an additional 25 minutes of work per patient (250 minutes) to be completed later. Over the next 2 to 3 hours, as evaluations are being completed, results of diagnostic tests become available and dispositions are developed, giving the provider time to catch up. However, more patients will arrive, and the provider and the ED will fall further behind.

This combination of batching and queuing commonly causes flow problems in the ED. By properly staffing the department to match the flow of patient arrivals, providers can keep up with their workload and smooth the flow of cases throughout their shift. This environment is less stressful and decreases the overall work for both providers and nurses by reducing the number of interruptions and service requests. Ramping up staffing to match increases in patient arrivals avoids the all-too-common nursing complaint, "Doctor, everything's back on the patient in room 3, and he and his family want to know when he can go home."

Incorrect Skill Mix

Whether staffing for low- or high-acuity cases, leaders should understand the proper mix of APPs and doctors required to run an efficient department. Insufficient APP capacity for low-acuity patients creates congestion and poor flow because patients must wait to see the APP. However, if doctors accommodate the excess demand, they are not working to their full capability. Furthermore, two APPs can sometimes replace one doctor, creating more capacity for less cost and identical quality. However, this substitution can create a flow problem if it results in APPs working above their skill level or requiring more physician oversight.

Understaffing for Low-Acuity Patients

Failing to maintain sufficient capacity for low-acuity cases or failing to open the low-acuity care pathway early enough in the morning can drive patients to the main ED and toward physician management. This patient misplacement creates a congestion of low-acuity cases. By staying ahead of the curve, department leaders can optimize the LOS in their ED; this, in turn, reduces the occupancy of low-acuity cases, freeing up treatment spaces for sicker patients. Leaders should stay ahead of the curve and properly staff for low-acuity patients to optimize LOS and in so doing reduce occupancy of low-acuity patients and free up treatment spaces for sicker patients.

Incorrect Assumptions About Physician Workflow and Productivity

Perhaps the most common misconception about workflow is that staggering shifts allows providers to remain equally effective throughout the shift. With staggered shifts, providers are very active for the first few hours. However, once relief arrives, the arriving provider takes on most of the new work, and the first provider becomes less productive (perhaps taking the time to catch up). By the time the third provider arrives, the first provider may stop seeing new patients altogether. This layered staffing is much less efficient than other models like pods, which allow direct provider-to-provider contiguous shift relief.

Poorly Designed Segmentation Schemes

Segmentation is important for optimizing productivity of providers working in the context of care delivery systems and teams. A three-stream model, for instance, in which Emergency Severity Index (ESI) 4 and 5 patients are taken to a specific area, where they can be attended to by an APP, nurse, and tech, can greatly enhance provider productivity. A super track can easily accommodate 2.5 patients per hour, enhancing typical nurse productivity fourfold and typical physician and APP productivity by 25% to 50% due to teamwork, reduced waste, compact layout, and better organization.

No Dedicated Front-End Process

Traditional EDs fall short when beds or nurses impede flow. EDs must be designed to overcome process-related bed constraints and always allow patient–provider interaction immediately on arrival.

DEFINING DEMAND

The elements of demand are relatively straightforward:

- Patient arrivals
- Acuity levels

Patient arrivals vary predictably throughout the day, week, year, and on holidays. Although patient arrivals cannot be forecasted for a specific hour or day, average arrival rates can be projected based on historic patterns, providing a likely range in the number of patients arriving at a given time.

Patient acuity drives the workload of providers and nurses. This factor can be predicted according to historical measures of acuity, such as ESI levels (triage stratification defining those with most and least urgent needs), admission rate, or resources used to provide care (such as average relative value units per patient visit). Contrary to conventional wisdom, ESI levels can vary substantially from day to day, and assessments of ESI levels can vary from triage nurse to triage nurse. This variation results from training and environmental factors (e.g., when the main ED is full and fast track is not, an ESI 3 might be assigned an ESI level 4 to expedite the initial provider interaction). Admission rates, which can also vary by provider, can change considerably on any given day, particularly in small, single-coverage EDs. All other things being equal, the most accurate way to predict future demand is through the study of these important variables.

Arrivals

Hour-of-Day Variation

The typical ED arrival pattern over a 24-hour period is remarkably predictable and universal, with few exceptions. The patient arrival rate in the ED drops during overnight shifts and begins to ramp up around 6 am or 7 am, peaking between 10 am and 10 pm. The fall to typical overnight lows usually occurs by 2 am. Many EDs experience a slight lull in patient arrivals during the midday, between the morning and afternoon rushes.

The typical ED realizes a patient arrival ratio between 4:1 and 6:1 during peak times and the slower overnight shift. For example, a busy ED with 24 patient arrivals during peak hours will characteristically have an overnight arrival rate of four to six patients per hour. Notable exceptions to the classic adult distribution are pediatric environments, which experience lower acuity and more arrivals in the evening between 5 pm and 10 pm owing to children's school hours and parents' work schedules. EDs in areas with few urgent care centers will also recognize this evening spike. Lastly, a drop-off in demand toward the late afternoon and early evening hours could be due to poor operational performance early in the day or significant penetration of urgent care centers in the area. See **Figure 21.1** for typical hourly arrival patterns.

Day-of-Week Variation

There are also typical day-of-week arrival patterns. The most typical low is Saturday and Sunday, with a peak on Monday and downward trending over the remainder of the weekdays. Pediatric arrival rates during the week are a notable exception, with significant volume increases on weekends, especially Sundays. Mondays are not only the busiest day of

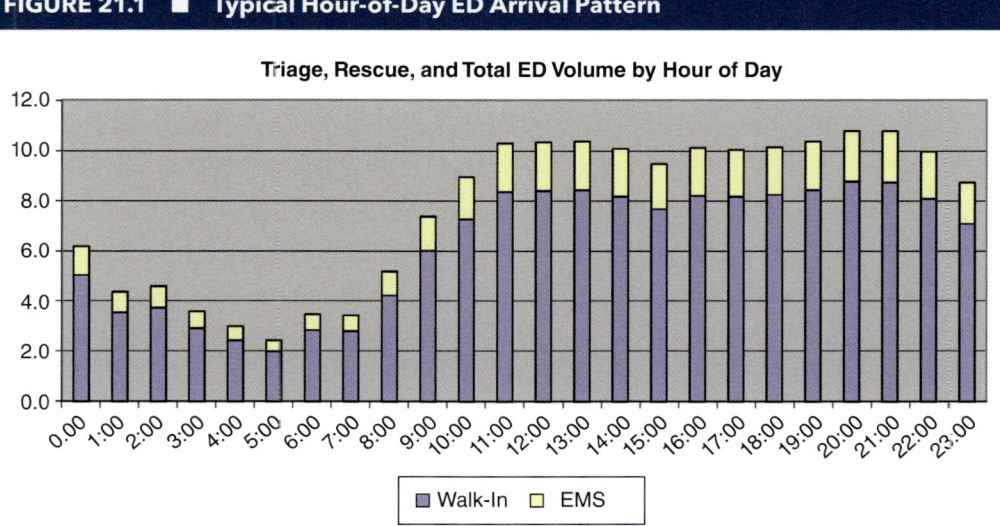

FIGURE 21.1 ■ Typical Hour-of-Day ED Arrival Pattern

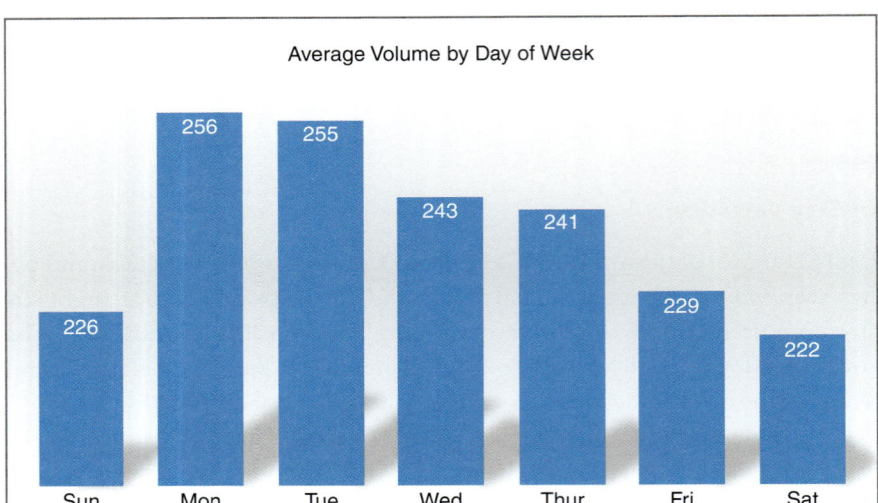

FIGURE 21.2 ■ Typical Day-of-Week Variation

the week in adult EDs, they are also typically the highest in acuity, a challenge that creates a double jeopardy for staffing and flow. See **Figure 21.2** for day-of-week variations.

Seasonal Variation

Most EDs encounter subtle changes in winter volume related to influenza and other challenges associated with colder weather. This seasonal volume flux may vary by up to 10% in the typical ED. However, some EDs in the southeastern and southwestern United States encounter much greater variation in volume—between 20% and 50%—as the local population swells during the winter ("snowbird") months. Pediatric EDs face similar spikes in volume during the winter owing to colds, flu, and respiratory syncytial virus infections. In fact, during the H1N1 swine flu epidemic, many pediatric EDs saw volume increases of over 100%!

Holidays

There are predictable peaks and valleys related to holidays. For example, Christmas morning and early New Year's Eve (before midnight) typically see dramatically reduced volumes, whereas the Tuesdays after Labor and Memorial Days are typically the busiest of the year. Some urban locations may experience low volume early on Sunday (with a population going to church and watching professional football), followed by busier evening.

Acuity

Patient-specific characteristics can drive additional demand. As an example, trauma patients tend to display wide variation in arrival times and require a large variety of provider and other resources. This variation is especially true in institutions with trauma designation. Ironically, a major trauma designation often creates a lower demand on the ED physician, who typically manages the airway and defers other procedures in this setting. In contrast, other resources, such as nursing, may have very high utilization. Alternatively, in health-care centers not designated as trauma centers, the ED provider must manage the entire extensive trauma workup, including multiple time-consuming procedures, counseling, and coordination of care. Very sick or elderly patients can have a similar effect on productivity owing to the likelihood of admission and critical care time.

DEFINING CAPACITY

The next important element of proper staffing requires defining productivity or service capacity. Service capacity is determined by calculating the following elements, which influence proper staffing:

- Average service rate
- Peak service rate
- Boarding

Average Service Rate

The average service rate is calculated by simply dividing the total number of arrivals during a period by the total staffing hours during that same timeframe. For example, an ED that has 48 arrivals and 24 hours of provider coverage per day averages two patients per provider hour. Although this number might seem to reflect a well-staffed ED, the variation of arrivals during the day might include three to four patients arriving during peak hours and zero to one patient arriving during the overnight hours. Thus, with single-provider coverage, this ED would perform very poorly at peak times because the peak arrival rate might significantly exceed the peak service rate.

Peak Service Rate

The peak service rate is calculated by first defining the peak arrival period, for example, 10 am to 10 pm, when it is likely the provider will be constantly busy and there may be an increasing number of patients in the waiting room (WR). The WR census is taken immediately before and after this time interval, and the difference is subtracted from the total number of patient arrivals over this period to determine the net number of patients seen. The net number is divided by the number of provider hours over the same period to calculate the peak service rate.

For example, assume there are five patients in the WR of a double-coverage ED at 10 am. Over the next 12 hours, an average of four patients arrives per hour (48 patients total). Then, at 10 pm, there are 11 patients in the WR waiting to be brought back. The result is 48 – 6, or a net of 42 patients managed during that time. Dividing 42 by the number of staffed hours in the 12-hour period (a total of 24) results in an estimate of 1.75 patients per provider hour. In this example, productivity represents the number of patients the providers were able to care for in the operational system and not the theoretical maximum, which could be determined through more advanced time studies. See **Figure 21.3** for the peak service rate calculation.

FIGURE 21.3 ■ **Peak Service Rate Calculation**

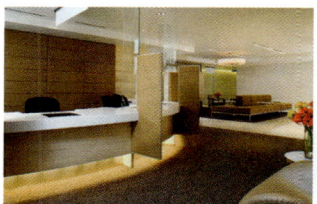
Waiting room count start

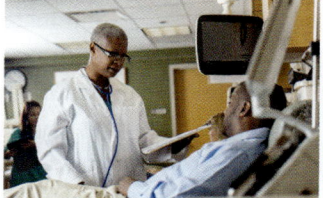
Total patients/ total physician hours

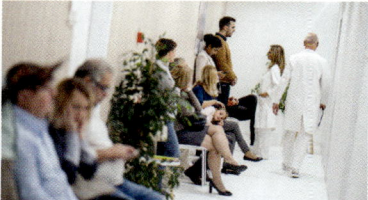
Waiting room count end

$$\frac{[\text{Total Arrivals} - (\text{WR Count End} - \text{WR Count Start})]}{\text{Total Provider Hours}}$$

Many provider groups use adjusted patient per provider hour (PPH), a calculation that adjusts for the utilization of APPs (including physician assistants [PAs] and nurse practitioners [NPs]) by multiplying by some factor to indicate lower productivity or lower cost. Commonly, provider groups apply a 0.5 multiplier for adjusted PPH.

In the example above, if one of the providers is an APP, the total provider hours are 12 + 12 × 0.5, or 18. Using the number of patients completed (42) divided by the adjusted hours (18) results in an adjusted PPH of 2.33 patients per provider hour. One benefit of using adjusted PPH to calculate productivity is the incentive, when appropriate, to staff the department with less expensive, highly productive, and quality APPs. The primary downside is that PPH can be confusing to anyone who is not intimately familiar with its use.

Patient Boarding

Although boarding rarely affects provider productivity directly (except in the case of critical intensive care unit patients requiring ongoing care), it indirectly affects provider productivity through the consumption of valuable resources, including nurses and beds. Therefore, ED physician leadership teams must work collaboratively with their nursing leadership and administrative counterparts to create schedules, contingency plans, and operational models that are responsive to the typical boarding and overcrowding challenges an ED faces.

Benchmarks

Provider productivity benchmarks are scarce, and there is no universal ideal. The American College of Emergency Physicians, the Society of Academic Emergency Medicine, and the American Academy of Emergency Medicine each have position statements regarding provider productivity. However, due to the disparate conditions of each facility and capacity of each provider, a specific productivity target is difficult to identify.

Most experts agree that provider productivity in the range of 1.6 to 2.4 patients per provider hour is reasonable. According to preliminary data provided by the Emergency Department Benchmarking Alliance (EDBA) in 2017, average adjusted provider productivity (daily patients divided by [physician hours + 0.5 × APP hours]) was 2.06 patients per adjusted hour. The EDBA did not publish straight PPH data. Many believe that an aging population and alternative care locations, such as urgent care centers, are pushing ED patient acuities higher and potential productivity lower. Simultaneously, financial stressors and provider availability are forcing EDs to become more efficient. As such, current productivity targets are not exhibiting meaningful trending changes.

Getting at True Capacity

Using average productivity or peak productivity calculations to estimate the peak achievable service rate (the number of patients that can be seen per hour) may be misleading for many reasons. The more scientific way to determine the maximum number of patients a provider can see per hour is to measure all the time-consuming activities required to evaluate, treat, discharge, transfer, or admit a patient—a process referred to as a "time study."

Several studies have documented the relationship between patient acuity and the time required to manage specific types of cases.[2-5] Unfortunately, all of these studies originated in Canada or Denmark and may not reflect the American ED experience. The only relevant US investigation was performed in a single ED setting with 12 different physicians that

TABLE 21.1 ■ ED Provider Service Times

	Minutes	
CTAS 1	73.6	
CTAS 2	38.9	
CTAS 3	26.3	
CTAS 4	15	
CTAS 5	10.9	Pts/Hr
Weighted Avg	26.0	2.3
120%	31.2	1.9

considered only a subset of patient encounters (e.g., laceration repairs). The most relevant international study was published by Dreyer et al in 2009.[2] Using the Canadian Triage and Acuity Scale (CTAS) shown in **Table 21.1**, the study measured the total time spent caring for more than 11,000 patients. Although CTAS and ESI triage systems have their differences, this study does show a very close correlation between increased acuity and the increased time required to treat. In this study, at 100% utilization, a physician would be able to treat almost six CTAS level 5 patients, four CTAS level 4 patients, two CTAS level 2 or 3 patients, and one CTAS level 1 patient. Intuitively, this result seems consistent with productivity targets in the US health system.

An important point to note about time studies is that they are seldom generalizable owing to the site-specific nuances of flow and productivity inherent to an individual ED. Variables such as nurse staffing, bed availability, ancillary turnaround time, ED information systems, human factors, educational mission, and other elements can dramatically affect individual provider productivity. Because of this local variation, the authors strongly recommend performing site-specific time studies to determine peak achievable productivity in an individual ED. Details on how to undertake a time study can be found in *The Definitive Guide to Emergency Department Operational Improvement*.[6]

OPTIMIZING SERVICE CAPACITY

Many elements contribute to provider productivity. Individual provider traits, training, and workflow efficiency can dramatically affect performance. The key to enhancing individual productivity is to incorporate a system that promotes throughput. If a provider continues to underperform, promote self-awareness by having the provider shadow a peer or vice versa. The most commonly noted factors for provider underperformance are personality or social factors, low motivation, distractions in the workplace, ordering practices (i.e., sequential workups or uncertainty in diagnosis or workup plan after initial assessment), and personal disorganization.

Documentation

There are great advantages to the Centers for Medicare and Medicaid Services' Meaningful Use Initiative. However, the implementation of electronic health records (EHRs), computer-based documentation, electronic order entry, and provider-driven results retrieval has detracted from direct patient care and consumed significant amounts of provider time. In fact, multiple studies demonstrate that time spent interacting with the EHR consumes 30% to 40% of the physician's clinical shift time.[5,7] This time demand exceeds the time spent directly caring for the patient. In one high-profile study, the authors discovered that providers spent only 28% of their time on direct patient care and 43% of their time on data entry, which requires an average of 4,000 clicks during a typical 10-hour shift.[7]

Scheduling Practices

Scheduling practices affect provider productivity on a macrolevel by limiting the overall productivity achievable in a 24-hour period. For example, many EDs prefer 10-hour shifts. Unfortunately, if one is limited to 10-hour shifts, the only scheduling method to cover a 24-hour period is with 30 hours of daily coverage (three shifts with 2-hour overlaps). In this scenario, an average daily volume of 60 patients per day achieves an average productivity of 2.0 patients per hour. Use of 8- or 12-hour shifts—creating a schedule without overlap or periods of double coverage—could result in a productivity of 2.5 patients per hour. Alternatively, longer shift duration can lead to lower productivity in the later hours of the shift, especially when there is significant shift overlap.

For example, in a 12-hour shift, a provider may stop seeing patients at hour 10. Similarly, the provider may see 3.0 patients for the first 4 hours, 2.0 patients per hour for the middle 4 hours, and 1.0 patient per hour for the final 4 hours. Although the average is still two patients per hour, patient flow will be very different in this scenario versus a scenario in which the provider consistently sees two patients per hour throughout the entire shift.

Finally, the total number of hours worked in a year can affect provider performance. Vukmir and Howell demonstrated that maximum productivity was achieved at 1,550 hours worked per year.[8] This productivity declined measurably when hours worked exceeded 1,800 hours annually.

Site-Specific Operations

Operations like flow and boarding can also affect provider productivity. Specifically, the ED's front-end approach and its ability to get patients in front of providers is the most important variable for enhancing clinician performance. Systems that rely on formal bed placement and nursing workflow to feed patients to providers are inherently less efficient than systems in which providers can direct and lead throughput in the department.

In the main ED, the key to enhancing provider productivity is teamwork through pods or zone-based care, which reduce walking, movement, and patient transportation and greatly enhance communication by limiting the number of interactions required by every member of the team.[9] For example, a 27-bed ED with three providers and nine nurses at peak times could have three providers, each with nine randomly distributed cases, and nine separate nurses with whom providers must work. Conversely, the same ED with three pods would have one provider and three nurses per nine-bed pod. Documentation areas are typically located centrally in each of the pods, enabling all caregivers to work near one another, which greatly enhances passive and active communication. Pods encourage teamwork and can help predict the needs of individual team members.

Furthermore, if nurses know when a patient is bedded in their zone, they immediately know which doctor or APP will manage the case. The nurse is likely cognizant of the provider's workup and procedure preparation preferences, which can contribute to the efficiency of patient management.

Nurse Staffing

As previously mentioned—but worth emphasizing—one of the most important variables in provider productivity is nurse staffing and availability. As financial and workforce availability constraints increase for hospitals and health systems, fewer nursing resources are available to provide direct patient care. With growing shortages and callouts, nurses are pulled from critical high-flow areas, such as FTs and provider-in-triage processes, to provide patient care in the main ED. The result is reduced productivity because the sickest patients become the highest priority; the less-seriously ill patients, who could contribute to high-flow rates, may leave as the capacity of providers deteriorates.

Skill Mix

Historically, APPs staffed fast-track and other lower-acuity areas of the ED. However, recent financial pressures and advances in APP training and capacity have resulted in APPs staffing higher-acuity patient areas that were traditionally managed by physicians only. Depending on the expertise of the APPs staffing a site, this practice may prove helpful or harmful. Although many APPs can be quite adept at managing or initiating management for higher-acuity patients, some APPs may find it more challenging, leading to increased diagnostic testing and longer LOS.

Typically, staffing for higher acuity patients requires closer physician supervision, which may reduce the physician's individual productivity and overall throughput. Furthermore, increasing ratios of APPs to physicians can cause a similar reduction in aggregate physician productivity and reduce overall department throughput. Although national physician-to-APP ratios trend toward 2:1, there are some locations that push the envelope and staff the ED in a manner consistent with the anesthesia model, with multiple nurse anesthetists per supervising anesthesiologist. This model creates significant challenges in the ED, including the APP management of high-complexity patients, variability in patient presentations, and the downstream need to communicate with admitting providers and consultants, some of whom prefer to be consulted directly by the attending physician.

An interesting emerging model for front-end ED operations involves an attending physician as the first point of contact in a vertical model supported by one or more APPs. In this model, the physician's role is to initially see and evaluate all patients, with the APPs executing the ongoing treatment, procedures, and ultimate disposition of the patient. This promising approach reduces ancillary testing, increases throughput, improves productivity, and enhances provider satisfaction through teamwork.

Optimizing Alignment

Optimal demand–capacity alignment contributes to improved flow, responsiveness, and maximized productivity of providers. Provider capacity should be aligned with demand, departmental resources (e.g., nurses and techs), and operational processes (e.g., split flow and super track).

Proper alignment with nursing resources ensures there are no significant bottlenecks related to relative imbalances of providers to nurses. For example, in EDs where the nursing and physician leadership do not align their schedules, the early morning hours may be insufficiently staffed. This imbalance creates a scenario in which providers might be ready to see patients, but there are insufficient nurses to support them or vice versa, leading to wasted resources.

Specialized processes require alignment of providers and nurses to drive flow in the department. For example, a department with three low-acuity arrivals per hour starting at 9 am should consider implementing a super track or other dedicated low-acuity process. However, if providers and nurses do not arrive to staff the area until 11 am, six patients will either be pushed into the main ED to compete with high-acuity patients or will have to wait in the WR until the low-acuity process opens. In either case, this resource misalignment represents a lost opportunity.

Scheduling Strategy

Once the proper alignment of resources is determined, the final step is to translate the perfect alignment into a feasible schedule. Although this step may seem straightforward, it is actually quite complex. Factors such as shift duration, shift start and stop times, and schedule rotations can result in a schedule that requires 10% to 20% more resources than the demand would suggest. Therefore, another form of misalignment may occur when there is a mismatch between staffing efficiency (achieving the closest alignment to the determined patient demand) and scheduling efficiency (achieving the best schedule fit to the determined hours needed).

For example, a 17,000-visit ED might have the demand for one physician 24 hours a day, 7 days per week, with 8 hours of APP coverage. However, if the available APPs are only willing to work 12-hour shifts, there will be 28 hours (12.5%) excess coverage weekly. This misalignment translates into an incremental, unnecessary expense of approximately $130,000 annually. An organization that has considerable flexibility in planned shift start times and durations will be able to develop schedules that tightly fit demand and minimize the amount of wasteful excess scheduled hours.

As a Google search for "emergency department scheduling program" will show, most modern EDs use sophisticated computerized programs to create their schedules. These programs incorporate shift requests, shift preferences, and rules for modifying individual shifts. Most apps rely on a traditional vacation or shift request approach. However, such processes are hindered by lag time; 60 days may pass between the time a provider makes a shift request and the publication of the schedule. Some directors solve this issue by using a progressive rotation that projects the schedule months in advance (e.g., four shifts on, four-shifts off). A single-coverage ED with 8-hour shifts (7 am-3 pm, 3 pm-11 pm, 11 pm-7 am) might have a shift rotation similar to the schedule shown in **Figure 21.4**, which includes a 24-day repeating cycle of shifts that could be rolled out indefinitely. An overlapping add–drop–trade process can accommodate vacation and other time-off requests.

FIGURE 21.4 ■ Shift Rotation Example

	Day of Month															
	1	2	3	4	5	6	7	8	9	10	11	12	13	14	15	16
Doctor #1	7a-3p	7a-3p	7a-3p	7a-3p	Off	Off	Off	Off	3p-11p	3p-11p	3p-11p	3p-11p	Off	Off	Off	Off
Doctor #2	Off	Off	Off	Off	7a-3p	7a-3p	7a-3p	7a-3p	Off	Off	Off	Off	3p-11p	3p-11p	3p-11p	3p-11p
Doctor #3	11p-7a	11p-7a	11p-7a	11p-7a	Off	Off	Off	Off	7a-3p	7a-3p	7a-3p	7a-3p	Off	Off	Off	Off
Doctor #4	Off	Off	Off	Off	11p-7a	11p-7a	11p-7a	11p-7a	Off	Off	Off	Off	7a-3p	7a-3p	7a-3p	7a-3p
Doctor #5	3p-11p	3p-11p	3p-11p	3p-11p	Off	Off	Off	Off	11p-7a	11p-7a	11p-7a	11p-7a	Off	Off	Off	Off
Doctor #6	Off	Off	Off	Off	3p-11p	3p-11p	3p-11p	3p-11p	Off	Off	Off	Off	11p-7a	11p-7a	11p-7a	11p-7a

CONCLUSION

Staffing optimization is a core skill for leaders in emergency medicine. Because providers are scarce and expensive resources, an efficient staffing design is integral to running a reliable ED with highly efficient throughput. Flow, patient satisfaction, and staff satisfaction suffer greatly when staffing is not optimized.

Mastery of queuing theory and the TOC, coupled with an operations improvement strategy, provides the foundation for success. Identifying demand and its variability allows the proper understanding of staffing needs. Defining staff capacity and optimizing productivity are necessary to accommodate demand in an efficient, effective manner.

REFERENCES

1. Noon CE, Hankins CT, Cote MJ. Understanding the impact of variation in the delivery of healthcare services. *J Healthc Manag.* 2003;48(2):82-97.

2. Anderson CK, Zaric GS, Dreyer JF, Carter MW, McLeod SL. Physician workload and the Canadian Emergency Department Triage and Acuity Scale: the Predictors of Workload in the Emergency Room (POWER) Study. *CJEM.* 2009;11(4):321-329.

3. Innes GD, Stenstrom R, Grafstein E, Christenson JM. Prospective time study derivation of emergency physician workload predictors. *CJEM.* 2005–7(5):299-308.

4. Graff LG, Wolf S, Dinwoodie R, Buono D, Mucci D. Emergency physician workload: a time study. *Ann Emerg Med.* 1993;22(7):1156-1163.

5. Fuchtbauer LM, Norgaard B, Mogensen CB. Emergency department physicians spend only 25% of their working time on direct patient care. *Dan Med J.* 2013;60(1):A4558.

6. Crane J, Noon C. *The Definitive Guide to Emergency Department Operational Improvement.* Boca Raton, Fla: CRC Press; 2011.

7. Hill RG, Sears LM, Melanson SW. 4000 clicks: a productivity analysis of electronic medical records in a community hospital emergency department. *Am J Emerg Med.* 2013;31(11):1591-1594.

8. Vukmir RB, Howell RN. Emergency medicine provider efficiency: the learning curve, equilibration and point of diminishing returns. *Emerg Med J.* 2010;27(12):916-920.

9. Valentine MA, Edmondson AC. Team scaffolds: how meso-level structures support role-based coordination in temporary groups. *Working Paper Harvard Business School.* Harvard Business School, Cambridge, MA. 2014.

NURSE STAFFING

CHAPTER 22

Denise Bayer, Donna Mason, Nancy Bonalumi

Ensuring the emergency department (ED) has appropriate staffing is one of the most critical and complex duties of the ED nurse director. For better or worse, there is no aspect of the department that is not influenced or affected by staffing. Research has consistently demonstrated a correlation between staffing and good patient outcomes, including patient safety, mortality, and satisfaction.[1,2]

The challenge for the ED nurse director is to create a staffing plan that will ensure high-quality patient care that results in positive outcomes, safe and effective care that leads to staff satisfaction and a positive work environment, and efficient care that meets both the customer service expectations and the financial needs of the organization. To do this, nurse directors must rely on their extensive knowledge of ED operations and their ability to apply staffing models and budgetary concepts related to labor cost. In present times, it is also necessary to not only understand ED staffing and labor costs but also to have knowledge of inpatient and critical care labor theories. The nurse director must build, sustain, monitor, and manage the staffing plan while forecasting future budget and volume demands. Staffing and scheduling is something most ED directors will spend a significant amount of time on; however, given its impact on every other aspect of ED operations, it is time well spent.

LEGISLATION, REGULATION, AND PROFESSIONAL STANDARDS

There have been many attempts to regulate nurse staffing at both the state and federal levels. The Centers for Medicare and Medicaid Services requires hospitals participating in Medicare to "have an adequate number of licensed registered nurses (RNs), licensed practical (vocational) nurses, and other personnel to provide nursing care to all patients as needed."[3] This requirement is as challenging as it is vague and open to considerable interpretation of the term "adequate" regarding licensed personnel. Since 2006, there have been multiple unsuccessful attempts to pass the Registered Nurse Safe Staffing Act at the federal level.[4] The lack of a federal statute has led several states to develop and pass legislation related to nurse staffing (**Table 22.1**).

The nurse director can turn to two professional organizations for staffing guidance: the American Nurses Association (ANA) and the Emergency Nurses Association (ENA). Both of these organizations provide resources to help nurses understand staffing principles and processes (**Table 22.2**).

The ANA supports a legislative model in which nurses are empowered to create flexible staffing plans specific to their unit. This approach aids in establishing staffing levels that are flexible and account for any "real-time" changes needed due to patient care needs and census and recognizes the need to view staffing beyond a simple nurse to patient ratio.[5]

TABLE 22.1 ■ State-Based Legislation Regarding Nurse Staffing			
Nurse Staffing Legislation	**Required Staffing Committee**	**Required Nurse-to-Patient Ratio**	**Required Public Disclosure of Staffing Levels**
• California • Connecticut • Illinois • Michigan • Minnesota • Nevada • New York • North Carolina • Ohio • Rhode Island • Texas • Vermont • Washington	• Connecticut • Illinois • Nevada • Ohio • Oregon • Texas • Washington	• California	• Illinois • New Jersey • New York • Rhode Island • Vermont

The ENA has worked for years to provide emergency nurses with meaningful tools to determine safe and effective staffing. The ENA position statement "Staffing and Productivity in the Emergency Department" states[6]:

- Registered nurses are essential to the delivery of quality, cost-efficient care.
- Patient care delivered by nurses educationally prepared with a BSN or higher leads to improved patient outcomes and nurse satisfaction.
- Regardless of ED census and acuity, a minimum of two RNs responsible for providing care in the ED at all times facilitate safe emergency care.
- Ongoing systematic evaluations of staffing and productivity are essential to the delivery of emergency care.

ED nurse directors must be aware of applicable state and federal legislation related to nurse staffing. In addition, they must be familiar with any contractual/labor union agreements with their hospital. Failure to comply with staffing legislation and/or contractual agreements can result in significant penalties and unit disruption.

Staffing Models

There are three basic staffing models: *acuity, financial,* and *ratio*. Emergency department nurse directors must know how each of these models is relevant for determining the appropriate staffing structure used in their ED. In most organizations, a blend of all three

TABLE 22.2 ■ Professional Nursing Organization Staffing Resources	
American Nurses Association	**Emergency Nurses Association**
• *Nurse Staffing 101: Principles for Nurse Staffing* • *ANA's Principles of Nurse Staffing, 2nd ed.*	• *Staffing and Productivity in the Emergency Department* • *Emergency Department Manager's Survival Guide*

models can be used when developing and monitoring the ED staffing plan. In addition, the nurse director must apply a primary, team, or functional nursing care model (discussed in detail below under "Nursing Care Models").

Acuity Staffing Model

The acuity staffing model is based on the assessed severity of patient illnesses and the intensity of nursing care required. There are many factors involved in patient acuity, including the time it takes to perform nursing tasks like assessments, medication administration, and discharge planning.

There is currently no real-time acuity-based staffing model for the ED. To approximate the acuity of the patients in the ED, a leader can consider the department's triage level and evaluation and management (E&M) billing level. The triage level is based on patient presentations on arrival, which may rapidly change. The E&M billing level may well be a better indicator of a patient's overall acuity during their ED stay; however, this factor is not determined until after the visit has ended and cannot be used prospectively. Both of these parameters should be reviewed and considered by analyzing what percentage of patients are assigned the various triage and E&M levels over a period of time. This information will help the nurse director estimate the overall acuity of the department.

Financial Staffing Model

The financial model is widely used and is historically how the ED staffing plan has been determined.[7] The financial model is expressed in hours per patient visit (HPPV) and is calculated by dividing the number of nursing hours in a period of time by the patient census for the same period of time (nursing hours/ED visits = HPPV). This model establishes the personnel cost for the department and is monitored in the monthly ED finance report. The ED nurse director must demonstrate skill in analyzing deviations from the budgeted personnel cost and how to advocate for changes to the personnel budget.

Hospitals often use national or regional benchmarks to determine the HPPV for the ED. However, it is important to understand that what is included in the nursing hours varies by facility. Elements that may or may not be included in nursing hours are reflected in **Box 22.1**. Nurse directors and staffing coordinators must understand what is included in the calculation of their nursing hours.

While the financial model does not account for all variations in patient acuity or the ebb and flow of the workload in the ED, it does serve a purpose. When first establishing a staffing budget/plan, the financial model guides the ED nurse director when benchmarking

---

BOX 22.1 ■ ELEMENTS OF NURSING HOURS

- Direct care hours
- Indirect care hours
  - Manager
  - Director
  - Educator
  - Administrative assistant/data analyzer
- Nonproductive time
  - Education
  - Orientation
  - Vacation
  - Sick
  - Leave of absence
  - Meeting/in-service time

the calculated HPPV against comparable facilities. In addition, once the staffing plan is established, it can be used to compare department performance to the budgeted plan. It is important to know when the ED is deviating from the established staffing plan to either the positive or negative. Being underbudget may lead to poor patient outcomes/care, decreased staff satisfaction/morale, and increased staff burnout. Conversely, being overbudget does not reflect good stewardship of resources, both human and financial.

Ratio Staffing Model

The nurse staffing ratio model is based solely on the number of patients or beds on a unit and the number of staff positions required based on the bed/patient volume. This model is solely based on the number of patients that can be assigned to a nurse and does not take into account the acuity of each case or a nurse's judgment of patient care needs. There are obvious limitations to this model. The ED might be forced to stop placing patients into ED beds when the nurse-to-patient ratio has been maximized regardless of patient acuity or care needs. This poses a significant concern in the ED when federal law requires hospitals to provide medical care or screening to patients who present to the ED, while state laws limit their ability to do so. This also poses a "back-end" problem when patients cannot be admitted because there is not enough staff on the inpatient units to provide care. This further backlog exacerbates the problem of "too many" patients for the ratio staffing model, as the ED must handle both the incoming volume and the need for inpatient care.[4,7]

Nursing Care Models

The nursing care model is the foundation for organizing and managing patients in the ED.[6,8] It will influence the number and type of staff needed, which impacts the cost to the organization. The nursing care model chosen by an ED will vary from hospital to hospital, and no one model is right for all.

Primary Nursing Model

The primary nursing model is the ideal when caring for all types of patients. In the primary nursing model, a specific nurse is assigned to a specific patient and assumes all responsibility for a case for the duration of that patient's visit. The primary nurse will work in collaboration with other team members and may delegate aspects of the patient's care as needed.[9]

The primary nursing model is believed to have a positive impact on patient satisfaction, nurse satisfaction, and nurse quality-indicator outcomes. It is therefore considered the most professional model, yet it is more costly than other types of nursing care due to the high percentage of RNs needed to support it.[10] Reviewing and monitoring nurse-sensitive patient outcome measures such as patient falls, catheter-associated infections, intravenous infiltrations, patient restraint use, pain management, sepsis identification, and return to the ED within 72 hours may be a useful tool to justify a primary nursing model.

Team Nursing Model

Team nursing models are commonly used in the ED. In the team nursing model, a team of health care providers (RN, licensed vocational nurse, ED technician, or nursing assistant) is responsible for the care of all patients in an assigned group. Depending on the size of the patient group, there may be more than one nurse assigned to the team. These models are generally observed to be cost-efficient and can be accomplished in a wide variety of ways.

An RN must always manage the patient plan of care while directing nonlicensed personnel in a variety of tasks.

Many EDs have created a variation of the team nursing model that includes a physician; this approach is referred to as an ED team or "pod" model. In this model, the ED team consists of a group of providers (usually one physician, one or two RNs, and one tech) who are assigned to a specific number of beds in a small geographic area of the department. This model results in increased collaboration among caregivers, improved overall efficiency, and increased staff and patient satisfaction.

Functional Nursing Model

The primary goal of functional nursing is to ensure that no patient goes without a vital component of care throughout a particular shift or visit. This type of nursing has been around since the Great Depression. It was the beginning of using nonlicensed personnel to assist in the care of soldiers during World War II. When hospitals saw their nursing staff decrease, it was more practical to teach ancillary personnel, such as nursing aides, to perform specific clinical tasks.

Instead of nurses serving many functions, several nurses are given one or two assignments to accomplish in a given time. For example, one nurse may be tasked solely with giving medications; another may perform all the assessments or initial care. With this approach, nurses are not assigned patients but rather specific groups of tasks. Although functional nursing arose out of necessity, it delivers a fragmented system of care, limits the development of the nurse–patient relationship, diminishes nurses' accountability and responsibility, and negatively affects the evaluation of nursing care. The functional nursing model is not commonly used in the ED setting.

OPERATIONAL CONSIDERATIONS

Operational aspects of the ED must be considered when developing a staffing plan.[6,8,11] While each department may have unique requirements, the more common aspects include:

- Unit geography
- Charge nurse role
- Triage
- Unit flow patterns
- Support staff
- Boarding of inpatients

Departments that offer specialized services (e.g., advanced trauma, burn, pediatric, chest pain, or stroke care) must consider the particular needs of these special patient populations when defining the ED's staffing requirements.

Unit Geography

Each ED has unique geographical challenges that must be considered when developing a staffing plan. Many departments are divided into separate areas, zones, pods, or teams. It is not realistic or safe to have one nurse manage patients in multiple geographically distinct areas. The staff members must be able to efficiently organize care and have ready access to all their patients. For example, if the staffing plan calls for nurses to care for four patients and the geographic area contains six beds, two nurses are needed to staff this area.

When determining the staffing plan, it is necessary to note the number of beds in each geographical area and the acuity of patients typically placed in those beds. Many departments have specific rooms for more critical patients. It may be reasonable to expect the nurses assigned to those rooms to have a smaller number of assigned patients than nurses assigned to lower-acuity areas.

Charge Nurse Role

The charge nurse is critical to a smoothly managed ED. In the staffing plan, it must be specified if the charge nurse will routinely care for patients or be dedicated to overseeing the operations of the department. A dedicated charge nurse in the ED will help ensure unit metrics are met, positive patient outcomes are achieved, and unnecessary/avoidable events are reduced and managed. Emergency departments of all sizes should have a dedicated charge nurse who focuses on maintaining and overseeing patient flow; the only exception may be in departments with an exceptionally low patient volume.

During high-volume and high-acuity episodes, charge nurses are often tempted to jump into the clinical fray to provide support for bedside nurses; however, doing so is not in the best interest of overall departmental operations and patient flow. In fact, critical episodes that often involve multiple nurses are the worst times for the ED to be without its charge nurse coordinating patient care and operational activities. Charge nurses cannot effectively drive patient flow or provide clinical and professional guidance for the rest of the nursing staff if they are consumed in direct patient care or attempting to cover triage.

Triage

Triage is an independent assignment. A charge nurse who is assigned to triage does not do justice to either role. A triage nurse who is also assigned to patient care or overall department coordination cannot respond expeditiously to arriving patients. In other words, triage is an indispensable front-door function, even when done in a rapid-pivot fashion. In low-volume EDs where limited nursing resources support 24-hour coverage by a dedicated triage nurse, newly arriving patients should be immediately placed in a treatment space so that a medical screening examination can occur.

Alternatively, the triage role can be preassigned to a nurse who has a lighter patient caseload or rotated among treatment-area RNs in preassigned blocks of time. Coverage of their patients (when called to triage) can also be preassigned to other clinical RNs with the expectation that arriving patients will be brought directly to any available treatment space. Preassignment reduces the potential for delays in responding to arriving patients.

Flow Patterns

Variability in patient flow impacts patient length of stay and demand for resources in the ED.[12] When developing a staffing plan for the ED, the nurse director should complete an analysis of the daily census by day of the week and patient arrivals by hour of the day. Analyzing this data can help the nurse leader predict staffing needs based on patient trends.

Support Staff

The use of support staff must also be considered when determining an ED staffing plan. Support staff include patient care technicians, phlebotomists, pharmacists, transporters, case managers, social workers, and other essential personnel. Support staff in the ED may report either to the ED director or to their primary department. In either case, the ED director must work closely with the director of the support staff's primary department to ensure adequate coverage, staff competency, and accountability.

Boarding Inpatients

Boarding inpatients in the ED can create serious space, operational, and staffing burdens. The ENA position statement "Crowding, Boarding and Patient Throughput" defines boarding as follows: "Boarded patients are those who have been admitted to an inpatient unit in the hospital but continue to wait in the ED for a bed to become available."[13] Boarding in the ED is a significant cause of crowding, and since it reflects a hospital throughput problem, these issues must be addressed on both the hospital and ED levels.

Emergency nurses frequently provide ongoing care, including critical care, to admitted patients for whom there are no available inpatient beds. This ED inpatient care occurs while the nursing staff continues to manage newly arriving patients. To address this problem, some hospitals provide roving admission nurses and hospital-staff inpatient nurses to care for patients boarding in the ED. Other programs to decompress overcrowded EDs include admission units, clinical decision units, and admit-to-inpatient hallway protocols. Safe nurse staffing for admitted patients, regardless of the location of care, is delivered by RNs with the same competencies as inpatient nurses and at the same staffing levels or nurse–patient ratios.

DEVELOPING AN ED STAFFING PLAN

After considering the historical data on patient census and arrival times, patient acuity, the chosen nursing model, and any legally mandated staffing requirements, the ED nurse director can develop a staffing plan. Whether constructing a plan from the ground up or simply modifying a system that is already in place, the steps will be the same.

Understanding Full-Time Equivalents

The first step is to understand the concept of full-time equivalents (FTEs). One FTE will work 2,080 hours in a year—based on working 40 hours per week for 52 weeks a year. In health care, it is common for employees to work only a fraction of an FTE; for example, many nurses work three 12-hour shifts (36 hours) per week. An employee who works 36 hours per week or 72 hours per 2-week pay period is a 0.9 FTE. Additionally, when calculating necessary FTEs, the plan must consider paid time off (PTO, discussed below under "Staffing Plan").

Note that the number of FTEs needed to staff a department is not the same as the number of employees needed to staff the department. Since many employees are hired to work less than 1.0 FTE, more employees than FTEs are required. As a result, the ED director should be permitted to hire the total FTEs (not employees) required to staff the department and approved in the department budget. When calculating FTE of employees, each 0.1 of an FTE is 8 hours in a 2-week pay period. **Table 22.3** demonstrates how to convert hours per pay period to FTE fractions. Converting hours to FTEs for ED staff may be especially challenging since there are so many different shifts and shift lengths.

TABLE 22.3 ■ Hours of Pay and FTE Status

HR/PP	80	76	72	68	64	60	56	52	48	44	40	36	32	28	24	20	16
FTP	1	0.95	0.9	0.85	0.8	0.75	0.7	0.65	0.6	0.55	0.5	0.45	0.4	0.35	0.3	0.25	0.2

FIGURE 22.1 ■ Daily Staffing Needs (Sample)

											Registered Nurses													Total H	FTE's
700	800	900	1000	1100	1200	1300	1400	1500	1600	1700	1800	1900	2000	2100	2200	2300	2400	100	200	300	400	500	600		
RN	RN	RN	RN	RN	RN	RN	RN	RN	RN	RN	RN	RN	RN	RN	RN	RN	RN	RN	RN	RN	RN	RN	RN		
RN	RN	RN	RN	RN	RN	RN	RN	RN	RN	RN	RN	RN	RN	RN	RN	RN	RN	RN	RN	RN	RN	RN	RN		
RN	RN	RN	RN	RN	RN	RN	RN	RN	RN	RN	RN	RN	RN	RN	RN	RN	RN	RN	RN	RN	RN	RN	RN		
RN	RN	RN	RN	RN	RN	RN	RN	RN	RN	RN	RN	RN	RN	RN	RN	RN	RN	RN	RN	RN	RN	RN	RN		
RN	RN	RN	RN	RN	RN	RN	RN	RN	RN	RN	RN	RN	RN	RN	RN	RN	RN	RN	RN	RN	RN	RN			
RN	RN	RN	RN	RN	RN	RN	RN	RN	RN	RN	RN	RN	RN	RN	RN	RN	RN	RN	RN	RN	RN				
		RN	RN	RN	RN	RN	RN	RN	RN	RN	RN	RN	RN	RN	RN	RN	RN	RN	RN	RN					
				RN	RN	RN	RN	RN	RN	RN	RN	RN	RN	RN	RN	RN	RN								
					RN	RN	RN	RN	RN	RN	RN	RN	RN	RN	RN	RN									
					RN	RN	RN	RN	RN	RN	RN	RN	RN	RN	RN										
						RN	RN	RN	RN	RN	RN	RN	RN	RN											
									RN	RN	RN	RN	RN	RN											
6	6	7	7	11	11	11	11	12	12	12	12	13	13	13	13	9	9	9	9	7	7	7	7	234	40.95
1	1	1	1	1	1	1	1	1	1	1	1	1	1	1	1	1	1	1	1	1	1	1	1		
1	1	1	1	1	1	1	1	1	1	1	1	1	1	1	1	1	1	1	1	1	1	1	1		
4	4	5	4	5	5	5	5	6	6	6	6	7	7	7	7	5	5	5	5	5	5	5	5		
				2	2	2	2	2	2	2	2	2	2	2	2	2	2	2	2						
			1	1	1	1	1	1	1	1	1	1	1	1	1										
	1	1	1	1	1	1	1	1	1	1	1	1	1	1											

										Emergency Technicians															
700	800	900	1000	1100	1200	1300	1400	1500	1600	1700	1800	1900	2000	2100	2200	2300	2400	100	200	300	400	500	600		
TECH	TECH	TECH	TECH	TECH	TECH	TECH	TECH	TECH	TECH	TECH	TECH	TECH	TECH	TECH	TECH	TECH	TECH	TECH	TECH	TECH	TECH	TECH	TECH		
TECH	TECH	TECH	TECH	TECH	TECH	TECH	TECH	TECH	TECH	TECH	TECH	TECH	TECH	TECH	TECH	TECH	TECH	TECH	TECH	TECH	TECH	TECH	TECH		
TECH	TECH	TECH	TECH	TECH	TECH	TECH	TECH	TECH	TECH	TECH	TECH	TECH	TECH	TECH	TECH	TECH	TECH	TECH	TECH	TECH	TECH	TECH	TECH		
TECH	TECH	TECH	TECH	TECH	TECH	TECH	TECH	TECH	TECH	TECH	TECH	TECH	TECH	TECH	TECH	TECH	TECH	TECH	TECH	TECH	TECH	TECH	TECH		
4	4	4	4	4	4	4	4	4	4	4	4	4	4	4	4	4	4	4	4	4	4	4	4	96	16.8

										Unit Secretaary															
US	US	US	US	US	US	US	US	US	US	US	US	US	US	US	US	US	US	US	US	US	US	US	US		
1	1	1	1	1	1	1	1	1	1	1	1	1	1	1	1	1	1	1	1	1	1	1	1	24	4.2

Staffing Plan

To develop a staffing plan, the ED nurse director must determine how many staff members are needed on duty each hour of the day. The worksheet shown in **Figure 22.1** is an example of how to document the number and type of staff needed throughout the day. In the sample provided, the ED requires 234 RN staff hours, 96 technician hours, and 24 unit secretary hours. This worksheet will also serve as the template for calculating daily schedule needs.

After determining the number of hours needed for each type of staff member, calculate the number of FTEs needed by multiplying the number of hours needed per day by 14 (the number of days in a pay period), then divide this number by 80 (the number of hours an FTE works in a pay period) (**Box 22.2**).

This calculation will give you the number of FTEs that are needed to cover the unit schedule; it will not include the number of FTEs needed to cover nonproductive time. Nonproductive time includes PTO (vacation leave, sick and personal time, education/orientation time), meetings, and any other time the staff is paid but not performing direct patient care. Some facilities have a standard percentage for calculating nonproductive time (e.g., 10%, 15%, or 20% of the total FTEs for the department). However, if the facility does not have a predetermined standard, the number of FTEs needed to cover nonproductive time can be calculated by taking the total number of *nonproductive hours* used by the department for 1 year and dividing it by 2,080; this calculation provides the number of additional FTEs that need to be added to the department. The total hours of nonproductive time should be accessible to the ED nurse director through the payroll system.

BOX 22.2 ■ RN FTE CALCULATION

234 hours per day × 14 days per pay period = 3,276 hours per pay period/80 hours (1 FTE in a pay period) = 40.95 FTEs

Hours per Patient Visit

The next step is to calculate the HPPV. Typically, EDs use HPPV as a financial target to ensure fiscal responsibility.[7] To calculate your HPPV, divide the total number of staff hours in a 24-hour period by the number of visits in the same 24-hour period. In this example, the ED is using 234 RN hours, 96 ED technician hours, and 24 unit secretary hours for a total of 354 staff hours per day.

It is very important at this point to know what is included in the budgeted HPPV, which varies from facility to facility. Does it include only direct patient care hours, or are indirect patient care hours—such as hours worked by the department director, manager, educator, administrative assistant—included? Most financial departments want to include all positions that are paid out of the cost center and therefore include both direct and indirect patient care positions. Indirect care positions should have their scheduled hours spread over a 14-day pay period for the purposes of calculating daily productivity. The actual, or paid, HPPV is used as the productivity standard and is often expressed, or referred to, as a percentage of compliance with the budgeted HPPV.

After developing the staffing plan and converting the staffing hours needed per day to HPPV, it should be compared to the budgeted HPPV. The two must be in alignment to achieve fiscal responsibility. A needed HPPV higher than the budgeted HPPV is considered over budget and requires a discussion with leadership/finance department to bring the budgeted and needed HPPV into alignment. Adjustments to the HPPV occur by changing the number of staff hours needed per day or changing the number of patient visits per day. It is the role of the ED director to negotiate required changes and create a balanced staffing budget.

Daily monitoring of compliance with the HPPV is necessary. The tool shown in **Figure 22.2** can be used to assist the department director with daily monitoring. In this sample, the ED is consistently running over budget. To meet this ED's budget, it is necessary either to reduce the dailing staffing or to increase the daily census. The charge nurse

- Is in the best position to know when the daily staffing should be flexed up or down based on the unit activity
- Should be trained in the dynamics of the productivity/HPPV standards in order to provide the necessary information about variation from the budget
- Should be involved in completing the tool and monitoring the daily performance of the unit

There are many causes of variations, including staff on orientation and boarding and high-acuity patients who require additional staff. The key to successful staffing is to know how your unit is operating and whether it is over or under budget. This permits the ED nurse director to speak effectively about what is causing variation.

FIGURE 22.2 ■ HPPV Compliance Monitoring Tool

Unit	Emergency
Month	Feb-12
Budgeted Productive Stat	2.85
Budgeted Daily Visits	135

Daily budgeted HR			2/1 wed	2/2 thu	2/3 fri	2/4 sat	2/5 sun	2/6 mon	2/7 tue	2/8 wed	2/9 thu	2/10 fri	2/11 sat	2/12 sun	2/13 mon	2/14 tue
	Daily Visits		97	106	87	100	128	116	101	118	98	94	108	107	116	96
234	RN		230	227	222	229	227	231	234	225	227	227	233	228	234	227
96	ED Tech		87.5	85.5	102	94	96	108	93.5	75	79	102	96	95	95	88
24	US		24	24	24	24	24	24	24	24	24	24	24	24	24	24
22	Admin		22	22	22	22	22	22	22	22	22	22	22	22	22	22
	Total hours		363	359	370	369	369	385	374	346	352	375	375	369	375	361
	Productive Stat		3.74	3.38	4.25	3.69	2.88	3.32	3.7	2.93	3.59	3.99	3.47	3.45	3.23	3.76

Position Control

Position control is a management tool designed to provide an accurate inventory of filled and vacant positions and ensure the schedule is balanced based on the unit staffing plan. In addition, position control will ascertain vacancies to help identify recruitment needs. Some facilities have a standard position control process used by the finance department. Ask for a copy of the document if the facility has one. If a position control does not exist, the ED director should create one for the department. The basic data elements that should be on all position control worksheets include lists of:

- All employees by shift, with their FTE status and the type of employee (e.g., RN, tech)
- The number of FTEs needed to staff each shift based on the unit staffing plan
- The budgeted number of FTEs

A position control spreadsheet can easily be created in Excel (**Table 22.4**).

TABLE 22.4 ■ Sample RN Position Control

Employee Number	Last Name	First Name	FTE	Shift	Shift Hours	Job Title
	Last name	First name	0.9	Day		Charge Nurse
	Last name	First name	0.9	Night		Charge Nurse
	Vacant		0.9	Day		Staff RN
	Last name	First name	0.9	Day		Staff RN
	Last name	First name	0.9	Night		Staff RN
	Last name	First name	0.9	Day		Staff RN
	Last name	First name	0.9	Day		Staff RN
	Last name	First name	0.9	Night		Staff RN
	Vacant		0.9	Night		Staff RN
	Last name	First name	0.9	Day		Staff RN
	Last name	First name	0.9	Day		Staff RN
	Last name	First name	0.9	Day		Staff RN
	Last name	First name	0.75	Day		Staff RN
	Last name	First name	0.75	Day		Staff RN
	Last name	First name	0.75	Day		Staff RN
	Last name	First name	0.75	Day		Staff RN
	Last name	First name	0.5	Day		Staff RN
	Last name	First name	0.5	Day		Staff RN
	Last name	First name	0.5	Day		Staff RN
	Last name	First name	0.01	Flex		Per diem RN
	Last name	First name	0.01	Flex		Per diem RN
Total FTE			**15.5**			
Budgeted FTE			**15.5**			

CONCLUSION

Proper staffing is the foundation of any nursing unit; without it, the ED will not achieve the clinical or financial outcomes needed and expected. Inadequate staffing models lead to compromised patient outcomes, excessive overtime, and increased staff burnout and frustration. This "perfect storm" will result in a poorly performing department. The first step to success is to ensure the ED nurse director and ED director have a thorough knowledge of the departmental personnel budget and staffing plan and tight control of vacancies and recruitment.

REFERENCES

1. Mensik J. *The Nurse Managers Guide to Innovative Staffing*. 2nd ed. Indianapolis, Ind: Sigma Theta Tau International; 2017.
2. Workforce Management, PCAS, and The RFP Process. (n.d.). Available at: https://www.nursingworld.org/practice-policy/work-environment/nurse-staffing/workforce-management-pcas-and-the-rfp-process/. Accessed August 19, 2020.
3. Centers for Medicare and Medicaid. Conditions of participation: nursing services. 2017. Available at: https://www.cms.gov/Regulations-and-Guidance/Guidance/Manuals/downloads/som107ap_a_hospitals.pdf. Accessed August 19, 2020.
4. Kinsella L. New safe staffing legislation introduced to congress. 2018. Available at: https://dailynurse.com/new-safe-staffing-legislation-introduced-to-congress/. Accessed August 19, 2020.
5. American Nurses Association. Optimal nurse staffing to improve quality of care and patient outcomes: executive summary. 2015. Available at: https://www.nursingworld.org/~4ae116/globalassets/practiceandpolicy/advocacy/ana_optimal-nurse-staffing_white-paper-es_2015sep.pdf
6. Emergency Nurses Association. Position statement: staffing and productivity in the emergency department. 2015. Available at: https://www.ena.org/practice-research/Practice/Position/Pages/StaffingandProductivityEmergencyDepartment.aspx. Accessed August 19, 2020.
7. Kirby K. Hours per patient day: not the problem, nor the solution. *Nurs Econ*. 2015;33(1):64-66. Available at: https://pubmed.ncbi.nlm.nih.gov/26214941/
8. Powell K. Staffing and scheduling. In: *ED Manager's Survival Guide*. 1st ed. Emergency Nurses Association, Schaumburg, IL; 2017: 66-69.
9. Molin AD, Gatta C, Gilot CB, et al. The impact of primary nursing care pattern: results from a before-after study. *J Clin Nurs*. 2018;27(5-6): 1094-1102. doi:10.1111/jocn 14135.
10. Kusk KH, Groenkjaer M. Effectiveness of primary nursing in the care and satisfaction of adult inpatients. *JBI Database System Rev Implement Rep*. 2016;14(6):14-22. doi:10.11124/jbisrir-2016-002390.
11. Jenson K. Staffing your emergency department efficiently, effectively and safely: core concepts. 2017. Available at: https://www.envisionphysicianservices.com/campaigns/breakthrough-series/presentation-materials/presentations/09-staffing-your-ed-core-concepts.pdf. Accessed August 19, 2020.
12. Nambiar KM, Nedungalaparambil N, Aslesh O. Studying the variability in patient inflow and staffing trends on Sundays versus other days in the academic emergency department. *J Emerg Trauma Shock*. 2017;10(3):121. doi:10.4103/jets.jets_139_16
13. Emergency Nurses Association. Crowding, boarding, and patient throughput. 2015. Available at: Available at: https://ena.org/docs/default-source/resource-library/practice-resources/position-statements/crowdingboardingandpatientthroughput.pdf?sfvrsn=5fb4e79f_4. Accessed August 19, 2020.

SUGGESTED READINGS

- *ANA's Principles of Nurse Staffing*. 2nd ed. American Nurses Association; 2012.
- *Emergency Department Manager's Survival Guide*. Des Plains, Ill: Emergency Nurses Association; 2017.

CHAPTER 23

PHYSICIAN AND NURSE PRODUCTIVITY ASSESSMENTS

Robert W. Strauss, Aviva Segal, Andrew M. Amaranto, Nancy Bonalumi

Emergency physician and nurse productivity are interrelated, as both depend upon the productivity of the other. In addition, efficiency requires the substantial involvement of hospital administrative resource allocation, the responsiveness of lab and radiology, access to inpatient beds, and the availability of consulting/admitting medical staff.

Budgets for staffing and support services are traditionally driven by volume, for nurse staffing, and hours per patient visit (HPPV). This approach assumes that all clinician types are equally productive; in other words, a physician is a physician and a nurse is a nurse. However, there are wide variations in the productivity of individual clinicians. A better way is necessary to measure individual productivity and determine how it is influenced by the level of support from all of the other necessary resources.

MOTIVATIONAL THEORY

Motivation and productivity are intimately related. As such, it is informative to expound briefly on the subject of motivation. In his book *The Surprising Truth about What Motivates Us*, author Daniel Pink summarizes research that suggests, "money is a motivator for purely mechanical tasks but as soon as some level of cognitive processing is required to complete the task, money is secondary to other factors."[1] This fact likely underlies the ease and difficulty of achieving effective productivity-based compensation for various tasks:

- It is easy to get physicians to complete documentation when there is little or no cognitive processing required, such as filling in all of the requested data points on a template.
- Alternatively, it may be quite difficult to motivate clinicians to participate in significant governance and leadership activities, which require substantial cognitive processing.

Generally, hospitals have not embraced productivity-based emergency department (ED) nursing compensation. Among the reasons for this resistance are:

- Nursing productivity is more difficult to measure, since there are often several nurses involved in the care of ED patients.
- The precedent of productivity-based ED nursing reimbursement would be noted by the entire hospital nursing staff.
- Very few successful models have been demonstrated.

This raises the question to which Daniel Pink refers, when considering nursing motivation, what are these other (motivational) factors? Autonomy, mastery, and purpose are the nonmonetary elements that motivate all people. For those new to organizational leadership, it is tempting to believe that success lies in hiring good people and getting rid of bad people until, sooner or later, the perfect team is in place. Unfortunately, it is not that easy; there simply are not enough perfect people in the world.

While very few people get out of bed in the morning planning to be disagreeable and disruptive at work, some seem purposefully antagonistic. A lack of effective engagement may arise when personal or organizational limitations interfere with the achievement of autonomy, mastery, and purpose most people seek in their working lives. Sophisticated leaders eventually discover that their job includes inspiring ordinary people to do extraordinary things.

> . . .the carrot and stick theory does not work at all once man has reached an adequate subsistence level and is motivated by higher needs.[2]

Among these higher needs is the drive to perform well among peers. Through years of competitive higher education, physicians and nurses naturally develop the ambition to achieve success. This desire makes feedback a powerful tool to motivate and change behavior. There are numerous studies in the quality and patient safety world that demonstrate improved behavior and adherence to best practice guidelines by simply providing individualized feedback to providers.[3,4] When measured against colleagues, physicians and nurses experience a natural drive to perform at least to the middle of the bell curve and, more often than not, exceed the norm.

The leader's job is to create a purposeful vision, provide the right balance between autonomy and oversight, ensure availability of the resources necessary, and provide consistent and constructive feedback for individuals to achieve mastery.

EMERGENCY PHYSICIAN PRODUCTIVITY

The Centers for Medicare and Medicaid Services (CMS) introduced the resource-based relative value scale (RBRVS) method of physician compensation in 1992. Reimbursement methodology is currently based on a measurement of the number and type of resources necessary to care for patients of differing levels of complexity.

The RBRVS System

The RBRVS system uses a complex set of rules tied to the content of the medical record. The level of reimbursement is determined by the medical record documentation, including the complexity of medical decision-making. Since the implementation of the RBRVS system, providers have learned to write down everything they've learned, done, and thought about the patient in order to obtain the reimbursement to which they are entitled.

Emergency physicians often document their patient care on a set of chief complaint-driven medical record templates that prompt complete content at the point of service. These templated and other effective documentation methodologies, such as scribes, have enabled emergency physicians to gradually regain their prior productivity levels (see Chapters 25 and 106).

The RBRVS system requires practitioners to thoroughly document according to a specific set of rules. For example, under RBRVS, an acute myocardial infarction, historically a high-paying final diagnosis, might only justify payment for a minor service visit if documentation is inadequate. To ensure effective documentation leading to appropriate reimbursement, most emergency physician groups have moved to systems of compensation based, at least in part, on the level of medical record documentation. This payment system transfers the risk of documentation deficiencies to the individual, where it properly belongs.

Relative Value Units

Though complex, bureaucratic, and frequently changing, the RBRVS system does provide a yardstick by which to measure provider productivity. Each level of "evaluation and management" (E/M) service complexity, from minor to extensive and critical care, is given objectively measurable medical record criteria and assigned a number of relative value units (RVUs). (RVUs are described in much greater detail in Section 8.)

Relative value units are therefore a proxy for documented work. When RVUs are totaled and divided by the hours worked by any individual provider, they yield the productivity metric: *RVUs per hour of staffing cost*. Whereas effective documentation results in optimum reimbursement, inadequately documented work leads to "downcoding" or underreimbursement for services rendered.

Coding Inaccuracy

Conversely, intentionally (or having the appearance of intentionally) "upcoding" or overcharging for a visit can lead to serious federal regulatory and financial penalties—if such "fraud and abuse" is discovered on an audit. The threats associated with overbilling are significant and include fines, liability, OIG declaration of fraud, and penalties, including exclusion from Medicare and state health care programs. As a result of these risks, many providers purposely err on the side of undercoding in order to avoid the possibility of government audits.[5] The single biggest problem with using level-of-service codes as a proxy for provider work is that this approach presumes that the documentation is complete and that the current procedural terminology (CPT or charge) codes are correct. Unfortunately, these assumptions are often incorrect.

The regulations are sufficiently complex that even certified medical coders disagree with each other's coding 17% to 69% of the time.[6] Further, there are several factors that prevent emergency providers from accurately documenting their patient care. For example:

- It is inherently impossible to record every thought, action, and conversation.
- Providers are interrupted every 3.5 to 6 minutes.[7-9]
- Many documentation systems lack content prompting (cognitive forcing strategies).
- Electronic medical records (EMRs) have cumbersome user interfaces.
- Providers fear audits, which bias the overall process in the direction of underestimating the true productivity.

In spite of the associated inaccuracies, the RBRVS/RVU system offers a close approximation of provider productivity. However, productivity can also be hampered by several inefficiencies that are not accounted for by the system, including inadequate staffing support, slow lab or radiology response, an outmoded physical plant, the lack of availability of inpatient beds, nonexistent psychiatric care facilities, consulting/admitting physicians that do not call back promptly, or any one of a number of other barriers that might negatively impact the provider's productivity.[10]

The RVU Productivity System

Table 23.1 lists the CMS total RVU and dollar values (at Medicare rates) for the five major E/M codes and critical care for the year 2019 which, when multiplied by the 2019 EM conversion factor, yield the corresponding dollar amounts. Using these metrics, many EM groups have moved their providers to productivity-based compensation systems. Such systems, discussed elsewhere in this text at greater length (see Chapter 86), explicitly clarify the relationship between individual provider documentation and productivity. To be effective and readily adopted by providers, these systems must follow the A-S-M-A principle:[11]

- **A (Agreeable)**—The plan participants (providers) must agree that the plan is fair, ethical, and demonstrates an accurate representation of their work effort. It is helpful to involve group members in the development of the plan.
- **S (Simple)**—Plan participants must be able to easily understand how the system works, including precisely how documentation leads to RVUs and payment. Plans fail early by trying to include too many components and modify too many behaviors.
- **M (Measurable)**—The plan must use objective agreed-upon measures. Providers are most likely to accomplish what they can understand and can be measured. Some poorly defined plans are based on subjective criteria and therefore create confusion.
- **A (Achievable)**—Choose realistic and accomplishable goals. If too difficult and unachievable, few will make an effort to change their practice.

Because the use of EMRs has generally slowed providers and negatively affected productivity, many EDs have implemented scribe programs. Comparable productivity with scribes has been noted to generate 20% more RVUs per hour of physician staffing.

Productivity-based compensation systems have not consistently increased productivity. Data suggest that there is a proportional relationship between the percentage of total compensation at risk and the degree of documentation improvement as shown in **Figure 23.1**. In one group of 46 EDs transitioning from hourly compensation with nontemplated records to 100% productivity-based compensation with templated records, the average increase in billable RVUs was 43%, with the increase in collected revenue averaging just over 20%.

Using the documented RVUs per hour of staffing approach, it is possible to compare the productivity of each provider and class of providers (emergency physicians, primary care physicians, nonphysician practitioners) to each other and to the group averages. The

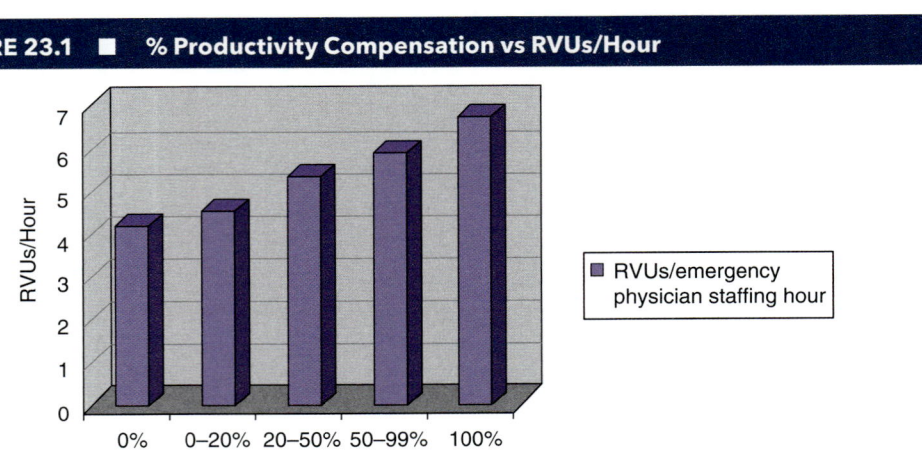

FIGURE 23.1 ■ % Productivity Compensation vs RVUs/Hour

TABLE 23.1 ■ CPT Codes and RVUs			
CPT Code	**Total RVU Value**	**2019 M-Care CF**	**$ Value at M-Care Rate**
99281	0.60	$36.04	$21.62
99282	1.17	$36.04	$42.17
99283	1.75	$36.04	$63.07
99284	3.32	$36.04	$119.65
99285	4.89	$36.04	$176.24
99291	6.28	$36.04	$226.33

product of RVUs per patient and patients per hour allows the providers to look at their own productivity numbers. Low RVUs per patient are typically due to a documentation deficiency problem, while too few patients per hour may be due to being too slow to pick up new patients, doing excessive workups, or both.

EMERGENCY NURSE PRODUCTIVITY

Is it true that "a nurse is a nurse is a nurse?" Hospital nurses have not received the same intense focus on individual productivity as emergency physicians. Yet nowhere in the hospital do physicians and nurses work in such close proximity and with such mutual dependency as in the ED. Physician assessments and treatment plans are coded and categorized, while nursing activities focus on carrying out these treatment plans without consideration for the "work output" or alteration of any applied codes. Measures such as length of stay, patient satisfaction, and patient outcome depend heavily on nursing productivity and efficiency. So why have productivity metrics rarely been applied to nursing?

Current Approaches

In general, it is accepted that directed incentives lead to improved performance. Extrinsic motivation (e.g., monetary incentives) have been shown to have a positive impact on performance.[16] Specialty units, career ladders, and certification pay differentials are nursing methods to "pay for performance" (see Chapter 87). These programs have been successful in motivating nurses to reach for higher benchmarks of professionalism. But do they specifically address and incentivize increased patient care productivity? These programs still presume that every nurse with a particular skill set functions at the same level once that nurse achieves minimal competency. But in truth, a nurse can become certified and can climb the clinical ladder without improving bedside efficiency.

Creative Approach

Let's assume a hospital's administration determines that, with correct incentives, the inpatient unit staff could discharge patients and admit new patients more quickly. These efforts are expected to significantly unburden the ED, which is overcrowded with boarders, has a "left prior to medical screening exam" (LPMSE) rate of 5%, and is frequently on diversion.

To address these problems, a proposal is made to create a bonus incentive for the inpatient nursing staff—$25.00 would be paid for every rapid discharge of an inpatient (<1 hour from discharge order). Another $25.00 would be paid for every rapid admission from the ED

(<1 hour from admission order). After brief consideration, this proposal is rejected because it would be too costly. A deeper consideration of the situation reveals the following fact pattern:

1. ED volume = 100 patients/day
2. % ED patients admitted = 20%
3. Time in ED from admission decision to leaving the ED = 4 to 8 hours
4. ED patients who LPMSE = 5 per day
5. Hospital on diversion weekly and loses three likely high-acuity admissions
6. Collection for discharged ED patients = $300
7. Collection from admitted ED patients = $7,000
8. Collection from high-acuity ambulance admissions = $10,000
9. Current daily loss (potential gain) from LPMSE and diversion patients = 4 × $300 + 1 × $7,000 + 3 × $10,000/7 = **$12,285/day**
10. Potential daily cost of incentive program = **$1,000**

Even a partially successful implementation of this trial program could:

- Incentivize the inpatient staff to become more productive.
- Improve patient satisfaction.
- Improve ED staff morale.
- Decrease ED staffing requirements.
- Enhance the hospital's reputation in the general and emergency medical services communities.
- Increase the hospital's collections and net revenue.

Clearly, the example above can be broadened, altered, or enhanced, but its ultimate lack of attention to other potentially critical bottlenecks is clear. The described set of goal-driven incentives are applied to inpatient nurses but fail to financially reward staff in other departments. Transporters' punctuality will affect admission times, inpatient nursing staff rely on housekeepers to clean admission rooms in a timely manner, and ED technicians and ED nurses are expected to carry out specific tasks prior to admission. Further, once inpatient nurses adapt to this new level of reimbursement, even-higher incentives may be needed to yield identical results.[12]

Intrinsic vs Extrinsic Motivations

The example highlights some of the shortcomings of financial incentives when applied to nursing. Monetary incentives are short-lived and may undermine intrinsic motivation. Intrinsic motivation has proven to be a stronger driving force of performance when the activity itself is the reward. Generally, those who become nurses are intrinsically motivated to help others. The job itself entails caring for people, identifying and satisfying their needs, and contributing to improving their health. Achieving those goals are the self-motivators that drive nursing performance.

What drives nurses' intrinsic motivation and, ultimately, their productivity? A recent study identifies nourishment, progress, and catalysts as driving motivational forces for nurses.[13] Nourishment refers to "interpersonal support, including respect, encouragement, emotional supports, and affiliation." Progress is the nurse's ability to find "meaning and accomplishment . . . forward movement and goal achievement." Catalyst refers to "events that directly facilitate the work such as clear goals, sufficient resources, allowing autonomy and a positive climate." Clearly, motivational forces extend well beyond financial incentives. Nursing managers have the ability to impact nursing productivity by intervening and enhancing these factors.

Determining Staffing Needs

Previously, EDs were permitted to hire and utilize a certain number of full-time equivalents (FTEs; staff), regardless of the cost and function of the individuals. Given the mandate of a specific number of FTEs, most ED nursing directors choose to staff their departments exclusively with registered nurses (RNs). This approach can give them the most educated, fully functional staff, using the argument, "Well, if I am going to get hit with an FTE limit, it might as well be an FTE with the broadest possible capabilities." In other words, it is better to choose an RN rather than a tech, who costs less but has a more limited scope.

More recently, the definition of FTEs has been modified to incorporate the specific roles and responsibilities of the employees. In these settings, while FTEs are still predetermined per department, there is a value attributed to different roles that an FTE can assume. For example, one RN FTE is equal to the cost of approximately three support staff FTEs. Managers should consider the value of support staff in assisting with nursing workloads. Some of the most efficient EDs have techs or paramedics supporting nurses by doing 30% or more of the nursing interventions as defined by the Emergency Nurses Association (ENA).[14-16]

The use of sophisticated, multifunctional nursing support staff who possess expanded technical skills must be consistent with the specific state's nurse practice act and is ideally guided by ENA's statement on delegating to non-RNs in the ED setting.[17] The balance between RN and supportive non-RN staff is vital to the overall efficiency of the department. These technicians can significantly extend the ability of RNs to provide safe, comprehensive, and more expediently delivered care.

Traditionally, hospitals have utilized hours per patient day to contain costs by allocating, tracking, and controlling budgeted hours per FTEs in the inpatient setting. In the ED, utilization of a similar model measuring HPPV did not take into account the specific factors that support or limit ED nurse efficiency. Inpatient boarding, patient volumes, and patient acuities all differ day-to-day and all directly impact nurse productivity. The same ED nurse in the same role will function very differently on different days when those and other critical factors impede or promote efficiency. Therefore, the allocation of FTEs can be more difficult to determine and track in the ED.

Newer data-driven analyses and programs, such as Truven Health Analytics, take additional measures into account to determine the best mixed staff ratios.[18] Patient visits, walkout rates, admission rates, lengths of stay, and hours worked per patient visit give a more precise calculation of needed staff. These combined data points deliver a more accurate picture of patient volume and acuity, which may change daily, monthly, or seasonally. Additionally, EDs can compare their staffing ratios to other hospitals with similar patient volumes, acuities, and so on. Financially, managers can utilize these data to approve overtime or hire additional travel staff during busier seasons.

BARRIERS TO EFFICIENCY

Imagine an auto assembly line in which the people installing the driver-side wheels are paid by the hour, and the people installing the passenger-side wheels are paid according to the number of wheels they install. The company's goal is to get more "quality built" cars off the assembly line per hour, but the two sets of interdependent workers have diametrically opposed incentives. One group has the opportunity to make more money by working harder, and the other group has the opportunity to have a better career "lifestyle" by working less hard for the same pay.

Emergency nurses and physicians today have an incentive mismatch that, until it can be reconciled, will continue to present a serious barrier to achieving greater ED efficiency. A second major issue relates to the nursing educational philosophy that promotes "collaborative practice."[19] Hospital-based nurses assume an independent duty to the patient in parallel to that of the physician, which can create an unnecessary redundancy. Such an approach clearly has benefit for critically ill patients and also provides an additional layer of information, safety, and assessment. However, if the nurse and the physician simply duplicate some of each other's work, the redundancy may not significantly contribute to the efficiency or quality of care, particularly for a large number of ED patients with noncritical or low-acuity presentations. Conducting and voluminously documenting an independent nursing assessment on noncritical patients not only duplicates effort but also removes the nurse from bedside care. Furthermore, physicians do not consistently read the entire nurses' notes.

Many EDs across the country utilize nurse extenders with expanded skill sets, allowing technicians and paramedics to assume increasing responsibility for technical tasks. Nurses would prefer to work synergistically with the physicians, be highly efficient, and reduce throughput times. However, the growing mountain of responsibilities, mandates, and documentation must be accomplished to satisfy the expanding hospital and regulatory demands.

A NEW PRODUCTIVITY MODEL

Inherently, ED physicians and nurses have a shared goal: positive patient health outcomes. Yet achieving that goal depends on multiple interrelated factors. Historically, physician and nursing productivity measurements have focused primarily on fiscal implications, while other initiatives, such as operational efficiency and patient satisfaction, have been addressed separately as if they were unrelated. With the mandatory implementation of the Hospital Consumer Assessment of Healthcare Providers and Systems data collection in 2007 and patient experience of care surveys, the patient's satisfaction is consistently measured. In many cases, CMS reimbursement is directly linked to a hospital's patient experience scores.

Barriers caused by incentive mismatches can be diminished by effective collaboration. Positive nurse–physician collaboration has been linked to improvements in the quality of care.[20] Nurses and physicians in the ED generally interact more frequently, creating the potential for clear communication, shared decision-making, and teamwork, all of which improve team collaboration and ultimately nurses' intrinsic motivation. It would be beneficial for medical schools, hospitals, and EDs to develop and implement simulated team-building/communication classes for physicians and nurses to ensure effective collaboration.[20]

Additionally, to address redundancy and duplicative documentation, the ideal solution lies in ensuring that what is necessary for safety and quality patient care continues to exist. Beyond that, "wasteful" documentation should be eliminated. Improving productivity and efficiency must begin with streamlining and standardizing processes and systems. It just makes sense to begin the ED assessment with:

- **What** people must do (processes) in order to be more productive (provide certain deliverables)
- **Who** should do it (right staffing ratios with appropriate responsibilities)
- **How** it should be done (standardized performance and efficiency)
- **Time** required to do it (cycle or "takt" time—from the German word *taktzeit*)
- **When and in what numbers** they do it (alignment of capacity with demand)

There are new methods and tools available that have the potential to revolutionize the way productivity is understood and measured. These tools account for the actual time it takes for patients to move through "current state processes," with physician and nurse hours allocated and distributed according to demand for services by hour of the day. These more sophisticated tools also capture length of stay and department-specific acuities, resulting in metrics that yield a more refined, sensitive, and accurate depiction of collective productivity.

Collective productivity, when translated into hour-by-hour staffing levels and budgeted FTEs, can be used to better serve patients and provide objectively measurable returns. This approach also gives greater consideration to "utilization," recognizing the significant interdependent roles that resources, acuity, and patient census have on output.

Utilizing computer modeling and queuing theory to analyze staffing brings greater clarity to the interdependence of emergency physician and nurse productivity. In a random arrival environment, such as the line for a ride at Disneyworld or patients presenting to the ED, queuing theory demonstrates that as the percent of a worker's utilization exceeds 85%, waits begin to increase exponentially. Given the historical ED staffing that results in staff working at or even over 100% of worker capacity, it is no wonder that most EDs have (had) a waiting and LPMSE problem.

Newer models of patient care within the ED, such as the implementation of "direct bedding," minimize the queuing effect of patients waiting to be seen. The triage process has been shortened, allowing both nurses and physicians to take care of patients more expediently. However, the need to calculate demand and capacity is still relevant, as sicker patients can still burden nurses and providers and create bottlenecks.

An alignment of demand and capacity therefore results in greater productivity. **Figures 23.2** and **23.3** illustrate how the factors of a usual physician workload of 2 patients per hour or 30 minutes per patient and the usual RN workload of 0.75 patients per hour or 80 minutes per patient are aligned. The bars represent workload in minutes during each hour of the day, including arrivals and length of stay for patients who are presently in process plus those who are still present from prior hours using a 240-minute average overall length

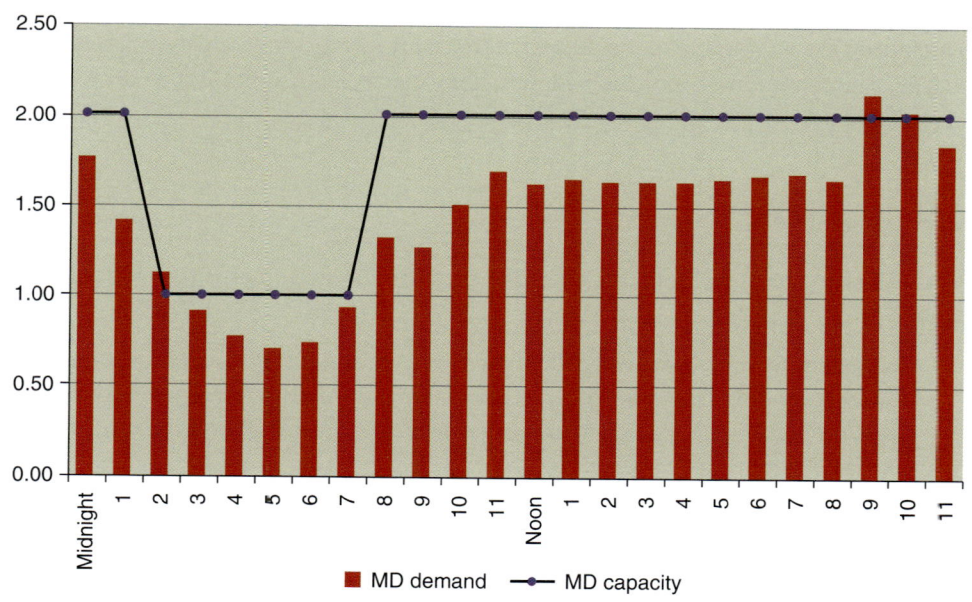

FIGURE 23.2 ■ MD Demand vs Capacity by Hour of Day

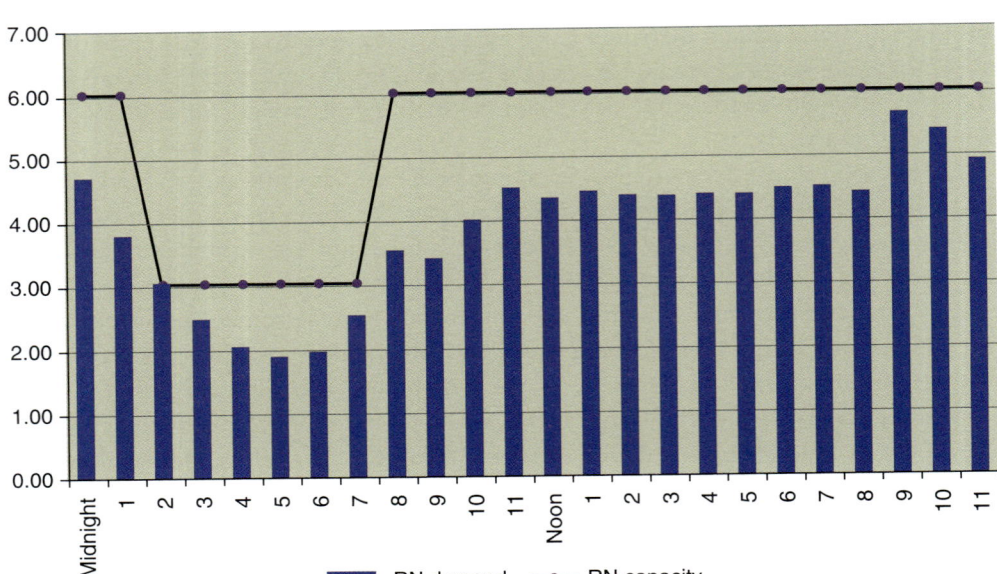

FIGURE 23.3 ■ RN Demand vs Capacity by Hour of Day

of stay.[21] The excel formulas can be modified as needed to include department-specific conditions and processes that affect workload and length of stay.

More sensitive tools calculate productivity (utilization) based on "takt" time (server cycle time) and queuing theory (see Chapters 33 and 34). If those calculations are applied in conjunction with Lean methodologies to reduce operational wastes, level workload, and minimize variation in practices and processes, the overall boost to ED productivity can be significant.[22]

To make the calculation of demand and capacity even more accurate and sensitive to department-specific acuities, Emergency Severity Index percentages (translated into minutes per patient) can also be incorporated into the formula for RN and physician time per patient by hour of the day.[21,23] Carrying the productivity paradigm shift even further, a comprehensive approach considers supporting and rate-limiting factors specific to a given ED, including the role and responsibilities of the charge or lead nurses, the current process for triage, segmentation of acuities, bed or space capacity, staff mix ratio, and provider-to-nurse ratio.

CONCLUSION

A measurement of multiple processes is necessary to develop effective systems, which require:

- Collaborative practice between emergency nurses and physicians, with decreased unnecessary duplicative practices, particularly related to low-acuity, low-risk patients
- Greater reliance on lower-cost human resources for technical tasks that can be delegated with proper oversight
- Philosophical underpinnings (an understanding of the why) of productivity, including supportive and restraining forces
- Measurement tools that demonstrate factors that positively and negatively impact the efficiency of individual staff members as well as the system

Ideally, the ED nurse director or medical director will measure the primary resources necessary to deliver patient care in the current environment and structure "what if" queries to determine what would happen if the resources were modified.

Enhanced productivity and efficiency require an approach that addresses both operational/fiscal accountability and behavioral sciences. It is necessary to implement a productivity plan with visionary leadership, efficiency tools, and initiatives that measure productivity; define the productivity of individuals supported or constrained by that system (individuals with the same job classification can have variable personal practices and speeds); and motivate and hold individuals accountable for accomplishing safety, efficiency, and productivity goals. Leaders must clearly communicate, educate, inspire, and coach up to acceptable levels of performance.

REFERENCES

1. Pink DH. *The Surprising Truth About What Motivates Us*. New York, NY: Penguin Publishing; 2009.
2. McGregor D. *The Human Side of Enterprise*. Cambridge, MA: MIT Press; 1957.
3. Trent SA, Havranek EP, Girde AA, Haukoos JS. Effect of audit and feedback on physician adherence to clinical practice guidelines for pneumonia and sepsis. *Am J Med Qual*. 2018;34(3):217–225.
4. Jain S, Frank G, McCormik K, Wu B, Johnson BA. Impact of physician scorecards on emergency dept resource use, quality, and efficiency. *Pediatrics*. 2015;136(3):e670-e679.
5. Arnett C, Emord J, Huntoon L, Charrow R. How Medicare Paperwork Abuses Doctors and Harms Patients. *The Heritage Foundation Lecture Series*. Published May 11 2020.
6. King MS, Lipsky MS, Sharp L. Expert agreement in Current Procedural Terminology evaluation and management coding. *Arc Int Med*. 2002;162(3):316-320.
7. Croskerry P, Cosby KS, Schenkel SM, Wears RL. Patient safety tip of the week March 8 2011. Yes, Physicians Get Interrupted Too! Available at: http://patientsafetysolutions.com/docs/March_8_2011_Yes_Physicians_Get_Interrupted_Too.htm. Accessed July 25, 2020.
8. Grey-Eurom, K. Creating Conflict Resolution in the Emergency Department. Emergency Medicine & Critical Care Review 2006. June 2006:12–13.
9. Wears RL, Caution, Interrupted: The Commentary. Published September 2004, in AHRQ - PSNet, Patient Safety Network. https://www.psnet.ahrq.gov/index.php/web-mm/caution-interrupted. Access July 25, 2020
10. ACEP News, January 2012, M. Granovsky and CMS, January 10, 2012.
11. Strauss RW, Rosenberg M, Barton ED, Mayer TA. Optimizing physician performance through incentives. In Strauss RW, Mayer TA, eds. *Strauss & Mayer's Emergency Department Management* (P. 487). Philadelphia, PA: McGraw-Hill; 2013.
12. Strang S, Park SQ, Strombach T, Kenning P. Applied economics: the use of monetary incentives to modulate behavior. *Prog Brain Res*. 2016;229:285-301.
13. Ahlstedt C, Lindvall CE, Holmström IK, Athlin ÅM. What makes registered nurses remain in work? An ethnographic study. *In J Nurs Stud*. 2019;89:32-38.
14. Emergency Physician-Nurse-Tech Care Team in Triage. Washington Hospital Center's ED Gold Team is "Worth Its Weight..." Maryland Patient Safety Center. 2010 Annual Conference Solutions Submission.
15. Patel PB, Vinson DR. Team assignment system: expediting ED care. *Ann Emerg Med*. 2005;46(6):499-506.
16. Schoenfeld E, Boniface K, Shokoohi H. ED technicians can successfully place ultra- sound-guided intravenous catheters in patients with poor vascular access. *M J Emerg Med*. 2011;29(5):496-501.
17. Gurney D, Gillespie G, McMahon M. Nursing code of ethics: provisions and interpretative statements for emergency nurses. *J Emerg Nurs*. 2017;43(6):98.
18. Truven Health Analytics. Available at: http://truvenhealth.com. Accessed February 20, 2019.
19. Nevada RN Formation. Nevada Nurse's Association. 2004;13(4).
20. House S, Havens D. Nurses' and physicians' perceptions of nurse-physician collaboration. *J Nurs Adm*. 2017;47(3):165-171.
21. Harris M. Little's Law: The science behind proper staffing. *Emerg Phys Monthly*. 2010.
22. Door-to-Doc Patient Safety Toolkit, published January 9, 2008 by AHRQ - PSNET (Patient Safety Network). https://psnet.ahrq.gov/issue/door-doc-patient-safety-toolkit. Accessed July 24, 2020
23. Crane J, Noon C. The Definitive Guide to Emergency Department Operational Improvement: Employing Lean Principles with Current ED Best Practices to Create the "No Wait" Department. Pub Routledge Productivity Press, New York, NY, ed. 2, 2020. Accessed December 30, 2020.

CHAPTER 24

PHYSICIAN ASSISTANTS AND NURSE PRACTITIONERS

Jeremy D. Tucker, Robert W. Strauss, Cary J. Stratford, Cyndy Flores, Marylou Killian, Randal Dabbs

The use of physician assistants (PAs) and nurse practitioners (NPs) continues to increase dramatically in emergency departments (EDs). A recent study of ED workforce providers using 2014 Medicare public use files demonstrated that PAs and NPs comprise 24.5% of the ED workforce.[1] Michael Menchine published the results of a survey reviewing the increased use of advanced practice providers (APPs), also known as advanced practice clinicians, revealed that the use of these clinicians increased from 28% to more than 77% between 1997 and 2006.[2] However, ED patient census has increased only 2% annually since 1996.[3]

The participation of APPs in emergency care fills critical needs, including addressing emergency physician (EP) shortages, responding to the increased demand for emergency care, and providing a less expensive high-quality provider. In light of this trend, it is crucial for the ED leader to have a clear working knowledge of the education, background, use of, and issues surrounding the use of these APPs.

The differences in the PA and NP educational models make it difficult to directly compare the two professions. Despite the divergences in their education, specific training, and licensing, PAs and NPs often work side by side in EDs, performing similar job functions.

In this chapter, the term *APPs* is used interchangeably with *PAs* and *NPs*.

PHYSICIAN ASSISTANTS

Historically, EPs had more experience with PAs than with NPs. This occurred as the evolution of emergency medicine (EM) as a physician specialty paralleled the evolution and development of the PA profession. Under the leadership of Dr. Eugene Stead II at Duke University, PAs began practicing alongside EPs.[4] Emergency physicians were among the earliest adopters of the evolving profession. The American College of Emergency Physicians (ACEP) worked in tandem with the American Academy of Physician Assistants (AAPA) and played an important part in the formulation and development of the PA profession from its beginnings.

Overview

According to the AAPA, there are more than 123,000 clinically practicing PAs, with just under 10% specializing in EM.[5] In fact, EM represents the largest specialty practice of PAs, arguably superseded only by all the PAs practicing in the surgical specialties and subspecialties combined. This incorporation of PAs into EM practice might well be traced to the early involvement of EPs in their training and development. Not surprisingly, this tandem evolution created a profession that fits well into the mindset and performance of EM practice.

Philosophy of Practice

Physician assistants practice medicine under the supervision of licensed physicians. This has been an unwavering tenet of the profession since its development over 50 years ago. The PA profession has long aligned itself with traditional medicine and the physicians who practice and supervise it. A national legislative effort from the AAPA, termed *Optimal Team Practice*, would ease the burden on supervising physicians without establishing independent practice.

Although PAs are dependent practitioners by law, they typically exercise considerable autonomy and clinical decision-making in many ED settings. The relationship between the physician and the PA is one of mutual trust, respect, and reliance. The EP trusts the PA to provide the same or similar quality care to patients and consult with a physician on those cases that are outside the PA's scope of practice. The PA trusts the physician to be available for supervision, to provide learned advice, and to accept care of patients with serious or complex problems.

In the best models of PA use in EM, this mutual trust and support is seamless. Because of their interdependent role, PAs remain extraordinarily flexible and responsive to the EP's oversight and practice. The efficiency of this model has led to its use in all medical and surgical specialties. The team is effective because of the similarities in physician and PA training, the PA profession's commitment to practice with supervision, and efficiencies created by using the strengths of each professional in the clinical practice setting.

PA Education and Training

As already noted, there are substantial similarities between the education of PAs and the education of physicians. Physician assistant instructors—who include physicians, PAs, and other professionals—provide a curriculum that follows the traditional medical model. Physician assistant students typically share classes and facilities in clinical rotations with medical students.

Most PA students entering graduate education possess a bachelor's degree. Some programs require prior health-care experience. Currently, there are over 260 accredited PA training programs throughout the United States, primarily located at teaching institutions and medical schools. The typical program, modeled after physician education, lasts 27 months or 3 academic years. Students graduate from PA programs with a master's degree, and all graduates must complete an accredited formal educational program and pass a national certifying exam to obtain a license.[6]

Another unique aspect of the PA profession is the defined educational experience. The Accreditation Review Commission accredits PA programs and will soon accredit postgraduate fellowships. Accreditation standards require competency-based curricula. Physician organizations that work closely with this accrediting agency include the American Medical Association, American Academy of Family Physicians, American Academy of Pediatrics, American College of Physicians, and the American College of Surgeons.

The initial year of PA education consists of a didactic curriculum with course work in anatomy and physiology, pharmacology, physical diagnosis, biochemistry, pathophysiology, microbiology, and medical ethics. The didactic curriculum is composed of approximately 400 hours of basic sciences and 580 hours of clinical medicine. The second year of PA education consists of clinical rotations in most major specialty areas, including EM. Prior to graduation, PA students complete an average of over 2,000 hours of clinical practice.

Postgraduate EM Training

There are more than 80 PA postgraduate training programs in the United States, at least 25 of which are specifically designed for EM. The typical program lasts 12 to 18 months and offers a certificate in specialty training. These postgraduate training programs follow didactic and clinical curricula similar to physician residency programs. Most EM postgraduate PA residency training programs limit the number of students and, in some cases, offer only one or two positions annually. There are continuing efforts to expand postgraduate opportunities in EM for PAs, including formal residency programs. Most EM PAs (as of the time of this publication) have not participated in formal postgraduate training programs.

Certification

In order to practice, the PA program graduate must pass the national certifying exam administered by the National Commission on Certification of Physician Assistants (NCCPA). In addition to being certified, PAs must meet licensing criteria for the states in which they intend to practice and have a supervising physician. All licensing authorities allow physicians to delegate prescriptive authority to the PAs they supervise. Similar to EPs, PAs must complete 100 continuing medical education (CME) credits every 2 years and pass the recertification exam every 10 years to maintain certification.

Since 2011, the NCCPA has offered an additional level of demonstrated competency in EM, called the Certificate of Added Qualifications (CAQ) in EM.[7] To obtain this certificate, the candidate must:

- Possess a state license
- Successfully pass the national certifying exam
- Document 3,000 hours of practice in EM
- Document 150 hours of continuing education specific to EM
- Complete advanced cardiac life support, pediatric advanced life support, advanced trauma life support, and an airway course
- Provide an EP's attestation indicating the PAs practice and expertise
- Successfully complete a mastery level examination in EM

Although the CAQ in EM certificate has only been offered since 2011, the majority of PAs who practice in the ED support its implementation. However, it may be decades before most PAs practicing in EM complete the competency. Since the CAQ requires extensive documented experience in EM practice, it is viewed as a mastery-level credential rather than an entry-level standard for newly graduated PAs.

NURSE PRACTITIONERS

Nurse practitioners are licensed, independent, advanced-practice registered nurses (RNs) who have completed a formal advanced education program beyond that of the RN. Nurse practitioners practice in ambulatory, acute, and long-term care settings as primary and/or specialty providers. Research has demonstrated that NPs provide safe, cost-effective, high-quality health care.[8]

Overview

The Emergency Nurses Association (ENA) originally developed the *Scope and Standards for the Emergency Nurse Practitioner* in 1999. The most recent (as of this publication) update of core competencies for NPs in emergency care was in 2016. The new standards were created in collaboration with the American Association of Nurse Practitioners (AANP), American Academy of Emergency Nurse Practitioners (AAENP), American Academy of Emergency Medicine (AAEM), and ACEP.[9]

The American Association of Nurse Practitioners estimates that approximately 4,500 certified NPs are currently working in emergency care in the United States.[1] The reported certifications include Family Nurse Practitioners (43%), Acute Care Nurse Practitioners (13%), Adult Nurse Practitioners (12%), Critical Care Nursing Specialists (9%), and Pediatric Nurse Practitioners (7%).[10] Additionally, behavioral health NPs are utilized in the ED to help alleviate the crisis of holding patients with behavioral health emergencies. In many hospitals, these APPs provide care under the supervision of the department of psychiatry.

Philosophy of Practice

The role of the NPs is very diverse. Nurse practitioners are educated under the nursing model, which is designed to provide holistic and preventive care and to engage the patients as the primary leaders in their own care and well-being. Nurse practitioners act as patient advocates to partner with the individual for mutually agreed-upon treatments and optimal health outcomes. Nurse practitioner education incorporates the medical model but remains distinct as a result of the emphasis on and foundation in the nursing perspective. Multiple studies have shown that NPs provide high-quality health-care services similar to those provided by primary care physicians and are able to diagnose and treat a wide range of medical problems.[11]

NP Education and Training

To be licensed as an NP, the candidate must first complete the education, training, and licensing necessary to become a registered nurse. Upon completing a graduate-level NP program (either a master's, post-master's certificate, or doctorate degree), the candidate must then pass the national board certification in their area of specialty. According to the American Association of Colleges of Nursing, there were 445 NP programs in 2017 in the United States.[12] Nurse practitioners are trained in a specialty area of life span: Family NP (FNP), Adult-Gerontology NP (AGNP), Pediatrics NP (PNP), Acute Care NP (ACNP), and Psych/Mental Health NP (MHNP).

The didactic portion of NP programs may be traditional classroom, online, or hybrid programs that include classroom and online learning. Requirements range from 39 to 52 credit hours. The clinical portions of the programs require between 500 and 860 supervised clinical hours depending on the specialty. Additionally, many programs require between 2,000 and 4,000 practice hours as an RN as a prerequisite for acceptance into the program.[13]

Postgraduate EM Programs

As of this publication, there are 10 academic programs in the United States that specifically prepare emergency nurse practitioners (ENPs). Nurse practitioners who did not attend one of these programs can develop additional competency to work in EDs through postmaster's fellowship programs, continuing education, and on-the-job training.

Certification

All states require national board certification before NPs are permitted to practice. The certifying bodies for NPs, the American Nurses Credentialing Center (ANCC) and the AANP require applicants to hold a master's degree, post-master's certificate, or doctoral degree to be eligible to test for certification. Certifications for NPs who work in the ED include FNP, ACNP, AGNP, and PNP. Recertification is required every 5 years.[10]

After completing the education program, the candidates must be licensed by the state in which they plan to practice. Each state board of nursing regulates the NP's practice and has its own licensing and certification criteria. In order to practice, the standards for NPs require licensure as an RN, completion of a graduate degree in nursing, and board certification by an accrediting body (e.g., ANCC, AANP).

In 2017, the American Association of Nurse Practitioners Certification Board (AANPCB), in collaboration with ACEP, AAENP, and AANP, developed a certification exam to validate the competencies of the ENP. This certification is in addition to the FNP certification. Eligibility to take the ENP exam includes the following[14]:

- The candidate must be licensed and hold a current certification as an FNP.
- The candidate must either:
  - graduate from an approved ENP educational program, *or*
  - complete an approved fellowship for APPs in EM, *or*
  - during the 5 years prior to application, have:
    - documentation of 2,000 clinical hours in emergency care *and*
    - proof of 100 hours of approved continuing education that is specific to EM, with 30 of these hours being education in emergency medical procedures.

SUPERVISION AND DELEGATION OF APPs

The skills (or competencies) of APPs can be categorized into three domains: patient management, professional roles, and procedural skills within the scope of practice.

Management of a patient's health or illness status encompasses those behaviors that are necessary to effectively diagnose and treat patients presenting for emergency care. Essential skills in this domain include obtaining the patient's history, performing a physical examination, developing a differential diagnosis, ordering and interpreting diagnostic studies, developing a plan of care for the patient, and ensuring appropriate follow-up. Advanced practice providers may also be utilized in triage and in the performance of medical screening exams.[15-17]

The *professional roles* of APPs include those activities that ensure that they are practicing as a member of the emergency care team in accordance with their legal and ethical professional responsibilities. These activities include, but are not limited to, being a member of medical staff, participating in quality improvement (QI) activities, and directing the work of other members of the health-care team.

The *procedural skills* of APPs, with proper training and supervision, allow them to become credentialed to perform most EM procedures. Procedures most commonly performed by APPs were identified in the delineation of practice during the development of the Certificate of Additional Qualification for EM and by the AANPCB for the ENP certification exam.[7] An analysis of the procedures from both documents show that the procedures commonly performed by PAs and NPs are identical.

The *scope of practice* for APPs may vary based on state laws and regulations, facility policies, the practice setting, the employment arrangement, and the knowledge and experience of the APP.[1]

Practice Delegation

Most states require a "practice agreement" that delineates the responsibilities delegated by the supervising physician to the PA or NP. These agreements define how the PA or

NP is to function in the practice setting. The location-specific practice agreements are developed to meet the specific needs of a specific ED. Some states require that specific forms are completed and filed, while other states simply describe the necessary requirements for these documents. The supervising physician should only delegate those practices and procedures that are within the APP's scope of practice, education, training, and competency.

The high-functioning EDs that use APPs have a culture of teamwork and collegiality among all providers. It is very important for the EP and the APP to understand each other's strengths, weaknesses, and practice styles. This, of course, takes time, communication, proper supervision, and a culture of collaboration.

APP UTILIZATION

The spectrum of utilization detailed on the Society of Emergency Physician Assistants (SEMPA) website is as follows[18]:

- Almost 75% of PAs surveyed work in the main ED.
- Approximately 17% work in fast track (quick care for minor complaints).
- About 1.5% work in triage.
- Approximately 6% work in an urgent care system.

These data are counter to the common belief that most PAs work only in low-acuity areas. In fact, most PAs work in programs that are customized fit to each system's specific needs. Indeed, this degree of flexibility is at the core of the success of PAs in clinical medicine.

Cost-Effectiveness

Since APPs earn 35% to 50% of a typical emergency physician (EP) salary and have a reduced cost of insurance and salary-based benefits, APPs can provide significant program cost savings. In primary care, it has been demonstrated that PAs can provide over 80% of the services traditionally provided by MDs.[19] In the ED, APPs can often provide most of the services of the EP with similar efficiency. It may be particularly cost-effective to utilize APPs for multiple aspects of care, including lacerations, provider-in-triage, observation care, minor care, and others. Furthermore, APPs have become the sole providers in some critical access EDs or urgent care centers, with EPs providing remote supervision.

The advantages of having APPs on staff extend beyond salary and benefit savings. The corresponding reduction in EP workload and improvement in departmental efficiency provide additional benefits to the practice in financial savings, better workflow, decreased burnout, and enhanced clinician satisfaction. Advanced practice providers have higher job satisfaction if they are well supported, believe their talents and expertise are used on higher-acuity problems, and work in an environment with increased efficiency. Satisfied APPs have improved retention and job satisfaction, which directly translates to improved quality, customer experience, and ED director satisfaction.

Frequently, the question arises whether it is better to supplement EP services with APPs or with non-EM-boarded physicians, who may be working part-time in the ED to supplement their income. While, in theory, it may seem reasonable to hire a physician who requires less supervision, there are several potential disadvantages to utilizing a non-EM physician instead of a dedicated APP:

- **Cost:** Almost invariably, non-EM physicians cost more.
- **Commitment:** Advanced practice providers are EM-career focused, whereas non-EM-boarded physicians are more focused on their primary specialty. This includes CME, integration with team, and so on.
- **Supervision:** Non-EM physicians still require supervision, quality reviews, and feedback.
- **Credentialing:** Increasingly, EDs require physicians to be EM board certified, making the dedicated emergency APP even more attractive.
- **Adaptability:** Advanced practice providers readily adapt to delegation and supervision.
- **Patient satisfaction:** Advanced practice providers are attentive to ensuring excellent patient experience scores and are willing to dedicate the time to patients and families as required in the department.

In summary, the APP is adaptable, committed to the profession, and willing to conform to a variety of systems with ease. Because of their commitment and adaptability, APPs actively participate in and often lead change in the department. These intangible elements are important considerations in APP versus non-emergency-medicine boarded physician utilization. With future health-care reform, declining reimbursements, and salary increases, the cost-benefit advantages of APP utilization may increase further.

Salary and Benefits

Data from the 2019 *Advanced Practice Provider Compensation and Pay Practices Survey Report* demonstrates a mean salary figure of $121,750 for NPs and $133,006 for PAs practicing in EM.[20] Of interest, the ED practice setting provided the highest salary for NPs and nearly the highest for PAs (**Table 24.1**); 48% of PAs report that compensation has productivity or performance ties.[20]

To compensate for overtime and productivity, some systems pay clinicians a salary for a set number of clinical hours, and then further compensate clinicians on an hourly basis for hours

TABLE 24.1 ■ Median Total Compensation for Nurse Practitioners and Physician Assistants Practicing Emergency Medicine[20]		
Practice Location	**Nurse Practitioners**	**Physician Assistants**
National	$118,986	$133,120
North Central	$112,216	$127,030
Northeast	$120,661	$123,667
South Central	$118,964	$128,490
Southeast	$116,381	$114,953
Rural	$130,565	$117,426
Urban	$118456	$124,753

worked above and beyond the contracted hours. Appropriately incentivized APPs are willing to do more than the minimum, including arriving early and staying late to provide clinical support or complete superior documentation, participating in leadership and committees, and so on.

Compensation Structures

There are many different compensation structures, including:

- *Hourly compensation*: Many providers are paid based on a flat hourly rate structure. Regulations for this type of payment require overtime payment for hours beyond 40 hours in a week. Daily overtime payments are required in those states with daily overtime rules (greater than 8 hours a day), which at last review included, Alaska, California, Nevada, Puerto Rico, and the Virgin Islands. Colorado has daily overtime laws for working over 12 hours in a day. Advanced practice providers in EDs and urgent care centers are more likely to be paid an hourly rate than a salary.
- *Salary*: Straight salary is a common method of APP payment. Generally, the salary form of payment does not require overtime pay under the Fair Labor Standards Act Section 13(a)(1).[21]
- *Base pay with bonus*: There are compensation models with base pay (hourly or salaried) combined with bonuses. Bonuses are usually designed to incentivize desirable behaviors and outcomes, including patient satisfaction scores, the number of patients per hour, relative value units (RVUs) per hour (based on productivity, expertise, or effort), and on-call availability.

Discretionary bonuses are those paid at the prerogative of the medical director, often for a job well done.

Performance Pay

Performance pay is intended to incentivize APPs to work more efficiently and with greater productivity in the department. These payments should recognize a provider's full contribution to the department and can include:

- Productivity (patients/hour, charges/hour, and/or RVUs)
- Patient experience of care measured by satisfaction score
- Minimal complaints from patients, colleagues, staff
- Minimal cases identified as quality concerns
- Department participation and effectiveness as a team player

Incentivizing excellent performance rewards the top providers while encouraging the slower (less productive) performers to become more efficient. Bonuses can be paid annually, quarterly, or with each check. It is uncommon to pay PA/NPs based on a 100% (pure) productivity model.

On-call systems provide rapid capacity to "up-staff" the ED and provide last-minute coverage for emergencies like staff members calling in sick. On-call duty (often called just "call") can be shared among interested participants or made mandatory, but unless it is appropriately incentivized, call is likely to be an unpopular component of the compensation package. There are various ways to compensate for call coverage, including hourly "call" pay; a flat rate per day of call (if on a regular salary); and an hourly bonus on top of normal pay (a shift differential).

Benefits

Generally, benefits are similar to those provided to employed EPs and typically cover insurances, pensions, vacation, and CME allotments. (Examples of typical benefits are listed below, with information available for PAs through SEMPA.)[22]

- *Insurance* (e.g., dental, short-term and long-term disability, term life)
- *Professional liability insurance*
- *Retirement plans* (e.g., 401k, 403b, IRA)
- *CME allotments*, including:
  - Time off and expenses. More than half of APPs have 1 week or more of paid time off specifically for CME.
  - CME benefits typically range between $1,000 and $3,000 a year, with 25% of PAs receiving $2,000 or more.
  - Many groups provide CME funding at rates similar to those for EPs. Travel costs are identical for all providers. Typically, APPs in EM obtain most of their CME at physician conferences, but CME tuition at these events is often discounted for APPs by a factor of 30 to 50%.
- *Professional membership dues*
- *Paid time off* (Most respondents indicated a range between 2 and 5 weeks beyond their CME allotment. However, 28% reported no vacation time. This may be explained by the large number of PAs who work for a per-diem hourly rate.)
- *Recertification costs* (Beyond annual CME [100 hours for PAs], there is a 10-year cycle for recertification by the Physician Assistant National Recertifying Examination offered by the NCCPA. The newly formulated CAQ in EM costs $350 with a recertification cycle of every 6 years. Physician assistants who participate in the CAQ in EM are still required to maintain their primary NCCPA certification.)

Malpractice and Insurance Considerations

It is a common misconception or concern that PAs and NPs are subject to greater malpractice exposure than their physician counterparts; however, this concern is not supported by experience.[23] In fact, the literature demonstrates the opposite. Research shows that APPs (in all specialties) experience a number of claims that is 10 times lower than that experienced by physicians, with near-identical rates between PAs and NPs.[24] Further, payments for physician claims are 1.3 to 2.3 times higher than the payments for APPs.

Professional Liability Insurance

Advanced practice providers are often added directly onto a group's professional liability policy, creating identical coverage based on the number of patient encounters. When purchased separately, APP premiums are typically less than those of EPs. A lower cost for coverage coupled with a lower incidence of claims provides an additional advantage to utilizing APPs.

Practice Variation and Unit-Based Utilization

Advanced practice providers may practice in a wide variety of emergency medical positions. Since supervising physicians develop and delegate responsibilities based on the unique needs of their departments, the flexibility of APPs practicing in the ED is a tremendous asset. In addition to working side-by-side with physicians in the direct provision of care in the main ED, there are myriad opportunities for APP practice in a broad variety of settings and with multiple responsibilities (**Box 24.1**).

Among the many reasons that APPs have partnered with EPs to assume multiple roles in the care of emergency patients are professionalism, quality, collaboration, efficiency, and cost-effectiveness. Prior to the broad use of APPs in the ED, most fast-track, observation, and provider-in-triage (rapid assessment) models only used physicians.

> **BOX 24.1 ■ EM PRACTICE OPPORTUNITIES FOR APPs**
>
> - Fast tracks
> - Observation units
> - Provider-in-triage
> - Super tracks
> - Hospital EDs
> - Free-standing EDs
> - Urgent care centers
> - Critical-access EDs
> - Emergency medical services (EMS)
> - Flight programs

Most systems utilize APPs in the main ED to evaluate and care for patients, perhaps those with lower acuity but that are nonetheless complex and utilize significant resources. Patients with generalized weakness, multiple complaints, or psychosocial challenges can be time-consuming and take the EP away from the most complex patients. By assigning APPs to some of the cases that require intensive workups, the EPs are freed up to oversee the entire department and focus on the highest-acuity patients.

Another example of appropriate APP use includes patients with multiple minor wounds that require detailed debridement and closure. These cases can easily occupy a clinician for an hour or more. Assigning an APP to these patients avoids tying up the most highly trained and expensive providers to address problems that do not require their expertise. PAs and NPs also serve roles in some advanced life support out-of-hospital systems, including aeromedical and interfacility critical care transfers.

ED DIRECTOR RESPONSIBILITIES

Leading and managing an ED is a critical and complex process, requiring constant attention to solid recruiting, effective on-boarding, mentoring, feedback, and supervision. The medical director is responsible for creating a vision and motivating the team to accomplish its primary responsibility: providing the best possible care for the patients while addressing the needs of the clinicians who are providing it.

Provider Recruitment

Recruitment of all ED providers is an ongoing process that requires a "step-ahead" approach. Prominent EM leader Kevin Klauer refers to the "plus 1" method.[25] He states, "There is a constant ebb and flow of providers due to changing professional goals, personal goals, family needs, illnesses, the rigors of shift work, physician burnout, and other unforeseen circumstances." Therefore, many directors will recruit for potential needs rather than waiting until an APP has resigned, leaving the group understaffed, overwhelmed, and in crisis.

The appropriate professional tone should be set throughout the recruitment process. Best-practice medical directors actively participate in a thorough pre-interview screening process, an interview that involves multiple stakeholders, a tour of the facility, an opportunity for the candidate to learn about the community, and substantial time for open-ended conversation about the practice. In other words, determining the "fit" of the job candidate is the responsibility of the medical director. Done well, this process avoids poor hiring practices and is most likely to ensure an integrated, high-functioning team.

When interviewing candidates, it is advisable to also include a senior APP as well as a nursing leader. Since training and experience are highly variable, it is important to do the following:

- Compare the candidate's experience against the job requirements.
- List all the anticipated procedures.
- Determine the candidate's comfort level with those procedures.
- Define further training requirements.

Recruiting experienced or emergency-trained APPs can be a challenge. There are a variety of ways to contact APPs with prior experience, such as through job-posting websites, classified ads, display ads in APP publications, and professional organizations (e.g., SEMPA, ACEP, AENP).

New Provider Orientation

Orientation is another critical process that frequently determines the success of new providers. If orientations are casual and superficial, new APPs will not know what is expected of them. As the saying goes, "You cannot live up to expectations you do not know." The components of a successful orientation processes include making sure the candidate is informed about:

- Professional expectations: showing up on time, respectful communications, chart completion, relationship with staff and other clinicians
- Supervision guidelines
- Organizational (hospital and group) resources and policies, including compliance standards
- "Citizenship" expectations (e.g., meeting attendance and participation)
- Educational resources

New clinicians should not be placed on their own in the ED without immediately available mentors. Clinical orientations are key and should include information on provider-specific strategies for addressing an individual's gaps, patient flow and electronic health record processes, and essential services like diagnostic imaging.

Supervision and Feedback

Newly graduated APPs and those with limited experience in the types of care provided at their new institution will often require additional training. Knowledge deficits should be determined before hiring rather than coming as a surprise during the provision of clinical care. Thorough background assessments will usually uncover knowledge and experience gaps. No matter when they are discovered, it is essential that the department leadership has an organized and effective plan for filling the gaps.

State laws, group protocols, and institutional policies have mandated different requirements for the oversight of APPs, which address chart co-signatures, the ratio of supervising physicians to APPs, methods of supervision, and guidelines for advancing from direct to proximate supervision.

Supervision

The primary principles of supervision are patient protection and open communication between the physicians and the APPs. While the term "proximate supervision" has various interpretations, most states minimally require the supervising physician to be available by "electronic communication" at all times. Proximate supervision could mean that the delegating practitioner exercises direct oversight by being present at all times, immediately available in person, or nearby and accessible by telephone or electronic means.

It is important that APPs know and comply with the hospital bylaws and department rules and regulations. The supervision strategies that are employed by the ED should ensure safe patient care, open communication, and opportunities for feedback and improvement. The leadership of the ED group must determine the appropriate supervision of the APP in each setting.

Mandated supervision of all patients: Some ED groups mandate that the physicians see and assess any patient who is evaluated by an APP. This is the most time-consuming and intensive method of supervision and degrades physician productivity. There may be additional reimbursement "captured" when the physician co-evaluates the Medicare patients previously seen by a PA (100% versus 85%). Negative aspects of this approach include:

- Continual interruptions that decrease the physician's productivity (and possibly reimbursement)
- Patient flow bottlenecks prolonging lengths of stay
- Frustration of competent APPs
- Physician frustration

Guideline-based supervision: Alternatively, groups often institute guidelines that specify which patients must be reviewed or seen by the supervising physician based on their acuity and presenting condition, or the experience of the APP. The goals for establishing guidelines are to manage risk, provide oversight, and perform real-time peer review of cases. Guideline-based supervisions provide situation-based communication that can help the EP to understand the comfort level of the APP with different types of patients. Examples of this may be, "triage categories 1, 2, horizontal 3s," "all chest pain patients," or a requirement that the EPs "review all axial spine images." While guidelines are appropriate and necessary, exhaustive lists with multiple restrictions can limit the efficiency of the APP.

Needs-based consults: Most groups perform needs-based consults with the supervising EP on an informal basis. Advanced practice providers with significant ED experience know when to seek a consultation with the supervising physician. Understanding the practice style of the EP also allows the APP to know which physician wants to be consulted on certain types of cases. However, if only needs-based consultations occur and no other guidelines are in place, some patients may be discharged without necessary oversight.

Chart reviews: Many groups also routinely perform APP chart reviews. Chart reviews can be performed prior to the patient leaving the ED, but required pre-discharge chart reviews delay discharge. Chart reviews can vary from a random sample to 100% chart review. Most states, hospitals, and groups have a mandatory physician co-signature requirement. While some groups may not review all charts, some level of chart review is strongly advised. It is important for the EP to understand that a co-signature is really saying you have reviewed the chart and agree with it. Charts can be reviewed after the fact as part of a QI process. This process must be HIPAA compliant and should allow the blinded review of APPs by other APPs and EPs. Broad review of and by multiple providers provides the director or management team a look at the strengths and weaknesses of the whole group, permitting focused improvement efforts.

Minimally experienced APPs: Hiring an APP who does not have EM experience can be successful. However, this situation requires robust on-boarding, training, and feedback processes, which should first identify strengths and weaknesses of the new employee. The training can then be tailored to address specific deficits. If suturing experience is lacking, a formal suturing course may be useful as well as direct one-on-one training with a senior APP. Directed CME may be helpful to a new APP. For instance, an APP with a gap in pediatric training can be sent to an affiliated pediatric ED to get intensive one-on-one training with pediatric EM physicians. Depending on experience and training, it may take 2 to 6 months before an inexperienced APP can work independently.

Meaningful Feedback

Advanced practice provider feedback is a critical part of developing consistent care and an effective team. Appropriate feedback helps to set goals and improve performance over time. All providers should get regular performance feedback, including a review of individual quality, efficiency, patient and staff satisfaction, utilization data, and peer group comparisons. This objective examination of the data allows the leader to discuss ways to improve. It is very important to give positive feedback at this time as well.

The process should include specific follow-up on any areas identified for improvement. Providers want feedback and taking time to address both the APP's concerns and those of the supervising physician leads to a more successful group that understands continuous performance improvement is an enduring goal. Feedback sessions should be bidirectional, giving the provider an opportunity to make recommendations and describe what is and is not working well. There are many ways to ensure feedback, including regular "rounding on providers," a Studer Group (health care consultants) process using a predetermined set of questions to determine the provider's satisfaction with the ED operation.[26-27] In all cases, the process should occur consistently and for all providers. Ideally, new providers should receive formal feedback at 1, 3, 6, and 12 months and every 6 months after that.

Regular off-site retreats incorporating educational topics identified by the group as well as team-building programs will enhance the team spirit. Lectures by EPs or consultant providers, procedure clinics, and simulations are beneficial to the APP (and all clinical staff). Simulation labs, particularly those with observational areas to observe and videotape APPs in action, can be used to assess and improve skills. Ongoing staff development has enormous value as it improves patient care, lowers risk, and enhances employee satisfaction and retention.

Creating a Healthy Culture

Experienced APPs are integral to optimizing the delivery of efficient, cost-effective, and quality care in the ED. However, turnover is common among APPs as a result of multiple opportunities (e.g., ease of transition from one institution or one specialty to another), unsatisfactory work conditions (e.g., a disproportionate share of evening shifts), poor relationships (e.g., EPs who are critical and do not provide appropriate feedback or supervision), and so on.

Frequent turnover leads to constant recruitment and on-boarding, inconsistent workflow, wide variations in care, and increased leadership effort. The goal of ED leadership should be to minimize turnover by increasing engagement and retention of the APPs in the department.

Fostering Inclusivity

An inclusive and respectful culture is the principal requirement for effective collaboration. The supervisory role, institutional and department policies, and the malpractice environment make it difficult to create and maintain an atmosphere where all clinicians are considered peers. This challenge can be overcome with regular group meetings during which all clinicians are encouraged to have a voice and provide input, and all input is respectfully considered.

Additionally, non-work-related social events that build a foundation of friendship and trust are invaluable to offset the high-stress moments of an ED. Another valuable example of inclusiveness is to include an APP leader on all new clinician interviews. This establishes the message from the very beginning that all team members have a voice and will be treated as peers.

Recognizing Positive Contributions

Recognition of positive contributions to the department is an important strategy for improved APP engagement. These acknowledgments and appreciations may be related to clinical outcomes, patient experiences, productivity, or team-building efforts with the nurses, medical staff, or EPs. These positive activities must be consistently and strategically identified and publicly displayed via a newsletter or communiques to the group and C-suite.

Communicating Consistent Expectations

Early and consistent communication of behavioral, operational, and relationship expectations prevents misunderstanding, uncertainty, and potential conflict. The leaders should set and exemplify a standard of professionalism, collegiality, and inclusiveness among all clinicians. The medical director should establish supervisory guidelines (see the earlier section "Training, Supervision, and Feedback") so that the APPs know when and how to consult with their physician supervisors and, in turn, the physicians are held accountable for being approachable, responsive, and amicable. These characteristics should be monitored by regularly surveying the group.

Providing Professional Growth and Leadership Opportunities

As do most clinicians, APPs seek opportunities to grow professionally, build leadership skills, and add value to their group. As a retention strategy, qualified APPs should be considered for any roles that allow them to teach, to serve as members or chairs of hospital or departmental committees, to manage special projects (such as flow or quality), and to serve in leadership positions (such as an assistant medical director or being the lead APP). The medical director should create paths that promote engagement and tenure within the group.

BOX 24.2 ■ LEADERSHIP ROLES HELD BY APPs

Departmental/institutional
- Project lead in department QI
- Reimbursement director
- Education champion
- Patient experience director
- Lead APP for the department
- APP scheduler
- Director of APP quality/risk
- Vice chair (assistant director) of department
- Medical staff committee chair

National/regional
- Government committees
- Committees within:
  - ACEP
  - AAEM
  - SAEM
  - ACOEP
  - ENA
  - SEMPA
  - ...and others
- Regional or national APP director

Box 24.2 provides examples of APP leadership opportunities that should be supported by the medical director.

Providing Constructive Feedback

Finally, APPs appreciate the opportunity to improve their performance by receiving their individual data on a regular basis, such as patient satisfaction scores, departmental metrics, productivity, and outcomes. Every effort should be made to gather this information and share it with the APPs of the department. Conscientious providers desire constructive professional feedback and education by their physician colleagues given in a positive and private manner. These efforts improvement engagement and patient care.

Whether your clinical team is composed of NPs, PAs, or both, the critical element that adds the most value is the relationship between the physicians and the APP. That relationship can be strengthened over time by implementing effective retention strategies.

CONCLUSION

The utilization of APPs in EM is well-established, and their value to emergency care will only continue to grow in the future. For the medical director, it is vital to understand employment and staffing models for APPs and to optimize the department's quality, efficiency, and cost of care. The importance of conscientiously on-boarding and retaining quality APPs cannot be overstated. Advanced practice providers are and should be treated as essential, skilled, and professional members of the team.

RESOURCES

- **AANP**: American Academy of Nurse Practitioners, www.aanp.org.
- **AAPA**: American Academy of Physician Assistants, www.aapa.org.
- **ACEP**: American College of Emergency Physicians, www.acep.org.
- **ANCC**: American Nurses Credentialing Center, www.nursingworld.org/ancc/
- **ENA**: Emergency Nurses Association, www.ena.org.
- **SEMPA**: Society of Emergency Medicine Physician Assistants, www.sempa.org.
- **NCCPA**: National Commission on Certification of Physician Assistants, www.nccpa.net.

REFERENCES

1. Hall MK, Burns K, Carius M, et al. State of the National Emergency Department Workforce: who provides care where? Ann Emerg Med. 2018;72(3):302-307. doi:10.1016/j.annemergmed.2018.03.032.
2. Menchine MD, Wiechmann W, Rudkin S. Trends in midlevel provider utilization in emergency departments from 1997 to 2006. Acad Emerg Med. 2009;16(10):963-969.
3. Centers for Disease Control and Prevention. Emergency department visits, 2016. 2017. Available at: https://www.cdc.gov/nchs/fastats/emergency-department.htm. Accessed December 12, 2018.
4. http://en.wikipedia.org/wiki/Eugene_A._Stead. Accessed October 4, 2012
5. American Academy of Physician Assistants. PA profile. Available at: https://www.aapa.org/download/31811/. Accessed December 28, 2018.
6. American Academy of Physician Assistants. Pre-requisites and training. Available at: https://www.aapa.org/career-central/becomea-pa/. Accessed December 28, 2018.
7. American Academy of Physician Assistants. Physician Assistant Certificate of Added Qualifications (CAQ) in Emergency Medicine. Available at: https://www.nccpa.net/emergencymedicine. Accessed November 21, 2018.
8. Jennings, S, Clifford S, Fox A, O'Connell J, Gardner G. The impact of nurse practitioner services on cost, quality of care, satisfaction, and waiting times in the emergency department: a systematic review. Int J Nurs Stud. 2015;52(1):421-435.
9. Campo T, Carmen MJ, Evans D, et al. Scope of practice for emergency nurse practitioners. Adv Emerg Nurs J. 2016;38(4):252-254.
10. American Academy of Emergency Nurse Practitioners Certification Board. 2016. Executive Summary of the 2016 Practice Analysis of Emergency Nurse Practitioners. Available at: https://www.aanpcert.org/resource/documents/emergency%20NP%20handbook.pdf. Accessed June 17, 2018
11. AANP, Quality of Nurse Practitioner Practice, https://www.aanp.org/advocacy/advocacy-resource/position-statements/quality-of-nurse-practitioner-practice Published 2015, Amer Assoc Nurse Prac. Accessed June 11, 2020
12. NP Schools. How do I become a nurse practitioner. 2018. Available at: https://www.nursepractitionerschools.com/faq/how-to-become-np. Accessed December 29, 2018.
13. AANP Certification Board. Qualification of Candidates https://www.aanpcert.org/certs/qualifications. Published 2020, Amer Assoc Nurse Prac., Accessed June 11, 2020

14. AANP Certification Board, Emergency Nurse practitioner Specialty Certification: ENP Certification Handbook, https://www.aanpcert.org/resource/documents/Emergency%20NP%20Handbook.pdf Published March 2018; AANPCB; Accessed June 11, 2020
15. Marriott T, "Maximizing Utilization of PAs & NPs: Rules, Realities, and Reimbursement," http://www.namss.org/Portals/0/ConferenceDocuments/2016Conference/2016%20Handouts/TU15%20-%20Maximizing%20Utilization%20of%20PAs%20and%20NPs.pdf , Accessed December 26, 2018
16. Phillips A, Klauer K, Kessler C, Emergency physician evaluation of PA and NP practice patterns, Jl Amer Acad PAs, 31:5, May 2018
17. Moor M, NP and PA Scope of Practice Vary Greatly in US Emergency Departments, Clin. Adv. June 12, 2018, https://www.clinicaladvisor.com/practice-management-information-center/ed-trends-in-np-pa/article/772423/ Accessed October 10, 2018
18. SEMPA, PA Clinical Practice Data, https://www.sempa.org/practice-management/clinical-practice-data/, Accessed December 18, 2018
19. Ballweg R, Sullivan EM, Brown D, VetroskyD, Physician Assistant: A guide to Clinical Practice. Pgs 665-666, Elsevier Saunders, Philadelphia 2013
20. Sullivan Cotter, 2019 Advance Practice Provider Compensation and Pay Practices Survey Report, https://sullivancotter.com/wp-content/uploads/2018/10/SAMPLE-2019-Advanced-Practice-Provider-Compensation-and-Pay-Practices-Survey-Report-Full.pdf. Published 2020, Accessed June 16, 2020.
21. Legal Information Institute, 29 U.S. Code § 213.Exemptions, https://www.law.cornell.edu/uscode/text/29/213 Published 2019, Cornell Law School, Accessed June 10, 2020
22. Society of Emergency Medicine Physician Assistants, Salary & Benefits Data, https://www.sempa.org/Static/360/Resources/Salary---Benefits-Data/index.html Published 2019, SEMPA, Accessed December 22, 2019
23. Nicholson JG., 'Physician Assistant Malpractice History: Comparing PAs to Physicians and Nurse Practitioners." https://expertpages.com/news/Physician_Assistant_Malpractice_History.htm Published 2016, Accessed October 25, 2018
24. Brock DM, Nicholson J, Hooker RS, "Physician Assistant and Nurse Practitioner Malpractice Trends." Med Care Res Rev. 2017 Oct;74(5):613-624.
25. Klauer K. The +1 approach to recruiting. Presented at the American College of Emergency Physicians–Emergency Department Directors Academy; 2018.
26. Hotko B. How to increase employee retention and drive higher patient satisfaction. Available at: https://www.studergroup.com/hardwiredresults/hardwired-results-01/rounding-for-outcomes. PostedAccessed November 29, 2018.
27. Kennedy-Oehlert J, "The Single Most Powerful Tactic for Creating Physician Engagement." The Studer Group, posted February 1, 2012, Accessed June 11, 2020

CHAPTER 25

SCRIBES

W. Clayton Alexander IV, Chelsey Geiger

Scribes have been in general use since antiquity, although the first use of a medical scribe is unknown.[1] More recently, a 1974 article in the *Journal of the American College of Emergency Physicians* written by Thomas Lynch of Decatur Memorial Hospital discussed using a licensed practical nurse as a scribe during busy times.[2] One of the earliest medical scribe programs to receive national recognition began in 1995 at the emergency department (ED) of then-named Harris Methodist Hospital in Fort Worth, Texas.[3] Harris Methodist won the USA Today/Rochester Institute of Technology Quality Cup, in part because of the innovation and quality of its scribe program. Emergency Medical Associates of New Jersey was an innovator and early adopter of medical scribes in 1990 through the organization's Clinical Information Manager program, which is still in use today.

HISTORY OF MEDICAL SCRIBES

Anyone who has completed a patient's medical chart by hand knows that the process is cumbersome and time consuming. Handwritten charts frequently result in an incomplete record, especially with regard to meeting diagnosis and charge coding criteria. Those relying on the information in handwritten medical records to provide subsequent care to patients struggle with poor legibility and frequent errors of omission. A busy and understaffed ED may increase the likelihood of these challenges. Poor or hurried documentation, including the use of unorthodox or unknown abbreviations, exposes the patient and physician to the risk of error. As an example, a physician once wrote on a chart, "D-75 P-25 IM" (Demerol and Phenergan) as a shortcut measure and relied on the nurse to decipher the cryptic phrase.

Some of the first scribes brought into the ED for full-time coverage were introduced to address handwriting issues and the patient safety issues they created. Scribes were tested for their command of medical vocabulary and good penmanship during the interview process. The 1974 article by Thomas Lynch discusses legible handwriting during busy times as a major benefit of the system.[2] In the beginning, as the scribes worked to write what they were told or heard, this "real-time" documentation was in itself a great benefit. As scribe programs evolved, new and unforeseen benefits became apparent. The assistance of a scribe made providers more efficient and enabled them to see more patients in the course of a shift. Fewer patient safety errors occurred, and providers felt overall less stressed during their work days.

The Electronic Medical Record and Its Impact

Though the formal use of scribes in the ED dates back to well before the widespread use of electronic medical records (EMRs), it is no coincidence that the widespread adoption of EMRs and the dramatic increase in the demand for scribes are closely related. EMRs also offer a potential upside for hospital systems. However, in a busy ED, the increased documentation requirements can have a nearly disastrous impact on the productivity of ED providers, who are constantly pressed to meet the multiple demands of patient satisfaction, quality of care, and regulatory requirements.[4]

In 2004, the push to replace handwritten charts in medicine with an electronic format was made clear by President George W. Bush's executive order encouraging EMR adoption by 2014.[5] However, simply having an EMR is not sufficient to receive the federal funds promised—the use of the EMR must meet the "meaningful use" standard and contribute to the efficient communication of a patient's medical history and information.[6] Furthermore, in 2015, effective use of the EMR was incorporated into Merit-Based Incentive Payment System (MIPS), which was designed to update and consolidate several CMS incentive programs.[7]

As of 2016, nearly all critical access hospitals had adopted an electronic record.[8] The challenge with the EMR is that the economic benefit accrues disproportionately to the relatively low-cost personnel, while the EMR's propensity to degrade productivity falls on the most expensive resource in the system, the providers. Physicians are burdened with increasing administrative tasks that decrease the time available to focus on patient care. In fact, only 28% of ED physicians' time is spent providing direct patient care, while nearly half of their time is spent on data entry.

According to the 2018 Medscape National Physician Burnout & Depression Report, one out of every two ED physicians reports feeling burned out. The burden of bureaucratic tasks, including charting and paperwork, and the increasing computerization of the practice are some of the leading contributors to burnout.[9] While there are clear benefits to the consistent use of the EMR system, the economic and quality-of-life case for EMRs is least compelling for the providers. Simply put, data input is not a good use of provider time.

The parallel growth of the scribe industry and the EMR adoption is undeniable. Scribes are a viable solution to offset the productivity losses and burnout rates associated with an EMR change. They also can serve as a catalyst to expedite adoption and minimize the negative impacts to performance when integrating a new EMR system.

WHO ARE SCRIBES?

The answer to the question of scribe demographics and qualifications depends on the geographic location of a program and the expectations and intended use of the scribe. Scribes are widely used in both academic and community hospital EDs, free-standing EDs, urgent care centers, and inpatient and outpatient settings. Scribe duties may be performed by traditional outsourced-contracted scribe companies, in-house or home-grown scribe programs, or medical staff members acting as scribes.[10-12] **Table 25.1** lists the various scribe personnel backgrounds with their strengths and weaknesses.

The scribe must know medical terminology and spelling and be able to sense the practice pace and rhythm of multiple physicians. He or she needs to be discrete in the presence of patients, comfortable talking to physicians, and technically proficient in whatever mode of documentation is in use. The scribe typically does not engage in any activity beyond passively documenting patient history; retrieving information and test results; recording multiple other patient-related encounters, including recheck discussions and consult discussions; and recording any other information that the provider dictates. Most scribes do not see being a scribe as a long-term employment opportunity, but rather as valuable growth experience on the way to another opportunity. This chapter focuses on this type of scribe.

TABLE 25.1 ■ Backgrounds of Various Scribes		
Scribe Demographic	Strengths	Weaknesses
Premedical student	Well educated and motivated, ideal for ED settings	Limited time availability; transient
Nursing student	Educated and motivated	Limited time availability; transient
College graduate	Educated and motivated; greater time availability	Lower tenure commitment; often require additional vocabulary training
EMT-P or equivalent	Comfortable around patients; highly motivated; stable	Less educated; often require additional vocabulary training
MA-C, LPN or equivalent	Career-seeking, vocationally trained, ideal for the outpatient setting	Less educated, often require additional training on documentation, may perform duties commiserate with licensure

For most, being a scribe is a logical step in the process of becoming a licensed health-care professional. The modest salary—between $9 and $18 per, varying by geographic region—is generally not the prime motivation behind the hours of hard work needed to become an asset to an emergency physician group.[12,13] Experience that may contribute to becoming a health-care professional is the short-term goal.

STARTING A SCRIBE PROGRAM

When considering the implementation of a scribe program, the two questions a physician group or hospital must ask itself are:

- How much of the startup process and ongoing management of the program do we want to take on ourselves?
- How will we measure success of the scribe program implementation, both financially and functionally?

In most cases, the fastest way to successfully implement scribe coverage is to hire a professional scribe company to design, roll out, and manage the program. Alternatively, the emergency medicine (EM) group can start its own scribe program, but that will take significantly more time and resources to accomplish. In the end, the answer to the question of "buy or build" hinges on the amount of time and money a group wants to invest in starting and managing a program. As this is written, the average cost of an outsourced scribe program is in the $20 per hour range, while the cost of in-house programs is more difficult to verify as administrative costs, such as oversight, training, hiring, firing, and continuing education, are more difficult to quantify. The financial challenge posed by the administrative costs of in-house programs can make a financial return difficult to achieve.[12]

The most important elements of a group-developed scribe program include defining leadership and providing appropriate training, as well as building clear reporting relationships with the physician who will oversee the program. Not all EM groups have a physician with that interest and competence. Another important element is human relations (HR) infrastructure, since a scribe program is HR intensive and requires a staff dedicated to managing recruiting, hiring, training, evaluating, counseling, and, when necessary,

TABLE 25.2 ■ In-House Scribe Programs

Advantages	Disadvantages
Program easily customized to group's wishes	Lack of scribe company experience necessary to understanding what works and what doesn't work, providing adequate user education, and focusing on and adapting to changes in regulatory requirements
Greater sense of family and scribe accountability to EM group	Program may cost more than scribe company if developed for just a few EDs
Greater flexibility in HR policies and benefits	Serious potential to negatively impact high-paid provider retirement plans
Less turnover due to generally higher scribe wages	Significant ongoing management time demands

terminating staff. Finally, a program for just one hospital requires essentially the same leadership expertise and HR infrastructure as a program for 100 hospitals, but the single-hospital program must shoulder the entire administrative cost of development, whereas the multihospital provider can spread that cost over many programs. **Table 25.2** lists some of the advantages and disadvantages of in-house programs.

Scribe program vendors are best evaluated by their track record. Industry benchmarks include filled shift rate (%), amount of training per scribe, and availability of quality reporting on scribe program quality and value to the customer. Take the time to call references and make an independent judgment about their consistency. Ask for references from people who discontinued their services, as these interviews will be the most revealing of the company's weaknesses. **Table 25.3** lists some advantages and disadvantages of outsourced programs.

In addition to the HR workload associated with scribe programs, groups choosing to build an internally managed program will also need to consider additional administrative burdens. These include legal and compliance support, scribe leadership development, continuing scribe education and training, reporting to ensure a financial return, and year-round scribe recruitment.[12]

TABLE 25.3 ■ Outsourced Scribe Programs

Advantages	Disadvantages
Less trial and error and therefore less cost; less risk of failure	Less customizable to meet granular specifics or requests of the group or individual provider
Less costs associated with the day-to-day management and turnover of a young, transient, low-wage population	Greater scribe loyalty to the scribe company than the EM group in some cases
Scribes are employed by vendor and therefore not a threat to retirement plans	Minimum-coverage plans are typically required by the outsourced company and are contractually enforceable
Program can generally be operational faster than an in-house program	For expanding EM groups, the scribe company owns the intellectual property of the program

TABLE 25.4 ■ Implementation Milestones

ED assessment and program design	• ED layout and physical space assessment • Observation of physician workflow and patient throughput
Coordination with hospital and ED management team	• Provider and nursing education on scribe use • Scribe EMR build design • Scribe onboarding plan • Procurement of hardware and accessories for scribe use
Recruitment and hiring	• Typically conducted at local universities and colleges • Hiring conducted by vendor or group, depending on program
Training and implementation	• HIPAA and compliance training required • Both classroom and on-shift training are necessary
Ongoing management plans initiated	• Quality assurance and value reporting • Continuous hiring year-round

Design and Training

While this chapter is not intended to be a "how to" on starting a scribe program, it is important to understand the process and implementation strategy (**Table 25.4**). Two main factors distinguish scribe programs from other ancillary medical businesses:

- The makeup of its workforce
- The high level of ongoing turnover

The workforce is predominately made up of preprofessional students (whenever they are available) who view this line of work not as a job, but rather as a unique opportunity that gives them a competitive advantage when applying to medical school or other health-related programs. The ongoing turnover of this workforce is significant—in most locations approaching 70% per year—and results in one-quarter to one-half of the workforce receiving acceptance to a professional school each year. This turnover rate translates into a significant cost burden, which is outweighed by the talent and motivation of the premedical demographic. **Table 25.5** lists some administrative cost categories of a typical scribe program.

The rollout of a new scribe program typically involves five stages (**Table 25.6**). The first two, which involve hospital management and staff, are 1) the assessment and design

TABLE 25.5 ■ In-House Scribe Program Costs

Cost Category	Percentage of Total Cost
Sales, general and administrative (recruiting, scheduling, payroll management)	24%
Training and onboarding	7%
Scribe wages	60%
Scribe administrative cost	3%
Scribe payroll tax	6%

TABLE 25.6 ■ Scribe Training and Assessment	
Pre-hire screening	Screen for typing ability, grammar and literacy, experience with medical terminology and professionalism.
Initial training	Conducted virtually and/or in a classroom setting. Includes medical terminology and spelling, SOAP note construction, common diagnoses and differentials, and E/M documentation requirements.
EMR training	Practice note creation in the EMR practice environment. Use mock patient scenarios to practice charting. Practice procedure documentation.
Floor training	Trainees are paired with veteran trainer scribes for a series of shifts. All previous training is put to practice in the ED.
Continuing scribe education (CSE)	Ongoing training on a monthly, quarterly, or annual basis. Includes review of previous topics, advanced topics, new documentation protocols, and/or professionalism topics.

and 2) coordination of the program. The third stage involves the recruiting and hiring of scribes. The fourth stage is the training and evaluation of the prospective scribes, while the fifth and final stage involves the implementation and postimplementation evaluation and adjustments.

Medical terminology and basic anatomy training are accompanied by documentation training and EMR familiarization. The final step in training is bedside experience during patient encounters. This step is the most critical and requires an experienced trainer to deal with patient privacy concerns and appropriately coach the new scribe—though patients generally do not report negative feelings toward having scribes present in the room.[14] The training of the scribes is, without question, the most time-consuming and expensive aspect of creating a new program and may reach expenses totaling over $6000 per fully trained scribe.[15]

Program Implementation

Introducing new personnel into the ED environment is never an easy task. The greatest challenge is working out the relationship between the scribe and the provider, providing the maximum benefit with the least disruption to normal workflow patterns. Many providers are uncomfortable with the idea of introducing a layperson into the provider–patient encounter. Colleagues who have learned to work comfortably with the scribes are often able to coach those who are struggling. The scribe may also have to be proactive and describe what services he or she can do for the providers to make their lives easier.

In the typical ED, the diverse staff members have developed a level of comfort with each other, which may be threatened by the presence of a "green" college student. Generally, within a week or two, the staff figures out where the scribes fit into this puzzle, and the scribes come to be seen as an asset to the patient-care process. In fact, staff usually recognize that scribes free the providers to be more available by substantially decreasing the administrative burden.

Within the scope of their position, scribes who are trained with an emphasis on teamwork can assist not only the provider but also others who work in the ED, including volunteers, technicians, charge nurses, the nurse director, and so on. Understanding this benefit can go a long way in gaining support for an ED scribe program. For example, nurses have someone:

- Who knows exactly where the provider is at all times
- Whom they can ask about a patient's disposition plan if the provider is busy
- To relay minor messages to the provider

A significant challenge of some EMRs is the capacity to accommodate the work performed by the scribe. In fact, some EDs have discontinued their scribe programs because of the impediments posed by the EMR or its deployment within the system. Specific system impediments include:

- Inaccurate attribution of the history, physical examination, and medical decision-making process
- Wrong attribution of the procedure performed by the physician
- Nonacceptance of scribe documentation when another team member is simultaneously entering information into the patient record
- Delays in medication administration
- Delays in results entered by the scribe affecting timing of necessary information appearing in the record

Once assimilated into the department—with every team member knowing what and what not to expect from a scribe—the scribes are soon seen as a solution to an inefficient and overworked ED staff. It takes time to get to this stage, but it does occur. Educating the staff about the scribe's role in advance will help avoid confusion and resistance.

The ED must have room for scribes to work. Scribes are hard-pressed to do their job and deliver their full benefit without a place to work and accessible computer terminals. Computer hardware supplied for the program is typically purchased, owned, and operated by the hospital, since hospital-licensed EMR software is installed on these devices and will be updated and maintained by the hospital information technology department.

While identifying the usual challenges to implementation is important, it is equally important to recognize when a scribe program may not be suited for an ED. Postponement of a scribe program is appropriate if a hospital is planning to purchase a new EMR system, complete an infrastructure remodeling project, or purchase additional computer terminals and tablets. Another challenge is the recruitment of qualified scribes in rural or remote geographical locations. Professional scribe companies and consultants can offer valuable guidance to EDs when encountering these kinds of logistical questions.

In the end, experience shows that premature implementation may cause significant dissatisfaction among the providers and other staff. Thus, it is imperative to ensure there is adequate preparation, education, and discussion to avoid resistance that could result in the permanent loss of program support from hospital administrators and nursing staff.

SCRIBE PROGRAM TIPS AND BEST PRACTICES

Regardless of whether the scribe program is managed in-house or is outsourced, the tips described next can help overcome common pitfalls and help set the program up for success.

Scribe Adoption

The most important factors in the success of a scribe program are provider motivation and willingness to adopt scribes. Groups should keep in mind that scribes are not for everyone. Placing scribes with a physician who isn't motivated to use them can be damaging to the overall adoption and cost the group unnecessary expense. Groups can overcome this problem by allowing individual providers to opt in or out of scribe coverage. While this option presents more challenges when staffing and scheduling scribe coverage, the benefits of provider buy-in outweigh the challenges. In many cases, these initial skeptics often opt in once they understand the financial rewards and improvements in peer productivity associated with scribe programs. While this isn't feasible in all cases, having champions of the program, especially at the onset, is instrumental for success.

Goals and Incentives

Failure to achieve program goals may occur when there is a misalignment between the goals of the program and the incentives or motivations for the providers. As an example, many groups implement scribes as a tool to increase provider productivity (the goal). An effective way to align the goal would be to tie a portion or all of a provider's compensation base to productivity. Another strategy is to set a productivity benchmark that providers have to maintain in order to "keep" their scribe. Alternatively, if there is no financial incentive for providers to see more patients, the use of scribes might enhance the quality of a busy shift without enhancing provider productivity. This misalignment would lead to the program falling short of its productivity goal. Regardless of what the goals are, it is important for groups to assess the motivating factors of the providers to ensure they align with the desired outcomes of the scribe program.

Shift Times

Each ED has unique nuances and different physical layouts, which presents an array of options for scheduling physician and advanced practice provider (APP) shifts. There are a few guiding principles that can help groups identify when and where to schedule scribes (**Table 25.7** and **Figure 25.1**).

Due to their ability to offload clinical documentation from various members of the care team, scribes are paired with both physicians and APPs.[11] While the effects of scribes with APPs as compared to physicians have not been widely studied, APPs report enhanced job satisfaction when using a scribe as well as improved bed turnover in the ED's rapid-assessment zone.[16] In academic settings, attending physicians are often paired with residents, who shoulder the majority of documentation. In that setting, scribes may be more

TABLE 25.7 ■ Guiding Principles for Scheduling Scribe Shifts

Scheduling Practice	Rationale
Schedule one scribe with one provider	Scheduling scribes with multiple providers can be inefficient, as providers may have to wait for a scribe, delaying documentation and care. This can also decrease the overall impact of a scribe program.
Closely align shift times	Scribes work best when starting and ending at same time as the provider, allowing the scribe and provider to ensure that all documentation is complete.
Schedule scribes when volumes ramp up and during peak hours	Scheduling scribes during the busiest hours of the ED can help providers manage a large influx of patients. As new patients enter the ED, scribes can help expedite workups and keep providers organized during these ramp-up times.
Leverage scribes when patient demand exceeds the current staff's capacity	Scribes can increase provider productivity, particularly when scheduled at times that patient demand is higher than the provider's capacity. Scribes may eliminate the need to expand provider coverage, i.e., adding a provider shift.

FIGURE 25.1 ■ Capacity-to-Demand Chart for Scribe Coverage

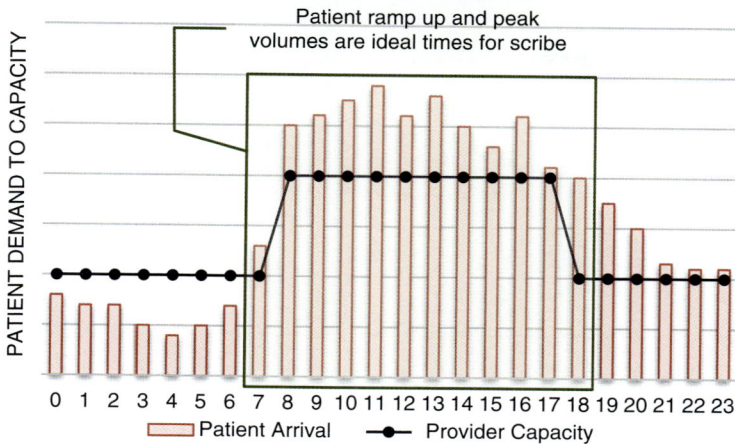

valuable when paired with APPs who are seeing a greater number of patients without the assistance of a resident or student.[12]

Scribe Program Evaluation

Establish a system to track and evaluate the operational performance of the scribe program. An annual or semiannual review is recommended for both outsourced and internally managed programs. It can be challenging to compare or benchmark the performance of a scribe program against the industry standard and Health Insurance Portability and Accountability Act (HIPAA) requirements. As an example, it is essential to assess the program reliability, measured by the filled shift rate (total number of shifts filled divided by the total number of scheduled shifts). Providers come to rely on scribes, and the impact of missed shifts can have a significant operational and financial impact to both the EM group and the hospital. In addition to reliability, other areas to evaluate include:

- Recruitment success
- Onboarding time
- Scribe retention
- Market wages
- HIPAA compliance rating
- Documentation accuracy
- 360-degree evaluations
- Communication skills

Value and Impact of Scribes

The scribe industry has continued to evolve since its early inception and is now an efficient solution to physician productivity and stakeholder satisfaction. Organizations start scribe programs to accomplish a variety of goals, including:

- Improving provider productivity
- Addressing increasing volumes or understaffing
- Enhancing the patient experience
- Decreasing walk-out rates
- Shortening length-of-stay times
- Enhancing quality of life to retain providers and prevent burnout

> **BOX 25.1 ■ VARIABLES NOT IMPACTED BY SCRIBES**
>
> **Facility**
> - Bed availability
> - Boarding times
> - Hospital capacity
> - Nurse staffing
> - Lab/radiology turnaround times
> - ED culture
>
> **Environmental**
> - Patient volume
> - Acuity
> - Payer mix
> - CMS reimbursement rates

Box 25.1 outlines some facility and external factors that will NOT be directly influenced by scribes. For example, scribes do not open up more beds on the floor to decrease boarding times. While this may seem obvious, EM group leaders should carefully examine their current ED inefficiencies or bottlenecks before implementing a scribe program in order to have realistic expectations of the possible improvements. Scribes are not a fix-all but rather serve as a catalyst for driving significant improvements when they are implemented correctly, and other constraints are removed.

On a fundamental level, scribes "create" time for providers. By offloading charting and nonclinical administrative tasks to a scribe, providers can redistribute their time, permitting them to focus on patient-care management.[16] The direct impact of scribes can be seen in provider productivity, documentation completeness, and patient throughput (**Table 25.8**).

TABLE 25.8 ■ Impact of Scribes on Metrics

Impact Area	Common Metrics
Productivity	PPH
	RVUs per hour
Documentation	Undocumented Services % (UDS %)
	RVU per patient
Throughput	Door-to-doc time
	Doc-to-disposition time
	Length of stay (discharged)
	Left without being seen (LWBS %)

Provider Productivity

Productivity is the product of two distinct items, provider capacity and patient volume. Scribes have a direct impact on productivity by expanding provider capacity. Scribes allow providers to see patients more quickly and improve the timeliness of patient care at the facility.[17] From a measurement standpoint, this impact can be measured by patients per hour (PPH) or relative value units (RVUs) per hour. The productivity gains with scribes can vary greatly among specific facilities; however, studies and third-party scribe companies commonly report PPH improvements between 10% and 20% or 0.2 to 0.5*.[16,18,19] Over a 10-hour shift for a provider seeing 2.0 PPH, adding a scribe could result in the ability to treat an additional two to four patients (* 0.5 if currently seeing 2.5 PPH and scribes lead to a 20% increased capacity).

The positive productivity impact of scribes is most notable during periods when patient demand exceeds provider capacity, which are commonly experienced in busier, higher-volume EDs.[20] As patient volumes go up without increasing provider hours, patient demand will exceed provider capacity. To realize the optimal productivity gains from scribes, groups should adjust staffing to account for increases in provider capacity either by 1) decreasing provider hours (**Table 25.9**[21]) or 2) not adding provider hours as volumes increase (**Table 25.10**).

Simply adding scribe hours without adjusting provider staffing will not necessarily translate to overall productivity lifts, unless there are multiple patients who leave prior to medical screening exam (LPMSE) that can now be seen. Alternatively, if no more patients are seen by the providers, increased productivity is largely predicated on the adjustments (decrease) to staffing to compensate for the capacity increases afforded by scribes.

Documentation

A well-trained scribe can document provider–patient encounters while the providers focus on treatment. During the history and physical exams, scribes accurately and completely capture the evaluation details in real-time, documenting elements required for billing. In some practices that do not have the benefit of real-time documentation, groups lose RVUs because of insufficient or incomplete documentation.

TABLE 25.9 ■ Staffing Cost Comparison With No Volume Change[a]

	Without Scribes	With Scribes
Patient volume	60,000	60,000
Physician hours	60	55 (−5)
APP hours	44	36 (−8)
Scribe hours	0	55
Patient to adjusted provider hour[b]	2.00	2.25
Net annual staffing savings		$182,500

[a] Assumes hourly physician rate of $200, APP rate of $75, and scribe rate of $20.[19]
[b] Adjusted provider hour: physician = 1, APP = 0.5.

TABLE 25.10 ■ Staffing Cost Comparison With Volume Change

	Without Scribes	With Scribes
Patient volume	60,000	67,000 **(+7,000)**
Physician hours	60	60 **(0)**
APP hours	44	44 **(0)**
Scribe hours	0	60
Patient to adjusted provider hour[b]	2.00	2.25
Net annual staffing savings		$87,000-$262,000

This table provides an example of how the productivity impact of scribes can be leveraged for staffing savings. This outlines two specific tactics: decreasing providing coverage with constant volume and preventing the addition of provider hours as volume increases.
[a] Assumes physician rate of $200, APP rate of $75, and scribe rate of $20.[19]
[b] Adjusted provider hour: physician = 1, APP = 0.5.

It is important to note that scribes do not influence the level of service but rather close gaps between the services rendered and documentation. For higher acuity/more complex patients, scribes capture thorough evaluation and management details, critical care times, and procedures that might otherwise have been inadequately documented, downcoded, or unbilled. These impacts can be measured with metrics such as RVU/encounter or undocumented service percentage.[22] Facilities that have had significant documentation gaps before instituting a scribe program can decrease the number of downcoded charts to well under 1%, which in turn increases the RVU/encounter metric and demonstrates the reimbursement advantages of scribe services.

The extent of scribes' impact is primarily predicated on a group's pre-scribe baseline (PPH, RVUs/patient, LPMSE, documentation completions, coverage hours, etc.), and these same metrics compared to the degree of utilization of scribes when the program is implemented.

Throughput

In addition to documentation, scribes can help expedite the timeliness of care and decrease overall wait times in an ED.[16] Experienced scribes can serve as flow facilitators, helping providers navigate throughout their shift. By monitoring patient intake, the tracking board, and imaging and lab results, scribes can prompt providers when information is available to move the patients to the next stage of their care, including additional communication, testing, assessment, and/or disposition (**Figure 25.2**).

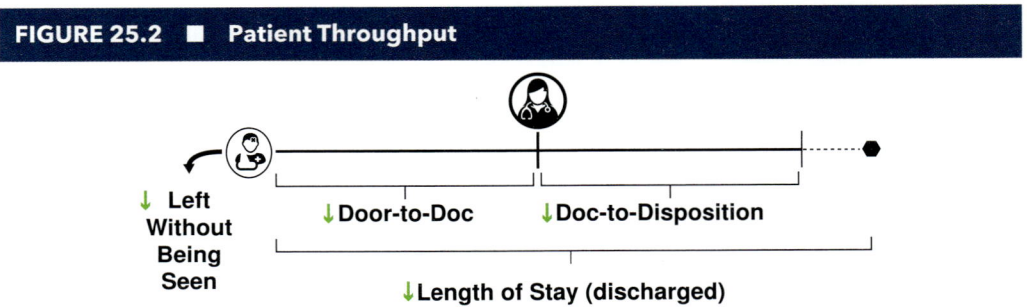

FIGURE 25.2 ■ Patient Throughput

Leveraging experienced scribes to serve as workflow facilitators is an underutilized aspect of their role. The prospect of a scribe—an entry-level, aspiring health-care provider—prompting a seasoned physician can be intimidating. Scribes may be hesitant to be assertive because they don't want to irritate the provider or be perceived as "pushy." To overcome this hesitation, providers and scribes should address the intimidating dynamic of this relationship and clearly define the type of information that is most useful to communicate throughout the shift. This discussion can empower and encourage scribes to be more assertive in workflow management and further maximize their positive impact.

The throughput metrics impacted by scribes are those largely controlled by provider timeliness and efficiency, such as door to doc, length of stay (discharged patients), and doc to disposition.[18] As mentioned earlier, there is an array of other factors that may serve as bottlenecks, but scribes are an effective catalyst for improving throughput. In fact, one study found that each scribe saved an average of 3.89 hours of patient wait time each shift.[18] As a result, there can be significant decrease in the number of patients leaving without being seen and significant improvement in the overall patient experience, both of which can have a significant financial impact for groups and hospitals.[23]

Other Benefits

Burnout alleviation: Another benefit of scribes is increased provider satisfaction, which could help curb the growing trend of burnout. According to a 2018 survey, more than half of all physicians report being burned out, with EM physicians near the top of the list.[24] The top contributing factor for burnout was having too many bureaucratic tasks, including charting and other administrative tasks.[9,25] Scribes have been shown to improve provider job satisfaction and can be part of an overall strategy to address or prevent burnout, turnover, and even prolong a provider's career.[17,26] Health-care leaders, who have recognized the serious problem of burnout within their organization, reported scribes as the top tool/initiative deployed to alleviate burnout and off-load clerical tasks.[25]

Scribes are not the only solution to solving provider burnout, but they do play a role in alleviating some of the top causes and improving overall job satisfaction for providers.

Patient experience scores: Most physicians and APPs verbalize the physical exam, history, and decision-making process to the scribe while in the patients' rooms. As a result of knowing that the providers are describing and accurately documenting their findings, most facilities have found that their patients are more satisfied with their care, resulting in increased patient experience scores.

Facility revenue capture: Because the evaluation and management (E/M) codes are so closely correlated with the care and documentation of the APPs, any increase in appropriate coding for professional fee revenue will also generate better revenue for the facility component as well.

Return on Investment

As EM groups struggle with the question of whether or not to add scribes, the discussion inevitably turns to the cost, or return on investment (ROI). As a baseline, groups should be intimately familiar with their current metrics of productivity, documentation, and throughput (**Table 25.8**). The cost of scribes can be paid by the hospital, group, provider, or a combination. When calculating the ROI, it is important to understand who is paying and how they financially benefit. The ROI will vary, as each department's goals differ; therefore, understanding some of the financial drivers of ROI can help groups evaluate this decision.

One of the largest costs for a group is the provider overhead. Therefore, the most effective and tangible way to realize optimal returns is through staffing efficiencies. By realizing an

TABLE 25.11 ■ Scribe Cost Compared to Physicians/APPs

Provider Hour	Scribe Hours
↓ 1 Physician hour (at $200 hour)	10
↓ 1 APP hour (at $75 per hour)	3.75

Assuming the total hourly cost of a scribe is $20.00, by decreasing a physician hour by 1 hour per day, it would pay for 10 hours of scribe coverage.

increased provider capacity when utilizing scribes, groups can replace costly provider hours with far less costly scribe hours (**Table 25.11**).

As it relates to integrating scribes into the staffing model, a good benchmark to use is a productivity increase of 0.25 PPH for each hour a provider is paired with a scribe. For example, if a group uses a productivity factor of 2.0 patients per physician hour to allocate staffing needs based on the patient demand, the capacity boost from scribes can be accounted for by adding a factor of 0.25 (equating to 2.25 patients per physician hour) for hours the physician is paired with a scribe. As mentioned earlier, immediate documentation performed by the scribe creates more accurate and complete medical records and can lead to increased RVUs and revenue. Using the 2019 CMS conversion factor of $36.04 and the cost of a scribe at $20 per hour, a practitioner or group would have to earn/save 0.55 RVUs per hour to be cost-neutral. The RVU per hour is a consolidation of productivity and documentation improvements and can be used to project scribes' impact on revenue (**Table 25.11–25.13**).

Several other potential cost and operational benefits occur when implementing scribes. Among these are savings in the cost of provider recruitment and better retention. Performance can also be impacted, particularly if there is focus on addressing bottlenecks and optimizing staffing. It is important to note once again that each facility is different, requiring a calculation adjustment based on the specific operational processes and staffing requirements of the specific institution.

HUMAN RESOURCE REQUIREMENTS AND OTHER COMPLIANCE ISSUES

Human Resources

All standard human resources regulations, including state workers' compensation laws, apply to scribes. When beginning a scribe program, it is necessary to have a thorough understanding of these laws and ensure provisions are in place to address the standards.

TABLE 25.12 ■ Pre- and Post-Scribe Analysis of PPH and RVUs per Patient

	Pre-Scribe	Post-Scribe	Change (+ %)
Daily volume	84	84	–
PPH	2.00	2.25	+0.25 (12.5%)
RVUs per encounter (documentation)	3.50	3.75	+0.25 (7%)
RVU per hour	7.00	8.44	+1.44 (20.5%)

TABLE 25.13 ■ ROI Calculation Using Scribes		
	Calculation	**Benefit <Cost>**
Step 1: Cost of scribes	Hourly rate = $20 × Scribe hours 37 per day	<$740>
Step 2: Calculate cost savings from adding 37 scribe hours and removing 5 physician hours	Provider hours without scribes: 84 (patients per day)/2.00 (pre-scribe PPH) = 42 Provider hours with scribes: 84 (patients per day)/2.25 (post-scribe PPH) = 37 Provider hours saved: 42 − 37 = 5 hours × $200	$1,000
Step 3: Calculate increased revenue from productivity and documentation lifts	Additional RVUs per day with scribes: 37 (scribe hours per day) × 1.44 (additional RVU per scribe hour) = 53.28 RVUs b. 53.28 * $36.04† (reimbursement per RVU) †CMS CY 2019 CMS conversion factor	$1,920
Net impact (per day)		**$2,180**

Table 25.12 is a case study example for a pre- and post-scribe impact analysis, the results of which are used as an example in **Table 25.13**, which demonstrates a simple template groups can be used to calculate the ROI from the scribe investment.

Whether employed by the group or another entity, leased or contracted, the laws govern how the providers should relate to individuals working under their direction in the ED. Because of the frequent gender and age differences and the close working relationship, issues related to a hostile workplace occur. This potential should be anticipated with appropriate education provided to both providers and scribes.

Health Insurance Portability and Accountability Act

By the nature of their duties, scribes have access to sensitive patient information, including that defined by the government as protected health information (PHI). Scribes have a duty to keep all patient information confidential by adhering to hospital compliance and confidentiality policies and the specific requirements of HIPAA. This duty arises from the relationship between the scribe vendor and the hospital and/or physician group. Under HIPAA regulations, the scribe vendor and its scribes are considered business associates to the covered entity, whether it be a hospital or a physician group. Recent amendments to HIPAA regulations now require all business associates to 1) maintain patient confidentiality by properly handling PHI and 2) hold each associate accountable for the possibility of civil and/or criminal penalties in the event of a breach.[27] The duties and responsibilities regarding the use of PHI are customarily addressed within a business associate agreement between the scribe vendor and the covered entity.

All scribes should undergo rigorous HIPAA training prior to being placed in a healthcare facility. Customarily, this training consists of either instructor-led classroom training or an internet-based training module in addition to specific instruction. Each scribe must understand the scope and purpose of HIPAA; the proper and improper use of PHI; and importantly, the civil and criminal penalties that may be imposed in the event of a breach. In addition to initial HIPAA training, scribes are usually required to complete annual training and to acknowledge each hospital's confidentiality policies.

The Joint Commission

As mentioned previously, scribes are often college students majoring in a pre-health profession or are post-baccalaureate students preparing to enter one of the health professions. As such, scribes are not licensed, registered, or credentialed health-care providers. In fact, scribes are prohibited from direct involvement in patient care by The Joint Commission (TJC) and other regulatory agencies; in other words, they may not independently interact with patients or engage in any form of "hands-on" care other than attending to documentation and workflow management.[24] Because a scribe's job description is limited to clerical services, scribes are not required to undergo a credentialing or other verification process as outlined by TJC standards for the medical staff. Despite this fact, in rare circumstances, some hospitals have required scribe programs to be reviewed and approved by their Medical Executive Committee or Medical Staff Office. In other cases, the hospital has required that the scribes fulfill all hospital contractor requirements, such as immunizations, drug testing, and background screenings, and they are expected to abide by hospital policy at all times.

Medicolegal Considerations

A number of medical and legal considerations apply to use of a scribe program.

Accuracy of Documentation

While scribes are trained to document thoroughly and accurately, each provider is charged with the duty to verify each patient record for its accuracy and completion. While the scribe is performing this clerical service on behalf of the provider, the provider is the only licensed health-care professional in the scribe–provider relationship. Thus, the provider is responsible for the information documented by the scribe in each patient record and must authenticate it through his or her attestation and signature prior to leaving the patient care area.[24]

Physician/APP Orders

As nonlicensed workers, scribes are prohibited from engaging in computer physician order entry (CPOE).[24] Some EMR platforms allow scribes to "pend" orders until those orders are authenticated and officially entered by the provider; this process must also be approved by the hospital or health system.

When using an EMR, each scribe and each physician has his or her own login for accessing a patient record. Effectively designed EMRs limit the scribe role to performing only certain approved tasks and accessing certain approved areas within the EMR. For optimal workflow and accuracy, the design of the scribe and provider notes should be nearly identical with the exception of CPOE features. These notes should be readily shared in order to engage in simultaneous review for efficient editing.[12] All providers must keep in mind that the patient record is a legal document for which they must take full responsibility at all times; therefore, thorough review prior to signature is essential.

HORIZONS

The demand for enhanced electronic documentation support is imminent, and onsite scribes as we know them will continue to evolve in scope and medium. Below are brief overviews of some of the emerging trends and solutions with comparisons to current on-site scribe services.

Virtual Scribes

With the technology advancements and growing adoption of telehealth services, the marketplace for "virtual scribes" has become increasingly attractive. Virtual scribes are located remotely, away from the ED, with audio/visual equipment allowing them to listen and/or watch patient encounters in real time or, in some cases, observe a recording of a patient visit. Using a remote EMR access or screen sharing platform, the virtual scribe is able to document the encounter, locate labs or previous records, and document follow-up care from the facility's EMR platform.[28] Some EMR systems also allow the virtual scribe to schedule follow-up appointments upon discharge.

Many organizations, such as Augmedix, Nuance, Scribekick, and ScribeAmerica, are offering an array of virtual scribe services to provide documentation assistance without the physical presence of another person in the room. These services comprise live audio and/or video feeds that allow scribes to simultaneously document the patient encounter into the EMR system. Virtual scribes can be especially advantageous in rural or hard-to-recruit markets and for smaller outpatient practices that don't need a full-time scribe beyond a few peak hours of the week.[28]

As artificial intelligence (AI) continues to evolve in health care, technology will allow clinician voice recognition with increasing accuracy. Further, future AI-driven documentation systems will contextualize the clinicians' words based on additional information in the patient's presentation. Virtual scribe programs will likely begin to incorporate AI tools to increase the efficiency of charting completion and accuracy, boosting the overall impact to the provider at a potentially lower price point.

Scribes vs Voice Recognition

With increasing financial pressures faced by hospital systems and physician groups, many are considering "cheaper" alternatives to onsite or virtual scribes. One of the prevalent alternatives is voice recognition systems, including Nuance Dragon or M*Modal. These platforms provide documentation assistance such as speech-to-text technology, allowing providers to dictate the record in lieu of typing. Other capabilities include voice-prompted EMR workflow, such as order sets and macros (short for "macroinstructions," programmed patterns) and navigation to sections within the patient record. These technologies continue to advance and expand the tools offered to providers to more efficiently manage the EMR systems.

In general, the overall cost of voice recognition is cheaper than scribes and it can more readily scale/ramp-up coverage. The ramp-up for scribe services can take anywhere from 1 to 3 months to recruit, onboard, and train an entire scribe team. Additionally, it could be argued that the service reliability is more consistent with voice recognition, as the quality of individual scribes is less consistent and is based on the training, tenure, and overall proficiency in the role.

It is challenging to make a direct comparison of scribes to voice recognition, as they are two different services. Documentation assistance is just one subset of the scribe's function and utility. One of the most significant and important advantages of scribes relates to workflow. Scribes allow providers to operate in a parallel workflow, meaning that during the encounter, the scribe can discern and document the relevant information real time in the record. On the other hand, voice recognition platforms necessitate the provider to allocate time after the patient encounter to dictate the record or stop to modify and edit text captured through real-time voice recognition. While the dictation may offer a more efficient mode of inputting information in the record, the overall impact it has on expanding provider capacity is marginal to that of a scribe.

As previously mentioned, another significant workflow advantage of scribes is their ability to gather and prepare information for the clinician's review. This can save precious minutes the provider would have spent reviewing the EMR, looking for results that may or may not be available.

Nurse Use of Scribes

Pairing scribes with nurses in the ED has been trialed in the past and is gaining momentum in recent years with the emergence of professional nurse scribe programs.[29] Scribes paired with ED nursing staff can support triage workflow in addition to trauma, fast track, and other areas of the department.

Provider in triage (PIT) models have been shown to positively impact a number of ED throughput measures, including wait times and length of stay; however, as productivity increases, nurse availability can become a bottleneck to patient flow given the heavy load of clinical and administrative tasks associated with each patient.[30,31] Supporting the triage nursing staff with scribes to offload documentation, patient paperwork, and other administrative or clerical work may allow nurses to better support the PIT model.

The same logic applies to ED nurse workflow outside of triage. The scribe working alongside an ED nurse utilizes a workflow similar to the workflow when paired with an ED physician, with some nuance. The scribe can complete nursing documentation and some of the nurse's other duties, for example, retrieving or organizing paperwork, restocking basic supplies, tidying patient rooms, and tracking test results. Nursing documentation support is particularly valuable to the ED nurse during rapid response events, when it becomes difficult to document the formidable number of treatment events in real-time. Scribe support for ED nurses may also allow them to keep pace with highly productive providers who treat a high number of PPH, reducing nursing bottlenecks to patient throughput and mitigating the need to add more nursing staff.

Since nursing documentation is not billable, the financial justification for a nurse–scribe model should correlate with other financial drivers in the ED. This could include traditional methods of financial return by enhancing provider productivity when nursing services are a bottleneck to full productivity potential. Additionally, scribes paired with nurses can better optimize nurse staffing models and lower overall costs of nurse labor, nurse attrition, and nurse understaffing. Recently, some nurse scribes have evolved beyond their documentation roles into nurse care team assistant (CTA) roles, attending to lower-level clinical duties equivalent to that of a patient care technician or nurse assistant. With the additional clinical support, nursing CTA programs improve nurse recruitment, ameliorate nurse attrition challenges, improve nurse satisfaction, and allow nurses to treat more patients, thus improving staffing ratios.[29]

Scribes and Hospital Medicine

While not as widely adapted as the ED scribe model, scribes are employed by some hospitals and hospital medicine physician groups to work alongside hospitalist providers, and sometimes nurses, in the inpatient setting. Scribes paired with hospitalists and other inpatient providers assist with documentation during patient rounding. When compared to the ED, scribes on the inpatient units spend more time independently, organizing paperwork and preparing charts prior to making rounds. Emphasis must be placed on a training program that is specific to inpatient documentation and workflow.[34] Similar to results of scribes in the ED setting, inpatient scribes also decrease the time physicians spend on documentation and dictation, leading to higher physician satisfaction and productivity.[35]

Hospital medicine scribes may improve the case mix index (CMI) through enhanced documentation of patient acuity, leading to higher-weighted diagnosis-related groups (DRG). Improving documentation through a strong clinical documentation improvement program or other documentation training has been linked to higher DRG and CMI.[36,37] It is likely that a similar improvement of physician documentation would occur through use of a scribe program.

In practice, a successful inpatient scribe program cannot be created by simply relocating scribes from the ED to another area of the hospital. A robust training program must be built to reflect the inpatient-specific workflows and clinical documentation components that differ from those in the ED setting. In many settings, hospitalists round on patients in an irregular schedule pattern, which could create an unreliable scribe staffing and scheduling model. To establish an inpatient scribe program, a schedule must be created that gives the scribes full, reliable shifts of work. Then, when inpatient scribes spend time away from the provider organizing and preparing charts, gathering and inputting results into the patient record, and completing other ancillary tasks geared toward workflow organization, it is both additive to the provider's workflow and allows a schedule of full shifts necessary to staff the scribe program.

CONCLUSION

The introduction of the EMR largely catalyzed the initial growth of the scribe industry. In the current landscape, the continuing pressure for groups to do more with less and the additional regulatory responsibilities for providers and health-care organizations have created a niche for scribes in the ED. While the current utilization of scribes is unknown, the use of scribes as cost-effective labor at the point of service will likely continue to expand.[38] The increased prevalence of the role has caught the attention of the academic community, leading to a better understanding about the impact scribes have on hospitals, patients, and providers. Evidence suggests that scribes may be able to improve provider productivity, patient throughput times, organizational revenue, and provider satisfaction, among others.

Whether a scribe program is built or purchased, it is important to beware of the unknowns when establishing a new scribe program—*caveat emptor* (buyer beware). A few dollars spent on expert advice on the front end can save thousands of dollars and months of misery on the back end. Proper planning and preparation are necessary as every ED is different; the workforce pool in every geographic market is different, and the skills and expertise necessary to train and manage all of the involved people are different.

One fact, however, will forever be true: Every minute of provider time shifted from documentation and non-value-added functions to medical decision-making and time with patients will consistently yield value for the health-care system. If the predictions about the coming US physician shortage are even close to true, we will be able to look back to this time and say, "But it would have been worse without scribes."

With appreciation to Jason B. Ruben, J. Alexander Geesbreght, and Ralph F. Baine, who contributed to the previous version of this chapter.

REFERENCES

1. Wikipedia contibutors. Wikipedia, The Free Encyclopedia. http://en.wikipedia.org/wiki/Scribe. Revised August 13, 2020. Accessed August 19, 2020.
2. Lynch TS. An emergency department scribe system. *JACEP.* 1974;3:303-303.
3. Geesbreght J. (January 10, 2010). Medical Director, Texas Health Harris Methodist.
4. Hill RG Jr, Sears LM, Melanson SW. 4000 clicks: a productivity analysis of electronic medical records in a community hospital ED. *Am J Emerg*

Med. 2013;31(11):1591-1594. doi:10.1016/j.ajem.2013.06.028. PubMed PMID: 24060331. Accessed April 17, 2018.

5. Incentives for the Use of Health Information Technology and Establishing the Position of the National Health Information Technology Coordinator, 69 FR 24059 (April 27, 2004).

6. Centers for Medicare and Medicaid Services. Fact Sheet—CMS finalizes definition of meaningful use of certified electronic health records (EHR) technology. Available at: https://www.cms.gov/newsroom/fact-sheets/cms-finalizes-definition-meaningful-use-certified-electronic-health-records-ehr-technology. Accessed April 18, 2018.

7. United States, Congress, CMS. MIPS Overview. Available at: https://qpp.cms.gov/mips/overview. Accessed May 21, 2018.

8. Office of the National Coordinator for Health Information Technology. Hospitals Participating in the CMS EHR Incentive Programs, Health IT Quick-Stat #45. 2017. https://dashboard.healthit.gov/quickstats/pages/FIG-Hospitals-EHR-Incentive-Programs.php. Accessed May 21, 2018.

9. Peckham C. Medscape National Physician Burnout & Depression Report 2018. *Medscape*. 2018. Available at: www.medscape.com/slideshow/2018-lifestyle-burnout-depression-6009235#13. Accessed May 21, 2018.

10. Sinsky CA. Moving our attention from keyboards to patients: a way forward for improving professional fulfillment and health care value. *Jt Comm J Qual Saf*. 2018;44(5):235-237.

11. Shultz CG, Holmstrom HL. The use of medical scribes in health care settings: a systematic review and future directions. *J Am Board of Fam Med*. 2015;28(3):371-381.

12. Martel ML, Imdieke BH, Holm KM, et al. Developing a medical scribe program at an academic hospital: the Hennepin County medical center experience. *Jt Comm J Qual Saf*. 2018;44:238-249.

13. Medical Scribe Salary. (n.d.) https://www.payscale.com/research/US/Job=Medical_Scribe/Hourly_Rate. Accessed July 1, 2018.

14. Dunlop W, Hegarty L, Staples M, et al. Medical scribes have no impact on the patient experience of an emergency department. *Emerg Med Australas*. 2017;30(1):61-66.

15. Arya R, Salovich DM, Ohman-Strickland P, et al. Impact of scribes on performance indicators in the emergency department. *Acad Emerg Med*. 2010;17:490-494.

16. Allen B, Banapoor B, Weeks EC, et al. An assessment of emergency department throughput and provider satisfaction after the implementation of a scribe program. Advances in Emergency Medicine. 2014. Vol. 2014, Article ID 517319, 7 pages. https://www.researchgate.net/publication/270629130_An_Assessment_of_Emergency_Department_Throughput_and_Provider_Satisfaction_after_the_Implementation_of_a_Scribe_Program

17. Hess JH, Wallenstien J, Ackerman JD, et al. Scribe impacts on provider experience, operations, and teaching in an academic emergency medicine practice. *West J Emerg Med*. 2015;16(5):602-610. PMC. Accessed June 4, 2018.

18. Friedson AL. Medical scribes as an input in healthcare production: evidence from a randomized experiment. *MIT Press Journals, American Journal of Health Economics*. 2017. Available at: https://www.journals.uchicago.edu/doi/abs/10.1162/ajhe_a_00103. Accessed June 1, 2018.

19. Heaton HA, Nestler DM, Jones DD, et al. Impact of scribes on billed relative value units in an academic emergency department. 2017; 52(3): 370–376. Available at: https://pubmed.ncbi.nlm.nih.gov/27988262/. Accessed June 6, 2018.

20. PhysAssist Scribes, Inc: Turnkey Model. Available at: https://www.scribeamerica.com/. Accessed June 11, 2018.

21. Katz B. 2017–2018 compensation report for emergency physicians shows steady salaries. 2017. Available at: www.acepnow.com/article/2017-2018-compensation-report-emergency-physicians-shows-steady-salaries/. Accessed June 1, 2018.

22. Schaeffer J. Rise of the scribes. For The Record. 2015. 27(1):10. Available at: http://www.fortherecordmag.com/archives/0115p10.shtml. Accessed June 11, 2018.

23. Bleustein C, Rothschild DB, Valen A, et al. Wait times, patient satisfaction scores, and the perception of care. *AJMC*. 2014. Available at: https://pubmed.ncbi.nlm.nih.gov/25181568/. Accessed June 14, 2018.

24. The Joint Commission. Medical Scribe FAQs. 2020. Available at: https://www.jointcommission.org/en/standards/standard-faqs/#q=documentation%20assistance%20provided%20by%20scribes. Accessed July 25, 2020.

25. Swensen S, Strongwater S, Mohta NS. Leadership survey: immunization against burnout. *NEJM*. 2018. Available at: https://catalyst.nejm.org/doi/full/10.1056/CAT.18.0209. Accessed June 15, 2018.

26. Gidwani R, Nguyen C, Kofoed A, et al. Impact of scribes on physician satisfaction, patient satisfaction, and charting efficiency: a randomized controlled trial. *Ann Fam Med*. 2017;15(5):427-433. Available at: www.annfammed.org/content/15/5/427.full.pdf.html. Accessed June 15, 2018.

27. Health Insurance Portability and Accountability Act of 1996 (42 U.S.C. 1320d-2).

28. Caliri A. The case for virtual scribes. Becker Hospital Review. 2019. Available at: https://www.beckershospitalreview.com/hospital-physician-relationships/the-case-for-virtual-scribes.html. Accessed June 27, 2019.

29. ScribeAmerica, LLC. Nurse care team assistants. Available at: https://www.scribeamerica.com/solutions-nurse-cta/. Accessed July 12, 2019.

30. Russ, S, Jones, I, Aronsky, D, et al. Placing physician orders at triage: the effect on length of stay. *Ann Emerg Med*. 2010;56(1):27-33.

31. Imperato J, Morris D, Binder D, et al. Physician in triage improves emergency department patient throughput. *Intern Emerg Med*. 2012;7(5):457-462.

32. Hooper C, Craig J, Janvrin D, et al. Compassion satisfaction, burnout, and compassion fatigue among emergency nurses compared with nurses in other selected inpatient specialties. *J Emerg Nurs*. 2010;36(5):420-427.

33. Hollingsworth J, Chisholm C, Giles B, et al. How do physicians and nurses spend their time in the emergency department? *Ann Emerg Med*. 1998;31(1):87-91.

34. Malouli W. Innovative use of scribes in the inpatient setting. *The Hospitalist*. 2010;2010(10).

35. Tegen A, O'Connell J. Rounding with scribes: employing scribes in a pediatric inpatient setting. *J AHIMA*. 2012;83(1):34-38.

36. Vandermark W, Blankenship J, Pfeifer J, et al. Improved case mix index due to embedding clinical documentation improvement specialists on an inpatient cardiology service at a tertiary medical center. *J Am Coll Cardiol*. 2015;65(10).

37. Rosenbaum B, Lorenz R, Luther R, et al. Improving and measuring inpatient documentation of medical care within the MS-DRG system: education, monitoring, and normalized case mix index. *Perspect Health Inf Manag*. 2014;11(Summer):1c. Available at: https://www.ncbi.nlm.nih.gov/pmc/articles/PMC4142511/. Accessed June 20, 2019.

38. The growth of medical scribes and what it means for healthcare. *MedCity News, Kaiser Health News*. December 7, 2015. Available at: https://medcitynews.com/2015/12/growth-of-medical-scribes/. Accessed August 28, 2020.

CHAPTER 26
VIOLENCE IN THE EMERGENCY DEPARTMENT

Christopher M. Ziebell, Jonathan D. Apfelbaum, Bill Schueler

The emergency department (ED) has always been a dangerous place, but a recent confluence of factors has created a crisis of violence that puts patients, physicians, and staff at risk. The majority of providers entering the medical field are unaware that they are entering a career with one of the highest risks of workplace assaults and threats. The number of nonfatal violent incidents per 1,000 providers is 16.2 for physicians, 21.9 for nurses, and 69.0 for mental health professionals compared to 12.6 for all occupations.[1,2]

Compared to outpatient clinics and offices, health-care facilities have substantially higher rates of nonfatal injuries from workplace violence, and the ED has one of the highest rates within health-care facilities.[3] Violence against staff in the ED is pervasive worldwide. In 2016, the estimated rate of injuries from all private-sector workers due to violence that required days away from work was 3.8 per 10,000 employees. For private-sector hospital workers, the rate of injuries was 15.9/10,000, and for nursing and residential care providers, the rate was 47.9/10,000.[4]

In 2011, the Emergency Nurses Association surveyed more than 7,000 ED nurses. Twenty-five percent of the respondents reported experiencing physical violence more than 20 times in the previous three years, and 20% reported being the recipient of verbal abuse more than 200 times during the same period. The stark reality is that these occurrences are vastly underreported.[5] According to a 2018 American College of Emergency Physicians (ACEP) poll of 32,714 emergency physicians, 44% to 48% report having been physically assaulted while at work.[6] Emergency physicians may actually experience less violence that other ED workers; multiple studies have reviewed the incidence of violence against nurses.[1,5,7-11] In the highest among these studies, 72% of ED nurses reported having been assaulted, and almost all ED nurses were verbally abused.

EPIDEMIOLOGY OF VIOLENCE IN THE ED

The leading factors associated with violent or abusive behavior in the ED include alcohol and drug use, followed by psychiatric disease, organic cognitive disease (e.g., dementia), and patient/family inability to deal with a crisis situation. Contributing environmental factors include a lack of security or police, security or police not responding in a timely fashion, and inadequately trained security staff. The ease of bringing weapons into the ED, lack of adequate staff, and around-the-clock public access also contribute.[1,3,12-14] The location of security either in triage or in patient care areas does not appear to correlate directly to a reduction in violence.[1]

Bound by the Emergency Medical Treatment and Active Labor Act (EMTALA), and as part of society's safety net, those working in EDs cannot choose their patients or

> **BOX 26.1 ■ FACTORS PRECIPITATING VIOLENCE IN THE ED**
>
> - Facility location
> - Local high-crime area
> - Crowding/high patient volume
> - Holding/boarding patients
> - Prolonged wait times
> - No-smoking policy affecting patients/families
> - Staff removing personal items from patients
> - Drug-seeking behavior
> - Patient/visitor under the influence of alcohol/illicit drugs
> - Psychiatric patients being cared for in the ED
> - Dementia patients being cared for in the ED
> - Poorly enforced visitor policy
> - Misconceptions of staff behavior by patients/visitors
> - Perception that staff is uncaring
> - Perceived prejudice from staff

refuse to serve those who are intoxicated, aggressive, or violent. Common reasons for aggressive behavior in the ED are highlighted in **Box 26.1**.[15]

Patients or family members who hear health-care workers laughing at the nurses' station may perceive the staff as uncaring or mistakenly believe that they are being mocked.[12] Further frustration is felt by patients who may have suboptimally treated chronic medical issues, lack access to reliable primary care, or are noncompliant with treatment recommendations.

The patient population in the ED also includes those with a predisposition toward violence, such as intoxicated or drug-seeking individuals, patients in police custody, and those with underlying dementia or psychosis.[1] Many emergency providers describe their impression that patient expectations have increased over time, which has contributed to increased levels of aggression.[16] Additionally, EDs are considered an integral part of our society and, as such, are at an increased risk of potential terrorist attacks according to a 2017 US Department of Homeland Security bulletin.[17]

Impact of Violence

While 19% of all workplace injuries happen in medical environments, health-care workers suffer 50% of all assaults.[2] In one study, 42% of emergency physicians who had been assaulted sought personal protection by carrying a gun, taser, or knife or by obtaining a security escort.[18]

Career Implications

Experiencing physical violence and verbal abuse compounds the stress health-care providers already experience in their day-to-day jobs. Consequences include the injuries themselves as well as psychological trauma. Victims of violence describe feeling anger, helplessness, isolation, shame, a negative attitude toward work, and difficulty maintaining concentration, as well as post-traumatic stress. Ninety-four percent of nurses experience at least one symptom of post-traumatic stress disorder (PTSD) after a violent event.[19] A reported 17% of emergency nurses who experience a violent event are likely to suffer from PTSD; furthermore, their symptoms can have a negative impact on their cognitive ability to perform their work.

Approximately 40% of ED workers appear to manifest at least one criterion of PTSD, and 36% exhibit symptoms that may later manifest as PTSD.[15] This rate is similar to that of military health-care providers delivering care in a combat zone. The overall result is diminished productivity and staff retention as well as decreased job satisfaction and an increased rate of burnout. Emergency department budgets are strained by employee days off work, increased turnover, and the medical and psychological expenses of workers' compensation. Ultimately, there is a negative financial impact to the hospital related to decreased patient satisfaction, increased litigation, and diminished reputation, as well as fines incurred from professional and regulatory agencies.[9,18-22]

Studies indicate concern among ED workers regarding job safety in response to violent events.[1,7] Up to 25% of ED doctors report feeling "sometimes, rarely, or never" safe at work, and nurses are dramatically less likely to feel safe at work than doctors.[1] Numerous surveys reflect providers' concerns that violence in the ED is a pervasive problem with increasing incidence.[1,8]

Multiple studies describe how workplace violence leads to increased turnover, reporting that between one-quarter and one-third of nurses consider leaving the ED after being exposed to violence.[19,20,22] Sixteen percent of emergency medicine physicians have considered leaving their hospital because of the fear of assault.[16] Recent emergency medicine journals have gone so far as to publish self-defense strategies.[23] All of this makes it harder to recruit and retain qualified staff to fulfill the mission of the ED.

Institutional Pressures

The increasing incidence and awareness of violence in the health-care workplace has been responsible for the development of state and federal standards. However, the federal Occupational Safety and Health Administration (OSHA) has set no federal occupational safety and health standards for workplace violence and does not require employers to have a workplace violence prevention program. However, the organization issued voluntary guidelines in 1996 and published an advisory guide in 2015, "Preventing Workplace Violence: A Road Map for Health Care Facilities."[11] OSHA may issue citations to employers for violating the "General Duty" clause of the OSHA Act, which requires each employer to "furnish each of his employees employment and a place of employment which are free from recognized hazards that are causing or likely to cause death or serious physical harm." To cite a business, OSHA must have evidence that:

- A condition or activity in the workplace presents a hazard to an employee.
- The condition or activity is recognized as a hazard by the employer or within the industry.
- The hazard is causing or likely to cause death or serious physical harm.
- A feasible means exists to eliminate or materially reduce the hazard.

While the nature of emergency medicine is such that personnel function in a chaotic environment, lack of effort to mitigate the risk to staff has resulted in hospitals being cited or penalized. The number of inspections has increased over the last several decades; however, the number of citations remains small. Between 1991 and 2014, there were only 18 citations issued for failing to address workplace violence.[4] As of 2018, however, OSHA's website had over 500 listings regarding health-care facilities/organizations being investigated or cited due to inadequate protection of their employees. As of 2015, nine states require certain medical facilities to have workplace violence prevention programs in place.[5,24,25]

Social Media

Social media has provided a useful forum to address workplace violence in health care, including Stanford internist and social activist Zubin Damania's Silent No More Foundation and Australia's EMS Violence Public Awareness campaign.[26,27] These programs bring first-hand accounts to light and are beneficial, in part, by encouraging legislators to increase criminal penalties for the assault of health-care professionals. While it is important to create awareness through such programs, inappropriate postings on social media regarding specific experiences have had career-ending consequences, especially when such posts violated HIPAA, federal or state law, or their employer's policies.[28]

Underreporting

Only 15% to 26% of physical assaults in the ED are formally reported, and verbal abuse is reported even less frequently.[29-31] Various reasons for the underreporting have been explored. Many providers who were surveyed discussed feeling that violence was just "part of the job." Others described experiences in which law enforcement personnel were reluctant to pursue charges or prosecute individuals accused of abuse. One nurse described a judge berating her in court, asking why she was pressing charges when violent encounters were an "expected" part of working the ED.[30]

A recurring perception is that hospital corporations respond inadequately to victims of workplace violence. Staff members may feel that efforts to improve patient satisfaction too often come at the expense of the institution's providers. Aspects of this insufficient response range from:

- Minimum or no preventative measures, with some facilities reluctant to place metal detectors or security guards, as they it might make their facility less "inviting"
- Inadequate staffing and other risk-mitigation measures[20,22,27,32,33]
- Perceptions among staff members that assaults may be perceived as evidence of poor job performance[5]

The absence of visual evidence of a physical injury and the presence of an ambiguous or onerous reporting policy can contribute to a provider's reluctance to document a violent event. Conversely, institutions that are committed to reducing ED violence, have accessible reporting policies, and have a positive track record of responding to incidents are associated with decreased rates of workplace violence.[3,12] As of 2016, 32 states have criminal statues making it a felony to assault medical personnel.[12,25]

CATEGORIES OF WORKPLACE VIOLENCE

Workplace violence has become so prevalent that it has its own definitions and categories, as shown in **Box 26.2**. It is broken down into four types based upon assailant.[24] The majority of ED violence falls into the first two categories, with patients and their friends or families being the assailants.[1-5]

BOX 26.2 ■ TYPES OF WORKPLACE VIOLENCE

Type 1: Workplace violence committed by a person who has no legitimate reason for being at the work site, including violence perpetrated by anyone who enters the workplace with the intent to commit a crime.

Type 2: Workplace violence directed at employees by customers, clients, patients, students, inmates, visitors, or other persons accompanying a patient.

Type 3: Workplace violence against an employee by a present or former employee, supervisor, or manager.

Type 4: Violence committed in the workplace by someone who does not work there, but has, or had, a personal relationship with an employee.

> **BOX 26.3 ■ PATTERNS OF VERBAL ABUSE**
>
> - Name-calling
> - Condescension
> - Manipulation
> - Criticism
> - Demeaning comments
> - Threats
> - Blame
> - Accusations
> - Withholding
> - Gaslighting
> - Circular arguments

Forms of Violence

Verbal Threats and Abuse

Verbal abuse can range from swearing, the use of slurs, and derogatory or belittling comments to threats of violence, legal action, or sexual harassment. Verbal abuse in the ED is so common that it often goes unnoticed.[34] The One Love Foundation describes 11 patterns of verbal abuse (**Box 26.3**).[35] While these categories were initially intended to describe verbal abuse in relationships, they are relevant in the ED because of the intimate nature of emergency care and the patterns of verbal abuse observed there.

Physical Assault

Physical assaults range from grabbing, punching, and kicking, all the way to rape and homicide, as highlighted in **Box 26.4**.[6] It should be standard practice for the manager/leader of the department to investigate every reported incident of violence within 24 hours, debriefing the victim and ensuring access to appropriate medical and psychological support.

Confrontation Outside of the ED

Outside-of-ED confrontations occur much less frequently. Such perpetrators are less likely to be intoxicated and more likely to be family members with unresolved issues. Security involvement and formal reporting of these encounters has rarely occurred.[1,4]

Stalking

Stalking, while infrequent, is particularly worrisome because it involves a different level of intent and motivation than that of an acutely intoxicated individual. Victims of stalking have tended to be females with less ED experience, and most stalkers have been patients.[1,4,5]

> **BOX 26.4 ■ FORMS OF WORKPLACE VIOLENCE**
>
> - Biting
> - Choking/strangling
> - Grabbing/pulling
> - Hair pulling
> - Hitting/punching/slapping
> - Throwing objects
> - Kicking
> - Pushing/shoving/throwing
> - Scratching
> - Sexual assault
> - Spitting
> - Assault with body fluids
> - Stabbing
> - Shooting

Sexual Assault

Research from the Institute of Alcohol Studies shows that 35% of ED workers have been victims of sexual harassment or assault at the hands of intoxicated individuals.[33] Masturbation, sexual advances, and intentional indecent exposure are common occurrences.[36] Though less common, there are numerous reports of patients sexually assaulting nurses during clinical encounters.[37,38] As in any other industry, health-care workers can also be victims of harassment at the hands of their coworkers.[39]

Perpetrators of Violence

Violence is more common in facilities with an annual census of over 60,000 patients.[40] Uniformly, all studies have shown that the most common perpetrators of violence against health-care professionals are patients, followed by family members, visitors, and coworkers.[1,3,4,12]

Intoxicated Patients

The majority of patients perpetrating violence against ED providers are intoxicated.[1,5,9,12] Each facility should prospectively develop standardized approaches to the intoxicated patient. Facility leaders should work with law enforcement to ensure their willingness to prosecute offenses committed in the ED if those same behaviors would be prosecuted in other public locations.

Geriatric/Demented Patients

Elderly and demented patients may become violent due to underlying organic neurologic issues. Their inability to grasp the consequences of their actions increases their potential to create a dangerous situation. Some of the highest rates of health-care workplace violence occur in long-term care centers. Because these patients may lack cognitive abilities, their violent behavior is appropriately perceived and addressed differently than the actions of intoxicated individuals.[2,4,25,41]

Psychiatric Patients

Second only to patients intoxicated by drugs or alcohol, psychiatric patients have the highest risk for violence in the ED setting. Therefore, other than the ED, psychiatric units have the highest rate of violence against staff. The perception of violence on these units includes patients who are suicidal or homicidal, psychotic, delusional, or have personality disorders.[2,5,6,41] The increasing challenges and delays associated with the timely disposition and placement of psychiatric patients has certainly contributed to increased patient frustration, agitation, and violence.

Family and Friends of Patients

Illness and injury can create substantial stress to both patients and their loved ones. Difficultly understanding the issues, anxiety, anger, and frustration in the setting of perceived delays or inequities in the health-care system can precipitate violent behavior, especially when coupled with intoxication or poor coping skills.[12,13,21,42]

Prisoners

People in custody have an obvious motivation to escape. Except for institutions with a "prison unit" or a "lock-down unit," the typical hospital environment may provide a flight opportunity. Numerous media reports show a high rate of violent incidents associated with inmate patients, including shootings and deaths. Studies have demonstrated a rate of nearly two attempted or successful escapes by prisoners per week from the ED or other hospital clinics.[2,43-45] Of ED-related shootings, 29% involve individuals in custody. Poorly trained security, especially regarding firearm retention, contributes to this risk. This concern is further illustrated by the fact that 50% of guns used in ED shootings are not brought in by the perpetrator, but rather involve the perpetrator taking the firearms from the security personnel.[45]

MANAGING VIOLENCE

Although a remarkable body of literature related to workplace violence, and specifically ED violence, has been published in recent years, there are few evidence-based recommendations. Most of the related literature is descriptive and does not demonstrate the impact of the various approaches. One systematic review states that many common-sense environmental changes are recommended and have been widely implemented—without strong supporting evidence.[46] Without endorsing specific interventions, OSHA has listed five "building blocks" necessary for the prevention of workplace violence, as shown in **Box 26.5**.[47]

Advocacy

Creating a safe environment for our staff and patients begins long before the potentially violent person enters the ED. Many states already have laws protecting persons who work in the ED. If your state does not have such a law, work with your hospital, your hospital association, your state ACEP chapter, your state's emergency nursing association, and other professional organizations to get these protections adopted in your state. The ACEP Board of Directors and several of its committees have taken a strong interest in workplace violence and represent another opportunity for advocacy. A compilation of ACEP resources regarding workplace violence can be found on the ACEP website.

Recognition of Potentially Violent Persons

Data Sharing

When allowed by law, sharing information related to violence lowers the incidence of subsequent violence.[48] This data-sharing process usually includes the creation of a supportive environment in which staff are encouraged to report when they are the victims of crime in the ED and press charges when appropriate. Even in states where ED workers do not have extra protections, simple assault is still a crime, and its victims are entitled to justice. Hospital and ED management should encourage the prosecution of crimes against staff to reduce the frequency of subsequent incidents.

BOX 26.5 ■ "BUILDING BLOCKS" FOR THE PREVENTION OF WORKPLACE VIOLENCE

- Management commitment and employee participation
- Worksite analysis
- Hazard prevention and control
- Safety and health training
- Recordkeeping and program evaluation

Entities can also share data internally. Systems for flagging charts and particular patients can alert future providers of an individual's potential for violence (see "Chart Flags" below). Providers can then proactively approach high-risk patients with de-escalation in mind and/or with the presence of appropriate security.

Screening Tools

In a review of more than 120 tools for assessing the risk of violent behaviors, predictive validity varied widely, with tools designed to assess targeted populations performing better than those designed to target the population at large.[49] Few of these tools were designed for the ED setting. Given the lack of validation and inability to generalize such tools to the ED population at large, the implementation of any specific tool for the screening of patients with violent potential cannot be recommended by the authors.

There are checklists and protocols that have been developed for assessing the environment to maximize safety.[50-52] These tools and the OSHA guidelines should be used by ED and hospital management to assess the safety of the workplace and ensure that reasonable steps have been taken to minimize the risk of developing violence. Such tools typically assess issues such as crowding, staffing, physical plant, privacy, staff training, potential hazards, security measures, and ED policies.

Chart Flags

Most modern electronic health record systems have a mechanism for putting alerts into an individual patient's chart. While these flags are typically used to alert providers to patients who carry infectious disease, they can be easily adapted to warn providers about individuals who pose a potential threat. This set of alerts allows the medical team to evaluate the patient's history for triggers and review previous interventions that have succeeded in de-escalating the individual.[53]

Such systems need to be carefully managed to ensure that patients are not inappropriately stigmatized. Instead, these systems should be used to enhance care while maximizing the safety of the environment. Each facility should develop specific policies related to any chart-flagging system. These policies should clearly identify who can apply the flag to the chart and how providers should behave when the flag is present. The policies should include specific training on approaching potentially dangerous individuals and the specific role of security and police in these situations. Facility policies and signage should also clearly indicate that individuals can be searched for potential weapons.

Methods of Protection

De-escalation Training

De-escalation training has been one of the cornerstone strategies to reduce violence in the ED. The approach is now being adopted by other sectors, such as law enforcement, where the desire to reduce violence-inducing conflict is powerful.

A recent Cochrane Review sought to validate the effectiveness of these training programs.[54] The review was limited in scope to the effectiveness of formal de-escalation on psychosis-induced behaviors. It is notable that of the 345 citations identified, zero showed statistical benefit to patients whose providers had received this training. Price studied the factors influencing the success or failure of de-escalation techniques in this population and found that coercive control techniques (e.g., reprimands, deterrents, and the like) appeared to increase aggression in individuals with mental health issues.[55] Thus, programs may need to be focused more on providing support to the disturbed individuals using techniques like problem solving, distraction, and reassurance.

It is worth noting that, although research has not yet proven the clinical benefit of de-escalation training for patients, there is some evidence that it benefits staff.[56] In the review article, it was noted that de-escalation training improved nurses' knowledge, skills, and confidence related to aggression management. This likely would result in a more confident and secure workforce and less staff turnover.

Simulation training has been shown to be an effective method of teaching mental health nurses to manage episodes of violence using simulated patients.[57] With training experiences, nursing students report increased confidence and knowledge regarding the management of potentially violent individuals. While this pilot program was geared toward nursing students headed toward a career in a mental health environment, one can reasonably conclude that ED nurses could be trained in a similar manner.

Technologies

One interesting study describes the results of placing body cameras on staff in a mental health unit.[58] Staff members who wore cameras reported that both staff and patients behaved better when the cameras were in use, and the incidence of aggressive interactions and restraints fell dramatically. This is consistent with the "Hawthorne effect," in which individuals modify their behaviors in response to being knowingly observed.

The ED team at Valley Hospital in Ridgewood, New Jersey, developed a "silent alarm" system that is activated by pressing a button on the lanyard holding their ID badge.[59] This alarm alerts other staff members to the need for backup and a show of force without alerting the patient to the security response. Technology should also include access control at ED entrances and exits. These include badge readers and combination keypads that limit who can enter or exit certain areas.

Security

In guidance from the Joint Commission (JC), there is a recommendation for each ED to have "a visible security presence."[60] Although the JC specifies that such a security presence should include individuals in uniform and in view, the roles of these individuals will be institution-specific. The Joint Commission does not have a specific recommendation about arming these officers but notes, "In some cases, these officers may have a 'strength instrument' that can be used during escalating situations."

When building a security plan, each facility should consider the environment in which they exist and the population they serve to determine whether security officers or sworn police officers are appropriate, as well as the extent to which the officers should be armed. In all cases, the JC does recommend that security personnel be trained in the prevention of violence as well as the proper way to respond to a violent incident.

One study on the effectiveness of conductive electrical weapons in the hospital setting found that the use or availability of these weapons did not decrease the overall rates of violence-related injury, though they may have decreased the severity of these violence-related injuries.[61]

Environmental Design

The environmental design has an impact on safety in the setting of ED violence. In the design phase, it is vital to pay attention to the entry zone, traffic management, clustering of patient rooms, centralization versus decentralization, and provisions for special populations.[62] The entry zone should have a security podium or office that provides visual control of the entrance as well as any areas where patients/families are waiting. These areas should include public restrooms and a patient drop-off zone. The triage area should be clearly marked and visible from the entrance. Traffic flow into and out of the ED clinical spaces should be planned, and routes should be clearly designated. Large departments may need to have rooms clustered into pods, so that the staff can maintain their line of sight. Smaller departments may have one centralized nursing station. Behavioral health patients may need to be cohorted together in departments that serve larger numbers, and every ED should be designed with the appropriate number of psych-safe rooms, that is, rooms that provide a safe, secure, and therapeutic environment.

There is no clear evidence that metal detectors enhance the safety of the ED or decrease violence. Most hospitals have multiple doors through which an armed individual could enter the building and potentially gain access to the ED. Having one metal detector at one entrance does little to protect against someone who is determined to enter the building with a weapon. Culturally, a visible metal detector may enhance the perception of safety among staff and patients, or it may have the opposite effect, as some may view its presence as an indication that they are in a dangerous environment.

MANAGING THE VIOLENT PATIENT

Assessing the Potential for Violence

One important predictor of future violence is the knowledge of past violence involving the individual perpetrator. Each health-care facility should develop a robust system for reporting incidents of violent behavior and should keep records.[63] Best practice includes having the means to push this information to the bedside clinicians at each future encounter to ensure that staff are prepared to minimize escalation and manage agitation.[64]

Staff education should ensure an understanding of the role played by mental health and cognitive disorders in predisposing patients to violence. Those with a history of drug or alcohol abuse may also be more predisposed. Those suffering significant pain or needing to use the bathroom may be agitated and prone to acting out. Emergency department policies should allow for hourly rounding to ensure patient comfort and the exchange of information related to wait times. There should be a form of entertainment, such as TV or internet access, for patients who are required to wait. Food should be readily available for those with no contraindication to oral intake.

De-escalation

When an individual in the ED becomes aggressive, staff need clear guidance procedures. Silent alarms and coded overhead pages can bring a designated response to help defuse the situation. The rates of actual violence and restraint use are both reduced when security officers and charge nurses with enhanced training respond to agitation events.[65] Thus, hospitals should actively plan for these situations and have clearly established response teams with specific roles in the de-escalation process.

Restraint and Seclusion

Medications do play an important role in aborting agitated behavior. Each ED should have a policy in place regarding the use of "chemical restraints." The department should be stocked with an appropriate supply of benzodiazepines, atypical antipsychotics, and ketamine. Hospital policies and delineated privileges should allow emergency physicians to utilize these medications for the management of agitated, potentially violent, or actively violent individuals. Policies describing the proper use of these drugs and the authority of ED physicians to administer them will eliminate confusion during a moment of crisis.

Rules

Each facility must develop a policy regarding the application of restraints. These policies should allow nurses to apply restraints ahead of a provider order when appropriate. While restraints applied for medical/nonviolent reasons have their own rules and indications, restraints to control behavior in agitated, combative, violent, or dangerous individuals should be applied according to specific national standards. The Centers for Medicare and Medicaid Services Conditions of Participation, §482.13, specify these rules at the federal level. Hospital policy needs to reflect these rules.[66]

Complications

The application of restraints may be complicated and associated with risks to both the patient and staff. Any facility that utilizes restraint as a necessary part of patient care should be prepared to manage the complications that can arise. These are dangerous moments for all involved, and the facility must properly train staff in techniques for safely applying the restraints as well as rescuing patients who develop complications. Possible complications from restraint application include asphyxia, aspiration, blunt trauma, catecholamine rush, enhancement of ill effects of psychotropic medications, rhabdomyolysis, thrombosis, and psychological distress.[67]

ACTIVE SHOOTER EVENTS

In Mar 2018, a 31-year-old disgruntled employee entered a hospital in Birmingham, Alabama, where he shot and killed a 63-year-old nursing supervisor, injured a 28-year-old employee, and then killed himself. Metal detectors at the hospital were in use at the time.[68] According to two studies, events like this one are increasing in frequency.[45,69] Fortunately, active shooter events are the rarest form of workplace violence that health-care workers face.[45,70]

In a study of 154 hospital shooting events from 2000 to 2011, the ED was the most common site (29% of the total).[45] Of the shootings in the ED, 23% involved the perpetrator taking a gun from an officer. Metal detectors haven't been proven to decrease violence in the ED. However, the study estimated that metal detectors could have prevented 49% of hospital shootings, but they were less likely to prevent a shooting event in the ED compared to other places in the hospital.

Another study supported by the Federal Bureau of Investigation reviewed 160 active shooter incidents from 2000 to 2013. The study included four health-care shootings, in which a total of 10 were killed and 10 wounded. Of the 160 incidents, 60% ended prior to the arrival of law enforcement, and more than two-thirds of these events ended in 5 minutes or less.

The 2017 Hartford Consensus study highlighted the public and health-care workers' perceptions of active shooter situations.[71] Health-care workers rated the risk of active shooter events in hospitals nearly double that of the public. The study hypothesized that the reason for this difference in perception was that the public views hospitals as sanctuaries of caring and healing. While both the public and health care workers similarly viewed the responsibility of law enforcement and firefighters to protect patients, the public felt that doctors and nurses should accept a very high degree of risk to help those who wouldn't be able to protect themselves from harm.

Specialized Training

Emergency departments should be on high alert after any active shooter event in the community. Active shooters are a recognized risk and should be included in emergency operations planning.[72] Hospitals should collaborate with community partners, such as law enforcement and EMS, in their active shooter response planning. This teamwork should carry through into drills and simulations, as all parties are likely to be involved in a real-life response. An ED will likely have to deal with an active shooter event before the arrival of law enforcement, and prior planning and training can assist in providing an optimal response. After their arrival, law enforcement will take over, but hospital personnel should do whatever it takes to assist them in restoring a safe environment.[73]

While active shooter events are difficult to predict, the goal is to maximize the number of lives that can be saved, and remove potential targets. Health-care workers who are not trained in the response to an active shooter can experience helplessness and denial, only making a bad situation worse. Hospitals should avoid a "one-size-fits-all" response. Given that difficult decisions will be made in the moment, health-care staff should neither be mandated to stay with patients nor mandated to leave. Attempts to continue to care for patients should be made but might be impossible without putting others at risk. Even with planning and training, zero risk is not achievable.[45]

Multiple accounts in the literature highlight what hospitals have learned from their own active shooter drills. One study highlighted that an active shooter could essentially go anywhere—to any building or any floor—and cause great damage.[73] One hospital included community partners in staff training, and one did not.[73,74] A hospital performed active shooter simulation within an empty unit, as the physical layout was familiar, provided a safe space for first-time exposure, and offered the best opportunity for on-duty staff to attend. Another hospital found that its active shooter drill helped staff prepare for the Boston Marathon bombing response.[75] A commonly taught response to active shooter events is the "Run, Hide, Fight" approach endorsed by the Department of Homeland Security.[76] While there are other approaches available, the purpose of all responses is to minimize harm and restore safety.

SUPPORTING THE VICTIMS OF VIOLENCE

Support of health-care workers as victims of workplace violence has room for improvement. A survey revealed that two-thirds of participating staff had experienced occupational violence in the preceding 12 months, yet less than half reported receiving postincident support.[77] Multiple studies have shown that nurses have mentally normalized and minimized violence.[22,78-81] Additionally, a perceived lack of support discourages the reporting of these incidents. The literature reveals that younger, less-experienced nurses are at a higher risk of violence; male nurses are more likely to experience physical assaults; and nurses are more exposed to violence than physicians over the span of their careers.[82]

Nurses have reported lasting effects after violent encounters, including hypervigilance, shock, embarrassment, confusion, sadness, anger, difficulty thinking and trusting, and keeping increased distance between themselves and patients.[81,82] Even violence-reduction measures, such as reporting and signage for inappropriate behavior, are not consistently supported or enforced, which contributes to feelings of abandonment by the staff. Physical violence can be considered high acuity and typically receives higher levels of attention and support. Nonphysical violence, such as verbal threats and aggression, tends to be minimized by health-care workers. Frequent, cumulative exposure to nonphysical violence may have major negative psychological consequences and might be more significant than the severity of a violent event.[22]

It's important to understand the neurobiological effects of violence; reactions to violence are subconscious.[78] The rational brain can cease to function in a violent encounter, and individuals become very reactive in their thinking and behavior. Individuals involved in violent encounters are less able to regulate their response and may not be able to assess their own needs. These responses should be considered normal and not a failure of the individual to utilize their training. The flight, or freeze response is also normal, and an individual would have to be well-trained and well-grounded to recognize that they were experiencing that reaction. Thorough de-escalation training has the potential to help health-care workers better understand their reactions to violence and assist them in modulating their current and future response to similar events.

Employee Assistance Programs

Victims of workplace violence tend to debrief with colleagues and seek support by other nonformal means.[79,82] Formal support can include the help of management and the use of an employee assistance program (EAP). Multiple studies highlight the shortcomings of these formal support mechanisms, including management blaming the victim for the violent encounter, a lack of response from leadership, and an expectation that violence comes with the job.[80,81]

An established peer-help program can support victims and lead to a decrease in turnover and sick leave, lower legal and medical expenses, and improved morale.[80] Utilizing a peer support program as a formal response to violence is a largely untapped resource and has a significant opportunity to bolster immediate postincident support for assaulted health care workers.[82]

The EAP, if available, is commonly offered after critical incidents as an additional resource to help health-care workers with the psychological aftereffects of violence. Even when this program is offered, many decline to use it.[78] Health-care workers often refuse support resources after violence because they may find it uncomfortable and embarrassing to be perceived as victims. This concept of the "wounded hero" highlights the difficulty of role reversal for many health-care workers, who are accustomed to helping others.[79] A strong EAP can support the victim's recovery by diffusing any associated stigma. The ultimate goal is to assist the worker in restoring psychological equilibrium.

Critical Incident Stress Management

Critical incident stress management (CISM) is a commonly used method to support health-care workers after critical incidents. Workplace violence has been described as a critical incident, and a study by DeFraia revealed assaults had one of the highest mean scores on the Critical Incident Severity Index Scale–Revised.[83,84] It is important to note that CISM is not psychotherapy, but "psychological first aid."[85]

Critical incident stress management can consist of a short, in-the-moment defusion followed by a more comprehensive debriefing. Recent literature highlights a controversy as to the effectiveness of CISM: a study published in the *European Journal of Trauma & Dissociation* suggests that eye movement desensitization and reprocessing (EMDR) may be effective. EMDR is a form of psychotherapy in which the patient is asked to recall distressing images. The patient is then directed to engage in a bilateral sensory input, such as hand tapping or moving the eyes from side to side. Researchers found that this method is more effective than CISM at preventing PTSD; however, EMDR is a form of individualized psychotherapy, and rapid deployment of this method after a critical incident might prove difficult.[86] Whatever the method used to support victims of workplace violence, it is important to remember that the consistent application of these mechanisms can offer the best outcomes.

CONCLUSION

Workplace violence in health care, and especially in the ED, is a complex, multifactorial problem without easy answers. Emergency providers face a high risk of violence due to EMTALA regulations and the ED environment itself. Every hospital has an obligation to protect its staff. In addition to performing a risk assessment, health-care organizations must educate and train their personnel in violence prevention as part of a comprehensive risk-reduction strategy. An essential component of these programs entails providing support to ED staff after an assault. Perpetrators of violence should be held accountable, and every effort must be made to ensure appropriate legal consequences.

When addressing ED violence, an "it doesn't/won't happen here" or "it's expected with the job" attitude is unacceptable. Workplace violence does happen with alarming regularity despite attempts to mitigate the risks. It's time for a societal and cultural shift; violence in our EDs is not acceptable and should never be considered "part of the job."

REFERENCES

1. Behman M, Tillotson R, Davis S, et al. Violence in the emergency department: a national survey of emergency medicine residents and attending physicians. *J Emerg Med*. 2009;40(5):565–579.

2. Blando JD, McGreevy K, O'Hagan E, et al. Emergency department security programs, community crime, and employee assaults. *J Emerg Med*. 2012;42(3):329–338.

3. Schnapp BH, Slovis BH, Shah AD, et al. Workplace violence and harassment against emergency medicine residents. *West J Emerg Med*. 2016;17(5):567–573.

4. U.S. Department of Labor, Bureau of Labor Statistics. 2016 Survey of Occupational Injuries & Illnesses Chart Data. US Department of Labor. 2017. Available at: https://www.bls.gov/iif/soii-chart-data-2016.htm. Accessed August 27, 2020.

5. *Emergency Department Violence Surveillance Study [Internet]*. Des Plaines, Ill: Emergency Nurses Association; 2011. Available at: https://www.ena.org/docs/default-source/resource-library/practice-resources/workplace-violence/2011-emergency-department-violence-surveillance-report. Accessed August 27, 2020.

6. American College of Emergency Physicians News Release: Emergency Department Violence. 2018. Available at: http://filecache.mediaroom.com/mr5mr_acep/178990/download/2018ACEP%20Emergency%20Department%20Violence%20PollResults.pdf. Accessed August 27, 2020.

7. Gates D, Ross C, McQueen L. Violence against emergency department workers. *J Emerg Med*. 2006;31:331–337.

8. Kansagra S, Rao S, Sullivan A, et al. A survey of workplace violence across 65 U.S. emergency departments. *Acad Emerg Med*. 2008;15:1268–1274.

9. Gacki-Smith J, Juarez AM, Boyett L, et al. Violence against nurses working in US emergency departments. *J Nursing Admin*. 2009;39(7–8):340–349.

10. Campbell JC, Messing JT, Kub J, et al. Workplace violence: prevalence and risk factors in the safe at work study. *J Occup Environ Med*. 2011;53(1):82–89.

11. US Department of Labor. Preventing Workplace Violence: A Road Map for Healthcare Facilities. Occupational Safety and Health Administration. US Department of Labor website. 2015. Available at: https://www.osha.gov/Publications/OSHA3827.pdf. Accessed August 27, 2020.

12. Gacki-Smith J, Juarez AM, Boyett L, et al. Violence against nurses working in US emergency departments. *J Healthc Protect Manag*. 2010;26(1):81–99.

13. Kowalenko T, Walters BL, Khare RK, et al. Workplace violence: a survey of emergency physicians in the state of Michigan. *Ann Emerg Med*. 2005;46(2):142–147.

14. Renker P, Scribner SA, Huff P. Staff perspectives of violence in the emergency department: appeals for consequences, collaboration, and consistency. *Work*. 2015;51(1):5–18.

15. Gillespie GL, Bresler S, Gates DM, et al. Posttraumatic stress symptomatology among emergency department workers following workplace aggression. *Workplace Health Saf*. 2013;61(6):247–254.

16. Knowles E, Mason S, Moriarty, F. "I'm going to learn how to run quick": exploring violence directed towards staff in the emergency department. *Emerg Med J*. 2013;30(11):926–931.

17. Homeland Security Terrorist Call for Attacks on Hospitals, Healthcare Facilities, Unclassified Bulletin, February 8, 2017.

18. Violence Against ED Workers a Growing Problem. *Emergency Physician Monthly*. 2012. Available at: http://epmonthly.com/article/violence-against-ed-workers-a-growing-problem/. Accessed August 27, 2020.

19. Copeland D, Henry M. The relationship between workplace violence, perceptions of safety, and professional quality of life among emergency department staff members in a level 1 trauma centre. *Int Emerg Nurs*. 2018;39:26–32.

20. Gillespie G, Gates D, Kowalenko T, et al. Implementation of a comprehensive intervention to reduce physical assaults and threats in the emergency department. *J Emerg Nursing*. 2014;40(6):586–591.

21. Laeeque SH, Bilal A, Babar S, et al. How patient-perpetrated workplace violence leads to turnover intention among nurses: the mediated mechanism of occupational stress and burnout. *J Aggress Maltreat Trauma*. 2018;27(1):96–118.

22. Wright-Brown SA-B, Sekula K, Gillespie G, et al. The experiences of registered nurses who are injured by interpersonal violence while on duty in an emergency department. *J Forensic Nurs*. 2016;12(4):189–197.

23. Johnson A. Proxemics training can prevent ED violence [In English: don't let things escalate]. *Emerg Med News*. 2018;40(5):13–15.

24. California Occupational Safety and Health Administration. Cal. Cod Regs. Subchapter 7, Group 2, Article 7, §3342. Violence Prevention in Health Care.

25. Occupational Safety and Health Administration. Workplace violence prevention and related goals. Occupational Safety and Health Administration. US Department of Labor website. 2015. Available at: https://www.osha.gov/Publications/OSHA3828.pdf. Accessed August 27, 2020.

26. Australia SA. *Video Highlights Violence against Australian Paramedics*. JEMS; 2015.

27. Jones R. Violence in Adelaide hospitals targeted in social media campaign. *ABC News*. 2017. Available at: http://www.abc.net.au/news/2017-02-09/emergency-department-violence-targeted-in-social-media-campaign/8256356. Accessed August 27, 2020.

28. Francis A. NY nurse fired for trauma room pic. A case of oversharing? *Techtimes*. 2014. Available at: https://www.techtimes.com/articles/10039/20140712/ny-nurse-fired-for-trauma-room-pic-a-case-of-oversharing.htm. Accessed August 27, 2020.

29. D'Ettorre G, Pellicani V, Mazzotta M, et al. Preventing and managing workplace violence against healthcare workers in emergency departments. *Acta Biomed*. 2018;89(4-S):28–36.

30. Wolf LA, Delao AA, Perhats C. Nothing changes, nobody cares: understanding the experience of emergency nurses physically or verbally assaulted while providing care. *J Emerg Nurs*. 2014;40(4):305–310.

31. Copeland D, Henry M. Workplace violence and perceptions of safety among emergency department staff members: experiences, expectations, tolerance, reporting, and recommendations. *J Trauma Nurs*. 2017;24(2):65–77.

32. Shaw G. Punched, assaulted, and worse: violence in today's ED. *Emerg Med News*. 2018;40(5):12–14.

33. Institute of Alcohol Studies. Alcohol alert. 2018. Available at: http://www.ias.org.uk/What-we-do/Alcohol-Alert/April-2018.aspx. Accessed August 27, 2020.

34. Joint Commission. Sentinel Event Alert. 2018. Available at: https://www.jointcommission.org/assets/1/18/SEA_59_Workplace_violence_4_13_18_FINAL.pdf. Accessed August 27, 2020.

35. Hughes JA. 11 common patterns of verbal abuse. 2018. Available at: https://www.joinonelove.org/learn/11-common-patterns-verbal-abuse/. Accessed August 27, 2020.

36. Chuck E. For nurses, sexual harassment from patients is 'Par for the Course'. *NBC News*. February 21, 2018. Available at: https://www.nbcnews.com/storyline/sexual-misconduct/nurses-sexual-harassment-patients-par-course-n848086. Accessed August 27, 2020.

37. Patient arrested for attack, sexual assault on metro nurse. *News9.com*. December 12, 2017. Available at: https://www.healthleadersmedia.com/nursing/patient-arrested-attack-sexual-assault-metro-nurse. Accessed August 27, 2020.

38. Nurse sexually assaulted by patient at hospital, police say. *WPXI.com*. February 7, 2018. Available at: https://www.ajc.com/news/national/nurse-sexually-assaulted-patient-hospital/DINPV6ouxcrqB9eNB2C5pJ/. Accessed August 27, 2020.

39. Jagsi R. Sexual harassment in medicine—#MeToo. *N Engl J Med*. 2018;378:209–211.

40. Medley DB, Morris JE, Stone CK, et al. An association between occupancy rates in the emergency department and rates of violence toward staff. *J Emerg Med*. 2012;43(4):736–744. (crowding = violence).

41. Tadros A, Kiefer C. Violence in the emergency department: a global problem. *Psychiatr Clin North Am*. 2017;40(3):575–584.

42. Gates D, Gillespie G, Kowalenko T, et al. Occupational and demographic factors associated with violence in the emergency department. *Adv Emerg Nursing J*. 2011;33(4):303–313.

43. Mikow-Porto V, Smith T. The International Association for Healthcare Safety and Security 2011 Prisoner Escape Study. *J Healthc Prot Manage*. 2012;27(2):38–58.

44. Midlow-Porto V. Violence in the ED reaches a crisis point. *Emerg Physicians Monthly*. June 2016. Available at: http://epmonthly.com/article/violence-ed-reaches-crisis-point/?utm_source=TrendMD&utm_medium=cpc&utm_campaign=EPMonthly_TrendMD_0. Accessed August 27, 2020.

45. Kelen G, Catlett C, Kubit J, et al. Hospital-based shootings in the United States: 2000–2011. *Ann Emerg Med*. 2012;60(6):790–798.

46. Weiland T, Ivory S, Hutton J. Managing acute behavior disturbances in the emergency department using the environment, policies, and practices: a systematic review. *West J Emerg Med*. 2017;8(2):647–661.

47. Occupational Safety and Health Administration. *Guidelines for Preventing Workplace Violence for Healthcare and Social Service Workers (PSHA Publication 3148-04R)*. Washington, DC: US Department of Labor; 2015.

48. Price J, Martin M, Dean J, et al. Violence intervention and prevention in emergency rooms: The Viper Study. *Emerg Med J*. 2017;34:887.

49. Singh J, Grann M, Fazel S. A comparative study of violence risk assessment tools: a systematic review and metaregression analysis of 68 studies involving 25,980 participants. *Clin Psychol Rev*. 2011;31(3):499–513.

50. Stowell K, Hughes N, Rozel J. Violence in the emergency department. *Psychiatric Clin N Am*. 2016;39:557–566.

51. Hamblin LE, Essenmacher L, Luborsky M, et al. Worksite walkthrough intervention: data-driven prevention of workplace violence on hospital units. *JOEM*. 2017;59(9):875–884.

52. Ramacciati N, Ceccagnoli A, Addey B, et al. Interventions to reduce the risk of violence toward emergency department staff: current approaches. *Open Access Emerg Med*. 2016;8:17–27.

53. Smith T. What every healthcare facility should do now to reduce the potential for workplace violence. *J Healthc Prot Manage*. 2016;32(1):41–47.

54. Du M, Wang X, Yin S, et al. De-escalation techniques for psychosis-induced aggression or agitation (Review). *Cochrane Database Syst Rev*. 2017;4(4).

55. Price O, Baker J, Bee P, et al. The support-control continuum: an investigation of staff perspectives on factors influencing the success of failure of de-escalation techniques for the management of violence and aggression in mental health settings. *Int J Nurs Stud*. 2018;77:197–206.

56. Halm M. Aggression management education for acute care nurses: what's the evidence? *Am J Crit Care*. 2017;26(6):504–508.

57. Martinez A. Implementing a workplace violence simulation for undergraduate nursing students: a pilot study. *J Psychosoc Nurs*. 2017;55(10):39–44.

58. Hardy S, Bennett L, Rosen P. The feasibility of using body worn cameras in an inpatient mental health setting. *Ment Health Fam Med*. 2017;13:393–400.

59. Whitman E. Best practices: frequent violence in the ED doesn't have to be part of the job. *Modern Healthcare*. September 24, 2016.

60. Preventing violence in the emergency department: ensuring staff safety. *Environ Care News*. 2009;12(10):1–11.

61. Gramling JJ, McGovern PM, Church TR, et al. Effectiveness of conducted electrical weapons to prevent violence-related injuries in the hospital. *J Emerg Nurs*. 2018;44(3):249–257.

62. Pati D, Pati S, Harvey TE Jr. Security implications of physical design attributes in the emergency department. *HERD*. 2016;9(4):50–63.

63. Harmon J. Workplace violence mitigation: the three-year model. *J Healthc Prot Manage*. 2016;32(1):56–62.

64. Ziebell C. *An Effective Case Management Program for the Emergency Department*. Dallas, Tex: IMX Summit, April 2015.

65. Martinez A. Managing workplace violence with evidence-based interventions: a literature review. *J Psychosoc Nurs Ment Health Serv.* 2016;54(9):31–36.

66. Centers for Medicare & Medicaid Services, HHS. § 482.13 condition of participation: patient's rights. *The GPO Website.* Available at: https://www.gpo.gov/fdsys/pkg/CFR-2010-title42-vol5/pdf/CFR-2010-title42-vol5-sec482-13.pdf. Accessed August 10, 2018.

67. Mohr W, Petti T, Mohr B. Adverse effects associated with physical restraint. *Can J Psychiatry.* 2003;48(5):330–337.

68. Reid T. Disgruntled worker killed nurse, injured employee at UAB Highlands, police say. *CBS 42.* Available at: https://www.cbs42.com/news/local/disgruntled-worker-killed-nurse-at-uab-hospital/1051624920. Accessed August 25, 2018.

69. Blair JP, Schweit KW. *A Study of Active Shooter Incidents, 2000–2013. Texas State University and Federal Bureau of Investigation.* Washington, DC: US Department of Justice; 2014.

70. Warren B, Bosse M, Tornetta P III. Workplace violence and active shooter considerations for health-care workers. *J Bone Joint Surg Am.* 2017;99:e88(1–5).

71. Jacobs LM, Burns KJ. The Hartford consensus: survey of the public and healthcare professionals on active shooter events in hospitals. *J Am Coll Surg.* 2017;225(3):435–442.

72. International Association of Emergency Medical Services Chiefs. Active Shooter Planning and Response in a Healthcare Setting. 2017. Available at: https://www.fbi.gov/file-repository/active_shooter_planning_and_response_in_a_healthcare_setting.pdf/view. Accessed August 11, 2018.

73. Rorie S. Implementing an active shooter training program. *AORN Connections.* 2015;101(1):C5-C6.

74. Mannenback MS, Fahje CJ, Sunga KL, et al. An in situ simulation-based training approach to active shooter response in the emergency department. *Disaster Med Public Health Prep.* 2019;13(2):345–352.

75. Best practices for active shooter response and prevention in hospitals. *Healthcare Life Safety Compliance.* 2017;20(12):10–12.

76. Department of Homeland Security. Active shooter preparedness. 2018. Available at: https://www.dhs.gov/active-shooter-preparedness. Accessed August 25, 2018.

77. Shea T, Cooper B, De Cieri H, et al. Postincident support for healthcare workers experiencing occupational violence and aggression. *J Nurs Scholarsh.* 2018;50(4):344–352.

78. Beattie J, Innes K, Griffiths D, et al. Healthcare providers' neurobiological response to workplace violence perpetrated by consumers: informing directions for staff well-being. *Appl Nurs Res.* 2018;43:42–48.

79. Ashton R, Morris L, Smith I. A qualitative meta-synthesis of emergency department staff experiences of violence and aggression. *Int Emerg Nurs.* 2018;39:13–19.

80. Flannery RB Jr. The Assaultive Staff Action Program (ASAP): 25 year program analysis. *Psychiatr Q.* 2016;87:211–216.

81. Stevenson K, Jack S, O'Mara L, et al. Registered nurses' experiences of patient violence on acute care psychiatric inpatient units: an interpretive descriptive study. *BMC Nurs.* 2015;14(1):1–13.

82. Edward K, Ousey K, Warelow P, et al. Nursing and aggression in the workplace: a systematic review. *Br J Nurs.* 2014;23(12):653–659.

83. Wuthnow J, Elwell S, Quillen J, et al. Clinical: implementing an ED critical incident stress management team. *J Emerg Nurs.* 2016;42:474–480.

84. DeFraia GS. EAP-based critical incident stress management: utilization of a practice-based assessment of incident severity level in responding to workplace trauma. *Int J Emerg Ment Health.* 2013;15(2):105–122.

85. Everly G, Mitchell J. A primer on critical incident stress management (CISM). The International Critical Incident Stress Foundation website. Available at: http://www.icisf.org/a-primer-on-critical-incident-stress-managementcism/. Accessed September 1, 2018.

86. Tarquinio C, Rotonda C, Houlle WA, et al. Early psychological preventive intervention for workplace violence: a randomized controlled explorative and comparative study between EMDR-recent event and critical incident stress debriefing. *Issues Ment Health Nurs.* 2016;37:787–799.

EMERGENCY DEPARTMENT FACILITY DESIGN

CHAPTER 27

Frank Zilm, James J. Augustine, Nancy Mannion Bonalumi

The physical environment of the emergency department (ED) is critical to the effective and safe operation of the service. The ability to move patients efficiently, provide safe and appropriate work and support spaces, and ensure the ability to respond to critical events require the right space elements and configuration. Each ED is a unique blend of patients, processes, and institutional characteristics. Successful planning requires a logical framework for analysis along with the commitment of health-care organization leaders.[1]

A key factor for the development of an effective ED design is discussion and planning among the ED leadership team. It should be understood that the ultimate design will be an indirect reflection of the effectiveness of the department's leaders. A critical first step is to ensure that consensus exists among all key stakeholders related to the mission and scope of the space. Incongruity among the stakeholders can lead to a design that is inefficient or impractical. The team must understand the present use and anticipated needs of the ED, while maintaining flexibility for unanticipated changes in the department's scope of services.

The ED leadership and clinical team should establish a primary contact for ease of interaction with the design and senior administrative team. The team leader must give appropriate consideration to the perspectives of all of the primary users of this space. Key support departments, such as security, registration, and diagnostic services, must also be able to voice their own concerns and considerations. Reaching out to other community partners like police and emergency medical services (EMS) may also be valuable for determining the maximum functionality of the design.

Designing for flexibility is critical to accommodate new care models that may be radically different through the coming years. Too tight a "fit" between anticipated operational patterns and the design solution could actually limit the life of the building. Designing with flexibility maximizes the alignment between best estimates of current needs and the requirements of future emergency care delivery.

THE PLANNING AND DESIGN PROCESS

The ED design should be developed and evaluated based on the mission statement and a set of objectives established during the planning process. These objectives should reflect the strategic goals and operational objectives of the service. It is also important to establish an achievable timetable for the process that maintains momentum while providing sufficient time for evaluating new process and facility concepts. The planning team should make key decisions in a logical sequence, avoiding premature decisions on key issues. The planning and design process is

> **BOX 27.1 ■ THE FIVE STEPS OF SPACE DETERMINATION**
>
> **Predesign**
> 1. Strategic/operational planning
> 2. Functional/space programming
>
> **Design**
> 3. Schematic design
> 4. Design development
> 5. Construction documents

a series of reflective tasks. It is not uncommon to "loop-back" and revise earlier decisions as the design evolves.

Determining space needs and developing a design solution is typically divided into five steps—two predesign steps and three steps in the design phase (**Box 27.1**).

Predesign

Predesign includes strategic/operational planning and functional/space programming.

- *Strategic and operational planning*: This process entails developing a goal statement for the ED design, projecting target workloads and patient mix, and identifying a desired patient processing and operation plan—all consistent with the present and future mission of the organization. Questions to consider include:
  - Are there new program/service lines being considered (e.g., stroke, chest pain center, trauma, urgent care, new medical/surgical units, or diagnostic services) that will impact the ED's volume and acuity?
  - What is the hospital's long-range plan, and how does the ED fit into it?
  - For process planning and modeling, what are the needs for areas such as adult, pediatric, trauma, mental health, observation, and specialty needs (e.g., cardiac intervention, sexual assault nurse examiners, and orthopedic).
- *Functional and space programming*: In this process, the strategic projections and process models based on volume, staffing, and treatment care plans are converted into specific space elements. The product of this phase of work includes a listing of all the space elements, diagrams illustrating the grouping and relationship of space elements, and a description of their key relationships to other services, such as imaging, surgery, intensive care, and other inpatient units. The clinical and design staff must begin to use the common definitions adopted during this phase of development (**Table 27.1**).

Design Phase

The design phase includes schematic design, design development, and construction documents:

- *Schematics*: Schematics entail the early translation of the functional and space program into layouts that show the department's physical organizational concepts, site access and circulation, and budget estimates. Alternative schematic designs are frequently developed and evaluated. This phase moves from simple "bubble" diagrams of areas into "single-line" drawings that depict the approximate scale and relationship of elements (**Figure 27.1**).

- *Design development*: This step involves the refinement of the preferred schematic design to show wall thicknesses, structural grid layouts, door and window locations, and placement of major fixed equipment (e.g., sinks, headwall units, imaging equipment, etc). The initial development of interior design concepts (materials, fixed or mobile cabinetry, the "image" of the services) is undertaken during design development. Drawings, an outline of written specifications, and a budget are products of this phase (**Figure 27.2**). Changes to the basic layout of the department and sizes of rooms become increasingly difficult during the later stages of this phase (**Figure 27.3**).
- *Construction documents*: These are technical documents intended to provide information about the construction requirements and costs. In addition to drawings, detailed specifications describe specific materials, equipment, and construction methods. A significant part of the architect's time and effort is directed to this phase of the process. Changes during this stage can result in significant delays in the execution of the project and additional fees.

Influencing the Design

The ability of ED leaders to influence design solutions is highest during the predesign and schematic phases. As a project moves into design development, it becomes increasingly difficult to make changes that impact the project timeline. Committing time and input into the strategic planning, programming, and schematic phases provides the best opportunity to influence the final design.

As noted earlier, the design process is a strategic and "reflective" sequence of events. The program and schematic design phases are a discovery process in which early assumptions

TABLE 27.1 ■ Key Architectural Terms and Definitions

Term	Definition
Net square feet (NSF)	The space within the walls of a room or the usable floor area assigned to a function in an open area (e.g., cubicles or workstations). The space includes casework, fixtures, and door swings but does not include wall thicknesses.
Departmental gross square feet (DGSF)	The space inside the centerline of the walls separating a department from adjoining areas; includes internal walls, corridors, and so on.
Building gross square feet (BGSF)	The total area of the facility, including outside walls, mechanical spaces, and canopies.
Net-to-gross factor or grossing factor	A multiplication factor applied to space to increase the allotment to accommodate elements not in the base number. A grossing factor is applied to space lists on NSF to take into account internal circulation and walls to give DGSF. Another factor is used to increase DGSF to BGSF and estimate the amount required for major vertical circulation and shafts and building circulation.
Construction costs	The capital cost for site, building, and major fixed equipment (cabinets, doors) for new and remodeling construction.
Project costs	The total costs associated with construction, including the construction costs, equipment, professional fees, legal, owner expenses, and other related expenses.

452 Emergency Department Management

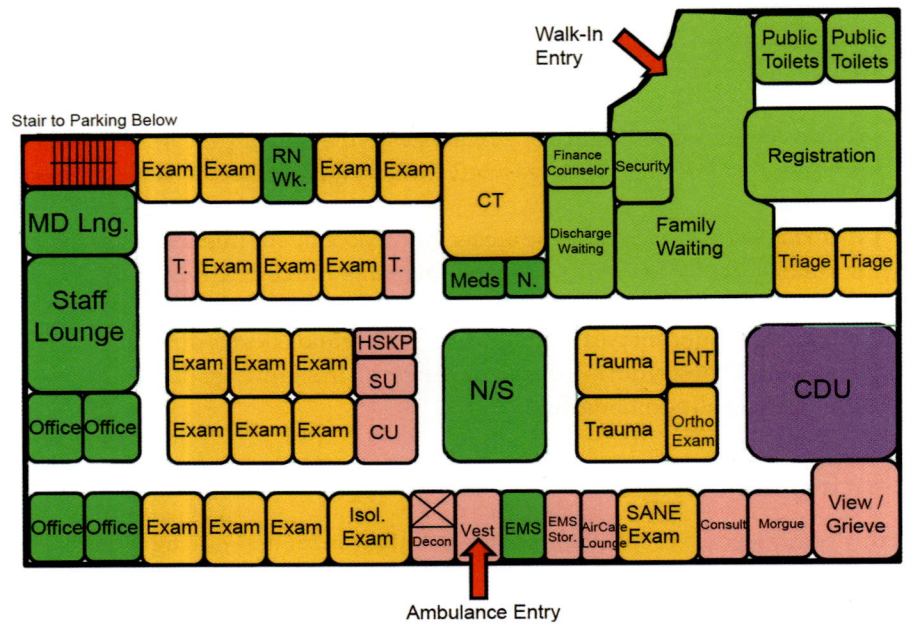

FIGURE 27.1 ■ Schematic of General Design Elements

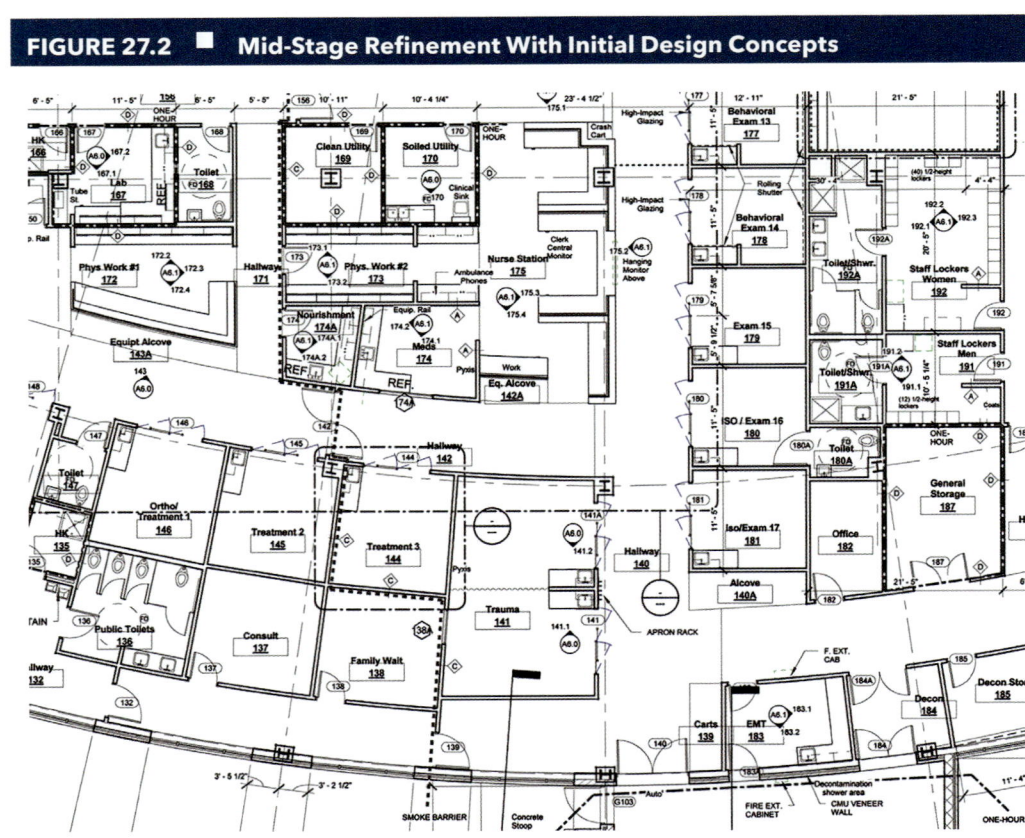

FIGURE 27.2 ■ Mid-Stage Refinement With Initial Design Concepts

FIGURE 27.3 ■ Late-Stage Technical Plans

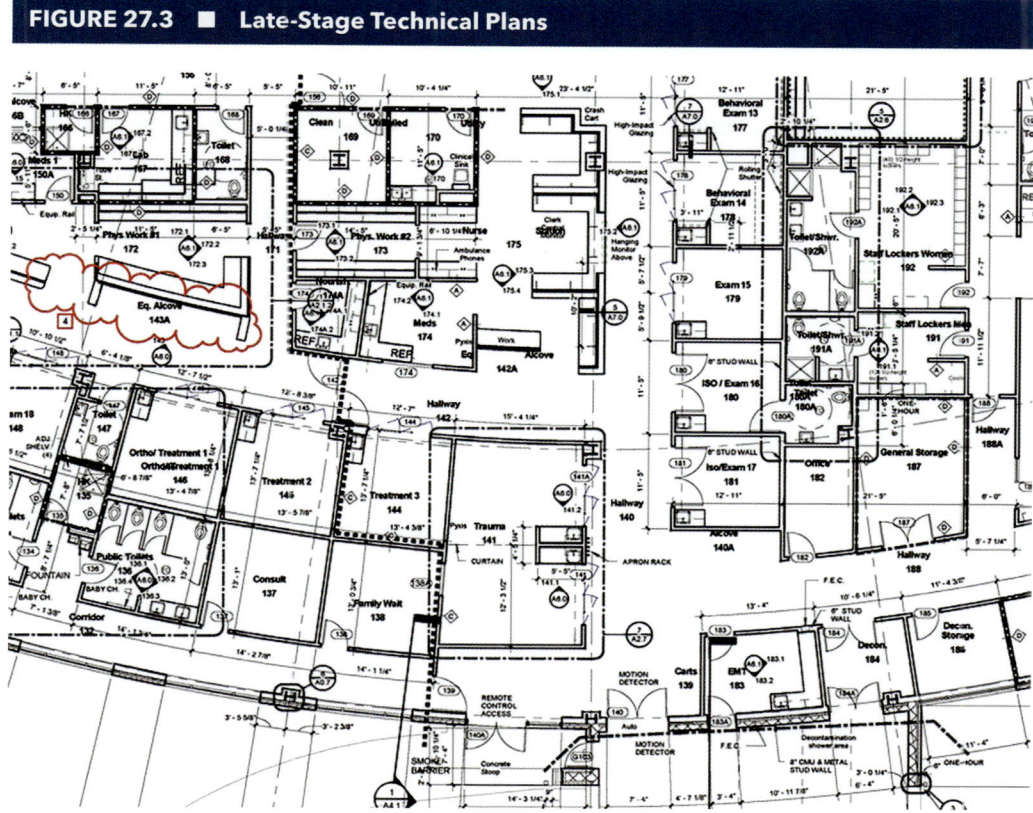

are tested and evaluated. New knowledge gained through early design may change previous assumptions regarding traffic patterns, the size of areas, clustering and organization of components, and access for key care personnel. Revising and redrawing multiple solutions during this phase should be expected and encouraged to ensure identification of the best plan.

Projecting Space Needs

One of the most important responsibilities of the design team is the "space program," which will be discussed in detail later in this chapter. Early planning frequently requires quick, gross estimates of total space requirements and budgets. A first step is determining how the service and volume of your department compare to those of peer/cohort EDs. The ED Benchmarking Alliance (EDBA) has developed definitions, performance measures, and data comparisons for EDs of similar volumes and acuities. This information allows the stratification of performance elements and design features to match the desired service characteristics. Using comparisons to similar institutions is essential in evaluating current operations and projecting future design needs (**Table 27.2**).

Factors That Stand Out

Certain factors stand out from the above data.

New EDs use more space and more patient care areas. The 12 years of EDBA data point to an increase in the physical area and number of patient care locations. These designs allow the staff to manage an older patient population with more chronic medical conditions,

TABLE 27.2 ■ EDBA Data Survey

Year	All EDs, visits per patient care space	Pediatric EDs, visits per patient care space	All EDs, visits per square foot
2017	1,510	1,723	2.9
2016	1,526	1,749	3.0
2015	1,515	1,731	3.0
2014	1,519	1,908	3.1
2013	1,553	1,886	3.1
2012	1,597	1,892	3.2
2011	1,610	1,815	3.2
2010	1,615	1,834	3.7
2009	1,677	1,697	3.5
2008	1,700	Not available	3.4
2007	1,710	Not available	3.9
2006	1,723	Not available	3.8

higher acuity, and longer length of stay (LOS). As a result of longer LOS, the average capacity of patient care spaces decreased from about 1,723 annual visits in 2006 to about 1,500 visits in 2017. The gross square footage and visits per square foot provide a crude proxy for how "compact" an ED is. Most EDs are sized for 2.5 to 5.0 annual visits per square foot, with average space utilization decreasing in 12 years from 3.9 to about 3.0 patient visits per square foot. This decline is primarily a result of overcrowding and the increase in overall size of the departments.

Visits per patient care space differ for adults and children and by total volume. Pediatric EDs, which tend to have shorter turnaround times, average about 1,723 visits per patient care space annually, a number that is significantly higher than the overall average of 1,500. This higher capacity is due, in part, to the lower use of imaging, electrocardiography, and other diagnostic resources in pediatric patients. It is critical that the ED leaders responsible for designing the department consider the use of these tools and understand the spatial proximities and transportation logistics that benefit both adult and pediatric patients who require these studies.

Lower ratios of visits per treatment area are also present in very large and very small hospitals, and the highest treatment space utilization can be found in hospitals that see 20,000 to 40,000 patients per year. Departments that report fewer visits per treatment space tend to report lower walkaway rates.

Advanced imaging per patient, especially in high-acuity EDs, is increasing. The use of advanced imaging imaging has increased to approximately 24 uses per 100 patients, especially in high-acuity EDs, trauma centers, and stroke centers. Computed tomography scanners for ED patients should be housed in a location that is in or near the ED to allow for timely imaging and safe patient transitions to and from the scanner.

The LOS of admitted and boarding patients affects overall ED LOS. The LOS of admitted patients has the largest impact on overall ED LOS. The boarding time of admitted patients is

> **BOX 27.2 ■ USE REALISTIC NUMBERS**
>
> **Beware of "magic" numbers:** It is important to recognize that benchmark and peer data are typically descriptive and not explanatory. Performance variations should be assessed along with median values. This information should inform the planning process and not dictate key metrics. One metric commonly cited to estimate the number of required treatment spaces is the annual visits per "bed." Historically, a ratio of 2,000 visits per bed has been used as a quick estimator of required bed needs. Over the past decade, as ED LOS has increased and hospitals have recognized the need to eliminate the wait for first contact with a provider, the ratio of visits per treatment space has dropped to 1,400 to 1,500 for nonteaching hospitals.

a key driver of overall ED bed needs. High-volume EDs often generate a higher percentage of admissions. Approximately 67% of all inpatient admissions are processed through the ED.

Predicting the Number of Beds

Key goals of the ED design team include determining the number of required treatment spaces and maximizing their efficiency. The two most significant variables in predicting needs are the average number of patients seen per day and the median LOS. (**Box 27.2** emphasizes the need to be realistic when interpreting and applying benchmark and peer data.)

Organizational models that emphasize "Lean" and similar operational improvement techniques can help reduce ED patient LOS. The use of nontraditional treatment spaces, such as results waiting areas, offers an opportunity to further decrease treatment space LOS and improve the patient experience. This results in the need for fewer treatment spaces. Planning leaders must be careful to consider the acuity and flow of patients in their department and not simply use benchmark data when making assumptions about a new or renovated ED.

Other process changes in patient management are a further driver of ED design during the predesign phase. EDs are providing care in chairs, recliners, and other upright spaces. It is unclear if patients benefit from "vertical care," but there are clearly many who are more uncomfortable in beds or on stretchers. For EDs using team triage models, spaces that can serve both for greeting and for rapid care (some using recliners because of their flexibility) are a very effective use of square footage.[2]

Building codes prohibit the use of hallway spaces for patient management. This is not tolerated in any hospital and should not be part of the planned process for managing patients in the ED. To the degree that the median LOS for a particular department varies from the "typical" ED, the ratio of visits per treatment space will change. A rural or community hospital without a major trauma service may experience a significantly lower median LOS, raising the ratio of annual visits per treatment space. Conversely, EDs with significantly longer median LOS may accommodate fewer visits per treatment area.

Current ratios of departmental gross square feet (DGSF) per treatment space typically range from 650 to 750 DGSF per treatment space (**Table 27.3**). If the quick estimate of treatment space results in 20 beds, the "order of magnitude" DGSF to support the service would be estimated at 13,000 to 15,000 DGSF. These estimates do not necessarily apply to academic departments, which have teaching and administrative space requirements that do not support direct patient care functions. Note that the visits per square foot for newer EDs are significantly lower than the EDBA measures for current facilities.

TABLE 27.3 ■ Recent ED Design Projects

Major Teaching ED	Target Annual Visits	Treatment Rooms	Visits/ Treatment Room	Treatment Room Avg. Net Sq. Ft.	ED Only			ED + Admin Space			Actual Built DGSF	Actual Built DGSF/ Bed
					DGSF ED only	DGSF/ Treatment ED only	Visits/ DGSF ED only	DGSF ED + Admin	DGSF/ Treatment ED + Admin	Visits/ SF with Admin		
●	121,000	88	1,375	140	54,200	616	2.2	62,703	713	1.9	63,000	716
	32,000	22	1,455	140	16,654	757	1.9	19,321	878	1.7	29,020	1,209
	60,000	41	1,463	154	27,400	668	2.2	32,240	786	1.9	36,340	886
●	70,000	50	1,400	140	26,288	526	2.7	29,993	600	2.3	32,000	640
	37,000	28	1,321	130	16,037	573	2.3	18,557	663	2.0	21,140	729
	40,000	21	1,905	140	15,696	747	2.5	18,423	877	2.2	30,100	1,115
●	90,000	73	1,233	160	45,986	630	2.0	49,653	680	1.8	64,500	872
	65,000	45	1,444	140	24,424	543	2.7	27,224	605	2.4	33,880	753
	65,000	39	1,667	150	26,186	671	2.5	30,013	770	2.2	37,700	838
	63,000	40	1,575	130	29,150	729	2.2	29,150	729	2.2	29,150	729
	33,600	21	1,600	150	14,200	676	2.4	16,576	789	2.0	26,680	861
●	65,000	42	1,548	120	25,786	614	2.5	27,991	666	2.3	24,800	590
	22,885	16	1,430	145	13,924	870	1.6	14,348	897	1.6	16,725	836
	65,000	42	1,548	140	25,786	614	2.5	27,991	666	2.3	34,800	829
●	45,000	32	1,406	140	25,853	808	1.7	41,596	1300	1.1	40,540	1,267
●	104,000	70	1,387	150	40,237	575	2.6	51,052	729	2.0		
●	110,000	76	1,447	140	32,656	430	3.4	37,561	494	2.9		
●	80,000	62	1,290	140	38,550	622	2.1	42,527	686	1.9		
●	47,000	35	1,343	140	20,984	600	2.2	23,774	679	2.0		
	64,000	35	1,829	140	22,789	651	2.8	26,756	764	2.4		
●	125,000	78	1,603	N/A	52,000	667	2.4	54,900	704	2.3		
●	185,000	164	1,128	N/A	1,05,800	645	1.7	105,800	645	1.7		
	60,000	44	1,364	N/A	25,260	574	2.4	28,360	645	2.1		
	45,000	33	1,364	N/A	23,000	697	2.0	22,351	677	2.0		
●	110,000	89	1,236	N/A	57,000	640	1.9	59,090	664	1.9		
	100,000	87	1,149	N/A	50,654	582	2.0	54,482	626	1.8		
	50,000	27	1,852	N/A	12,400	459	4.0	12,935	479	3.9		

●	125,000	103	1,157	N/A	81,500	755	1.5	84,446	782	1.5	
	50,000	23	1,786	N/A	26,500	946	1.9	27,900	996	1.8	
●	135,000	63	1,985	N/A	67,500	993	2.0	69,411	1021	1.9	
	55,000	42	1,310	N/A	33,554	799	1.6	33,554	799	1.6	
	120,000	82	1,463	N/A	40,000	488	3.0	42,853	523	2.8	
		High	1,985			993	4.0		1300	3.9	1267
		Low	1,128			430	1.5		479	1.1	590
		Average	1,471			661	2.3		735	2.1	858

Caution is important at this planning stage. Early numbers and projections can quickly become established as "facts" despite their cursory nature. It is highly recommended that a range of estimates be developed that can provide boundaries based on market forces (like the closure of a competitor hospital), hospital service-line changes (e.g., the addition of an interventional cardiac lab), overall market growth (a Sunbelt issue), ED LOS, and changes in hospital administration or direction.

Detailed Analysis

Classic systems-approach methods can be useful in the planning process. One typical goal of these tools is to ensure that space components do not constrain the flow of patients through the emergency service. This planning approach should be achieved through a careful analysis of current and anticipated variables that affect the service. The application of this information through the use of techniques like queuing theory and simulation modeling will help the planners make informed decisions.

Typically, the elements that influence the emergency service are divided into two groups:

- *External variables* that place demand on the department or are outside the control of the emergency service
- *Internal variables* that include organization, staffing, space, and technology elements used to respond to the demand

Examples of external variables include the arrival pattern of patients, the acuity mix of care required, hospital strategies and service-line changes, and strategic actions of other providers in the service area. It is important to focus on these factors first because they reflect the basic purpose of an emergency service's existence: *the patients*. In today's complex health-care environment, these components are the hardest to determine.

Space requirements should be estimated based on peak demand. One key element in determining peak periods is the arrival patterns of patients. An analysis of seasonal variations, day of week, and time of day should be undertaken to determine the maximum period of projected patient arrivals. This is typically expressed in arrivals per hour during the peak period. In addition to these arrival patterns, assumptions regarding the mix of patient acuity and special needs (behavioral health patients, pediatrics, and others) can be identified as part of the external analysis.

Perhaps the most difficult component of the external analysis involves projecting the annual visit target. Factors that contribute to the complexity include changing utilization rates, population demographics, indigent care, and the actions of other providers in the ED's service area. One technique that can be used to address the uncertainty in forecasting is developing a range of projections based on alternative assumptions and then testing the facility implications of the alternative projections. Scenario planning techniques can be a valuable approach in developing alternatives.

Other external variables include existing and future service lines. Important service lines that influence ED volume and acuity include trauma center status, cardiac services (especially interventional care), stroke center status, orthopedics, pediatrics, mental health, and planned urgent and primary care. The presence of these service lines will drive the need for space that is dedicated to those patient services. Many hospitals now attempt to decompress the main ED by building and staffing urgent care centers, satellite EDs, and primary care centers. If these programs actually change patient behavior, the result will be higher acuity in the main ED and moderation of volume growth.

In addition to understanding the arrival patterns of patients on peak days, the mix, typically defined by the Emergency Severity Index (ESI) or other triage acuity measurement, is important in determining the appropriate type of treatment spaces and the acceptable levels of queuing for the patient population. Ideally, the planning team should be able to break down the percentage of patients (and their LOS) requiring trauma/resuscitation spaces, general exam rooms, behavioral treatment spaces, and low-acuity treatment areas. It is reasonable to assume that any major capital investment in the ED will be a once-in-a-decade occurrence. Forecasting workload and patient mix at least 5 years into the future should be used, at a minimum, to determine treatment space needs.

Initiating a major building project provides a unique opportunity to explore new operational models. Sufficient time should be taken to identify, prototype, and site-visit new models of care delivery. Flow and patient throughput are enhanced by universal room design, and patient care areas must be designed for infection control, noise reduction, and staff efficiency. At the department level, the design must facilitate ambulance reception, toileting availability and cleanliness, and space designed for the safe processing of mental health patients.

Staffing of the ED is a unique internal variable. There are similarities between institutions, but essentially every ED has a unique staffing mix and organizational culture. Staffing mix, ratios of nursing and physician care, presence of a dedicated pharmacist, presence of trainees and physician extenders, and the teams that are part of an academic teaching hospital all drive design needs. The more disciplines present in the department, the greater the need for space that is dedicated to staff maintenance and functionality.

The Programming Process

The major products of the programming phase include:

- Identification of the desired physical organization
- Listing of all space elements
- Identification of key functional (performance) requirements

The most important task of the programming phase is determining the required number of treatment spaces. The previously described external and internal analyses are synthesized into the number and mix of room types. The variability of patient arrival patterns, patient acuity, service needs, and LOS can make this a difficult task. However, a number of analytical tools can support this process.[1,3]

Deterministic Modeling

Deterministic modeling, which can be done on Excel spreadsheets, estimates room requirements by calculating the total minutes of treatment space needed and then dividing this number by the minutes of care that can be provided by each room. The art of this approach rests on the judgment the planning team uses to estimate the maximum utilization that can be achieved during given time periods. The higher the assumed utilization, the greater the probability that patients will experience delays in access to rooms.

If this approach is used, the analysis should focus on the peak demand period—peak month, day of week, and hours of care (typically 11 AM to 11 PM for adult EDs). In this scenario, a reasonable assumption for the maximum utilization of treatment spaces would be in the range of 80% to 85%. If the period of analysis is the entire 24-hour period, then a lower utilization target should be used (50%-60%) to reflect the underutilization of space during low-census times of the day.

Simulation Modeling

Simulation modeling is a much more sophisticated approach for incorporating variations in arrival patterns and LOS. A major benefit of this tool is its ability to replicate actual arrival patterns, statistical distributions of LOS, and patient flow decisions. The output capabilities of these tools include their ability to estimate potential queuing for access to treatment space, room utilization, and other operational issues. New organizational and operational procedures can be tested to determine their actual performance and space implications. Accurate operating assumptions are critically important to this approach and require careful coordination with the laboratory and imaging leaders of the hospital to ensure that accurate input variables are built into the models.

Simple simulation models can be built quickly. Conversely, the analysis of staffing and operational options, while providing more robust information for decision making, can be data intense and require significant staff time and programming effort. However, more accurate assumptions and analysis will lead to a more appropriate configuration. Unfortunately, pressure to resolve space problems or proceed within the overall project timetable can limit the ability to execute a complex simulation model. For the best planning process, the ED strategic design teams should be using these techniques in the predesign phase.

Once the desired organizational model and number of treatment spaces are identified, the next step is developing a space listing of all areas of the emergency service. A typical space listing will show the individual rooms, the net square footage of each area, and note any special requirements for the space (**Table 27.4**).

Regulations, Codes, and Standards

Most states have adopted recommendations defining minimum room sizes and other requirements as established by the Facilities Guidelines Institute (FGI).[4] The planning team should review their state's version of the FGI Guidelines for the Design and Construction of Hospital and Health Care Facilities to ensure compliance. Experts on local fire codes must be involved in the design to fulfill these requirements to the letter. Occasionally, state health organizations, disaster planners, and standard-setting agencies also issue design elements that must be addressed.[3-7] A hospital can always request a variance from space guidelines when there is a logical and compelling reason to do so. The state agency that has legal jurisdiction over building code enforcement will have the ultimate responsibility for approving or denying variances.

TABLE 27.4 ■ Typical Space Listing

	Emergency Service Area/Room	NSF/Unit	# of Units	Total NSF	Subtotal	Comments
Ambulance entrance						
1	Ambulance canopy					Four ambulance bays; enclose with doors
2	Ambulance entrance vestibule	180	1	180		Includes space for gurney storage
3	Decontamination room	120	1	120		
4	EMT storage	60	1	60		
5	Decontamination storage supplies	120	1	120		
6	EMT/police workroom	140	1	140		Charting/break area
Public entrance						
7	Security office	140	1	140		Desk area in waiting room
8	Entry vestibule	140	1	140		
9	Stretcher/wheelchair storage	80	1	80		
10	Reception	80		160		Includes one station
11	Triage/registration rooms	120	1	120		
12	Registration interview cubicles	60	1	60		Backup space; assumes bedside registration
13	Registration work area	80	1	80		Split near triage/registration area and in core
14	Financial counseling/co-pay	100	1	100		Alcove area near exit
15	Waiting—open seating	18	20	360		Small clusters of seating 1.5 seats per treatment
16	Family waiting rooms	170	1	170		Seating for 8 in each room
17	Pediatric play area	80	1	80		
18	Computer terminal	35	1	35		Public access
19	"Hot" office	100	1	100		Social work finance, mystery, etc.
20	Public telephones	10	1	10		
21	Vending alcove	80	1	80		
22	Public toilets	120	2	240		
	Subtotal				1,955	

	Emergency Service Area/Room	NSF/ Unit	# of Units	Total NSF	Subtotal	Comments
Critical care/trauma						
23	Trauma/resuscitation	340	1	340		Design for standard occupancy for two patients
Acute clinical area						
24	Treatment	180	3	540		
25	General exam rooms	150	17	2,550		Adapt one room into behavioral
26	General exam–psychiatry	140	0			Swing with general exam
27	Eye/ENT	150	1	150		
28	Subcharting alcove	10	12	120		
29	Subwaiting	60	2	120		Mix of chairs and wheelchair waiting
30	Patient toilet	55	4	220		
	Staff work areas					
31	Clerks/secretarial	60	2	120		
32	Monitor output	20	1	20		
33	Pneumatic tube station	20	1	20		
34	Communications alcove	20	1	20		
35	Computer workstations–central	30	12	360		To be confirmed
Other support areas						
36	Radiographic/fluoroscopy unit	240	1	240		
37	Digital cassette loader/reading	80	1	80		
38	CT	340	1	340		
39	Tech work area	80	1	80		
40	Portable units alcove	40	1	40		Imaging and ultrasound
41	Clean utilities	100	0			In line 45
42	Soiled utilities	80	2	160		
43	Orthopedic supply area	80	1	80		Equipment supply and alcove cart
44	Medication	80	1	80		
45	Nourishment	80	1	80		

(Continued)

TABLE 27.4 ■ Continued

	Emergency Service Area/Room	NSF/Unit	# of Units	Total NSF	Subtotal	Comments
46	Clean supply/equipment storage	460	1	460		
47	Janitor closet	60	1	60		
48	Cart alcove	20	1	20		Crash cart
	Subtotal				**6,300**	
Staff support						
49	Lockers—female	3	40	120		Half-height lockers—locate with toilet area
50	Lockers—male	3	20	60		Half-height lockers—locate with toilet area
51	Lounge	140	1	140		
52	Staff toilets	60	1	60		
53	Staff toilets	80	1	80		
54	Office, Director	140	1	140		
55	Office Medical Director	140	1	140		Shared with Mcare
56	Office, Nurse Manager	140	1	140		
57	Conference/education	400	1	400		Seating for 20
58	Trauma coordinator	100	1	100		
59	Equipment storage	140	1	140		
60	On-call room	80	1	80		Off of physician lounge area
61	Shower	60	1	60		
62	Communications closet	100	1	100		
	Subtotal				**1,760**	
	Total NSF				10,015	
	NSF administrative support				1,760	Includes staff support space
	NSF emergency services				8,255	
	Net-to-gross factor					
	Emergency service			1.60	13,208	
	Emergency administration			1.35	2,376	
	Total DGSF			**15,584**		
					708	Per treatment space

Some states—in an attempt to control health-care costs—require issuance of a certificate of need (CON) before a major hospital construction project can proceed. The CON is issued if the state approves the paperwork the hospital has submitted. A well-developed and documented space program will be an important part of the required documentation.

Nonclinical Care Space

Net square footage is the sum of the usable areas within a building, including the interiors of rooms. However, the sum of the net square footage for all of the areas in the department does not reflect the total space required for the service. Adjustments for corridors, structural elements, and mechanical systems must be added to the net square footage to estimate the total DGSF. The final footprint is site dependent and considers factors such as traffic access, security, weather patterns, and adjacencies to key service areas. An additional factor for public circulation, stairwells, and support spaces may be required for a project. This is called a "building grossing factor."

Determining the size of the treatment space is a necessary component of programming. One of the first considerations is determining the role and placement of family/significant others. If the philosophy is that the family/significant others belong at the bedside, then treatment rooms will be built to allow for chairs and movable space. If the ED staff determines that families belong away from the patient, then space needs to be redistributed from the treatment area to a family waiting room. Simple, full-scale mock-ups of space can be very useful in confirming the appropriate room size. Decisions regarding patient support issues, such as toileting, security, and isolation, are other factors that can help dictate the size and dimensions of patient rooms. Staff should visit recently completed EDs and ideally test room dimensions with simple, full-scale mock-ups.

Freestanding EDs and Micro-Hospitals

Freestanding emergency facilities have emerged over the past decade as a viable care model. There are currently two types of freestanding facilities:

- *Hospital-based freestanding EDs* are associated with a hospital but provide separate, distinct services. As provider-based facilities, they are typically reimbursed for ED services at the rate that would be paid to the larger hospital, including the facility fee. Some private insurers are challenging the facility fee charge.
- *Independent freestanding EDs* are recognized in a limited number of states providing emergency services without being associated with any hospital. Most are classified by Medicare as outpatient clinics, resulting in a lower reimbursement level for fees and testing.

The Emergency Benchmarking Alliance data for freestanding EDs indicate a lower-acuity pattern, with only 8% of patients being admitted, and a slightly better throughput time than what is seen with hospital-based EDs with similar volumes. A sample of existing freestanding EDs indicates a slightly higher area per bed than for similar hospital-based services, primarily due to the dedicated diagnostic and support services.

Freestanding EDs in rural areas are currently being encouraged by the American Hospital Association through a proposed new Medicare classification, the "Rural Emergency Medical Center Model."[8] This proposal would create a fee structure based on ED services with additional reimbursement to compensate for the low volumes typically seen in rural settings. Criteria for this designation would exclude acute inpatient beds. Additional outpatient services and skilled nursing could be provided as part of a Rural Emergency Medical Center Act. To date, an act of this type has not yet been passed by Congress, but efforts will continue to bolster emergency medical care in rural, sparsely populated areas.

> **BOX 27.3 ■ CRITICAL DESIGN QUESTIONS**
>
> - Does the design provide efficient patient flow and visitor access?
> - Are staff work areas, supplies, and medications located to maximize staff efficiency?
> - Are work areas designed to implement information technologies, maximize staff interaction, and utilize appropriate visual connectivity?
> - Can the ED staff up and down during the day to respond to patient demand without creating unnecessary queues, inefficient staff ratios, or unsafe care?
> - Can the ED functionally respond to high-risk potential events?
> - Is the design flexible to accommodate future growth through internal adaptation or expansion?
> - Is the design efficient from a square foot/treatment perspective?
> - Are room designs flexible to accommodate service-line changes?
> - Is there a communication system that will serve the patient and staff needs?

An evolution of the freestanding emergency services is the "micro-hospital." Components of this type of facility typically include emergency care, outpatient imaging, ambulatory surgery or procedure areas, and observation beds. The implementation of micro-hospitals has been concentrated in suburban areas of major cities to expand hospital markets into new areas. Acquisition of land to allow the future conversion of a micro-hospital into a full-scale hospital has allowed hospital systems to incrementally expand services as the surrounding community grows or in response to strategic shifts on the location of specialty services.

The potential for adapting micro-hospitals to rural settings could help alleviate the crisis caused by the closures of critical-access hospitals, particularly if the provision of observation beds would comply with regulations proposed for inclusion in a Rural Emergency Medical Center Act. A micro-hospital in a rural setting can provide treatment for chronic diseases, dental care services, and social spaces to combat isolation as a sustainable health-care delivery model.

ED DESIGN GEOMETRY

Contemporary emergency designs can be grouped into three general design concepts: traditional ballroom layouts, pod clusters, and inner core/linear layouts. To incorporate appropriate design priorities into these concepts, critical questions like those presented in **Box 27.3** must be asked and answered.

Traditional Ballroom Layout

Until recently, the predominant ED design model was the ballroom layout, which wraps patient care stations around a central working area (**Figure 27.4**). This model allows maximum visibility of patients and easy control of the department. Ideally, there is a separation between EMS ingress and public access and close proximity to key services, particularly imaging. As workload volumes increase and more departments provide private patient rooms, the functional limit of the ballroom model is typically reached at 16 to 18 rooms. A larger unit loses the ability to maintain visual observation of all patient care areas, and the size of the staff work area starts to increase.

FIGURE 27.4 ■ Traditional Ballroom Layout Model

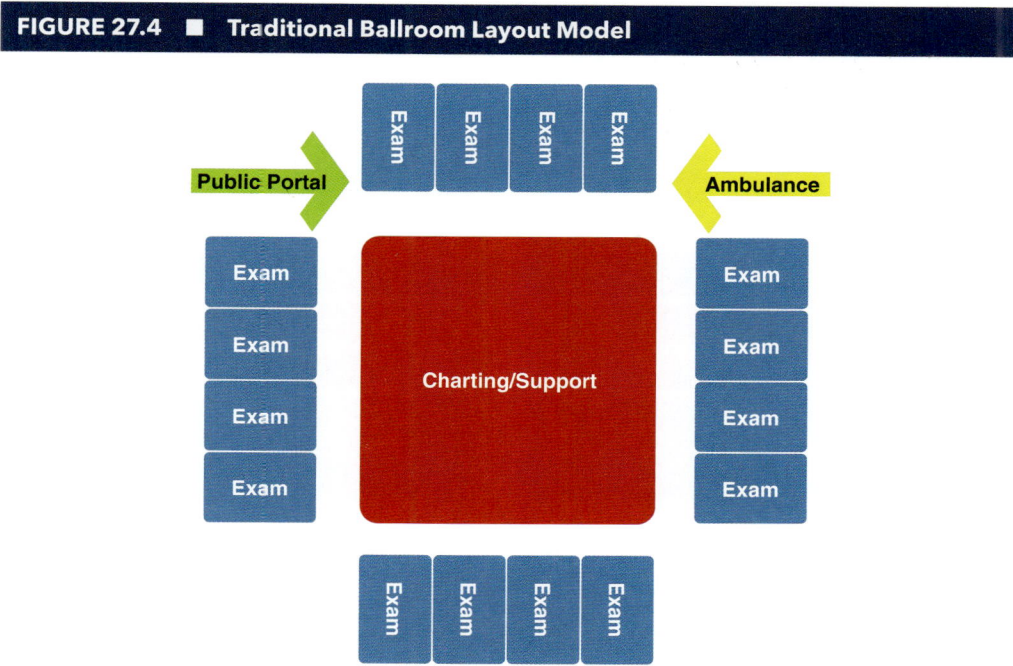

The Pod Design

One response to these issues is the pod design, which clusters 8 to 12 examination rooms together with appropriate support areas and internal circulation to other pods (**Figure 27.5**). This concept maintains efficient staff travel and creates a balance between support space and treatment areas. The pod design further allows the expansion and contraction of bed spaces based on volume needs. However, when patient volume and workloads rapidly change, an inability to efficiently staff pods may become a limitation

FIGURE 27.5 ■ The Pod Model

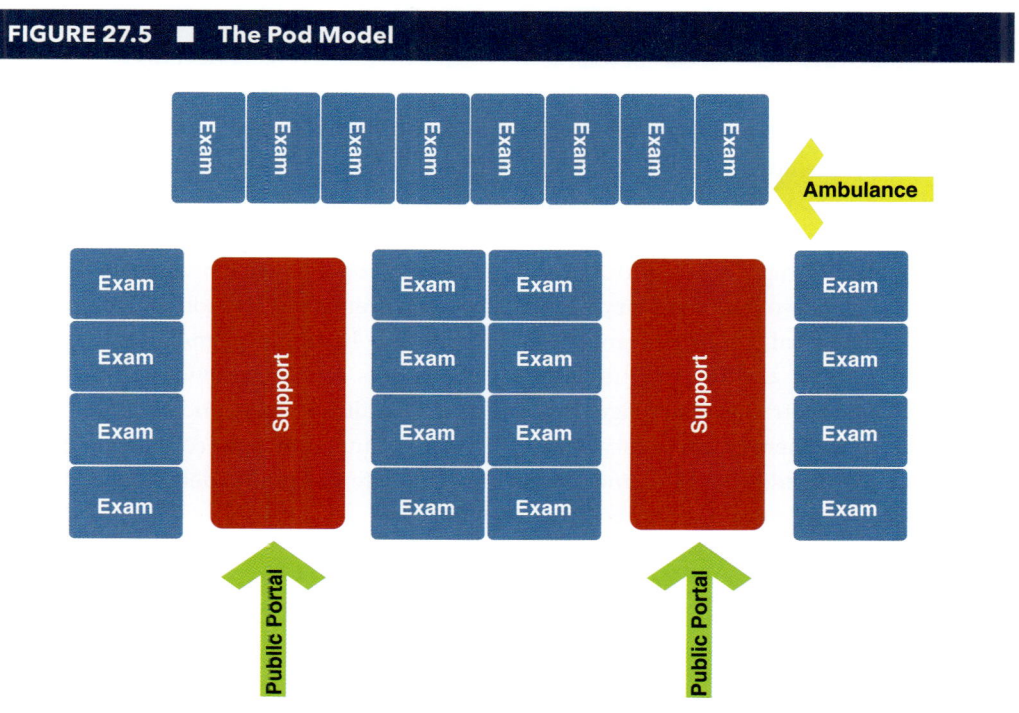

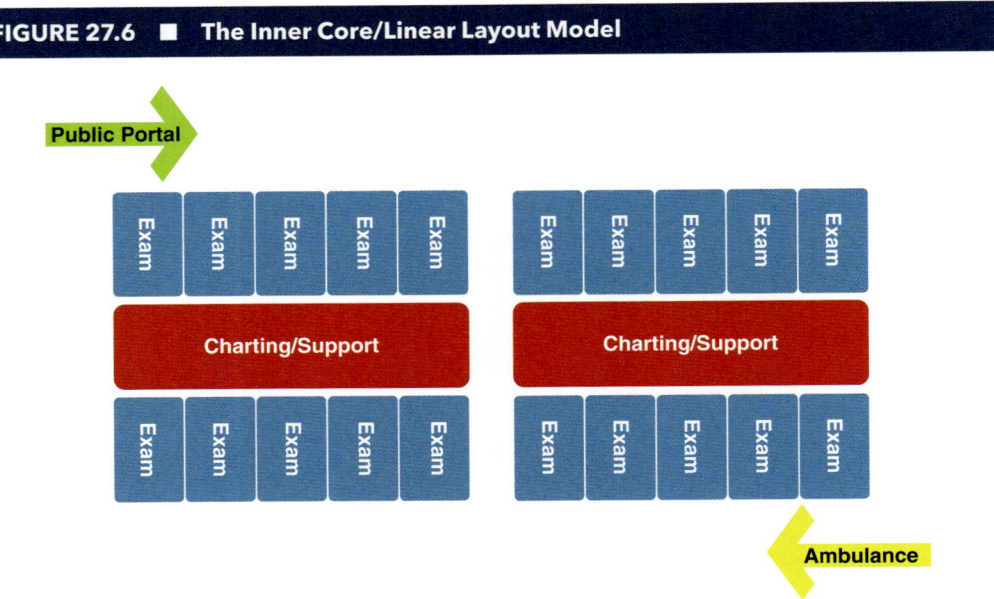

FIGURE 27.6 ■ The Inner Core/Linear Layout Model

of this design model. Additional issues may arise if pods are assigned to specific services, such as pediatrics, fast track, behavioral medicine, or observation. The ability to reassign pods can quickly degenerate into political turf battles with each group focusing on optimizing its own work area.

Inner Core/Linear Layout

A third organizational concept is emerging as a solution to the changing hourly volumes, staff efficiency, and expanding needs associated with growth. The inner-core concept organizes treatment rooms around a staff work area. Rooms are dual entry, with patients and family accessing treatment spaces from a perimeter corridor (**Figure 27.6**). Conceptually, staffs work in decentralized zones that support 10 to 12 examination rooms. These zones are staffed up and down to match the typical increase or decrease in patient volume throughout the day. If positioned correctly within the institution's overall space, expansion of the ED could be achieved logically and efficiently.

Each institution should evaluate these and other space and organization concepts while considering their stated goals and the realities of site and budget constraints. Early stages of schematic design can test alternative organization models. It is essential to allow adequate time to fairly evaluate a variety of options. Decisions should not be made prematurely. The institution's leadership team should identify critical milestones for each phase of the process, thereby helping to avoid unnecessary time pressure and premature decision-making.

New operational processes and technologies are being implemented to achieve higher throughput and shorter times between arrivals to first provider contact.[4] The reconfiguration of traditional triage, internal results waiting areas, and intake areas for the quick management of low-acuity patients are generating new space conformations. The planning team should carefully and thoroughly evaluate these new delivery modes and their impact on facility and design requirements.[1,9]

DISASTER SCENARIOS AND SECURITY ISSUES

Hospitals are an integral element of community preparedness for major events, including disasters. As such, the design of an ED must account for space and safety needs that might result from these scenarios.[10]

> **BOX 27.4 ■ DISASTER SCENARIOS**
>
> **Lean process planning and event scenarios:** The application of new operational techniques that incorporate the design of an ED for dangerous and disaster events. Planning will consider space needs for safe and adequate care and may include the application of results waiting and intake chair areas, which may allow for significant improvements in throughput times and space requirements. The planning team should ensure that the desire to minimize space through internal waiting and other techniques does not jeopardize the ability to protect staff, the hospital, and other patients from contagious diseases, violence, or other threats.

High-risk events that could occur in the ED should be considered during the programming phase and continue through design (**Box 27.4**). This process involves considering any risk issues identified by the facility's hazard vulnerability analysis and community preparedness efforts. Hospital leadership, hospital security, community emergency and security personnel, and other appropriate agencies should be contacted to determine potential threats. These potential dangers include chemical, biologic, radiologic, nuclear, and explosive incidents as well as mass shootings and direct threats to the emergency service. The risk of each threat and its facility requirements should be assessed.

An ED's ability to accommodate patient surges resulting from these special events is an important consideration. Planning for these situations can provide clear benefits for staff efficiency and safety. If addressed early in the design process, quarantine zones, the conversion of public spaces into treatment areas, and security issues can be addressed with minimal effect on space and project costs.

Disaster preparedness includes planning for the appropriate size and number of patient care spaces. Additionally, recent events have required next-generation EDs to address the risk to staff and patients from threats, including contagious diseases, community violence, and extreme weather events. Recent incidents of mass violence, some even targeted at hospitals, highlight the responsibility to appropriately design the receiving areas and entrance to the ED.

Biologic, chemical, and radiologic events require significant facility design considerations to facilitate patient care while protecting the hospital staff. In these incidents, the at-risk patients must be guided through the ED utilizing a dedicated and safe flow process that includes decontamination areas and/or cohort quarantine zones within, or adjacent to, the

> **BOX 27.5 ■ CRITICAL PRIORITIES FOR SAFE DESIGN**
>
> - Does the design provide the safest possible environment for ED staff? The ability to flow patients directly into an appropriately designed receiving area, quarantine zone, quick lockdown of staff areas, and the design of traffic access to limit public vehicle arrivals under direct threat scenarios are examples of issues that may be appropriate considerations for an ED design.
> - Does the design protect the hospital from airborne contamination, toxic aerosols, liquid chemical or biologic agents, and other risks through the segregation of mechanical systems and limitation of patient transport through the hospital?
> - Does the design enable the ED to maintain operations and absorb the surges in patient flow through the use of support spaces? Does the design support the provision of safe patient care, the conversion of adjacent areas for ED use, and other techniques that allow a functional transition from normal operations to a surge situation?

ED. Another important consideration is the inclusion of a multipurpose utility dirty room for patient evaluation, decontamination, and care.

Potential risk situations point to three crucial priorities in the assessment of a department's design (**Box 27.5**). Early consideration of these issues can result in a flexible design with minimal initial construction cost implications.[5-7,11-15]

CONCLUSION

The design of the ED is a product of its leaders' ability to project future demands, systems of care delivery, and service requirements for emergency care. An effective design allows flexibility over years in delivering quality care and a safe operation. Each emergency service program is a unique blend of patients, processes, and institutional characteristics. Designing the ED with flexibility maximizes the "sweet spot" between best estimates of needs and requirements of future emergency care delivery.

REFERENCES

1. Zilm F. Estimating emergency service treatment bed needs. *J Ambul Care Manage*. 2004;27(3):215-223. doi:10.1097/00004479-200407000-00005.

2. Sheahan M. Designing emergency departments to maximize staff communication. 2017. Available at: https://www.buildingbetterhealthcare.com/news/article_page/Improving_staff_communication_through_emergency_room_design/130569. Accessed June 2017.

3. *Health Buildings Note 15-10: Accident & Emergency Departments Planning and Design Guide*. 2013. Norwich, United Kingdom: United Kingdom Department of Health. ISBN: 0113229828.

4. Facility Guidelines Institute. *Guidelines for Design and Construction of Hospitals and Outpatient Facilities*. Chicago, Ill: American Society for Healthcare Engineering; 2014.

5. Zilm FD, Berry R, Pietrzak MP, Paratore A. Integrating disaster preparedness and surge capacity in emergency facility planning. *J Ambul Care Manage*. 2008;31(4):377-385. doi:10.1097/01.jac.0000336556.54460.25.

6. Whitcomb J, Trioano P, Coogan P, et al. Reforming the ED: a new vision for emergency medicine. *Physician Exec*. 2010;36(6):28-30.

7. Menes K, Tintinalli J, Plaster L. How one Las Vegas ED saved hundreds of lives after the worst mass shooting in U.S. history. 2017. Available at: http://epmonthly.com/article/not-heroes-wear-capes-one-las-vegas-ed-saved-hundreds-lives-worst-mass-shooting-u-s-history/. Accessed November 03, 2017.

8. Ensuring Access in Vulnerable Communities: The Rural Emergency Medical Center Act of 2018. 2018. Available at: https://www.aha.org/system/files/2018-05/rural-emergency-medical-ctr-act-2018.pdf. Accessed Jun 15, 2018.

9. Gharaveis A, Hamilton DK, Pati D, Shepley M. The impact of visibility on teamwork, collaborative communication, and security in emergency departments: an exploratory study. *HERD*. 2018;11(4):37-49. doi:10.1177/1937586717735290.

10. Henrich S, Cirrincione N. Preventive measures: designing for safety in the ED. 2018. Available at: https://www.healthcaredesignmagazine.com/trends/operations-facility-management/preventive-measures-safety-security/. Accessed February 21, 2018.

11. Zilm F. Designing for emergencies. Integrating operations and adverse-event planning. *Health Facil Manage*. 2010;23(11):39-42.

12. Ciottone GR, Biddinger P, Darling R, et al. *Disaster Medicine*. 2nd ed. Philadelphia, Pa: Elsevier; 2016.

13. Georges G. Design that meets Ebola at the door. *HCD Magazine*. 2016. Available at: http://www.healthcaredesignmagazine.com/trends/architecture/design-meets-ebola-door/. Accessed April 19, 2016.

14. Resilient design protects hospitals from natural disasters. 2015. Available at: https://www.hhnmag.com/articles/3643-resilient-design-protects-hospitals-from-natural-disasters. Accessed March 10, 2015.

15. Langlands B, Vincent D, Carr C. A case for the low-acuity patient treatment station: reducing the length of stay for emergency department visits. 2018. Available at: https://www.fgiguidelines.org/fgi-bulletin-6/. Accessed February 13, 2018.

ADDITIONAL READINGS

- Huddy J, Sanson TG. *Emergency Department Design: A Practical Guide to Planning for the Future*. Dallas, Tex: American College of Emergency Physicians; 2016.

CASE STUDIES

Case Study One: Tampa General Hospital

Frank Zilm, Frank Zilm & Associates, Inc.

Disaster Planning

Tampa General Hospital provides an excellent example of how to integrate disaster planning into a building design. During the programming of their new emergency service, a daylong workshop was conducted with representation from the emergency and trauma services, security, infection control, outside agencies responsible for disaster preparedness, and other high-risk stakeholders, including an adjacent military base and airport. The workshop attendees successfully identified potential threats and their implications for the ED.

The building design incorporated ideas from the Department of Homeland Security's ER One study, discussions with the state authority having jurisdiction, and unique ideas developed by the project architects. As a result, conducting mass decontamination, moving high-risk contagious patients, and responding to surges in arrivals were all integrated into the design with a minimal impact on capital costs. Although the ED was designed with 77 standard treatment spaces, the department could be expanded during surge events to absorb up to 270 patients by doubling the standard exam room capacity and using concealed medical gas panels in the waiting, office, consultation, and corridor areas.

The ability for mass decontamination was facilitated by converting a valet parking lot underneath the ED into a dedicated decontamination area. A route was also designed to move high-risk patients into the ED holding area without passing through the main department. The holding area could then be converted into a cohort treatment zone.

Design considerations for an ED should be based on its role in the community (e.g., a level 1 trauma service), alternative resources available to meet community needs, and the nature of high-risk events that could occur over the life of the facility.

Case Study Two: Robert Wood Johnson University Hospital

Jon Huddy, Huddy HealthCare Solutions, LLC

External and Internal Expansion

The Robert Wood Johnson University Hospital (RWJUH) is part of the RWJBarnabas Health system in northern New Jersey. This high-volume (designed for 120,000 visits), university-affiliated, urban ED serves a diverse patient population, including local neighborhood residents (adults and children) as well as level 1 trauma patients from across the New Jersey, New York, and Pennsylvania tri-state region. The project included the addition of 6,880 square feet to "infill" an existing ambulance drop-off bay and three phases that covered an additional 53,120 square feet in the ED. The addition of 45 patient spaces was delivered by:

- Sizing 21 of the private adult ED spaces and three trauma rooms for a second stretcher for surge/overflow
- Providing additional capacity utilizing results-pending spaces (vertical recliners and chairs) and imaging holding bays (designed as ED care spaces with gases and so on)

In the event of an extreme surge or disaster, the RWJUH ED is equipped with a total of 126 patient care spaces.

Clinical Leadership

The project was led by ED physician and nursing leaders with an initial focus on operational redesign. Robert M. Eisenstein, MD, chief of emergency medicine, had instituted an innovative "split emergency severity index 3 patient flow model" in the old, cramped ED that worked to expedite throughput. This initial "split-flow" model was used as a basis for the creation of a "care initiation" flow concept that became the basis for the architectural project. Dr. Eisenstein explains, "The focus on patient flow patterns at the outset of the project allowed our clinical team to establish expectations for rapid patient access. I can't overemphasize the role of the ED physician and the need to lead the process from the very beginning of any architectural redesign project." Nancy Bonalumi (clinical consultant for Huddy HealthCare Solutions) was involved in early process analytics and workflow development. She adds, "Having ED physician and nursing leadership on the same page and focused on the same patient care goals is the first step in a project's ultimate success."

Defined Patient Flow

Upon entering the RWJUH ED, pediatric patients and their families are rapidly separated from the adult patients and placed in a pediatric-specific internal staging area. Walk-in and EMS-arriving ESI level 1 and 2 patients are expedited to the main ED or resuscitation trauma suite. All other adult patients are immediately assessed in the care initiation area (CIA). Emergency Severity Index 5s, 4s, and an estimated 40% of ESI 3s (lower acuity) remain in the CIA area for their entire stay. The remaining 60% of ESI 3s (higher acuity) start in the CIA to expedite their diagnostics, then continue to the main ED for their remaining care. The adult CIA has 13 private assessment rooms and 15 vertical recliners in its results-pending area. This area is adjacent to the EMS arrival corridor, and nonurgent patients arriving via ambulance are diverted to the CIA to avoid filling the main ED with lower-acuity patients. The department includes two general radiology rooms and a CT scanner that is accessible from the main ED and directly from the resuscitation/trauma suite.

Staff Communication

Faith Orsini, assistant vice president of construction services at RWJBarnabas Health, led the organization's design and construction efforts and was the link between the clinicians and design and construction teams. She attributes the success of the ED project to:

> . . . a detailed, clear construction plan developed in tandem with the clinical staff, hospital administration, EMS, design team, and contractors. This three-year, multiphased construction project was situated on a tight urban campus and was in a location within the hospital that encompasses five different buildings. The collaboration of the team allowed our ED to remain operational, treating over 100,000 patients each year while construction was in full swing. Integrating the clinical and EMS staff into the effort was a key to our success, allowing us to limit the impact of the construction on our patients.

Patient Wayfinding

The complexity of the interior renovations across numerous original buildings built at different times required the team to design around support columns and existing pipe and mechanical shafts. Interior design was a critical part of developing recognizable wayfinding for families and patients. Nicole Cocolin, president of DCC Design Group, led the interior design effort and said the team was focused on:

> . . . developing an internal design for the CIA and overall ED that supported efficient patient, family, staff, and material flow while honoring the privacy and well-being of

patients and their families. The use of curvature and translucent elements encouraged "treatment-to-care station" adjacencies, strategically promoting visibility, and clarifying wayfinding. The design objective was to lower patient anxiety levels, which are otherwise elevated when trying to navigate emergency care facilities without clear direction.

Project Data

The total cost of the project included $52 million in construction expenses and an additional $5 million in equipment and other costs. The construction costs included relocating multiple departments to clear space for the internal expansion of the ED as well as a great deal of site construction, including the lowering of the city street (by a few feet) to allow easier access to the new ambulance bay and public walk-in area.

Bed Types and Numbers				
Rooms	**Specific Room Types**	**#**	**Subtotal**	**Total**
Private rooms	Pediatric universal	14		
	Pediatric behavioral health	2		
	Care initiation area–Exam	13		
	Adult/pediatric trauma	3		
	Decontamination/Ebola/isolation	1		
	Adult behavioral health	12		
	Adult exam rooms	36	81	
Surge-flex capacity	Pediatric vertical/results pending	6		
	Care initiation area–Results pending	15		
	Adult pediatric trauma flex	3		
	Adult overflow/flex	18		
	Imaging holding bays (exam spaces)	3	45	
Total				126

CHAPTER 28

EFFECTIVE MARKETING OF THE EMERGENCY DEPARTMENT

John H. Proctor

Marketing is so basic that it cannot be considered a separate function. It is the whole business seen from the point of view of . . . the [patient].

—Peter Drucker, renowned management theorist and writer

The primary "customers" of the emergency department (ED) are patients (and their families) who are sick, injured, and afraid. Many patients choose the ED over other options due to its convenience; as no appointment is necessary, the ED "door is always open" and no one is turned away. In most circumstances, the patient can choose the venue for immediate care, so ED leaders must continue to implement process improvements that enhance their capacity to manage a growing population of patients. The competition for ED patients includes freestanding EDs, urgent care centers, specialty hospitals, retail clinics, and extended-hour primary care offices. Health-care service delivered remotely via telehealth technology is an emerging competitor to traditional emergency care. None of these competitors offer the comprehensive emergency and inpatient care services of a hospital-based ED. An effective marketing strategy can help ensure that patients are managed in the appropriate emergency care venue.

Figure 28.1 illustrates the growth strategy of an emergency physician group organized around four pillars: *resources, processes, value to customers,* and *financial performance*. The figure focuses on the customer as the heart of the organization's growth strategy. A successful organization builds a marketing initiative based on the customer's expectations, but there are other foundational aspects that must be in place to effectively meet and exceed customer expectations.

ATTRACTING MORE PATIENTS

The ability to expand the targeted customer base and increase revenue is essential to the success of any business enterprise. However, amid the challenges of crowding, inpatient holds, and diversion, many EDs resist the prospect of actively attracting more patients. To address these challenges to intentional growth, effective ED leaders collaborate with their facility leadership through operational and physical plant improvements to attract more business while still achieving quality, satisfaction, and improved throughput. Successful marketing initiatives depend on the organization's ability to deliver on what it promotes.

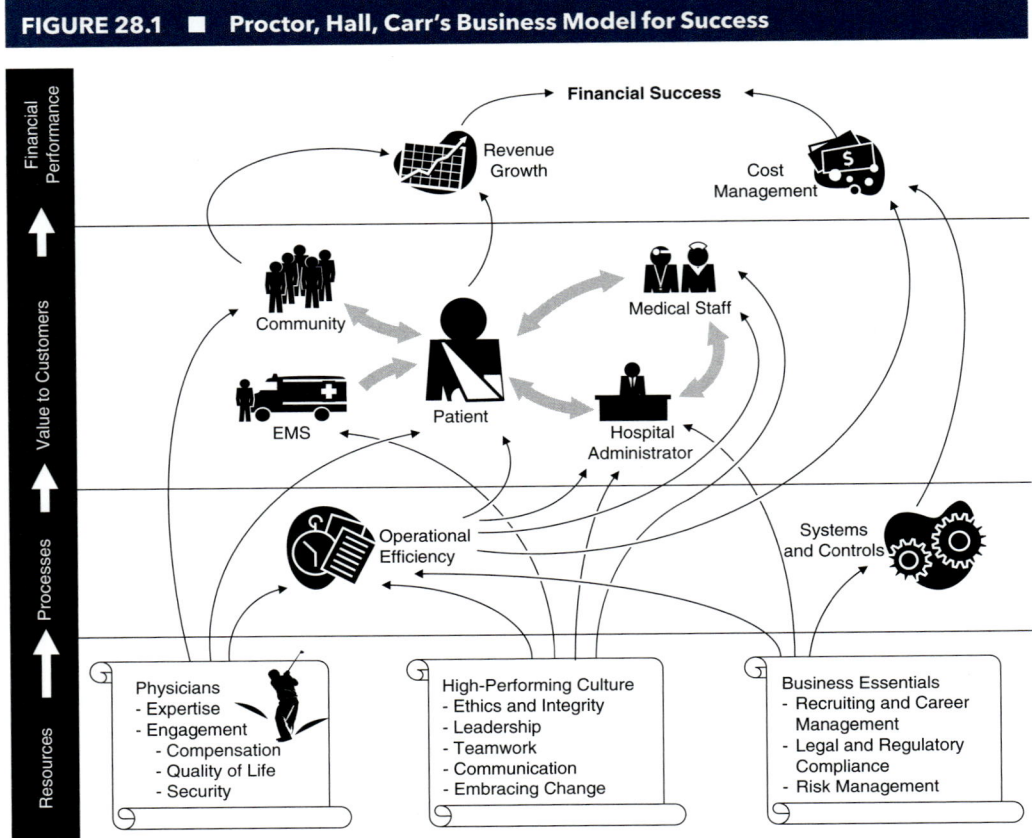

FIGURE 28.1 ■ Proctor, Hall, Carr's Business Model for Success

Source: The Business of Emergency Medicine, 2004.

Expanding Appropriate Access for Patients

In view of the operational and growth barriers, some organizations limit uncompensated or poorly compensated primary care delivery in the ED. Alternative access to care for the un(der)insured is accomplished by some ED leaders who develop networks with primary care providers and facilities. This approach expands the out-of-ED primary care for the underinsured, providing a more appropriate setting for the care of these patients.

Simultaneously, a successful marketing strategy seeks to attract a growing patient base from segments that help drive fiscal success for the department, the group, and the hospital. This approach includes outreach efforts to entice and efficiently deliver care to patients from attractive demographic areas and regional employers (**Box 28.1**).

BRANDING

The ED and each of its staff members are integral to the branding efforts of the larger hospital system. Successful branding of a medical institution produces a powerful, timeless image for patients and the hospital referral base.

> **BOX 28.1 ■ MARKETING ESSENTIALS**
>
> - Identify the target market.
> - Understand what they want.
> - Know what they don't want.
> - Determine how to effectively capture their attention.

FIGURE 28.2 ■ Cleveland Clinic Logo

Cleveland Clinic

The ED can most effectively support the brand through delivery of high-quality performance. The ED can further expand the institution's brand image into the community through organic growth. Examples might include partnering with the hospital (system) to develop new facilities, such as affiliated urgent care centers and free-standing EDs. Conversely, poor ED performance or reputation can produce a profound negative impact on the enterprise's branding effort, and further community expansion may be hampered.

The Cleveland Clinic provides an example of successful branding efforts in the health-care space. The institution is recognized as a national leader and model of quality health care with 7 million patients from all US states and 135 countries. Multiple specialties within the organization score in the top 5 of *US News & World Report's* annual rankings, and it capitalizes on its superior quality reputation through images and messaging that consistently communicate its brand (**Figure 28.2**). Additionally, the Cleveland Clinic inculcates its providers and workforce with a message emphasizing a patient-centric focus on quality and care, further driving its brand strength.

While an ED's performance and reputation are integral parts of the larger enterprise's branding campaign, few EDs brand themselves as stand-alone organizations. An ED's marketing strategy must include the principles of the larger branding campaign and its logo (**Figure 28.3**).

Marketing methods change over time, but effective branding generates a resilient connection to the consumer. When given the opportunity, consumers choose the particular health-care brand that they believe will provide the most efficient, compassionate, and highest-quality care.

FIGURE 28.3 ■ Expanded Brand Marketing

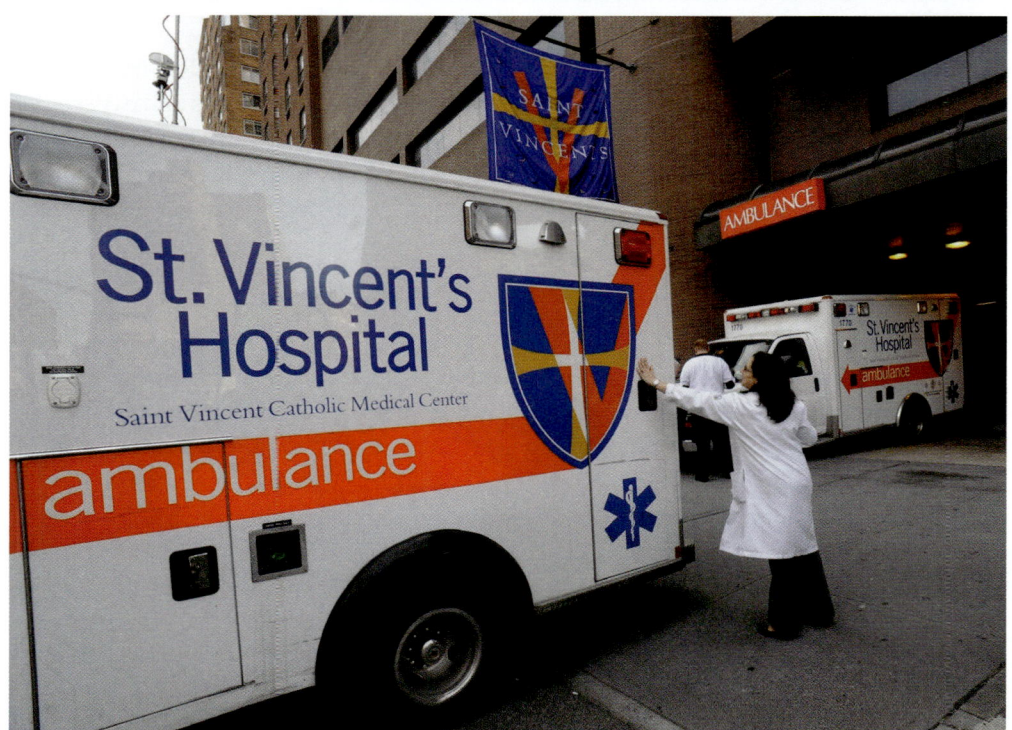

INTERNAL AND EXTERNAL MARKETING

Effective marketing requires identifying targeted customers to whom specific services are to be delivered. Organizations such as Walmart utilize widespread advertising, but they do not attempt to be all things to all people. Walmart primarily targets price shoppers, not all shoppers. Casting a wide net through scattergun advertising usually is indicative of a poor marketing approach that is fiscally unsound and generates poor return on investment. Furthermore, an overly broad approach may attract the misaligned customers who can distract from the service/product delivery process or subvert the organization's mission. For example, ED marketing strategies should avoid targeting patients seeking routine primary care or annual vaccinations.

By virtue of the specialists' training in emergency medicine, the obvious target markets are acutely ill and injured patients. However, other key market segments emerge when considering the patient's decision-making process in selecting a particular ED. Furthermore, the mere presence of large numbers of patients does not ensure the fiscal strength of the department or the emergency physician group. Hospital-related stakeholders, such as medical staff and administration, significantly influence the growth and viability of the ED and, as such, are another key target market.

There are two primary target markets: internal customers and external customers. There is some overlap in their expectations, allowing use of some similar tactics to attract their positive attention. However, unique expectations within each group require specific tactics.

Internal Markets

The ED has three key internal target market segments:

- Patients
- Medical staff
- Administration

Patients

Marketing to patients goes beyond simply attracting them to the ED. Regardless of the patients' enticements to select a particular ED, once they arrive, their needs and expectations must be met; the anticipated product must be delivered. Strategically created messages (**Box 28.2**) delivered effectively throughout the encounter may help determine the patient's or designee's response to satisfaction surveys. Specifically, effective messages help to:

- Shape the patients' perceptions of their experience
- Determine the likelihood of their return in the future
- Increase the likelihood of recommending the ED to others

Research shows that satisfied patients (customers) share their good experiences with four to six acquaintances, whereas *dissatisfied* customers report their discontent to nine to 15 acquaintances, with 13% telling more than 20 people.[2] The ubiquity of social media

---

BOX 28.2 ■ KEY WORDS AT KEY TIMES[1]

"... carefully chosen words healthcare professionals use to 'connect the dots' and help patients, families and visitors better understand what we are doing—and most importantly, *why*."

greatly expands the opportunity for patient-to-public communication. The highly satisfied patient is a powerful marketer for the ED. Conversely, the message from a mildly dissatisfied ED patient may have broad reach and thereby become an even more powerful conduit for negative online reviews and commentary.

Medical Staff

It is important that hospital staff members recognize and appreciate the caliber of the ED and the qualities that set it apart from its competitors. Proper internal marketing also drives collaboration and respect for the ED and its caregivers. Emergency department leaders must communicate routinely and effectively with their colleagues about their physicians' scope of practice; operational efficiency; and ED processes that support others' practices, including the use of collaborative care pathways and transition orders.

The maturation of hospital medicine (i.e., hospitalists) allows a more synergistic and consistent approach to patient care between emergency physicians and hospital medicine physicians. This synergy, including effective and thorough patient handoffs, is essential to efficient, safe patient care and can enhance patients' perceptions of the hospital experience.

Administration

It is vitally important that key administrative leaders perceive that the mission, values, and objectives of the ED physician group align with the hospital system. They should also recognize the value of partnering with the existing group rather than collaborating with competitors who are vying for an opportunity to contract with the hospital.

Rather than leveraging the virtues and value of the group when faced with crisis or encroachment by competitors:

- The proactive ED physician leaders and group will utilize effective internal marketing efforts. Specifically, key administrative leaders will create and maintain an intimate knowledge of the benefits of the partnership.
- The reactive group will be forced to attempt to convince the administration and staff of their many positive attributes (after the fact).

Emergency department groups are misguided to assume that performance results—and even friendly relationships—convey the intended message to key hospital decision makers. The ED group must routinely and proactively communicate the benefits and results of their initiatives in a compelling way.

External Markets

The key external targets include emergency medical services (EMS), the referring physician base, and the community.

Emergency Medical Services

EMS professionals have significant discretion to determine the ultimate destination for many out-of-hospital patients. Effective communication and respectful, collaborative relationships with EMS professionals engender mutual trust and encourage them to direct EMS traffic to a preferred ED.

Referring Physicians

While members of the referring physician base sometimes also serve on the medical staff of the facility, they are an external source of ED patient referrals. Therefore, the ED group must customize its marketing efforts to this important segment to bolster their confidence in, and encourage their referrals to, the ED and facility.

Community

The community's impression of a particular ED influences the referral decisions of outside physicians, payer network inclusion and exclusion selection, and the loyalty of patients, who "vote with their feet." For every 10 US inhabitants, there are four ED visits annually.[3] Because of the nature of emergencies, every member of the community is a potential ED customer.

ENGAGING KEY STAKEHOLDERS AND RESOURCES

The most effective marketing strategies include all key stakeholders in their formulation (including community members and previous patients). The stakeholders contribute their specific knowledge to the plan to ensure it is comprehensive and that it is coordinated for execution across the organization. For example, ED leadership has a critical stake in delivery of services; finance allocates funding for operational, capital, and other projects; supply management delivers goods or services to the providers; and legal counsel oversees contractual and other regulatory concerns. Marketing personnel lead the comprehensive efforts to ensure proper segment targeting, appropriate messaging, and management of the marketing budget. Effective marketing aligns, prioritizes, and sequences the organization's marketing activities.

The facility's budget includes funds appropriated for marketing efforts. Most EDs are responsible for at least 50% of a facility's admitted patients. Marketing the ED's capabilities and particular strengths (e.g., cardiovascular services, efficient urgent care, stroke center accreditation, trauma care) allows the department to become an integral part of the facility's strategic marketing plan.

Unfortunately, many direct marketing budgets focus on enhancing the overall perception of the system or facility rather than on the most likely reason that consumers come to a hospital—the ED. Some institutions proudly cite spending less than one penny of every expense dollar on marketing and advertising. ED–specific marketing typically represents only a small percentage of an organization's total marketing budget. More funding is usually devoted to high-margin services, such as cardiovascular and/or neurovascular care. As a result, EDs must often implement less expensive direct-to-patient marketing methods.

In addition to proper funding, it is important to prioritize and properly schedule marketing activities. Failure to develop a well-organized marketing plan could result in an inability to deliver promised services. For example, promoting an ED as part of a certified stroke center without first achieving patient management and protocol consensus among all providers undermines the marketing initiative and is likely to result in uncoordinated care, an unmet promise to the community, and poor patient outcomes. Alternatively, good project management ensures that action steps are prioritized and sequenced properly and that competing initiatives do not deplete required resources.

APPLICATION OF ED MARKETING TACTICS

Each organization must determine a strategy for reaching specific market segments and addressing the needs of those customers (**Box 28.3**). Some approaches are particularly applicable to growth strategies, such as tactics that elucidate a positive image to current and potential patients and generate valuable word-of-mouth advertising. Other tactics

BOX 28.3 ■ ED MARKETING STRATEGIES

Direct interaction with patients
- Operational performance
- Patient callbacks
- Rounding
- Brochures and business cards
- Comment cards and satisfaction surveys

Traditional advertising
- Newspapers and mailers
- Billboards
- Radio and television

Mobile and web-based partnerships
- Medical staff
- EMS
- Community

are designed to augment the ED's existing reputation and improve its visibility within the community.

Direct Interaction With Patients

The success of any ED marketing tactic requires sufficient attention to the patient experience. Patient satisfaction survey results clearly indicate the importance of respecting the patient's time and communicating clearly during the visit. As such, optimizing operational efficiency is core to any ED's marketing success (**Figures 28.4** and **Table 28.1**).

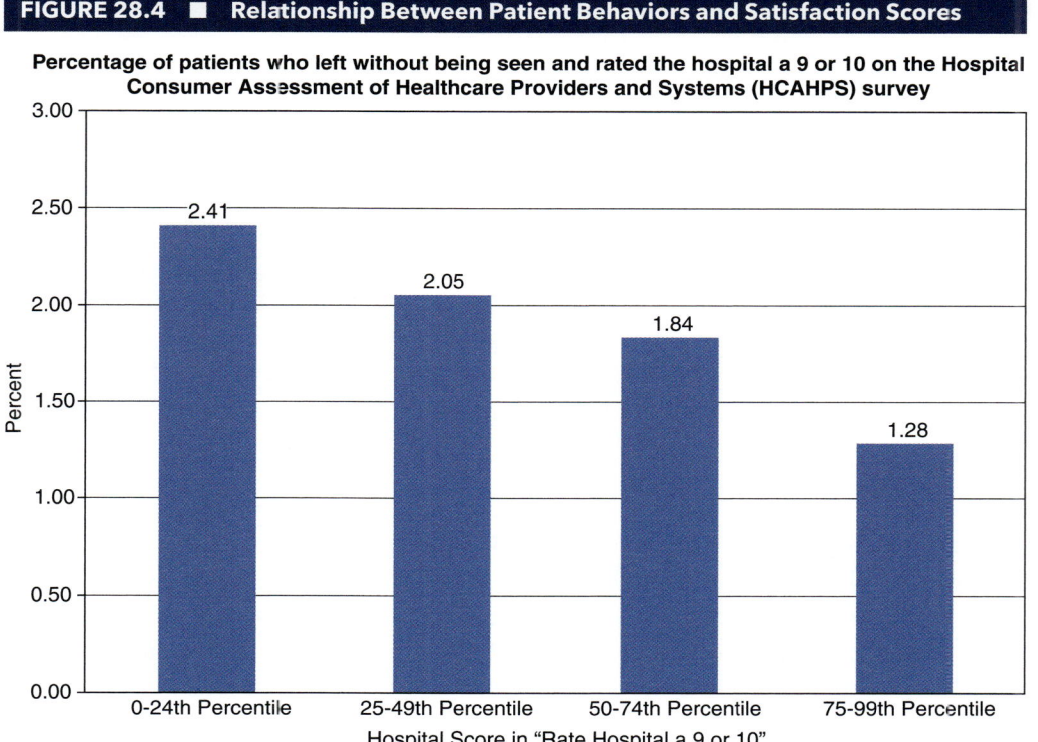

FIGURE 28.4 ■ Relationship Between Patient Behaviors and Satisfaction Scores

Percentage of patients who left without being seen and rated the hospital a 9 or 10 on the Hospital Consumer Assessment of Healthcare Providers and Systems (HCAHPS) survey

- 0-24th Percentile: 2.41
- 25-49th Percentile: 2.05
- 50-74th Percentile: 1.84
- 75-99th Percentile: 1.28

Hospital Score in "Rate Hospital a 9 or 10"

Reflects data from >3500 EDs reporting to the Centers for Medicare & Medicaid Services

Source: Reprinted with permission from the Studer Group.

TABLE 28.1 ■ Optimizing Key Patient Intervals

Patient arrival to room
- Immediately acknowledge the patient's arrival.
- Assist the patient when they are exiting their private vehicle.
- Offer valet services.
- Perform rapid triage-bedside registration or team triage in treatment areas.

Room to provider
- Promote the speedy arrival of nurses, physicians, and advanced practice clinicians.
- Interact empathically with the patient and their family and friends.
- Limit repetitive questions.

Provider to disposition
- Ensure efficient essential services (lab, radiology).
- Provide effective access to patient health care records.
- Communicate regularly with the patient regarding the treatment plan and timeline.
- Communicate diagnostic findings and encourage questions.
- Provide creature comforts, such as pillows, blankets, food, beverages, television.

Disposition to departure
- Clearly communicate disposition and follow-up plans.
- Communicate directly with the patient's personal physician, whenever feasible.
- Thank the patient for choosing your ED and encourage them to come back when needed.
- Give the patient a business card with the physician's name and contact information.

Whenever possible, it is important to understand and then exceed patients' expectations. Exceeding expectations produces loyalty and generates word-of-mouth advertising. Patients who are *very* satisfied with ED services may generalize their experiences and associate the hospital with that positive experience, thereby increasing their likelihood to use other services. Patient loyalty is particularly relevant to an ED's growth because:

- Retaining existing patients is easier and more cost-efficient than attracting new ones.
- Retained loyal patients are more likely to recruit new patients among their friends and family members.
- Increasingly, patient satisfaction survey results are publicly reported and accessible.
- Stakeholders use these survey results to gauge the quality of the ED and the strength of their partnership with emergency providers.

Patient Callbacks

Two patient callback methods provide opportunities to directly market the ED to patients. First, during a clinical callback, an ED health-care professional encourages the patient to follow up on the clinical aspects of the visit through follow-up appointments, prescriptions, and progress. The ED representative reiterates discharge instructions and answers questions while simultaneously letting the patient know that the ED staff cares about the patient's well-being.

The second callback method queries the patient's overall experience and satisfaction with the visit and the likelihood that the patient would recommend the ED and facility. A variety of people can perform these calls. Both forms of callbacks, when performed in a timely and effective manner, provide the opportunity to strengthen the patient's connection to the hospital, reinforce the use of other services, and perform service recovery, if needed.

> **BOX 28.4 ■ AIDET COMMUNICATION FRAMEWORK**
>
> - Acknowledge
> - Introduce
> - Duration
> - Explanation
> - Thank you

Rounding

A number of health-care organizations adopt the principles of Quint Studer, founder and CEO of the Studer Group, to hardwire a patient interaction methodology called AIDET (**Box 28.4**). Best practice institutions include patient rounding—a brief physician or nurse interaction to gauge and document the effectiveness of provider communication.

ED change-of-shift rounds provide a structured approach to patient hand-offs. Like "huddles," this variety of rounding may include physicians and nurses and other personnel, including case managers, technicians, and volunteers. Face-to-face transitions mitigate risks associated with shift changes and improve patients' perceptions of their care.

Brochures and Business Cards

Brochures presented upon or soon after the patient's arrival can provide information about the ED experience and highlight specific features of the department (**Box 28.5**). Business cards (**Figure 28.5**) can also provide an opportunity to connect patients more closely with their emergency physician and the facility.

Comment Cards and Satisfaction Surveys

End-of-visit patient surveys—either paper-based or electronic—afford patients an opportunity to convey their overall satisfaction level along with their specific observations. Surveys can provide immediate feedback to the ED staff and allow patients to receive prompt service recovery when appropriate. Because it is uncommon for an ED to use this feedback to benchmark against other facilities, surveys are seldom used as official measurements of patient satisfaction. Furthermore, while some of the "real-time" surveys are electronic, those that are paper-based require manual information extraction.

> **BOX 28.5 ■ TOPICS FOR AN ED BROCHURE**
>
> - Welcome
> - Mission
> - The visit
>   - Registration
>   - Medical examination
>   - Test results
>   - Admissions
>   - Discharge
> - Family involvement
> - Patient responsibilities
> - What we offer
> - Facility awards and accomplishments
> - Optional
>   - Leadership team photos and credentials
>   - Emergency providers photos and credentials
>   - Pain management policy

FIGURE 28.5 ■ **Business Card Example**

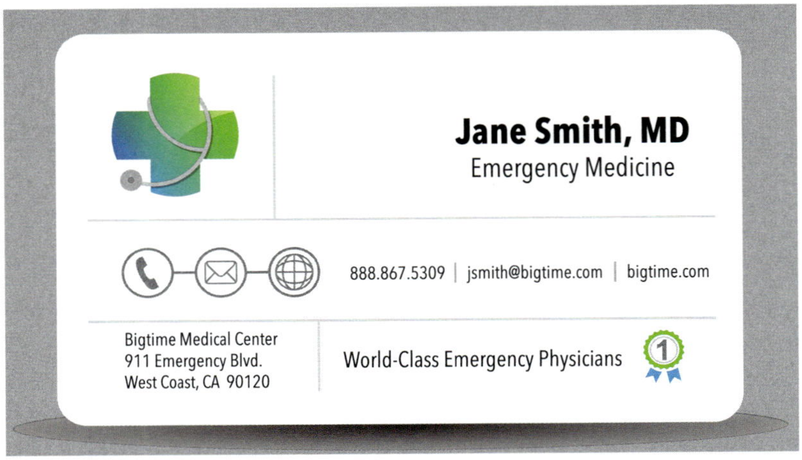

Vendor-facilitated patient satisfaction surveys are the most common method for gauging the patient experience. To leverage these results in the marketing strategy, it is necessary to:

- Achieve a robust understanding of the vendor's methods (e.g., phone-based surveys, mailed surveys, paper or electronic surveys, etc), statistical analysis techniques, the questions asked, and the sample sizes.
- Effectively script providers with key phrases that align with and positively reinforce the patient survey questions.
- Provide timely, individualized feedback of satisfaction survey results to providers and ED staff for specific questions that focus on them.
- Establish a patient-centered culture of excellence that conveys a commitment to quality, care, and compassion.

Superior performance on patient satisfaction surveys is very useful in marketing campaigns to create and influence a positive perception of the ED in the community.

Traditional Advertising

Traditional advertising remains an effective approach to ED marketing.

Newspapers and Mailers

A facility's systematic communication with the public influences the community's perception. One such venue is print media, most notably community newspapers. Appropriate content for newspapers includes:

- Announcements of additions and changes to the ED provider staff
- Awards and accomplishments of the ED and its staff
- Capital investments and facility expansions
- Process improvement initiatives with positive results
- Public service announcements
- Public health communiqués

Mailers, using similar content as newspapers, use marketing databases or hospital mailing lists to target key demographics or zip codes.

Billboards

Strategically placed billboards target key market segments to increase awareness and showcase distinct attributes or programs at the ED (**Figure 28.6**).

FIGURE 28.6 ■ Example of Billboard Advertising

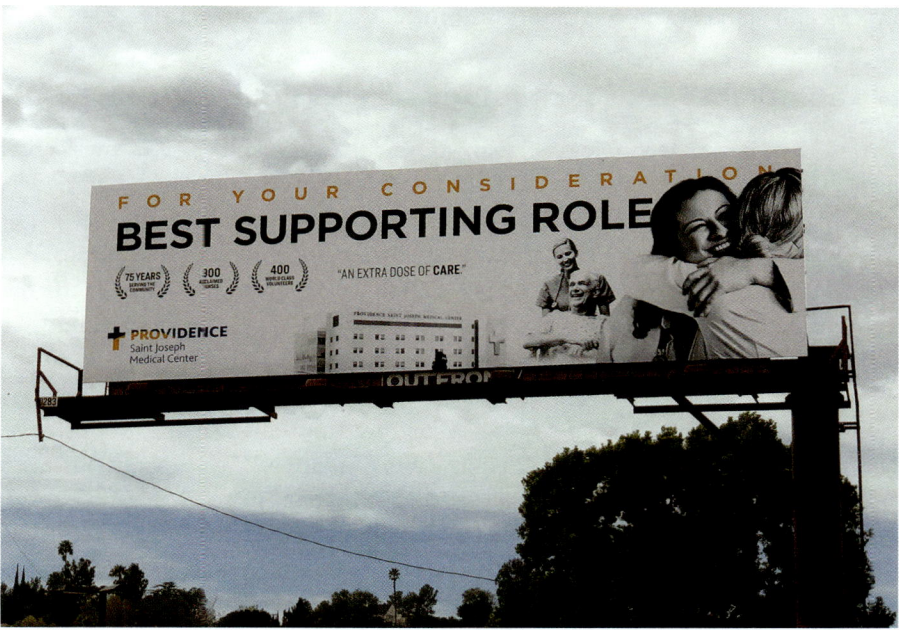

Radio and Television

Radio and television commercials provide an opportunity to purchase exposure for the ED's marketing message. However, there are many no-cost opportunities to promote the ED/facility using these media in the context of community outreach and education. For example, members of the ED team can network with radio and TV health-care content creators/producers to provide subject matter expertise. Developing effective media relationships results in multiple ED provider opportunities to present public information whenever there is a radio or television segment with emergency medicine implications.

Many hospitals employ a marketing professional or department that can promote ED leadership presentations to the media. Example topics include flu management, hypothermia, and carbon monoxide alerts during cold-weather months and fireworks safety, heat-related illnesses, bug- and snakebites, and drowning hazards during hot-weather months. Current news events, such as a heat wave, may generate these opportunities. Community access radio and television are especially popular in some markets and often seek content and presenters. Regular educational spotlights, such as "Ask an Emergency Physician" segments, call-in shows, and so on, are effective promotional programs. The ED leader must collaborate with hospital administration before making media statements on behalf of the hospital.

The American College of Emergency Physicians (ACEP) provides an abundance of emergency care-related materials via its sponsored website www.emergencycareforyou.org (**Box 28.6**). This

BOX 28.6 ■ ACEP-SPONSORED HEALTH NEWS SITE

- Adult emergencies
- Child emergencies
- Disasters
- Holiday and seasonal
- Home safety
- Infectious diseases
- Prevention
- Senior safety
- Travel safety

resource may be useful to an emergency physician preparing for a media event or appearance. Additionally, the social media tab on the website includes a direct link to the emergency medicine portion of Health Radio, an Internet radio site devoted to topical health-care issues.

Mobile and Web-Based Technologies

Mobile and web-based technologies, such as social media, blogs, text messaging, and websites, offer powerful access to both focused and broad markets. ED leaders may strategically deploy these technologies to develop dialogue with existing and potential consumers of emergency care. ED leaders also use these technologies to communicate with other key internal and external marketing segments, including medical staff, referring physicians, EMS, and even new recruits.

Change in Technology

The use of fixed landlines continues to decline, limiting their use and importance as an outreach tool for activities such as follow-up calls (i.e., after-care clinical and satisfaction assessment). According to the *International Telecommunication Union Report* and database, the number of fixed-line phone subscriptions per 100 inhabitants in the United States fell from 58 to 40 between 2005 and 2014.[4] During that same period, the *2016 United Nations Statistical Yearbook* reports that cell phone subscriptions per 100 US inhabitants increased from 68 to 110.[5] Increasingly, the phone numbers documented during the ED registration process are the patient's or patient's guardian's cell phone.

According to the 2018 *Mobile Fact Sheet* produced by the Pew Research Center, 95% of American adults use cell phones (up from 89% 5 years earlier).[6] In the same study, smartphone users increased from 51% to 77%. The Pew Research Center's report, *Cell Phone Activities in 2012*, reveals that 80% of respondents use phones for texting (**Table 28.2**).[7]

Marketing Opportunities

Cell phones and Internet-enabled smartphones, in particular, provide significantly expanded marketing opportunities. According to CTIA—The Wireless Association, smartphone use in the United States rose from 78 million in 2010 to 273 million in 2017, a growth of 250% over 7 years.[8] Mobile marketers contend that the open rates and timeliness of opening texts far exceed other forms of web-based and traditional communication. The Pew Research Foundation's research indicates that 52% of smartphone owners gather health information on their phones, compared with 6% of Americans who don't use smartphones.[9]

To use mobile device access properly and effectively, the ED marketing group must have a strategy designed specifically for key segments and well-planned objectives. For example, studies on texting indicate high "conversion" rates for turning text recipients into consumers of goods and services. Worthington, et al demonstrated success in the text-based campaign's "call to action."[10] The researchers found it difficult to communicate with the targeted patients

TABLE 28.2 ■ Cell Phone Activity Usage[7]

Activity	Percentage
Send or receive text messages	81%
Access the Internet	60%
Send or receive e-mail	52%
Participate in a video call or video chat	21%

through traditional means like educational sessions, mailers, flyers, and so on. However, they found that only 11% of these patients did not have a cell phone or text messaging capacity. After obtaining the patient's permission for this form of communication, they sent two to three brief text messages each week with evaluation questions to assess behavioral change. Fifty-nine percent of the participants always or almost always took actions suggested in the text messages. Other health-care-related studies, such as those for smoking cessation programs and HIV drug compliance, have successfully used similar mobile messaging and text-based interactions.[11]

Hence, an ED group's mobile marketing strategy should include both text-messaging tactics along with content support for the hospital enterprise's social media presence.

Marketing Program Steps

Important steps for an effective, text-based ED marketing program include:

- Create a database early.
  - With the patient's written consent, collect cell phone numbers even before the program is in place.
  - Obtain the patient's permission to communicate via text messaging.

- Integrate text and other forms of mobile marketing.
  - Use text messages to "drive hits" to websites via smartphones or other means.

Through mobile analytics, an organization can glean specific information about those who respond to text messages. The organization can then populate its database with names, addresses, types of phones, and so on, to further stratify marketing segments and create segment-specific messages.

Hospitals and EDs are just beginning to explore the usefulness of mobile messaging. Mobile messaging can reach many internal and external market segments to communicate thanks, offer reminders, assess services, request calls and follow-up actions, provide links to other resources and payment options, and so on. ED leaders must ensure these messages are user-friendly and align all messages—regardless of format—with the organization's overall marketing strategy.

Despite its pervasiveness, it is unlikely that a particular ED will create and maintain its own social media presence. The ED's social media strategy should be supportive of and aligned with the hospital system's overall social media presence. An independent ED's social media campaign risks departing from the compliance policies and overall messaging strategy of the greater enterprise. In particular, patient-specific comments can have important regulatory and legal consequences. Nonetheless, the ED's active collaboration in the development of ED specific/promotional content adds significant value to overall social media effectiveness.

If the emergency providers are not direct employees of the hospital, the provider group must ensure that its social media practices regarding HIPAA compliance and other aspects of public commentary align with those of the facility or hospital system.

Partnerships

Partnerships with medical staff, EMS, and the community are powerful tools for marketing the ED.

Medical Staff

Since patients often rely on the direction of their personal physician or physician group to choose an ED, the medical staff is a high-value market segment. Cultivating the medical staff's trust and respect for the ED drives its reputation among medical groups and the medical community as a whole. Recommended approaches include the following:

- Integrate emergency physicians into the medical staff committees and leadership structure.
- Form interdisciplinary committees with key medical staff departments/leaders to facilitate dialogue regarding challenges and opportunities for the ED.
- Participate as a speaker for CME or other medical staff educational venues to promulgate the ED and its approach to patient care.
- Ensure open, direct communication (e.g., cell phone, face-to-face, and other means of contact) between medical staff and EM group leadership to discuss and address specific patient care or other ED issues.
- Ensure regular and predictable presence by ED leadership outside of the clinical setting.
- Collaborate closely with medical staff to develop ED care pathways, transition orders, and other processes.
- Attend key interdepartmental meetings (e.g., medicine, surgery, and others).
- Conduct periodic medical staff satisfaction surveys.

Emergency Medical Services

Emergency medical services–transported patients comprise an essential percentage of the ED population. As mentioned earlier, EMS professionals should be considered an integral part of the emergency care team. The ED team and its leaders must make a concerted effort to develop collaborative partnerships, which include daily, patient-centered interactions and ongoing professional roles and activities in conjunction with the EMS organizations (**Box 28.7**).

Community

Keeping in mind that annually there is more than one ED visit for every three people (often with family members) and that about half of all patients admitted to the hospital come through the ED, the ED's reputation strongly influences the community's perception of the hospital. Community leaders and business owners must trust the capabilities of the hospital and its ED. As discussed earlier, radio, television, and other forms of media afford access to the community. Further, ED personnel can promote the department and demonstrate its value by participating in civic organizations, churches, schools, and business groups. Emergency department groups can also market through participation in health fairs, lectures, and other community events.

BOX 28.7 ■ FOSTERING AN ED-EMS TEAM APPROACH

- EMS directorship
- EMS board membership
- Educational lectures and dinners
- Structured celebration of annual EMS week
- Organized approach to ED crowding and diversion
- Greet and acknowledge arrival
- Listen or seek out information and observations
- Provide a comfortable workspace for documentation
- Offer coffee and snacks

CONCLUSION

The things we fear most in organizations—fluctuations, disturbances, imbalances—are the primary sources of creativity.

—Margaret J. Wheatley, EdD,
author and management consultant

This chapter reviews the purpose of marketing for the ED, its internal and external customers, and outlines specific tactics for creating positive, far-reaching marketing messages. The authors recommend an organized, comprehensive ED marketing strategy that is founded in a culture of commitment to clinical quality, care, compassion, and service excellence in order to attract patients and drive growth.

REFERENCES

1. Robinson BC, Cook K, Studer Q. *The HCAHPS Handbook: Hardwire Your Hospital for Pay-for-Performance Success.* Pensacola: FL. Fire Starter Publishing; 2010.

2. The Research Institute America, Inc. *Greater Emphasis Placed on Business Etiquette to Build Sales, The White House Office of Consumer Affairs.* Washington, DC: American Institutes for Research; 1986.

3. Centers for Disease Control. *National Hospital Ambulatory Medical Care Survey.* Atlanta, GA: US Department of Health and Human Services, Centers for Disease Control and Prevention, National Center for Health Statistics; 2015.

4. International Telecommunication Union. World Telecommunication/ICT Development Report and Database. Fixed Telephone Subscriptions (per 100 People). The World Bank Group. 2019. Available at: https://data.worldbank.org/indicator/IT.MLT.MAIN.P2?locations=US&name_desc=false&view=chart/. Accessed May 12, 2019.

5. *Statistical Yearbook 2016 Edition, Fifty-Ninth Issue.* New York, NY: Department of Economic and Social Affairs, Statistics Division, United Nations; 2016:298.

6. Mobile fact sheet. Pew Research Center. 2018. Available at: http://pewinternet.org/fact-sheet/mobile/. Accessed May 12, 2019.

7. Duggan M. Cell phone activities 2012. Pew Research Center. 2012. Available at: http://www.pewinternet.org/2012/11/25/cell-phone-activities-2012/. Accessed May 12, 2019.

8. The State of Wireless. The CTIA website. 2018. Available at: https://api.ctia.org/wp-content/uploads/2018/07/CTIA_State-of-Wireless-2018_0710.pdf. Accessed May 12, 2019.

9. Fox S, Duggan M. Mobile health 2012. Pew Research Center. 2012. Available at: http://www.pewinternet.org/2012/11/08/mobile-health-2012/. Accessed May 12, 2019.

10. Worthington L, Braunscheidel EM, Lachenmayr L, et al. Text2bhealthy: a pilot nutrition texting program targeting parents of school-aged children. *J Acad Nutr Diet.* 2012;112(9):A78.

11. Free C, Knight R, Robertson S, et al. Smoking cessation support delivered via mobile phone text messaging (txt2stop): a single-blind, randomised trial. *Lancet.* 2011:378(9785):49-55.

CHAPTER 29

MULTICULTURAL APPROACH TO EMERGENCY DEPARTMENT PATIENTS

Lynne Richardson, Gallane Abraham, Marlaina Norris, Theresa Tavernero

Of all the forms of inequality, injustice in health care is the most shocking and inhumane.

—Martin Luther King Jr

America, which was founded on the promise of liberty and opportunity for all, is growing increasingly diverse (**Figure 29.1**). These shifting demographics are keenly felt in the emergency department (ED). Even in fairly homogeneous communities, the ED must be prepared to care for any patient, regardless of race, ethnicity, religion, country of origin, primary language, sexual orientation, gender identity, or socioeconomic status. Providing high-quality emergency care to all patients requires cognizance of the complex interactions between culture and health, as well as an awareness of the pervasive existing disparities in health care for certain groups.

The Institute of Medicine has included "equitable" as one of the six components of quality clinical care.[1] Most physicians and nurses believe that they deliver equitable care to their patients, but very few have data to substantiate that belief. Whether motivated by professional pride, a commitment to social justice, or a desire to optimize clinical and financial performance, ED directors must be able to *demonstrate* that their clinicians and staff provide equitable care. Achieving this requires attention to the issues that are discussed in

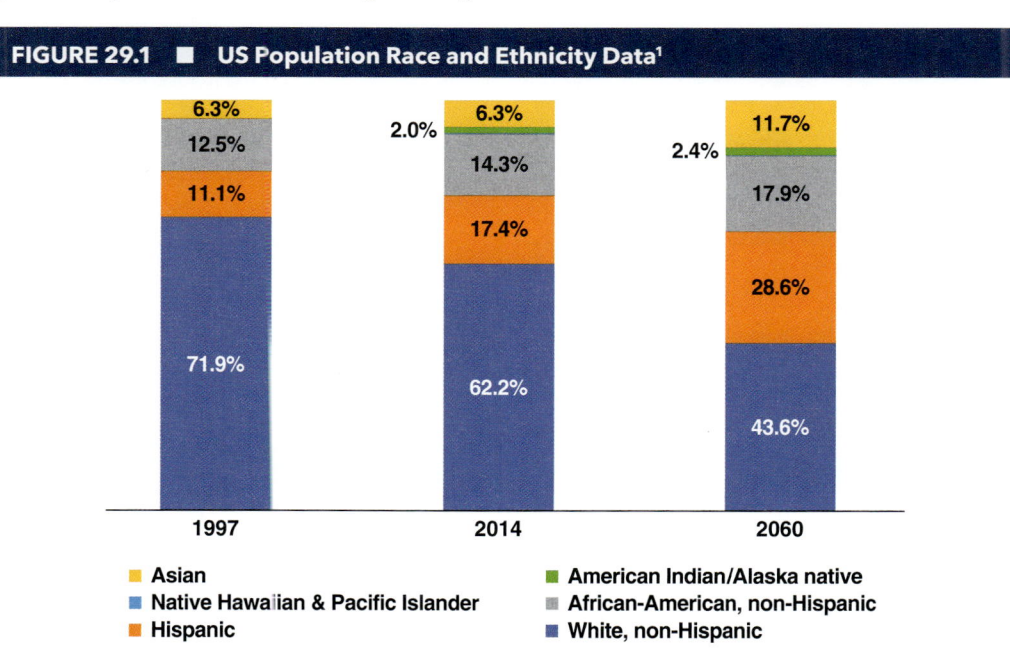

FIGURE 29.1 ■ US Population Race and Ethnicity Data[1]

TABLE 29.1 ■ Important Definitions
Health disparities: Observed, preventable differences in the burden of disease, injury, morbidity, and mortality that are experienced by socially disadvantaged populations.
Health-care disparities: Observed differences in care that are not due to differing clinical needs, patient preferences, or the appropriateness of the intervention.
Culture: Beliefs and behaviors that are learned and shared by members of a social group.
Cultural competence: The ability to function effectively in the context of cultural differences. Cultural competence requires knowledge, attitudes, and skills.
Transgender and gender nonconforming (TGGNC): Transgender people have a *gender identity* that does not align with the sex they were assigned at birth. Gender-nonconforming people have a *gender expression* that does not conventionally align with the person's assigned sex at birth.
LGBT: Lesbian, gay, bisexual, and transgender.

this chapter: existing disparities in health care, cultural competence, workforce diversity, and the need for accurate, group-specific data on patient race and ethnicity (**Table 29.1**).

UNDERSTANDING HEALTH-CARE DISPARITIES

Racial and ethnic disparities in health have been well described, with data showing that African Americans, Hispanics, and Native Americans suffer disproportionately from many conditions, including cardiovascular disease, stroke, diabetes, asthma, influenza, and pneumonia. Racial and ethnic minorities have excess morbidity and mortality, as well as decreased life expectancy, at every economic level.[2,3] The causes of racial and ethnic health disparities are multifactorial, reflecting differences in biological vulnerability to disease as well as differences in social resources, environmental conditions, and health-care use.[4-6] Since 2002, the Agency for Healthcare Research and Quality has annually tracked core measures of quality and access. As shown in **Figure 29.2**, the 2017 National Healthcare Quality and Disparities Report reveals

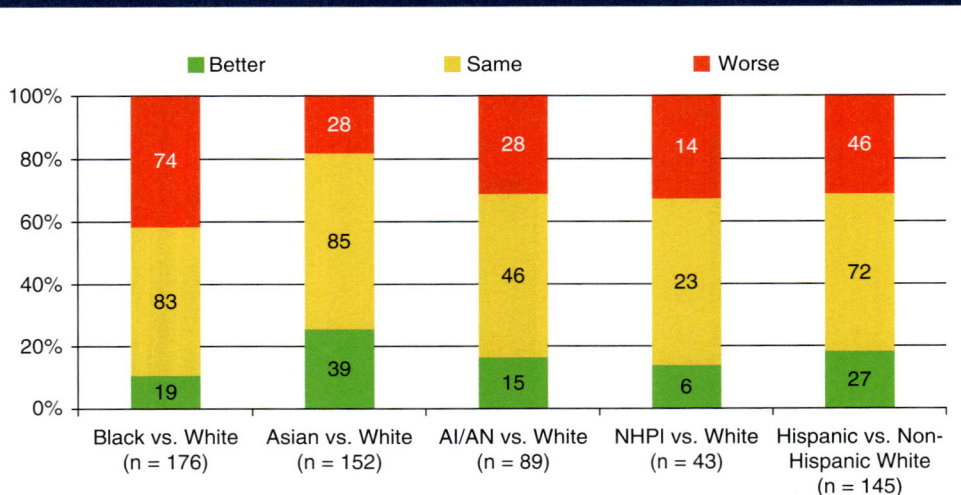

FIGURE 29.2 ■ Racial and Ethnic Disparities in Core Quality Measures[7]

Key: AI/AN = American Indian or Alaska Native; n = number of measures; Improving = disparity is getting smaller at a rate greater than 1% per year; No change = disparity is not changing or is changing at a rate less than 1% per year; Worsening = disparity is getting larger at a rate greater than 1% per year.

that few of the disparities faced by African Americans, Native Americans, and Hispanics are narrowing.[7]

There is substantial and troubling evidence that health disparities are, in part, attributable to the inferior quality of care delivered to members of racial, ethnic, and cultural minorities compared to that received by whites. The 2003 Institute of Medicine report "Unequal Treatment" concluded that "stereotyping, biases, and uncertainty on the part of health-care providers can all contribute to unequal treatment."[8] Of particular relevance to emergency physicians and nurses are the types of situations that promote these biases: time pressure, incomplete information, and high demand for attention and cognitive resources.[8]

Although the idea that unequal care is provided to racial and ethnic minority patients is anathema to most emergency physicians and nurses, the conditions known to promote the use of stereotypes and encourage biases are precisely the conditions in which emergency providers work. The ED, with its unique role in the health-care safety net, provides care to diverse populations; thus, ED providers are frequently required to care for patients from a race or culture different than their own. In any cross-cultural clinical encounter, there is an element of subjective variability that stems from provider attitudes and beliefs, which may shape the interpretation of information given by the patient. Providers must rapidly establish rapport, efficiently obtain relevant information, and quickly make judgments about the patient's condition. The entire ED decision-making process is nested in uncertainty and occurs under considerable time pressure within a busy, complex, demanding environment. The nature of ED clinical encounters, particularly in the setting of ED crowding, time pressure, constrained resources, and rapid complex cognition, is known to result in negative outcomes due to stereotypes, prejudice, and a lack of information.[9,10]

Providers do not have to be aware of these attitudes or consciously endorse stereotypes for these factors to influence diagnostic and treatment decisions.[11] Provider behavior that reveals implicit or explicit prejudices may evoke mistrust in minority patients.[12,13] Patients may also hold beliefs, attitudes, or stereotypes toward the health-care system that, independent of clinician behavior, adversely affect provider–patient communication. These cultural barriers may lead to dissatisfaction and poor health outcomes.[14]

Emergency care involves multiple decision-makers, a dynamic that increases the probability of conflict (**Table 29.2**).[9] Racial and ethnic disparities have been documented in the treatment of asthma, psychiatric conditions, and pain; in access to emergency

TABLE 29.2 ■ Aspects of Emergency Care Susceptible to Disparities
Ambulance destination decisions made by prehospital personnel
Triage assessments made by nursing personnel
Diagnostic testing ordered by physicians or physician extenders
Timing and intensity of analgesia and other ED therapy
End-of-life care
Referral patterns to specialists and follow-up care
Disposition decisions
Priority for hospital admission and monitored bed assignment
Prescription choices for discharged patients

care; and in diagnostic approaches to headache and chest pain.[15-21] Other not-yet-quantified disparities in ED care may also exist.

Clinician and staff biases may be triggered by patient characteristics other than race and ethnicity, such as religion, country of origin, English proficiency, disability, sexual orientation, gender identity, or socioeconomic status. Providers may react negatively to certain social conditions, such as homelessness; certain medical conditions, such as HIV/AIDS and sickle cell anemia; and certain behavioral conditions, such as schizophrenia and substance abuse.[22-27] Transgender and other gender-nonconforming individuals report difficulties in obtaining high-quality, respectful medical care.[28-30] To deliver equitable treatment, clinicians and staff must be prepared to provide high-quality care to all persons who seek help in the ED.[31]

PROMOTING CULTURAL COMPETENCE

One important strategy to eliminate disparities in ED care is to ensure the cultural competence of all staff members. Cultural competence, simply defined, is the ability to interact effectively with people from different cultures and people who may have differing norms and values, patterns of communication, beliefs about health and illness, and approaches to decision-making. Patient variations in symptom recognition, thresholds for seeking care, ability to describe symptoms, and expectations of care may influence patient and physician decision-making.[32,33] These differences may lead to misunderstanding, misjudgment, and stereotyping, all of which interfere with the delivery of quality care.[8,34] To acquire sufficient cross-cultural knowledge and skills to manage these differences, ED staff must start with an honest and insightful examination of their feelings, beliefs, and values to detect internalized attitudes that may compromise their ability to care for certain groups of patients.[35]

The American health-care system may be perceived as ethnocentric in the way it imposes its approaches to illness, injury, and healing without considering the traditional beliefs and health practices embraced by many ED patients. Cultural competence requires attention to the differences in values, norms, customs, and beliefs that patients bring. Emergency providers should treat all such beliefs with respect. For example, many groups hold beliefs about the cause and nature of illness based on body imbalance. Among many Asians, the balance is between yin and yang; other cultures think of disease as an imbalance between "hot" and "cold," and treatment must restore the balance.[36] Emergency protocols for fever, for example, such as removing excess clothes or giving popsicles, may be seen as harmful by some cultures.

Expression of pain varies widely across cultures. Clinicians should be careful about undertreating stoic patients and avoid dismissing very expressive vocalizations of pain as overly dramatic. Even conventions about what is polite vary between groups. In Western cultures, people who don't look you directly in the eye may be regarded as evasive or untrustworthy, but in many cultures, avoiding eye contact is a sign of respect, especially when dealing with someone in authority. Tremendous cultural variation also exists regarding touching, especially involving the opposite sex. Gestures that are common in American culture (such as beckoning someone with a finger) may be considered offensive in others. A simple compliment such as "your baby is so pretty!" may terrify a young Hispanic, Asian, or African mother who believes that by calling attention to her child's beauty, you are summoning the envious "evil eye." Traditional healing practices, such as rubbing or coining, may be mistaken for abuse by naïve providers. Cutting or shaving hair, drawing or receiving blood, and wearing sacred symbols are all situations in which a provider's lack of cultural knowledge may lead to misunderstanding or even conflict with patients.

Although ED staff cannot become experts on every culture, they can learn about groups that constitute a significant segment of their patient population, and they should understand the areas likely to lead to misunderstanding in clinical settings. Many problems can be avoided by informing patients and families about what is being done and paying attention to their verbal and nonverbal reactions. Emergency department staff must avoid open displays of disapproval, disrespectful behaviors, and judgmental attitudes toward patients. Sincerity and genuine respect are the key elements of cultural competence. These traits are universal and are understood by all.

Some well-meaning but inept educational efforts in the area of cultural competence serve only to reinforce stereotypes. Clinicians must remember that there is variability within every group and that an individual may not adhere to traditional customs. Assuming that an individual holds certain health beliefs just because they belong to a particular racial or ethnic group is stereotyping. To determine a patient's values and beliefs, simply ask the patient. Several credible resources for training on cultural competence are listed in **Table 29.3**.

TABLE 29.3 ■ Cultural Competence Training and Health Equity Resources

RESOURCES ON CULTURAL COMPETENCE

A Physician's Practical Guide to Culturally Competent Care: A free online educational program designed for physicians, physician assistants, and nurse practitioners and accredited by the American Medical Association. Available at: https://cccm.thinkculturalhealth.hhs.gov/.

Culturally Competent Nursing Care: A Cornerstone of Caring: A free online educational program designed specifically for nurses and accredited by the American Nurses Credentialing Center. Available at: https://ccnm.thinkculturalhealth.hhs.gov/.

Cultural Competency Curriculum for Disaster Preparedness and Crisis Response: A free online educational program designed for first responders of disaster preparedness and crisis response, including emergency medical technicians, psychologists, psychiatrists and social workers. Available at: https://thinkculturalhealth.hhs.gov/education/disaster-personnel.

Kaiser Permanente–Provider's Handbook on Culturally Competent Care: Provides clinicians with an overview of the cultural and epidemiological differences that characterize major cultural groups, with a focus on common characteristics that have implications for health care organizations and practitioners.

African American Populations: http://residency-ncal.kaiserpermanente.org/wp-content/uploads/2018/12/African-American-Handbook.pdf

Latino Populations: http://residency-ncal.kaiserpermanente.org/wp-content/uploads/2018/12/Latino-Handbook.pdf

Lesbian, Gay and Transgender Populations: http://residency-ncal.kaiserpermanente.org/wp-content/uploads/2018/12/LGBT-Handbook.pdf

Individuals with Disabilities: http://residency-ncal.kaiserpermanente.org/wp-content/uploads/2018/12/Disability-Handbook.pdf

Diversity and Inclusion in Quality Patient Care: Your Story/Our Story–A Case-Based Compendium: Written by emergency medicine leaders, this book focuses on bias in health care and provides a variety of case examples related to the unconscious bias and microaggressions encountered in clinical settings. Available for purchase at: https://www.springer.com/us/book/9783319927619

RESOURCES ON CARING FOR PERSONS WITH LIMITED ENGLISH PROFICIENCY

Guide to Providing Effective Communication and Language Assistance Services: A web-based interactive tool that can assist health organizations in planning, implementing, and evaluating language access services to better serve their patients with limited English proficiency and decrease disparities in access to health care. Available at: https://thinkculturalhealth.hhs.gov/education/communication-guide.

Improving Patient Safety Systems for Patients with Limited English Proficiency: A Guide for Hospitals: Provides hospital quality and safety leaders guidelines and strategies for identifying, reporting, and addressing medical errors that occur as a result of language barriers in limited English proficiency and culturally diverse patients. Available at: https://www.ahrq.gov/sites/default/files/publications/files/lepguide.pdf.

(Continued)

TABLE 29.3 ■ Continued

RESOURCES ON CARING FOR TRANSGENDER AND GENDER NONCONFORMING PERSONS

Affirmative Care for Transgender and Gender Nonconforming People: This document was developed by the National LGBT Health Education Center to help prevent the issues and concerns from TGNC patients that often arise at the front desk and in waiting areas due to a lack of awareness and education. Available at: https://www.lgbthealtheducation.org/wp-content/uploads/2016/12/Affirmative-Care-for-Transgender-and-Gender-Non-conforming-People-Best-Practices-for-Front-line-Health-Care-Staff.pdf.

Providing Quality Care to Lesbian, Gay, Bisexual, and Transgender Patients: This resource summarizes important LGBT terminology and explains the health-care disparities faced by this vulnerable population. People, and explaining the importance of effective and affirming communication. Available at: https://www.lgbthealtheducation.org/wp-content/uploads/legacy/providing-quality-care-to-lesbian-gay-bisexual-and-transgender-patients/story_html5.html.

Achieving Health Equity for LGBT People: Provides an overview of LGBT health disparities, demographics, terminology, and key strategies for bringing high-quality care to LGBT people at medical centers and other health-care organizations. Available at: https://www.lgbthealtheducation.org/wp-content/uploads/Achieving-Health-Equity-for-LGBT-People-1.pdf.

Caring for LGBT Older Adults: A module that aims to bring recognition to the presence of LGBT elders and provides clinician recommendations on how to address their unique medical, psychological, and social service needs. Available at: http://lgbthealtheducation.org/wp-content/uploads/Module-6-Caring-for-Older-LGBT-Adults.pdf.

INSTITUTIONAL RESOURCES ON HEALTH EQUITY

Improving Quality and Achieving Equity: A Guide for Hospital Leaders: Provides the rationale for addressing health-care disparities with a focus on quality, cost, risk management, and accreditation and recommends activities and resources that can help hospital leaders initiate an agenda for action. Available at: https://mghdisparitiessolutions.files.wordpress.com/2015/12/improving-quality-safety-guide-hospital-leaders.pdf.

Creating Equity Reports: A Guide for Hospitals: Provides practical information on how to collect data on race, ethnicity, language, and socioeconomic status and how to use those data to develop an equity report. Available at: https://mghdisparitiessolutions.org/wp-content/uploads/2015/12/guide-creating-equity-reports.pdf.

In addition to familiarity with differences in beliefs, behaviors, and values, cultural competence requires knowledge of ethnic and racial differences in disease prevalence and the efficacy of treatment. Lack of accurate, group-specific information may adversely affect the quality of diagnostic decision-making for minority patients.[9] For example, African Americans have twice the incidence of subarachnoid hemorrhage compared to whites living in the same community, a fact that should guide decisions about which patients with headache should receive a CT scan.[37] Coronary artery disease in individuals from Bangladesh, India, and Pakistan has a much earlier onset, greater prevalence, and higher mortality than in whites; these are facts that should influence management of a 35-year-old Bangladeshi man with chest pain.[38,39] Emergency physicians who prescribe antihypertensive medication should know that among African Americans, thiazide diuretics provide greater systolic blood pressure reduction, greater stroke reduction, and greater heart failure reduction than other antihypertensive agents.[40] True cultural competence requires knowledge as well as skills.

The United States has been described as a nation of immigrants, a description supported by a report from the American Community Survey that identified more than 380 languages that are currently spoken in American homes, a phenomenon that affects every

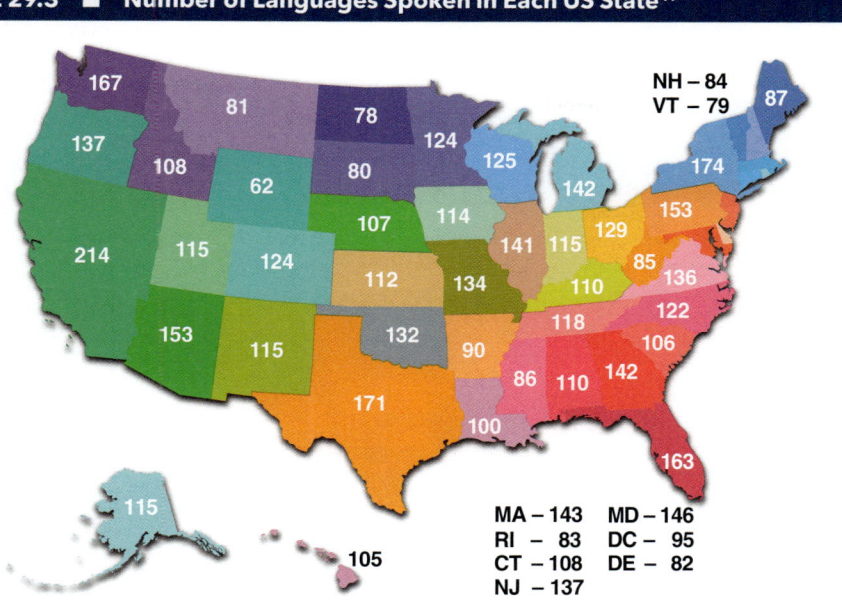

FIGURE 29.3 ■ **Number of Languages Spoken in Each US State**[41]

state (**Figure 29.3**).[41] Individuals who do not speak English as their primary language and who do not speak and understand English very well are defined as having limited English proficiency (LEP). Patients with LEP have significantly more ED visits and hospitalizations than patients who do not require interpreter services.[42-44] Lack of interpreter services or culturally and linguistically appropriate health education materials is associated with patient dissatisfaction, poor comprehension and compliance, and ineffective or lower-quality care.[45,46]

Providing ED patients with adequate discharge instructions in an appropriate language and ensuring that they are understood by patients and family members are paramount to patient safety. Since 2001, the US Department of Health and Human Services has promulgated National Standards for Culturally and Linguistically Appropriate Services in Health Care (CLAS). Compliance with standards five to eight (**Table 29.4**) regarding linguistic services for patients with LEP is mandated for all health-care organizations.[47,48]

With respect to ED care, cultural competence is needed at the organizational level as well as at the level of individual practitioners. Prehospital personnel, front office staff, and clinical support staff must be as adept at cross-cultural communication as ED clinicians. Emergency departments often take the lead in emergency preparedness planning in their communities: they must plan for communication with and organize services for LEP populations in the event of a disaster.[49] A "culturally competent" system is one that incorporates, at all levels, the importance of culture, vigilance toward the dynamics of cultural differences, expansion of cultural knowledge, and adaptation of services to meet culturally unique needs.[50]

Increasing the diversity of the ED workforce could contribute substantially to decreasing health-care disparities and improving care for all patients.[51] Although they are more than 31% of this nation's population, African Americans, Hispanics, and Native Americans

TABLE 29.4 ■ CLAS[47]

1. Provide effective, equitable, understandable, and respectful quality care and services that are responsive to diverse cultural health beliefs and practices, preferred languages, health literacy, and other communication needs.
2. Advance and sustain organizational governance and leadership that promotes CLAS and health equity through policy, practices, and allocated resources.
3. Recruit, promote, and support a culturally and linguistically diverse governance, leadership, and workforce that are responsive to the population in the service area.
4. Educate and train governance, leadership, and workforce in culturally and linguistically appropriate policies and practices on an ongoing basis.
5. Offer language assistance to individuals who have LEP or other communication needs, at no cost to them, to facilitate timely access to all medical services.
6. Inform all individuals of the availability of language assistance services clearly and in their preferred language, verbally and in writing.
7. Ensure the competence of individuals providing language assistance, recognizing that the use of untrained individuals and/or minors as interpreters should be avoided.
8. Provide easy-to-understand print and multimedia materials and signage in the languages commonly used by the populations in the service area.
9. Establish culturally and linguistically appropriate goals, policies, and management accountability and infuse them throughout the organizations' planning and operations.
10. Conduct ongoing assessments of the organization's CLAS-related activities and integrate CLAS-related measures into assessment measurement and continuous quality improvement activities.
11. Collect and maintain accurate and reliable demographic data to monitor and evaluate the impact of CLAS on health equity and outcomes and to inform service delivery.
12. Conduct regular assessments of community health assets and needs and use the results to plan and implement services that respond to the cultural and linguistic diversity of populations in the service area.
13. Partner with the community to design, implement, and evaluate policies, practices, and services to ensure cultural and linguistic appropriateness.
14. Create conflict and grievance resolution processes that are culturally and linguistically appropriate to identify, prevent, and resolve conflicts or complaints.
15. Communicate the organization's progress in implementing and sustaining CLAS to all stakeholders, constituents, and the public.

make up less than 9% of nurses, 10% of physicians, and fewer than 2% of individuals with senior leadership roles in health-care management.[52-54] Much anecdotal evidence suggests that lack of leadership and workforce diversity in health-care organizations results in policies, procedures, and delivery systems inappropriately designed to serve diverse patient populations.[51,52] Emergency departments should strive to recruit a workforce that reflects the populations being served.

ACHIEVING EQUITY IN HEALTH CARE

Collection of accurate data on race, ethnicity, and language preference is the first step in determining whether the care provided is equitable. Lack of basic demographic data on patients seen in various settings has been repeatedly identified as a key barrier to tracking and eliminating disparities. Because they provide an important perspective on the health-care systems of the communities they serve, EDs play a key role to play in this regard. All ED practices are required to track certain quality measures. If accurate data about patient race, ethnicity, and language preference are also collected, the practice can systematically identify disparities in care across various demographic groups, determine which subpopulations are more likely to receive poorer quality care, and then target those subpopulations for specific quality improvement interventions.[55] Because minorities often lack access to other sources of care, they have higher rates of ED use and may be more likely to have unscheduled returns and readmissions.[7,56] Emergency department-based interventions to address these issues may play a key role in achieving institutional quality benchmarks. Such data can also help to develop tailored, patient-centered, culturally appropriate services to more effectively market ED services to local communities.[57]

Many organizations have initiated voluntary programs to collect race, ethnicity, and language data, and there are several policy, statutory, and regulatory initiatives that would require all health-care organizations to do so. The National Academy of Sciences, the National Academy of Medicine, and the "meaningful use" criteria for electronic health record systems (now part of the Merit-Based Incentive Payment System enacted with MACRA) all endorse the inclusion of race, ethnicity, and primary language as part of the basic demographic data collected about each patient. Patient race, ethnicity, and preferred language data should be self-reported; the widespread but unfortunate practice of clerical or clinical personnel assigning race or ethnicity classifications based on the patient's appearance or surname should be discontinued. Some practices may be reluctant to collect race, ethnicity, and language data or uncertain about how to train staff to inquire. Studies have shown that patients do not object to being asked for such data when it is collected properly (**Table 29.5**).[58]

Pitfalls

When disparities in health care are discussed, denial is a common response because most ED physicians and nurses believe that they provide equitable care. Examining clinical data will provide empirical evidence, rather than mere opinion, regarding the presence of disparate care in a particular setting. Complacency and the belief that "everyone is treated the same" are characteristic of those who mistakenly believe that the norms and values of the dominant culture are universally applicable, rather than recognizing and valuing differences between cultures and customizing care to meet each patient's needs.

TABLE 29.5 ■ Sample Script Regarding Race, Ethnicity, and Language[58]
"Now I'm going to ask a few questions about your race and ethnic background. We collect this information from all our patients and use it to track quality of care. This information goes into your medical record and it is confidential."
"First, how would you describe your racial background?"
"Next, how would you describe your ethnicity, such as your family background or ancestry?"
"What language do you usually speak at home?" (If English, skip remaining questions)
"Would you say you speak English very well, well, not well, or not at all?" (If "very well," skip remaining questions)
"In what language would you feel most comfortable *speaking* with your doctor or nurse?"
"In what language would you feel most comfortable *reading* health care instructions?"

TABLE 29.6 ■ Ways to Eliminate Clinical Disparities[9]

Increase awareness: Emergency physicians, nurses, and other ED staff must be made aware of disparities in ED care on both individual and departmental levels. Individuals who are unaware of the possibility of inequities in their treatment of patients are not motivated to change.

Zero tolerance for stereotypical remarks: In some clinical environments, remarks that label or denigrate patients are tolerated. Whether openly prejudicial or subtly stereotypical, such comments by staff members may engender inappropriate stereotyping in clinical decision-making. Such expressions should be regarded as unprofessional and unacceptable.

Collect accurate patient data on race, ethnicity, and language preference: Train ED personnel to obtain self-reported data from patients or family members.

Use patient data to identify disparities in ED care: Through existing quality assurance and performance improvement programs.

Develop interventions to ensure equitable care: Targeted interventions should be implemented to address identified disparities. Ongoing quality assurance and performance improvement efforts can be used to measure the impact of the interventions.

Give individual and practice-wide feedback: Regular reporting of individual clinician data may help overcome the lack of awareness or tendency toward denial. Identify successful providers and develop specific metrics based on best-performing providers.

Use of evidence-based clinical guidelines and pathways: It has been shown that use of evidence-based protocols decreases clinical disparities by decreasing uncertainty and minimizing physician variation.

Institutional report cards: Also called equity reports, institutional report cards summarize an organization's ability to provide nondisparate care while monitoring progress over time.

Training in cultural competence: All ED personnel should be adept at communicating with and caring for patients from differing backgrounds and cultures. Specific training in the skills and knowledge necessary to practice in a culturally competent manner should be provided to all ED staff members.

Appropriate linguistic services: The provision of culturally competent care requires that properly trained interpreters be available to assist with patients who are not fluent in English.

Workforce diversity: Increased workforce diversity among physicians, nurses, and other ED staff would serve to ensure that the providers of emergency care more closely resemble its consumers. A diverse workforce promotes cultural competence through interactions with diverse colleagues.

Opportunities for Success

To improve patient outcomes, create a timeline and build an infrastructure to initiate and sustain efforts to achieve equitable care (**Table 29.6**). Develop diverse, multidisciplinary teams to manage the process of improving patient care: 1) measure quality performance indicators at practice and individual levels, 2) give feedback (practice and individual), 3) set goals (practice and individual), and 4) publicly track progress with quarterly score card or equity report.[55]

CONCLUSION

Significant and persistent health-care disparities result in excess mortality and morbidity for members of some groups. EDs have an important role to play in providing data to monitor the equitableness of care delivered in the ED and beyond. EDs should collect accurate data on race, ethnicity, and language preference and use these data, along with existing quality and patient satisfaction initiatives, to identify areas of disparity.

Cultural practices and behaviors of racial and ethnic minorities affect health. These groups may have special needs, as do patients with disabilities, patients with certain medical and behavioral diagnoses, gender-nonconforming individuals, and patients who are socioeconomically disadvantaged. These special needs must be addressed to provide appropriate and effective ED care. Like clinical competence, developing cultural competence requires mastery of a body of knowledge and the acquisition of cognitive and interpersonal skills.

Culturally competent clinicians will be aware of data on group-specific disease prevalence and treatment efficacy, and they will not allow personal biases to interfere with the care they deliver to patients. Efforts should be made to improve cultural competence and workforce diversity among every ED's clinical, administrative, and support staff.

REFERENCES

1. Committee on Quality of Health Care in America, Institute of Medicine. *Crossing the Quality Chasm: A New Health System for the 21st Century*. Washington DC: The National Academies Press; 2001:35. Available at: https://www.ncbi.nlm.nih.gov/books/NBK222274/pdf/Bookshelf_NBK222274.pdf. Accessed September 9, 2018.

2. National Center for Health Statistics. *Health, United States, 2017: With Special Feature on Mortality*. Hyattsville, MD; 2018. Available at: https://www.cdc.gov/nchs/hus/. Accessed October 4, 2018.

3. Williams DR, Jackson PB. Social sources of racial disparities in health. *Health Aff (Millwood)*. 2005;24(2):325-334. Available at: https://scholar.harvard.edu/files/davidrwilliams/files/2005-social_sources_of-williams.pdf. Accessed September 9, 2018.

4. Artiga S, Hinton E. Kaiser Family Foundation May 2018. Issue Brief. Beyond health care: the role of social determinants in promoting health and health equity. 2018. Available at: http://files.kff.org/attachment/issue-brief-beyond-health-care. Accessed October 4, 2018.

5. Committee on the Review and Assessment of the NIH Strategic Research Plan and Budget to Reduce and Ultimately Eliminate Health Disparities. Health disparities: concepts, measurements, and understanding. In: Thomson GE, Mitchell F, Williams MB, eds. *Examining the Health Disparities Research Plan of the National Institutes of Health: Unfinished Business*. Board on Health Sciences Policy. Institute of Medicine of The National Academies. Washington, DC: The National Academies Press; 2006:21-33 Available at: https://www.ncbi.nlm.nih.gov/books/NBK57043/pdf/Bookshelf_NBK57043.pdf. Accessed September 9, 2018.

6. Williams DR, Mohammed SA. Discrimination and racial disparities in health: evidence and needed research. *J Behav Med*. 2009;32(1):20-47. Available at: https://www.ncbi.nlm.nih.gov/pmc/articles/PMC2821669/pdf/nihms168906.pdf. Accessed September 9, 2018.

7. *2017 National Healthcare Quality and Disparities Report*. Content last reviewed November 2018. Rockville, MD: Agency for Healthcare Research and Quality. Available at: http://www.ahrq.gov/research/findings/nhqrdr/nhqdr17/index.html. Accessed December 4, 2018.

8. Smedley BD, Stith AY, Nelson AR, eds. *Unequal Treatment: Confronting Racial and Ethnic Disparities in Health Care*. Washington DC: The National Academies Press; 2003. Available at: https://www.nap.edu/catalog/12875/unequal-treatment-confronting-racial-and-ethnic-disparities-in-health-care. Accessed September 9, 2018.

9. Richardson LD, Irvin CB, Tamayo-Sarver JH. Racial and ethnic disparities in the clinical practice of emergency medicine. *Acad Emerg Med*. 2003;10(11):1184-1188.

10. van Ryn M. Research on the provider contribution to race/ethnicity disparities in medical care. *Med Care*. 2002;40(1 suppl):I140-I151.

11. LaVeist TA, Nickerson KJ, Bowie JV. Attitudes about racism, medical mistrust, and satisfaction with care among African American and white cardiac patients. *Med Care Res Rev*. 2000;57(suppl):146-161.

12. Dovidio JF, Kawakami K, Gaertner SL. Implicit and explicit prejudice and interracial interaction. *J Pers Soc Psychol*. 2002;82(1):62-68.

13. Balsa A, McGuire TG. Prejudice, clinical uncertainty and stereotyping as sources of health care disparities. *J Health Econ*. 2003;22(1):89-116.

14. James T. The patient–physician clinical encounter. In: Martin LM, Heron S, Moreno Walton L, Jones WA, eds. *Diversity and Inclusion in Quality Patient Care*. Cham, Switzerland: Springer International Publishing; 2016:69-81.

15. Rand CS, Butz AM, Kolodner K, Huss K, Eggleston P, Malveaux F. Emergency department visits by urban African American children with asthma. *J Allergy Clin Immunol*. 2000;105(1 pt 1):83-90.

16. Strakowski SM, Lonczak HS, Sax KW, et al. The effects of race on diagnosis and disposition from a psychiatric emergency service. *J Clin Psychiatry*. 1995;56(3):101-107.

17. Todd KH, Samaroo N, Hoffman JR. Ethnicity as a risk factor for inadequate emergency department analgesia. *JAMA*. 1993;269(12):1537-1539.

18. Tamayo-Sarver JH, Hinze SH, Cydulka RK, Baker DW. Racial/ethnic disparities in analgesic prescribing in the emergency department. *Am J Public Health*. 2003;93(12):2067-2073.

19. Lowe RA, Chhaya S, Nasci K, et al. Effect of ethnicity on denial of authorization for emergency department care by managed care gatekeepers. *Acad Emerg Med*. 2001;8(3):259-266.

20. Harris B, Hwang U, Lee WS, Richardson LD. Disparities in use of computed tomography for patients presenting with headache. *Am J Emerg Med*. 2009;27(3):333-336.

21. Pezzin LE, Keyl PM, Green GB. Disparities in the emergency department evaluation of chest pain patients. *Acad Emerg Med*. 2007;14(2):149-156.

22. Pierce A. Vulnerable populations: the homeless and incarcerated. In: Martin LM, Heron LS, Moreno Walton L, Jones WA, eds. *Diversity and Inclusion in Quality Patient Care*. Cham, Switzerland: Springer International Publishing; 2016:151-160.

23. Doran KM, Vashi AA, Platis S, et al. Navigating the boundaries of emergency department care: addressing the medical and social needs of patients who are homeless. *Am J Public Health*. 2013;103 (suppl 2):S355-S360.

24. Castaneda-Guarderas A, Glassberg J, Grudzen CR, et al. Shared decision making with vulnerable populations in the emergency department. *Acad Emerg Med*. 2016;23(12):1410-1416.

25. Glassberg JA, Tanabe P, Chow A, et al. Emergency provider analgesic practices and attitudes toward patients with sickle cell disease. *Ann Emerg Med.* 2013;62(4):293-302.

26. Farley-Toombs C. The stigma of a psychiatric diagnosis: prevalence, implications and nursing interventions in clinical care settings. *Crit Care Nurs Clin North Am.* 2012;24(1):149-156.

27. Van Nieuwenhuizen A, Henderson C, Kassam A, et al. Emergency department staff views and experiences on diagnostic overshadowing related to people with mental illness. *Epidemiol Psychiatr Sci.* 2013;22(3):255-262.

28. Jalali S, Sauer LM. Improving care for lesbian, gay, bisexual, and transgender patients in the emergency department. *Ann Emerg Med.* 2015;66(4):417-423.

29. Chisolm-Straker M, Jardine L, Bennouna C, et al. Transgender and gender nonconforming in emergency departments: a qualitative report of patient experiences. *Transgend Health.* 2017;2(1):8-16. doi:10.1089/trgh.2016.0026.

30. Chisolm-Straker M, Willging C, Daul AD, et al. Transgender and gender nonconforming patients in the emergency department: what physicians know, think, and do. *Ann Emerg Med.* 2018;71(2):183-88.e1.

31. Nivet MA, Fair M. Defining diversity in quality care. In: Martin LM, Heron LS, Moreno Walton L, Jones WA, eds. *Diversity and Inclusion in Quality Patient Care.* Cham, Switzerland: Springer International Publishing; 2016:3-10.

32. Cooper-Patrick L, Gallo JJ, Gonzales JJ, et al. Race, gender, and partnership in the patient-physician relationship. *JAMA.* 1999;282(6):583-589.

33. Van Ryn M. Research on the provider contribution to race/ethnicity disparities in medical care. *Med Care.* 2002;40(1 suppl):I140-I151.

34. Scott CJ. Ethnicity culture, and the delivery of health-care services. In: Bernstein E, Bernstein J, eds. *Case Studies in Emergency Medicine and the Health of the Public.* Boston, MA: Jones and Bartlett Publishers; 1996:129-151.

35. Richardson LD. Patients' rights and professional responsibilities: the moral case for cultural competence. *Mt Sinai J Med.* 1999;66(4):267-270.

36. Galanti G. *Caring for Patients From Different Cultures.* 2nd ed. Philadelphia, Pa: University of Pennsylvania Press; 1997:P12-P14, 26-28.

37. Broderick J, Brott T, Kothari R, et al. The Greater Cincinnati/Northern Kentucky Stroke Study: preliminary first-ever and total incidence rates of stroke among blacks. *Stroke.* 1998;29(2):415-421.

38. Yusuf S, Reddy S, Ôunpuu S, Anand S. Global burden of cardiovascular diseases: part II: variations in cardiovascular disease by specific ethnic groups and geographic regions and prevention strategies. *Circulation.* 2001;104(23):2855-2864.

39. Anand SS, Yusuf S, Vuksan V, et al. Differences in risk factors, atherosclerosis, and cardiovascular disease between ethnic groups in Canada: the Study of Health Assessment and Risk in Ethnic Groups (SHARE). *Lancet.* 2000;356(9226):279-284.

40. ALLHAT Officers, Coordinators for the ALLHAT Collaborative Research Group. Major outcomes in moderately hypercholesterolemic, hypertensive patients randomized to pravastatin vs usual care: The Antihypertensive and Lipid-Lowering Treatment to Prevent Heart Attack Trial (ALLHAT-LLT). *JAMA.* 2002;288(23):2998-3007.

41. US Census Bureau. Detailed languages spoken at home and ability to speak English for the population 5 years and over: 2009-2013. 2015. Available at: http://www.census.gov/data/tables/2013/demo/2009-2013-lang-tables.html. Accessed April 28, 2016.

42. Njeru JW, St Sauver JL, Jacobson DJ, et al. Emergency department and inpatient health care utilization among patients who require interpreter services. *BMC Health Serv Res.* 2015;15:214.

43. Gallagher RA, Porter S, Monuteaux MC, Stack AM. Unscheduled return visits to the emergency department: the impact of language. *Pediatr Emerg Care.* 2013;29(5):579-583.

44. Ngai KM, Grudzen CR, Lee R, Tong VY, Richardson LD, Fernandez A. The association between limited English proficiency and unplanned emergency department revisit within 72 hours. *Ann Emerg Med.* 2016;68(2):213-221.

45. Crane JA. Patient comprehension of doctor-patient communication on discharge from the emergency department. *J Emerg Med.* 1997;15(1):1-7.

46. Carrasquillo O, Orav EJ, Brennan TA, Burstin HR. Impact of language barriers on patient satisfaction in an emergency department. *J Gen Intern Med.* 1999;14(2):82-87.

47. National Standards for Culturally and Linguistically Appropriate Services in Health Care. 2001. Available at: https://thinkculturalhealth.hhs.gov/assets/pdfs/EnhancedNationalCLASStandards.pdf. Updated 2013. Accessed November 22, 2018.

48. Chan YY, Alagappan K, Bilal S, Hargrave J, Bentley S, Martin ML. Interpreter services. In: Martin LM, Heron S, Moreno Walton L, Jones WA, eds. *Diversity and Inclusion in Quality Patient Care.* Cham, Switzerland: Springer International Publishing; 2016:55-67.

49. Kingston AM, Morien M, Hinrichs SH. Bioterrorism preparedness: the challenge of disparate populations. In: Satcher D, Pamies RJ, eds. *Multicultural Medicine and Health Disparities.* New York, NY: McGraw Hill; 2006.

50. Betancourt JR, Green AR, Carrillo JE, Ananeh-Firempong O II. Defining cultural competence: a practical framework for addressing racial/ethnic disparities in health and health care. *Public Health Rep.* 2003;118(4):293-302.

51. Smedley BD, Stith AY, Colburn L, Evans CH. *The Right Thing to Do, The Smart Thing to Do: Enhancing Diversity in Health Professions.* Washington DC: National Academy Press; 2001:9-12. Available at: https://www.ncbi.nlm.nih.gov/books/NBK223633/pdf/Bookshelf_NBK223633.pdf. Accessed November 8, 2018.

52. Sullivan Commission on Diversity in the Healthcare Workforce. Missing persons: minorities in the health professions. 2004. Available at: http://health-equity.lib.umd.edu/40/1/Sullivan_Final_Report_000.pdf. Accessed November 8, 2018.

53. American Medical Association. *Physician Characteristics and Distribution in the US.* 2015 ed. 2015. Available at: https:///C:/Users/LDRMD/Downloads/Underrepresented_by-Specialty.pdf. Accessed September 4, 2018.

54. Pamies J, Hill GC, Watkins L Jr, McNamee MJ, Colburn L. Diversity and the health-care workforce. In: Satcher D, Pamies RJ, eds. *Multicultural Medicine and Health Disparities.* New York, NY: McGraw Hill; 2006:405-414.

55. Health Research and Educational Trust. *Improving Health Equity Through Data Collection and Use: A Guide for Hospital Leaders.* Chicago, Ill: Health Research & Educational Trust; 2011. Available at: http://www.hret.org/health-equity/index.shtml. Accessed September 9, 2018.

56. Niska R, Bhuiya F, Xu J. *National Hospital Ambulatory Medical Care Survey: 2007 Emergency Department Summary. National Health Statistics Reports. No 26.* Hyattsville, MD: National Center for Health Statistics; 2010. Available at: https://www.cdc.gov/nchs/data/nhsr/nhsr026.pdf. Accessed November 8, 2018.

57. New York State Toolkit to reduce health care disparities: improving race and ethnicity data. 2014. Available at: https://www.albany.edu/sph/cphce/mrt_nys_toolkit_to_reduce_healthcare_disparities.pdf. Accessed September 9, 2018.

58. A toolkit for collecting race, ethnicity, and primary language information from patients. Health Research and Education Trust. 2011. Available at: http://www.hretdisparities.org/Howt-4176.php. Accessed December 2019.

CHAPTER 30

EMERGENCY DEPARTMENT MANAGEMENT ESSENTIALS

Robert W. Strauss, Jay Kaplan, Jeffrey Eye

Emergency departments (EDs) must consistently deliver exemplary results within a highly regulated and unpredictable environment. Department leaders must provide a prescriptive, predictable, and reliable service and simultaneously demonstrate agility and responsiveness to conditions that fall outside of the standard workflow while also increasing productivity. To accomplish these goals, leaders must facilitate and develop:

- Strong strategic plans
- Positive departmental culture and identity
- Robust clinical and administrative processes
- Quality performance measures and improvement
- Effective learning and innovation systems

Effective ED leaders perform their duties within their institution's and service line's organizational infrastructure—integrating meetings, processes, relationships, and tools. Successful ED leaders proactively define and organize their department processes. Failing that, the department may simply organically and entropically evolve and change from day to day.

A number of factors influence the ED infrastructure, including organizational culture, size, mission, past performance, leadership style, affiliations, physician and nursing engagement, and inherent incentives. Regardless of form, it is within and through the department's infrastructure that the department leadership and clinical professionals:

- Define the identity and direction of the department.
- Create work systems.
- Measure and address performance.
- Prepare for future challenges.

A well-defined service-line infrastructure does not inherently drive better performance; rather, it is an organizational tool that must be used by passionate professionals. In other words, systems are only successful if they are consistently used by people committed to reaching defined outcomes. A well-managed department requires leaders who are knowledgeable, set goals, create vision, define plans, engage staff, evaluate results, hold people accountable, and have the initiative to act. A thoughtfully implemented infrastructure provides the construct and organizational discipline by which to channel departmental resources toward achieving the desired results.

LEADERSHIP AND ALIGNMENT

It is rare to find an organization with aspirations of mediocrity; yet, many function as if that is the aim. The absence of identity, strategic direction, standards of practice, and accountability make it impossible to efficiently move a complex system toward any exceptional purpose. These must be developed and managed by the ED's leaders. A clear organizational chart with defined reporting relationships is vitally important.

Cohesive Leadership

Patients are unaware of the fragmented siloed compartments. Instead, they experience care in a continuous arc from entry to discharge. ED staff weave a social fabric in which patients and families receive care and that fabric answers the fundamental questions patients have: "Is it safe here? Is everyone working together to help me?" The action of each agent in the system impacts the clinical care and the experience of the patient, and it only takes one person to rupture that fabric.

The best EDs are viewed as complete and seamless systems. They align goals with expectations. These high-performance EDs overcome the stereotypical divisions of labor between nursing, medical, diagnostic, and business units, all with conflicting incentives and direction. Rather, these EDs are led by a cohesive and aligned leadership that creates and shares a vision of an integrated department. When there is a group of directors identified as leaders, they must develop and communicate a clear and consistent plan to guide the department. This is often referred to as "dyad" or "triad" leadership, with medical director, nursing director, and (if so defined) administrative director speaking with one voice.

It has been said that the relationship between the ED medical director and ED nursing director is like a marriage. If it is good, it can be really good; if it is dysfunctional, everyone suffers. There must be agreed-upon goals, mutual appreciation, lots of give and take, and continuous communication resulting in collaboration on and clarity of direction. Medical and nursing leadership are covered in more detail elsewhere in this text, but any discussion of organizational infrastructure must recognize that infrastructure has to be built on effective and unambiguous leadership. While disagreements may and likely will occur behind closed doors, the medical and nursing directors must continuously work toward consensus and have one message to all staff once consensus has been reached.

Leadership Caveats

Several caveats are important to mention before discussing the tools needed for ED excellence. These cautionary notes pertain to physician and nurse leadership, the charge physician, and the charge nurse.

Physician and Nurse Leadership

First, the physician and nurse leaders of the department must be given the resources to be successful. Regardless of the staffing model, the physician functioning as the medical director must be given the protected time necessary to carry out leadership duties as well as clinical responsibilities. It is impossible for a physician to work a full clinical load of 12 to 16 shifts a month and still have the time to attend meetings, develop staff, participate in operational and clinical improvements, communicate with other institutional leaders, manage complaints, and devote thoughtful attention to the direction of the department. Not only the medical director but also the nursing director is expected to carry multiple responsibilities. Too often, the nursing director/

manager is expected to "do it all," and there may be no job more difficult to do well than being an ED nursing director.

While some of the duties of the leaders may be delegated, many require direct involvement. Medical and nursing directors should not be just figureheads. They must be intimately involved in all aspects of departmental operations and all major decisions, innovations, and process changes. Many believe those leaders should also continue to have a clinical presence in the department.

The organization must also have the appropriate assistants and systems to support the tasks of leadership, management, education, staffing, budgeting, and concurrent problem-solving. Because neither the medical director nor the nursing director can be on the unit 24 × 7, it is crucial to have continuous real-time management of the department, which can be provided by the on-duty charge physician and charge nurse.

Charge Physician

When more than one physician is on duty at any given time, it is appropriate to designate a lead physician. The role of that "charge physician" is to:

- Work with the charge nurse to maintain efficient ED patient and information flow.
- Be the chain-of-command liaison for patient issues, such as patient complaints, nurses having questions about medical treatments or discharges, and so on.
- Help to coordinate patient movement when wait times are exceeding the established thresholds.
- Assign which physician will see the next critical patient or any patient when physicians are soon to go off shift.
- Initiate additional triage orders before placing patients in rooms if needed by the triage/float nurse.

If the charge physician role is not defined, then the ED charge nurse unfairly shoulders the burden of patient flow in the ED. Without a collaborating charge physician, providers may wait passively for patients to be placed in examination rooms for their medical evaluations.

Charge Nurse

Charge nurse leadership is also critical. The nursing director and the ED staff must be able to rely on the charge nurse to ensure that expectations for both flow and staff behaviors are consistently met. This responsibility might include processes such as:

- Quick registration
- Provider at triage
- Rapid triage and immediate bedding of patients when ED space is available
- Rounding on patients every 30 to 60 minutes to ensure they are kept informed regarding any delays and that their comfort measures are addressed
- Rapid transfer to an inpatient bed once the bed has been assigned.

When different nurses rotate through the charge position, there is no consistency of direction and no one with the authority to hold others accountable.

One ED made dramatic improvements by promulgating and supporting a set of leadership principles for the charge physician and charge nurse. The list (shown in **Box 30.1**) was created by the lead staff, who then provided their signatures as a commitment.

> **BOX 30.1 ■ CHARGE PHYSICIAN/CHARGE NURSE COMMITMENTS**
>
> 1. I will choose to have a **positive attitude**.
> 2. I will **address issues as they occur** (either 1:1 or as a group) and will *mediate conflict*.
> 3. I will **practice the art of listening** to peers and customers.
> 4. I will **be accountable** to accept, set, and promote expectations and will help to **hold my CCC colleagues accountable**.
> 5. I will **show mutual respect**.
> 6. I will **support my CCC colleagues** as a **unified** group.
> 7. I will **maintain confidentiality** in all aspects of my role.
> 8. I will be **committed to ongoing leadership education and learning**.

EFFECTIVE MEETINGS

Optimal ED outcomes require attention to both systems and people. Those with a vested interest in success must have regular meetings with a clear focus on improving clinical outcomes and patient perception of the ED experience. The meetings must focus both on optimizing performance processes and on creating an environment in which providers want to work and patients want to receive care.

Aligning personnel with clinical excellence as well as with patient and staff satisfaction can be successful if the providers are engaged. But great and efficient systems fail without the "buy-in" of the health-care professionals—the systems will either not be used or will fall into disarray. Conversely, great people without the great systems to support them will become frustrated and leave.

Basic Rules

The second law of thermodynamics relates to entropy, implying that any system will move toward disorganization and chaos without a constant pressure toward order. This law applies to ED systems. To continue to improve performance and apply pressure toward order, certain meetings are crucial. Before discussing the types and content of these gatherings, let's review the rules of effective meetings (discussed in greater detail in Chapter 9):

1. *Agenda*: An "action" agenda should be sent out in advance so that attendees are clear about the content, meeting goals, and responsibilities of each member present. The agenda is the roadmap that will focus the discussion on the critical issues to be addressed.

2. *Start on time*: Start on time. If a participant arrives late, some leaders will interrupt the meeting to catch them up, thus wasting the time of those who came on time and rewarding inappropriate behavior. After the meeting, the leader should privately remind the late-arriving member of the group's commitment to start on time. Each member of the team should commit to arriving on time or alerting the leader in advance if he or she will be late or absent.

3. *Begin with a positive orientation*: Perhaps start the meeting with a positive recent occurrence (e.g., a patient compliment, recognition of a specific individual, or a great patient outcome) or a reflection that connects to the group's purpose. Then

orient the participants to the purpose of the current agenda. Engage the group by describing how a successful conclusion will lead to improvement of a critical aspect of the ED, its operations, and the patients' or providers' experience—signaling to those present the importance of the work to be accomplished.

4. *Confirm action items*: Always leave the meeting with a review of the next steps or action items, including who is responsible for each item and by when the item is to be accomplished. By clarifying responsibility and gaining each participant's personal commitment, accountability is established and the leader and other members learn to expect task completion.

5. *End on time*: A meeting scheduled to last 1 hour ideally concludes the major agenda items within 50 minutes, leaving the final 10 minutes to evaluate the meeting, discuss the need for subsequent meetings or responsibilities, and address a critical off-agenda or "parking lot" issue.

By ending a few minutes early, those present will be pleased with the "gift" of extra time. By ending late, attendees will be frustrated with the poor leader management and the infringement on their time.

The Final 5 Minutes

Some leaders spend 5 minutes at the end to have the participants grade the meeting on a 1 to 5 scale, with 5 being a great session that ran smoothly, invited input from all, and accomplished its goals. This final point is crucial to long-term success. It is all too common that people leave a meeting thinking, "Well, that was a waste of my time!" Immediate feedback to the leaders of the session and to all attendees engenders improved outcomes and more efficient use of everyone's time.

Critical Meetings

Several critical types of meetings involving the ED and its leadership may need to occur at regular intervals.

Quarterly (or Monthly) Meetings

Executive leadership: Typically, the only times the C-suite (CEO, COO, CNO, CMO—the Chief Executive, Operating, Nursing, and Medical Officers) hears about the ED are when there are unfortunate outcomes, patient complaints, or prolonged poor performance. In most organizations, the ED is the highest-volume department (or perhaps second only to the primary care clinics). The reputation of the acute-care facility in the community is substantially shaped by the experiences of patients in the ED. This is one reason why regular meetings between executive leadership and ED leadership are essential.

The purpose of these meetings with the executive leadership is to create alignment with the greater organizational strategy and to critically analyze the ED's associated strategy. Hospital administration and ED leaders must collaborate to set clear expectations about the ED's direction and performance.

It is appropriate for the ED leadership to present information regarding the critical metrics and the resources required to carry out the goals of the organization. The ED leaders can also promote the ED by informing the executive team of the positive outcomes and performance of the department. This can provide balance to the executives' perceptions of the ED if they have received negative comments. Stressing the ED's accomplishments is thus an important part of an internal public relations campaign to "manage up" the department.

At the beginning of the meeting, the leaders should openly listen to any perceptions of the ED held by the administration leaders. Once the negative issues, if any, are presented, the ED leaders can work to ensure that the administration leaders understand the challenges of the department, how they are being met, and what is being done to overcome any obstacles to great patient care. It is essential to describe these obstacles objectively without embroidering on them as an excuse for not having accomplished the organizational goals.

Such clear and frequent communication of concerns, expectations, and progress will prevent little fires from becoming catastrophic conflagrations. Texting and e-mailing executive leadership can be helpful, but electronic messages *must not* replace face-to-face formal meetings. It is recommended that formal meetings with senior leaders should occur *at least* quarterly. In times of rapid change, major program development/implementation, or exponential growth, monthly meetings with senior administrators are necessary to ensure that the ED is:

- Listening to administrative goals and vision
- Communicating progress
- Receiving necessary resources and assistance
- Establishing, measuring, modifying, and accomplishing defined performance expectations

In addition to formal meetings, ED leaders should establish regular communication protocols with senior leaders, which might include the following:

- *C-suite walking rounds*: These occasional visits can provide invaluable opportunities for touching base with hospital leaders.
- *E-mail updates*: Although regular e-mail updates can be valuable, it is important to determine if your administrative leadership welcomes this form of communication. In every case, it is important to avoid using e-mail to "vent," complain, or blame.
- *Phone calls*: The phone remains one of the best ways to share quick, critical information of importance to the recipient.
- *Elevator speech*: ED leaders should always be prepared for brief, unexpected interactions with senior hospital leadership (e.g., in the elevator, in a hallway, in the lunchroom).

Monthly Meetings

Emergency performance improvement committee: The ED patient experience relates to many systems and departments. An operational meeting that reviews and refines all of these elements is vitally important. If led well, this complex multidisciplinary meeting can have profoundly positive results and lead to great improvements. Various names for this committee include Emergency Performance Improvement Committee (EPIC), ED Joint Practice Council, Emergency Services Committee, and ED Steering Committee. Names may vary, but the goal of this team is always the same: to continuously coordinate and improve all aspects of care and caring provided in the ED, including service delivered by all of the interfacing services.

Goals: The specific goals of the EPIC meetings must be patient centered and ensure that the work environment functions efficiently so that all ED staff can enjoy giving that care. It is essential that this meeting is led by ED leadership and ideally includes representatives from the multidisciplinary teams responsible for patient care, including:

- Inpatient units
- Laboratory services

- Diagnostic imaging services
- Admitting and registration staff
- Hospitalists
- Intensivists (if a separate service)
- Information technology (IT)/informatics service
- Housekeeping/environmental services
- Residency programs (if an academic center)

Each service is given time to talk about its involvement and interaction with the ED and its approach to providing service to ED patients. To ensure coordination of care, it is important that each ancillary ("essential") support service hears what the others are doing, rather than have each present their information and then leave. It is also critical that at least one member of the C-suite attend the meeting. The objectives are to ensure that all participants and systems function together as a seamless work system so that patients receive the highest quality care; and both the patient and clinicians are seen as customers or consumers of the services provided by the other departments.

Collaboration: An effective collaborative process eliminates silos and encourages all members of the committee to consider what they and their divisions can do to most effectively meet the needs of the other parties as they provide care to the patients. The goal is to break down the traditional barriers and create a collaborative partnership with all services focused on meeting the patients' needs. Some form of consistent and agreed-upon measurement method, such as an ED scorecard, can be reviewed at this meeting. The metrics will help to ensure that those departments that provide diagnostic studies and other services to ED patients take responsibility for meeting the targets that have been mutually defined.

This is an appropriate time to review the departmental action plan (see further information below). The broader perspective of the plan will demonstrate to the committee members how their work influences the outcomes of the department and its stakeholders and will validate the importance of their participation on this council.

Service excellence team: A service excellence team (which may also be called a work environment group or combined unit council) engages all of the staff and providers in the efforts to make the ED both a better place for patients to come for care and a better place for staff and physicians to work. Whereas the cross-departmental, operationally focused, EPIC meeting focuses mainly on process and what should happen, the service excellence team emphasizes the work environment and the patient experience. Defining how specific services are delivered and perceived leads to the formation of behaviors, patterns, and ultimately culture. To achieve success, the team must identify and address the common forms of resistance among staff who may not understand the importance of the patients' perceptions.

Many ED personnel mistakenly believe that patients and other clinicians only care about the quality of the care. They would assert that they must only demonstrate clinical competence; that patients will automatically be satisfied if appropriate care is provided; and that someone else is responsible for creating a great practice setting.

The reality is that it takes more than quality care to satisfy the many stakeholders who interact with the ED. Unfortunately, some members of the ED team may not possess the skill set, the desire, or have the time to employ quality *caring* while providing quality *care*. This committee should comprise high-performing clinical staff and providers, those who are among the best at their job and who understand the mandate to simultaneously deliver quality care and caring. Ideally, the ED leadership plays a facilitating role instead of directing the solutions and dialogue. As facilitators, the responsibility of the leaders is to ensure that the members remain aligned with the values of the organization/department and receive training relative to designing effective processes.

In this meeting, the group can brainstorm and consider: "What would it take to generate the best place for us to work and the best place for our patients to come for care?" Brainstorming entails a "freethinking process" without the constraints of current thinking, processes, or resources. Then the committee can create a list of what is working (and not working) in the department and determine what solutions can be used and/or invented to make things better. This committee can address and solve highly emotional, inefficient, or frustrating processes that ED staff deal with on a daily basis. Broad participation on this team can be empowering. Participants recognize that an efficient and caring work environment will not happen spontaneously but rather through intentional and consistent effort.

Effective service excellence teams should present the list of suggestions, solutions, and recommendations they have generated to the ED management team (EPIC) and senior leadership. When staff members transition from shift workers to engaged and empowered owners of processes, rapid changes for improved quality and service are facilitated. Participants in this committee may self-nominate or be chosen by ED leadership and invited. Broad representation is essential, and physician attendance at such meetings is mandatory. Committee membership should require a 1-year commitment. It is prudent to set the schedule and time of the meeting in advance and avoid schedule conflicts to allow for consistent attendance.

Staff meetings: A goal of any hospital senior leadership team is to create a consistent environment and set of processes for all patients. Another goal is to create a workspace in which recruitment and retention of excellent people are paramount. Many ED providers are individualistic and have individualized approaches to caring for patients that do not always entail working together as a team. However, to accomplish a consistent approach to the provision of excellent emergency care, a regular (monthly) discussion of uniform processes, outcomes, and behaviors is necessary.

Staff members must be well versed in the design of the processes and the desired/expected outcomes. Sharing performance data, including improvements and continuing gaps, helps staff understand the impact of individual actions on the collective performance of the department. The agenda should be sent out in advance and typically include discussions of service and quality results, peer review, and operational efficiencies and opportunities. If these meetings include only a single, rather than multiple, discipline(s), nurse leaders should be invited to a portion of the physician staff meeting and physician leaders invited to a portion of the nursing staff meeting.

While monthly ED staff meetings are important, it is equally important for the physician and nurse teams to meet on a regular basis. Technology allows regular meetings to be accomplished virtually. Nonetheless, it is important to have occasional, at least a quarterly, meetings with all available physicians and nurses in the room so that the departmental vision may be communicated.

Weekly Meetings

A weekly or biweekly ED management team meeting ensures effective functioning and responsive management of issues and opportunities. An ED management team meeting is not a "catch-you-on-the-fly-while-you-the-medical/nursing-director-are-seeing-patients" get-together. It is a formal meeting where the agenda is defined and minutes are kept in order to create accountability and define the action steps that are needed for the coming week(s).

These management meetings are appropriately led by either the ED medical director or nursing director and attended by nursing and physician leadership, the clerical/registration supervisor of the ED, and occasionally senior hospital leadership. Depending on the volume and complexity of the ED, meeting frequency may be at least biweekly or even weekly. The purpose of these meetings is to ensure proactive management of department processes rather than relying on retrospective attempts to solve problems. Topics covered may include:

- Metrics with review of the scorecard (see later) including both clinical quality and service results
- Intradepartmental issues such as staffing, stocking of supplies, tools, and equipment
- Opportunities identified in rounding or in staff meetings
- Morale, relationships between different members of the team, and recognition and reward of high performers
- Interdepartmental subjects such as relationships with inpatient units (e.g., acceptance of admitted patients)
- Flow issues related to lab or imaging, turnaround times, and patient flow
- Information technology's assistance in concurrent and retrospective patient data

Daily Meetings

Some meetings should occur on a daily basis. These include staff huddles, "medical minutes," tracking board rounds, and nursing supervisor rounds.

Staff huddles: Huddles are stand-up meetings held in the ED at the beginning of a shift. During the huddles, the current operational state of the ED and the hospital and the daily areas of focus are reviewed. Much as a coach meets with the team prior to the game, the huddles allow the ED team to regularly evaluate current conditions, review the game plan, and receive some words of encouragement. Starting the shift as a team—with a huddle—aligns everyone and solidifies expectations.

It is important that the physicians attend these meetings whenever possible, even if their shift has already started. Integration of the nursing and physician work systems in the ED is vital to achieving operational excellence. If the ED nurse manager or clinical supervisor is not available to lead these meetings, the charge nurse manages the agenda. It is important that the managers/leaders of the department are present for these meetings several times a week and that they interact with both day and night staff members as they begin their shifts. Most leaders find that a standardized agenda permits a brief gathering while accomplishing the goal of informing and motivating staff as well as reminding them about behaviors that are being coached. The following standardized agenda addresses most necessary huddle issues:

1. ***Current state of the ED:*** The number and acuity of patients in the ED, the number of (boarded) patients awaiting inpatient bed placement, and staffing/assignments for the day (shift)
2. ***Current state of the hospital inpatient services:*** The number of available inpatient and specialty unit beds, occupancy rate, and staffing issues
3. ***Current or expected concerns:*** For example, IT outages, scheduled radiology maintenance, community events
4. ***Current metrics review:*** Patient satisfaction (e.g., door-to-provider times, decision to admit-to-bed assignment times, bed assignment-to-ED discharge times)
5. ***Patient outcomes:*** Wins, saves, feedback from callbacks of patients treated and released
6. ***Current focus (for the day or month):*** Processes and behaviors, such as scripts, quick triage and immediate bedding on the front end, half-hourly rounding on patients, and completion of whiteboards
7. ***Other information:*** Brief information that staff may need to know to help them have a great shift and provide patients outstanding care

The "medical minute": To start off the shift with a strong sense of physician and nurse collaboration, the concept of the "medical minute" may be incorporated into the stand-up meetings or huddles. At the shift change, an attending or senior resident gives a 60-second "lecture." Anything goes, but this discussion must be limited to 60 seconds. Topics can include a new drug; exclusion criteria for pulmonary embolus, transient ischemic attack versus stroke; or a recent patient case with an interesting clinical presentation and diagnosis. Staff typically appreciate this, and it may stimulate discussion later if a patient presents to the ED whose care involves the topic of the day.

A culture of learning and innovation can be created in 60 seconds. This brief educational process sparks questions and reminds staff that the science of health care is continually changing. It also allows staff to see their peers as teachers and experts. This perception inevitably impacts patient interactions and promotes "managing up" coworkers, which has a positive impact on patients' perceptions of teamwork, competence, and communication. One physician wrote:

> *The medical minute is also a great opportunity to gently guide staff in [positive] ways. For example, after discussing [pelvic inflammatory disease] during our medical minute, I had nurses prompting me immediately to complete pelvic exams (instead of avoiding them!). Nurses and technicians love getting medical teaching. They work in the ED because they are naturally drawn to this varied and fascinating patient population and pathology, but they haven't had the years and years of academic study that we have. Sharing what we know and how we think is good for morale and I believe will increase the quality of the care we provide.*

From a practical standpoint, the best way to start this process is to "hardwire" it by consistently presenting it at the 7 am (shift change) meeting; it may be difficult to consistently implement this program at the evening stand-up meeting time as it is often much busier. Once the medical minute concept is introduced, nurses may be asked to create a list of topics they would like covered.

Tracking board rounds: Periodic appraisal of the status of the ED's capacity, patient demand, and patient flow facilitates more efficient ED operations. The charge nurse (flow coordinator) and emergency physician(s) review all patients currently in process (including potential admissions), in the waiting (reception) room, and ready for discharge. Patients no longer requiring a stretcher can be placed in alternative treatment spaces (including a results pending area). Note that when several physicians are staffing the ED simultaneously, many organizations pair the charge nurse (flow coordinator) with a charge emergency physician.

Either the charge nurse or charge physician may call for the analysis. One positive effect of this practice is that increasing physician awareness and involvement increases their sense of responsibility for patients not yet in rooms. This awareness generates proactive patient movement, decreasing the sometimes overwhelming "tsunami" wave of patients waiting to be seen.

Nursing supervisor rounds: Most inpatient units are staffed for current census rather than for the expected number of admissions from the ED. Additionally, inpatient staff scheduled to work may be "called off" (told not to come in) 2 hours before the beginning of a shift. To address potential incongruent inpatient demand/capacity needs, scheduled board rounds with the administrative/inpatient nursing supervisor can assist ED patient flow, identify patients whose admission to the hospital is likely but not yet ordered, and alert the inpatient nursing leadership of probable admissions and the need for currently scheduled (or increased) inpatient staff. Regularly scheduled rounds can also help nursing supervisors avoid inappropriately telling the staff to stay home. It is recommended that these rounds take place at a minimum of every 3 hours and 2½ hours prior to shift change.

MEASUREMENT SYSTEMS

Creating a specific ED scorecard/dashboard is necessary for operational improvement.

"Bowling" in the ED

The sport of bowling can be used to create an excellent analogy:

- When rolling the ball down the alley, the goal is to knock all the pins down.
- If there were no pins at the far end of the alley, no one would go bowling.
- If someone said "let's go bowling but not keep score," it would not be as much fun and improvement would not be perceived or enjoyed.
- When a throw does not lead to getting a strike by knocking all the pins down, in the next new frame the bowler usually thinks "What can I do to throw differently so I knock more pins down this time and improve my score?"

This works in bowling . . . but too often in health care, unfortunately:

- We throw the ball down the alley (and repeat our process) again and again.
- We have no clear pins (goals) for which we are aiming.
- We do not keep score (keep and evaluate metrics).
- If someone asks "Why are you doing it the way you are doing it?" our response can only be "Because we have always done it this way."

When there are no goals and score is not kept, processes occur by habit, and improvement is not sought, change does not occur—no one owns or takes responsibility for the process. When change is desired, leaders must do the following:

- Set up the pins (i.e., define targets and goals).
- Aim and follow-through (i.e., attempt to achieve the goals).
- Keep score (i.e., measure success by reviewing the key metrics).
- Ascertain the current score (i.e., determine the baseline).
- Allow bowlers to know their scores (i.e., provide feedback results in a timely manner).
- Encourage higher scores (i.e., share tools necessary to improve).

Balanced Scorecards

A balanced scorecard is an excellent way to organize goals into a clear and understandable framework. For example, the "The Balanced Scorecard—Measures that Drive Performance" by Robert S. Kaplan and David P. Norton[1] defines the following four perspectives addressed by the balanced scorecard and the questions they answer:

- *Customer perspective*: How do customers see us?
- *Innovation and learning perspective*: Can we continue to improve and create value?
- *Internal business perspective*: What must we excel at?
- *Financial perspective*: How do we look to shareholders?

Pillars

The five pillars used by many health-care organizations (defined by Quint Studer in his book *Hardwiring Excellence*)[2] are:

1. Service
2. Quality
3. People
4. Finance
5. Growth

Some hospitals have added the additional pillars of community and medical staff. These organizational frameworks are then consistently used to discuss process improvements and initiatives for the institution—from the senior leadership to the day-to-day staff. Once this foundational (organizational) concept is accepted, an integrated ED scorecard can be organized.

Too often, hospitals have multiple independent scorecards with one for quality, another for finance, one for patient satisfaction, and yet another for patient safety. It is recommended that organizations create a single executive ED scorecard to track all of the key metrics for the ED (**Table 30.1**). Care needs to be exercised to focus on the *key* metrics rather than *all* of the metrics. Rather than passively tracking the statistics, the goal is to define the baseline statistics, create target goals, create an action plan to accomplish those goals, and measure and share progress.

Effective action plans have action steps tied to goals on the scorecard and containing the following *SMART* characteristics: Steps must be:

- **S**pecific, with outcomes that are...
- **M**easurable, with...
- **A**ssigned with accountability for each of the steps. The steps must also be...
- **R**esults-oriented with...
- **T**imelines defined for completion.

The action plan creates a summary document that guides performance improvement and operational oversight. It is vital to provide ED professionals with ongoing communication and feedback. Additional communication tools and mechanisms that can be helpful include the following:

- *Mini-incident care variance report*: A tool to document the little things that get in the way of having a great workday in the ED (**Figure 30.1** and **Figure 30.2**).
- *Stoplight report*: A method to define for ED staff and physicians what you are doing to address their issues: green for what you have already addressed, yellow for what is in process, and red for what you cannot do currently and defining why (**Figure 30.3**).
- *Communication boards*: Post in the staff lounge the current results of the balanced scorecard.
- *Newsletters*: Monthly documents that communicate departmental issues as well as educational and social information.

TABLE 30.1 ■ ED Goals and Metrics Sheet

Facility _____

	Metrics	Baseline	Goal	March	April
Service Service	Patient satisfaction—Overall percentile		85 percentile		
	Patient satisfaction—Physician section percentile		85 percentile		
	Patient satisfaction—Nurse (or other key) section percentile		85 percentile		
	Discharge phone calls % contacted		60%		
Quality	Patient arrival to bed		15 minutes		
	Bed to physician/advanced practice provider		15 minutes		
	Length of stay times				
	ED discharges		150 minutes		
	ED fast-track vol.		60 minutes		
	ED admissions		240 minutes		
	Imaging/lab turnaround time measures		30 minutes		
	Admit order to patient, leaves ED for inpatient bed		60 minutes		
	Patient boarding—Number and hours		0/0		
	Core measures—Acute MI–percutaneous coronary intervention within 90 minutes		100%		
	Core measures—Admit decision time to ED departure		100%		
	Inpatient metric—% patients discharged by 12 noon				
People	% vacancy rate RN/LPN		10%		
	% or number shifts below minimum core staffing		10%		

(Continued)

TABLE 30.1 ■ (Continued)

Finance	% ID copied on patient chart	100%		
	% Left prior to medical screening examination	1.0		
	Co-pays and deductibles collected per month(s)	25,000		
Growth	Patient visits–% change for the month comparing the month this year to last year			
	Patient visits–% change for the year to date comparing this year to last year			
	Patient admissions–% change for the month comparing the month this year to last year			
	Patient admissions–% change for the year to date comparing this year to last year			

FIGURE 30.1 ■ Mini-Incident Care Variance

"My work-life was challenging today because…"

_____ Lab turnaround time
_____ Consultation response time
_____ X-ray turnaround time

- ❑ Private MD
- ❑ On-call service
- ❑ Psychiatry
- ❑ Pharmacy
- ❑ Nurse/tech/MT
- ❑ House supervisor
- ❑ Dietary issues
- ❑ Housekeeping issues
- ❑ Stocking of supplies
- ❑ Missing equipment
- ❑ Broken equipment
- ❑ Attitude of staff
- ❑ Attitude of physician
- ❑ Other

Turn in to director when completed.

Comments

FIGURE 30.2 ■ Mini-Incident Care Variance

MINI-INCIDENT REPORT

- ❏ Supply issues
- ❏ Lab issue
- ❏ Radiology issues
    - ❏ Plain films
    - ❏ CT
    - ❏ US
    - ❏ Other _____
- ❏ Blood bank
- ❏ Nursing units
- ❏ Registration
- ❏ Respiratory
- ❏ Pharmacy
- ❏ Behavioral health
- ❏ Social worker
- ❏ MD
    - ❏ ECC _____
    - ❏ Other _____
- ❏ EMS
    - ❏ Cabarrus
    - ❏ Rowan
    - ❏ Stanly
- ❏ Security/LEO
- ❏ EVS
- ❏ Facilities
- ❏ IS

"WASN'T THAT FRUSTRATING?!"

Date _____
Shift _____

Comments (description of issue)
_____
_____

You will receive feedback via email if you provide your name _____

Place in manager's mailbox or give to a PCC.

FIGURE 30.3 ■ Stoplight Report

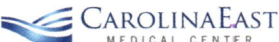

Stoplight Report

Department: _____ Month: _____

	GREEN - COMPLETED		
Date	Improvement / Item / Opportunity	Solution	Date Completed

	YELLOW - IN PROGRESS		
Date	Improvement / Item / Opportunity	Status	Status Date

	RED - UNABLE TO COMPLETE AT THIS TIME		
Date	Improvement / Item / Opportunity	Status	Status Date

EMERGENCY DEPARTMENT

Use only non-abrasive cleaners, CaviWipes, Expo, Isopropyl alcohol, soap & water and disinfectants Ok with 6 year warranty from www.ahutton.com

CONCLUSION

A sound organizational infrastructure with committed and knowledgeable leadership is a requirement in the rapidly changing health-care environment. EDs are scrutinized by senior hospital leadership who see the importance of the ED as the front door to the hospital. Emergency care leaders and managers must maintain a foundation on which to build improvement efforts—systems and methodologies to help create a consistent high-quality, highly-caring clinical environment. The processes shared in this chapter are a beginning. As noted, author Tom Peters states in his book *The Circle of Innovation*[3]:

> *If the other guy's getting better, you'd better be getting better faster than that other guy's getting better, or you're getting worse.*

REFERENCES

1. Kaplan RS, Norton DP. The balanced scorecard—measures that drive performance. Harvard Business Review. January to February 1992. https://hbr.org/1992/01/the-balanced-scorecard-measures-that-drive-performance-2.
2. Studer Q. Hardwiring Excellence. Pensacola, Fla: Fire Starter Publishing; 2014.
3. Peters T. The Circle of Innovation. New York, NY: Vintage Books; 2010.

CHAPTER 31

THE VIEW FROM THE C-SUITE

Thom A. Mayer, Steve Narang, Robert W. Strauss, Charles Stokes, John Brennan, Michael Born

Leadership is a matter of how to be, not what to do.

—Frances Hesselbein[1]

What you are stands over you and thunders so that I cannot hear what you say.

—Ralph Waldo Emerson[2]

The bonds between patients and their physicians and nurses, as well as those among the emergency department (ED) team, are the most critical in emergency medicine and nursing. Other than those bonds, no single relationship is more important than the one between the ED leadership team and the senior leadership of the hospital and the health-care system. As this text makes clear, leadership *matters*. Hospitals are complex, adaptive systems that cannot operate, much less innovate, without visionary leadership.[3,4] It did not take the challenges of the severe COVID-19 pandemic to focus on the importance of leadership to an ED, but it did epitomize why leadership matters, as well as exemplify the cataclysmic nature of change in health care.[5,6]

Dynamic paradigms create dynamic tensions, as the rules become less important than the relationships that produce the desired results. Like all meaningful and lasting changes, these are driven by intrinsic motivation not extrinsic forces, but all substantive change initially involves resistance, which must be overcome to make meaningful progress.[7] More details on the science of change management are presented in Chapter 3.

This chapter reflects the collective voices of CEOs from some of the most successful health-care systems across the country. It is a synthesis from conversations concerning the best practices of how a powerful partnership between ED leaders and senior health-care leadership can be both meaningful and transformational. Of necessity, some duplication of insights in different sections and in the authors' personal reflections exists, all of which simply reemphasize the importance of those points. The C-suite and particularly the CEOs' views and actions, in the words of Steve Narang, MD, CEO of Inova Fairfax Medical Campus, come "straight from the airway of the organization," meaning they reflect the most fundamental aspects, which is the *A* of the fundamental resuscitative concept of the ABCs of airway, breathing, and circulation (S. Narang, personal conversation with the author TM, June 14, 2020.) "Straight from the airway of the organization" wonderfully illustrates Hesselbein's insight on "how to be," as well as Emerson's on "what you are" as opposed to "what you say." What comes "straight from the airway" through the actions of leaders can and should be assessed by the team each day.

SENIOR LEADERSHIP AND ED LEADERSHIP TEAMS

The CEO of the hospital leads the senior leadership teams of medical organizations and typically reports either to the chair of the board (see Chapter 5) or to the CEO of the healthcare system.[8] The team also typically comprises the:

- Chief operating officer (COO)
- Chief medical officer (CMO)
- Chief nurse executive (CNE)
- Chief financial officer

Other members of the leadership teams may include the chief experience officer, chief quality officer, chief safety officer, chief information officer, and others. Together, this group of senior leaders is often referred to as the C-suite, which is not a pejorative term but widely used shorthand referring to senior leadership.[9]

The ED leadership team should include the nursing director and the medical director and increasingly includes a hospital administration representative as well. Depending upon leadership team preferences and structure, the ED leadership team works with and reports to a specific, assigned member of the senior leadership team. The most common reporting relationships for the ED team are to the CEO or COO, but some report to the CMO, CNE, or both.

Without exception, specific goals and objectives for ED operations are identified, as well as metrics by which to monitor success. The frequency of team meetings and reporting of metric success vary by organization. In all cases, one of the key aspects of the relationship between the senior leadership team and the ED leaders is the "alignment of strategic incentives," meaning ensuring that both groups have a clearly aligned perspective on how the ED fits into the broader strategic objectives of the organization.[10,11]

REACHING THE FUTURE EXTRAORDINARY STATE

Thomas Kuhn's *The Structure of Scientific Revolutions* stressed the importance of "paradigm shifts," in which ways of framing scientific discussion changed as the paradigms by which they are understood shifted in response to the science.[12] Health-care leadership is in the midst of a paradigm shift from the ordinary precepts of a relatively stable environment to the extraordinary state of rapid change.

Functional Silos vs Dyad-Triad Leadership

Several chapters in Section 2 discuss the concept of moving from functional silos to dyad leadership, in which nursing and physician leaders cocreate an environment focused on teamwork for the good of the patient. Ideal systems and processes are based on the principle that they must be good for the patient and good for those caring for the patient. Functional silos were first described by Phil Ensor, who was describing manufacturing processes, but the term applies well to traditional health-care systems in which physician, nursing, and administrative leaders report through separate pathways and structures, resulting far too often in working at cross purposes and without an integrated set of values, systems, and processes.[13,14] In functionally siloed EDs, it is common to hear:

That's not a nurse problem, that's a doctor problem.
That's not a doctor problem, that's a nurse problem.
That's not an ED problem, that's a radiology/laboratory/hospital medicine, etc., problem.
That's not our problem; talk to the people upstairs.

All language has meaning, and this "finger-pointing–not my responsibility" language indicates a fragmented, functionally siloed organization that will always have distractions from patient care and team dynamics. To accomplish the organization's and the department's strategic goals as an integrated team, the team must be led by collaborative leaders who are committed to tearing down the walls of functional silos. ED leadership is by nature and necessity a team sport.[15]

One of the most important developments that ensures deep respect among team members is the concept of dyad leadership, which is discussed in more detail in Chapters 6 and 12. Dyad leadership is a close, collegial, and collaborative partnership in which physician and nurse leaders combine as a team to use their respective skills, abilities, and training for the good of the ED team and the patients for whom they care (see Chapter 20).[16,17]

Inova Health System has recently extended that concept to triad leadership, which adds a hospital administration partner to the physician–nurse dyad in order to navigate the hospital and health-care system boundaries.[18] It recognizes that all EDs are, by their very nature and the processes that define them, complex, adaptive systems that require a team-based, dyad or triad approach to function effectively. The systems approach is at the heart of dyad–triad leadership, based on psychological and practical safety across complex boundaries, leading to adaptive and cooperative leadership. When someone asks, "Who is in charge of the ED?" dyad and triad leaders proudly answer, "*We* are!"

This adaptive approach addresses the substantial challenges facing the ED team, all of which occur within the context of constant innovation. Robert Greenleaf's model of servant leadership serves well in dyad and triad models, particularly in its emphasis on the necessity of being "servant first, then leader," as well as having a "scientist's mind, but a servant's heart."[19,20]

Dyad and triad models have joint goals and accountability with a clear division of responsibility. Effective team leadership in a dyad or triad model has some additional characteristics applicable to the ED, including:

- Alignment of strategic incentives (see above)
- A no-blame game zone characterized by mutual trust and support
- Members working to the top of their licenses
- Joint accountability for mutually developed metrics
- Eliminating, versus perpetuating, functional silos
- Joint recruitment of team members
- Team celebration of wins
- Mutually developed, specific plans for improvement
- Boundaryless EDs

Branding and Culture

Not only is the ED the front door or gateway to the hospital, it is also the gateway to the entire brand and culture of the health-care system. EDs account for the majority of inpatient admissions in most hospitals and health-care systems, which range from lows of 40% to as high as 90% of the total admissions, driving revenues and fueling efficiency.[21] But as health care transforms from a volume-based system and reimbursement model to one based on value, simply looking at admissions is a one-dimensional lens to view the ED's contribution to the hospital and health-care system.

Filling beds and using resources effectively and efficiently are clearly important, but perhaps less so in the long term than viewing the ED through a lens that balances short-term issues of volume with long-term issues of value. Charles Stokes, former CEO of two organizations that separately won the Malcolm Baldrige National Quality Award, notes "Many health-care leaders spend their days transitioning their organizations to a value-based focus . . . but they pray at night for volume!"[22]

Branding

While the term branding is often associated with marketing of products, Professor Leonard Berry of Texas A&M University's Mays Business School was among the first to understand its importance in the service industry.[23,24] Further, he and others appropriately viewed health care as a quintessential service industry, in which medicine, nursing, and personal service interact in unique ways. Berry and Seltman explored this in their work which examined the *brand* of the Mayo Clinic.[25,26] While branding is sometimes treated as being synonymous with marketing strategy, tactics, or use of evocative logos, its meaning in health care has evolved far beyond this in important ways. (While logos are a part of effective branding strategies, in this discussion, the focus is both more intense and more personal than a simple logo.) Health care—and ED care, in particular—is a personal service business, where the stakes are often as high as they can get—and are certainly to be perceived as such for ED patients and families. Branding is inextricable from the culture of the organization.

Branding in health care is bonding through trust between patients, their families, and the hospital or health-care system. It is a promise that the hospital will deliver whatever is needed, whenever it is needed, to everyone who needs it—every patient, every time. Branding connects experience with the values of the organization and the people comprising the patient experience itself. The intense, unplanned, and unexpected exposure in ED care is primarily with the team members providing the service in a culture of caring, in which the brand is "discovered" each time a patient or family member interacts with nurses, physicians, and the essential services staff comprising the team, who provide "moments of truth," as Jan Carlzon calls them—one person and one touch at a time.[27]

Emergency care occurs in highly emotional moments in which an organization with a highly developed culture (brand) establishes a complex relationship and connection with the patient, part of which is emotional, experiential, intellectual, financial, and so on. But ED care is always personal, which affords a unique opportunity for the ED to become a central part of the health-care system's brand. Data from the ED Benchmarking Alliance indicate that ED visits occur at a rate of 467 visits per 1,000 population, meaning that nearly half of the community will be touched by the ED over time.[23] That is a powerful branding opportunity, which should be understood as such and cultivated to the maximum extent.

Effective branding occurs when people drive by the hospital and express thoughts such as:

- That's where I was born.
- That's where our children were born.
- That's where they did my surgery.
- That's the ER where they took care of my . . .
  - ☐ Broken arm
  - ☐ Heart attack
  - ☐ Stroke
  - ☐ Motor vehicle accident
  - ☐ Knee injury
  - ☐ Baby when she had a fever

Branding as Trust

At its core, effective branding comes down to a culture of *trust*.[28,29] In their time of greatest need, the people who deliver the clinical care and personal service become trusted resources—and trust brings people back, again and again, when the need arises, even if it is a distinct and less-emergent need.

Branding is less consumer focused as much as it is patient and family focused. It is not (just) a financial transaction, but an opportunity for a relationship, both now and for the future. Very few areas of the health-care system offer the volume of opportunity to brand, as well as the *intensity* of the opportunity to brand as the ED, whose leadership team must understand, embrace, and communicate that great opportunity to their teams. Branding during the ED encounter and with its team creates opportunities for the entire hospital and health-care system, since the trust generated often extends to future medical needs, including obstetrics, pediatrics, adult general medical, and surgical problems. ED leaders should communicate to the team members the massive impact their work has on branding the hospital and health care system to the community and the region.

Simplicity in Branding

In branding, *simplicity* is essential. For example, here are some ways the authors' health-care systems succinctly state their cases:

- Inova—"Privileged to serve, providing world-class health care—every time, every touch"
- WellStar—"More than health care. PeopleCare"
- Memorial Hermann—"Charting a better future. A future that's built upon the HEALTH of our community"

Effective ED leaders understand that their teams are not just the front door to the hospital but also the gateway to the branding and culture of the entire system, creating unique opportunities to establish ongoing relationships built on trust, thousands, tens of thousands, or even hundreds of thousands of relationships per year—one at a time.

Hiring Right: Qualifications vs Qualities

As both the front door to the community and the gateway to the brand of the hospital and health-care system, the team members (and their leaders) who deliver the service largely define the commitment to service and clinical quality for the entire organization. *Hiring right* for leadership skills at all levels is essential to having a successful ED and includes screening, interviewing, hiring, coaching, and mentoring team members.[30,31] The effectiveness of this process will guide the team's current success, but even more importantly lays the foundation for the future of the organization. Doing so entails moving from an exclusive focus on qualifications to a more contextual focus on qualities.

Checking with colleges and previous employers is a standard part of the hiring process, but what about checking with the colleagues with whom they attended school and the employees they supervised? The CV lists an applicant's academic honors, but are their actions guided by honor? Their education is apparent, but what about the ethics by which it was attained? Their transcripts and performance evaluations tell of their intelligence, but isn't their integrity equally if not more important? While many tangibles may be listed on a form, isn't the single most important issue the trust they have engendered with others?

Hiring right requires moving from what has often been an exclusive focus on qualifications to a contextual consideration of the qualities they embody. It requires consideration of both columns. Think about this—if it were necessary to change the attributes in one versus the other column, which would be easier to change? And which would provide more leverage to leadership? Without question, the attributes in the "Qualities" column are far more difficult, if not impossible, to change, and yet they are the keys to leadership success, not the qualifications alone. Qualifications deliver a *team of experts*, but qualities deliver *an expert team* which is far more important.

Box 31.1 lists some of the most important qualities needed in ED leaders, including physicians, nurses, and administrators, developed as a consensus among the authors. It is an

> **BOX 31.1 ■ ESSENTIAL QUALITIES OF ED LEADERS**
>
> - Honesty
> - Integrity, Ethics
> - Courage
> - Composure
> - Boldness
> - Compassion
> - Passion
> - Innovation
> - Approachable
>
> - Humility
> - Predisposed to excellence
> - Visionary leadership
> - Objectivity
> - Servant's heart
> - Curious mind
> - Consistency and constancy
> - Change leadership skills
> - Listening and communication skills

impressive list and not easily attained by simply being smart. Taken together, they comprise the *character* of the leader, without which success rarely occurs and certainly cannot be sustained.[32]

Discussing Qualities With Prospective Leaders

The following are some suggested questions the authors have found useful in the journey of discovering the character of leaders. Based on experience, it is usually wise to first establish a rapport with the interviewee prior to asking these questions (which should also be vetted with human resources)[33]:

- Who are your mentors and why?
- Which qualities do you value most in your team and why?
- What's the best thing I will hear about you and from whom will I hear it?
- What's the worst thing I will hear about you and from whom will I hear it?
- When was the last time you were moved to tears at work? Please tell me the story if you are comfortable.
- What are you *most* proud of in your career? Why?
- What are you *least* proud of in your career? Why?

Conversations With Colleagues

Whenever possible, make an effort to speak not only with those listed as references but with others who have worked with or reported to the person most recently and also throughout the course of their career. Questions might include:

- How does this person make others on the team feel?
- What are the facial expressions of the team members when they see this person's name on the schedule?
- What qualities best describe this person?
- How did you feel when they told you this person would be leaving?
- If you could help this person improve in some way, small or large, what would it be?

Metrics vs Relationships

At the C-suite and board of directors' level in nearly every medical system, there has been a dramatic emphasis on metrics as the measure of success. Patient experience, flow, safety, and other measures of effectiveness and efficiency have often been the major, if not sole, ways of determining how well EDs are functioning. Concepts such as pillar management, balanced scorecards, and others are ways in which measurements have been matched to the organization's stated purposes, mission, vision, and values.[34-36] In some cases, this exclusive focus on metrics has seemed like "metrics mania without means."[37] These organizations may have a maniacal focus on producing numbers without providing the resources requisite to deliver those metrics, including a willingness to change culture, processes, and systems that stand in the way of the team attempting to meet the metrics. A fundamental question is whether the metrics and surveys are being used as a tool or a club. Are they a *tool* that helps the team develop systems and processes capable of delivering results—or are they used as a *club* to beat the team into compliance?

The maniacal focus on merely metrics has given way in health-care systems that have seen the importance and advantages of focusing on the people leading teams capable of developing and sustaining the relationships that lead to top-level results. These leaders realize that while metrics are important they should never be more important than the people and the relationships that produce them.

As **Figure 31.1** indicates, relationship-based cultures require movement *from* . . . "move the meat," "treat 'em and street 'em," hit the metrics, deliver about the 90th percentile Press Ganey or other patient experience score to broader issues of alignment with system, the hospital campus, and the people whose skills and abilities allow the team to achieve the target metrics. It is not necessarily the results alone, but how the results are produced by a talented, motivated, enthusiastic, and appreciated team, which brings people together in aligned strategic and tactical incentives. Teams that bring people together to produce outcomes have moved from a purely *results-based* culture to a *relationship-based* culture.[38,39] These teams are inclusive of all lenses, all perspectives, and all people, which recognize that there are no *more* important people on the team, so there are no unimportant perspectives from the team members.[40]

The issue of hospital boarding, a major issue for many EDs, is an example that demonstrates moving to *relationships* capable of delivering results. Chapters 45 and 46 address boarding and solutions for it. Succinctly stated, many hospitals have allowed inpatient units to be protected from accountability for boarding metrics. Conversely,

FIGURE 31.1 ■ Rules-Based vs Relationship-Based Cultures

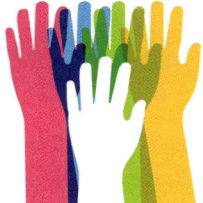

- "My way or the highway!"
- "I don't care what it takes — get it **done**!"
- "The doctors hit their metrics. Why can't the nurses?"
- "We've always done it that way!"
- "That's not in the protocol."

- All voices, all lenses
- Inclusive teams
- Teamwork across boundaries
- Relationships before results
- How results are delivered as important as the results themselves
- New, inventive protocols

many Emergency departments are held solely accountable and criticized for boarding and numerous related metrics that boarding negatively affects, including:

- Flow metrics
- Patient experience metrics
- Safety metrics
- Staff satisfaction/engagement scores
- ED diversion hours

When the combined and collaborative ED and senior leadership teams, including inpatient leaders, come together in a relationship-based manner, they can devise solutions that cut across boundaries and deliver better results, while simultaneously developing cross-functional and boundaryless stakeholder relationships.

In the authors' experiences, there is a curious but dramatically positive side effect of this cultural transition—focusing on people and relationships first and then results. The emphasis of high-performing organizations are "every time, every touch." They are willing to change the culture, systems, and processes that get in the way of relationships with the nearly universal result of better and more sustained metrics. It is not *why* focusing on culture, systems, processes, hardwiring flow, and fulfillment are done—but it is a fortunate byproduct of that wise strategic investment.

Reigniting Passion and Fulfillment

There is an increasing recognition among many successful leaders and their teams that focusing exclusively on systems and processes is insufficient to produce the depth of change and innovation necessary to meet the current and future challenges of health-care systems. This is not to say that systems and processes are not important, but rather that they are *necessary, but not sufficient* conditions. Necessary because they must be addressed for success to occur, but not sufficient because they are not enough in and of themselves to produce success in the complex, adaptive systems in which the work is done.[41]

The movement is *to* a commitment to focus on a culture of professional fulfillment and to develop personal passion and resilience, as well as the relationship and metrics which each embody (**Figure 31.2**). The three elements of this broader concept are:

1. A culture that focuses not just on traditional metrics but also on cultivating the passion of the team members and their professional fulfillment
2. A commitment to hardwiring flow *and* professional fulfillment, as well as the courage to change systems and processes in order to do so
3. A commitment to reigniting the passion of the team members as well as strengthening their personal resilience[42]

Chapters 125 and 126 address the important subjects of burnout and compassion fatigue, respectively. Effective leaders understand the importance of continuously reenergizing the members of the team by ensuring the culture, systems, and processes of the organization embody the commitment to reignite passion and build their personal and professional resilience. Resilience is simply adaptive capacity, which grows when the focus is on "how to be" and "who you are" and less on "what you do" and "what you produce." Reigniting passion occurs when the team is encouraged to bring people together in mutually nurturing relationships and align not just organizational but personal incentives as well.

Leaders in the ED and the C-suite should invest in people caring for patients—and then get *them* to invest in each other. The calculus of that investment results in exponential, not arithmetic returns, particularly when all voices, all lenses, and all perspectives are considered.

FIGURE 31.2 ■ Successful Health-Care Environment

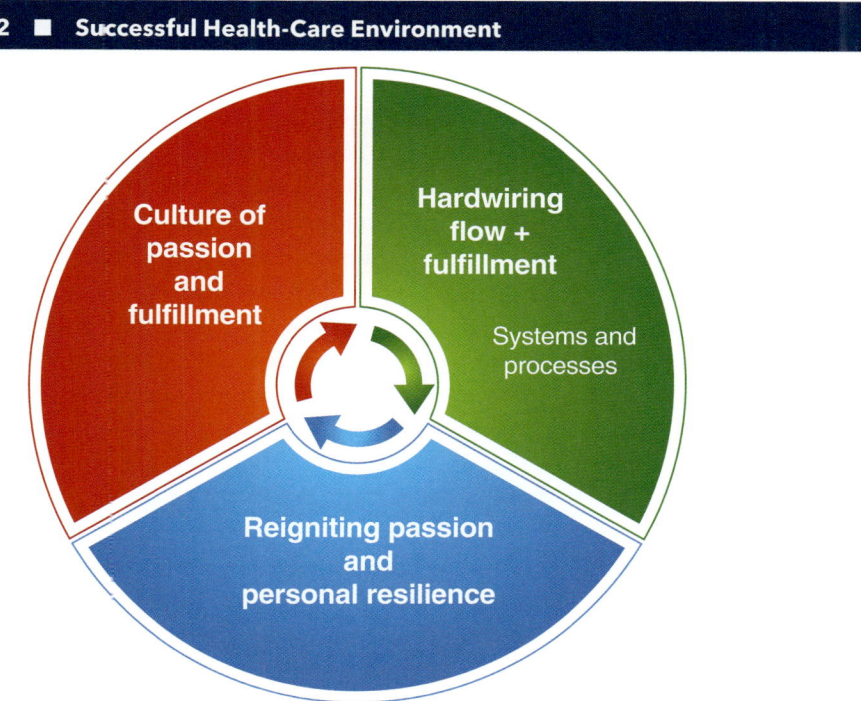

From Triple Aim to Quadruple Aim

Creating the culture and commitment to passion and personal resilience drives the necessary and sufficient conditions to ensure both relationships and results. This broader lens through which to view health care and EDs is related to the movement from the Institute for Healthcare Improvement (IHI) Triple Aim Initiative to the more inclusive "Quadruple Aim" of hospitals and health-care systems. Don Berwick and his colleagues at the IHI delineated the Triple Aim in order to focus on one primary and two supporting goals: Improve the health of the general population by improving the patient's experience (including quality and satisfaction) while reducing the cost of care.[43]

As admirable and essential as these aims may be, unless these goals are matched to the appropriate resources necessary to attain them, the result is increased frustration for those providing that care. In fact, without improving the means to attain these laudable goals, increased burnout could reasonably be the unintended consequence, as described by Robert Merton in 1936.[44] Recognizing this, Bodenheimer and Sinsky proposed that a fourth aim be added: "Improving the work life of clinicians and staff."[45]

With the focus on the Quadruple Aim, we have a more reliable compass by which to guide health care's legitimate progress while acknowledging the need for consideration of and investment in those who create that progress.

Developing More Integrated Roles

For decades, ED care has focused on delivering acute, episodic, unscheduled care to thousands of patients per year. That care ranges from the highest levels of acuity and the broadest spectrum of illnesses and injuries to more minor issues, although they rarely seem minor to the patients and families. As Chuck Stokes astutely points out, as artificial intelligence doubles the rate of new knowledge acquisition every 18 months, those entering (or staying) in health care will need to "reinvent themselves" since the work will of necessity be changing to keep pace with the knowledge (C. Stokes, personal communication to the author TM, June7, 2020.) For some, this will mean redoubling their efforts in their chosen areas; for others, it may mean subspecializing or diversifying their practices.

Others may choose to reinvent themselves by broadening their practices from strictly episodic care to something like a health-care navigator role, developing mechanisms to seek more detailed feedback and follow-up with patients through telephonic, electronic, or social media platforms, going far beyond simple follow-up phone calls. Still others may reinvent themselves through changing venues and retraining into other areas of health care, from education to research to hospital medicine to urgent care, and so on.

It will be important for ED and senior leaders to recognize this phenomenon, develop mechanisms to help this reinvention process, and encourage team members to remain in health care to make a contribution, even if the area of contribution changes over time.

PERSONAL LEADERSHIP PERSPECTIVES

This section reflects the collective wisdom of the chapter's coauthors, captured from interviews as they reflected on their views as CEOs of some of the leading health-care systems in the world and the importance of the ED to their respective institutions. Quotation marks are used somewhat sparingly, largely to emphasize key phrases or concepts.

The Best of the Best

Charles "Chuck" Stokes, former CEO of Memorial Hermann Health System and North Mississippi Medical Center; past chairman, American College of Healthcare Executives

Because of the very nature of the ED, it is a place for extraordinary experience where extraordinary leaders often develop. In every ED I have seen, the people who work there are by nature predisposed to excellence—they want to be and usually are the "best of the best." Having trained as a critical nurse, my experience has been that the preparation for the worst eventualities creates a mindset of problem solving in the midst of deep personal interaction that helps create great leadership. Having clinical talent over a broad range of entities gives those physicians and nurses the capacity for much wider and more in-depth understanding of the systems nature of health care. They see how pieces of the puzzle fit because they have worked with all of those pieces closely, both clinically and operationally. They know the system because they touch the entire system.

While many qualities make great leaders, among the most important are relationship skills, a high degree of emotional intelligence, and an almost innate intuitiveness for how people act and what their needs are during stress and crises. There is also a kind of swagger about them, a sense of confidence that they can and will handle anything thrown at them. That confidence—but never arrogance, which is a fine line—makes them stand out when they operate across boundaries and with different stakeholders across the health-care system. In leadership, confidence breeds confidence and great ED leaders are excellent at that. Since they consider themselves the best of the best and ready to handle anything that comes through the door, they also recruit the best; they aren't afraid to recruit people who will challenge them. Emergency physicians are a special breed; since by nature they use time efficiently, they are very good at succinct, focused briefings on difficult issues, and they see things from both strategic and tactical perspectives. That is probably a combination of nature and training.

Patient safety and the creation of high reliability organizations (HROs) have been particular areas of passion, and EDs provide one of the best examples of how those principles can be applied in high-volume, high-risk, and problem-prone situations, where procedures that have important consequences are performed regularly. ED nurse and physician leaders gravitate toward HRO concepts and implement them effectively. Probably because they are so "forward facing" every day with large volumes of patients, ED leaders understand they are the *brand* of the hospital and health-care system and combine a consumer-focused and personal service mentality toward their patients, despite the fact they have never met them before and, in most cases, will not have long-term relationships with them. By differentiating themselves through expertise and compassion, they differentiate the institution's excellence.

There is a long history of emergency nurse and physician leaders moving to senior leadership positions as CNEs, CMOs, chief information officers, and presidents of the medical staff, with some becoming COOs and CEOs. For all the reasons stated previously, that trend is likely to continue and accelerate, which will be a welcome situation for hospitals and health-care systems.

Every Patient, Every Time, Every Touch

Steven Narang, MD, MCHM, President, Inova Fairfax Medical Campus, Inova Health System, former CEO of Banner-University Medical Center

It is impossible to overstate the importance of culture to health-care organizations, not the slogans on the walls, but the actions and the relationships between people that embody the culture in action. That is what is meant by "straight from the airway of the organization!" In resuscitations, teams follow airway, breathing, circulation or the ABCs, and the airway is always first and most important. Nearly everyone early in their training had the experience with a trauma patient of rushing to stop the bleeding, only to be reminded to focus on the airway first. Straight from the airway means that what we *do* speaks much more loudly than what we *say*. The words and the actions of the team reflect culture and values of the *airway*.

The ED is a critical unit in every hospital, and the ability to lead the ED is essential. Inova Health System focuses on "Every patient, every time, every touch." The ED is a level I trauma center, seeing over 100,000 patients each year, including a busy pediatric ED. What better place to exemplify that concept, touching not just over 100,000 patients, but their families, their neighbors, and the community as well. A somewhat one-dimensional way to view the ED is as a gateway to patients, admissions, filling the beds, and driving volume, along with the traditional measures of efficacy, efficiency, and effectiveness. While those are important considerations, a deeper concept of gateway related to brand and connection with the patient experience is emerging, with a commensurate move from patient as consumer to patient as a blend of customer and partner in the provision of health care.

Leadership requires changing from a "move the meat, treat 'em and street 'em," mentality focused excessively on turnaround times, flow metrics, and patient satisfaction scores to a more contextual focus on *how* the metrics were obtained. Leaders, particularly ED leaders, should reflect those values in their daily actions, where the culture invests in people, not just results, as well as develop lenses to look at *ourselves* at least as often, if not more so, than looking at results alone. All of this occurs in the midst of an environment that by design requires the ED team to add value to the patient experience while understanding that every patient's care will be transitioned to other providers—either to an admitting team or back to the patient's physician(s)—in the case of those who are discharged from the ED. The intensity of caring for patients who did not expect to be in the ED is followed by a handoff of that care to other team members. That is not just a transfer of care, it is a *transfer of trust* that requires a unique set of talents, which ED leaders are charged with mentoring.

Hesselbein's and Emerson's insights are correct in that *who we are as people* who happen to be in a leadership positions cannot be overemphasized. It is a question more of *being enough* versus *doing enough*, which can be a tough transition for results-focused leaders to make if they are not coached to balance results with relationships. It requires a delicate balance between confidence and humility. On the one hand, leadership in health care, but particularly in the ED, requires the experience and confidence to act aggressively and with clarity in times of crisis. In this sense the sheer volume of patient experience in the ED is a pure blessing, as it generates the confidence, born of frequency and intensity, to deal with ambiguity and uncertainty. That confidence arises in part from an ability to see 1,000 mistakes being made and learning something meaningful from each of them, which accelerates leadership development. Coupled with the humility and a commitment to humble inquiry, confidence creates places of trust and safety, where leaders feel sufficiently safe to go to others and openly ask, "I need your help. What's your take on this?" This captures an *all lenses, all voices* approach that is essential to progress. Focusing on building *enough spaces for everyone to speak* moves away from a hierarchical approach to a more inclusive one, where if there is deference it is deference to expertise, not position. One of the most important lessons is self-reflection—the capacity to pause, reflect, and reconsider how the leader can improve.

Innovation is essential, particularly in these radically changing times, but innovation can only occur at the speed of trust. If team members have not connected across boundaries with confidence, humility, and genuine efforts to capture varying perspectives, innovation will largely be individual and not a team effort, regardless of how talented the team members may be.

The nurse–physician bond is unique in the ED as there is nowhere nurses and physicians work as closely together for long periods of time under such stressful circumstances and with so many patients, none of whom were known to the team previously. Valuable unique bonds arise from this experience, but unique strains also arise from this proximity. Perhaps the single most important factor governing the success of an ED is the relationship between the nurses and physicians. With nurse and physician leaders, but also among all the team, the transition from me-centered to patient-centered to team-centered is in constant flux and to varying degrees. One test of the success of ED leaders is how well their team members have been able to make that transition, as well as how effective they have been at making the patient part of the team.

Leadership requires the skill of convening, or pulling people together in a culture that invests in people at all levels, since there are no unimportant members of the team. Teams are not simply groups of people who work together—teams are groups of people who trust each other. "One Team" is an important approach, but this can only occur when the time, effort, and energy have been invested to build trust.

Very few providers have been patients in the same ways their patients are, so a deep sense of empathy is needed. The etymology of empathy is instructive in that it derives from the Greek words *em* and *pathos*, meaning in-feeling, but the term has come to mean the ability to understand or imagine the feelings of others, while not being paralyzed from actions needed to help them. Empathy is an essential foundation of the movement to patient-centered care, as well as precision, personalized medicine. ED leaders and their staff have a unique resource in this regard, due to the sheer volume of patients and their experiences to which they are exposed. If ED team members exercise the discipline of trying to get an "in-feeling" of what the patient is going through, they have a distinct advantage, not only in patient care but in leadership as well, as it builds the sense of how to be, not just what to do.

Fanatical Focus on the Patient

John Brennan, MD, MPH, Executive Vice President and Chief Clinical Integration Officer, WellStar Health System, former President and CEO, Barnabas Health System, Newark Beth Israel Health Center, and Children's Hospital of New Jersey

Having done both jobs, it is clear that what makes a good ED leader also makes a good CEO/CMO/hospital–medical system leader. Human qualities always trump qualifications; it is nice if a leader has both, but if you have to choose one, it is the qualities of the individual that will sustain them as a leader and inspire others to follow them. Among the qualities, integrity, character, intensity, ferocity, kindness, humility, and the right "dose of patience for the situation" are most important. Each situation is different, which is innately known to ED nurse and physician leaders because of the patients for whom they care, so having patience when patience is called for (and can be afforded) is on one end and a having a "healthy impatience" for times when change needs to be rapid and decisive is on the other. Good leaders need both. And please note that among the qualities is kindness; no leader in the ED or at the senior leadership level can succeed if they are not fundamentally kind. Passion for people and compassion in the details help move kindness from an innate predisposition to pragmatic application.

Results matter, but relationships matter more. Successful ED leaders are past masters at developing relationships, even when they fundamentally disagree with those with whom they work across the boundaries of the hospital, the health-care system, and the community. Class, style, and grace are overused words, but they are the correct words to describe great leaders who develop relationships even while disagreeing on methods or pathways.

The ability to brief a topic with an almost military precision is essential for leaders, including providing objective insights from each perspective, while never failing to provide clarity on what is being recommended. Because they see the broadest possible diversity and acuity of patients, ED leaders, if they are paying attention to their patients, are able to see the playing field in a unique way, which gives them a key leadership attribute—perspective.

Everyone says some variation of "patient first," but far fewer people and organizations actually do it. From experience in leading both EDs and health-care systems, ED leaders are unique in a nearly "fanatical focus on the patient." It shows when they brief the team on problems and possible solutions—the story is always told from the patient's perspective first—and then and only then from the perspective of those caring for the patient, which is a refreshing change, since many people approach the senior leadership team with a narrow focus on their desires and demands, often without regard to how that fits into the broader landscape. The ED *is* the broader landscape, since the ED team sees patients across all specialties. In addition, some health-care leaders have a long list of why things *can't be done*, whereas ED leaders seek a clear perspective on the department's goals and objectives while finding ways to *make things happen*.

Three Essential Qualities

Michael Born, MD, MBA, former CEO, Swedish American Hospital

Moving from being the Chair of the Department of Emergency Medicine to CMO to CEO requires the dynamic tension of reinventing oneself while accentuating the qualities developed needed to get there. The biggest challenge of reinvention is moving from an advocate for individual patients to responsibility for advocacy for all patients. It is a "problem of the apostrophe," since clinicians advocate for the *patient's* needs, and leaders are charged with *patients'* needs.

Three qualities are essential to all those jobs: boldness, the ability to work across boundaries, and a deep sense of intellectual and psychological curiosity. It is virtually impossible to lead at any level in health care without a bold and courageous spirit, unafraid of the depth and acuity of challenges. Leadership is not for the timid or faint of heart. A fear of failure or getting caught in the paralysis of analysis are not consistent with success anymore; in fact, they never were. Having almost "maniacal courage" is an asset, but it must be tempered by a realization that not everything can be fixed on the first day on the job. With courage comes both confidence and composure in even the most stressful situations, both of which are contagious.

The breadth of clinical entities seen in the ED fosters the development of clinical curiosity, as well as the need to be curious about the psychological impact on the experience of the patient. Because change management is essential to leadership, only an intellectual curiosity to understand human and organizational change can fuel effective innovations. Without some level of resistance and reluctance, no real change is occurring, only window dressing. An understanding of dealing with resistance and possessing the integrity to do is a daily part of the work. Making the right "diagnosis" for the reluctance and resistance to change is essential, since doing so will determine the right solutions in a context of complexity. Curiosity is also essential since hospitals and EDs are complex adaptive systems, and only a curious mind and spirit can effectively lead a system. Boundary management skills are essential in the ED, since it is seemingly nothing *but* boundaries. Working across those boundaries effectively while keeping the patients' needs at the center of the enterprise is a skill worth developing.

Both ED and senior leadership teams require an ability to see the whole field, much like a quarterback in football or a point guard in basketball. Situational awareness and an ability to discern patterns out of seemingly small details are the basis of having a working understanding of problems. Seeing the whole field also involves elements of being able to understand multiple perspectives simultaneously and then balancing those perspectives in making decisions. The paradoxical concept of becoming "the problem physician or nurse" is also important, meaning developing the reputation for being a person to whom others bring their problems because of the leader's ability to help solve them or at least frame them in a way that a path to a negotiated solution can occur. Investing in the team members is an important part of leadership and the Quadruple Aim concept is central to that investment.

Successful ED and senior health-care leaders both live, act, speak, and write in the *active voice*. Terse, declarative language implies the leader will take similar actions—direct and to the point. Passivity in a leader, in particular a reluctance to make difficult decisions, is poison.

Finally, leaders need to have the courage and intellectual honesty to be their own worst critics, both personally and in assessing the ED's performance, whether results or relationship based in nature, similar to Admiral Stockdale's concept of "brutal optimism."

CONCLUSION

The working relationship between the ED leadership team and the hospital's senior leadership is one of the most important in all of health care, particularly given the ED's position as the gateway to the brand and culture of the entire medical system. In the midst of dramatic change, leaders are also evolving from functional silos to newer and more effective models of dyad and triad leadership, in which nurses, physicians, and administrators are working together across boundaries for the good of the patient and the good of those taking care of the patient.

As leaders better understand the importance of recruiting and retaining talented teams, it is critical to *hire right* by focusing not exclusively on qualifications and emphasizing qualities of the team members and then coaching and mentoring to build from them. Part of the transformation is to move from an excessive focus on metrics and results to a commitment to teams which can develop and nurture inclusive relationships capable of producing excellent outcomes. These teams focus not just on hardwiring flow through improved systems and processes but also on developing a culture of passion and fulfillment for the team and building the personal resilience of its members. Through these efforts, better bonds and relationships can be built, and in President Abraham Lincoln's words, "Just as our case is new, we must think anew, and act anew."[46] The future is ours to build, and its foundation consists of bedrock relationships capable of promoting the growth of the team members under the guidance of confident, yet humble, leaders at both the ED and senior leader levels.

REFERENCES

1. Hesselbein F. *My Life in Leadership: The Journey and Lessons Learned Along the Way.* San Francisco, Calif: Jossey-Bass; 2011.

2. Emerson RW. *Letters and Social Aims.* New York, NY: Wentworth Press; 2019.

3. Drucker P. *Managing in the Next Society.* New York, NY: St. Martin's Press; 2002.

4. Mayer T. Developing leadership and communication skills. Paper presented at: American College of Emergency Physicians Emergency Department Directors Academy; February 5, 2020; Dallas, Tex.

5. Dzau VJ, Kirch D, Nasca T. Preventing a parallel pandemic: a national strategy to protect clinicians' well-being. *N Engl J Med.* 2020;383:513–515.

6. Hartzband P, Groopman J. Physician burnout, interrupted. *N Engl J Med.* 2020;382:2485–2487.

7. Gagne M, Deci EL. Self-determination theory and work motivation. *J Organiz Behav.* 2005;26:331–362.

8. Mayer T. Rewarding the champions and corralling the stragglers: performance review and aligning incentives. Paper presented at: American College of Emergency Physicians Emergency Department Directors Academy; February 5, 2020; Dallas, Tex.

9. Groysberg B, Kelly LK, MacDonald B. *The New Path to the C-Suite.* Harvard Business Review; 2011. Available at: https://hbr.org/2011/03/the-new-path-to-the-c-suite. Accessed July 28, 2020.

10. Drucker P. There's more than one kind of team. *WSJ.* 1992. Available at: https://www.wsj.com/articles/SB10001424052748704204304574544312916277426. Updated November 18, 2009. Accessed July 26, 2020.

11. Kaplan RS, Norton DP. The Office of Strategy Management. *Harvard Business Review.* 2005. Available at: https://www.wsj.com/articles/SB10001424052748704204304574544312916277426. Accessed July 26, 2020.

12. Kuhn T. *The Structure of Scientific Revolutions.* Chicago, Ill: University of Chicago Press; 2012.

13. Ensor P. Organizational renewal—tearing down the functional silos. *Target.* 1988:4–14.

14. Gleeson B. The silo mentality: how to break down the barriers. *Forbes.* 2013. Available at: https://www.forbes.com/sites/brentgleeson/2013/10/02/the-silo-mentality-how-to-break-down-the-barriers/#13701e708c7e. Accessed July 26, 2020.

15. Katzenbach JR, Smith DK. *The Wisdom of Teams: Creating the High Performance Organization.* New York, NY: Harper Collins; 2003.

16. Zismer DK, Brueggeman J. Examining the "dyad" as a management model in integrated healthcare systems. *Phys Exec J.* 2010;36:14–19.

17. Sanford K, Moore S. *Dyad Leadership in Healthcare: When One Plus One is Greater than Two.* Philadelphia, Pa: Wolters Kluwer; 2015.

18. Gilgore S. Inova is making structural changes: here are the details. *Washington Business Journal.* October 18, 2019. Available at: https://www.bizjournals.com/washington/news/2019/10/18/inova-is-making-structural-changes-here-are-the.html. Accessed July 26, 2020.

19. Greenleaf R. *Servant Leadership: A Journey into the Nature of Legitimate Power and Greatness.* New York, NY: Paulist Press; 1977.

20. Mayer T. Patient experience skills. Paper presented at: American College of Emergency Physicians Emergency Department Directors Academy; February 5, 2020; Dallas, Tex.

21. Emergency Department Benchmarking Alliance. Annual Report 2018. Available at: https://www.edbenchmarking.org. Accessed July 28, 2020.

22. Stokes C. Engaging the organization in patient safety. Address to the American College of Healthcare Executives Congress; March 22, 2019; Chicago, Ill.

23. Berry LL. *Discovering the Soul of Service: The Nine Drivers of Sustainable Business Success.* New York, NY: The Free Press; 1999.

24. Berry LL. *On Great Service: A Framework for Action.* New York, NY: The Free Press; 1995.

25. Berry LL, Seltman KD. *Management Lessons From Mayo Clinic: Inside One of the World's Most Admired Service Organizations.* New York, NY: McGraw-Hill; 2008.

26. Berry LL, Seltman KD. Building a strong services brand: lessons from Mayo Clinic. *Business Horizons.* 2007;50:199–209.

27. Carlzon J. *Moments of Truth: New Strategies for Today's Customer-Driven Economy.* New York, NY: Ballinger Books; 1987.

28. Kemp E, Jillipalli R, Becerra E. Healthcare branding: developing emotionally based consumer brand relationships. *J Serv Mark.* 2014;28(2):126–137.

29. Elrod JE, Fortenberry JL. Driving brand equity in health services organizations: the need for an expanded view of branding. *BMC Health Serv Res.* 2018;18:23–28. doi:10.1186/s12913-018-3679-4. Accessed July 28, 2020.

30. Mayer T, Cates RJ. *Leadership for Great Customer Service: Satisfied Employees, Satisfied Patients.* 2nd ed. Chicago, Ill: Health Administration Press; 2014.

31. Mayer T, Cates R. *Leadership for Great Customer Service: Satisfied Patients, Satisfied Employees*. 1st ed. Chicago, Ill: Health Administration Press; 2004.
32. Wilson RA, ed. *Character Above All—Ten Presidents from FDR to George Bush*. New York, NY: Simon and Schuster; 1996.
33. Mayer T. *Battling Healthcare Burnout: Learning to Love the Job You Have While Creating the Job You Love*. San Francisco, Calif: Berrett-Koehler; Expected on 2021.
34. Studer Q. *Hardwiring Excellence: Purpose, Worthwhile Work, Making a Difference*. Gulf Breeze, Fla: Fire Starter Press; 2003.
35. Kaplan RS, Norton DK. *The Balanced Scorecard: Translating Strategy Into Action*. Boston, Mass: Harvard Business School Press; 1996.
36. Centers for Medicare and Medicaid Services. *Hospital Compare*. Available at: https://www.cms.gov/medicare/quality-initiatives-patient-assessment-instruments/hospitalqualityinits/hospitalcompare. Accessed July 26, 2020.
37. Mayer T. *Battling Healthcare Burnout: Learning to Love the Job You Have While Creating the Job You Love*. San Francisco, Calif: Berrett-Koehler; 2021.
38. Block P. *Stewardship: Choosing Service Over Self-Interest*. San Francisco, Calif: Berrett-Koehler; 1996.
39. Peters T. *The Excellence Dividend: Meeting the Tech Tide With Work That Wows and Jobs That Last*. New York, NY: Vintage Books; 2018.
40. Beaton A. The Doctor and the 'Badasses' keeping NFL players safe from the Coronavirus. *Wall Street Journal*. 2020. Available at: https://www.wsj.com/articles/the-doctor-and-the-badasses-keeping-nfl-players-safe-from-the-coronavirus-11590580800. Accessed June 19, 2020.
41. Rogers CR. The necessary and sufficient conditions of therapeutic personality change. *J Consult Psychol*. 1957;21:95–103.
42. Mayer T. *Getting Back to the Job You Love: Reconnecting With Passion to Battle Burnout*. Healthcare Executive. 2020:40–43.
43. Berwick DM, Nolan TW, Whittington J. The triple aim: care, health, and cost. *Health Aff*. 2008;27:759–769.
44. Merton RK. The unanticipated consequences of purposive social action. *Am Sociol Rev*. 1936;1:894–904.
45. Bodenheimer T, Sinsky C. From triple to quadruple aim: care of the patient requires care of the provider. *Ann Fam Med*. 2014;12:573–576.
46. Lincoln A. Annual Message to Congress-Concluding Remarks. Washington, DC. 1862. Available at: http://www.abrahamlincolnonline.org/lincoln/speeches/congress.htm. Accessed July 26, 2020.

CHAPTER 32
EMERGENCY MANAGEMENT OF DRUG AND SUPPLY SHORTAGES

James J. Augustine, John H. Proctor

Drug and medical supplies have been plagued by tremendous shortages during the COVID-19 pandemic, preventing ready access to the critical elements of care providers need to manage their infected patients. The emergency department (ED) has been at the heart of shortage issues, with ED leaders forced to manage a critical lack of personal protective equipment (PPE), testing materials, treatments, disinfection agents, and equipment. The pandemic response unveiled significant gaps in the supply chain, particularly related to the manufacturing of critical materials.

The majority of drug shortages involve lifesaving interventions for high-acuity conditions. For several of these drugs, no therapeutic alternative is available. Multiple governmental, regulatory, and commercial organizations must engage with ED leaders to create comprehensive strategies that address the growing challenge of medication and medical equipment shortages. Although further work is needed to understand the impact of drug and medical equipment shortages on patient outcomes, the primary issues contributing to the problem include manufacturing issues, unanticipated demand, and the declining production of older drugs in favor of newer, more profitable ones.

CASE STUDY

Over the past 10 years, recurrent shortages of self-injectable epinephrine (EpiPen) have created life-threatening problems for patients. The shortage has resulted from a variety of manufacturing issues and has not been reliably communicated to patients, the general public, providers, payers, or regulators. Simultaneously, the price of the product to has increased significantly. The shortage has been more severe for the pediatric population.

The EpiPen shortage affects all members of the emergency care industry. Patients, parents of children with severe allergies, and agencies find that they are unable to obtain EpiPens at an affordable price—or at any price at all. In addition to the anxiety about obtaining the product is uncertainty about whether an EpiPen is effective beyond its printed expiration date.

To avoid potential catastrophe, patients and parents without an available EpiPen are taught to call emergency medical services (EMS) early after an allergic exposure, even if the patient is minimally symptomatic or asymptomatic. First responders, including fire and EMS agencies, may not carry an EpiPen because of its cost or availability or may only have only an adult product when a child is the patient. Protocols have been rewritten to allow for any form of available epinephrine to be administered in life-threatening patient encounters, requiring multiple training programs and messaging to the EMS providers.

Emergency providers are faced with patients who would have otherwise been treated with an EpiPen earlier in their clinical course but now may be in extremis without any prehospital treatment. Providers trying to give discharge instructions to the family of a patient who has survived an allergic reaction also cannot provide a reliable path of medication availability, reassurance, and patient education.

Across the many elements of the emergency care system, the prolonged, unpredictable, and poorly communicated shortage of a very effective evidence-based lifesaving medicine causes high levels of anxiety, morbidity and mortality, complexity at all levels of the emergency system, expense and complex workaround processes, distrust in the regulators who are overseeing the availability of critical supplies, and anger toward the producers of products that are irregularly available and suddenly prohibitively expensive.

A BRIEF HISTORY OF MEDICATION AND SUPPLY SHORTAGES

Medication shortages affect many health-care delivery spaces, including oncology and anesthesia, but the emergency care system is particularly at risk for the inherent patient safety issues caused by such situations.

The crisis of shortages involves all classes of emergency medications, including those that sedate, control pain, restore heart function, treat anaphylaxis, and apply to common emergencies in children. Due to the relatively high cost and the short shelf lives of emergency medications, the US is faced with inadequate reserves of critical drugs. While hospitals have typically maintained more robust supply chains and alternatives for care, the problem is now profound for hospitals as well.

Critical medications often have no alternatives. Some medications come in preferred formulations that are safer to use in emergency settings. Without access to the preferred or most clinically appropriate treatment, ED personnel may be forced to use alternative drugs that are less effective, have a higher risk profile, and are poorly vetted in the medical literature. In both the out-of-hospital setting and the ED, some of these medicines have no substitutes, or personnel may not have the ability to render alternative therapies.

A number of issues exacerbate the challenge of shortages, including:

- Surges of patients, such as occurred in the COVID-19 pandemic
- Medications unavailable for the lay public to use for self-rescue, such as EpiPens
- Stocks of emergency medications that are inadequate due to their relatively high cost and short shelf lives
- No alternatives for critical medications
- Hospital rules, regulations, or protocols that limit substitution with alternative medications
- Budgets that ineffectively address medication and supply shortage issues
- Hospitals that cannot resupply or exchange medications with EMS providers due to some legal interpretations of anti-kickback rules

MARKET FORCES

The health-care field must be able to manage patient surges and rapidly evolving community needs. The COVID-19 pandemic caught ED personnel in the middle of a rapid increase in patients requiring respiratory care, while many other areas of the hospital shut down due to staff concerns about safety. There are many forces within the market that can produce rapid changes in the need, availability, and cost of critical supplies. All have contributed to the

FIGURE 32.1 ■ 2017 Hurricane Maria Damage in Puerto Rico

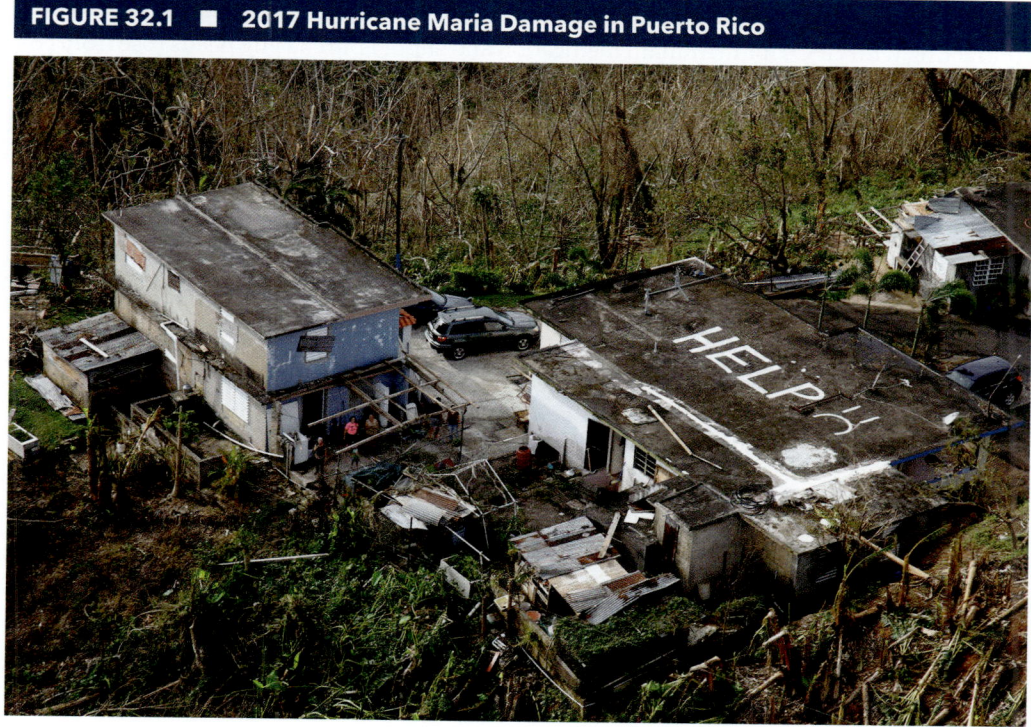

shortage of emergency medications, including monopolies, group purchasing organizations (GPOs), and artificially short expiration dates.

Monopolies

In some cases, the national supply chain for a particular medication or medical device is controlled by only one or two manufacturers. An interruption in the controlling manufacturers' production can produce an abrupt, unforeseen shortage. Hurricane Maria's 2017 landfall in Puerto Rico significantly damaged the Puerto Rico-based manufacturing plant of Baxter International, which dominated the US saline bag market (**Figure 32.1**). The subsequent shortage of saline led to service disruptions across the US.

Group Purchasing Organizations

The preponderance of US hospitals and hospital systems acquire medications and other supplies through contracts with GPOs. These intermediaries offer catalogues of products from manufacturers to facilities, simplifying the communications and price negotiations (**Figure 32.2**).

FIGURE 32.2 ■ Group Purchasing Organization Model

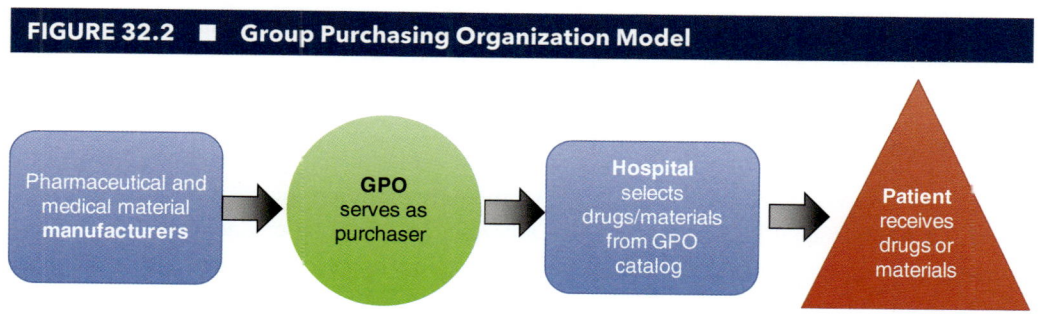

According to the Healthcare Supply Chain Association, the percentage of hospitals contracting with GPOs for their main medication and supply purchasing needs rose from 68% in 2000 to 98% in 2014.[1] The four largest GPOs in the United States account for 90% of the market for medical supplies.[2] The 1972 Anti-Kickback Statute (AKS) amended the Social Security Act to ban the use of kickbacks, bribes, and rebates in return for items or services. The AKS was designed to combat fraud, enhance competition, and promote price transparency. However, in 1987, GPOs received a safe harbor exemption from the statute, meaning they would not be prosecuted by the AKS if their business practices were potentially prohibited by the law.

Group purchasing organizations earn profit margins in two principle manners:

- Vendor fees paid to GPOs by medication and medical supply manufacturers in return for product placement in GPO catalogs of products available to hospitals
- Premium fees paid by manufacturers to GPOs for rights as the sole supplier of a particular medication or medical device

In return for these fees, the GPO may receive a discounted fee schedule for the products supplied to the hospital by the contracting GPO.

These organizations contend that, through scale and efficiencies, hospitals realize medication and supply cost savings through an intermediary GPO. This contention is debatable. In 2010, the US Senate Committee on Finance found no empirical, peer-reviewed data to support the claim of facility savings through GPO contracts.[3] In a 2011 study involving 8,100 hospitals, the purchase price was 10% lower for three of four transactions directly with manufacturers, rather than through a GPO.[4]

In 2005, GPO organizations created the Healthcare Group Purchasing Industry Initiative (HGPII) to promote open and competitive purchasing processes. Group purchasing organization membership in HGPII is voluntary, and its published code of conduct does not address the potential impact of GPOs on medication, supply, and medical device shortages.

Expiration Dates

Peer-reviewed literature suggests that many drugs maintain their potency well past the manufacturer-imposed expiration date.[5,6] This phenomenon is variable, drug-specific, and influenced by external environmental factors, including temperature, light exposure, and humidity. Some pharmaceutical manufacturers, upon request and for a fee, will batch-test products to determine their potency and other potential problems like particulate formation, solution stability, and degradation. This testing is costly, and a determination must be made about whether it is more cost-effective to batch-test existing drugs or purchase new ones. Certain clinical and legal risks may limit the value of batch-testing products that technically are expired.

REGULATORY AGENCY INVOLVEMENT

The United States has a number of agencies that have authority over elements of the medical supply change. Their responsibilities include maintaining the quality and safety of health-care equipment, technologies, devices, and medications.

The Food and Drug Administration

The US Food and Drug Administration (FDA) currently maintains a task force focused on the issue of drug shortages. In 2017, through its Center for Drug Evaluation and Research, the FDA worked with manufacturers to mitigate over 100 potential drug shortages; in 2018, the agency conducted a public forum, *Identifying the Root Causes of Drug Shortages and Finding Enduring Solutions*. Despite these efforts, ongoing critical shortages of essential medications persist.

The Drug Enforcement Administration

The US Drug Enforcement Administration (DEA) works across constituents, including hospitals and manufacturers, to avoid and mitigate drug shortages. The DEA's efforts apply principally to potential shortages of certain injectable products that contain morphine, hydromorphone, meperidine, and fentanyl. Manufacturers of these products must register with the DEA, which exerts some influence on allocations and quotas for the production of injectable narcotics.

The Centers for Disease Control and Prevention

The US Centers for Disease Control and Prevention (CDC) Strategic National Stockpile (SNS) is the nation's largest supply of potentially lifesaving pharmaceuticals and medical supplies for use in a public-health emergency that is severe enough to exhaust local supplies (**Figure 32.3**). The pandemic exposed the reality that even large stockpiles and seemingly healthy supply chains can be depleted rapidly by a nationwide crisis. The domestic supplies of critical materials also rely on foreign manufacturing and the presence of effective logistical chains. Those were broken in the early days of the pandemic, and any supplies that were being produced in other countries were also being sought by the many nations that had equal health-care demands. In more localized surge events, the SNS will be the first source of needed materials and has performed well in events like hurricanes and winter storms. Stockpiled products include:

- Antibiotics
- Chemical antidotes
- Antitoxins
- Vaccines
- Antiviral drugs
- PPE
- Ventilators
- Other medical supplies

FIGURE 32.3 ■ CDC Strategic National Stockpile

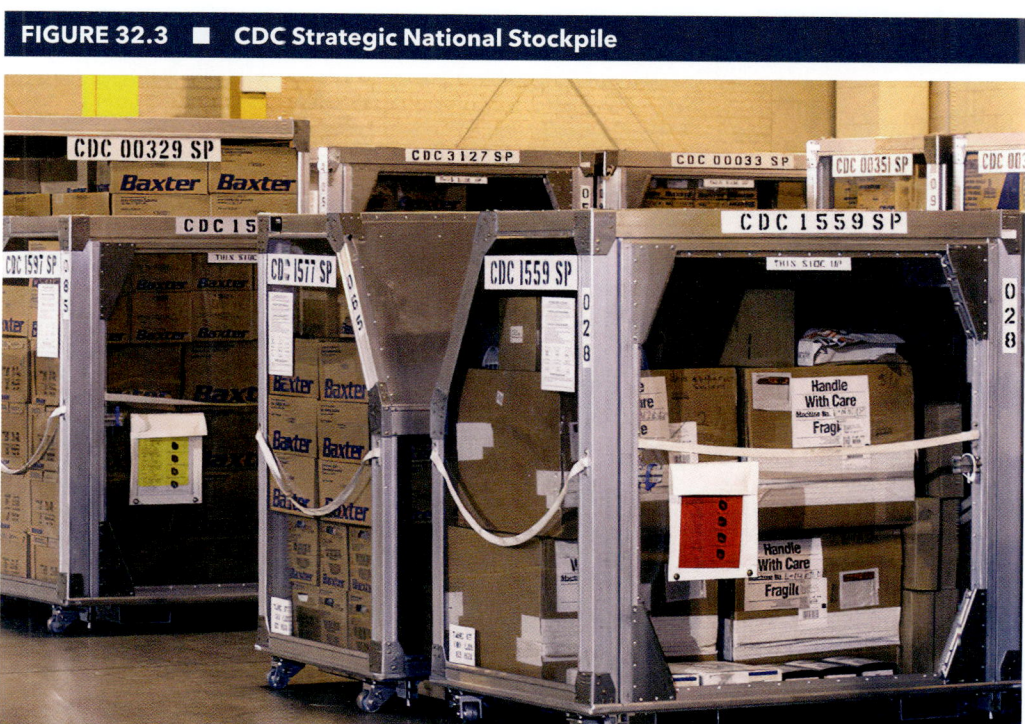

12-Hour Push Package

If a community experiences a large-scale public health incident in which the disease or agent is unknown, the first line of support from the stockpile is a 12-hour "push package (**Figure 32.4**) that contains a broad range of pharmaceuticals and medical supplies. Contents are prepacked and configured in transport-ready containers for rapid delivery anywhere in the United States within 12 hours of the federal decision to deploy. Each package contains 50 tons of emergency medical resources.

CHEMPACKs

CHEMPACKs are containers of nerve-agent antidotes placed in secure locations at local levels around the country to allow rapid response to a chemical incident. These medications treat the symptoms of nerve-agent exposure and can be used even when the actual toxin is unknown.

The Federal Trade Commission

The Federal Trade Commission (FTC) works for consumers to spot and prevent fraudulent, deceptive, and unfair business practices. In this role, the FTC actively monitors business activity related to the interplay between rival pharmaceutical, medical supply, and device manufacturers, including the role of GPOs in product pricing. The FTC monitors pricing competition between commercial and generic drug manufacturers and the financial impact of the importation of medicines and other medical supplies from foreign countries.

State and Regional EMS Organizations

Emergency medical services agencies are particularly susceptible to shortages of medications that have potentially lifesaving benefits. Many EMS organizations work collaboratively

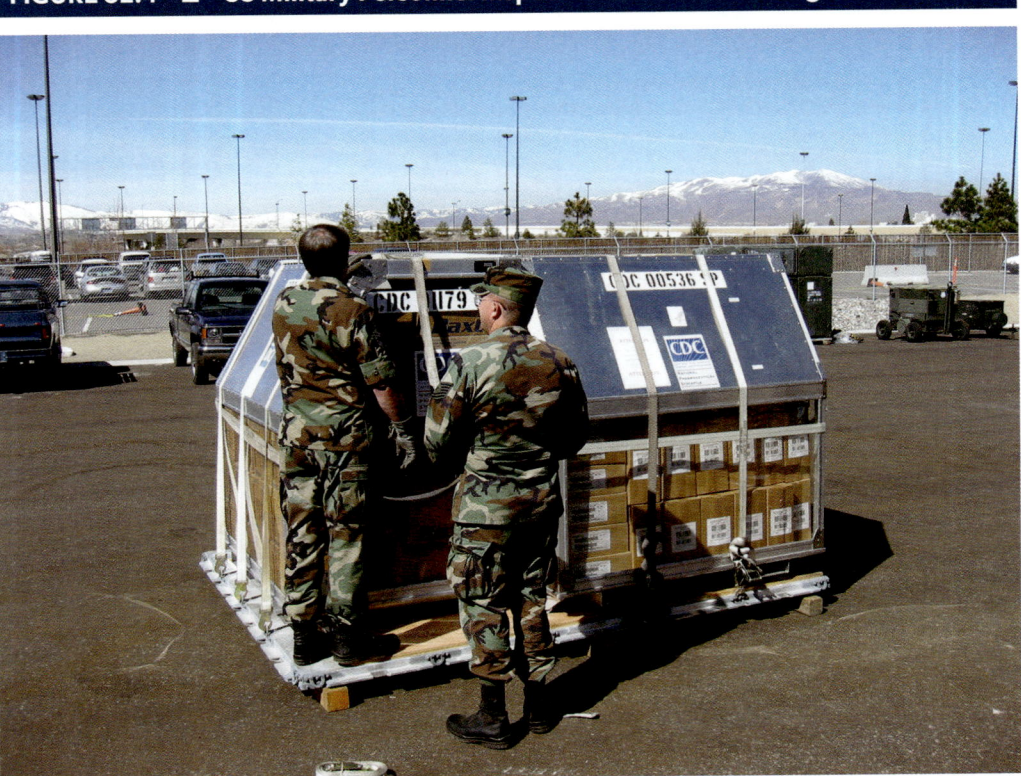

FIGURE 32.4 ■ US Military Personnel Inspect 12-Hour Push Packages

with other constituents to address the clinical implications of medication and equipment shortages. Emergency physician advocates and hospital organizations can support the efforts of EMS personnel to obtain critical supplies of epinephrine, atropine, bicarbonate, magnesium sulfate, and other essential out-of-hospital medications.

Some EMS agencies maintain incident action plans (IAPs) and incident management teams (IMTs). These strategies and personnel are put in place to allow for phased activation of a shortage mitigation-and-response plan. A phased approach allows health-care leaders to react based on the dynamics of each situation and ensures that EMS agencies and hospitals act cooperatively with local, regional, and state response strategies.

Other Governmental and Regulatory Agencies

Medication and supply shortages can reach crisis levels, compelling intervention by a state's office of the governor, emergency management agency, and boards of pharmacy, health, EMS, and medicine. A state disaster declaration by a governor triggers additional incident actions, including the deployment of IMTs and potential federal relief and support.

PROFESSIONAL ORGANIZATION INVOLVEMENT

The American Society of Health-System Pharmacists

The American Society of Health-System Pharmacists (ASHP) is a professional organization that represents pharmacists who serve in acute and ambulatory care settings. On its website, ASHP publishes best practices, guidelines, and tools related to drug shortages. Additionally, the organization maintains a listing of current shortages, discontinued drugs, and other valuable resources (**Table 32.1**). During its 2017 Drug Shortage Roundtable, the ASHP identified the main causes of drug shortages:

- Manufacturing quality concerns
- Lack of a supply cushion to adjudicate shortages
- Insufficient notification by manufacturers to alert the FDA of an impending shortage and its anticipated duration

The American Medical Association

The American Medical Association (AMA) Council on Science and Public Health Report 2-A-18 reviews causes of drug shortages and requires an annual AMA report on the issue of shortages, including any role of GPOs. In addition, the AMA is actively studying the potential repeal of the safe harbor for GPOs.

TABLE 32.1 ■ ASHP Drug Shortage Updates[7]	
Generic Name	**Revision Date**
0.9% Sodium chloride (<150 mL bags)	June 23, 2020
25% Dextrose injection	September 9, 2020
Acyclovir injection	September 22, 2020
Albuterol sulfate metered dose inhalers	October 7, 2020
Amiodarone injection	September 16, 2020
Amphotericin B injection	October 6, 2020
Azithromycin injection	October 5, 2020

National EMS Professional Organizations

The National Association of State EMS Officials maintains drug-shortage options and strategies for its members and collaborates widely on the issue. The National Association of EMS Physicians provides informational documents on drug shortages and a list of pharmaceutical backorders pertinent to the provision of out-of-hospital care.

SHORTAGE CHALLENGES

Emergency department leaders have options for managing acute shortages of supplies, equipment, medications, and technologies. They may be implemented in phases as the nature of the crisis becomes visible. When patient care is impacted or staff are put at risk, the progressive implementation of management strategies using a broad range of resources may be necessary.

Drug and equipment shortages can be predictable or unforeseen, transient or chronic, readily addressed via a substitute or formidable due to the lack of alternatives, and relatively innocuous or life-threatening relative to the medical condition(s) involved. Given this variability, a concrete strategy to address shortages is in order.

CONOPS

A medication or supply shortage "concept of operations" or CONOPS outlines a general strategy for deployment in the event of a national emergency.[8] It is activated to address the goals outlined in this section. CONOPS allows for the following three phases of activation:

- Phase 1 of this plan is activated in response to the *potential* for significant medication or equipment shortages impacting patient care.
- Phases 2 and 3 are activated in stages based on the impact of a shortage on operations and patient care in the field and in hospitals. This approach affords organizations the flexibility to react based on a dynamic situation and ensures that ED, EMS agencies, and hospitals act cooperatively with local, regional, and state response strategies.

The CONOPS strategy includes a sequential set of steps for preparedness and action. Emergency agencies work with county health departments, hospitals, and state regulators to develop solutions for patient safety relative to emergency medical care, workforce protection, and continuity of operations.

Goals

The goals of the equipment and drug shortage CONOPS plan are:

- To create a system whereby medicines and medical equipment are available for patient care when and where they are needed—at a reasonable cost to the system
- To outline the command structure in accordance with the National Incident Management System (NIMS)
- To integrate out-of-hospital and hospital-based supplies and patient care
- To ensure patient safety
- To reduce the budget impact of shortage events

Assumptions and Constraints

CONOPS have been constructed on the assumption that shortage events will continue into the foreseeable future. The plan is constrained by imperfect and rapidly changing information related to the nature of medication production and distribution—an ongoing international issue. The plan assumes that the state EMS oversight agencies and the state board of pharmacy will support regional efforts to address the shortages.

Planning assumptions regarding emergency system operations include the following:

- Patients' needs for emergency medicines will increase.
- Emergency providers are placed at risk if there are insufficient supplies of protective equipment, ventilators, and other medical devices and drugs needed for patient care.
- Traditional suppliers are unable to deliver adequate supplies in a timely manner.
- Federal government proclamations are not going to impact the availability of supplies and medicines if the supply chain is broken.

Five-Step Management Process

Physician and organizational leaders must develop, in collaboration with key stakeholders, an effective response to potential and real drug and medical equipment shortages. One such five-step plan follows (**Box 32.1**).

Active Stock Management

Organizations must address supply, utilization, rationing, and the storage of supply and medication stocks. The organization must develop the list of supplies and medicines critical to the provision of care and the individual management plan for each material. It is critical that a lead person actively manages all stocks, maintains the physical stock such that medicines with short expiration windows are used first, and provides reports to upper-level management on use, supply, and strategies for optimizing the stocks of important goods. In the early days of PPE shortages, strategies were developed to reuse equipment, with disinfection at critical intervals. That process needed to be developed and implemented by the ED leaders in a very short period of time. Plans regarding reuse or restocking must also include the method of rapid delivery (human, transport system, etc.).

Partnerships

Collaboration with fellow regional health-care providers and leaders is a strategy to enhance alternative supplies for potential or real medication or supply shortages. In the emergency care system (and applying the NIMS nomenclature), this collaboration is referred to as *mutual aid*. Others health-care entities may maintain reserve stock that they are willing to share or relationships with out-of-region providers who can contribute to the solution.

Deployment

Following the active stock management plan, supplies and drugs in limited supply must be stored and deployed *just in time* and based on patient need. Key considerations include

---

BOX 32.1 ■ FIVE-STEP MEDICATION/MEDICAL DEVICE SHORTAGE MANAGEMENT PROCESS

1. Active stock management
2. Partnerships
3. Deployment
4. Use of expired medications
5. Alternate medicine sources

avoiding supply or medication degradation due to environmental exposure, loss due to waste or diversion, and nonuse prior to expiration date.

Expired Medications

As described previously, medical science suggests that many drugs maintain their potency past the manufacturer-imposed expiration date.[5,6] This phenomenon is variable, drug-specific, and influenced by external environmental factors like temperature, light exposure, and humidity.

Alternate Medicine Sources

Organizations can address certain drug shortages through local or regional compounding pharmacies. The average price for compounded medicines is 8 to 10 times higher than sourcing through traditional methods. Compounded drugs have a limited shelf life of approximately six months. Federal officials suggest the use of accredited compounding pharmacies to ensure quality.

CONCLUSION

Shortages affecting emergency care have grown dramatically since 2008. The lack of all forms of supplies was a stressful element of ED management in the early months of the COVID-19 pandemic and exposed many gaps in the medical supply chain. Medication shortages will impact lifesaving interventions and high-acuity patient conditions with limited or no therapeutic alternatives. The impact of drug and supply shortages on staff safety and confidence is equally substantial. Accordingly, a well-conceived strategy for the management of shortages is an essential duty of organizational leadership. Multiple constituents are vital when planning for medication and equipment shortages, including governmental and regulatory agencies, professional societies, and pharmaceutical and medical device manufacturers. Furthermore, it is important to understand that the FDA, CDC, and other governmental agencies may not be prepared to provide significant resources in the event of a large-scale shortage event.

REFERENCES

1. A Primer on Group Purchasing Organizations: Questions and Answers. The Healthcare Supply Chain Association. Washington, DC. Available at: https://www.hiscionline.org/Files/gpo_primer.pdf. Accessed October 20, 2018.
2. Bruhn WE, Fracica EA, Makary MA. Group purchasing organizations, health care costs, and drug shortages. *JAMA*. 2018;320(18):1859–1860.
3. Kohn LT. *Group Purchasing Organizations: Research on their Pricing Impact on Health Care Providers*. U.S. Government Accountability Office. 2010. Available at: https://www.gao.gov/new.items/d10323r.pdf. Accessed October 21, 2018.
4. Litan RE, Singer HJ, Birkenbach A. An empirical analysis of aftermarket transactions by hospitals. *J Contemp Health Law Policy*. 2011;28(1):23–38.
5. Cantrell L, Suchard JF, Wu A, et al. Stability of active ingredients in long-expired prescription medications. *Arch Intern Med*. 2012;172:1685–1687.
6. Greene J. Short expiration dates may exacerbate drug shortages. *Ann Emerg Med*. 2018;71(2):A13–15.
7. ASHP.org. Drug Shortages List. 2020. Available at: https://www.ashp.org/Drug-Shortages/Current-Shortages/Drug-Shortages-List?page=CurrentShortages. Accessed October 9, 2020.
8. Augustine J. Emergency departments need plan to deal with drug shortages. *ACEP Now*. 2017;36(8):20–21.

OPERATIONS: FLOW

SECTION 3

CHAPTER 33

PATIENT THROUGHPUT: WHY IT MATTERS, HOW IT IS DONE

Kirk Jensen, Thom A. Mayer, With Jay Kaplan, Stephanie Baker

Flow is an important concept, as it addresses making processes, people, place, and performance in the emergency department (ED) more efficient and effective, thus resulting in greater satisfaction and better outcomes for both patients and staff. This chapter briefly introduces the key concepts involved in flow, which other chapters examine in more detail. Most important, it presents a vocabulary or taxonomy of flow and highlights the key operational management principles that are essential for understanding the more detailed concepts and applications presented in other chapters.

UNDERSTANDING FLOW

The concept of flow can be found in a number of industries, but it is particularly important in service operations like health care, restaurants, and hotels. The concept of flow plays a critical role in the "Lean" approach to health-care operations and services—a method that originated in Japanese manufacturing to streamline processes and improve productivity while always focusing on the needs of the customer.

Flow in Emergency Medicine

Theories, methodology, and applications of flow have been increasingly refined over the years and adapted for use in medicine. "Flow" in emergency medicine can be defined as the efficient movement of patients through the network of services that constitute ED operations (from arrival to evaluation, diagnosis, treatment, and discharge or admission to the hospital) while adding value and eliminating waste.[1]

The essence of flow as it pertains to health-care service operations is that all of the steps in the process are highly coordinated and orchestrated in such a manner that patients progress smoothly through the continuum of care. Like water flowing in a river, patients should move continuously through health-care processes toward desired outcomes and end points. Delays caused by inefficient or uncoordinated processes impede patient movement through the system just as rocks, sharp curves, and other obstacles can impede the flow of water.

Flow is easy to misunderstand. For instance, ED managers can be tempted to map their processes and declare, "Here is our flow." Having a process is not synonymous with having flow; in fact, a great deal of work and effort is usually required to fine-tune the process. Because flow initiatives emphasize efficiency, it is tempting to think that flow simply entails shaving time off of critical processes. While taking steps to improve flow often does involve making processes more efficient, such steps should only be taken if they lead to better patient care. Simply stated, improving flow both reduces waste and adds value. For some patients and conditions, these improvements mean allocating *more* time to diagnose and treat conditions properly.

Another perspective, and an important one, is the psychological concept of flow, which can be found in studies originated by psychologist Mihaly Csikszentmihalyi in the mid-1970s. Csikszentmihalyi describes flow as being deeply and constructively engaged or immersed in a task or action, with a resultant sense of clarity, where feedback is immediate and clear, challenges are matched with skills, a feeling of intense focus develops, self-consciousness disappears, time seems transformed, and the results are at an extremely high level of performance (**Figure 33.1**). In other words, when flow exists, people are able to carry out their roles with an energized focus and a

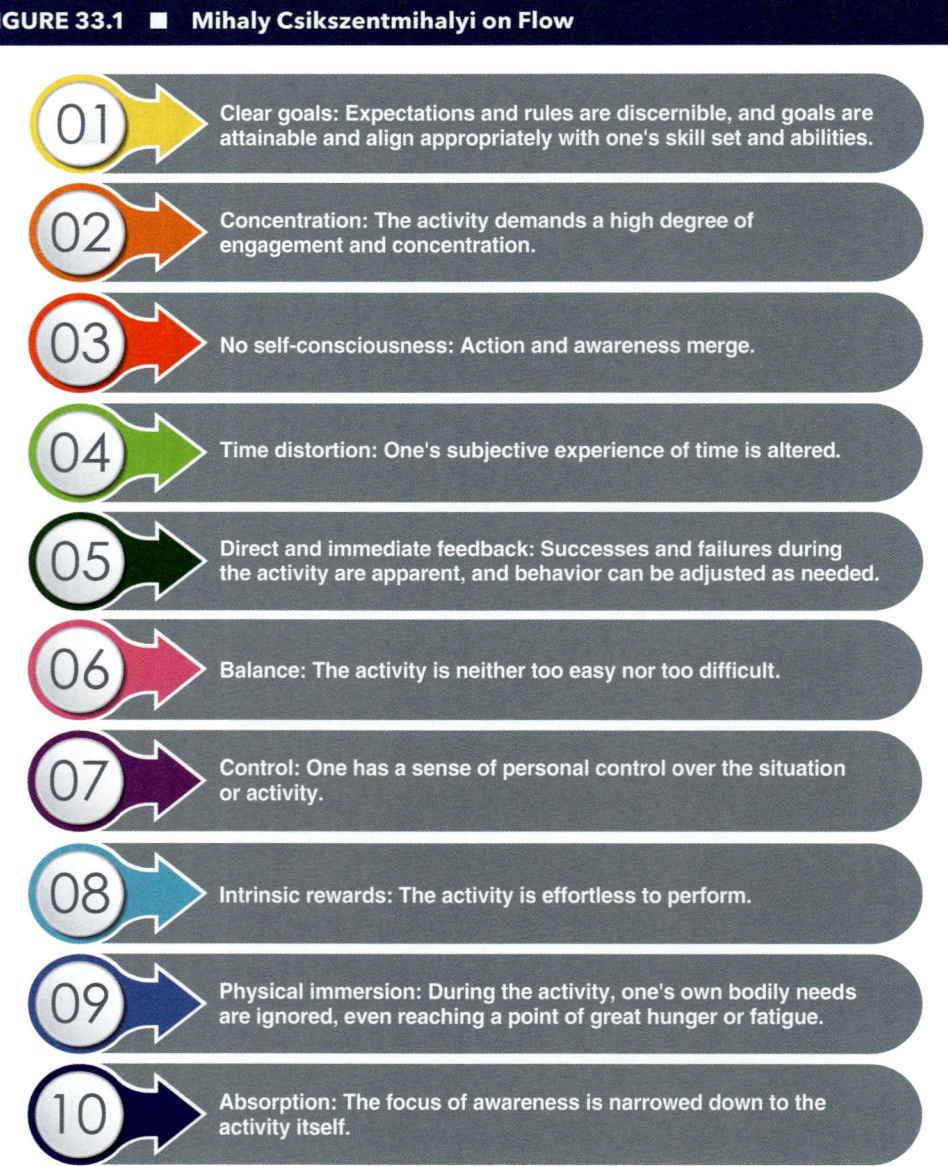

FIGURE 33.1 ■ Mihaly Csikszentmihalyi on Flow

01 Clear goals: Expectations and rules are discernible, and goals are attainable and align appropriately with one's skill set and abilities.

02 Concentration: The activity demands a high degree of engagement and concentration.

03 No self-consciousness: Action and awareness merge.

04 Time distortion: One's subjective experience of time is altered.

05 Direct and immediate feedback: Successes and failures during the activity are apparent, and behavior can be adjusted as needed.

06 Balance: The activity is neither too easy nor too difficult.

07 Control: One has a sense of personal control over the situation or activity.

08 Intrinsic rewards: The activity is effortless to perform.

09 Physical immersion: During the activity, one's own bodily needs are ignored, even reaching a point of great hunger or fatigue.

10 Absorption: The focus of awareness is narrowed down to the activity itself.

deep sense of fulfillment.[2-4] This feeling of "being in the zone" is what ED leaders and staff seek to attain when working to optimize departmental flow.

The Seven "Rights" of Flow

Effectiveness and efficiency capable of adding value and eliminating waste arise from ensuring that leaders have systems that are designed to produce the right application of the seven "rights" (**Figure 33.2**).

- The **right resources** ensure that only the necessary costs are applied to the problem, whether clinical or administrative.
- The **right patient** ensures that core measures are used to define what measures will be used to gauge success for this patient.
- The **right environment** means that the "MVP" of the health care system, the bed, is used to the best advantage, and only for as long as the bed adds value.
- The **right reasons** are the evidence-based-protocols (grounded in evidence-based medicine [EBM])— based on randomized controlled trials whenever possible and open to iterative change as further evidence develops.
- The **right team** ensures that all those involved in the patient's care are operating at the top of their license and are best deployed to add value.
- The **right time** means that flow metrics are in place and monitored over time, so that flow and efficiency are maximized.
- Finally, **every patient, every time, every person** is an embodiment of the commitment to patient safety and high-reliability organizations.

FIGURE 33.2 ■ Flow and the Seven "Rights"

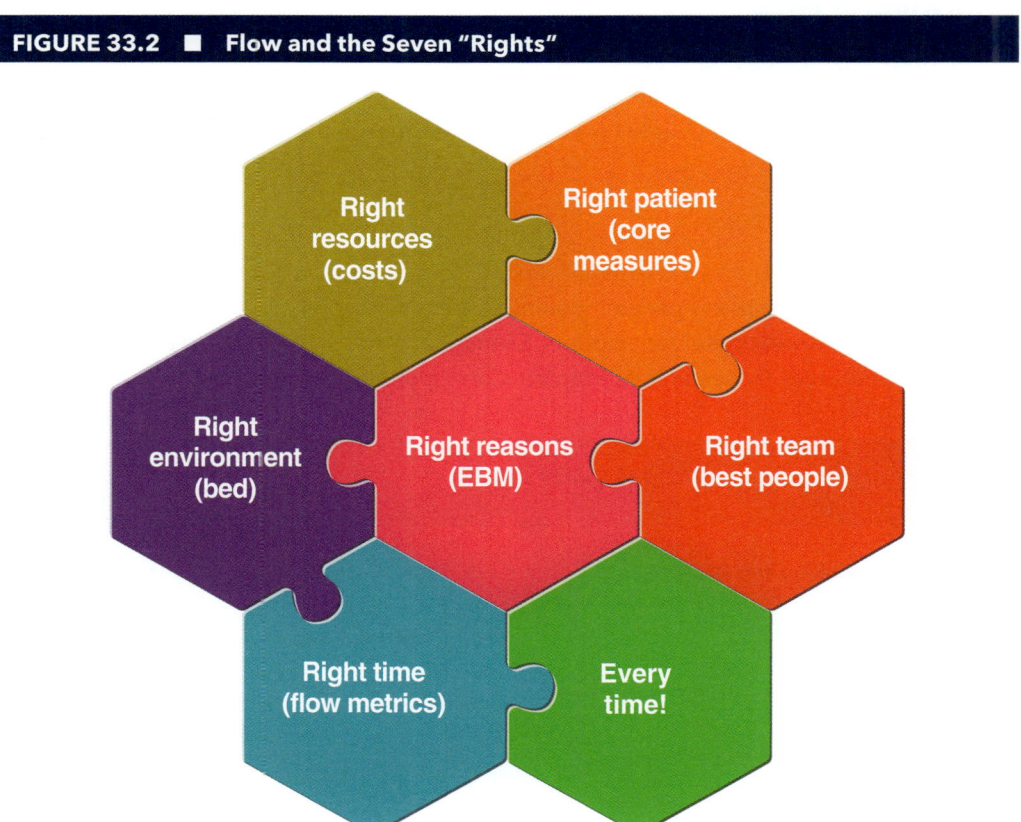

The Importance of Flow

Consider the following case study. In an ED averaging 40,000 patient visits each year, an initiative to improve flow cut the average length of stay by 1 hour (from 2-3 hours). Doing so provided 40,000 additional hours of service capacity in that department. At 2 hours per visit, that improvement in throughput provided the capacity for 20,000 additional patient visits annually, utilizing essentially the same staff and resources.[2] If net collected revenue is $100 per patient in professional fees and $400 in professional fees, this flow improvement would result in an increase of net revenue of $2 million for the physician group and $8 million for the facility fees, as well as $3,000 to $7,500 per admitted patient.

This example illustrates an important observation about flow and throughput: Flow can be affected positively or negatively by small changes in the number of patients moving through the department or small changes in service capacity. Changing those capabilities at particular points in the process can negatively affect the ED through delays or positively enhance it by smoothing flow and reducing bottlenecks. Processes can determine whether patients experience satisfying encounters or frustrating delays and whether staff feel energized, focused, and engaged or rushed and at risk of making mistakes.

The reason small changes in volume or capacity can have ripple effects is mathematical: As these variables change, they influence the system exponentially and not linearly. Mathematicians can describe the theory and demonstrate the effects, but the important implication for attaining smooth flow is that small changes can lead to big impacts.

Principles of Flow

The lessons businesses and service organizations have learned about flow over the past half century fall into several categories listed in **Box 33.1**. By being familiar with these concepts and applying the insights gained from research, flow can improve dramatically in the ED.[5-7]

Demand and Capacity

As **Figure 33.3** makes clear, "demand" and "capacity" are important concepts in flow. "Demand" means how many people—potential customers or, in health care, patients—want or need the services an organization offers. Demand in health care can also be viewed as the amount of resources those patients require. Correspondingly, "capacity" is the amount of

---

BOX 33.1 ■ PRINCIPLES OF FLOW

- **Systems thinking and appreciation:** a network of components that work together to achieve common aims
- **A theory of knowledge:** an understanding of the ED, the hospital, and their processes
- **Key drivers of system performance:**
    - Demand-capacity management
    - Queuing
    - Variation
- **High-leverage interventions:** the theory of constraints
- **Method of improvement:** Lean, Six Sigma, etc.
- **Where waiting exists:** apply *The Psychology of Waiting Lines*

FIGURE 33.3 ■ Adjusting Physician/Advanced Practice Provider Staffing

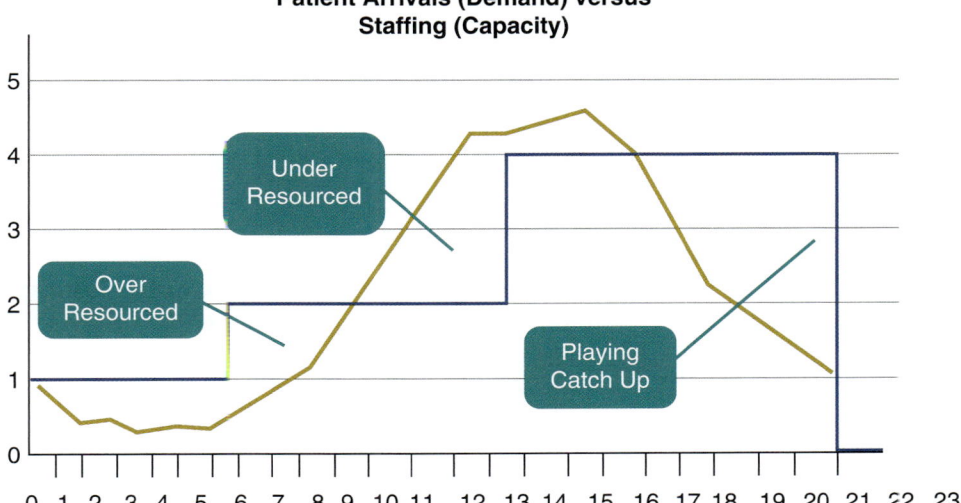

resources available to evaluate, diagnose, and provide treatment and service. The interplay between these variables determines how smoothly the process flows.

Demand is created by the arrival of incoming patients who require various levels of treatment. The demand for services created by patients will be met by various servers in the ED, including beds, nurses, doctors, and advanced practice providers (APPs). Therefore, it is important to determine the specific demands patients will have on each type of server. The challenge faced by professionals staffing an ED is that demand can fluctuate on a daily and hourly basis. That being said, there are methods for characterizing demand within a service environment like an ED to account for this type of variation. In this sense, even though demand is uncertain, it is somewhat predictable, allowing managers to align or match capacity to meet it.

One has to appreciate that there are trade-offs between cost, throughput, productivity, length of stay, patient waiting times, and safety. Recognizing these trade-offs is the key to staffing an ED that meets throughput targets while simultaneously providing high-quality care to patients, a satisfying work environment for staff, and financial stability for the department.

A sophisticated demand/capacity analysis should be based on arrivals and acuity by hour of the day and day of the week, and even by season of the year—as well as on service times and targeted performance measures. With the appropriate use of such demand/capacity management analytics, the ED operations team is best equipped to answer the following questions:

- How many physicians, APPs, and scribes do I need to meet the demand of incoming patients?
- How many nurses do I need to meet the demand of incoming patients?
- How many beds do I need in my department?
- Do I have the right staffing level, staffing mix, and staffing hours?
- Are those staff members functioning at the top of their level of training/licenses?
- How do scribes affect physician productivity?
- Is there an opportunity to operationalize fast-tracking or some other front-end patient flow model?

What happens when demand exceeds capacity in an ED is obvious: longer delays, more patients leaving without being seen, increased errors, and decreased patient and staff satisfaction. Although what happens when capacity exceeds demand may not come as readily to mind, this imbalance can lead to wasted resources. Furthermore, since health care is a service not a product, a hospital or ED team cannot store unused capacity; if resources are idle or underutilized for several hours, that lost productivity can never be recovered. The better capacity is matched to the demand, the smoother the flow will be through the department and the greater the efficiency will be throughout the system.

Flow in Real Time

Knowing what is going on moment to moment and hour by hour in the department is vital. Without a dashboard to reflect real-time demand and capacity (**Figure 33.4**), the ED will operate blindly.

Forecasting

The flow of patients into an ED appears random and unscheduled, which might seem to make prediction impossible, but prediction is not impossible because unscheduled flow into a system follows predictable patterns, a phenomenon mathematicians have studied and described.[8,9] These patterns can be modeled (**Figure 33.5**). Forecasting methods can predict how many patients will come to the department, when they will come, and what services they will need. Doing so positions leaders to manage flow.

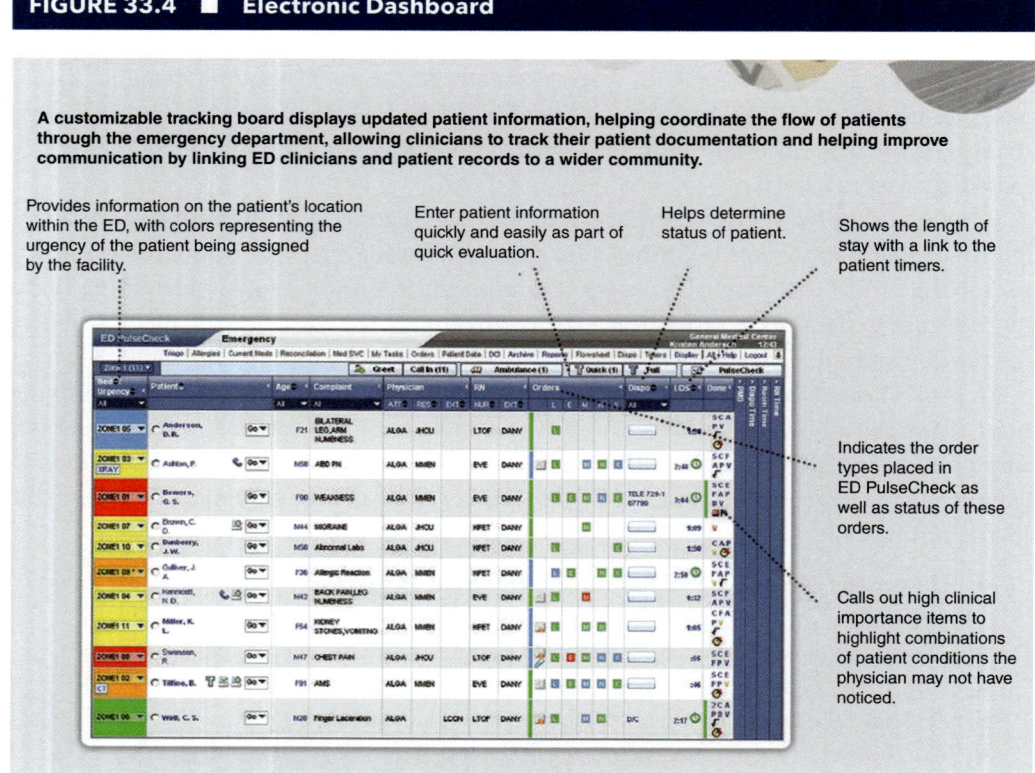

FIGURE 33.4 ■ Electronic Dashboard

FIGURE 33.5 ■ Modeling Forecasting Patient Arrivals and Staffing to Demand

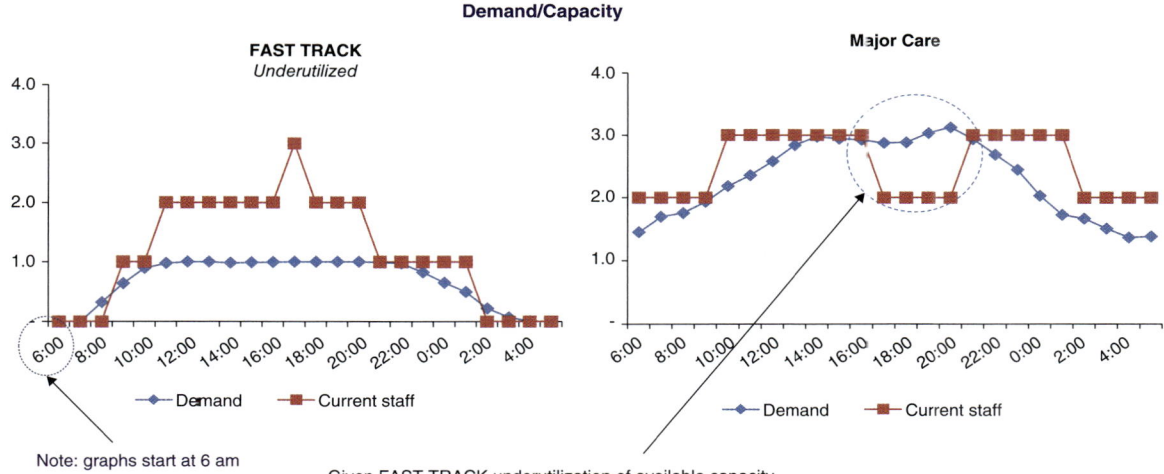

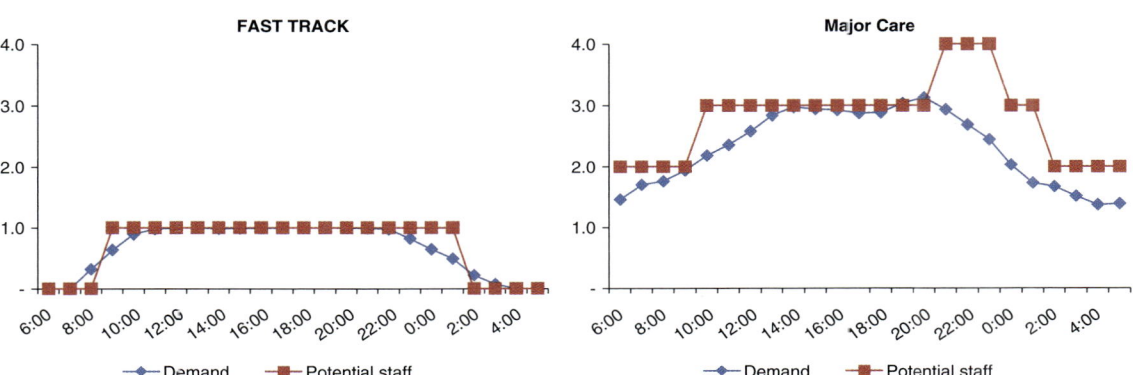

- Move FAST TRACK double coverage into Major Care, start shift slightly later (anytime between 11AM and 4PM—graphs show 4PM-2AM)
  - Develop a system to incorporate additional midlevel capacity in Major Care, including utilizing Kids Care real estate as a results waiting area for Major Care patients
  - Develop a system in which this NP could swing to FAST TRACK if deep laceration or other procedure slows down FAST TRACK throughput

Queues

A queue is a group of people waiting for a service (or a product). People generally think of lines when they envision queues, but patients sitting in chairs in an ED waiting area, patients in ED beds awaiting care by a physician, physicians waiting for diagnostic test results, admissions waiting for an inpatient bed—all represent queues. Any key server (e.g., doctors, nurses, technicians, beds . . .) can, at a given moment, be embedded in a queue. Engineers and mathematicians have studied queues for many years, and businesses have applied that knowledge to managing queues.[10,11]

A critical attribute of a queuing system, as mentioned earlier, is that as the utilization of a service (or server) increases in a queuing system (any system with unscheduled queue for a service), the waiting for each customer of that server becomes longer until, at a critical point (discussed in more detail in Chapter 34), the waiting time lengthens

FIGURE 33.6 ■ Queue Behavior as a Function of Utilization

On the surface, it might seem that health care managers would seek 100% utilization of servers; however, increases in utilization are *only achieved* by increases in the length of the waiting line and the average waiting time. This is because as utilization approaches 100% waiting times increase in a *highly non-linear fashion*.

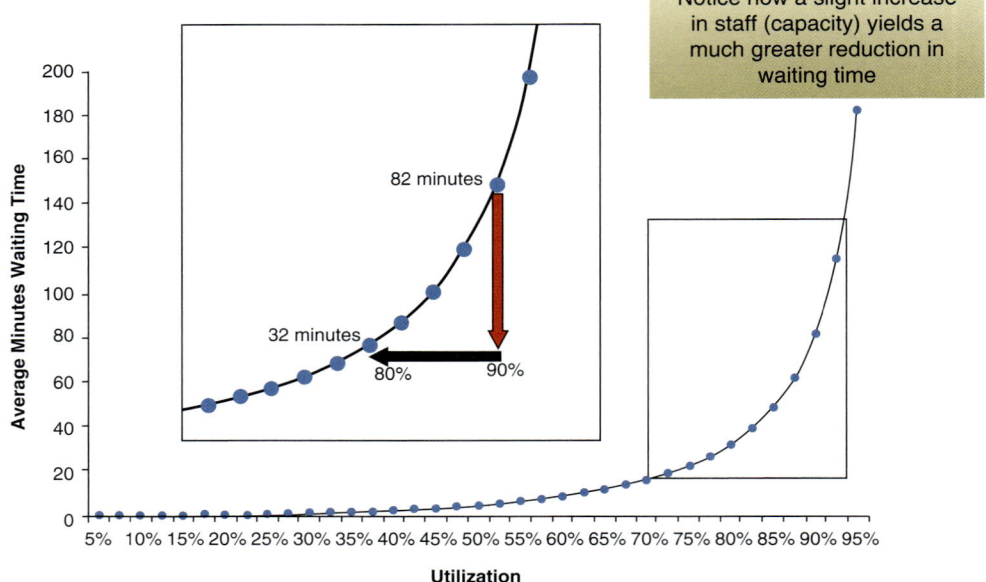

dramatically. But the math works both ways: Small increases in capacity or decreases in demand in highly stressed systems can reduce waits and delays significantly (**Figure 33.6**).

Constraints

A constraint is something that hinders performance of an organization enough to keep it from accomplishing its goal.[12] Waiting lines/queues form when capacity exceeds demand at a given server (e.g., doctors, APPs, nurses, beds). When this happens, bottlenecks begin to form. The bottleneck defines the speed and limits the flow of entities (e.g., patients) through a system. If a resource has a demand that exceeds its capacity, then it is a constraint on the system. A resource in an ED can be a physician, nurse, or any staff member, a piece of equipment (such as a CT scanner), or even a bed. If a resource is a constraint, then a queue will form at the point where that resource delivers its service. This bottleneck and the delays that occur will impact the entire system.

Variation

A system with unscheduled, random flow, such as an ED, inevitably experiences variation. Its most obvious form is fluctuation in the number of patients. But variation takes a number of other forms. Even when overall volume is not excessive, several patients arriving around the same time with complicated conditions can cause delays and variation in flow. Different procedures and illnesses require different amounts of time and resources by various providers. Physicians, nurses, and technicians bring different skill sets and approaches to ED patients. Clinicians with the same professional credentials may have different levels of training, experience, and skills and take different amounts of time to diagnose and treat patients.

FIGURE 33.7 ■ The Importance of Variation

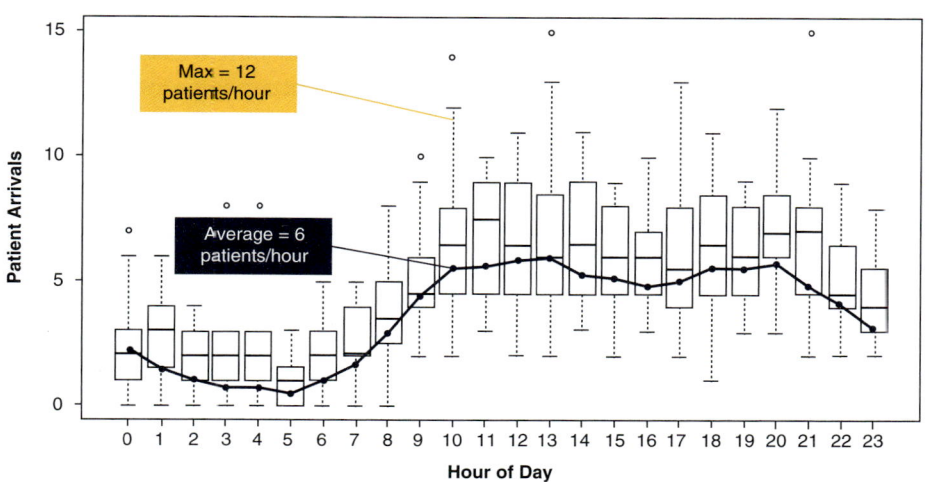

A key and nuanced concept is differentiating value-added versus non-value-added variations (**Figure 33.7**). Intelligently using value-added variation can dramatically improve flow in the ED. Variation in the processes employed at triage is necessary as the demand–capacity curve changes through the course of the day. In the morning hours, triage bypass is an effective strategy. However, when all the ED beds are full, triage bypass gives way to standing orders to begin evaluation and therapy.[13] If there are prolonged periods of time identified by a demand–capacity analysis, when beds will predictably be unavailable, placing a team of caregivers at triage can be beneficial.[14]

FIGURE 33.8 ■ The Psychology of Waiting Times[15]

- Unoccupied time feels longer than occupied time.
- Preprocess waits feel longer than in-process waits.
- Anxiety makes waits seem longer.
- Uncertain waits are longer than known, finite waits.
- Unexplained waits are longer than explained waits.
- Unfair waits are longer than equitable waits.
- The more valuable the service, the longer a person will wait.
- Solo waits feel longer than group waits.

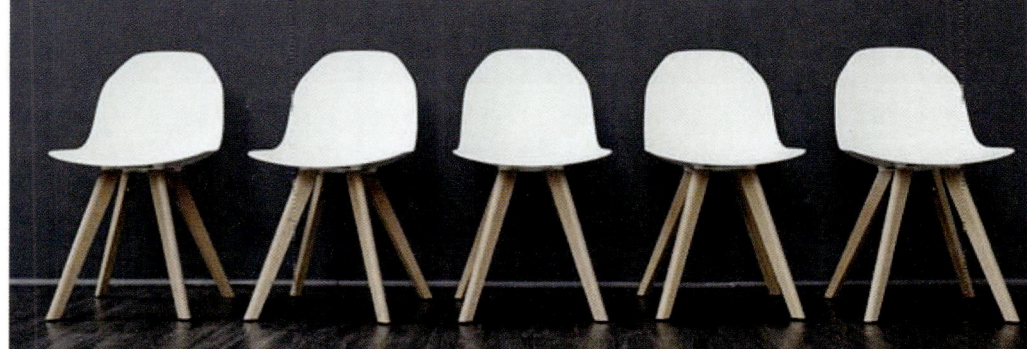

The Psychology of Waiting

When waiting is unavoidable, making use of principles arising from the study of waiting—about the psychology of how people perceive waiting and how those perceptions can be managed—can be a valuable tool for mitigating patient anxiety and dissatisfaction. Applying these principles can make waiting times seem shorter to people by occupying their attention, communicating effectively, and treating them fairly. Maintaining a reputation for delivering excellent clinical care helps as well; research has determined that people will wait longer and more patiently for service they deem of high quality (**Figure 33.8**).[15]

For a deeper discussion of the principles of the psychology of waiting and how they can be applied in the ED, see Chapter 42.

STRATEGIES TO IMPROVE FLOW

Equipped with a basic understanding of the components of flow, an ED can take advantage of strategies and tactics that have proven effective for a wide variety of industries.

Measuring and Forecasting Demand

Measuring demand and forecasting the need for service is an innovative way of thinking. How many patients will enter the department? When will they come? What will they need? Does one have the capacity to meet this demand? To be useful, the answer to these questions must be framed in an appropriate interval. For example, the hourly arrival and severity rate will indicate how many physicians, APPs, nurses, technicians, and beds are needed at that hour. The daily arrival rate is an indicator of how many staffing hours and beds are needed over the 24-hour period. Even the seasonal volume is helpful for certain parts of the United States when framing the need for resources (**Table 33.1**).

Dashboards should be used to track volumes and case complexity. When enough data are compiled over time, patterns become apparent that can drive decision-making. Specific numbers may fluctuate, but the general patterns should remain predictable and useful. The pattern for one day of the week may not be the same as another, just as the pattern for June will likely be different from the pattern for November.

Dashboards are useful for tracking data (such as patient volumes, severity, ambulance arrivals, and resource utilization) both in real time and over time. Understanding the patterns of these data elements allows a department to use this information to optimize the deployment of staffing, services, spaces, and supplies; provide better, more reliable patient care; and maintain a healthier work environment. For instance, this information

TABLE 33.1 ■ Balancing Demand and Capacity	
Who is coming?	Demand
When are they coming?	Demand
What will they need?	Demand
Will the resources be available?	Capacity
Will they be available at the time and in the quantity needed?	Capacity
Will the resource result in improved outcomes?	Demand/capacity match

can be used to predict the number and complexity of patients who will come in on Tuesday morning versus Tuesday evening and how many are likely to be admitted to the hospital. The ability to predict these variables can be leveraged to improve flow, safety, and satisfaction.[16]

Data that are compiled on volume, chief complaints, and needed resources can be projected into the future (forecasted) to facilitate planning ahead. For example, if an ED is confident that, on average, 12 patients will come to the ED between 6 am and noon and around 45 patients between 4 pm and 10 pm, then it can better align physicians, nurses, beds, and other resources to this demand. In addition, as flow improvement initiatives are undertaken, demand and capacity must be continuously measured and monitored, as bottlenecks "move" within the system.[17]

Monitoring Flow in Real Time

The dashboard not only enables the analysis of historical data, it also enables staff to see what is happening right now. Even though historical patterns can be discerned well enough to make generally reliable predictions, because of the unscheduled nature of demand, there will certainly be time periods when ED demand exceeds (or falls short of) projections. A real-time dashboard, particularly an electronic one that is widely visible to staff throughout the department, makes it possible to quickly realize when the anticipated 12 patients that morning are exceeded, thereby signaling the need to adjust capacity to accommodate this surge. The transparency of this spike enables a better reaction and response. Even a simple, nonelectronic dashboard can work, as long as it lists patients and where they are in the process of diagnosis and treatment. An electronic dashboard that is accessible via multiple monitors can supply additional information and insights that can prove invaluable for operational excellence.

Managing Queues, Constraints, and Variation

Real-time dashboards are particularly valuable for managing queues, offloading constraints, and smoothing variations. Bottlenecks can appear and change over time. A critical bottleneck in the morning (e.g., beds or staff) may not be the critical bottleneck in the evening. With real-time monitoring and analysis of patterns, the what, when, where, and why bottlenecks are occurring can be analyzed, and plans for helpful responses can be put into action.

If physicians or nurses are likely to become constraints, then one way to reduce that possibility is to make sure they are only performing critical tasks, such as patient evaluations, procedures, and dispositions—in short, doing what only they can uniquely do. Putting it another way, doctors should not be spending their time entering data on computers; nurses should not be using time to look for supplies. Clinicians should be primarily focused on providing direct patient care.

Preparing for potential spikes in patient volume is essential. Smartly leveraging the deployment of APPs, scribes, and technicians can be critical strategy. It can be helpful to use non-ED hospital areas that typically serve admitted patients during daytime hours to accommodate volume surges during the busy evening periods in the ED. Cross-training some staff members to perform duties of other team members (e.g., training unit coordinators to perform technicians' functions) enables patient needs to be better met when a key clinical team member is fully engaged in direct patient care. Coaching, transparent metrics, and education can help reduce variations in training and skills among similar providers. Standardizing processes for similar conditions is another helpful strategy for mitigating non-value-added variations.

Segmenting Patient Flow

Directing patients into service or operational streams based on the acuity of their conditions—so that similar conditions or resource needs are grouped into one stream where resources are available and processes are standardized—improves the efficiency of patient flow and the effectiveness of care.

There are several approaches to segmentation or streaming. Most EDs use two or three patient-flow streams, and some even use four. Many traditional EDs use two basic streams (low acuity and high acuity), while more advanced approaches (commonly found in higher-volume EDs) also incorporate mid-acuity flow. A fourth stream would be trauma and critical care. Five-level triage systems, such as the Emergency Severity Index, the Canadian Triage and Acuity Scale, the Australian National Triage Scale, and the British Manchester Triage System, can also be used to segment patients.[18-21]

An effective triage process helps the work of flow segmentation. To sort effectively, triage needs to be limited to a quick assessment after which the patient can be directed into the appropriate care stream, where a more complete examination can take place. Sorting patients needing critical care (or multiple resources) and nonurgent patients (needing relatively few resources) is admittedly easier than sorting those who fall within the middle streams, but efficiently sending these groups into the right treatment pathway aids smooth flow.

When patient volume and acuity justify its deployment, *team triage* is a good way to fully enhance and operationalize the effectiveness of patient and resource segmentation. A team in this model would include several clinician and technical support staff members. Depending on the size of the department, it might include one or two physicians or midlevel providers, one or two nurses, a registrar, a technician, and one or two scribes. The team combines assessment, diagnosis, and treatment, performing the latter two with patients who can be quickly and easily treated and discharged and directing others into the proper pathways (including directly to a bed for those who need one).

Fast Tracking

Fast tracking (or low-acuity tracking) is a technique designed to diagnose and treat patients whose conditions require few resources and who are relatively easy to treat. It is important to emphasize that "fast track" is best used as a verb and not a noun. It is an approach and set of processes to most effectively treat lower-acuity patients and not a place where they must be treated. It is a process whereby an ED can smooth flow by efficiently assessing, treating, and discharging patients who fit the criteria outlined here. In fact, with an effective segmentation, triage, and fast-track process, an ED can treat as much as 40% of its patients in this way.[22]

Applying the Psychology of Waiting

Understanding the psychology of waiting can make it possible to maintain patients' overall satisfaction with their visit in spite of encountering delays. Giving patients something to occupy their attention while they are idle diverts their focus from the fact that they are waiting. Even having them register while they're waiting can accomplish this task. Frequent communication and rounding on patients who are waiting and keeping them well informed is another effective strategy. When patients are kept apprised of how long processes are taking, reasons for delays, and next steps, they are generally more willing to wait.

Using a Management and Performance Improvement Methodology

Efforts to improve flow will be more effective if they make use of one of the performance improvement methodologies that have been developed and put to use in businesses and services in recent decades, including Lean and Six Sigma. Health-care organizations, in particular, have made use of Lean, which emphasizes adding value to processes and eliminating waste.[23-25] Streamlining processes by examining every step to determine whether it adds value results in smoother organizational flow.

Emphasizing Teamwork

An ED staff that works together as a team—as is true in most other aspects of life—is more effective than a group of individuals who work in an unsynchronized fashion. Teamwork should be the focus of continuous performance improvement. Training staff in *how* to work effectively as a team is imperative to maximize the likelihood of success. There are a number of established, proven programs for doing so. In Lean terms, effective teamwork eliminates waste and adds value to processes. For example, processes that are repeated or overlooked because they are not coordinated can lead to system-wide waste. Good teamwork can eliminate those duplications and oversights.

Coaching and mentoring should be an ongoing, essential part of any ED focused on patient flow, safety, and service. Honest evaluations that point out both strengths and weaknesses as well as targeted practical strategies should be an integral part of that process. As important as teaching teamwork and coaching are, hiring the right people in the first place is foundationally important. A strong team of high-performing clinical and nonclinical staff goes a long way toward successfully implementing measures to improve flow.

PITFALLS

Initiatives to improve flow often fail because departments or systems start out with enthusiasm but try to implement too many projects, or work on the wrong projects, or work with the wrong people. It is not uncommon for teams to fail to sustain their improvement efforts over time. Though it is wise to set short-term goals, the overall performance improvement initiative is seldom a brief process—it takes time, and the will and persistence to stay the course. Analyzing and understanding current practice and operational patterns before testing new ones is also important. Testing ideas on a small scale and prototyping the new best practice in the department before undertaking a full-scale deployment is another component in success. One more prescription for failure includes adjusting processes or introducing new ones without training staff to work effectively as a team once the new protocols are underway.

CONCLUSION

Understanding the science of operations management and what drives smooth flow through health-care systems provides the insights and tools needed to make successful patient flow in the department a reality. Tracking data; analyzing the patterns discernible in the data; using those patterns to predict patient volume, patients' conditions, and the resources they will require; monitoring flow as it occurs; and adjusting when necessary will lead to smoother flow and improve patient satisfaction. When patients are satisfied, flow is smooth, and workplace conditions optimized, then the staff is going to be satisfied too. Such a department will be a good place to visit—and a great place to work.

REFERENCES

1. Mayer T, Jensen K. *Hardwiring Flow: Systems and Processes for Seamless Patient Care*. Gulf Breeze, Fla: Fire Starter Publishing; 2009.

2. Csikszentmihalyi M. *Flow: The Psychology of Optimal Experience*. New York, NY: Harper & Row; 1990.

3. Csikszentmihalyi M. *The Evolving Self: A Psychology for the Third Millennium*. New York, NY: Harper Collins; 1993.

4. Csikszentmihalyi M. *Finding Flow: The Psychology of Engagement With Everyday Life*. New York, NY: Perseus Books Group; 1997.

5. Jensen K, Kirkpatrick DG. *The Hospital Executive's Guide to Emergency Department Management*. Marblehead, Mass: HCPro Inc.; 2010.

6. Jensen K, Mayer T, Welch SJ, Haraden C. *Leadership for Smooth Patient Flow*. Chicago, Ill: Health Administration Press; 2007.

7. Pines JM, Batt RJ, Hilton JA, Terwiesch C. The financial consequences of lost demand and reducing boarding in hospital emergency departments. *Ann Emerg Med*. 2011;58(4):331-340.

8. Hwang J, Christensen CM. Disruptive innovation in health care delivery: a framework for business model innovation. *Health Aff (Millwood)*. 2007;27(5):1327-1335.

9. Litvak E, Bisognano M. More patients, less payment: increasing hospital efficiency in the aftermath of health care reform. *Health Aff (Millwood)*. 2011;30(1):76-80.

10. Asplin B, Magid DJ. If you want to fix crowding, start by fixing your hospital. *Ann Emerg Med*. 2007;49(3):273-274.

11. Ballard DW, Price M, Fung V, et al. Validation of an algorithm for categorizing the severity of hospital emergency department visits. *Med Care*. 2010;48(1):58-63.

12. Goldratt E, Cox J. *The Goal*. Great Barrington, Mass: North River Press; 1992.

13. Kokiko J, Mayer TA. Advanced triage/advanced interventions: improving patient satisfaction. *Topics Emerg Med*. 1997;19(2):19-27.

14. Mayer T. Innovations initiating early patient care through team triage and treatment. *Urgent Matters*. 2005;2(1). Available at: http://urgentmatters.org/346834/318774/318802/318805. Accessed June 2, 2013.

15. Maister D. The psychology of waiting lines. 1985. Available at: http://davidmaister.com/articles/5/52/. Accessed June 2, 2013.

16. Mayer T. Drive service excellence to the next level: moving patient satisfaction scores from the 4s to the 5s is key. *Health Exec*. 2010;25(6):54-56.

17. Verdile VP. Sutton's law need not apply. *Ann Emerg Med*. 2011;58(4):341-342.

18. Wuerz RC, Milne LW, Eitel Dr, Travers D, Gilboy N. Reliability and validity of a new five-level triage instrument. *Acad Emerg Med*. 2000;7(3):236-242.

19. Beveridge R, Clarke B, Janes L, et al. Canadian emergency department triage and acuity scale: implementation and guidelines. *Canad J Emerg Med*. 1999;(suppl):S2-S28.

20. Welch SJ, Davidson SJ. The performance limits of traditional triage. *Ann Emerg Med*. 2011;58(2):143-144.

21. Matias C, Oliviera R, Duarte R, et al. The Manchester Triage System in acute coronary syndromes. *Rev Port Cardiol*. 2008;27(2):205-216.

22. Wiler JL, Gentle C, Halfpenny JM, et al. Optimizing emergency department front-end operations [in English, Portuguese]. *Ann Emerg Med*. 2010;55:142-160.

23. Mayer T. Applying the principles of lean management to health care. Paper presented at: the American College of Emergency Physicians Scientific Assembly; October 13, 2011; Denver, Colo.

24. Spear SJ. Learning to lead at Toyota. *Harvard Bus Rev*. 2004;82(5):78-86.

25. Jensen K, Crane J. Improving patient flow in the emergency department. *Healthc Financ Manage*. 2008;62(11):104-106.

ADDITIONAL READINGS

- ACEP: Emergency Medicine Practice Committee of the American College of Emergency Physicians. Emergency department crowding: high-impact solutions. 2016. Available at: https://www.acep.org/Legislation-and-Advocacy/Practice-Management-Issues/Boarding/Crowding/Emergency-Department-Crowding---High-Impact-Solutions/.

- Advisory Board. *Building the Clockwork ED: Best Practices for Eliminating Bottlenecks and Delays in the ED*. Washington, DC: HWorks, An Advisory Board Company; 2000.

- Advisory Board. *The High-Performance ED Optimizing Capacity and Throughput to Meet Ever-Growing Demand*. Washington, DC: HWorks, An Advisory Board Company; 2008.

- Baker S. *Excellence in the Emergency Department: How to Get Results*. Gulf Breeze, Fla: Fire-Starter Publishing; 2009.

- Crane JT, Noon CE. *The Definitive Guide to Emergency Department Operational Improvement: Employing Lean Principles With Current ED Best Practices to Create the "No Wait" Department*. New York, NY: Productivity Press; 2011.

- Emergency Nurses Association. Staffing guidelines. 2017.

- Falvo T, Grove L, Stachura R, et al. The opportunity loss of boarding admitted patients in the emergency department. *Acad Emerg Med*. 2007;14(4):332-337.

- Forster AJ, Stiell I, Wells G, Lee AJ, van Walraven C. The effect of hospital occupancy on emergency department length of stay and patient disposition. *Acad Emerg Med*. 2003;10(2):127-133.

- Institute for Health care Improvement. Optimizing patient flow: moving patients smoothly through acute care settings. *Innovation Series*. Chicago, IL: Institute for Health Care Improvement; 2003.

- Holden RJ. Lean thinking in emergency departments: a critical review. *Ann Emerg Med*. 2011;57(3):265-278.

- Horowitz LI, Green J, Bradley EH. US emergency department performance on wait time and length of visit. *Ann Emerg Med*. 2011;55(2):133-141.

- Jensen K. Emergency department crowding: the nature of the problem and why it matters and improving patient satisfaction through flow. In: *Patient Flow: Reducing Delay in Health Care Delivery*. 2nd ed. New York, NY: Springer; 2013:97-106, 429-446.

- Jensen K and Mayer T. *The Patient Flow Advantage: How Hardwiring Hospital-Wide Flow Drives Competitive Performance*. Gulf Breeze, Fla: Fire-Starter Publishing; 2015.

- Litvak E, Buerhaus PI, Davidoff F, et al. Managing unnecessary variability in patient demand to reduce nursing stress and improve patient safety. *Jt Comm J Qual Patient Saf*. 2005;31(6):330-338.

CHAPTER 34

PATIENT FLOW PRINCIPLES

Charles Noon, Jody Crane, Mark B. Kauffman

In contrast to a goods-producing operation that has a physical product as its output, health care is considered a *service operation*. Service operations are designed to meet the needs of the customer rather than produce a physical good *for* a customer. Examples of services might include an airline moving a customer from one location to another or an investment firm facilitating an exchange of financial instruments. In health care, customers are transformed from sickness to wellness or, in many cases, informed of a physiological issue and provided guidance on improving their health.

The concept of achieving high-velocity flow with value-creating activities became a pillar of the Lean movement that took hold in the 1980s, first in manufacturing and later in service industries. In health care, improved flow benefits all key stakeholders. Patients are better served by ready access to medical treatment. Caregivers benefit by doing what they do best: providing high-quality care without the distractions that are symptomatic of poor systemic flow. Health-care organizations benefit by serving a greater number of customers without adding facilities or excessive staff.

"LEAN" FLOW

In health care, a value-added activity is any action that moves patients closer to resolving their medical needs. When compromised, these activities decrease the quality of care. In keeping with this view, any process that does not benefit the patient is considered "non–value added." Examples of *value-added* activities include an examination by a provider, physician, or nurse; a procedure; or a necessary diagnostic test. *Non–value-added* activities include transportation, registration, and waiting. The concept of "Lean flow" (derived from the Lean management methodology) means moving a patient from one value-added activity to the next with minimal delays. There are clear benefits associated with Lean flow for both patients and staff.[1]

Prompt assessment and treatment can minimize the risk of an adverse event or further deterioration. Pain management, for example, is easier and more effective when started early in the patient's visit. Similarly, an early evaluation by a medical professional results in swifter patient transitions. For example, the parents of a febrile infant will remain anxious until a physician can evaluate their child and render a diagnosis. In short, the same efficiencies resulting from Lean flow techniques can minimize patients' length of stay, ensure faster treatments, decrease the duration of anxiety and pain, and enhance the satisfaction of all involved.

Decreasing Waste

For the emergency department (ED) staff and physicians, Lean patient flow reduces waste. For example, the longer a patient must wait to complete treatment, the more services and evaluations will be required by the nursing staff. Long turnaround times for lab tests, imaging, and other service providers can unnecessarily extend a physician's shift.

Another form of waste occurs whenever a health-care worker is idle. In contrast to a manufacturing operation that can keep workers busy by building inventory, a service operation cannot recover productive time that is lost because of inertia. Consider a physician managing a pod of eight patients, all of whom are waiting for diagnostic results, admission, or a provider's help. Even when there are patients in the waiting room, the physician is unable to treat them because of a lack of Lean flow.

Lean flow also has the advantage of requiring fewer treatment spaces. Too often in EDs with poor flow, treatment spaces are used as "holding" spaces. Hence, poor flow and its accompanying delays can have three negative effects:

- First, poor flow can result in costly capital expansions by wrongly appearing to be a "space constraint" when, in fact, it is a flow problem.
- Second, requiring more treatment spaces than necessary requires staff members to cover more rooms spread over a larger area, thereby incurring wasted movement or, in the case of mandated ratios, more staff to care for the same number of patients.
- Third, covering wide treatment areas adversely affects nurse and physician communication because of the greater likelihood that they will be in different areas of the ED treating patients, getting supplies, or arranging transport.

INHIBITORS OF PATIENT FLOW

Lean flow does not happen naturally for several reasons:

- The cause of flow dysfunction is sometimes subtle and can be difficult to see and understand. There are many "servers" that all play a role in furthering ED care. High levels of variation due to the wide scope and nature of the services make it difficult to manage flow since the points of congestion are rarely stationary.
- The measures for improving flow usually require changes in staff process design, work assignments, shift schedules, and degree of engagement. Such changes are never easy within a dynamic and complex system like an ED. A proactive approach addressing processes that promote and hinder flow is crucial.

For Lean flow to occur, patients should be able to proceed swiftly from one value-added step to the next. This means minimizing any non–valued-added bottlenecks that occur between such steps.

Non-Value Activities

When a physician orders an x-ray for a patient, the act of ordering the test is considered value added. The next value-added activity would be performing the x-ray. Before that can occur, however, the patient will likely experience some idle waiting during transport to the radiology unit. The non–value-added activity (the transport) should be identified and challenged for elimination (perhaps through a portable x-ray) or reduced (by a more compact layout).

Idle Waiting

Another cause of delays, idle waiting, can occur for several reasons:

- First, there may be no clear signal to the server that there is a patient waiting for service. This can be remedied by establishing better signals for managing the work.

- Second, service requests are sometimes batched before service is started. For example, this often is the practice in the lab and may be remedied with process changes or fewer batch-intensive technologies.
- The third major cause of idle waiting is when a queue develops in front of a busy server.

QUEUING THEORY

Queuing theory is the study of waiting lines, and its roots date back to the early 20th century.[2] Understanding queuing theory can make a substantial difference when targeting improvement efforts related to flow.

A basic queuing system consists of a "server" who provides a service to "customers." A triage nurse is an example of a server, and an arriving ED patient is an example of a customer. If the triage nurse is busy triaging other patients, the arriving patients would essentially wait in a queue until it is their time for service. Queuing theory helps define the causes of waiting and permits ED leaders to estimate a system's performance under certain conditions.

Two key parameters for estimating the behavior of a queuing system are the rate of arrivals and the rate of service. The rate of arrivals corresponds to the incoming requests for service. For this example, the rate of triage arrivals might be six patients per hour. The rate of service, also measured in requests per hour, reflects the rate at which the server could process requests if they were constantly backed up waiting for service. For the triage example, suppose it takes a triage nurse an average of 12 minutes to perform the triage service (chair to chair). The triage rate (or "service rate") is, therefore, five patients per hour.

It is clear that if the arrival rate continually exceeds the service rate, a queue will develop in front of the server. For the previous triage example, the queue will likely grow by one patient per hour because the arrival rate of six exceeds the service rate of five. One might conclude that a queue will develop only if the average arrival rate exceeds the average service rate, but queues can form even when the arrival rate equals or is less than the service rate.

For the triage example, suppose that the average arrival rate is only four patients per hour, but the service rate remains five cases per hour. If the patients arrive every 15 minutes and triage takes exactly 12 minutes, then there would be no waiting. In this case, the triage nurse would be busy providing triage for 12 out of every 15 minutes, which implies a utilization of 80%. As efficient as this may sound, the situation is totally unrealistic. Patients do not arrive at perfectly fixed intervals, and the time it takes to triage each case often varies considerably.

Consider a more realistic scenario. Assume that the *average* rate of arrivals is still four patients per hour, but the patients arrive in a random pattern. This is referred to as a "Poisson" arrival process. (The French mathematician Siméon-Denis Poisson developed the theory that characterizes independent, random arrivals from a large population.) In such cases, consecutive arrivals may occur close together or very far apart.

Arrival Time Variation

Arrivals to an ED are the result of random, independent events happening to individuals within a large population. **Figure 34.1** shows example arrival timelines with an average rate of four patients per hour, with and without variation. It should be obvious now that

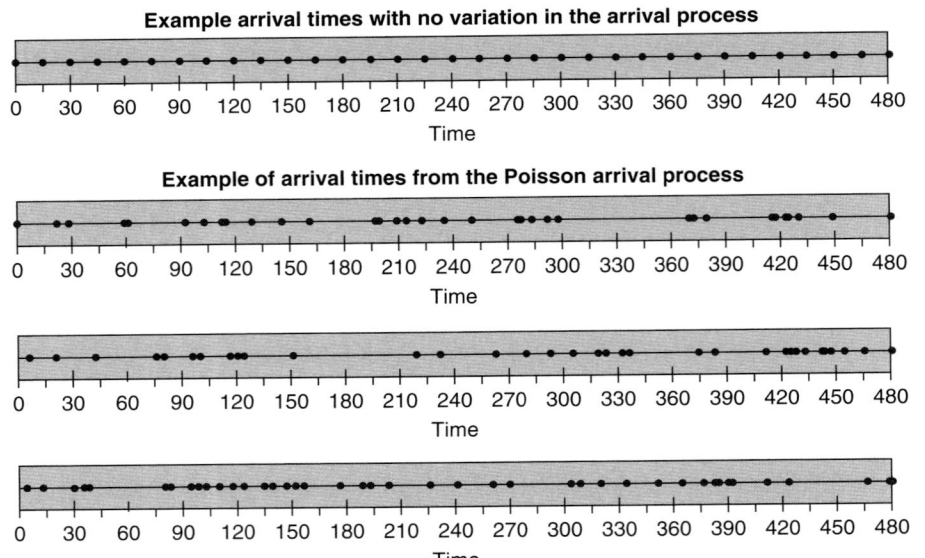

FIGURE 34.1 ■ Arrival Times With and Without Variation

if two patients arrive very close in time, one of them will incur some amount of waiting. The average rate of arrivals may still be four per hour, but the exact timing and number of patients for any given hour are subject to considerable fluctuation.

Service Time Variation

Variation in service time derives from the fact that patients or procedures do not all take the same amount of time. A patient with a psychiatric issue, for example, may take 20 minutes to triage, while a patient requiring a medication refill might take just a few minutes. Rather than assuming exactly 12 minutes (as in the previous example), it is more realistic to assume that the time it takes to provide the triage service is variable and can be characterized using an *exponential* distribution.

An exponential distribution is a good approximation for services that have a wide range of times. **Figure 34.2** illustrates an exponential distribution of service times with an average of 12 minutes. Clearly, if a patient requires a lengthy triage process, subsequent arrivals may have to wait. What is unclear, however, is how this queuing system will perform in the long run. There are various ways to estimate the behavior of a queuing system, but for this discussion, a spreadsheet model called QueueCalc (freely downloadable online) will be used.[3,4]

With the parameters of one server, an arrival rate of four patients per hour, a service rate of five cases per hour, and the assumptions of Poisson arrivals and exponential service times, the resulting average wait prior to triage would be 0.8 hours, or 48 minutes! In addition, the average number of patients waiting for triage would be 3.2. This differs considerably from the situation associated with no variation in arrivals or service times. However, the average utilization remains 80%, as there are still four arrivals per hour, and the triage process takes an average of 12 minutes. As before, there will still be an average of 48 minutes of triage work required per hour.

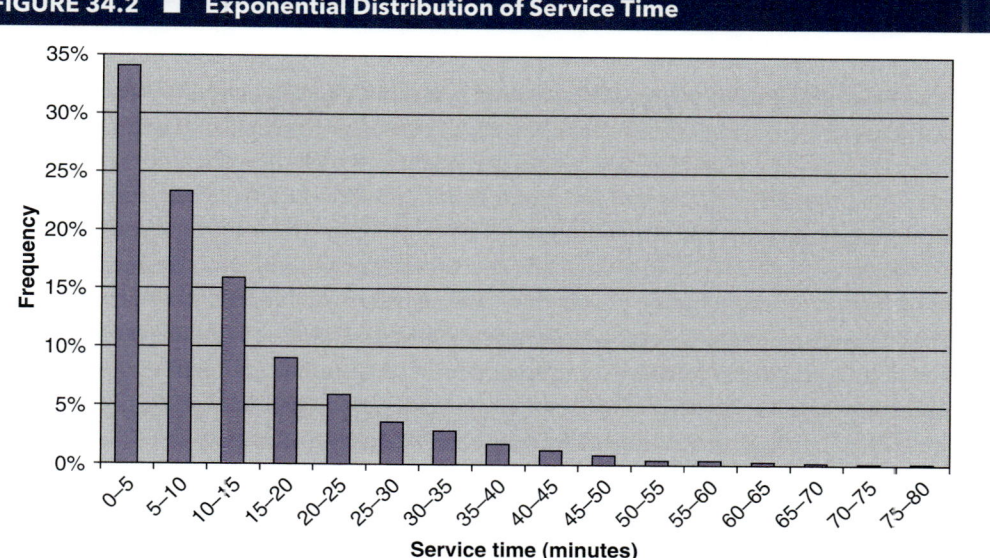

FIGURE 34.2 ■ Exponential Distribution of Service Time

A SIMPLE QUEUING SYSTEM

There are three major elements that contribute to the amount of waiting within a simple queuing system: *variation*, *utilization*, and the *degree of server sharing*.

Variation

The role of variation in queuing systems should be obvious. Waiting increases as the system changes from one with no fluctuations to one with many. As noted earlier, there are two sources of variation in a simple queuing interface: the arrival process and the service process.

Arrival Process

For the arrival process, variation is measured by looking at "interarrival" times, or the elapsed time between consecutive arrivals. When new patients are arriving every 15 minutes, the interarrival times are all exactly 15 minutes. Observing and gathering arrival data for such a system would demonstrate that the interarrival times were distributed with an average of 15 and a standard deviation of 0. However, with Poisson arrivals, the interarrival times would vary considerably and be characterized by an exponential distribution with an average of 15 minutes and a standard deviation of 15 minutes. In general, a good measure of the variation of a process is the coefficient of variation (CoV), which is calculated as the standard deviation divided by the average. In the latter case, the CoV of the arrival process would be equal to 1.0, implying a high degree of variation.

Service Process

The variation for the service process is measured similarly. Without variation, each triage encounter would take exactly 12 minutes. The average would be 12, and the standard deviation would be 0. In the case of highly variable service times, the average triage time is 12 minutes and the standard deviation (by definition of an exponential distribution) is also 12 minutes, thus giving a CoV of 1.0 for the service time distribution.

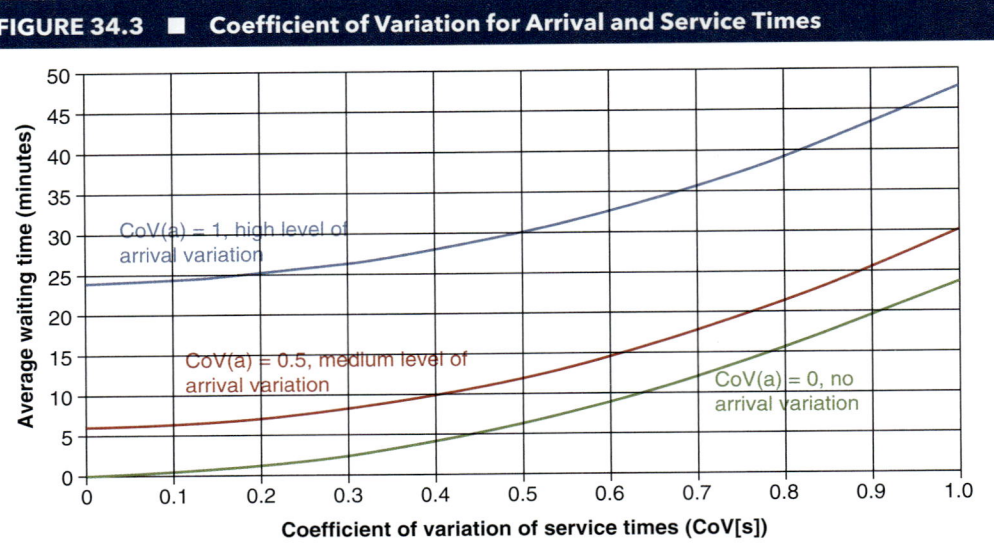

FIGURE 34.3 ■ Coefficient of Variation for Arrival and Service Times

Arrival and service processes are unlikely to have either zero variation or very high levels of variation, as the examples might suggest. Queuing systems have respective variations, as measured by CoV, which are somewhere between 0 and 1.0. **Figure 34.3** shows average waiting times for a queuing system with one server, an arrival rate of four patients per hour, and a service rate of five cases per hour, under three levels of arrival process variation, CoV(a), and a range of service process variation, CoV(s). As an example, note that if the CoV(a) arrival time variation is 0.5 and the CoV(s) service time variation is 0.5, the average wait time for arriving patients will be 12 minutes.

Utilization

Utilization can be estimated using the following three values:

- The average rate of arriving patients
- The average service time in minutes
- Available minutes of server capacity

The average rate of arriving patient times multiplied by the average service time represents the amount of arriving work per period of time. The available server capacity is simply the number of servers multiplied by 60 minutes. Utilization, as a fraction of 1.0, is simply the amount of arriving work divided by the available minutes of server capacity. In the earlier triage example (four patients per hour, each needing 12 minutes of triage server time), the amount of arriving work is 48 minutes per hour. With only one triage nurse, the available server capacity is 60 minutes. Taken together, the estimate of the utilization is 0.80, or 80% by dividing 48 by 60. Note that if there were two triage nurses on duty, the available server capacity would be 120 minutes each hour. If the amount of arriving work remained at 48 minutes, the utilization of the servers would be 0.40, or 40%, calculated as 48 minutes divided by 120.

Figure 34.4 shows the average waiting time as a function of utilization for one server with a service rate of five patients per hour. As the arrival rate ranges from 0 to 4.8, the utilization will range from 0 to 0.96 (96%). A key observation is that waiting tends to increase *dramatically* as the utilization starts to approach 100%, especially in environments with high variation.

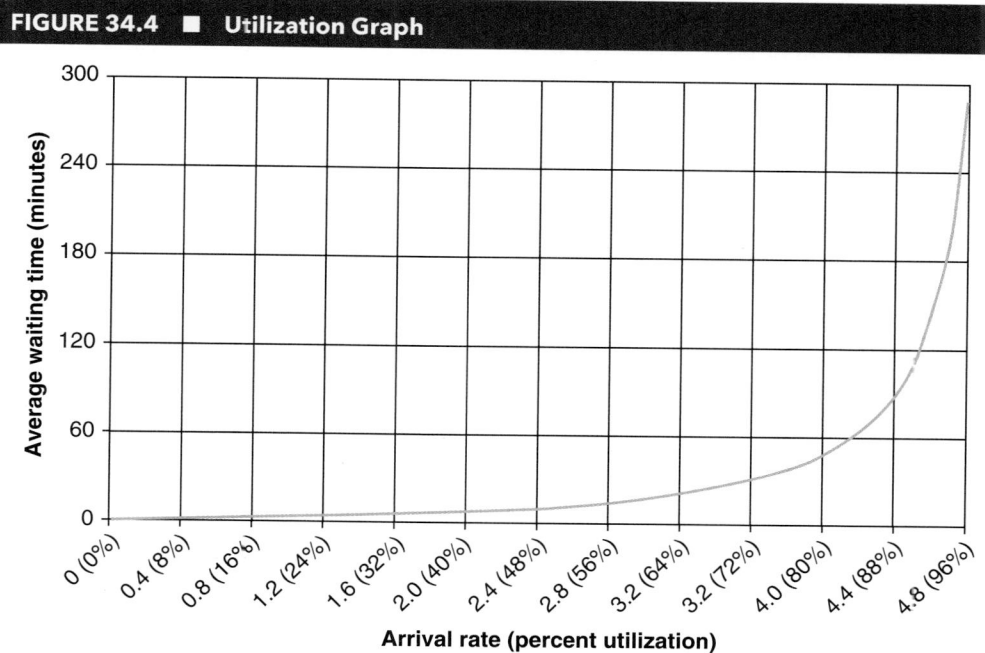

FIGURE 34.4 ■ Utilization Graph

The Degree of Server Sharing

The examples in this chapter have described queuing systems with one server; in reality, many queuing systems rely on a "pool" of servers so that any one of them can be used to provide the requested service. Suppose that during a busy part of the day, the arrival rate is eight patients per hour. If the service rate per triage nurse is still only five cases per hour, at least two triage nurses will be required to stay on top of the demand. With two nurses available to triage during those hours, the utilization of the nurses will be 80% since there are now 96 minutes of arriving work and 120 minutes of available capacity.

If both triage nurses are busy, patients will wait in a single queue. Assuming the same high levels of arrival, CoV(a) = 1, and service variation, CoV(s) = 1, as before, QueueCalc could be used to show that with two servers, an arrival rate of eight cases, and a service rate of five patients per server, the average wait will be approximately 22 minutes. This compares favorably to the 48-minute wait time described earlier with many of the same assumptions regarding variation and server utilization.

Table 34.1 shows the average waiting times associated with various combinations of server utilization and number of servers under the assumption of high levels of arrival

TABLE 34.1 ■ Average Waiting Time vs Number of Servers and Utilization*

Number of servers		Utilization of Servers									
		50%	55%	60%	65%	70%	75%	80%	85%	90%	95%
1	Average waiting time in minutes	12	15	18	22	28	36	48	68	108	228
2		4	6	7	9	12	16	22	32	52	111
3		2	3	4	5	7	9	13	20	33	73
4		1	2	2	3	5	6	9	14	24	54

*Each server has a service rate of five patients per hour, and the arrival rate is set to produce the given utilization. Arrival process and service distribution are assumed Poisson and exponential, respectively.

and service variation. This concept of making more than one server available to handle a combined stream of tasks is referred to as the *pooling* of servers. Pooling can be used to reduce average wait times or accommodate greater patient volumes through higher server utilization.

STRATEGIES FOR IMPROVING FLOW

Remember that it is crucial to provide clear and unambiguous signals (visual cues) to servers regarding requests for service (waiting patients). If there is no immediate and ongoing signal to a server, patients may wait unnecessarily and clinician productivity will be lost. Lean methods for visual management can be applied directly in health care with great results.[5]

Reduce Variation

It is clear that variation in either the arrival or service process of a queuing interface is a major cause of waiting. For walk-in service operations, there is not much that can be done to decrease variation at the front door unless the arrivals are scheduled. Although this may sound far-fetched and counter to the classic view of emergency care, there are now online services that enable patients to schedule ED appointments ahead of time.

Carefully studying routine activities and identifying sources of unreliability can reduce variation in service times. For example, the time it takes a caregiver to acquire supplies should vary only minimally. This can be accomplished by ensuring that reliable quantities of supplies are in a known location and that the procedures for acquiring them are properly communicated to the staff. Lean tools, including process mapping, workplace organization, and standard work, can be used to identify and deploy best practices. The methodology and tools of Six Sigma, with its focus on reducing variation, can be used to measure and reduce nonstandard occurrences within a process.

Reducing variation in one queue can mitigate time disparities in the next queue. From the example earlier, suppose that after triage, the next patient activity is an evaluation by a physician. If the triage service time varies tremendously, the pattern of triaged patients arriving for the physician evaluation will vary in the same way. If, on the other hand, the triage service takes a reliable, almost constant amount of time, then clinical examinations will occur at more consistent intervals. Hence, if the service time variation is reduced, it will have the effect of shortening the queues in front of that server and the servers that follow.

Reduce Server Utilization

In a high-variation environment like an ED, waiting will increase as server utilization rises. As noted earlier, the rate of increase (waiting) is especially high if servers are already busy with other cases. However, waiting times can decrease dramatically with only modest reductions in utilization. Understanding the capacity of key servers can help leaders target efforts effectively.

Reducing Rate of Arrivals

The rate of arrivals to a server can be reduced either by determining that some arrivals should not have occurred in the first place or by diverting some patients to other servers. For example, some ED cases do not necessitate a full triage in the classic sense. Low-acuity, ambulatory patients may require nothing more than a quick screening. This practice effectively reduces the number of patients seen by the triage nurse.

Suppose a lower-acuity patient is seen initially by a provider. A blood sample is drawn, and rather than sending that patient to a bed, the the clinician directs the patient to a "results waiting area," essentially a room with a number of comfortable chairs. With this practice, diverting the arrivals to the chairs (servers) reduces the rate of arrivals to beds (servers).

Reducing Service Times

Carefully studying the process and eliminating as much waste as possible can reduce service times. The most common types of waste in ED operations are "movement" and "overprocessing." Waste in the form of movement occurs whenever a caregiver is moving from one location to another within an ED, whether to attain supplies, equipment, information, other staff, or simply to see the next patient. Overprocessing occurs when more activities are performed than needed to provide safe, quality care for the patient. Too many handoffs, redundant information gathering, and excessive testing are all examples of overprocessing. Classic Lean tools, including value-stream mapping, process-sequence mapping, spaghetti diagrams, and standard work can be used to identify waste and reduce or eliminate it.[5-7]

Adding Servers

Adding servers will reduce server utilization, but this step should be taken only after other approaches have been applied. In the earlier example with one triage nurse, arrival rate of four, service rate of five, and high levels of arrival and service variation CoV(a) and CoV(s) = 1, the average wait time was estimated to be 48 minutes. If a second triage nurse is added, the server utilization is reduced to 40%, and the average waiting time drops to less than 3 minutes. While the addition of a second triage nurse dramatically improves patient waiting times, the cost to perform triage would effectively double.

Checking the Alignment

Before simply adding servers, it is important to carefully evaluate the alignment of capacity with demand over time. Capacity misalignment is evident when a queuing interface routinely performs well at a particular time of day and relatively poorly at other times.

Note that although the ED arrival process is random (as noted by Poisson), the average rate of arrivals by hour of day is fairly predictable. This means that if the average number of arrivals between 3:00 and 4:00 pm has averaged four patients this year, there's a pretty good chance that it will average four patients next year, too (unless there are overall changes to the market or a volume change brought on by epidemiological reasons, such as a pandemic). However, any changes are likely reflected across all hours of the day as a proportional increase or decrease.

To illustrate the concept of capacity alignment, assume that the average rates of arrival by hour of day are as displayed in **Figure 34.5**. This ED is staffed with two triage nurses with a service rate of four patients per hour. When viewed in this way, the utilization of the triage nurses will rise very close to or exceed 100% during busy periods, but productivity will drop as low as 25% during the overnight period.

A computer simulation can demonstrate how such a system performs with high levels of variation.[5] Given a sufficient time for accurate measurement, the resulting average wait for all patients before triage is 45 minutes. The average wait for patients arriving from 7:00 to 9:00 pm is greater than 70 minutes, whereas the average wait for patients arriving between 5:00 and 7:00 am is less than 5 minutes. In this case, the somewhat predictable periods of good (minimal waiting) and bad (considerable waiting) queuing performance are indicative of capacity misalignment.

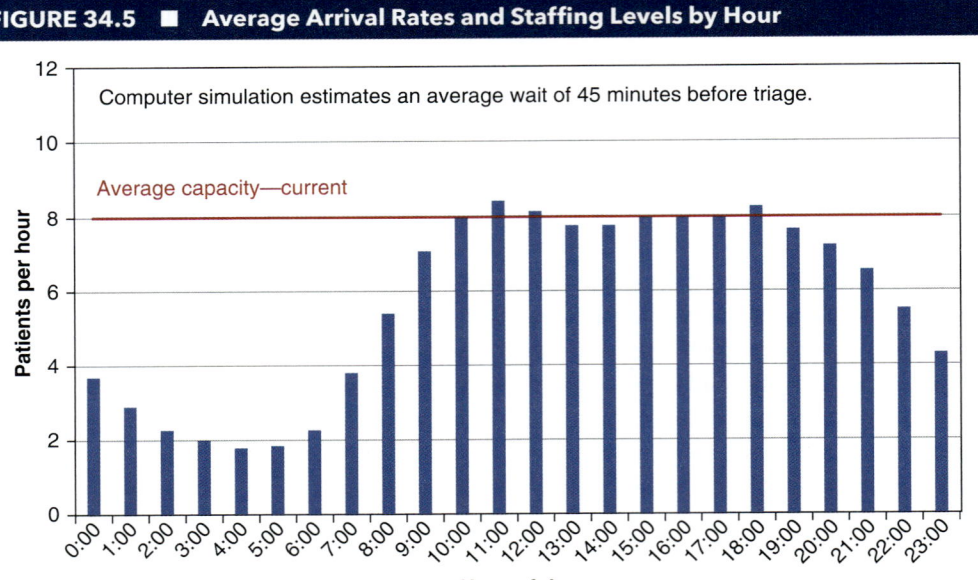

FIGURE 34.5 ■ Average Arrival Rates and Staffing Levels by Hour

If the triage staffing pattern is changed by dropping down to one nurse on the overnight shift and staffing up to three nurses during the peak time (**Figure 34.6**), there is a more even pattern of utilization across the 24-hour period. Running the computer simulation with this staffing plan results in an average waiting time before triage of 16 minutes. The message here is that the alignment of capacity (staffing) should always be checked before adding additional caregivers. In this example, a 64% reduction in the average waiting time was achieved without adding server hours.

It is beneficial to analyze the alignment of all key servers, including physicians, midlevel providers, nurses, technicians, and even hospitalists and support personnel. Within the analysis, it is important to include elements like callouts, lunch breaks, and differences in service rates among individuals.

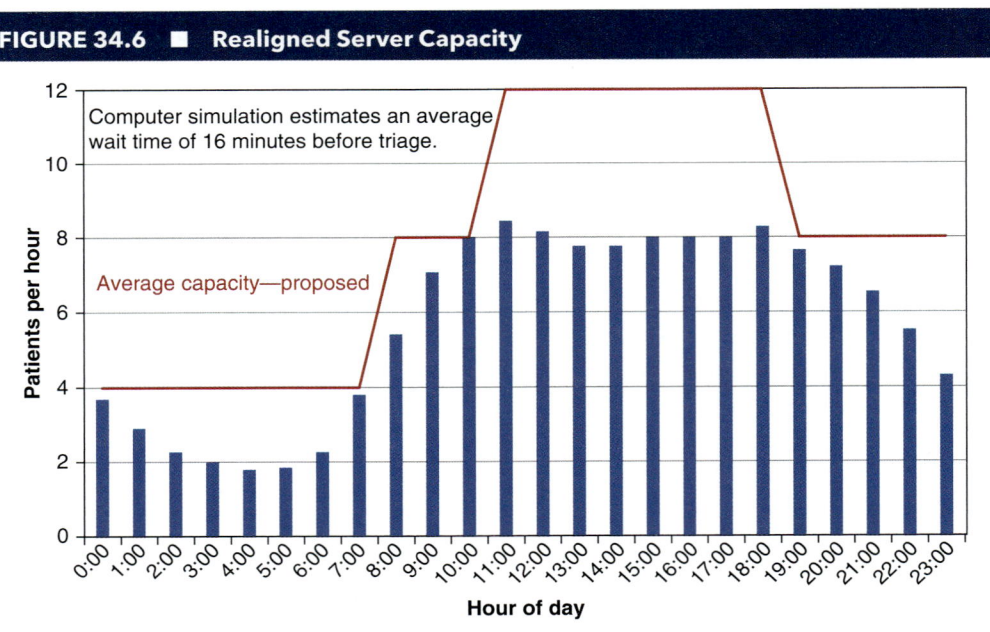

FIGURE 34.6 ■ Realigned Server Capacity

For example, if an ED schedules 10 nurses during peak periods, but two typically call out sick, the effective capacity is really only eight nurses. And if the nurses take their 30-minute lunch breaks in pairs over a two-hour period, the effective capacity is six nurses during those lunch hours. Taken together, the ED loses about 40% of its nursing capacity during lunch breaks. The system will very likely build up a queue for nursing services that will linger for many hours. It is also important to consider productivity differences among staff members. Suppose most emergency physicians can treat two patients per hour, but one physician can only treat patients at the rate of 1.2 patients per hour. If the slow physician is working a shift (even if with another doctor or two), it may negatively affect the overall physician capacity to the point that a predictable queue will develop.

Promote Pooling

Opportunities for pooling arise when a server remains idle despite that fact that a patient is waiting for a service that the idle server could provide. For example, suppose it is the job of the ED technicians to draw blood for tests. Because of typical variation in arrivals and service times, there will be occasions when patients are waiting for their blood to be drawn because the technicians are backed up. During these situations, some of the nurses may be idle because their patients are waiting for diagnostics. Pooling could be implemented by having an idle nurse draw blood whenever the technicians are backed up. This sounds easy, but there are many challenges:

- First, it requires instilling a culture that certain activities are "everyone's work." This conflicts with a natural desire to have well-defined jobs, or in some cases, a union-imposed set of work rules.
- Second, clinicians often value their independence and may assume pooling will only reward the underperformers and result in more work for the others.
- Third, specialization usually promotes greater quality and productivity, elements that may decline within a "generalist" approach.

In the face of such challenges, however, there are ways to make pooling work systematically. The use of clear signals to indicate the presence of an awaiting task has tremendous advantages. For example, a rack might be placed at the nurses' station labeled "Patients Waiting for Lab Draws," and whenever there is an order in the rack, any properly trained team member is eligible to draw the blood. To make this process as simple as possible, the necessary supplies must be close at hand in order to minimize the time and hassle for the assistant. In this example, the work rules could establish that a nurse should not be standing idle if there are blood draws in the queue. Visual controls are a classic Lean method for directing the way work is performed. When used to promote pooling, the result is a strong move toward the Lean principles of greater efficiency, reduced waste, and decreased waiting.

NETWORK OF QUEUES

Any individual who provides a service in the ED, whether the activity is value-added or not, is a server. At any time, the physician may have a queue consisting of a mix of new cases, patients waiting for a procedure (e.g., laceration repair), and those awaiting test results. Unlike the triage nurse, the physician will have multiple requests for service emanating from each patient. These revolving responsibilities make it difficult to perform a time study because physicians may be constantly switching their focus. A nurse in the main treatment area may also have multiple requests for service from patients as they progress through their course of care. An ED technician may have a wider variety of service requests, some directly related to patient care, like drawing blood or transport, and others indirectly related, such as restocking supply carts or turning over rooms.

In addition to the human workers in the ED, equipment can also be viewed through the lens of service; for example, beds, scanners, monitors, and stretchers all provide a service to the patient. Ancillary services, transport, housekeeping, consulting physicians, inpatient floors, and other types of support can also be considered servers in this broadened view of patient care.

It is also helpful to keep in mind that every interval of patient waiting implies the existence of a queue and, therefore, a server. For example, a patient with an order for a CT scan with contrast may incur intervals of waiting related to transport, scanning, and image reading. These intervals imply the following human servers: nurse, transporter, CT technician with scanner, and radiologist.

It is important to recognize that virtually any server can hinder the progress of the patient. Think about a typical day in the ED. Are there predictable periods in which physicians are waiting for nursing activities to be completed, and other parts of the day when it is the other way around? If so, patient flow will always be limited by the greatest relative bottleneck (e.g., the nurse or the physician, depending on the time of day). The practice of continually identifying and addressing bottlenecks has its roots in the theory of constraints.[8] The integrated nature of care activities also brings to light the importance of enlightened collaboration among ED personnel and staff in other areas of the hospital.

When looking at one's own ED through a "queuing lens," there are key considerations that must be addressed. Chief among them are concerns about server utilization and the levels of variation in patient arrivals and service times. For a particular server, it is necessary to understand the requests for service over the course of a shift by asking these questions:

- What are the various categories of requests?
- Do the requests arrive in a steady fashion, or are there bunches or gaps in the arrival pattern?
- How long does it take to perform a particular task (from start of a task until the start of the next waiting task), and how much do the task times vary?

Answers to these questions, along with objective supporting data on arrival rates and service times, will help determine the nature of the queuing interface and identify opportunities for improvement.

As patient care is mapped through a network of queues, ED leaders must be mindful of the number of backlogs that can hold up patient progress. Beyond simply eliminating unnecessary steps and activities, simulation shows that reducing the number of queues can promote overall flow. For example, rather than having a sequence of queues consisting of triage, registration, and bed placement, bedside registration could occur while patients await ancillary results. Another flow-enhancement approach is to reduce the number of handoffs. A process with fewer steps will flow better, even if service times remain unchanged. Decreasing queues reduces the number of spaces required to "park" patients while they are in process and decreases the likelihood of one server idly waiting on another.

Segmentation, another solution to a network of queues, occurs when a patient stream is divided and directed to different care areas. A classic example of segmentation is to split off "fast-track" patients from the main ED. Depending on acuity, patients are directed to the appropriate care area. In general, segmentation is a form of antipooling. Poorly planned and rigid segmentation can create situations in which one care area is extremely backed up and the other is virtually empty. To overcome this antipooling effect, segmentation should be accompanied by an intense focus on streamlining the respective care areas and their associated processes. In this "fast-track" example, it is important to study the individual arrival rates of lower-acuity patients and adjust the open and close times of the low-acuity area accordingly. If higher productivities are achieved and variation is reduced, the flow through the segmented system will be better than through an unsegmented system.[5,9]

CONCLUSION

The mathematics of queuing are like the laws of gravity. When certain conditions exist, such as high variation coupled with high utilization, queues will most certainly develop. The challenge is to apply the right tools in the right manner to counteract the "laws of queuing." Elements of queue improvement are embedded throughout the remainder of this book. A solid foundation of queuing theory and Lean flow methodologies is necessary to implement best practices.

Mastering the technical elements of queuing is only part of the solution. Efficient flow can only be achieved if the workers themselves have an appreciation for the value of Lean flow and an understanding of their role in making it happen. By design, Lean methods focus on the value-creation process with the customer at the center. Lean management focuses on making flow happen through visibility, accountability, and relentless attention to process detail.

REFERENCES

1. Holden RJ. Lean thinking in emergency departments: a critical review. *Ann Emerg Med.* 2011;57(3):265.
2. Erlang AK. The theory of probabilities and telephone conversations. *Nyt Tidsskrift for Matematik B.* 1909;20:33-39.
3. Gross D, Shortle J, Thompson J, Harris C. *Fundamentals of Queuing Theory.* 4th ed, Hoboken, NJ: John Wiley & Sons; 2008.
4. Sakasegawa H. An approximation formula $Lq = a.p^3/(1-p)$. *Ann Inst Stat Math* 1977;29(1):67.
5. Crane JT, Noon CE. *The Definitive Guide to Emergency Department Operational Improvement.* New York, NY: Productivity Press; 2011.
6. Zidel T. *A Lean Guide to Transforming Healthcare.* Madison, WI: ASQ Quality Press; 2006.
7. Graban M. *Lean Hospitals.* New York, NY: CRC Press; 2009.
8. Goldratt EM, Cox J. *The Goal.* Great Barrington, Mass: North River Press; 1984.
9. King DL, Ben-Tovim DI, Bassham JE. Redesigning emergency department patient flows: an application of lean thinking to health care. *Emerg Med Australasia.* 2006;18:391.

CHAPTER 35

IMPROVING THE FRONT-END PROCESS TO ADD VALUE

Jody Crane, Sally Sulfaro

The concept of medical triage originated in the Napoleonic Wars through the work of Dominique Jean Larrey. His work was later systematized by the French in World War I when the goals of triage were to identify those who were likely to live or die, regardless of the care they received, and those whose outcome might improve with immediate care.[1]

EMERGENCY TRIAGE

Triage has evolved to address care in the emergency department (ED), in which medical resources are more plentiful than they were on World War I battlefields. The modern form of triage, which has become a basic element of every ED in the country, raises these questions:

- Have EDs acquiesced to the concept that they will never meet the demand of arriving patients?
- Has triage evolved over time as a way to control the demand of patients and the workload of providers, ignoring the inherent operational inefficiencies?

As triage in the ED has evolved, it has been delegated to nurses who have largely developed, performed, and taught the practice of triage. The fundamental flaw is that a single person (nurse or physician) can certainly assign an acuity level but cannot consistently predict what tests another evaluation practitioner will order. In a high-volume ED, the triage nurse may try to anticipate the resources needed, even though they do not know which of the physicians working will eventually see the patient. Thus, triage itself is flawed because of the inherent lack of inter-rater reliability (the degree of agreement among different raters), which has not been eliminated from current processes.

The Triage Debate

The process of triaging patients in the ED evokes a broad range of opinions. Many consider triage a complete waste of time, asserting that it can be viewed as nothing but a way to determine who can wait the longest to be seen. Others believe that triage is a vital aspect of the traditional ED encounter, which ensures that the sickest patients with the greatest need have quick access to the correct resources. This is especially important when the ED has predictably long wait times.

Proponents of traditional triage assert that it provides one central place to collect all of the critical data required by (a) physicians and nurses so they can have an efficient patient encounter and (b) regulatory agencies to ensure the visit is in compliance with quality standards.

Opponents of traditional triage, on the other hand, argue that it does not add value from the patient's perspective—that every step that precedes seeing a provider only delays care. Skeptics might add that all of the data collected in triage can be collected at other points during the patient encounter. According to this argument, the only real advantage of triage is that is enables the ED to[2]:

- Recognize patients requiring immediate intervention
- Prevent delays in care that result in poor outcomes
- Stream all patients through efficient pathways to meet their needs
- Expedite the movement of patients from the door to the physician or midlevel provider

Increasing ED Complexity

As the number of EDs has shrunk, average ED patient volume has increased to meet the escalating patient demand. With growing volumes, inadequate resources, and overcrowding caused by admission delays, multiple bottlenecks have developed.[3] These bottlenecks in patient flow are the most frequently cited causes of "sentinel events" (i.e., events that can cause an unexpected outcome or death and trigger an investigation), and they have driven the need for rapid yet reliable classification of acuities and efficient movement of patients through ED systems.[4]

As a result of the growth in ED volumes, the aging (higher-acuity) population, and the associated patient care inefficiencies, there has been a dramatic rise in alternative care facilities (e.g., urgent care centers and clinics), which typically manage lower-acuity patients. As volume and acuity increase, most EDs have become less efficient. To address these shortcomings, many EDs have developed refined treatment pathways for certain subgroups of patients using a process known as "segmentation." Segmentation creates customized pathways for certain types of patients and employs an experienced clinician at the front door to "stream" or direct the patient through a particular pathway that entails the fewest inputs necessary for that category of patient.

The Emergency Medical Treatment and Active Labor Act (EMTALA) enacted in 1986 has helped prevent the treatment delays that formerly happened when financial screening was part of the registration process. The recent push to get patients in front of physicians in a more timely manner has transformed financial screening and associated paperwork from a traditionally front-end, obtrusive process into a largely back-end process, much to the satisfaction of patients.

Accurate Patient Classification

Triage should be designed to expedite treatment by ensuring the rapid evaluation of all patients who arrive at the lobby (formerly known as the "waiting room"), the most dangerous place in the department.[5] Performing triage effectively requires redesigning processes and reinventing roles, for example:

- Creating virtual spaces (computer representations of ED spaces and flow) to proactively prevent the development of multiple queues in the department
- Relocating or reassigning medical, nursing, and registration staff as needed to keep the department flow operational when there is a demand–capacity mismatch

It should be emphasized that when an appropriate treatment space and a provider are available, *the best front-door triage is none at all*. Often referred to as "pull to full," "direct bedding," "quick pass," or "hot bedding," the best way to minimize the time between arrival and treatment is the direct placement of patients in an open treatment space followed by a timely clinical evaluation.

When there will be a delay in provider evaluation, a more involved nursing evaluation may be necessary. More traditional nursing triage evaluations are required more frequently at some EDs than at others, depending on demand and capacity. However, additional capacity can be created using a number of process efficiencies *that begin at the front door,* such as:

- Aligning of demand and capacity
- Using parallel flow instead of sequential flow
- Having a cluster of providers
- Keeping vertical patients vertical and moving instead of "parking" them in beds while test results are pending
- Eliminating "wasted" steps and entire processes that do not facilitate flow or add value from the patient's perspective

Front-door processes can no longer be considered isolated segments of patient throughput, and the former gatekeeper (the triage nurse) has necessarily become the flow facilitator.

CLASSIFICATION SYSTEMS

There are several ED triage classification systems, the most common of which are three-level triage and Emergency Severity Index (ESI) five-level triage.

Three-Level Triage

The popular three-level (emergent/urgent/nonurgent) model bases acuity decisions on lists of chief complaints and presenting conditions for each category. In practice, triage nurses have subjectively applied this model with unideal inter-rater reliability.

ESI Five-Level Triage

Evidence-based, five-level triage models yield a more reliable and objective classification of acuities than older models.[6] ESI is a resource-based triage model in which the sickest patients (ESI levels 1 and 2) are identified based on presenting chief complaint and danger-zone vital signs. ESI 3, 4, and 5 patients are deemed to not require immediate life-saving intervention and are further delineated based on anticipated resource utilization (**Figure 35.1**).

The ESI triage system has the additional appeal of allowing triage nurses to apply critical reasoning rather than simply adhere to lists of conditions. By incorporating the term *consider*, the system provides latitude in application of the algorithm. It permits the triage person to move patients to a higher-acuity level using guidelines for entities such as pediatric fever and danger-zone vital signs. Specifically, ESI permits acuity decisions based on the full clinical picture, rather than on subjective pain scores and decisions to place a certain patient in the last available bed.

While it might seem that segregating acuities into five rather than three levels should foster a system that is more sensitive to acuity differences, the reality is that, unless level 3

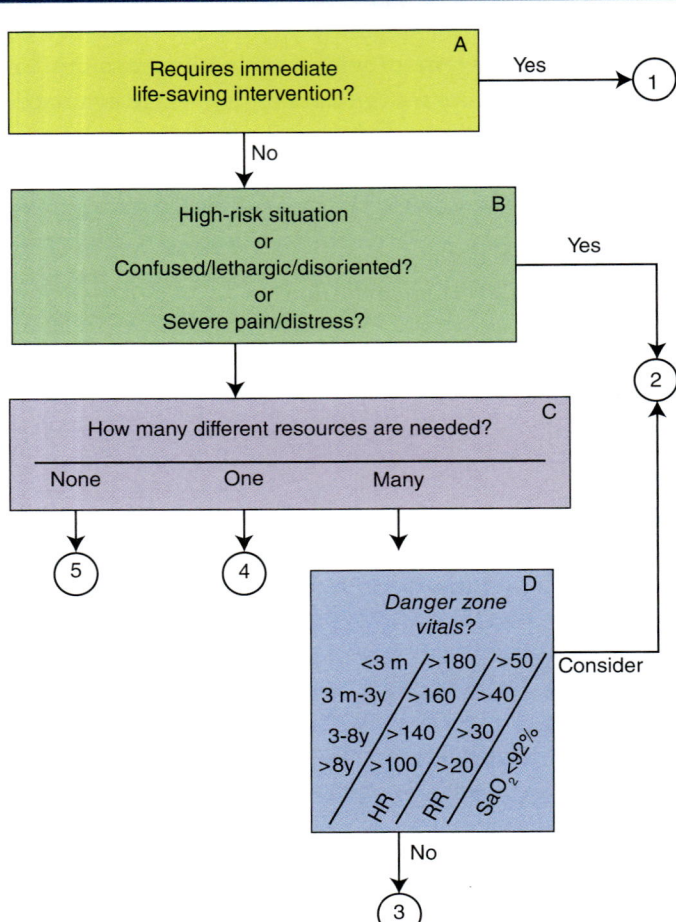

FIGURE 35.1 ■ Emergency Severity Index Five-Level Triage Algorithm

patients are further subdivided, the net result is a three-level triage system that yields the acuity distributions as shown in **Figure 35.2**.

In **Figure 35.2**, note the quantified separation of acuities into three major groups: ESI levels 1 and 2 (group 1), ESI level 3 (group 2), and ESI levels 4 and 5 (group 3). EDs with fast tracks that serve ESI level 4 and 5 patients commonly observe that ESI level 3 patients have to wait longer to receive a physician evaluation, and these patients are most apt to be placed into the lobby when the ED is saturated. Widespread experience with this distribution method has led to the development of split-flow models that provide safer and faster evaluation and care for the largest population of ESI acuities (or "the tweeners").[7] These patients not only have greater urgency and potential for reassignment to higher-acuity triage levels, they also require more involved medical decision-making.

An additional issue with the ESI system is the significant heterogeneity of ESI 3 patients, whose needs range widely (**Box 35.1**). While "horizontal 3s" require a bed or treatment space for at least their initial evaluation and treatment, "vertical 3s" can often be seen in nonhorizontal treatment spaces, particularly in effective split-flow models. Despite considerable experience with the ESI system and a wealth of literature describing its use, there has never been a study to assess whether ESI-triaged patients actually require the number of resources projected, nor has there been a study addressing inter-rater reliability.

Even though the five-level ESI system is often more reliable than the three-level system, there are still considerable variations in how the tool is applied. Some of these discrepancies

FIGURE 35.2 ■ ESI vs Traditional Three-Level Triage

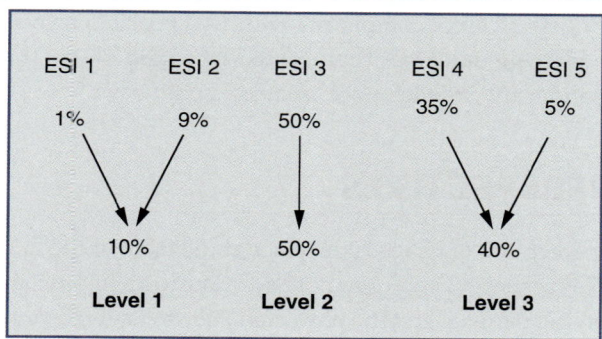

are related to a lack of user education, and others are due to the system's flexibility (previously mentioned). Situational variation occurs when the ED is congested and triage nurses downgrade patients (e.g., from ESI level 3 to ESI level 4) to ensure that they are seen faster. Similarly, when the fast track is overwhelmed, patients may be up-triaged from level 4 to level 3, modifying the system "on-the-fly." While this kind of clinical judgment is in the best interests of the patient, it can skew the application of ESI and the resulting average acuity scores.

Other Triage Systems

Several other triage systems are used worldwide, the most prominent of which are the Canadian Emergency Department Triage and Acuity Scale (CTAS)[8] and Manchester Triage System (MTS).[9] Significantly, each uses a five-level scale. The MTS allows clinicians to assess the urgency of each case and prioritize care accordingly. Both the CTAS and the MTS are chief-complaint based with two levels of modifiers: general complaint (e.g., pain, level of consciousness), and chief complaint, which is specific (e.g., headache, suicidal ideation, elbow injury). Both tools expressly indicate that the scales are used to determine the appropriate time to treatment. The MTS is not designed to judge whether a patient is appropriate for an

BOX 35.1 ■ ESI LEVEL 3 VARIATIONS

Vertical ESI 3s

- Sitting, standing
- Nonsevere pain
- Extremity lacerations
- <1 liter of fluids, oral
- Headache (not worst in life)
- No active vomiting/diarrhea
- Back pain, no fever
- Vaginal spotting
- Minor epistaxis
- Nondisplaced musculoskeletal injury

Horizontal ESI 3s

- Needs to lie down
- More severe pain
- Complex lacerations
- >1 liter of IV fluids
- Severe headache
- Active vomiting or diarrhea
- Altered mental status
- Needs monitoring
- GI bleeding
- Propriety

ED evaluation; instead, it helps "ensure that those who need care receive it appropriately [and] quickly . . . also to monitor care and to drive care pathways. A complementing feature of the MTS is that it lists 50 chief complaints with five possible levels within each. Thus, there is a finite set of triage outcomes represented by a grid of 250 that enhances patient streaming, segmentation, and standardized treatment pathways."[9]

PROVIDER PERSPECTIVES

The current public perception of triage is the place at the front of the ED where people must qualify to enter. In this respect, triage does not add value to an ED encounter and is merely a barrier between arriving patients and the physician. However, if triage expedites movement from the front door to a doctor, it carries value. Value, in terms of the Lean methodology, is anything a customer would be willing to pay for; in health care specifically, value is anything that moves the patient closer to wellness. More simply stated:

- Lean *management* focuses on adding value and eliminating waste as the patient moves through the service transitions and queues of the ED.
- Lean *triage* focuses on getting the patient to the physician more quickly and eliminating delays.

Provider perspectives on triage range from, "Just skip it and bring the patient back," to "I need the vital signs, medical history, allergies, and current medications charted." Providers who share the first perspective tend to be the ones who readily float to the front of the department to evaluate cases during "bed-locked" episodes. Those who prefer a more detailed triage approach cite provider efficiency and patient safety when explaining why patients should undergo a comprehensive triage process prior to receiving a clinical examination. Some have become so accustomed to the amount of information provided by comprehensive triage that they consider it necessary; they want as much information as possible before seeing the patient.

Some triage staff have difficulty letting go of the habit of asking the battery of questions needed to fill in all the blanks on the electronic medical record (EMR). Wary of overlooking critical information, many are initially resistant to moving patients from arrival to the physician more quickly. This concern is reinforced by clinicians who prefer for the complete assessment to already be done by the time they enter a patient's room. Upon initiation of direct bedding, an already overwhelmed ED nurse may express concern about taking on the added responsibility of triage.

For doctors and nurses, the value of maintaining traditional front-door triage is control of the work pace demanded by increasing volumes. However, it has only been within the past few years that innovative Lean methodologies have offered alternatives to moving patients through overcrowded and bed-locked EDs.

THE FLEXIBLE FRONT END

EDs must be prepared to shift front-end processes based on the needs of the department. These needs are usually dictated by bed and provider availability. When appropriate treatment space is available and there is a provider who can see the patient quickly, direct bedding of the patient should be done without intervening triage. This more rapid process often requires a nurse to ask just enough questions to determine what type of treatment space and level of care are indicated, commonly referred to as a "quick look" assessment.

When treatment space is unavailable or there will be a delay to see a provider, an established process of triage may be done at the front of the ED. It is during these times that patients might have to be placed into the lobby post-triage. During these periods, the department should have written standards for periodic reassessment of lobby patients. Additionally, a predetermined staff member (pulled from the treatment area) can use physician-approved, registered nurse–initiated protocols to expedite care so that patients are more likely receive their test results by the time they are placed into a bed. This system must be considered with great care, since these protocols often require additional support staff.

PATIENT IDENTIFICATION AND SEGMENTATION

Triage is not a place for the inexperienced or the indecisive.

—Thom Mayer and Kirk Jensen, *Hardwiring Flow: Systems and Processes for Seamless Patient Care*[10]

Triage Pitfalls

A pitfall of nurse triage education is cognitive shortcuts (heuristics). Examples include "representative restraint," "premature anchoring," and age and gender bias.

Representative restraint is the concept that if it does not fit the pattern, it cannot be "X." This problem occurs when a practitioner only recognizes prototypical presentations while dismissing the atypical. Triage examples include ruling out an atypical acute coronary syndrome presentation when a patient is younger than usual or complains of left elbow pain, and dismissing potential appendicitis in an afebrile patient.

Premature anchoring is another cognitive shortcut that can be problematic during triage. This pitfall occurs when a person fixates on certain features, such as constipation in an elderly person complaining of abdominal pain, without further consideration of other possible causes.[11]

Age and gender biases create the potential for discounting presentations and assuming lower acuity. These biases, such as the perception that women are less likely to present with acute coronary syndromes, are examined in multiple published works and are another example of triage-related heuristics.

Misclassifications occur with any triage system. Experts fully expect that judgment, informed by evidence-based practice, can be used to make triage acuity decisions without the benefit of in-depth evaluation or diagnostic studies. Therefore, the accuracy of a triage decision should be measured against the type and extent of subjective and objective findings (minimum data set) that another experienced triage nurse would elicit and factor into a decision.

Newer "split-flow" models quickly assign ESI 3 patients to higher- or lower-acuity triage areas based on expected resource utilization. This assignment may be followed by transfer of care between locations or department tracks, if needed. In these split-flow models, low-resource 3s may receive care in the lower-acuity portions of the ED (i.e., fast-track or super-track), while high-resource 3s may be streamed to the higher-acuity portion of the ED.

Patient Identification

The primary purpose of triage is to identify patients in need of life-, limb-, or organ-saving intervention. Most newer front-end systems place a highly skilled, experienced nurse at the first point of contact, which is where the most risk resides. This "quick-look" or "pivot" nurse is charged with performing a rapid assessment based on a patient's appearance, chief complaint, and possibly vital signs.

Patient Segmentation

The secondary goal of triage, after identifying emergent cases, is to stream patients to the appropriate location that will be most efficient for their needs (**Figure 35.3**). Advanced ED operational configurations segment cases into streams of patients who are likely to need the same types of testing and treatment. The need for different segmentation schemes is largely driven by volume and acuity, although other factors, such as trauma and teaching designations, have a role in determining the number and type of treatment pathways.

Vital signs are helpful but seldom necessary for streaming, except when the segmentation scheme is based on ESI levels. If the patient does not look ill after the quick-look assessment, the next question becomes: *"What is the best place for this patient to receive high-quality, efficient care?"*

These advanced triage systems are designed with specific areas designated for:

- Patients who need basic care and are likely to go home (low-acuity, vertical patients)
- Patients who need more significant diagnostics and interventions (mid-acuity, vertical patients)
- Patients who are likely to need intensive evaluation and management (high-acuity, horizontal patients)

As previously mentioned, the volume and acuity mix of an ED will largely determine how many patient segments are practical. For example, an ED that typically experiences

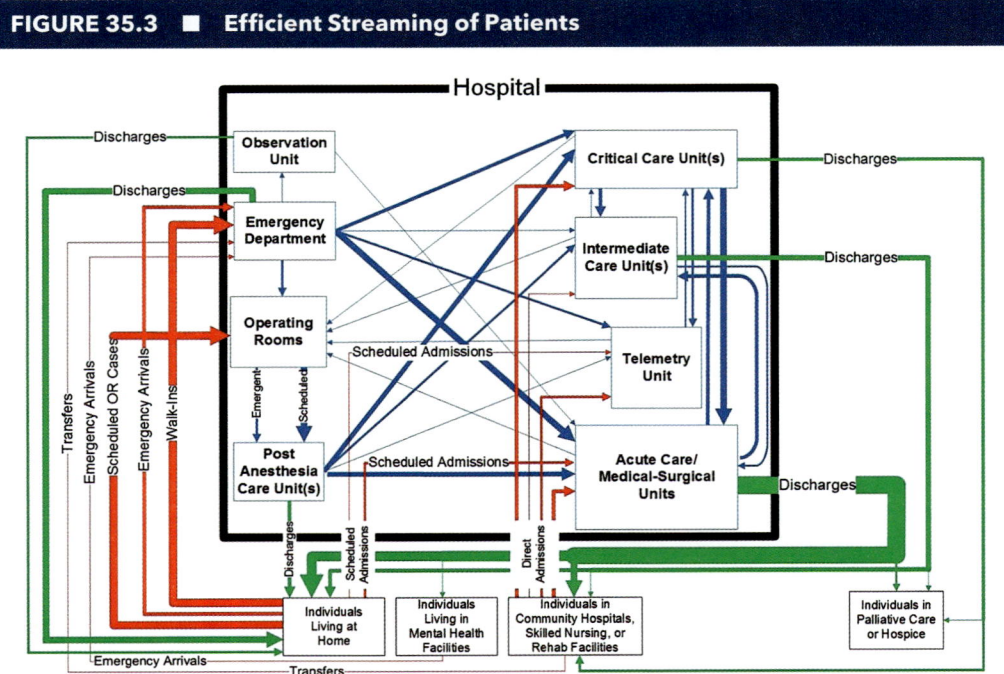

FIGURE 35.3 ■ Efficient Streaming of Patients

Key: **Blue arrows:** Flow within hospital | **Red arrows:** Flow into hospital | **Green arrows:** Flow out of hospital | **Width of arrows:** Typical flow volumes

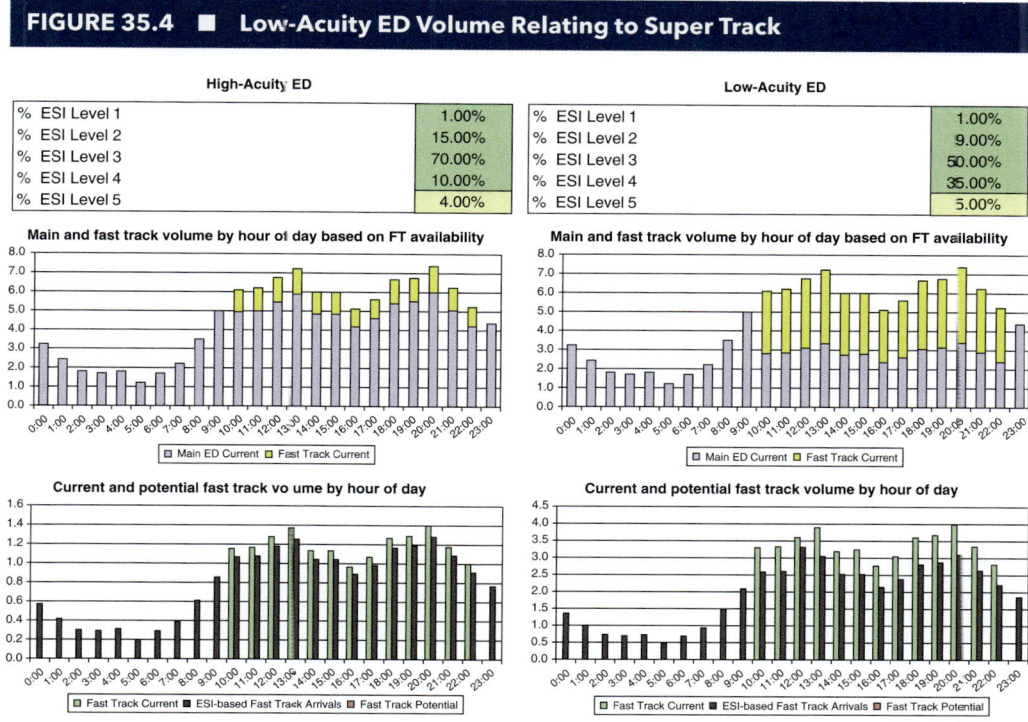

FIGURE 35.4 ■ Low-Acuity ED Volume Relating to Super Track

40,000 high-acuity patient visits a year will not need a triage-based low-acuity treatment area (super track), but it would likely benefit from an intake team that includes a physician and mid-level provider in triage (because of the low numbers of ESI 4 and 5 patients and the high numbers of ESI 3 patients). Alternatively, an ED with 40,000 mostly low-acuity visits annually would have the volume to support a super track with a peak arrival rate of three to four ESI level 4 and 5 patients per hour (**Figure 35.4**).

Over-segmentation can negatively affect flow. For instance, if an ED has separate pediatric, adult, fast-track, and behavioral health patient areas, it will be common for providers in some areas to be idle while patients in other areas are experiencing queues and delays. It is important to develop proper segmentation based on volume and acuity to ensure smooth flow and efficient use of staff.

REGISTRATION

Traditional sequential flow models place registration prior to triage. There are still a few EDs in which full registration, including obtaining payer information, takes place before triage and the medical screening examination. This process is counter to the intent of EMTALA and delays nurse triage and door-to-doctor time. In the event that a patient walks out before receiving a medical screening examination, particularly if they claim a delay in care or denial of services, full registration could be seen as proof that the hospital knew of the patient's inability to pay. Therefore, early full registration can expose EDs to potential allegations of noncompliance with EMTALA regulations.[12]

Fortunately, this order of events has been reversed in most EDs. An abbreviated registration process that obtains limited identifiers and yields an account number allows providers and nurses to begin care. This "quick registration" or "preregistration" process may be necessary to rapidly order diagnostics, obtain records, and access medications. Quick registration does not, however, have to happen prior to the quick-look assessment.

Ideally, full registration is performed after the medical evaluation or even delayed until the time of disposition. Registration should never interfere with the clinical process or flow. Rather, it should blend seamlessly yet deliberately within the patient experience. The preferred flow sequence places the triage nurse at the forefront for arriving patients and performs quick registration in tandem with, or immediately after, the quick-look assessment. In these instances, registration personnel are located in a shared clinical work area, where they can:

- Complete the registration after the physician evaluation.
- Observe discharges and ambulance arrivals.
- Process paperwork on patients admitted from the ED.
- Collect co-pays following medical screening.
- Reduce the number of patients who leave before paying.

Some of the most progressive EDs are eliminating registration clerks altogether by incorporating the quick registration into the pivot nurse workflow.

EFFECTING AND MEASURING CHANGE

While common barriers to change include deep-seated cultural biases and "the way we have always done it" attitudes, it is possible to transform the front end of most EDs.

The Challenge of Change

Transforming front-end ED processes requires a team of well-supported workers who are passionate about triage and efficient, high-quality patient care. Small tests of change can be effective in creating an open-minded environment in which experimentation is the rule rather than the exception. Once the team has transformed the front end, its members will take pride in their workplace and what they have accomplished. They will have positively affected patient care and made a palpable difference in staff satisfaction. It takes six to eight weeks of vigilant change management to overcome resistance. If resistance outlasts vigilance, the prognosis for sustained progress is poor.

The major cultural barrier to transforming triage is the perception that triage is a place where all of the documentation occurs in preparation for the physician encounter. This necessary documentation includes vital signs, weight, history, allergies, and assessment—sometimes including review of systems—and any risk screens deemed necessary by the hospital (such as fall risk, domestic violence, smoking, recreational drug use, and pneumonia vaccination). The addition of hospital medication reconciliation within the National Patient Safety Goals by The Joint Commission several years ago nearly overwhelmed emergency nurses with documentation requirements and undoubtedly increased ED lengths of stay. The Joint Commission recently modified the drug reconciliation standard to allow healthcare organizations to document current medications in a usable format.

Metrics

The minimum data set for triage has not been consistently defined. The traditional ED metric for the time from front door to triage has been less than 10 minutes. Triage time varies greatly based on the amount of information collected and the presence or absence of an EMR. Traditional triage processes coupled with EMRs typically result in significant bottlenecks. The best triage formats allow an experienced triage nurse to determine the minimum data set, use free text to enter it, and proceed with acuity-level documentation without cognitive forcing (a system of thinking designed to avoid diagnostic errors).[13] Even the best triage processes will take 2 to 3 minutes, while many "non-best"' processes take 10 minutes or more. Furthermore, lengthy, traditional triage processes make it difficult to achieve the 30-minute door-to-doctor gold standard. Therefore, most EDs have modified their front-end process to ensure the least time between the patient's entrance and the physician encounter.

CONCLUSION

Triage and all the other front-end ED processes must form a fluid macrosystem that moves patients from the door to the doctor as quickly and seamlessly as possible. Effective triage processes use methods to rapidly identify, classify, segment, and assign patients to locations and providers that match their clinical urgency and required level of care. Efficient front-end flow requires a mobile, "spring-loaded" ED nurse equipped with a valid, reliable triage algorithm. Patient flow must no longer be driven by registration; rather, triage should be performed in tandem with registration, and provider evaluations should be performed simultaneously with nurse assessments just inside the front door.

REFERENCES

1. Iserson KV, Moskop JC. Triage in medicine, part I: concept, history, and types. *Ann Emerg Med.* 2007;49(3):275-281.

2. Fitzgerald G, Jelinek GA, Scott D, Gerdtz MF. Emergency department triage revisited. *Emerg Med J.* 2010;27(2):86-92.

3. Niska R, Bhuiya F, Xu J. *National Hospital Ambulatory Medical Care Survey: 2007 Emergency Department Summary. National Health Statistics Reports No. 26.* Washington, DC: US Department of Health and Human Services; 2010.

4. Patient safety in the ED: a guide to identifying and reducing errors in the emergency department. *Hospitals and Health Networks Magazine.* 2006. Available at: www.hhnmag.com. Accessed January 23, 2011.

5. Jensen K, Crane J. Improving patient flow in the emergency department. *Healthc Financ Manage.* 2008;62(11):104-106.

6. Gilboy N, Tanabe P, Travers DA, Rosenau AM, Eitel DR. *Emergency Severity Index, Version 4: Implementation Handbook.* Rockville, Md: Agency for Health Care Research and Quality; 2005. AHRQ Publication No. 05-0046-2.

7. Crane J. The journey toward a Lean ED. 2007. Available at: https://docplayer.net/11002171-The-journey-toward-a-lean-ed-jody-crane-md-mba.html. Accessed December 17, 2018.

8. Murray M, Bullard M, Grafstein E; CTAS National Working Group and CEDIS National Working Group. Revisions to the Canadian Emergency Department Triage and Acuity Scale implementation guidelines. *CJEM.* 2004;6(6):421-427.

9. Manchester Triage Group. *Emergency Triage.* Oxford, England: Blackwell; 2006.

10. Jensen K, Mayer T. *Hardwiring Flow: Systems and Processes for Seamless Patient Care.* Pensacola, Fla: Fire Starter Publishing; 2015.

11. Sulfaro S. Charting the course for triage decisions. *J Emerg Nurs.* 2009;35(3):268-269.

12. Department of Health and Human Services. *Clarifying Policies Related to the Responsibilities of Medicare-Participating Hospitals in Treating Individuals With Emergency Medical Conditions.* Washington, DC: Centers for Medicare and Medicaid Services. 42 CFR Parts 413, 482, 489 [CMS-1063-F] RIN 0938-AM 34. Available at: http://www.cms.gov/EMTALA. Accessed January 31, 2011.

13. Sulfaro S. Initial presentation to triage: does it matter? *J Emerg Nurs.* 2010;35(2):182-183.

CHAPTER 36

FRONT-LOADING FLOW

Thom A. Mayer, Kirk Jensen, Robert W. Strauss
With John Howell, Alan Lo

There is a tide in the affairs of men,
Which, taken at the flood, leads on to fortune: Omitted, all the voyage of their life
Is bound in shallows and miseries. On such a full sea are we now afloat,
And we must take the current when it serves
Or lose our ventures.

—William Shakespeare
Julius Caesar, Act IV, Scene III, lines 218-224[1]

Diseases desperate grown
By desperate appliance are relieved,
Or not at all.

—William Shakespeare
Hamlet, Act IV, Scene III, lines 9-11[2]

In one of the earliest episodes of the television program *ER*, Dr. Mark Greene finds himself in a situation many, if not all, emergency physicians and nurses have faced. The rooms of the emergency department (ED) are all filled, occupied by "hospital boarders"—patients who have been evaluated and treated by the ED staff and have been admitted to the hospital, but for whom there are no inpatient beds currently available. Nor is there any expectation that such beds will become available for many, many hours. As a result, the ED is in total gridlock.

The ED charge nurse approaches Dr. Greene and tells him that the waiting room is completely full of patients who are getting increasingly agitated and angry, most already having waited several hours for care. After thinking for a moment, he says, "Then come with me and let's go take care of them!" He and the nurse begin making their way from patient to patient, walking through the waiting room, evaluating complaints, treating those who need medications, discharging those with minor illnesses and injuries, and staging those with more serious conditions. This continues throughout the night until all the patients have been seen and the waiting room is emptied, just as dawn arrives. Another nurse approaches them and says, "Good news, we will be getting some beds in a couple of hours!" Dr. Greene and the charge nurse just smile at each other, content in a job well done on behalf of their patients.

The episode arose from the personal experience of one of the chapter authors (T.M.), who had just spent such a night in the ED and served as a script consultant to *ER* in its early seasons. From experiences such as these arose a growing leadership philosophy to develop and implement systems to "front-load flow" in the ED, particularly during times when patient demand predictably exceeds available capacity.[3,4] These demand–capacity mismatches have become both widespread and predictable, particularly in large-volume EDs.[5] Data from the Emergency Department Benchmarking Alliance, which represents over 41 million annual ED visits, indicate that over 25% of EDs with volumes greater than 40,000 visits have some form of physician or advance practice provider (APP) in triage.[5] The stressors and pressures on ED personnel, including caring for high-volume and high-acuity patients in an increasingly capacity-constrained environment with dramatic demand–capacity mismatches, surely qualifies. But understanding the inexorable reality of those stressors and pressures can give rise to creative and innovative processes designed to benefit patients and those who care for them.

DEFINING THE TERMS

Mayer and Jensen have defined *flow* as "adding value or eliminating waste as patients move through the service transitions and queues in ED patient care."[6] *Front-loading* means creating value-added processes or services prior to the patients' arrival and the assumption of their care by the ED team assigned to that area. From the patients' perspective, front-loading flow means getting the patient and the doctor together as quickly as possible.[6] One of the most important questions in the ED is, "What do patients *want?*" They simply want "GB[3]":

- **G**et **b**ack (to see the doctor/APP and nurse)
- **G**et **b**etter (relief from their symptoms or concerns)
- **G**et "**b**oogeying" (get on with their lives, whether discharged or admitted)[7]

Front-loading flow strategies attempt to meet each of those needs by expediting flow despite significant constraints and variations. An additional important question that isn't asked often enough is: Does triage *add value?* Does it:

- Improve throughput?
- Increase safety?
- Improve patient experience?
- Improve quality?
- Provide useful, actionable information?
- Increase revenue capture?

If the answers to these questions aren't "yes," then triage needs to be redesigned, and front-loading flow solutions may need to be implemented.[6,7]

Demand–capacity management is a flow-based tool that recognizes prospectively the arrival of patients, their likely needs, and the ability of the ED staff to meet or exceed those needs, as well as what to do when demand exceeds capacity (**Table 36.1**).[7-9] (Chapters 33 and 34 discuss patient throughput and patient flow principles in more detail.) The focus of this chapter is primarily on front-end aspects of such care and the role that ED providers at triage may play.

TABLE 36.1 ■ Demand–Capacity Analysis	
Questions	**Demand-Capacity Aspect**
Who is coming?	Demand prediction (volume and acuity)
When are they coming?	Demand timing (hour of day, day of week, and by month/season)
What are they going to need?	Capacity anticipation
Will the resources be adequate? (staff, space, services, and supplies)	Capacity management
If resources are not adequate, how will the care process and capacity be adjusted?	Using demand-capacity to add value to processes, optimizing flow, throughput, and capacity

THE FLOW "CASCADE"

The problem of ED crowding and its subsequent effect on front-loading aspects of care is a serious problem, which shows no signs of dissipating.[10,11] The number of visits is rising, while the number of EDs available to provide care to those patients continues its steady decline.[9-11] Solutions to effectively decrease inpatient length of stay (LOS), improve handoffs from the ED to the inpatient units, and provide more efficient inpatient care are detailed in Chapters 43 and 46. The adoption of such strategies is just beginning to take hold in many EDs, while others have a rich experience with them. The increase in patient care demands (volume and acuity) continues to outstrip capacity in many EDs. Moreover, as patient visits continue to rise and the shortage of primary care physicians escalates simultaneously, front-loading flow is now and likely will be necessary to ensure timely, effective, efficient, and safe ED operations.[6-11]

Front-Loading Flow Means Admitting Failure

Front-loading flow by moving resources "forward" in (toward the beginning of) the course of patients' care should be recognized for what it is: a failure to be able to "unlock the back door of the ED" to use its beds for evaluation and treatment. However, this "failure" (moving resources forward) is done for the good of the patient as well as the good of the entire ED staff.[7,12] So, while the solutions presented here have demonstrated value, it is wise to focus on "unlocking the back door" efforts at the same time, as Chapters 40 and 41 delineate.

The bottlenecks of patient flow move and change during the course of a single day, depending on the time of day, patient arrivals, patient acuity, and a multitude of other factors. Likewise, the processes used must also adjust to meet the changing needs of the patients and providers over the course of time.

A great deal has been written about the need to reduce variability in health care.[12-14] A Lean-based definition of flow requires a clear understanding that the goal is to accommodate and manage natural variability but design out (or "manage out") unnatural or unnecessary disparities that simply tolerate or increase waste.[15,16] The flow cascade concept recognizes this essential reality and adapts processes to add value and decrease waste. There are many advantages to front-loading flow, depending on the circumstances and the processes used (**Box 36.1**).

BOX 36.1 ■ THE ADVANTAGES OF TEAM TRIAGE

- Front loads flow for the patient
- Speeds up door-to-doctor times
- Decreases the number of patients who leave without being seen
- Improves the patient experience
- Improves the provider experience
- Increases patient safety ("Great Catch!")
- Adds reputational value
- Creates a bearable waiting-room experience
- Captures revenue by increasing capacity
- Increases flow by increasing capacity
- Speeds time to admission
- Decompresses emergency medical services issues
- Positions the ED as an innovation center
- Creates hope!

The elements of the flow cascade include:

- Triage bypass/direct bedding
- Bedside registration
- Advanced triage/advanced initiatives
- Team triage and treatment (T3)
- Provider at triage
- Emergency severity index (ESI) level 3 fast tracks
- Results waiting rooms
- "Ultratracking" ESI 4s and 5s

Triage Bypass/Direct Bedding

Triage bypass was first initiated in the late 1980s at several institutions, including Inova Fairfax Hospital in Virginia and Christiana Medical Center in Delaware. These large volume, high-acuity EDs recognized that there were predictable hours in the morning, typically from about 7:00 am and lasting for a few hours, when there were actually staffed and open ED beds in which patients could be placed without being triaged. Triage, in effect, was an unnecessary or wasted step, since detaining patients at the triage area provided no added value and simply delayed getting them to the nurses and doctors who were waiting to care for them. Robert Cates, chairman emeritus of the Department of Emergency Medicine at Inova Fairfax Hospital, describes the genesis of the concept:

> *I was scheduled to give a lecture at a large medical center back in the days when you had to go to the airline ticket counter to get your boarding pass. I was running late when I got to the airport and was distressed to see the "cattle gates" up, in which the ropes force you to go through the "maze" before getting to the ticket agent. Fortunately, no one was in line, so I cut around the ropes and went straight to the agent at the counter.*
>
> *She looked at me and said, "Sir, we have a policy here at this airline that states that I cannot take care of you unless you have gone through the line." I looked back and there was no line, but having been happily married for a number of years, I take direction from women well. I quickly hustled back around the ropes and entered the maze; after making some left and right turns, I was quickly back at the same agent, who then smiled and said, "Next!" It suddenly hit me, "That's what we do every morning at triage! We make people go through a maze when there is no need to."*[17]

Triage bypass effectively recognizes that waste is created when patients are put through a "maze," going from triage to the waiting room to registration back to the waiting room, only to then be called back to precisely the same open room that they could have been placed in directly from triage (or from the waiting room without going through triage).

Triage bypass is also referred to as direct bedding, immediate bedding, mini-triage, direct to room, or "pull until full."[18-20] Although this approach requires the ability to perform bedside registration, it has been found to improve patient turnaround and satisfaction; decrease wait times, LOS, and the number of patients who leave without treatment (LWOT)—all without eroding patient safety.[19-22] In fact, triage bypass is a seemingly simple and eminently logical way to front-load flow by getting the patient and the clinical team together quickly, which is precisely what the patient wants.[23] However, as with any meaningful change initiative, there are always "pockets" of resistance no matter how logical and well-intended the change may be (see Chapter 3).

The primary resistance to change in triage bypass typically comes not from triage nurses, the registration team, or the treating emergency physician but rather from primary care nurses, who may perceive a loss of control over their rooms, which are now being filled directly by the triage nurse. The traditional system empowers the primary care nurse or the charge nurse to determine when and when not to bring patients back to fill the rooms, a dynamic that inherently has the potential to create unnecessary patient care delays.

In effect, this "triage bypass" is a sea change of control for the primary care or zone nurse and requires a reassessment of goals, roles, and processes. Many institutions have found it hard to sustain this change. Nonetheless, "triage bypass" can be a highly effective strategy to improve flow by adding value (getting the patient in a room and seen by the ED team faster) and decreasing waste (avoiding triage and registration), at least during the hours when there are beds readily available. It derives from a simple concept that, nonetheless, requires substantial leadership to implement effectively: "Triage is a process, not a place."[24]

Bedside Registration

Bedside registration has also been utilized since the late 1980s and typically involves an initial rapid registration (often called quick registration or "Quick-Reg"), comprising the patient's name, date of birth, social security number, and presenting complaint. (Some EDs add vital signs to this list.) The patient is then placed into a patient care room where registration personnel can complete the detailed process of full registration when the patient is not undergoing care. This in-room registration is typically accomplished using a portable computer on a rolling cart. This process allows the staff to immediately begin patient treatment, including ordering lab tests, imaging studies, and medications.[22-25] Fundamentally, this concept allows parallel processing of the patient with multiple activities occurring simultaneously, as opposed to the more traditional sequential processing. Most large-volume, high-acuity departments use bedside registration for their patients. When first introduced, it was common for ED staff to challenge this "new" approach until they realized that just such a process has always been used in EDs to register trauma codes, chest pain cases, and most patients who arrive by ambulance.[23] The vast majority of EDs currently use some form of bedside registration.

Advanced Triage/Advanced Initiatives

Triage bypass uses ED beds at those times when they are immediately and readily available and relies on bedside registration to affect the strategy. But once all ED beds are filled, how can flow be front-loaded when there are no appropriate treatment beds? Advanced triage/advanced initiatives (AT/AI) were developed specifically to address situations in which the likely diagnostic and/or treatment regimens are known, but in which there are no spaces in the treatment area to begin the evaluation or care. While AT/AIs are also known by many names, they share a fundamental strategy. Using standardized evaluation and treatment protocols (usually supported by standing physician order sets), AT/AIs allow the nurses at triage to initiate diagnostic, therapeutic, or management regimens for specified patients based on presenting complaints and vital signs.

Now widely used, AT/AI shortens patient turnaround time and, when combined with appropriate scripts, can be an important contributor to patient satisfaction (see Chapter 11).[25] At one point, The Joint Commission briefly criticized this strategy on the basis that each and every physician order required prior physician contact with the patient and approval of the order. However, once the self-apparent folly of this approach was pointed out (e.g., if a physician is busy with a trauma code and another patient has a cardiac arrest, should the nurse withhold CPR until the physician can evaluate the patient?), EDs quickly turned back to AT/AI as a highly effective strategy.[26] Data from multiple reports are clear that AT/AI:

- Decreases LOS
- Decreases time to pain relief
- Increases patient comfort
- Decreases time to antibiotic therapy in community-acquired pneumonia
- Decreases time to open artery in chest pain patients presenting to triage[23-27]

TEAM TRIAGE AND TREATMENT

Triage bypass addresses times when beds are available, while AT/AI addresses situations in which beds are not available but treatment for minor illnesses or injuries can be initiated. Team triage takes the flow cascade to still another level, addressing times when beds may not be available for prolonged periods.

In the first several years of the 21st century, United States safety-net hospitals almost constantly faced the problems of ED crowding. National averages for ED crowding in 2001 were at 21%, whereas safety-net hospitals were overcrowded up to 80% of the time.[28,29] To address this situation, the Robert Woods Johnson Foundation created the Urgent Matters grant program in 2002, which sought innovative and creative solutions to crowding in large-volume, high-acuity EDs.[3]

One of the 10 national $250,000 grants was awarded to Inova Fairfax Hospital, which at the time was a 72,000 visit ED and a level I trauma center and with a dedicated pediatric ED. The ED faced crowding 79% of the time on a consistent basis. The grant was for the nation's first development and implementation of a concept called "Team Triage and Treatment" or "T3."[30] Using statistical process control methods, the peak hours of ED crowding and boarding were determined to be a predictable 10-hour period from 10:00 am to 8:00 pm. The program deployed emergency physicians, nurse, technicians, scribes, and registrars to front-load the triage area for this 10-hour period. This team used two to five designated treatment beds (depending on patient flow) in or immediately adjacent to the triage area to begin—and in many cases to complete—the ED evaluation at the initial point of contact for the patient.

Critical Components of Team Triage

First, it is essential that this program utilizes a *team* approach rather than simply placing an emergency physician or mid-level provider (MLP) at triage. The physician, nurse, and other members of the team must work closely together in a designated space and according to clearly delineated protocols. Without an emergency nurse dedicated to team triage, blood drawing, intravenous lines, and medication administration would fall either to the triage nurse or to already overstressed and overworked ED nurses who would have to abandon their other duties to care for these patients.

Second, after a quick registration is completed at traditional triage, lab and imaging tests can be administered so that patients never wait to have full registration completed.

Third, the ED technician is also a critical part of the team, since T3 functions occur within a discrete area with dedicated staff. By performing designated procedures, technicians free up the physician and nurse to perform their responsibilities.

Fourth, scribes are essential to the team (see Chapter 25) by allowing the emergency physician to maintain flow in the T3 area. A key attribute of team triage is ensuring that the emergency physician is available to provide bedside patient care and, to the maximum extent possible, freed from charting and electronic medical record (EMR) responsibilities.

The Successful Implementation of Team Triage

The results of T3 at Inova Fairfax were dramatic.[30,31] While patient velocity (patients seen per hour of physician coverage) in the ED generally was 1.9 during the study period, the T3 physicians averaged 3.7 patients per hour. Patient satisfaction improvements were dramatic, rising from the 60th percentile to the 97th percentile and with a 100% patient loyalty rating (likelihood to return or recommend). While the 212-minute reduction in LOS for T3 patients is perhaps not surprising (from 330 to 118 minutes), even more impressive was the 46-minute mean decline in LOS for patients *not* seen at T3 (a 15% reduction from 330 to 284 minutes). This supports the long-held but never previously documented concept that, if crowding can be avoided, it has an impact on the entire ED flow.

Of specific interest is that 34% of patients had their entire ED evaluation and treatment completed while in the triage area. An additional 18% of patients had their ED workup completed and were admitted directly to an inpatient bed from team triage. Patient safety incidents declined 80%, showing the important improvement in risk reduction from front-loading flow.

It is important to recognize the slogan "triage is not a place for the weak and timid," meaning that just as the best and most experienced nurses should be allowed to work at triage, the same principle applies to emergency physicians. Because judgment is necessary to determine segmentation into appropriate value streams and because overordering imaging and laboratory studies can defeat the purpose of team triage, the best and most efficient physicians should work at team triage whenever possible. The ideal team triage physician possesses three critical attributes: sensitivity (sick/not sick?), specificity (is this test, treatment or procedure necessary?), and speed.

Because of ED staff shortages, more recent iterations of team triage have used an emergency physician and scribe dedicated to team triage, with ED nurses and technicians "pulled" into the area as needed to support the diagnostic and therapeutic orders from the emergency physician. This version of team triage has also been successful and is currently in use at Sentara Northern Virginia Medical Center, where it has resulted in LOS reductions of 15.5%, decreased door-to-doctor times, a reduction of LWOT from greater than 8% to less than 1%, and an increase in patient satisfaction and capacity.[31] A physician incentive compensation plan has also contributed to improved outcomes.

Obstacles to Team Triage

While improvements with team triage can be dramatic, there are predictable obstacles to overcome when implementing and sustaining such a program.

Expense

The costs of deploying a five-member team can be substantial, requiring a significant investment on the part of the physician group and the hospital. In particular, the cost of having a dedicated emergency physician in team triage for 6 to 12 hours per day (depending on demand–capacity curves and their prediction of times when ED beds will not be available for sustained times) may be prohibitive for some physician groups. Alternatives include using MLPs in team triage or variants of providers at triage. Nonetheless, the return on investment (ROI) for team triage exceeded 200% in a high-acuity level I trauma center, taking into account the reduction in LWOTs (and therefore increased patients), increased admissions, decreased risk, and improved functional capacity. The reduction in LWOTs is an important part of this equation, as is the increase in hospital admissions. Generally speaking, if ED crowding results in persistent delays of three or more patients per hour for more than

TABLE 36.2 ■ Applying Disney Concepts to the ED	
Concept	**Application to the ED**
"Onstage" vs "offstage"	Physicians and nurses in team triage or provider at triage are easily visible to the waiting room.
Equitable queues	Differential queues due to acuity require scripting.
Expectation creation	Creating evidence-based time estimates for flow creates an expectation that must be met or improved.

5 to 6 hours, team triage is a highly effective strategy to decompress the department and improve its standing in the community.[29-31]

Culture Shifts and Visibility

Team triage is a culture change of dramatic proportions, and physician and nursing leaders must be prepared for the change from "Let the patients wait; they're not *that* sick" to "Get out front and get things moving!" Without committed and effective leadership, this cultural change is doomed at the start.

A part of this cultural change is the highly visible nature of the program, since the waiting room and the triage/team triage areas are typically in the direct line-of-sight of anyone in the waiting room. While triage nurses have been used to this, emergency physicians may have to adjust to this "on-stage" concept, as Disney refers to it (**Table 36.2**).[32]

Resistance Among Physicians

While a third of patients may have their evaluation and treatment completed at team triage, the remainder are eventually moved to rooms in the main ED. There is typically some resistance from the emergency physicians "in the back" to receiving partially treated patients. (Nurses are typically less resistant, probably because it is more common for them to transfer care.) However, this resistance can be overcome by simply pointing out that transferring care from one emergency physician to another routinely occurs at change of shift. In addition, team triage greatly reduces risk, as the data clearly show. The potential disadvantages or drawbacks are listed in **Box 36.2**.

Although there are many refinements and alternative options to team triage, it remains an attractive option for large-volume, space and capacity-constrained EDs, which routinely

BOX 36.2 ■ POTENTIAL DISADVANTAGES TO PROVIDER IN TRIAGE

- It doesn't work. (It didn't work for us in our setting.)
- Moving resources from fast track to the front doesn't work.
- It interferes with resident education.
- I don't like getting patients another doc has seen. (Do you take sign-outs?)
- Two docs means more malpractice risk.
- If nursing staffing is short, this is the first place to pull from.
- It increases reliance on ED techs, scribes, and registrars.
- If you don't develop scripts, the patient doesn't know they got special treatment.

face situations where demand exceeds capacity for several hours of the day. It should be noted that members of T3 teams often report increased job satisfaction.[29-31]

VARIATIONS OF TEAM TRIAGE

Since the initial report of the T3 concept in 2003, the approach not only has become much more widespread but also has been parent to many effective variations (**Table 36.3**). Variations include:

- Emergency severity index level 3 fast tracks[33]
- Using providers at triage[33,34]
- "Ultratracking" ESI level 4s and 5s[3]

Team triage, both at its inception and in subsequent iterations, is not weighted toward the care of ESI 1-2 (more severe acuity, who are typically recognized quickly and sent to the acute care area of the ED) or level 5 (minor) patients. Team triage at Inova Fairfax Hospital is comprised of nearly 90% of ESI level 3 and 4 patients.[29,30] Alternative ways of dealing with these cases are presented next.

Team Triage Variants

Anne Arundel Medical Center in Annapolis, Maryland, is a busy community ED with an annual volume exceeding 50,000 patients. Because of recognized capacity constraints at peak-load flow times of the day, the ED staff implemented a variant of team triage as shown in **Table 36.3**.

During peak flow times, an emergency physician, nurse, and ED technician are deployed at the triage area to evaluate and begin the treatment of patients at times when rooms are not immediately available. The emergency physician does a complete evaluation, and order sets are implemented according to previously established treatment protocols.

Once the evaluation is completed, the patient is placed into the next available treatment area and is accepted for follow-up care by an APP. The APP then completes the workup, considers the results of the lab and imaging studies as well as the patient's clinical course, and, in most cases, makes a disposition of the patient. In cases where the patient's clinical course changes or the results of the workup require further physician involvement, an ED physician reevaluates the patient.

Ken Gummerson, medical director at Anne Arundel, also uses a "middle-linebacker shift" in which a dedicated emergency physician is not assigned to a specific area but rather plugs any "holes" that may exist at the time.[34] This is an example of real-time demand–capacity management utilizing the emergency physician.

TABLE 36.3 ■ Team Triage Types	
Team triage and treatment	Physician, nurse, scribe, ED tech, and registrar at triage during set hours of the day
Threshold-based team triage	Teams deploy to triage when certain thresholds for waits are reached, depending on ED flow
Anne Arundel team triage	Physician sees patient at triage, begins workup, and transfers to mid-level practitioner (MLP) in the ED
Physician/provider at triage	Physician or MLP at triage, with or without nursing, tech, or scribe support, depending on local factors

> **BOX 36.3 ■ DESCRIPTIONS OF FRONT-LOADING FLOW PROGRAMS**
>
> - Physician at triage
> - Provider at triage
> - Immediate care physician
> - Immediate care provider
> - Rapid care assessment
> - Rapid medical evaluation
> - Rapid intake and treatment zone (RITZ)

Provider at Triage

As described, team triage is usually intended to indicate that a physician and a team of providers are available at the triage area during certain hours of the day or certain days of the week. "Provider at triage" is somewhat less descriptive and may include an APP at triage, with or without a nurse, tech, scribe, or registrar. (Chapter 37 describes this concept in more detail.) As **Box 36.3** indicates, there are many ways to describe these programs, including "provider at triage," "immediate care physician," "immediate care provider (an APP)," "rapid care assessment," and "rapid medical evaluation."

All of these approaches share the basic goal of bringing patients and providers together as rapidly and safely as possible upon patient arrival to the ED. In addition, all programs share a "parallel processing approach" to these patients, in which either physicians or APPs work closely with their nursing and support colleagues to front-load care. A data-intense approach that allows all ED providers to visualize and monitor patient flow is essential to success. Whether the provider at triage is an emergency physician or APP will depend on volume, acuity, risk factors, financial issues, and local circumstances. However, the use of both emergency physicians and APPs has been successful.[35,36]

Emergency Severity Index Level 3 Fast Tracks

For EDs that choose not to deploy a team of providers at triage, other "front-loaded" options have been developed to address issues of flow.[36]

"Fast tracks" (a noun) were originally developed as a specific area of the ED in which patients with minor illnesses and injuries were treated. Current approaches consider "fast tracking" (a verb) as a way in which patients with certain identifiable clinical entities are processed in a highly evidence-based fashion. Thus, patients with numerous high-acuity illnesses or injuries are now "fast-tracked" in EDs based on their presenting symptoms. (Chapter 37 addresses this in more detail.)

The concept is critical to understanding ways in which flow is front-loaded. For example, some EDs do not deploy personnel to the triage area to evaluate and treat patients but instead create a "split flow" or segmented flow.[37] In this way, they create processes by which patients with ESI level 3 acuity can be "split" and moved through the system in an expedited fashion.

One of the difficulties with the creation of an ESI level 3 fast track is an attribute of the ESI system itself. The triage categorization scheme of ESI fails to account for the reality that there are both "horizontal" level 3s (patients who are sicker and require a bed or horizontal surface for the majority of their care) and "vertical" level 3s (whose care can often be provided in a treatment chair or space, as opposed to a bed or stretcher.

Vertical level 3 patients are much more amenable to a fast-track process than those who are horizontal and have more needs. Triage protocols should recognize this and restrict patients sent to an ESI level 3 fast track to vertical patients.

Results Waiting Areas

What, typically, is the most rate-limiting component of the ED? Is it the physician? The nurse? A simple answer might be "the team." However, the true rate-limiting step or bottleneck for most EDs is "the bed." Do all ED patients need a bed? The answer is "no," since some low-acuity patients may be seen in chairs, whether in a room or a hallway, depending on availability. Perhaps more importantly, do patients who require a bed need it for their entire LOS in the ED? Patients with critical illnesses or injuries, those with protracted vomiting, and those who require monitoring usually do require a bed for their entire stay. But for many patients, the bed adds value only for the period during which the nurse and physician evaluate and initially treat the patient. Recognizing this temporary need and the capacity constraints that the bed (or other horizontal surfaces in the ED) represents, many departments have developed "results waiting rooms" where patients wait until their diagnostic studies are completed. Properly set up, these rooms have comfortable chairs and are readily visible to nurses and other qualified ED personnel in case problems arise. The results waiting rooms are often positioned next to the triage area in the front of the ED. These patients must also be tracked so that there is a clear understanding of where they are located.

The Pivot Nurse Concept

During his early work on applying Lean principles to ED operations, emergency physician Jody Crane applied the concept of a "pivot nurse" at triage, whose duties included pivoting to direct patients to the appropriate value stream through segmentation of care.[37] A patient might be directed to the SuperTrack area (see below) or to other areas of the ED, depending on their acuity, likely resources needed, and the processes necessary to deliver their care. In some settings, the pivot nurse also rounds on patients to determine their progress through the system, but in large-volume EDs, they are usually extremely busy directing traffic at triage.[38]

SuperTrack or Ultratrack

"SuperTrack" or "ultratrack" is a concept first implemented at Mary Washington Hospital in Fredericksburg, Virginia. SuperTrack "is thus a fast track that is located at or near triage for the purpose of promptly treating patients who require very low resource utilization."[37] Typically it utilizes two to three beds or chairs, has an adjacent results waiting area, and is staffed with a physician or MLP, a nurse, and potentially an ED technician, depending on the number and flow of patients.

The concept is an example of segmenting patient flow and creating a separate process and area for those with very low-acuity problems. Patient flow data should help determine whether (and when) such a concept is needed. For obvious reasons, these programs are usually utilized in large-volume EDs (greater than 50,000 annual visits), since these EDs have enough high-acuity patients to fill the beds in the main treatment areas, while simultaneously having a "critical mass" of lower-acuity patients to necessitate a separate and dedicated flow pattern and process. This concept again illustrates that variations in process can add value for this specific group of patients by reducing waiting times, decreasing LOS, and improving patient satisfaction.

PUTTING IT ALL TO WORK

When considering the "how" of front-loading flow, these are useful steps to take in implementation[38]:

1. *Build a powerful guiding coalition.*
   Front-loading flow is a team approach that requires input from all team areas, including nurses, physicians, APPs, ED technicians, registration, and scribes. Identify a "champion" from each area who can be tasked with designing the changes.
2. *Identify the bottlenecks to effective flow.*
   Use data from the EMR and all other sources to determine, in detail, where the bottlenecks and constraints lie. List them in detail by time of day, day of week, and type of patient, as well as possible sources for the delay.
3. *Use the demand–capacity questions to interpret the data.*
   The five questions in **Table 36.1** should act as a guide to determine where demand–capacity mismatches occur and how to address them. Continuously update the data over time.
4. *Anticipate resistance.*
   Without resistance, there is no real change. Anticipate the sources of such resistance, both by area and by individuals, and develop solutions to that resistance. (If key influencers are expected to resist, consider putting them on the steering committee.)
5. *Customize the solution.*
   Front-loading flow is not a "one size fits all" phenomenon. Each aspect listed in the chapter should be considered compared to the actual bottlenecks (supported by data, not just opinion) to determine which are most likely to work.
6. *Anticipate the C-Suite.*
   Think ahead about what the leaders of the organization will say about the program, avoid functional silos, and develop a case for the good of the patient—but also for what the ROI of the program will be, since there will be costs involved.
7. *Keep vertical patients vertical—and moving.*
   Use the "vertical versus horizontal" concept to help the team keep vertical patients in motion through the system, since these patients value speed (time) versus "real estate" (a bed or horizontal surface).
8. *Triage is not for the faint of heart.*
   Triage requires considerable judgment, acumen, and patient experience skills. It is not a place to "hide" poor performers. Particularly during the rapid-cycle testing phase, but throughout implementation of the program, use the best A-team members to front-load flow.
9. *Adapt the program as needed.*
   If the original trials don't show the anticipated success, reassess the data for accurate bottleneck sources and be prepared to adapt the details of the program.
10. *Beware of moving bottlenecks.*
    It is common for bottlenecks at one area to "move" to another area when the first one is fixed. Having team triage or a provider at triage when there are substantial delays in imaging or lab tests will only move the delay from "door to provider" to "diagnostic tests to decision." Take a global approach to identifying sources and causes of all delays, not just front-end constraints.

CONCLUSION

As emergency patient visits rise and the number of functional EDs contract, it will become increasingly important for department leaders to consider ways such care can best be provided. For most moderate-to-large-volume EDs, particularly those that serve a safety-net function for their communities and that regularly experience crowding, front-loading flow will become a necessity. Triage bypass, bedside registration, AT/AI, team triage, providers at triage, level 3 fast tracks, results waiting rooms, and SuperTracks or ultratracks are all options ED leaders should consider. Depending on local circumstances and resources, these programs may improve the lives of their patients and the lives of those who care for them.

REFERENCES

1. Shakespeare W. *Julius Caesar*. Act 4, Scene 3, lines 218–224.
2. Shakespeare W. *Hamlet*. Act 4, Scene 3, lines 9–11.
3. Jensen K, Mayer TA, Welch SJ, Haraden C. *Leadership for Smooth Patient Flow: Improved Outcomes, Improved Service, Improved Bottom Line*. Chicago, Ill: Health Administration Press; 2007.
4. Mayer T. Applying the lessons of Lean in healthcare. Presented at: American College of Emergency Physicians Scientific Assembly, October 8, 2012; Denver, Colo.
5. Emergency Department Benchmarking Alliance, 2017 Annual Report. Available at: www.edbenchmarking.org. Accessed August 27, 2018.
6. Mayer T, Jensen K. *Hardwiring Flow: Systems and Processes for Seamless Patient Care*. Gulf Breeze, Fla: Fire Starter Press; 2009:20–21.
7. Mayer T. Rewarding the champions, corralling the stragglers. Presented at: The ACEP Leadership and Advocacy Conference; May 5, 2018, Washington, DC.
8. Resar R, Nolan K, Kaczynski D, et al. Using real-time demand capacity to improve hospital wide flow. *Jt Comm J Qual Patient Saf*. 2011;37:217–227.
9. Nawar ED, Niska RW, Xu J. National Hospital Ambulatory Medical Care Survey—2005 emergency department summary. *Adv Data*. 2007;386. Available at: https://pubmed.ncbi.nlm.nih.gov/17703794/. Accessed October 3, 2012.
10. Wiler JL, Gentle C, Halfpenny JM, et al. Optimizing emergency department front-end operations. *Ann Emerg Med*. 2010;55:142–160.
11. Smith AC, Barry R, Brubaker CE. *Going Lean: Busting Barriers to Patient Flow*. Chicago, Ill: Health Administration Press; 2007.
12. Mayer TA, Cates RJ. *Leadership for Great Customer Service: Satisfied Employees, Satisfied Patients*. 2nd ed. Chicago, Ill: Health Administration Press; 2014.
13. Busse R, Scheeryogg J, Smith PC. VariaEU countries—results from the HealthBASKET project. *Health Econ*. 2008;17:S1–S8.
14. Litvak E, Buerhaus PI, Davidoff F, et al. Managing unnecessary variability in patient demand to reduce nursing stress and improve patient safety. *Jt Comm J Qual Patient Saf*. 2005;6:330–338.
15. Jensen K. Better patient flow means breaking down silos. Available at: http://www.ihi.org/knowledge/Pages/ImprovementStories/BetterPatientFlowMeansBreakingDowntheSilos.aspx. Accessed October 3, 2012.
16. Mayer T, Jensen K. The business case for patient flow. Unique approaches to patient flow improve the patient experience and the bottom line. *Healthc Exec*. 2012;27(4):50, 52–53.
17. Mayer T, Cates RJ: *Leadership for Great Customer Service: Satisfied Patients, Satisfied Employees*. Chicago, Ill: Health Administration Press; 2004.
18. Spaite DW, Batholomeaux F, Guisto J, et al. Rapid process redesign in a university-based emergency department: decreasing waiting time intervals and improving patient satisfaction. *Ann Emerg Med*. 2002;39:168–177.
19. Bertoty DA, Kuszajewski ML, Marsh EE. Direct-to-room: one department's approach to improving ED throughput. *J Emerg Nur*. 2007;33:26–30.
20. Chan TC, Killen JP, Kelly D, et al. Impact of rapid entry and accelerated care at triage on reducing emergency department wait times, length of stay, and rate of left without being seen. *Ann Emerg Med*. 2005;46:491–497.
21. Welch S, Augustine J, Camargo CA, et al. Emergency department performance measures and benchmarking summit. *Acad Emerg Med*. 2006;13:1074–1080.
22. Welch SJ, Augustine J, Li D, et al. Volume-related differences in emergency department performance. *Jt Comm J Qual Patient Saf*. 2012;39:395–402.
23. Press I. The emergency department: a special case. In: *Patient Satisfaction: Understanding and Managing the Experience of Care*. 2nd ed. Chicago, Ill: Health Administration Press; 2006:217–245.
24. Mayer T, Jensen K. *Hardwiring Flow: Systems and Processes for Seamless Patient Care*. Gulf Breeze, Fla: Fire Starter Press; 2009:45.
25. Gorelick MH, Yen K, Yun HJ. The effect of in-room registration on emergency department length of stay. *Ann Emerg Med*. 2005;45:128–133.
26. Strauss R, Mayer T. Scripts using evidence-based language to improve service. In: *Strauss and Mayer's Emergency Department Leadership*. New York, NY: McGraw-Hill; 2013.
27. Cooper JJ, Datner EM, Pines JM. Effect of an automated chest radiograph at triage protocol on time to antibiotics in patients admitted with pneumonia. *Am J Emerg Med*. 2008;26:264–269.
28. The Healthcare Advisory Board. *The Clockwork ED*. Washington, DC: The Advisory Board Companies; 2004.
29. Robert Wood Johnson Foundation. Urgent Matters program: bursting at the seams. Available at: https://hsrc.himmelfarb.gwu.edu/sphhs_policy_facpubs/250/. Accessed October 3, 2012.
30. Mayer T. Team triage and treatment improves ED outcomes. Available at: https://smhs.gwu.edu/urgentmatters/sites/urgentmatters/files/enewsletter_volume2_issue1_TeamTriage_Mayer.pdf. Accessed October 3, 2012.
31. Howell J, Mayer T, Druckenbrod G, et al. A qualitative study to improve the efficiency of a high volume, high acuity academic emergency department: physician in triage and physician incentive compensation decrease length of stay, improve patient satisfaction and increase capacity. *Jt Comm J Qual Patient Saf*. 2013. In press.
32. Connellan T. *Inside the Magic Kingdom: 7 Keys to Disney's Success*. Boston, Mass: Bard Press; 1997.
33. Holroyd BR, Bullard MJ, Latoszek K, et al. Impact of a triage liaison physician on emergency department overcrowding and throughput: a randomized controlled trial. *Acad Emerg Med*. 2007;14:702–708.
34. Partovi SN, Nelson BK, Bryan ED, et al. Faculty triage shortens emergency department length of stay. *Acad Emerg Med*. 2001;8:991–995.

35. Tom P. Provider at triage. Presented at: The American College of Emergency Physicians Scientific Assembly; 2010.
36. Mayer T, Jensen K. *Hardwiring Flow: Systems and Processes for Seamless Patient Care*. Gulf Breeze, Fla: Fire Starter Press; 2009:62.
37. Crane J, Noon C. *The Definitive Guide to Emergency Department Operational Improvement*. New York, NY: CRC Press; 2011.
38. Mayer T, Quick Doc: Providers in Triage, presented at the American College of Emergency Physicians Scientific Assembly 2020, Dallas, October 29, 2020.

ADDITIONAL READINGS

- ACEP: Emergency Medicine Practice Committee of the American College of Emergency Physicians. Emergency department crowding: High-impact solutions. 2016. Available at: https://www.acep.org/globalassets/sites/acep/media/crowding/empc_crowding-ip_092016.pdf
- Advisory Board. *Building the Clockwork ED: Best Practices for Eliminating Bottlenecks and Delays in the ED*. Washington, DC: HWorks, An Advisory Board Company; 2000.
- Advisory Board. *The High-Performance ED Optimizing Capacity and Throughput to Meet Ever-Growing Demand*. Washington, DC: HWorks, An Advisory Board Company; 2008.
- Institute for Healthcare Improvement. Optimizing patient flow: moving patients smoothly through acute care settings. *Innovation Series*. Chicago, Ill: Institute for Healthcare Improvement; 2003.
- Holden RJ. Lean thinking in emergency departments: a critical review. *Ann Emerg Med*. 2011;57(3):265–278.
- Jensen K, Mayer T. *The Patient Flow Advantage: How Hardwiring Hospital-Wide Flow Drives Competitive Performance*. Gulf Breeze, FL: Fire Starter Publishing; 2015.
- Mayer T, Jensen K. *Hardwiring Hospital-Wide Flow to Drive Sustainable Competitive Performance*. Management in Healthcare. Vol. 2. Issue 4. Henry Stewart Publications; 2018: 1-15.Rabin E, Kocher K, McClelland M, et al. Solutions to emergency department 'boarding' and crowding are underused and may need to be legislated. *Health Aff*. 2012; 31(8): 1757–1766.
- The Joint Commission. Approved: standards revisions addressing patient flow through the emergency department. Joint Commission Perspectives. 2012;32(7):1–5.
- Warner LS, Pines JM, Chambers J, et al. The most crowded US hospital emergency departments did not adopt effective interventions to improve flow, 2007-2010. *Health Aff*. 2015;34(12):2151–2159.
- Wiler JL, Gentle C, Halfpenny JM, et al. Optimizing emergency department front-end operations. *Ann Emerg Med*. 2010;55:142–160.

CHAPTER 37

THE ROLE OF EMERGENCY DEPARTMENT FAST TRACKS

Kirk Jensen, Thom A. Mayer, Robert W. Strauss,
With Alison Atwater, Susan Bednar

A woman has a minor injury at work, a cut to the heel of her hand. She wraps it in a bandage but worries that it might become infected. "I'd better go to the emergency department," she thinks. It's a quick drive, but once she gets there, she finds herself sitting in the waiting room, seemingly forever. "It *can't* take that long to treat a cut!" she grumbles. But her wait goes on and on, and she doesn't know why. After waiting for hours, she finally gets treatment. The next day, one of her coworkers hears this story and says, "You should have gone to the emergency department that I go to! They have a 'fast track' and I always get in and out quickly."

ORIGINS OF THE FAST-TRACK CONCEPT

In the early 1980s, several high-volume and forward-thinking emergency departments (EDs) had an essential insight. They recognized that low-acuity patients were being treated in the same physical space as the high-acuity patients with the same processes, procedures, and protocols. The lower-acuity patients were often considered subordinate to patients with more time-sensitive problems. Those with less urgent complaints often had long wait times, as the emergency physicians and nurses were prioritizing treatment for those with potentially life- or limb-threatening conditions. In addition, most ED nurses and physicians were drawn preferentially to the acute patients, who were largely the reason these talented and highly trained professionals had chosen the adrenaline-fueled environment of the ED.

The pioneering institutions and their leaders understood that all EDs treat a wide spectrum of acute and subacute illnesses, and that lower-acuity patients (70%-80%) often significantly outnumber those with more serious conditions (20%-30%). Recognizing that low-acuity cases were uniformly relegated to the "back of the line," a few innovators set out to solve the problem. With these central observations and goals in mind, a number of EDs developed an alternative track or system of care. The goal was to treat patients with lower-acuity illnesses or injuries using a process that was separate from yet parallel to the approach used for the higher-acuity cases. This separate process typically took place in a physically distinct area, often called a "fast track," where these patients were evaluated and treated using a simplified approach.

"Fast track" was not simply a *place* in which low-acuity patients were seen; more importantly, it became a *system and set of processes* by which these highly predictable cases were managed. A key insight was that this was a defined group of patients that could be segmented and managed (i.e., a "fast track" designed with staff, space, supplies, and defined service hours). The fundamental approach was a Lean system designed to add value and eliminate waste. The evolution of fast-track programs was one of the earliest ways EDs

> **BOX 37.1 ■ THE FUNDAMENTAL CONCEPTS OF THE FAST-TRACK DEMAND–CAPACITY MANAGEMENT SYSTEM APPROACH**
>
> - The number of low-acuity patients is predictable (demand prediction).
> - The times of day that these patients arrive are predictable (demand timing).
> - The patient's clinical problems are highly predictable (demand anticipation).
> - The resources needed to evaluate, treat, and make a clinical disposition are predictable (capacity recognition).
> - For low-acuity patients requiring laboratory or imaging studies, there are predictable conflicts or competition with the acutely ill or injured patients for the ED's scarce resources (capacity competition). These competing demands for resources, known as bottlenecks or constraints, must be eliminated, eased, or managed.

learned to leverage the key operational strategies of demand–capacity management and patient segmentation/streaming/split-flow.

Merriam-Webster defines *fast track* (noun) as "a course of expedited consideration" and *fast-track* (verb) as "to speed up the processing, production, or construction in order to meet a goal."[1] The adoption of these fundamental operational approaches has led to the concept of fast-tracking as a distinct process by which patients can be processed promptly and appropriately. Currently, most moderate- and large-volume EDs have created a separate area for these patients to be evaluated and treated (fast track as a *noun*—a place). However, fast track is most meaningfully viewed as a set of processes rather than simply a location where such patients are seen.

The fundamental concepts of this demand–capacity management system approach are listed in **Box 37.1**.

CURRENT APPROACHES

The risks associated with ED volume surges and overcrowding have been well-documented and include long wait times, staff dissatisfaction, poor patient experience, decreased productivity, and patient safety concerns.[3] Developing an area within the ED where lower-acuity patients are fast tracked can optimize flow and alleviate overcrowding.

Fast Track Versus Fast-Tracking

Traditionally, the ED's primary function has been to provide care for patients with life-threatening medical conditions. Multiple approaches to fast-tracking acutely ill patients are increasingly implemented in EDs using evidence-based operational, diagnostic, and therapeutic protocols. Fast-tracking uses the science of patient segmentation and standardized operational best practices to deliver a defined set of treatment pathways (encompassing flow, diagnostic, and therapeutic components) to an identified cohort of patients, usually with a dedicated ED staff working in a specified area.

EDs provide care to a significant number of patients who present with less serious, nonemergent conditions, which constitute between 10% and 66% of all ED visits.[4] Current approaches to deploying fast tracks usually involve defining a designated area in or near the main ED where care is provided expeditiously to a specific cohort of lower-acuity patients.

Fundamental Drivers of Fast Tracks

To be successful, ED fast tracks must deliver a focused patient care journey that involves rapid identification, minimal diagnostics, efficient processes, and accelerated time lines to achieve defined operational goals. Simply put, fast tracks are designed to increase value to patients through four fundamental mandates:

- Decrease the turnaround time (TAT) for lower-acuity patients who present to the ED.
- Provide a dedicated group of emergency physicians and nurses who are not distracted by other, higher-acuity patients.
- Ensure that care is guided by evidence-based protocols geared toward optimizing speed and quality of care.
- Provide an improved patient experience that is reinforced by evidence-based language for fast-track patients.

Benefits of Fast Tracks

A well-planned and well-operated fast track can increase both patient and staff satisfaction by eliminating wasted time and effort and easing the backlog of cases that arise during times of rapid patient influx. Long wait times, delays in care, capacity mismatches, and delays in admissions are all among the reasons for decreased patient satisfaction in the ED.[5]

By reducing these delays, fast tracks improve throughput, efficacy, and the patient experience. One study that evaluated patients' satisfaction with their length of stay (LOS), time spent with the provider, and the skills and personal manner of the provider found significant improvement in overall satisfaction after the initiation of a fast track.[5] In addition, this approach can alleviate the stress on staff that often results from backlogs and poor service quality.

Right Patient, Place, and Provider

The criteria used to determine who should be treated in the fast track are typically based on an assessment of the time and resources needed to treat the patient. Accurate triage is a vital factor that is frequently undervalued when developing and managing a successful fast track. It is essential to implement a triage practice that is reliable, valid, and based on the anticipated resources necessary to complete the patient's care. For the triage process to succeed, all staff (physicians, nurses, nurse practitioners [NPs], and physician assistants [PAs]) must possess a thorough understanding of the purpose of triage, the process of triage, and the use and leveraging of triage categories. Triage scales and systems must communicate the acuity and resource needs of patients assigned to each category. The goal is to get the right patient to the right place to be seen by the right provider in the right amount of time, and fast-track programs are an integral part of that process.

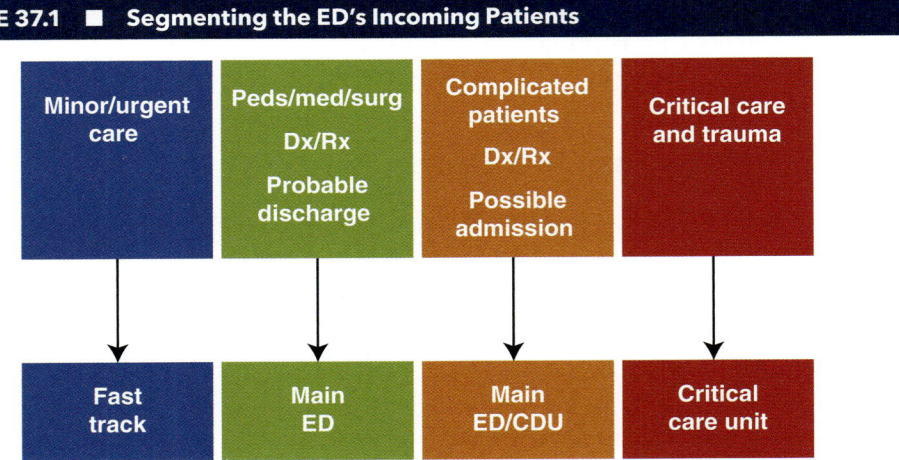

FIGURE 37.1 ■ Segmenting the ED's Incoming Patients

This can be achieved by:

- Reviewing guidelines necessary to develop a fast-track system within the ED
- Understanding the importance of defining and tracking measurable goals
- Implementing a successful fast-track program
- Avoiding common pitfalls
- Establishing a triage system based on resource allocation

DEPLOYING A FAST TRACK

The role of the fast track is to segment and serve low-acuity patients with conditions that are relatively easy to treat. The fast track is *not* a casual add-on or overflow unit; it is a "carve out"—a key component of the patient flow segmentation portfolio and solution set. Its key tactics are to:

- Optimize and maximize patient selection.
- Match the hours of operation to patient demand.
- Optimize space and capacity.
- Deploy the right clinical mix of providers for productivity.
- Devise the right evidence-based language (scripts) to optimize the patient experience.

To summarize, patients with simple or discrete problems should be fast-tracked through the ED, utilizing resources that are matched to service needs (**Figure 37.1**). The fast track allows an ED to carve out a stream of patients with limited diagnostic or therapeutic needs and expedite their care. This has a positive effect on the throughput of *all* patients in the ED. Fast-tracking requires space, staff, supplies, entry criteria, and protocols.

Improving Front-End Flow

Implementing a fast track requires the ability to leverage key actions and commit to enhancing front-end ED flow to maximize service capacity.[6] The following actions outline a potent approach to improving flow, safety, and the patient experience:

- Measure the patient demand by hour, and design a system to that demand.
- Ensure the triage processes enhance flow and avoid bottlenecks by segmenting low-acuity patients.
- Design and fully deploy a fast-track approach to uncomplicated patients.

- Commit to the "right stuff"—the right space, the right staffing mix, and the right staff.
- Establish a designated area for patients who are awaiting test results.
- Devise and implement a reliable method for tracking patients and results.

WILL A FAST TRACK HELP?

Fast tracks are designed specifically to decrease the throughput time of lower-acuity patients. Therefore, before deploying these resources, it is wise to determine if there is sufficient demand for such a service. This need can be determined by asking the following questions:

- Do the volume and types of patients seen in the ED warrant the development of a fast-track service?
- Are there too many ED patients who leave prior to receiving a medical screening exam?
- Does the hospital use a patient experience tool, and how is the ED service rated by the lower-acuity patients?
- How do the hospital leadership and the ED staff approach clinical operations and performance improvement?

Answers to these questions will require some data mining to assess the opportunities for improvement, the patient population (volume and acuity), and the current throughput of patients with specific diagnoses. These data determine the potential value of a fast-track delivery model listed in **Box 37.2**. Deploying a fast track that does not solve institution-specific patient flow issues can lead to frustration, dissonance, and wasted resources. For example, if a high percentage of the ED's patient population is elderly (with multiple morbidities that require numerous resources), implementing a fast track may not be the best use of that department's assets.

Key Performance Metrics and Entry Criteria

One common performance metric establishes the goal of managing 90% of ED fast-track patients with a total LOS of 60 minutes or less.[7] Achieving this standard improves wait times, shortens LOS (possibly for all patients), and leads to fewer patient "walkouts."[8] Decreasing LOS is a patient and staff satisfier. Therefore, if volume and acuity permit, it is appropriate from an operations management perspective to focus on chief complaints that require fewer

---

BOX 37.2 ■ ADVANTAGES OF FAST TRACK SYSTEMS

- Decreased patient wait times
- Increased flow by improving throughput for lower-acuity patients
- Decreased number of patients left without being seen (LWBS)
- Decreased unnecessary hospital admissions by providing timely care
- Decreased testing and costs (by evidence-based protocols)
- Improved quality and reliability through evidence-based approaches
- Ensured that specific providers are available for a specific group of patients
- Improved patient experience
- Improved staff engagement
- Improved accountability for defined parameters of success for a focused group of patients

resources and can be taken care of expeditiously (**Table 37.1**). Another approach to defining patients who are appropriate for the fast track is to cohort the Emergency Severity Index (ESI) 4s and ESI 5s (some EDs add specific "vertical" ESI 3s).

TABLE 37.1 ■ Potential ED Fast-Track Triage Guidelines

Policy: Patients with minor illnesses and injuries will be fast tracked to expedite their care.

Guidelines

1. Patients are triaged and designated as fast-track patients.
2. The mid-level practitioner examines and treats patients under the direct supervision of the ED physician.
3. The goal is for the mid-level practitioner to discharge patients in an average of 1 hour.
4. Complicated illness or injury may require specialty services, such as orthopedics, dentistry, or ophthalmology evaluation. If patient management can be expedited in fast track, patients receive care and are discharged as soon as possible from fast track.
5. Patients requiring intensive treatment, such as conscious sedation, are moved to the main treatment area for further management or admission.

Complaints that should be triaged to fast track:

- Eye problems: injury and infection
- Ear problems: injury and infection
- All throat problems (excluding respiratory distress)
- All dental problems
- Lacerations
- UTI symptoms (unless the patient is elderly or presents with vomiting, hypotension, or abdominal pain)
- STIs with no abdominal pain
- URIs including cough, cold, sinusitis, bronchitis (pulse oximetry >95)
- Insect bites/stings
- Animal bites
- Rashes
- Burns (restricted to one major body part)
- Soft-tissue injuries
- All occupational needle sticks
- Insect/mite infestations
- Nasal injuries (excluding epistaxis)
- Isolated minor trunk injuries
- Isolated extremity injuries (excluding open fractures or injuries requiring conscious sedation)
- Prescription refills
- Vaginal complaints: itching, discharge, lesions, foreign body (with no associated abdominal pain)
- Level 4 and 5 patients (according to 5-level triage acuity system)

Complaints that should NOT be fast tracked:

- Repeat ED visits
- Patients requiring conscious sedation
- Patients with positive loss of consciousness
- Cardiac/acute chest pain workups

WHAT IS THE GOAL?

Once it is decided that a fast track would be beneficial or that the performance of the current fast track could be optimized, the next (often overlooked) step is to define the goals and determine how success will be measured. A successful fast track relies on three strategic goals:

- Maintain high-quality, safe care (as measured by evidence-based standards).
- Achieve improved patient experience and staff engagement.
- Attain optimal patient flow with a short TAT/LOS.

Well-run fast tracks take a group of nonemergent ED patients requiring limited resources and apply a targeted intervention that decreases throughput time and improves satisfaction. This model can easily fail when goals are not well defined and capacity is not matched to demand. For example, if a fast track that is designed to handle lower-acuity patients routinely manages complex patients who require multiple resources, the entire process slows down—increasing TAT, decreasing patient satisfaction, and frustrating health-care staff. It is particularly important for leaders, managers, caregivers to have a clear and concise understanding of what the ED's fast track is—and what it is not (**Box 37.3**).

Once the fast track is operational, it is imperative to put systems in place that provide performance data to monitor objectives, productivity, outcomes, and patient satisfaction surveys. The information technology systems (electronic health records) can track the most common diagnoses seen in the fast track. Templates can be developed to improve the ease and speed of documentation. Advanced voice-activated technology and medical scribes can be used to lessen the documentation workload and optimize the delivery of patient care.

Typical fast-track quality indicators Include:

- Throughput times (subdivided, e.g., by diagnosis, resources used, practitioner
- Patient experience scores
- Staff engagement

A valuable tool for assessing outcomes, tracking productivity, and identifying opportunities for improvement was developed by two acute care NPs at Rush University

---

BOX 37.3 ■ FAST TRACK DEFINED

What it IS:
- A specific patient-centric product line
- A focused resource matching demand to capacity
- An enthusiastic A-Team focused on results
- Matches hours to patient arrival and acuity
- Dedicated to matching the right patients to the right resources

What it is NOT:
- An overflow unit
- A casual add-on
- A place for B-Team members
- A swing shift
- An obstacle to care

> **BOX 37.4 ■ ASSESSING FAST-TRACK OUTCOMES**
>
> 1. Identify the variable that you can impact.
> 2. Organize a team.
> 3. Clarify current knowledge: What do you want to improve and why?
> 4. Understand and anticipate variation.
> 5. How will you improve it?
> 6. Plan the implementation.
> 7. Follow the plan.
> 8. Review/analyze the data.
> 9. How will you use what you found to improve practice?

in Chicago (**Box 37.4**). This tool provides a structure for for problem-solving and tracking productivity, putting this framework into action.

Delivering quality care to lower-acuity patients should not negatively affect the care given to the higher-acuity or critically ill patients. Multiple studies have shown that the development of a fast track does not diminish the quality of care delivered to high-acuity patients.[9] In fact, the implementation of these programs has been shown to reduce the time between a critically ill patient's arrival and their clinical assessment.[10] Additionally, a survey of patients and staff at Dartmouth-Hitchcock Medical Center found a significant improvement in both staff and patient satisfaction following the development of a fast track.[11]

IMPLEMENTING OR REFINING A FAST TRACK

Once a decision has been made to develop or refine a fast track and goals have been set, the next step is to organize an implementation team.

Developing a Team

Members of the fast-track implementation team should include key stakeholders and those who come into regular contact with the fast track:

- Registration staff
- Patient care technicians
- Nurses
- Nurse's aides
- Physicians
- Nurse practitioners
- Physician's assistants
- Essential services (lab and imaging)
- Administrators
- Patients (optional)

These key stakeholders can help determine the design, location, hours of operation, and structure of the fast track. It is essential to ensure that all appropriate participants have a voice in the design and implementation of the program. These considerations are similar whether one is establishing a new fast track, working with an already existing model, or seeking to optimize performance, capacity, throughput, or satisfaction.

Using a Lean Framework

The simplest and most easily implemented definition of Lean in health care is "adding value and eliminating waste as patients move through the service transitions and queues of patient care."[6] Lean structure includes the following components:

- Creating value
- Eliminating waste
- Promoting flow
- Achieving continuous improvement
- Developing people

Lean theory assumes that frontline workers know the system intimately and often have the answers to problems that regularly arise. Rather than managers having sole control over the process, frontline workers are given the autonomy and accountability to adapt and improve the system. Lean organizations empower their staff by teaching them to improve their workplace and giving them the tools to do so.[12] The bottom line is that the more frontline workers are engaged and empowered, the more they become vested in the results. In turn, this participation and commitment increases the team's ability to create a successful fast track.

Location, Location, Location

A key variable to consider is the location of the fast track in the ED. The designated fast-track area should consist of a defined number of treatment spaces modeled on the projected volume of patients that will be seen. With the help of the team, it is also crucial to stock the area with the equipment and supplies that will be used most often, eliminating wasteful visits to the stockroom. Essential service personnel (e.g., laboratory, radiology, registration) should be included in the planning.

Locating the fast track near the main ED is often a best practice, since this allows open communication between the triage nurse, charge nurse, charge physician, and other clinicians. An adjoining location is particularly important when a fast-track patient requires more resources than expected and further care must be coordinated with the main ED. One study found that 5% of patients triaged as "nonurgent" required admission to the hospital after evaluation in the ED.[3]

Communication is also essential when volume exceeds typical patient arrival patterns. For instance, if an unusually large number of either low- or high-acuity patients arrive in the ED, the charge nurse, the health-care providers in the fast track, and the staff in the core treatment area can collectively allocate the best resources and providers to deliver efficient care to all ED patients. A fast track that is in close proximity or adjacent to the main ED allows for frequent communication and the simple shifting of patients or resources as emergent needs dictate.

Hours of Operation

A critical variable to consider is the hours of operation. An evaluation of the volume and acuity by hour of the day and day of the week will help determine the demand for fast-track hours of operation. The hourly capacity of the fast track should be based on the hourly demand of eligible patients. Typically, fast tracks are open during peak volume times, with overlapping day and evening shifts, and coincide with increases in main ED staffing

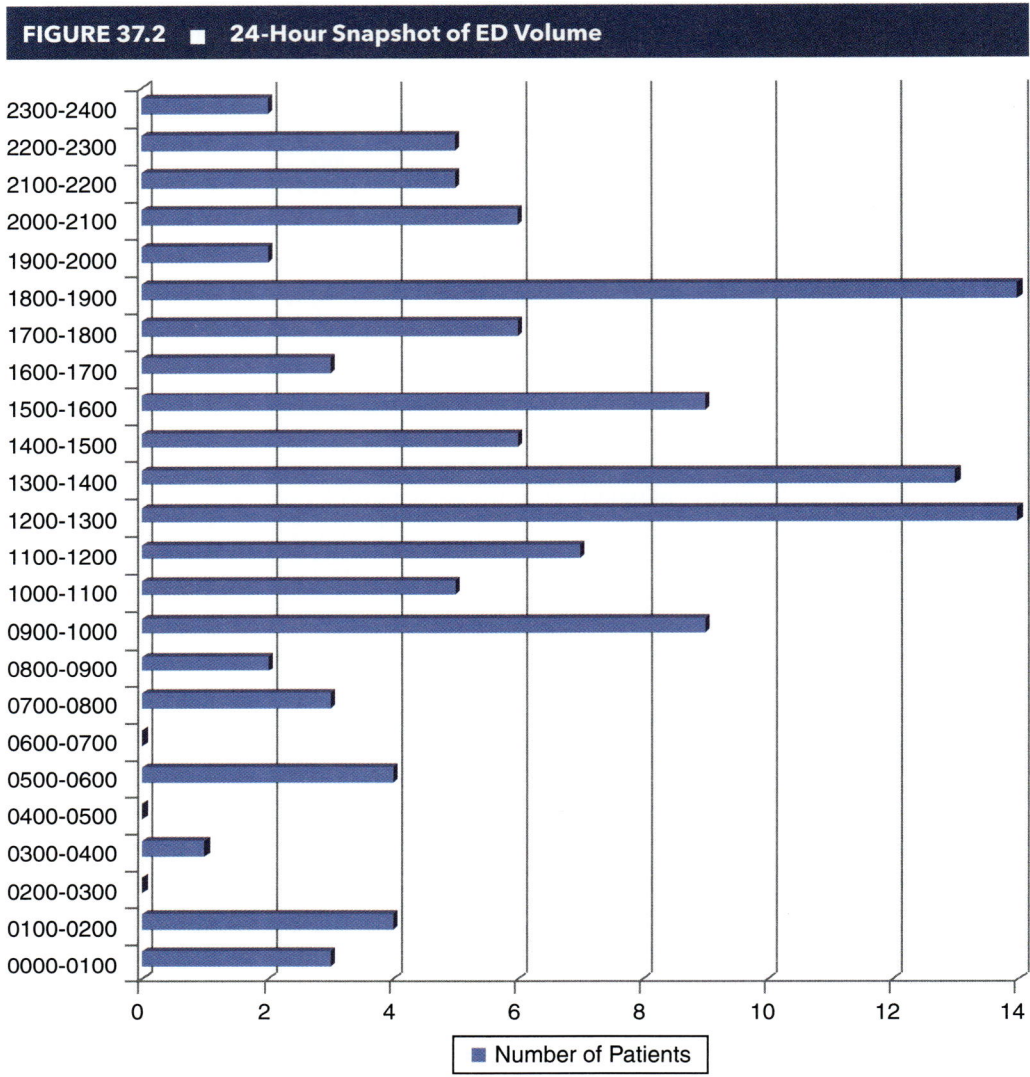

FIGURE 37.2 ■ 24-Hour Snapshot of ED Volume

patterns (**Figure 37.2**). Utilizing key questions, the arrival of the patients who will benefit from a fast track is a realistically predictable operational metric (**Box 37.5**).

Provider Staffing

The number and type of staff used in a fast track can be calculated by taking into account patient volume, patient acuity, the projected fast-track LOS, and the number of treatment spaces. Efficiency and throughput are critical to patient care in a fast track.

BOX 37.5 ■ KEY QUESTIONS TO STUDY PATIENT ARRIVALS

- How many patients are coming?
- When are they coming?
- What are they going to need?
- Is our service capacity going to match patient demand?
- If not, what are we going to do about it?

Fueled by the shortage of emergency physicians and the proliferation of NP and PA programs, fast tracks are increasingly staffed by nonphysician providers (advance practice providers [APPs]). Patients have become accustomed to receiving high-quality care from a variety of nonphysician providers. The educational backgrounds of APPs often position them to be ideal fast-track providers in collaboration with, and in some cases independent of, ED physicians. Other fast-track models of care include staffing by an emergency physician, family medicine physician, or a resident. One patient survey found that only 36% were willing to wait longer to see an MD (rather than a PA); of that group, only 5% were willing to wait more than 60 additional minutes.[3]

Regardless of whether the fast track is staffed by resident physicians, NPs, or PAs, it is important for all clinicians to have access to a supervising physician. Physician consultation may be necessary for several reasons, including atypical presentations, unexpected complexity, or simply the need for a second opinion.

Triage Criteria

A successful fast track ensures that patients are appropriately assigned. These patients must be stable, without obvious threats to life or limb. The number of diagnostic and therapeutic resources likely to be used should be incorporated into the triage decision.[14] Patients requiring single, rapidly performed diagnostic tests (e.g., x-ray) are appropriate for the fast track. Alternately, the use of multiple resources (e.g., computed tomography, specialty consultation, intravenous hydration) requires substantial time and is usually inappropriate for the fast track. Further delays occur as the provider both waits for and responds to the results. Patients who require multiple diagnostic and therapeutic resources will typically exceed the desired LOS for fast-track patients; their care should be provided in the main treatment area.

Thus, a successful fast track begins at triage. The Emergency Nurses' Association and the American College of Emergency Physicians have endorsed the use of multilevel acuity scales, including the ESI and the Canadian Triage and Acuity Scale.[15,16] These tools are evidence based and have been shown to have high inter-rater reliability, ensuring that patients are triaged objectively based on clinical condition rather than on subjective staff perceptions. These triage systems use multilevel acuity scales that integrate resource utilization and allow the triage nurse to segment and stream patients.

A triage nurse must be both knowledgeable and experienced in order to safely meet the demands of this role. While it can be easy to identify an obviously critically ill patient, segmenting patients on the lower end of the acuity scale requires expertise and judgment. All ED nurses should be exposed to the ESI scale during orientation and be familiar with the department's triage process. Similarly, all ED providers must understand the implications of receiving a patient designated as ESI level 1 or 2 and the need for immediate intervention. When training nurses for triage, it may be helpful to use the Agency for Healthcare Research and Quality materials on version 4 of the ESI scale.[17] Successful completion of a triage competency and skills checklist may be used to conclude the formal orientation.

Patient Experience Opportunities

Fast-track (as a verb) also entails opportunities to improve patient satisfaction. The team members must all use evidence-based language (scripts) to reinforce the fact that they are dedicated to delivering excellent care. Evidence-based language is language that has been shown to be effective. Examples include:

Based on your symptoms, I can triage you to our fast-track unit, which has a dedicated team of people who can take care of you now.

Hello, I'm Isak, your nurse, and I'll be taking care of you here in our fast-track unit, where we have a team of professionals to care for you now.

Mrs. Smith, I'm Dr. Rodriguez, and I'm the emergency physician who will be taking care of you today. I'm sorry this happened to you, but I'm delighted to be your doctor and to be working with a team of people who are focused on getting you better as quickly as possible here in our fast-track unit.

Mr. Jones, I'm happy to say that we had a goal of completing your care in less than 60 minutes in fast track, and we were able to do so in just 45 minutes. Have we met your expectations and answered all your questions?

Thanks for choosing our fast-track unit. We hope you will feel comfortable recommending it to others when they need emergency care.

Each fast-track unit should regularly review what evidence-based language has worked well. At staff meetings, the team can review the scripts and augment the discussion with letters and e-mails praising the service.

CONCLUSION

As many as 60% of ED patients present with nonurgent complaints. The wide variability of acuities places increased responsibility on department leaders to create a triage function that ensures that every patient is seen rapidly, regardless of the seriousness of their presentation.

The Fast-Track Strategy

The development of a fast track is one strategy that can be used to effectively manage the sheer volume of patients in many EDs. Fast tracks function as parallel systems within the ED with a unique set of goals.[19] Monitoring productivity and outcomes is essential to sustain and improve a fast track. The unit may be thought of as a small operation within a larger one, which uses service operations management approaches to provide and monitor high-quality care. Efficient flow of all ED patients is supported by The Joint Commission, which requires hospitals to identify and correct impediments to this critical process. Educational resources like Urgent Matters (sponsored by the Robert Woods Johnson Foundation) allow and encourage EDs across the country to share workplace solutions related to flow.[18]

Prioritizing patients with fast-track complaints over patients who are more acutely ill can appear to go against the traditional rationale behind triage and emergency medicine (*take the sickest first*). Thus, it is essential to clearly communicate the rationale behind the fast track before it can become a source of conflict among providers.

Ensuring Success

A well-designed fast track embodies a set of streamlined processes designed to service a defined group of patients. The effective fast track is operationalized with staff, space, supplies, and specific service hours that run parallel to and independent of the delivery system in place for acute patients.

Successful implementation of a fast track requires department leaders to clearly communicate patient care goals and create an environment of mutual respect, trust, and commitment. It also requires the provision of necessary resources to ensure sufficient capacity and desired capabilities. A strong program can be achieved by engaging key staff in the development, monitoring, and continuous improvement of the program.

REFERENCES

1. Merriam-Webster. Fast track. 2017. Available at: http://www.meriam-webstercollegiate.com/dictionary. Accessed September 15, 2018.
2. Rui P, Kang K. National Hospital Ambulatory Medical Care Survey: 2015 Emergency Department Summary Tables. 2016. Available at: http://www.cdc.gov/nchs/data/ahcd/nhamcs_emergency/2015_ed_web_tables.pdf. Accessed September 15, 2018.
3. Wiler JL, Gentle C, Halfpenny JM, et al. Optimizing emergency department front-end operations. *Ann Emerg Med*. 2010;55(2):142-160.
4. Rodi S, Grau M, Orsini C. Evaluation of a fast track unit: alignment of resources and demand results in improved satisfaction and decreased length of stay for emergency department patients. *Qual Manag Health Care*. 2006;15(30):163-170.
5. Veronesi J. Musing on emergency department patient satisfaction. *Top Emerg Med*. 2005;27(4):258-264.
6. Mayer T, Jensen K. *Hardwiring Flow: Systems and Processes for Seamless Patient Care*. Gulf Breeze, Fla: Fire Starter Publishing; 2009.
7. Considine J, Kropman M, Kelly E, Winter C. Effect of emergency department fast track on emergency department length of stay: a case-control study. *Emerg Med J*. 2008;25(12):815-819.
8. Guido K. Making an ED fast track exactly that—fast and efficient. *J Med Pract Manage*. 2007;23(3):197-198.
9. Cooke M, Wilson S, Pearson S. The effect of a separate stream for minor injuries on accident and emergency department waiting times. *Emerg Med J*. 2002;19(1):28-30.
10. Darrab AA, Fan J, Fernandes CM, et al. How does fast track affect quality of care in the emergency department? *Eur J Emerg Med*. 2006;13(1):32-35.
11. Nash K, Zachariah B, Nischmann J, Psencik B. Evaluation of the fast track unit of a university emergency department. *J Emerg Nurs*. 2007;33(1):14-19.
12. Holden RJ. Lean thinking in emergency departments: a critical review. *Ann Emerg Med*. 2011;57(3):265-278.
13. Mundinger MO, Kane RL, Lenz ER, et al. Primary care outcomes in patients treated by nurse practitioners or physicians: a randomized trial. *JAMA*. 2000;283(1):59-68.
14. Wiler JL, Rooks SP, Ginde AA. Update on midlevel provider utilization in US emergency departments, 2006 to 2009. *Acad Emerg Med*. 2012;19(8):986-989.
15. American College of Emergency Physicians and Emergency Nurses Association. Joint ACEP/ENA Policy Statement: standardized ED triage and acuity categorization. 2017. Accessed January 1, 2020.
16. ACEP. Clinical practice and management: triage scale standardization. Approved January 2017. Available at: http://www.acep.orgessed. Accessed September 15, 2018.
17. Agency for Healthcare Research and Quality. ESI version 4. 2017. Available at: http://www.ahrq.gov/research/esi/esi1.htm. Accessed September 15, 2018.
18. Quattrini V, Swan B. Evaluating care in ED fast tracks. *J Emerg Nurs*. 2011;37:40-46. Urgent Matters. Available at: http://www.urgentmatters.org/. Accessed June 2, 2013.

ADDITIONAL READINGS

- ACEP: Emergency Medicine Practice Committee of the American College of Emergency Physicians. Emergency department crowding: high-impact solutions. 2016. Available at: https://www.acep.org/Legislation-and-Advocacy/Practice-Management-Issues/Boarding/Crowding/Emergency-Department-Crowding---High-Impact-Solutions/.
- Advisory Board. *Building the Clockwork ED: Best Practices for Eliminating Bottlenecks and Delays in the ED*. Washington, DC: HWorks, An Advisory Board Company; 2000.
- Advisory Board. *The High-Performance ED Optimizing Capacity and Throughput to Meet Ever-Growing Demand*. Washington, DC: HWorks, An Advisory Board Company; 2008.
- Ardagh MW, Wells JE, Cooper K, Lyons R, Patterson R, O'Donovan P. Effect of a rapid assessment clinic on the waiting time to be seen by a doctor and the time spent in the department, for patients presenting to an urban emergency department: a controlled prospective trial. *N Z Med J*. 2002;115:U28.
- Arya R, Wei G, McCoy JV, et al. Decreasing length of stay in the emergency department with a split emergency severity index 3 patient flow model. *Acad Emerg Med*. 2013;20(11):1171-1179.
- Baker S. *Excellence in the Emergency Department: How to Get Results*. Gulf Breeze, Fla: Fire Starter Publishing; 2009.
- Bish PA, McCormick MA, Otegbeye M. Ready-JET-go: split flow accelerates ED throughput. *J Emerg Nurs*. 2016;42(2):114-119.
- Considine J, Kropman M, Kelly E, Winter C. Effect of emergency department fast track on emergency department length of stay: a case control study. *Emerg Med J*. 2008;25:815-819.
- Cooke MW, Wilson S, Pearson S. The effect of a separate stream for minor injuries on accident and emergency department waiting times. *Emerg Med J*. 2002;19:28-30.
- Crane JT, Noon CE. *The Definitive Guide to Emergency Department Operational Improvement: Employing Lean Principles with Current ED Best Practices to Create the "No Wait" Department*. New York, NY: Productivity Press; 2011.
- Darrab AA, Fan J, Fernandes CM, et al. How does fast track affect quality of care in the emergency department? *Eur J Emerg Med*. 2006;13:32-35.
- Emergency Nurses Association. Staffing guidelines—Emergency Nurses Association. Position Statement—Staffing and Productivity in the Emergency Department. 2017.
- Fernandes CM, Christenson JM, Price A. Continuous quality improvement reduces length of stay for fast-track patients in an emergency department. *Acad Emerg Med*. 1996;3:258-263.
- Higginson I1, Whyatt J, Silvester K. Demand and capacity planning in the emergency department how to do it. *Emerg Med J*. 2011;28(2):128-35. doi:10.1136/emj.2009.087411.
- Ieraci S, Digiusto E, Sonntag P, et al. Streaming by case complexity: evaluation of a model for emergency department fast track. *Emerg Med Australas*. 2008;20(3):241-249.
- Kelly AM, Bryant M, Cox L, Jolley D. Improving emergency department efficiency by patient streaming to outcomes-based teams. *Aust Health Rev*. 2007;31:16-21.
- Kilic YA, Agalar FA, Kunt M, Cakmakci M. Prospective, double-blind, comparative fast-tracking trial in an academic emergency department during a period of limited resources. *Eur J Emerg Med*. 1998;5:403-406.

- Kwa P, Blake D. Fast track: has it changed patient care in the emergency department? *Emerg Med Australas.* 2008;20:10-15.
- O'Brien D, Williams A, Blondell K, Jelinek GA. Impact of streaming "fast track" emergency department patients. *Aust Health Rev.* 2006;30:525-532.
- Oredsson S, Jonsson H, Rognes J, et al. A systematic review of triage-related interventions to improve patient flow in emergency departments. *Scand J Trauma J Resusc Emerg Med.* 2011;19:43.
- Poon S, Schuur J, Mehrotra A. Trends in visits to acute care venues for treatment of low-acuity conditions in the United States from 2008 to 2015 [published online ahead of print September 4, 2018]. *JAMA Intern Med.* doi:10.1001/jamainternmed.2018.3205.
- Rogers T, Ross N, Spooner D. Evaluation of a 'See and Treat' pilot study introduced to an emergency department. *Accid Emerg Nurs.* 2004;12:24-27.
- Rodi SW, Grau MV, Orsini CM. Evaluation of a fast track unit: alignment of resources and demand results in improved satisfaction and decreased length of stay for emergency department patients. *Qual Manag Health Care.* 2006;15:163-170.
- Sanchez M, Smally AJ, Grant RJ, Jacobs LM. Effects of a fast-track area on emergency department performance. *J Emerg Med.* 2006;31:117-120.
- Vaghasiya MR, Murphy M, O'Flynn D, et al. The Emergency Department Prediction of Disposition (EPOD) study. *Australas Emerg Nurs J.* 2014;17(4):161-166.
- Wiler JL, Rooks SP, Ginde AA. Update on midlevel provider utilization in US emergency departments, 2006 to 2009. *Acad Emerg Med.* 2012;19(8):986-989.

CHAPTER 38
OPTIMIZING PATIENT THROUGHPUT

Joseph Twanmoh, Kirk Jensen, P. K. Howard, Robert W. Strauss

The time from initial physician contact to disposition decision is a critical interval in the flow of a patient through the emergency department (ED). Patient flow can be described by a classical service operations model (**Figure 38.1**):

- *Input*: Arrival to provider evaluation (door to physician)
- *Throughput*: Doctor to diagnosis and disposition decision (physician to decision)
- *Output*: Disposition decision to actual disposition (decision to disposition)

The throughput interval between the physician contact and the patient's deposition represents the segment of the visit during which patients receive their assessments, diagnostic testing, therapeutic interventions, diagnosis, and disposition decision. In addition, it is the time in which patients and their family members get their most important questions answered:

- "What's wrong?"
- "Is it serious?"
- "What needs to be done?"
- "Do I get to go home or will I be admitted?"

The input interval (i.e., the time between arrival and seeing a clinician) and output interval (i.e., the time from disposition to departure) are two segments of the patient visit in which the registration and nursing staff play key roles. During the physician-to-disposition decision interval, physicians and advanced practice providers (APPs) assume a primary role. Although nurse-initiated orders and triage protocols may expedite care during this

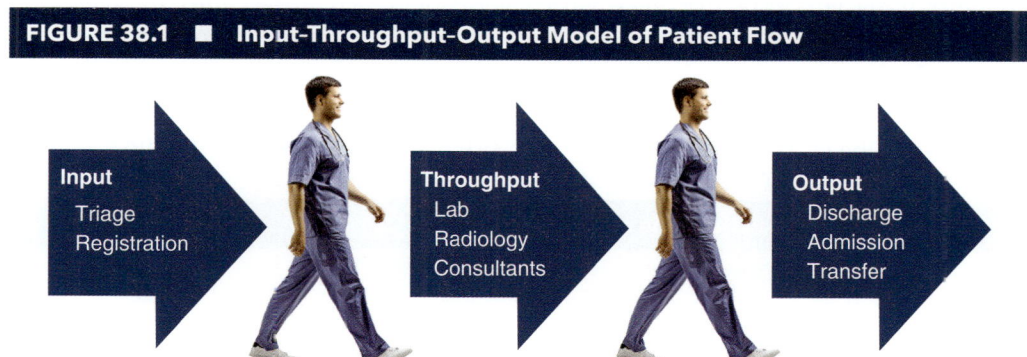

FIGURE 38.1 ■ Input-Throughput-Output Model of Patient Flow

Input: Triage, Registration
Throughput: Lab, Radiology, Consultants
Output: Discharge, Admission, Transfer

throughput interval, the physician or APP primarily directs throughput. They start the evaluation and workup, and make a disposition once all necessary diagnostic test results, consultations, and treatments have been completed.

CRITICAL SERVERS

The term *throughput* will be used throughout this chapter to refer to the phase during which physicians/APPs evaluate patients and make their disposition decisions. *Provider* will be used to encompass medical providers: physicians and APPs unless otherwise specified. *Nursing staff* will refer to registered nurses, licensed practical nurses, and unlicensed assistive personnel. *Beds* will refer to any type of treatment space, including hallway stretchers and chairs that may be used for the initial evaluation and treatment or while awaiting test results.

Matching demand to capacity is essential to achieve effective patient flow. In any ED, there are three main critical resources: beds, nursing staff, and physicians/APPs. A deficit in any one of these three critical resources or *servers* (i.e., physicians/APPs, nursing staff, or beds) will significantly compromise the effectiveness and productivity of the other two.

This observation is further illuminated by applying the theory of constraints (TOC) to ED operations and services. Applying the TOC helps to identify the multiple bottlenecks to patient care and flow (**Figure 38.2**).[1] Some constraints or bottlenecks are more significant than others, backing up flow throughout the entire process or system. Once these critical constraints are identified, it is essential to either ease ("elevate" in TOC terms) or eliminate them. If the tightest or critical bottlenecks are not effectively addressed, efforts to improve flow through the system will have limited success.

For example, imagine a frequently congested and overwhelmed four-lane highway, with two traffic lanes in each direction. Recognizing the problem, county road planners decide to increase traffic capacity by widening the highway to three lanes in each direction. However the highway also has a bridge in the middle that, due to budgetary constraints, remains unchanged: two lanes in each direction. Traffic will always back up no matter how many lanes are built before or after the bridge. Total transit time will not improve and may, in fact, worsen.

Nurses understand that if there are not enough physician resources, the ED becomes crowded and dysfunctional with long waits. Nurses can draw blood for labs, start intravenous solutions (IVs), and ask for medication orders; ultimately, however, patients cannot be diagnosed, admitted, or discharged without significant physician engagement. Similarly, physicians recognize that when a majority of ED beds are occupied by "boarders" (i.e., admitted patients), then nurses and beds are effectively taken out of service. In this setting, physicians may be unproductive and unable to see new patients.

A common misperception is that critical resources and servers are fixed in the throughput phase. As a result, attention is often primarily focused on speeding up

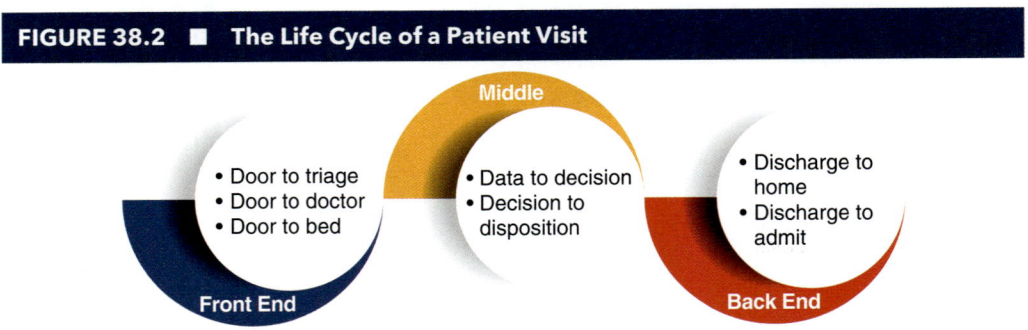

FIGURE 38.2 ■ The Life Cycle of a Patient Visit

essential services such as laboratory and radiology (lanes before the bridge). While these services can represent bottlenecks to flow and will be addressed later, the workflow and capacity of beds and the clinical team often represent the critical constraints (the bridge) to patient flow, and these must be addressed first.

In addition to considering physicians/APPs, nurses, and beds as critical servers, it is equally important to ensure that all of these servers are "operating at the top of their license," meaning they are functioning at a level consistent with their training and expertise. For example, allowing trained EMTs to start IVs and perform other functions frees up nurses to utilize their critical thinking skills for the benefit of the patient. Having an APP do the laceration repair and wound care instead of the emergency physician frees up the doctor to drive flow. As efforts to optimize throughput are deployed, "operating at the top of their licenses" should be a key driver.

PATIENT FLOW CHALLENGES

Box 38.1 lists common circumstances that often challenge the health-care team during the throughput phase and affect the performance and productivity of the critical servers.

Hospital Boarders

ED boarding (retaining admitted patients in the ED until they can be transferred to hospital inpatient beds) and its deleterious effects on patient safety, patient experience, and ED crowding have been studied extensively and produce predictably negative effects in all domains. Boarding is unlikely to completely go away, and simply increasing the number of beds is seldom an available solution. From a patient flow standpoint, boarders produce two undesirable outcomes. They consume nursing staff and occupy beds, reducing the functional capacity of two of the ED's three critical servers, and produce downward pressure on the third.

All EDs have waiting rooms that serve as a buffer for patient influx into the treatment areas. Even high-performance EDs have patients in their waiting rooms from time to time due to natural variations in patient arrivals and complexity. From the perspective of numerous hospital personnel, the ED functions as a triage area and waiting room for unscheduled inpatient admissions. For many hospitals, ED admissions can represent 60% or more of hospital admissions. The ED determines where and to which service patients should be admitted, and patients often wait in the ED for their inpatient beds to be available.

> **BOX 38.1 ■ CHALLENGES TO ED PRODUCTIVITY**
>
> - Hospital boarders in the ED
> - Server mismatches: allocation and deployment of critical resources
> - Misuse of key resources
> - Unfilled shifts
> - Bed closures due to construction or renovation
> - The single-server bottleneck
> - The implications of the utilization curve
> - Using average volume for planning purposes

Approaching hospital administration with demands that the ED never house boarders is unlikely to be a successful management strategy. Instead, one should determine how much boarding one's department can tolerate without negatively impacting patient care, flow, and safety. Except in very small EDs, managing one noncritical boarder for several hours will not significantly impact throughput or wait times. But, how would two boarders, or three, or more affect throughput? At some point, a threshold is crossed where boarding becomes untenable for both the patients and the providers. That threshold is facility- and acuity-dependent but can be identified through the use of data. When the numbers of boarders per day and length of stay (LOS) per day are studied, a pattern emerges. This "boarder threshold" is the place to begin discussions with hospital administration on "boarder relief," the point at which the ED needs additional beds and nurses to continue to function efficiently and safely. A variety of solutions are possible. Inpatient nurses could come down to the ED to manage patients. Boarders could be moved to a temporary holding location or an express admitting unit. ED staff could annex a nearby area to treat admitted patients. The solutions will depend primarily on the resources and space available.

Allocation and Deployment of Critical Resources

Allocation mismatch refers to improper matching of beds, nurses, and physicians. In larger EDs, patient care areas are often closed down late at night as volume decreases and opened back up during the day as volume ramps up. Staffing for both physicians and nurses increases during the day. But, do these critical servers ramp up and ramp down together in a coordinated fashion, and are physician and nursing staff schedules synchronized, or are they unplanned and disconnected?

Schedule mismatch occurs when the nursing and physician schedules are not synchronized in terms of hours and capacity. Two examples:

- ED patient volume predictably rises at 10:00 am. An additional physician or APP is scheduled to meet that demand. However, if additional nurses do not arrive until 11:00 am, at which time another treatment area is opened, then the 1 hour of physician staffing without appropriate nursing support represents a wasted resource, and a bottleneck will be created.
- The scheduled nurse and APP start their fast-track shifts at the same time, but the APP is responsible for reviewing culture results and x-ray variances during the first hour and does not see patients.

Misuse of Key Resources

Increased Patient Volumes

The volume of ED patients in the United States has steadily risen and now exceeds 130 million patients annually. Beyond the increase in volume, there has been a significant shift in the acuity and composition of patients. Trauma is a smaller component of the emergency medicine patient cohort with a corresponding rise in complex medical conditions. ED patients classified as 4 and 5 on the Emergency Severity Index (ESI) are decreasing, while ESI 3 patients are increasing.[2] As the population ages, the number of geriatric patients seen in EDs has risen, driving higher acuity and complexity.

These higher-acuity patients increasingly visit the ED for a myriad of complex medical and social challenges, including chronic diseases and mental health issues. These patients seldom have access to primary care and may not have anywhere else to go. In such cases, the ED is the only health-care safety net.

Vertical Versus Horizontal ESI 3 Patients

Historically, EDs have operated on a dedicated-bed model, where each patient was assigned a bed and stayed there for the duration of their visit. This model may have worked well 10 or 20 years ago. However, the traditional model of a dedicated bed for each patient is not consistent with rising ESI 3 patient volumes. Recently, EDs have begun using the vertical patient concept, where nonacute patients (vertical patients) are not necessarily placed in a bed for their entire stay but rather are quickly assessed (often in a chair, perhaps in a bed) and then moved to and managed in a "results-pending" environment. "Keeping vertical patients vertical" frees bed spaces for incoming or complex patients. The challenge is distinguishing vertical from horizontal patients. Within the ESI 3 category, patients may be "vertical 3s" or "horizontal 3s" depending on the need for resources, including a bed (**Table 38.1**).

Maximizing bed capacity by identifying the vertical patient who will not require a prolonged in-bed dwell time is vital to optimal patient flow. Assuming that virtually all admitted patients will require a bed, it is essential to determine which of the remaining patients are potential vertical patients. Patients who are elderly, frail, or have multiple comorbid conditions or problems require a dedicated treatment bed. Many of the remaining patients may be able to be treated as vertical patients for at least a portion if not for their entire stay. Consider the effect on bed capacity if half or a third of ED patients discharged home could be treated in vertical treatment spaces. The bed capacity constraint could be greatly reduced.

TABLE 38.1 ■ Segmentation Scheme for ESI 3 Patients

Vertical	Horizontal
Able to sit up	Needing to lay down
Not in severe discomfort	Likely to be admitted
Not anticipating prolonged workup or procedure	Need for extensive fluids (>1 L)
Nontraumatic flank pain	Complex wound closure (needs plastics)
Headache	Impaired (alcohol or drugs)
Pregnant with vaginal bleeding	Need for contrasted CT/imaging
Vomiting/diarrhea needing hydration	Abdominal pain
Back pain, ambulatory, minor mechanism, afebrile	Needs cardiac monitoring
Mild asthma	Short of breath, especially >50 old
Respiratory complaint with oxygen saturation >92%	Weak and/or dizzy
Chest pain <30 years of age without cardiac history, normal electrocardiogram	Gastrointestinal bleeding
Vaginal spotting	Syncope or near syncope
Isolated extremity swelling	Sickle cell patients
Minor epistaxis	

ESI criteria alone are insufficient to define vertical versus horizontal patients because of inconsistencies in the following:

- Nature of ESI 3 patients
- Application of ESI criteria
- Evaluations performed by various providers
- Hand-offs from one provider to another

Inevitably, there are well-defined difficulties that can be avoided by developing clear guidelines to define patient placements, evaluations (order sets), and hand-offs.

Unfilled Shifts

Unfilled shifts on the schedule, whether due to staffing shortages or to unanticipated illness, adversely affect throughput. Patient arrivals represent natural variation; patient volume predictably rises in the morning and falls off late at night. Staffing can be adjusted around that predictable variation. Unfilled shifts represent artificial variation. If they are unpredictable and unplanned for, unfilled shifts are detrimental to patient care. Open shifts on a schedule or sick calls should be actively managed, since even ideal plans for staffing to patient volume and demand are of little worth if there are insufficient nursing staff or providers to fill the schedule.

On a short-term basis, staffing shortages can be managed with a variety of short-term solutions, such as incentives to work extra shifts, mandatory overtime, and travelers/locum tenens practitioners (generally professionals who take short-term assignments in hospitals with staffing needs). A backup call system may be used to address sick-call vacancies (excessive sick call often requires a change in human resource management and policy). On a long-term basis, recruiting, retention, and engagement are best practices to manage nursing staffing shortages.

Bed Closures

Fortunately, bed closures due to construction or renovation are usually known well in advance. The best strategy is to find a way to replace these beds on a provisional basis. Temporarily annexing other space, including unused hallway space, can achieve this goal. Thinking that the clinical team can just work a bit harder and faster to make up for a shortage in beds is an example of tempting but flawed reasoning, for it is operationally and mathematically unsound.

The Single-Server Bottleneck

Single-server bottlenecks can occur anytime one – and only one – individual is responsible for a task. This bottleneck occurs when demand significantly exceeds that server's capacity. In any system, a single server can and will get overwhelmed at times. Because one critically ill patient can significantly impact flow by creating a backlog of cases, the overwhelmed provider may spend the entire shift just trying to catch up.

The single-server bottleneck is prevalent in many ED settings, not just those with solo physician coverage. Consider departments that might have just one triage nurse, a single provider in fast track, or a single phlebotomist in the ED who can become overwhelmed, resulting in longer throughput times. Segmentation of space and resources, such as deploying a fast-track or dedicated areas for pediatric or geriatric patients, can create other areas or processes where single servers may exist.

While patient demand on average may justify staffing by a single person, simply being resigned to critical and lengthy bottlenecks in single single-server lines is unacceptable. Instead, develop processes to buffer single servers when demand overwhelms capacity. For instance, an average triage volume of four to five patients per hour may justify only a single nurse. However, five or even 10 patients could arrive in 10 minutes, completely overwhelming the most experienced triage nurse. The lone triage nurse needs immediate backup to manage the influx of patients, some of whom may be quite ill. Advance planning for this occurrence could include pulling another nurse (or two) to assist. Another option is directly bedding some patients to off-load demand from the triage nurse (and, thereby, alleviating pressure on a constraint).

As departments become larger, sub-segmentation of patient flow and throughput is often useful or necessary. Consider a department that treats 100,000 patients per year in one large rectangular treatment area. Walking from one end to the other to see patients would result in significant wasted time each day, and communicating with staff members at either end would be difficult. In this and similar settings, it is necessary to develop patient care approaches, such as pods, specialty areas, and the like, that move dedicated resources (space, staff, services, supplies, and so on) closer together while also providing clear visual sight lines to allow for robust and effective communication.

An additional challenge is that queue management becomes exponentially more complicated as multiple areas are segmented off, particularly when patient populations are subdivided. For example, consider a department with just two areas, a low-acuity area and a high-acuity area, as well as a provider in triage. Some days, there may be a surfeit of low-acuity patients. Other days, there may be a preponderance of high-acuity patients. If one of the designated patient areas becomes full and patients must wait for a bed in that specific area, physician time to disposition time will increase. Just as nursing staff and physicians need to be agile and flexible, beds need to be flexible to meet the variable acuity of patients on any given day. Assuming that the low- and high-acuity areas are adjacent, it can be helpful if some beds can flex between high and low acuity.

Implications of the Utilization Curve

Queuing theory predicts that as utilization for any given server begins to reach capacity, wait times for that server will inevitably rise. As beds fill, patients wait longer for the next available bed. As a clinical team cares for more patients, the queue for that team's services gets longer. At some point, team members become too busy to see the next patient or even to reevaluate their existing ones. All patients, particularly those are undergoing pre-evaluations, will experience longer wait times. Since all systems have limited resources, it is imperative to determine what processes are in place to effectively deploy critical resources in times of need.

Using Average Volume for Planning Purposes

Because the arrival of patients is random and is an example of "natural variation," it is predictable within a range. One obvious way to misjudge staffing is to go by the average of hourly arrivals. More than 50% of the time, the average number of arrivals over a span of hours is unlikely to be the actual number of arrivals in any particular hour.

An appreciation of the variation in patient arrivals (from the mean) is critical to optimal demand–capacity planning.

Many staffing plans are based on nearly 100% staff utilization during peak periods. However, both queuing theory and experience have shown that consistent utilization over 85% often overwhelms staff resources and creates system failure. When the ED is under-resourced and operating at the high end of the utilization curve, wait times for critical servers and lengths of stay will become excessive. Adding to the complexity, staffing plans based purely on average patient arrivals seldom factor in patient acuity.

Few departments have the data management and statistical support to develop sophisticated demand–capacity curves based on volume and acuity. Without these modeling systems, most leaders attempt to improve the existing system by redeploying the current staffing, usually an inaccurate and inadequate process. When performing an analysis, key questions include:

- When do backups or waits occur?
- Which critical resource is the biggest bottleneck to flow?
- What changes, or adjustments in resources, can be applied?

EXPEDITING TESTING

Many bottlenecks occur within the complex testing procedures endemic to all EDs. However, testing procedures can often be expedited through innovative planning.

Laboratory Testing

The majority of ED cases require laboratory tests, including virtually all ESI 1, 2, and 3 patients. Intuitively, it would seem that if laboratory turnaround is quicker, overall throughput and LOS would improve. Implicit to that assumption is that laboratory testing is the rate-limiting factor in the decision to admit or discharge. In fact, this is true for some but not all patients who have laboratory tests ordered. Since not all decisions to admit or discharge depend on laboratory results, there will seldom be a significant reduction in LOS with incremental reductions in average laboratory turnaround time. The decision to have zero versus any laboratory tests drawn other than point-of-care testing (POCT) is a much bigger determinant of patient LOS.

The percentage of laboratory outliers (i.e., those with unusually long test times) appears to be more important than the average laboratory turnaround time for determining the LOS.[3] One study of 11 community hospitals compared average laboratory turnaround times and outlier percentages with ED LOS. While helpful, the fast turnaround of some tests failed to offset the delays caused by slower studies. Because these outlier tests have the largest impact on patient LOS, it is advantageous to address the longest test times, instead of the average.

In addition, attributing all laboratory work turnaround time to the laboratory ignores the aspects of the process that are most influenced by the ED. The laboratory process consists of three phases:

- Preanalytic (order entry to laboratory accessioning)
- Analytic (processing)
- Postanalytic (verification and release)

The analytic and postanalytic phases are highly automated and typically very consistent. Markedly abnormal laboratory test results may take somewhat longer than the normal results due to the general process in place for confirmation of results. The greatest opportunity for improving laboratory turnaround time is in the preanalytic phase, consisting of the following steps:

1. Order entry
2. Order acknowledgment or receipt
3. Specimen acquisition
4. Specimen transport to laboratory
5. Laboratory accession

Point-of-Care Testing

Efficient laboratory POCT can save a significant amount of time when compared to standard bench laboratory testing. These methods include:

- *Preanalytic time*: The specimen goes directly from the patient to the analyzer.
- *Testing time*: The analysis is done directly on whole blood, eliminating the centrifuging process to separate serum.
- *Analyzer time*: Analyzer time is usually only 1 to 5 minutes.

However, will POCT actually reduce patient LOS? POCT is most valuable when it involves end-point tests—those tests that lead directly to a decision and move the patient along the throughput process. Examples include:

- *Strep screen*: enables a decision to discharge the patient with or without antibiotics
- *Negative pregnancy test*: often results in a decision to perform a radiologic procedure

From a throughput perspective, many POCTs are not end-point tests. For instance, troponin results seldom shorten LOS, as shown in a multicenter trial.[4] The decision to send a patient to the cardiac catheterization laboratory is not necessarily troponin dependent. The decision to admit is usually not determined by a single troponin, though it may impact the admission location.

Generally, the decision to admit or discharge requires the comprehensive review of all laboratory test results. Therefore, when some tests must be sent to the central laboratory, such as liver function tests or serum drug levels, most clinicians will wait until all the laboratory test results are available before finalizing a decision to admit or discharge. This is not to minimize the value of point-of-care laboratory testing. The early information from POCT may have significant impact on the care of a patient, such as the early diagnosis of hyperkalemia, hypokalemia, or hyperglycemia or confirmation of a non-ST-segment elevation myocardial infarction or sepsis. And, in some cases, these results do lead to immediate disposition decisions.

Effective Electronic Medical Records and Orders

Effective electronic medical records (EMRs) with well-developed order sets simplify and shorten the first phase of the process: order entry. Conversely, poorly organized EMRs or order sets can create delays, particularly if the physician has to spend time searching for the correct test. Ordering the wrong test, such as ordering a computed tomography (CT) of the chest instead of a CT angiogram of the chest, leads to rework and wasted time. In addition, verbal orders are increasingly frowned upon and for generally good reason. There is always the risk of an error when orders are verbally relayed, particularly in a noisy and hectic ED environment.

The busy environment and inconsistent processes found in EDs often lead to variations of physician-only order entry. For instance, time-sensitive treatments for an acute stroke or major trauma often require the physician to assess the patient while verbally giving orders to a nurse. It would be less efficient for a physician to find a nearby workstation, sign on, and enter orders for a critical patient. Time from order entry to order acknowledgment is often a source of delay. Consider a nurse working in an ED with a 4:1 patient to nurse ratio:

- Patient 1 has sepsis and requires immediate laboratory work, a chest x-ray, a fluid bolus, and antibiotics.
- Patient 2 (new) has chest pain and requires rapid assessment.
- After completion of those urgent tasks, the nurse notices orders placed 10 and 25 minutes earlier on the other two previously assessed patients.
- Patient 3 has abdominal pain and there are orders for laboratory work, including a urinalysis, IV fluids, pain medicine, and a CT scan of the abdomen/pelvis.
- Patient 4 is an elderly female complaining of weakness. There are orders for laboratory work, IV fluids, and a urinalysis.

In this particular ED scenario, there is a patient care technician who can draw blood and start IVs. However, the nurse might ask the technician to assist with patients 3 and 4, and this technician is shared among three nurses and, unbeknownst to the requesting nurse, the technician is urgently required to assist with a patient who has become confused and combative.

Perhaps 30 minutes later, the staff is able to work on establishing an IV and obtaining blood work on patient 3, who turns out to be a "difficult stick." Then, after completing the task on patient 3, the technician proceeds to get blood work and establish an IV on patient 4. Sixty or more minutes after the order is entered, blood specimens are sent via pneumatic tube to the laboratory, where they sit for another 15 minutes before accessioning occurs. At 90 minutes after order entry, the physician calls the laboratory wondering why it is taking so long to get results. The laboratory tech confirms that the specimen is in the laboratory and results will be coming soon. Laboratory tests are processed and completed 45 minutes after accessioning. The turnaround time was 2 hours. The physician comments to the nurse that "Lab is really slow today."

In this scenario, the preanalytic phase took at least 75 minutes, while the analytic and postanalytic phase took 45 minutes. Sixty minutes of the preanalytic phase were under the control of the ED and 15 minutes were the responsibility of the laboratory. From the opportunity standpoint in this setting, developing consistent and reliable processes in the ED can save far more time than trying to address minor delays in laboratory accession. Rather than looking at raw global numbers, for example, 2 hours' turnaround time from the laboratory, doing an in-depth analysis and looking at the turnaround time in each segment of the process will often yield the greatest results.

Imaging Services

The radiology turnaround time process consists of:

1. Pretesting phase:
    a. Patient stable for transport to radiology
    b. Completion of preliminary blood work, if necessary
    c. Patient transport
2. Study performed
3. Patient transported back to the ED
4. Study available for viewing—ED provider reviews
5. Radiologist interpretation available—ED provider reviews

Like laboratory services, there is a preanalytic pretesting phase. However, unlike laboratory services, patients must often be physically transported to the study location by a staff member. In some institutions, the patient transport can represent a significant delay in radiology turnaround time. Also, the postanalytic phase is not automated and may require the radiologist to interpret the images. Some studies will autopopulate the EMR, while others must be actively tracked to ensure that interpretive readings have been performed. If the hospital uses a nighttime teleradiology system, the service might not be tied into the hospital EMR, in which case obtaining the reading or querying the radiologist becomes even more complicated.

From a management perspective, accountability is clearest when the "home" radiology department owns the entire process: preanalytic, analytic, and postanalytic phases. Transport, testing, and results reporting are all under the radiology department's umbrella. When monitoring metrics and performance, it is important that analysis be reported on all three phases, which creates transparency and identifies outliers.

The transport process may be shared between radiology and the ED, or a dedicated transporter may be used. Either way, clear lines of responsibility should exist defining who is responsible for transport in most conceivable situations, including those times when staff members are busy. Transporters can be pulled to move patients to other units. Effective process improvement requires monitoring of the preanalytic phase and clear lines of responsibility and accountability.

EXPEDITING PHYSICIAN CARE

Physicians often get blamed for slow patient throughput, particularly with increased attention to metrics such as patients per hour or LOS by physician. Because the patient evaluation begins and ends with the provider, the metric clock starts with the medical evaluation and ends with the clinician's disposition decision. Because physicians are one of the critical servers, and the most expensive component of the system, optimizing the use of physicians and APPs is paramount.

From an economic perspective, it is appropriate for all members of the clinical team to work at the "top of their licenses," focusing on activities or tasks that only that clinical team member can do. Using clinical team members to perform nonclinical activities is a poor use of their time, while performing direct patient care activities is the more effective use of their time.

Improving EMRs

While EMRs have addressed many of the shortcomings of paper records, EMRs do still have multiple shortcomings. Depending on which system is in use, navigating screens can be unintuitive and frustrating. Finding the correct imaging study or laboratory result can be challenging when an infrequently ordered test is performed. Chart documentation can require significant keyboarding, or if using voice dictation, charts must be carefully proofread to avoid transcription errors. Moving from a known system to a new system because of upgrades or working at a new institution can lead to all of these inefficiencies simultaneously.

Customization is usually required for an efficiently operating EMR. Screens should be designed to be as intuitive as possible, and the number of screens navigated to complete a task should be kept to a minimum. A computer click only takes a second, but getting through multiple screens adds up to minutes, and repeating that hundreds of times in a shift adds up to hours.

Dedicated computer workstations for team members are necessary. Workstations on wheels may be helpful as the ability to have access to the EMR without having to repeatedly go back to a workstation can further optimize efficiency.

Using Scribes

The use of EMRs has substantially increased the demand for medical scribes. In a busy ED, scribes can increase physician productivity by several patients per shift.[5,6] Assuming that peak patient volumes occur 12 hours per day, if there is double or triple physician coverage, the increased productivity could translate into 12, 18, or more additional patients seen. The average cost for scribes has been $20/hour or more at some sites, and the investment usually pays for itself.[7]

An appropriately trained scribe may act as a prompter to a physician when test results are back. When scribes are working with a single physician during a shift, the scribe is usually aware of the demands on a physician's time and when a patient is ready for disposition. For instance, consider a physician who has finished performing a procedure on a patient and is determining what to do next (e.g., see a new, noncritical patient or reevaluate existing patients). By maintaining an awareness of flow, scribes can recommend a course of action. For example:

- If all tests are back on a particular patient, the next step may be to make disposition.
- Alternatively, if some tests on existing patients are still pending, seeing a new patient may be most efficient.

In addition, scribes can communicate information to the physician while minimizing interruptions, distractions, and wasted time – all of which can lead to errors. Some physicians use scribes to communicate noncritical information (i.e., *not* clinical orders) until their tasks have been completed. The use of scribes with physician assistants and nurse practitioners is less common. This is generally due to the cost differences between physicians and APPs. However, from a throughput perspective, it can make operational and flow sense to pair scribes with APPs. Scribes may be particularly beneficial if the rate-limiting factor for the APP is EMR documentation and the APP is capable of managing patients at the same rate as a physician.

Enhancing Individual Performance

There will always be some variability in physician productivity and speed. Not every physician will take the same amount of time to evaluate a patient or perform a procedure. However, for an ED to run efficiently, a defined minimum standard of performance should be met. Motivation may vary; some physicians are eager to see the next patient, while others may prefer to attend to their current workload before picking up another case. There may even be a few who are content to sit back and allow others to "pick up the slack," biding their time until the shift is over.

Fortunately, physicians and APPs are mostly a competitive group when it comes to performance and ranking that is within their control. The self-perception of wanting to be above average, when used appropriately and respectfully, can be helpful in modifying behavior and keeping group performance high and within a narrow range. Standard performance metrics for physicians are patients per hour or relative value units (RVUs) per hour, with RVUs taking into account some measure of differences in patient acuity.

Comparing all physicians and APPs to each other can identify high versus low productivity performers. Simply sharing this information with individuals often results in performance (productivity) improvement by alerting clinicians who are below average in productivity. Seeing one's own name on the left side of a bell curve can create a visceral reaction, and public disclosure of such information within the group can ratchet up the pressure. Incentive-based payment systems are commonly used to align incentives and motivate physicians to work efficiently and effectively.

EXPEDITING NURSING CARE

Compared to physician workflow, nursing may be more task oriented. Nursing efficiency can be highly impacted by a number of constraints. The physical layout of the department is a key contributor to nursing efficiency and effectiveness. In Lean terms, moving area-to-area seeking equipment or supplies wastes time and energy. It can be eye-opening to attach a pedometer to key staff members and review the results. Wasted movement also applies to physicians, APPs, and anyone else who delivers care on the front line.

"5S" the ED

5S is a Lean term that stands for[8]:

- Sort
- Straighten
- Shine
- Standardize
- Sustain

Efficiency requires:

- Eliminating unneeded items from the department
- Keeping frequently used items where they are needed, at the point of service
- Moving items that are only occasionally needed to a centrally convenient location

Organize patient and supply rooms in a consistent manner to enhance efficiency. Restocking should occur with enough regularity that supplies do not run out. Equipment should always be fully operational and returned to a designated location. In short, efficiency depends on a work environment that is in a state of constant readiness.

These concepts may all seem intuitive and basic, yet the following is a list of commonly found operational inefficiencies:

- Inoperable otoscopes or ophthalmoscopes in patient rooms
- Working otoscope but no ear speculums in a patient room
- Printers running out of prescription paper
- Printers running out of regular paper
- Hunting for hemoccult cards or tongue depressors
- No appropriately sized exam gloves in the room
- No nearby pyxis medication dispenser in the treatment area, requiring a nurse has to walk to another area to get needed medications
- Routine supplies in different locations in different rooms

While these may seem like trivial and merely aggravating matters, having to leave the bedside to get or find something is a waste of valuable time, attention, and energy. Doing that dozens of times in a shift creates inefficiency, additive waits, and unnecessary frustration, or in Lean terms, substantial "non-value-added time." Efficient organization is key to maximizing clinician productivity.

Eliminating Single-Server Bottlenecks

It is common for nurses to have a fixed patient (bed) assignment, such as a 4:1 patient to nurse ratio or a geographic assignment. This patient allocation can create a "single-server bottleneck."

Example 1: A nurse is managing four patients within a fixed area. Two patients have recently been admitted and have new orders, and the other two patients were discharged and replaced by two new patients.

Example 2: A physician sees the two new patients and enters orders for IVs, meds, laboratory tests, and x-rays. The nurse now has multiple tasks spread across four patients simultaneously:

- Patients A and B: assess patient, acknowledge orders, administer meds, start IV, draw blood, label specimens, and send to laboratory.
- Patients C and D: reassess patient, address additional orders, call report, call transport, and get patient ready for transport.

At this particular hospital, the nurses have 1 hour to get the patient upstairs once admission orders have been placed. Thus, rather than focusing on any new ED cases, the nurse's priority will be transferring the admitted patient upstairs. Without backup or a workable plan, the nurse in this particular scenario will inadvertently create a single-server bottleneck, and throughput time will suffer. There are different ways to manage this problem. Team nursing, in which two nurses together care for twice as many patients, may be effective. This approach permits a nurse who may have more time and fewer immediate demands to help a nurse who has more to do.

Another form of team nursing utilizes the "divide-and-conquer" approach. One or more nurses may assist with the initial patient assessment, while another nurse provides primary care to address the initial flurry of orders. A charge nurse without a patient assignment, or a float nurse, can also act as a resource when an individual nurse is overwhelmed. Whatever system is used, the goal is to avoid the single-server bottleneck associated with fixed patient or geographic assignments.

Monitoring time from order to execution will identify delays related to the nursing resources. When significant delays are recognized, resources must be reallocated to improve patient flow and reduce LOS. Demand–capacity mismatches and the impact of variability in patient complexity and workflow are the most common culprits. At times, if flow metrics are calculated for individual nurses, outliers may be correlated with individual performance. Because nursing staffs tend to be much larger than physician staffs, the management of these data can be complex, particularly if nurses have different assignments on different shifts or changing assignments within a shift.

A simpler but perhaps less precise method uses data to validate perception and drive change. For instance, the nurses in most EDs can discern the fast doctors from the slow ones. Similarly, nurses and physicians may know who the perceived outliers are on the nursing staff. Running the data on the perceived slow-moving performers against the average may help determine whether or not the perceptions are correct. Sharing that information with the individual staff member may be a powerful tool for change.

Incentive-based pay for nursing has not been widely adopted. Existing nursing payment systems across departments in a hospital fall into a relatively narrow range. This avoids interdepartmental competition that would occur if the pay in one department were substantially higher than in another. If unequal incentives existed, nurses might transfer to the higher-paying department, complain about pay inequity, and potentially create labor unrest. Physician pay, on the other hand, is often based on measurable units of production and varies by specialty. Because of this, financial incentive systems are technically and culturally much easier to implement for physicians than for nurses.

CONCLUSION

The time from the initial patient–physician contact to the patient disposition decision is the segment of the patient visit in which the specific efficiencies of the ED are tested. This interval begins and ends with the physician/APP. The ED and hospital leaders must assess and work to improve performance and workflow efficiency. ED and hospital leaders should assess the current workflow and create improvements, where needed, by establishing an optimal work environment with realistic goals and by providing usable metrics with group and individual feedback.

The critical drivers of optimal workflow require appropriate matching of the three most critical servers—beds, nursing staff, and physicians/APPs—to patient demand and acuity. As the challenges of matching these servers to patient needs are addressed, department leadership can then focus on ancillary service times, particularly during the preanalytic phase. The final piece of this throughput puzzle requires reviewing individual performance to address low-performing outliers.

Close review of this throughput interval can also reveal how well the ED interfaces with the other departments in the hospital, such as the laboratory, imaging services, and information technology. Since much of the ED's success depends on other hospital departments, improving some aspects of throughput can only occur by working collaboratively with others to effect change. Consequently, it is essential that the ED leaders have generated sufficient interdepartmental good will and credibility to optimize the physician-to-disposition decision throughput interval.

Successful change requires ED leaders to share a compelling vision. The leaders must believe fully in the value that accomplishing these goals will provide. This information should be presented to the frontline staff and to senior management in a way that will resonate with them. Once specific goals have been shared and baseline metrics provided, the ED leaders should empower a multidisciplinary team to study the process, create countermeasures to re-engineer and improve flow, and provide the tools and resources needed to make, measure, and sustain the change.

REFERENCES

1. Goldratt EM. *The Goal.* 3rd ed. Great Barrington, Mass: The North River Press; 2004.
2. Poon S, Schuur J, Mehrotra A. Trends in visits to acute care venues for treatment of low-acuity conditions in the United States from 2008 to 2015. *JAMA Intern Med.* 2018;178:1342-1349.
3. Holland LL, Smith LL, Blick KE. Reducing laboratory turnaround time outliers can reduce emergency department patient length of stay. *Am J Clin Pathol.* 2005;124:672-674.
4. Ryan RJ, Lindsell CJ, Hollander JE, et al. A multicenter randomized controlled trial comparing central laboratory and point-of-care cardiac marker testing strategies: the Disposition Impacted by Serial Point of Care Markers in Acute Coronary Syndromes (DISPO-ACS) trial. *Ann Emerg Med.* 2009;53:321-328.
5. Arya R, Salovich DM, Ohman-Strickland P, et al. Impact of scribes on performance indicators in the emergency department. *Acad Emerg Med.* 2010;17:490-494.
6. Walker K, Ben-Meir M, O'Mullane P, et al. Scribes in an Australian private emergency department: a description of physician productivity. *Emerg Med Australas.* 2014;26:543-548.
7. Beckers Hospital Review: Are Medical Scribes Worth the Investment? 2013. Available at: https://www.beckershospitalreview.com/patient-flow/are-medical-scribes-worth-the-investment.html. Accessed December 24, 2019.
8. Womack JP, Daniel TJ. *Lean Thinking.* 2nd ed. New York, NY: Free Press Division of Simon and Schuster, Inc; 2003:348, 361.

ADDITIONAL READINGS

- ACEP - Emergency Medicine Practice Committee, Published May, 2016, accessed: July 13, 2020. Change the url to: https://www.acep.org/globalassets/sites/acep/media/crowding/empc_crowding-ip_092016.pdf

- Advisory Board. *Building the Clockwork ED: Best Practices for Eliminating Bottlenecks and Delays in the ED*. Washington, DC: HWorks, An Advisory Board Company; 2000.

- Advisory Board. *The High-Performance ED Optimizing Capacity and Throughput to Meet Ever-Growing Demand*. Washington, DC: HWorks, An Advisory Board Company; 2008.

- Baker S. *Excellence in the Emergency Department: How to Get Results*. Gulf Breeze, Fla: Fire-Starter Publishing; 2009.

- Emergency Nurses Association. *Staffing Guidelines*. 2017.

- Holland LL, Smith LL, Blick KE. Reducing laboratory turnaround time outliers can reduce emergency department patient length of stay. *Am J Clin Pathol*. 2005;125:672-674.

- Husk G, Waxman D. Using data from hospital information systems to improve emergency department care. *Acad Emerg Med*. 2004;11(11):1237-1244.

- Horowitz LI, Green J, Bradley EH. US emergency department performance on wait time and length of visit. *Ann Emerg Med*. 2011;55:133-141.

- McClelland MS, Lazar D, Sears V, et al. The past, present, and future of urgent matters: lessons learned from a decade of emergency department flow improvement. *Acad Emerg Med*. 2011;18:1392-1399.

- Murphy SO, Barth BE, Carlton EF, et al. Does an ED flow coordinator improve patient throughput? *J Emerg Nurs*. 2014;40:605-612.

- Morgan R. Turning around the turn-arounds: improving ED throughput processes. *J Emerg Nurs*. 2007;33:530-536.

- Retazar R, Bessman E, Ding R, et al. The effect of triage diagnostic standing orders on emergency department treatment time. *Ann Emerg Med*. 2011;57:89-99.

- Wilson M, Nguyen K. *Bursting at the Seams: Improving Patient Flow to Help America's Emergency Departments*. Urgent Matters White Paper. 2004.

CHAPTER 39

ROLE OF OBSERVATION UNITS/RAPID TREATMENT

Michael Ross, Louis Graff, Stephen Bohan, Keith DellaGrotta

Rising medical expenses have increased public sentiment for improved health-care value, and observation medicine can be an effective tool toward that end. To avoid unnecessary inpatient admissions when uncertainty exists around the severity of a patient's medical condition, observation allows physicians more time and resources to determine whether a longer hospital stay is warranted.

Observation medicine is classified as an outpatient service by the Centers for Medicare and Medicaid Services (CMS) and is described as clinical management with the purpose of determining the need for inpatient admission. The CMS states that an observation patient should require less than 24 hours of care—and rarely, up to 48 hours—to make a decision to admit as an inpatient.[1]

Observation units address certain shortcomings of traditional emergency department (ED) patient evaluation and management. Failure to diagnose and treat serious disease is an important problem for many patients who are inadvertently discharged home. Based on their initial evaluation alone, emergency physicians miss 2% to 5% of acute myocardial infarction (MI), 10% to 20% of acute appendicitis, and 20% to 40% of ectopic pregnancy.[2-5] To avoid the problem of inadvertently missing the diagnosis of acute serious disease, emergency physicians often must lower their threshold for admitting patients, which results in many patients being found to have no serious disease during hospitalization.

For example, of patients admitted for a chief complaint of chest pain, over two-thirds are found to have no serious coronary artery disease.[1] On the other hand, of the patients who are actually suffering an MI, one-third will present without chest pain, and half will have a nondiagnostic electrocardiogram.[6,7] Such atypical symptoms for acute MI become a growing problem as the population ages.

Yet as health-care costs consume a larger fraction of total national spending, the use of acute care hospitalization to evaluate patients with low probability of serious disease has become unacceptable to third-party payors and the public.[8] Decreasing avoidable admissions while maintaining quality of care continues to be a central issue in controlling national health-care costs through programs such as accountable care organizations.[9,10] Patients and third-party payors expect as many patients as possible to be managed on an outpatient basis with acute care hospitalization utilized only for patients with acute serious disease.

BENEFITS OF OBSERVATION UNITS

About one-quarter to one-third of hospitals in the United States have observation units, with more than half managed by emergency medicine (EM).[11-13] The ED observation units (EDOUs) are a tool that clinicians may use to decrease diagnostic uncertainty for serious conditions such as chest pain, syncope, transient ischemic attacks (TIAs), and abdominal pain, while remaining cost-effective by avoiding unnecessary admissions.[3,14-16] The unit can also be used to extend the treatment window of acute conditions, again avoiding admission and decreasing costs. This has been shown for conditions such as asthma, atrial fibrillation, and congestive heart failure.[17-19]

Observation medicine has developed over the past several decades as emergency physicians improved diagnostic accuracy.[3,15,16] Patients with a difficult diagnostic condition (e.g., abdominal pain, chest pain, or grand mal seizure) are not discharged home until the physician has a high degree of certainty that they do not have a serious disease that might require further inpatient diagnostic or treatment interventions.

With EDOUs, emergency physicians have also improved their therapeutic success rate. Most patients who fail an acute trial of clinical therapy (such as those with asthma or acute congestive heart failure) can be successfully managed with the use of ED observation beds. These units have allowed emergency physicians to assume a greater role in providing acute care to the patient. Given the relatively short time available to make a definitive disposition in traditional emergency practice, many patients have to be admitted for further evaluation because they have the potential for serious disease or have not been adequately stabilized. If these patients can be evaluated over 24 hours in ED observation beds, diagnostic and therapeutic yield increases, and many such patients can be discharged home. Surveyed emergency providers expressed satisfaction with observation units, stating these units augment their clinical decision-making capacity and the quality of care provided for patients.[20] Savings to health-care payers can be substantial, ranging from $1,000 to $3,000 per patient.[21,22] Patient satisfaction is also often enhanced by active management and the avoidance of a hospital admission.[23,24]

IMPLEMENTATION STRATEGY

The successful introduction of an ED observation program (see **Box 39.1**) requires an ED to substantially change its infrastructure. The American College of Emergency Physicians (ACEP) has maintained a policy on "Emergency Department Observation Services" that encompasses the essentials of unit design and operations (see **Box 39.1**).[25]

As a first step, the mission of an EDOU must be clearly defined after collaboration with various hospital departments, the medical staff, and ED personnel. A dedicated physician medical director is also critical to success. For a smaller ED, this could be the ED director; however, for a busier ED, this should be a separate position. Observation is a service that is provided in addition to traditional ED evaluation and treatment for patients in the department for 12 to 24 hours, rather than the usual 2 to 6 hours. Therefore, the ED must develop additional space and staff.

Because the complexity of patient care is increased by the prolonged stay, patient care requires the development and implementation of specific policies and procedures. Mechanisms to provide food, medications, and physician oversight must be defined.

> **BOX 39.1 ■ ACEP POLICY ON ED OBSERVATION UNITS[11,24]**
>
> ED patients frequently require services beyond their initial care to determine the need for inpatient admission. These distinct and reimbursable services may include but are not limited to further diagnostic evaluation, continued therapy, or management of acute psychosocial issues.
>
> To promote quality of care and safety for ED observation patients, ACEP supports the following principles:
>
> - Observation of appropriate ED patients in a dedicated ED observation area (instead of a general inpatient or acute care ED bed) is a "best practice" that requires a commitment of staff and hospital resources.
> - An emergency physician and emergency nurse should direct ED observation areas with clearly defined administrative responsibilities for the unit.
> - Written policies and procedures for the ED observation area should be approved by appropriate ED and hospital medical staff representatives.
> - ED observation area policies should address the following:
>   - Patient criteria for admission into the unit, discharge from the unit, and admission to an inpatient bed.
>   - A clear statement of which physician bears clinical responsibility for each patient in the area.
>   - A clear delineation of emergency physician and nursing staff roles and responsibilities throughout the day, including how care will be transferred between providers.
>   - Circumstances that require notification of the physician who is responsible for the patient.
>   - Maximum allowable length of stay in the unit and means to address outliers.
>   - A description of how utilization and relevant quality measures will be monitored and reported.
> - ED observation areas should have adequate space, staffing, equipment, and supplies appropriate for the conditions being managed.
> - Mechanisms should be in place to expedite patient discharge or transfer to an inpatient bed, when appropriate.

Most EDOU programs have protocols for common specific conditions. The quality management program needs to be expanded to evaluate and continuously improve the processes of care for these patients. Responsibility for the various management entities needs to be clearly delineated. In addition, the ED should have a utilization review program to review the care provided in the unit and to prevent inappropriate admissions.

Compliance with payer requirements is an important aspect of implementation of an observation unit. "Place in outpatient observation services" is considered by CMS as the correct terminology for the order for observation. It is important that orders include the word "outpatient" and the word "observation" and not include the word "admit." Level of care designation (outpatient observation versus inpatient admission) has become a major focus for third-party payor audits, including federal government audits such as those by the RACs (Recovery Audit Contractors) and MACs (Medicare Administrative Contractors). Observation services are no longer a discretionary alternative to acute care hospitalization but instead are now a mandated level of care for patients who do not have criteria for hospitalization, as often judged by a primary nurse utilization review (e.g., InterQual criteria) or by a secondary physician utilization review.

TABLE 39.1 ■ Hospital Settings in which Observation Services Are Provided		
Setting	**Description**	**Characteristics**
Type 1	Protocol driven, observation unit	Highest level of evidence for favorable outcomes Care typically directed by ED
Type 2	Discretionary care, observation unit	Care directed by a variety of specialists Unit typically based in ED
Type 3	Protocol driven, bed in any location	Often called a "virtual observation unit"
Type 4	Discretionary care, bed in any location	Most common practice Unstructured care Poor alignment of resources with patient needs

Facility Design

Observation medicine is practiced in various settings across hospitals nationwide (**Table 39.1**). Patients can be placed in observation status in an inpatient bed on a floor mixed with other admitted patients or in a dedicated observation unit often managed by emergency practitioners. Of these settings, EDOUs have been shown to provide the best patient care in a more efficient and cost-effective manner, especially if guided by condition-specific protocols.[26]

The design of the ED observation area should be consistent with its function. Patients are there for 12 to 24 hours and need access to appropriate amenities such as a sink, table, cabinet, and bathroom. Suggested national architectural guidelines for such a unit include a centralized nursing station, ideally 100 square feet of clear floor space per treatment area, a nurse call bell, oxygen, vacuum, and air.[27] Most EDs with observation units have one or two beds per 10,000 patient visits.[11] This number may vary based on local medical staff practice, hospital resources, and institutional case mix. Because observation services are outpatient services, they do not need to meet standards of an inpatient or licensed bed.

Another means of estimating the number of required EDOU beds is through the use of benchmark data, using the percent of the ED census that might be observed and the average number of patients per bed per day (**Table 39.2**). For example, higher-acuity EDs often admit about one-quarter of their patients and observe roughly 7% to 8% in an EDOU. When these units are optimally managed—with length of stays of roughly 15 hours—they average 1.1 patients per bed per day. This number takes into account census variations during off times and weekends. Simply applying these numbers to a hypothetical 50,000 visits per year, the ED yields 3,500 patients per year (7% of 50,000), or 9.58 patients per day. Using the benchmark estimate of 1.1 patient per bed per day would estimate that this 50,000 visit/year ED would need an average of 9 beds (9.58 patients per day/1.1 patient per bed per day). These estimates can be adjusted up or down for each variable to better match the ED characteristics.

Monitoring capabilities in the observation unit depend on the types of patients treated there. Monitoring is not needed for patients free of cardiovascular risk or hemodynamic instability, such as those being evaluated for abdominal pain or treated for asthma. For them, the observation unit bed functions in a way similar to a hospital med-surg bed. In contrast, monitoring is needed for patients at risk of sudden cardiovascular events or hemodynamic instability, including those being evaluated for chest pain, syncope, congestive heart failure, or atrial fibrillation. In those cases, the observation unit bed requires equipment similar to

TABLE 39.2 ■ EDOU Characteristics (18 Teaching Hospitals Sample)	
Average number of ED patients observed	4,430 (±3,478)
Average number of beds in the EDOU	13.3 (±7.4)
Percent of EDOUs located within/adjacent to ED	82.3%
Percent of "closed" units (EM only)	93.8%
Average ED length of stay for EDOU patients	4.2 hours (±1.6 hours)
Average EDOU length of stay	15.7 hours (±3.8 hours)
Percent discharged from EDOU	82.4% (±4.3%)
Percent of ED census that is admitted (inpatient)–a surrogate of case mix acuity	22.9% (±8.7%)
Percent of ED census that is observed	7.2% (±6.7%)
Number of EDOU beds per ED beds	4.25 EDOU beds/1 ED bed
Number of EDOU beds per ED visits	1 EDOU bed/7,461 ED visits
Number of EDOU patients/EDOU bed/day	1.14 patient/bed/day

a telemetry bed or step-down unit. Monitoring capabilities for such patients may include arrhythmia alarms, oximetry, blood pressure, pulse, respiratory rate, and advanced monitoring techniques such as ST-segment analysis.

Staffing

According to ACEP's policy on EDOUs, "observation of appropriate ED patients in a dedicated ED observation area, instead of a general inpatient bed or an acute care ED bed, is a 'best practice' that requires a commitment of staff and hospital resources."[25] One such resource is additional nursing staff, as services are needed outside of those provided in traditional ED evaluation and management. In general, one nurse is needed for every eight nonmonitored beds, and one for every four monitored beds.

Additional physicians/advanced practice providers (APPs) are needed to staff an observation program. Approximately one additional FTE of physician or APP staffing will be required for every 3,000 patients observed. A 2003 survey reported that units were staffed with an average 4.2 patients per nurse and 21.4% used APPs.[11] In most cases, emergency physicians split time on a given shift between overseeing the observation unit and taking care of patients in the ED. This makes sense for the average observation unit, which is around 10 beds in size. However, observation units large enough to support a dedicated physician shift can be more financially advantageous, especially if the physician belongs to a different legal entity, and can therefore provide separate observation billing and coding services (discussed later in this chapter under "Funding and Reimbursement").[28]

An observation unit may be "open" if any hospital physician or specialist is credentialed to place patients in the unit, or it may be "closed" if patient care in the unit is limited to a particular group of clinicians at the exclusion of others. An "open" observation unit may be politically the only acceptable model for the hospital's medical staff, but it makes standardized, efficient, high-quality patient care much more difficult and is not the best practice model.

Unit Management

Successful EDOU performance requires strong physician and nursing leadership. The EDOU leadership must actively interact with other hospital departments and collaboratively develop and implement protocols. Medical and nursing education in the ED is necessary to ensure the staff understands observation medicine as separate and different from typical EM services.

Policies and Procedures

Policies and procedures are needed for the observation unit beyond those required for usual ED patient services. There are two issues to consider: guidelines for the unit as a whole, and guidelines and protocols for specific patient conditions. Unit guidelines are needed to detail the following:

- Administrative direction (for nurses and physicians) of the unit
- Admitting privileges and processes
- Monitoring quality and utilization as described in ACEP policy (see **Box 39.1**)

The policies and procedures should be consistent with the goals of the observation unit: to provide continual care, in contrast to the episodic care provided in a traditional ED. Documentation and orders should be aimed at all personnel providing services to the patient, clarifying what should be done and the patient's ultimate disposition.

As discussed previously, many EDOUs have protocols with written guidelines for common specific conditions.[16,30] This approach decreases variability and improves consistent quality of care. These EDOUs have standards for medication and nonmedication orders.

In addition, many EDOUs have standards for risk stratification, defining which patients are appropriate for outpatient observation care and which are appropriate for acute care hospitalization (see an example for asthma patients in **Figure 39.1**). In addition, these standards may have inclusion and exclusion criteria to define which patients:

- Require observation and management beyond the initial ED intervention
- Are high risk and require acute care hospitalization
- Can be safely discharged home based on specific criteria
- Should be admitted to the hospital

Comprehensive protocols limit variation and allow all the providers in the group to provide more consistent, efficient, and quality patient care. Further information may be found through ACEP, which has published a toolkit for managing ED observation services (available online at https://www.acep.org/by-medical-focus/observation-medicine/observation-services-toolkit/).[31]

When a patient is assigned to the EDOU, the ED record should include the medical decision-making, including communications with others involved in the patient's care (e.g., primary care physician) and the goal of the EDOU stay. A copy of this record should be available to the EDOU team. A written order assigning the patient to ED observation is a mandatory requirement and marks the time the EDOU stay began.

The EDOU protocols ideally contain structured, protocol-specific order sets. Progress notes should be interdisciplinary and unified, with frequency dictated by the patient's condition. Discharge notes can be templated to the specific syndrome, noting clinical course, final diagnosis, and disposition (home versus admit) with reasons for the decision. Additionally, the notes should contain standard discharge instructions similar to traditional

FIGURE 39.1 ■ Observation Orders for Asthma Patients

The Hospital of **Central Connecticut**

Asthma/COPD Observation
Physician Orders

ALLERGY STICKER

Date/Time:	Refer to Observation For Service of Dr. ______

DO NOT USE ABBREVIATIONS: μ, mcg, u, iu, QD, QID, QOD, B.I.W., T.I.W., MgS04, MS04, MS, HISS, RISS, AD, AU, AS
Please check box to activate the order. Cross out (X) any blank spaces prior to signing orders.

Non-Medication Orders	**Medication Orders**
Date/Time	Date/Time
☐ **Cardiac Monitoring: Indication** ______	☐ IV fluids: ______
DX: Asthma / COPD	@ ____ ml/hr x ____ liters
☐ Vitals: Every 4 hours	☐ Methylprednisolone ☐ 40 mg ☐ 125 mg (check one) IV x 1
Diet (Check One): ☐ Regular/house ☐ Clear Liquids ☐ NPO	☐ Prednisone ______ mg PO twice daily
☐ Carbohydrate Controlled (1800 kcal/day, no conc. Sweets)	**Nebulizer Orders (check one)**
☐ 2 gram Na ☐ Pureed ☐ Other: ______	☐ Albuterol neb 2.5 mg Nebs every ____ hours (every 4 or 6 hours)
Acitivity (Check One): ☐ Ambulate ad lib ☐ OOB to BR	PRN SOB/Wheezing
☐ Ambulate with assist ☐ Other: ______	☐ Albuterol 2.5 mg / Ipratropium 0.5 mg Nebs
☐ Intake and Output q shift	every ____ hours (every 4 or 6 hours) PRN SOB/Wheezing
☐ Insert Saline lock	
Labs at ______ (check box(es)): ☐ CBC ☐ lytes	☐ Acetaminophen 650 mg PO/PR every 6 hrs PRN
☐ other labs: ______	pain score 1-4 **and/or** Temp > 101F
☐ O2 (circle): ____ per liter nasal; Other ____	☐ For smokers: Nicotine (Nicoderm)
☐ Notify MD for: HR < 55 or > 100	☐ 7 mg ☐ 14mg ☐ 21 mg (check one) patch topically Daily
RR < 12 or > 25	**Other Medications:**
Temp < 96F or > 100.4F	
SBP < 100, SBP > 170, DBP > 120	
SaO2 < 90%	
☐ Peak flow pre and post every neb treatment	

MD Signature: ______________ Beeper #: ______ Date: ______ Time: ______

HCC Form #1911 Revised 7-10 **Asthma/COPD Observation Physician Orders**

ED discharges. Appropriate Current Procedural Terminology (CPT) codes for EDOU patients are listed in **Figure 39.2**; they vary according to whether the patient enters and leaves ED observation on the same calendar day or on different days.

Quality, Performance, and Utilization Review

In general, observation of patients with high-service intensity or high severity of illness is not an optimal use of the EDOU because these patients are unlikely to be discharged, and the unit may not be designed for their optimal care. These patients should be admitted directly to the acute care hospital. It is also inappropriate to place patients in the EDOU who have

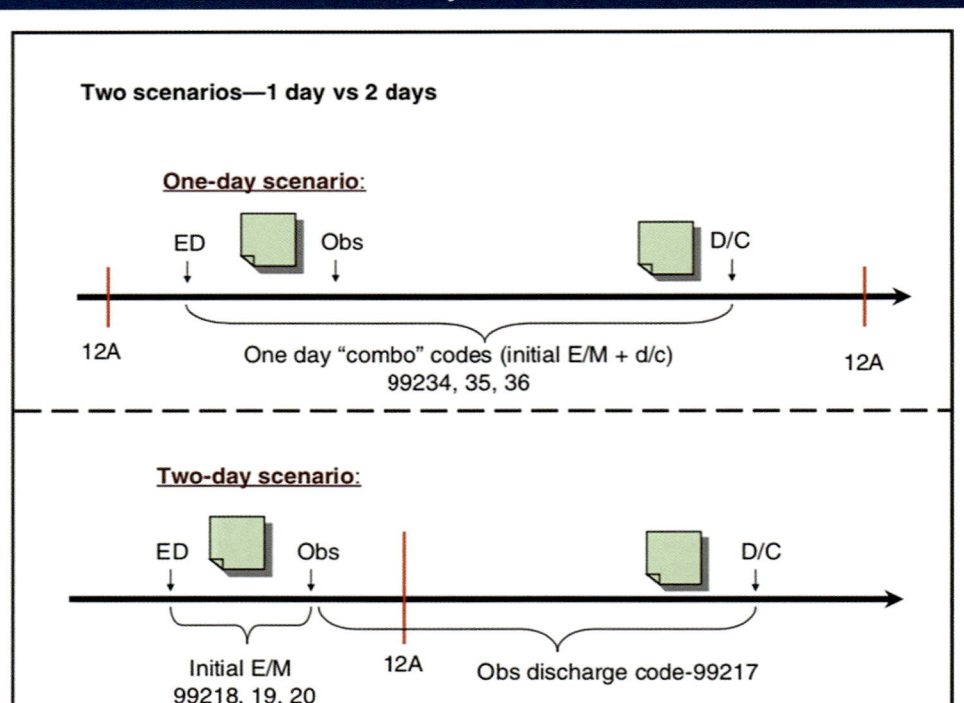

FIGURE 39.2 ■ The CPT Codes for Physician Reimbursement

minor complaints or because it is convenient for the private physician. On a monthly basis, the CQI/UR (continuous quality improvement/utilization review) program should review the appropriateness of all observation patients in relation to the admitting guidelines.

An active CQI/UR program is essential to ensure high-quality patient care. When emergency physicians provide observation services, they assume additional responsibilities. The processes of patient care require careful evaluation and constant improvement. Leadership needs to develop and implement protocols to reduce variability in quality and utilization between clinicians. Useful quality indicators include all of the following:

- Physician and nursing documentation
- Timeliness of care
- Patient experience
- Accurate individual provider diagnosis ("rule in" or "rule out" for significant diseases). This can be compared with overall rates for the unit.
- EDOU return visit rates
- Significant EDOU events, such as missed diagnoses (often identified by return visit audits)
- Deaths within 48 hours of EDOU stay
- Admissions to an intensive care unit from the EDOU

Roughly 7% of discharged EDOU patients may return for a related visit, with about half of these (4%) leading to admission. Return rates are highest for treatment of painful conditions such as back pain or chronic pain.[32]

A vigorous utilization review program examining the appropriateness of observation status assignments is critical to the success of the unit and good patient care. Units with chief complaint/disease-specific protocols lend themselves to tracking condition-specific utilization data to facilitate leadership monitoring and feedback to individual clinicians on their performance. To collect this information, key data elements must be identified within a hospital database or, if unavailable, collected separately.

A sample EDOU utilization database would include a patient identifier, age, and gender; reason for observation (EDOU admission diagnosis); date time elements (ED arrival, EDOU arrival, and EDOU departure); and final disposition. From these basic elements, monthly reports of most common conditions, length of stay in the ED and EDOU, and percent of admission can be followed. Additional data elements would optimally include 7-day return visits and cardiac imaging used, which tends to represent a significant portion of EDOU services.

Funding and Reimbursement

Additional services are provided to ED patients who are observed—including more nursing and physician services—than the average patient in the ED. Consequently, additional funding must be provided to offset costs.[29]

Starting in 2016, Medicare modified its payment policy to cover the majority of costs associated with an observation stay as a single bundled payment called a comprehensive APC (C-APC 8011). Doing so simplified the billing process that encompasses all levels of observation and made it less likely that patient out-of-pocket expenses would be more than the average inpatient deductible. The C-APC pays for such related observation services as diagnostic tests (such as stress tests), imaging, laboratory tests, treatments, and intravenous medications. It is important to note that the lump-sum payment does not cover self-administered medications. Also, a hospital can bill the APC only if there is no associated major or T-status procedure (e.g., cardiac catheterization, endoscopy, or appendectomy). In these situations, the hospital would bill the appropriate procedure APC in place of an observation APC, thus preventing double billing.[33]

Physician payment for observation services occurs using CPT codes specific for observation services. These include three groups of codes: the 1-day codes (99234, 99235, 99236), the 2-day codes (99218, 99219, 99220), and the interim day code (99). According to CMS, physicians of the same specialty (identified by specialty code) and group (identified by tax ID number) will be treated as a single individual (in terms of billing procedure). As such, an ED and EDOU physician cannot bill two E/M (evaluation and management) codes (such as an emergency E/M code and an observation E/M code) on the same calendar day.

The CPT clarifies that both services are captured by the observation family of codes, since the care was initiated in the ED and completed in the EDOU. As such, the initial ED care would be billed using the observation codes for initial evaluation and management instead of using the emergency codes. The subsequent and additional work of caring for the patient in the EDOU is covered using the observation discharge codes. Observation codes, unlike emergency codes, recognize and pay for the work of discharging the patient. Payment for the initial evaluation using observation codes is roughly comparable to emergency care payments.

The economic impact of the observation unit must be viewed from a larger perspective than direct charges and payments. The observation unit may have great value for a hospital in a competitive health-care market and may be important when strategically developing contracts and pricing with managed care plans.

EMERGENCY MEDICINE PRACTICE IMPACT

The development of ED observation services is another step in the maturation and development of EM. In the 1970s, the presence of physicians in the ED 24 hours per day, 7 days per week created the opportunity for the development of observation services. In 1983, prospective payment and hospital admission criteria were implemented. These programs created powerful incentives for ED observation services. Patients were not to be admitted to the acute care hospital without clear documentation of the presence of serious disease. Extended ED evaluation and therapy were often needed to determine which patients really needed such care.

With a 10- to 12-hour period of ED observation, many studies have shown that as many as 80% of potential short-term hospital admission patients can be safely discharged home. There have been randomized clinical trials on many conditions—such as chest pain, asthma, TIA, syncope, and atrial fibrillation—which have confirmed the superior value of observation over hospitalization.[15,18,34,35]

For example, TIA patients randomized to observation compared to acute hospitalization had lengths of stay 26 hours rather than 67 hours, costs of $890 rather than $1,547, and comparable short- and long-term outcomes.[16] Further retrospective, prospective, and case studies also show the value of observation medicine for conditions such as cellulitis, nonspecific abdominal pain, electrolyte abnormalities, intoxication, and traumatic conditions.[36-40] The breadth of conditions managed by observation medicine will likely only increase as the medical field matures.

CONCLUSION

ED observation services are rapidly becoming a crucial element of the modern health-care system. The creation of observation units may represent the final stage in the evolution of the ED from a nursing triage station to a definitive patient care unit. The creation of observation units may also enhance the image of ED physicians beyond acute care clinicians as primary caregivers, short-stay specialists, and hospital "gatekeepers," which will underscore their importance in the managed care systems of the future.

REFERENCES

1. Centers for Medicare and Medicaid Services. Observation services. In: *Medicare Claims Processing Manual*. US Department of Health and Human Services. Revised December 12, 2017.
2. Pope JH, Aufderheide TP, Ruthazer R, et al. Missed diagnoses of acute cardiac ischemia in the emergency department. *N Engl J Med*. 2000;342(16):1163–1170.
3. Graff L, Radford MJ, Werne C. Probability of appendicitis before and after observation. *Ann Emerg Med*. 1991;20(5):503–507.
4. Cacioppo JC, Diettrich NA, Kaplan G, et al. The consequences of current constraints on surgical treatment of appendicitis. *Am J Surg*. 1989;157(3):276–281.
5. Goldman L, Cook EF, Brand DA, et al. A computer protocol to predict myocardial infarction in emergency department patients with chest pain. *N Engl J Med*. 1988;318(13):797–803.
6. Canto JG, Shlipak MG, Rogers WJ, et al. Prevalence, clinical characteristics, and mortality among patients with myocardial infarction presenting without chest pain. *JAMA*. 2000;283(24):3223–3229.
7. Welch RD, Zalenski RJ, Frederick PD, et al. Prognostic value of a normal or nonspecific initial electrocardiogram in acute myocardial infarction. *JAMA*. 2001;286(16):1977–1984.
8. Martin AB, Hartman M, Washington B, et al. National healthcare spending in 2017. *Health Aff*. 2018;38(1).
9. Kautter J, Pope GC, Trisolini M, et al. Medicare physician group practice demonstration design: quality and efficiency pay-for-performance. *Health Care Financ Rev*. 2007;29(1):15–29.
10. Berwick DM. Launching accountable care organizations—the proposed rule for the Medicare Shared Savings Program. *N Engl J Med*. 2011;364(16):e32.
11. Mace SE, Graff L, Mikhail M, et al. A national survey of observation units in the United States. *Am J Emerg Med*. 2003;21(7):529–533.
12. Wiler JL, Ross MA, Ginde AA. National study of emergency department observation services. *Acad Emerg Med*. 2011;18(9):959-965.
13. 2011 Emergency Department Summary Tables. National Hospital Ambulatory Care Medical Survey. Table 27. Available at: https://www.cdc.gov/nchs/data/ahcd/nhamcs_emergency/2011_ed_web_tables.pdf. Accessed September 13, 2018.
14. Graff LG, Dallara J, Ross MA, et al. Impact on the care of the emergency department chest pain patient from the chest pain evaluation registry (CHEPER) study. *Am J Cardiol*. 1997;80(5):563–568.
15. Shen WK, Decker WW, Smars PA, et al. Syncope evaluation in the emergency department study (SEEDS): a multidisciplinary approach to syncope management. *Circulation*. 2004;110(24):3636–3645.

16. Ross MA, Compton S, Medado P, et al. An emergency department diagnostic protocol for patients with transient ischemic attack: a randomized controlled trial. *Ann Emerg Med.* 2007;50(2):109–119.

17. McDermott MF, Murphy DG, Zalenski RJ, et al. A comparison between emergency diagnostic and treatment unit and inpatient care in the management of acute asthma. *Arch Intern Med.* 1997;157(18):2055–2062.

18. Decker WW, Smars PA, Vaidyanathan L, et al. A prospective, randomized trial of an emergency department observation unit for acute onset atrial fibrillation. *Ann Emerg Med.* 2008;52(4):322–328.

19. Peacock WF, Remer EE, Aponte J, et al. Effective observation unit treatment of decompensated heart failure. *Congest Heart Fail.* 2002;8(2):68–73.

20. Martin GP, Wright B, Ahmed A, Banerjee J, Mason S, Roland D. Use or abuse? A qualitative study of emergency physicians' views on use of observation stays at three hospitals in the United States and England. *Ann Emerg Med.* 2017;69(3):284–292.

21. Baugh CW, Bohan JS. Estimating observation unit profitability with options modeling. *Acad Emerg Med.* 2008;15(5):445–452.

22. Baugh CW, Venkatesh AK, Bohan JS. Emergency department observation units: a clinical and financial benefit for hospitals. *Health Care Manage Rev.* 2011;36(1):28–37.

23. Rydman RJ, Roberts RR, Albrecht GL, et al. Patient satisfaction with an emergency department asthma observation unit. *Acad Emerg Med.* 1999;6(3):178–183.

24. Rydman RJ, Zalenski RJ, Roberts RR, et al. Patient satisfaction with an emergency department chest pain observation unit. *Ann Emerg Med.* 1997;29(1):109–115.

25. American College of Emergency Physicians. Emergency department observation services. *Ann Emerg Med.* 2008;51(5):686.

26. Baugh CW, Venkatesh AK, Hilton JA, et al. Making greater use of dedicated hospital observation units for many short-stay patients could save $3.1 billion a year. *Health Aff.* 2012;31(10):2314–2320.

27. American Institute of Architects Committee on Architecture for Health with assistance from the US Department of Health and Human Services. *Guidelines for Construction and Equipment of Hospitals and Medical Facilities, 1992-1993.* Aurora, Ill: American Institute of Architects Press; 1993.

28. Baugh CW, Suri P, Caspers CG, Granovsky MA, Neal K, Ross MA. Financial viability of emergency department observation unit billing models [published online May 16, 2018]. *Acad Emerg Med.*

29. Graff LG, Wolf S, Dinwoodie R, et al. Emergency physician workload: a time study. *Ann Emerg Med.* 1993;22(7):1156–1163.

30. Ross MA, Compton S, Richardson D, et al. The use and effectiveness of an emergency department observation unit for elderly patients. *Ann Emerg Med.* 2003;41(5):668–677.

31. Brillman J, Mathers-Dunbar L, Graff L, et al. Management of observation units. American College of Emergency Physicians. *Ann Emerg Med.* 1995;25(6):823–830.

32. Ross MA, Hemphill RR, Abramson J, et al. The recidivism characteristics of an emergency department observation unit. *Ann Emerg Med.* 2010;56(1):34–41.

33. Ross MA, Granovsky M. History, principles, and policies of observation medicine. *Emerg Med Clin North Am.* 2017;35(3):503–518.

34. Roberts RR, Zalenski RJ, Mensah EK, et al. Costs of an emergency department-based accelerated diagnostic protocol vs hospitalization in patients with chest pain: a randomized controlled trial. *JAMA.* 1997;278(20):1670–1676.

35. Rydman RJ, Isola ML, Roberts RR, et al. Emergency department observation unit versus hospital inpatient care for a chronic asthmatic population: a randomized trial of health status outcome and cost. *Med Care.* 1998;36(4):599–609.

36. Yusuf S, Hagan JL, Adekunle-Ojo AO. Managing skin and soft tissue infections in the emergency department observation unit. *Pediatr Emerg Care.* 2019;35(3):204–208.

37. Marshall JR, Katzer R, Lotfipour S, et al. Use of physician-in-triage model in the management of abdominal pain in an emergency department observation unit. *West J Emerg Med.* 2017;18(2):181–188.

38. Crilly CJ, Allen AJ, Amato TM, et al. Evaluating the emergency department observation unit for the management of hyperglycemia in adults. *Am J Emerg Med.* 2018;36(11): 1975–1979.

39. Mong R, Arciaga GJ, Tan HH. Use of a 23-hour emergency department observation unit for the management of patients with toxic exposures. *Emer Med J.* 2017;34(11):755–760.

40. Hagiwara Y, Inoue N. The effect of an observation unit on pediatric minor head injury [published online April 24, 2018]. *Pediatr Emerg Care.* doi:10.1097/PEC0000148700000000.

EXPEDITING ADMISSIONS

Francisco Javier Andrade Jr, Robert W. Strauss, Stephen A. Colucciello

CHAPTER 40

Efficient emergency department (ED) patient flow provides multiple benefits to patients, staff, and the hospital. To ensure optimal flow, ED leaders must pay direct attention to three critical aspects of patient management:

- Door-to-provider (arrival-to-practitioner) times
- Provider (evaluation) to disposition decisions
- Disposition decision to *actual* disposition (e.g., discharge, transfer, admission)

Interruptions in or barriers to any of these components can lead to prolonged delays, dissatisfaction, and financial loss.

A well-known problem and major barrier to clinical flow occurs when admitted patients are held in the ED (i.e., "boarded") due to inpatient capacity issues. Boarding inpatients in the ED delays care, results in overcrowding, and consumes resources that are meant for new cases.[1] When a hospital is full, patients who need inpatient care are often boarded in examination rooms or hallways until an appropriate bed is available. This common practice ties up space, equipment, and personnel that would otherwise be available to meet the needs of incoming patients. Critically ill patients often wait the longest for admission because beds in the intensive care unit (ICU) are in particularly short supply.

An extensive body of literature describes the negative impact of ED boarding, including increased length of stays, delayed medication administration, medical errors, and even increased death rates (**Box 40.1**).[2,3] This critical problem can only be resolved through the collective recognition and collaboration of institutional leaders at multiple levels, including hospital administrators, health-care board members, ED leaders, and inpatient service managers. The solution requires a unified effort to alleviate the bottleneck caused by emergency patients waiting for inpatient beds. A singular focus on the ED, however, inappropriately assigns the problem to an individual department and fails to fully address

---

BOX 40.1 ■ RAMIFICATIONS OF ED CROWDING

- Ill patients wait longer for evaluation and care.
- Complications increase.
- The rates of death are higher during periods of crowding or longer boarding.
- ED lengths of stay increase for all (not just admitted) patients.
- More patients leave prior to receiving a medical screening examination.
- Medical errors increase.
- Patient satisfaction scores plummet, which impacts hospital reimbursement.
- Patients must wait longer to receive pain medication.
- Hospital stays are longer for patients who waited longer in the ED.
- The number of ambulance diversions increases.
- The number of negligence claims is higher in patients who wait.

the adverse impact on patients, providers, and the institution. As such, it is critical to understand that ED boarding is a hospital problem—not an *ED* problem. Until this collective responsibility is understood, the efforts of a single department are unlikely to result in significant success.

ADMISSIONS STRATEGIES

Progressive patient-centered institutions endeavor to remove these bottlenecks by creating admission protocols that move patients quickly from the ED to inpatient beds. These practices rely on identifying and addressing communication barriers, breaking down "silo" thinking, mitigating unambiguous admitting protocols, optimizing electronic medical record capabilities, minimizing service (e.g., laboratory tests, imaging, and transportation) delays, and most importantly, focusing on what is best for the patient (**Box 40.2**).

Early Decision to Admit

In most cases, an experienced emergency physician knows whether hospital admission is required within minutes of seeing the patient.[4] While some diagnostic testing may be necessary to ascertain the type of medical service, bed, or unit needed, it is rarely necessary to review the results of every laboratory and diagnostic test to make this determination.

Members of the admitting service may express concern about tests that have not been performed or whose result is not yet available. Because an unexpected finding might warrant a bed reassignment for an already admitted patient, some suggest waiting until all test results are received before beginning the admission process. Occasionally, an in-house physician may have other incentives for suggesting additional tests or consultations:

- ED admissions can be disruptive to a hospitalist's (i.e., admitting provider's) workflow, and asking for additional tests delays the admission.
- Slowing the process could delay the admission until after the current admitting physician has signed out to an oncoming clinician.
- Additional consultations might result in another patient being admitted.

When a case is thoughtfully considered, experienced emergency physicians almost always choose the right bed and right service. Early admission can greatly benefit patients, who are likely to be far more comfortable once settled into an inpatient unit where they have prompt access to definitive care.

BOX 40.2 ■ STRATEGIES TO EXPEDITE ADMISSIONS

- Early decision to admit
- Early bed request
- Proper bed selection
- Expedited testing
- Early notification of the admitting team
- Speaking the language of the admitting physician
- Admitting officer in the ED
- Admitting agreements
- Express admitting units and holding areas
- Holding orders
- ICU lean protocols
- Expediting nursing reports
- Adopt-a-Boarder programs
- Utilization of ED dashboards

Early Bed Request

As soon as the emergency physician discerns the required level of care, an order should be placed for an inpatient bed. In most hospitals, it can take 30 minutes or longer to assign a patient to a clean, available bed. Early bed requests, therefore, become an important strategy for quickly moving cases out of the ED and into the inpatient setting. By using the early request approach, the bed management process occurs *during* the ongoing diagnostic evaluation (i.e., parallel processing), rather than after the patient has been examined (i.e., sequential processing).

This approach allows the emergency provider to communicate (via the electronic medical record) the appropriate information to expedite the patient's transition from the ED to the admission unit. The emergency physician must simply know:

- an inpatient bed is needed,
- the type of inpatient bed that will best serve the patient's needs (e.g., critical care unit, telemetry, medical–surgical unit, isolation ward), and
- which service should admit the patient.

Proper Bed Selection

In some cases, emergency and inpatient physicians may disagree regarding the type of bed or unit that will best meet the patient's needs. In addition, certain nursing units may restrict the number of cases that require substantial resources (e.g., ventilators) or certain interventions or monitoring, such as two-hour neuro-checks. To address these specific admission criteria, effective organizations collaborate to develop written consensus protocols for bed selection.

Some hospitals have nurses who have been specially trained in bed management and can assist in this selection process by using published criteria and their knowledge of the specific admitting rules for each unit. These "clinical care managers" effectively select the best units for each patient's needs, a process that results in fewer bed reassignments after admission. These managers can also adjudicate any disagreements between providers and protocol-driven admission limitations.

Codified protocols result in more streamlined assignments, fewer variations in bed selection, fewer disagreements and patient delays, and fewer refusals based on changing criteria or the perception that a patient is "too sick" for a certain unit. Detailed, unit-specific protocols can help address elements such as telemetry, isolation, vasoactive drips, and transplant status.

Expedited Testing

While diagnostic testing may be necessary to determine a patient's admission requirements or bed location, a complete battery of laboratory tests is seldom necessary to make such decisions. However, when specific studies are necessary to guide the appropriate disposition, the turnaround time can be the rate-limiting step to admission.

Point-of-care (POC) laboratory studies may be an excellent solution to this problem and allow for earlier decision-making. In some settings, this approach has decreased testing turnaround times by 60 minutes or more.[5,6] For instance, a clinician who is caring for a patient with suspected diabetic ketoacidosis can obtain POC electrolytes, glucose, venous arterial blood gases, and a dip urine for ketones at the bedside. In this example, POC testing can help the provider make the diagnosis, provide treatment, initiate an inpatient consultation, and request a bed within minutes of the patient's arrival.

Similarly, an electrocardiogram (ECG) and a POC troponin test may allow the provider to rapidly determine the appropriate admitting service for patients with chest pain. A portable chest x-ray, ECG, dip urine test, and POC electrolyte measurements can help determine the destination for many medical admissions. Although it is rarely necessary to wait for a leukocyte count before making an admission decision, the test is an expressed "concern" by some inpatient teams.

EARLY NOTIFICATION OF THE ADMITTING TEAM

It is often helpful to involve the admitting team early, though some practitioners require more complete information before making admission decisions. Alternatively, other practitioners may prefer to avoid late calls and request early notification about patients who are likely to require admission. As a rule, the ED physician should be able to answer the following questions with confidence when notifying an admitting team:

- What is the reason for the consultation (e.g., admission, recommendations)?
- Does the patient require critical care?
- Does the patient require emergent interventions or procedures?

A formal agreement can define the consistent and appropriate timing of the consultation and eliminate the confusion and frustration often associate with variations. For example, it is reasonable for a clinician to require chest x-ray results before admitting a patient with suspected pneumonia. However, it may be unnecessary to wait for a complete blood count (**Box 40.3**).

BOX 40.3 ■ CONSULTING AN ADMITTING GROUP

The emergency physician sees most patients who are admitted to the ED's hospitalist group and performs a history and physical examination. If the patient requires admission, the emergency physician will order studies that are central to the evaluation before calling the admitting team.

Timing of Consultation and Diagnostic Testing

The admitting team should be called as soon as it becomes clear that the patient requires admission, even before diagnostic testing is complete. However, if a chest x-ray, ECG, or dip urinalysis is central to a patient's evaluation and management, these studies should be completed prior to calling the admitting physician. If it is likely that POC laboratory tests, including a bedside troponin measurement, will significantly accelerate the evaluation, these tests should be ordered before calling the inpatient physician.

Bed and Admitting Orders

The emergency physician should discuss the type of the bed needed with the inpatient team. Under most circumstances, the admitting team can expedite the process by placing orders and evaluating the patient on the inpatient floor instead of the ED. However, any admitting physician who chooses to see the patient in the ED should do so within 30 minutes to prevent boarding.

Transfer to Floor

Stable patients may go to their room when a bed is available, assuming the inpatient team agrees, where they can be evaluated by the admitting team. This does not apply to patients who must be transferred to the ICU or operating room.

Patients Transferred From Outside the Hospital

Clinically stable patients who are transferred from a clinic, private office, or outside hospital should be admitted directly to a floor bed without being seen in the ED. An ED stop wastes time and money (unless the patient requires an emergency intervention or the hospital has capacity issues).

TABLE 40.1 ■ Speaking the Language of the Admitting Practitioner		
Specialist	**Poor Communication**	**Effective Communication**
Psychiatrist	He's pretty crazy!	Agitated paranoid schizophrenic with active delusions and command hallucinations requiring chemical sedation in the ED
Orthopedist	A badly broken ankle	An unstable displaced tri-malleolar fracture
Oncologist	Her white count is low and she is sick.	She has a neutropenic fever

Speaking the Language of the Admitting Physician

Successful emergency clinicians have learned to effectively present their patients to the admitting physician in a clear, reliable, and compelling manner (**Table 40.1**). It is substantially more difficult to be convincing when a patient "probably" requires hospitalization but has an atypical or "soft" presentation. Effective protocols, a history of trust, and consistent integrity are essential when communicating about complex or unclear cases.[7] When speaking to the admitting physician, clinicians can set the stage for excellent care by beginning their presentation with, "I have a nice patient who requires admission because of [insert diagnosis]."

Admitting Officer in the ED

Some large hospitals place a medical admitting officer—the "quarterback"—in the ED to expedite medical admissions. The ED admitter is commonly a hospitalist or a resident from an inpatient service. Well-organized programs discourage the admitting officer from performing exhaustive and redundant evaluations in the ED; instead, they expect the clinician to concentrate on the logistics of the patient's medications and admission orders. Extensive additional testing, a comprehensive reevaluation, and exhaustive admission orders should be deferred until the patient arrives on the inpatient unit.

Admitting Agreements

ED leaders should advocate for a "no-delay" expedited workflow. Occasionally, office-based physicians ask the ED to hold their patients until they have completed their daily administrative responsibilities and are free to admit their patients from the ED. This nonpatient-centered process can result in multihour delays. In addition, the admitting team may have other priorities that further delay care. For example, on-call surgeons may be in the operating room for prolonged periods—a limitation that can significantly affect how quickly they respond to the ED.

To address these potential delays, EDs should collaborate with admitting services to develop agreements that allow the ED to send stable patients to the floor for a subsequent evaluation by the admitting team. Computed tomography- or ultrasound-proven surgical conditions are easier for the surgeon to accept. This collaboration can lead to the use of holding/bridging orders (see Holding Orders) that define and provide workarounds to potential holdups. A written policy can help ensure an appropriate (rather than exhaustive) ED workup and determination of stability (**Box 40.4**).

BOX 40.4 ■ CONSULTING AGREEMENT FOR DIRECT ED ADMISSIONS

Most stable ED patients who require admission to the hospital should be evaluated by the admitting team in the inpatient nursing unit rather than in the ED. In such cases, the emergency physician will place brief holding orders after a discussion with the admitting team, who should submit more comprehensive orders after evaluating the patient on the floor.

Some hospitals now expect ED physicians to admit patients to the hospital for medical conditions that obviously require inpatient care (e.g., congestive heart failure, pancreatitis). In these cases, the ED physician enters an "ED hospitalist" admission power plan that is specific to the admitting diagnosis. The admitting team then reviews the ED physician's orders and calls him/her if they have any questions. It is safest for the emergency physician to place the admission orders under the name of the actual admitting physician to avoid the appearance of admitting the patient themselves. While emergency physicians often write "holding" or "bridging" orders, they should avoid writing "admitting" orders, which carry their legal responsibility into the inpatient area.

Eligible Patients

Clinically stable adult patients going to a floor or monitored bed who are being admitted from the ED.

Diagnostic Exclusion Criteria

1. Active or recent chest pain, unless the ECG and initial enzyme tests have been completed
2. Undiagnosed abdominal pain, unless abdominal imaging has been completed
3. Any undiagnosed neurological condition (e.g., focal weakness, confusion, paresthesia), unless neuroimaging (e.g., computed tomography or magnetic resonance imaging) has been completed
4. Patients who require intensive or progressive care
5. Patients who require an emergent operation or procedure

Procedure

1. **Involvement of an emergency medicine attending, if needed:** The midlevel emergency medicine provider (e.g., resident) should notify the emergency medicine attending of any potential direct admissions from the ED.
2. **Notification of the admitting team:** The emergency physician will consult the admitting team. Some institutions have a direct "no call" admissions process, in which the inpatient clinicians only speak with the ED team if they have specific questions regarding the patient.
3. **Selection of an inpatient nursing unit:** The emergency physician will order a bed after discussing the bed type and the nursing unit needed (e.g., monitored, unit, floor, or isolation) with the admitting team. If the admitting physician does not select the bed type, the emergency physician will make the decision based on clinical criteria.
4. **Completion of direct admission orders:** The emergency physician will enter a bed request and holding orders, if appropriate, immediately after speaking with the admitting team.
5. **Evaluation by the admitting team:** The admitting team is encouraged to see the patient in the ED while the patient is waiting for the in-house bed. The team may write new orders in the ED or change the bed type as clinically indicated.
6. **Transfer to floor:** Patients with a ready bed will be transferred if they have not already been evaluated by the inpatient team.
7. **Additional diagnostic evaluation:** Once a bed has been ordered, additional diagnostic studies, such as laboratory tests or imaging, may be ordered by the admitting team. However, the patient's transfer to an inpatient bed must not be delayed by these additional tests or procedures unless the results are likely to change the patient's disposition.
8. **Disagreements:** If there is a disagreement regarding a patient suitability for this direct admissions process, the midlevel ED provider should discuss the case with the ED attending.

Express Admitting Units and ED Holding Areas

Busy EDs need to decompress before boarders begin to stress available resources. Once the department is backed up by waiting patients, the staff must attend not only to "active" cases but also to the inpatient boarders. This consumes resources and further overloads providers. Boarders also prevent new patients, who may be in the waiting room, from receiving the attention and care that they require.

Express admitting units and holding areas may provide a solution to the problem by accepting patients into a nearby but a geographically separate unit. The size of these units varies according to the number of ED admissions per day, typically between 5 and 12 beds (although some large EDs may have 25-30 beds). In these units, patients' concerns are often addressed by the inpatient team, whereas patients in ED holding units are typically managed by emergency clinicians until the admitting physician assumes responsibility.

Using "holding orders," stable ED patients who require admission can be moved to the intermediate staging area while they await further evaluation or an available bed. Protocols for either type of unit should include a time-limited expectation for the completion of admitting orders. It is important to note that clinicians must be mindful to avoid "out of sight, out of mind" lapses in care when managing patients in these units. As such, it is imperative for the nursing staff to ensure timely reevaluations, clinical continuity, and provider responsiveness.

Holding Orders

Holding orders (i.e., "bridging orders") can decrease the time to admission and are a routine part of modern emergency practice in many large hospitals.[8] Note that holding orders are *not* admission orders, they are *time-limited* orders that permit stable patients to move safely from the ED to an inpatient setting or a holding unit (**Box 40.5**).

Historically, experts strongly discouraged emergency physicians from writing admission orders. The concern was that signing orders outside the control and scope of the ED could unnecessarily extend the emergency physicians' medicolegal liability to the inpatient setting. However, current data suggest that properly written holding orders pose little additional medical or legal risk to the emergency physician. The orders should have a time limit and clarify that the inpatient team and admitting physician are responsible for all further orders. In addition, the admitting team (*not* the emergency physician) must be notified of any changes in the patient's condition.

BOX 40.5 ■ KEY COMPONENTS OF ED ADMISSION ORDERS

Temporary Holding Orders (Non-ICU)

- Vital signs/oxygen saturation/cardiac monitoring
- Activity level
- Diet
- Nursing communication indicating these are holding orders (timed orders)
- Notification of further communication requirements (who and when)

- As needed (optional):
    - Urinary catheter or nasogastric tube maintenance protocol
    - Additional support (e.g., oxygen on nasal cannula or non-rebreather mask)
    - Intravenous fluids
    - Medications
    - Antiemetic agents, analgesia, and so on

Boarding patients in an overcrowded ED may carry more medicolegal risk than properly constructed holding orders. The American Academy of Emergency Medicine states:

The Academy believes that it is acceptable for emergency physicians to write Holding Orders, which define any necessary treatment and assessment parameters required in the interval until completion of admission orders.[9]

In its October 2017 policy revision, the American College of Emergency Physicians states:

There are circumstances in which, in the interest of patient care, patient safety, and operational efficiency, an emergency clinician may be asked to and may choose to write transition orders. Transition orders are meant to include essential treatment and assessment parameters on the patient's initial admission to an inpatient bed; they should be time limited and should serve as a bridge before complete admission orders are provided by the admitting physician (or designee).[10]

ICU LEAN POLICY

Critically ill patients who remain in the ED divert human resources, monitoring, and care from other patients. There is a clear correlation between the duration of time an ICU patient remains in the ED and subsequent mortality, especially for stays longer than 6 hours.[2,11,12]

The common goal for any ICU lean policy is to decrease the time between protocol activation and the patient's arrival in the ICU to less than 60 minutes (**Box 40.6**). An essential aspect of this approach is a ready (or quickly available) bed. Some ICUs have developed a "bed ahead" policy in which one empty bed is always available and reserved for ED admissions. As soon as that bed is full, they begin working on transferring another patient out of the ICU.

Intermountain Medical Center in Salt Lake City, Utah, developed a lean production protocol called "ED-ICU Priority One" to expedite the movement of critically ill patients out of the ED.[13] When a patient meets certain criteria, the Priority One protocol is activated. A critical care team comes to the ED to accept the handoff and then transports the patient directly to the ICU. The intensivist writes the ICU orders when the patient arrives in the unit. The ED length of stay for these patients went from 300 minutes before this effective intervention to less than 60 minutes after the protocol was established.

Although there are various iterations of this policy, successful protocols permit the patient to go directly to the ICU after a phone consultation with the intensivist and appropriate ED stabilization. This approach eliminates the need for the intensivist to come to the ED.

Typical indications for automatic ICU consultations and ICU lean protocols include intubation, extreme respiratory distress, persistent hypotension (especially if vasopressors or transfusion is required), hypothermic resuscitation postcardiac arrest, early goal-directed therapy for sepsis, and "provider discretion." These indications can be triggers for a "Code Critical Alert," which warns multiple stakeholders about an impending ICU admission.

BOX 40.6 ■ ICU LEAN

1. Request an ICU bed.
2. If an ICU bed is available, determine the need for a consultation based on a critical (i.e., intensivist) or noncritical (i.e., general admission) code criteria.
3. If the patient **IS** critical:
   - Page the intensivist, and discuss the patient's status.
   - Ask the ED secretary to page the admissions team.
4. If the patient is **NOT** critical:
   - Page the appropriate admitting physician.
   - Ask the secretary or nursing staff to page the inpatient care team for transfer to the medical ICU.

Expediting Nursing Reports

Just as emergency physicians' efforts to admit a patient may be impeded by the admitting team's inability to accept the case, emergency nurses' efforts may also be delayed when attempting to provide reports to the inpatient staff. In many hospitals, inpatient nurses are extremely busy and may not be able take an ED report when the patient is ready to be transferred. This may occur for a variety of reasons, including limited staff, staff on break, change of shift, high acuity, recent "code," and so on.

Standardized reports can negate the need for verbal reports (**Figure 40.1**). Instead of a telephone conversation, which requires both nurses to be available and unencumbered at the same time, the ED nurse can communicate the hand-off through a standardized report, which can be sent to the floor electronically or via fax. The ED nurse can simply notify the

FIGURE 40.1 ■ An Electronic Patient Report Sample

Emergency Department

Patient Sticker _____

Admitting Diagnosis: _____ **Admitting Physician:** _____

Date: _____ Pt. room number: _____ Time faxed: _____
Report by: _____ at phone number _____
Estimated transport time: _____ Transported by: ☐ RN   ☐ EDT
Equipment needed: ☐ monitor   ☐ pulse ox   ☐ oxygen   ☐ IV pump ☐ other _____
Precautions: ☐ suicide   ☐ respiratory isolation   ☐ contact   ☐ immunocompromised ☐ droplet
☐ other _____

Allergies: _____
Past medical history: _____
Past surgical history: _____
Home medications: _____

Oxygen source: _____ at _____ L/min ☐ NA O_2 sat _____ %
VS: T_____ P_____ R_____ BP_____ cardiac rhythm _____
IV: #1 site _____ size _____ solution _____ rate _____ DC credit _____
     #2 site _____ size _____ solution _____ rate _____ DC credit _____
Other: ☐ Foley catheter   ☐ NG tube   ☐ other _____

Lab results: CK: _____ MB: _____
                                                      Troponin: _____
                                                      PT: ____ PTT: ____ INR: ____
Other abnormal labs: _____
Radiology: ☐ chest   ☐ KUB   ☐ pelvis   ☐ obstruction series   ☐ c-spines   ☐ head CT   ☐ abd CT
☐ helical CT   ☐ other _____
Abnormal radiology results: _____

Medications give: Name: _____ dose: _____ route: _____ effect: _____
                  Name: _____ dose: _____ route: _____ effect: _____
                  Name: _____ dose: _____ route: _____ effect: _____
                  Name: _____ dose: _____ route: _____ effect: _____
Interventions still needed: meds _____
IV _____
other _____

Comments: _____

unit secretary on the inpatient unit to expect a report. If questions arise, the floor nurse may call the ED nurse for clarification. If there are no questions or issues that delay transport, the patient can be transferred to the floor 15 minutes after the report is sent. Alternatively, if there are problems that prevent the patient from being transported, the ED nurse and the nursing supervisor can be called simultaneously. The nursing supervisor can immediately address the issue that is causing the delay, thereby removing the barrier to patient flow. This protocol prevents a single person from backing up the system, a safeguard that decreases boarding times and increases bed-flow efficiency.[14]

ADOPT-A-BOARDER PROGRAM

The Adopt-a-Boarder program, which was first instated by the Inova Medical Group and Stony Brook University Hospital, has since been embraced by many of the largest hospitals in the United States.[15] The underlying premise of the program is that admitted patients can routinely spend hours in the ED hallway while waiting for an inpatient bed. A high-volume ED may occasionally be forced to "board" 10 or more patients in the hallway. In some institutions, these patients can wait for 12 hours or more.

While some institutions may deny that boarding is a problem, the reality is that most US hospitals board patients in hallways every single day—in the *ED* hallway! Clinical care and patient satisfaction can be improved by sharing this burden with the inpatient wards. Physician Peter Viccellio, an originator of the Adopt-a-Boarder program, suggests asking the following questions:

- Instead of having all 10 patients wait in a single hallway in the ED, what if 1 patient was placed in each of 10 different hallways on inpatient wards?
- Would these patients get better care in the ED or in the inpatient unit?
- Would the patients be more satisfied with their boarding stay in the inpatient unit?

Multiple studies have examined these questions. The universal answer is that admitted ED patients uniformly prefer the inpatient hallway to the ED hallway, where they report receiving more personal attention and better care. Nearly all patients report being happier when they are physically closer to an inpatient bed.

Studies show that an Adopt-a-Boarder program can accelerate inpatient bed turnover. Many patients who are destined for an inpatient hallway bed may instead go straight to their inpatient rooms; beds may be cleaned in a fraction of the usual time. Patient satisfaction with the program was extremely high at all the hospitals studied. With the increasing importance of the patient experience and its reimbursement implications, Adopt-a-Boarder initiatives may benefit most hospitals, their patients, and their staff.

ED DASHBOARDS

Many hospitals are using technology to help guide decisions and improve flow. The Johns Hopkins Hospital, which uses ED dashboards to monitor flow and make improvements, notes that "the use of visual information reduces information overload and increases the understanding of data and the ability to remember information."[16] This, in turn, aids decision-making and improves compliance with clinical guidelines, ultimately resulting in better outcomes. Johns Hopkins clinicians report that their electronic dashboard also provides valuable information that enables hospital workgroups to improve flow and processes. Even better, once the changes have been implemented, institutions can use the technology to monitor the impact of the changes at all admission levels.[16]

In large hospitals, these dashboards can include patients who are scheduled or ready to be transferred to the institution. In such circumstances, transferred patients can go directly into their inpatient bed instead of waiting in the ED.

CONCLUSION

Expediting admissions requires a change in culture—from top to bottom. Admitting services and nursing units seldom intuitively recognize the advantages that sound protocols can have on patient care, flow, and satisfaction. Such revolutions in care must be driven by the central question, "What is best for the patient?" With this patient-first approach, administrative, ED, and inpatient leaders can forge programs that effectively expedite the flow of patients and improve care while addressing the needs of the providers.

REFERENCES

1. Kellermann AL. Crisis in the emergency department. *N Engl J Med.* 2006;355:1300-1303.
2. American College of Emergency Physicians. ACEP Task Force Report on Boarding. https://www.acep.org/globalassets/uploads/uploaded-files/acep/membership/sections-of-membership/intnatl/news/2008boardingreport.pdf?_t_id=&_t_q=ACEP%20task%20force%20boarding&_t_tags=andquerymatch,language:en|language:7D2DA0A9FC754533B091FA6886A51C0D,siteid:3f8e28e9-ff05-45b3-977a-68a85dcc834a|siteid:84BFAF5C52A349A0BC61A9FFB6983A66&_t_ip=&_t_hit.id=ACP_Website_Application_Models_Media_DocumentMedia/_18e8e81e-560c-4725-81fa-5c2162e2bc8f&_t_hit.pos=0
3. Bernstein SL, Aronsky D, Duseja R, et al. The effect of emergency department crowding on clinically oriented outcomes. *Acad Emerg Med.* 2009;16(1):1-10.
4. Wiswell J, Tsao K, Bellolio MF, Hess EP, Cabrera D. "Sick" or "not-sick": accuracy of system 1 diagnostic reasoning for the prediction of disposition and acuity in patients presenting to an academic ED. *Am J Emerg Med.* 2013;31(10):1448-1452.
5. Hsiao AL, Santucci KA, Dziura J, Baker MD. A randomized trial to assess the efficacy of point-of-care testing in decreasing length of stay in a pediatric emergency department. *Pediatr Emerg Care.* 2007;23(7):457-462.
6. Murray RP, Leroux M, Sabga E, Palatnick W, Ludwig L. Effect of point of care testing on length of stay in an adult emergency department. *J Emerg Med.* 1999;17(5):811-814.
7. Innes G. Successful hospitalization of patients with no discernible pathology. *CJEM.* 2000;2(1):110-120.
8. Patterson J, Dutterer L, Rutt M, Marsteller K, Jacoby J, Heller M. Bridging orders and a dedicated admission nurse decreases emergency department turnaround times while increasing patient satisfaction. *Ann Emerg Med.* 2007;50(3):351-352.
9. http://www.aaem.org/positionstatements/admissions.php. Accessed November 29, 2018.
10. American College of Emergency Physicians. ACEP policy: writing admission and transition orders. http://www.acep.org/Content.aspx?id=29860&terms=admission. Accessed February 12, 2018.
11. Chalfin DB, Trzeciak S, Likourezos A, et al. Impact of delayed transfer of critically ill patients from the emergency department to the intensive care unit. *Crit Care Med.* 2007;35:1477-1483.
12. Reznek MA, Upatising B, Kennedy SJ, Durham NT, Forster RM, Michael SS. Mortality associated with emergency department boarding exposure: are there differences between patients admitted to ICU and non-ICU settings? *Med Care.* 2018;56(5):436-440.
13. Weich SJ. Priority one protocol relieves ED of critical care burden. *Emergency Medicine News.* April 2009:15-18.
14. Potts L, Ryan C, Diegel-Vacek L, Murchek A. Improving patient flow from the emergency department utilizing a standardized electronic nursing handoff process. *J Nurs Adm.* 2018;48(9):432-436.
15. Mayer M. Adopt-a-boarder. Views from the Field. 2013. Inova Fairfax Hospital. https://smhs.gwu.edu/urgentmatters/news/views-field-inova-fairfax-hospital. Accessed November 21, 2019.
16. Martinez DA, Kane EM, Jalapcur M, et al. An electronic dashboard to monitor patient flow at the Johns Hopkins Hospital: communication of key performance indicators using the Donabedian model. *J Med Sys.* 2018;42(8):133.

CHAPTER 41

DECISION TO DISCHARGE: FINISHING STRONG

Jody Crane, Robert W. Strauss, Suzanne Stone-Griffith, Thom A. Mayer

Great is the art of beginning, but greater is the art of ending.

—Henry Wadsworth Longfellow

Successful strategies to improve emergency department (ED) flow require specific attention to the management of patient disposition (outflow). Department flow is based on the "input-throughput-output" model introduced to emergency medicine in 2003 by Brent Asplin.[1] In many EDs, the most significant barriers to flow exist in the outflow of patients from the department. Based on the Theory of Constraints, we know that output obstruction (boarding patients) constrains all other upstream elements of ED flow. Mayer and Jensen notes, "It's difficult to open the front door of the ED (input) unless and until the back door of the ED (output) can be opened."[2]

All elements of flow must be optimized from patient arrival through disposition. Because flow can break down at any time, all three phases must be optimized and constantly maintained. When any one phase becomes problematic, contingencies must be in place to overcome the obstruction. Perfecting flow requires leveraging strategic partnerships with other hospital leaders, including administration, medical staff, nursing leaders, the bed board, and others to continuously improve flow processes.

These improvement efforts are best viewed through the lens of a Lean leadership approach, in which adding value and eliminating waste at each stage of the process are central tenets of the hospital's approach.[2-4] This is complicated by the simple but often unrecognized fact that the ED performs patient dispositions, including admissions and discharges around the clock. However, hospitals typically do not discharge patients or transfer them between inpatient units in the late evening or early morning hours.

Outflow improvement requires strong hospital leadership, sustained commitment, and the mobilization of significant institutional resources. However, improvement in outflow does not by itself enhance the patient experience. Other organizational inefficiencies can undermine the credibility of ED leadership and impair further improvement efforts. Therefore, ED flow improvements require a combination of highly coordinated internal and external efforts to smoothly "flow" patients through the system. Without this consistent and organized focus, patients will experience long waits, either due to inefficiency or hospital flow constraints, which in turn often result in hospital crowding and ED boarding of inpatients. Prolonged delays result in poor clinical outcomes, dissatisfied patients, and financial losses.[2-5]

A wealth of data confirms that ED boarding leads to increased morbidity and mortality. In 2007, Chalfin et al looked at 100,000 critical care patient visits and found that boarding in the ED for more than 6 hours led to an increase in inpatient length of stay (LOS) by 1 day, an increase in ICU mortality by 27%, and an increase in inpatient mortality by 35%.[6]

In 2011, Singer et al showed the mortality rate increased 80% (from 2.5% to 4.5%) for patients boarding in the ED for more than 12 hours when compared to those boarding less than 2 hours.[7] In the same study, inpatient LOS increased from 5.6 days when boarding less than 2 hours to 8.7 days for patients boarding in the ED for more than 24 hours. Another study of nearly 14 million ED visits found a greater risk of short-term death and admission in patients who presented during shifts with longer waiting times.[8] Finally, there are excellent reviews in the literature about the impact of boarding and ED crowding.[9-11]

Due to the significant impact of outflow congestion on quality and the increased emphasis on transparency, a number of national organizations, such as The Joint Commission and the National Quality Forum, are measuring and holding hospitals accountable for ED LOS.[12,13] It is imperative that each health system and every hospital embrace these measures as a means to drive operational and quality improvement within their organizations.

KEY METRICS AND MILESTONES

Emergency department metrics have been used to measure flow since before emergency medicine became a specialty. The specific application of metrics continues to evolve to drive operational improvement. In 2006, the ED Benchmarking Alliance published a paper listing a set of metrics in the ED.[14] This list has been updated several times. The availability of objective, improved, and timely metrics is dramatically increasing as access to data and information is rapidly expanding.

Consistent measurement methods are necessary to compare data. However, many organizations develop elements of ED performance with self-reported information that is not objectively reproducible. This measurement variation makes it difficult to benchmark performance, including outflow metrics. Further complicating effective data comparisons is the fact that there are a wide variety of metrics based on individually customized processes and technologies. With the Centers for Medicare and Medicaid Services endorsement of several new outflow measures, it is likely that there will be increased standardization.

Common Outflow Metrics

As technology standards become more widely accepted, data will continue to be more efficiently translated into usable information. **Table 41.1** presents a list of generally accepted and emerging metrics used to measure outflow performance.

The most commonly measured outflow interval is called the disposition decision to departure. This outflow metric is generally divided into two groups of patients: those who are treated and released and those who are treated and admitted. In both cases, the metric is generally defined as the time period from the physician disposition order to the

TABLE 41.1 ■ Outflow Performance Metrics

Generally accepted measures	More detailed measures
Disposition to departure for patients treated and released	Decision to admit to bed request
Disposition to bed assignment for admitted patients	Admitting orders completed to departure
Bed assignment to departure for admitted patients	Ready for inpatient transport to departure
Boarding hours for admitted patients	Bed request to clean bed available

patient's actual departure from the ED bed. For treated and admitted patients, the interval is somewhat more difficult to define because of the various admission processes used in each facility, including the time for the:

- Emergency physician placing the order to admit (In many institutions, this occurs only after approval by the admitting physician, and often well after the decision is made by the emergency physician.)
- Admitting physician accepting the patient (though the patient may remain in the ED)
- Hospital bed desk assigning the patient an inpatient bed
- Patient being moved to (or residing in) a holding bed
- Staff changing the patient to a new status in the electronic health record (EHR)
- Patient leaving the ED

While many institutions have a difficult time defining the actual disposition time for admitted patients, most cite the moment when the ED physician enters his or her decision (order) to admit the patient into the system. The disposition decision time can be defined by a documented time in the medical record, a time stamp on a call, a page to a receiving physician, or the time bridging orders are placed in institutions that use these orders to facilitate the admission process. Also, the departure time should be consistently defined as the time when the patient physically departs, as documented in the ED information system or the hospital bed tracking system.

Like many metrics, it is often helpful to break the process down into its component parts so that each may be assessed for discrete bottlenecks. For instance, the typical admission disposition time may be further broken down as follows:

- Physician decision to admit to the:
  - System notification, that is, entry of an order to admit
  - Physician handoff—communication with an admitting physician to the
    - Entry of admission or bridging orders
    - Bed request to the
      - Bed assignment to the
      - Bed ready to
      - Departure
      - Nursing handoff—inclusive of preparation and communication to the
      - Final preparation and movement of the patient, including the
      - Preparation of report
      - Communication of report via fax, phone, EHR, or auto print
      - Organization of personnel and equipment for patient departure, including monitors, transportation personnel, etc
      - Change entered into bed-tracking system

To optimize performance, each component requires close scrutiny. The disposition-to-bed-assignment interval encompasses the physician handoff, the bed request, and the bed assignment. The bed-assignment interval encompasses the handoff between the ED nurses and inpatient nurses, any transport-related logistics, and the completion of the patient's clinical workup and treatment. Times should be measured both by the ED and the unit to which the patient is admitted (e.g., intensive care units [ICUs], monitored units, medical-surgical floors), because the processes for each of the units may vary. While defined metrics—such as those listed in **Table 41.1**—can be used to assess and address flow issues within an institution, benchmarking across multiple institutions is more difficult, as definitions and local practice, technology, or systems often defy cross-institutional analysis.

For example, teaching institutions seldom allow bed requests until the receiving service evaluates and accepts the patient. (In these institutions, the fundamental question of the value added versus the waste created by such policies should be carefully scrutinized. Is there truly a value added to the teaching mission and, if so, is it worth the waste (disposition delays) created for the patient and for the ED?) In this type of situation, it may be less meaningful to track ED physician disposition to bed request and more meaningful to track the timeliness of consult or admitting service evaluation:

- Call to admitting service to response by or arrival of the admitting resident
- Arrival of admitting resident to admitting orders
- Percentage of patients evaluated by, but not admitted to, admitting service

Some institutions use hospital bed-tracking software to signal that the sending unit is ready to move the patient. This time stamp may be flawed by the inaccurate entry of information. When used effectively, the time between "ready to move" and "departure" may isolate system inefficiencies both within and beyond the ED.

Environmental services (EVS) issues are sometimes identified by using "bed request to clean bed available" as a measurement interval. A newer metric evaluates the "percentage of beds assigned clean." This approach stresses the creation of a pull system by striving to always have a clean bed available for the next admitted patient. While EVS efficiency can be a potential bottleneck, it is important to properly diagnose the problem. A common misperception is that long EVS turnaround times (TATs) are solely related to EVS performance. However, the most common cause of prolonged EVS TAT may involve the batching of hospital discharges at shift changes, and EVS performance could be best in class.

Performance Measures and Rapid-Cycle Testing

Only by measuring performance and instituting a series of rapid-cycle tests (RCTs) can an institution improve. This focus, which starts with senior leadership, drives performance through a hospital-wide committee of all key stakeholders. The philosophy of "owning your own queue" should be stressed to all members of the team. As examples:

- *Inpatient and ED physicians* should collaboratively own the physician component of the outflow queue, cooperating to drive efficient evaluations in the ED. Alternatively, the physicians can create an efficient bridging order protocol when timely evaluations by the inpatient physicians are not feasible.
- *Nursing supervisors and unit charge nurses* should own the bed-assignment process. As a subcomponent of that metric, inpatient and ED nurses own the bed assignment-to-departure interval. The nurses should be held accountable by their respective managers, who ideally have a common supervising administrator driving cooperation among the areas.
- *Hospital administration* must own bed management to smooth the needed resources across the organization, ensure reliable staffing, regularly address bed demand and availability, and relentlessly pursue the LOS reductions necessary to meet the demand of admitted patients in a timely, responsive manner.

Hospital administration must also be relentless about responding to and resolving boarding in the ED. Addressing this issue involves the design of alert systems that trigger specific interventions when overcrowding reaches predetermined levels and further involves accountability measures to ensure those responsible are executing the plan. A simple question for hospital leaders is: "If this were a member of your own family, would this delay be acceptable?" If the answer is no, the process should be changed (see Chapter 43).

All parties involved in the improvement and RCT efforts must clearly understand the definitions of the pertinent terms. While originally proposed as the taxonomy for inpatient flow, the definitions must be accepted and understood by ED staff as well.

- *Available bed* is a bed that is cleaned, staffed, and ready to accept a patient.
- *Discharge* is a patient who has actually left the bed.
- *Capacity* is defined as discharges plus available beds.
- *Admission* is a patient who has been placed in an available inpatient bed or will be placed in a potentially available inpatient bed.
- *Hospital boarder* is an admitted patient residing in the ED.
- *Inpatient* is a patient who resides on an inpatient unit.

For example, a patient who has been "discharged" but is still in an ED bed would not be considered a discharge until they actually leave the bed. Similarly, both on the inpatient and the ED units, an "available bed" only refers to a bed that is cleaned, staffed, and ready to accept a patient. Beds that do not fit these criteria should not be used to solve flow.

It is important to mention that there is no standardized definition of the term *boarding*. The generally accepted benchmark and, anecdotally, the most common practice is "admission" plus 1 hour starts the boarding clock. Some sites use "admission" plus 2 hours. A small minority start the clock immediately upon disposition (admission plus zero hours). Some allowance is reasonable, as there is a certain amount of time required to find an inpatient bed, make the provider and nurse handoffs, and finally move the patient upstairs.

DISCHARGES

There are essentially three distinct destinations for patients who have been evaluated in the ED: *discharge home, transfer to another facility,* and *hospital admission*. Because there are unique challenges to optimizing each of these disposition pathways in the ED, they are discussed separately in the following text.

Challenges to Patient Discharge

The process of discharging a patient home is perhaps the simplest and most straightforward disposition from the ED. Yet, there are challenges. Perhaps the most significant of these is addressing inertia—creating a compelling motivation to move the patients out of the ED. Often, the discharged patient is the lowest priority of the staff. The new unknown patient may be unstable and require substantial staff attention, while the *known* patient who is ready for discharge is usually stable and does not require immediate attention. Further, the act of discharging a patient inherently creates more work. For these reasons, staff members may instead turn their attention to other urgent work prior to discharging the current patient.

Another form of discharge delay is the patient waiting for one simple test to come back, such as a urinalysis. Because of the drivers previously mentioned, it can be relatively easy to avoid work by not fulfilling a simple task, such as collecting the urine.

The primary goal in the ED is to stabilize critically ill patients, and while it may be somewhat counterintuitive, our next most important goal is to discharge patients. Most EDs fall into the trap of getting everyone seen; however, the *actual* goal of efficient flow requires the assessment and discharge of patients. To address the challenges to patient discharge, the fundamental mission, vision, and values of the ED and the entire hospital must reflect a commitment to flow. Staff at every level in every unit should be recruited, onboarded, trained, promoted, and rewarded for improving flow and other aspects of the patient experience (see Chapters 2 and 78).

Misaligned Incentives

All nurses and many physicians are paid on an hourly basis and have little incentive to improve throughput (other than their considerable innate professionalism). Further, competing variables, such as staffing constraints, can undermine the pursuit of performance excellence and instead lead to a focus on self-preservation. Overwhelmed, overworked, and understaffed nurses and physicians are unlikely to engage in the promotion of patient flow. Attention to efficient patient flow requires a properly supported ED staff that understands the importance of ensuring timely patient evaluations. Excellent leadership can overcome the negative incentives by painting the right vision and holding staff accountable. Additionally, throughput incentives encourage and inspire staff to focus on efficiently processing patients.

Many physicians are paid based on performance methodologies, such as relative value units. These reimbursement arrangements provide a financial incentive to increase productivity by increasing the number of patients evaluated and the completeness of documentation. Productivity-based payment methodologies can effectively incentivize physicians to process patients efficiently. However, the lack of a similar payment methodology among team members (see Chapters 86 and 87).

Patients with inadequate family, social, or financial support systems further complicate the discharge process. Patients with special needs frequently require case management intervention while still in the ED to arrange for special care at home and coordinate the availability of equipment. Unfortunately, most EDs do not have 24-hour access to dedicated case managers, and inpatient case management workers are rarely available to consult on ED patients. This lack of discharge resources may lead to patient admissions or prolonged waits for those who could otherwise be sent home if they had adequate community and personal resources. A busy ED without adequate discharge resources further backs up as patients wait longer for an an evaluation because they cannot be placed in a bed currently occupied by a patient with a complex and prolonged discharge.

Behavioral Health Challenges

Many hospitals and communities are facing the challenges associated with behavioral health and substance or alcohol issues. Since most of these patients are "discharged," the prolonged evaluations, observations, and placement problems are significant contributors to ED boarding and crowding. Many of these patients spend hours under observation, waiting for a documented improvement in mental capacity. Emerging "best practice" strategies to manage these patient populations include:

- "In-house/ED" mobile crisis support evaluators
- Behavioral telemedicine evaluation and management
- Time-sensitive initial evaluations that expedite patient placement
- Discharge coordinators in the ED for patients with special needs (including the elderly, for whom early studies are promising[15]).

Substance abuse poses another barrier to discharge. The requirement for and complications associated with medical clearance often contribute to delayed behavioral patient management and placement. Nonstandard and inconsistent industry definitions of medical clearance create additional confusion. For example, there is often controversy between emergency and behavioral practitioners about the acceptable blood alcohol level required to prompt further evaluation and discharge. Creating safe and efficient dispositions of these patients requires a high degree of collaboration and consensus.

Facilitating Patient Discharge

Many institutions have experimented with innovative programs to facilitate patient discharge. There are several promising processes, including implementation of a float nurse, stratification of discharges by complexity and number of resources required, discharge rooms or lounges, results waiting areas, ED navigators, and discharge kiosks. These programs show great potential, but there are no published studies that prove them beneficial.

Discharge Float Nurse

The ED discharge float nurse has a primary responsibility to discharge patients who are ready to go home. This strategy frees up the primary nurse to focus on other duties, patient assessments, and management. Another benefit is that if there are no discharges, the float nurse can assist other nurses to provide primary care for their patients.

The major argument against this strategy is that it either requires additional staffing or removes a nurse from the staffing pool/mix with the potential of further burdening the primary nurses. By this reasoning, if instead of creating a float nurse position, an additional nurse were added to the regular working pool, all nurses would be less burdened and more efficient in their patient management and responsive in their discharges. Furthermore, if the discharge nurse position were strictly adhered to and the nurse becomes the only pathway to discharge, the process would be more susceptible to another bottleneck.

Simple vs Complex Discharges

Discharges may be stratified into simple and complex discharges, with simple discharges handled by a technician following the provider instructions. If the provider has given the instructions directly to the patient and printed the discharge materials, a technician often can complete the process. The nurse may then focus on the more complex discharge instructions and needs.

Discharge Room, Lounge, or Results Waiting Area

A discharge room or lounge is another way to increase the efficiency of discharges and decrease the queue of waiting patients. The discharge area is staffed by a nurse and others, such as financial coordinators, who can attempt to collect copays, verify insurance, and enroll uninsured patients into special government programs. Involving registration personnel in the discharge process can be very effective, since up to 25% of patients are found to have inadvertently provided inaccurate information. In addition, some EDs collect copays or full payment as a part of the discharge process, which can be a significant source of fair payments. The patient proceeds to the discharge area after the final physician instructions, where the nurse rechecks vital signs and provides discharge instructions and prescriptions.

Results waiting areas are typically used for patients in a "front-loaded" SuperTrack or ultratrack area. This is an ideal option for patients likely to be discharged who are waiting only for the result of a laboratory test or image and do not need active management by a nurse. The rooms are comfortable and potentially allow multiple patients to wait for their results in a space separated from the preassessment waiting room.

Discharge rooms or lounges are typically used for patients with somewhat more complex medical problems than those in the results waiting area. Effective discharge rooms have developed processes to ensure communication between the discharge nurse, who is somewhat unfamiliar with the patient, and the primary nurse or physician who managed the case. Communication devices eliminate the wasted time required for the discharge nurse to find previous caregivers.

An obvious advantage of a dedicated discharge room is that the evaluation and treatment room is vacated in a timelier manner, thereby freeing up additional room time for patient care. The disadvantages are that the dedicated discharge room requires both additional staffing and an available room that is not used for patient care.

ED Navigators

Emergency department navigators assist with discharge follow-up appointments for primary care physicians (PCPs), specialists, and outpatient testing. These appointments can sometimes be made prior to the patient's discharge. These navigators can also make follow-up calls to help avoid unnecessary repeat visits and improve patient satisfaction.[16]

Discharge Kiosks

Good discharge planning can positively affect the immediate postdischarge period and improve the patient experience. As an example, the innovation of e-prescribing and prescription kiosks facilitates the acquisition of discharge medications. Discharge kiosks are increasingly available in EDs across the nation. These kiosks electronically obtain the prescription from the EMR, reference the patient's insurance information, and dispense the prescribed medications with one swipe of a credit card.

TRANSFERS

Efficient transfers to and from the ED enhance efficiency. The increasing complexity and demands of acute care pathways (e.g., acute ST-elevation myocardial infarction, stroke designations to manage cerebrovascular accident, and trauma designations) coupled with cost constraints and limited resources are changing the way care is delivered in the ED. Health systems cannot staff specialists at every facility, a limitation that has led to the adoption of the "hub-and-spoke" models chosen by many organizations. These models rapidly transfer patients requiring acute interventions from secondary to tertiary sites. To accomplish this redistribution of care, hub-and-spoke facilities have created sophisticated, efficient networks with protocol-driven transfer systems. These interfacility transfer systems may also be used to return nursing home and other long-term care facility patients back to their residences.

Specialized Transfers

The primary reason to transfer a patient is to access a higher level of care. EMTALA was enacted to ensure that sending and receiving facilities are held accountable for maintaining appropriate standards. It is critical that specialized protocols are thoughtfully developed to ensure that transfers are driven by what is best for the patient.

Pediatric Patients

Many pediatric transfers require specialized transportation services, such as pediatric or neonatal critical care teams. Prolonged preparation for these transfers can result in delays. To expedite these transfers, many organizations draft special transfer agreements with receiving facilities to ensure the smooth flow of critically ill patients. Further delays may occur because of overcrowding in the tertiary care receiving facilities.

Behavioral Health

Behavioral health inpatient capacity varies widely based on a number of factors, including location (urban, suburban, rural), access to behavioral health specialists and units, availability of specialized units (detox, pediatric psychiatric units), and community state support. Due to increased financial pressure, many communities are encountering behavioral bed closures in the face of increasing patient demands.

Few community EDs have sufficient resources, and most are experiencing increasing pressure to discharge these patients to underresourced community clinics or board them in the ED (sometimes for days) while they await inpatient treatment by mental health professionals (see Chapter 50). Patients requiring detoxification from drug and alcohol abuse can pose further logistical issues for EDs. These patients frequently require complicated inpatient and transfer destination decisions and clearance.

Nursing Homes and Long-Term Acute Care Hospitals

Disposition to nursing homes and other long-term acute care hospitals requires careful planning, including:

- Facility acceptance procedures
- Paperwork and documentation completion and access
- Real-time knowledge of bed availability
- Reliable, responsive transportation

In recent years, changes in observation status and government payment policies have led to unique challenges for elderly patients. Medicare policy requires most of these patients to be admitted to a hospital for 3 days in order to approve the payment for a long-term care facility. However, increased scrutiny over inpatient versus observation designations place the hospitals in a "Catch-22" situation. Consider a patient who is admitted to a hospital in advance of transfer to a long-term facility. If the admission does not meet hospitalization criteria, reimbursement for the entire stay may be retrospectively denied. However, if the hospital admits the patient under observation status, the eventual nursing home stay will not be covered under Medicare because the patient did not meet the "3-day criterion." The end result is increased pressure on emergency physicians to find alternatives to admitting these patients, again resulting in prolonged ED stays.

Other Special Transfers

Issues of guardianship and forensic evaluations for suspected victims of abuse also create special transfer challenges. Some communities have addressed these challenges by developing specialized resources. However, many dispositions prove difficult to solve, requiring patients to spend days in the ED. Where special prolonged LOS situations exist, it is appropriate to separate the data from the patients, who can significantly skew overall performance measures. The LOS is prolonged not only for these patients but also for others who experience a crowded ED with overburdened resources.

ADMISSIONS

The outflow of admitted patients from the ED is complex and incorporates elements of the nursing handoff, the physician handoff, and inpatient bed (and hospital flow) management. Successful management of these elements is critical to moving the patient to an inpatient unit efficiently and effectively. Aligning all of these key variables requires the relentless attention of senior leadership and the engagement of frontline staff and middle management.

Nursing Handoffs

Delays

As the first key element, the nursing handoff is frequently plagued with politics, incentive misalignment, and resource constraints. The process is often complex, with a number of failure points and bottlenecks. Increasing financial constraints placed on systems has caused many institutions to utilize "core staffing" to reduce inpatient staffing or use real-time demand capacity techniques to "right-size" staffing based on current rather than anticipated demand. This conservative approach can result in a lack of staffed inpatient beds causing the delay of patient transfers to and from critical care units and from the ED to inpatient units. Further, overwhelmed staff may by necessity delay taking a report, receiving bed assignments, and discharging patients.

Just as in the ED, discharging inpatients requires significant work. Placing even more pressure on the inpatient nurses, many of the discharges and admissions occur as staff conclude a shift or attempt to take scheduled breaks from their shifts, that is, between noon (lunch) and the 3 pm shift change and between 5 pm (dinner) and the 7 pm shift change. These breaks further limit the time during which nursing reports can be given and taken.

In an attempt to address these problems, some facilities have formal "no admit zones," times during shift change (or breaks) when the ED cannot provide patient information or transfer patients to the units. This attempt to protect the nurses whose shifts are ending increases the pressure on the nurses whose shifts are beginning and on the ED. While the hazards associated with nursing change of shift are well-documented in the literature many are linked to communication breakdowns for which there are few proven solutions.[17,18] There are no studies linking patient safety and transfer of patients between areas of the hospital during shift change. Many ED staffs argue that their patients *never* stop coming, so others should be continuously open to accept the same constant flow.

However, it should be noted that the ED providers and nursing staff also participate in this uneven flow of admissions. For example, emergency physicians, who continue to see new patients during and near the end of their shifts, will attempt to admit several patients at once. As do emergency nurses, who also may not admit patients for significant periods of time because of prolonged sign-outs (handoffs).

Solutions

The current best practice is "call and send": First, the transferring ED nurse calls report to the inpatient unit. If the floor nurse is unavailable, then the charge nurse takes report and the patient is sent upstairs. If the charge nurse is unavailable, then the floor has 15 minutes to call back. If there is no call back, then the report is faxed or the floor alerted that the EMR report has been entered and the patient is moved. Although this system is widely used, direct nursing handoffs are preferred, when possible.

Another recent trend involves the ED nurse directly transporting all of the patients to the floor. While this is resource intensive, it does obviate the need to discuss clinical issues over the phone and allows reports to be given face-to-face at the bedside. Other hospitals have the inpatient nurses come to the ED to retrieve their patients and receive reports at the bedside. However, while this practice does provide direct transfer of care, it does not overcome the motivational issues that delay patient receipt.

Another emerging practice involves handing off admitted patients to an ED flow coordinator, who acts as a bridge between the ED and the nursing units. The flow coordinator "packages" the patient, transports, provides bedside review of the ED nursing summary, and assists the nursing floor with settling the patient into that floor. In this approach, the patient's needs are met and the nurses on the floor have support for inpatient paperwork during the times of high transition volumes.

Physician Handoffs

Academic Medical Centers

An effective physician handoff is essential to ensure efficient patient movement. In the name of "education," some academic medical centers introduce significant physician delays that often exceed the nursing delays. In these institutions, after the decision to admit is made, members (sometimes multiple) of the admitting physician team are required by policy to evaluate the patient in the ED before the bed can be formally requested. This reevaluation process inserts a queue for the additional evaluation that usually occurs prior to (rather than simultaneously with) the bed request. Even worse, there can be multiple queues in the inpatient physician evaluation, from intern to junior to senior resident and finally to the attending, all requiring approval for admission.

As academic medical centers increasingly face competitive financial and service pressures, it is unlikely that the traditional processes will continue. There is limited or no value added to these processes, even from an educational and training perspective.[2-5] As an academic medical center best practice, attending-to-attending conversations begin the admission and bed request processes, allowing resident assessments to occur in parallel with the bed placement process. This parallel process significantly reduces queuing, communication, and decision-making delays.

Hospitalists

In community hospitals, primary care providers (PCPs) have increasingly chosen to focus their work in their offices, leading directly to a dramatic increase in the use of hospitalists. Consistent presence of hospitalists has substantially changed the physician handoff process. Traditionally, the ED physician called the PCP, who was often not immediately available. Once contacted, the PCP provided admitting orders by phone to the ED or inpatient nurse. Now, though the initial contact with the hospitalist may occur more quickly, there may be other delays. Some hospitalists insist on evaluating the patient prior to admission, creating queues in the ED. This delay can be exacerbated if staffing does not match the peak demand for admissions. As a result, admitted patients residing in the ED or on the inpatient unit can wait several hours for a hospitalist evaluation. As the relationship between emergency physicians and other specialists evolves, many hospitals are developing processes that allow for much faster and more efficient communication between these groups.

Bridging or Transitional Orders

In the past, most emergency physicians considered it unacceptable to write any type of admission orders. The practice was frowned upon. It could increase malpractice risk, confuse the transition of patient care, and lead to inadequate care because inpatient management is not a competency of emergency physicians. However, in order to facilitate flow, many ED physicians are choosing to write transitional orders or continuation of care orders that are timed and limited to facilitate safe and effective patient movement from the ED to the inpatient units. This practice has recently been endorsed by the American College of Emergency Physicians and The American Academy of Emergency Medicine.[19,20]

It is now considered a "best practice" for emergency physicians to write brief, time-limited bridging orders when the accepting physician is not immediately available to write them. This practice allows bed assignments to occur without waiting for the inpatient physician assessment. The minimum set of bridging orders includes admitting diagnosis, admitting attending, NPO status, and "Call the admitting physician when the patient arrives to the floor."

Bed Management

The third key element in the admission transition is bed management. It requires leadership at the highest levels of the hospital and health-care system to address several critical components to ensure bed availability. Effective bed management starts with a timely decision to discharge and then an efficient discharge. It requires timely reporting of dirty beds, efficient EVS services, effective bed management from the individual units and the nursing supervisor, and the optimization of short-stay strategies such as observation and clinical decision units (CDUs).

Timely inpatient discharges are usually a significant issue in both community hospitals and academic medical institutions. Because this process is quite complicated, it requires a focused, efficient physician and nursing workforce; sufficient nursing resources; and a commitment to organizational goals.

Discharging Patients in Academic Medical Centers

Executing early discharges is more difficult in academic medical centers due to teaching obligations and their inherent interference with flow. Many academic medical centers have predictable patterns of rounding and discharge. As an example, teaching rounds consume most of the morning and may continue until the beginning of didactic conferences. Interns and residents may not be able to get to their competing responsibilities of reevaluations, new admissions, and discharges until later in the afternoon, even though the discharge decision may have been made hours before. Best practice requires a specific team focus on timely inpatient discharges, including rounding with case management and nursing leadership and preparing for the discharge 24 to 48 hours ahead of time.

Be-a-Bed-Ahead Programs

For over 10 years, some hospitals have used an evidence-based approach to identifying and assigning beds, based on the principles of demand–capacity management.[2-4] These programs use statistical process methodologies to predict:

- Time, acuity, and the level of service needed for patients needing beds from all areas of the institution (including ED admissions)
- Transfers within the institution and from other hospitals
- Admissions from the operating rooms

Instead of waiting until the bed request is made, Be-a-Bed-Ahead programs prospectively identify a bed for the next patient and advise the charge nurse on those units that the case will be assigned to them. These programs have dramatically improved hospitals' ability to more efficiently and proactively utilize their resources.[21]

Optimized Rounding Practice

Another practice that contributes to optimal bed availability during high census is reverse-order rounding. Historically, rounding begins with the ICU, then moves to progressive care units, and finally to medical and surgical floors. In reverse-order rounding, practitioners begin with patients requiring the lowest level of care (resources) and work toward the highest level of care. In this manner, interfacility movement is optimized as filled or overutilized high-resource units (telemetry, ICU) can offload patients as beds become available. This practice is often adopted by the hospitalist working closely with EDs, post-anesthesia care units (PACUs), and other hospital areas that routinely require access to patient beds.

Bed Hiding

Once the patient is discharged, some institutions tolerate "bed hiding," the nonreporting of "dirty" rooms (the patient has been discharged from the room, but the room has not been cleaned and put back in service on the bed board). This slow reporting delays room cleaning by EVS, and consequently, the transfer of a patient from the ED to the inpatient unit. To counter this practice, some institutions have adopted several best practices:

- Unit manager or charge nurse is held accountable for managing bed flow and ensuring rapid turnaround of beds.
- Nonclinical staff (volunteers, transporters, or other staff) are responsible to report the newly evacuated bed as dirty.
- Order to discharge creates an automatic electronic alert to EVS and the nursing supervisor.

Discharge Lounges

To create rapid bed turnover and availability, it is necessary to reduce "batching" and ensure the availability of key resources. Many hospitals have implemented discharge lounges to vacate patient rooms earlier. In concept, moving the patient from the clinical space allows those rooms to be cleaned more efficiently for the next admission. There are limited reports of success; however, most of these discharge lounges have not been proven to expedite patient flow or free inpatient resources, and there are no published data supporting the routine use of this strategy.

Bed Huddles

Managers responsible for inpatient bed availability must vigilantly address admissions and manage beds in real time to ensure capacity. Hospitals that actively address demand–capacity consistently conduct daily huddles to predict the likely admissions from all sources and the anticipated discharges. This information is used to determine the net surplus or deficit of beds, which then triggers specific responses from the individual floors to facilitate offloading of critical care beds and early discharges, when necessary. The data can also be used to predict staffing and right-size nursing capacity. However, this staffing practice should be used with great caution as unanticipated ED census and acuity lead to congestion because empty beds on the units may not be adequately staffed.

During high-census periods, a best practice employs two (or more) nursing huddles—one in the morning and one in the evening. Some hospitals are also instituting "no meeting periods," with the goal of having all managers on the floors to expedite patient discharges. Depending on the frequency of demand–capacity mismatches, no meetings are routinely scheduled during certain hours, or meetings during high-census, low-capacity periods are canceled.

The hospital's strategy of bed resource management has significant implications for bed availability. Some hospitals allow charge nurses or unit managers to assign beds on their units. Other hospitals allow nursing supervisors to handle the entire process. And still others employ a hybrid system, in which the nursing supervisor assigns the unit and the unit charge nurse assigns the bed. Unit-level control creates greater potential for delaying notification of a potentially available bed unless specific accountability mechanisms exist.

Generally, the simplest process with the fewest number of steps and people and the most accountability results in the best performance. The best outcomes occur when there is a "bed czar" (a role often assumed by the nursing supervisor). To be effective, the bed czar should immediately be aware of admission needs, consistently assess inpatient resources, and have the authority to independently assign beds. While this loss of control is often unsettling at the unit level, it significantly decreases the potential to "game the system."

Senior Management Responsibility

All successful hospital and bed-flow systems have support from executive teams, with institutional leaders holding managers accountable for recognizing and addressing the queues of patients heading to individual units. There are many competing demands for the inpatient beds, particularly from units that are not open 24 hours per day and 7 days a week, such as PACU and the cath lab. However, it is imperative that ED patients continue to move to inpatient units with the same priority as other patients from other areas of the hospital.

Any hospital patient being held in an area or bed that is not their final inpatient destination poses safety and risk issues for the patient as well as hospital leaders. Executive teams must be fully engaged in problem solving and own strategic process changes to mitigate holding patients in any area of the facility. Robust hospital throughput measures should be developed and routinely monitored to ensure optimal performance.

Clinical Decision Units and Observation Units

Another important strategy that enhances inpatient capacity is the use of low-acuity admission pathways, including CDUs and observation units (see Chapter 39). This alternative to inpatient placement is equivalent to developing an ED inpatient fast track that facilitates the flow of low-acuity patients and increases bed availability for high-acuity patients.

The most successful observation units are administered by or in collaboration with the ED leadership and may be run either by emergency physicians or hospitalists. Further, they are "closed" units with admissions initiated only by emergency physicians and hospitalists, regardless of the patient's attending physician. Effective units have well-defined evidence-based and protocol-driven patient care pathways and admit patients whose workups are generally predictable and exclude patients with complicating factors.

The observation unit should be staffed by a committed team that possesses a working knowledge of clinical observation medicine as well as a clear understanding of observation versus admission criteria. The units may limit consultations, which often prolong the patient LOS. Patients requiring multiple consultations are more appropriately admitted to inpatient units. Ideally, the observation units are located in or near the ED, allowing rapid and efficient movement of patients and access to providers (24/7), radiology, cardiac stress testing, and echocardiography. Most hospitals that implement decentralized observation units without a dedicated location find it difficult to maintain standard patient diagnostic and treatment pathways and, as a result, suffer from a longer average LOS.

CONCLUSION

Efficient outflow from the ED entails a commitment from senior leadership, middle management, and frontline physicians and nurses. Success requires leaders to:

- Define measurable goals.
- Create commitment to the goals.
- Establish a dashboard with specific metrics.
- Develop incentives that align stakeholders.

- Hold the stakeholders accountable to those metrics.
- Keep the patient in focus.

In the coming years, as national reporting and the requirement for transparency evolve, admitted patient LOS will be a core measure that reflects the strength of the organization. Organizations that ensure rapid and effective patient discharges, transfers, and admissions expand their capacity and shorten their overall LOS. These institutions create the greatest opportunity for financial viability.

REFERENCES

1. Asplin BA, Magid DJ, Rhodes KV, et al. Conceptual model of emergency department crowding. *Ann Emerg Med*. 2003;42(2):173–180.
2. Mayer T, Jensen K. *Hardwiring Flow: Processes and Systems for Seamless Patient Flow*. Pensacola, Fla: Fire Starter Publishing; 2009.
3. Crane JT, Noon CE. *The Definitive Guide to Emergency Department Operational Improvement: Employing Lean Principles With Current ED Best Practices to Create the "No Wall" Department*. CRC Press; 2011.
4. Toussaint JS, Berry, LL. The promise of Lean in health care. *Mayo Clin Proc*. 2013; 88(1):74–82.
5. Mayer T, Jensen K. The business case for patient flow: unique approaches to patient flow improve the patient experience and the bottom line. *Healthc Exec*. 2012;27(4):50,52–53.
6. Chalfin D, Trzeciak S, Likourezos A, et al. Impact of delayed transfer of critically ill patients from the emergency department to the intensive care unit. *Crit Care Med*. 2007;35(6):1477–1483.
7. Singer AJ, Thode HC Jr, Viccellio P, et al. The association between length of emergency department boarding and mortality. *Acad Emerg Med*. 2011;18(12):1324–1329.
8. Guttmann A, Schull MJ, Vermeulen MJ, et al. Association between waiting times and short-term mortality and hospital admission after departure from emergency department: population based cohort study from Ontario, Canada. *BMJ (Online)*. 2011;342:d2983.
9. Public Health and Injury Prevention Committee. *Public Health Impact of ED Crowding and Boarding of Inpatients*. American College of Emergency Physicians; 2009.
10. Hoot NR, Aronsky D. Systematic review of emergency department crowding: causes, effects, and solutions. *Ann Emerg Med*. 2008;52(2):126–136.
11. ENA. "Crowding, Boarding, and Patient Throughput" ENA Position Statement. 2017. Available at https://www.ena.org/docs/default-source/resource-library/practice-resources/position-statements/crowdingboardingandpatientthroughput.pdf. Accessed July 19, 2020.
12. NQF. REMCS: Emergency Department Crowding and Boarding, Healthcare System Preparedness and Surge Capacity. 2012. Available at: http://www.qualityforum.org/Publications/2012/12/REMCS__Emergency_Department_Crowding_and_Boarding,_Healthcare_System_Preparedness_and_Surge_Capacity.aspx. Accessed July 17, 2020.
13. The "Patient Flow Standard' and the 4-Hour Recommendation. Joint Commission Perspectives®. Vol. 33, Issue 6:1–4. 2013. Available at: https://www.jointcommission.org/-/media/deprecated-unorganized/imported-assets/tjc/system-folders/topics-library/s1-jcp-06-13pdf.pdf?db=web&hash=3863CF4FC9DA41CB1A07BD519C2EE9A8. Accessed July 17, 2020.
14. Welch S, Augustine J, Camargo CA, et al. Emergency department performance measures and benchmarking summit. *Acad Emerg Med*. 2006;13(10):1074–1080.
15. Guttman A, Afilalo M, Guttman R, et al. An emergency department-based nurse discharge coordinator for elder patients: does it make a difference? *Acad Emerg Med*. 2004;11(12):1318–1327.
16. Baker S. *Hardwired Newsletter*. The Studor Group Website. 2012. Available at: http://www.studergroup.com/newsletter/Vol1_Issue12/Issue12_article1.html. Accessed December 29, 2012.
17. Riesenberg LA, Leitzsch J, Cunningham JM. Nursing handoffs: a systematic review of the literature. *Am J Nurs*. 2010;110(4):24–34.
18. Patterson ES, Wears RL. Patient handoffs: standardized and reliable measurement tools remain elusive. *Jt Comm J Qual Patient Saf*. 2010;36(2):52–61.
19. Writing admission and transition orders. American College of Emergency Physicians Policy Statement. 2019. Available at https://www.acep.org/patient-care/policy-statements/writing-admission-and-transition-orders/. Accessed July 19, 2020.
20. Position Statement on Admission Orders. AAEM. 2020. Available at: https://www.aaem.org/resources/statements/position/position-statement-on-admission-orders. Accessed July 19, 2020.
21. Mayer T. (Adopt a boarder) Views from the Field Urgent Matters Newsletter. 2013. Available at: https://smhs.gwu.edu/urgentmatters/news/views-field-inova-fairfax-hospital. Accessed July 19, 2020.

CHAPTER 42

MANAGING WAITS: THE PSYCHOLOGY OF WAITING

Kirk Jensen, Christina Dempsey

Patience, n. A minor form of despair, disguised as a virtue.

—Ambrose Bierce, *The Devil's Dictionary*

Waiting is a significant part of life. M.I.T operations researcher Richard Larson, widely considered to be the world foremost expert on lines, estimates that Americans spend 37 billion hours each year waiting in line.[1] Some of that waiting may not register as troublesome—the average American sits at stoplights for six months and spends five years waiting in line over the course of a lifetime. But people notice many types of waiting and become annoyed. A survey by the NCR Corporation identified the nine most frustrating waits. Registering a car or renewing a driver's license topped the list, followed by checking out at a retail store. Third on the list was registering at a hospital or clinic.[2] This ranking alerts emergency care providers about the importance of understanding and managing waits in the emergency department (ED) as they relate to the patient experience.

UNDERSTANDING PATIENTS' PERSPECTIVES

Emergency care providers can certainly become numb to the experiences and concerns of waiting patients. Waiting seems a normal part of the process. Clinicians are busy. Interruptions are frequent. The triage process and capacity constraints dictate that some patients seeking care will wait, and some patients will wait longer than others. But *patients* aren't indifferent to having to wait, and the length of waits correlates directly with patient experience outcomes, as **Figure 42.1** shows clearly. The longer patients have to wait, the unhappier they are, and patient experience scores will reflect that reality.

Timeliness of care—particularly the amount of time patients wait to be treated by a physician or an advanced practice provider (APP)—has a strong correlation with patients' overall perception of the care experience.[3-5] However, wait time alone is not the key driver of patient experience in the ED. While waiting is important, the most significant influences on patient perceptions of the ED are their connection to their caregivers, the information they were provided during their visit, and the quality of the communication they received while waiting and being treated (**Figure 42.2**).

Despite demographic differences and differences in outcome measures, patients' perception of their experience in EDs across the world demonstrates an overall dissatisfaction with long waits for care. These negative perceptions of waits are responsible for sweeping changes in the delivery of care, reimbursement, and provider behavior. In the United Kingdom, for example, researchers found that "perceived waiting time was consistently

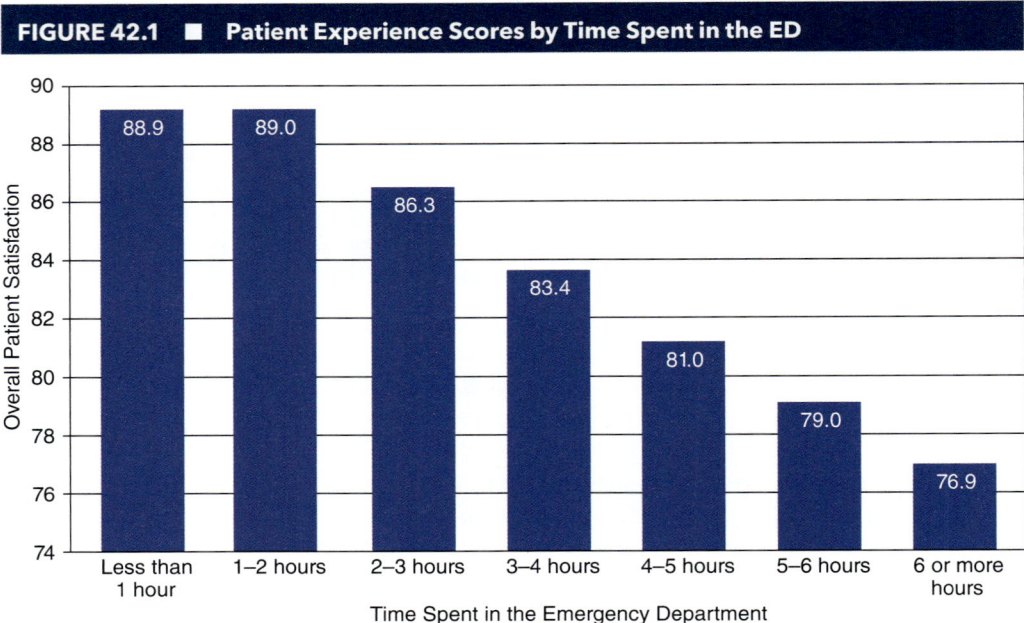

FIGURE 42.1 ■ Patient Experience Scores by Time Spent in the ED

associated with overall satisfaction" and that "dissatisfaction with waits was reflected in an increasing number of patients who left without being seen." Further, for every 2.8 patients who are seen, an additional one will leave without being seen in a British ED.[6]

How Long Is Long?

A key factor in the psychology of waiting is why a patient perceives a wait as excessive. Health-care researchers have established different measures of a "long wait." In England, the National Health Service defines excessive waiting as more than 4 hours in the ED (from arrival to departure).[6] In Canada, the government defines it as a "situation in which demand for service exceeds the ability to provide care within a reasonable time, causing physicians and nurses to be unable to provide quality care."[7] In the United States, a survey outlined five possible definitions of excessive waits **(Box 42.1)**.[8]

The Importance of Perception

No matter what definition is used, providers must understand the patient's perception of waiting time. The patient's perspective is important because it often differs from the perspective of health-care providers. *Perception* is emphasized here because it can differ from the actual experience. Patients' perception of time may not be accurate when estimating the time spent in the ED waiting room or exam room or waiting to see the physician. Although the degree of inaccuracy may not be great, the impact could be.

A year-long study in a Pennsylvania hospital measured actual time in the ED using real-time "passive locating systems" in conjunction with patient experience surveys.[9] The study identified the correlations between self-reported and actual time spent in the ED. On average, patients overestimated the time they spent by approximately 20 minutes. Those patients who overestimated their time had significantly lower experience scores than those who underestimated across every area of experience. Since 2.2 times as many patients overestimated as underestimated, ED scores were lower overall than they should have been. (This phenomenon, the observation that it is common for customers to overestimate the time actually spent on waiting for a service is seen in multiple service industries and settings.[10])

FIGURE 42.2 ■ Factors Influencing "Likelihood to Recommend"[11]

Category	Factor	Correlation to Likelihood to Recommend
Personalized Care	Staff cared about you as a person	0.79
Information	Kept informed about delays	0.72
Pain Control	Pain controlled	0.72
Empathy	Doctor's concern for your comfort	0.72
	Doctor kept you informed	0.71
	Staff kept family/friends informed	0.71
	Nurses' kept you informed	0.71
Discharge Prep	Information re-self care at home	0.71
	Nurses' attention to your needs	0.70
	Doctor listened to you	0.69
	Courtesy toward family or friends	0.69
	Nurses listened to you	0.68
	Courtesy of the doctor	0.68
	Wait in treatment area to see doctor	0.66
	Courtesy of the nurses	0.65
	Nurses' concern for your privacy	0.63
	Allow family/friend to be with you	0.62
	Waiting time pre-treatment area	0.58
	Helpfulness person first asked re-condition	0.58
	Comfort of the waiting area	0.57
	Concern for comfort blood draw	0.53
	Courtesy person took blood	0.53
	Wait for radiology	0.53
	Privacy re-personal/insur info	0.52
	Ease giving personal/insur info	0.52
	Courtesy person re-personal/insur Info	0.51
	Waiting start noticed your arrival	0.51
	Concern for comfort during tests	0.50
	Courtesy of radiology Staff	0.48

An important finding of the Pennsylvania study for understanding the psychology of waiting was that there was no significant difference between the actual time spent in the ED for those patients who overestimated and those who underestimated. This finding highlights how critical *perception* is in the determination of the patient experience. Further, it suggests ways of dealing with waiting to improve the patient experience of care.

The strongest correlations in the Pennsylvania study involved getting the patient into the treatment area or to the physician. In other words, patients don't seem to mind waiting in the actual treatment area as much as they mind waiting in the waiting room.[10] Another finding of the study came when researchers analyzed patient perception of interaction with each category of health-care provider.

BOX 42.1 ■ FIVE US DEFINITIONS OF EXCESSIVE WAITS

1. Patients waiting more than 60 minutes to see a physician
2. All ED beds filled more than 6 hours a day
3. Patients placed in corridors more than 6 hours a day
4. Emergency physicians feeling rushed more than 6 hours a day
5. Waiting room filled more than 6 hours a day

TABLE 42.1 ■ Patient Experience by Provider Type[9]									
Provider Type	Arrival	Nurses	Doctors	Tests	Family/ Friends	Insurance	Personal Issues	Overall Assessment	Overall Score
Licensed practical nurse									
Registered nurse									
Doctor									
Greeter									
Triage nurse									

Note: Shaded areas indicate significant differences in the scores of the highest and lowest scoring provider of that type. Each staff member received a score for each component of patient experience, including an overall mean score (calculated as the mean scores from all patients the provider interacted with/managed).

Table 42.1 shows differences in patient experience scores according to each provider type. Shaded areas are components between the highest and lowest provider of a type. Two components of experience had the most significant differences for each type of provider (doctors, nurses, greeters). The significant differences were found in the patient experience components of time from arrival to entry to treatment area and "personal issues."

Table 42.2 describes the top five priorities of ED patients.[11] These rankings reveal that being treated as human beings is more important to patients than the quality of the facilities and equipment in the ED. In fact, patients report they are willing to wait for care "as long as they are kept informed about the wait time." Those patients who reported that they received "good" or "very good" information about delays reported nearly the same overall perception of their care experience whether they spent more than four hours or less than one in the ED.

An implication of these findings is that not all waiting is perceived negatively. To illustrate, consider the following scenarios. Observe the experience of a child waiting beside an oven with a glass door, watching and smelling cookies baking, anticipating the result. Consider the experience of adults waiting at a table in a fine restaurant, engaged in conversation, and anticipating the meal to come. The important observation applicable to the psychology of waiting in an ED is to "reframe" how patients experience their waits. Researchers who have studied that psychology have developed sets of principles, as described in the rest of this chapter.

TABLE 42.2 ■ National Emergency Department Priority Index			
Survey Item	Mean	Correlation	Priority Rank
How well you were kept informed about delays	71.3	0.726	1
How well your pain was controlled	77.9	0.72	2
Degree to which staff cared about you as a person	82.0	0.795	3
Overall rating of care received during your visit	83.0	0.897	4
Nurses' concern to keep you informed about your treatment	83.1	0.702	5

THE PSYCHOLOGY OF WAITING

As with many other principles of flow, much can be learned from observing how successful businesses have applied the psychology of waiting to their operations. The closest analogy to the care provided in EDs is a business that provides a service (an experience), not a tangible product (a consumed good). Health care is a service business, rather than a consumer products business that makes things, for example, gadgets that people use or pizza that they take home and consume. In a service industry, the consumers' (patients') experience is significantly influenced by how they perceive that service (wait, relationship with caregivers, and care provided).

Examples of businesses providing services that demonstrate best-in-class management of waits include the Disney resorts (the entertainment–experience economy . . .), first-class hotels (the Ritz-Carlton and others . . .), and exemplary mass-market chains like Starbucks. While care provided in the ED does not involve theme park rides or a magical experience, there are takeaway lessons from these businesses that ED leaders should consider. Two principles of service are worth noting:

- Customers will be satisfied if the service exceeds their expectations; customers will be dissatisfied if the service does not meet their expectations.
- It is difficult to recover from an initial perception of poor service. If service does not meet customers' expectations on the front end, then the service provider must work particularly hard to subsequently change the customer's perception.

Disney and others maintain that customers need to have as many as 12 positive experiences with a service provider in order to overcome the negative effects of one bad encounter or experience.[12,13] Thus, problems with service on the front end of a visit will require significant compensatory effort. In many EDs, there is a bottleneck at the front end, creating an unexpected or undesired wait. So if a patient's experience with service in the ED begins with unmet expectations, it can be difficult to improve that patient's perception of service later. In fact, for patients admitted to inpatient units, their emergency experience colors their perception of the entire hospital stay.

One of the foundational documents in the study of the psychology of waiting is David Maister's work.[14] Maister identified eight principles describing how people experience waiting, which are listed in **Box 42.2**. By understanding these principles, a leader can implement changes in an ED to manage and improve the patient experience.

Unoccupied Time Feels Longer Than Occupied Time

When someone has something engaging to do, time seems to pass more quickly. This principle is easy to see in action at Disney World or Disneyland because Disney Parks masterfully

---

BOX 42.2 ■ HOW PEOPLE EXPERIENCE WAITING

1. Unoccupied time feels longer than occupied time.
2. Pre-process waits seem longer than in-process waits.
3. Anxiety makes waits seem longer.
4. Uncertain waits feel longer than known, finite waits.
5. Unexplained waits feel longer than explained waits.
6. Unfair waits seem longer than equitable waits.
7. The more valuable the service, the longer the customer will wait.
8. Waiting alone feels longer than waiting in groups.

keeps customers' time occupied. Something is always going on. Customers waiting in line are entertained through the use of videos, characters in costume, detailed sets drawing attention, preshows, and so on, so the time spent waiting for a popular attraction does not seem so long.

Emergency departments can use Wi-Fi and televisions in the waiting room, as well as stock current magazines and relevant health information. Patients can also fill out registration forms in the waiting room as they wait for the next step—doing so fills the time and shortens the process. An ED should also ensure there is room for friends and family to wait with the patients. Further, having staff regularly "round" throughout the waiting area to update patients and families helps provide the information so important to waiting patients and a feeling of progress.

Preprocess Waits Feel Longer Than In-Process Waits

This concept is related to the previous concept that occupied time feels shorter than unoccupied time. This principle supports the idea of beginning the "occupied" time or process as soon as possible. Waiting seems shorter when the process begins shortly after arriving, that is, when the patient is beginning his or her care process immediately.

How a good restaurant treats customers is instructive. Having a menu immediately available enrolls the customer in the process. The waiter may be tied up with other tables, but as soon as the customers are seated, someone brings them water, hands them menus, asks if they want anything to drink, and describes "specials"—the engagement starts right away. All of these small interactions move the process along and provide customers with a sense that the experience for which they came is unfolding. Restaurants have also applied this principle—and accidentally discovered an entire new service line—by providing a bar with immediately available seating while customers are waiting for their tables. (Bars in restaurants were originally deployed solely as a device to manage customer waiting.)

The service offerings and missions may be different, but there are parallel lessons for the ED. In a well-run ED, patients move sequentially through the process. Less well-run EDs keep patients waiting unoccupied in the waiting room until nurses or doctors are ready for them, which is counterproductive. If a triage nurse meets the patient quickly to gather information and then moves that patient to a treatment space or room, the patient is involved in the unfolding care process, and the wait will seem shorter. When patients have a sense that they are moving through the system of treatment, waiting seems more tolerable. Using team triage is another effective way to introduce emergency care process quickly. Additionally, results-waiting lounges or rapid diagnostic units help patients move from the waiting room to other areas, which is perceived by the patients as progressing through the process rather than waiting in a waiting room or returning to the same waiting room after triage or diagnostic testing.

Anxiety Makes Waits Seem Longer

Suppose a traveler flying from New York to Los Angeles, changing planes in Chicago, learns that their first flight has been delayed. Immediately that passenger worries about making the connecting flight in Chicago. The passenger continues to worry while boarding the plane and during takeoff. But if the flight attendant makes a simple announcement that connecting flights in Chicago are being held because of the delays, then the passenger can relax and enjoy the flight free from worry about missed connections and the ensuing difficulties. The time seems to pass more quickly—and more pleasantly—than it would if that passenger continually worried about missing the connection.

By definition, a high percentage of patients have anxiety before they even arrive in the ED. Few people start their days planning on or hoping to get sick or injured. Once compelled to seek emergency care, the additional stress of long waits increases their anxiety. Contacting them regularly and simply letting them know why they have to wait, how long they'll likely have to wait, and what they can expect once the waiting is over eases their anxiety and makes their waits seem shorter. Using well thought-out and sincerely delivered "scripts" to address typical questions and common scenarios can be effective at relieving anxiety (see Chapter 74).

Patients and providers may have different ideas of what "adequate patient contact and communication" means. Surveys of ED staff indicate that they think contacting patients once an hour or more is sufficient. Surveys of ED patients, on the other hand, show that they often prefer communication every 20 to 30 minutes. Studies of real-world experience in the ED demonstrate that "hourly rounding" is satisfactory for most patients. Establishing a policy of regular contact and making sure that staff adheres to it gives patients a sense that they do not have to wait long. Further, anxiety and pain often begin the well-known fight or flight response. When adrenaline is high, understanding, compliance with treatment, and comprehension in general are reduced. Therefore, as Maslow's Hierarchy of Needs suggests, making patients feel safe is a foundational objective in the quest to reduce anxiety and improve the patient experience. It is not simply about keeping them safe—it is making them *feel* safe in your care.

Uncertain Waits Are Longer Than Known, Finite Waits

Like anxiety, uncertainty makes waiting feel longer. To counter uncertainty in the ED, providers should regularly contact patients who are waiting and let them know how much longer they are likely to have to wait and what will happen during the course of their visit. Providing a time frame and preview relieves anxiety. When a patient or family member asks how much longer a computed tomography (CT) scan will take, answering "as soon as we can" or "we are really busy today" can inadvertently create the impression of a long and uncertain wait.

It is necessary to move beyond patient satisfaction. A positive patient experience involves more than being nice or making people happy. People want to feel safe, secure, and valued. This effort is about making patients feel safe in our care, connecting with them on a personal level, and managing the team up to enhance the patient's perception of safety and quality.

Excellent service businesses take advantage of the psychology of expectations. Disney regularly indicates a wait will be 45 minutes when it is known (based upon their analysis of process flow) the time will actually be 30 minutes. Restaurants frequently use this tactic when they inform customers how long they will wait for a table. If a provider in the ED tells the patient waiting for the CT a definite time that is actually a bit longer than the scan will likely take, the patient experience will be better for two reasons:

- An uncertain wait was converted into a finite wait.
- The actual time frame was less than the patient was told, exceeding his or her expectations.

As a result, the wait actually seems shorter. If an ED's processes are effective enough to regularly fulfill a promised service interval—guaranteeing patients they will be seen within 30 minutes, for example—then waiting does not seem long. A department must be certain, though, that it can deliver before making such a promise ("under-promise, over-deliver").

Unexplained Waits Feel Longer Than Explained Waits

In the airline analogy, a passenger who arrives at the gate with plenty of time to spare but does not see the plane at the gate as the departure time approaches and does not receive any clarifying information from airline representatives begins to worry. Time, once again, seems to drag. Worry and anxiety surge. However, if an airline representative supplies passengers with definite information on the plane's arrival and subsequent departure, then the explanation changes uncertainty to certainty and the passenger can determine if there is time to make the connecting flight or if other arrangements must be made. The traveler can either relax or address the known issue.

Health-care providers should explain to ED patients why they are waiting by:

- Telling them what is happening in the department that is causing them to wait
- Describing what will happen next
- Giving them a concrete idea of how long the wait for that step will be

For example, if the ED is dealing with several trauma cases, then providers can let patients in the waiting room know what is going on and how handling those cases will likely affect the time those patients will have to wait before treatment.

Anxiety, uncertainty, and unexplained waits are related. One technique that can address all three is patient rounding. A study by the Studer Group on the impact of rounding in the ED found that the number of patients who left without being seen decreased by 23.4%, falls in the ED decreased by 60%, use of call lights fell by 34%, and approaches to the nursing station declined by 40%.[15] Rounding makes waiting times seem shorter, increases patient experience scores, and even improves patient safety. Adding specific questions to rounding in the study had a significant impact on patient experience ratings:

Tell me what is important to you for your care today.
Tell me what a good visit would look like for you today.
I've never taken care of you before; when you aren't in the ED, what do you like to do?

Find a way to connect with the patient that has nothing to do with the reason they've come to your ED. Connecting with patients on a personal level makes them feel cared about not just cared for and begins to build trust that is necessary for compliance and the perception of safety. Patients who receive information about their ED visit rate their experience more highly. One study looked at the impact of information describing ED operations and evaluation times, which was distributed to patients upon their arrival. Those who received the information rated the following attributes higher than the control group: physician skill and competence, physician concern and caring, and their own likelihood of using the same ED again.[16]

Physician communication is also highly correlated with better patient adherence to diagnostic and treatment plans. There is a 19% higher risk of nonadherence among patients whose physician communicates poorly than among patients whose physician communicates well. With physician training, the odds of patient adherence were 1.62 times higher than when a physician received no training.[17]

Unfair Waits Are Longer Than Equitable Waits

"Unfair versus equitable waiting"—this concept may sound abstract, but people encounter this notion frequently in everyday life. Americans, as a society, have a highly refined sense of *equity theory*. If people are in line for a product or service and someone who arrived later is called forward for service earlier, those waiting are likely to be resentful. It feels similar to observing another person "cut in line" in front of the group. The perception of the wait, and the level of service, deteriorates.

This sense of unfairness leads most service industries to prefer the "snake line," the single queue leading to several service stations, rather than several lines leading to several service stations. Service providers and customers know that the snake line is fair—no one can go before someone who arrived earlier. And the single queue leading to multiple servers mitigates against high levels of either natural or artificial variation in the customers of the service queue and prevents "queue chaos." In actual practice, while the single queue leading to multiple servers is usually the most efficient, one will often see multiple lines feeding multiple servers in the United States because people often prefer "line jockeying" and a sense of control, scoping out the line that seems to move more quickly and joining it. In England, by contrast, people instinctively maintain queue discipline, allowing their service industries and customers to leverage the operational efficiencies of a single queue delivering customers to multiple servers.

This principle and its practical effects have implications not just for patient experience but for patient flow. An ED fast track, if poorly designed and implemented, can create the same sense of unfairness. If the entrance and waiting areas are the same, patients with higher acuity, who may have arrived earlier, may resent observing patients and "jumping the queue" ahead of sicker patients who may have been waiting longer. This process leads to a negative perception of the care experience. Service queues with obviously unequal service times (e.g., the fast track and the main ED) should have separate waiting areas, if possible, to facilitate the perception of service operations in the ED.

There are clearly times and situations where multiple service lanes leading to multiple service stations make good sense. A familiar operations example of this is appropriately segmenting patient flow to a fast-track or clinician-in-triage model. Deploying service lines in addition to the main ED leverages different service delivery systems and thereby improves operations and efficiencies.

The More Valuable the Service, the Longer the Customer Will Wait

As an example, a college student will wait a certain period of time, perhaps 5 or 10 minutes, for a late teaching assistant. That same student might wait much longer for a late professor because the perceived "value of the services" is greater. Therefore, the "customer"—students in this case—will willingly wait longer. This principle can be seen in action at a rock concert by a celebrated band. Usually the band doesn't come on at the start but is preceded by a lesser known (and sometimes little known) warm-up act. But fans are willing to wait because they perceive the subsequent service (experience) provided as valuable.

This same principle holds true in health-care and emergency medicine. Patients will tolerate a longer wait if the facility is recognized as one providing excellent care or special capabilities. The converse is also true—patients will be less tolerant of waits if the facility is not perceived as a high-quality hospital or ED. This tolerance is somewhat generationally dependent. Baby boomers demonstrate a greater tolerance for waits than millennials do.

Reputation, of course, is built on performance over time. Just as businesses intentionally promote their brands, a hospital ED can enhance its reputation ("brand") by marketing its capabilities and quality via broad community-wide promotions and smaller tasteful displays in the waiting room. For instance, the ED might promote its staff with photographs and biographies of physicians, APPs, and nurses, describing training, background, qualifications, and interests. In the long run, brand identity and brand appeal (reputation) will depend on the quality of the service provided. The best way to make patients more tolerant of waiting is to ensure the ED is considered the best place to be in an emergency.

Solo Waits Feel Longer Than Group Waits

Misery loves company, the old saying goes, and when people wait for a service, it is easier to wait with friends and family than it is to wait alone. Time passes more pleasantly. A sense of community develops—it becomes a shared situation and a shared experience. Friends, family, and significant others can alter the waiting dynamic. This principle can be turned to a facility's advantage by creating waiting areas that are conducive to group activity. The first step is to encourage patients to have family and friends wait with them. Additionally, waiting areas can be designed to facilitate a sense of community by providing enough room and a warm and welcoming environment—clean, comfortable, and pleasant. These initiatives pay dividends in patient experience outcomes.

AN ALTERNATIVE APPROACH

American design researcher Donald Norman has approached the psychology of waiting with subtle refinements to David Maister's principles by studying how design influences behavior and how people interact with their environment.[18] Like Maister, Norman has proposed eight principles, shown in **Box 42.3**. Norman's emphasis on emotions ("emotions dominate") points out the importance of regular contact with patients and the expression of concern over their needs. The prioritized rankings (from the patient's perspective) in **Table 42.2** should inform the process design. Patients (and their significant others) want to know that the providers care about them as people.

Patients want to be kept informed. Repeatedly responding to these desires greatly increases the chances of satisfying patients and family members. Providers should immediately clarify ("eliminate confusion") where patients and family members are to go, what they are supposed to do, and what will happen. The layout of the department should enhance this clarity rather than present the patients and their family members with a visually confusing labyrinth.

"Start strong and end strong" is a fundamental principle in any service. People remember "first things" and "last things"—how a service encounter starts and how it finishes. This concept is true in all relationship, personal business, and service encounters. If the experiences of the front and back end of the ED visit are well organized and hospitable, patients will have a better impression of the facility.

The memory of an event is often more important than the experience itself. Real-time diaries of events comparing how people feel about their experiences with what actually happened reveal that what is most important is the memory of the event. The more health-care providers can create a powerful, positive memory in a patient's encounter, the more likely patients are to perceive and rate the service favorably.

OPPORTUNITIES FOR SUCCESS

There are various ways to improve the patient experience with wait times. These include implementing patient flow principles, taking advantage of patient psychology, and avoiding pitfalls.

BOX 42.3 ■ NORMAN'S EIGHT PRINCIPLES FOR WAITING

1. Emotions dominate.
2. Eliminate confusion; provide a conceptual model, feedback, and explanation.
3. The wait must be appropriate.
4. Set expectations, then meet or exceed them.
5. Keep people occupied; filled time passes more quickly than unfilled time.
6. Be fair.
7. End strong, start strong.
8. Memory of an event is more important than the experience.

Observing the Principles of Flow

Not surprisingly, patient flow affects patient experience outcomes. The Pennsylvania study mentioned earlier found that patients who arrived between 7 am and 3 pm reported a more positive experience with the ED than those arriving later in the day. The Centers for Disease Control and Prevention has reported that 62.9% of adult ED visits occur after traditional business hours. Thus, a less crowded (more efficient) department means more satisfied patients. Day of week also affects the experience of care. Mondays (typically the busiest days) have the lowest mean experience score. As the week progresses, the experience scores increase daily until their highest point, on the weekend.

The key operational principles of patient flow are described in other chapters within this textbook and include:

- Triage is a process, not a place (see Chapters 35 and 36).
- Fast track is a verb, not a noun (see Chapter 37).
- The patient should be seen and evaluated by the physician or APP as quickly as possible (see Chapter 24).

The more ED leaders and managers implement the general principles of flow, the more likely they are to create conditions conducive to successfully managing waiting and enhancing the patient experience.

Taking Advantage of Psychology

In designing and refining ED processes, leaders and managers should pay attention to and benefit from the principles described in this chapter. They should give patients something to occupy their time, communicate and connect with them regularly, keep them informed, and focus on what the patients need and want. Queues should be arranged so that patients have a sense of fairness about their treatment. Providers should encourage patients' families and friends to wait with them, and the facility should be designed to promote group awareness.

Pitfalls

Patients cannot tell what health-care providers are feeling or thinking. About 90% of communication is nonverbal. If doctors and nurses convey unhappiness over ED conditions, or if patients sense the service providers are distracted or not interested in them as people, patient experience scores can plummet. Applying the principles outlined here without sincerity or integrity will not be effective. Nor will an initiative be effective without addressing the underlying conditions of the department. The principles of the psychology of waiting are meant to be applied to manage necessary or unavoidable waits. They are not a substitute for effective operations and process management. If approached from the perspective of coordinating and improving all aspects of the patients' experiences, the principles of the psychology of waiting can be a helpful strategy in the quest to deliver a satisfactory and even superb patient experience.

CONCLUSION

While waiting is a fact of life in modern society, members of the ED staff do not have to sit back helplessly when patients have to wait. There are well-described and time-tested tools and principles to manage and improve the experience of waits. Emergency department leaders can use the principles outlined here to fill the time in ways that make the waiting less uncertain, less anxious, and more dynamic. Providers should keep patients occupied and keep them informed. All staff should let patients know that they care about them as people—and mean it. Working to provide the best service possible will give a facility a reputation as a place of high-quality care and excellent service. Patients can experience waits in any ED, but by deploying the ideas outlined in this chapter, EDs can promote best practices and avoid any needless suffering associated with waiting.

REFERENCES

1. Stone, A. Why waiting is torture: gray matter. *New York Times*, August 18, 2012. Accessed December 11, 2018. https://www.nytimes.com/2012/08/19/opinion/sunday/why-waiting-in-line-is-torture.html

2. The wait we hate the most: Consumers driven to frustration. *Atlanta (Business Wire)*. January 22, 2007. Accessed December 11, 2018. https://www.businesswire.com/news/home/20070122005736/en/Wait-Hate-Consumers-Driven-Frustration

3. Bursch B, Beezy J, Shaw R. Emergency department satisfaction: what matters most? *Ann Emerg Med*. 1993;22(3):586-591.

4. Thompson DA, Yarnold PR, Williams DR, et al. Effects of actual waiting time, perceived waiting time, information delivery, and expressive quality on patient satisfaction in the emergency department. *Ann Emerg Med*. 1996;28(6):657-665.

5. Boudreaux ED, D'Autremont S, Wood K, et al. Predictors of emergency department patient satisfaction: stability over 17 months. *Acad Emerg Med*. 2004;11(1):51-58.

6. Cooke M, Fisher J, Dale J, et al. *Reducing Attendances and Waits in Emergency Departments: A Systematic Review of Present Innovations*. London, UK: National Co-Ordinating Centre for NHS Service Delivery and Organisation R & D; 2004.

7. Drummond AJ. No room at the inn: overcrowding in Ontario's emergency departments. *Can J Emerg Med*. 2002;4(2):91-97.

8. Derlet RW, Weiss SJ, Ernst AA, et al. Development of an emergency department overcrowding scale: results of the National ED Overcrowding Study (NEDOCS). *Acad Emerg Med*. 2002;9:366.

9. Fulton B, Baxley L. Wait times and satisfaction in the ED: a new, high-tech perspective. *Partners*. 2011;15(Jan-Feb):4-10.

10. Hornik J. Subjective vs. objective time measures: a note on the perception of time in consumer behavior. *J Cons Res*. 1984;11(1):615-618.

11. Press Ganey Associates, Inc. *Emergency Department Pulse Report*. South Bend, Ind: Press Ganey; 2010.

12. Bateson JEG. *Managing Services Marketing: Text and Readings*. Fort Worth, Tex: Dryden Press; 1995.

13. Zemke R, Schaaf D. *The Service Edge: 101 Companies That Profit From Customer Care*. New York, NY: New American Library; 1989.

14. Maister D. The psychology of waiting lines. In: Czepiel JA, Solomon MR, Suprenant CF, eds. *The Service Encounter: Managing Employee/Customer Interaction in Service Business*. Lexington, Mass: Lexington Books; 1985:113-123.

15. Meade CM, Kennedy J, Kaplan J. The effects of emergency department staff rounding on patient safety and satisfaction. *J Emerg Med*. 2010 Jun;38(5):666-74.

16. Krishel S, Baraff LJ. Effect of emergency department information on patient satisfaction. *Ann Emerg Med*. 1993;22(3):568-572.

17. Zolnierek KB, Dimatteo MR. Physician communication and patient adherence to treatment: a meta-analysis. *Med Care*. 2009;47(8):826-834.

18. Norman DA. Designing waits that work. *MIT Sloan Management Rev*. 2009;50(4):23-28.

ADDITIONAL READINGS

- ACEP: Emergency Medicine Practice Committee of the American College of Emergency Physicians. Emergency Department Crowding: High-impact Solutions. 2016. Available at: https://www.acep.org/Legislation-and-Advocacy/Practice-Management-Issues/Boarding/Crowding/Emergency-Department-Crowding---High-Impact-Solutions/.

- Advisory Board. *Building the Clockwork ED: Best Practices for Eliminating Bottlenecks and Delays in the ED*. Washington, DC: HWorks, An Advisory Board Company; 2000.

- Advisory Board. *The High-Performance ED Optimizing Capacity and Throughput to Meet Ever-Growing Demand*. Washington, DC: HWorks, An Advisory Board Company; 2008.

- Baker S. *Excellence in the Emergency Department: How to Get Results*. Gulf Breeze, FL: Fire-Starter Publishing; 2009.

- Csikszentmihalyi M. *Flow: The Psychology of Optimal Experience*. New York, NY: Harper and Row; 1990.

- Horowitz LI, Green J, Bradley EH. US emergency department performance on wait time and length of visit. *Ann Emerg* Med. 2011;55(2):133-141.

- Jensen K, Mayer T. *The Patient Flow Advantage: How Hardwiring Hospital-Wide Flow Drives Competitive Performance*. Gulf Breeze, FL: Fire-Starter Publishing; 2015.

- Jensen K. Improving patient satisfaction through flow. In: *Patient Flow: Reducing Delay in Healthcare Delivery*. 2nd ed. New York, NY: Springer; 2013: 97-106, 429-446.

- Mayer T, Jensen K. *Hardwiring Flow: Systems and Processes for Seamless Patient Care*. Gulf Breeze, FL: Fire-Starter Publishing; 2009.

- Mayer T. Drive service excellence to the next level: moving patient satisfaction scores from the 4s to the 5s is key. *Healthc Exec*. 2010;25(6):54, 56.

- Mayer T, Cates R. *Leadership for Great Customer Service: Satisfied Employees, Satisfied Patients*. 2nd ed. Health Administration Press; 2014.

- Stone A. Why waiting is torture. *New York Times*. August 18, 2012.

HOSPITAL-WIDE PATIENT FLOW AND THE EMERGENCY DEPARTMENT

CHAPTER 43

Jody Crane, Christina Dempsey, Kirk Jensen, Barbara Weintraub, Robert W. Strauss, Thom A. Mayer

Flow in the emergency department (ED) is both a product of and a contributor to the flow of patients throughout the entire hospital. The process of patient flow begins when the patient crosses the threshold into the ED and does not end until the patient leaves the hospital. When addressing the flow problems in the ED, an approach that views the ED as an entity independent from the hospital is not a viable approach.

Bottlenecks in the ED, operating room (OR), and the postanesthesia care unit (PACU); issues with the availability of telemetry beds; longer lengths of stay (LOS); complications and "adverse events"; and poor satisfaction of patients, physicians, and staff may all be manifestations of poor patient flow in the hospital. Contributing factors to poor patient flow include:

- Peaks and valleys in the inpatient census driven by the elective schedules of the OR, catheterization lab, and other procedural areas of the hospital (variable demand)
- Staffing and scheduling preferences with little or no correlation to clinical needs of patients (demand–capacity mismatch)
- Poor admission and discharge practices
- Variable ED volume
- Lack of coordinated care
- Lack of availability of long-term care and psychiatric beds

In addition, the variable availability of ancillary services presents significant flow problems for both inpatients and the ED. The notion that hospitals are (fully) staffed and function at full capacity 24 × 7 × 365 is just not reality. This variability causes ancillary services, such as nuclear medicine, physical therapy, case management, and some imaging capabilities, to be less available on weekends and after hours. This decreased capacity results in longer LOS when these services are needed but unavailable.

Improving patient flow requires collaboration and a multidisciplinary effort. When making decisions about change, it is necessary to first gather data to drive decisions and create a foundation of collaboration among physicians, nurses, and hospital leadership. These decisions must be based on relevant, recent, and actionable data as well as a commitment by the hospital and physicians to hold each other accountable.

Some ways hospitals can improve patient flow include:

- Matching capacity to demand
- Smoothing the flow of elective admissions
- Addressing the drivers of admission and discharge efficiency for inpatients
- Creating effective dashboards by which to measure success

Experience with hospital-wide flow committees has shown that three key issues commonly emerge[1]:

- Selected improvement projects are often not aimed at the true patient flow bottlenecks.
- Changes resulting from those selected projects may improve only in part of the system but may not optimize flow in other parts of the system.
- Many hospitals lack the resources, will, and ability to execute the changes needed to improve flow across the system.

CONCEPTS OF FLOW IN THE HOSPITAL

The concepts of Lean management, queuing theory, and the theory of constraints (see Chapter 34) also apply to inpatient flow. When considering hospital-wide flow, one must understand the key "servers"—beds, nurses, and physicians—and the demand on those servers relative to their capacity to care for patients. Understanding these aspects of system flow requires consideration of overall arrivals to the hospital measured by daily bed demand—the number of admissions per day multiplied by the average LOS. Comparing this figure to the hospital's licensed bed capacity allows prediction of the system's performance.

Clear and consistent definitions are essential to flow improvement by the various stakeholders[1]:

- An *available bed* is defined as one that is cleaned, staffed, and ready to accept a patient.
- A *discharge* is a patient who has actually left the bed.
- *Capacity* is defined as discharges plus available beds.
- An *admission* is a patient who has been or will be placed in an (potentially) available inpatient bed.
- An *ED boarder* is an admitted patient residing in the ED.
- An *inpatient* is a patient who resides on an inpatient unit.

Factors Affecting Demand

Typically, new hospital inpatient bed demand is characterized by the sum of admissions from the OR, the ED, and all other outpatient sources. Both the scheduled surgical case load and the number of surgical patients requiring admission are known. This same information is unavailable for the ED and the other outpatient services. The admissions from these services require estimating the likely inpatient bed needs based on historical data.

There are a number of very complex regression analysis tools that may be used to predict these patterns. However, the simplest and yet still fairly accurate method is to take a rolling average over a number of like days. Great care must be taken to ensure that this rolling average properly estimates the likely volume of the day in question. The period of the rolling average must be long enough to capture enough data points and recent enough to capture short-term fluctuations, including seasonal (influenza) or dynamic volume fluctuations (steady volume increases). Using a rolling average of the previous four same days (e.g., the previous four Mondays) to predict potential unscheduled admissions from ED patients and outpatients on Monday is a reasonable approach.

Using the formula in **Box 43.1**, if a hospital has 100 licensed beds, 25 admissions per day (13 OR cases, 10 predicted ED, and 2 predicted direct admits), and a LOS of 4.5 days,

BOX 43.1 ■ UTILIZATION FORMULA

$$\frac{A \times LOS}{BC} = U$$

A = admissions per average day; LOS = average length of stay; BC = bed capacity; U = utilization

utilization (demand) will be (25 patients × 4.5 days)/100 beds, or 113%. Once hospital utilization exceeds 85%, ED boarding ensues.[2] In this example, a minimum of 13 patients will be held in the ED while they await inpatient beds. In reality, this number will be much higher due to variation in ED arrival and inpatient discharge times and the fact that all beds are not available for all patients (some are for pediatric, neonatal ICU, critical care, telemetry, and other specialized units).

Setting Improvement Goals

Queuing theory can be used to help set improvement targets. If 85% (ideal utilization) is the percent that is likely to provide beds for all admissions in a timely manner, the target LOS that will allow the hospital to run at or near 85% inpatient utilization can be calculated using a variation in the utilization formula (**Box 43.2**).

In the previous example, (100 beds/25 patients) × 85% = 3.4 days. This then serves as the target for LOS efficiency improvement. Unfortunately, most hospitals see an 85% occupancy rate as a call for action to cut staff and close beds. This maneuver can lead to perpetual ED boarding *by design,* as the utilization of the hospital becomes artificially inflated, and the capacity is artificially decreased. In fact, fiscally conservative practices leading to bed closures and subsequent insufficient inpatient capacity are the most common cause of boarding seen in the United States.[2]

Theory of Constraints

Another important principle for inpatient flow is the theory of constraints. When applied to inpatient flow, this theory holds that to move patients through the hospital, the constraining resource (the bottleneck) must be determined. Once determined, a way must be found to offload that resource to enhance flow. Working on any other resource will not significantly enhance overall throughput. This applies in every area of the hospital. Simply mapping flow and understanding all the competing resources and the demands placed on them can very effectively target improvements.

Two examples of determining the underlying constraint:

Example 1: If cardiac telemetry beds are in short supply, it may seem logical to add more. However, if after mapping flow, it becomes clear that the true constraint is cardiac-stress testing, adding beds will further prolong LOS and increase the demand for a scarce resource.

Example 2: Similarly, if beds in the ICU seem in short supply, the reflex response is to add more ICU beds. However, if the true constraint is telemetry beds, then adding ICU beds will simply cause further congestion, since a larger ICU will increase the demand for telemetry beds. In this second example, the preferred solution is reduction of LOS in telemetry areas or the addition of telemetry beds. These solutions will simultaneously increase ICU bed capacity, since transfer to the telemetry unit would be available as needed.

BOX 43.2 ■ UTILIZATION FORMULA

$$\frac{IU \times BC}{A} = LOS$$

A = admissions per average day; LOS = average length of stay; BC = bed capacity; IU = ideal utilization

Now, consider both examples together. The ICU has inadequate capacity because of the staff's inability to transfer patients to the telemetry unit. The telemetry unit has inadequate capacity because of its inability to obtain timely cardiac stress testing. The combination of these two "backed up" units leads to inpatient boarding in the PACU and the ED, patient and staff dissatisfaction, and additional staffing requirements. The solution to all these problems is simply to create additional cardiac stress-testing capacity.

INPATIENT CAPACITY AND OVERCROWDING

In many cases, the ED boarding of patients who are waiting for inpatient beds is the primary cause of ED overcrowding. Inpatient beds are seldom assigned in advance (held) for ED patients, despite the relative predictability of the number of admissions that will come from the ED. Lack of inpatient bed availability is caused by several factors, including:

- Peaks and valleys in the inpatient census—with peaks resulting in patient placement on inappropriate units and longer LOS delayed discharges
- Untimely physician rounding patterns
- Insufficient discharge planning and case management
- Hidden beds
- Staffing level determination

Daily Cycles

The daily census highs and lows often result from volume variations in the elective OR schedule coupled with the variable nature of ED admissions. These surges in elective OR volume fill the inpatient units on and after the peak surgery days (generally Monday, Tuesday, and Wednesday) and leave those beds unavailable for urgent or emergent patients who may require inpatient specialty beds. Patients who require admission must then be placed "off-service" or must board in the ED waiting for a bed. This consequence of longer LOS in the hospital is often seen with orthopedic and ICU patients.

Placing patients in "off-service" beds has several negative ramifications. Patients who are placed in inappropriate beds (medicine patients in surgery beds, surgery patients in medicine beds, non-ICU patients in ICU beds) often:

- Stay longer in the hospital
- Have a higher risk of complications and adverse events
- Are less satisfied (lower patient satisfaction scores)

Patients placed in off-service beds are frequently taken care of by nurses who may not be as comfortable managing that type of patient—and may not be trained to do so. For example, orthopedic nurses have specific specialty training in orthopedics. Placing a patient with a small bowel obstruction or acute renal failure on an orthopedic nursing unit does a disservice to both the patient and the nursing staff. When an "any bed available" approach is adopted (any open bed is acceptable when holding patients in the ED or PACU), physicians are forced to round in multiple areas of the hospital, lengthening their rounding period and delaying the physicians' availability to the OR, the clinic, their practices, their personal lives, and so on.

Therefore, a primary goal of improved flow is to ensure that patients are placed in the right bed, at the right time, with the right nursing staff. This approach not only improves flow, it also improves quality, safety, and comfort for both patients and providers.

Delayed Discharges

Delayed discharges are another common problem plaguing the inpatient units of the hospital, resulting in the "daily dump" of patients late in the day. The delays may be related to rounding patterns of physicians, inadequate case management, poor discharge planning, or underreporting of available beds. Occasionally, the delay is a symptom of overworked nurses who would rather keep a patient than receive a new admission (who may or may not be appropriate for the receiving unit).

Untimely Physician Rounding Patterns

There are two issues here: one obvious and the other more nuanced. Physicians are not necessarily available to discharge patients when the patients are clinically ready. They may be engaged in surgery, rounding in another hospital, or seeing patients in their offices. The result is that patients may unnecessarily occupy an inpatient bed, while another patient is waiting for that bed.

A less obvious cause of bed unavailability relates to the order in which physicians round on and discharge their patients. Physicians usually begin their patient rounds seeing the sickest patients first. These patients are often in the ICU, step-down units, or units with a higher nurse-to-patient ratio. In other words, these patients are already receiving the highest level of care in the hospital—nursing, monitoring, and so forth. While it may seem counterintuitive, seeing the sickest patient first when the hospital's utilization is very high may actually delay appropriate disposition for that patient and others who are waiting to receive care.

This delay is the result of a cascade or "domino effect." It is of little value to discharge a patient from a high-acuity bed to an unavailable low-acuity bed. When a lower-acuity bed is unavailable, attempting to move patients to a unit requiring fewer resources will not succeed until that lower-acuity bed becomes available. Simple changes in rounding sequence that focus first on patients ready for discharge make inpatient beds available to those waiting in the ED or higher-acuity (critical care) units. Then rounding on the ICU patients after the lower-acuity patients are discharged or transferred allows a more streamlined flow of patients through the hospital. Because of the positive cascade effect, critical care beds are available more quickly. This process potentially reduces LOS and improves satisfaction while maintaining the quality of patient care.

Discharge Planning/Case Management

Another reason for late discharges is insufficient discharge planning and case management. Rarely is discharge a surprise to either the physician or the nurses caring for the patient. Ironically, the most common question asked by patients when hearing that they will be admitted to the hospital from the ED is, "When can I go home?" Unfortunately, that may be the last time until the day of discharge that "going home" is discussed with the patient. This lack of planning often increases the patient LOS and the number of late discharges.

Discharge planning for patients undergoing elective admissions (e.g., surgery, cardiac ablation) should begin before the patient enters the hospital and reinforced throughout the encounter, including during preadmission testing, morning admission, the anesthesia interview, and the postoperative visit. Furthermore, the progress note for every post-procedure day should factor in the discharge needs of the patient. Patients and their families want to be included in the treatment plan. Contrary to popular belief, discussing discharge with patients on a daily basis does not make them feel rushed out of the hospital. In fact, it makes them feel that they are a part of the treatment team and have the ability to make decisions and understand their home-care needs.

Hidden Beds

"Bed hiding" is perceived to be a common issue underlying an inpatient unit's lack of available staffed beds. Because nurses often feel short staffed and overworked, there may be a tendency to prioritize those patients ready for discharge last, thus preventing a new admission on that nurse's shift. Unfortunately, this and other practices that delay discharge result in poor patient satisfaction and comments such as, "At 9 am, the doctor told me I could go home, and it was 4 pm before they let me leave." It also delays inpatient admission for those boarding in the ED or PACU.

Admitting a patient to an inpatient bed is no small task. It requires a great deal of time and effort on the part of the nurse to complete the necessary admission forms, educate the patient regarding the unit and admission needs, and answer questions, all while taking care of other patients in the ED. The tendency may be to wait until the next shift or "let the ED handle it," rather than discharge a patient only to receive another one. This problem can be averted with:

- Dedicated admitting or discharge nurses
- An express admission unit
- Clarification that discharges are not the sole responsibility of the nursing staff
- Correct staffing of environmental services (EVS) staff

Automating the discharge protocol further expedites the process. Once the discharge order is received:

- The discharge nurse provides instructions and prescriptions.
- Discharge transport is automatically notified.
- EVS personnel are automatically notified to clean the room.
- EVS personnel notify the "bed board" that the room is available.

Many hospitals actually decrease the level of EVS in the afternoon shift, precisely when the demand for it rises.

Determining Staffing Level

When considering the following day's staffed bed availability, most hospitals use the midnight census to determine staffing levels on the inpatient unit. With the trend toward more observation and short-stay hospitalizations, hospital stays are shorter. An inpatient bed may actually turn over twice (or more) in a given 24-hour period. Therefore, the midnight census may give a false depiction of the productivity of the nursing staff and the complexity of patient care in today's inpatient units. Bed turns should be calculated using inpatient units to determine the real census for staffing and budgetary purposes. Staffing should then be based on the real patient census throughout the 24-hour period, including the acuity of the patient population served.

Weekly Cycles

Key variations throughout the week are primarily related to scheduled and unscheduled admissions. A component of this variability is that weekend services in most hospitals are very different from those provided during weekdays, yet illness is a 24/7 problem. Pending patient procedures and treatments build up over the weekend, placing excessive demands on services near the beginning of the week. This "batching" of demand subsequently drives an imbalanced occupancy, which usually peaks on Tuesday and Wednesday and does not decrease until the following weekend. This variation can be documented; the capacity can be matched to the demand and be used to help forecast the need for services.

Operating Room Scheduling

Variation in demand coupled with decreased services on the weekend is further complicated by the system-induced variation in imbalanced OR scheduling. This lack of OR capacity is partially due to working through the queue that built up during the weekend. The remainder lies in the preference of surgeons to front-load their schedules early in the week. At first glance, it would seem this preference is primarily related to the surgeons' desire to have their weekends free; however, as noted below, this early week scheduling preference is grounded in some fundamental flow/capacity issues.

While the origins of the OR schedule imbalance are multifactorial, the impact on the hospital census is clear—the census peaks midday on Tuesday, when it is frequently 10% to 15% higher than the weekend low. Hospitals that are not at peak bed capacity can flex staffing to accommodate this variation, but this practice is rare and impractical. A better approach, and the *only* approach for hospitals at capacity, is to:

- "Smooth" the variation from all admission sources as much as possible.
- Look closely at the weekend demand, performing work the day that it is needed.

The OR has a significant impact on the flow of patients throughout the hospital. The typical peaks and valleys in the elective surgery schedule drive the corresponding patterns in the inpatient census. During the peak days, usually early in the week, electively scheduled patients fill the inpatient units. As a result, when urgent or emergent patients come to the ED, these specialty beds may not be available.

Smoothing OR flow: The common practice of performing elective total joint replacements early in the week is illustrative. Thoughtful surgeons may wish to discharge the patient before the weekend, as ancillary services like physical therapy are usually less available then. As a result, early in the week, the orthopedic inpatient unit is filled with patients who will require an average 3-day stay. When the hip fracture patient requiring an orthopedic bed presents to the ED on Tuesday evening, there may not be an available bed. That patient must then be placed off-service or boarded in the ED waiting area. In addition, the patient may be placed on the pending (add-on) surgical list without a scheduled procedure time. The patient may even be bumped day to day, increasing the risk of complications and unpaid avoidable days for the hospital. These fluctuations decrease the predictability of nurse and physician scheduling (**Figures 43.1 and 43.2**).

Smoothing the flow of elective admissions and ensuring that adequate capacity is available for the demand (i.e., beds for urgent and emergent patients) results in less variation, that is, smaller ranges between high and low volumes. Smoothing admission flow also increases the capacity of both the OR and the inpatient units, a significant benefit to the ED.

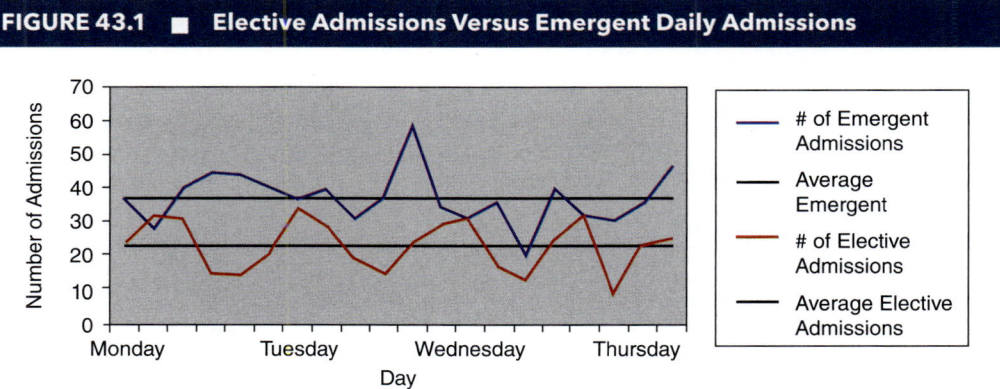

FIGURE 43.1 ■ **Elective Admissions Versus Emergent Daily Admissions**

FIGURE 43.2 ■ Elective Surgical Versus Urgent/Emergent Volume

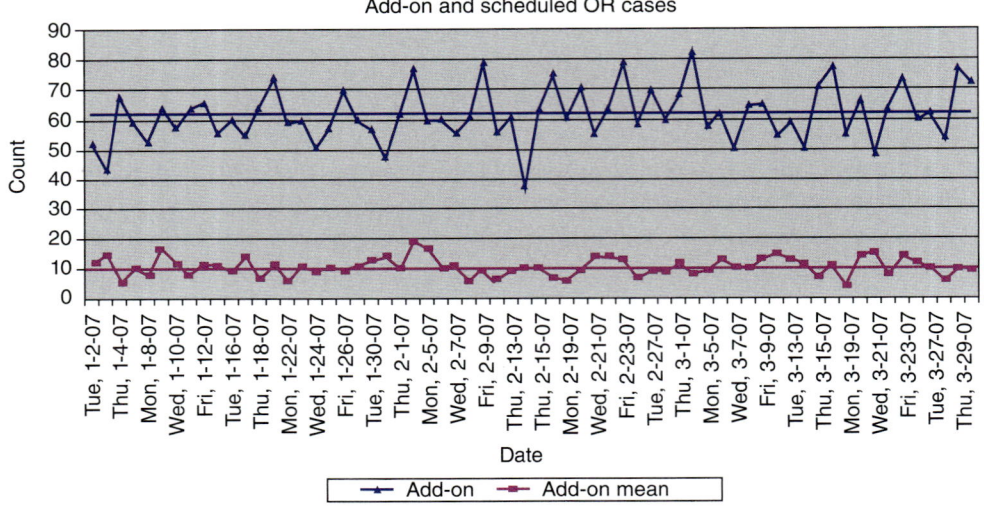

Upper line = elective surgical volume
Lower line = urgent/emergent volume

The OR block schedule is typically based on the surgeons' utilization and preferences, without considering the flow of patients on the inpatient units. Smoothing the elective OR schedule incorporates the flow of inpatients, ensuring they are predictably admitted and discharged to the appropriate inpatient units. This smoothing process makes staffing, rounding, and overall care more predictable, with shorter stays and improved satisfaction (**Figures 43.3** and **43.4**).

This type of smoothing process requires substantial collaboration between the hospital and the surgeons. Surgeons must be willing to change the days of the week or hours that they work. To facilitate this change, hospitals must provide the surgeons with relevant data related to patient placement, patient satisfaction, nursing overtime, and physician office issues.

FIGURE 43.3 ■ Inappropriate Patient Placement

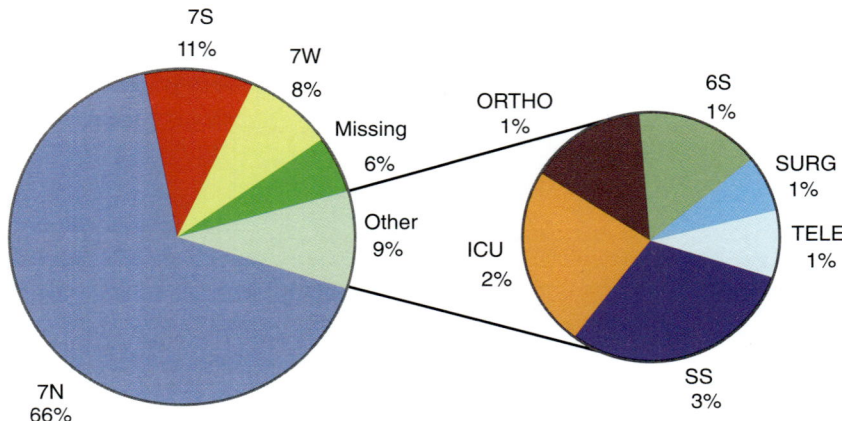

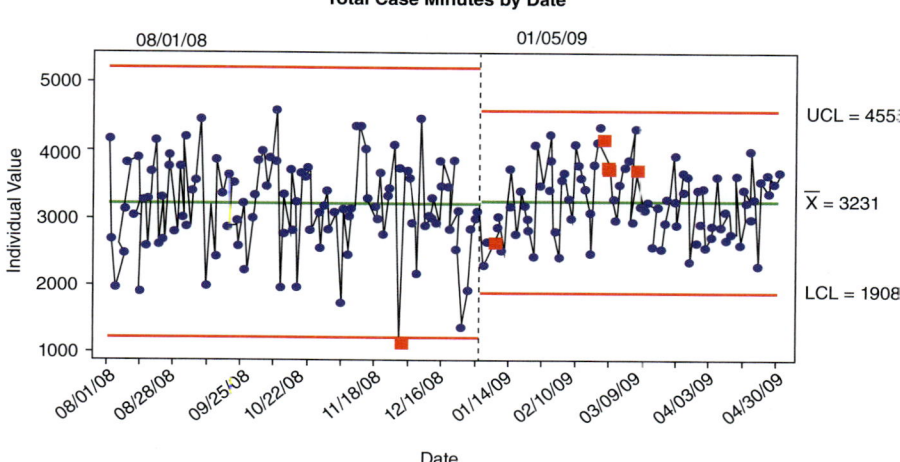

FIGURE 43.4 ■ Variability Reduced by Smoothing

For its part, the hospital must agree to provide the necessary ancillary support services on the weekend to ensure that the quality of care remains consistent throughout the patient's stay. The hospital will have to adjust staff schedules, a process that may not require hiring more personnel but rather smoothing the schedule. With services more consistently spread throughout the week, the hospital no longer has to hire additional physical therapists to handle the peak loads.

If the process is well designed and successful, surgeons will find that access to the hospital and the OR is improved. The collaboration required to accomplish these changes serves as a foundation for better physician–hospital relationships, as well as improved efficiencies and quality.

Using the correct data: Smoothing the elective schedule requires recent, relevant, reliable, and actionable data. The most frequent obstacle in this process is review of the wrong data. For example, surgical scheduling and information systems are often based on the time from the surgeon's incision to dressing rather than the time from patient entry to departure. Faulty data inaccurately represent the true time that a patient occupies an OR and an inaccurate calculation of average case duration. Inaccurate information leads to errors in scheduling and block allocation that further inhibit smoothing initiatives. When actual and scheduled case durations match, scheduling is more accurate and predictable, the flow of patients to their destination units is improved, and bed availability is enhanced (**Figure 43.5**).

Results from smoothing the flow of elective admissions are compelling (**Figures 43.6** and **43.7**). Reducing fluctuation:

- Opens more functional capacity in the OR and on inpatient units
- Places patients in the appropriate bed and unit, reducing LOS
- Improves patient and physician satisfaction
- Increases functional capacity by reducing the volume variations
- Improves patient flow through the ED
- Improves ED patient satisfaction

Intensive Care Unit and Telemetry Units

In many hospitals, the ICU and telemetry units are throughput bottlenecks. Due to the typical surgical schedule (described earlier), most ICUs are near or at capacity at the beginning of

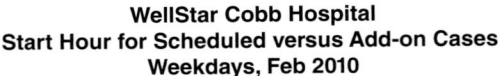

FIGURE 43.5 ■ Accuracy of Actual Versus Scheduled Case Duration

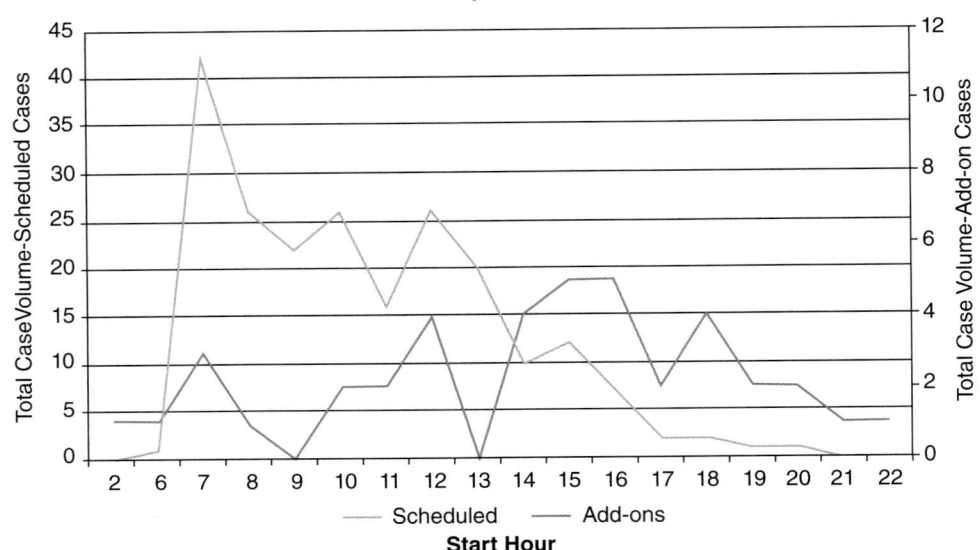

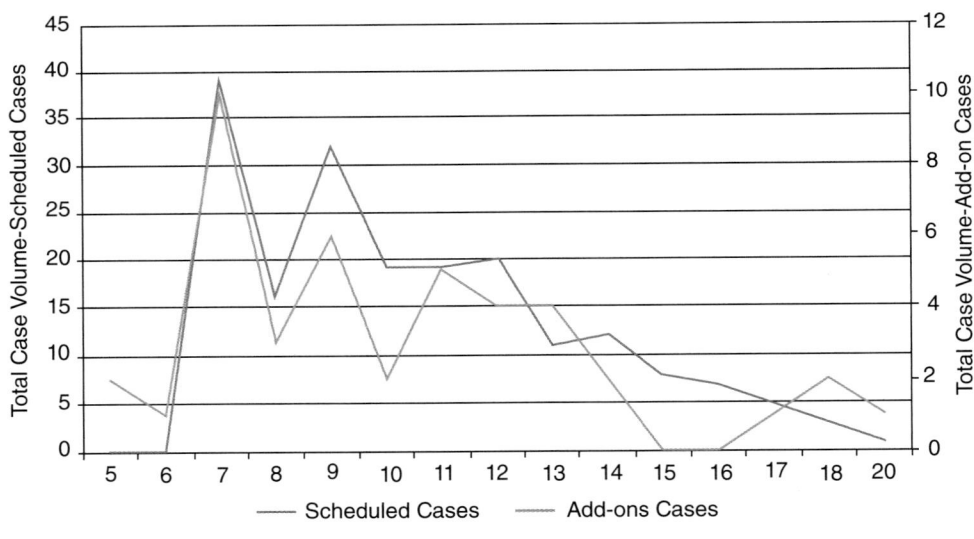

the week. The ICU flow is also impeded by nonstandard admission and discharge criteria, leaving each patient's LOS contingent on individual physician preferences and practice patterns. This nonstandard approach causes uncertain and often excessive LOS, limiting bed capacity. Bottlenecks in telemetry also impede the movement of patients out of the ICU and the ED, further limiting throughput in both units. Closed ICUs managed by a single group of physicians can increase efficiency, as this practice increases the likelihood of consistent admitting, management, and discharge practices. When closed units are impractical, utilization of standard protocols and patient care pathways can also achieve this consistency.

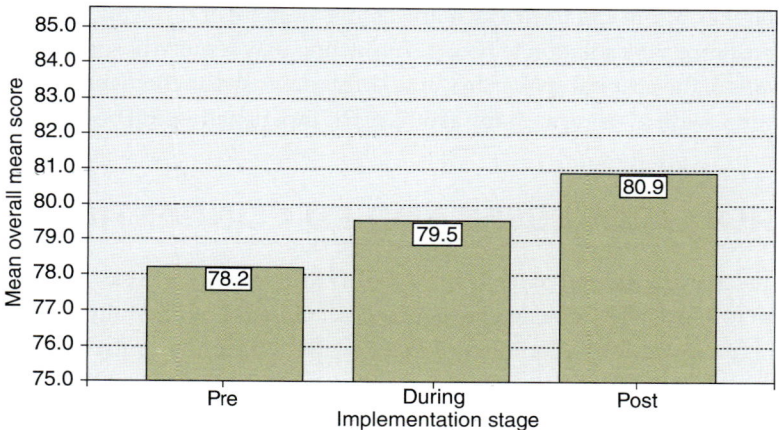

FIGURE 43.6 ■ Improvement in Patient Satisfaction After Smoothing Volume

The lack of telemetry capacity is frequently the cause of inpatient bottlenecks (review the examples given in the earlier section "Theory of Constraints"). The root cause is usually inefficient processes that prolong the patient LOS, thereby consuming more telemetry resources than necessary. Typical causes of delays in telemetry availability include:

- Physician rounding and discharge practice inconsistencies
- Insufficient availability of stress testing
- Excessive consulting requiring multiple signoffs to discharge the patient
- Lack of standardized admission and discharge protocols

Frequently, hospitals also keep patients on telemetry units far longer than clinically indicated. Establishing clear criteria for instituting and discontinuing monitoring of otherwise stable patients should be part of every hospital's management scheme.

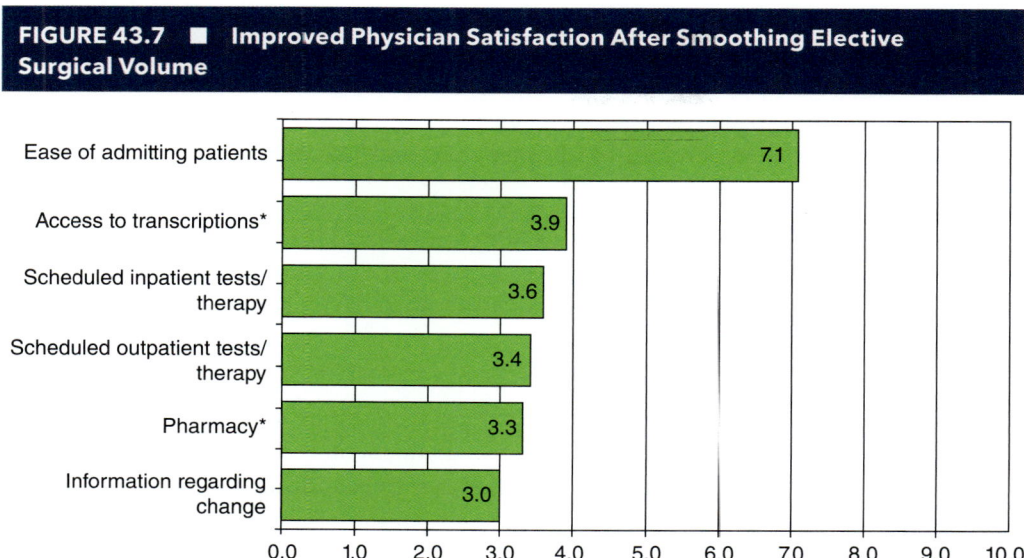

FIGURE 43.7 ■ Improved Physician Satisfaction After Smoothing Elective Surgical Volume

* The most noticeable shifts (scores which changed >=+/- 3.0 points) tended to involve patient flow issues.

Unavailable Long-Term Care

A final, noteworthy cause of inpatient constraints involves "downstream" bottlenecks due to the unavailability of long-term and psychiatric care facilities outside the hospital. Patients waiting for long-term care can utilize as many as 10% or more of the available inpatient beds. In such circumstances, the solution to hospital crowding may require hospital leaders to focus outside the walls of the hospital proper. In Canada, this downstream bottleneck is a major cause of hospital overcrowding, using as many as 30% of the inpatient hospital beds in certain cities.

ADMISSION PROCESSES AND ED CONGESTION

Delays in transferring admitted patients from the ED to inpatient units can cause major delays in the ED. The resolution to these delays requires collaborating with multiple leaders outside the ED. Some causes of admission delays are partially within the control of the ED leader, though actions taken to address them will generally involve institutional leadership as well.

Bed Assignment Issues

Bed assignment issues include practices that exacerbate shortages of inpatient beds as well as strategies that can be used to find and latch onto beds needed by admitted ED patients.

Batching Inpatient Bed Reports

Delays related to reporting and readying available inpatient beds were discussed earlier. Additionally, paper (rather than electronic) bed assignment negatively affects bed availability; unit secretaries may tend to batch their paper reports of available beds, leading to delays within those units. Similarly, batching of EVS and bed-desk notification of "dirty" beds may cause beds to be held until after a shift change. In short, batching occurs for several reasons, including a lack of bed processing guidelines and staff convenience (i.e., putting off time-consuming admissions until the next shift).

When batching occurs, a cascade of events follows, all of which lead to incremental delays in patient flow and patient care, for example:

- Medications and meals are prepared for patients who are no longer there, creating inefficiencies and delaying medications and meals for other patients.
- Simultaneous notification to housekeeping of a "batch of beds" delays the cleaning of "stat" and other beds.
- Batching is "anti-smoothing," as it creates peaks and valleys of resource requirements.

The uninformed observer might place the blame on housekeeping's shoulders, but the root cause usually lies elsewhere: batching or staffing mismatches. These issues underscore the importance of all departments, including clerical and EVS staffs, working together as a team, with each party recognizing its own role and perceiving the others as important to the overall effort.

"Bed-Ahead" and "Pull" Systems

Emergency department patients may experience delayed bed assignments through a "last-in-line" phenomenon. In other words, regarding inpatient bed assignments, EDs may have a low priority when compared to other services. By justification or rationalization, it is sometimes asserted that ED boarders are already in the system and are getting a high level of care. Further, the PACU closes at a certain time, while the ED is available 24/7. This reasoning places other patients ahead of the ED patients.

Hospitals often change the bed assignment process at different times of day. During the day shift, the registration/bed desk may be responsible for bed assignments. However, during the evening (the ED's high admission time) and overnight, the nursing supervisor may assume responsibility for assigning beds. Hospitals should ensure that the bed assignment process operates consistently 24 hours a day, 7 days a week.

As an example, Inova Fairfax Hospital, a tertiary care teaching hospital, instituted a "Be-a-Bed-Ahead" program in 2004. It was designed to ensure that the bed board was actively managed. Beds were "preassigned" to patients, from both the ED and the ORs. This resulted in fewer delays for both groups of patients. Other health-care systems have subsequently deployed this strategy with great success. In the Be-a-Bed-Ahead system, patient assignment coordination is exemplified by a "pull" system. Staff in the inpatient units work to identify beds that can be used for anticipated ED admissions.

Bed Huddles

Bed huddles are a practice that improves the current bed situation. Inpatient-unit staffs meet daily or during each shift to consider the net bed surplus/deficit, that is, by calculating and comparing the anticipated admissions from all sources and the anticipated discharges. In the case of a projected deficit, all floor managers are assigned the task of finding the required numbers of beds and staffing necessary to meet the anticipated demand for the day. This process may be combined with expediting discharges when necessary.

Some facilities make the morning bed huddle a priority and create "no-meeting zones" from 9:00 am until 10:30 am. During that time, all managers, nursing supervisors, and even hospitalists focus solely on discharging patients from the hospital. Successfully executing such a strategy requires commitment from the highest levels of leadership, particularly from the chief nursing officer.

Batching ED Patient Reports

Although ED arrivals and subsequent admissions are random, they are predictable. Even so, inpatient beds are generally not allocated to the projected ED patients who will undoubtedly be admitted every day. Some emergency physicians exacerbate the bottleneck by waiting to notify the hospitalist until there are "a few" admitted ED patients to be seen—another form of batching. The emergency physician may think this is a courtesy to the hospitalist, especially at night when there are fewer in-house hospitalists. Unfortunately, it has the opposite effect by delaying care for the patient, creating longer LOS and decreased satisfaction. Batching also creates an unnecessary queue, decreasing the efficiency of the hospitalist who generally performs evaluations in a linear fashion, evaluating one patient, then the next, and then the next.

Another form of batching occurs when the hospitalist waits to evaluate or admit several ED patients at once and then sends them to the inpatient unit en masse. This batching overloads the inpatient unit and extends the LOS for each patient in the ED. Directing hospitalist admissions to designated units is an effective way to establish a "pull system" for patients. With this system, hospitalists are responsible for a designated floor or floors and become very familiar with the nurses and care provided there. This familiarity enables patients to be pulled from the ED to the floor more quickly, allowing additional workups to occur on the inpatient unit rather than in the ED. To work, this system requires collaboration and trust between the ED physicians and the hospitalists. It has proven to be effective in moving patients from the ED to the inpatient units more quickly.

The Nursing Report

A complicated aspect of patient admissions is the patient handoff between the nurses of the ED and the inpatient units. Sharing patient transfer information is particularly difficult in institutions that do not have a culture committed to expediting ED admissions. Emergency nurses frequently cite this handoff as the most frustrating aspect of admission because of the intermittent refusal to take report by inpatient nurses. In fact, some institutions forbid calling report during shift changes on the inpatient side, citing that this is a dangerous time for nurses on the inpatient units. Some units have resolved this concern by allowing the charge nurse for the respective floor to take report during a shift change.

Other "rule-based" report delays can be addressed by creating alternative systems for times when delays occur. One such alternative system is faxed reports. While not a replacement for verbal sign-out, faxed or scanned reports can facilitate the movement of the patient from the ED to the inpatient wards. Faxed reports are generally used when the communication between the ED and inpatient nursing staff is likely to be delayed by 15 or more minutes. In these cases, the ED nurse faxes the report and moves the patient to the inpatient unit, where the bedside report is given. While this is technically a "push" mentality, it may be necessary in hospitals that have not developed a pull culture on the inpatient units.

The ED Role

Of course, ED leaders and staff themselves play key roles in preventing ED congestion and bed-assignment delays.

Early Bed Assignment

The ED staff can take steps to prevent delays in bed assignments. For instance, as soon as an ED physician knows that a patient is going to be admitted to the hospital, he or she can immediately request a bed. Physicians can notify the nursing supervisor, who can coordinate the bed-request submission. If the hospital has bed placement coordinators, the ED staff can contact them as soon as the decision to admit has been reached.

Anticipating Admissions

Beyond considering the patients currently being evaluated, anticipating admissions is the key to preventing delays in bed assignments. Both the number of patients who will present to the ED and the number who will need to be admitted can be predicted and should be forecasted.

Tracking and analyzing data over time allows ED leaders to project the approximate volume of patients who will require admission by time of day, day of the week, and week and month and season. This information provides the ED, administration, registration, and inpatient units with a process by which they can plan admissions. Indeed, some systems, such as Be-a-Bed-Ahead, reserve beds for anticipated admissions at various times during the day based on observed trends.

OPPORTUNITIES FOR SUCCESS

The principles of flow discussed in this book apply to hospital-wide flow as much as they do to flow in the ED. Using a real-time dashboard to track the current situation and compiling the data and analyzing patterns will help match capacity to demand, whether smoothing OR schedules or anticipating ED admissions. Gathering data that can demonstrate trends is essential when attempting to convince administrators, physicians, nurses, and others that change from the status quo is necessary and urgent. Emphasizing teamwork, a coordinated effort throughout the hospital is critical; flow initiatives are not likely to succeed without it.

Dashboards should track both inpatient and ED data. The inpatient dashboard should include inpatient census, LOS by inpatient unit, occupancy rate, and bed turnovers. For the ED, the dashboard should track daily volume, time from a patient's arrival to seeing a doctor, and LOS in the ED (divided into its components), including time of:

- Decision to admit to bed assignment
- Bed assignment to ED departure
- ED boarding hours
- Number of patients who leave without being seen

The dashboard should be visible to staff throughout the facility so that trends can be spotted early and corresponding actions can be taken to reduce any developing bottlenecks. A key tool to flow improvement on a hospital-wide basis as well as in the ED is forecasting the number of patients who will come to the ED, require hospital admission, and need urgent or emergent surgery.

PITFALLS

Hospitals commonly make the mistake of using or reacting to the wrong data when determining the existing flow bottlenecks. Common mistakes include:

- Reviewing average volumes
- Using comparative data from other hospitals
- Implementing flow projects that other hospitals have used successfully

While it might be reasonable to rely on strategies that others have used successfully, it is critical to track institution-specific data, uncover local bottlenecks, and implement and measure individualized improvements locally. Programs that do not precisely address actual bottlenecks in one's own facility will not improve overall flow.

A related issue is that some hospitals focus only on the ED rather than on the hospital as a whole. The ED processes directly or indirectly influence and are influenced by other departments' processes. Implementing measures to improve flow in the ED without working to optimize flow in the larger hospital system will ultimately not succeed. Embarking on a flow improvement project without a broad institutional commitment is another common reason for failure. Hospitals must devote sufficient money, time, and personnel to flow improvement. If senior administrators do not fully support the initiatives, they will not succeed.

CONCLUSION

Successfully optimizing patient flow in the ED depends on optimizing patient flow throughout the hospital. To optimize flow, it is critical to:

- Ensure coordination among departments.
- Obtain convincing data based on tracking volume, time, and other factors.
- Persuade physicians, nurses, and others that change is necessary and can succeed.

The techniques of flow can be successfully used to:

- Anticipate the need for and numbers of beds.
- Secure those beds.
- Smooth scheduling in the OR.
- Improve processes involved in admission and discharge.
- Result in greater patient and staff satisfaction.

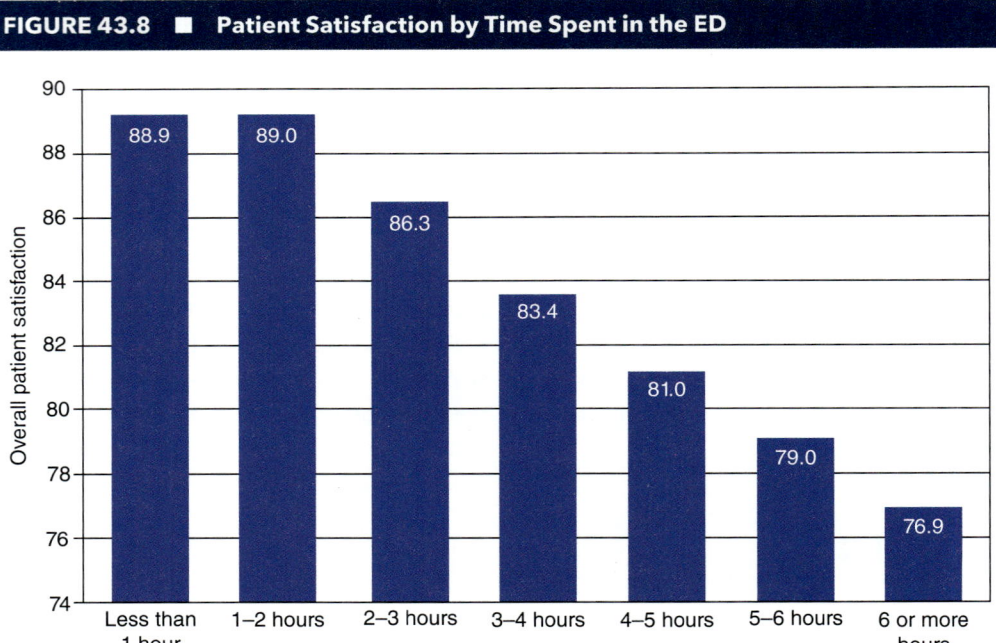

FIGURE 43.8 ■ Patient Satisfaction by Time Spent in the ED

Represents the experiences of 1,501,672 patients treated at 1,893 hospitals nationwide between Jan 1 and Dec 31, 2009.

Figures 43.8 to **43.11** demonstrate this point graphically. Successfully improving flow creates a department where patients prefer to go when they need urgent care and where physicians, nurses, and other health-care professionals prefer to work.

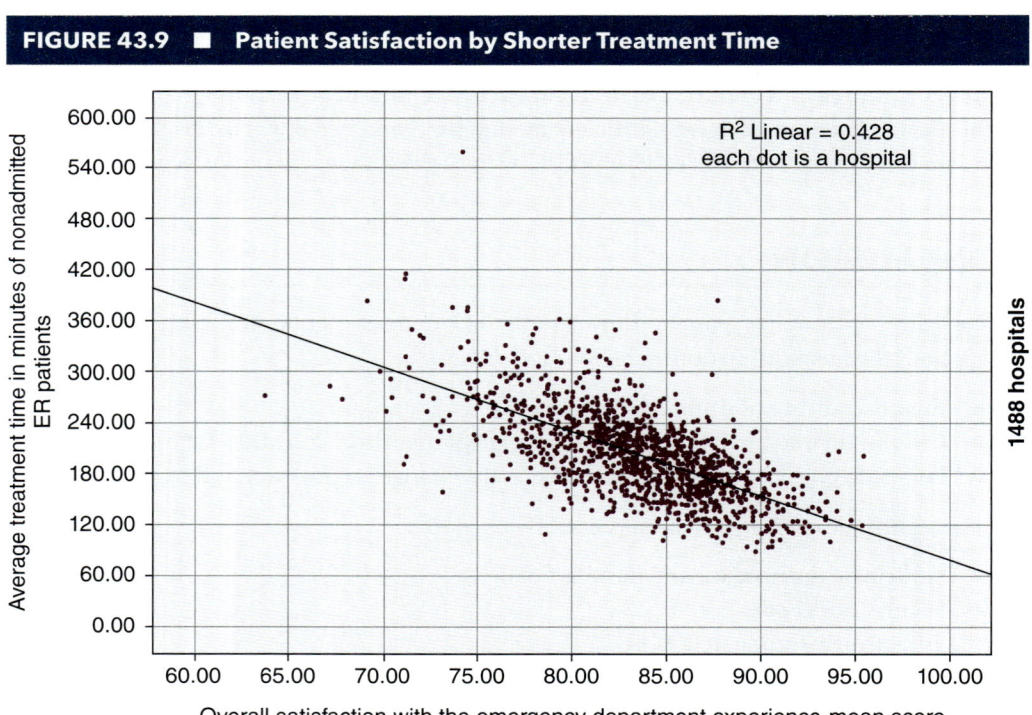

FIGURE 43.9 ■ Patient Satisfaction by Shorter Treatment Time

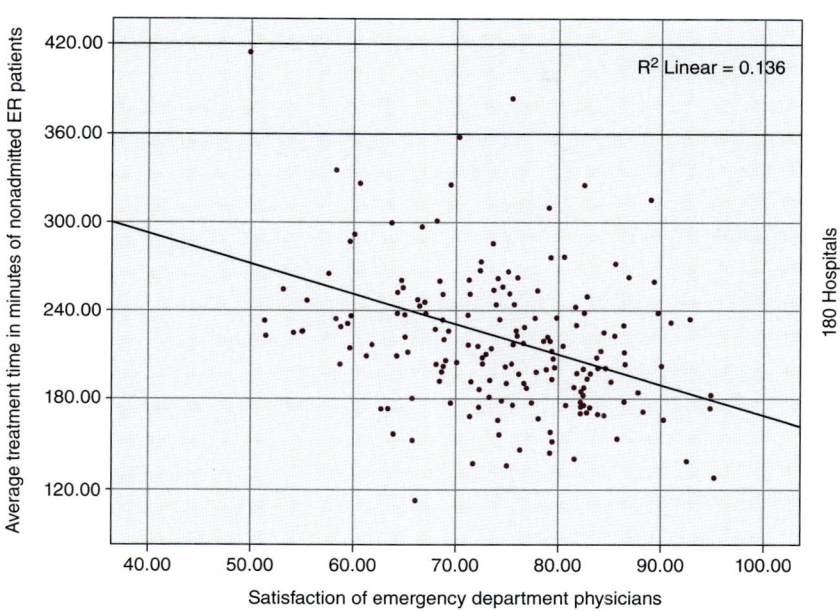

FIGURE 43.10 ■ Physician Satisfaction by Shorter Treatment Time

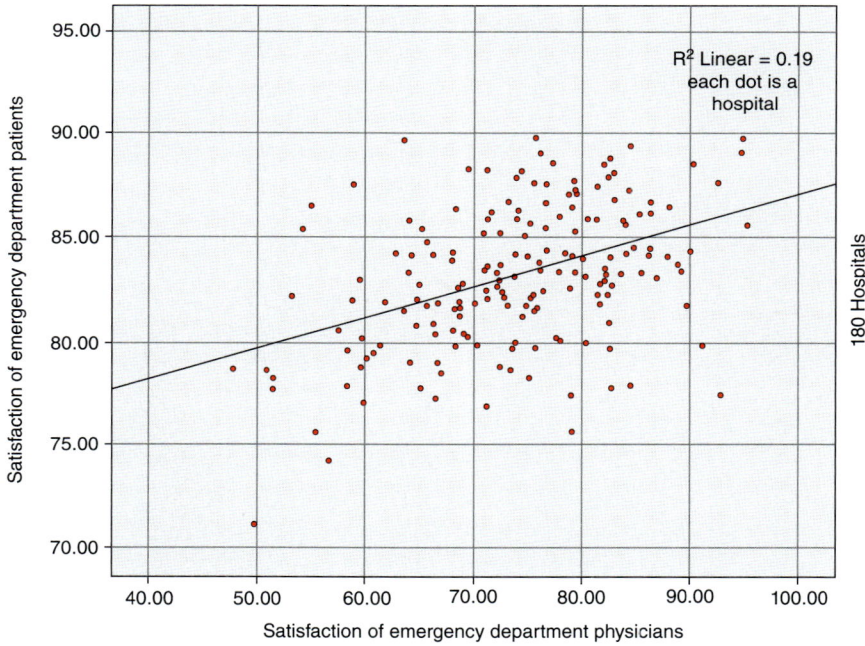

FIGURE 43.11 ■ Patient Satisfaction by Physician Satisfaction

REFERENCES

1. Resar R, Nolan K, Kaczynski D, et al. Using real-time demand capacity management to improve hospitalwide patient flow. *Jt Comm J Qual Patient Saf.* 2011;37(5):217-227.

2. Sabarwhal AD, Mason MG, Lapin R. Cardiac telemetry guidelines improve bed utilization and resources. *Patient Saf Qual Healthc.* 2008. Online journal. Available at: http://psqh.com/sepoct08/cardiac.html. Accessed June 4, 2013.

CHAPTER 44

EFFECTIVE RESPONSE TO FULL CAPACITY

Eric J. Morley, Sandra Schneider, Peter Viccellio

Crowding is a serious problem in emergency departments (EDs) in the United States and abroad.[1-5] It is considered by many emergency physicians to be the greatest safety risk for patients, more so than timeouts for procedures, handwashing, antibiotic timing for pneumonia, and the unavailability of specialty consults.[6]

Multiple studies and the US Government Accounting Office agree that the primary cause of crowding in the US is the practice of boarding: the holding of patients already admitted to the hospital in the ED.[7-12] This practice has been associated with an increase in errors, costs, and morbidity and mortality; delays in care; and a decrease in the initiation of protocolized care in patients with severe sepsis and septic shock.[13-28]

WHY CROWDING OCCURS

Hospitals resort to boarding patients in the ED when there is a shortage of beds or nurses on the inpatient floors. A hospital's failure to anticipate and plan for sufficient inpatient capacity can lead the ED to become the repository for these excess patients. Crowding increases as the number of patients requiring admission increases. Simultaneously, previously admitted patients remain in the ED for excessive amounts of time waiting for an inpatient bed to become available. These patients compete for nursing and other resources, further adding to delays in care. Unfortunately, the practice of boarding patients in the ED has become pervasive, and boarding times have become prolonged, leading to multiple ED handoffs (doctor-to-doctor and nurse-to-nurse).

Some hospitals have realized that the management of inpatients residing in the ED may be associated with greater expense and lower reimbursement.[29-31] Admissions from the ED are largely medical; surgical patients have a higher contribution margin (greater profit). As a result, hospitals may prioritize elective surgical admissions over "routine" ED admissions. Some teaching hospitals attract national and international referrals, yet they are often physically located in low-income neighborhoods. Such institutions, in the face of a constrained supply of inpatient beds, may prioritize the allocation of their beds to the better-insured referrals, thereby limiting the number of ED patients who can be admitted. At the extreme of this practice are hospitals that geographically limit beds to specific specialties (calling them "centers of excellence"), limiting resources for cases that are perceived as less profitable.

CONSEQUENCES OF ED CROWDING

Unfortunately, the consequences of boarding include a prolonged length of stay (LOS) and greater cost to the hospital.[12,32] Several studies have shown that patients boarded in the ED have a longer overall hospital stay.[33,34] Other studies have shown that hospital charges are substantially greater for patients who are boarded in the ED.[15] Recently, Massachusetts developed a statewide plan to reduce boarding and end ambulance diversion, described later in this chapter. Preliminary data from those hospitals that have reduced boarding show increased profit margins.

Decreased bed availability in the ED reduces the number of patients who can be treated and released. Patients who are made to wait too long for an ED examination room often leave before they are seen, thereby reducing ED revenue.[32] In fact, left-prior-to-medical-screening-examination (LPMSE) rates are thought by some to be a surrogate for a measure of crowding.[35] Although the reason for this phenomenon is unknown, it is hypothesized that a waiting room crowded with visitors as well as ED patients prompts some ambulatory patients to leave before registering. Finally, ED crowding can have a consistent, negative effect on LPMSE rates.[36]

The cost of crowding and boarding extends into the community. Ambulance diversion is a common consequence of crowding, as EDs attempt to reduce the inflow into their departments. Ambulance diversion results in patients being taken to different ("new") EDs, where their records and prior test results are not immediately available. The duplication of tests, transfer of information and, in many cases, the transfer of patients back to "their" hospitals add costs and further inefficiencies. Ambulance response and turnaround times increase when ambulances are taken out of service for additional and more prolonged transports, preventing them from offloading their patients quickly and further increasing costs often borne by the community. In one case, diversion was estimated to add over $1 million in costs per year.[37]

Decreased Satisfaction and Increased Errors

Crowding and boarding both reduce patient satisfaction and potentially decrease the chance the patient will choose that hospital for future care.[38,39] This loss of future customer loyalty could be important long term. As health reform continues to develop in the United States, patient experience will be reported publicly and will be a factor in hospital reimbursement.

As mentioned earlier, crowding and boarding are associated with an increase in medical errors. The sheer number of patients in the ED at one time increases nurse-to-patient ratios. The greater the number of patients assigned to each nurse and physician, the greater the chance for error. Many procedures used throughout the hospital to reduce errors, such as pharmacy oversight and unit dosing, are often unavailable to inpatients housed in the ED. High stress, interruptions, noise, and distractions have been known to increase errors in other settings. A recent study found that working in an overcrowded ED leads to tension and frustration among nurses.[40]

To the disadvantage of the patient, specialists who provide care for boarded patients often do so from a distance. Alternatively, some EDs have the emergency physician provide the inpatient care, though it is seldom part of their scope of practice. Neither of these methods serves the best interests of the patient. The patients themselves are also affected by overcrowding; one study found that the perception that other ED patients are likely to die increased post-traumatic stress disorder in ED patients treated for acute coronary syndromes.[41]

OPTIONS TO ADDRESS CROWDING

It is argued that endemic boarding signifies the need to expand hospital capacity. However, accessing the required capital and financing personnel costs may not be feasible in tight economic times. Furthermore, the expansion of ED capacity often reduces the department's pressure on inpatient services, prolonging inpatient stays and ironically leading to more ED beds filled with boarding inpatients, longer ED LOS, and *worsening* crowding. One study showed that ED expansion did not affect ambulance diversion and led to increased LOS and boarding times.[42] A more recent study found that ED expansion did not alter LPMSE rates but negatively impacted boarding times.[43] Expansion alone was shown to decrease patient satisfaction and increase door-to-provider times, the duration of stay, and patients' LPMSE.[44] Both studies indicate that increasing capacity shifts the burden of admitted patients to the already-overwhelmed ED.

An observation unit, ideally run by the ED, may be the exception. By reducing inpatient LOS for certain patient populations, an observation unit can unload both the ED and inpatient units and, because of its 24/7 operational mentality, move patients through the system more quickly and efficiently.[45,46]

Hospital Solutions to Crowding

Full-Capacity Protocol

The "full-capacity protocol" (FCP) is a straightforward solution to crowding that has proven to be safe and effective.[47] By this protocol, when the ED and hospital are at capacity, appropriate (non-intensive care unit [ICU]) patients are sent to the inpatient floor to wait for a bed to become available. Instead of the patient waiting (boarding) in the ED, the patient waits on the inpatient floor. Nursing ratios are often worse in the crowded ED than on the inpatient floors, where patients are distributed throughout the hospital. Furthermore, patients seem to prefer boarding in hallways on inpatient floors more than remaining in crowded EDs.[48-52]

A recent study evaluated the effects of an FCP and various ED performance measures.[53] This particular FCP requires non-ED staff to gather in the ED to help remove barriers and enable patients to go to the floor. This FCP had a positive effect on the LPMSE and ambulance diversion rates despite increased patient volume and admissions during the study period.

Smoothing Admissions

The smoothing of elective admissions, particularly elective surgery, has demonstrated some of the greatest improvements in capacity. Many services in the hospital are only available Monday through Friday, encouraging the practice of admitting the majority of elective patients early in the week. This asymmetry in flow drives a lack of capacity early in the week and excess capacity late in the week and over the weekend. When elective surgical services are more evenly distributed over a full 5-day (or even a 7-day) schedule, inpatient and ICU capacity increase and overall throughput improves, with demonstrably decreased boarding in the ED.

Early and Weekend Inpatient Discharges

In some regards, hospitals have a hotel-like function, including the turnover of beds for the next patient. Delayed discharges from the floor lead to increased LOS in the ED and in access block for ED patients.[54] In one study, shifting the average inpatient discharge times to 4 hours earlier eliminated ED boarding.[55] Inefficiencies in the discharge process often occur on weekends. In one simulation-based study, smoothing out inpatient discharges had a dramatic effect on LOS and boarders in the ED.[56]

ED Solutions to Crowding

Triage, Tracking, and Testing Solutions

Emergency departments can improve their own processes to increase patient flow and access. Beginning at triage, bedside registration and triage bypass can save valuable minutes and improve flow. Moving nonemergent patients to a fast track or utilizing a "split-flow" process isolates low-acuity, low-resource-intensive patients from the crowded conditions. Increasingly, patients undergo extensive testing and imaging prior to admission. Determining clear expectations for turnaround times for these tests and monitoring performance can reduce wait times. Protocols and order sets, often initiated in triage, can reduce the time spent waiting for results.

Scribes

Physicians spend significant time working in electronic medical records (EMRs). One study performed in a community hospital found ED physicians spent 44% of their time in the EMR and only 28% in direct contact with patients.[57] Scribes can be used to decrease this burden by writing notes, gathering laboratory information, and obtaining medical records. A recent randomized trial showed the use of scribes in an Australian ED increased physician productivity by 15.9% and decreased median LOS by 19 minutes.[58] Scribes may also be valuable for nonphysician providers.

Completion of Workup

"Packaging" the patient often requires the completion of nondeterminative tests in the ED, many of which could be performed on the inpatient unit. Consultation in the ED can be valuable, but the demands on specialists in both teaching and private settings can delay their response and, therefore, patient admission to an available bed. Protocols that bypass a specialty workup in the ED with direct admission to the service can save minutes to hours and increase bed availability. Monitoring consultants' response times can further decrease the wait.

Provider in Triage

When crowding is severe, some facilities have moved a physician or advanced practice provider into the triage area. This process has been shown to decrease the number of patients who LPMSE, reduce wait times, and decrease LOS in the ED.[59] It is important to note that the effects of these programs may be modest and must be weighed against the expense of putting a trained emergency medicine provider in triage (PIT). It is also important to note that if volume increases as a result of the PIT strategy, boarding may worsen and ED bed capacity could be further reduced. Therefore, front-end strategies should be used in conjunction with efforts to reduce the root cause of the inpatient boarding, thereby definitively relieving the downstream bottleneck.

Triage Out

Some hospitals defer the care of patients to other non-ED settings after an initial screening examination. These programs entail performing a medical screening examination and recommending that patients without an "emergency medical condition" seek care elsewhere. This effort has been directed mostly at uninsured patients, and the safety of such practices has not been clearly established. Unless there is a specific referral site for them, these patients may be left completely without care; ultimately, their illnesses will progress, creating pain and suffering for the patient and increasing the cost burden to society.

CREATING CHANGE

The Centers for Medicare and Medicaid Services (CMS) recognizes the negative impact of crowding on patient care. As a result, CMS developed four throughput measures for which hospitals are responsible.[60] The metrics are:

1. Door to diagnostic evaluation by a qualified medical professional
2. Time in the ED from entry to discharge for treat-and-release patients

3. Time in the ED from entry to discharge for admitted patients
4. Time from the decision to admit until discharge for admitted patients

In addition to these required metrics, monitoring specific factors within and outside the ED can be useful (**Table 44.1**).

Change requires buy-in from all parties; unfortunately, a crisis is sometimes needed to capture the attention of stakeholders and mobilize them to act. Too often, crowding is blamed on "unnecessary" visits or ED inefficiency. In many areas of the country, boarding inpatients in the ED has become a byproduct of the "normalization of deviancy." This occurs when unacceptable practices and conditions become routine.[61,62] This term was used to explain the *Challenger* shuttle failure. The defect in the O-ring had been known for years but had become accepted as normal since no alternative seemed apparent. Solutions to the O-ring problem were no longer sought. In an analogous fashion, boarding has become the norm at many institutions.

At a local level, change will not occur until the hospital leadership recognizes the problem, determines that a change must occur, and then joins with the ED leaders to resolve the issues.

Examples of Effective Change

Stony Brook Hospital in New York

In 2001, the FCP was instituted, which allowed up to two inpatients to be placed in the hall of each inpatient unit if the ED was at capacity.[47] This protocol was authorized in 2000 by the Commissioner of Health of the State of New York. Since then, the FCP has become routine practice.

The Stony Brook protocol has resulted in a decrease of hospital LOS from 6.2 to 5.4 days for patients placed in the hall. Of the patients sent to the inpatient unit halls, 25% are immediately placed into a bed and another 25% wait less than 1 hour for a bed. The rest

TABLE 44.1 ■ Metrics for ED Flow	
Organizational Component	**Metrics**
ED performance	Patient/hour/physician
	Door-to-provider time (time from entry to ED to first encounter with a provider)
	Time to antibiotics for pneumonia
	Door to thrombolytics or balloon time
	Left-without-being-seen rate
	Time to ECG (time from entry to ED to ECG interpretation)
	Time of entry until discharge for treat-and-release patients
Ancillary services	Time of order to CT result
	Time of order to CBC result
	Time of order to chest x-ray result
	Time of consult order to completion of consult
Hospital performance	Percentage of discharges leaving before noon
	Boarding time (number of patients held in ED × amount of time held)
	Percentage of admissions in ED >2 hours after decision to admit
	Number of patients boarding/number of empty beds
	Time from decision to admit to patient leaving the ED

wait between 8 and 10 hours; 1 in 30 wait for 1 day.[47] Other studies show this practice is safe, increases the department's capacity, and is preferred by patients compared to waiting in the hall of the ED.[48,53,62,63] This practice has been highlighted as a benchmark practice by the Joint Commission and has been instituted in other locations.[64]

State of Massachusetts

Emergency physicians worked within the Massachusetts Medical Society to address the issue of ED crowding, boarding, and ambulance diversion. The EDs of the state decided to abolish ambulance diversion. At the same time, hospitals were required to create a "Code Help" policy, which established rules that required hospitals to relieve congestion in the ED within a two-hour window or activate an internal disaster plan. As a result, institutions have improved flow, increased patient satisfaction, and increased their profit margins.

Mental Health Patients: A Special Concern

The boarding of mental health patients waiting for admission is of special concern. Although these patients may have normal vital signs and show no outward signs of illness, they must frequently wait for extraordinarily long periods due to the limited number of available behavioral health beds and the bureaucracy surrounding patient transfers. In one area of the country, patients must have a court order issued on the same day to complete a behavioral health transfer. Court orders can only be obtained Monday through Friday until 4:00 pm. Mental health inpatients are routinely discharged from the inpatient units after 5:00 pm, leaving the potentially available bed open for 16 hours or more. Waits of 7 or 8 days are not uncommon. Compounding this inefficient care, drug therapy beyond sedation is rarely initiated in the ED for behavioral health patients. CMS District 1 is considering extending EMTALA to psychiatric hospitals, requiring them to admit patients without regard to payment.

Many patients awaiting psychiatric beds do not receive treatment specific to their illness. This may be because the emergency physician is uncomfortable starting new medications, may not be able to consult with a psychiatrist to determine the correct medication, or may be asked to withhold medication until the patient is evaluated. The majority of hospitals do not have 24/7 access to a psychiatric consultant and rely on nonphysicians to perform mental health evaluations. As boarding times increase, it may be in the patient's best interest for emergency physicians to restart/continue home psychiatric medications. When feasible, emergency physicians should develop protocols for initiating treatment in the ED for common psychiatric conditions in conjunction with local psychiatrists if available.

International Efforts to Address Crowding

Access Block

Internationally, there have been attempts to address crowding and long waits in EDs. In the United Kingdom and Australia, the term "access block" is used for ED crowding. Access block is defined by the Australian College of Emergency Medicine (ACEM) as "the situation where patients who have been admitted and need a hospital bed are delayed from leaving the ED because of lack of inpatient bed capacity."[65] The ACEM goes on to describe access block as "the single most serious issue facing EDs in Australia, as it negatively affects the provision of safe, timely, and quality medical care to patients."[65]

Carrot and Stick

In 2004, England's Department of Health for the National Health Service created a target of 4 hours for patients to leave the ED and tied this performance to incentives and penalties for hospitals. Unfortunately, the program resulted in increased spending, increased admissions, and no clear mortality benefit.[66] Further, hospital staff complained of increased workload pressure and anger at an imposition of a target.[67] Expecting the ED to do more with the same resources is not reasonable. It is likely that other systematic fixes listed above would have had a greater impact.

CONCLUSION

There has been an effort in the US to educate legislators, regulators, and the public about ending the practice of boarding patients in the ED. The recent throughput measures established by CMS are a first step. Other organizations that may play a role in placing pressure on hospitals include The Joint Commission and the Department of Health and Human Services. The problem of boarding and crowding in EDs is only a symptom of a fragmented and broken system. While regulatory pressure will help create an environment for change, conclusive change on a local level will only occur when the hospital, the medical staff, and the payers come together to rebuild our health-care delivery system.

REFERENCES

1. Richardson D, Kelly AM, Kerr D. Prevalence of access block in Australia 2004–2008. *Emerg Med Australas*. 2009;21(6):472–478.

2. Lowthian JA, Cameron PA. Emergency demand access block and patient safety: a call for national leadership. *Emerg Med Australas*. 2009;21(6):435–439.

3. Ay D, Akkas M, Sivri B. Patient population and factors determining length of stay in adult ED of a Turkish University Medical Center. *Am J Emerg Med*. 2010;28(3):325–330.

4. Cha WC, Shin SD, Song KJ, Jung SK, Suh GJ. Effect of an independent-capacity protocol on overcrowding in an urban emergency department. *Acad Emerg Med*. 2009;16(12):1277–1283.

5. Bittencourt RJ, Hortale VA. Interventions to solve overcrowding in hospital emergency services: a systematic review [in Portuguese]. *Cad Saude Publica*. 2009;25(7):1439–1454.

6. Sklar DP, Crandall CS, Zola T, Cunningham R. Emergency physician perceptions of patient safety risks. *Ann Emerg Med*. 2010;55(4):336–340.

7. General Accounting Office. Hospital Emergency Departments: Crowded Conditions Vary Among Hospitals and Communities. 2003. https://www.gao.gov/new.items/d03460.pdf. Accessed July 13, 2020.

8. Bair AE, Song WT, Chen YC, Morris BA. The impact of inpatient boarding on ED efficiency: a discrete-event simulation study. *J Med Syst*. 2010;34(5):919–929.

9. Carr BG, Hollander JE, Baxt WG, Datner EM, Pines JM. Trends in boarding of admitted patients in US Emergency Departments 2003–2005. *J Emerg Med*. 2010;39(4):506–511.

10. Canadian Health Services Research F. Myth: Emergency room overcrowding is caused by non-urgent cases. *J Health Serv Res Policy*. 2010;15(3):188–189.

11. Henneman PL, Nathanson BH, Li H, et al. Emergency department patients who stay more than 6 hours contribute to crowding. *J Emerg Med*. 2010;39(1):105–112.

12. Lucas R, Farley H, Twanmoh J, et al. Emergency department patient flow: the influence of hospital census variables on emergency department length of stay. *Aca Emerg Med*. 2009;16(7):597–602.

13. Weissman JS, Rothschild JM, Bendavid E, et al. Hospital workload and adverse events. *Med Care*. 2007;45(5):448–455.

14. Kulstad EB, Sikka R, Sweis RT, Kelley KM, Rzechula KH. ED overcrowding is associated with an increased frequency of medication errors. *Am J Emerg Med*. 2010;28(3):304–309.

15. Krochmal P, Riley TA. Increased health care costs associated with ED overcrowding. *Am J Emerg Med*. 1994;12(3):265–266.

16. Pines JM, Hollander JE, Localio AR, Metlay JP. The association between emergency department crowding and hospital performance on antibiotic timing for pneumonia and percutaneous intervention for myocardial infarction. *Acad Emerg Med*. 2006;13(8):873–878.

17. Sikka R, Mehta S, Kaucky C, Kulstad EB. ED crowding is associated with an increased time to pneumonia treatment. *Am J Emerg Med*. 2010;28(7):809–812.

18. Pines JM, Shofer FS, Isserman JA, Abbuhl SB, Mills AM. The effect of emergency department crowding on analgesia in patients with back pain in two hospitals. *Acad Emerg Med*. 2010;17(3):276–283.

19. Mills AM, Shofer FS, Chen EH, Hollander JE, Pines JM. The association between emergency department crowding and analgesia administration in acute abdominal pain patients. *Acad Emerg Med*. 2009;16(7):603–608.

20. Schull MJ, Morrison LJ, Vermeulen M, Redelmeier DA. Emergency department gridlock and out-of-hospital delays for cardiac patients. *Acad Emerg Med*. 2003;10(7):709–716.

21. Hwang U, Richardson LD, Sonuyi TO, Morrison RS. The effect of emergency department crowding on the management of pain in older adults with hip fracture. *J Am Geriatr Soc*. 2006;54(2):270–275.

22. Pines JM, Pollack CV Jr, Diercks DB, Chang AM, Shofer FS, Hollander JE. The association between emergency department crowding and adverse cardiovascular outcomes in patients with chest pain. *Acad Emerg Med*. 2009;16(7):617–625.

23. Bernstein SL, Aronsky D, Duseja R, et al. The effect of emergency department crowding on clinically oriented outcomes. *Acad Emerg Med*. 2009;16(1):1–10.

24. Carr BG, Kaye AJ, Wiebe DJ, Gracias VH, Schwab CW, Reilly PM. Emergency department length of stay: a major risk factor for pneumonia in intubated blunt trauma patients. *J Trauma*. 2007;63(1):9–12.

25. Sprivulis PC, Da Silva JA, Jacobs IG, Frazer AR, Jelinek GA. The association between hospital overcrowding and mortality among patients admitted via Western Australian emergency departments. *Med J Aust*. 2006;184(5):208–212.

26. Richardson DB. Increase in patient mortality at 10 days associated with emergency department overcrowding. *Med J Aust*. 2006;184(5):213–216.

27. Hickey F. Casualty overcrowding and increased mortality; is it time to say no? *Ir Med J*. 2006;99(8):248-249; author reply 249.
28. Gaieski DF, Agarwal AK, Mikkelsen ME, et al. The impact of ED crowding on early interventions and mortality in patients with severe sepsis. *Am J Emerg Med*. 2017;35(7):953-960.
29. Handel DA, Hilton JA, Ward MJ, Rabin E, Zwemer FL Jr, Pines JM. Emergency department throughput, crowding, and financial outcomes for hospitals. *Acad Emerg Med*. 2010;17(8):840-847.
30. Schneider SM, Asplin BR. Form follows finance: emergency department admissions and hospital operating margins. *Acad Emerg Med*. 2008;15(10):959-960.
31. McHugh M, Regenstein M, Siegel B. The profitability of Medicare admissions based on source of admission. *Acad Emerg Med*. 2008;15(10):900-907.
32. Falvo T, Grove L, Stachura R, Zirkin W. The financial impact of ambulance diversions and patient elopements. *Acad Emerg Med*. 2007;14(1):58-62.
33. Liew D, Liew D, Kennedy MP. Emergency department length of stay independently predicts excess inpatient length of stay. *Med J Aust*. 2003;179(10):524-526.
34. Richardson DB. The access-block effect: relationship between delay to reaching an inpatient bed and inpatient length of stay. *Med J Aust*. 2002;177(9):492-495.
35. Weiss SJ, Ernst AA, Derlet R, King R, Bair A, Nick TG. Relationship between the National ED Overcrowding Scale and the number of patients who leave without being seen in an academic ED. *Am J Emerg Med*. 2005;23(3):288-294.
36. Carter EJ, Pouch SM, Larson EL. The relationship between emergency department crowding and patient outcomes: a systematic review. *J Nurs Scholarsh*. 2014;46(2):106-115.
37. Schneider S, Zwemer F, Doniger A, Dick R, Czapranski T, Davis E. Rochester, New York: a decade of emergency department overcrowding. *Acad Emerg Med*. 2001;8(11):1044-1050.
38. Pines JM, Iyer S, Disbot M, Hollander JE, Shofer FS, Datner EM. The effect of emergency department crowding on patient satisfaction for admitted patients. *Acad Emerg Med*. 2008;15(9):825-831.
39. Collis J. Adverse effects of overcrowding on patient experience and care. *Emerg Nurse*. 2010;18(8):34-39.
40. Chen LC, Lin CC, Han CY, Hsieh CL, Wu CJ, Liang HF. An interpretative study on nurses' perspectives of working in an overcrowded emergency department in Taiwan. *Asian Nurs Res (Korean Soc Nurs Sci)*. 2018;12(1):62-68.
41. Konrad B, Hiti D, Chang BP, Retuerto J, Julian J, Edmondson D. Cardiac patients' perceptions of neighboring patients' risk: influence on psychological stress in the ED and subsequent posttraumatic stress. *BMC Emerg Med*. 2017;17(1):33.
42. Han JH, Zhou C, France DJ, et al. The effect of emergency department expansion on emergency department overcrowding. *Acad Emerg Med*. 2007;14(4):338-343.
43. Mumma BE, McCue JY, Li CS, Holmes JF. Effects of emergency department expansion on emergency department patient flow. *Acad Emerg Med*. 2014;21(5):504-509.
44. Sayah A, Lai-Becker M, Kingsley-Rocker L, Scott-Long T, O'Connor K, Lobon LF. Emergency department expansion versus patient flow improvement: impact on patient experience of care. *J Emerg Med*. 2016;50(2):339-348.
45. Hung GR, Kissoon N. Impact of an observation unit and an emergency department-admitted patient transfer mandate in decreasing overcrowding in a pediatric emergency department: a discrete event simulation exercise. *Pediatr Emerg Care*. 2009;25(3):160-163.
46. Kelen GD, Scheulen JJ, Hill PM. Effect of an emergency department (ED) managed acute care unit on ED overcrowding and emergency medical services diversion. *Acad Emerg Med*. 2001;8(11):1095-1100.
47. Viccellio A, Santora C, Singer AJ, Thode HC Jr, Henry MC. The association between transfer of emergency department boarders to inpatient hallways and mortality: a 4-year experience. *Ann Emerg Med*. 2009;54(4):487-491.
48. McGowan H, Gopeesingh K, O'Kelly P, Gilligan P. Emergency department overcrowding and the full capacity protocol cross over study: what patients who have experienced both think about being an extra patient in the emergency department or on a ward. *Ir Med J*. 2018;111(7):788.
49. Richards JR, Ozery G, Notash M, Sokolove PE, Derlet RW, Panacek EA. Patients prefer boarding in inpatient hallways: correlation with the national emergency department overcrowding score. *Emerg Med Int*. 2011;2011:840459.
50. Viccellio P, Zito JA, Sayage V, et al. Patients overwhelmingly prefer inpatient boarding to emergency department boarding. *J Emerg Med*. 2013;45(6):942-946.
51. Walsh P, Cortez V, Bhakta H. Patients would prefer ward to emergency department boarding while awaiting an inpatient bed. *J Emerg Med*. 2008;34(2):221-226.
52. Bartlett S, Fatovich DM. Emergency department patient preferences for waiting for a bed. *Emerg Med Australas*. 2009;21(1):25-30.
53. Willard E, Carlton EF, Moffat L, Barth BE. A full-capacity protocol allows for increased emergency patient volume and hospital admissions. *J Emerg Nurs*. 2017;43(5):413-418.
54. Khanna S, Boyle J, Good N, Lind J. Early discharge and its effect on ED length of stay and access block. *Stud Health Technol Inform*. 2012;178:92-98.
55. Powell ES, Khare RK, Venkatesh AK, Van Roo BD, Adams JG, Reinhardt G. The relationship between inpatient discharge timing and emergency department boarding. *J Emerg Med*. 2012;42(2):186-196.
56. Wong HJ, Wu RC, Caesar M, Abrams H, Morra D. Smoothing inpatient discharges decreases emergency department congestion: a system dynamics simulation model. *Emerg Med J*. 2010;27(8):593-598.
57. Hill RG Jr, Sears LM, Melanson SW. 4000 clicks: a productivity analysis of electronic medical records in a community hospital ED. *Am J Emerg Med*. 2013;31(11):1591-1594.
58. Walker K, Ben-Meir M, Dunlop W, et al. Impact of scribes on emergency medicine doctors' productivity and patient throughput: multicentre randomised trial. *BMJ*. 2019;364:l121.
59. Abdulwahid MA, Booth A, Kuczawski M, Mason SM. The impact of senior doctor assessment at triage on emergency department performance measures: systematic review and meta-analysis of comparative studies. *Emerg Med J*. 2016;33(7):504-513.
60. CMS. Hospital Outpatient Quality Reporting Program. 2018.
61. Banja J. The normalization of deviance in healthcare delivery. *Bus Horiz*. 2010;53(2):139.
62. Guthrie BD, King WD, Monroe KW. Parental preferences for boarding locations when a children's hospital exceeds capacity. *Ann Emerg Med*. 2009;53(6):762-766.
63. Garson C, Hollander JE, Rhodes KV, Shofer FS, Baxt WG, Pines JM. Emergency department patient preferences for boarding locations when hospitals are at full capacity. *Ann Emerg Med*. 2008;51(1):9-12, 12.e11-e13.
64. The Joint Commission, "Case Study: Reducing Overcrowding in the ED with the Full Capacity Protocol." The Joint Commission Benchmark, July/August 2009, pgs 3-4.
65. ACEM. Statement on Access Block. 2014.
66. Jones P, Schimanski K. The four hour target to reduce emergency department 'waiting time': a systematic review of clinical outcomes. *Emerg Med Australas*. 2010;22(5):391-398.
67. Mortimore A, Cooper S. The "4-hour target": emergency nurses' views. *Emerg Med J*. 2007;24(6):402-404.

CHAPTER 45

DEFEATING BOUNCE BACKS: MANAGING HIGH-UTILIZER PATIENTS

Blaine Hannafin, Kimberly Anderson, Gigi Baniqued, Karen Murrell

A 50-year-old man well known to a community emergency department (ED) in Northern California frequently presents with complaints of asthma and requests to refill his rescue inhaler. Visits are typically brief, with the patient reporting improvement after a single nebulization treatment. A new high-utilizer committee reviews the patient's chart and finds that he has had 33 ED visits in the previous 12 months. However, further investigation among partner EDs shows a combined census of 105 ED visits. The committee digs deeper, and the patient's insurance plan administrator and medical director agree to meet. A review of the insurance company's claims records reveals the full scope of the problem: a staggering 227 ED visits over the preceding 12 months. In some cases, his visits were at two different hospitals on the same day.

The concept of high-utilizer patients is a known phenomenon to physicians and staff working in emergency departments (EDs) across the country. Other common names like "super users" and "frequent flyers" are often described.[1,2] Despite how widespread this phenomenon seems, published literature is variable in how the problem is defined, framed, and addressed by health systems.[3] Physicians and staff often experience a sense of hopelessness and a feeling that the care they deliver will not impact or benefit these high utilizers or avert another preventable ED visit.

Emergency departments were not designed to provide continuity of care or address social determinants of health. As a result, frequent use of EDs is considered an inefficient and costly use of health-care resources.[4] Even with the myriad ED management challenges, it is clear that high-utilizer patients are a phenomenon worth discussing, and several strategies to address inefficient utilization have been successful.[1,2,5] The variability in definition and approach to this challenge is not indicative of an unsolvable problem but rather a reflection of the heterogeneity of the high-utilizer population and the complexities they pose to health-care systems.

Specific to this population, the ED should reconsider its reactive "treat and street" mantra and instead develop a proactive model to expand its purpose and optimize its internal and external resources. While doing so goes against some of the foundational teachings of emergency care, it can also pay rewarding dividends to the health-care organization that engages in this practice by offering a more realistic chance of meeting the challenging needs of these patients.

Case Study: Part 1 of 3

A 64-year-old woman, RL, is well known to a community ED. She frequently presents by ambulance for chest pain or chronic obstructive pulmonary disease (COPD) symptoms.

Despite her frequent ED visits, she is rarely admitted to the hospital. The ambulance crew knows her well and has expressed frustration about handling her calls. She is also well known to the ED providers and staff, who feel a sense of hopelessness that the patient will return no matter what care they provide. The care delivered during her visits, including the diagnostics and patient messaging and education, varies greatly. On average, she presents to the ED about twice per week, typically during normal business hours.

DEFINING THE UNDEFINABLE

No standard definition of ED high utilizers exists, and published reports use different parameters to define them.[1,6] A review of the literature reveals variability in both the time frame used to assess baseline ED visits (6-12 months) and the absolute visit frequency.[6-8] Though a cutoff of four or more visits is sometimes used, this number is arbitrary and yields very different populations depending on its facility-specific application.[6]

The lack of a standard definition makes evaluating publications challenging as differing methodologies and population mixes do not allow for comparable analysis.[8] Compounding this challenge is that each ED has varying volumes and acuities, and thus, its high-utilizer population will likewise be distributed differently. Each health system also serves various proportions of commercial, Medicare, Medicaid, and uninsured members. These differences affect the population mix within a high-utilizer cohort regardless of what definition is used.

Based on the inconsistent definitions of high utilizers and differences that are unique to each community and practice environment, it is recommended that each health-care facility embrace an operational definition for ED high utilizers (**Box 45.1**). Such a definition would avoid an overly restrictive set of objective measures. While variability and comparisons would remain a challenge, an agreed-upon operational definition embraced by each health-care facility, regardless of payor mix and ED volume, can lead to a consistent understanding and approach to the high-utilizer patient population.

Creating a local definition for high utilizer that is suited to a facility's needs can be a daunting task. Beginning with a simple, if arbitrary, starting point such as the top 100 utilizers of a facility's emergency services can illuminate the combination of disease burden, visit patterns, and social challenges that are present in this group.

Population

While no one characteristic is universally present in high utilizers, these patients tend to have a higher burden of medical, psychiatric, and social challenges and report lower

---

BOX 45.1 ■ PROPOSED DEFINITION OF HIGH UTILIZERS

High utilizers may be broadly thought of as patients who frequently present to the ED for services. However, for the purpose of population management, they may be better thought of as the subset of *impactable* patients frequently using ED services. Patients with *impactable* circumstances who can obtain services outside the hospital may reasonably expect to avoid future ED visits.

The word *impactable* is important, as not all patients will avoid ED visits simply by connecting them to services. There is no visit minimum or visit maximum cutoff, as differing facilities may experience different visit distributions depending on their annual visit census. For example, the authors' home facility in suburban Sacramento, California, sees about 130,000 ED visits per year and will have a different strategy than a low-volume ED in a community without many resources.

The challenge is assessing high utilizers in the context of a facility's innate resources, without using an overly pessimistic barometer for assessing their modifiability. It is the authors' experience that many more patients are impactable than our gut instincts would otherwise suggest.

socioeconomic status.[1] Housing instability has been independently associated with not having a usual source of care and is also found among the high-utilizer population.[4]

Studies have attempted to describe the top users of ED care in different health settings in both North America and Europe. Those studies describe a diverse and heterogeneous population that frequently challenges some of the underlying stereotypes that ED staff may have traditionally held. For example, there is a long-held belief that simply obtaining coverage for uninsured high ED utilizers will solve the problem.[6] However, one study demonstrated that obtaining health insurance coverage minimally impacted ED use by high utilizers.[6] Clinicians frequently reference substance abuse as a reason for high ED utilization and, while prevalent, it is frequently comingled with many other confounders and is not itself a specific predictor of frequent ED use. One study found a strong majority of frequent ED utilizers (defined as seven or more visits in a year) did not have substance abuse.[6]

Interestingly, there is a subpopulation of relatively young patients among high utilizers. While not well described in the literature, their prevalence can be seen broadly in Centers for Disease Control and Prevention ED statistics for ages 18 to 44.[9] In fact, the ED visits are higher in this population than in the subsequent age group of 45 to 64 years old, in which this trend dates back more than 15 years.[9]

Data are conflicting around ED utilization post Affordable Care Act implementation for patients who receive Medicaid. Most studies show an initial increased ED utilization that decreases over time as deferred needs are eventually met, and patients become familiar with the health-care system. What is clear is that all EDs have a cohort of high utilizers whose challenges will be related broadly to the composition of the community and the patient's life circumstances and access to care.

Figure 45.1 shows high-utilizer visit distributions for the top 100 patients at each of five medical centers identified at Kaiser Permanente. Regardless of annual ED census (**Figure 45.2**), the shape of each curve follows a similar sideways boot shape, with the highest utilizers located to the left.

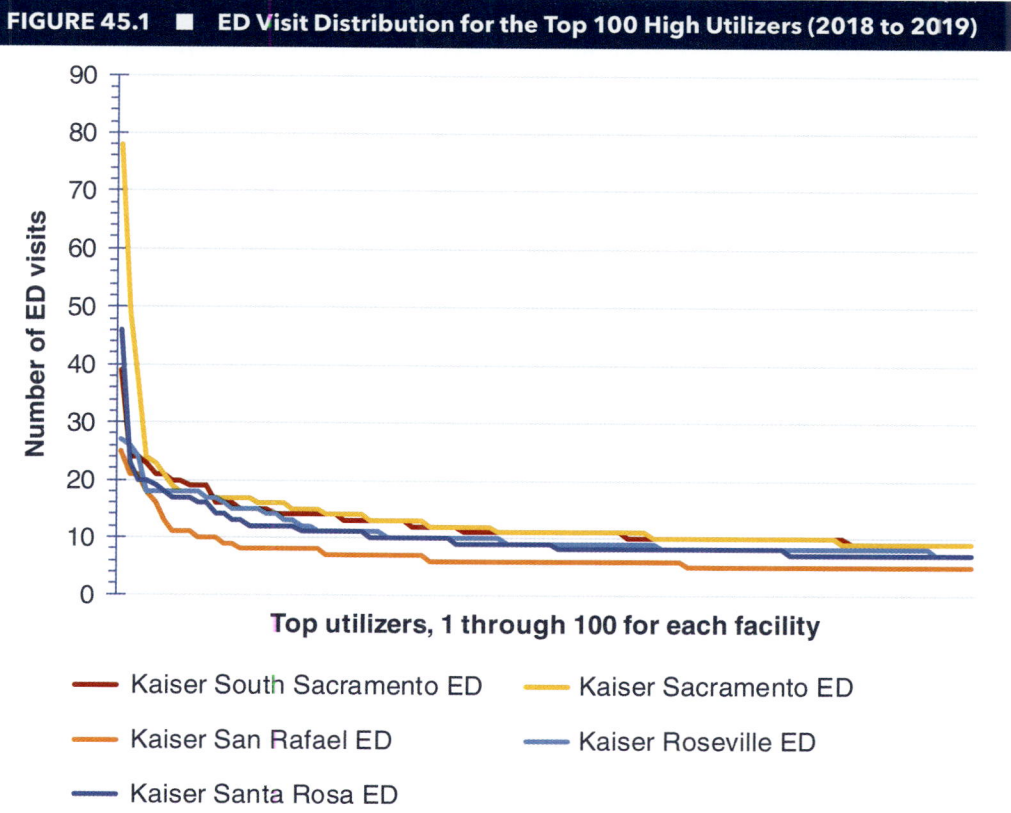

FIGURE 45.1 ■ ED Visit Distribution for the Top 100 High Utilizers (2018 to 2019)

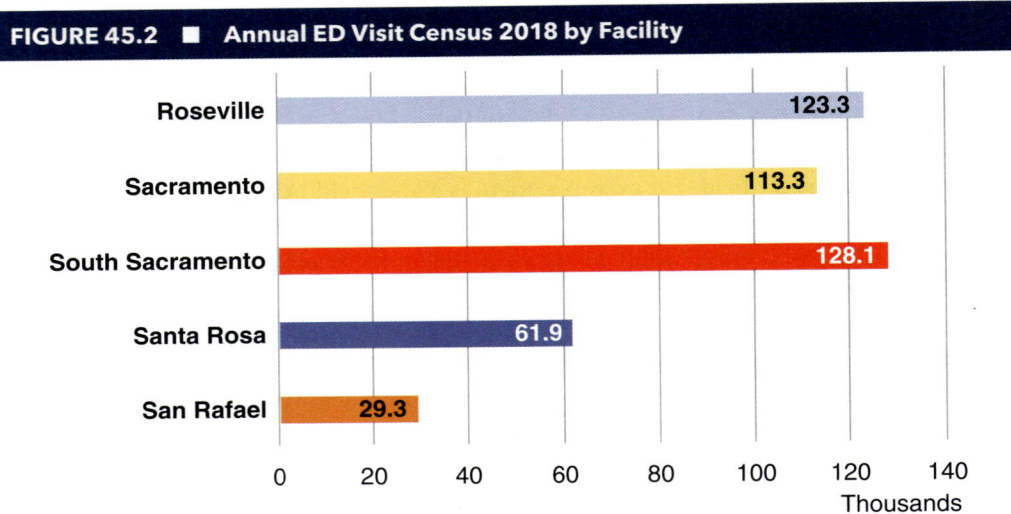

FIGURE 45.2 ■ Annual ED Visit Census 2018 by Facility

Stratification Methodology

There are two broad methods used to stratify high-utilizer populations: rigid vs soft and nonimpactable vs impactable populations.

Rigid Approach

The rigid stratification methodology is based solely on objective measures, which may include ED visit count per defined time interval. Medical, psychiatric, or substance abuse conditions may be used to include, exclude, and further define the population. The advantages to the rigid method include an objectively predefined patient population that is easily quantified by routine application of the *rigid* definition rather than relying on subjective measures or clinician judgment. This method is well suited to environments that have access to well-defined treatment or follow-up algorithms.

A rigid set of criteria also lends itself to the reliable and reproducible creation of a control group. While not every ED must undertake the challenge of operationalizing a program, the business case for an ED high-utilizer program can be bolstered by creating intervention and control groups, demonstrating the difference in outcomes based on the impact measures. Using a rigid definition lends itself to this analysis and helps prevent selection bias that may be introduced with more subjective criteria. A successful program with well-defined criteria may then be suitable to spread to other facilities in a health system.

The disadvantage of the rigid model is its tendency to exclude patients who fall outside the rigid confines of its definition. For example, a new patient with a rapidly accelerating visit count may initially be below the arbitrary preidentified cutoff but nevertheless identified by ED staff as likely needing extra attention. Such clinical premonition is common among clinicians and ED staff, who are frequently able to correctly guess that a patient "will be back again." This would also apply to a patient who is new to a hospital and may not yet have an electronic health record that is populated with data points that would be used to identify frequent ED use.

Conversely, a rigid definition may inadvertently include patients whose circumstances are not readily impactable or patients with acute illness with appropriate and time-limited utilization patterns. Significant resources and time may be spent trying to address behaviors that cannot or should not be changed, when those same resources might be better spent on impactable individuals who are more likely to benefit from them.

Rigid inclusion criteria are common, and the system/hospital definitions are often unique as they take into consideration the specific community, facility, resources, and practice environments that are unique to each facility. However, that very uniqueness within a health system may isolate its care-coordination programs into distinct silos that do not cross communicate well.

Soft Approach

Soft stratification methodology divides high utilizers into impactable and nonimpactable populations, with the nonimpactable population being patients who are most likely to not have alterable visit patterns due to life-limiting medical ailments truly requiring higher-level care in the ED and hospital. These soft definitions are more fluid, may take into account clinical judgment, and consider differing levels of service and support found among different health systems. Thus, the definition would include the particularities of the ED and its community rather than being externally imposed on a facility.

In addition to tailoring the definition to the facility, the soft definition can be tailored to the available ED resources and talent. It can leverage the clinical experience of providers, nurses, and social workers in identifying the high-utilizer patients and the strategies that are likely to be most effective in meeting their needs. A clear example would be using the staff's clinical premonition that a patient will likely have repetitive visits to the ED as one avenue to identify patients who may need additional time, investigation, or services. In the age of data-driven infrastructure and decisions, the role of clinical expertise is frequently downplayed. However, it is our experience that taking advantage of clinical experience and intuition from engaged staff can successfully guide where the greatest impact will be for effort put forth. It also further engages staff, as they feel they have some control and input into the work.

One disadvantage of a soft criteria is that, without guidance, the program may focus on the wrong types or quantities of patients. The soft criteria will not, on its own, provide a manageable subset of patients of limited quantity or complexity. When the authors' own program initially asked for provider and staff referrals, a significant influx of potential patient referrals came through. However, many of the referred patients had nonimpactable medical illnesses, circumstances, or utilization patterns that occurred *in other health systems*. While the staff engagement was excellent and heartfelt, distinguishing the signal from all the referral noise became a challenge.

Another consideration of a soft criteria is creating a credible impact analysis. It cannot be overemphasized that it is important to make a good-faith effort to measure the impact of this work. Simple pre- and postintervention measures for high utilizers may be enough, but a comparison group that considers disease burden and regression to the mean is more robust. While a rigid criteria can yield a well-defined population, a soft criteria can yield a more heterogeneous and ill-defined population for which creating a comparison group is much harder.

Nonimpactable Population

These patients are defined by intense medical needs that are not likely or reasonably expected to be met outside of a hospital (**Box 45.2**). In an environment with limited time and resources, it is prudent to focus on the areas where the impact will be the greatest.

> ### BOX 45.2 ■ EXAMPLE: NONIMPACTABLE HIGH UTILIZER
>
> A 25-year-old woman has a history of severe anemia, thrombocytopenia, immune thrombocytopenic purpura, and malignant histiocytoma of the spleen. She was repeatedly referred to the ED for bleeding or very low hemoglobin. Although she had a hematologist and access to the outpatient ambulatory transfusion unit, her illness was so severe that she would often self-present or be referred to the ED for severe symptoms. Her hematologist insisted that he'd "never seen anything like it." It was neither reasonable nor prudent to try to address this patient's intense medical needs anywhere other than the hospital.

Impactable Population

These patients have impactable circumstances with potentially avoidable ED visits. Social needs are frequently encountered in this population, including:

- Housing (homeless) or transportation insecurity
- Intimate partner violence[10]
- Inadequate support systems
- Minimal financial resources

Low-acuity medical complaints are more common, including medication refills, work excuses, minor injuries, or illness among the impactable population. Many of these patients have psychiatric diagnoses, most notable anxiety and/or depression. One longitudinal study in Washington over a 15-month period revealed that of the highest utilizers (visit count range 78-134), 100% of the patients had probable mental illness, 90% had a substance abuse problem, and 20% were homeless.[11] Some patients may not have access to regular medical care or have existing health insurance but are unsure of how to properly make use of it. In order to impact this population, dividing them into distinct categories that form the basis of care plans and/or interventions has been found to be extremely successful (see **Box 45.3**).

MEETING PATIENTS' NEEDS

In the fast-paced setting of the ED, the true drivers of repetitive visits may not be easily detected, acknowledged, or acted upon. Some of these patients are unaware of their drivers (lack insight) or are unwilling to share the reason with the ED staff. An example of an unspoken reason for multiple ED visits might be a particularly difficult social situation, such as intimate partner violence.[12] A patient's needs, either real or perceived, are ultimately what drive a patient to the ED. If those needs remain unmet or unrecognized, the visit pattern is likely to continue.

Interventions

The creation of a high-utilizer committee offers a venue for thorough assessment and can provide a more detached and broad view of a patient's needs and visit patterns.

BOX 45.3 ■ COMMON DRIVERS OF IMPACTABLE PATIENTS

- Access to health care
  - Uninsured
  - Insured, access challenges
    - Patient unsure of how to access care
    - Patient unable to get timely access to care
    - Housing insecurity/homeless
- Transportation insecurity, unable to get to appointments or fill prescriptions
- Intimate partner violence
- Easy access to specialized care in ED
- Secondary gain
  - Medication, food, work excuses, attention, socialization
- Risk aversion
  - The perception that symptoms are severe enough for the ED
  - The perception that they will receive better care in the ED
- Untreated psychiatric illness

Clustering

When considering a facility's high utilizers, it may be helpful to segment the population into clusters that contain individuals who are similar and dissimilar to those in other clusters. Creating patient clusters can help quantify the patterns of disease intensity and social and psychiatric challenges thet are present.

Clustering can also be done by payor, as some payors will have case management programs that can be leveraged to help address their members' challenges or provide continuity or community navigation after discharge. This approach also helps establish what existing resources are on hand, what additional hospital/community resources are required, and what care pathways can be developed to address the challenges of each cluster.

Interventions can also be clustered to better assess what tools, resources, and workflows exist to meet the challenges present in the high-utilizer population. For example, a facility may have certain resources or workflows surrounding homelessness or palliative care. Defining and consolidating these processes into a cluster presents an opportunity to streamline overlapping or redundant workflows and makes the potential population strategy easier to decipher. Clustering in this manner also reinforces consistent patient messaging.

As described in previous sections, the high-utilizer population is diverse. A high utilizer need not belong to a single cluster, and not every patient will fit into a cluster that has a corresponding workflow or resource attached to it. Clustering will also not eliminate the need to perform chart reviews and develop interventions in conjunction with an interdisciplinary team. From a pragmatic point of view, it may be wise to begin high-utilizer work with a cluster that staff have a strong desire to address and for which resources are available. Early success is important to initiating momentum, creating a sustainable program, and maintaining the engagement of providers and staff.

Multidisciplinary Management

A multidisciplinary group that consists of physicians, nurses, pharmacists, case managers, social workers, a data analyst, a project manager, and representatives from community resources should develop strategies. Members of the insurance industry are also critical partners since they are financially motivated to decrease utilization but may not have the ability to address high-utilizer patients in real time during an ED visit. Insurance carriers also provide case management and other services that can be used to help address this patient population.

Communicating effectively with community resources, such as clinics, primary care provider offices, housing programs, and so on, to arrange referrals, interventions, and ensure follow-up can provide additional relief for patients and the ED as well as a feedback loop to the high-utilizer program (ecosystem). Regular bilateral reporting can help determine which resources are having a positive impact and which are not.

Community Partnerships

Community partnerships are not only pivotal for addressing the continuity of care but are also necessary to ensure sustainable solutions that meet the patient's long-term social needs. For example, an ED may provide a meal, taxi voucher, and clothing, which may temporarily mitigate a patient's need during an episodic encounter. However, the typical patient's needs go far beyond the short-term ED intervention and require additional resources only found in the community.

Challenges

Creating an infrastructure to communicate, design programs, create follow-up protocols, and develop and disseminate care plans across health systems and other community partners is essential to program success. However, there are many challenges, including inconsistencies in electronic health record systems and diverse policies for information sharing across health systems.

In all cases, the goal for the high-utilization team is to connect patients to services that will effectively and efficiently meet their needs. A thoughtful, resource-knowledgeable, empathetic health-care worker may be able to uncover the patient's hidden needs and motives and then provide appropriate services. The health-care worker does not necessarily need to have substantial clinical background but may simply be the one who has the passion and desire to help this complex patient population.

For example, some community health workers are trained laypersons who have walked in the shoes of these high-utilizer patients. This understanding in and of itself creates an immediate trust that may effectively engage high-utilizer patients and enable the health-care worker to uncover and address their social and behavioral needs.[1] While addressing these needs on a case-by-case basis can be done, using the stratification and clustering method will allow the high-utilizer team members to stretch their capacity and focus time on cases that require more intensive management.

DEVELOPING AN ECOSYSTEM

Case Study: Part 2 of 3

A social worker interviews the patient, who lives at home with her daughter, son-in-law, and two grandchildren. She is insured and does attend outpatient appointments with her primary care physician. The patient's family is financially secure. There is no concern for abuse or neglect. After speaking with the patient, family, ambulance crew, and primary care physician, it becomes clearer that her presentations to the ED are multifactorial. She does have severe COPD and diabetes but also appears to be lonely and enjoys the company of the ED staff and the hospital meatloaf that is served during her visits. Additional input is obtained from pulmonary critical care specialists and the outpatient pulmonary wellness program. An interdisciplinary care plan is created to encourage consistency of care and address the patient's medical and social needs.

Formal and Informal Leadership

It is critical to engage senior institutional leaders who understand and champion a high-utilizer initiative. Their approval and support will give the members of the team legitimacy and the authority needed to make necessary changes and partner with existing programs. Informal leaders who are passionate about this cause can also add tremendous value to the team's success by participating in the development and implementation of solutions and offering diversification of thought.

Care Coordination Partnerships

Most facilities already have care-coordination programs in place for non-ED populations. Some of these programs are focused on quality, hospital readmission, disease-specific care, or payor-specific presentations (such as Medicaid). An ED high-utilizer initiative should seek to partner with existing care-coordination programs to avoid redundancy and leverage existing infrastructure and resources. Integrated health systems like Kaiser Permanente in Northern California have an additional advantage, as clinicians working in primary care, inpatient units, and EDs all use the same electronic health record, increasing the likelihood that providers from different parts of the care spectrum will participate in an interdisciplinary plan. However, while partnerships with existing care plans can yield synergy, these programs are not likely, by themselves, to have the expertise or local knowledge of an ED's operations, resources, population, and payor mix. Thus, to address the challenges of high utilizers, the ED itself must be engaged, invested, and participating in the solution.

Governance

The ideal governance of a high-utilizer initiative would tie into the existing oversight infrastructure to foster cross-collaboration and communication across programmatic initiatives. A case management or care-coordination committee would be an appropriate governing body. An ED high-utilizer program is most likely to succeed as part of a larger ecosystem that can collectively manage patients' needs. If that infrastructure does not already exist, an ED high-utilizer workgroup may have to start in the ED and gradually create these collaborative relationships with key constituents. More than most, these patients require a collaborative plan that involves a broad variety of caregivers, including outpatient, inpatient, and ED providers.

Ethical Principles of Engagement

A health program that primarily focuses on decreasing utilization without providing solutions to address the needs of its target population could find itself on an ethical slippery slope. Individuals developing these programs must first define the values and goals of the effort before embarking on patient interventions. To prevent the unfair stereotyping of frequent utilizers, these ethical principles should be agreed upon by both the core group participating in the effort and the broader ED staff. One suggestion is to use patient-centered language, making it clear that these individuals should be connected to services that meet their unique needs.

Composition of Team

A multidisciplinary team should include emergency physicians, nurses, and social workers with extensive knowledge of community resources and clinicians from behavioral and primary care. Care coordinators, pharmacists, and individuals who understand the broader care delivery infrastructure should also participate. Specialists can be included on a case-by-case basis. An information technology consultant should participate as needed to help implement creative technological solutions, such as an electronic medical record alert to notify the ED team of arriving patients. A consultant or project manager with dedicated time alloted to help develop processes and workflows, bring teams and community partners together, and spearhead the management of the high-utilizer initiative is an essential part of these initiatives.

Data Analysis

It is essential to invest in data infrastructure.[2] Data on ED high utilizers, based on either the hard or soft criteria detailed previously, can help identify potential case reviews. Program leadership can then use the data to determine the measures and methods by which the initiative's impact and effectiveness will be tracked. Early agreement on the quantitative measures will avoid subsequent skepticism by senior hospital leadership who may otherwise regard the program with reservation. The team should use a feedback system to measure both the intended and unintended consequences of the program.[8]

Metrics on ED and inpatient utilization are important. A program may also look at quality metrics, such as control of chronic conditions like diabetes and hypertension as well as health screenings and opioid prescribing. Access and compliance with mental health appointments are also key for many patients and should be included in metrics, if appropriate.[13] Specific metrics will vary depending on the facility, scope of work, and availability of an analyst.

Intrafacility Partnerships

Many hospitals and health systems have an abundance of teams and committees, each with a specific mission. New ED high-utilizer teams would be well advised to quantify and partner with *existing* programs that involve care coordination, case management, or population management. Working with existing groups to define common inclusion and exclusion criteria will lead to common language and effective crossover to other groups. Alternatively, a siloed work environment cannot effectively address high utilizers' complex needs. The ED high-utilizer team should strive to break down these barriers and cross-collaborate on shared patient care planning whenever possible.

Extrafacility Partnerships

As with intrafacility partnerships, involving medical offices and forming relationships with community programs can be an added benefit when trying to connect patients to services. These can include clinical facilities, community housing, substance abuse treatment, or community faith groups.

Partnerships with health insurance entities deserve special mention since they have a fiduciary responsibility to address inefficient resource consumption. These entities will often have case managers or utilization managers who are willing to collaborate with ED high-utilizer programs. Ideally, the health plan call center can serve as a partner to address frequent utilizers' needs if and when they call. Health plans also have information on contracted physician groups, primary care clinics, and transition care or urgent care clinics for non-ED patient follow up.

Call centers can help direct ED patients to these extrafacility resources during discharge, which also aids in follow-up and can prevent a bounce-back visit. While face-to-face coaching for complex patient follow-ups is essential, it can be effectively supplemented by a simple handout highlighting follow-up options.

Ongoing Team Meetings

The team should meet consistently to identify which patients require intervention. The development of workable and achievable care plans may entail meetings with community clinics and insurance companies and discussions with primary care and community navigators. In-depth and nuanced discussions with multiple stakeholders will create more effective final care plans. When appropriate, the patient can be involved. Setting aside time to discuss methods for sharing ideas, performing assessments, and implementing improvements helps create a sustainable, innovative infrastructure and achieve optimized results.

Care Plan Elements

Care plans should primarily focus on *actionable* steps to take and not simply describe what has occurred. An effective action-oriented care plan anticipates the patient's next ED arrival and offers specific guidance. Care plans are designed to address three key elements: medical issues, social determinants, and behavioral health challenges, all customized for the patient. By addressing all three dimensions, the entirety of the patient's needs are fulfilled. The ultimate goal of the team is to determine the underlying causes of the frequent ED visits and address those causes in a compassionate way.

Unilateral

Clear care plans are directive, with well-defined recommendations and action items. Unilateral plans decrease the cognitive burden on clinicians who may not be familiar with the broader context of the patient's visits and help decrease testing redundancy, poly-prescribing, and ED length of service.

Bilateral

These care plans are typically developed by the ED in conjunction with another service, for example, outpatient services or behavioral health. Like unilateral plans, bilateral plans provide clear and consistent guidance for ED visits but, in addition, address the patient's needs in less costly, more effective venues like clinics. Outpatient behavioral health or primary care may offer electronic or telephonic contact for patients. These same outpatient services may offer a period of regularly scheduled visits.

Multilateral

These care plans involve the ED and multiple other parties and may include outpatient social services or case managers, primary care, medical specialists, behavioral health, community resources, and third-party community health workers. Similar to unilateral and bilateral plans, multilateral plans have a set of action-oriented ED recommendations designed to create a consistent treatment experience during and after the ED visit. Efforts to connect the patient to outpatient and community resources may be facilitated by a case manager, social worker, navigator, or community health worker. Outpatient services are tailored to a meet the patient's specific needs. The plan should carefully document and assign action items, and the team should revisit the case to make sure all items have been executed. At follow-up, the plan can be amended to address changing needs.

Because of the heterogeneous nature of the patient population, no single template will work for everyone. Care plans are high-effort, high-reward initiatives. Effective teams flexibly select creative yet simple interventions for each patient that address the individual's particular medical and social needs.

Behavioral Health

Since behavioral health patients make up a large segment of the high-utilizer population, special mention is warranted. Each patient should have an identified provider of care and set appointments for follow-up. There should be an agreement that if the patient arrives to the ED during office/clinic hours, the patient can be sent directly to the clinic after receiving a medical screening in the ED. When possible, a peer navigator should help connect the patient to community and health-care resources. Each plan should incorporate the following:

- Behavioral and emotional cues that the patient identifies to prevent an unnecessary revisit
- A review of the patient's coping strategies while in the ED

- Assessment of the living situation with a specific emphasis on the type of housing (If the patient lives in a shelter, the plan should discuss and incorporate its hours of operation and alternatives when the shelter is closed. Specific contact information for caregivers, if applicable, should be included.)
- Transportation availability
- Collateral contacts (e.g., family or friends) who can be contacted
- Medical issues and medications

Documentation: Centralized, Actionable, and Relevant

After developing a care plan, the team should decide on a naming convention and centralized location in the electronic medical record that is easily accessible. Housing the care plans under common names allows the coordination of plans and accessibility for all providers caring for the patient. Frontline clinicians will not look for difficult-to-access plans.

Care plans must be action oriented and highly relevant. Information that is buried or exists in a narrative format is less likely to be found or followed. Bullet pointed, succinct, and sequential recommendations that have clear relevance to clinicians are more easily seen, understood, and followed. Effective constructed plans help guide and advance the patient's care plan and reduce the cognitive burden on providers.

Health Information Exchange

Well-designed health information exchange (HIE) systems enable providers to share patient information across the spectrum of care delivery and outside the facility footprint. Continuity of care for patients can reduce unnecessary testing and the length of stay and provide an avenue for analyzing visit patterns across multiple locations. This can often result in increased patient satisfaction. Third-party software programs are available to push out real-time alerts to ED staff when high utilizers register, centrally warehouse care plans, and share interdisciplinary interventions with partner hospitals.

These HIE networks have been required by law in the state of Washington and have been shown to significantly decrease ED utilization. The state reported a 14% reduction in ED visits by super-utilizer patients and a 24% reduction in the number of opioid prescriptions written. These programs are currently being considered by other states, including Oregon and Virginia.[14]

Outcomes

Outcomes for ED high-utilizer programs typically focus on objective measures, such as ED visit frequency and length of service. It is easy to determine cost both per visit and per hour of care delivered. Because of the intensity of efforts, plans should be individualized, as it is impossible to develop plans for large volumes of patients without losing the action-oriented and highly relevant recommendations that make them effective.

Centers for Medicare & Medicaid Services data show that the top 1% of utilizers nationally account for 22% of expenditures in health care. Data for Medicaid patients demonstrate just 5% of beneficiaries account for 54% of total costs.[2] Another study published in the *Annals of Emergency Medicine* in 2011 reports that when 30 high utilizers of the ED were cared for in an appropriate and timely way outside of the ED, the number of visits dropped from 904 in one year to 104 the next year, and costs dropped from $1.2 million to $129,792.[15] Supported by mutiple studies with consistent results, it is clear that a functional high-utilization program can have a positive organizational financial impact.

Case Conclusion: Part 3 of 3

The team creates a plan of care in conjunction with the ED staff, primary care physician, case management, and outpatient pulmonary wellness group. Her chart is flagged electronically so that ED providers are aware of her plan and can consult and proceed with its recommendations. During ED visits, she is rapidly evaluated by her care team, which reports that the plan has greatly reduced the burden of chart review and increased consistency of care. When discharged, the patient is taken (with her permission) to the pulmonary wellness gym, which is staffed by respiratory therapists uniquely suited to teach her how to better self-manage her COPD. Simultaneously, her outpatient social worker increases her telephonic outreach and makes an effort to meet the patient at appointments. She is noted to make friends with other patients and staff and begins to schedule outpatient visits to the pulmonary gym and wellness program. Postintervention, the patient's ED visits drop from 70 visits in one year down to six in the subsequent 12 months.

CONCLUSION

Development of a high-utilizer team with integrated care plans can benefit patients, clinicians, and institutions. This process requires an interdisciplinary and detailed strategy. The variability in the definition of and approach to high utilizers are not indicative of an unsolvable problem; rather, they confirm that no one health system has a "one-size-fits-all" solution. Emergency department leaders must reach beyond their own parochial views and seriously question the specialty's "treat and street" mantra that contributes to repetitive and fragmented care of high utilizers and, more importantly, misses the true underlying reasons for all those visits!

The authors would like to acknowledge Ana Macias, MPH, MLIS, manager of library services for the Kaiser Permanente Library System, for assisting with the literature search

REFERENCES

1. Lin MP. ED-based care coordination reduces costs for frequent ED users. *Am J Manag Care*. 2017;23(12):772–776.
2. Centers for Medicare & Medicaid Services. *Targeting Medicaid Super-Utilizers to Decrease Costs and Improve Quality*. Baltimore, MD: Department of Health & Human Services; 2013.
3. Wu JE. A practical method for predicting frequent use of emergency department care using routinely available electronic registration data. *BMC Emerg Med*. 2016;16:12.
4. Mitchell MS. Cost of health care utilization among homeless frequent emergency department users. *Psychol Serv*. 2017;14(2):193–202.
5. Capp R, Misky GM. Coordination program reduced acute care use and increased primary care visits among frequent emergency care users. *Health Aff*. 2017;36(10):1705–1711.
6. Doupe MB. Frequent users of emergency departments: developing standard definitions and defining prominent risk factors. *Ann Emerg Med*. 2012;60(1):24–32.
7. Kanzaria HK. Persistent frequent emergency department use: core group exhibits extreme levels of use for more than a decade. *Health Aff*. 2017;36(10):1720–1728.
8. Van den Heede K, Van de Voorde C. Interventions to reduce emergency department utilisation: a review of reviews. *Health Policy*. 2016;120(12):1337–1349.
9. Centers for Disease Control and Prevention. Emergency department visits. 2018. National Center for Health Statistics. Available at: https://www.cdc.gov/nchs/fastats/emergency-department.htm. Accessed November 25, 2020.
10. Bonomi AE. Health care utilizationk and costs associated with physical and nonphysical-only intimate partner violence. *Health Serv Res*. 2009;44(3):1052–1067.
11. Center for Health Care Strategies, Inc. Super-utilizer summit: connon themes from innovative complex care management programs. 2013. Center for Health Care Strategies. Available at: https://www.chcs.org/media/FINAL_Super-Utilizer_Report.pdf. Accessed November 25, 2020.
12. Kothari CR. Missed opportunities: emergency department visits by police-identified victims of intimate partner violence. *Ann Emerg Med*. 2006;47(2):190–9.
13. Bryk JF. Improvement in quality metrics by the UPMC enhanced care program: a novel super-utilizer program. *Popul Health Manag*. 2018;21(3):217–221.
14. Anderson S. Emergency department information exchange can help coordinate care for highest utilizers. 2017. ACEP Now. Available at: https://www.acepnow.com/article/emergency-department-information-exchange-can-help-coordinate-care-highest-utilizers/2/. Accessed November 25, 2020.
15. Waller R. Research abstracts: biopsychosocial intervention of high frequency emergency department utilizer. *Ann Emerg Med*. 2011;228.

ADDITIONAL READINGS

1. Seaberg D, Elseroad S. Patient navigation for patients frequently visiting the emergency department: a randomized, controlled trial. *Acad Emerg Med.* 2017;24(11):1327-1333.

2. Frost DW. Using the electronic medical record to identify patients at high risk for frequent emergency department visits and high system costs. *Am J Med.* 2017;130(5):601.e17-601.e22.

3. Gingold DB-M. Impact of the affordable care act medicaid expansion on emergency department high utilizers with ambulatory care sensitive conditions: across-sectional study. *Am J Emerg Med.* 2017;35(5):737-742.

4. Johnson TL. For many patients who use large amounts of health care services, the need is intense yet temporary. *Popul Health.* 2015;34(8):1312-1319.

5. Kimmel HJ. Real-time emergency department electronic notifications regardinghigh-risk patients: a systematic review. *Telemed J E Health.* 2019;25(7):604-618.

6. Lyons TW. Patients visiting multiple emergency departments: patterns, costs, and risk factors. *Acad Emerg Med.* 2017;24(11):1349-1357.

7. Maeng DD. Patterns of multiple emergency department visits: do primary care physicians matter? *Perm J.* 2017;21:16-063.

8. Ondler CH. Resource utilization and health care charges associated with the most frequent ED users. *Am J Emerg Med.* 2014;32(10):1215-1219.

9. Ruger JP. Analysis of costs, length of stay, and utilization of emergency department services by frequent users: implications for health policy. *Acad Emerg Med.* 2004;11(12):1311-1317.

10. Ruger JP. Analysis of costs, length of stay, and utilization of emergency department services by frequent users: implications for health policy. *Acad Emerg Med.* 2004;11(12):1311-1317.

11. Capp R, Misky GM. Coordination program reduced acute care use and increased primary care visits among frequent emergency care users. *Health Aff.* 2017;36(10):1705-1711.

12. Duseja RB. Revisit rates and associated costs after an emergency department encounter. *Ann Intern Med.* 2015;162(11):750-758.

13. Herring AA. High-intensity emergency department visits increased in California, 2002-09. *Health Aff.* 2013;32(10):1811-1819.

14. Kanzaria HK. Persistent frequent emergency department use: core group exhibits extreme levels of use for more than a decade. *Health Aff.* 2017;36(10):1720-1728.

15. Lam CN. Increased 30-day emergency department revisits among homeless patients with mental health conditions. *West J Emerg Med.* 2016;17(5):607-6012.

16. O'Keeffe CM. Characterising non-urgent users of the emergency department (ED): a retrospective analysis of routine ED data. *PLoS One.* 2018;13(2):e0192855.

17. Ronksley PE. Variations in resource intensity and cost amonghigh users of the emergency department. *Acad Emerg Med.* 2016;23(6):722-30.

18. Ruger JP. Analysis of costs, length of stay, and utilization of emergency department services by frequent users: implications for health policy. *Acad Emerg Med.* 2004;11(12):1311-1317.

19. Solberg RG. The prehospital and hospital costs of emergency care for frequent ED patients. *Am J Emerg Med.* 2016;34(3):459-463.

20. Tadros AL. A 5-year comparison of ED visits by homeless and nonhomeless patients. *Am J Emerg Med.* 2016;34(5):805-808.

CHAPTER 46

INNOVATIVE STRATEGIES TO ENHANCE FLOW

Thom A. Mayer, Kirk Jensen

Health care is in the midst of "cataclysmic" change. Yet, change is *always* cataclysmic to those being asked to change. Shifts in a staff's workplace, resources, metrics, and daily processes can cause serious turbulence, particularly in a service-oriented business with scientifically measurable outcomes. Adding the need to "do more with less," as the Institute for Healthcare noted in defining patient flow, creates a harsh prescription for those who are actually involved in beside care, unless the right tools are available. One of those tools is the ability to hardwire hospital-wide flow.[1]

Becoming high-quality, low-cost providers of care is a constant challenge for all health-care leaders and managers. In fact, the dissonance between their perception of the *resources available to them* and the *metrics expected of them* is a primary cause of burnout.[2] Hospital performance expert Paul Batalden summarizes health care's current dilemma (adapting the thoughts of Arthur Jones) this way[3]:

Every system is perfectly designed to get precisely the results it gets.

Is the emergency department (ED) achieving targeted results in for turnover rates, patient experience scores, patient safety markers, clinical guideline compliance, and so on? If so, a great system has been "perfectly designed" to get those results. For most, however, there is a substantial divide between target metrics, current performance, and deployment of the resources requisite to obtain that performance. Batalden's fundamental insight is that the very nature and fabric of the system itself (not just the system's components) must change if different results are to be expected. The sad fact is, however, that too few health-care leaders and managers are ready to completely change the processes by which care is provided to get the better results to which all aspire.

One reason for that dilemma is that health care is extremely complicated. Indeed, no less a leader than Peter Drucker notes, "The hospital is altogether the most complex human organization ever devised."[4] Although he was clearly correct, consider this: To an observer, US Navy and Marine operations off the flight decks of nuclear aircraft carriers involve a dizzying, complex, and confusing array of personnel and aircraft movements. But, closer examination reveals that those operations are subject to detailed, highly consistent processes provided by a cascade of people with disparate levels of education and training; yet, all of variables result in predictably safe and efficient flights.[5] Perhaps health care is not so unique when it comes to the complexity of operations provided by those with varying educational backgrounds.

DEFINING PATIENT FLOW AND INNOVATION

Innovation is an area of considerable focus for health-care systems across the country, including some of the highest-ranking ones such as Duke, IFMC, WellStar, The Cleveland

Clinic, Harvard, and Johns Hopkins. Innovation is necessitated by the need to fix systems that are broken or are failing to meet performance objectives.

Innovation

A simple definition of *innovation* is "a new idea, process, device, or method." When used in the current health-care environment, innovation is often viewed as the application of better solutions to meet new requirements, unarticulated needs, and a dramatically changing environment in which there are multiple moving targets.

In this sense, innovation has less to do with changes *within* a system and more to do with the much more difficult and challenging changes *of* the system. If fundamental changes to the system itself are required to obtain improved results, then innovation requires the ability to tolerate risk—in this case, the very real risk of failure. Unless innovation teams have a tolerance for failure, they probably aren't really innovating. Instead, they may be adopting "best practices" at a slightly earlier time and a slightly faster rate than the competition. That may result in small improvements in metrics, but this approach usually lacks the imprimatur of true innovation.

Armed with a healthy tolerance for failure, what is a failure rate that results in meaningful innovation but does not entail the futility of too much failure? Experience with hundreds of EDs in numerous health-care systems indicates that failure rates of 25% to 30% are probably necessary to result in meaningful innovations capable of driving dramatic improvement. (Chapter 3 is devoted to a more detailed discussion of change and innovation.)

Flow

Patient flow in health care can be defined as "adding value and eliminating waste in processes, services, or behaviors by increasing benefits and decreasing burdens of moving patients through our service transitions and queues."[6] This definition of patient flow is applied in the Lean management philosophy that originally evolved from Japanese manufacturing systems. (In a Lean system, everything that does not add value is considered waste and is stripped away from the process.) Indeed, while some organizations have a deep commitment to Lean concepts, formal Lean training is not necessary to use this practical definition of flow.

However, "value" in health care requires a more practical definition than the one traditionally assigned—one that can be used by bedside clinicians to make decisions based on their assessment of value. In most formulations, value is defined as a ratio of outcomes divided by the cost to attain those outcomes: (value=outcomes/cost). The literature on defining health-care outcomes is increasingly helpful in setting metrics around desired states, although it is still very much in evolution. "Cost" remains a troublesome and vague concept to most clinicians—it works on the macroeconomic level of health care but offers less utility for most clinicians. For example, what is the *cost* of obtaining an MRI scan for a patient? When we have asked physicians and nurses that question, the responses varied from, "I don't know—I never thought about that," to "Several thousand dollars." However, the latter answer isn't really the *cost* of one additional MRI scan, it's the *charge*, including both the facility fee and the professional fee component. The actual marginal cost of an MRI, once the scanner has been purchased and is operational and the radiologist is there to interpret it, is substantially lower than most appreciate. Unless and until we can reliably determine true costs versus charges,

FIGURE 46.1 ■ Defining Value

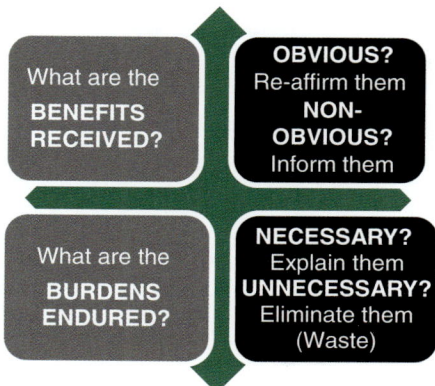

any formulation of value as a ratio of outcomes divided by costs is incomplete and misleading.

For that reason, value in the flow equation is defined as a ratio of *benefits received versus the burdens endured* in the process of receiving those benefits. This concept drives value to the bedside in a way clinicians can understand and substantially affect (**Figure 46.1**). Defining flow in this way helps ED leaders, managers, and bedside clinicians understand that they are "flow detectives" in search of ways to increase value while also identifying and eliminating waste. Empowering staff to add value and cut waste results in a much broader and more enthusiastic acceptance of flow.

Using this practical definition of value and waste helps the team understand that there are six "rights" that comprise effective flow:

- The right **resources** (cost-effectiveness) for . . .
- The right **patient** in the . . .
- Right **environment** (bed) for . . .
- The right **reasons** (evidence-based) at . . .
- The right **time** (flow metrics) . . .
- **Every time** (reliability and consistency)

Why Improve Flow?

Communicating to the health-care team the reasons for moving to flow-based processes requires two fundamental insights. First, changing systems and processes requires the input of those actually providing the service; their voice must be heard at every stage of the redesign. As the saying goes, "If they're not with you on the takeoff, they won't be with you on the landing." Flow initiatives that don't include the active input of the staff simply will not work in either the short or the long term. Conversely, if people feel they have been the authors of redesigned processes and systems, they are far more enthusiastic. Most people don't mind change, they mind *being changed*.[8]

Intrinsic motivation is a far better catalyst for change than extrinsic drivers.[9] Certainly, the team needs to understand the realities of our changing health-care environment, particularly as the move from volume-based to value-based reimbursement systems continues. It will be the job of leaders and managers to make that clear. But, it is also important that staff realize that the way they're working isn't working well for the ED team or their patients.

TABLE 46.1 ■ Flow: a Case Study

ED Patients	Results
40,000 ED visits × 1 hour reduction in length of stay	40,000 hours of increased ED capacity/year
40,000 hours of increased ED capacity/2 hours per ED visit	20,000 potential new visits per year
20,000 new ED visits × $100/visit in physician revenue ($150-$200/visit?)	$200,000 new revenue for the group
20,000 new ED visits at $400/visit for the hospital	$800,000 new revenue per year for the hospital
New hospital admissions at $3,000-$7,500 per admission	1 more admission per day (365 × $3,000-$7,500/patient admission = $1,095,000-$2,737,500 year)

Start with the refreshing insight that choosing to change systems, processes, and behaviors provides ways that are better for both the patients and the ED team. The benefits include:

- Improved financial return by increasing capacity
- Shortened time intervals by eliminating waste
- Identification and removal of bottlenecks
- Improved patient and clinician experience
- Increased safety by reducing non-value-added variation
- Improved clinical outcomes and reliability
- Reduced costs by decreasing non-value-added steps

Although improving patient flow is better for the hospital as a business (**Table 46.1**), it is also beneficial to patients and employees because it creates additional capacity while making patient care easier.

KEY FLOW TOOLS AND INSIGHTS

Demand-Capacity Management

In a capacity-constrained environment, ED leaders and managers must utilize the concept of demand–capacity management (DCM), which focuses on five core questions:

- Who's coming?
- When are they coming?
- What are they going to need?
- Will we have it?
- What will we do if we don't?

The answers to each of these questions should be based not on opinion or personal experience but on data dashboards that are rigorously collected and analyzed over time. The answer to "Who's coming?" clarifies how many patients should reasonably be expected to arrive on each clinical unit or entity, based on historical data and trends. "When" tells the team the times of day and days of the week that these patients should be expected. "What" tells us their specific acuity needs, again based on historical data.

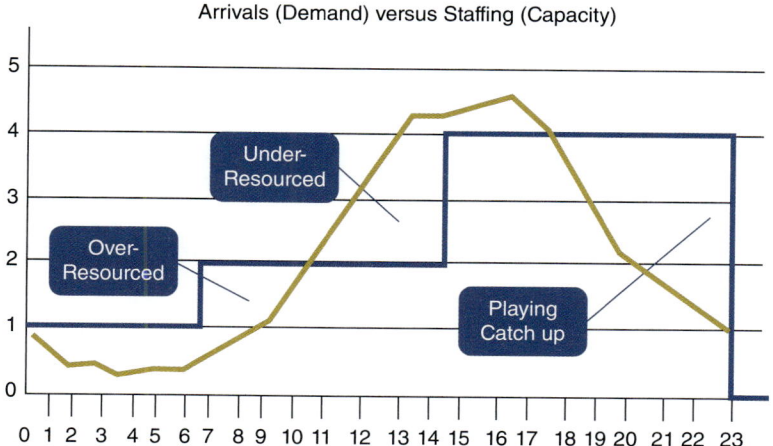

FIGURE 46.2 ■ **Demand-Capacity Management**

For example, if a hospital's cardiothoracic surgeons all have their "block time" on Monday and Tuesday, the ICUs can reliably predict their staffing needs will be high from Monday afternoon through at least Wednesday, and the ED can expect delays in obtaining beds during those times. "Will we have it?" recognizes that using data to predict capacity is a fundamental skill for success in health care. At times, the ED's capacity will be simply insufficient. Examples include patients boarding in the ED instead of being admitted to the hospital, closing beds due to nursing shortages, inadequate behavioral health resources, and long delays for outpatient appointments. Finally, "What will we do if we don't?" recognizes that when demand exceeds capacity, it's important to develop contingency or surge plans for the demand–capacity mismatch; otherwise, patients will face delays and, potentially, poor outcomes and safety issues.

Figure 46.2 shows graphically what many of your clinicians have experienced: Understaffing produces underresourced units that will eventually have to "play catch-up" with patient arrivals and acuity. These basic (but often ignored) insights should be augmented by the use of information technology (IT) systems that not only graphically illustrate these concepts but also guide efforts to change staffing to adjust for DCM mismatches. As **Figure 46.3** shows, using DCM tools can help shift rather than increase staffing to more appropriately meet demand issues. Sophisticated IT departments should be able to develop similar DCM tools.

"Pull" vs "Push" Systems

Understanding the difference between the classic "push" system seen in most hospitals and a "pull" system is an important aspect of hardwiring flow. Most hospitals have functioned in a "push" system, where the unit wanting to transfer or admit a patient has the responsibility to push as hard as possible to move the patient to the next phase of care. This is in sharp contrast to a "pull" system, which is designed to motivate the entire inpatient team to proactively "pull" patients onto the unit they serve whenever they have capacity. This is a key flow insight, since it relies on the intelligent use of health care's most important resource: the hospital bed (see below).

How can it be determined if a hospital is a "push" versus a "pull" system? One of the best diagnostics is to monitor the words and actions of the staff.

FIGURE 46.3 ■ Demand-Capacity Tools

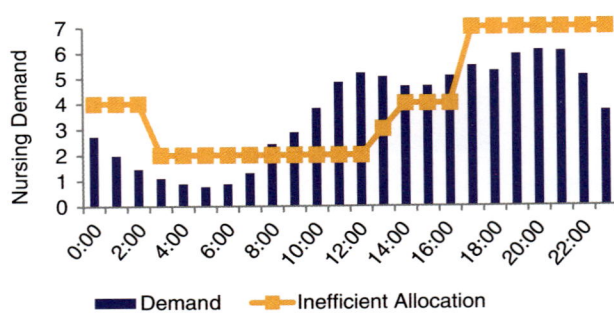

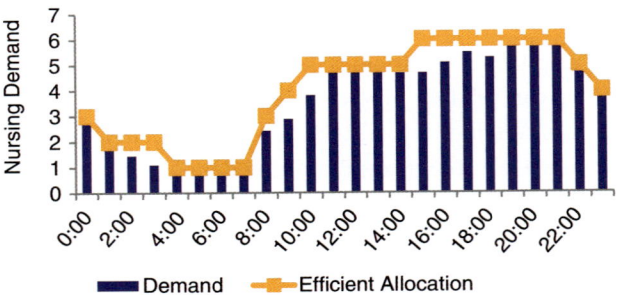

"Push" Systems Language

- Do you have a bed?
- Can you take a patient?
- We have six boarders. Can you help us?
- We're on rounds. We can't talk right now.
- This is not a good time for us to take a patient.

"Pull" Systems Language

- I looked at the bed board and saw you have 10 boarders in the ED. We can take two, one now and one in 20 minutes.
- What can we do to help?
- We won't have an ICU bed for another hour, but I'll send a nurse down now to help out.
- We're on rounds, but I'll have a nurse break out to take report and get that patient up here ASAP.
- We have three beds open in Cardiac Short Stay. Do you have any ED patients who are likely to be coming to us? We can take them now.

Leaders who are committed to flow should ensure that the cultures of the hospital and each of its units are based on a "pull" ("We have capacity. Give us patients.") versus a "push" philosophy ("What do I have to do to get someone to take a patient?").

Theory of Constraints and Bottlenecks

One of the most fundamental concepts in chemistry is that of the "rate-limiting step," which is the phase of a chemical reaction that occurs most slowly and therefore limits the speed of the reaction as a whole. Similarly, bottlenecks and constraints exist throughout health care as rate-limiting steps to flow. It is up to ED leaders to identify and eliminate them.

Several fundamental aspects include:

- Constraints limit performance.
- Focusing on the elimination of constraints improves performance.
- In health care, capacity cannot be stored, but it can be intelligently managed.
- An hour lost at the bottleneck is an hour lost to the whole system.
- An hour saved at a nonbottleneck is of no benefit for the system or the patient.

A simple definition is that a constraint or bottleneck is *anything that significantly limits the performance of an organization or process in moving toward its goal*. Constraints fall into two categories: a weakness in the system or a scarce resource. A physician or lab technician who performs a certain service may be the only one available to do so, which can easily become a constraint on the system.

The *theory of constraints* is a management philosophy that focuses on eliminating bottlenecks to improve the fluid flow of products or services. Management guru Eliyahu Goldratt uses a chain analysis: a focus on "chain strength" that strengthens the weakest link (i.e., the constraint).[9] The journey of a patient into, through, and out of the hospital is actually a journey through a network of queues, each with its own set of bottlenecks. Here are succinct definitions to distinguish between bottlenecks and nonbottlenecks:

- A bottleneck is any resource whose capacity is equal to or less than the demand placed upon it.
- A nonbottleneck is any resource whose capacity is greater than the demand placed upon it.
- The capacity of the system is thus the capacity of the bottleneck: The slowest process or resource ("rate-limiting") in the service chain governs throughput. Remember that patient care comprises a network of queues and service transitions. A related implication is that you can reduce the time spent at the nonbottleneck but not reduce time spent within the overall system.

The following five sequential steps may help eliminate bottlenecks and constraints while addressing the need for change:

1. *Identify the system constraint/bottleneck*: The key here is to identify the part of the system that constitutes the weakest link. Start by looking at the processes that have the highest utilization and those that take the longest time to complete. If you are unsure what these are, draw a value stream map to help identify the bottleneck.
2. *Exploit the constraint*: Make every effort to improve a process before adding new resources or making expensive changes. This is accomplished by reducing variations and eliminating waste.
3. *Subordinate everything else*: Managers should focus their efforts on improving the bottleneck. Remember, improving a *nonbottleneck* is a mirage. Align every other part of the system to alleviate the constraints even if this reduces the efficiency of nonconstraint resources: standard work, support, process buffers.
4. *Elevate the constraint*: If we are unable to eliminate the constraint with steps 2 and 3, then we must consider adding resources or reinventing the process. If not, this constraint will continue to limit system performance.
5. *Repeat Step 1, but beware of inertia*: Managing constraints is an *iterative process*, since once you "break" a bottleneck/constraint, another step in the process will become the new bottleneck/constraint, and so on. Inertia occurs because we get frustrated by the fact that changes made at one step often affect another step,

creating another bottleneck to fix, which may cause us to give up on this seemingly endless effort and just let things lapse back to the way they were. The challenge is to never get complacent and to recognize that improving any system is a continuous but rewarding process.

Who Are the Hospital MVPs?

It's a provocative question, isn't it? Are the most valuable players (MVPs) the doctors? The nurses? The essential services support staff? Of course, someone might appropriately claim, "It's the entire *team!*" While that insight is accurate, we have a slightly different answer. It turns out that the "who" is actually a "what." Consider the highly successful restaurant chain, The Cheesecake Factory.[9] How are they able to deliver high-quality, attractive meals in the right quantity so consistently that customers literally wait for hours to eat there? There are a number of important answers to that question, but one of the most critical is that the core of their ability to serve customers is . . . the table.[10] The faster they are able to turn tables (consistent with delivering quality food and service), the more customers they can accommodate and the more revenue they generate.

What's the health-care analogy? "Table turns" in health care are dependent upon . . . beds. *Beds are the MVPs of our system.* In a system where doing more with less is a necessity, it is not just the number of beds that is important but also the intelligent use and deployment of those beds to add value and reduce waste. The ability to deliver effective "bed turns" depends on many factors, some seemingly beyond our control, but others quite amenable to modulation. First, at the heart of the effort is a fundamental understanding that, for most health-care systems, the bed is a potential bottleneck. For example, hospital boarders in the ED pose clear constraints that affect the patient experience, outcomes, and safety. Beds are perhaps our most capacity-constrained resource (we seemingly can't build them fast enough, and the transition to value-based as opposed to volume-based reimbursement will change the fundamental fabric of reimbursement.)

These challenges drive the hospital to encourage a better and more strategic use of beds. Many hospitals have developed "Everyone out by 11 am" programs to facilitate early discharges to create additional capacity for incoming patients, whether from the ED, operating rooms (ORs), ICUs, or transfer facilities.[11] Some of these programs have been highly successful, while others have not.

The Science of Service Operations: Hardwiring Tactics

Patient flow requires a disciplined approach through the following steps:

1. Use the demand–capacity questions to gain a fundamental understanding of patient demand and the department's capacity to meet those demands.
2. Commit to the right staffing mix, the right staff, and the right number of staff to meet expected demands.
3. Make sure patient intake (e.g., triage in the ED) enhances flow by adding value and eliminating waste.
4. Develop a consistent and reliable system to segment patient flow into value streams designed to meet their needs.
    - Keep vertical patients vertical and moving.
    - Vertical patients value speed; horizontal patients value beds.
5. Match service delivery options to incoming patient streams.
    - Remove all work that does not add value.
    - Ensure that physicians, nurses, and advanced practice providers (APPs) work at the top of their licensed skills.

ACCELERATING FLOW

Figure 46.4 lists the best strategies for ensuring that input to the hospital admission process is guided by flow principles.

Early Decision to Admit

Data from the Emergency Department Benchmarking Alliance, which represents over 40% of all ED visits, show between 12% and 35% of ED patients will be admitted to the hospital, with the higher levels occurring in high-volume EDs and trauma centers. Even in lower-volume departments, ED admissions contribute 60% to 80% of total hospital admissions, indicating they are an important source of potential flow improvements.[11]

In most cases, an experienced emergency physician-nurse team knows immediately whether a patient will need admission based on their initial assessment. Yet, instead of calling immediately for inpatient bed placement, most ED teams are forced to wait until lab and imaging studies are complete. This is a classic example of sequential instead of parallel processing and is an enemy of smooth flow. To be sure, diagnostic testing is sometimes necessary to determine the type of bed that is required. That said, in the majority of cases, diagnostic testing and the patients' progression *confirm* rather than *determine* the need for admission.

Simply stated, delaying admission until every lab test and x-ray is back is an unrealistic expectation in hospitals committed to patient flow. Yet, early consultation is often resisted, usually because it is perceived as disruptive to the flow of the admitting team: "We're on rounds–we can't be bothered with *more patients*!" However, if there is no resistance to change, there is probably no meaningful change involved. Fundamentally, an early decision to admit

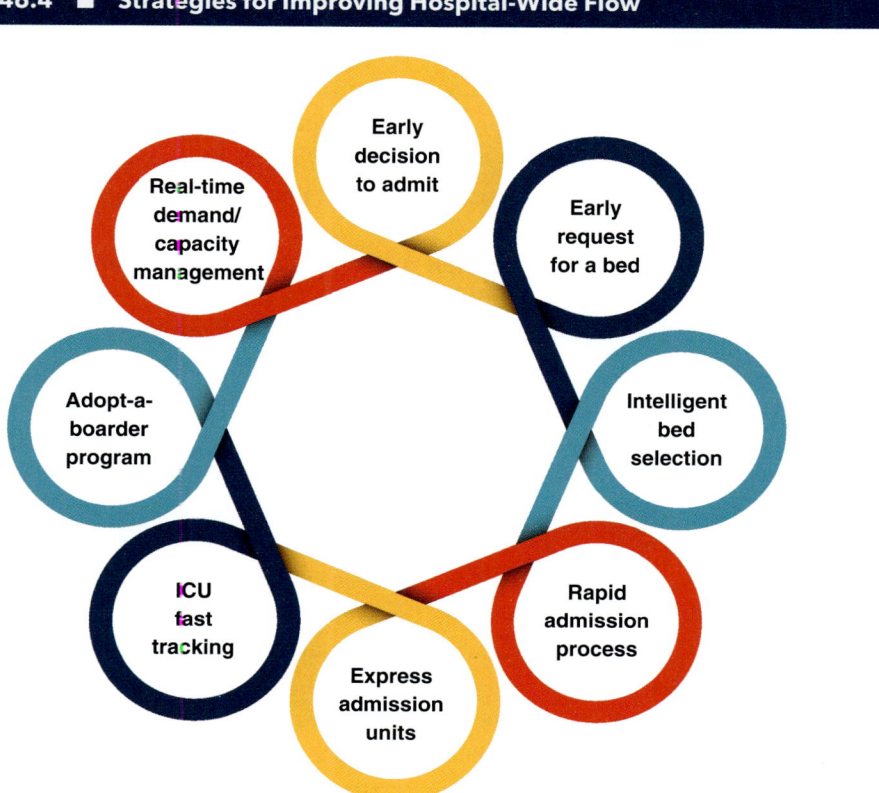

FIGURE 46.4 ■ Strategies for Improving Hospital-Wide Flow

is another example of the "rights" discussed previously: right resources, right patient, right bed, right reasons, right time, every time.

Intelligent Bed Management

As important as it is to obtain a bed for a patient in the timeliest manner possible, it is also important to select the "right" bed for your patients. This is an example of segmenting patients into the "right" value stream for their clinical demands. Intelligent bed management uses both real-time and historical data to determine where the patients' needs can best be met. These decisions should be guided by a *written agreement* between nurses and physicians and should include key factors such as telemetry, isolation, vasoactive drip, and other resources. There are both process goals and outcomes goals to intelligent bed management programs:

Process Goals

- Adding accuracy
- Improving cooperation and teamwork
- Reducing variation

Outcomes Goals

- Efficiently and effectively place the patient in the right nursing unit, capable of the right skills, with the right staffing.
- Facilitate the acceptance of the patient by that nursing unit ("pull vs push").

Of course, there are caveats to intelligent bed management, including the fact that admitting physician preferences will need to be taken into consideration. In addition, this approach requires a multidisciplinary team to develop, implement, and improve the system and an agreement negotiated in the spirit of diplomacy in the best interests of the patient.

Express Admitting Units and ED Holding Areas

For hospitals whose data predictably show delays in bed placement (usually those with more than 10 hospital boarders per day), one strategy is the creation of express admitting units (EAUs), also known as ED holding areas. We recommend the term EAU because it more accurately describes the unit's purpose; furthermore, the term "holding area" has a negative connotation for patients and staff alike.

The purpose of an EAU is to decompress the boarder burden before "gridlock" ensues. EAUs are intended to provide stable patients with a pleasant waiting area while their laboratory, imaging, and clinical assessments determine their precise and appropriate bed placement. Patients should have time-limited transition orders in place, most of which can be predetermined based on the most common clinical problems admitted to the unit.

These units can be located anywhere within the hospital, but the most efficient ones are physically contiguous to the ED. Most EAUs range from 5 to 15 beds, depending on the number of hospital boarders; however, some very large hospitals with substantial boarding issues have units as large as 25 to 30 beds. Key components of streamlined EAU operations include EAU nurses who are relentless in their pursuit of (1) admitting orders from the inpatient team and fast-tracking the preliminary diagnostic and treatment plan, (2) "bird-dogging" laboratory and imaging results, and (3) informing the admitting teams when they are complete.

EAUs can be a very effective flow strategy for hospitals that have a consistent boarder burden but cannot achieve inpatient bed expansion. Both patient and staff satisfaction are typically high in these units, and inpatient length of stay is usually reduced.

Transition Orders

As patients transition from ED to inpatient care, one important issue is the gap in responsibility and the orders that will guide the patients' care. Transition orders (also known as "GAP," bridge, or holding orders) can significantly decrease the time to admission and ED length of stay while freeing up ED beds for arriving patients. To be clear, transition orders are *not* admitting orders; they simply allow for a transition of care from the ED to the inpatient team, giving that team a specified amount of time to evaluate the patient, develop a treatment strategy, and create a set of orders that reflect that strategy. Transition orders are *time-limited* orders for stable patients that permit them to be safely moved to an inpatient bed or EAU. Transition orders should make clear that the admitting team is responsible for actual admission orders, and the admitting team should be informed of status updates and diagnostic test results.

In the past, considerable resistance arose from some emergency physicians regarding the possibility of increased medicolegal liability in writing such orders. However, both the American College of Emergency Physicians and the American Academy of Emergency Medicine have developed position statements supporting transition orders if they are carefully and thoughtfully developed. Our closed-claims experience from a large emergency physician group is that there is actually more medicolegal risk from boarding patients in the ED than in writing time-limited, focused transition orders.

Adopt-a-Boarder and Full-Capacity Protocols

At some hospitals with persistent and recalcitrant boarding issues, as many as 10 to 20 patients may wait 12 to 24 hours in an ED hallway while awaiting inpatient bed placement. Data from several different centers show that these patients have worse outcomes, longer stays, increased safety issues, and poorer patient experience scores. In response to these issues, two institutions independently developed solutions to this problem. The logic driving these innovations was that, instead of having 10 (or more) patients waiting in the hallways in the ED, why not place one patient each in 10 different inpatient units, diffusing the boarder burden across multiple areas of the hospital?

At Inova Fairfax Medical Campus (IFMC) and Stony Brook University Hospital in New York, these policies were put in place, and other similar programs have been developed at Duke University Medical Center, William Beaumont Army Medical Center, and the University of California-Los Angeles (UCLA). The results have been predictably positive:

- Admitted ED patients very much preferred the inpatient hallway to the ED hallway.
- Adopted boarders felt they got more personal attention and better care in the inpatient hallways than in the ED.
- Nearly all patients stated that they were happy to be closer to their inpatient bed.
- Studies from Stony Brook, IFMC, and UCLA showed that the Adopt-a-Boarder program accelerated bed turnover.
- Many patients who were destined for an inpatient hallway bed instead went straight to their inpatient rooms because beds were cleaned in a fraction of the normal time, probably due to pressure on EVS to assist in getting the patients out of the hallways.

ICU Fast-Tracking

Intensive care unit patients in the ED consume significant nursing and physician resources and divert monitoring and care from other patients in the department. There is also a correlation with the duration of time an ICU patient remains in the ED and subsequent mortality, especially for stays longer than 6 hours.[12] This can cause delays and poor outcomes, since up to 5% to 10% of ED patients are admitted to the ICU. For these and other reasons, several proactive hospitals have developed the concept of "ICU fast-tracking," which recognizes that certain ED patients will undoubtedly be admitted to the ICU and deploys appropriate resources to provide for their needs. The policy indicates that a "critical care alert" can be called for patients who meet any of the following inclusion criteria:

- Sepsis/sepsis syndrome
- Acute respiratory failure requiring mechanical ventilation
- Resuscitation post-arrest
- Unstable hemodynamics requiring vasopressor intervention
- Intracranial hemorrhage with evolving neurological deficits or airway compromise

When it is determined that a patient has met the inclusion criteria, a critical care alert is called; this process drives the following protocol:

- A 30-minute response time (from notification to arrival in ED) is required by the patient's physician or the intensivist.
- The critical care unit will respond within 30 minutes of notification with both a bed assignment and a team for transporting the patient to critical care.
- All immediate diagnostic radiology needs should be completed prior to transport.
- The patient's ED nurse will accompany the team to the critical care unit to provide bedside report.

Such a policy and protocol predictably results in safer, more timely care and, in many cases, decreased length of stay for ICU patients.

Flow, Surgery, and Anesthesia

Our friend and colleague, Eugene Litvak, has written eloquently and persuasively that surgical smoothing is one of the primary keys, if not *the* primary key, to success in improving patient flow for surgical and nonsurgical patients.

The OR has a significant impact on the flow of patients through the hospital.[13,14] The peaks and valleys typically seen in the elective surgery schedule drive corresponding patterns in inpatient census. During the peak days, usually early in the week, these electively scheduled patients fill the inpatient units, which restricts bed availability when urgent or emergent cases present to the ED. These fluctuations in the OR volume and resulting variability in the inpatient census also make it very difficult to provide predictable scheduling for nurses and physicians. Smoothing the flow of elective admissions ensures that separate and adequate capacity is available to meet the demands of elective and urgent/emergent patients even during peak days. It also increases capacity in both the OR and the inpatient areas of the hospital.

The block schedule in the OR is typically based on surgeons' schedules and preferences. Rarely is the schedule based on what happens in the inpatient units of the hospital. Smoothing the elective schedule incorporates the inpatient units into the OR scheduling process by adjusting the block schedule based on utilization and postoperative patient placement. These thoughts should help guide the process.

- There must be give and take by both the hospital and the surgeons in order to make smoothing work. In some cases, surgeons must be willing to change the days of the week or hours that they work. In order to facilitate this, it is imperative that the data around patient placement, patient satisfaction, nursing overtime, and physician office issues be provided to the surgeons being asked to change.

- Results from smoothing the flow of elective admissions and thereby reducing peaks and valleys are compelling. Reducing this fluctuation opens more functional capacity in the OR and in inpatient units.
- Further, with smoothing based on the destination unit of the patient, fewer patients are placed off-service, which leads to a reduction in length of stay. Additionally, placing patients in the appropriate bed and unit improves not only patient satisfaction but also physician satisfaction.

Table 46.2 summarizes many of these concepts into strategies to smooth surgical flow.

ED Flow

Much of the original work on patient flow came from the ED, where processes were ripe for improvement. A brief summary of these improvements is presented here.[15-17] Emergency departments (and health-care systems generically) can be viewed as a series of inputs, throughputs, and outputs. **Figure 46.5** summarizes effective flow strategies for each of these phases.

The "output" strategies have been discussed above in more detail, but a brief summary of the other strategies follows. On "input," value is added by getting the patient and the caregivers (particularly the doctor) together as quickly as possible. Triage bypass/bedside triage does that by taking patients directly to the ED treatment area during hours in which beds are available, considerably improving patient-to-bed and bed-to-provider flow metrics. When all beds are full, the triage nurses are empowered through physician-written standing orders to begin simple treatments and diagnostic testing. In EDs where hospital boarders cause long delays for beds, a team triage and treatment program puts an emergency physician (or an APP) along with a nurse, technician, and registrar in the triage area to initiate (and sometimes complete) treatment. First used at IFMC, such programs have shown dramatic results across patient flow, safety, core measure compliance, and patient experience scores.

In the "throughput" phase, segmenting patient flow into fast tracks, super tracks, and ESI 3 fast tracks can all improve flow and the patient experience. The use of "results waiting

TABLE 46.2 ■ Fundamental Change Concepts for Surgical Smoothing	
Dedicate a room for unscheduled surgeries.	Synchronize case start times.
Develop and enforce scheduling procedures.	Designate "on-call" staff to help alleviate unexpected high-demand situations.
Place cases of unpredictable length in a separate room or schedule them for the end of the day.	Use an RN perioperative facilitator to streamline and manage the room transition process.
Stagger surgery case start times.	Use admission/discharge criteria to ensure appropriate postoperative patient placement.
Standardize room set-up and prepare commonly used drugs, equipment, and supplies ahead of time.	Use an OR cleaning and turnaround strategy.
Complete all preoperative work before the start time.	Use historical data to establish surgical schedules (i.e., case length).

FIGURE 46.5 ■ Flow Cascade

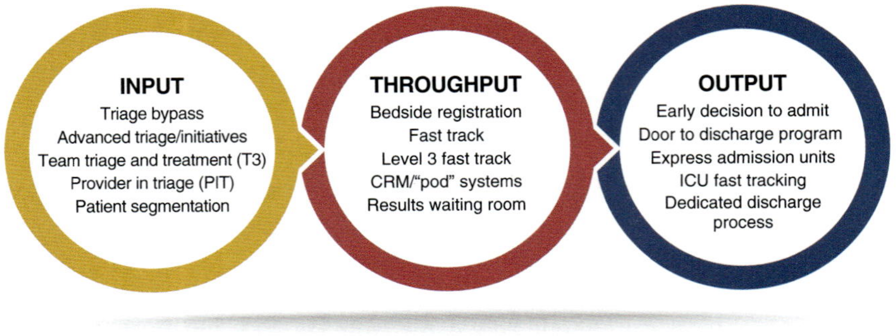

INPUT
Triage bypass
Advanced triage/initiatives
Team triage and treatment (T3)
Provider in triage (PIT)
Patient segmentation

THROUGHPUT
Bedside registration
Fast track
Level 3 fast track
CRM/"pod" systems
Results waiting room

OUTPUT
Early decision to admit
Door to discharge program
Express admission units
ICU fast tracking
Dedicated discharge process

rooms" and "standing EDs" are examples of treating the ED bed as the "MVP of the ED" by having patients occupy beds only as long as it adds value. Afterwards, patients can wait in a designated area, thereby making beds available for other patients.

CONCLUSION

By hardwiring hospital-wide flow and encouraging a healthy spirit of innovation, EDs can deliver high-quality, low-cost care. Involving clinicians in these important process improvements not only makes patients' lives better, it can also make our lives easier. Because improving flow always involves cross-functional work across boundaries, these necessary skills help health-care teams work together for the betterment of everyone involved.

REFERENCES

1. *IHI Innovation Series. Optimizing Patient Flow: Moving Patients Smoothly Through Acute Care Settings*. Boston, Mass: Institute for Healthcare Improvement; 2003. Available at: http://www.ihi.org/resources/Pages/IHIWhitePapers/OptimizingPatientFlowMovingPatientsSmoothlyThroughAcuteCareSettings.aspx. Accessed January 1, 2020.
2. Mayer T. Learning to love the job you have while creating the job you love—burnout and resiliency. The James Mills, Jr Lecture, American College of Emergency Physicians Scientific Assembly, Las Vegas, Nev; 2016.
3. Batalden P. In a speech at Dartmouth College. Available at: http://www.ihi.org/education/ihiopenschool/blogs/_layouts/15/ihi/community/blog/itemview.aspx?List=9f16d15b-5aab-4613-a17a-076c64a9e912&ID=45. Accessed January 1, 2020.
4. Drucker P. *Managing in the Next Society*. New York, NY: St. Martin's Press; 2002:119.
5. Weick KE, Sutcliffe KM. *Managing the Unexpected: Assuring High Performance in an Age of Complexity*. San Francisco, Calif: Jossey-Bass; 2001.
6. Mayer T. Jensen K. *Hardwiring Flow: Systems and Processes for Seamless Patient Care*. Gulf Breeze, Fla: Fire Starter Press; 2009.
7. Nietzsche F. *Basic Writings of Nietzsche*. Kaufmann W, trans, New York, NY: The Modern Library; 2000.
8. Mayer TA, Cates RJ. *Leadership for Great Customer Service: Satisfied Employees, Satisfied Patients*. Chicago, Ill: Health Administration Press; 2014.
9. Goldratt E, Cox J. *The Goal: A Process of Ongoing Improvement*. 3rd ed. New York, NY: Routledge; 2016.
10. Gawande A. Big Med. *New Yorker Magazine*. August 12, 2012. Available at: https://www.newyorker.com/magazine/2012/08/13/big-med. Accessed January 1, 2020.
11. Johnson M, Sensie L, Capasso V. Improving patient flow through a better discharge process. *J Healthc Manag*. 2012;57(2):89-93.
12. Chalfin DB, Trzeciak S, Likourezos A, Baumann BM, Dellinger RP; DELAY-ED Study Group. Impact of delayed transfer of critically ill patients from the emergency department to the intensive care unit. *Crit Care Med*. 2007;35:1477-1483.
13. Emergency Department Benchmarking Alliance. EDBA 2015 Report. 2017. Available at: http://www.edbenchmarking.org/. Accessed January 1, 2020.
14. Litvak E, Fineberg HV. Smoothing the way to safety, high quality, and economy. *N Engl J Med*. 2013;369:1581-1583.
15. Litvak E. Don't get your operation on a Thursday. *Wall Street Journal*. December 2, 2013. Available at: https://www.wsj.com/articles/don8217t-get-your-operation-on-a-thursdaydon8217t-get-your-operation-on-a-thursday-1386024395. Accessed January 1, 2020.
16. Jensen K, Mayer T, eds. Emergency department solutions to flow: fundamental principles. In: *The Patient Flow Advantage: How Hardwiring Hospital-Wide Flow Drives Competitive Performance*. Gulf Breeze, Fla: Fire Starter Press; 2015.
17. Jensen K, Mayer T, eds. Advanced emergency department. In: *The Patient Flow Advantage: How Hardwiring Hospital-Wide Flow Drives Competitive Performance*. Gulf Breeze, Fla: Fire Starter Press; 2015.

OPERATIONS: EMERGENCY DEPARTMENT DIVERSIFICATION

SECTION 4

CHAPTER 47
POISON CENTERS AND MEDICAL TOXICOLOGY

Diane P. Calello, Lewis S. Nelson

Over the last two decades, an increasing number of emergency physicians have developed an area of specialty expertise in medical toxicology. Emergency medicine significantly contributes to the growing subspecialty of medical toxicology, as emergency physicians now account for more than 80% of board-certified medical toxicologists.[1] Emergency physician/medical toxicologists typically divide their time between their practices of emergency medicine and medical toxicology, as the latter has limited opportunities for clinical contact and tends to be poorly reimbursed, particularly given the long-standing trend toward regionalization of poison control centers (discussed later in this chapter). The practice of medical toxicology includes:

- Teaching medical toxicology and related topics (e.g., clinical pharmacology) to medical students, emergency medicine and other (e.g., pediatric, internal medicine) house staff, other health-care professionals (e.g., pharmacists, nurses, paramedics), and through continuing medical education
- Research in medical toxicology, both clinical and basic science
- Medical direction of or consultation for a poison center
- Bedside consultation and/or inpatient medical toxicology service, outpatient/telehealth patient care
- Assistance of or employment within governmental agencies, such as the Centers for Disease Control and Prevention (CDC) and Food and Drug Administration (FDA)
- Consultation regarding forensic and medicolegal issues

Practice diversification into medical toxicology provides an opportunity for the emergency physician to develop a subspecialty niche while continuing to confront the challenges of a diverse emergency medicine practice.

DEVELOPMENT OF POISON CONTROL CENTERS

Poison centers developed in the early 1950s as a means of centralizing information about potentially toxic drugs and chemicals. As the number of available drugs and chemicals multiplied after World War II, individual physicians found it increasingly difficult to keep fully informed on product information and treatment recommendations for the growing number of potentially toxic agents available around the home and workplace.

Simultaneously, household poisoning became increasingly recognized as a problem, especially among young children. A 1952 study showed that potentially poisonous ingestions accounted for more than 50% of childhood accidents.[2] Responding to these developments, the first poison center opened in Chicago, Illinois, in 1953 as a collaborative effort among several local pediatric departments to meet the informational needs of local pediatricians.

Over the next few years, the poison center concept rapidly spread across the United States. These first centers provided toxicity information on drugs and household products and made management recommendations to health-care professionals. The National Clearinghouse for Poison Control Centers, established in 1957, helped standardize poison center informational resources by disseminating 5″ × 8″ index cards containing poison information to the various centers. In turn, the poison centers collected demographic data on toxic exposures that were tabulated by the Clearinghouse. As more centers opened, it became apparent that poison center services were useful to the public, and over time, the public became the most frequent user at many centers.

By 1978, there were 661 poison centers in the United States. Many of these centers consisted of a part-time telephone service located in the back of the emergency department (ED) or pharmacy, often staffed by anyone who was free from other responsibilities.[3] A 1970 survey of those varied poison centers revealed wide disparities in the level of care, documentation, access, utilization, laboratory capability, and public education.[4] In 1978, the American Association of Poison Control Centers (AAPCC) introduced standards of regional poison center designation to upgrade poison center operations and offer a national standard of service. Obtaining this designation required poison centers to be staffed by full-time poison specialists dedicated exclusively to poison center activities 24 hours a day. Such centers were required to have a medical toxicologist as their medical director and to serve a catchment area of between 1 and 10 million people.[5]

In response to these rigorous guidelines for poison centers, a rapid consolidation among centers resulted. By 2002, the entire population of the United States was covered by 64 poison centers certified by the AAPCC.[6] Recently, a combination of federal and state budget shortfalls have led to the closure of several poison centers despite meeting AAPCC criteria. As of 2020, there are 55 poison centers in the United States, serving the 50 states and its territories such as Puerto Rico.

Unfortunately, poison center funding is often threatened in times of economic contraction. A comprehensive report by the Institute of Medicine (IOM) in 2004 weighed the efficacy of several options for the number and distribution of poison centers.[7] They determined that a single national center would:

- Not readily appreciate local epidemiologic variations
- Eliminate the availability of timely local bedside consultation
- Be vulnerable to logistical problems, such as surge capacity, power failures, and natural disaster

A system with one poison center per state would have similar deficiencies in larger states and might be economically inefficient in states with smaller or more rural populations. The IOM report concluded that a system of regional centers would reliably balance local availability of expertise with financial efficiency.

POISON CENTER OPERATIONS

According to the 2018 report by AAPCC, poison centers managed over 2 million exposures a year, and on average poison centers managed 5,723 human exposure cases a day (averaging 104 cases per center). This report estimates that US poison centers experience a new encounter involving human poison exposure every 15 seconds (14 minutes per center).[8]

Contacting a Poison Center

Initially, each center maintained its own phone system, with many using a combination of local and toll-free access to facilitate calling across long distances. In 1999, a national toll-free number (1-800-222-1222) was introduced to standardize access to poison centers and provide complete coverage to the United States.[9] The national number routes callers according to geographic location to the appropriate regional poison center. One unintended consequence of the introduction of portable mobile phone technology is that it is the phone's registered area code, not the current location of use, that determines to which poison center a call is routed. More recently, poison centers have expanded their means of access to include text messaging and social media, such as Facebook and Twitter, and many maintain additional phone numbers for callers wishing to contact a specific center despite geographic location outside of the catchment area and for administrative communication between centers.

Specialist Staffing

During the early years of poison centers, staffing was often provided by personnel with little special training in toxicology. Some of the staff consisted of nurses or pharmacists who were designated to answer the *poison phone* when time permitted them to be away from their primary responsibilities. Other staff may have had no formal health-related education and answered poison calls as part of a telephone crisis hotline.

Professionalization of the staff occurred as part of the growth and development of poison centers. The personnel who currently answer the telephone at poison centers are referred to as specialists in poison information (SPI). Eligible candidates for such a position are required to have a degree in nursing (BSN, NP), pharmacy (RPh or PharmD), or medicine (MD, DO, or be a PA). A 1994 survey of SPIs revealed that 56.3% were nurses, 36.1% were pharmacists, and 7.6% were classified as other.[10]

Newly hired SPIs undergo extensive didactics and closely supervised internship-style training. Since 1983, the AAPCC has offered a credentialing examination for SPI to enhance the rigor and standards of poison centers. Candidates for the certification examination must have handled at least 2,000 poison exposure calls. The average full-time SPI handles 3,500 to 5,000 human exposure calls a year.

Poison centers are operated under the medical direction of a medical toxicologist, who is by definition a physician. The first medical directors were predominantly pediatricians whose emphasis was on unintentional childhood ingestions.[11] Over the years, more emergency physicians have taken leadership roles in poison centers. In 1989, only 30% of medical directors had emergency medicine board certification.[12] As of 2009, emergency physicians account for more than half.[13] Medical directors of regional poison centers spend on average 45% of their professional time allotted to poison center activities.

Poison centers also employ an administrative (managing) director as well as one or more public health educators. Managing directors usually have an advanced degree in pharmacy, pharmacology, or nursing. Their duties typically include budgetary, scheduling, quality, and outreach responsibilities. A rigorous credentialing examination offered by the American Board of Applied Toxicology is available for nonphysician managing directors.

Public health educators who work for poison centers often have an advanced degree in education. The majority of an educator's time is spent away from the poison center, delivering presentations and providing educational materials throughout the region served by the poison center. The purpose of education programs is to prevent poisonings, promote the safe use of medications, and increase public awareness and utilization of poison centers. The challenges include the need to effectively reach people with low health literacy and complicated demographics, such as the aged and non-English speakers, and provide a consistent message using understandable terms and multiple languages.

INFORMATION AND MANAGEMENT GUIDANCE

Daily operations of the poison center include:

- The 24-hour delivery of sophisticated information and current treatment advice to health professionals (physicians, nurses, paramedics, pharmacists, hazardous materials response teams, etc.) and the lay public
- Data collection and public health surveillance
- Professional education and training
- Public education

Telephone calls and other contacts are initially received by the SPI who collects basic demographic and toxic exposure data. For the vast majority of information inquiries, the SPI can adeptly answer the callers' questions.[14] Major advances in the storage and retrieval of poison information permit the poison specialist to have immediate access to data on the vast majority of toxic or potentially toxic products used by physicians and consumers. These include the POISINDEX database (Micromedex, IBM), safety data sheets, toxicology resources in the National Library of Medicine, and a variety of toxicology textbooks and journals.

Poison centers also use a variety of consultants in selective situations such as cases of life-threatening toxicities or when the caller specifically requests a consultant. The primary consultant, who must be continuously available per AAPCC criteria, is the medical toxicologist, who may be the medical director, assistant medical director, or other faculty members associated with the poison center. At poison centers with medical toxicology fellowships, the medical toxicology fellows actively participate in both telephone and, at an affiliated hospital, bedside consultations. Qualified backup for the fellows is always available from medical toxicologists.

Nonmedical consultants include botanists, mycologists, zoologists, herpetologists, entomologists, and marine biologists who may assist in the identification of poisonous fungi, plants, and animals.[15] Close cooperation with local hyperbaric experts may expedite the provision of hyperbaric therapy. Poison centers may also call on other medical specialists such as neurologists, nephrologists, and cardiologists to assist with particularly problematic cases. In cases that involve potential chemical terrorism, bioterrorism, or other public health risks, contact with hazardous materials experts, the CDC, and health departments may also be necessary.

Management Recommendations

One of the most important decisions of the poison center is whether to treat the patient at home or refer them to the hospital. These recommendations are often derived from evidence- or consensus-based guidelines.[16] In 2018, approximately 65% of the calls to the poison center originated in a non-medical facility (usually the home), and 31% of these cases were referred to a health-care facility for management.[9] These statistics have changed in recent years to reflect the increasing complexity of poisoning calls, with more patients managed in health-care facilities. Fortunately, the remainder can be safely treated at home for a nominal societal cost compared with an ED visit. Thus, poison centers have the potential to provide tremendous savings to the health-care system.

Recommendations for patients who are already hospitalized include assisting with differential diagnoses, determining appropriate utilization of tests, analyzing test results, and advising on treatment modalities. Follow-up telephone calls to the home or hospital on all potentially consequential or complicated exposures is another important facet of poison center operations.[17] During follow-up calls, the poison specialist or medical toxicologist seeks to establish whether recommendations have been properly followed, appraises their impact, and/or counsels on appropriate treatment strategies. The hours and days immediately following a poisoning are also the most effective times for patients and families to institute poison prevention strategies.[18]

Data Collection

In addition to providing information to the caller, an important function of the poison center is to collect epidemiologic data on toxic exposures. The National Poison Data System (NPDS), developed by the AAPCC, provides continual updates in near real time and is linked with public health departments and the CDC to provide automated alerts of epidemiological anomalies.

In 2018, 2.5 million calls (including exposures) were reported to the NPDS database from 55 participating poison centers.[9] These included human exposure cases as well as information requests and animal exposures. The collected data provide toxin-specific demographic and morbidity and mortality information. They also provide for surveillance of iatrogenic medication errors[19] and adverse effects from marketed products, drugs, and other chemicals, although these cases are clearly underreported.[20,21] Regulatory agencies and industry use this information to monitor product safety. Public health agencies use these data for toxicosurveillance of potential burgeoning population-based illness through both syndromic analysis and product exposure (e.g., increased cough medication exposure calls portend influenza). Analysis of the database may uncover important new toxicological trends,[21,22] as well as focus preventative and treatment strategies on the more frequently encountered highly toxic problems.[23]

The integrity of the database requires routine reporting of cases encountered by health-care professionals, particularly in the ED setting, where the patient may first be evaluated. A close relationship between the ED and regional poison center is essential to maintain the optimal flow of information between the poison center and the ED reciprocally. Collaborative efforts among emergency medicine colleagues situated in both sites exemplify a team approach to provide optimal patient care. Some states and metropolitan areas have gone so far as to mandate the reporting of poisoning, particularly those involving controlled substances.[24,25]

Education

Poison centers also serve as important educational resources for health professionals and the general public. These agencies offer a unique training environment for the teaching of medical toxicology and related aspects such as clinical pharmacology and substance use to physicians, pharmacists, and nurses, while in school, training, and/or practice.[26-28] The large array of clinical cases, vast informational resources, presence of board-certified medical toxicologists, and ongoing research endeavors offer a rich environment for learning. During such rotations, residents and students usually take part in poison center follow-up calls, supervised handling of poison center calls, didactic conferences, bedside toxicology teaching, and research projects. Poison centers also may offer continuing education programs for local physicians, pharmacists, nurses, and other health professionals.[29] Most fellowship programs in medical toxicology are closely affiliated with a regional poison center.

Public education is another important poison center responsibility. As required by the AAPCC, poison centers employ educators who work extensively with schools, faith-based organizations, and a variety of outreach organizations to address poison prevention issues and orient people to the functions of the poison center. Target groups are those most at risk for unintentional poisoning or who historically have not utilized poison center services: (families with) children younger than 6 years, recent immigrants and refugees, senior citizens, rural communities, and socioeconomic groups with poor access to health care, including individuals who use substances and those with low health literacy.[30-37]

Areas of emphasis include education on the handling and storage of drugs and household chemicals, understanding safety packaging, performing first-aid interventions, and accessing poison prevention services.[38] Close cooperation with the conventional and social media and participation at community health fairs are also important components of public education operations.[39,40] Multiple techniques and formats have demonstrated efficacy, including pamphlets, stickers, magnets, textbook covers, teach-the-teacher programs, advertisements, instructional videos, interactive media, and smartphone apps.[41-44]

POISON CENTER FUNDING

The health burden of poisoning is increasing.[45] In 2008, poisoning surpassed motor vehicle collisions as the most common cause of unintentional death among people 35 to 54 years old and is the most common cause of unintentional death for all ages.[46] Those statistics stand in stark contrast to the funding difficulties poison centers have encountered during the last two decades.[47] Maintaining stable funding resources has been problematic and has contributed to the closure of poison centers that were otherwise delivering state-of-the-art health care.

Funding Sources

Funding sources for poison centers vary considerably among centers. Because poison center services to the public are nonreimbursable, operations tend to rely on a variety of benefactors from both the public and private sectors. Some poison centers received several different sources of funding, including non-Medicaid federal funding; Medicaid support; funding from the state, county, or city government; and private hospital support. Other types of support included donations from corporations (24% of centers), insurers/HMOs (4%), industry contracts (27%), grants (50%), and support from the host institution (50% of centers).[48] One method of estimating the cost-effectiveness of poison centers is to evaluate the cost per call as a metric. This metric is not reported on a national scale due to its subjective nature and reliance on varied health-care delivery models. However, it is clear that calls to poison centers provide savings in terms of reducing unnecessary medical visits and other costs. One study suggested that each call to the poison center could be considered to have saved $175.[49]

State funding mechanisms include state legislative appropriations, state departments of health block grants, excise taxes on residential and business telephone use,[50] and surcharges on ED and/or inpatient admissions at the parent hospital of the poison center. Private funding sources include philanthropic organizations, direct mail solicitation of contributions from poison center users, contractual arrangements with private industry, partnerships with chain drug store corporations, and underwriting by hospitals and universities.[14,51,52] To generate needed revenue, some poison centers have organized affiliate member hospital programs that charge annual fees to member hospitals and fee-for-service to nonmember hospitals for poison services.[53,54] The IOM recommended in 2004 that Congress appropriate $100 million annually to fund the core services provided by US poison centers.[7] As of 2020, the proposed 2021 fiscal budget was $22.8 million.[55]

Decreasing Costs

The rationale to fund poison centers stems, in part, from the poison center's ability to decrease health-care costs by discouraging unnecessary ED visits for unintentional exposures to nontoxic and/or minimally toxic substances.[56] Poison centers routinely advise parents to keep their children at home when the exposure is not thought to be significantly toxic.[16] Nearly 87% of telephone inquiries to the poison center involve nontoxic or minimally toxic exposures.[9]

The SPI is quite adept at supervising basic decontamination strategies or deciding that no treatment is required when the exposure is judged to be minimally toxic over the telephone.

When the poison control center is used for patients with exposures that only require dilution or reassurance, overall medical costs can be decreased by 75% to 80%.[33,57-59] Decreasing unnecessary hospital admissions and unnecessary use of the emergency medical services (EMS) system creates further cost savings. Recent studies from places as dissimilar as New Jersey, Kentucky, and Brazil found that poison center consultation decreased the length of stay for hospitalized poisoned patients by an average of 1 to 3 days.[60-62] A study from Austin, Texas, showed transportation rates decreased to 16% when EMS providers consulted with the poison center for human exposures.[63]

Regional poison centers reduce unnecessary ED visits. A large cross-sectional survey of callers to a single PCC who were managed at home and not referred to a health-care facility found that a substantial portion would have called 911, visited the ED, or called their physician if the PCC was not available. The authors estimate that over the study period 14.4 to 16.8 thousand ED visits were prevented, with a savings of health-care costs between $16.6 and $24.4 million dollars annually.[57]

One of the most informative studies on the cost impact of the poison center was the result of the unfortunate closing of the poison center in Baton Rouge, Louisiana, which served the entire state.[64] The costs for unnecessary outpatient services resulting from *self-referral* to health-care facilities increased significantly after the poison center closed. Self-referral of poison exposure cases to health-care facilities quadrupled during this period. A cost analysis showed that the annual expenditures from unnecessary outpatient usage was estimated to be $1.4 million, more than triple what the state had previously appropriated to the poison center.

Emergency physicians who are involved with a poison center, either as director or consultant, are able to have a significant impact on improving appropriate patient use of the ED. Such physicians bring to the poison center an important perspective on the needs of the department and its patients. Decreasing unnecessary visits to the ED may have a role in:

- Decreasing waiting times in the ED
- Increasing availability of EMS for the transport of truly sick and injured patients
- Increasing the quality of ED care to patients in need of emergency services

Studies in several states have attributed a health-care savings of $7 to $36 for every dollar spent on poison centers.[7,65,66] As noted, the IOM report in 2004 recommended increasing federal funding to $100 million to fully capitalize on the potential savings of poison centers.[7] Unfortunately, ongoing fiscal concerns leaves many poison centers in financial jeopardy.[67,68] State funding, which provides the majority of poison center operating costs in most states, has been similarly curtailed.[69] Thus, poison centers, like many other public health programs during a recession, will have to continue to provide more services with less resources.

DEVELOPMENT OF MEDICAL TOXICOLOGY

Analogous to emergency medicine, medical toxicology is one of medicine's newest subspecialties. The specialty is dedicated to the evaluation and treatment of poisoned and envenomated patients.[70] The core content includes medical expertise in the management of patients with unintentional and intentional overdoses of medication and drugs, substance use and withdrawal, exposure to industrial and other hazardous chemicals, envenomation and natural substance exposures, and public health aspects of substance exposure.[71,72] The first physicians to develop a strong interest in medical toxicology were pediatricians who became active in addressing the problems of childhood poisonings during the 1950s and 1960s, a period that predates the origins of organized emergency medicine. With the development of the specialty of emergency medicine, emergency physicians, including those specializing in pediatric emergency medicine, have played an increasingly visible and important role in the development of medical toxicology. A survey of medical toxicologists revealed that 82% were board certified in emergency medicine, 8% were board certified in pediatrics, and 10% were board certified in preventive medicine.[1]

In 1968, the American Academy of Clinical Toxicology (AACT) was founded by a group of clinical toxicologists to improve the national standard of care of poisoned patients.[73] Clinical toxicologists include both physicians and nonphysicians, such as pharmacists and nurses. Medical toxicology first established itself as a medical subspecialty in 1974 when the AACT established the American Board of Medical Toxicology (ABMT). This board was founded to recognize the physician practitioner of medical toxicology. A certifying examination was implemented, and by 1992, 212 physicians were board certified by the ABMT.[74]

Because the ABMT developed outside the jurisdiction of the American Board of Medical Subspecialties (ABMS), an attempt was made in the early 1990s to obtain formal ABMS recognition for the specialty. Despite the relatively small number of medical toxicologists, the ABMS granted formal subspecialty recognition to medical toxicology in 1992. Medical toxicology board certification is now offered through the Medical Toxicology Sub-board, a joint effort of the American Boards of Emergency Medicine, Pediatrics, and Preventive Medicine. Beginning in late 1994, the sub-board-sponsored certifying examination in medical toxicology was offered to eligible candidates. Those eligible now include only those who complete an Accreditation Council for Graduate Medical Education-accredited fellowship in medical toxicology. The American Board of Emergency Medicine administers the sub-board examination to all candidates, regardless of their primary specialty, and provides certificates for those not primarily board certified in pediatrics or preventive medicine.

Training Programs

As the field of medical toxicology has matured, training programs have developed around the world. Currently, there are 28 fellowship programs in medical toxicology in the United States. The majority of these programs are operated under the auspices of academic departments or divisions of emergency medicine. Board eligibility in a medical specialty is the primary prerequisite, and fellowship programs take a minimum of two years to complete. Although many candidates have trained in emergency medicine, given the broad scope of medical toxicology, graduates of pediatrics, occupational medicine, internal medicine, neurology, psychiatry, pathology, and other residency programs have also engaged in medical toxicology fellowship training.

Scope of Practice

About 79% of medical toxicologists are affiliated with a poison center, and most continued to work primarily in EDs.[1] However, the skill set of a medical toxicologist is highly practical and may be applied over a diverse range of practice settings. A survey of medical toxicologists attempted to better define the scope of practice.[1] According to this survey, the respondents practiced medical toxicology most often in the setting of research, education, and consultation (often via telephone for a poison center). Alternatively, direct patient care was provided more often while practicing their primary specialty. In contrast to most other subspecialties, there are currently few incentives for individual providers to transition completely to a medical toxicology practice. Despite the high value to patients, most outpatient practices are of low volume, inconsistent referral patterns, and often address issues that are not likely to be toxicological in origin. Inpatient consultations, while similarly valuable, often do not integrate well into an emergency physician shift schedule and reimbursement is often poor. These barriers will need to be addressed in order for medical toxicology to develop into a stand-alone subspecialty.

Some medical toxicologists have developed expertise in specific niches, such as snakebite management, hyperbaric medicine, or medical review officer, and others have focused on issues of health-care safety and quality or health policy. There has been widespread adoption of aspects of addiction medicine into the specialty, particularly regarding opioid use disorder and alcohol withdrawal management (see Chapter 60).[75] Furthermore, many medical toxicologists actively assist attorneys and legal authorities in both civil and criminal litigation in addition to regulators and governmental agencies regarding issues that are relevant to the specialty.

POISON CONTROL IN THE ED

Several studies have analyzed interactions between emergency physicians and poison centers. Research shows that emergency physicians frequently called poison centers for:

- Acute symptomatic drug overdose—53%
- Occupational exposure—15%
- Chronic poisoning—13%
- Adverse drug reactions—5%[76]

The most common reasons for calling the poison center include the desire for toxicity information and management recommendations. Thirty-two percent of physicians called the poison center for consultation with a medical toxicologist, whereas less than 10% of physicians called the poison center simply to report a case to the AAPCC database. A Washington State study revealed similar reasons for emergency physicians to call and noted an average of 19 cases reported per emergency physician per year.[77]

Many EDs and hospitals now have access to electronic toxicology resources like POISINDEX. In surveys of these facilities, respondents suggested that direct access to POISINDEX decreased their use of the poison center.[76,78] Additionally, a vast variety of toxicological information is now rapidly available online. Because the poison center may no longer be the primary source of information, even for severely ill patients, there is increasing concern about the validity of the AAPCC database. Health-care providers who choose to rely on POISINDEX or other sources of information may not be privy to important local epidemiological trends that the poison center can provide. A survey study about emergency physician's perceptions of poison centers showed that 78% believe their calls to the poison center contribute to better patient management.[79]

Several studies have suggested that a notable number of in-hospital poisoning deaths were not reported to the poison center.[80,81] In a review of 121 in-hospital poisoning deaths in Rhode Island, only 27% were reported to the poison center.[80] A similar study in California revealed only 4% of medical examiner-determined poisoning deaths were also reported to the poison center.[81] This underuse of the poison center has generated significant concern.[82] Increased emphasis on the other resources of the poison center, including prompt consultation with a medical toxicologist, is required to optimize use of the poison center.

In an attempt to reconcile a modest growth in the number of practicing medical toxicologists and the decreased reporting of poisonings, the American College of Medical Toxicology developed a collaborative registry in 2009. The Toxicology Investigators Consortium (ToxIC) Registry is a growing database of cases treated at the bedside by medical toxicologists. The aggregate data are often more detailed than can be readily gathered by telephone at poison centers and has contributed to both quality research and toxicovigilance.

FUTURE TRENDS

Although the field of medical toxicology has grown significantly in the last few years, the financial stress affecting poison centers has become more acute. Health-care reform, with its emphasis on cost containment, may provide the much-needed long-term financial commitment to poison centers in recognition of their ability to curb unnecessary healthcare expenditures. Managed care providers may recognize that poison centers play a useful *gatekeeper* role by determining when an appropriate need exists for hospital-based medical evaluation of patients with a possible poisoning exposure.[83]

The 2004 report by the IOM discounted the feasibility of a single, national poison center and endorsed the maintenance of the regional system of poison centers. Nevertheless, further consolidation of poison centers is most likely inevitable. Although the presence of 60 regional poison centers had been suggested as an optimal number of centers nationwide,[84] the number of adequately funded centers is already low and ultimately may be considerably lower. These trends suggest that the number of positions for medical toxicologists in poison centers is declining while other opportunities for medical toxicologists, such as direct care of toxicological patients on a fee-for-service basis, are evolving.[53]

There has been inconsistent enthusiasm among medical toxicologists to establish regional toxicology treatment centers in the United States. Such centers have existed in several European cities including Copenhagen, Edinburgh, London, Birmingham, Paris, Brussels, and Marseilles for many years, but have not as of yet established a firm footing in this country.[85] As distinguished from regional poison centers, which offer telephone consultative services, toxicology treatment centers serve as referral centers for patients requiring advanced toxicology evaluation and treatment. The goals of the toxicology treatment center include enhancing the care of poisoned patients, strengthening toxicology training, and facilitating research.[86]

Toxicology treatment centers would be staffed by board-certified medical toxicologists and provide direct inpatient, outpatient, and consultative services. Somewhat akin to trauma centers, the toxicology treatment center requires financial commitments, EMS cooperation to optimize its operations, and a critical mass of appropriate patients and willing clinicians.

CONCLUSION

A career combining medical toxicology and emergency medicine is an exciting vocational alternative for emergency physicians seeking a subspecialty niche. Medical toxicology offers the opportunity to develop an expertise in a well-defined discipline firmly rooted in basic science that has fallen outside the confines of traditional medical specialties. Because the emergency physician is the first to recognize so many toxicological problems, practice diversification into medical toxicology is but a small step. Medical toxicology as a medical subspecialty is still in its infancy. Nurturing by its many different practitioners (including the considerable number of emergency physicians involved in this field) will undoubtedly influence its growth and development in the years ahead.

REFERENCES

1. White SR, Baker B, Baum CR, et al. 2007 survey of medical toxicology practice. *J Med Toxicol*. 2010;6(3):281–285.
2. Crotty JJ, Verhulst HL. Organization and delivery of poison information in the United States. *Pediatr Clin North Am*. 1970;17:741–747.
3. Scherz RG, Robertson WO. The history of poison control centers in the United States. *Clin Toxicol*. 1978;12:291–296.
4. Lovejoy FH Jr, Alpert JJ. A future direction for poison centers. A critique. *Pediatr Clin North Am*. 1970;17(3):747–753.

5. Manoguerra AS, Temple AR. Observations on the current status of poison control centers in the United States. *Emerg Med Clin North Am.* 1983;2:185–197.
6. Watson W, Litovitz T, Rodgers G, et al. 2002 annual report of the American Association of Poison Control Centers Toxicologic Exposure Surveillance System. *Am J Emerg Med.* 2003;21:353–421.
7. Insitute of Medicine Committee on Poison Prevention and Control, Board on Health Promotion and Disease Prevention. *Forging a Poison Prevention and Control System.* Washington, DC: National Academies Press; 2004.
8. Gummin DD, Mowry JB, Spyker DA, et al. 2018 Annual Report of the American Association of Poison Control Centers' National Poison Data System (NPDS): 36th Annual Report. *Clin Toxicol.* 2019;57:1220–1413.
9. Krenzelok EP, Klick RN, Burke TV, Mrvos R. Capitalizing on a current fad to promote poison help: (1-800-222-1222). *Clin Toxicol.* 2007;45:787–790.
10. Mrvos R, dean BS, Krenzelok E, Herrington L. A demographic profile of the specialist in poison information. *Vet Hum Toxicol.* 1994;36(4):330–331.
11. Robertson WO. National organizations and agencies in poison control programs: a commentary. *Clin Toxicol.* 1978;12:297–302.
12. Manoguerra AS. The status of poison control centers in the United States, 1989: a report from the American Association of Poison Control Centers. *Vet Hum Toxicol.* 1991;33:131–150.
13. Litovitz T, Benson BE, Youniss J, Metz E. Determinants of U.S. poison center utilization. *Clin Toxicol.* 2010;48:449–457.
14. Poynton MR, Bennett HK, Ellington L, et al. Specialist discrimination of toxic exposure severity at a poison control center. *Clin Toxicol.* 2009;47:678=682.
15. Chyka PA, Butler AY. Utilization of expert consultants by poison centers in the United States. *Vet Hum Toxicol.* 1995;37:369–370.
16. McGuigan MA. Guideline for the out-of-hospital management of human exposures to minimally toxic substances. *J Toxicol Clin Toxicol.* 2003;41:907–917.
17. Litovitz TL, Elshami JE. Poison center operations: the necessity of follow-up. *Ann Emerg Med.* 1982;11:348–352.
18. Demorest RA, Posner JC, Osterhoudt KC, Henretig FM. Poisoning prevention education during emergency department visits for childhood poisoning. *Pediatr Emerg Care.* 2004;20:281–284.
19. Scalise JA, Harchelroad F, Krenzelok EP. Poison center utilization in nosocomial toxicologic exposures: a prospective study. *Vet Hum Toxicol.* 1989;31:584–587.
20. Chyka PA, McCommon SW. Reporting of adverse drug reactions by poison control centers in the US. *Drug Saf.* 2000;23:87–93.
21. Gryzlak BM, Wallace RB, Zimmerman MB, Nisly NL. National surveillance of herbal dietary supplement exposures: the poison control center experience. *Pharmacoepidemiol Drug Saf.* 2007;16:947–957.
22. Wolkin AF, Patel M, Watson W, Et al. Early detection of illness associated with poisoning of public health significance. *Ann Emerg Med.* 2006;47:170–176.
23. Krenzelok EP, Allswede MP, Mrvos R. The poison center role in biological and chemical terrorism. *Vet Hum Toxicol.* 2000;42:297–300.
24. Cimino JA. New York City's Poison Control Center. *Public Health Rep.* 1968;83(5):396–398.
25. Texas Controlled Substances Act. 1989. Available at: http://www.statutes.legis.state.tx.us/docs/hs/htm/hs.481.htm. Accessed June 17, 2020.
26. Lovejoy FH, Edlin AL, Goldman P. Utilization of the poison center for teaching of clinical toxicology to medical and pharmacy students, housestaff, and health care professionals. *Clin Toxicol.* 1979;15:393–400.
27. Davis CO, Cobaugh DJ, Leahey NF, Wax PM. Toxicology training of paramedic students in the United States. *Am J Emerg Med.* 1999;17(2):138–140.
28. Hantsche CE, Mullins ME, Pledger D, Bexdicek KM. Medical toxicology experience during emergency medicine residency. *Acad Emerg Med.* 2000;7(10):1170.
29. Chafee-Bahamon C. Poisor center outreach to hospitals through area conferences. *Vet Hum Toxicol.* 1985;27(6):481–483.
30. Baraff LJ, Guterman JJ, Bayer MJ. The relationship of poison center contact and injury in children 2 to 6 years old. *Ann Emerg Med.* 1992;21(2):153–157.
31. Vassilev ZP, Shiel M, Lewis MJ, Marcus SM, Robson MJ. Assessment of barriers to utilization of poison centers by Hispanic/Latino populations. *J Toxicol Envircn Health A.* 2006;69(18):1711–1718.
32. Kroner BA, Scott RB, Waring ER, Zanga JR. Poisoning in the elderly: characterization of exposures reported to a poison control center. *J Am Geriatr Soc.* 1993;41(8):842–846.
33. Zaloshnja E, Miller T, Jones P, et al. The potentail impact of poison control centers on rural hospitalization rates for poisoning. *Pediatrics.* 2006;118(5):2094–2100.
34. Belson M, Kieszak S, Watson W, et al. Childhood pesticide exposures on the Texas-Mexico border: clinical manifestations and poison center use. *Am J Public Health.* 2003;93(8):1310–1315.
35. Vassilev ZP, Marcus S, Jennis T, Ruck B, Swenson R, Rego G. Rapid communication: sociodemographic differences between counties with high and low utilization of a regional poison control center. *J Toxicol Environ Health A.* 2003;66(20):1905–1908.
36. Schwartz L, Howland MA, Mercurio-Zappala M, Hoffman RS. The use of focus groups to plan poison prevention education programs for low-income populations. *Health Promot Pract.* 2003;4(3):340–346.
37. Kelly NR, Groff JY. Exploring barriers to utilization of poison centers: a qualitative study of mothers attending an urban Women, Infants, and Children (WIC) clinic. *Pediatrics.* 2000;106:199–204.
38. Spiller HA, Mowry JB. Evaluation of the effect of a public educator on calls and poisonings reported to a regional poison center. *Vet Hum Toxicol.* 2004;46(4):206–208.
39. LoVecchio F, Katz K, Watts D, Pitera A. Media influence on Poison Center call volume after 11 September 2001. *Prehosp Disaster Med.* 2004;19(2):185.
40. Krenzelok EP. The use of poison prevention and education strategies to enhance the awareness of the poison information center and to prevent accidental pediatric poisonings. *J Toxicol Clin Toxicol.* 1995;33:663–667.
41. Krenzelok E, Mrvos R, Mazo E. Combinind primary and secondary poison prevention in one initiative. *Clin Toxicol.* 2008;46(2):101–104.
42. Yudizky M, Grisemer P, Shepherd G, Ray M, Garrison J. Can textbook covers be used to increase poison center utilization? *Vet Hum Toxicol.* 2004;46(5):285–286.
43. Timpe EM, Wuller WR, Karpinski JP. A regional poison prevention education service learning project. *Am J Pharm Educ.* 2008;72(4):87.
44. American Association of Poison Control Centers launches smartphone application to celebrate poison prevention week [press release]. Alexandria VA. March 24 2011.
45. Spiller HA, Singleton MD. Comparison of incidence of hospital utilization for poisoning and other injury types. *Public Health Rep.* 2011;126(1):94–99.
46. Olaisen RH, Rossen LM, Warner M, Anderson RN. Unintentional injury death rates in rural and urban areas: United States, 1999–2017. *NCHS Data Brief No 343.* 2019.
47. Giffin S, Heard SE. Budget cuts and U.S. Poison Centers—regional challenges create a nationwide problem. *Clin Toxicol.* 2009;47(8):790–791.

48. Mrvos R, Dean BS, Krenzelok EP. Poison center funding—who should pay? *J Toxicol Clin Toxicol.* 1994;32(5):503–508.

49. Miller TR, Lestina DC. Costs of poisoning in the United States and savings from poison control centers: a benefit-cost analysis. *Ann Emerg Med.* 1997;29(2):239–245.

50. Bobbink S. Consolidating a poison network via total state funding [abstract]. *Vet Hum Toxicol.* 1993;35:324.

51. Trestrail JH, McCoy FJ. Direct mail solicitation of contributions from poison center users—success or failure?. *Vet Hum Toxicol.* 1985;27:506.

52. Krenzelok EP, Dean BS. A program of poison center services to business and industry. *Vet Hum Toxicol.* 1987;29(2):172–173.

53. Dean BS, Tibbs IS, Krenzelok EP. Toxicology consultation fees to health care facilities: a successful revenue generating program for poison centers. *Vet Hum Toxicol.* 1992;34:166–167.

54. Chafee-Bahamon C, Lovejoy FH. Member hospital network for poison control. *Vet Hum Toxicol.* 1984;26:20–23.

55. Department of Health and Human Services, Health Resources and Services Administration. Fiscal Year 2021. Available at: https://www.hhs.gov/about/budget/index.html. Accessed May 31, 2020.

56. Zaloshnja E, Miller T, Jones P, et al. The impact of poison control centers on poisoning related visits to EDs—United States, 2003. *Am J Emerg Med.* 2008;26(3):310–315.

57. Tak CR, Malheiro MC, Bennett HKW, Crouch BI. The value of a poison control center in preventing unnecessary ED visits and hospital charges: a multi-year analysis. *Am J Emerg Med.* 2017;35(3):438–443.

58. Polivka BJ, Casavant M, Baker SD. Factors associated with healthcare visits by young children for nontoxic poisoning exposures. *J Community Health.* 2010;35(6):572–578.

59. Kearney TE, Olson KR, Bero LA, Heard SE, Blanc PD. Health care cost effects of public use of a regional poison control center. *West J Med.* 1995;162(6):499–504.

60. Galvão TF, Silva MT, Silva CD, et al. Impact of a poison control center on the length of hospital stay of poisoned patients: retrospective cohort. *Sao Paulo Med J.* 2011;129:23–29.

61. Vassilev ZP, Marcus SM. The impact of a poison control center on the length of hospital stay for patients with poisoning. *J Toxicol Environ Health A.* 2007;70(2):107–110.

62. Bunn TL, Slavova S, Spiller HA, Colvin J, Bathke A, Nicholson VJ. The effect of poison control center consultation on accidental poisoning inpatient hospitalizations with preexisting medical conditions. *J Toxicol Environ Health A.* 2008;71(4):283–288.

63. Bier SA, Borys DJ. Emergency medical services' use of poison control centers for unintentional drug ingestions. *Am J Emerg Med.* 2010;28(8):911–914.

64. King WD, Palmisano PA. Poison control centers: can their value be measured? *South Med J.* 1991;84:722–726.

65. LoVecchio F, Curry S, Waszolek K, Klemens J, Hovseth K, Glogan D. Poison control centers decrease emergency healthcare utilization costs. *J Med Toxicol.* 2008;4(4):221–224.

66. Blizzard JC, Michels JE, Richardson WH, Reeder CE, Schulz RM, Holstege CP. Cost benefit analysis of a regional poison center. *Clin Toxicol.* 2008;46(5):450–456.

67. Woolf AD, Karnes DK, Kirrane BM. Preserving the United States' Poison Control System. *Clin Toxicol.* 2011;49:284–286.

68. Poison centers federal appropriations cut by nearly 25 percent in proposed FY 2011 continuing resolution: damaging impact to states' ability to help citizens [press release]. Alexandria VA. April 13 2011.

69. Youniss J, Litovitz T, Villanueva P. Characterization of US poison centers: a 1998 survey conducted by the American Association of Poison Control Centers. *Vet Hum Toxicol.* 2000;42(1):43–53.

70. American College of Medical Toxicology. About Medical Toxicology. Available at: https://www.acmt.net/overview.html. Accessed June 17, 2020.

71. Schier JG, Rubin C, Schwartz MD, et al. Public health partnerships in medical toxicology education and practice. *Am J Prev Med.* 2010;38:667–674.

72. Nelson LS, Baker BA, Osterhoudt KC, Snook CP, Keehbauch JN. The 2012 core content of medical toxicology. *J Med Toxicol.* 2012;8:183–191.

73. Rumack B, Ford P, Sbarbaro J, Bryson P, Winokur M. Regionalization of poison centers: a rational role model. *Clin Toxicol.* 1978;12:367–375.

74. Donovan JW, Goldfrank LR. Medical toxicologist practice characteristics, specialty certifications and manpower needs [abstract]. *Vet Hum Toxicol.* 1992;34:336.

75. Laes JR. The integration of medical toxicology and addiction medicine: a new era in patient care. *J Med Toxicol.* 2016;12:79–81.

76. Caravati EM, McElwee NE. Use of clinical toxicology resources by emergency physicians and its impact on poison control centers. *Ann Emerg Med.* 1991;20:147–150.

77. Robertson WO, Caffrey A. Washington Poison Center as perceived by our state's emergency physicians. *J Med Toxicol.* 2008;4(1):16–17.

78. Wax PM, Rodewald L, Lawrence R. The arrival of emergency department based POISONDEX: perceived impact on poison control center utilization. *Am J Emerg Med.* 1994;12:537–540.

79. Misra S, Haulman J, Robertson WO. Washington ER physicians' perceptions of poison centers. *Vet Hum Toxicol.* 1993;35:164–165.

80. Linakis JG, Frederick KA. Poisoning deaths not reported to the regional poison control center. *Ann Emerg Med.* 1993;22:1822–1828.

81. Blanc PD, Kearney TE, Olson KR. Underreporting of fatal cases to a regional poison control center. *West J Med.* 1995;162(6):505–509.

82. Goldfrank LR. Data, epidemiology, and the future strength of emergency medicine [editorial]. *Ann Emerg Med.* 1993;22:1859–1960.

83. Bonfiglio F, Rainey, Seger D. Health care reform - managed care or managed chaos: what's in store for poison centers? *Vet Hum Toxicol.* 1994;36:354.

84. McIntire MS, Angle CR. Regional poison-control centers improve patient care [editorial]. *N Engl J Med.* 1983;308:219–220.

85. Donovan JW, Martin TG. Regional poison systems - roles and titles [editorial]. *J Toxicol Clin Toxicol.* 1993;31:221–222.

86. American College of Medical Toxicology. Center for Poison Treatment Facility Assessment Guidelines. Available at: https://www.acmt.net/resources_guidelines.html. Accessed June 17, 2020.

PEDIATRIC EMERGENCY MEDICINE: IMPROVING QUALITY AND READINESS

Sujit S. Iyer, Winnie T. Whitaker, Katherine Remick, Thom A. Mayer

CHAPTER 48

Pediatric visits account for approximately 20% of all emergency department (ED) visits in the United States.[1] Although the majority of these patients (83%) are seen in general EDs, approximately 69% of EDs report managing fewer than 15 children per day. Because children account for a relative minority of ED visits, pediatric-specific needs may be easily overlooked. Respiratory diseases, injuries, and poisoning account for nearly 60% of all acute pediatric complaints, followed by nervous system disorders and GI disease—the largest proportion of visits (40%) for children under 5 years of age.[2] The Healthcare Cost and Utilization Project (HCUP) demonstrated that while 96% of pediatric ED visits result in treat-and-release, infants under 1 year of age account for over 20% of admitted pediatric ED patients.[2]

In an attempt to address standards for pediatric emergency care in EDs across the country, the American Academy of Pediatrics (AAP) and the American College of Emergency Physicians (ACEP) issued the *Joint Policy Statement—Guidelines for Care of Children in the Emergency Department* in 2009.[3] In 2013, the national Emergency Medical Services for Children (EMSC) program, in collaboration with AAP, ACEP, and the Emergency Nurses Association (ENA), launched a national assessment to determine the capacity of EDs to care for children.[4] The results of this assessment, based on responses from 4,146 EDs (83%), demonstrated a median weighted pediatric readiness score of 69 based on a 100-point scale. Unfortunately, while 94% of children are within 30 minutes of an ED, only 55% of pediatric patients are within 30 minutes of a *pediatric-ready* ED (90 or higher on a 100-point scale).[5]

PEDIATRIC VERIFICATION PROGRAMS

Pediatric verification programs for hospitals and EDs have been associated with decreased mortality and universally use the 2009 policy statement as an outline to assign pediatric ED verification.[6] The following 11 states now offer pediatric verification/recognition programs: Alaska, Arizona, California, Delaware, Illinois, Montana, New Jersey, Ohio, Tennessee, Utah, and West Virginia. An additional 13 states and the District of Columbia have programs in development, including Colorado, Connecticut, Florida, Indiana, Kansas, Kentucky, Michigan, New Mexico, New York, Oklahoma, Pennsylvania, South Carolina, and Texas. The presence of pediatric verification is associated with a 20-point increase in weighted pediatric readiness scores as well as decreased patient mortality.[7] Additionally, during simulated pediatric resuscitations, providers from pediatric-ready facilities appear to perform at a higher level than those from other EDs.[8,9]

The National Pediatric Readiness Project (NPRP) is an ongoing collaborative effort by the AAP, ACEP, ENA, and the EMSC program. The goal of NPRP is to create and support local, regional, state, and national efforts to improve pediatric emergency care. These efforts are not focused on inpatient, high-cost, or rare resources. Rather, every ED can and should be pediatric ready.

It is important to keep in mind that while some EDs may have low annual volumes of pediatric visits, the public does not necessarily differentiate one department from another. Many rural and low-volume EDs serve as a safety net for their communities. State and national efforts are in place to help support lower-volume sites (see NPRP toolkit in **Appendix 48.2**). Given that most of the lower-volume and rural EDs will transfer pediatric patients to high-resource areas for subspecialty care or inpatient management, comprehensive medical centers and children's hospitals can play a role in both outreach and education.

COMPONENTS OF A PEDIATRIC PROGRAM

Just as there are multiple members of the pediatric emergency medicine (PEM) team, there are also multiple components of any successful PEM program, including leadership, team members, and the systems in which they practice.

Administration and Coordination

Pediatric emergency care coordinators (PECCs) can be physicians or nurse leaders who ensure an ED stands ready to meet the needs of children of all ages. In 2006, the Institute of Medicine (now the National Academy of Medicine) called for PECCs to oversee all aspects of pediatric emergency care (**Box 48.1**).[10] Departments that report the presence of a PECC appear to have higher levels of pediatric readiness.[4]

While PECCs have a strong interest and/or additional training in pediatric emergency care, their responsibilities are more likely to be impactful when administrative time is allotted to this role. Unfortunately, without clear evidence demonstrating the impact of PECCs on pediatric outcomes, hospital administrators and ED leadership may fail to carve out the necessary financial support. High rates of turnover in this position can undermine the success of such programs.

BOX 48.1 ■ RESPONSIBILITIES OF PECCs

Responsibilities:
- Act as liaison to other committees and departments
- Establish pediatric competency training and evaluation for staff
- Oversee clinical quality and performance improvement efforts for children
- Ensure pediatric equipment, supplies, and medications are available and staff are trained on use and location
- Ensure department policies include pediatric-specific elements
- Train staff on pediatric-specific safety measures
- Collaborate with physician or nurse PECC to facilitate efforts

Considered PECC roles for larger EDs:
- Medical community outreach (e.g., EMS agencies, pediatricians)
- Family and community education programs
- Regional disaster planning
- Systems-based quality improvement programs with referring and transferring sites

Another innovative approach to share resources is the establishment of regional networks of pediatric quality improvement (QI). Most recently, the federal EMS for Children program launched the Pediatric Readiness Quality Collaborative (PRQC), a national initiative that includes pediatric champions from 146 EDs across 17 states, representing 5% of annual pediatric ED visits in the United States. Each pediatric champion is paired with a comprehensive regional center or training site to facilitate local QI efforts targeting pediatric readiness and, ultimately, pediatric quality measures. The results from the PRQC may help to support a more permanent presence for PECCs in EDs across the country.

Workforce

The workforce required for a PECC includes physicians, advance practice providers (APPs), nurses, and child life specialists.

Physicians

The type and training of physicians that staff a PEM section will vary per the size of the department and the ability to recruit fellowship-trained pediatric emergency physicians. In lower pediatric volume departments, coverage is often provided solely by general emergency physicians, and the PECC may be the only person with specific training and additional expertise in PEM. In departments with 24-hour pediatric coverage and a large patient volume, the majority of the section members may be trained and certified in PEM. Some centers have hybrid EDs in which the pediatric volumes are sufficient to justify a distinct pediatric presence but insufficient to financially sustain 24-hour coverage with dedicated pediatric providers.

In this model, pediatric specialists cover high-volume times of day, and general emergency physicians cover during off-peak overnight and early-morning hours. As such, it is prudent to allow members of the general emergency physician group who are interested in, committed to, and willing to participate in acute pediatric care to join the section. It is the role of the PECC to ensure that both pediatric and nonpediatric emergency providers are competent in established pediatric treatment protocols and willing to meet the educational, quality, and patient-safety criteria of the section.

Generally, EDs that manage between 15,000 and 24,000 pediatric patients per year can justify a distinct pediatric section. In the absence of a hospital subsidy, 24-hour coverage can occur somewhere between 20,000 and 25,000 pediatric patients per year (with some internal subsidization from the rest of the practice). For EDs that provide focused pediatric coverage, an appropriate staffing pattern can be determined by using arrival and flow data to match department capacity to patient demand. Arrival data for pediatric ED patients typically peak in the afternoon and evening and taper off between midnight and midmorning. These data help determine the hours when dedicated pediatric emergency physicians and other pediatric-trained staff should begin coverage, with additional hours added as patient volume grows. Double coverage during peak evening hours provides better patient care than single around-the-clock coverage.

Advance Practice Providers

It is becoming commonplace to supplement physician coverage in EDs with APPs, such as nurse practitioners and physician assistants. APPs with pediatric training can be invaluable in the pediatric ED. Multiple studies have shown these clinicians to be efficient, cost-effective team members, and when compared to physicians, no significant differences have been found in diagnostic accuracy, recidivism, or the correct interpretation of radiographs.[11,12] All APPs working in the pediatric ED should maintain certification in either the American Hospital Association-AAP Pediatric Advanced Life Support (PALS) course or the ACEP-AAP Advanced

Pediatric Life Support (APLS) course, pursue continuing education in the field of PEM, and participate in mock or simulated resuscitations. The function of APPs in the pediatric ED will likely vary, and their flexibility should be maximized to match the needs of the department.

Since pediatric EDs tend to have a large proportion of lower-acuity visits, one model is to have APPs manage these patients independently to promote throughput. This approach has been shown to reduce lengths of stay and left without being seen rates.[13] For this to be carried out safely, clearly defined criteria for APP consultation with the emergency physician must be established, even for conditions in which autonomous care would normally be expected.

Some EDs utilize APPs much like residents, where APPs work alongside a physician but do not practice independently. Instead, they staff 100% of their patients with the attending physician. One study comparing relative productivity between pods staffed by a pediatric emergency physician and a nurse practitioner versus those staffed with a pediatric emergency physician and a resident found that the nurse practitioner care model had greater productivity, measured by relative value units.[14]

Having a pediatric-trained APP act as the provider-in-triage not only results in a decrease in door-to-provider time, but can also lead to more accurate assignation of patient acuity level and expedited ordering of crucial diagnostic tests and initiation of proper treatments.[15] Compared to a triage nurse with less pediatric experience, the APP may more easily recognize situations such as respiratory distress in an infant with bronchiolitis or the need for an ultrasound to rule out intussusception in a vomiting patient. Analgesics are also given in a more timely manner when an APP is involved in care.[16] When there are no or few children waiting to be triaged, the APP can also quickly evaluate and provide disposition to low-acuity pediatric patients. Concerns about excessive resource utilization by APPs are unfounded; in fact, recent studies have shown that APPs order fewer diagnostic tests than physicians.[17,18]

Nurses

Nursing care rendered to pediatric patients is critical to the success of a dedicated pediatric program. Nurses must be comfortable with the care of children and adept at procedures like inserting peripheral intravenous (IV) lines, drawing blood, and placing urinary catheters, all while having some baseline training in techniques to ease the anxiety and discomfort of children and their families. The nuances of pediatric triage require special attention, as critical presentations unique to pediatrics, such as midgut volvulus, neonatal seizures, sepsis, and decompensated congenital heart disease, can sometimes be subtle. It is vital for all nurses caring for children to be familiar the normal range of vital signs for neonates, infants, toddlers, school-age children, and adolescents, as what is acceptable for one age group can be significantly abnormal for another.

In most cases, nurses spend a great deal more time with individual patients than do emergency physicians. Furthermore, more nursing time is often needed with children than with adults. Nurse staffing patterns must take all of the following factors into account:

- It takes longer to obtain vital signs in an uncooperative child.
- Simple procedures, such as peripheral IV placement or urine acquisition, are usually more difficult to perform in infants and young children.
- It can be challenging to administer oral medications successfully to infants and unwilling children.
- Interaction with and education of parents is a necessity and requires added amounts of clinical time.

Like physicians and APPs, the nursing staff should become PALS-certified, with the hospital financially supporting such efforts. In addition, pediatric nursing courses, such as the Emergency Pediatric Nursing Course sponsored by ENA, can raise the quality of pediatric emergency nursing. The PECC can be a liaison to the pediatric inpatient floors, the pediatric ICU, and the trauma service, where additional resources may be available.

Child Life Specialists

Child life programs are recommended to help enhance the patient experience and quality of pediatric care. Certified child life specialists (CCLSs) are professionals with bachelor's or master's degrees who have undergone a rigorous training process, including college-level coursework in child life, at least 600 hours of a supervised clinical internship, and a certification exam.[19] These professionals relate to children on a developmentally appropriate level and foster trust in the medical team by answering questions, explaining procedures and diagnoses, and using distraction techniques to alleviate anxiety and pain. For example, CCLS involvement with children undergoing laceration repair in the ED has been shown to lessen emotional distress.[20]

The provision of child life services has demonstrated similar improvement in patient experience regarding day surgery, radiology, and other clinical settings.[21-23] According to a 2014 AAP policy statement, the "provision of child life services is a quality benchmark of an integrated patient- and family-centered health-care system, a recommended component of medical education, and an indicator of excellence in pediatric care."[19]

Currently, there are estimated to be more than 400 child life programs in hospitals delivering pediatric care in the United States.[18] The AAP recommends providing one full-time CCLS per every 15 pediatric inpatients in the hospital setting, ideally with child life services available 7 days a week. In hospitals with low pediatric volumes, a single CCLS might be able cover all units, including the ED, inpatient, and outpatient settings. In larger hospitals, more than one CCLS may be needed for each unit to ensure every-day coverage.[19] It has been suggested that child life services can set an ED apart from its competitors and should be considered in departments that see at least 15,000 to 20,000 pediatric patients a year.[24]

QUALITY AND PROCESS IMPROVEMENT

QI and process improvements (PIs) are integral to ensuring pediatric best practices are implemented effectively. A sustainable pediatric QI process in a general ED should be integrated into existing departmental metrics, reliant on evidence and support from local and national organizations, and integrated with efforts of local pediatric hospitals and specialists.[25]

The Donabedian framework of structure/process/outcome measures is a good reference for choosing meaningful metrics that reflect the entire pediatric experience.[26] Examples include pediatric equipment and supply lists (structure), time to treatment for pain with fractures or steroids with asthma (process), and bounce-back or transfer rates for children (outcome). National experts have developed proposed pediatric quality measures that can be used to guide a general ED's focus.[26] Through the nationally funded EMSC program, each state has a dedicated program manager who can be found online to help guide pediatric care improvements and strengthen relationships between tertiary children's hospitals, community EDs, and out-of-hospital emergency services.[27]

Communication with referring pediatric practices as well as regional pediatric centers is an essential part of the quality-assurance process. Most children's hospitals employ coordinators or liaisons who can provide feedback on transferred cases, and all Level I pediatric trauma centers have coordinators and educators dedicated to community outreach and education. As most pediatric patients are discharged home from the ED, a reliable system of communicating with outpatient pediatricians is vital for safe follow-up. Regular chart reviews, annual staff competencies, and on-site education by local pediatric specialty hospitals are all vital parts of ensuring staff knowledge and maintaining quality. On-site education from local pediatric specialists can help supplement mandatory staff competencies in common procedures and conditions, such as sedation, splinting, pain and anxiety control, and lacerations.

Policies and Procedures

In order to ensure that pediatric patients continue to receive the highest standard of care, EDs must adhere to standard policies and procedures. While standard triage policies, provider expectations, and clinical protocols for pediatrics are necessary, there is no need for any department to create them from scratch. Evidence-based clinical decision tools and policies from tertiary children's hospitals exist for every major pediatric condition (see **Appendix 48.2**). It is the general ED's responsibility to ensure that every local policy is reviewed for the inclusion of pediatric-specific needs. Additionally, it may be necessary to develop unique local guidelines for managing certain patient situations, such as an unaccompanied minor, optimization of family-centered care, and recognition and evaluation of child maltreatment. Failure to fully integrate pediatric needs into local policies and procedures increases safety risks and unnecessary variations in care.

For underresourced sites, the presence of interfacility transfer guidelines and agreements are critical to ensure that children have access to the right care at the right time. Based on results from the 2013 NPRP assessment, only 70% of EDs use established interfacility transfer guidelines.[28] Telemedicine can also be used to avoid costly and unnecessary transfers when local resources are unavailable.[29] Lastly, disasters must always be planned for, yet less than 50% of EDs report addressing pediatric-specific needs in their local disaster preparedness plans. Resources are now available online to incorporate pediatric needs into hospital disaster preparedness plans (see **Appendix 48.2**).

Patient Safety

Health-care professionals are arguably at greater risk of making medical errors when caring for pediatric patients; risk factors such as weight-based medication dosing, varied developmental stages, and limited ongoing provider experience may result in delays in treatment or failure to recognize a child at risk. In 2006, the National Academy of Medicine highlighted the following gaps in day-to-day infrastructure that heightened the risk to children:

- Most general EDs and EMS agencies do not require specialized pediatric training for clinical staff.
- Most EDs do not have the full scope of pediatric equipment, medications, and supplies for children.
- A paucity of research exists on best practices, clinical outcomes, and patient safety for children.

The cognitive load associated with estimating pediatric weight, calculating weight-based doses, and converting doses from milligrams to milliliters prior to administration is associated with an increased risk of errors.[30,31] Stressful situations, such as pediatric resuscitations, are further associated with an increase in error that approaches 25%. Standardized dosing order sets and increasing awareness (i.e., time-out) around the administering phase of the medication process may help decrease dosing errors.[32] While an exact scale-based determination of weight is preferred, color-coded medication safety systems can help reduce drug errors in children.[33] Based on the 2013 ED assessment for pediatric readiness, one-third of EDs do not have a standard process to ensure that pediatric patient weights were measured and recorded in kilograms.[28]

Physical Plant

When designing an ED that will contain a specialized pediatric section, it is important to consider several factors. First, the facility should be designed so that high levels of care can be delivered in the most cost-effective manner. It is not necessary to have an independent section to care for pediatric patients, but separating children from adult patients who may become agitated or abusive is of the utmost importance; witnessing a major medical resuscitation can be a traumatic experience for a small child. This separation can be achieved by clustering the pediatric rooms in one area or by using a designated hallway of rooms for children.

Treatment areas should be separated by walls, not curtains, and rooms should be closed off from outside noise and visual stimuli. Vocalizations of fear or crying from a nearby child can easily frighten other children. Further, it is disconcerting for family members waiting outside the treatment area to hear a child crying and feel helpless to comfort them.

Each of the rooms used to treat children requires the supplies necessary to perform routine pediatric examinations (e.g., diapers, child-size gowns, wipes). Rooms used to care for sicker children specifically require airway management supplies and monitoring equipment designed for children. Care should be taken to childproof the room to ensure patient safety; utilize outlet covers when appropriate, and do not keep potentially dangerous medical supplies or equipment in low drawers or shelves. The room should be decorated using bright colors, designs, and pictures to camouflage the sterile, medical look of an examination room.

A major resuscitation room or trauma room should be available and stocked for pediatric use. It can be the same resuscitation room used for adult patients as long as the pediatric equipment is stored separately and is quickly accessible. An important consideration in a pediatric resuscitation is control of the thermal environment. This may entail availability of an overhead warmer or a bank of heating lamps that can be used when a neonate or infant needs to be resuscitated.

Ideally, the ED should also have a children's waiting room that is segregated from the area used by adult patients. The pediatric waiting area should be capable of isolating children from any adult patients who are exhibiting violent behavior, while at the same time allowing parental observation or supervision. The waiting area entrance should include a highly visible, secure vestibule with security cameras when possible. It should also contain children's books, coloring books, and activity blocks so that the children may entertain themselves. It is also advisable for the pediatric waiting area to have its own television for viewing child-appropriate programming. Such a setup may also allow the ED staff to show educational videos about common pediatric problems.

Equipment, Supplies, and Medications

Emergency and resuscitation equipment specifically sized for children must be present, clearly labeled, and easily accessible. It is vital that the pediatric equipment, even if not used on a daily basis, has a prominent place in the ED and can be quickly located; staff anxiety around a pediatric resuscitation can be compounded if critical equipment or supplies are needed and cannot be found. Thoughtful management of storage requires the entire team (particularly the nursing and tech staff) to be aware of and continually monitor equipment location, its working order, and the expiration dates. One staff member should be assigned at the beginning of each shift to check the equipment. All common pediatric supplies, including small ear speculums, formula and oral hydration fluids, small-gauge catheters, and infusion pumps, must be consistently available.

A pediatric crash cart of medications should be available to move to any of the rooms in which a pediatric patient may be seen. The contents of the cart may vary among institutions,

TABLE 48.1 ■ Medications Used in Pediatric Patients in EDs	
• Atropine • Adenosine • Amiodarone • Antiemetic agents • Calcium chloride • Dextrose (D10W, D50W) • Epinephrine (1:1,000, 1:10,000 solutions) • Lidocaine • Magnesium sulfate • Naloxone hydrochloride • Procainamide • Sodium bicarbonate (4.2%, 8.4%) • Topical, oral, and parenteral analgesics • Oral sucrose	• Activated charcoal • Antimicrobial agents (parenteral and oral) • Anticonvulsant agents • Antidotes (common antidotes should be accessible to the ED) • Antipyretic drugs • Bronchodilators • Corticosteroids • Inotropic agents • Neuromuscular blockers • Sedatives • Vaccines • Vasopressor agents

but basic supplies are outlined in **Table 48.1**. Length-based systems (e.g., Broselow tape), medical software, or other pediatric dosing systems should be routinely used to safely administer correct dosages to children (see **Appendix 48.1**).

WORKFORCE DEVELOPMENT AND DEPARTMENTAL STANDARDS

Although the development and evolution of emergency medicine has attempted to ensure a sufficient supply of emergency physicians to meet demand, there is ample evidence that the specialty is still understaffed. Furthermore, at least three additional factors have made it difficult to meet the needs of pediatric emergency patients.

First, while emergency medicine residencies are three to four years in length, most trainees spend 13% or less of their training time on pediatrics, even though approximately 34% of all ED patients are children.[34] Second, even though board certification in PEM has been in place for over 20 years, there are only approximately 1,900 board-certified pediatric emergency physicians in the United States, and 40% of them are over the age of 50. Current fellowship training programs only produce about 160 new pediatric EM fellowship-trained graduates per year. This is a tremendous limitation to staffing any ED with 24/7 board-certified PEM physicians.[35,36] Third, 50% of EDs care for fewer than 10 pediatric patients per day, making planning and preparation more difficult yet even more essential.[35]

Although the availability of staff with extensive pediatric-specific training and experience will always be limited, the commitment to using these resources and the development of a PECC to improve workforce competencies are only limited by the focus of department leadership.

Evolution of PEM and Practice Diversification

Pediatric emergency medicine evolved into a true subspecialty in the early 1980s, when ACEP and the AAP established PEM sections. At the same time, formal fellowship training programs in PEM were developed; these fellowships were initially one or two years in length, primarily based at free-standing children's hospitals, and almost exclusively offered to graduates of pediatric residencies. Subspecialty certification became available through either the American Board of Pediatrics (ABP) or the American Board of Emergency Medicine (ABEM) in 1992. Fellowship training programs now consist of specific tracks for graduates of emergency medicine (two years) or pediatric (three years) residency training programs.

To expand providers, many hospitals have hired general practitioners or advanced pediatrics nurse practitioners who have intense training in PEM protocols and have worked closely with a PEM-boarded physician. It is necessary to analyze practice variation and resource utilization when looking to expand independent providers who will care for pediatric patients by themselves.[11,37,38]

As a natural outgrowth of these advances, the question about whether to create a dedicated pediatric ED commonly occurs. It is necessary to consider several factors before launching an investment into this type of practice diversification.

Advantages of Pediatric Practice Diversification

Improved quality: Studies have shown that a focused initiative to improve protocols, equipment, and staff training leads to better pediatric outcomes if properly designed and implemented.[39] This can have a tremendous impact on the overall ED population as well as staff satisfaction.

Opportunities for partnership: Many regions of the country are lucky to have a large tertiary care children's hospital. While it may appear as a market competitor, most of these centers have infrastructure and a commitment to improve staff education and community knowledge of pediatric best practices. For community EDs, this often results in free training from experts, access to protocols, and a streamlined system for patient referrals.

Improved EMS relationship: An institutional dedication to improve pediatric care can help alleviate the stress of an out-of-hospital physician who may have to decide on the proper destination for a child who is not a trauma or high-acuity patient.

Improved community relationship: Community pediatricians and families clearly recognize that children are not simply small adults. A focus on explaining departmental improvements, staff training, pediatric-focused supplies, and a good communication plan with outpatient providers can go a long way in increasing the market share of this population.

Barriers to Pediatric Practice Diversification

Volume: Although the patient populations of many EDs are comprised of 30% children, other facilities may see higher pediatric volumes during winter respiratory illness and a paucity the rest of the year. A sustainable pediatric-specific ED requires a sufficient volume to cement protocols, validate and test training, and create a financial model that is worth the costs.

Resistance to change: The science of change management is addressed elsewhere in this book, but the natural human resistance to change is the most common barrier. Most nurses and physicians have had some experience working with children and may not perceive any gaps in their care. Additional training, new protocols, and a different culture should be presented as an opportunity to reduce variation and stress in the care of pediatrics and, in some instances, reduce workload for providers.

Investment cost: The investment cost of pediatric-specific supplies, training, branding, and aesthetic changes to treatment rooms all sum to a substantial up-front cost. This cost must be balanced with market forces and growth of the pediatric community in the area, the improved reputation to local EMS providers and general pediatricians, and the marketing advantage of keeping families all centered and tied to one facility. The measure of these benefits must be discussed with hospital administration well before any investment in practice line diversification.

EDUCATION

While education is a mandatory component in improving the department's pediatric standards, an effective education plan must 1) incorporate the clinical frequency in which pediatric knowledge is tested, 2) leverage local resources and expertise, and 3) appoint a champion to ensure gaps are being filled in the clinical workspace and clinician education is maintained year-round.

A minimum training standard for all staff includes credentialing for common pediatric resuscitation programs, including APLS, an emergency nursing pediatric course, and many others. However, educational outreach efforts from local children's hospitals have recently included onsite simulation in community hospitals that have led to more meaningful analyses of gaps in clinical performance and a developed action plan to improve staff performance and pediatric readiness.[40] This type of work highlights the need for community EDs to leverage the educational tools at local children's hospitals as well as the state level. In addition to routine education on resuscitation and procedures, EDs should consider utilizing tailored education on conditions that staff may not feel comfortable managing, such as nonaccidental trauma, psychiatric emergencies, or technologically dependent children.[41] The development of the Child Protector app to help educate community providers in real time on signs of child abuse is a high-quality example of this work (**Appendix 48.2**).[42]

The federal EMSC program organizes and leads pediatric-centered education through state partnership managers. While each state has different initiatives, the overall mission to improve pediatric quality measures is dependent on engaged community ED partners. Resources include out-of-hospital personnel training, evidence-based protocols, education focused on technologically dependent children, and more.[27]

Departmental education should also include the implementation of evidence-based protocols geared toward reducing unnecessary variation, improving the delivery of evidence-based care, and easing transfers to referral children's hospitals. An abundance of these resources are available for free online, but EDs may consider adopting the preferences and practices of the local referring hospital (see **Appendix 48.2**). Furthermore, the implementation of protocols can only be achieved with multidisciplinary education, an analysis of current workflow, and a meaningful audit of process measures that tie back to the preferred standard.

Lastly, pediatric education should cover the nuances of caring for children and their families, as well as the human factors that can be hard to measure but are nevertheless important to implement. This includes child life education on pediatric language based on milestones, appropriate distraction techniques based on age, proper assessment and treatment of pain in children, and education of families. The Simply Sayin' app, developed by a family and local children's hospital, has been widely used to help explain medical terminology and procedures in appropriate language and even to educate staff on how to prepare children for procedures.[43]

CONCLUSION

While there is great variation in resources and experience in pediatric care for community EDs, the simple fact is that most children will go to those EDs for their care. The evolution of pediatric readiness, online education, and standard evidence-based guidelines has made it even easier to bridge the gap between pediatric inexperience and expertise. The opportunities to go even further by creating a specialty pediatric ED, receive recognition with pediatric verification programs, and collaborate with tertiary care children's hospitals can be extremely rewarding and fruitful for a department's growth. However, none of this can occur without departmental leadership, staff buy-in, and the development of supported and sustainable PECCs.

APPENDIX 48.1: PEDIATRIC READINESS CHECKLIST

General Equipment

- Patient-warming system
- IV blood/fluid warmer
- Restraint device
- Weight scale in kilograms (not pounds)
- Tool or chart that incorporates weight (in kilograms) and length to determine equipment size and correct drug dosing
- Age-appropriate pain scale assessment tools

Monitoring Equipment

- Blood pressure cuffs: neonatal, infant, child, adult-arm, adult-thigh
- Doppler ultrasonography devices
- ECG monitor/defibrillator with pediatric and adult capabilities including pads/paddles
- Hypothermia thermometer
- Pulse oximeter with pediatric and adult probes
- Continuous end-tidal CO_2 monitoring device

Vascular Access

- Arm boards: infant, child, adult
- Over-the-needle catheter gauges 14, 16, 18, 20, 22, 24
- Intraosseous infusion needles or device: pediatric, adult
- IV administration sets with calibrated chambers and extension tubing and/or infusion devices with ability to regulate rate and volume of infusate
- Umbilical vein catheters: 3.5F, 5.0F
- Central venous catheters (any two sizes): 4.0F, 5.0F, 6.0F, 7.0F
- IV solutions: normal saline, dextrose 5% in normal saline, dextrose 10% in water

Fracture Management Devices

- Extremity splints: femur splints, pediatric and adult
- Spine-stabilization devices appropriate for children of all ages

Respiratory

- Endotracheal tubes: uncuffed 2.5 mm, 3.0 mm; cuffed/uncuffed 3.5 mm, 4.0 mm, 4.5 mm, 5.0 mm, 5.5 mm; cuffed 6.0 mm, 6.5 mm, 7.0 mm, 7.5 mm, 8.0 mm
- Feeding tubes: 5F, 8F
- Laryngoscope blades: straight 0, 1, 2, 3; curved 2, 3
- Laryngoscope handle
- Magill forceps: pediatric, adult
- Nasopharyngeal airways: infant, child, adult
- Oropharyngeal airways: 0, 1, 2, 3, 4, 5
- Stylets for endotracheal tubes: pediatric, adult
- Suction catheters: infant, child, adult
- Tracheostomy tubes: 2.5 mm, 3.0 mm, 3.5 mm, 4.0 mm, 4.5 mm, 5.0 mm, 5.5 mm
- Yankauer suction tip

- Bag-mask device, self-inflating: infant 450 mL, adult 1000 mL
- Masks to fit bag-mask device adaptor: neonatal, infant, child, adult
- Clear oxygen masks: standard infant, child, adult; partial nonrebreather infant; nonrebreather child, adult
- Nasal cannulas: infant, child, adult
- Nasogastric tubes: infant 8F, child 10F, adult 14 to 18F
- Laryngeal mask airway: 1, 1.5, 2, 2.5, 3, 4, 5

Specialized Pediatric Trays and Kits

- Lumbar puncture tray (including infant/pediatric 22 G and adult 18 to 21 G needles)
- Supplies/kit for patients with difficult airway (supraglottic airways of all sizes, laryngeal mask airway, needle cricothyrotomy supplies, surgical cricothyrotomy kit)
- Tube thoracotomy tray
- Chest tubes: infant 10 to 12 F, child 16 to 24 F, adult 28 to 40 F
- Newborn delivery kit, including equipment for resuscitation of an infant (umbilical clamp, scissors, bulb syringe, towel, hat)
- Urinary catheterization kits and urinary (indwelling) catheters: 6 F to 22 F

APPENDIX 48.2: ONLINE PEDIATRIC RESOURCES

TABLE 48.2 ■ Online Resources for Pediatric Policies, Education, and Support

Category	Title/Description	Location
Pediatric Readiness	Pediatric Readiness Project—Survey and resources	https://www.pedsready.org/
Pediatric Readiness	National Pediatric Readiness Toolkit—Package of improvement tools and resources	https://emscimprovement.center/domains/hospital-based-care/pediatric-readiness-project/readiness-toolkit/
Pediatric Disaster Planning	Pediatric Disaster Preparedness Toolbox	https://emscimprovement.center/resources/toolboxes/pediatric-disaster-preparedness-toolbox/
Pediatric State Partnerships	EMSC State Partnership Coordinators	https://emscimprovement.center/categories/state-partnerships/
Pediatric State Partnerships	EMSC Regionalization of Care	https://emscimprovement.center/programs/sproc/
Evidence-Based Pathways	Dell Children's Medical Center	https://www.dellchildrens.net/for-healthcare-professionals/evidence-based-care-guidelines/
Evidence-Based Pathways	Texas Children's Hospital	https://www.texaschildrens.org/departments/safety-outcomes/clinical-standards
Evidence-Based Pathways	Cincinnati Children's Hospital	https://www.cincinnatichildrens.org/service/j/anderson-center/evidence-based-care/recommendations
Prehospital Pediatric Protocols	Texas EMSC State Partnership	https://www.bcm.edu/departments/pediatrics/sections-divisions-centers/texasemsc/resources/ppr-toolkit/eb-prehospital-protocols

Simulation	IMPACTs Project–Community outreach onsite pediatric simulation education	https://medicine.yale.edu/lab/impacts/
Smartphone Apps	Simply Sayin' Medical Jargon	https://itunes.apple.com/us/app/simply-sayin-medical-jargon-for-families/id645810680?mt=8
Smartphone Apps	Child Protector–Assists in the evaluation of children with potential abuse	https://itunes.apple.com/us/app/child-protector/id1019023917?mt=8
Smartphone Apps	Pedi STAT–Rapid reference for pediatric medications and resuscitation guidelines	https://itunes.apple.com/us/app/pedi-stat/id327963391?mt=8
Free Open Access Med-education (FOAM) Podcasts	Pediatric Emergency Playbook podcast	http://pemplaybook.org/
FOAM Podcasts	EMRAP podcast	https://www.emrap.org/hd/playlist/pediatricsPL
FOAM Blogs	PEMBLOG–Online blog from Cincinnati Children's ED	http://pemcincinnati.com/blog/

REFERENCES

1. Whitfill T, Auerbach M, Scherzer DJ, et al. Emergency care for children in the United States: epidemiology and trends over time. *J Emerg Med*. 2018;55(3):423–434.
2. Moore BJ, Stocks C, Owens PL. Trends in emergency department visits, 2006–2014. *HCUP Statistical Brief* 2017;227.
3. American Academy of Pediatrics, Committee on Pediatric Emergency Medicine, American College of Emergency Physicians, Pediatric Committee, Emergency Nurses Association Pediatric Committee. Joint policy statement—guidelines for care of children in the emergency department. *Pediatrics*. 2009;124(4):1233–1243.
4. Gausche-Hill M, Ely M, Schmuhl P, et al. A national assessment of pediatric readiness of emergency departments. *JAMA Pediatr*. 2015;169(6):527–534.
5. Ray KN, Olson LM, Edgerton EA, et al. Access to high pediatric-readiness emergency care in the United States. *J Pediatr*. 2018;194:225–232.e1.
6. Remick K, Kaji AH, Olson L, et al. Pediatric readiness and facility verification. *Ann Emerg Med*. 2016;57(3):320–328.e1.
7. Rice A, Dudek J, Gross T, et al. The impact of a pediatric emergency department facility verification system on pediatric mortality rates in Arizona. *J Emerg Med*. 2017;52(6):894–901.
8. Kessler DO, Walsh B, Whitfill T, et al. Disparities in adherence to pediatric sepsis guidelines across a spectrum of emergency departments: a multicenter, cross-sectional observational in situ simulation study. *J Emerg Med*. 2016;50(3):403–415.e1–e3.
9. Auerbach M, Whitfill T, Gawel M, et al. Differences in the quality of pediatric resuscitative care across a spectrum of emergency departments. *JAMA Pediatr*. 2016;170(10):987–994.
10. The National Academies of Sciences, Engineering, and Medicine. Emergency Care for Children: Growing Pains [Internet]. 2006. Available at: https://www.nap.edu/catalog/11655/emergency-care-for-children-growing-pains. Accessed September 6, 2018.
11. Pavlik D, Sacchetti A, Seymour A, et al. Physician assistant management of pediatric patients in a general community emergency department: a real-world analysis. *Pediatr Emerg Care*. 2017;33(1):26–30.
12. Pirret AM, Neville SJ, La Grow SJ. Nurse practitioners versus doctors diagnostic reasoning in a complex case presentation to an acute tertiary hospital: a comparative study. *Int J Nurs Stud*. 2015;52(3):716–726.
13. Muller K, Chee Z, Doan Q. Using nurse practitioners to optimize patient flow in a pediatric emergency department. *Pediatr Emerg Care*. 2018;34(6):396–399.
14. McDonnell WM, Carpenter P, Jacobsen K, et al. Relative productivity of nurse practitioner and resident physician care models in the pediatric emergency department. *Pediatr Emerg Care*. 2015;31(2):101–106.
15. Love RA, Murphy JA, Lietz TE, et al. The effectiveness of a provider in triage in the emergency department: a quality improvement initiative to improve patient flow. *Adv Emerg Nurs J*. 2012;34(1):65–74.
16. Jennings N, Gardner G, O'Reilly G, et al. Evaluating emergency nurse practitioner service effectiveness on achieving timely analgesia: a pragmatic randomized controlled trial. *Acad Emerg Med Off J Soc Acad Emerg Med*. 2015;22(6):676–684.
17. Begaz T, Elashoff D, Grogan TR, et al. Differences in test ordering between nurse practitioners and attending emergency physicians when acting as provider in triage. *Am J Emerg Med*. 2017;35(10):1426–1429.
18. Liu H, Robbins M, Mehrotra A, et al. The impact of using mid-level providers in face-to-face primary care on health care utilization. *Med Care*. 2017;55(1):12–18.
19. Committee on Hospital Care and Child Life Council. Child life services. *Pediatrics*. 2014;133(5):e1471–e1478.
20. Hall JE, Patel DP, Thomas JW, et al. Certified child life specialists lessen emotional distress of children undergoing laceration repair in the emergency department. *Pediatr Emerg Care*. 2018;34(9):603–606.

21. McGee K. The role of a child life specialist in a pediatric radiology department. *Pediatr Radiol.* 2003;33(7):467–474.

22. Brewer S, Gleditsch SL, Syblik D, et al. Pediatric anxiety: child life intervention in day surgery. *J Pediatr Nurs.* 2006;21(1):13–22.

23. Schlechter JA, Avik AL, DeMello S. Is there a role for a child life specialist during orthopedic cast room procedures? A prospective-randomized assessment. *J Pediatr Orthop Part B.* 2017;26(6):575–579.

24. Child life services can provide competitive edge. *ED Manag Mon Update Emerg Dep Manag.* 2004;16(10):115–117.

25. Macias CG. Quality improvement in pediatric emergency medicine. *Acad Pediatr.* 2013;13(6 suppl):S61-S68.

26. Alessandrini E, Varadarajan K, Alpern ER, et al. Emergency department quality: an analysis of existing pediatric measures. *Acad Emerg Med.* 2011;18(5):519–526.

27. EMSC. State Partnership Grants [Internet]. Available at: https://emscimprovement.center/categories/state-partnerships/. Accessed August 1, 2018.

28. Gausche-Hill M, Ely M, Schmuhl P, et al. A national assessment of pediatric readiness of emergency departments. *JAMA Pediatr.* 2015;169(6):527.

29. Committee on Pediatric Workforce, Marcin JP, Rimsza ME, Moskowitz WB. The use of telemedicine to address access and physician workforce shortages. *Pediatrics.* 2015;136(1):202–209.

30. Luten R. Error and time delay in pediatric trauma resuscitation: addressing the problem with color-coded resuscitation aids. *Surg Clin North Am.* 2002;82(2):303–314, vi.

31. Luten R, Wears RL, Broselow J, et al. Managing the unique size-related issues of pediatric resuscitation: reducing cognitive load with resuscitation aids. *Acad Emerg Med.* 2002;9(8):840–847.

32. Doherty C, McDonnell C. Tenfold medication errors: 5 years' experience at a university-affiliated pediatric hospital. *Pediatrics.* 2012;129(5):916–924.

33. Feleke R, Kalynych CJ, Lundblom B, et al. Color coded medication safety system reduces community pediatric emergency nursing medication errors. *J Patient Saf.* 2009;5(2):79–85.

34. Tamariz VP, Fuchs S, Baren JM, et al. Pediatric emergency medicine education in emergency medicine training programs. SAEM Pediatric Education Training Task Force. Society for Academic Emergency Medicine. *Acad Emerg Med.* 2000;7(7):774–778.

35. Pitts SR, Niska RW, Xu J, et al. National hospital ambulatory medical care survey: 2006 emergency department summary. *Natl Health Stat Rep.* 2008;(7):1–38.

36. Althouse LA, Stockman JA. Pediatric workforce: a look at pediatric emergency medicine data from the American Board of Pediatrics. *J Pediatr.* 2006;149(5):600–602.e1.

37. Chang Y-C, Ng C-J, Chen Y-C, et al. Practice variation in the management for nontraumatic pediatric patients in the ED. *Am J Emerg Med.* 2010;28(3):275–283.

38. Seow V-K, Lin AC-M, Lin I-Y, et al. Comparing different patterns for managing febrile children in the ED between emergency and pediatric physicians: impact on patient outcome. *Am J Emerg Med.* 2007;25(9):1004–1008.

39. Walls TA, Hughes NT, Mullan PC, et al. Improving pediatric asthma outcomes in a community emergency department. *Pediatrics.* 2017;139(1):e20160088.

40. Whitfill T, Gawel M, Auerbach M. A simulation-based quality improvement initiative improves pediatric readiness in community hospitals. *Pediatr Emerg Care.* 2018;34(6):431–435.

41. Barr RG, Barr M, Rajabali F, et al. Eight-year outcome of implementation of abusive head trauma prevention. *Child Abuse Negl.* 2018;84:106–14.

42. Children's Mercy Kansas City—Child Protector App [Internet]. Available at: https://www.childrensmercy.org/childprotector/. Accessed August 27, 2018.

43. Simply Sayin'—Medical Jargon for Families on the App Store [Internet]. App Store. Available at: https://itunes.apple.com/us/app/simply-sayin-medical-jargon-for-families/id645810680?mt=8. Accessed August 27, 2018.

CHAPTER 49

UNDERSEA AND HYPERBARIC MEDICINE

Thom A. Mayer, Joseph P. Dervay, Norma L. Cooney

From birth, man carries the weight of gravity on his shoulders. He is bolted to earth. But man has only to sink beneath the surface and he is free.

—Jacques Yves Cousteau

Undersea and hyperbaric medicine (UHM) is among the newer subspecialties of emergency medicine, although the origins of hyperbaric therapy are much older. The history of the clinical use of hyperbaric medicine is tied closely with diving. Dating back to ancient times, there is some evidence that Hippocrates referred to the effects of diving accidents in his work. Aristotle made reference to Alexander the Great's use of a manned, pressurized submersible in the Siege of Tyre in 332 BC. During the middle of the 17th century, British physician Nathaniel Henshaw used pressurization to treat various diseases, and in 1662, he built a pressurized room he referred to as a "Domicilium."[1]

In 1834, French physician Junod first observed how pressurization could increase circulation to internal organs. A few years later in 1837, orthopedic surgeon Charles Gabriel Pravaz began using the technique to treat pulmonary diseases and other disorders. Nearly 40 years after that, New York physician Andrew Smith used the terms "caisson disease" and "compressed air illness" to describe the cases of decompression sickness (DCS) he encountered during the construction of the Brooklyn Bridge. The nickname "the bends" was used to describe the Brooklyn Bridge workers' stooped posture after leaving the pressurized construction site.

HISTORY OF HYPERBARIC MEDICINE

Hyperbaric medicine moved into the operating room in 1877 when the first hyperbaric operating theater was built for hernia repairs. In 1878, French physiologist Paul Bert discovered that nitrogen gas bubbles released from tissues and blood during or after decompression caused DCS and showed the advantages of using oxygen instead of air in the hyperbaric treatment environment. In 1885 during the construction of the Hudson River Tunnel in New York, a medical lock was successfully used to treat caisson disease; prior to the development of this approach, 25% of these patients died. After the installation and initiation of hyperbaric treatments, the death rate fell from one worker per month to two workers in 15 months.[2]

In 1912, the first United States Navy (USN) decompression tables were developed by French and Stillson for the USN Bureau of Construction and Repair. The decompression tables were instituted to reduce the probability of DCS. Since then, several subsequent generations of tables have been developed. In the 1920s, physician Orval Cunningham used hyperbaric oxygen therapy (HBOT) to treat Spanish influenza and cardiac disease. He observed higher mortality in patients from higher elevations. Specifically, the survival rate was greater for patients living at sea level when compared to those living in the Rocky Mountains. Postulating that these differences were due to the differential effects of the partial pressure of oxygen, he built a series of hyperbaric facilities of ever-increasing size

FIGURE 49.1 ■ Divers Alert Network Flag

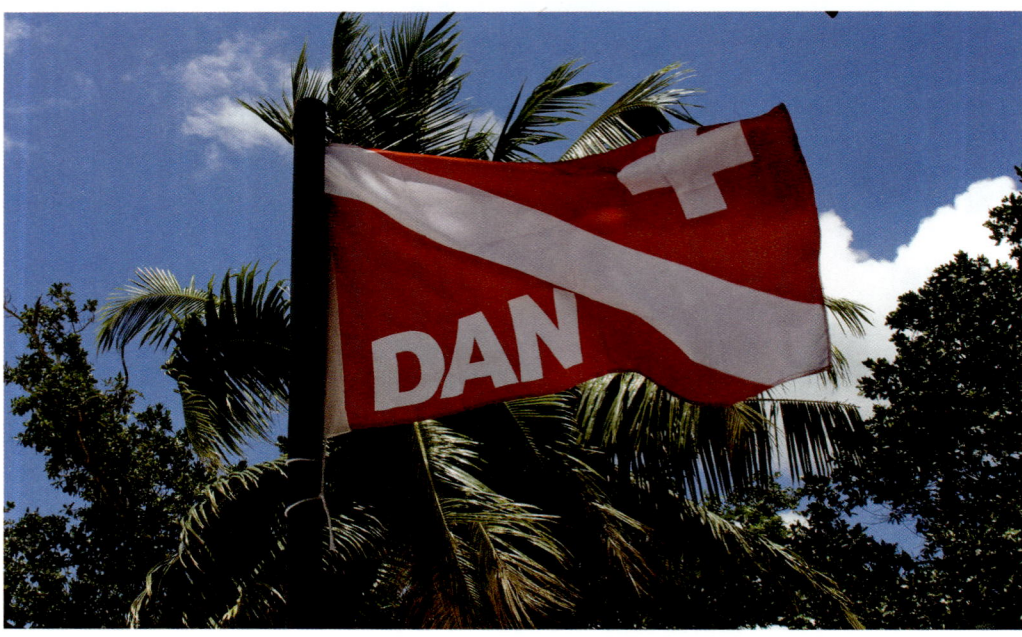

to treat patients with various illnesses and diseases, culminating in a five-story facility in Cleveland, Ohio, to house and treat patients with pressurized air. However, despite his enthusiasm for the treatment, Cunningham refused to cooperate with medical researchers who sought to document his claims. Later, his facility and methods fell into disrepute, and his chamber facility was dismantled in 1937.[3]

In that same year, Behnke and Shaw showed conclusively that nitrogen was the cause of DCS among air divers. They were the first to use HBOT to successfully treat the condition.[4] Nonetheless, pressurization facilities capable of delivering HBOT were not prominently in use until the more widely recognized birth of hyperbaric medicine in the mid-20th century. In 1956, Dutch surgeon Ite Boerema began to use pressurized oxygen to treat pediatric patients with cyanotic congenital heart disease and performed cardiac surgery in a pressurized chamber. He was also the first to treat clostridial myonecrosis successfully with HBOT in 1961.[5] By 1962, Smith and Sharp had successfully used HBOT to treat patients with carbon monoxide poisoning. In 1964, Goodman and Workman published the USN's updated treatment tables for DCS utilizing oxygen.[6]

The widespread use of hyperbaric therapy to treat decompression diving accidents led to the more widespread expansion of pressurized oxygen therapy. Scuba divers who developed symptoms upon ascent were treated with 100% oxygen in treatment chambers with increased atmospheric pressure. Not only was this treatment highly successful, but networks were established to refer divers with DCS to the nearest HBOT facilities, including the most widely recognized organization, Divers Alert Network (http://www.dan.org) (**Figure 49.1**).

HYPERBARIC MEDICINE TRAINING

Undersea and hyperbaric medicine is a diverse specialty providing opportunities in many areas where the treatments have been proven efficacious. Current efforts are underway to explore additional areas of research, including resuscitation, sepsis, traumatic brain

> **BOX 49.1 ■ REASONS TO PURSUE UHM**
>
> - Broadens the emergency physician's practice and knowledge base
> - Addresses specific clinical entities amenable to hyperbaric oxygen treatment
> - Provides alternate/additional income sources for the individual or the practice
> - Develops the emergency physician group as a referral service
> - Provides a clinical practice alternative
> - Integrates the group into the medical staff and hospital fabric

injury (TBI), and vascular diseases. As hyperbaric medicine developed beyond treatment of pressurization illnesses, there were many efforts to assess its utility for treating a wide variety of acute diseases. At least partially for that reason, many of the initial hyperbaric services fell under the categories of anesthesia, critical care, and trauma services at academic institutions. More than 500 medical centers in the United States and Canada currently operate clinical hyperbaric chambers.[7] At a number of large accredited hyperbaric facilities, emergency physicians provide medical direction for the hyperbaric programs.

Hyperbaric oxygen therapy is also widely used for conditions other than DCS and is approved by Medicare for 14 discrete indications. Many of the conditions are diagnosed and treated by emergency medicine physicians, thus making UHM a popular and logical option for practice diversification.[7] Several reasons to pursue diversification in UHM are listed in **Box 49.1**.

Fellowship Programs

As of 2020, there were 11 fellowship training programs in UHM approved by the Accreditation Council on Graduate Medical Education (ACGME), each of which are 12 months in length (**Box 49.2**).[8] Louisiana State University, New Orleans, under the direction of Dr. Tracy LeGros, has the largest ACGME UHM fellowship in the United States, with five positions. Prerequisite training for entry into a UHM program is contingent upon completion of an ACGME-accredited residency program. Fellows have come from a variety of backgrounds, including emergency medicine, surgery, anesthesiology, preventive medicine, internal medicine, family medicine, pediatrics, and neurology.

A 1-year fellowship program qualifies graduates to take the examination for a subspecialty certification in UHM. The examination is cosponsored by the American Board of Emergency Medicine (ABEM) and the American Board of Preventive Medicine (ABPM), the latter of which develops and administers the examination.

> **BOX 49.2 ■ ACGME-APPROVED FELLOWSHIP TRAINING PROGRAMS IN UHM**
>
> - Duke University Medical Center
> - Hennepin County Medical Center
> - Louisiana State University New Orleans
> - State University of New York Upstate Medical Center
> - University of California San Diego
> - University of Pennsylvania Medical Center
> - University of Texas Southwestern Medical School
> - USAF School of Aerospace Medicine, Lackland AFB
> - Kent Hospital, Warwick, Rhode Island (Osteopathic only)

While fellowship training and board certification in UHM are not yet requirements for supervising a hyperbaric program, such training is highly sought, particularly for HBOT program medical directors. Most physicians practicing hyperbaric medicine in the United States are not currently board certified in the subspecialty. The "grandfather path" to certification was phased out in 2010. Fellowship training and board certification are the most comprehensive and appropriate methods of obtaining a full scope of knowledge and appreciation for UHM and all it encompasses. Several hospitals and academic medical centers provide "mini-fellowship" training sessions and scientific courses in hyperbaric medicine.

National Oceanic and Atmospheric Association Training

The National Oceanic and Atmospheric Association (NOAA) offers a 12-day course called Physicians Training in Diving Medicine.[9] The goals of the program are to train physicians in a range of diving medical emergencies. After completing the NOAA course, a physician should have the knowledge to manage diving emergency cases and safely operate a hyperbaric chamber.

The Undersea and Hyperbaric Medical Society

The Undersea and Hyperbaric Medical Society (UHMS) (www.uhms.org) is an international, nonprofit organization serving over 2,400 members from more than 50 countries. The UHMS is a recognized source of professional scientific information for diving and hyperbaric medicine physiology worldwide. The organization is involved in many arenas, including advocating standards of practice through the implementation of treatment guidelines, position statements, and clinical hyperbaric facility accreditation; conducting workshops and training courses; holding an annual scientific meeting; and publishing a bimonthly scientific journal, the *Undersea and Hyperbaric Medicine Journal*.

Accreditation and Operations

Those involved with managing a hyperbaric facility should be well versed in accreditation processes; ancillary staffing and training; equipment installation, operation, and maintenance; facility and patient safety; and standards of care. The supervision of treatments and the related reimbursements are areas of recent change and controversy. Within the past few years, insurance carriers have set strict guidelines regarding the supervision and immediate availability of physicians during treatments. This proximate supervision contrasts with the less-stringent protocols that were previously mandated. Furthermore, the limitation of billing by and reimbursement to nonboarded physicians is under discussion. Specifically, the movement to prohibit payment for hyperbaric oxygen treatment services unless the treating physician is boarded in UHM by ABEM or ABPM is being seriously reviewed by insurers.

As EDs branch out and develop hyperbaric services, the longitudinal evaluation of patient care and outcomes requires thorough investigation. While some conditions are managed emergently with only a few treatments, others require several weeks of care and follow-up. Proper charting and documentation regarding the medical necessity of treatment are important considerations.

There are two parts to the HBOT service: 1) the facility component, which is the hospital side (typically employing the nursing and technical staff and purchasing and maintaining the treatment chamber), and 2) the professional component, which is the physician (supervision of patient treatment). Both entities must work effectively together and coordinate activities and documentation. Although emergency medicine physicians may manage a hyperbaric medicine practice, the management, policy, and operational components are substantially different from a standard ED practice.

MECHANISM OF ACTION AND INDICATIONS

Hyperbaric oxygen therapy is a treatment modality used to manage a variety of illnesses. The treatment's mechanism of action was initially postulated to simply be increased oxygen tissue perfusion at increased pressure. However, it is now known that the mechanism of action is much more complex and is dependent on a cascade of cell-signaling events.[10]

Treatment protocols are dependent on the specific UHM indication for each case. Arterial gas embolism and DCS are collectively known as "decompression illness." The rationale for treatment of an arterial gas embolism is to compress the gas bubbles, drive them out of circulation, restore blood flow, and hyperoxygenate ischemic tissues. The treatment's mechanism of action for the other UHM indications—such as carbon monoxide poisoning, osteoradionecrosis, refractory wounds (e.g., diabetics, skin grafts), peripheral ischemia, thermal burns, and mixed or anaerobic infections like necrotizing fasciitis—are complex and beyond the scope of this chapter.

However, it is well established that HBOT is known to reduce edema, increase epithelization and graft take, suppress toxin production, enhance neutrophil function and antibiotic potentiation, increase neovascularization, ameliorate ischemic-reperfusion injury, increase osteogenesis, increase collagen deposition, reduce inflammation, and increase granulation.[11]

Current UHM treatment is dictated by the evidence-based guidelines for each specific disease process. Treatment for an emergent indication, such as carbon monoxide toxicity, may range from one to three treatments; a chronic condition like as osteoradionecrosis may necessitate 40 to 60 treatments. Treatment protocols are not standardized across all hyperbaric centers. Typically, hyperbaric oxygen treatments are at two to three times normal atmospheric pressure (14.7 psi), or 2 to 3 atmospheres absolute, for variable periods of time.

The Centers for Medicare and Medicaid Services approves certain medical conditions for reimbursement by Medicare. Commercial insurance carriers generally recognize the listed conditions (although the specifics of reimbursement require regional/local review). The National Coverage Determination for hyperbaric therapy denotes currently covered conditions. The UHMS Committee Report lists indications for HBOT that have sufficient data to support such use, with some variation (**Box 49.3**). Because of the recognized utility of HBOT in wound care of various types, many hyperbaric programs operate in close cooperation with wound care centers, including general, plastic, trauma, and orthopedic surgeons.

There are a number of other diseases for which "off-label" HBOT has been attempted, with variable results, including Lyme disease, epidural abscess, inflammatory bowel disease, and psoriasis. Hyperbaric oxygen therapy has also been attempted in a wide variety of neurological disease entities. The mechanism of action is not clearly understood and is much more complex than simply increased tissue oxygen levels. These neurologic conditions include autism, multiple sclerosis, cerebral palsy, stroke, migraines, and concussion.

Although very few large studies have been completed for most of these conditions, the US Department of Defense has investigated the therapeutic value of HBOT in concussed patients; the results are varied. The management of TBI is not a current indication for the treatment, but studies are ongoing. As clinical trials continue, the specific role of HBOT in a variety of clinical entities, some beyond the currently recognized indications, will undoubtedly become more clearly elucidated.[12,13]

> **BOX 49.3 ■ INDICATIONS FOR HBOT THERAPY**
>
> **Medicare**
> - Acute carbon monoxide intoxication
> - Decompression illness
> - Gas embolism
> - Gas gangrene
> - Acute traumatic peripheral ischemia
> - Crush injuries and suturing of severed limbs
> - Progressive necrotizing infections
> - Acute peripheral arterial insufficiency
> - Preparation and preservation of compromised sign grafts
> - Chronic refractory osteomyelitis, unresponsive to conventional medical and surgical management
> - Osteoradionecrosis as an adjunct to conventional treatment
> - Soft tissue radionecrosis as an adjunct to conventional treatment
> - Cyanide poisoning
> - Actinomycosts, only as an adjunct to conventional therapy when the disease process is refractory to antibiotics and surgical treatment
> - Diabetic wounds of the lower extremities if all of these apply:
>   - You have to type 1 or type 2 diabetes and have a lower-extremity wound that's due to diabetes
>   - You have a wound classified as Wagner grade III or higher
>   - You've failed an adequate course of standard wound therapy
>
> **UHMS**
> - Air or gas embolism
> - Carbon monoxide poisoning
> - Clostridial myositis and myonecrosis (gas gangrene)
> - Crush injury, compartment syndrome, and other acute traumatic ischemias
> - Decompression sickness
> - Arterial insufficiencies
> - Severe anemia
> - Intracranial abscess
> - Necrotizing soft-tissue infections
> - Osteomyelitis (refractory)
> - Delayed radiation injury (soft tissue and bony necrosis)
> - Compromised grafts and flaps
> - Acute thermal burn injury
> - Idiopathic sudden sensorineural hearing loss

ESTABLISHING A UHM SERVICE

Needs-Based Formulas

Various models and formulas are used to estimate the number of hyperbaric programs needed within a given geographic or service area. One model, developed by Perry Baromedical Services (Riviera Beach, Florida), estimates the need for one HBOT per day per 100,000 people in a referral area (e.g., in an urban metropolitan area). Another model, developed by Hyperbaric Oxygen Treatment Systems (HOTS; San Diego, California), estimates a need of 4.25 treatments per year per 1,000 people.

For example, in a metropolitan area containing 1 million people, the Perry model would yield an estimated need of 10 HBOTs a day. The HOTS model would yield approximately 4,250 treatments a year, or 12 treatments a day. In our experience, both models yield a very conservative estimate of the potential need for HBOT in a community. The formulas may

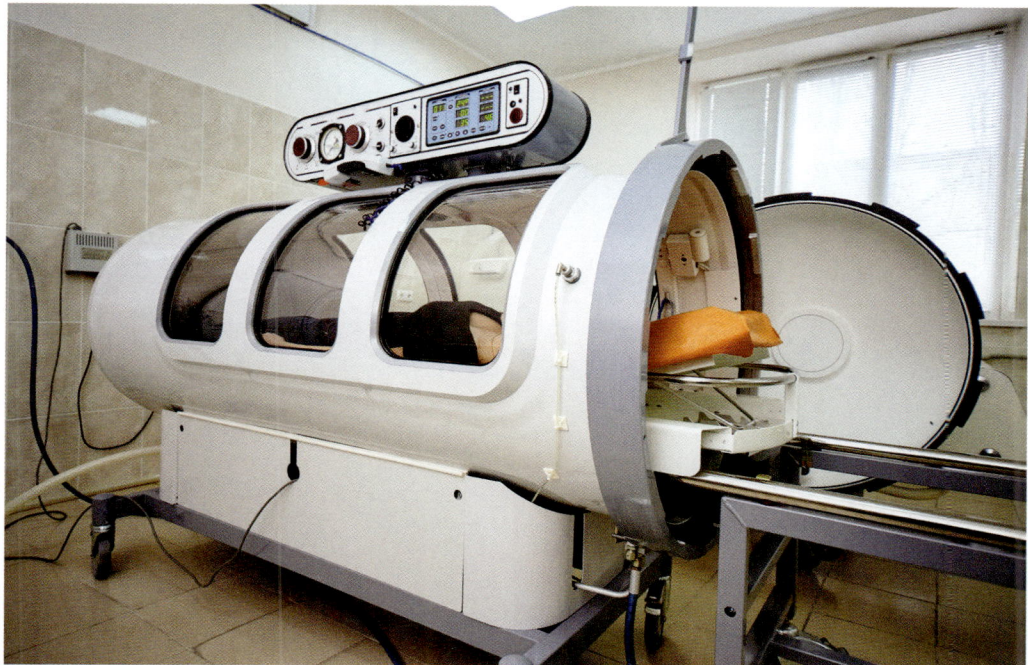

FIGURE 49.2 ■ Monoplace Hard-Shelled Chamber

be useful in providing a "worst-case scenario" (low baseline utilization) for determining patient flow and financial viability of a hyperbaric service. Patient flow can be favorably influenced by an effective marketing system, positive clinical interactions, and positive patient results (the best possible marketing technique). Educating the local medical community on the clinical benefits of HBOT and developing strong working relationships will go far in enhancing the use of this valuable treatment modality.

Monoplace vs Multiplace Chambers

In most cases, the initiation of a new hyperbaric program occurs with the purchase and implementation of one or more "monoplace" chambers, with each capable of treating a single patient (**Figure 49.2**). Hard-shelled monoplace chambers cost in the range of $175,000 to $250,000. Alternatively, new multiplace chambers typically cost millions of dollars, depending on how many patients are to be treated at any given time (**Figure 49.3**). In addition, monoplace chambers can typically be staffed with a smaller clinical staff (medical director, hyperbaric technician, wound care/HBOT nurse, and a nursing director). Multiplace units, on the other hand, require the additional staff discussed earlier as well as an inside observer to monitor the patients (typically a nurse or paramedic). Many programs launch their service with two monoplace chambers, since the same staff can often work and monitor two chambers, at least doubling the treatment capacity and amortizing the staffing costs over more patient treatments.

Marketing the Program

An effective and comprehensive marketing program can often be the determining factor in establishing a successful hyperbaric service. Marketing should be a continuous process. It is logical to begin by marketing within the institution and then broaden the program to a local and regional level.

FIGURE 49.3 ■ Multiplace Hyperbaric Chamber

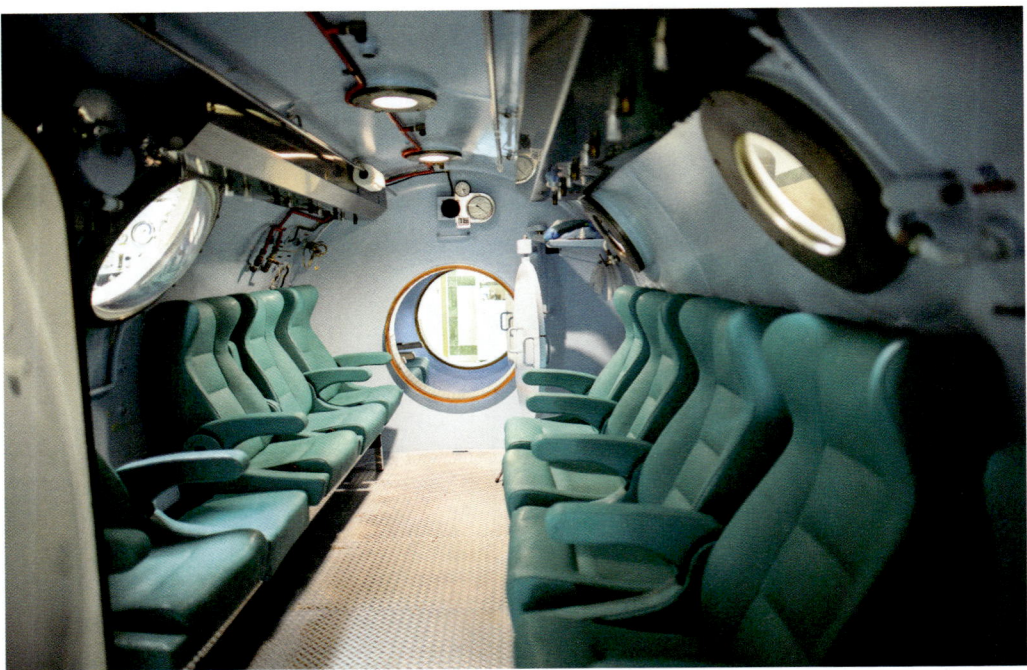

The primary target marketing audiences are potential referring physicians, based upon the clinical indications listed previously. Referrals are therefore most likely to come from general, vascular, and plastic surgeons, as well as maxillofacial surgeons, otolaryngologists, orthopedic surgeons, and radiation oncologists. Providing lectures to the medical staff is a time-honored technique to generate referrals.

The most successful marketing tool is the provision of high-quality service and the return of successfully treated patients to their referring physicians. Positive feedback on the results of therapy, including pictures and specific outcomes, are an important tool in growing the practice. Local and regional marketing also can involve direct contact with targeted specialists. Newsletters and direct mailings can be productive as well. Regional marketing should include direct contact with other emergency departments, poison control centers, firefighters, burn units, and wound care centers. Program directors may develop relationships with rescue dive teams, dive shops, dive clubs, or diving contractors when the hospital is located near an area of significant diving activity. Whenever possible, access to local and regional press and television sources should be cultivated as well.

In these efforts, a high level of professionalism and a strict adherence to making no claims other than those supported by scientific evidence and accepted clinical practice should be made. Whenever possible, participation in clinical research trials is encouraged.

CONCLUSION

Undersea and hyperbaric medicine is a growing and emerging subspecialty of emergency medicine. The treatment indications are continuing to increase based on current research studies. Education among colleagues and other specialties are vital for the longevity and survival of this subspecialty. Hyperbaric oxygen therapy has been shown to reduce morbidity and mortality for specific disease processes; for some patients, it is a lifesaving adjunctive therapy. Presently, physicians from nearly every specialty practice hyperbaric medicine. The strength of this diversity is the knowledge brought to underwater and hyperbaric medicine from all areas.

Hyperbaric medicine provides a unique perspective from the physician's standpoint. This area of medicine is still developing and offers many advantages to those who are dedicated to the care of patients who may benefit from its use. While there are capital, intellectual, and time costs associated with developing or expanding such a service, it is an effective strategy for ED diversification.

REFERENCES

1. Henshaw N. *Aero-Chalinos*. Dancer; 1664.
2. Fontaine JA. Emploi chirurgical de l'air comprine. *Union Med*. 1879;28:445-451.
3. Cunningham OJ. Oxygen therapy by means of compressed air. *Anesth Analg*. 1927;6(2):64-66
4. Yarbrough OD, Behnke AR. Treatment of compressed air illness utilizing oxygen. *J Indust Hyg Toxicol*. 1939;21:213-218.
5. Boerema I, Kroll JA, Meijnem E, et al. High atmospheric pressure as an aid to cardiac surgery. *Arch Chir Neerl*. 1956;8:193-211.
6. Tibbles PM, Edelsberg JS. Hyperbaric oxygen therapy. *N Engl J Med*. 1996;334(25):1642-1648.
7. Moon RE. Hyperbaric oxygen therapy indications. Undersea and Hyperbaric Medicine Society. 14th ed. 2019. Available at: https://www.uhms.org/images/UHMS-Reference-Material.pdf. Accessed July 19, 2020.
8. Fellowships in Undersea in Hyperbaric Medicine. Undersea and Hyperbaric Medial Society. 2020. Available at: https://www.uhms.org/education/credentialing/fellowship-programs.html. Accessed July 19, 2020.
9. National Oceanic and Atmospheric Administration. Physicians training in diving medicine course. 2020. Available at: https://www.omao.noaa.gov/learn/diving-program/diving/noaa-diving-medicine. Accessed July 19, 2020.
10. Thom SR, Bhopale VM, Mancini JD, et al. Actin S-nitrosylation inhibits neutrophil beta2 integrin function. *J Biol Chem*. 2008;283(16):10822-10834.
11. Gill AL, Bell CNA. Hyperbaric oxygen: its uses, mechanisms of action and outcomes. *QJM*. 2004;97(7):385-395.
12. Ling G. Personal correspondence with the author (TM). February 7, 2018.
13. Wilkie R. Under Secretary of Defense for Personnel and Readiness, letters to The Honorable John McCain and the Honorable William Thornberry, January 29, 2018.

CHAPTER 50

BEHAVIORAL HEALTH IN EMERGENCY CARE

Abhi Mehrotra

The passage of the Community Mental Health Act in 1963 precipitated the deinstitutionalization of patients with mental illnesses.[1] This trend resulted in a significant decrease in the number of inpatient and residential psychiatric beds. The legislation was intended to spur the creation of mental health centers in every community; however, a lack of adequate funding restricted the growth of the projected community capacity. **Figure 50.1** demonstrates the drastic decline in state and county psychiatric hospitals from 1970 to 2014.[2]

According to recent national trends, more than 10% of emergency department (ED) visits are for a mental, behavioral, or neurodevelopmental disorders as a primary diagnosis.[3] This number likely underestimates the number of patients who are evaluated for behavioral health-related complaints due to the separate classification of injuries, ingestions, and comorbid presentations. In addition to the lack of available psychiatric beds, nearly half of that capacity is occupied by forensic patients (i.e., those who are charged with or convicted of a crime).[4] This use of psychiatric beds places even more strain upon the availability of inpatient beds for those seeking emergency behavioral care.

On average, patients with psychiatric complaints spend more time in the ED than patients with nonbehavioral conditions. This problem may be broken down into the following two categories:

- Delays in psychiatric assessment
- Delays in disposition/placement (once determined that inpatient hospitalization or community resources are required)

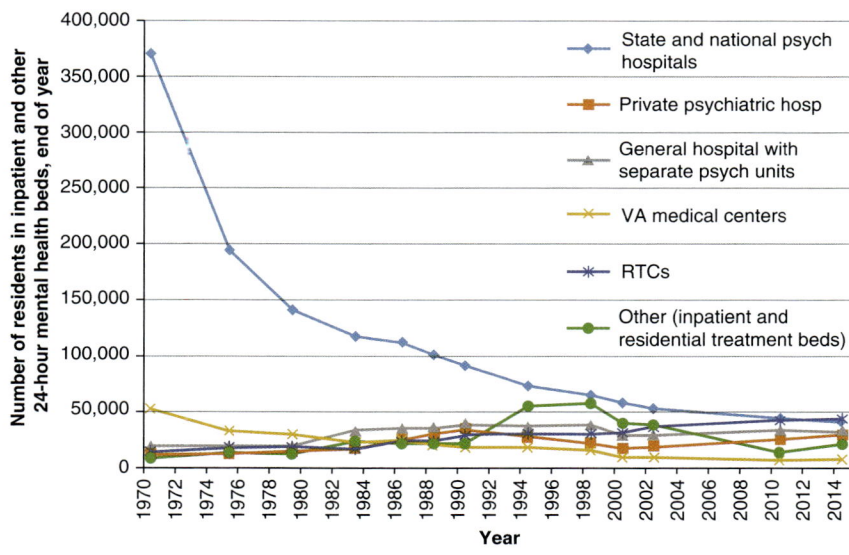

FIGURE 50.1 ■ Trends in Psychiatric Inpatient Capacity[2]

FIGURE 50.2 ■ Breakdown of the Problem

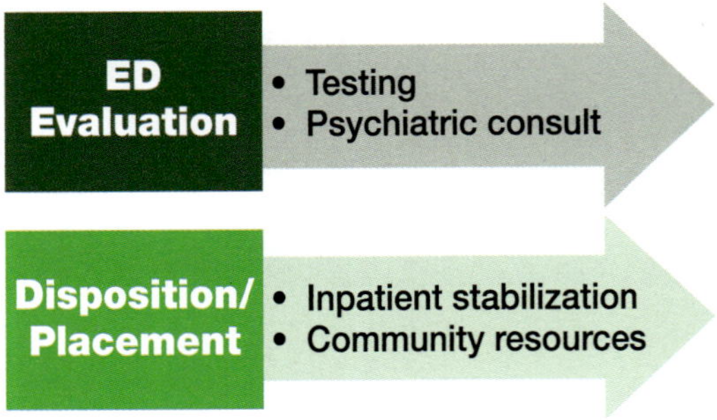

ED Evaluation
- Testing
- Psychiatric consult

Disposition/Placement
- Inpatient stabilization
- Community resources

Lengths of stay for psychiatric admissions are significantly longer than for nonpsychiatric patients. Understanding the impact of these delays can help guide solutions to these issues. The delays in psychiatric assessment and boarding of behavioral health patients impact the workflow of the entire ED.[5] Additionally, the lack of bed turnover adds to the opportunity cost, thereby estimating a cost to the department of more than $2,000 per patient (**Figure 50.2**).[5]

Special behavioral populations add to the complexity of the problem; for example, patients who are pediatric, developmentally delayed, geriatric, or have substance use disorders present challenges and resource requirements beyond those of the general behavioral patient needs. The volume of these vulnerable populations is increasing as well. In the time period from 2011 to 2015, there was a 28% increase in patients ages 6 to 24 years arriving to the ED and diagnosed with a psychiatric complaint.[6]

IMPACT OF THE EMERGENCY CARE ENVIRONMENT

In 2014, the American College of Emergency Physicians (ACEP) released the white paper "Care of the Psychiatric Patient in the Emergency Department—A Review of the Literature."[7] It provides a summary of the literature, broken down into seven areas. They can be broadly categorized as:

- ED evaluation
  - Evaluation of psychiatric patients in the ED
  - Medical clearance of psychiatric patients in the ED
- Disposition/placement
  - Boarding of psychiatric patients in the ED
  - Best practices for reducing ED boarding of psychiatric patients
  - Medical management of psychiatric patients in the ED
  - Disposition of psychiatric patients in the ED
  - Community resources for emergency psychiatric patients

The atmosphere and culture of the commonly designed ED can inadvertently add to the destabilization of many patients who present with behavioral health problems. Emergency department staff are trained to be professional, efficient, effective, and unemotional. In many cases, the patients and their families can interpret this behavior as uncaring, distant, and brusque. Many ED staff members, from physicians to aides, see behavioral health clients as requiring a significant investment of time and resources that could be better invested in patients with *true* medical or surgical emergencies.

To further underscore the magnitude of the problem, a 2008 survey by ACEP of ED medical directors revealed that 99% of their EDs admitted psychiatric patients every week.[8] Twenty-three percent of the 328 respondents (1,400 surveys distributed) had no community psychiatric resources available. Finally, a significant majority (62%) reported that patients boarding in the ED prior to admission or transfer received no psychiatric services. With record volumes of patients coming through the ED (145.6 million visits in 2016 as reported by the Centers for Disease Control and Prevention), holding behavioral health patients for extended lengths of time with no treatment is not sustainable.[9] This untenable situation is made worse by the increasingly limited capacity of inpatient beds and community resources.

Potential Solutions

In 2015, the ACEP Emergency Medicine Practice Committee released a white paper on the subject of solutions to boarding of psychiatric patients.[10] The committee notes that individual solutions will vary and that a combination of solutions may be necessary at the local, regional, and state levels. The solution concepts the paper described are specific and may be categorized by evaluation (telepsychiatry services, patient navigation, mobile crisis units) and disposition (regional evaluation, bed registries, and discharge protocols).

A useful construct for solutions comes from a *Health Affairs* article by Alakeson, Pande, and Ludwig, which describes the following seven steps to reduce boarding (and potential ED utilization) of behavioral health patients:[8]

1. Quantify and monitor the problem.
2. Improve the ED care of psychiatric patients.
3. Make more efficient use of existing capacity.
4. Implement low-cost collaboration.
5. Work with law enforcement.
6. Invest in comprehensive community crisis services.
7. Invest in continuity of care.

Using this schema, the first three items are somewhat within the control of the local ED management team and are therefore the focus of the following discussion. Of course, implementing items 4 through 7 provides even further improvement but requires multistakeholder collaboration beyond the ED.

Quantify and Monitor the Problem

The measures chosen for tracking improvement will determine the areas of attention. The measures should be aligned with the main objectives of the hospital.

Length of Stay

One of the most useful statistics is ED length of stay (LOS) for both admitted and discharged patients. Understanding the intervals of delays, including the times from arrival to psychiatric assessment and psychiatric assessment to discharge/placement, can help identify where to direct improvement efforts.

When non-ED stakeholders understand these issues, it is easier to gather support for and implement specific aspects of improvement. To the extent that ED beds are used for observation and holding of behavioral patients, the overall LOS for these and all patients will increase. Consistently obtaining and reviewing this statistic for behavioral health patients improves recognition and understanding of these delays and helps to create targets for improvement. Hospitals generally help collect these data as the Centers for Medicare & Medicaid Services tracks LOS for admitted and discharged patients. While not currently publicly available, the metric is broken out for psychiatric patients.

Use of Restraints

A second important measure is frequency and duration of restraints, required by The Joint Commission. Placing a patient in restraints is associated with risk, demeaning to the patient, and may indicate the need for improved alternate methods of care. While it may not be possible to completely eliminate restraints, reducing their use to as few cases as possible is a good indicator of quality of care.

Readmissions

Measuring rehospitalizations within 30 days is a third important metric. It is common for clinicians to think of rehospitalizations for behavioral health issues as inevitable. Yet a number of processes can be employed to reduce the frequency of readmissions. Additionally, rehospitalizations in different institutions range from a low of 6% to 8% to a high of 35% or more. The breadth of this range suggests much can be done to reduce the incidence of rehospitalizations. In some hospitals, two-thirds or more of the rehospitalizations of behavioral health patients are for chronic medical conditions such as coronary artery disease, chronic obstructive pulmonary disease, and diabetes. In some cases, the behavioral health issues exacerbate the medical issues, and conversely, exacerbation of medical problems can aggravate the behavioral issues. The ED staff should address both general and behavioral health issues to most effectively reduce readmissions.

Improve the ED Care of Psychiatric Patients

There are potential improvements in both categories, evaluation and disposition. Regarding ED evaluation, a number of potential options are available to deploy depending upon the bottlenecks discovered when assessing the ED operations; these include:

- *Standardizing medical clearance*—Many hospitals require medical clearance in the ED prior to behavioral health assessment and treatment by the psychiatric service. Medical clearance is generally defined as ensuring that the patient does not have a serious medical condition requiring immediate attention. A number of anecdotes exist about clients (patients) who have arrived at EDs and been shunted into behavioral health care only to later demonstrate serious general health issues, such as an myocardial infarction or an organic cause of altered mental status. At the same time, it is counter therapeutic to require an unnecessarily extended physical examination and testing for a person suffering primarily from behavioral health issues. Diagnostic evaluation should be directed as determined by the treating physician rather than by nonspecific guidelines, including routine testing.
- *Creating treatment protocols*—Specific protocols and guidelines for both routine and nonroutine evaluations can facilitate more effective flow between the ED and the psychiatric facility.
- *Conducting risk assessment*—Using standardized scales can facilitate communication between providers as well as facilitate a structured approach to behavioral health problems. This is especially true for patients expressing suicidality. One tool available is ICAR2E: Identifying Suicide Risk, a smartphone application developed by ACEP.[11] While no tool is a replacement for psychiatric

evaluation, a standardized approach to risk assessment can facilitate communication with other health care providers.

- *Telepsychiatry*—In facilities with limited access to behavioral health professionals, telepsychiatry may be an effective avenue to more rapid psychiatric evaluation. A number of commercial vendors are available, as well as specific, state-sponsored efforts. Reducing the time to psychiatric evaluation has been shown to decrease the need for admission.[12]

After the evaluation is complete, there is often an unproductive time spent waiting for placement at a psychiatric facility. While patients are boarding, clinicians can begin the following therapeutic interventions to both shorten the time before treatment and improve the patient's condition:

- *Telepsychiatry*—An additional benefit of utilizing telemedicine is utilizing the consultant to recommend initial treatment while the patient is waiting for placement. Ultimately, this early management can lead to de-escalation of symptoms and shorter stays on the inpatient side.
- *Medical management*—Starting medical management benefits the patients and the department. Earlier medical treatment is likely to lessen the necessity for restraints and may calm agitated patients, facilitating a more therapeutic environment for all.
- *Case management*—Case managers have a more expansive knowledge of the resources available in the community and are often better able to arrange a disposition plan.

Make More Efficient Use of Existing Capacity

Operationalizing a "Lean" approach to the evaluation and assessment of behavioral health patients can facilitate improved throughput. It is first necessary to understand the bottlenecks, their causes, and the reasons for their existence before implementing solutions. Some of the potential methods to manage capacity constraints include:

- *Behavioral health section*—Depending upon the volume and acuity of behavioral patients, creating a distinct section of the ED dedicated to behavioral health patients may create efficiency. This approach can address safety concerns and create a more calming environment. If the behavioral patient volume is inadequate or separate ED space is unavailable, utilizing this approach may worsen operational bottlenecks and has the potential to create further stigma for behavioral health patients.
- *A psychiatric emergency service (PES)*—A designated PES requires a significant financial commitment and takes time to set up, but it can significantly improve care delivery (see Case Two below).
- *Community paramedicine programs*—Some emergency medical service (EMS) agencies partner with hospitals to help patients find the right environment for their care needs. The program requires substantial community care coordination among the EMS service, the ED (when urgent evaluation is required), community clinics, and dedicated psychiatric facilities.
- *State bed registry*—This mechanism matches the real-time demand for and supply of beds and other necessary community resources. These registries can eliminate the frequent duplicative work of finding an inpatient bed for patients in the ED. Many states have developed or are in the process of developing these registries.[13] Ideally, these programs will provide real-time accurate data. Registries are a positive step in the direction of matching demand and capacity.

CASE STUDIES

Two case studies are provided to demonstrate successful process changes to enhance care to mental health patients.

Case One – The Carilion Approach: Mental Health Patients Boarding in the ED

It is advisable to stop thinking of these patients as ED patients or *boarders* and instead consider them mental health inpatients waiting for transfer to their inpatient beds. This is an important distinction that changes the language of administrators and providers to better conceptualize this pervasive problem.

Understanding the current relationship between prolonged mental health patient stays and the boarding of hospitalized patients in the ED is a key step in the process improvement of overall LOS and quality of care. The Carilion Clinic in Roanoke, Virginia, has instituted a broad array of enhancements that address many of the process improvements previously discussed in this chapter and provides proof that such steps can have profound effects on the management of mental health patients.

Process Changes

Over a single year, changes in arrival processing, throughput, and disposition of mental health patients cut the average boarding times of these patients by 50%, from 15 hours to 7.5 hours (**Figure 50.3**). The average number of days per month that mental health patients spent in excess of 13 hours in the ED was reduced from more than 15 days per month to less than 1 day per month (**Figure 50.4**).

It was essential to make existing capacity more efficient and improve law enforcement collaboration as examples of processes that were difficult to conceptualize but were key in making the changes into effective and efficient management of these patients. The experience at the Carilion Clinic demonstrates several concrete examples of these changes.

Mapping the Process

The Carilion Clinic began by mapping the ED process in its then-current state. Opportunities for improvement and reductions in redundancy became readily apparent

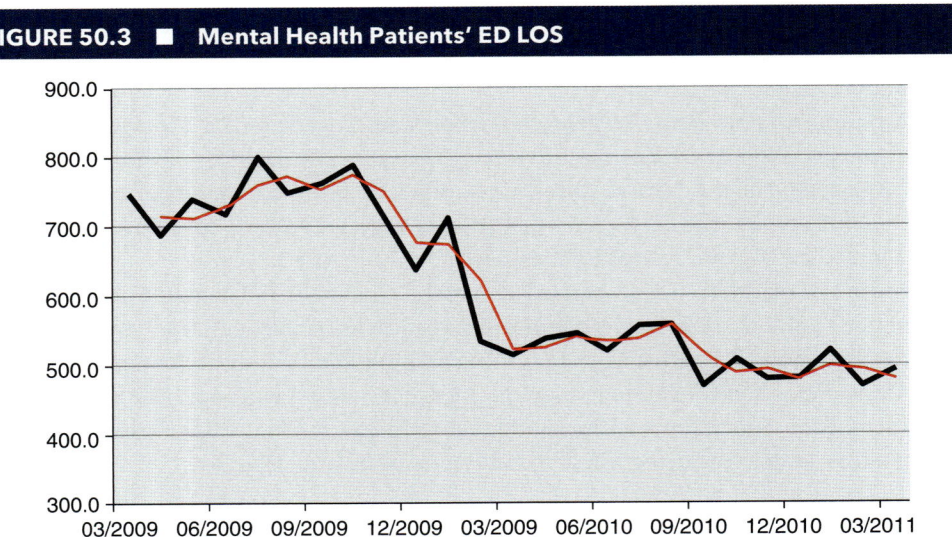

FIGURE 50.3 ■ Mental Health Patients' ED LOS

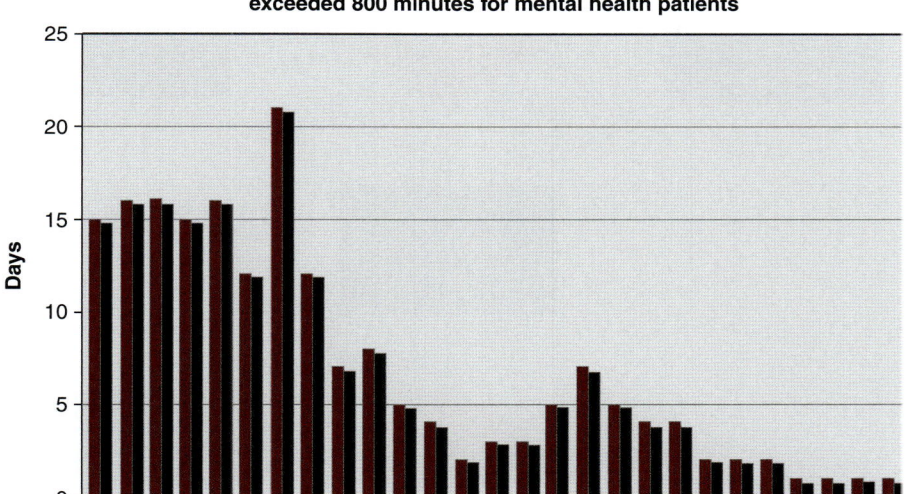

FIGURE 50.4 ■ ED LOS Exceeding 800 Minutes

when diagrammed. The creation of an idealized form became a clear road map for all parts of the system to follow, to be used every time a mental health patient entered the ED.

While it may be difficult to define when *boarding* begins, efforts to improve all phases of the mental health patients' care positively affect boarding times. Mental health patients in the Carilion Clinic ED are identified immediately on arrival, and all of these patients receive a Level 1 triage category (based on Emergency Severity Index system of a five-level triage). This categorization signifies to all team members that the moment a mental health patient enters the system, they are high-risk patients, and require multiple resources. In addition, standardizing intake for these patients and creating a dedicated ED mental health unit results in safe and reliable placement (**Figure 50.5**).

Standard order sets and processing of mental health patients are initiated by the nursing team. Patients who meet the criteria for rapid medical clearance are immediately taken to the dedicated emergency psychiatric area where they are met by core nursing staff. Expanding the ED team to include dedicated nurses who direct and staff this zone creates champions for this unique patient population. This dedicated staff is more familiar with the many complicated legal and social aspects of caring for mental health patients.

The volume of excess nursing time required to manage so many boarders in the ED, along with the lost revenue from decreased ED capacity, were used as arguments for increasing expenditures to expand staffing with additional mental health nurse practitioners and nursing staff (especially on weekends). Expanded weekend rounding made additional beds available for ED patients during peak times.

The community and law enforcement were also engaged to assist in the reduction of ED crowding and boarding times. The sheriff's department in multiple jurisdictions committed to improved response times for transporting patients on mental health holds. The long waits for available officers to transport patients to other facilities were greatly reduced. County and city magistrates and police departments were invited to provide additional solutions for managing frequent mental health patients and those with substance abuse problems.

Managing Repeat Mental Health Patients

One solution was directed to improving care for frequent *attenders* to the ED, particularly those with alcohol addiction and suicidal ideation. Magistrates and police had also become

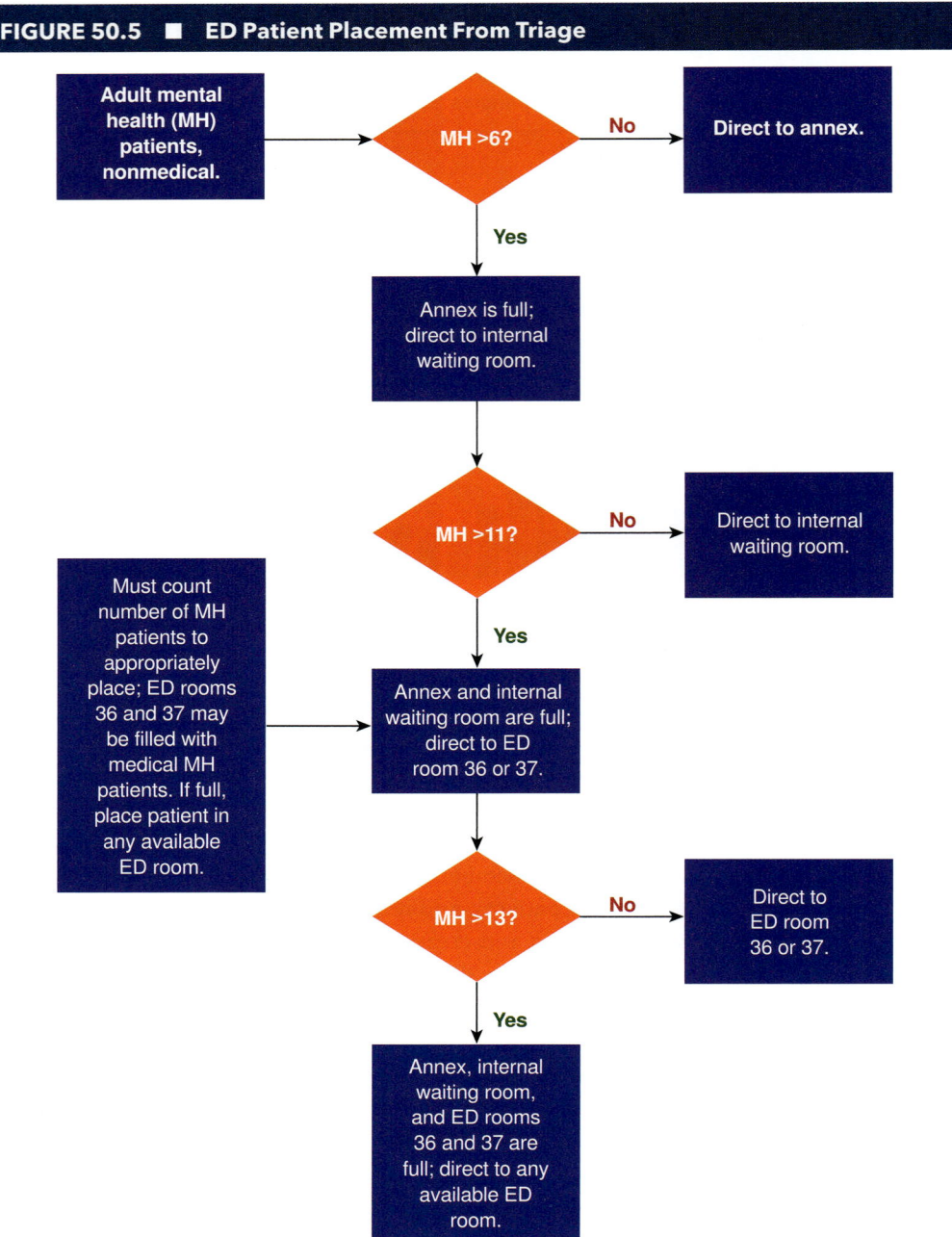

FIGURE 50.5 ■ ED Patient Placement From Triage

frustrated by the recurrent requests for ED and protective custody orders for this population. Such patients are particularly challenging in the ED because many have an initial level of intoxication that makes it difficult to assess or admit them to an inpatient mental health unit. Frequently, upon gaining sobriety, some of these patients deny their suicidal ideation.

Now, those entered into the program are identified at triage; if found to be intoxicated with suicidal ideation, they are provided a medical screening examination and then, when appropriate, remanded to the city police department for safe holding. Upon achieving sobriety and potential release, if the patients are still voicing suicidal ideation, they are returned to the ED for further mental health evaluation. However, if already established with a mental health community partner, the patients are directed to outpatient facilities. Frequent attenders to the ED for mental health problems who do not have substance abuse problems are also entered into coordinated care plans that allow for automatic admissions and discharges from the ED based on certain criteria.

Expanded Mental Health Coverage

Mental health patients are complex and frequently suffer from chronic medical problems, many of which are poorly controlled because of the patient's mental instability. Prolonged waits for inpatient mental health beds can result in the deterioration of comorbidities, further prolonging ED stays or resulting in a medical admission. The Carilion Clinic elected to expand physician coverage by adding a daily physician rounder responsible for mental health patients in the ED. The addition of this physician coverage for two hours each day:

- Improved initiation of outpatient medications and treatment plans
- Reduced the number of mental health patients being admitted due to medical deterioration
- Improved care coordination with the inpatient mental health teams

Another collaborative care improvement in the ED focused on patients with overdoses or uncontrolled chronic medical problems who had mental health complaints. Previously, the emergency physician was required to perform medical clearance and monitoring, commonly 4 to 6 hours for most mild or moderate overdoses, and then proceed with the psychiatric consultation. These patients now undergo an assessment for medical clearance and mental health-related complaints in parallel.

Case Two – The University of North Carolina Approach: Developing a PES

The University of North Carolina (UNC) Department of Emergency Medicine chose the approach of developing a PES to address the issues of time to evaluation. Despite having an available psychiatric residency program, the UNC ED saw a year-over-year increase in the volume of behavioral health patients as well as an escalating LOS (**Figure 50.6**). Because the volume of patients requiring a psychiatric consultation overwhelmed the infrastructure and operations of the ED, department leaders chose to collaborate with the hospital to create the PES team. The UNC program chose to address the time to evaluation as its primary focus.

Prior to the institution of the PES, the mental health patient flow process utilized the traditional consult model in which all patients were evaluated and discussed with an attending psychiatrist. The same consulting service was also managing and rounding on boarding patients in the ED, limiting their capacity to assess new mental health patients. The

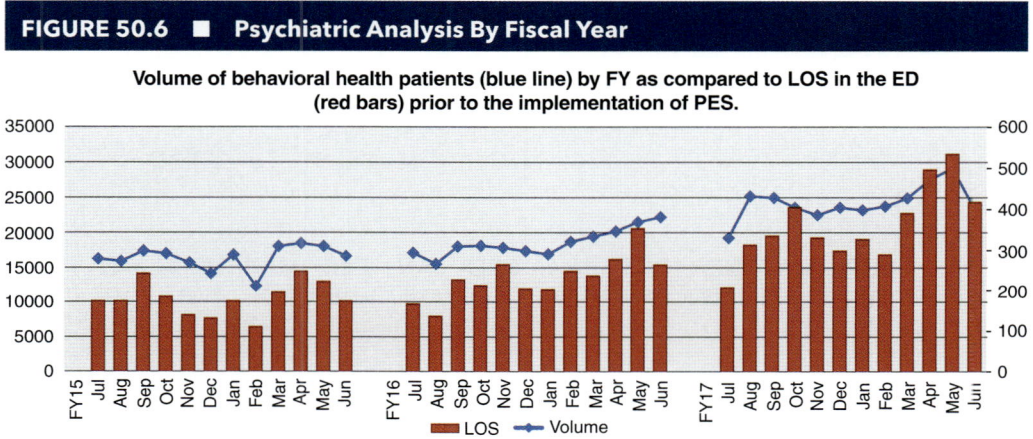

FIGURE 50.6 ■ Psychiatric Analysis By Fiscal Year

Volume of behavioral health patients (blue line) by FY as compared to LOS in the ED (red bars) prior to the implementation of PES.

situation became untenable, causing a poor experience and morale for patients, ED staff, and consulting staff and creating significant capacity constraints for the medical (nonbehavioral health) patients.

Implementing the PES

The PES began in July 2017. The PES team consisted of coverage that included a(n):

- Physician for 8 hours
- Licensed clinical social worker (LCSW) for 24 hours
- Advanced practice provider (APP) for 16 hours
- Clerical staff member for 8 hours

This was a total of 56 hours of coverage per day; the prior model had 88 hours of coverage deployed in a different model. The team was directed to focus on the time between emergency physician assessment and consultant evaluation. Once the consultant evaluation was complete and recommendations for treatment provided, the clerical support person would assist with placement.

In addition, the emergency physicians would follow up on the recommendations of the team while patients who were mental health inpatients were boarding in the ED. **Figure 50.7** demonstrates the results of the focus on door-to-evaluation times, demonstrating the time from ED arrival to PES evaluation. The remarkable performance improvement demonstrates the positive impact of changes in workflow while maintaining focus on important metrics. The PES model changed how patients were assessed and allowed the LCSWs and APPs to evaluate patients and practice to their full abilities. The attending psychiatrist was no longer the bottleneck.

Impact on Other Factors

While the directive given to the PES team was to focus on door-to-evaluation times, other benefits to the ED ensued. As a state, North Carolina had poor access to inpatient psychiatric beds. The expectation was that time to evaluation might improve, but the time from disposition to placement would not improve due to the limited inpatient resources. The experience was contrary to the expectation, as demonstrated in **Figure 50.8**. The ED LOS

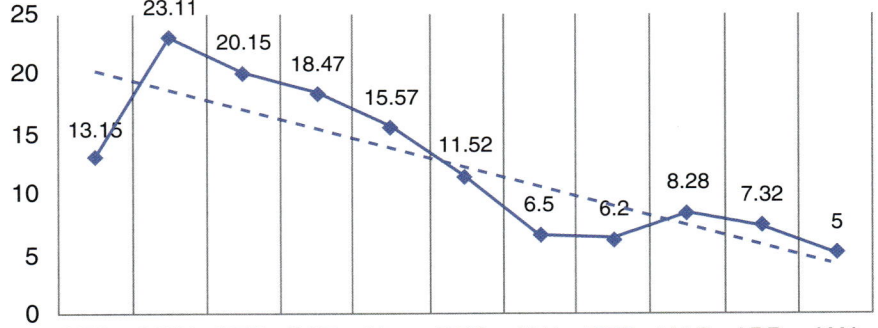

FIGURE 50.7 ■ Reduction in Evaluation Times With PES

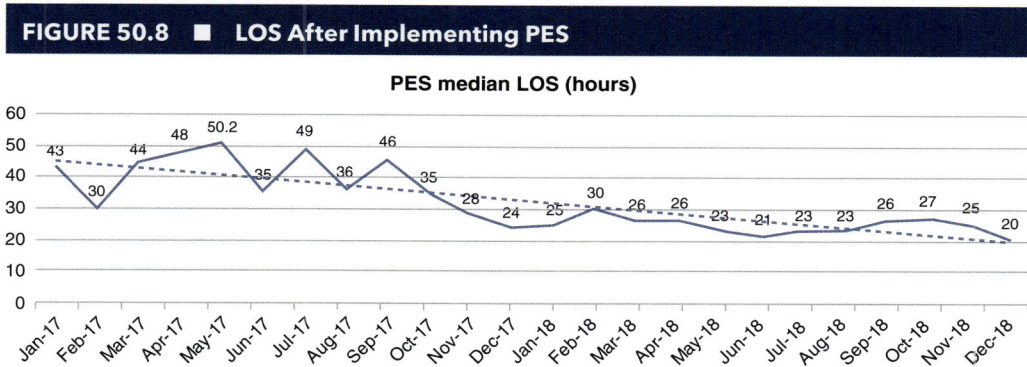

FIGURE 50.8 ■ LOS After Implementing PES

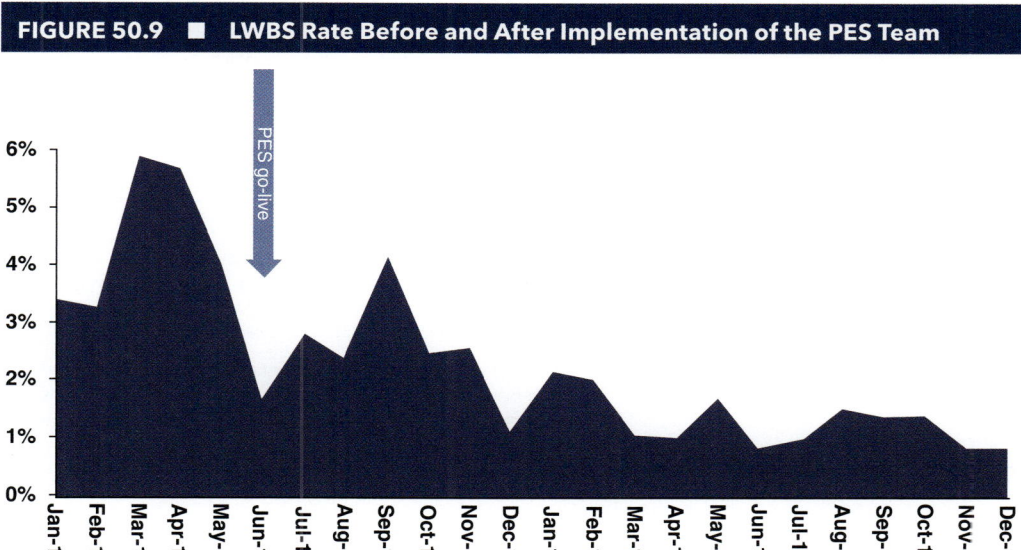

FIGURE 50.9 ■ LWBS Rate Before and After Implementation of the PES Team

for behavioral health patients improved by greater than the amount of reduction in arrival to evaluation times. The reasons are multifactorial, but simply stated, the overall process improvement had positive unintended consequences.

Finally, the overall ED door (arrival)-to-evaluation times metric also showed improvement. The ED had experienced a rise in the left without being seen (LWBS) rate in early 2017 due to the capacity constraints caused by behavioral health patient boarding. The implementation of the PES team led to a significant reduction in the LWBS rate, which has been maintained (**Figure 50.9**).

CONCLUSION

Improving the flow and treatment of behavioral health patients in the ED has received very limited attention and support. A strategy to quantify the problem, enhance the care of this vulnerable population, and make more efficient use of existing capacity are discrete steps that can improve improve the management of psychiatric patients *and* the overall flow of the ED.

REFERENCES

1. National Council for Behavioral Health. Community Mental Health Act. Available at: https://www.thenationalcouncil.org/about/national-mental-health-association/overview/community-mental-health-act/#:~:text=On%20October%2031%2C%201963%2C%20President, of%20optimism%20in%20mental%20healthcare. Updated 2020. Accessed August 8, 2020.

2. Lutterman T, Shaw R, Fisher W, et al. Trend in psychiatric inpatient capacity, United States and each state, 1970 to 2014. 2017. Available at: https://www.nasmhpd.org/sites/default/files/TACPaper.2.Psychiatric-Inpatient-Capacity_508C.pdf. Accessed August 8, 2020.

3. Axeen S, Menchine M, Santilanes G, et al. National trends in mental health-related emergency department visits by children and adults, 2009–2015. USC Leonard D. Schaeffer Center for Health Policy & Economics. 2020. Available at: https://healthpolicy.usc.edu/research/national-trends-in-mental-health-related-emergency-department-visits-by-children-and-adults-2009-2015/#:~: text=Results, to%20 20.4%25%20(p%20%3C%20. Accessed August 8, 2020.

4. Fuller DA, Sinclair E, Lamb HR, et al. Emptying the 'New Asylums' a beds capacity model to reduce mental illness behind bars. 2017. Available at: https://www.treatmentadvocacycenter.org/storage/documents/emptying-new-asylums-exec-summary.pdf. Accessed August 8, 2020.

5. Nicks BA, Manthey DM. The impact of psychiatric patient boarding in emergency departments. *Emerg Med Int*. 2012;2012:360308. 2012. Available at: https://pubmed.ncbi.nlm.nih.gov/22888437/. Accessed August 8, 2020.

6. Kalb LG, Stapp EK, Ballard ED, et al. Trends in psychiatric emergency department visits among youth and young adults in the US. *Pediatrics*. 2019;143(4).

7. Wiler JL. Care of the psychiatric patient in the emergency department—a review of the literature—A White Paper. American College of Emergency Physicians. 2014. Available at: https://www.acep.org/globalassets/uploads/uploaded-files/acep/clinical-and-practice-management/resources/mental-health-and-substance-abuse/psychiatric-patient-care-in-the-ed-2014.pdf. Accessed August 8, 2020.

8. Alakeson V, Pande N, Ludwig M. A plan to reduce emergency room 'boarding' of psychiatric patients. 2010. Available at: https://pubmed.ncbi.nlm.nih.gov/20820019/. Accessed August 8, 2020.

9. Augustine JJ. The latest emergency department utilization numbers are in. *ACEPNews*. October 20, 2019. Available at: https://www.acepnow.com/article/the-latest-emergency-department-utilization-numbers-are-in/. Accessed August 8, 2020.

10. Farley HL, Troutman GA, Brown A, et al. Practical solutions to boarding of psychiatric patients in the emergency department. American College of Emergency Physicians. 2015. Available at: https://www.macep.org/Files/Behavioral%20Health%20Boarding/Practical%20Solutions%20to%20Boarding%20of%20Psych%20Patients%20in%20EDs.pdf. Accessed August 8, 2020.

11. ACEP. iCAR2E: a tool for managing suicidal patient in the ED. American College of Emergency Physicians. Available at: https://www.acep.org/patient-care/iCar2e/. Updated 2020. Accessed August 8, 2020.

12. Seidel RW, Kilgus MD. Agreement between telepsychiatry assessment and face-to-face assessment for Emergency Department psychiatry patients. *J Telemed Telecare*. 2014. Available at: https://journals.sagepub.com/doi/10.1177/1357633X13519902. Accessed August 8, 2020.

13. Department of Health and Human Services. National Mental Health Services Survey (N-MHSS0): 2017. 2018. Available at: https://www.samhsa.gov/data/report/national-mental-health-services-survey-n-mhss-2017-data-mental-health-treatment-facilities. Accessed August 8, 2020.

CHAPTER 51

HOSPITAL MEDICINE

Robert W. Strauss, Thom A. Mayer, Michael Corvini, Hammad Rizvi

> ... [T]he forces promoting the use of the [hospitalist] model are sufficiently compelling ... improved clinical outcomes, lower costs, better education for physicians, and greater satisfaction on the part of patients.[1]
>
> —Robert M. Wachter, MD, and Lee Goldman, MD

The evolution, or more appropriately the revolution, in the management of inpatient care is a valuable example of how health care has adapted to meet the needs of patients and those who care for patients (clinicians and institutions). Born of the quest for consistent quality and increased efficiency, hospital medicine (HM) has transformed a large segment of the hospital-based health care delivery system. It has simultaneously relieved primary care physicians (PCPs) of the increasingly complex burden of balancing inpatient care with that of office-based practice.

WHAT IS HOSPITAL MEDICINE?

The Society of Hospital Medicine (SHM), defines a HM clinician or "hospitalist" as one whose primary professional focus is the general care of hospitalized patients and who engages in teaching, research, and enhancing the performance of hospitals and the health-care system.[2] The role of the hospitalist is to coordinate care during the hospital stay, often referred to as inpatient services. The specialty is broad in scope, with the majority of hospitalist physicians trained in internal medicine, family medicine, or pediatrics. Hospital medicine fellowships are increasing in number as HM has become a desirable "career path."

Work in the hospitalist field normally requires board certification in a primary care specialty. Clinicians who become hospitalists generally work only in the hospital and do not maintain an outside practice. Their role characteristically starts with the patient's evaluation after being informed by the emergency department (ED) clinician (or PCP in the case of direct admissions) that hospitalization is required. The hospitalist then works to provide the most appropriate treatment and patient experience, monitor the patient's progress, provide daily supervision, manage postdischarge planning and follow-up, and ultimately discharge the patient to the next level of care. Currently, HM includes multiple subspecialties, some of which are listed in **Table 51.1**.

The Why

The exponential advances in medicine, technology, evidence, and information have required medical institutions and providers to implement innovative approaches to quality and efficiency.[3] Hospitalists directly impact inpatient care by simultaneously improving the patient experience and appropriately utilizing hospital resources—a necessity in an increasingly cost-constrained environment.[4] This reassignment of responsibilities has

TABLE 51.1 ■ Hospital Medicine Subspecialties

Hospitalist Type	Care Provided
Hospitalists	Adult inpatient care
Pediatric hospitalists	Pediatric inpatient care
Surgicalists	Inpatient care for surgical patients
Intensivists	Intensive care unit care
Nocturnists	Night care for inpatients
Laborists	Obstetrical care

significantly improved patient care and overall hospital performance, while decreasing length of stay (LOS).[5]

Hospital medicine continues to grow primarily because it provides "value" by raising satisfaction and quality while lowering costs. Hospitalists can also save the hospital from financial penalties levied by regulatory agencies resulting from inappropriate admissions, costly readmissions, and health care-acquired conditions (HACs). Hospital medicine continues to overcome new challenges and find new opportunities to refine inpatient care through the collaborative expansion of relationships with other providers. Hospital medicine has captured the attention of multiple organizations interested in expanding their capacity to provide broad solutions to health-care organizations. Some have taken the form of small regional and large national hospitalist groups. Others involve moderate-to-large practice management companies that provide more diversified health-care solutions.

EVOLUTION OF HM

The last two decades have witnessed the fastest growth of HM, with now more than 50,000 practicing hospitalists.[6] In the mid-1990s, physicians Robert Wachter and Lee Goldman coined the term "hospitalist," describing clinicians who focus their efforts on managing the care of inpatients.[7] As Medicare changed reimbursement to a fixed-payment system, PCPs still attended to traditional recovery stays in the hospital on a fee-for-service physician schedule.[8]

Through the simultaneous delivery of quality and efficiency, HM has proven its ability to transform satisfaction and performance in a large segment of the health-care delivery system while simultaneously relieving PCPs of the increasing inpatient burden. Over the years, inpatient care has become increasingly complex and challenging, with mandates to address LOS, patient experience, and readmission benchmarks among many other value-based metrics. It has become increasingly difficult for PCPs with their own office workflow challenges to be responsive to the real-time demands of the acutely ill hospitalized patient while still conducting office hours. In addition, outpatient reimbursement has decreased, requiring PCPs to see more office patients and further limiting their ability to efficiently round at the hospital.

When hospitalists emerged as a solution to these problems, other challenges arose. Burnout and insufficient transitions of hospital care to community physicians were among the top concerns. Over time, the hospitalist structure evolved into different scheduling models to provide the best patient care. Block scheduling still remains the predominant model for most programs (e.g., 7 days on followed by 7 days off), but there are several other approaches that help inherent physician burnout and continuity of care.[9]

With the advent of advanced electronic medical records (EMRs), such as EPIC and Cerner, as well as many HIPAA-compliant communication modalities, transitions of care have improved significantly. Within the HM specialty, some practice management companies have found that the seamless integration of an HM program results in valuable synergism. A prime example is the collaboration with the ED.

THE VALUE OF HM

Hospital medicine programs offer extraordinary value to various stakeholders, including patients, PCPs, subspecialists, emergency physicians, and hospitals. Hospitalists, like emergency physicians, interact with all clinicians, staff, departments, and the sickest of patients. An effective service-oriented group provides coordinated care that enhances the health of patients and supports their colleagues.

Patients

Hospitalists practice exclusively within the hospital setting and offer unprecedented availability on an as-needed, real-time basis. Hospitalists also possess significant inpatient medical expertise as well as fluency in the nuances of coordinating care, including the role of consultants. This combination of availability and expertise has translated into improvements in quality, safety, efficiency, and satisfaction.

Primary Care Practitioners

Primary care physicians have benefited from the evolution of HM in several ways. Most PCPs have experienced an improvement in their quality of life, as the presence of hospitalists has obviated the challenge of dividing their time between the office and the hospital. Many PCPs have found that focusing exclusively on their private practice has allowed them to build volume, refine their business practices, improve the patient experience, and increase revenue. Hospitalists have also provided a convenient solution to the time-intensive and poorly reimbursed requirement of being "on call" to provide care to the growing population of unassigned and uninsured patients.

Subspecialists

When hospitalists serve as the attending of record for patients requiring specialized services, subspecialists are relieved of the arduous task of coordinating care and writing lengthy admission and discharge notes. Freedom from these responsibilities allows these providers to focus exclusively on their roles as consultants and increase their consultation volumes. Subspecialists who receive performance-based compensation have also benefited from the ability of hospitalists to decrease complications, LOS, and cost per case while improving the overall quality of care.

Emergency Departments

The expertise and availability of hospitalists results in significant efficiency gains for EDs. By reducing inpatient LOS and increasing early discharges, hospitalist programs can improve throughput and eliminate downstream delays. A prompt response to ED admission requests can further improve department efficiency. Using demand–capacity analyses to align hospitalist resources and hardwire flow in the transition from ED to inpatient care is a best practice.

An efficient hospitalist service can significantly improve ED throughput metrics, decrease boarding, decrease left without treatment (LWOT) percentages, improve patient experience, and improve clinical outcomes. The recovery of lost volume from LWOTs and the improved public perception from enhanced inpatient and ED patient experience can result in increased ED volume and collections.

A collegial and collaborative relationship between emergency physicians and hospitalists facilitates the challenging task of determining a patient's need for hospitalization and accurately assigning an inpatient or observation status. Hospitalists can also serve as the primary resource for rapid-response and code teams, allowing emergency clinicians to focus on the care of patients in the ED.

Nurses

The availability and consistency of hospitalists facilitates communication and teamwork, enhancing the working relationship between clinicians and nurses. Innovative patient-care models, including geographic rounding, bedside physician/nurse rounding, and multidisciplinary rounding, have leveraged the collaborative relationship between hospitalists and nurses to result in significant gains in quality, safety, efficiency, and patient and staff satisfaction.

Hospitals

Among their many advantages, effective hospitalist programs reduce LOS, increase efficiency, provide evidence-based and cost-appropriate care, align incentives, enhance outcomes, foster consistent management strategies, and improve the patient experience. It is important to note that the direct collections from a hospitalist service typically do not exceed the costs. Consequently, hospitals must provide financial support to hospitalist services in the form of a subsidy. However, hospitalist services are generally justified on the basis of the financial ROI (indirect revenues) made by the hospital. This dynamic makes it important to examine both financially quantifiable and nonquantifiable values provided by hospitalist services.

Quantifiable Financial Benefits

Hospitalist services provide financially quantifiable value to hospitals through a combination of reducing expenses and increasing revenue.

Reducing Expenses

Hospital costs reliably increase as LOS increases. Conversely, hospital reimbursement is driven by diagnosis-related groups (DRGs) and does not generally increase with LOS. In this environment of relatively fixed reimbursement based on diagnosis, a hospitalist service that decreases LOS will reduce overall hospital expenses.

Hospitalist services also reduce hospital expenses by decreasing the cost per case through lean resource utilization. Clinically adept hospitalists utilize evidence-based care plans to avoid unnecessary and expensive diagnostic tests and therapies and are able to defer nonessential testing to the outpatient setting. For example, by coordinating with a PCP, a hospitalist can often defer nonemergent magnetic resonance imaging (MRIs) to the outpatient setting. This reduces the cost of care, reduces the MRI demand, decreases LOS, and redirects testing to the outpatient environment, where costs are typically lower and capacity is typically greater. Of note, studies have suggested that more efficient care, including the earlier use of resources, also reduces LOS, independent of overall expenditure, making the timing of resource utilization an influencing factor on LOS.[10-12]

Another important example of lean resource utilization is antibiotic stewardship. Hospitalists significantly reduce expenses by decreasing inappropriate initial antibiotic utilization and limiting the duration of therapy. Effective antibiotic stewardship programs improve individual patient quality and safety as well as overall public health.

Effective hospitalist programs reduce insurance company denials by playing a pivotal role in determining the status of hospitalized patients. Maximizing status accuracy reduces the direct and indirect costs of status-based payer denials. When denials do occur, hospitalists participate in substantiating medical necessity and appealing denials.

Hospitalist programs also help hospitals avoid costly penalties. Collaboration with other clinicians (emergency physicians, PCPs and post-acute care facilities) can reliably reduce readmissions and associated penalties. By following best-practice protocols, hospitalists can also significantly reduce HACs and the associated penalties.

Increasing Revenue

A highly effective hospitalist service can increase revenue through the expansion of market share. The consistent provision of high-quality care, coupled with an optimized patient experience and exemplary communication with PCPs, can result in increased referral volume.

In hospitals that are functioning at or near full capacity, decreasing inpatient LOS can further enhance revenue. In situations of unmet patient demand, improved inpatient throughput can create additional "virtual" inpatient bed availability, capturing revenue that would otherwise be lost.

This additional bed availability also allows the ED to evaluate patients who might have otherwise LWOT. Considering that some of these patients will require hospitalization, a small decrease in LWOT volume coupled with a corresponding increase in ED and hospitalization volumes can result in significant financial gains for the hospital.

Surgical hospitalist/acute care surgery programs can dramatically improve response time for ED and inpatient surgical emergencies and consultations, enhancing surgical smoothing, which is a critical determinant of hospital profitability.

The inpatient specialization of hospitalists facilitates the development of exemplary documentation practices. This improves the capture of DRGs, including associated comorbidities; increases case mix index (CMI); and enhances facility reimbursement.

Nonquantifiable Benefits

Hospitalists perform various off-service and add-on encounters. They often develop and lead rapid-response and code teams, observation medicine services, hyperbaric medicine/wound care services, and others. Hospitalist services also form the backbone of clinician education initiatives. Hospitalists serve as faculty for graduate medical education programs, including residency programs and medical school clerkships. They also frequently provide in-service programs and informal education to clinicians, nurses, ancillary staff members, and hospital administrators.

An exemplary hospitalist program can make significant contributions to the overall culture and leadership of a hospital by serving as a platform for the promotion of hospital values and improvement initiatives. Individual hospitalists can become leaders or members of the medical staff and hospital committees. Hospitalist groups can also leverage their central position in hospital operations and medical staff relations to be a catalyst for the integration and alignment of multiple service lines and departments.

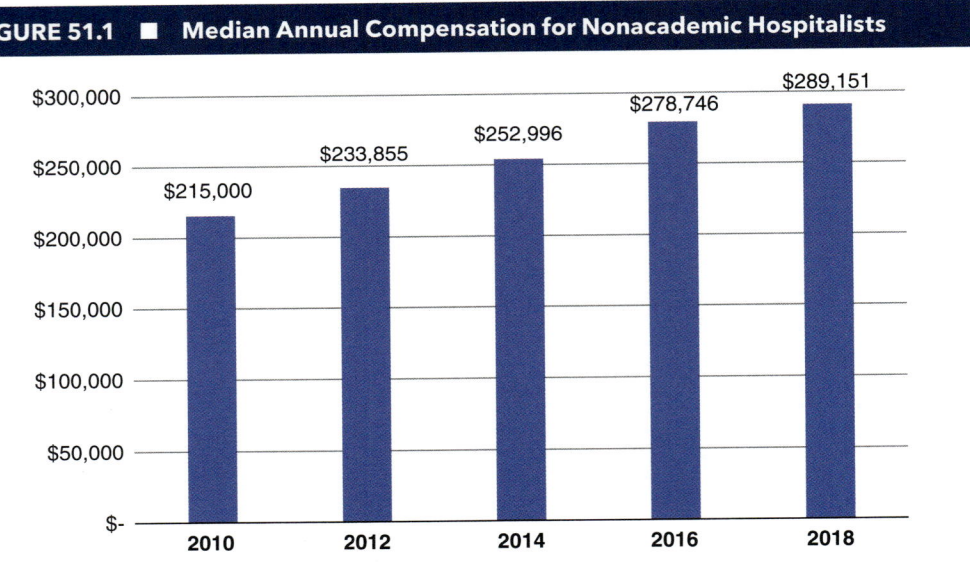

FIGURE 51.1 ■ Median Annual Compensation for Nonacademic Hospitalists

THE COST OF HM

The cost of hospitalist programs typically exceeds the direct reimbursement for their services, necessitating subsidization. As market forces have driven salaries upward and reimbursement downward, subsidy requirements have increased. Based on 2018 survey data from the Medical Group Management Association, the median nonacademic adult hospitalist compensation was $289,151, an increase of 35% from 2010 to 2018 (**Figure 51.1**).[13] In the same report, the SHM states the median amount of subsidy support per full-time equivalent (FTE) for adult hospitalists in 2017 was $176,657, up 12.1% from 2016.[13] There are significant regional variations in the degree of subsidy support, with the midwestern US requiring the most per FTE and western US requiring the least (**Figure 51.2**).

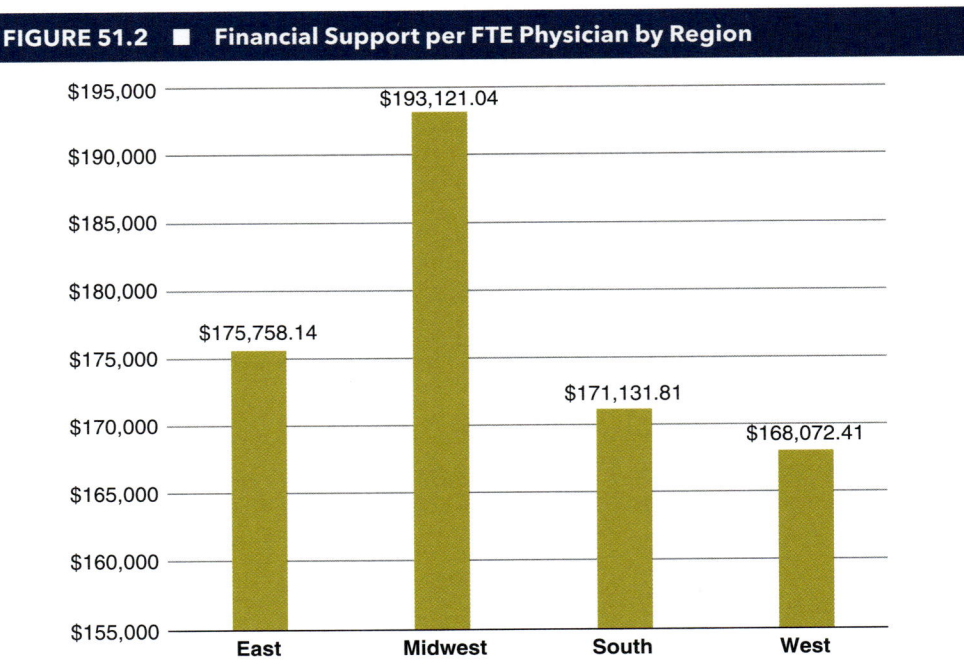

FIGURE 51.2 ■ Financial Support per FTE Physician by Region

The ROI

Even in the face of escalating subsidy requirements, the financially quantifiable value that hospitalist programs provide creates a substantial ROI.

Length of Stay Reduction

In order to calculate the savings yielded through LOS reduction, it is first necessary to determine the number of bed stays saved and then multiply the number of annual bed days saved by the daily cost of operating a bed. The daily cost of operating a bed varies per facility and is usually tracked by hospital administrations. These savings can be estimated through two related formulas:

$$Length\ of\ stay\ savings = Bed\ days\ saved \times Cost\ per\ bed$$

$$Bed\ days\ saved = Average\ length\ of\ stay\ reduction \times Annual\ admissions$$

Cost Per Case Reduction

Given the escalating costs of health care, lean resource utilization can lead to significant cost savings for hospitals. The savings yielded through cost per case reduction can be approximated by this formula:

$$Cost\ per\ case\ reduction\ savings = Annual\ admissions \times Cost\ per\ case \times Percent\ reduction\ in\ cost$$

Cost per case is variable and is typically tracked closely by hospital administrations.

Improved Case Mix Index

Whereas reduced LOS and reduced cost per case drive ROI by decreasing expenses, improved CMI enhances ROI by increasing revenue. Through a combination of optimal documentation practices and collaboration with case managers and clinical documentation specialists, hospitalists can maximize appropriate capture of DRGs, including comorbidities. These practices can increase CMI and hospital collections. The increased revenue can be estimated through the following formula:

$$Increased\ collections = Improvement\ in\ point\ value\ of\ CMI \times Average\ collections\ per\ point\ of\ CMI$$

CMI is typically tracked closely by hospital administrations; small changes can have profound impacts on reimbursement.

Increased Volume

Increased volume is another potential source of revenue enhancement. A hospitalist program increases hospital volume through two primary mechanisms. First, hospitalist programs can increase referrals and market share. The increased revenue derived from increased volume can be estimated by the following formula:

$$Increased\ revenue = Number\ of\ additional\ hospitalizations \times Average\ collection\ per\ hospitalization$$

The average collection per hospitalization represents a blended average of the collections for admissions and observations. These figures vary per facility and are usually tracked by hospital administrations.

Second, as described earlier, hospitalist programs can increase volume when hospitals are operating close to maximum capacity by decreasing LOS to create additional "virtual" bed capacity. Hospitals tend to run efficiently at occupancy rates of 85% or less (see Chapter 34). As hospital occupancy exceeds 85%, however, emerging inefficiencies may result in slower or delayed admission processing, boarding of patients in the ED, and greater numbers of ED patients who leave without treatment. As ED LWOT percentages increase, the potential for additional revenue capture through increased hospitalizations increases.

While it is theoretically possible that every bed day saved will result in an additional hospitalization, this is typically not the case. The actual number of additional hospitalizations created by LOS reduction is largely determined by the overall number of LWOT patients and the acuity of illness among this population. To account for this variability, the predicted impact of LOS reduction on revenue generation can be modulated by the use of an "impact modifier."

The impact modifier is typically considered to be 0% in hospitals operating below 85% occupancy, negating any potential revenue enhancement. As occupancy approaches 100%, however, depending on the estimated acuity of illness in the LWOT population, the impact modifier can be increased and the opportunity for revenue enhancement can become significant.

The increased revenue produced by expanding virtual bed capacity can be estimated through the following formula:

$$\text{Increased revenue} = \text{Bed days saved} \times \text{Impact modifier} \times \text{Average collection per hospitalization}$$

Cost/ROI Analysis

While LOS reduction, cost per case reduction, improved CMI, and increased volume are the four most commonly used elements of hospitalist program ROI improvement, it is worth noting that they are not the only sources of financially quantifiable value. Reduction in denials, readmission penalties, and HAC penalties also contribute to the ROI. Additionally, hospitalist services confer substantial nonfinancially quantifiable value. See the ROI example in **Table 51.2**, which uses hypothetical data to demonstrate the four primary components of hospitalist program ROI and the overall ROI. Actual HM ROI will vary depending on local variables and should include other factors like denial reductions, readmission penalties, and HAC penalties.

Changing Perceptions

As the hospitalist model of care delivery has progressed from novel to ubiquitous, the perception of HM ROI has also changed significantly. When hospitalist groups first replaced nonhospitalist groups, large deltas in ROI components made the business model extremely attractive. However, now that HM has become the standard, ROI variability between groups has become less substantial, and performance variations among hospitalist groups have become the basis of comparison.

Simultaneously, deteriorating hospital profit margins have created an intense focus on cost containment, and escalating hospitalist salaries have increased subsidy requirements. Performance-based reimbursement has also emerged as a major determinant of hospital revenue. The need for a hospitalist group to deliver a substantial ROI by effectively decreasing costs and increasing revenue has become more important than ever.

THE STRUCTURE OF HM

Hospital medicine programs have consistently demonstrated substantial value and, as a result, have grown. When developing or expanding a program, the question is usually what type of a hospitalist program should be implemented.

Contracts

There are multiple contracting structures in place, including hospital employment and contracting with practice management groups **(Box 51.1)**. Each structure confers advantages and disadvantages. For instance, a hospital-employed program might create better hospital-hospitalist engagement but might have difficulty recruiting and managing metrics. Practice management groups tend to have a regional and/or national presence and use multiple successful methodologies in these domains, making them an attractive option for some hospitals.

Some smaller hospitals and rural facilities have the ED groups extend their management to include the hospitalist program in their facilities. Telemedicine programs also play a role in these smaller facilities because recruitment can be particularly challenging in remote areas. Telemedicine programs have many challenges, such as varying reimbursements by state and third-party payors and the lack of on-site availability for patient emergencies. For the latter, many telemedicine hospitalist programs incorporate an on-site emergency medicine (EM) physician or intensivist to respond to urgent encounters that require bedside support.

The Role of the Hospitalist

Case study: A 78-year-old woman with a past medical history of hypertension, congestive heart failure, and moderate dementia is determined by the ED physician to have worsening shortness of breath related to acute on chronic congestive heart failure. The emergency physician admits her to the hospitalist service, and she arrives on the cardiac floor with a cardiology consultation request.

Over the next 4 days, the patient is treated and stabilized. At least once every day, she is seen by the same hospitalist, and her care is discussed at the multidisciplinary rounds. After a physical therapy evaluation, the patient is found to be significantly deconditioned, and a transfer to a skilled nursing facility for transitional care is recommended. After completion of the medication reconciliation, the hospitalist communicates the plan of care with the family and PCP.

Ultimately, a detailed discharge summary is completed, and the patient is transitioned to the nursing home. Once the patient returns home from post-acute care, she follows up with her PCP, who has all the information about her hospital course.

BOX 51.1 ■ HOSPITALIST CONTRACTING STRUCTURES

- Hospital employees
- Contracting with companies solely providing hospital medicine services
- Contracting with groups or companies with multiple specialties, including hospital medicine, anesthesia, radiology, surgical services, obstetrical services, and others
- Employed by ED groups diversifying into hospital medicine at a single site

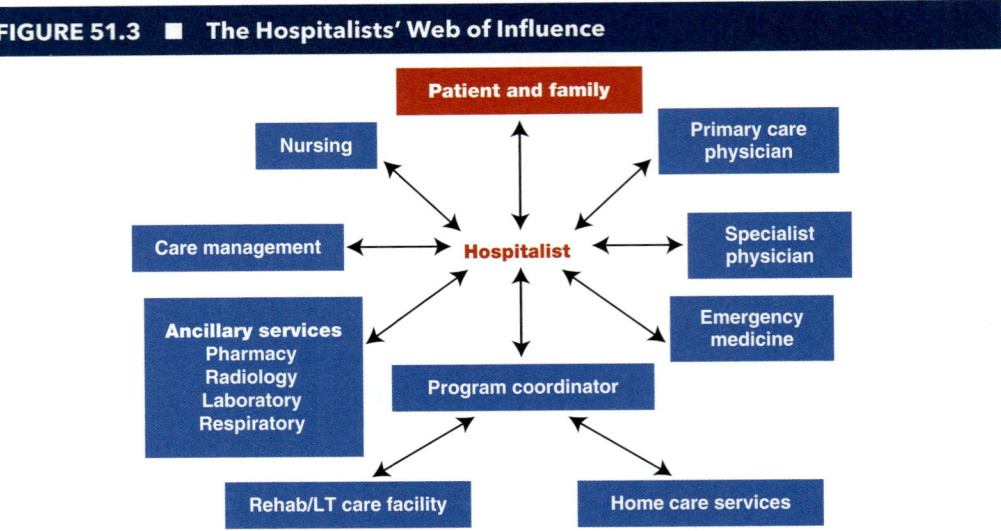

FIGURE 51.3 ■ The Hospitalists' Web of Influence

Some programs utilize hospitalists as the quarterbacks of their patient management team because they influence and interact with multiple key stakeholders, including ED clinicians, PCPs, specialists, case managers, patients, families, nursing staff, home care and post-acute care specialists (**Figure 51.3**).

Hospitalist services that are new to a facility may be viewed suspiciously by some members of the medical staff who fear that this service will lower their revenue by replacing the PCP's management of patients in the hospital and referring their private patients to other community providers upon discharge. Over time, however, PCPs and consultants usually develop strong relationships with the HM group and realize that their patients are best handled by hospitalists.

Hospitalists are positioned to efficiently manage admissions and serve as consultants—efficiently moving the patient from the point of entry to a bed on the inpatient floor. A common hospitalist performance metric is "discharge before 11 a.m." This rating spotlights that hospitalists can coordinate the care of their patients in the most efficient manner; how quickly the patient leaves the facility is just as important as how fast they leave the ED. Private practice PCPs have limited ability to efficiently respond to discharge requests.

Observation care is another area where each hour matters; once again, hospitalists are often best suited for the management of these patients. In fact, SHM estimates that approximately 59% of observation care for Medicare patients is provided by hospitalists.[14]

Advanced Practice Providers

Physician supply-and-demand issues are prevalent in HM as well as other medical and surgical specialties. As a result, advanced practice providers (APPs) are filling roles in hospitalist programs based on their permitted scope of service (**Figure 51.4**).[13] For example, some facilities allow APPs to function autonomously, and the hospitalist program may have them carry their own service with lower-acuity patients or even as dedicated providers for an observation unit with minimal physician oversight. In other facilities, the scope of the APP may be limited substantially; in these programs, they may be utilized more as care "extenders" (focused on discharges and transitions of care).

Coordination of Care

A day in the life of a hospitalist includes many tasks beyond the direct care of their patients. Daily multidisciplinary rounds are required to discuss barriers to inpatient care and discharge

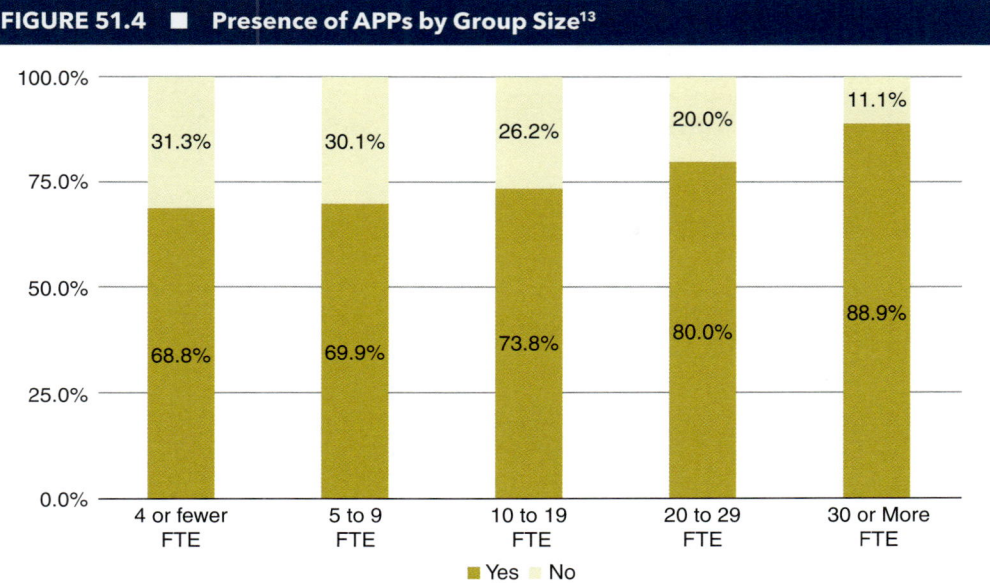

FIGURE 51.4 ■ Presence of APPs by Group Size[13]

KEY FINDINGS
- In teaching hospitals, Hospitalist Management Groups (HMGs) that provided teaching services only were less likely to employ nurse practitioners/physician assistants than HMGs that provided nonteaching services only.
- As group size increased, so did the presence of nurse practitioners/physician assistants.
- Use of nurse practitioners/physician assistants in academic HMGs increased from 52.1% in 2016 to 75.7% in 2018.
- A majority of nurse practitioner/physician assistant work was billed under their own provider number (78.0%) in 2018
- Respondents from the region of the West continue to have a very low adoption of nurse practitioners/physician assistants.

planning. These rounds typically include, but are not limited to, nursing staff, case managers, hospitalists, social workers, physical therapists, and palliative care personnel.

Large hospitalist programs often transition to geographic rounds, a best practice that ultimately leads to the better coordination of care while decreasing LOS and increasing patient satisfaction. This type of segmentation permits the team to spend more time with patients and less on continually reconstituting the team when moving unit to unit.[15] Teams may find it more efficient to perform multidisciplinary rounds in a meeting room (or at the nurses' station). At other times, collaborative bedside rounds are preferable to create a high-impact patient–family experience. A best practice is to identify bottlenecks during rounding and utilize lean tools to eliminate them.

Staffing and Scheduling

The number of hospitalists that see a patient from admission to discharge is often viewed as a marker of continuity of care. Provider continuity on day shifts (7 a.m. to 7 p.m.) is directly correlated with LOS and readmission metrics because most of their duties involve rounding on existing patients while doing some new admissions (**Figure 51.5**).[13] Block scheduling (7 on and 7 off) is associated with fewer handoffs. This scheduling pattern has become a common feature of HM programs and corresponds to a well-functioning program. However, the continuity of care during night shifts (typically from 7 p.m. to 7 a.m.) is less of a concern because night-provider duties are predominantly related to admitting new patients and cross-covering floor patients for urgent issues.

As a hospitalist program becomes larger, its coverage model (capacity) expands to match the demand from the ED. Typically, EDs are busiest in the afternoon and early evening hours. In order to add more staffing resources in a growing hospitalist program, an evening hospitalist swing shift often matches the increased ED workload. Different models assign the swing-shift hospitalist solely as an "admitter" or to both admit new patients and round on existing patients.[13]

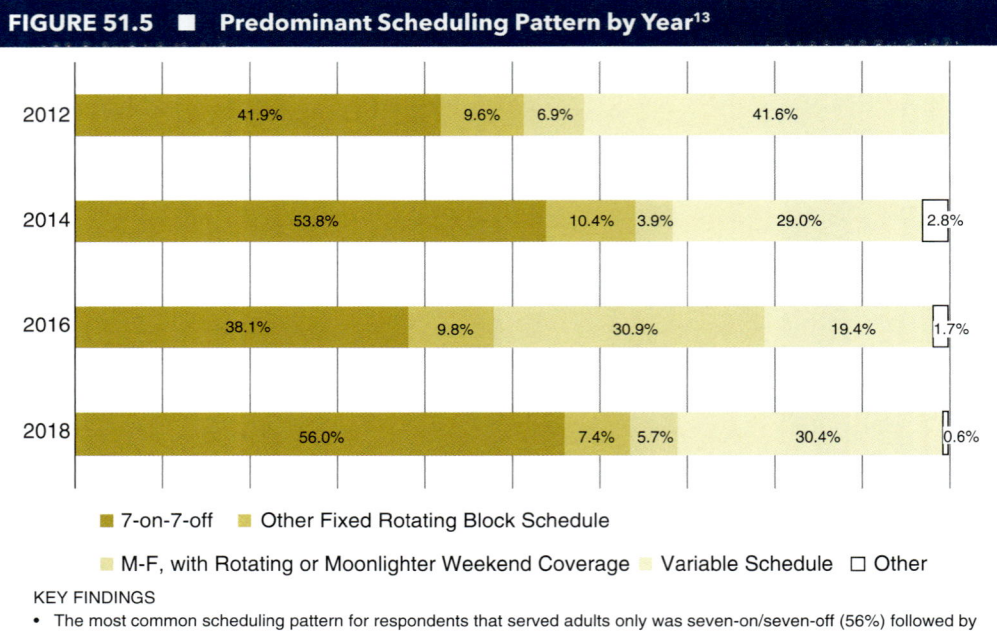

FIGURE 51.5 ■ Predominant Scheduling Pattern by Year[13]

- 7-on-7-off
- Other Fixed Rotating Block Schedule
- M-F, with Rotating or Moonlighter Weekend Coverage
- Variable Schedule
- Other

KEY FINDINGS
- The most common scheduling pattern for respondents that served adults only was seven-on/seven-off (56%) followed by variable scheduling (30.4%).
- The most common scheduling pattern for respondents that served adults only from the region of the West was variable scheduling (57.1%). Also, none of the 63 respondents from the West employ M–F scheduling.
- As compared to the 2016 SoHM Report, M–F scheduling has decreased substantially regardless of HMG demographics (30.9% in 2016 vs 5.7% in 2018).

Operational Metrics

Successful hospitalist programs closely monitor encounter volumes to address surges and trends (**Box 51.2**). There are three basic types of clinician–patient encounters—initial, subsequent, and discharge—all of which must be used to define the hospitalist's efforts.

Average Daily Census

While average daily census is a metric that generally describes a program's size, it does not account for all billable opportunities, including new admissions, discharges, critical care, consultations, and procedures.

Average daily "billable encounters" may be a more useful metric to determine staffing for a hospitalist program. Additionally, it is important to recognize and account for nonbillable work that is not factored into average daily encounters. As an example, a patient admitted by

---

BOX 51.2 ■ HOSPITAL QUALITY METRICS

- Mortality rate
- Continuity of care (number of hospitalists that care for a patient from admission to discharge)
- Consult utilization
- Readmission rate
- Health care-acquired conditions
- Patient experience
- Citizenship (hospital committee participation)
- Documentation (case mix index, coding, undocumented services rate)

the hospitalist after midnight may be evaluated again by the same hospitalist or the daytime hospitalist the following morning. Because only one encounter per day is reimbursed, the additional time-consuming evaluation is not a billable event (except in the case of an emergency or a procedure). The maximum benefit of a hospitalist is typically seen when the clinician's workload averages 1.5 encounters per patient per day, depending on workflow variables, such as EMR, ICU responsibilities, subspecialty support, and so on.

Just as in the ED, inpatient volumes may fluctuate dramatically. Relative value units (RVUs) based on Medicare's reimbursement schedule may be used to incentivize hospitalists for busy shifts.

Length of Stay

There are a few different ways to evaluate LOS:

- *Unadjusted (raw) LOS:* an LOS not adjusted for acuity or outliers
- *CMI-adjusted LOS:* an LOS adjusted CMI; thorough documentation can justify longer LOS based on higher acuity
- *Geometric LOS:* an LOS accounting for outliers, which can be helpful if a small number of patients have a very long LOS

AN INTEGRATED APPROACH TO PATIENT CARE

The modern health-care environment is exceedingly complex. Patients progress through an arc of care that spans outpatient, inpatient, and post-acute settings. Multiple departments and disciplines provide critical services, and various clinical and nonclinical providers deliver the care itself. The complexity of this environment has given rise to the need for an integrated model of care delivery, where multisetting, multidepartmental, multidisciplinary, and multiprovider care is carefully coordinated.

Not all EDs and hospitalist groups enjoy a collaborative and integrated relationship. Commonly expressed hospitalist concerns about their ED colleagues include:

- Batched admissions
- Incomplete workups
- Inappropriate admissions

Similarly, ED clinicians express consistent concerns about their HM colleagues, including:

- Delaying evaluations and admissions
- Resisting admissions
- Requesting unnecessary additional studies

These issues represent shared challenges that can be overcome by close collaboration and an integrated approach to patient care. But before that can be accomplished, a constructive, respectful awareness of how EM compares to HM is necessary.

Similarities

While EM and HM certainly have their differences, they are more alike than different. Rather than "apples and oranges," they are more like red and green apples (i.e., different versions of the same thing).

Emergency medicine and HM are the "acute care team," together managing the acute care of hospital patients. Both manage the care of the vast majority of admitted patients and both respond to emergencies in the hospital. Any differences between the two specialties are minor compared to the differences they have with the specialties that operate outside of the acute care setting.

Emergency department and hospitalist clinicians are the hospital's "home team." Both groups work exclusively within the hospital and know its operations and processes better than any other group of clinicians. Together, they interact with what can be considered the "away" team, which includes all clinical stakeholders who function outside of the hospital.

Differences

Granted that EM and HM have more similarities than differences, it is important to examine differences, which can be grouped into four key areas: primary responsibilities, the time line, information processing, and general personalities.

The primary responsibilities of emergency and hospitalist clinicians differ. Generally speaking, EM physicians are responsible for stabilizing patients, making a primary diagnosis and administering treatment, and determining a disposition. Hospitalists maintain the patient's stability, refine the primary diagnosis (or make a second one), develop and update a comprehensive treatment plan, and coordinate the actions of the multidisciplinary team. While these fundamental differences are certainly an oversimplification, understanding them can help bring consciousness to the motivations and behaviors of the clinicians and identify opportunities for alignment.

The time lines of EM and HM differ significantly. In EM, patient encounters are numerous, come in rapid succession, are relatively brief, and tend to involve unstable presentations that require swift intervention. Consequently, the time line is measured in seconds and minutes.

In contrast, hospitalist patient encounters are less numerous, come in slower succession, are more prolonged, and tend to involve stable issues that require careful consideration. Accordingly, the time line is measured in hours and days. While this is an oversimplification, recognizing these important differences can help foster mutual understanding and respect.

Styles of Thinking and Personality

Research in the field of cognitive psychology has identified two primary modes of thinking, classified as "System 1" and "System 2." System 1 thinking is fast, effortless, automatic, and unconscious; it is thinking that has great utility in facilitating rapid assessments and swift decisions. System 2 thinking is slow, effortful, deliberate, and conscious; it has great utility when seeking new or missing information and when making complex decisions. While clinicians in each specialty must utilize both types of thinking, EM clinicians tend to rely more on System 1 thinking and a higher degree of parallel information processing. HM clinicians tend to use more System 2 thinking and a higher degree of serial information processing.

Both nature and nurture influence the personalities of the clinicians who practice EM and HM. The nature of each field tends to attract clinicians with certain natural personality traits. One particular set of personality archetypes considers the EM clinician as the "doer" and the HM clinician as the "thinker." While this is a generalization, recognizing the distinction can help promote healthy relationships among the individual clinicians and the departments.

The Problems With Poor Coordination of Services

Utilizing hospitalists allows hospitals greater opportunity to control patient flow by effectively managing inpatient care discharges in a timely manner while simultaneously influencing a multitude of efficiency, satisfaction, and cost issues. For example, consider a patient who is ready to go home at noon, yet the PCP may not be able to get to the hospital to discharge the patient until 5 or 6 p.m. This delayed discharge unnecessarily occupies a bed and consumes resources.

As described earlier, the similarities between emergency physicians and hospitalists should lead to strong collaborations. The functions and goals of the two groups are intertwined, and the hospital's success frequently depends on these relationships. Unfortunately, in some hospitals, there is little trust and even an adversarial dynamic between the ED and hospitalist groups.[16]

The conflict is most likely to occur when the two services become more focused on their own convenience rather than on what is best for the patient. The conflict is further exacerbated by each team addressing its own metric performance in isolation, that is, without consideration for the other team's success. For example:

- Emergency physicians wait until they are no longer seeing new patients to communicate admissions to the hospitalist. Emergency physicians will describe the needs of the new "unknown" patient as being more urgent than the disposition of the already known "stabilized" patient.
- Hospitalists have periods during which they will not receive new patients. Transitions of care, morning rounds, and responding to acute issues may delay early discharges and increase the likelihood of ED boarding.
- Batched admissions frustrate all caregivers.

Ultimately, the two greatest consequences of a noncollaborative relationship between the emergency physician and hospitalist are poor patient-care coordination and deteriorating interservice communication and trust. The differences in the driving force for each department, as well as the differences in the incentives (productivity vs quality), can lead to poor communication, poor transitions, slower throughput, subpar patient care, increased frustration and dissatisfaction, increased liability, and wasted time and resources. As a group, these differences can result in additional time spent testing, reevaluating, negotiating, defending, and even arguing. Although this is wasted time for everyone, patients suffer most and are caught in the middle of the conflicting departments.

The Advantages of Integration

The tools for effective inpatient flow are the most important determinants of high-performing HM programs.[17,18] Effective hospitalists collaborate with multiple services to manage patients efficiently. They stay informed about:

- Demand
    - Routine ED daily admission request
    - Current ED boarded patients
    - Requests for transfers to the hospitalist service
    - Consultation requests
    - PCP requests for direct admission
- Capacity
    - Current available beds and types (med-surg, telemetry, etc)
    - Transfers from one unit to another
    - Potential discharges
    - Current barriers to flow for the day

When there are barriers to patient discharge, hospitalists should focus on the bottlenecks. If the barrier is related to a surge in volume (demand), medium-to-large hospitalist programs should have a backup schedule to increase staffing when indicated.

> **BOX 51.3 ■ CLINICAL VIGNETTE ONE**
>
> In the early evening, an emergency physician contacts the on-call hospitalist to notify him of three new admissions.
>
> **Emergency physician:** Hi, Carl. I'm sorry, but I've got three for you.
>
> **Hospitalist:** Three admissions? Are you kidding me? It's 6:35 p.m. Why couldn't you have given me any of these the past 2 hours so I could actually work on them? Now I have to hand them over to the night doc, and he will not be happy! And I'm going to be here for a couple of extra hours just so you can get out at 7 p.m. sharp!
>
> **Emergency physician:** Everyone's results literally just got back, and I am calling you now. We're *all* busy! I hope these admissions won't sit here forever. I really need orders to get them upstairs. Here are the patients . . .
>
> **Hospitalist:** You don't even have all the workups done yet. Why are you washing your hands so quickly? Why can't you get that CT scan done while the patient is in the ED? It's so much easier.
>
> **Commentary:** A malignant relationship between ED and HM could result in several assumptions about each other's workflow. Occasionally, the evaluations of several patients are completed around the same time, and it is easier to make a single phone call to discuss the admissions. Whenever possible, "batching," particularly at the end of the shift, should be avoided. This is more easily accomplished by establishing a "pull" mechanism from the hospitalist admitter. A hospitalist is unlikely to start an admission 25 minutes before the end of the shift. Nonurgent ED testing, better performed once the patient is admitted, creates ED bottlenecks. Unfortunately, two problems are evident in this dialogue: a lack of trust and poor coordination of care. An integrated model that coordinates patient care and clinician schedules might stagger shifts (so ED physicians and hospitalists are not leaving at the same time) and leverage bridge orders to help throughput.

A strong relationship with the ED is essential for mutual success and a coordinated and seamless continuum of care. For examples, see **Boxes 51.3, 51.4,** and **51.5:** Vignette 1 shows what can go wrong in the EM-HM relationship; Vignettes 2 and 3 illustrate how hospitalists and emergency physicians can be mutually supportive of the patients and each other.

An integrated approach to patient care has significant cultural, clinical, operational, and financial advantages. One of the most powerful drivers of success in the multidimensional hospital setting is the organizational culture of integration, which promotes collaborative problem solving and innovation. This creates an atmosphere of shared enthusiasm and builds forward momentum. Enhanced communication and cooperation among multiple service

> **BOX 51.4 ■ CLINICAL VIGNETTE TWO**
>
> **Problem:** Today, in the middle of flu season, there are 35 holds reported by the ED. An urgent text message has been sent to the entire hospital medical staff to encourage the expedited discharge of patients who are ready to leave.
>
> **Solution:** The hospitalist medical director meets with the ED medical director in the morning to review a strategy to drive throughput. The hospitalist informs the ED about 18 potential discharges and asks the ED to do "skeleton bridge orders" for any admissions that can be completed before noon. This will allow the hospitalist team to concentrate on early discharges and make room for the holding patients to come to the floors. The bridge orders entered by the ED on the new patients will help move along the bed-assignment process without disturbing the hospitalist workflow. These bridge orders have been developed collaboratively by both services and consist of observation vs inpatient status, diet, and PRN medications. The complete orders are entered by the hospitalist upon evaluation on the floors.

> **BOX 51.5 ■ CLINICAL VIGNETTE THREE**
>
> **Problem:** 20 patients are in the waiting room on a Friday afternoon, when there is no more room in the ED. The hospital is full and several discharges are pending. Several ED patients have LWOT.
>
> **Solution:** The ED doc contacts the on-call hospitalist to communicate the problem at hand. There are also two admissions ready to handoff. Once the ED doc completes sign-out, the hospitalist asks how many others may need to be admitted. There will be at least six more admissions in the next several hours, four of which are very straightforward and are just waiting for minimally consequential imaging and labs. The hospitalist who heading to the ED anyway asks for handoff on those four patients as well so she can start seeing them and placing orders. This integrated and coordinated delivery model helps improve the patient experience, decrease LWOTs, and facilitate throughput.

lines and departments decreases the potential for error and creates the opportunity for improvements in care delivery.

Clinical Pathways

A common example of this collaboration is the implementation of clinical pathways. Effective integration also creates opportunities for enhanced operational efficiency. Close collaboration between the ED and hospitalist service, for example, can result in improved throughput metrics for both departments. These cultural, clinical, and operational improvements can produce significant downstream financial gains.

The Parties Involved in Integration

An integrated approach to patient care should involve all settings, departments, disciplines, and providers; however, this goal can be difficult to achieve. The emergency and HM departments are typically two of the hospital's most critical constituents, and their relationship often sets the tone for integration. This synergy represents a challenge and an opportunity. An understanding of the structure of EM and hospitalist groups, as well as their similarities and differences, can set the stage for successful integration.

Leadership and Operations

Leaders should schedule regular joint meetings (at least monthly) to provide a structured review of common issues and problem cases to identify areas for improvement. Effective discussions occur when all participants are focused on advocating for the patients.

> **BOX 51.6 ■ ADVANTAGES OF A COLLABORATIVE RELATIONSHIP WITH HOSPITALISTS**
>
> - ED throughput
> - ED overcrowding
> - ED hold times
> - Left without being seen rates
> - ED utilization
> - Timely responses from hospitalists
> - Satisfaction and stability
> - Communication and trust
> - Less "negotiating" on admissions
> - Patient handoff improvements between emergency physicians and hospitalists
> - Decreased conflict

Meetings should be led jointly by the service-line leaders with particular attention to metrics without reproach or blaming. Separately, the service-line leaders should meet frequently to discuss issues and select topics to include in the interdepartmental meeting agendas.

Collaboration between EM and HM requires setting common patient-focused goals and metrics and addressing associated challenges (**Box 51.6**). It is a best practice for ED and HM clinicians to round or "shadow shift" on the other service to gain a deeper understanding of how their respective programs work. It is particularly valuable to define and agree on criteria for the handoff of common and low-acuity diagnoses. Throughput is expedited, and all clinicians can rely on a consistent approach. Other examples to address include:

- If incomplete ED workups are an issue, collaboratively defining what is and is not necessary for particular diagnoses can expedite care and transitions.
- If patient experience is an area of focus, it may be eye-opening for providers to understand that the patient's evaluation of one area is affected by their experience while in another service area. For instance, if a patient stays too long in the ED, the entire hospital evaluation may be tainted, regardless of the inpatient experience.

Models of ED and HM Group Engagement

The two primary models for ED and HM groups are hospital-employed and contracted groups. In a hospital-employed group model, the department and clinicians are directly employed by the hospital. In a contracted group model, the department and clinicians are engaged as employees or independent contractors by a private group or corporation that contracts with the hospital to provide those services. Contracted groups can vary in size, from small private groups (one or a few hospital contracts) to large, multistate organizations with numerous contracts. Contract groups can specialize in a single service line or manage multiple service lines, including both EM and HM. Regardless of configuration, cooperation between the two groups is critically important.

CONCLUSION

The goal is a customer-focused, quality-committed, and efficiency-minded partnership between the emergency physicians and hospitalists. Once these clinicians are all rowing in the same direction, efficiency is improved. Successful organizations support the patient-flow process by training nurse leaders, conducting operational assessments, implementing lean, deploying marketing resources, and hardwiring customer satisfaction techniques.

For programs to function well, the emergency physicians and hospitalists should have similar incentives. However, for great success, the groups will share the same goals and metrics and will be guided by leadership that has substantial experience and problem-solving expertise.

The trend of small and large emergency groups expanding into HM will most likely continue. Even smaller companies working together may take advantage of shared goals, such as expedited patient admission, improved throughput, attention to quality, and so on. Because of the costs and risks associated with starting a hospitalist group, smaller EM companies increasingly find it difficult to create a new (or take responsibility for and manage an existing) hospitalist program. Larger companies have some advantages because they often have broad management experience and the capacity to leverage and deploy resources on a broader level.

REFERENCES

1. Wachter RM, Goldman L. The emerging role of "hospitalists" in the American health care system. *N Engl J Med*. 1996;335(7):514–517.
2. Society of Hospital Medicine. What is a hospitalist. 2020. Available at: https://www.hospitalmedicine.org/about/what-is-a-hospitalist/. Accessed January 15, 2020.
3. Li JMW, Feinbloom D. Certification in hospital medicine: what does this mean to hospitalists? To employers? To patients? *Medscape*. 2007. Available at: https://www.medscape.org/viewarticle/560235. Accessed January 15, 2020.
4. Chen LM, Birkmeyer JD, Saint S, et al. Hospitalist staffing and patient satisfaction in the national Medicare population. *J Hosp Med*. 2013;8(3):126–131.
5. Salim SA, Elmaraezy A, Pamarthy A, et al. Impact of hospitalists on the efficiency of inpatient care and patient satisfaction: a systematic review and meta-analysis. *J Community Hosp Intern Med Perspect*. 2019;9(2):121–134.
6. Wachter RM, Goldman L. Zero to 50,000: the 20th anniversary of the hospitalist. *N Engl J Med*. 2016;375(11):1009–1011.
7. Watcher RM, Goldman L. The hospitalist movement 5 years later. *JAMA*. 2002;287(4):487–494.
8. Watcher RM. The state of hospital medicine in 2008. *Med Clin North Am*. 2008;92(2):265–273.
9. George R. Scheduling patterns in hospital medicine. *The Hospitalist*. 2017. Available at: https://www.the-hospitalist.org/hospitalist/article/150382/scheduling-patterns-hospital-medicine. Accessed May 12, 2020.
10. Kaboli PJ, Go JT, Hockenberry J, et al. Associations between reduced hospital length of stay and 30-day readmission rate and mortality: 14-year experience in 129 Veterans Affairs hospitals. *Ann Intern Med*. 2012;157(12):837–845.
11. 10 tips for optimizing length of stay. *Care Logistics Blog*. 2017. Available at: https://www.carelogistics.com/blog/2017/8/8/5txje43de7biprm5gclgy9q06gfk2r. Accessed May 12, 2020.
12. Whalley R. Why not home, why not today. *Better Care Support Programme Brochure*. 2017. Available at: https://www.local.gov.uk/sites/default/files/documents/NEW0164_DTOC_Brochure_Online_Spreads_1.0.pdf. Accessed May 12, 2020.
13. Society of Hospital Medicine Practice Analysis Committee. *2018 State of Hospital Medicine Report*. Philadelphia, PA: Society of Hospital Medicine; 2018.
14. Society of Hospital Medicine Public Policy Committee. *The Hospital Observation Care Problem: Perspectives and Solutions From the Society of Hospital Medicine*. 2017. Available at: https://www.hospitalmedicine.org/globalassets/policy-and-advocacy/advocacy-pdf/shms-observation-white-paper-2017. Accessed May 11, 2020.
15. O'Leary KJ, Wayne DB, Landler MP, et al. Impact of localizing physicians to hospital units on nurse–physician communication and agreement on the plan of care. *J Gen Intern Med*. 2009;24(11):1223–1227.
16. Covey SMR. *The Speed of Trust: The One Thing That Changes Everything, Simon & Schuster*. New York, NY: Free Press; 2018.
17. Resar R, Nolan K, Kaczynski D, et al. Using real-time demand capacity management to improve hospitalwide patient flow. *Jt Com J Qual Patient Saf*. 2011;37(5):217–227.
18. Jensen K, Mayer TA, Welch SJ, et al. *Leadership for Smooth Patient Flow*. Chicago, IL: Health Administration Press; 2007.

CHAPTER 52
DISASTER PLANNING AND RESPONSE

Knox Andress, Dan Hanfling

Always plan ahead. It wasn't raining when Noah built the ark.

—Richard Cushing, American Prelate of the Roman Catholic Church

Preparing for response to disaster events presents a unique challenge to emergency department (ED) leaders for a number of reasons. Most often it is assumed that disasters are something that happen "somewhere else." The likelihood that any given ED will have to respond to a disaster event remains relatively low. Issues of overcrowding, staffing shortages, violence in the workplace, and financial constraints are all much more likely daily stresses that might be encountered by ED management.[1-4] Yet the incidence of disaster events, whether due to natural causes such as extreme weather or as a result of intentional acts of terrorism, has increased over the past decade.[5] "Trends affecting the modern world are resulting in social changes that raise the probability of more and worse disasters in the 21st century . . . and stem from ever-increasing industrialization and urbanization . . ."[6]

The notion that it "won't happen here" really does not apply any longer. Moreover, there are plenty of false assumptions often mistakenly held by ED leaders regarding disaster events (**Box 52.1**).[7] So, it is important to understand the key elements related to disaster preparedness and response in the ED. Indeed, the ED manager in the leader role in this arena is often very much sought after by hospital administrators, government leaders, and the general public (**Figure 52.1**). In the nearly two decades since the September 11, 2001, attacks and the anthrax mailings, followed by the failures of the levees in New Orleans, the 2009 H1N1 pandemic, and the hurricanes of 2017, hospitals have come a long way in their efforts to prepare for disaster events.[8]

BOX 52.1 ■ MYTHS REGARDING DISASTER EVENTS

- EMS will conduct triage, provide stabilizing care, and if required, decontaminate patients at the scene.
- Casualties will be transported by ambulance to the ED.
- Casualties will be evenly distributed between hospitals.
- Hospitals will be contacted by EMS officials regarding the nature, type, and number of casualties that are expected.
- The most serious casualties will arrive to the ED first.

> **FIGURE 52.1 ■ Disaster Planning and Response Expectations**
>
> The American College of Emergency Physicians (ACEP) encourages emergency physicians to:
>
> 1. Assist their institutions and community to prepare for disasters.
> 2. Continue to work during disaster situations.
> 3. Use all available methods to protect themselves, their families, their coworkers, and their patients from risks.
> 4. Work with institutional and public leaders to effectively communicate public health and safety information to coworkers and the public.
> 5. Be prepared to assume the role of crises triage officer to allocate scarce resources, when necessary.
>
> ACEP will, when possible and appropriate during disasters, use its resources to disseminate current, scientifically based information from national experts.

However, disaster planning alone does not guarantee successful management of an emergency. In particular:

> *It is very easy to assume that if there has been disaster planning, there will be successful . . . management. After all, that would seem to be the ultimate purpose of planning ahead of time. Unfortunately, however, research has shown that is far from being the case; there often is a big gap between what was planned and what actually happens in a major disaster crisis . . .*[9]

Reviewing and implementing the key concepts delineated in this chapter will go a long way to ensuring that the ED is ready to face the multitude of requirements necessary for a successful disaster response.

WHAT IS A DISASTER?

A "disaster" can be defined in a number of ways, but what is most relevant to ED operations is that it creates a situation in which the ability to provide safe and timely health-care service delivery is exceeded by the demand for such care. As a result, the ability to allocate resources is altered significantly. Disaster events can occur as a sudden, no-notice event, such as a terrorist attack. Or they may be anticipated, as is the case with many weather emergencies. Finally, they may also take on more of a sustained time line, as might be experienced in the context of an emerging infectious outbreak. Disaster events may be considered "external disasters"—those that occur in the community—or "internal disasters" due to interruption of key services in the health-care facility.

An internal disaster is said to occur when a physical impediment to taking care of patients exists, such as would be the case in a fire, flood, or bomb threat. It may also occur as a result of the absence or loss of specific resources needed to manage patient care, such as the wholesale failure of laboratory services, telemetry, or other system services. Planning for such events must be predicated upon developing an "all-hazards" systems approach to response. In other words, there will be certain commonalities in the response regardless of the cause of the disaster. A well-developed plan will accommodate for such differences, while streamlining those processes that are consistent across most, if not all, events.

Developing an "All Hazards" Approach

The process for ensuring that an "all-hazards" approach will be utilized begins with the participation in performing a hazard vulnerability analysis (HVA).[10] This is a process that requires multidisciplinary participation and engaged discussion about the threats that exist in the community. Input from medical leaders, public health officials, and public safety officials helps to ensure that a wide range of concerns are considered. The process entails rank ordering those threats based on the likelihood of occurrence and the consequences of such events. It also takes into account the baseline preparedness of the community to meet those threats.

Risk is calculated by considering the two primary elements of hazard probability and hazard impact.[11] The probability equates to the likelihood of event or hazard occurrence and can be calculated based on historical incident frequency or estimated based on other risk factors. Impact is the damage or severity caused by the hazard and its effects on human life, business, infrastructure, and environment. Many times a function of the hospital safety officer and hospital emergency preparedness/management committee, the HVA results "drive" threat-specific incident planning (**Figure 52.2**).[12]

Developing an Emergency Operations Plan

Planning and coordination for the ED as part of the overall hospital response should be outlined in the hospital's "all-hazards" emergency operations plan (EOP). This document,

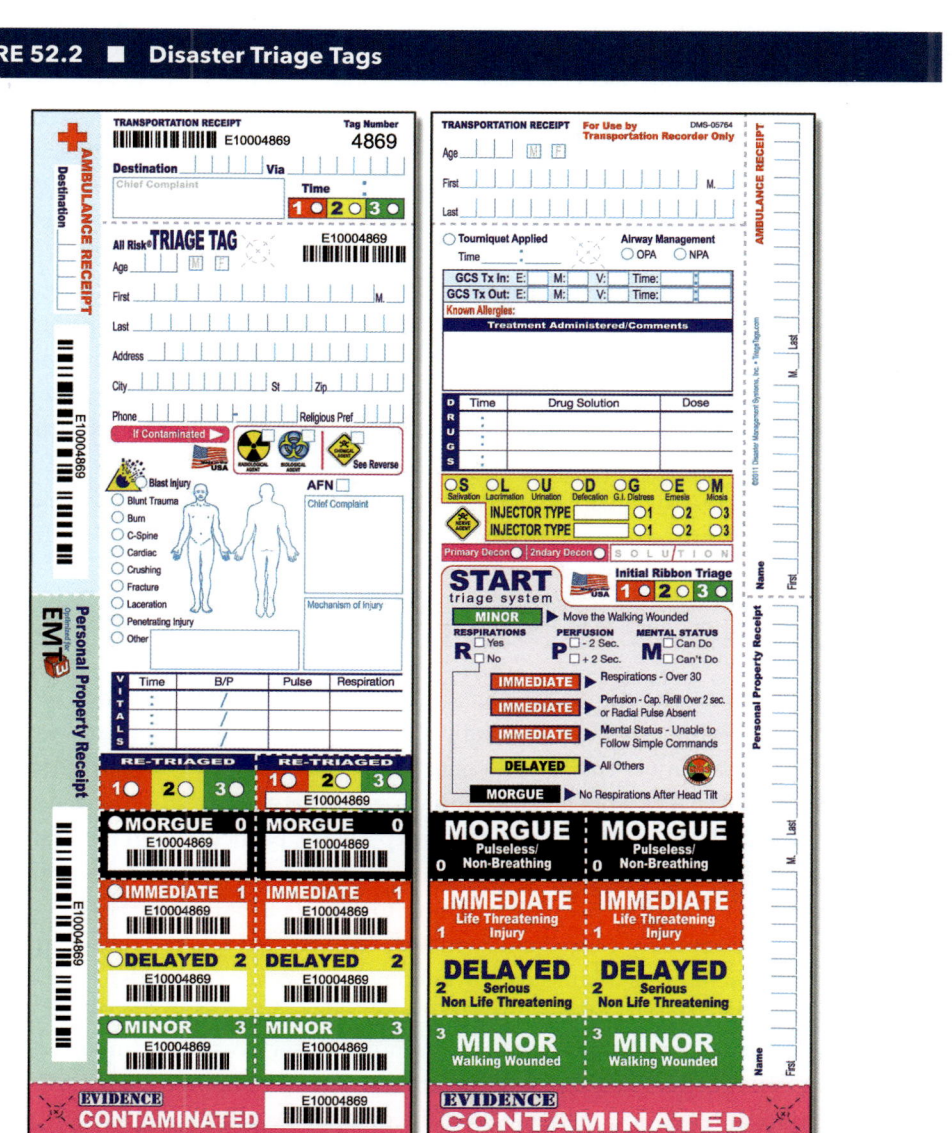

FIGURE 52.2 ■ Disaster Triage Tags

a requirement of The Joint Commission, assigns priority to specific hazards or threats that the hospital is likely to encounter, and it outlines the strategy for emergency response and recovery. The EOP, therefore, is strongly guided by the development of the HVA, which identifies and prioritizes hazards and risks for hospital planning. Although hospitals must be prepared for a variety of disaster and emergency-causing situations, most events place similar demands on the hospital in that they require leadership, coordination, communication, and other key response activities.

Because of these similarities, it is not necessary to develop totally separate plans and procedures for every different disaster imaginable. Thus, hospitals are encouraged to view disaster planning from an "all-hazards" approach; separate plans for different disasters can confuse staff and cause an unnecessary strain on budgets and storage capabilities. Preparedness and response plans should address the commonalities among the different types of disasters that could occur. For example, a plane crash and a bomb blast both result in an influx of patients who are in need of triage and rapid surgical interventions, even though the cause of their injuries is different.[13] Thus, the core of the hospital disaster preparedness plan is common to all events, with supplements included for those events needing specific responses, such as a contamination event requiring the addition of a decontamination team to the hospital's disaster response.

The hospital EOP outlines the four phases of emergency management and describes associated activities for preparedness, mitigation, response, and recovery.[14] These components of the EOP reflect the need for coordination of communications, resources, and assets, safety and security, staff responsibilities, utilities, patient clinical care, and patient and family support activities during an emergency. The document also provides guidance for the use of the incident command system (ICS), a means by which large-scale events can be managed in a coordinated fashion.

Regardless of the cause of the disaster, the common underlying situation remains the same—available resources will be stretched thin and the fundamental principles upon which health care is delivered will have to be adjusted. This suggests that the prevailing conditions of care delivery during a disaster event are significantly more complex and different than those encountered on a busy Saturday night in the ED. It therefore presupposes the importance of having a dedicated process in place by which plans are developed, implemented, and tested. Suffice it to say, disaster plans alone are not effective unless they are supported by a team of providers who have worked together to craft the result.

DEVELOPING AN ED DISASTER PLAN

The ED disaster plan should be developed and exercised in the context of the hospital's overarching EOP. While there will be many elements that are congruent and may overlap, it is important to remember that in a disaster event, the entire hospital must coordinate its response to the crisis. It is a mistake to simply expect that the ED will manage everything. While the ED will likely bear the brunt of the experience, particularly in the first few hours (or days) of a sudden-onset event (especially an external disaster that occurs without notice in the community), the entire hospital will have to alter its usual practices related to patient care delivery.[15-17] Eventually, ED patients will have been treated and stabilized, and decisions regarding their discharge or admission will be completed. While the sudden influx of patients has been attended to, disaster operations in the remainder of the hospital may still be ongoing.

It is important to emphasize that the continuity of services is an important planning assumption that must be incorporated into any ED disaster plan. While the ED must react and respond to the casualties generated by the disaster event, it must also be prepared to maintain access to care for the cardiovascular, respiratory, pediatric, traumatic, and other illnesses and injuries that will continue to occur. For this reason, it is important to plan for the simultaneous management of incoming disaster victims in addition to caring for those patients currently in the department or waiting to be seen.

One of the key elements in this plan must be to ensure rapid and effective communication of information regarding the onset of an event. This alert and notification may come into the ED by way of emergency medical services (EMS) communications, although it is just as likely be reported by the media on the radio, Internet, or television news. It may also come as information conveyed as part of a regional "bed status" information system that is deployed in any given community. Regardless, development and implementation of reliable communications channels with the public safety agencies that support the ED is critically important. This should include both a radio network that links regional hospitals together with each other on a regional network, as well as an information management platform that allows for the development of real-time situational awareness of an ongoing event.

Following notification that an event is unfolding, it is incumbent upon the lead emergency physician and ED charge nurse to evaluate the information that is available in order to make a determination as to whether the ED disaster plan should be initiated. In doing so, there are some key data points that they must know (**Box 52.2**). While gathering such information, plans must be initiated in order to clear out the department as much as is feasible so as to prepare for incoming patient arrivals. Patients who are likely to be admitted, even if in the midst of their workup, should be admitted and moved into the hospital. Those whose workups can be deferred or delayed should be discharged. Responsibility for making these and other critical decisions should rest with the on-duty doctors and nurses. Planning for implementation of the disaster plan during off hours, nights, and weekends will ensure that the on-duty staff understands that they are the critical decision makers in the early stages of any disaster event, until such time as more senior clinical and administrative leaders arrive to the hospital.

Other key tasks that must be accomplished soon after the notification that a disaster has occurred include the identification and designation of key players and preidentified designated treatment zones in the ED. One of the most important of these is the selection of the triage team and the location of their efforts. Triage should ideally be managed by the most senior and experienced members of the physician and nursing staff, and if staffing permits, combining physician and nursing efforts together works best. The location of the triage area should ideally be outside of the ED, yet close enough so that patient movement for initial stabilization and treatment can commence quickly. With the exception of those facilities in temperate climates that might allow triage outside on the ambulance bay, it might be best to locate the triage process in the ED waiting area or some other large space in close proximity to the department.[18]

BOX 52.2 ■ KEY QUESTIONS TO ASK WHEN ALERTED ABOUT A POTENTIAL DISASTER EVENT

- How many patients and what types of injuries are expected?
- Is there any immediate risk to the emergency department, its patients, and staff?
- Have other area hospitals been notified, and have patients been transported by EMS agencies?
- Does the event involve exposure to potentially dangerous chemicals or other contaminants?
- When are the first patients expected to arrive?

FIGURE 52.3 ■ Sample HVA Tool

EVENT	PROBABILITY	SEVERITY = (MAGNITUDE - MITIGATION)						RISK
		HUMAN IMPACT	PROPERTY IMPACT	BUSINESS IMPACT	PREPARED-NESS	INTERNAL RESPONSE	EXTERNAL RESPONSE	
	Likelihood this will occur	Possibility of death or injury	Physical losses and damages	Interruption of services	Preplanning	Time, effectiveness, resources	Community/Mutual Aid staff and supplies	Relative threat*
SCORE	0 = N/A 1 = Low 2 = Moderate 3 = High	0 = N/A 1 = Low 2 = Moderate 3 = High	0 = N/A 1 = Low 2 = Moderate 3 = High	0 = N/A 1 = Low 2 = Moderate 3 = High	0 = N/A 1 = High 2 = Moderate 3 = Low or none	0 = N/A 1 = High 2 = Moderate 3 = Low or none	0 = N/A 1 = High 2 = Moderate 3 = Low or none	0 - 100%
Electrical Failure								0%
Generator Failure								0%
Transportation Failure								0%
Fuel Shortage								0%
Natural Gas Failure								0%
Water Failure								0%
Sewer Failure								0%
Steam Failure								0%
Fire Alarm Failure								0%
Communications Failure								0%
Medical Gas Failure								0%
Medical Vacuum Failure								0%
HVAC Failure								0%
Information Systems Failure								0%
Fire, Internal								0%
Flood, Internal								0%
Hazmat Exposure, Internal								0%
Supply Shortage								0%
Structural Damage								0%
AVERAGE SCORE	0.00	0.00	0.00	0.00	0.00	0.00	0.00	0%

*Threat increases with percentage.

RISK = PROBABILITY * SEVERITY

It is important to note that not all patients will be arriving from a disaster scene by ambulance. Many more may be transported by private vehicle or other means of conveyance. And not all will be delivered directly to the predesignated triage area. So the location of the triage function must take into account the possibility that patients will be coming to the hospital seeking care and may be presenting to different parts of the facility. For those patients who do arrive by EMS, it is likely that they will have some sort of "triage tag" affixed to their body (often tied around their wrist or ankle) (**Figure 52.3**).

When utilized properly, the triage tag will convey basic information about the patient's injury and initial out-of-hospital treatments. It would be useful for the ED to stock additional triage tags that can be applied to patients immediately upon their arrival to the department. This serves the purpose of ensuring a total count of disaster victims presenting for care. It also helps to initiate the documentation process, until such time that registration can verify patient identification and the patients can be entered into the ED information system or patient care record system. It would also be useful to have a digital camera available in the triage area in order to photograph the faces of all incoming disaster victims, particularly those whose injuries may preclude them from being easily identified. Use of these photos might help in the identification of victims and would expedite the reunification of family members with their loved ones.

Note that while privacy laws under the Health Insurance Portability and Accountability Act (HIPAA) govern the day-to-day operations related to information sharing in the ED, significant caveats have been developed when considering information sharing during a disaster. Confusion over this matter has been addressed by the US Department of Health and Human Services (HHS), which essentially notes that for the purposes of patient identification and information sharing, it is recognized that critical patient care information can and should be shared during a disaster event. While HIPAA itself cannot be waived, certain provisions can be waived, provided the disaster is declared by the president of the United States and a public health emergency is declared by the secretary of HHS.[19] However, not every disaster will rise to the level of a Presidential Declaration, as evidenced by mass homicide events perpetrated by gun violence, such as the Orlando Pulse Nightclub shooting (June 12, 2016) and the Mandalay Bay Las Vegas shooting (October 1, 2017). Given such circumstances, interpretations of the law have been proffered by HHS that extend the emphasis on making common sense decisions regarding the sharing of such information.[20]

Disaster Triage and Patient Flow

While there are a number of triage systems that are employed to evaluate victims of disaster, particularly those with traumatic injuries, the most commonly used methodology is START triage, which is based upon rapid evaluation of respiratory status, circulation, and mental status.[21] Two newer triage systems include the SALT and Sacco triage methods.[22-26] Regardless of the methodology applied, it is important to remember that the triage process is only the first of many opportunities to identify and prioritize patients for immediate care. Secondary triage and definitive triage decisions will be made subsequent to the initial sorting of patients and should involve specialists and consultants when they are available. The importance of making the right triage decision cannot be overstated. Using hospital resources for victims who do not require immediate attention (overtriage) certainly is of no benefit to patients who may present subsequently in the disaster event. Such mistakes potentially threaten to delay the recognition and care of that small minority of patients with urgent and salvageable life-threatening injuries who are at immediate risk of death (undertriage).[27]

The ED charge physician and nurse should consult with each other regarding the initial placement of disaster victims within the department. As additional responders come to the ED upon hospital-wide notification that the external disaster plan has been put into effect, coordination and management of these additional responders will be important. The department can be quickly overrun by those who want to help but have no specific role. Crowd control, both inside and outside the ED, will become critically important. The ED staff should make assignments of disaster-victim teams that are comprised of an emergency physician or anesthesiologist to manage the airway and resuscitation, a respiratory therapist, a surgeon (if surgical injuries are anticipated), and two bedside nurses (at least one should be an ED nurse).[28-30] Ideally, these teams will remain with the patient through their entire ED course—initial stabilization, management, and ultimate disposition, including admission to the operating room, intensive care unit, or medical–surgical floor. This allows for continuity of care, particularly when there are enough medical staff members to provide it. In the event of fewer staff members being available, adjustments to this approach can be made.

A related consideration in managing the flow of disaster patients into and through the ED is the adherence to the principle of ensuring "unidirectional" patient flow.[31] Patients should ideally be managed using a minimal of laboratory and imaging studies, when possible. There are certain bottlenecks that have been identified in the simultaneous management of disaster patients, particularly those presenting as a result of mass casualty events. Radiography, especially the use of the computed tomography scanner, is often one such rate-limiting step in the diagnostic process.[32] Waiting for laboratory studies may be another. Patients need to be managed as expeditiously as possible, with the understanding of the patients and ED staff that the assignment of definitive diagnoses may be delayed. Patients who must undergo radiological studies should be moved from the radiology department directly to an inpatient unit and not back to the ED. Furthermore, the use of point-of-care testing in the ED may help cut down on turnaround times for certain studies.[33,34]

Demobilization and Recovery

At a certain point in the course of the disaster response, efforts will need to be initiated to prepare for the gradual and eventual return to normal operations. This needs to be anticipated during the course of the disaster response and will be based upon resource utilization needs, number of patients in the ED, acuity of illness or injury, available staff to manage patient needs, and information regarding the disaster event. Planning for demobilization and recovery is an important step in offsetting some of the psychological stresses that are sure to accompany any disaster response.[35,36] Nonetheless, mental health considerations must be taken into account when preparing for recovery, because they may delay the ability to get back to usual operations in an expedited manner.

Providing resources for counseling, stress debriefing, and allowing time away from the ED can be useful strategies that may facilitate the recovery process. Logistical resupply will also be important and may be undertaken as part of a hospital or regional effort to recover from the disaster response.

Decontamination and Isolation

There are a number of specific issues related to the management of potentially contaminated patients, particularly those who may be exposed to chemical or radiological agents.[37,38] Because of the risk such patients pose to the integrity and safety of the ED and the hospital, ensuring that these patients are decontaminated prior to definitive medical management is important. In the case of chemical contamination, patients might need to be treated outside of the hospital so as to limit the risk of hospital contamination.[39] With radiological contamination, decontamination is important, but lifesaving interventions should not be delayed; the radiological contamination is unlikely to be immediately life threatening.[40,41]

A best practice for hospital-based decontamination is the use of "fixed" shower facilities that are immediately contiguous to the hospital and close to the ED. In a worst-case scenario, water can be initiated from inside the facility, and patients can begin to disrobe and wash themselves, while staff don personal protective equipment and prepare for the receipt of such patients. This is preferable to the use of tent-based systems, given the complexity of setup, the time required to establish water flow, and the considerations regarding storage and preventive maintenance of such systems. Decontamination capabilities specific to the management of pediatric and special needs populations must also be developed.[42-43]

In a biological disaster response—such as to the Ebola virus disease outbreak in 2014–2015 or to a pandemic influenza—issues related to isolation surge planning and the use of infection control practices may make the response difficult.[44-47] Unlike events due to sudden, no-notice causes, a biological event may result in a campaign-style response, with patients presenting for care over weeks, not just hours or days. Effective screening tools to help identify patients at risk for disease, and protocol-based decisions regarding the need for laboratory and radiological studies, will all be useful adjuncts to streamline care. In the setting of response to an overwhelming biological emergency, suspension of some of the regulations governing ED management, including the Emergency Medical Treatment and Labor Act may occur, thereby helping to decompress overcrowded, overloaded EDs during crisis.[48]

Children and Vulnerable Populations

In disaster events in which there are a large number of pediatric patients, contingency plans to address pediatric care must be in place. It is not practical or ethically justifiable to assume that pediatric patients will simply be transferred to a children's hospital or pediatric ED (just as it is unlikely that trauma patients will all be transferred to a trauma center). The ED must ensure the availability of basic equipment and supplies necessary to manage ill or injured children.[49] In the likely event that there is a shortage of experienced pediatric emergency physicians and nurses to manage these cases, a partnering system that employs the use of pediatricians from the community should be explored. Furthermore, parents should be utilized as bedside assistants whenever possible, assuming that they themselves are not in need of immediate assistance. In the case where parent and child are both requiring hospitalization, it would be considered a best practice to attempt to keep the family together during the ED evaluation and, if required, during hospitalization.

Pediatric patients represent one category of vulnerable population that EDs and hospitals need to plan for during a disaster event. History teaches us that the most vulnerable in the population may be disproportionately affected by disaster events and the disruption of access to health-care service delivery. Previous events, such as hurricanes Katrina and Sandy and the storms of 2017, demonstrate surge impacts of vulnerable populations, especially geriatric and dialysis patients, who can overwhelm EDs and hospitals.[50] Other vulnerable population types that need to be planned for include institutionalized patients, such as nursing home residents; the impoverished, disabled, or homebound; and those who may not speak English. Having awareness of vulnerable populations in the area can aid in ED and hospital disaster planning for those who may present when infrastructure such as electricity or potable water is lost. The HHS EMPOWER tool provides awareness of electrically dependent and dialysis populations within a user-defined jurisdiction.[51] Use of this information, in conjunction with local health department officials, may limit the impact such populations may pose to the ED surge response during a storm event.

DEVELOPING A SURGE RESPONSE PLAN

In the past few years, planning and modeling for the impact a severe pandemic might have on hospitals has highlighted the significant gaps in the ability for health-care systems to manage an overwhelming need for personnel, medications, oxygen, ventilators, bed space, and other requirements.[52] Planning for a hospital surge overload, in which there are extraordinary demands for resources—including personnel, equipment and supplies, space and locations—is a complex, time-consuming, and costly process. While a lot of attention has been paid to surge capacity planning over the past few years, another important and evolving concept is the recognition that a surge response is not an all-or-nothing phenomenon.[53-55] Reaction to a disaster event necessitating a surge capacity response will result in the implementation of this plan along a continuum ranging from "conventional surge" to "contingency surge" to "crisis surge" response.[56]

"Conventional" surge includes providing patient care in manners and means using staff, equipment, pharmaceuticals, and supplies that are consistent with daily operations and usual practices. Planning for a conventional surge would include having processes and procedures to determine ED and hospital bed saturation. It comprises steps taken to cancel elective surgery and clinics, begin early or expedited discharge, and place the hospital on ambulance diversion.

"Contingency" surge planning incorporates the usage of staff, space, equipment, and supplies in a manner that is not consistent with daily practice but maintains or has minimal impact on patient care and patient care practices. Contingency planning would include strategies to provide patient care in areas or departments of the hospital that have the infrastructure to support but are not traditionally used in such a manner. Examples would include providing high-acuity care on a step-down unit or postanesthesia care unit where monitoring is available. Planning for contingency staffing would include strategies for assigning those from the hospital to duties they can safely conduct with appropriate oversight, such as having a floor nurse provide patient care in the intensive care unit.

In "crisis" surge capacity planning, the use of staff, space, equipment, and supplies is not consistent with usual standards of care but provides sufficiency of care in the catastrophic setting. Crisis surge capacity equates to the best possible care given the resources available and circumstances at the time. Examples would include providing inpatient care in locations not usually used for patients such as a tent, meeting room, or offsite in an alternate care location such as a hurricane shelter structure. Crisis surge staffing plans might include the use of nonclinical employees to provide clinical care, uncredentialed staff from other hospitals, or possibly the use of volunteers.

CRISIS STANDARD OF CARE IN DISASTER

Given the scope and scale of the disaster event, it may be possible that the surge in demand for patient care services significantly exceeds the resources available to meet such need. A catastrophic disaster, whether sudden in onset or sustained over time, may result in the prolonged shortage of available medical resources. It is recognized that events ranging from severe pandemic illness, use of improvised nuclear detonation, multipronged conventional terrorist attack with infrastructure disruption, and other horrific scenarios could lead to the rationing of health care.[57] Even in nondisaster settings, hospitals have recently been subject to the limited availability of key medications, including narcotic agents, influenza vaccine, paralytic medications (succinylcholine), and induction agents (propofol) used regularly in anesthesia, N-acetylcysteine used as an antidote in acetaminophen overdose cases, and chemotherapy agents (bleomycin, daunorubicin).[58-60]

In light of this "new normal," it is important for ED leaders to be familiar with work conducted by the National Academy of Sciences, Engineering and Medicine, which addresses the issue of standards of care in the setting of disaster events.[61] It delineates a process for creating an operational approach to the allocation of scarce resources in the clinical setting and is based upon the conventional/contingency/crisis surge response framework described previously.

There are a number of key planning and response assumptions that go along with this shift in the standard of care, including the very important fact that such an event occurs at the regional, if not state or national, level, as a result of which critical resources are unavailable elsewhere in the region or state, and a similar approach to allocating scarce resources is being invoked by other health-care delivery systems. Some key items that might be in short supply include ventilators, access to dialysis for renal replacement therapy, blood products, and key medications. Patient transfer to other facilities would not be possible or feasible. Also, it is assumed that all available local, regional, state, and federal resource caches of key equipment, supplies, and pharmaceuticals have already been distributed and no further immediate resupply of such stocks is foreseeable.[62,63]

As a result of the developing crisis, the delivery of medical services during the disaster will be governed by individual-based rather than population-based medical outcomes, thereby ensuring that clinical decisions support the ethical maxim in which the greatest good is provided for the greatest number of patients. In cases of scarcity, maximizing the medical benefit of limited available resources will be the ultimate goal. The Crisis Standards of Care reports[64,65] posit a uniform approach to rationing resources in a catastrophic disaster, ensuring maximal attempts at conservation, substitution of suitable alternatives to medications and equipment, adaptation of such alternative treatment modalities, and potential reuse of durable medical goods normally expended after single use (ensuring that careful attention is paid to infection prevention practices) (**Table 52.1**). Only after all such efforts are thoroughly exhausted would a reallocation approach for redistribution of those resources in shortest supply be invoked.

TABLE 52.1 ■ Framework for Management of Scarce Resources[61]		
Strategy	**Definition**	**Example**
Conservation	Using less of a resource by lowering the dosage or changing utilization practice	Minimize use of O_2 nebulizers
Substitution	Use of an equivalent device, drug, or staff member in the absence of what is usually available	Use morphine in place of fentanyl
Adaptation	Use of a device, drug, or staff member that would not be considered equivalent, but may still allow for delivery of sufficient care	Use of bag-valve-mask in place of ventilator
Reuse	Using appropriate disinfection/sterilization technique to reuse items that would normally be considered for single use only	Endotracheal tube, Foley catheter, central line
Reallocation	Taking a resource from one patient and providing it to another, based on transparent use of prognosis scoring	Ventilator reallocation based on sepsis-related organ failure assessment

UNDERSTANDING AND USING THE ICS

The response to an emergency incident requires the coordination, communication, and efficient use of multiple systems and resources. Many emergency events require initial single agency resources to integrate with other community response organizations. A hospital fire alarm will result in local fire officials responding to the hospital facility. Reports of a hospital shooting will initiate a law enforcement response, with numerous authorities arriving to assess and neutralize the threat. Both scenarios require close coordination with hospital officials in order to communicate effectively and coordinate resources for the response. The ICS is a standardized method and best practice for disaster, emergency, and daily incident management that facilitates response agency integration (**Box 52.3**).[66]

Incident command system was initially developed by a local, state, and federal interagency task force and FIRESCOPE (Firefighting Resources of California Organized for Potential Emergencies), a common operating plan to assist in combating California wildfires. FIRESCOPE was developed after the disastrous Southern California wildfires in 1970, which burned more than a half million acres, destroying 700 structures and taking 16 lives.[67] Challenges were noted by multiple agencies responding to the California wildfires, including inadequate communication technology or conflicting terminology; lack of a standardized management structure, which impeded fire responders' integration, ability for command and control, and workload efficiency; lack of personnel accountability; and lack of a systematic planning process.

After hearing of the successes of the use of FIRESCOPE and ICS in the Southern California wildfires, California hospitals began to explore ICS implementation in order to assist improving upon their own chaotic disaster and emergency responses.[68] In 1981, the State of California Emergency Medical Services Authority and Orange County Emergency Medical Services collaborated with local hospitals to create the first edition of the Hospital Emergency Incident Command System. Subsequent versions have been released in 1993 and

> **BOX 52.3 ■ INCIDENT COMMAND SYSTEM FEATURES**
>
> 1. **Predictable, responsibility-oriented chain of command:** ICS response roles have standardized titles, missions, responsibilities, and a clear reporting structure. In ICS there is one incident commander who has overall responsibility for the incident and who may activate other ICS positions as needed. The command positions include incident commander, public safety officer, liaison officer, and safety officer. Section chiefs include operations, planning, logistics, and finance.
>
> 2. **Use of a common nomenclature:** All agencies utilizing ICS use the same titles and functional roles for command staff positions. Common nomenclature assists when outside or different agencies are coordinating and responding to a common threat.
>
> 3. **Modular and flexible organization:** ICS allows for only those responses, roles, or sections needed to be activated. Similarly, roles and/or sections can be scaled back or taken out of service as the event culminates.
>
> 4. **Unified command structure:** ICS supports all response agencies in their establishment of unified incident objectives and strategies.
>
> 5. **Incident-action-planning (IAP):** ICS provides for an IAP to establish incident response goals and measurable objectives facilitating the response evaluation.
>
> 6. **Unity of command:** Each person reports to only one individual in ICS.
>
> 7. **Span of control:** Each manager or leader controls a defined set of response roles which is limited to what can feasibly and realistically be managed. The ideal is five to seven people per ICS leader role/supervisor.

1998, and the latest version, shortened in name to the Hospital Incident Command System, was released in 2014 (**Figure 52.4**).[69]

This event management tool has been incorporated into many hospital EOPs and implemented nationally and internationally during hospital emergency and disaster response.[70] The current version highlights the importance of establishing chain of command and incident action planning, and it includes specific tools that help establish accountability for specific command positions, including the development of "job action sheets" that serve as a checklist of "what to do," and encourages the adoption of common language for promoting interoperable communications (**Box 52.4**).[71]

In 2003, President George W. Bush issued Homeland Security Presidential Directive 5 and directed the secretary of Homeland Security to develop and administer the National Incident Management System (NIMS).[72] National Incident Management System was established to provide a response template for local, state, national, and tribal jurisdictions in domestic all-hazards incident management, including terrorism and nonterrorism events. A key component and requirement of the NIMS implementation is ICS adoption. Homeland Security Presidential Directive 5 requires all federal departments and agencies to adopt NIMS and makes NIMS compliance a requirement for states receiving federal preparedness assistance.

Ensuring Resource/Logistics Support

Planning for resource and logistical support will be an important component of the hospital EOP, and much of this planning is often done in conjunction with ED clinical and administrative input. Use of the hospital HVA can guide the development of selected stockpiles or disaster response kits. In addition, it is useful to develop backup agreements with alternate source vendors and suppliers. Examples of using the HVA to prioritize resource needs include the hypothetical hospital built on a flood plain, which chooses to

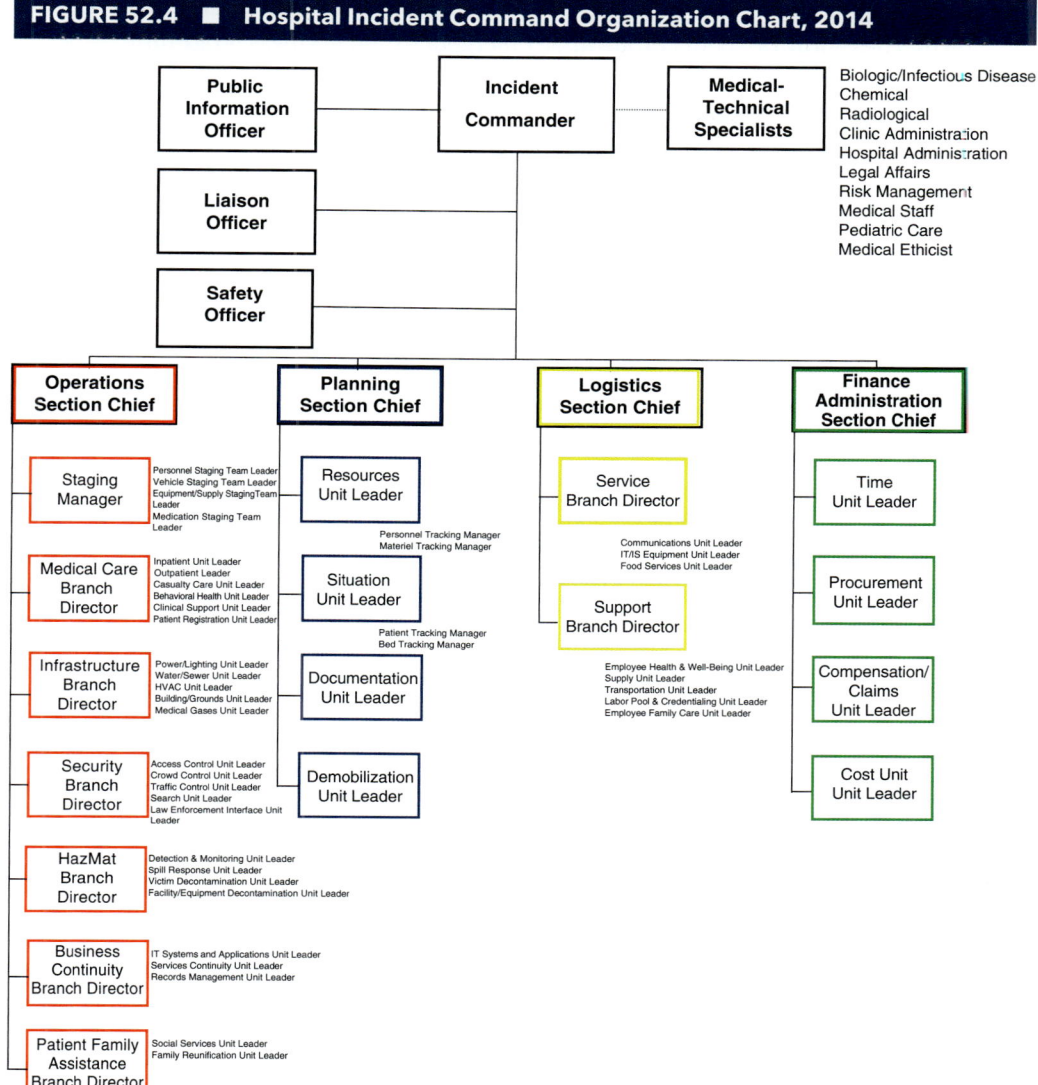

FIGURE 52.4 ■ Hospital Incident Command Organization Chart, 2014

BOX 52.4 ■ 2014 HICS REVISIONS

- A Patient Family Assistance Branch has been added under the Operations Section to address patient family needs during a response.
- An Employee Family Care Unit Leader has been included in the Support Branch within the Logistics Section to assist health-care staff and clinicians by providing support for their families.
- Greater emphasis has been placed on incident action planning, including the introduction of new, more practical tools.
- The HICS Forms have been revised to be more consistent with those used by the Federal Emergency Management Agency.
- A new chapter addressing HICS implementation during off hours and for small and rural hospitals has been added to the HICS Guidebook.

invest in an inventory of high-water clearance vehicles. Another example would be that of a hospital that lies within a Chemical Stockpile Emergency Preparedness Program jurisdiction (those communities that have chemical weapons stockpiled in depots). Such hospitals might choose to have additional nerve agent antidote available for use in case of an emergency.

The Joint Commission requires its member hospitals to maintain a resource directory as part of its EOP. The resource directory lists names and contact data for hospital operational needs, including equipment, medical gas, food, communications, IT support, and other pertinent vendors. It also requires that hospitals prepare to stand alone for 96 hours, without any resupply or support from external agencies.[73]

Coordinated Planning With the Community

Large-scale disaster events—including the 1995 Oklahoma City bombing, the September 11, 2001, World Trade Center and Pentagon attacks, the anthrax mailings, Hurricane Katrina, H1N1, the 2011 Joplin, Missouri, tornado, and the response to the 2017 Las Vegas mass shooting—all demonstrate the importance, and in Katrina's case, the failure of hospital and community planning for disaster and emergency response.[74] Indeed, one of the most important changes in disaster planning in the 15 years since funding first became available has been the development and maturation of hospital coalitions.[75-77] Hospital response to an external or internal emergency or disaster event is always a community impacting event, and rarely, with the exception being internal disasters, is it limited to a single hospital or health-care facility.

Coordinated disaster planning within local and regional jurisdictions has been integral to community disaster health for many years and today has evolved into formal health-care coalitions (HCCs). Health-care coalitions are local or regional collaborations of hospitals, EMS providers, public health, emergency management, and other provider types focused on "all-hazards" disaster and emergency preparedness. Initiated by the HHS/Assistant Secretary for Preparedness and Response Healthcare Preparedness Program, Cooperative Agreement, HCCs are structured and incentivized through federal funding to provide or facilitate resources and organization that may be required to plan, prepare, respond, and recover from a disaster event impacting the HCC and community.[78] Past HCC disaster responses have ranged from the anthrax attacks in the metropolitan Washington, DC region[79]; the Mississippi River bridge collapse in Minneapolis, Minn; the Houston, Tex, area responses to Hurricane Harvey[80]; and the Shreveport, La, coalition organization for Hurricane Katrina.

Coalition development is guided by the implementation of four program capabilities that guide how health-care systems within a coalition prepare for, respond to, and recover from disasters impacting community health. Capability implementation is coordinated with coalition hospitals, EMS providers, emergency management, public health, and other partner organizations that would support the health system in a disaster or catastrophic event. Not only do HCCs coordinate and respond to community disasters affecting population health, they also are a focal point for regional planning, training, exercises, and education. The benefit of ED leadership engaging with HCCs is ensuring that a coordinated plan evolves over the response to any given event. Operational HCCs can provide real-time situational awareness and serve as an additional resource to ED leaders by providing access to intelligence and operational updates, access to subject matter experts, and serve as a conduit to express the need for additional material and/or pharmaceutical resources that can be conveyed to state public health authorities.

In addition to coordinating with HCCs and understanding the requirements of the Joint Commission, ED leaders should be familiar with the fact that the Center for Medicare and Medicaid Services (CMS) has recently instituted a regulatory requirement for preparedness across an expanded array of health-care provider types.[81] This includes basic preparedness, including the development of plans, policies, and procedures, including those for communications, as well as testing and exercising such plans. Specific provider types in this preparedness rule include dialysis centers, skilled nursing facilities, and other outpatient facilities. The intent of the rule is to avoid the wholesale closure of such facilities and movement of their patients to EDs in the absence of continued service delivery. Multiple past disaster events have demonstrated such facilities as being the weak link in the chain for health-care service delivery during disaster events, particularly prolonged ones related to severe weather events. ED leaders, knowledgeable about the CMS preparedness rule, can help promote its compliance in conjunction with HCC leaders.

Communication deficits are not uncommon during critical events and are frequently reported after disaster exercises as a point for improvement. The importance of communications planning is most evident in the Congressional report "Katrina: A Failure of Initiative," which noted that timely delivery of medical care and coordination of hospital evacuations suffered from a lack of advance preparations and inadequate communications, among other difficulties.[78] The report demonstrates systemic failures at the local, state, and federal levels with an underscoring how failed hospital communications, and the inability to connect with local and state authorities, threatened the safety of medical staff and the lives of their patients. Hospitals were frequently without electronic communications as a result of wide-scale flooding. With the failure of infrastructure, including the loss of emergency electrical power and depletion of batteries, many hospitals could not communicate their functional status, existing capability, or requests for assistance.[78]

Another example of failed communications is described in the reports that detailed the EMS and hospital response to The Station Nightclub fire in 2003 in Warwick, Rhode Island, which resulted in 215 injured being transported to hospitals. Communication between EMS, hospital staff, and on-scene responders was reported insufficient. Some hospitals reported not receiving advance notification of incoming EMS units or the casualties they transported resulting in inadequate hospital preparations. In addition, EMS units, apparently self-directed, were creating problems tracking patient location.[82]

Emergency communication systems include functional hardware and supporting software that can dispatch messages to a variety of internal and external stakeholders. Mode examples include cell phones, text, satellite radios, 700 and 800 MHz radio, voice-over-internet protocol, and amateur (ham) radio and supporting equipment. Communication planning should include redundancies in equipment, power supply, and a variety of modes. This is important because one or more modes of communication may fail in a disaster event. The other key component to the communication system is the message and audience. Audiences include internal and external message recipients. With regard to ED and hospital planning, internal recipients include the hospital leadership and staff, while external messages go to patients, patient families, and the community at large.

CONCLUSION

Preparation and planning for response to a disaster event requires a significant amount of coordination of resources, personnel, equipment, and supplies. And it takes time to accomplish. This chapter provides the basic elements required to create a usable ED disaster plan and puts the implementation of this plan within the context of a hospital-wide and community-wide response. The time and effort put into figuring out how to respond to a disaster event, however unlikely it may seem, will be useful many times over in making the ED stronger, better organized, more cohesive, and if needed, ready to meet the challenges of a community disaster.

REFERENCES

1. Garcia TC, Bernstein AB, Bush MA. Emergency department visitors and visits: who used the emergency room in 2007? *NCHS Data Brief,* No 38. 2010 May;(38):1-8.

2. Kellermann AL. Crisis in the emergency department. *N Engl J Med.* 2006;355(13):1300-1303.

3. Behnam M, Tillotson RD, Davis SM, Hobbs GR. Violence in the emergency department: a national survey of emergency medicine residents and attending physicians. *J Emerg Med.* 2011;40(5):565-579.

4. Bayley MD, Schwartz JS, Shofer FS, et al. The financial burden of emergency department congestion and hospital crowding for chest pain patients awaiting admission. *Ann Emerg Med.* 2005;45(2):110-117.

5. Parker R, Little K, Heuser, S. Development actions and the rising incidence of disasters. IEG Evaluation Brief 4. The World Bank. 2007.

6. Quarantelli EL. Disaster crisis management: a summary of research findings. *J Manage Studies.* 1988;25(4):373-385.

7. Auf der Heide E. The importance of evidence-based disaster planning. *Ann Emerg Med.* 2006;47(1):34-39.

8. Niska RW, Shimizu IM. Hospital preparedness for emergency response: United States, 2008. Statistics Report No 37. *Natl Health Stat Report.* 2011;(37):1-14.

9. Quarantelli EL. Disaster crisis management: a summary of research findings. *J Manage Studies.* 1988;25(4):373-385.

10. HHS/ASPR TRACIE. Topic collection: hazard vulnerability/risk assessment. Available at: https://asprtracie.hhs.gov/technical-resources/3/hazard-vulnerability-risk-assessment/1. Accessed May 17, 2018.

11. Campbell P, Trockman SJ, Walker AR. Strengthening hazard vulnerability analysis: results of recent research in Maine. *Public Health Rep.* 2011;126(2):290-293.

12. California Emergency Medical Services Authority. The Hospital Incident Command Guidebook (HICS). 2006:18. Available at: https://emsa.ca.gov/disaster-medical-services-division-hospital-incident-command-system/. Accessed June 19, 2011.

13. Andress K. Hospital emergency management. In: Birnbaum E, Powers R, eds. *International Disaster Nursing.* Cambridge University Press; 2009:48-55.

14. The Joint Commission. Hospital Emergency Operations Plan, Standard EM.02.01.01.5; 2011.

15. Bloch YH, Schwartz D, Pinkert M, et al. Distribution of casualties in a mass-casualty incident with three local hospitals in the periphery of a densely populated area: lessons learned from the medical management of a terrorist attack. *Prehosp Disaster Med.* 2007;22(3):186-192.

16. Raiter Y, Farfel A, Lehavi O, et al. Mass casualty incident management, triage, injury distribution of casualties and rate of arrival of casualties at the hospitals: lessons from a suicide bomber attack in downtown Tel Aviv. *Emerg Med J.* 2008;25(4):225-229.

17. Ashkenazi I, Kessel B, Olsha O, et al. Defining the problem, main objective, and strategies of medical management in mass-casualty incidents caused by terrorist events. *Prehosp Disast Med.* 2008;23(1):82-89.

18. Baker MS. Creating order from chaos: part I: triage, initial care, and tactical considerations in mass casualty and disaster response. *Mil Med.* 2007;172(3):232-236.

19. US Department of Health and Human Services. Is the HIPAA privacy rule suspended during a national or public health emergency? Available at: https://www.hhs.gov/hipaa/for-professionals/faq/1068/is-hipaa-suspended-during-a-national-or-public-health-emergency/index.html. Accessed May 17, 2018.

20. HHS/ASPR TRACIE. HIPAA and disasters: what emergency professionals need to know. Available at: https://cchealth.org/ems/pdf/aspr-tracie-hipaa-emergency-fact-sheet.pdf. Accessed May 17, 2018.

21. Kahn CA, Schultz CH, Miller KT, Anderson CL. Does START triage work? An outcomes assessment after a disaster. *Ann Emerg Med.* 2009;54(3):424-430.

22. Lerner EB, Schwartz RB, Coule PL, et al. Mass casualty triage: an evaluation of the data and development of a proposed national guideline. *Disaster Med Public Health Prep.* 2008;2(suppl 1):25S-34Ss.

23. Lerner EB, Schwartz RB, Coule PL, Pirrallo RG. Use of SALT triage in a simulated mass-casualty incident. *Prehosp Emerg Care.* 2010;14(1):21-25.

24. Sacco WJ, Navin DM, Fiedler KE, et al. Precise formulation and evidence-based application of resource constrained triage. *Acad Emerg Med.* 2005;12(8):759-770.

25. Sacco WJ, Navin DM, Waddell RK, et al. A new resource-constrained triage method applied to victims of penetrating injury. *J Trauma.* 2007;63(2):316-325.

26. Navin DM, Sacco WJ, McGill G. Application of new resource-constrained triage method to military-age victims. *Mil Med.* 2009;174(12):1247-1255.

27. Frykberg ER. Principles of mass casualty management following terrorist disasters. *Ann Surg.* 2004;239(3):319-321.

28. Klein JS, Weigelt JA. Disaster management lessons learned. *Surg Clin North Am.* 1991;71(2):257-266.

29. Feliciano DV, Anderson GV, Rozycki GS, et al. Management of casualties from the bombing at the centennial Olympics. *Am J Surg.* 1998;176(6):538-543.

30. Mahoney EJ, Harrington DT, Biffl WL, Metzger J, Oka T, Cioffi WG. Lessons learned from a nightclub fire: institutional preparedness. *J Trauma.* 2005;58(3):487-491.

31. Bradt D, Aitken P, FitzGerald GJ, Swift R, O'Reilly G, Bartley B. Emergency department surge capacity: recommendations of the Australasian Surge Strategy Working Group. *Acad Emerg Med.* 2009;16(12):1350-1358.

32. Korner M, Krotz MM, Wirth S, et al. Evaluation of a CT triage protocol for mass casualty incidents: results from two large-scale exercises. *Eur Radiol.* 2009;19(8):1867-1874.

33. Brock TK, Mecozzi DM, Sumner S, Kost GJ. Evidence-based point-of-care tests and device designs for disaster preparedness. *Am J Disaster Med.* 2010;5(5):285-294.

34. Kost GJ, Hale KN, Brock TK, et al. Point of care testing for disasters: needs assessment, strategic planning, and future design. *Clin Lab Med.* 2009;29(3):583-605.

35. Benedek DM, Fullerton C, Ursano RJ. First responders: mental health consequences of natural and human-made disasters for public health and public safety workers. *Annu Rev Public Health.* 2007;28:55-68.

36. Tham KY, Tan YH, Loh OH, Tan WL, Ong MK, Tang HK. Psychiatric morbidity among emergency department doctors and nurses after the SARS outbreak. *Ann Acad Med Singapore.* 2004;33(suppl 5):78S-79S.

37. Hick JL, Hanfling D, Burstein JL, Markham J, Macintyre AG, Barbera JA. Protective equipment for healthcare facility decontamination personnel: regulations, risks and recommendations. *Ann Emerg Med.* 2003;42(3):370-380.

38. Hick JL, Penn P, Hanfling D, et al. Training healthcare facility decontamination teams. *Annals Emerg Med.* 2003;42:381-390.

39. Fenzl M, Jolliff H, Topinka M. Chemical exposure preparedness for emergency departments in a Midwestern city. *Am J Disaster Med.* 2008;3(5):273–281.

40. DiCarlo AL, Maher C, Hick JL, et al. Radiation injury after a nuclear detonation: medical consequences and the need for scarce resources allocation. *Disaster Med Public Health Prep.* 2011;5(suppl 1):32S–44S.

41. Hick JL, Weinstock DM, Coleman CN, et al. Health care system planning for and response to a nuclear detonation. *Disaster Med Public Health Prep.* 2011;5(suppl 1):73S–88S.

42. Freyberg CW, Arquilla B, Fertel BS, et al. Disaster preparedness: hospital decontamination and the pediatric patient: guidelines for hospitals and emergency planners. *Prehosp Disaster Med.* 2008;23(2):166–173.

43. Bulson J, Bulson TC, Vande Guchte KS. Hospital-based special needs patient decontamination: lessons from the shower. *Am J Disaster Med*. 2010;5(6):353–360.

44. Hanfling D, Hick JL. Hospitals and the novel H1N1 outbreak: the mouse that roared? *Disaster Med Public Health Prep.* 2009;3(suppl 2):100S–106S.

45. Tham KY. An emergency department response to severe acute respiratory syndrome: a prototype response to bioterrorism. *Ann Emerg Med.* 2004;43(1):6–14.

46. Chen SY, Ma MH, Su CP, et al. Facing an outbreak of highly transmissible disease: problems in emergency department response. *Ann Emerg Med.* 2004;44(1):93–95.

47. Schultz CH, Mothershead JL, Field M. Bioterrorism preparedness I: the emergency department and hospital. *Emerg Med Clin North Am.* 2002;20(2):437–455.

48. Roszak AR, Jensen FR, Wild RE, Yeskey K, Handrigan MT. Implications of the Emergency Medical Treatment and Labor Act (EMTALA) during public health emergencies and on alternate sites of care. *Disaster Med Public Health Prep.* 2009;3(suppl 2):172S–175S.

49. Thompson T, Lyle K, Mullins SH, Dick R, Graham J. A state survey of emergency department preparedness for the care of children in a mass casualty event. *Am J Disaster Med.* 2009;4(4):227–232.

50. Gotanda H, Fogel J, Husk G, et al. Hurricane Sandy: impact on emergency department and hospital utilization by older adults in Lower Manhattan, New York (USA). *Prehosp Disaster Med.* 2015;30(5):496–502.

51. HHS EMPOWER map 2.0. Available at: https://empowermap.hhs.gov/. Accessed April 29, 2018.

52. Bartlett JG. Planning for avian influenza. *Ann Intern Med.* 2006;145(2):141–144.

53. Hick JL, Hanfling D, Burstein JL, et al. Health care facility and community strategies for patient care surge capacity. *Ann Emerg Med.* 2004;44(3):253–261.

54. Hanfling D. Equipment, supplies and pharmaceuticals: how much might it cost to achieve basic surge capacity? *Acad Emerg Med.* 2006;13:1232–1237.

55. Bonnett CJ, Peery BN, Cantrill SV, et al. Surge capacity: a proposed conceptual framework. *Am J Emerg Med.* 2007;25(3):297–306.

56. Hick JL, Barbera JA, Kelen GD. Refining surge capacity: conventional, contingency, and crisis capacity. *Disaster Med Public Health Prep.* 2009;3(suppl 2):59S–67S.

57. Gostin LO, Hanfling D. National preparedness for a catastrophic emergency: crisis standards of care. *JAMA.* 2009;302(21):2365–2366.

58. Steinbrook R. Drug shortages and public health. *N Engl J Med.* 2009;361(16):1525–1527.

59. Hampton T. Experts look for ways to lessen impact of drug shortages and discontinuations. *JAMA.* 2007;298(7):727–728.

60. Current drug shortages. US Food and Drug Administration. Available at: https://www.fda.gov/Drugs/DrugSafety/DrugShortages/default.htm. Accessed May 3, 2018.

61. Institute of Medicine (IOM). *Guidance for Establishing Crisis Standards of Care for Use in Disaster Situations: A Letter Report.* Altevogt BM, Stroud C, Hanson SL, Hanfling D, Gostin LO, eds. The National Academies Press; 2009.

62. Centers for Disease Control and Prevention. Strategic National Stockpile Program. Available at: https://www.cdc.gov/phpr/stockpile/index.htm. Accessed May 3, 2018.

63. Centers for Disease Control and Prevention. Chempack Program Description, Public Health Preparedness and Response for Bioterrorism, Continuation Guidance–Budget Year Five, June 14, 2004. Available at: https://www.cdc.gov/phpr/documents/coopagreement-archive/fy2004/chempack-attachj.pdf. Accessed May 19, 2018.

64. Institute of Medicine (IOM) *Crisis Standards of Care: A Systems Framework.* Hanfling D, Altevogt BM, Viswanathan K, Gostin LO, eds. The National Academies Press; 2012.

65. Institute of Medicine (IOM). *Crisis Standards of Care: A Toolkit for Indicators and Triggers.* Hanfling D, Hick J, Stroud C, eds. The National Academies Press; 2013.

66. US Federal Emergency Management Agency (FEMA). Incident Command System (ICS) Review. 2008. Available at: https://training.fema.gov/emiweb/is/icsresource/assets/reviewmaterials.pdf. Accessed April 29, 2018.

67. Chase R. FIRESCOPE: A new concept in multiagency fire suppression. US Department of Agriculture. 1980:2–14. Available at: http://www.fs.fed.us/psw/publications/documents/psw_gtr040/psw_gtr040.pdf. Accessed April 29, 2018.

68. California Emergency Medical Services Authority (EMSA). Hospital Incident Command System (HICS) Guidebook. 2014. Available at: https://emsa.ca.gov/disaster-medical-services-division-hospital-incident-command-system-resources/. Accessed April 29, 2018.

69. California Emergency Medical Services Authority (EMSA). Hospital Incident Command System, History and Background. Available at: https://emsa.ca.gov/HICS-history-and-background/. Accessed May 19, 2018.

70. Tsai M, Arnold J, Chuang C, Chi C, Liu C, Yang Y. Implementation of the hospital emergency incident command system during an outbreak of severe acute respiratory syndrome (SARS) at a hospital in Taiwan, ROC. *J Emerg Med.* 2005;28(2) 185–196.

71. California Emergency Medical Services Authority (EMSA). Hospital Incident Command System–FAQ's, October 2014. Available at: https://emsa.ca.gov/disaster-medical-services-division-hospital-incident-command-system-faq/. Accessed May 3, 2018.

72. DHS Homeland Security Directive-5. Management of domestic incidents. Available at: https://www.dhs.gov/sites/default/files/publications/Homeland%20Security%20Presidential%20Directive%205.pdf. Accessed May 17, 2018.

73. The Joint Commission. Hospital Emergency Operations Plan, Standard, EM.02.01.01. 2011.

74. Maldin B, Lam C, Franco C, et al. Regional approaches to hospital preparedness. Biosecurity and bioterrorism: biodefense strategy, practice and science. *Biosecur Bioterror.* 2007;5:43–53.

75. Courtney B, Toner E, Waldhorn R, et al. Healthcare coalitions: the new foundation for national healthcare preparedness and response for catastrophic health emergencies. *Biosecur Bioterror.* 2009;7(2): 153–163.

76. Center for Biosecurity of UPMC. Hospitals Rising to the Challenge: The First 5 Years of the Hospital Preparedness Program and

Priorities Going Forward. Prepared for the US Department of Health and Human Services under Contract No. HHSO100200700038C. March 2009.

77. Burkle FM Jr, Hsu EB, Loehr M, et al. Definition and functions of health unified command and emergency operations centers for large-scale bioevent disasters within the existing ICS. *Disaster Med Public Health Prep.* 2007;1(2):135–141.

78. A Failure of Initiative–Final Report of the Select Bipartisian Committee to Investigate the Preparation for and Response to Hurricane Katrina, 2006. US Government Printing Office. Available at: https://katrina.house.gov/. Accessed May 3, 2018.

79. Special Report 109–322–Hurricane Katrina: A Nation Still Unprepared Special Report of the Senate Committee on Homeland Security and Governmental Affairs, 2006. US Government Printing Office. Available at: https://www.gpo.gov/fdsys/pkg/CRPT-109srpt322/pdf/CRPT-109srpt322.pdf. Accessed May 3, 2018.

80. Mahoney E, Harrington D, Biffl W, Metzger J, Oka T, Cioffi W. Lessons learned from a nightclub fire: institutional disaster preparedness. *J Trauma.* 2004;58(3):487–491.

81. Centers for Medicare and Medicaid Services. Emergency Preparedness Rule. Available at: https://www.cms.gov/Medicare/Provider-Enrollment-and-Certification/SurveyCertEmergPrep/Emergency-Prep-Rule. Accessed July 14, 2020.

82. NIST Engineering Laboratory. The Station Nightclub Fire. Available at: https://www.nist.gov/el/station-nightclub-fire-2003. Accessed July 14, 2020.

CHAPTER 53

MILITARY EMERGENCY MEDICINE

Vikhyat S. Bebarta, Linda L. Lawrence

Military emergency medicine has seen significant changes since the 1990s and has been redefined in positive ways by the past decade of war. The changes have had an impact beyond the military services through research, academic partnerships, and international collaboration. Just as military medicine heavily influenced the development of emergency medical services (EMS) and out-of-hospital care (which subsequently led to the need for the specialty of emergency medicine), the military continues to advance the clinical practice of emergency medicine, especially in the realms of trauma care, critical care, and patient transport. While the day-to-day clinical practice of military providers is similar to that of civilian providers, it is the unique opportunities for diversification and the operational experiences that make of military emergency medicine so rewarding.

ADVANTAGES OF THE MILITARY HEALTH SYSTEM

The military health system (MHS) and the Defense Health Agency maintain 56 hospitals and 365 clinics, and the MHS/TRICARE system provides coverage for 9.7 million beneficiaries, including active-duty personnel, retirees, and their families.[1] Similar to the civilian health-care system, the MHS has seen a reduction in military emergency departments (EDs). From a high of 164 EDs in 1998, there were 50% fewer by year 2000 and several more closures in the past decade, all due to fiscal reductions.[2]

There are numerous advantages to practicing military emergency medicine, as summarized in **Box 53.1.** And in contrast to the civilian population, MHS beneficiaries have universal health insurance, which significantly enhances their access to primary, specialty, and emergency care. In addition, military beneficiaries have no copay or need for preauthorization when visiting a military ED. Overall, the MHS focuses on patient-centered

---

BOX 53.1 ■ ADVANTAGES OF PRACTICING MILITARY EMERGENCY MEDICINE AND NURSING

- Universal health insurance for employees and dependents
- Patient-centered primary care teams
- Access to prescription drugs, immunizations, and public health and injury presentation services
- Psychiatric support services
- Sexual assault support services
- Defined and committed on-call physicians
- Disaster preparedness
- Defined and supportive medicolegal climate

care with a team approach that provides a greater level of support for emergency medicine providers and their patients.

Military beneficiaries have access to prescription drugs, immunizations, and many public health and injury-prevention services. The military goes through great lengths to promote on-the-job safety and injury prevention at all levels. These safety efforts include tough motorcycle helmet laws, required motorcycle safety courses, child safety seat requirements, and aggressive random screening programs and education to prevent alcohol- and drug-related accidents. In addition, military beneficiaries have access to a number of wellness programs including alcohol and drug treatment, smoking cessation, and access to fitness centers with a multitude of free programs that promote healthy lifestyles. Despite a zero-tolerance climate for sexual harassment and assault, the military recognizes the need for victims to have confidential access to treatment and thus have model programs.

As discussed in more detail later in this chapter, military emergency medicine benefits from a defined and committed group of on-call physicians, most of whom are military physicians, with the exception of certain subspecialties and tertiary care services.

Disaster preparedness is a strength of military hospitals because it is integral to operational readiness training. Typically, disaster response plans are more advanced than their civilian counterparts. Military hospitals place greater emphasis on preparedness training for all health-care workers and include regular drills for chemical, radiation, and biological threats (**Figure 53.1**). Training drills are also coordinated with states and communities, and the Department of Defense (DOD) remains a key partner in the National Disaster Medical System. Emergency physicians have become important leaders in the realm of disaster response, and many military emergency physicians will at some point in their career find opportunities to participate in disaster response and humanitarian support activities (**Figure 53.2**).

The medicolegal climate is much more favorable in the military, where government employees are not subject to personal liability lawsuits. In cases of alleged malpractice, the claimant files suit against the federal government instead of the individual provider. Each

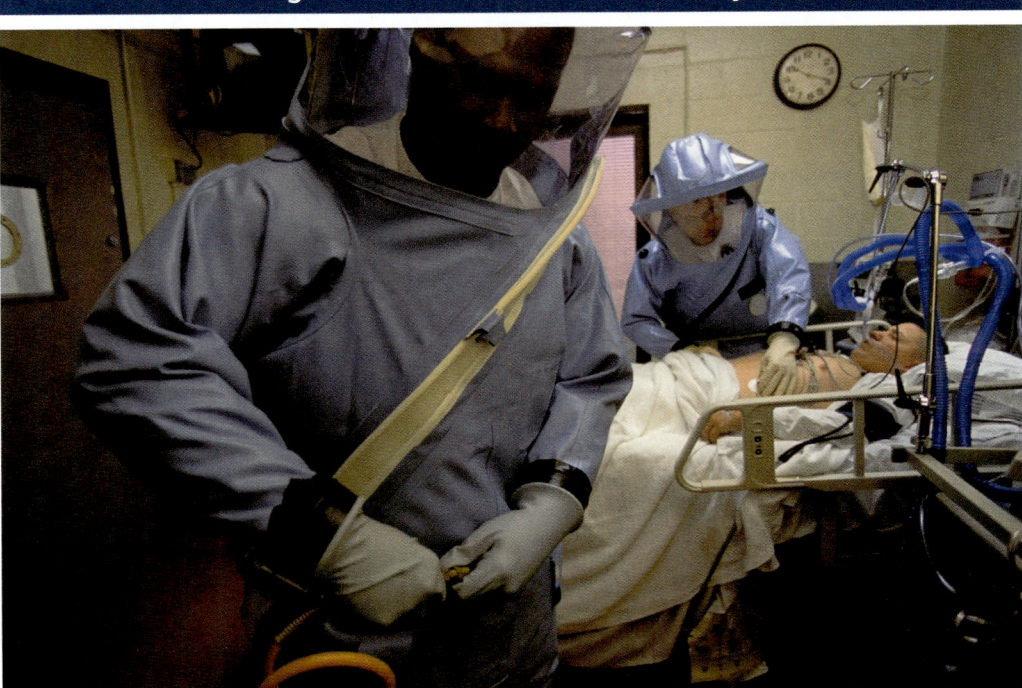

FIGURE 53.1 ■ Biological Warfare Exercise, Frederick, Maryland

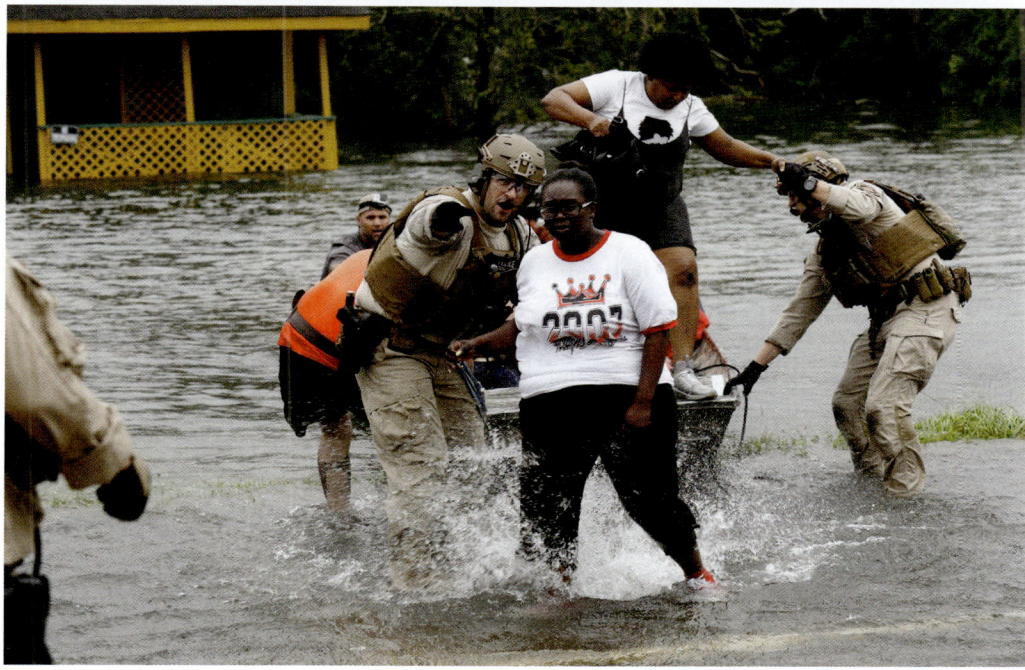

FIGURE 53.2 ■ Military Aircrew Rescue Team Evacuates Stranded Residents Trapped by Flood Waters, Beaumont, Texas

service has a process to identify significantly involved providers and perform standard-of-care reviews after an adverse outcome. These rigorous reviews are used in a separate process to determine if a claim is settled and whether the physician should be reported to the national practitioner databank. The process for determination to report affords due process to the physician and fair opportunities for physician input at several stages of the process. In addition, the DOD has a comprehensive patient safety program focused on identifying system trends and opportunities for improvement. The program promotes collaboration across all three services—US Army, US Navy, and US Airforce—and fosters trust, transparency, teamwork, and communication.[3]

Practice Pathways

Change and diversity are the rule for military emergency physicians because several career paths exist and one can cross pathways throughout their military career, however short or long. The typical length of an assignment is two to four years, with assignments at academic programs often lasting longer. Active-duty emergency physicians are all board certified or board eligible, and entrance now requires emergency medicine residency training to work in a military ED. In some overseas bases, 24/7 urgent care centers or low-volume EDs may be staffed with a mix of emergency medicine physicians and other providers. Although patient acuity may be lower at these facilities, the need for services to support the generally healthy base population drives the 24/7 access. While retention has improved in some services, overall the clinical workforce remains somewhat junior with the majority of emergency physicians completing one assignment and then leaving active-duty service.

In each service, a senior emergency physician is appointed as the chief consultant/specialty advisor to the service surgeon general and will serve as the voice of expertise and advocacy on all issues regarding emergency medicine. The consultant/specialty advisor assists the service senior-level management functions in managing the career field and serves as a clinical subject matter expert. Managing the career field includes important roles, such as developing manpower standards, annually projecting graduate medical education (GME) training requirements to include fellowship training and the selection of trainees, assisting the recruiting service with screening prospective candidates, and serving as advisor in the corps development and assignment process of emergency physicians.

Over the past decade, responsibility has increased significantly. The consultant/specialty leader has become a critical advisor in the deployment of emergency physicians to support combat operations and advocating for the proper training, equipment, and further development and refinement of the emergency physician role in the operational mission.

As a subject matter expert, the consultant/specialty advisor monitors the quality of care and ED operations, keeps abreast of advances in clinical practices and technology, assists in service policy, and supports facility-specific planning and implementation. The consultant/specialty advisor also assists in the evaluation of proposed research protocols, collaborates on technical and clinical innovations, and oversees standard-of-care determinations, medicolegal reviews, and medical incident investigations when necessary.

While each service has its own command channels and budgeting and resource-allocation programs, the emergency medicine consultant/specialty advisor sets an example of collaboration in promoting the specialty of emergency medicine within the MHS and externally.

CLINICAL PATHWAYS

There are several clinical pathways in military emergency care, each of which provide unique opportunities.

Emergency Physicians

The most common clinical pathway is an assignment to a military community hospital. Nonacademic military hospitals are similar to smaller community hospitals or, for some of the overseas locations, they may be more synonymous with a critical access hospital. The patient population is is particularly diverse, as military family members and retirees maintain access to ED care regardless of insurance status. In addition, military hospitals are active in the local EMS systems and may provide care to civilians in emergent situations. One military academic ED, the San Antonio Military Medical Center (SAMMC) in Texas, holds a level 1 trauma center designation. It's also a cardiac care referral center, and it supports a 24/7 stroke team. The Madigan Army Medical Center in Washington State is a level II, but most community military hospitals lack any official trauma designation, though they function at a level III.

Typically, a military emergency medicine department will be staffed by board-certified and board-eligible emergency physicians and may be augmented by emergency medicine physician assistants (EMPAs), many of whom are fellowship trained. Given the typical tour length of two to four years, it is common to have at least a 20% to 25% provider staff turnover each year. While this might appear problematic, most EDs have excellent processes, and the similarities in practice and systems from one military ED to another promote easy orientation. In addition, the high operational tempo and frequent deployments over the past decade have resulted in increased provider staffing, which may create more flexibility. The demand for emergency physicians exceeds the active-duty authorizations, so all services rely on hiring civilian emergency physicians through either contracts or general schedule (GS) federal employee system.

Emergency Nursing

Similar to civilian EDs, military emergency nursing skills are quite varied, but the recent trend is to promote more standardization and a clearer set of competency-based roles. The military recognizes the need for specialization and encourages nursing staff to obtain the certified emergency nurse (CEN) credential. That has not always been the case and, like the evolution of specialty-trained emergency physicians, the importance of specialty training and dedicated career paths for emergency nurses continues to mature. The past decade has further defined the importance for emergency nurses to maintain a skill set and competency to support the operational mission. All services now have specialized duty codes for specialty trained and CENs. However, since the recruitment of military nurses is predominantly focused on generalized nurses, initial specialty training commonly occurs through on-the-job training in military EDs.

To better support the need for robust training programs and clinical nursing oversight, the use of clinical nurse specialist (CNS) positions are becoming more prevalent. The CNS requires master- or doctorate-level advanced training along with demonstrated clinical experience and proficiency. The role of the CNS is vital to supporting department-level nurse training programs, quality and process improvement initiatives, and research and administrative and leadership roles.

Overall, the past decade has emphasized the importance of keeping nurses with specialized skills more involved in direct patient care, which has helped to promote a career path that keeps emergency nurses within the ED and provides more opportunities for advanced fellowships. Military emergency nurses have also played significant roles in the provision of combat casualty care, further driving the need for specialization and core competency in trauma and critical care. Maintenance of trauma knowledge and skills occurs through training affiliations with civilian trauma centers, simulation, and institutional training programs. The trauma nursing core course is another highly desired and often required training for military emergency nurses.

Medical Technicians/Hospital Corpsmen

Enlisted medical technicians or hospital corpsmen are vital to the ED team and have larger roles and broader scope of responsibility than typically seen by medical technicians in civilian EDs. Policy varies slightly by service as to the scope of practice for enlisted staff, but all services require additional training for the medical technicians working in the ED. ED technicians assist the nursing staff and work directly with them in rendering patient care. Some of the advanced skills taught to technicians include insertions of intravenous catheters, simple wound management, and splinting. A pathway exists in each service for advanced training to serve as independent duty medical technicians or corpsman with the ability to render fuller scope of medical care to active-duty personnel, especially in the operational environment. All care is closely monitored and supported by physician medical direction and comprehensive policies.

Depending on the location, the ED may support a base EMS. Emergency medical technicians (EMTs) will range in certification—the EMT-Basic, Advanced EMT, and Paramedic—with certification from the National Registry of EMTs. Off-line and online medical control is provided by the emergency physician, and each base EMS service will have a designated medical director. Due to the importance of EMS services both at bases and deployed, each service has EMS (i.e., out-of-hospital) fellowship-trained emergency physicians to serve as service consultants.

Organizational Structure of Military EDs

While the chief of the ED may be an emergency physician or a nurse, physicians are typically assigned that role. In those cases where a nurse is assigned as the chief of the ED, the medical director has an increased role in the oversight of clinical care and policies. What is unique is that the ED chief has administrative control over all the staff. This model promotes a stronger sense of teamwork and shared responsibility. Emergency physicians at all levels are encouraged to participate in administrative positions within the ED and the hospital from the earliest stages of their career. The almost unparalleled opportunity to develop leadership and management skills prepares the emergency physician to be very competitive for future senior leadership positions within the MHS or be highly sought after when after leaving the military for civilian emergency medicine practice. Indeed, with the increasing emphasis on accountability for measured results in civilian EDs, emergency physicians and nurses with experience in military leadership positions are extremely attractive candidates for medical and nursing director opportunities.

Patient care follows the same standards of care as any civilian ED, and all military hospitals maintain accreditation through The Joint Commission. The organization and resource management of military hospitals affords some positive aspects that reduce liability and promote quality of care. While the senior medical service level alignment of Army, Navy, and Air Force differs slightly, at the hospital level, there is less variance and all have a team-based patient-centered care focus. Fortunately, most patients have a primary care physician. Access to primary care is reasonable, especially in more recent years because the military has pushed toward a patient-centered medical home model with outcomes being tracked by each service surgeon general and the MHS. One of the metrics is ED/urgent care utilization by beneficiary with a goal to reduce unnecessary ED visits. Another key metric is continuity of care with the assigned primary care provider, and because most of the primary care providers are part of the same hospital, urgent follow-up can usually be obtained with good transitions of care.

Nonetheless, some perceptions remain that military EDs are inundated with a disproportionate percent of low-acuity patients. Emergency department utilization by military beneficiaries is very similar to rates reported for US and Canadian populations, with a rate of 40 visits per 100 population.[4] A 2009 study funded by Tricare Management Activity through Deloitte Consulting asked for reasons why beneficiaries utilize EDs. In response, 89% cited "problem critical and I felt it needed attention that only ER can deliver."[5] Regardless, perceptions remain realities and the practicing military emergency physician recognizes the need to remain current in procedural skills, which require higher acuity patients. The respective service's senior leadership also recognizes the important need for operational currency and is committed to maintaining robust clinical platforms for critical care and surgically based specialties.

Despite military EDs lacking a standardized electronic medical record (EMR), all outpatient clinics share a universal EMR that can be reviewed across services. Inpatient EMRs are now present at all military hospitals. This affords the emergency physician ready access for medical information on most patients, which helps to optimize transitions of care and reduce the need for unnecessary diagnostic studies. However, there are some patients, particularly the elderly and veterans, who receive their care outside the military system but have access to military emergency care. The MHS is working with the Veterans Health Administration (VHA) in the development of a universal EMR that will include an ED module. Fortunately, computerized prescription and lab order entry have been readily available for several years, along with systems to reduce medication errors.

The team approach is again noted with on-call specialty support. While the breadth of specialty support can vary, depending on the size of the hospital when services are available, there remains a clear line of authority for ensuring on-call support availability. No issues of insurance or reimbursement threaten clinical decision-making. Ordering of diagnostic tests centers on the right test at the right time. And the presence of EMR and good digital records allows easy access to prior studies. Knowing outpatient follow-up care can usually be easily arranged and that there is a relatively compliant patient population, the emergency physician can partner with specialists to make the best treatment decisions and sometimes avoid unnecessary admissions or prolonged periods of observation. However, most military hospitals share similarities with smaller community hospitals in that some of the more limited and higher acuity specialties are unavailable. For example, neurosurgery, cardiothoracic surgery, and pediatric subspecialties typically require referral. Thus, military EDs typically have well-established relationships with local tertiary referral centers and maintain ambulance transport services or contract with local ambulance transport services.

A decade of war has brought a renewed focus to MHS on the need for clinical currency at all staff levels driving the need to recapture care, especially in the surgical fields. During the early years of the Iraq and Afghanistan conflicts, staffing was extremely limited due to deployments. For some military hospitals, services were being cut and academic programs were in jeopardy of reaccreditation. Fortunately, it was recognized that to sustain their ability to remain competent in the core operational mission and for providers, nurses, and other health-care staff to remain competent, military hospitals would need to remain viable. A recent relook at ED, surgical, and inpatient flow in the Air Force Medical Service (AFMS) has allowed increased access and the ability to recapture patients who previously may have been deferred to network civilian hospitals. In a look at AFMS admission patterns, it was identified that approximately 50% of hospital admissions come from the ED. At most military hospitals, adequate inpatient bed availability exists and thus "boarding" is not a problem. Because the ED serves as a vital portal for recapture of care, especially for beneficiaries who don't receive their routine care at the military hospital, it has become more imperative that EDs maintain good flow and quality of care. This further drives the responsiveness of a team approach for on-call specialty support and access to inpatient care.

The 2012 MHS Stakeholders Report cites the following:

We will operate our MTFs (military treatment facilities) at full capacity to support readiness and the backbone of our clinical systems — our GME programs. Over the past five years, the amount of care provided to DOD beneficiaries has continued to increase, but the majority of that increase has occurred in the private sector. There is an opportunity to pull some of that additional workload back into military treatment facilities so that our providers can remain current in the skills they need for readiness and so that our trainees can have a rich clinical experience.[6]

This commitment is important in defining the future practice of military emergency medicine and, even if combat operations wind down, ensuring it will remain necessary to keep a comprehensive practice for military emergency physicians to maintain the full spectrum of currency.

With over a decade of recent combat in Iraq in Operation Iraqi Freedom and Afghanistan in Operation Enduring Freedom, traumatic brain injury and post-traumatic stress disorder remain the hallmark "invisible wounds" of those wars. Long deployments and intense combat conditions in both theaters have generated an increased demand for mental health services by both the members and their families, and the need for mental health services will only increase in the coming years as the US deals with the effects of more than a decade of conflict.[7] Despite executive orders to increase access to mental health services and mental health staffing within DOD and VHA, access to mental health services can be strained. Priority is given to active-duty patients, and the MHS has very few inpatient mental health facilities driving the need to coordinate care in an already overtaxed civilian mental health-care network. Military dependents and retirees must rely almost exclusively on the civilian mental health network, making the provision of care to mental health patients one of the greater challenges for the military emergency medicine physician. Mental health care and resource challenges illustrate the significance of the national crisis in American health care. Military solutions will further compete with an underresourced and underfunded civilian emergency health-care system in dire need of significant reform.

ACADEMIC PATHWAYS

Military leaders recognize the importance of maintaining their own academic medical facilities to support GME programs. Some of these are service specific, others are joint service training programs. Recently, more emergency medicine residency training positions have developed in collaboration with local civilian emergency medicine residency programs to meet the growing demand for more emergency physicians in the military's overseas contingency operations and to maintain currency platforms for faculty.

Military academic hospitals typically have multiple residency programs and thus a broader scope of subspecialty care. The patient population at these hospitals includes more military retirees and is found in geographic locations with denser military beneficiary populations. In addition, many academic military EDs receive civilian emergencies by ambulance. All military emergency medicine residencies are accredited through Accreditation Council for Graduate Medical Education by review of the residency review committee for emergency medicine. All graduates have eligibility to seek board certification through the American Board of Emergency Medicine, and the military strongly promotes specialty certification and maintenance of certification.

Faculty positions are highly sought and competitive. Some of emergency physicians start an academic career right out of residency, while others perform an operational or clinical tour first. In addition, some faculty will move in and out of the academic career path during their military service, thereby broadening their experience and clinical skills through operational or overseas tours or other career-broadening opportunities to include fellowship training. Program director positions are competitive and are seen as a pinnacle position in the academic career path. Emergency medicine residency program director positions have become joint opportunities, regardless of the service affiliation for that academic institution. This provides greater opportunities to select the most qualified applicant for the position from the three military branches. Services also recognize the importance of program director positions and will typically ensure individuals remain in place for at least 4 years, regardless of how long they have been assigned at the institution.

Even if not formally integrated with a local civilian emergency medicine residency, most military emergency medicine residency programs have some degree of collaboration with civilian programs to help round out specialty training and provide diversity in patient populations. The Uniformed Services University of the Health Sciences (USUHS) in Bethesda, Maryland, has a School of Medicine and all students are required to perform a clerkship in emergency medicine with many rotating in military EDs. Students at USUHS also receive operational field training and basic combat medical skills early in their education, affording several opportunities for military emergency physicians to serve as instructors. Academic emergency physicians also have opportunities for faculty appointments and educational opportunities at USUHS and civilian academic institutions through the previously discussed partnerships.

Research

Research and scholarly activity are required in academic programs. The past decade of combat has been both a curse and a blessing for research. The high deployment tempo for all emergency physicians, including academic emergency physicians, provided challenges to sustain research efforts. However, combat operations also drove the need for innovation, focused the military research agenda, increased military funding opportunities, and exploited the clinical strengths of emergency physicians. In addition, military leaders identified ways to better manage deployments of key academic faculty, such as program directors and lead researchers, so as not to jeopardize residency accreditation or funded research programs.

The rapid and sustained growth of clinical research performed by military emergency physicians over the last 10 years has been due to several factors. Primarily, the chief consultant of emergency medicine of each military branch has emphasized subspecialty training, research funding support, and support of clinical researchers. They have also encouraged emergency physicians to participate in joint military branch efforts and multispecialty research groups.

In addition, emergency physicians have clinical expertise innate to deployed and combat casualty care: disaster management, broad and acute medical and trauma management expertise, ultrasound proficiency at the bedside and in austere environments, medical and out-of-hospital system knowledge, and expertise in chemical weapons, toxins, and venoms. Thus, emergency physicians have led research efforts in these areas, which have previously been without physician specialty leadership. Emergency physicians have been recruited to military research agenda committees, grant review panels, and editorial boards. These factors and the current encouragement of emergency care research have led to the integration of emergency care within the military. As new physicians are mentored and trained in the military environment, emergency care research will expand.

Specific examples include research conducted by emergency physicians who have specialized in medical toxicology. Some have led efforts to examine the effects of opioids, pain, chemical weapon toxicity, and venom. Ultrasound fellowship-trained emergency physicians in the military have used ultrasound to evaluate trauma resuscitations, septic shock resuscitations, and care in rugged environments without the aid of radiography. Physicians trained in out-of-hospital care have conducted research to revolutionize how the military trains, uses, and deploys combat medics, and because of this work, they now lead out-of-hospital medic training for all branches. Recently, critical care trained emergency physicians have collaborated with intensivists and emergency physicians to systematically improve care between their units and to improve care in critically ill patients transported by critical care air transport teams (CCATTs) in combat and humanitarian operations.

Research funding is critical to sustain practice-changing research. Overseas contingency operations and its resultant clinical care gaps over the last 10 years have led to sustainable and efficient efforts to provide intramural and extramural research funding. The military provides specific funding for GME resident-related research. Although the funding amounts are limited, they allow for execution of small, defined projects that address military clinical gaps. In addition, each military branch provides intramural funding for its own investigators. As an example, the AFMS provides funding for USAF researchers to address its specific clinical problems related to peacetime and deployment. A large program of joint military funding is competitively awarded by way of grants to military and civilian investigators. The process is similar to that of the National Institute of Health (NIH) and other federal agencies, which support research and award multiyear research funding for important clinical problems the military needs addressed. This funding is highly competitive because it is divided by all branches, all specialties, among military and civilian researchers. Nonetheless, the emergency physicians with specialty training have been successful in obtaining military research funds through all of the previously discussed sources.

Finally, military emergency physicians have become incorporated in the military research agenda. Emergency physicians lead and develop research for out-of-hospital care and training. They are researchers in the US Army Institute of Surgical Research (USAISR), developing novel resuscitation techniques. Military EMS and ultrasound fellowship program directors collaborate with other specialties as coinvestigators and subject matter experts. The En Route Care Research Center (ECRC), located in the USAISR, is led by an emergency physician. Military emergency physicians have been recruited to grant review committees, multispecialty joint research boards, combat casualty care steering committees, and local institutional research boards, and institutional animal care and use committees. Annually, military emergency physicians present approximately 30 to 50 research abstracts at emergency care and other specialty meetings and are recruited to editorial boards, emergency medicine organizational boards, and civilian grant review panels. They receive funding from NIH for investigator-initiated investigations. They receive national research awards from military multispecialty organizations; emergency medicine societies such as the American College of Emergency Physicians (ACEP) and the Society of Academic Emergency Medicine, and civilian multispecialty associations such as the American Medical Association.

Because of the growth of military emergency care research and specialty training of emergency medicine, emergency physicians are embedded into the corporate process of military medicine, combat casualty care, critical care, and toxicologic research. They also collaborate with civilian institutions such as the University of Colorado Center for COMBAT Research or other universities on proposals and innovations, leveraging the operational expertise of the military investigator and the scientific expertise of the academic researcher. Emergency physicians will continue to be integral to military clinical research, collaborating with other specialties, all military branches, and academic centers to address the gaps in military clinical emergency and combat casualty care.

Fellowship Training

Another opportunity to seek an academic path and develop an area of subspecialty competency is through fellowship training. Each service offers fellowship training opportunities annually through the Joint Service Graduate Medical Education Selection Board; opportunities vary each year by identified needs within each service. Some emergency physicians will pursue fellowship training immediately after residency, while others will apply later in their career. The expanded role of emergency physicians in the operational setting has driven even greater fellowship training opportunities and the development of military fellowship training programs in areas of EMS, ultrasound, and austere and wilderness medicine. For training positions not at military sites, most often the fellow is civilian sponsored and thus continues to earn full military pay and benefits even though the training occurs at a civilian institution.

Medical toxicology is a subspecialty that fills unique needs beyond support to academic programs. Each military branch has two to four fellowship-trained 2-year programs that are also academic programs. Since there are no physician specialists in the military for toxicologic exposure, pharmacology, chemical agents, and envenomations, medical toxicologists provide clinical support as experts to outpatient clinics, hospitals, allied health professionals, disaster managers, and deployed providers.

Most military medical toxicologists support an inpatient consultative clinical service. As an example, at the SAMMC and tertiary care referral center, the toxicology service is the busiest in the military and provides inpatient bedside consultation 24 hours a day, treating overdoses, smoke inhalation (SAMMC is the only DOD-certified burn center), adverse drug events, occupational chemical exposures, envenomations, and other toxicologic emergencies. All of the DOD toxicologists also provide a telemedicine consult service, which provides specialty consultation 24 hours a day to providers in deployed settings and smaller military facilities across the world. The toxicologists respond to consults usually within 1 hour of initial contact.

Military medical toxicologists also provide expert consultation when deployed, acting as the theater consultant for the specialty to revise practice guidelines, modify response to potential threats, and treat critically ill patients with overdose, chemical exposures, and envenomations at the bedside in combat theater. Military toxicologists also provide opinions for medicolegal cases, quality care reviews, and military-wide approaches to mitigate substance abuse across all branches. Toxicologists provide specialty education to fulfill the curriculum needs for the local emergency medicine residencies but have a larger educational demand from nonemergency medicine residencies to fill their gaps in the didactic curriculum. For example, the toxicologists at SAMMC annually lecture to internal medicine, psychiatry, pediatrics, trauma surgery, critical care, nephrology, and neurology departments. Finally, military toxicologists conduct preclinical and clinical research that addresses gaps in military medicine. They conduct studies on chemical exposures, opioid toxicity, drugs of abuse, resuscitation, envenomations, and other related toxicologic emergencies.

Critical care fellowship opportunities have been new in the past 4 years, resulting from operational needs for more critical care providers in deployed locations. Some emergency physicians with critical care training have been assigned to civilian trauma programs where they assist with the currency training of military staff who rotate through on a regular basis. In the US Air Force, emergency medicine physicians have taken the lead in CCATT, driving the desire for more critical care emergency medicine physicians to support the training and oversight of this program. In addition, critical care trained emergency physicians augment hospital intensive care unit (ICU) staff and easily split time between ED and ICU, strengthening each department.

Several military physicians will train in sponsored positions in civilian institutions such as the Rocky Mountain Poison and Drug Center (toxicology), University of Colorado (sports medicine, global health, research, ultrasound), and University of Maryland (critical care).

In addition to physician training, the military has a long history of training physician assistants and is a role model for subspecialty training of EMPA and their integration into the practice of emergency medicine. Each service branch offers general physician assistant training programs and specialty training for emergency medicine. Emergency medicine physician assistants have a respected role in practice of emergency medicine in both EDs and the deployed environment. The San Antonio Medical Center's Department of Emergency Medicine sponsors one of the oldest EMPA training programs in the country.

In fact, the entire physician assistant movement grew out of the experience of Navy corpsmen, who returned from service in the Vietnam War with highly trained skills but no venue other than the military in which to utilize them. Dr. Eugene Stead, then Chair of Medicine at Duke University, recognized this situation and approached the Dean of the School of Medicine with a plan to create a new allied health specialty to use these highly trained and experienced people. The first class of physician assistants was comprised solely of former Navy corpsmen at Duke in 1965.

Finally, many military emergency physicians pursue an academic path whether they serve 4 years or 30 years in the military. The military offers leadership opportunities in combat and in stateside hospitals early in the career of emergency physicians. While many serve leading academic roles in the military, many also leave the service to enter civilian programs and mature into program directors, research directors, department chairs, institutional deans, health-care CEOs, and specialty organization leaders (e.g., ACEP president).

OPERATIONAL EMERGENCY MEDICINE

Operational emergency medicine opportunities and responsibilities differ among the respective services, yet the demand for emergency physicians has been so great during the past decade of combat that it has driven many "joint" tasking opportunities. In each service (including the Marines, which are supported by the Navy medical service), emergency physicians have become highly sought after by combatant commanders to fill critical medical billets. The high demand for emergency physicians and other specialties in the medical services has resulted in refined processes that identify emergency physicians to deploy. It has also brought greater standardization and predictability into the process, which benefits both the member and the department in being able to plan and leverage other resources. Many military emergency physicians will identify deployment as a highlight of their career, despite the personal and family sacrifices and strain.

Each of the military medical services significantly has transformed models for the delivery of operational medical support since the Persian Gulf War in the early 1990s to the more recent conflicts in Iraq and Afghanistan. Transformation has led to lighter, leaner, more mobile medical teams that can reach closer to the point of injury, allowing the rendering of critical care in the "Golden Hour." Indeed, the "Golden Hour" concept, first developed by Dr. R. Adams Cowley, has given way to the "Platinum 30 Minutes," largely as a result of advances in military medicine, many of which have now been adopted in civilian emergency medicine. Casualty survival rates have soared to an all-time high of 98%, and since 2007, the actual survival of combat casualties in Iraq and Afghanistan has exceeded results obtained in the leading trauma centers in the United States.[8] Critically injured patients have been evacuated from point of injury back to stateside tertiary trauma facilities in less than 72 hours, receiving repeated life-stabilizing operations and resuscitation along the way.[9]

Medical advancements on the combat field have significantly changed civilian trauma practices and vice versa. The military has partnered with highly respected academic institutions to help provide currency training to medical staff and collaborate in research. These relationships have often been forged through civilian faculty who once served in the military or may still serve in the military reserves or US National Guard and continue to deploy. Emergency medicine has been an essential partner in these relationships because trauma is a multidisciplinary practice.[10] Civilian training and research partnerships are essential. Even after conflicts have been resolved, those partnerships will help keep military emergency physicians and other medical staff current and competent.

The following provides information on some of the operational opportunities available to military emergency physicians. As mentioned previously, combat care is continuously striving to improve and innovation is the norm. In addition, geographic locations may drive different demands for medical support, which are carefully planned with combatant commanders. Thus, the information provided is dynamic and unclassified but still highlights the diverse opportunities for emergency medicine in supporting operational mission.

Forward Field Surgical Teams

Each military branch has created a specific version of mobile, expeditionary field surgical teams based on the core mission of that branch. Emergency physicians are included on these teams to work alongside surgical staff in providing resuscitative care and damage-control surgery in austere environments. Recognizing the need to bring advanced resuscitation and surgical care closer to the point of injury, many of these teams travel with combat units and are far forward on the battlefield. Resources are limited and resupply can be a challenge, leaving the physician to make clinical decisions with limited diagnostic studies and training in the use of specialized equipment designed specifically for the austere environment.

Level III Theater Hospitals

Regionalization of trauma care on the battlefield mirrors the civilian trauma center designation. However, the military classification system uses higher numbers (i.e., level III) to designate greater capability and resources—a numbering system that is the reverse of the civilian system. Theater hospitals are relatively fixed facilities with EDs, ICUs, operating rooms, and basic ancillary services to include blood bank and computed tomography scan. The Navy has two hospital ships with a capability that would rival many academic institutions. The size and number of staff assigned to theater hospitals vary depending on the mission. The ED is typically staffed with emergency physicians, emergency nurses, and medical technicians. Mass casualty situations, which are common in combat, often drive an "all hands on deck" approach requiring repeated training of nonemergency medicine staff to help support those efforts. Prior to the 21st century, patients remained in theater hospitals for days or sometimes weeks, but due to advances in air evacuation (AE), the most critically injured now may be moved within hours of presentation.

Theater hospitals provide both medical and trauma care, though most operational units have their own primary care assets, keeping the acuity in the ED high. Care is provided to US and coalition service members, contractors, and local nationals, including injured children, which provides the opportunity for the emergency physician to practice the full spectrum of emergency care (**Figure 53.3**). Emergency physicians routinely use fibrinolytics for cerebrovascular accidents and myocardial infarctions, administer vasopressors for sepsis, and anticoagulants to pulmonary embolisms. Trauma cases can be some of the most challenging, with multisystem organ injury and concurrent blast injury and amputations.

Recognizing the need for a systematic and integrated approach in the management and coordination of battlefield trauma, the Joint Trauma System (JTS) was developed in 2005 under the USAISR.[10] The JTS, now under the DOD Center of Excellence for Trauma, is responsible for the development of the DOD Trauma Registry, which tracks patients,

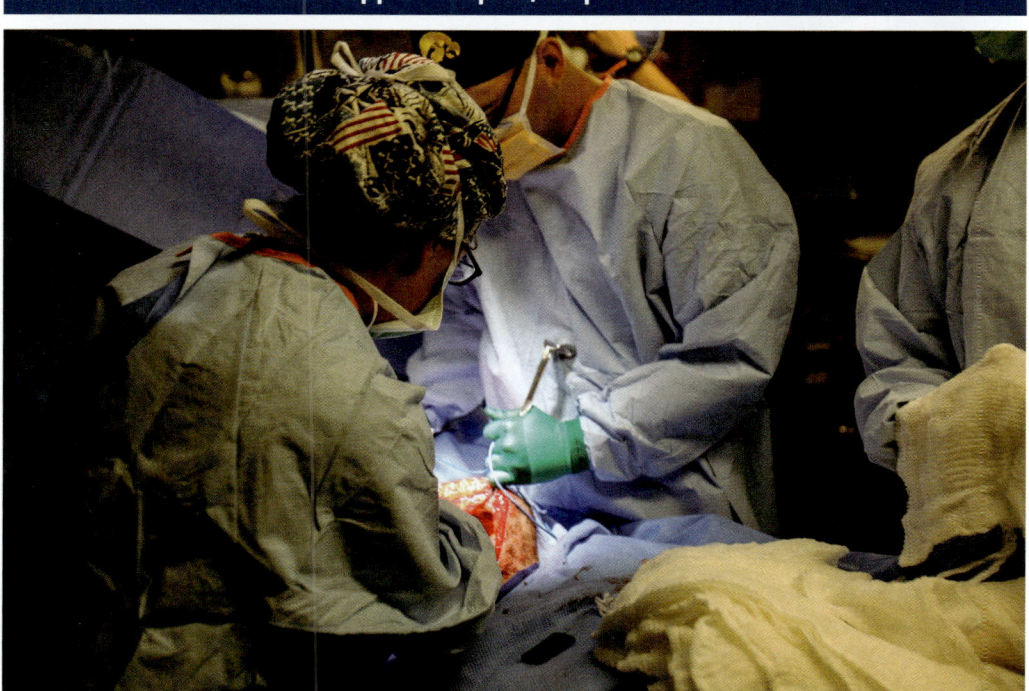

FIGURE 53.3 ■ **Combat Support Hospital, Iraq**

injury patterns, and treatment leading to development of clinical practice guidelines, new resuscitative medicine protocols, and predeployment training for Joint Theater Trauma System teams. In addition, weekly conferences occur, which provide real-time feedback and continued refinement and collaboration between specialties.

EN ROUTE CARE

One of the greatest medical advances during the past decade has been in en route care, which is the treatment of patients during transport from point of injury until evacuation to the United States. Emergency physicians serve in many of the leadership roles in military en route care, and most teams are led by an emergency physician. In prior conflicts, patients could not be moved in the AE system until they were stable. The development of the CCATT allowed the transport of patients requiring ongoing stabilization and critical care monitoring to move to a higher level of definitive care and out of theater much more rapidly, resulting in higher survivability rates and better long-term outcomes.[11]

The CCATT teams are composed of a critical care physician (emergency physician, anesthesiologist, intensivist, cardiologist, or surgeon), critical care nurse, and respiratory therapist.[12] The team carries specialized equipment that essentially allows monitoring and treatment of the patient in flight at the same level of an ICU (**Figure 53.4**). The CCATT teams are stationed around the theater and in Germany and will be added as a supplement to primary medical AE crews. The CCATT crew move in and out of theater transporting patients as directed. In addition, the CCATT team can be augmented to treat severely burned patients, complicated pulmonary patients, and patients requiring extracorporeal membrane oxygenation and other extracorporeal life support.[12-15]

The CCATT members are screened and selected based on demonstrated performance and competency. Currency and competency are maintained through attendance at the Center for the Sustainment of Trauma and Readiness Skills run by Air Force staff in collaboration

FIGURE 53.4 ■ Medical Transport Flight From Bagram Airfield, Afghanistan

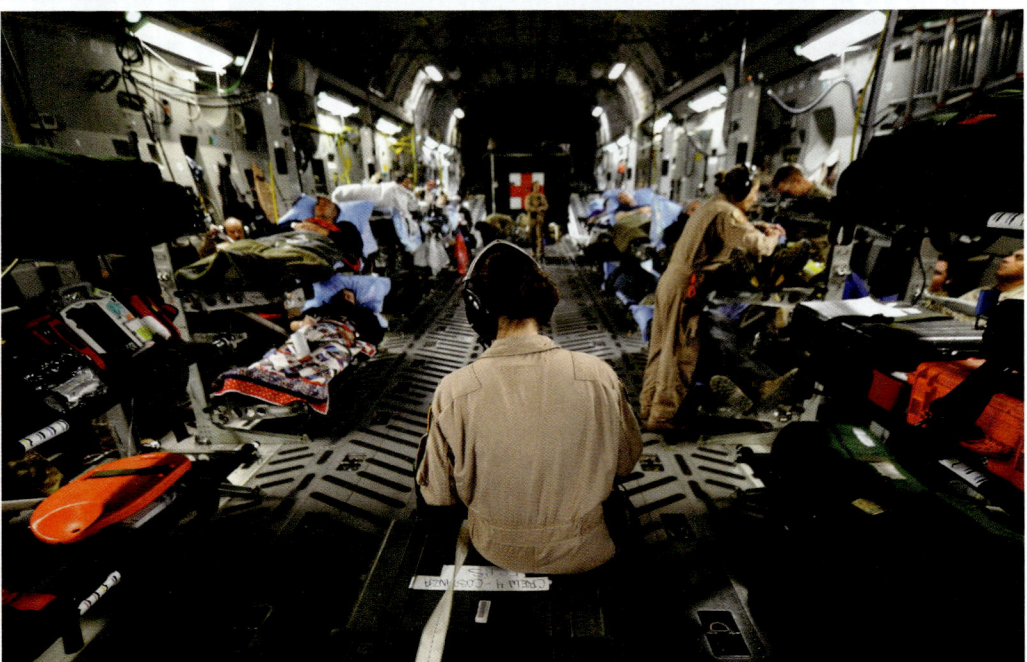

with the University of Cincinnati, which is a very sophisticated program of training and validation coupled with quality monitoring of all missions and ongoing improvement efforts. Lessons learned, innovation and research in en route care are redefining this capability for the civilian sector and for use in humanitarian and disaster response management. Other programs—such as UCHealth Memorial Hospital Central in Colorado Springs, Colorado—have a joint collaboration with the US Army and with the US Air Force to sustain trauma skills for deployable trauma teams and CCATTs.

Tactical Critical Care Evacuation Team

One of the most recent advances has been the development of the Tactical Critical Care Evacuation Team (TCCET). A DOD JTS Study reviewed patients who died of combat wounds from 2001 to 2009.[16] The study found that 51% of injuries were potentially survivable if the casualty had been closer to damage control resuscitation. Unlike CCATT teams, which fly more commonly on fixed wing aircraft and thus are limited in their ability to go forward, the TCCET teams travel predominantly on rotary wing aircraft such as the Black Hawk helicopter (**Figure 53.5**).[12] The teams are comprised of an emergency medicine physician, certified nurse anesthetist, and an ED nurse, intensive care nurse, or critical care nurse, who are all tasked to provide damage control resuscitation from point of injury. The team composition is modified based on the mission and often the emergency physician will transport a patient alone.

If CCATT is considered a flying ICU, then TCCET can be thought of as a flying ED in the very tight, space-constrained, and noisy environment of a helicopter. Training is more comprehensive and includes combat survival training. Deployment of TCCET teams has proven very promising with just under 1,000 intratheater evacuations in less than 2 years (**Figure 53.5**).[17] However, since 2018, the roles of TCCET are being transitioned to CCATT team members who will receive additional training, with the specific TCCET ultimately being phased out in the coming years.

FIGURE 53.5 ■ Flight Medic Attends to a Wounded Soldier, Afghanistan

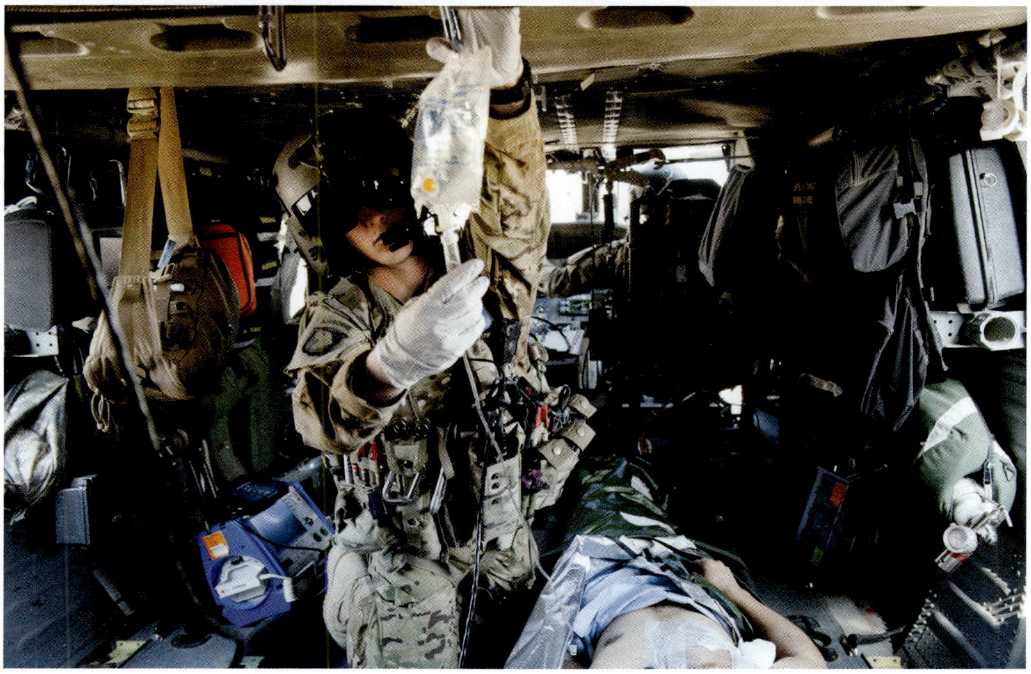

Support to Special Operations Forces

US Special Operations Forces have always had some of the more advanced medical teams, but the past decade has redefined their role, composition, and capabilities. Emergency physicians hold critical positions on many of these teams and are also lead instructors in training special force operators in point-of-injury combat care. A specific role of operational emergency medicine has been developed by the US Air Force to focused emergency physicians for special tactics and special operations units. Physicians are selected through a careful screening process and usually are assigned to special force units. Clinical competency is maintained through extensive initial and sustainment training as well as dedicated time to work within a local ED. Initial training can take up to a year, but 2 to 3 years are needed to develop a seasoned member. This highly competitive new field has led to the growth of emergency physicians in special operations units.

Nation-Building Efforts

One of the strategies used in winning the hearts and minds of nations and promoting peace is through nation-building efforts. Establishment of medical systems and capabilities is one of the more common venues. For many third-world countries, the basics in medical care that include out-of-hospital care, resuscitative medicine, and functioning hospitals are often lacking. Therefore, the military will often deploy teams to partner with local nationals to train and help develop more robust medical systems. For obvious reasons, emergency physicians have had opportunities to serve on these teams.

Humanitarian and Disaster Response

In addition to combat support, operational medicine also provides support to humanitarian and disaster relief efforts both within the United States and internationally. During recent US disasters—such as 2006 Hurricane Katrina or international events such as the 2010 Haiti earthquake—emergency physicians from Army, Navy, and Air Force have served in key leadership roles and as part of medical response teams. Many of the advances in combat care have led to development of more expeditionary and robust medical response packages. One example is the Air Force Expeditionary Medical Support Health Response Team, which is a scalable package, easy to assemble, and can provide immediate care within 15 minutes, a functioning emergency room in 2 hours, operating room capability in 4 hours, and ICU capability in 6 hours.

Operational Positions Outside Emergency Medicine

Each service has requirements for physicians to support line units (i.e., combatant units). Some of these roles include battalion surgeon, Special Forces battalion surgeon, Ranger Battalion surgeon, Brigade surgeon, and Flight surgeon. And emergency physicians are highly sought after to fill them. They serve in these roles to provide direct medical care to soldiers, sailors, and air force members, as well as to train and provide oversight to the many levels of medics, physician assistants, and other physician extenders who care for line unit members.

Such roles lead to significant leadership opportunities for the emergency physician who may be providing oversight care to upward of 1,000 military members. When an operational unit is deployed, the physician goes with them, overseeing and providing all care in the combat zone. A tour in an operational billet can provide career diversity, adventure, and challenges for an emergency physician. Assignments are usually 2 to 4 years in length. Emergency physicians also are encouraged to work in local military or civilian EDs to maintain currency for patient populations, such as pediatric and geriatrics, which they do not often see in their military roles.

ACCESSION/EMPLOYMENT OPPORTUNITIES

The most common pathway by which emergency physicians enter military service is through the Health Professions Scholarship Program (HPSP). The HPSP pays for medical school tuition, books, health-care insurance, small living allowance, and sometimes an accession bonus in exchange for 1-year service commitment postresidency training. Given the significant amount of debt many medical students accrue, military medicine can be a welcome alternative. In addition, the 3 to 4 years of military service after completion of internship/residency typically provide excellent opportunities to develop leadership skills, obtain combat experience, or launch an academic career. Other pathways to active-duty military service include attendance at a service academy or the US Reserve Officers Training Corps scholarship for undergraduate education or direct accession.

The reserve components of the US Armed Forces are military organizations whose members generally perform a minimum of 39 days of military duty per year and, when necessary, augment the active-duty military. The reserve components are also referred to collectively as the Guard and Reserves and afford the emergency physician the opportunity to keep a civilian practice, maintain the ability to live where he or she desires, but still have the opportunity to serve in the military and earn a retirement. While many choose this pathway after a period of active-duty service, others choose to join for career diversity and a desire to participate in operational tours. Length of operational tours and requirements for Guard and Reserves vary by service and position. The Individual Mobilization Augmentee Reserve program allows the service to retain highly trained physicians while providing a flexible training schedule to the service member.

Lastly for those who do not want to wear the uniform or be vulnerable for deployments, several military EDs still have contract or GS positions, providing great opportunities for emergency medicine physicians to work in the military full or part time.

A good reference to learn more about military emergency medicine opportunities or get connected with leaders in military emergency medicine is through the Government Service Chapter of the American College of Emergency Physicians (GSACEP). The GSACEP is open to all physicians who work in federal EDs or serve in the DOD and is an alternative to state chapter membership for the ACEP.

CONCLUSION

The perception of emergency medicine as a specialty has meaningfully improved over the last 20 years. It is now recognized and respected as a highly valued specialty in both combat and operational settings. Today emergency physicians are senior leaders, such as hospital CEOs, chief medical officers, academic deans, department chairs, and hold key military medical service headquarters positions such as command surgeons and combatant commanders. The military academic path has improved retention and development of emergency physicians as respected researchers and senior leaders in academic medicine as well. However, the greatest success has been in the emergency physicians' operational roles during the past decade of combat and the casualties and wounded warriors for whom they improved care.

The past 2 decades of combat have redefined military emergency medicine and helped to define the future. Military emergency physicians were recruited by combatant commanders and military leaders for their operational clinical skills and now have become leaders in major operational medical commands. Emergency physicians remain one of the most sought after physician specialties by the senior operational line commanders. Even if the United

States successfully reduces our presence in conflict, the MHS recognizes the importance for physicians to maintain clinical currency, competence, and satisfaction of practice and to do so requires the MHS to maintain robust clinical settings. Collaboration with civilian academic centers will continue to grow on an accelerated path, and innovation and research will remain a high priority. While EDs are the safety net to our health-care system, military emergency physicians are critical to the backbone of operational medical platforms for worldwide humanitarian and combat operations.

Military emergency medicine provides unparalleled opportunities for the emergency physician. Even if military service is limited to a single tour, the emergency physician will accrue experience and develop leadership acumen that place the officer above most peers at a similar career stage. The diversity of career opportunities and ability to move in and out of paths can provide the highest level of professional satisfaction.

REFERENCES

1. Jansen DJ. Military medical care: questions and answers. Congressional Research Service (CRS) Report #RL33537. 2014. Available at: https://fas.org/sgp/crs/misc/RL33537.pdf. Accessed December 30, 2012.
2. Backhus SP. Military treatment facilities: emergency department utilization. US General Accounting Office Report #GAO/HEHS-00-63R. 2000. Available at: http://archive.gao.gov/f0302/163395.pdf. Accessed December 30, 2012.
3. About the patient safety program. Health.mil. Available at: https://www.health.mil/Military-Health-Topics/Access-Cost-Quality-and-Safety/Quality-And-Safety-of-Healthcare/Patient-Safety. Accessed December 30, 2012.
4. DeLorenzo RA. ED use of military beneficiaries. *Am J Emerg Med*. 2009;27(9):1104–1108.
5. Green B, Rosenfale D, Majerol M. Innovations in the Military Health System—Deloitte. Available at: https://www2.deloitte.com/content/dam/insights/us/articles/4818_Innovations_military_health/DI_Innovations-military-health.pdf. Accessed December 9, 2020.
6. Defense Health Agency. 2018 Stakeholders Report. Availab;e at: file:///C:/Users/thomm/Downloads/2018%20Stakeholder%20Report%20Final_Jan_2020.pdf. Accessed December 9, 2020.
7. The White House Office of the Press Secretary. Executive order–improving access to mental health services for veterans, service members, and military families. 2012. Available at: https://obamawhitehouse.archives.gov/the-press-office/2012/08/31/executive-order-improving-access-mental-health-services-veterans-service. Accessed December 9, 2020.
8. Fulton L, Shanderson L. Military health system efficiency: a review of the history and recommendations for the future. *Mil Med*. 2012;177(6):686–692.
9. Lairet JR, Bebarta VS, Burns CJ, et al. Prehospital interventions performed in a combat zone: a prospective multicenter study of 1,003 combat wounded. *J Trauma Acute Care Surg*. 2012;73(2 suppl 1):S38–S42.
10. Blackbourne LH, Baer DG, Eastridge BJ, et al. Military medical revolution: military trauma system. *J Trauma Acute Care Surg*. 2012;73(6):S388–S394.
11. Mason PE, Eadie JS, Holder AD. Prospective observational study of United States (US) Air Force Critical Care Air Transport team operations in Iraq. *J Emerg Med*. 2011;41(1):8–13.
12. Blackbourne LH, Baer DG, Eastridge BJ, et al. Military medical revolution: deployed hospital and en route care. *J Trauma Acute Care Surg*. 2012;73(6 suppl 5):S378–S387.
13. Fang R, Allan PF, Womble SG, et al. Closing the "care in the air" capability gap for severe lung injury: the Landstuhl Acute Lung Rescue Team and extracorporeal lung support. *J Trauma*. 2011;71(1 suppl):9S1–S97.
14. Renz EM, Cancio LC, Barillo DJ, et al. Long range transport of war-related burn casualties. *J Trauma*. 2008;64(2 suppl):S136–S144;S144S–S145.
15. Allan PF, Osborn EC, Bloom BB, et al. The introduction of extracorporeal membrane oxygenation to aeromedical evacuation. *Mil Med*. 2011;176(8):932–937.
16. Eastridge BJ, Hardin M, Cantrell J, et al. Died of wounds on the battlefield: causation and implications for improving combat casualty care. *J Trauma*. 2011;71(1 suppl):S4–S8.
17. Critical Care Air Transport Teams. Available at: https://www.ccatt.info/index.php/ccatt. Accessed December 10, 2020.

FREESTANDING EMERGENCY DEPARTMENTS

CHAPTER 54

Thom A. Mayer, Gillian Schmitz, James Augustine, Frank Zilm

Freestanding emergency departments (FSEDs) are an area of innovative practice diversification in emergency medicine. Although these facilities have existed for over 40 years, like many innovations, FSED diversification initially saw delayed acceptance, followed by explosive growth, then decline in certain sectors—as well as controversy. There are at least 800 and perhaps as many as 1,000 FSEDs in the United States, the majority of which are now affiliated with hospitals.[1]

One Massachusetts General Hospital study reported that by 2017 there were as many as 669 FSEDs seeing nearly 9 million patients annually, comprising 6% of all emergency department (ED) visits.[2] Emergency department visits have grown by 32% in the last decade, while the total number of EDs has declined by nearly 5%.[3] This average growth per ED of almost 40% has placed enormous pressure on hospitals and health-care systems to meet the needs of the patients seeking emergency care. Add to this the increasing scrutiny of multiple stakeholders and the rising demand for alternatives to traditional ED care, and the need for FSEDs and micro-hospitals becomes readily apparent.[4,5]

In recent years, FSEDs have emerged by[6,7]:

- Providing an alternative to acute care EDs for patients with more minor illnesses and injuries
- Providing an attractive practice alternative for emergency physicians and nurses
- Protecting emerging markets for hospitals and health-care systems
- Providing enhanced access for the increasing demand of emergency services
- Developing sites and services designed to differentiate hospitals from their competitors
- Growing market share
- Developing a profitable medical business
- Meeting competitive threats from other hospitals
- Providing referrals for physicians
- Increasing referrals for hospital services
- Attaining branding of the hospital or health-care system and brand loyalty

MEDICAL FACILITY TAXONOMY

Although FSEDs urgent care centers (UCCs), hybrid models, and micro-hospitals are distinct entities with some similar features, they also have many discrete, distinguishing attributes (**Figures 54.1** and **54.2**). They share the provision of some level acuity of episodic, undifferentiated, unscheduled care at their core.

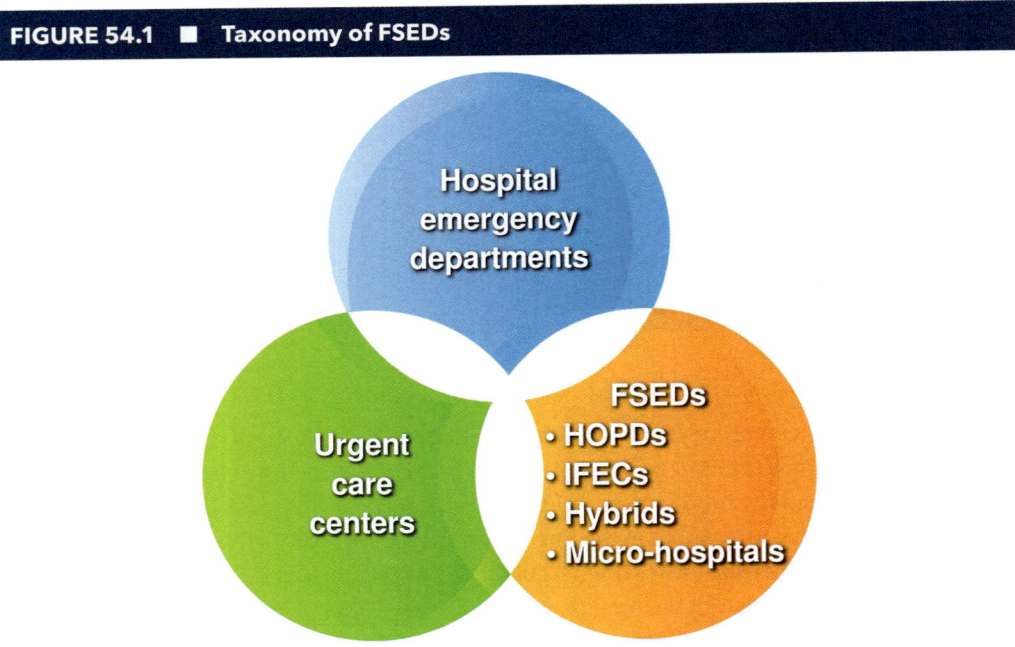

FIGURE 54.1 ■ Taxonomy of FSEDs

Freestanding Emergency Departments

In order to provide clarification to its members and the public, in 2015, the American College of Emergency Physicians (ACEP) published a paper titled *Freestanding Emergency Departments and Urgent Care Centers*.[8] ACEP also issued a policy statement in 2014 on FSEDs, which was reapproved in 2018 and 2020.[9] The policy defines an FSED as "a licensed facility that is structurally separate and distinct from a hospital and provides emergency care." Freestanding emergency departments are further divided as either hospital outpatient departments (HOPDs), also known as off-site hospital-based or satellite EDs, or independent freestanding emergency centers (IFECs). IFECs may be owned by nonphysician investors,

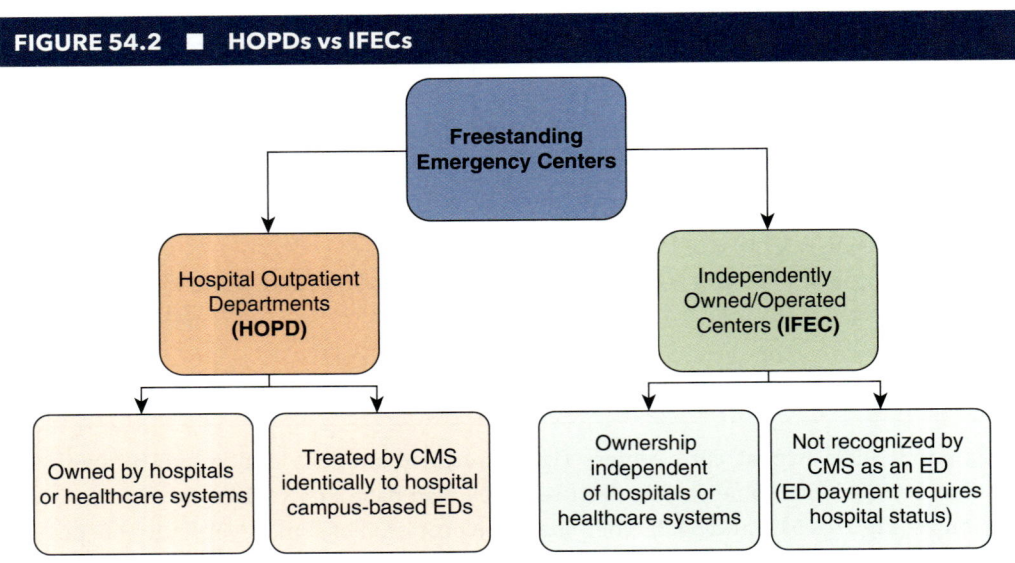

FIGURE 54.2 ■ HOPDs vs IFECs

physician entrepreneurs, or some combination of both. ACEP's policy statement notes that FSEDs should[9]:

- Be available to the public 24 hours a day, 7 days a week, and 365 days per year.
- Be staffed by appropriately qualified emergency physicians.
- Have adequate medical and nursing personnel qualified in emergency care to meet the written emergency procedures and needs anticipated by the facility.
- Be staffed at all times by a registered nurse with a minimum requirement of current certification in advanced cardiac life support (ACLS) and pediatric advanced life support.
- Have policy agreements and procedures in place to provide effective and efficient transfer to a higher level of care if needed (e.g., cardiac and stroke catheterization labs, surgery, intensive care units.
- Receive the same level of reimbursement for both the physician and technical component fee as a traditional hospital-based ED.

ACEP further states that:

> ... all FSEDs must follow the intent of the Emergency Medical Treatment and Labor Act (EMTALA) statute and that all individuals arriving at a FSED should be provided an appropriate medical screening examination by qualified medical personnel, including ancillary services, to determine whether or not the individual needs emergency care.
>
> The FSED should provide stabilizing treatment within the capability of the facility and should have a mechanism in place to arrange an appropriate transfer to the definitive care facility, if appropriate, for the patient to receive necessary stabilizing treatment regardless of the patient's ability to pay or method of payment.[9]
>
> FSEDs should have the same standards as hospital-based EDs for quality improvement, medical leadership, medical directors, credentialing, and appropriate policies for referrals to primary and specialty physicians for aftercare. Value-based payments should consider the intrinsic differences between FSEDs and hospital-based EDs.[9]

The majority of FSEDs operate 24 hours a day, and some states mandate that they do so (which can also have an impact on reimbursement). Regulations on hours of operation vary from state to state, but most require continuous operation. Admission rates at hospital EDs vary widely, generally from 10% (rural communities with little primary care access) to 40% (tertiary or quaternary care facilities). Typically, FSEDs admit between 5% and 15% of their patients.[10]

As the health-care market continues to evolve, adapt, and become increasingly competitive, it is likely that FSEDs will change to meet these societal and industry pressures. Kaiser Permanente recently developed 24 FSEDs with the capability of holding observation patients, whether seen at their facility or transferred from nearby hospital-based EDs not contracted with Kaiser. In Virginia, two competing health-care systems have opened FSEDs less than two miles from each other.

Achieving Accreditation

Because they are considered to be licensed through the hospital ED and are an extension or satellite department, HOPDs are certified through the same process as the hospital ED, which is usually done through The Joint Commission or Det Norske Veritas. An ACEP task force on FSED accreditation with the goal of assuring "high quality standards for patient care" resulted in the creation of a partnership effort between ACEP and the Center for

Improvement in Healthcare Quality to provide an accreditation process for FSEDs (and particularly, but not exclusively, for IFECs).[11] Following verification and surveys, a three-year accreditation is granted, the survey fee for which is $2,500, with discounts available for facilities with ACEP member emergency physicians.

Emergency Medical Services Issues

Regulations on accepting emergency medical services (EMS) patients vary widely, although many FSEDs accept EMS patients, with the possible exception of those requiring trauma activations in designated trauma systems. For those FSEDs accepting ambulance traffic, on average only 5% to 10% of their volume is accounted for by EMS, as opposed to 15% to 35% in a typical hospital ED.[12] All FSEDs that accept ambulances must have clearly developed EMS transfer arrangements in place to ensure rapid, safe, and efficient transfer of patients who require hospitalization. Sometimes those transfers are most expeditiously provided by private ambulances, since first response public EMS units have a primary responsibility to remain available in service to their "first due" geographic areas.

In some cases, even for high-acuity patients such as those with acute ischemic strokes and ST-elevation myocardial infarctions (STEMIs), a carefully planned and well-executed system in place can result in exceptional performance.[13] In every case, when EMS traffic is accepted, careful planning is needed to assure seamless and timely transfer of patients, with accountability for quality and time metrics for such patients, coordinated with the local EMS agency.

Hospital Outpatient Departments

The majority of currently operating FSEDs are hospital-owned as opposed to physician or investor-owned. This is largely because the hospital has a number of strategic advantages that are not typically available to physicians such as:

- Better access to capital
- Broader administrative support capability
- Greater human resources and better employee benefit packages
- Preferred equipment purchase and space finish-out construction pricing
- The undisputed ability to charge and be paid a facility fee in addition to an ED CPT Evaluation and Management (E/M) code series (99281-99285 and critical care) professional fees
- An existing facility provider number that can be extended to the FSED from the first day of operations
- Preexisting contracts with the major payers in the area
- The *halo effect* of the hospital or health-care system's reputation for quality

The typical hospital-owned FSED is in every respect identical to a hospital-based ED except for the proximity to an operating room, delivery room, cardiac catheterization lab, and inpatient beds. Most state's laws and all of the hospital accrediting entities require that FSEDs have, among other things, sophisticated laboratory and imaging availability, ACLS capability, around-the-clock, an on-call specialty roster, and standing hospital transfer agreements. Most hospital-owned FSEDs use the same physician group that staffs the hospital's hospital-based EDs. As will be discussed shortly, reimbursement factors such as the inability of IFECs to participate in Centers for Medicare and Medicaid Services (CMS) reimbursement programs have also driven a movement toward HOPDs.

Many FSEDs have expanded their capabilities by adding short-stay and observation services at their facilities, which better serve the needs of patients who require extended time and care.

Urgent Care Centers

UCCs are the middle of the spectrum of unscheduled, walk-in care facilities that treat lower acuity illnesses and injuries. These facilities occupy a space between extended-hours primary care practices and FSEDs. Although they are not typically staffed by board-certified or board-eligible emergency physicians or experienced emergency nurses, exceptions exist. Some are staffed by family medicine physicians or advanced practice providers (APPs). Laboratory and imaging services onsite are usually limited to basic studies, including plain film radiography.[14]

Hybrid Models

Largely in response to payer concerns regarding the cost of care provided to patients with low-acuity illnesses or injuries in FSEDs, some facilities developed hybrid clinical practice models, offering both FSED and UCC services in the same facility (although in distinct geographic areas). In most models, patients are triaged in a central area, following which they are directed to either the UCC or FSED area, depending on their chief complaint, Emergency Services Index (ESI) category, or likely needs. For example, patients with chest and abdominal pain are evaluated in the FSED area, while those with minor trauma are evaluated and treated in the wing.

Staffing varies by site and state regulation, but emergency physicians typically staff the FSED area, while APPs are often used in the UCC. Nursing coverage may be shared or separate, usually depending upon volume, but with a common nurse manager. Essential services (laboratory and imaging services) are commonly shared, depending largely on regulatory issues.

Urgent care center patients are billed at a separate rate, usually resulting in a much lower cost for the patient or insurer. Freestanding emergency department patients are billed just as ED patients would normally be billed, with both an E/M code for the physician component and an ambulatory payment group code for the hospital/facility component, resulting typically in a higher, but reimbursable bill.

Micro-Hospitals

A recent health-care trend is the micro-hospital, which includes an FSED and possibly a surgical center, along with short-stay beds for observation of medical and postprocedure patients (**Figure 54.3**). These facilities currently target and are located primarily in affluent, high-growth urban areas, but this model may have a role in rural settings as communities struggle to keep critical access hospital services.

As with freestanding EDs, these facilities must meet full licensure in their states and potentially meet certificate of need (CON) requirements in those states requiring them. It may be possible to have the micro-hospital designated as a specialty hospital where states allow this classification. Some states may require services and staffing, such as pharmaceutical, laboratory, obstetric and gynecological services, medical staff mixes, and credentialing.

The early generations of micro-hospital have been affiliated with larger health systems such as St. Vincent's neighborhood hospitals in Indianapolis, Indiana, although Texas and other areas of the country have a significant physician-owned building presence. Due to the small number of beds (8–12), these sites do not have the same support service needs as a community hospital and can therefore generate the same billing revenue with a lower overhead. Supplies are frequently provided in a just-in-time model, laundry is outsourced, and laboratory testing is primarily point-of-care testing.

FIGURE 54.3 ■ Micro-Hospital Example

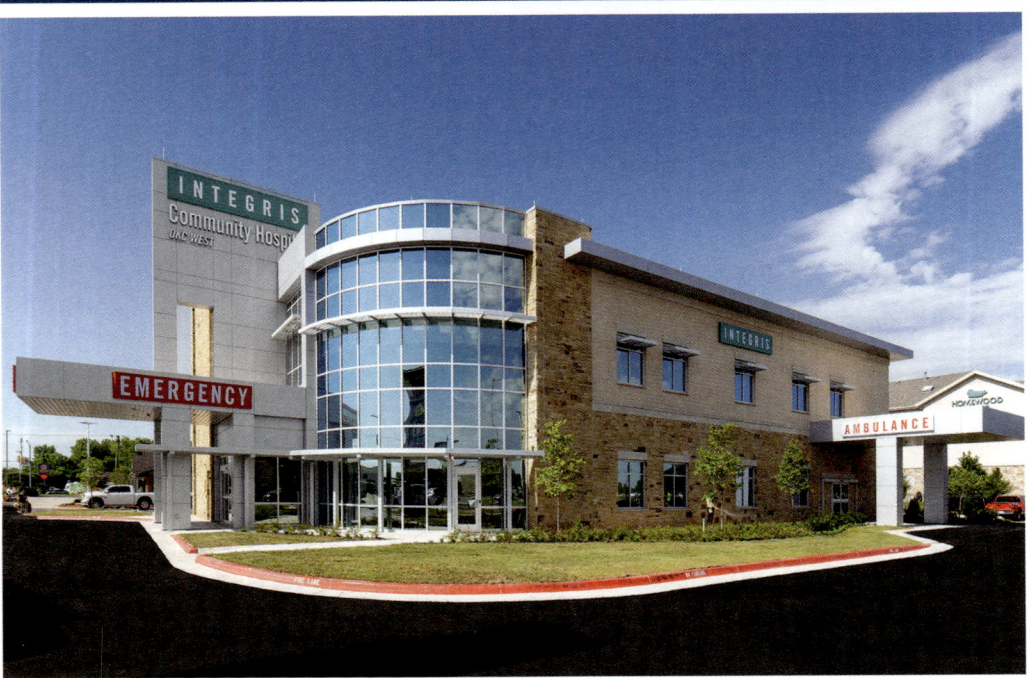

It should be noted that recent Medicare rulings regarding the definition of a hospital could impact the financial viability of the micro-hospital approach to care. A key definition of what constitutes the bulk of services dedicated to inpatient care could jeopardize qualification for reimbursement at hospital rates. Another unknown is the bigger strategic question regarding national health policies. Any shift to a capitated care financial model could result in aggressive efforts to reduce low-acuity utilization of emergency services.

HISTORY OF FSEDs

In 1977, Fairfax Hospital and the Fairfax Hospital Association (now the Inova Health System [IHS]), located in the planned community of Reston, Virginia, became the first US healthcare system to open an around-the-clock FSED that accepted ambulance traffic of all kinds.[15] Fairfax Hospital was staffed by the same emergency physicians from the local level I trauma center. Known as Access of Reston (now Inova Emergency Care Center of Reston), this FSED rapidly drew a high volume of patients (more than 40,000 per year), including high-acuity patients (15% of whom arrived by ambulance). It is still in operation today, with over 40 years of history and having seen hundreds of thousands of patients. Inova now operates six FSEDs with a total annual volume of approximately 150,000.

As the FSED phenomenon grew, states began to require hospitals and health-care systems to obtain a CON to remain open (**Figure 54.4**). Virginia, as an example, requires a COPN and treats FSEDs as off-site extensions of the hospital EDs under which they are licensed and subject to the same payer contracts and regulations.

The initial growth of FSEDs was relatively slow and largely limited to health-care systems that were either protecting markets or attempting to grow market share in key strategic areas, although some were located in underserved and/or rural areas. By 2007, there were 80 FSEDs nationwide, but that number grew to 225 by 2009 and to over 400 by 2018. Investor-owned FSEDs began to expand, particularly in states that did not have

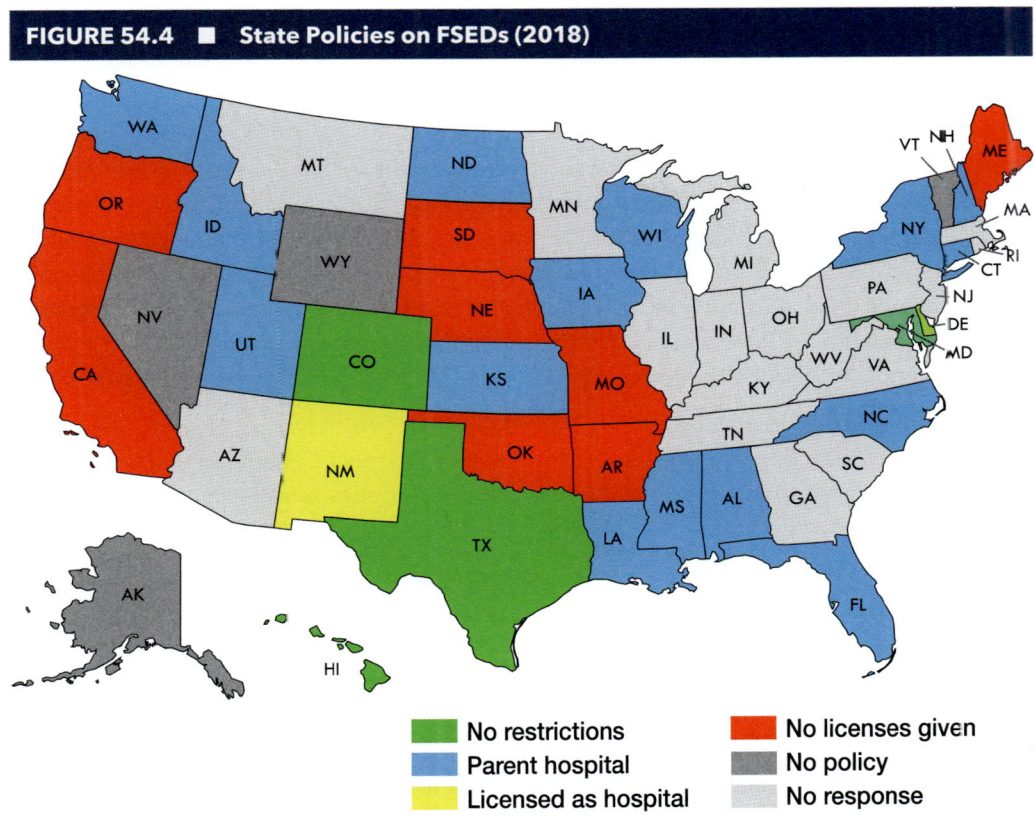

FIGURE 54.4 ■ State Policies on FSEDs (2018)

- 🟩 No restrictions
- 🟦 Parent hospital
- 🟨 Licensed as hospital
- 🟥 No licenses given
- ⬛ No policy
- ⬜ No response

significant regulations nor CON requirements for FSEDs, including Texas, Arizona, and Colorado.[16,17] In 2009, the Texas Legislature explicitly permitted FSEDs to operate, which led to explosive growth in that state.[18] However, at least two investor-owned FSED companies (Adeptus and Neighbors Health) filed for Chapter 11 bankruptcy protection in 2017 to 2018, resulting in the closure of a significant number of FSEDs.[10,19] Current estimates are that there are about 300 FSEDs of various types in operation, although that number is likely to continue to change, with most experts predicting a further contraction of sites. In addition, many investor-owned FSEDs have affiliated with or become hospital-owned, largely for billing and insurance reasons that will be discussed.

Freestanding Emergency Department Regulations

The following describes the current status of FSED regulations in the United States, although that status is in constant flux[20,21]:

- 32 states have FSEDs of some type.
- 21 states have FSED-specific policies and regulations.
- 29 states have no specific regulations applying to FSEDs.
- 9 states explicitly allow for FSED development without a hospital partner.
- 23 states have FSEDs operating as HOPDs (although only 11 states require that they do so).
- 24 states subject FSEDs to CON processes.

As will be discussed next, FSEDs that are not affiliated with a hospital (IFECs) are not allowed to participate in CMS reimbursement programs, which has resulted in a dramatic restructuring of the FSED landscape.[17] In addition, IFECs were initially not subject to the EMTALA statutes, although some states are seeking to address this.

THE ECONOMIC REALITIES OF FSEDs

The growth (and subsequent contraction) of FSEDs has led to major controversy in both the emergency medicine peer-reviewed literature and the lay press.[22-25] The majority of this controversy is related either to the putatively high cost of care or the choice of location of FSEDs in predominantly affluent areas. The phrase "form follows finance" is helpful in understanding the economics of FSEDs, implying, as it does, that the manner in which facilities are designed, located, and structured (*form*) is driven in part (perhaps largely) by the economics of reimbursement (*finance*). ED reimbursement is discussed in detail in Section 8, but a brief primer is instructive in understanding this concept.

Emergency department reimbursement is broadly comprised of two components[26]:

- *Professional fees*: coded by the CPT codes in the E/M codes and procedure codes
- *Facility fees*: largely governed by Ambulatory Payment Classifications (APCs), which cover the costs of room charges, medical supplies, and some, but not all, diagnostic tests

The current reimbursement system has the E/M and APC codes tightly *crosswalked*, linking the relative acuity and resources used to care for the patient for both the professional and facility fee components. It is important to note that the facility fees (and reimbursement for them) are typically at least three times (and may be as high as five times) the amount of the professional fees for any given patient. This drives the "form" for the HOPDs in that the acuity of patients seen in FSEDs may be lower than that of patients seen in the hospital ED, but they are billed and reimbursed by the same schedule. If the payer mix of the FSED is more favorable than that of the ED, this provides substantial revenue for the physicians and the hospital. Emergency physicians in fee-for-service practices who rely on professional fee billing as the sole revue source begin to show break-even profitability at around 30 to 40 patients per day (13,000–16,000 annual visits), depending on patient acuity (and therefore E/M codes) and payer mix. Below those levels, ED physicians have the options of either negotiating for a "start-up subsidy" from the hospital or treating it as an investment in future growth. HOPDs with annual volumes in the 20,000 to 24,000 range are a "sweet spot" from an operational and revenue perspective, since single emergency physician coverage can be augmented with APP hours at peak times.[27]

In the case of IFECs, this reimbursement calculus is even more important since the investors capture *both* the professional and facility fee components. It is highly likely that this reimbursement reality has played a major (and understandable) role in the explosive growth of these facilities, particularly since the facility component is typically three to five times the professional fee or E/M component. Freestanding emergency department patients typically generate $800 to $3,000 in total revenue, making such patients a substantial revenue generator if the payer mix is favorable. Break-even profitability typically occurs in IFECs at about 12 to 15 patients per day.[27] While there are fewer data available for hybrid models, the urgent care section breaks even financially at 40 to 50 patients per day.

As was discussed, IFECs are not governed by federal EMTALA statutes since they do not participate in CMS reimbursement. (During the COVID-19 pandemic, CMS issued guidelines to allow Medicare and Medicaid patients in the states of Colorado, Delaware, Rhode Island, and Texas to be seen in IFECs under an 1135 Waiver.)[28] Many medical insurance companies have promulgated policies that restrict full reimbursement of patients seen in IFECs that

TABLE 54.1 ■ Financial Comparison of UCCs vs FSEDs		
	Urgent Care Center	**FSED (HOPD & IFEC)**
Net Revenue	$100–$135	$350–$500 + facility fee
Co-Pay	$35–$50	$75–$100
Facility Fee	No	Yes
Squre Footage	2,500–4,000	5,000–20,000
Hours	12–18 per day	24/7/365
Docs	Family medicine	Emergency medicine + APPs
Lab	Basics-send outs	CLIA, CBC, D-Dimer, cardiac
Imaging	Plain films	MRI, CT, ultrasound
EMS	No	Generally yes

do not participate in CMS, driving many of them to pursue affiliation with a hospital to become, in effect, HOPDs, which is another example of form following finance.[29,30] One large national insurance company issued a screed claiming that FSEDs cost 22 times more than UCCs or physicians' offices, conveniently ignoring the fact that many FSED patients require resources not available in either place.[31]

A key aspect driving payers is the dramatic difference in charges between UCCs and FSEDs, which are summarized in **Table 54.1**. Freestanding emergency department professional fee charges may run to $350 to $500, depending upon acuity, in addition to the facility fee. Urgent care center charges are often $100 to $200, but this includes the facility fee. Patient co-pays are typically $25 to $50 for a UCC and $75 to $100 for an FSED visit. Many insurance companies use their patient portals and websites to direct patients to UCCs instead of FSEDs, even for more serious symptoms.

PROS AND CONS OF FSEDs

The emergence of FSEDs, like any truly disruptive innovation, is viewed positively as an opportunity or a negatively as a threat depending on one's viewpoint and local issues. Broadly speaking, these opportunities and threats come from the perspective of:

- Patients
- Providers (physicians and nurses primarily)
- Hospitals and health-care systems
- Payers

Patient Perspective

For patients, FSEDs offer several positives, including greater choice in care, more accessible locations, better access to parking, shorter wait times, and short total length of stay since the distractions of acutely ill and injured patients are less common. Other benefits include

TABLE 54.2 ■ Positives and Negatives of FSEDs From the Patient Perspective	
Positives	**Negatives**
More choice (ED vs FSED)	Confusion as to costs; perceiving FSED to be UCC with lower rates
Better location	Potential limited access to certain services (advance imaging)
More accessible parking and ease of access	Potential lack of on-call specialists willing to come to the FSED
Shorter waiting times	Potential billing for ambulance transport to hospitals
Doctors and nurses less likely to be distracted with acutely ill or injured patients-more satisfied	
Decreased total length of stay	

nurses and doctors with more time and less distractions in providing care, resulting in higher staff satisfaction in most cases and often greater willingness of on-call physicians to accept follow-up appointments (**Table 54.2**).

The largest negative from the patients' perspective is related to billing. Some patients may not recognize that the facility bills at FSED/ED rates may confuse it with a UCC, which may have different co-pays and coverage, particularly if private insurers refuse to cover FSED services. However, transparency with the patient (upfront if requested) usually prevents this confusion. Other potential negatives are the lack of specialized imaging services (e.g., ultrasound [US] or magnetic resonance imaging [MRI]) and possible inability to get on-call specialists to come to the FSED (although these specialists are often happier to come to the FSED than the ED itself). Additionally, and, for those patients requiring admission and ambulance transport to the hospital, the potential for ambulance "back-transport" charges exist if not addressed systematically.[32,33]

Clinician Perspective

Table 54.3 lists the many positives learned from long experience with FSEDs. Due to fewer patients with high-acuity illnesses and injuries, such as strokes, STEMIs, cardiac arrests, or

TABLE 54.3 ■ Advantages of FSEDs From Clinicians' Perspective	
More time with patients	Greater sense of teamwork
Fewer distractions	Less burnout
Greater satisfaction	Potential improved pay
Career opportunity-extension	Potential for ownership
More autonomy	On-call physicians likelier to gladly accept patients
Less stress	More satisfied patients
Less malpractice risk	

major trauma, physicians and nurses generally have more time with their patients in FSEDs, leading to higher patient experience scores, as well as higher physician, nurse, and staff engagement and commitment to the mission of the FSED. There is palpably less stress, less malpractice exposure, and more autonomy, all of which leads to less likelihood of burnout and the possibility of extending one's career longer in a more rewarding environment. Often, on-call physicians are more amenable to accepting patients in follow-up, for many reasons, including the likelihood of the better reimbursement of FSED versus ED patients.[34]

In practice, the negatives from the providers' perspective are less commonly experienced. However, arguments can be made that procedural skills may decline over time, boredom with more minor acuity patients may set in, emergency physician and nursing shortages in the main ED may be exacerbated, and that the market may become oversaturated with FSEDs, causing closures. In reality, each of these can be addressed, although recruitment of the most highly qualified emergency physicians and nurses to FSEDs is a very real phenomenon, at least for the hospital EDs from which they are recruited.

Hospital and Health-Care System Perspective

For proactive hospitals and health-care systems with sufficient capital (and vision), FSEDs, when properly planned and executed, have many benefits. They allow for greater access to care, protection of highly valued markets, referral of admissions, and the ability to brand into the community. They provide an attractive practice option for the workforce (particularly emergency physicians and nurses, but all the essential services staff as well). Freestanding emergency departments also provide the ability to "off-load" some patients, thereby decreasing ED crowding and meeting competitive threats from other hospitals which value the target market.[32,33] The expressed negatives of FSEDs largely come from hospitals that do not pursue this strategy and include the arguments that FSEDs do not lower cost (and may raise them when compared to UCCs); do not increase access to safety-net patients; "skim" profitable, positive reimbursement, low-acuity patients from the main ED; create unfair competition for patients; and "steal" talent from the ED. (In fact, careful analysis shows that once EMS patients, in particular those with trauma, cardiac, and stroke, are removed, the acuity mix of EDs and FSEDs is nearly identical.)[35]

Payer Perspective

In ED reimbursement, a variant of the golden rule is that, "Those who have the gold will do almost anything to keep it." In the case of the payers, it can be argued that, true to "form follows finance," many of them have reacted to the FSED movement with strategies designed to reduce or restrict payment in these settings. This is particularly true for IFECs, whether investor or physician-owned. It is quite clear that based on current regulations, charging E/M and APC codes for true FSEDs is clear, straightforward, and completely legal and ethical. Nonetheless, some payers have pursued strategies to deny coverage to FSEDs generically, but more specifically for IFECs, on the grounds that they are precluded from CMS reimbursement and regulations. One study showed that most insurance companies have pursued a strategy of refusing to negotiate with FSEDs—and with IFECs in particular.[36] Indeed, many IFECs have moved toward hospital affiliation to become HOPDs in an effort to overcome this impediment.[37] These issues have also been influenced by the "surprise billing" controversy.[38]

However, some progressive payers, particularly those closely aligned with provider networks (including but not restricted to hospitals), have seen the important role that FSEDs can serve in the value-based purchasing and population health era. Thus, the payer perspective is changing and that change is likely to accelerate.

OPERATIONAL AND FINANCIAL CONSIDERATIONS

While rules and regulations governing FSEDs vary from state to state, regardless of location, leadership must consider the following issues:

- *Staff composition (number and roles):* The full scope of essential services available in a hospital, such as pharmacists, respiratory therapists, social workers, laboratory and imaging staff, as well as central distribution, will not be immediately available in an FSED. Decisions made about the staff mix require regular reevaluation as the service requirements change, including developing contingency plans to cover the potentially needed services. Role flexibility (within written job descriptions) and cross-training of staff are keys to efficiency.
    - For hospital-owned FSEDs, staff can potentially float between the hospital-based ED and the FSED. This flexibility allows both facilities to adjust staffing to patient volumes at each site; this is particularly effective if parallel processes (same forms, same computerized systems, etc.) are in place.
- *Orientation of new staff members:* The skill set required to succeed in an FSED is similar facilities to but not the same as the skill set required to work in the ED. An orientation specific to the FSED is required. For hospital-owned FSEDs, it is necessary to consider if the acquisition of skills is better met at the FSED or at the sponsoring hospital where volumes and acuity are higher and the new staff member has the opportunity to be exposed to more types of patients.
- *Pharmacy:* The range of readily available medications may be different in the FSED. Without an on-site pharmacy, nurses may require special training to address preparation of specific medications. How will inventories be maintained and automated dispensing cabinets restocked? How will practitioners manage patients when the standard treatment of a particular condition requires medications that are not available on-site, that is, methotrexate for an early ectopic pregnancy or rabies vaccine for a bat exposure?
- *Supplies/equipment:* The supply stores in an FSED are more limited than a hospital, making it necessary to determine the type of equipment and the quantities of supplies (including linens, patient care items, and nourishments) as well as how inventories (par levels) of supplies will be maintained. Are all supplies disposable? If not, how are sanitizing and sterilization accomplished? Will patients who need equipment or supplies that are unavailable at the FSED be transferred to a facility that has the needed resource?
- *Security:* With limited resources, how will staff respond if a violent patient walks into the FSED? Security issues for FSEDs are the same as in any hospital-based ED. There are people who will seek care 24 hours per day, and sometimes those individuals have tendencies toward violence, theft, or other criminal activity or substance abuse. Some EDs use on-site security, especially during high-risk hours. Others have dedicated alarm systems to the local police and internal lockdown procedures to protect the staff. In any case, the leaders have the same responsibilities to provide a safe work and care environment in an FSED.
- *Critical care transport and noncritical transports:* It is estimated that only 5% to 10% of patients presenting to an FSED require transfer to an acute care facility.[39] Will transfer be accomplished by a contracted private ambulance service or by EMS? Ideally, patients requiring admission will be transported to the sponsoring hospital of a hospital-based FSED, but what if another facility is closer? How will the patient who walked into the FSED with a STEMI or stroke be managed and transported?

There is little published information on the precise start-up costs for either FSEDs or FSECs. However, estimated start-up costs range from a low of $2.5 million (FSEDs in existing medical office buildings) to much larger numbers (if sites are procured and built).

ARCHITECTURAL ISSUES

The evolution of FSEDs as a care type has created opportunities for exciting building images and efficient layouts that are hard to achieve in the traditional hospital-based environment. Many FSEDs seek to stimulate a strong branding image and state-of-the-art environments to support the functional care of patients and to create an image of high quality (**Figure 54.5**). The two major categories of facilities, IFECs and hospital-owned FSEDs, may present different goals and building requirements.

Space Requirements

Regulations and requirements for freestanding EDs are under the responsibility of each state's authority having jurisdiction for health-care licensure. Some states may require a CON for a project. Most states utilize the Facility Guidelines Institute's *Guidelines for Design and Construction of Outpatient Facilities*, which publish specific requirements for FSEDs every 4 years.[40] These recommendations are a good starting point for identifying needs and can be used as a framework for establishing an individual project's requirements. Note that DGSF = departmental gross square feet. This is typically equivalent to building gross square feet (BGF).

As discussed in Chapter 27, the single most important element in sizing an emergency service is the number of treatment spaces. For a freestanding ED, this would include a

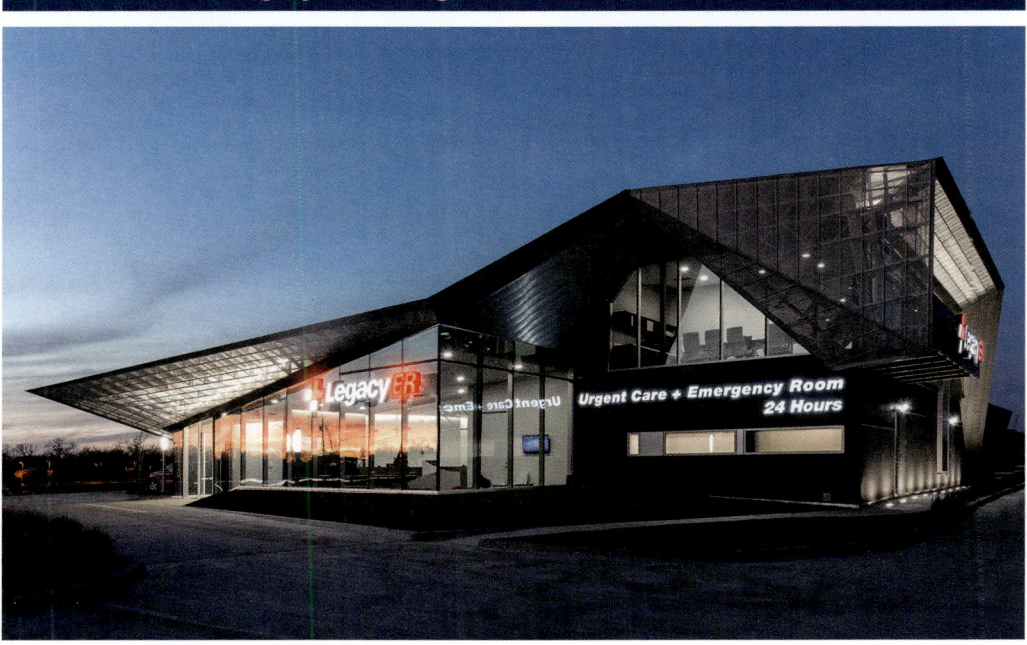

FIGURE 54.5 ■ Legacy ER and Urgent Care, Allen, Texas

Courtesy of 5G Studio Collaborative

combination of trauma/resuscitation, treatment, standard exam, and results waiting areas. In addition, some FSEDs have added larger rooms with private restrooms for observation status patients or for those who require overnight treatment and/or evaluation. One of the frequent selling points of this type of care is the short time from patient arrival to contact with a provider. To ensure sufficient treatment spaces to permit this rapid flow, the planning of a freestanding ED must anticipate the character of patient arrival patterns, mix of care, and length of stay to assure sufficient capacity. Typical hospital-based EDs are currently designed for 1,400 to 1,500 annual visits per treatment space. Freestanding facilities may be able to exceed this ratio due to the generally lower acuity of the patients being served (shorter lengths of stay) and less obstructions to patient flow, such as inpatient boarders, more efficient point-of-care labs, and shorter turnaround times for imaging and radiology interpretation. Many freestanding EDs are utilizing a split-flow model for patient management, which could include results waiting spaces to reduce the time patients occupy treatment rooms.

Once the basic operational flow model and the number of treatment spaces are defined, a space listing of all areas in the project is developed to determine the total net square feet and the estimated BGF. An early method for estimating the building area is to use a ratio of square feet to treatment areas. For hospital-based EDs, the ratio would typically fall in the range of 750 to 850 gross square feet per treatment space. Freestanding EDs, typically smaller than hospital-based services, experience a wider range of area per treatment space due to the need for diagnostic and other support services that may be outside the hospital base services. For example, small hospital-based EDs may not have in-department computerized tomography (CTs) scanning, whereas most freestanding services will include CTs and may have MRIs.

A major element that can affect space estimates is the possible colocation of medical office space. This is a common strategy for hospital-based facilities that are seeking to integrate demand from a new service area into their system.

Another key strategic planning decision is the possible expansion of services. This could include the ED and the possible expansion to a micro-hospital or satellite hospital facility. Acquisition of sufficient land to accommodate other structures and parking should be evaluated in the early stages of planning and budgeting. In addition, in some cases, there may be a consideration to use vertical expansion for further services, so local regulations on height restrictions should be considered.

Most current freestanding EDs are being designed with a traditional ballroom configuration with treatment space wrapped around charting and support areas. If the facility has a split-flow operational model, some of the treatment spaces may be separated near the entry/triage area to facilitate rapid movement.

The Micro-Hospital

Typical micro-hospitals have 14,000 to 20,000 square feet of space. If physician offices or other services are provided, the building can range from 30,000 to 60,000 gross square feet. One of the large Texas-based providers, Emerus, emphasizes a design that places imaging near the entry and seven to eight large emergency treatment rooms. As opposed to traditional small community access hospital with long nursing unit wings, micro-hospital building designs frequently are rectangular and multistoried (**Figure 54.6**). Current regulations for observation care in most states require windows from patient rooms, but the small number of rooms eliminates the need for a linear building geometry.

As with freestanding emergency service planning, careful consideration of the development of other related office and care buildings should be incorporated into the early planning of micro-hospitals.

FIGURE 54.6 ■ Floor Plan Example

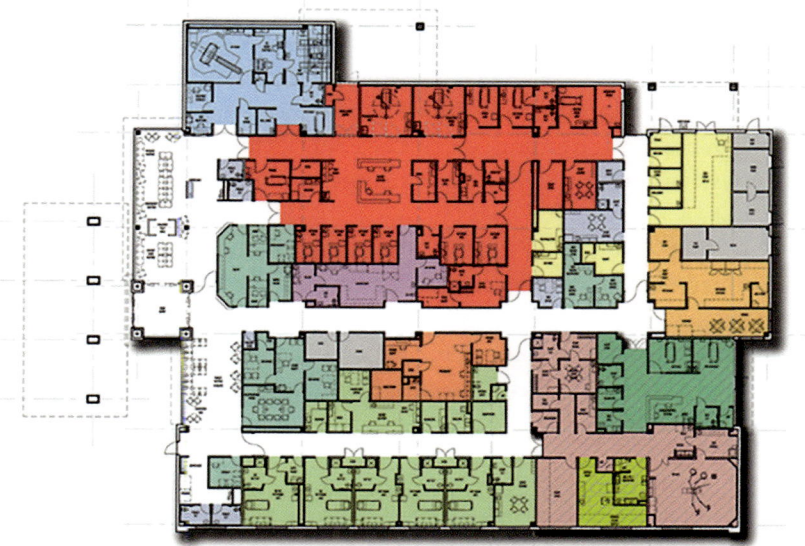

Courtesy of E4H Environments for Health Architecture

HORIZONS OF FSEDs

It is likely that FSEDs will be an enduring part of the health-care system in those states that allow them. However, it is equally likely that investor-owned facilities will seek some sort of hospital affiliation to avoid the issue of nonparticipation with CMS reimbursement programs. This will likely result in fewer FSEDs, with most of them evolving as HOPDs. However, the emerging phenomenon of physician-owned IFECs has been very successful in specific health-care markets, particularly in Texas. The attractiveness of physicians (and nurses) owning their own practice will be balanced by the willingness to be entrepreneurial and tolerate the risk of borrowing start-up capital, advertising the facility, and building the patient base during the start-up phase.

Freestanding emergency departmentss with CT, MRI, and US capability may find ways to amortize the costs of this equipment by providing overflow capability to nearby hospitals, whose use of those services on-site are stressed to and above capacity, although one state (Texas) has statutorily proscribed such access.

It remains to be seen if the emergency physician and nursing staffing shortages can be ameliorated as talented professionals migrate to FSED practices and if lower stress levels translate into less burnout.

CONCLUSION

If the overall cost of care is ever to be reduced, an essential part of the puzzle is almost certainly disruptive innovations like FSEDs. Whether hospital- or physician-owned, these facilities will continue to serve the market for convenient, high-quality, cost-effective acute episodic care provided in a practice environment that is less chaotic than the typical hospital ED. While entrenched interests will likely continue to try to hobble such facilities through various means, ultimately "the market will be served."

APPENDIX 54.1: HOPDs: A CASE STUDY

The Inova Healthplex (IHP) in Springfield, Virginia, was the third FSED added to the IHS's already considerable experience in this area. The site was carefully chosen to meet the needs of an important service area. Three Inova hospitals surround the area in Springfield: Inova Mount Vernon, Inova Alexandria, and Inova Fairfax Hospital, the area's level I trauma facility, and a major academic training center. The FSED facility is part of a medical complex that includes physician offices, an outpatient surgery center, and a full-service imaging center.

The FSED accepts all levels of EMS traffic except patients with major trauma and cardiac arrests. Specifically, chest pain patients are evaluated at the center, although 63% of the STEMI patients evaluated and transferred for angioplasty have been ambulatory patients. A dedicated transfer program for patients to be admitted to the hospital was developed with a private ambulance company, Physicians Transport Service (PTS), which includes critical care transport capability. For the past several years, a PTS unit has been based at the IHP.

The FSED volume rose to above 30,000 patients per year within the first 2 years of operation. By mid-2009, the IHP had experienced significant growth in patient volume. Average volume in June through September 2009 was 106 patients per day, an increase from 89 patients per day during the same period in 2008. In 2012, the patient volume remained above 100 patients per day. While such increases in volume are good, the growth led to challenges with patient flow, increased length of stay (LOS), and admission boarding delays. Partnering with the nursing and administrative teams, the physician group staffing the facility viewed this as an opportunity to improve patient flow processes, as well as patient satisfaction, team satisfaction, and overall teamwork.

An Operations Approach to Improvement and Flow

The state of flow and volume was mapped using flow maps, patient arrivals by time and acuity, by day of the week. A thorough assessment of staffing patterns and hours and clinical productivity (including relative value unit generation) was undertaken and plotted against the forecasted demand for services. Four areas of improvement were recommended:

1. Lower overall LOS by implementing a patient flow and service plan.
2. Create a separate treatment area for low-acuity patients.
3. Create a boarding/surge policy and plan.
4. Implement an enhanced compensation plan tied to specific progress on *metrics that matter*.

First, highly specific monthly LOS goals and flow-directed ED metrics were set for the group. Information was extracted from the electronic medical record. A patient flow operations plan was implemented, which included the development and deployment of a rapid intervention and treatment zone (RITZ) for patients with ESI level 5, 4, and selected 3s. Staffing was also increased during peak hours.

Second, a high percentage of IHP patients (>50%) are ESI 4s and 5s. These patients were treated in the RITZ, reducing stress on the main ED and improving overall patient flow. This RITZ process allowed the staff to *fast-track* and *super-track* these patients. Scripts were developed to ensure the patients knew that they were being seen in a new way, in a new area, with a specific focus on patient flow.

Third, as volume increased, so did the number of patients needing admission to the hospital. Boarding patients became a predictable problem. A boarding policy was implemented that included specific triggers and defined action plans, which allowed the staff to ease the boarding burden and handle boarders more efficiently. The ambulance service was an important part of this effort, as they also increased their staffing to improve flow. Patient and staff satisfaction both increased.

Fourth, while the legacy compensation plan had a meaningful productivity component, clinicians found it overly complex and too far removed from daily performance. A new productivity-based compensation plan was implemented that more clearly and frequently tied compensation to *line of sight* improvement in results. The compensation plan directly rewarded efficient LOS outcomes and patient safety behaviors.

Delivering the Results that Matter

The results at IHP exceeded expectations and can be attributed to the combined leadership of the nursing, administrative, and physician teams, who engaged the staff in planning an outside-the-box approach to flow and service excellence. The staff thus helped design and fully embraced a solid, data-driven plan. Results include:

- LOS sequentially dropped from a baseline of 200 minutes to 150 minutes, then to 120 minutes, and finally to a sustained level below 110 minutes.
- Patient satisfaction scores rocketed upward, from the 60th percentile to the 99th percentile.
- Courtemanche and Associates, a leading medical research and consulting firm, named the IHP as the nation's "best freestanding emergency department," an award the staff and leadership team richly deserved.

This case study shows that innovative and creative solutions are possible, particularly in FSEDs, where tradition and commitment to old, inefficient processes are perhaps more easily overcome.

APPENDIX 54.2: PHYSICIAN-OWNED FSECs: A CASE STUDY

Physician-owned FSECs are currently primarily a Texas phenomenon. At least 31 FSECs are either in operation or in the build-out phase of development. The Texas insurance code has some of the strictest payer requirements in the country, with 16 requiring prompt payment within 45 days of the receipt of a clean claim. Otherwise the payers are held strictly liable to pay billed charges, attorneys' fees, and an 18% per-annum penalty. Texas physician-owned FSECs have used these provisions to demand and receive payment for the hospital-based ED E&M CPT codes 99281–99285 and the critical care codes, 99291 and 99292. The typical Texas physician-owned FSEC plaintiff's argument is that:

- Patients are seen much faster in their (FSEC) facility than in a hospital-based ED.
- Medical care is identical in every respect and often provided by a physician who, on another night, might have provided the same service in a hospital-based ED setting.
- Equipment, supplies, and patient care processes are the same.
- The Health Care Finance Administration 1500 claim was properly coded and clean as defined by the insurance code.

Texas juries have found for the FSEC plaintiffs and in so doing have highlighted the irrationality of the rules that prevent the development of these kinds of facilities in other states.

Many physician-owned FSECs are well-equipped with on-site laboratory and imaging services. Cardiac monitoring and minor surgical and orthopedic equipment and instrumentation are comparable to that of a hospital-based ED. When a patient requires hospital admission, securing the appropriate on-call specialist is generally not a problem. As is the case in any other private practice, the physician-owned FSEC emergency physician refers to the specialist who they believe will provide the best service. The specialist usually helps with problem dispositions in order to keep the preferred provider status for the well-paying FSEC referrals. There is no need to beg and cajole for specialty backup, and referring physician abuse is largely unheard of.

Many middle-aged emergency physicians or emergency physicians who are disenchanted with their current practice environment have looked at the possibility of opening an FSEC as a way to gain more control over their practice environment and the types of patients they see. Unfortunately, the current payer challenges in states other than Texas and the financial stresses of starting this type of a capital-intensive business create substantial impediments. The physicians who have been successful say that it may take years to succeed. If considering the development of an FSEC, it would be wise to talk to emergency physicians who have pursued this endeavor and recognize the necessary level of commitment. Start-up costs range from $750,000 in strip center (mall) lease space to $3 million in a high-visibility retail site. Despite the challenges to physician-owned FSECs, maturation of accountable care organizations (ACOs) may remove some of the barriers to these innovations. When customer satisfaction, value, and cost savings accrue to the ACO, it will be in the ACO's interest to support entities that can deliver better customer service and lower cost.

Developing a Hybrid Model

In 2006, three Texas EM physicians with extensive experience working in various FSECs decided to launch their own venture. This type of enterprise takes months or years of planning involving financing, performing market research, overseeing construction build out, licensing, advertising, hiring, and so on. Their facility opened approximately 24 months after they began their planning. The FSEC is a 6,000-square-foot freestanding structure that operates as a hybrid model, with an urgent care center down one hall and a full-service FSEC down the other. This structure with different provider numbers on each side of the facility enables patients with urgent care problems to be billed using office visit codes, while those with ED visit criteria are billed using the CPT 9928* ED code series. Only patients who meet predefined criteria are charged as an *ED* patient (with separate facility/ancillary and professional bills). The advantage to this operational and billing structure is a broader range of services that:

- Allows a higher visit volume from day one
- Retains the ability to bill the CPT 9928* code series for patients who would otherwise have to been seen in a hospital-based ED

The facility has four urgent care rooms (typical doctor office examination rooms) and five ED rooms with extensive specialty equipment (resuscitation; critical care; ear, nose, and throat; gynecology, etc.). The total build-out expense was approximately $1,200,000.00, exclusive of the land cost. Marketing and monthly operating expenses are budgeted at $150,000/month, excluding provider payroll. The operating capital provision is an additional $2,000,000. Initially, the facility was staffed with a carefully selected staff of four people:

- Registration clerk
- CT/radiology technician
- RN
- MD

The technician, RN, and MD were all cross-trained to perform basic clinical procedures (such as phlebotomy and starting an intravenous line) and perform laboratory tests. As volume increased, paramedics or medical assistants were added to absorb the additional volume, which eventually peaked at 70 visits per 12-hour day.

Due to patient self-selection, the acuity of this type of facility tends to be lower than in a hospital-based ED. Nonetheless, the FSEC must be prepared to provide the same high-acuity care when necessary. Typical admission rates are between 2% and 5% versus a hospital ED's 15% to 20%.

While the financial risks and planning obstacles are significant, the payoff for an FSEC can be well worth the risk and effort. For emergency patients, the facility receives a facility fee similar to any hospital ED, which is usually in the $150 to $600 range, depending on the services provided. Although acuity and charges are typically lower than that of a hospital-based ED, a typical FSEC acute care patient's collections may average $1,000 to $1,500 per encounter, while an urgent care visit averages $150 to $250 per encounter. These numbers vary widely according to payer policies, managed care contracts, and the services offered.

REFERENCES

1. Hsia R, King J, Carr BG. Don't hate the player; hate the game. *Ann Emerg Med*. 2017;70(6):875–883.
2. Emergency Medicine Network. Massachusetts General Hospital, Freestanding Emergency Departments. 2017. Available at: http://www.emnet-usa.org/research/studies/nedi/nedi2017/freestanding-eds/. Accessed July 6, 2020.
3. Emergency Department Benchmarking Alliance. 2017 Annual Report. Available at: www.edbenchmarking.org. Accessed July 10, 2020.
4. Stand-alone emergency departments. Medpac. Report to the Congress: Medicare and the Healthcare Delivery System. 2017:245–264.
5. Microhospitals: Healthcare's newest patient access point. Building Design and Construction. February 7, 2017.
6. Pitts SR, Carrier ER, Rich EC, et al. Where Americans get acute care: increasingly, it's not at their doctor's office. *Health Aff (Millwood)*. 2010;29(9):1620-1629.
7. Simon EL, Griffin PL, Jouriles NJ. The impact of two freestanding emergency departments on a tertiary care center. *J Emerg Med*. 2012;43(6):1127-1131.
8. Board of Directors, American College of Emergency Physicians. Freestanding emergency departments and urgent care centers. 2015. Available at: https://www.acep.org/globalassets/uploads/uploaded-files/acep/clinical-and-practice-management/resources/administration/fsed-and-ucs_info-paper_final_110215.pdf. Accessed July 6, 2020.
9. American College of Emergency Physicians. Freestanding Emergency Departments: Position Statement. 2020. Available at: https://www.acep.org/globalassets/new-pdfs/policy-statements/freestanding-emergency-departments.pdf. Accessed July 6, 2020.
10. Pulsinelli O. Emergency center company to close Houston HQ. 2018. Available at: https://www.bizjournals.com/houston/news/2018/11/02/emergency-center-co-to-close-houston-hq-cut-jobs.html#:~:text=Neighbors%20Health%20will%20close%20its,part%20of%20its%20bankruptcy%20process.&text=Houston%2Dbased%20Neighbors%20Health%20LLC,corporate%20headquarters%20and%20billing%20office. Accessed July 6, 2020.
11. Center for Improvement of Healthcare Quality. Freestanding Emergency Department Certification. 2019. Available at: https://www.cihq.org/fsec.asp. Accessed July 6, 2020.
12. Augustine J. Emergency medical service arrivals, admission rates to the emergency department. *ACEP Now*. 2016.
13. Chang J, Lykidis P. Top 10 factors to consider when building a freestanding emergency department. Becker's Hospital Review. 2014.
14. ACEP Emergency Medicine Practice Management Committee. Freestanding Emergency Departments. 2015. Available at: www.acep.org.
15. Hellstern R, Mayer T, Mahor K, et al. Freestanding emergency departments. In: Strauss RJ, Mayer TA, eds. *Emergency Department Management*. McGraw-Hill; 2014.
16. Kellermann AL, Hsia RY, Yeh C, et al. Emergency care: then, now, and next. *Health Aff (Millwood)*. 2013;32(12):2069-2074.
17. Pines JM, Zocchi MS, Black BS. A comparison of care delivered in hospital-based and freestanding emergency departments. *Acad Emerg Med*. 2018;25(5):538–550.
18. Texas Insurance Code, Section 20A.18B—Prompt Payment of Physicians and Providers. Available at: www.tdi.state.tx.us/hprovider/ppresource.html. Last Revised May 2010.
19. Adeptus Health files for bankruptcy. Becker's Hospital CEO Report. 2017. Available at: https://www.beckershospitalreview.com/finance/adeptus-health-files-for-bankruptcy.html. Accessed July 6, 2020.
20. Harish N, Wiler JL, Zane R. How the freestanding emergency department boom can help patients. *NEJM Catalyst*. 2016. Available at: http://catalyst.nejm.org/how-the-freestanding-emergency-department-boom-can-help-patients/. Accessed July 6, 2020.
21. Schur JD, Yealy DM, Callaham ML. Comparing freestanding emergency departments, hospital-based emergency departments, and urgent care in Texas: apples, oranges, or lemons. *Ann Emerg Med*. 2017;70(6):858–861.
22. Ho V, Metcalfe L, Dark C, et al. Comparing utilization and costs of care in freestanding emergency departments, hospital emergency

22. departments, and urgent care centers. *Ann Emerg Med.* 2017;70(6): 846–857.

23. Kivela P. Original allegations about data integrity by emergency physicians. *Ann Emerg Med.* 2017;70(6):862–863.

24. Olinger D. Free-standing ERs abound in affluent Colorado neighborhoods. *Denver Post.* 2016. Available at: http://www.denverpost.com/news/ci_28874739/freestanding-ers-aboundaffluent-colorado-neighborhoods. Accessed July 6, 2020.

25. Walters E, Lin J. In wealthy ZIP codes, freestanding ERs find a home. *Texas Tribune.* 2015. Available at: http://www.texastribune.org/2015/08/21/freestanding-emergency-rooms-rise-texas/. Accessed July 24, 2016.

26. Granovsky M. Advanced billing and coding. In: Strauss R, Mayer T, eds. *Strauss and Mayer's Emergency Department Management.* 2nd ed. Dallas, Tex: American College of Emergency Physicians Press; 2020.

27. Mayer T. Freestanding emergency departments: threat, opportunity, or both? Presented at: the American College of Emergency Physicians' Scientific Assembly, Denver, October 29, 2019.

28. Centers for Medicare and Medicaid Services. CMS issues guidance allowing independent freestanding emergency departments to provide care to Medicare and Medicaid beneficiaries during the COVID-19 crisis. Available at: https://www.cms.gov/newsroom/press-releases/cms-issues-guidance-allowing-independent-freestanding-emergency-departments-provide-care-medicare. Accessed July 6, 2020.

29. Patidar N, Weech-Maldonado R, O'Connor SJ, et al. Freestanding emergency departments are associated with higher Medicare costs: a longitudinal panel data analysis. *J Healthc Org Prov Fin.* 2017;54:1–8.

30. La Pointe J. Freestanding emergency departments cost 22 times more than doctor's offices. RevCycle Intelligence. Available at: https://revcycleintellignece.com/news/freestanding-emergency-departments-cost-22-times-more-than-doctor. Accessed July 6, 2020.

31. UnitedHealth Group. Freestanding emergency departments: treating common conditions at emergency prices. Available at: https://www.unitedhealthgroup.com/content/dam/UHG/PDF/2017/Freestanding-ER-Cost-Analysis.pdf. Accessed July 6, 2020.

32. Blackwell T, Mayer T, Robinson K, et al. Practice diversification in EMS. In: Strauss RW, Mayer TA, eds. *Strauss and Mayer's Emergency Department Management.* 2nd ed. Dallas, Tex: American College of Emergency Physicians Press; 2021.

33. Cone D, Brice JH, Delbridge TR, Myers JB, eds. *Emergency Medical Services: Clinical Practice and Systems Oversight.* 2nd ed. Overland Park, Kans: National Association of Emergency Medical Services Physicians; 2018.

34. Draper E. Free-standing ERs draw patients, critics and legislation. Available at: https://www.denverpost.com/news/ci_25349086/freestanding-ers-draw-patients-critics-and-legislation. Accessed July 6, 2020.

35. Sullivan AF, Bachireddy C, Steptoe AP, et al. A profile of freestanding emergency departments in the United States, 2007. *J Emerg Med.* 2012;43(6):1175–1180.

36. Shaw G. Freestanding emergency departments in Texas closing one after another. *Emerg Med News.* 2018; 40:185–189.

37. Simon EL, Dark C, Kovacs, et al. Variation in hospital admission rates between a tertiary care and two freestanding emergency departments. *Am J Emerg Med.* 2018;36(6):967–971.

38. American Hospital Association. Fact sheet on surprise billing legislation. Available at: https://www.aha.org/fact-sheets/2020-02-14-fact-sheet-surprise-billing-legislation#:~:text=11%20approved%20the%20Ban%20Surprise,to%20address%20surprise%20medical%20bills.&text=For%20amounts%20paid%20above%20%24750, Ways%20and%20Means%20Committee%20Feb. Accessed July 6, 2020.

39. Davis C, Zacchinga L. Thinking about developing a freestanding emergency department? Four reasons to reconsider. Becker's Clinical Leadership and Infection Control. 2018. Available at: https://www.aha.org/fact-sheets/2020-02-14-fact-sheet-surprise-billing-legislation#:~:text=11%20approved%20the%20Ban%20Surprise,to%20address%20surprise%20medical%20bills.&text=For%20amounts%20paid%20above%20%24750, Ways%20and%20Means%20Committee%20Feb. Accessed July 6, 2020.

40. Health Facilities Guideline Institute. Guidelines for Design and Construction of Outpatient Facilities. 2018. Available at: https://fgiguidelines.org/guidelines/2018-fgi-guidelines/. Accessed July 6, 2020.

CHAPTER 55

SPORTS MEDICINE

James M. Ellis Jr, Stephanie N. Bailey

Emergency physicians are widely recognized for their diverse training encompassing virtually all elements of acute-care medicine, as well as many elements of primary care. This breadth of expertise can be utilized when considering practice diversification opportunities, which may be particularly helpful when addressing the common problem of "burnout" among emergency physicians (see Chapter 125). This situation has been attributed to a wide variety of causes, including shift work, lack of resources, anxiety regarding potential poor outcomes, and emotional exhaustion.[1-7] In addition, emergency physician groups may look for avenues of expansion to obtain additional income and engage in areas of personal interests and expertise. Sports medicine offers an important opportunity for these groups, as emergency physicians are well trained and comfortable with the acute evaluation and treatment of athletic injuries and illnesses (**Figure 55.1**).

Although sports medicine is traditionally considered the domain of orthopedic surgeons, it has become more accessible to physicians in other specialties. Primary care sports medicine fellowships are increasing in popularity for physicians trained in family medicine, pediatrics, physical medicine and rehabilitation, and emergency medicine. Over the last 20 years, the number of primary care sports medicine fellowship programs available for emergency physicians has grown significantly. Sports medicine, in the context of this chapter, is broader than simply providing medical oversight to a sports team. Most physicians think the subspecialty is limited to the expertise traditionally expected

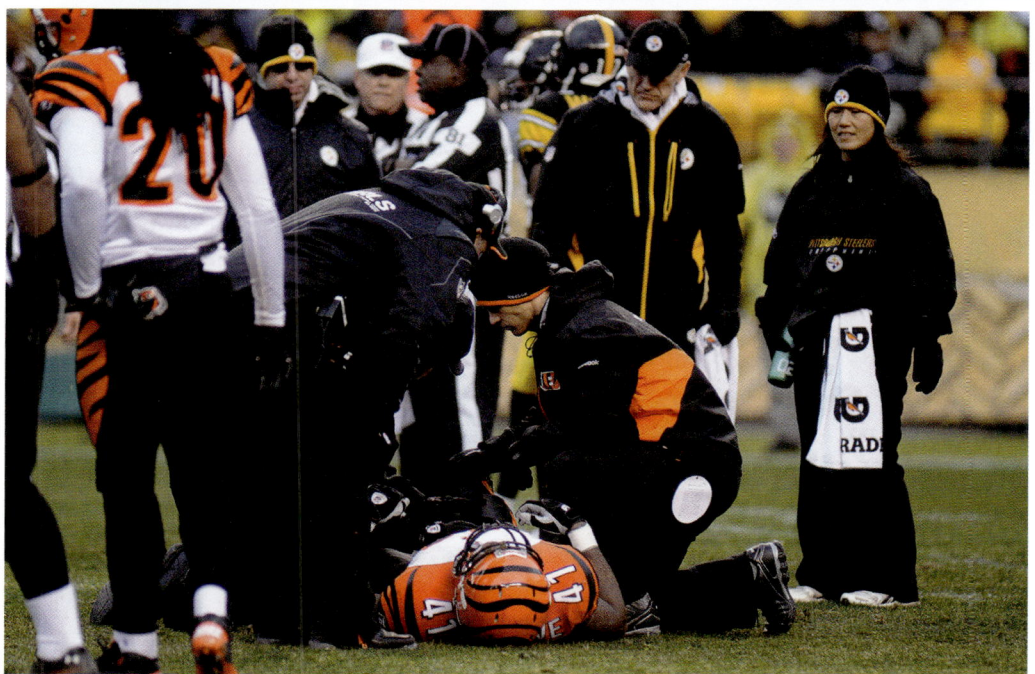

FIGURE 55.1 ■ Training Staff Attends to Injured Cincinnati Bengals Player

of orthopedic surgeons, including acute injury care, physical rehabilitation, and injury prevention. While the role of a team physician does include musculoskeletal expertise, it also includes the following additional aspects of primary and acute care management:

- Concussion and traumatic brain injuries
- Cervical spine injuries
- Heat illness and acclimatization
- Cardiovascular disease, arrhythmias, and athlete's heart changes
- Sleep apnea
- Performance-enhancing medication use
- Performance and conditioning
- Nonmusculoskeletal trauma/truncal trauma
- Allergic reactions
- Dermatologic diseases
- Infectious diseases, including methicillin-resistant *Staphylococcus aureus*

Spectators and athletes alike often sustain primary orthopedic injuries; however, general medical problems, including life-threatening emergencies, are also common. At many sporting events, care of the athlete has typically been the responsibility of an orthopedist, while emergency medical services (EMS) and/or registered nurses have delivered spectator care. All too often, spectator care receives minimal physician involvement. Frequently, providers are chosen to treat spectators based on their acquaintance with the event organizers rather than on their knowledge or ability. With an increased emphasis on risk management and professional liability, the careful selection of these clinicians has become more important.

The biggest obstacle for providers in sports medicine has been *reimbursement*. In many cases, members of the medical community are called upon to simply donate their time. They may receive compensation in another form, such as advertising in an arena or at an event. The question of reimbursement must be considered carefully before diversification into sports medicine can become a viable strategy for emergency clinicians. When negotiating compensation, it may be of helpful to stress the need for quality medical care in the setting of diverse and potentially complicated clinical scenarios. Given our litigious society, close attention must also be paid to risk management.

THE ROLE OF TEAM PHYSICIANS

The origin of sports medicine and the assignment of team physicians arose directly from the specialty of orthopedic surgery. Classically, the definitive management of many orthopedic injuries was the province of the orthopedic surgeon, whether that treatment was operative or nonoperative. Although the unquestioned experts in the field of musculoskeletal injuries, orthopedic surgeons are often faced with athletes whose injuries and medical needs exceed the specialty of orthopedics. Primary care sports medicine physicians are increasingly becoming integral to the management of nonoperative orthopedic injuries, nonmusculoskeletal traumatic injuries, and primary care needs.

Current Expectations

Team physicians have a variety of other responsibilities, including:

- Preseason physicals
- Diagnosis and treatment of medical illnesses
- Concussion evaluation and management

- Acute stabilization of cervical spine injuries
- Laceration repair
- Cardiovascular health
- Nutrition
- Acute electrolyte abnormalities
- Thermal illnesses

As teams have recognized the need for a broader scope of medical care, the greater utilization of internists, family practitioners, and emergency physicians has fulfilled these requirements. Physicians trained in primary care have a very broad scope of training but do not have the depth of knowledge and experience possessed by emergency physicians in managing severe injuries requiring advanced trauma life support, sudden cardiac death necessitating advanced cardiac life support, and other life-threatening emergencies. Airway management and cardiac arrhythmia recognition and treatment are invaluable skills that often distinguish emergency physicians from other providers.[8] By completing a primary care sports medicine fellowship and gaining a Certificate of Added Qualification (CAQ) in the subspecialty, the emergency physician becomes the best-qualified provider of nonoperative sports medicine.

Training and Experience

Emergency physicians are able to address injured athletes at virtually any level, including high school, college, and professional sports. Those who desire practice diversification with sports medicine may want to consider formal fellowship training. A CAQ in primary care sports medicine is becoming a standard expectation for collegiate and professional team physicians; however, if the physician is interested more broadly in venue coverage, event medicine, or just coverage of high school sports, this added training may not be a necessity.

There are currently close to 90 sports medicine fellowships in the US (**Figure 55.2**), and over 20 of these programs have graduated a fellow initially trained in emergency medicine. While additional training is ideal, the background and training of emergency physicians provides them with substantial knowledge in this field. This knowledge may be augmented

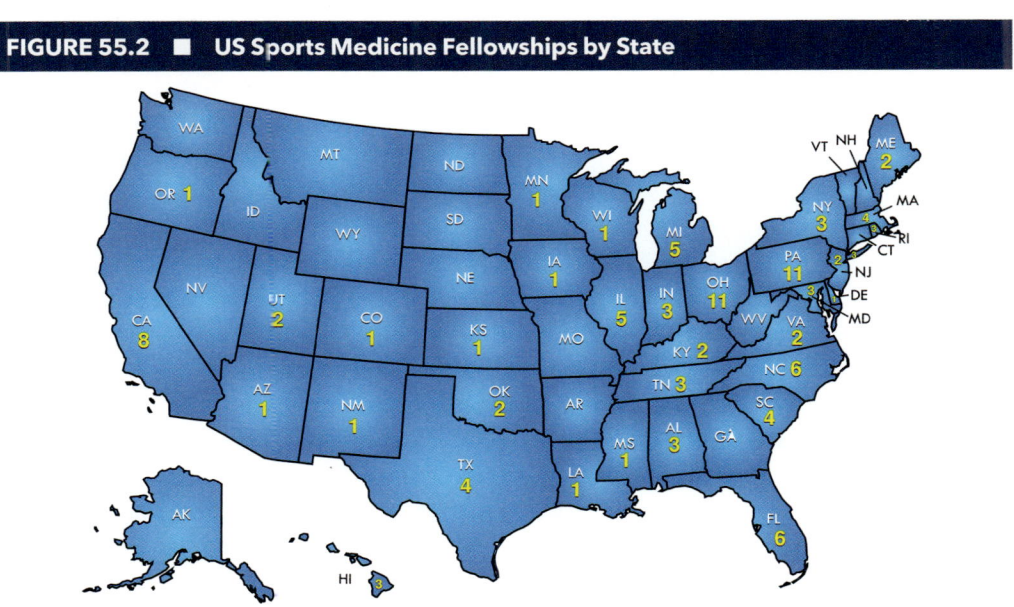

FIGURE 55.2 ■ US Sports Medicine Fellowships by State

by selected readings from the orthopedic literature. This may be all that is necessary for a team physician at the high school level. At the collegiate and professional ranks, higher levels of expertise and fellowship training may be required. For example, the National Football League (NFL) requires its new primary care physicians to have sports medicine fellowship training and a CAQ.

Most teams request a single person to be primarily responsible for the medical care so that they may have one provider to approach with concerns, problems, or feedback. Although a single lead physician is often requested or required by the team, multiple physicians within a sports medicine, orthopedic, and/or emergency medicine group may be utilized for coverage, offering substantial advantages. A nonoperative physician who is the lead team physician should have an agreement with an orthopedic surgeon for the referral of complicated injuries. The orthopedic surgeon is an integral part of the medical team, ensuring appropriate injury treatment, intervention, and potential operative management with continuity of care. The relationship between the orthopedic surgeon and the emergency physician providing sports medicine coverage is a key one.

The Medical Plan

To effectively organize a team's medical care, the practitioner should begin with a written medical plan that includes policies and procedures for all situations. This document should outline the expectations and details of the team physician's role. The protocols include preseason physicals, referrals, on-call availability during practices, an emergency action plan (EAP), and attendance at the games. Anyone interested in becoming a team physician should have direct contact with the team's decision-maker (e.g., athletic trainer, principal, head coach, athletic director, chancellor, owner, or current team physician). All parties should agree on the plan and be aware of its related procedures.

To prepare for the team's medical problems beyond those of sports medicine, an emergency physician typically develops a referral base for specific illnesses or injuries—similar to the referral base used in the day-to-day practice of emergency medicine. The team may desire to select its own panel of physicians or ask the team physician to undertake this process.

The Providers

The availability of the team physician must be defined. This includes expected on-site coverage of home and/or away games; the management of injuries and illnesses during the team's practices; and possibly night, weekend, and holiday coverage. The medical plan should include the method of 24/7 contact for the team physician or at least delineate the understanding of emergency coverage during nighttime hours.

The pathway for obtaining referrals should also be included in the plan. The team may refer their own panel of physicians, somewhat like a managed care organization. Alternatively, the team may request the team physician to contact these providers and initiate a relationship. While the orthopedic surgeon may be the most integral part of this referral process, it is necessary to incorporate other available subspecialists. Sports cardiologists, sports psychologists, physical therapists, and pulmonologists are just a few examples of providers who may be required. Residents may also be helpful in covering games or practices if acceptable to the team. Their expertise may be limited based on their level of training, yet they may be adequate under the appropriate supervision.

TABLE 55.2 ■ Factors Affecting Spectator Usage of Venue Medical Services

Factor	More Use	Less Use
Environment	Heat	Cold
Seating arrangement	Unseated event	Seated event
Age (no alcohol)	Older	Younger
Event	Football, concert	Baseball, basketball
Alcohol	Available	Unavailable

Designating a hospital in the EAP further expands the scope of care. As hospitals attempt to increase their market share, a partner hospital may wish to provide additional services and equipment. Although the attractiveness of this type of agreement is dependent upon the hospital and its marketing plan, it could prove advantageous for a hospital to "sponsor" a team. The level of sponsorship and commitment varies according to the hospital's desire to help and the possibility of a benefits package that the team could offer.

Athletic trainers are another integral part of the medical team. They often are present on the field during all practices and games; therefore, they are typically the first medical professional to learn of an injury. Athletic trainers are able to triage these injuries and rehabilitate many nonoperative injuries. A working relationship with the team's athletic trainer is a necessity for determining the progress of injured players and the need for further intervention.

Policies, Procedures, and Protocols

A team's medical plan should include the policies, procedures, and protocols for games, practices, and potentially nonathletic-related injuries and illnesses. An EAP should address most of these issues for practice and game scenarios. The way in which that athlete is cared for should be consistent with the treatment of other athletes with similar injuries. For example, an athlete with a concussion should undergo the same return-to-play protocol as any other player. All athletes should be treated with the same urgency and concern. Continuity and consistency are critical.

The medical plan addresses how to manage multiple conditions seen in athletic competition, including psychological and pharmacologic problems as well as rehabilitation and biomechanics. The only exception to following a typical treatment protocol is the avoidance of any substance banned by the sport's governing body. For example, oral corticosteroids are banned by the World Anti-Doping Agency (WADA); without a medical exemption form, an athlete with asthma may fail a drug test if treated with prednisone. There are also sport-specific protective devices and braces that may be prohibited. A thorough understanding of the sport and its governing body's rules is imperative to avoid penalties.

Equipment and Supplies

The allocation and availability of equipment and supplies should be clearly defined. The knowledge of available resources will lead to the development of certain policies, procedures, and protocols. For example, training rooms at the professional level will have the most up-to-date equipment and may have multiple imaging modalities. Training rooms at the high school level often have very few resources, as funding must be allocated to water coolers/bottles, athletic tape, and physical therapy tools. If there is a stable injury that requires imaging, the athlete may be evaluated by the professional team physician in the training room. At a scholastic event, in which the team physician may not have the same level of expertise, a plan to transport the athlete to obtain imaging may be required.

The emergency physician is trained to be effective in a variety of clinical scenarios; this is a necessary skill for practicing sideline sports medicine. Based upon the resources on-site, the physician may decide to procure a medical bag stocked with emergency equipment, medications, and wound-care supplies. The physician's comfort level for treating injuries on the sideline, the availability of on-site resources, and common sport-specific injuries will dictate which supplies are most helpful.

Emergency Action Plan

A written EAP should be developed, posted, and practiced for each sporting venue. The plan should include details on how to activate an emergency response system, designated personnel and their specific roles, method of transportation, designated hospital, and who should accompany the patient to the hospital. A good EAP should have one consistent strategy yet be flexible enough to accommodate any injury, illness, or natural disaster. The National Athletic Trainers' Association has an excellent publication with a template for an EAP that prepares the athletic trainer and team physician for emergency situations.[9]

How to activate the local emergency system should also be defined. This may require utilizing the local 911 system unless EMS or a properly equipped transport service is on-site. Many venues require an ambulance dedicated to the field of play to be on-site during games. The EAP describes the proper assessment, treatment, and stabilization of the athlete to ensure the best outcome in the event of injury or illness. This may include designating different hospitals based upon injury type, transport time, and necessary level of care. For example, concern for an intracranial hemorrhage may require transportation to a trauma center with neurosurgical coverage, while a pneumothorax can be appropriately managed at a smaller facility.

A critical component of the EAP is having an automated external defibrillator (AED) on-site. Multiple personnel should be trained on the AED, and the location of the device should be clearly labeled and posted on the EAP. The AED may be stored in a central location; however, it may be more useful if in the possession of the sideline medical team. Early defibrillation has been shown to improve survival in cases of sudden cardiac death; therefore, an AED is more beneficial if readily available on the sideline.[10]

Travel

The team physician may be expected to travel locally, nationally, and internationally with their team. There are many details to consider when traveling; therefore, early preparation is critical to having a well-organized trip. It is typically the medical team's role to ensure their athletes and staff members are aware of any local health concerns prior to travel. While traveling locally, this may include being prepared for a variety of weather conditions. For international travel, this is often far more complex and must include concerns about travel-related illness. Prior to departing, athletes should be instructed to obtain recommended immunizations for illnesses common to the region of travel, such as hepatitis A. They should also be versed in warnings regarding local infections and how to prevent them, such as utilizing bug spray and/or long clothing to prevent mosquito-borne illnesses. Malaria prophylaxis may also be suggested in endemic areas.

The physician should also be knowledgeable about the purity of drinking water and the cleanliness of food in the planned travel region. Traveler's diarrhea, which is common in international travelers, is most often the result of a bacterial infection due to contaminated food and water.[11] In areas with uncertainty regarding the potability of water sources, it is necessary to ensure all athletes have access to bottled water, do not use any ice made from a local water source, and refrain from eating fresh fruits or vegetables washed in contaminated water. The team physician should travel with medication or be knowledgeable about how to procure medication to treat traveler's diarrhea and other common illnesses while abroad.

Training in emergency medicine makes a team physician well suited to care for any acute traumatic or medical illness; however, resources may be difficult to obtain while traveling. Because of this, the physician may decide to travel with a medical kit. The contents of the kit will be specific to the sport covered, travel destination, and available space. While traveling internationally, it should be assumed that there will be no supplies on-site. The physician should plan to be as self-sufficient as possible and should pack efficiently. They should be equipped to treat simple illnesses and wounds; however, more severe injuries may require a trip to a hospital or clinic. The physician should be knowledgeable about the clinics and hospitals in the area and be prepared to accompany their athletes to the hospital if needed.

For domestic travel, the physician should also check local laws regarding treating athletes outside their state of medical licensure. This will be state-dependent; therefore, the laws of the destination state's medical board should be understood prior to traveling. The physician must also ensure their professional liability insurance will cover them while out of their home state or country.

Documentation

As with all patient encounters, every visit with an athlete must be documented. Where, how, and how long these records are maintained will vary based upon the location in which the athlete is treated. If a visit occurs in a formal hospital or clinic setting, a note is typically written in the hospital's electronic medical record system. The physician must determine how to document an evaluation if the patient is seen outside of a formal clinical setting. Where and how to store the medical records must also be considered. There may be an electronic medical record already in place; however, at the scholastic or collegiate level, each athlete may simply have a physical file secured by the athletic trainer in the training room. The medical record obviously must remain Health Insurance Portability and Accountability Act-compliant, and it must be determined who has access to these records. If there is not a formal documentation process in place, the physician may decide to keep their own notes in a secure location.

Knowledge of Rules

Each sport has its individual rules, regulations, and physical requirements for participation.[12] For example, some sports require the referee to clear an injured athlete for medical intervention. If medical assistance is offered on the field of play without following the proper guidelines, the athlete can be disqualified, or the team may be penalized. A number of sports have developed specific policies related to bleeding patients in an effort to address concerns regarding HIV and hepatitis B and C exposures. It is imperative that the team physician understands all of these rules as to not cause penalties to the athlete.

In Olympic sports, National Collegiate Athletic Association sports, and almost all professional sports, there are banned substances that cannot be used by the athlete. Rules vary by sport, including specific dosages, medications allowed while out of competition season, and medical exemptions. An updated list with these specifics can be found online on the websites for WADA and the US Anti-Doping Agency. These policies require the sports physician to be up-to-date on these substances or risk the athlete's suspension as they undergo year-round spontaneous testing.

In the realm of professional sports, the NFL provides an excellent, proactive approach to medical care of the athlete. In 2003, the NFL mandated that a physician with expertise in rapid-sequence induction/intubation must be on the sideline at every NFL game, serving as the airway management physician (AMP). The organization's 2018 guidelines, which required the provider to have performed a minimum of eight intubations in a trauma resuscitation environment at a level I or II trauma center, resulted in over 75% of AMPs being emergency physicians. Emergency physicians Thom A. Mayer (medical director of the NFL Players Association) and Joe Waeckerle (long-time Kansas City Chief's team physician) were instrumental in accomplishing these necessary improvements. The expert role of AMP has been expanded to encompass all aspects of airway management for NFL players at league games. The AMP must be independent from an individual NFL team (i.e., the home team) and is required to manage airway issues for both teams. Of the 32 NFL teams, the overwhelming majority use emergency physicians in this role.

Another recent opportunity for emergency physicians is the NFL's Visiting Team Medical Liaison Program (VTML). This program aims to improve access to high-quality care for the visiting team without overburdening the home team's medical resources. If the visiting team requires medical care while traveling, a liaison ensures the athletes are treated with the same level of care provided to the home team. The VTML offers assistance with local referrals for ancillary testing, specialty access, and prescription medications, which may be difficult to obtain when traveling to a state where the visiting team physicians are not licensed.

Range of Care

The best team physicians understand the athletes themselves, their desire to achieve peak performance, and their potential for injury. The physician must have knowledge of any preexisting conditions (specifically asthma, sickle cell trait, diabetes, previous concussions, and any cardiac conditions) that may require an individualized treatment plan. Complete treatment plans include a list of appropriate equipment and supplies that will be utilized in various situations, including games and practices.[13,14] More complex medical conditions may require assistance from a specialist. Rehabilitation and physical therapy are critical for getting injured athletes back on the field as quickly and safely as possible. Emergency physicians should understand the basics of rehabilitation; however, this component of treatment is often referred to the athletic trainer, physical therapist, or physiatrist, with the team physician overseeing the athlete's progress.

TEAM CONTRACTS

Emergency physician groups have an advantage over other independent physicians because they typically have access to a larger provider base. Larger physician groups have the ability to pursue more acquisitions; however, a person/group seeking these relationships must recognize the substantial commitment required to be a team physician. Scholastic teams who do not have physician medical coverage already in place are the most approachable. College and professional teams require a greater commitment and more comprehensive coverage. Selection at this level usually requires a history of excellent performance with a high school, college, or professional team as well as formal sports medicine training. Coverage for one team should not be compromised to obtain a relationship with another.

When approaching a team about becoming the team physician, it is important to stress your interest, background or participation in the sport, broad expertise, knowledge and understanding of the injuries unique to that sport, and the ability to handle a wide variety of emergencies. In particular, it may be helpful to expound on your expertise in:

- Neurosurgical problems, including head and cervical spine injuries
- Heat-related illnesses, including heat stroke
- Cardiac conditions with cardiac arrhythmias
- Cardiac arrest and other critical care
- Intra-abdominal trauma
- Airway management and asthma
- Sickle cell disease

A number of articles in the literature deal with sudden death in athletes requiring airway management, defibrillation, and traumatic stabilization.[15-25] These situations are all clearly the expertise of the emergency physician.

Contract Management and Maintenance

Once an agreement exists, it must be maintained and managed. Sports team leaders want a single contact and clear protocol when a problem occurs. The team physician should stress the availability of quality providers and assure the team that their needs will be met even for their most minor problems. A quality-assurance program should be part of every medical plan, and its results should be shared with the team to demonstrate the services and expertise that are being provided. Emergency physicians are well trained and generally deliver outstanding care to teams; however, sports organizations may have unrealistic expectations or goals in regard to their medical treatment. The physician's ability to provide excellent "customer service" and meet the team's needs will ensure that the relationship is a successful one.

Liability

The training of the emergency physician lowers the likelihood of liability when compared to other providers who have no training in trauma and cannot manage the breadth of possible injuries and illnesses common to emergency medicine. However, it is the responsibility of providers to discuss liability coverage with their malpractice carrier. They must ensure that sports medicine falls within the scope of their policy's coverage or purchase increased coverage. This decision may also be based on the athletes to whom they are providing care. A professional athlete may stand to lose millions of dollars due to a small mistake, causing liability coverage at the professional level to be far more expensive.

Reimbursement

There are many ways a physician or physician group may negotiate reimbursement for their services. Unfortunately, this reimbursement often falls far below an emergency physician's typical compensation. Team physicians may wish to negotiate a flat yearly rate or bill hourly for their time. Nonemergency team physicians who are able to see their athletes in clinic may be able to generate additional income from such visits, imaging, in-office procedures, and surgeries. This "spin-off" income rarely generates appropriate compensation for the time these practitioners spend with the team. Emergency physicians, with limited "spin-off" opportunities, may choose to bill for each athlete encounter. When considering this approach, the physician/group must assess whether the group or hospital contract permits this type of arrangement.

CONCLUSION

Sports medicine represents an increasingly attractive and appropriate opportunity for emergency physicians. Providing this service at the professional or nonprofessional level may offer an enjoyable alternative to typical shift work. Sports medicine is attractive because of the opportunity to attend sporting events and/or pursue close personal contact with athletes and the organizations they represent. Since appropriate compensation is still difficult to attain, participation requires significant motivation and successful negotiations. The interested physician or group enhances the likelihood of success with primary care sports medicine fellowship training, experience, association with an orthopedic group, attention to quality, and the ability to develop written plans that address the specific requirements of the event/team.

REFERENCES

1. Whitley, TW, Allison, EJ, Gallery, ME, et al. Work-related stress and depression among practice emergency physicians: an international study. *Ann Emerg Med*. 1994;23:1068–1071.
2. Keller KL, Koenig WJ. Management of stress and prevention of burnout in emergency physicians. *Ann Emerg Med*. 1989;18:42–47.
3. Hall KN, Wakeman MA, Levy RC, et al. Factors associated with career longevity in residency-trained emergency physicians. *Ann Emerg Med*. 1992;21:291–297.
4. Cydulka RK, Korte R. Career satisfaction in emergency medicine: the ABEM longitudinal study of emergency physicians. *Ann Emerg Med*. 2008;51:714–722.
5. Kuhn G, Goldberg R, Compton S. Tolerance for uncertainty, burnout, and satisfaction with the career of emergency medicine. *Ann Emerg Med*. 2009;54:106–113.
6. Popa F, Arafat R, Purcarea V, et al. Occupational burnout in emergency medicine—a nationwide study and analysis. *J Med Life*. 2010;3:325–331.
7. Kuhn G, Goldberg R, Compton S. Tolerance for uncertainty, burnout, and satisfaction with the career of emergency medicine. *Ann Emerg Med*. 2009;54:106–113.
8. Terry GC, Kyle JM, Ellis JM Jr, et al. Sudden cardiac arrest in athletic medicine. *J Athl Train*. 2001;36(2):205–209.
9. Andersen J, Courson RW, Kleiner DM, et al. National Athletic Trainers' Association position statement: emergency planning in athletics. *J Athl Train*. 2002;37(1):99–104.
10. Drezner JA. Preparing for sudden cardiac arrest—the essential role of automated external defibrillators in athletic medicine: a critical review. *Br J Sports Med*. 2009;43(9):702–707.
11. Simon LM, Rubin AL. Traveling with the team. *Curr Sports Med Rep*. 2008;7(3):138–143.
12. Starkey C. Injuries and illnesses in the national basketball association: a 10-year perspective. *J Athl Train*. 2000;35(2):161–167.
13. Mellion MB, Walsh WM, Shelton GL. *The Team Physicians Handbook*. St. Louis, Mo: Mosby; 1990.
14. Howe WB. What I take to the game. *Phys Sportsmed*. 1990;18:61–66.
15. Toler JD, Petschauer MA, Mihalik JP, et al. Comparison of 3 airway access techniques during suspected spine injury management in American football. *Clin J Sport Med*. 2010;20(2):92–97.
16. Jaworski CA. Advances in emergent airway management. *Curr Sports Med Rep*. 2002;1(3):133–140.
17. Roberts WO. Sideline airway access: emergency cricothyrotomy. *Phys Sportsmed*. 2000;28(4):113–114.
18. Swartz EE, Boden BP, Courson RW, et al. National Athletic Trainers' Association position statement: acute management of the cervical spine-injured athlete. *J Athl Train*. 2009;44(3):306–331.
19. Drezner JA. Preparing for sudden cardiac arrest—the essential role of automated external defibrillators in athletic medicine: a critical review. *Br J Sports Med*. 2009;43(9):702–707.
20. Drezner JA, Courson RW, Roberts WO, et al. Inter-Association Task Force recommendations on emergency preparedness and management of sudden cardiac arrest in high school and college athletic programs: a consensus statement. *J Athl Train*. 2007; 42(1):143–158.
21. Harmon KG, Drezner JA. Update on sideline and event preparation for management of sudden cardiac arrest in athletes. *Curr Sports Med Rep*. 2007;6(3):170–176.
22. Courson R. Preventing sudden death on the athletic field: the emergency action plan. *Curr Sports Med Rep*. 2007;6(2):93–100.
23. Kramer E, Dvorak J, Kloeck W. Review of the management of sudden cardiac arrest on the football field. *Br J Sports Med*. 2010;44(8):540–545.
24. Drezner JA, Rogers KJ. Sudden cardiac arrest in intercollegiate athletes: detailed analysis and outcomes of resuscitation in nine cases. *Heart Rhythm*. 2006;3(7):755–759. Epub Mar 28, 2006.
25. Roberts SD, Mustafa M, Penrod M, et al. Event and sideline management of sudden cardiac death. *Curr Sports Med Rep*. 2002;1(3):141–148.

CHAPTER 56

GERIATRIC EMERGENCY DEPARTMENTS

Kelly J. Ko, Adriane Lesser, Vaishal Tolia, Kevin Biese, Mark Rosenberg, Robert W. Strauss

The number of emergency department (ED) visits made by adults aged 65 and older increased by over 5 million visits between 2001 and 2015, mirroring the broader growth of this age group within the United States.[1] Given that the total number of geriatric patients is anticipated to more than double by 2060, it is imperative that medical leaders adapt and prepare for this demographic shift.[2] In an encouraging trend, EDs across the country are providing more focused care for older adults, as evidenced by the recent emergence of geriatric emergency departments (GEDs).

The following is a simple case demonstrating a typical ED stay for a geriatric patient.

A 78-year-old woman falls on the lower steps of her staircase and injures her ankle. She is functionally independent at home, and her daughter lives two blocks away. She presents to the community hospital, where she is triaged, placed in an exam area, and seen by a clinician. The patient's x-rays are negative, and she is sent home with instructions to follow up with her family physician and an orthopedist.

Although this would be a typical scenario in many EDs across the country, this same patient would be evaluated and managed differently in a GED, as shown here:

The 78-year-old female patient presents similarly to a GED, undergoes an initial risk assessment for her injury, and is then taken back to a geriatric bed. She is seen quickly and evaluated by a geriatric-trained nurse and ED physician. (A key focus of GEDs is reducing "door-to-doctor time.") After a thorough evaluation, an x-ray is ordered. When the patient returns from radiology, she is seen by an interdisciplinary geriatric team (e.g., nurse navigator, social worker, or case manager) and receives relevant risk screenings for issues like dementia, delirium, dietary problems, depression, and falls.

The case manager and nurse navigator arrange for discharge planning and transition to home under the guidance of the geriatric nurse specialist and ED physician, who manage any acute issues. Following discharge, the home health team is notified to perform an assessment and teach the patient safe mobility and fall-prevention techniques. Afterward, the nurse navigator follows up with the patient on days 1, 3, 7, and 30.

This brief case example illustrates one of the key goals of a GED, which is to utilize the ED visit as an opportunity to identify potential risk factors that can be mitigated either during the ED encounter or following discharge. Geriatric emergency departments are designed to assess older adults from multiple perspectives, including assessments of their acute medical needs, underlying syndromes (e.g., falls, delirium), and social requirements. In doing so, GEDs can improve the care of older patients both during and after an ED visit.[3]

While not all EDs have the same dedicated resources, many of these critical tasks can be completed by utilizing existing resources within the broader health system. For example, many hospitals already have access to physical therapists, social workers, case managers, and pharmacy consultants—at least for part of the day. When developing a GED, department leaders can focus on providing these additional services during hours in which they are already available while expanding those hours when possible.

Additionally, the primary care nurse, nurse navigator, or social worker can complete the geriatric screenings mentioned in the previous example. A home health team or community paramedic can arrange the home assessment. Many of these tasks can be completed by existing staff within the health system.

GERIATRIC PATIENTS ARE DIFFERENT

The medical needs of older adults are characterized by chronic illnesses that often require a wide range of hospital- and community-based providers. The ED is a busy, fast-paced, and frenetic environment designed for rapid patient evaluation and turnover. Unfortunately, the distractions and unpredictability of this setting can be disorienting to older adults and potentially interfere with the effectiveness of their care.

When compared to younger patients, older adults have greater acuity, longer ED lengths of stay, and more complications post discharge. The additional time spent in the ED may have adverse effects on geriatric patients; one study determined that every additional hour spent in the ED increases the risk of complications by 3%.[4] Furthermore, patient outcomes following an ED encounter may also be deleterious, as research suggests that older adults experience increased rates of adverse outcomes after discharge.[5-9]

Despite these factors, the ED remains the only option for many older adults throughout the nation, regardless of clinical, social, or insurance status. Thus, it is necessary to ensure that the needs of this vulnerable population are addressed during each medical encounter.

GED Guidelines

The imperative for quality geriatric emergency medicine (GEM) care has been recognized as a clinical priority by national geriatric and emergency medicine organizations, including the Academy of Geriatric Emergency Medicine, Geriatric Emergency Medicine Section of ACEP, and American Geriatrics Society (AGS). Two key resources demonstrate that priority: first, the creation and endorsement of the 2014 GED guidelines, and second, the world's first accreditation program for GEDs. Both initiatives have led to the development of two central documents that are critical for operationalizing a GED.

Through a partnership with the American College of Emergency Physicians (ACEP), AGS, Emergency Nurses Association (ENA), and Society for Academic Emergency Medicine, the first consensus document on best practices was created in 2014 for the acute care of older adults in the ED.[10] The guidelines put forth key recommendations regarding best practices that can effectively improve the care of geriatric patients in the ED. One of the goals is to help recognize those who will benefit from inpatient care and identify those who can be safely discharged with follow-up care (**Table 56.1**).

GED Accreditation

While the number of GEDs emerging across the country has rapidly increased over the past decade (0 in 2007 to 150+ in 2017), a high degree of variability exists in the services they provide. Specifically, there has not been any standardization or formal accounting of the quality of care being delivered in facilities that self-designate as GEDs. To address this issue, the ACEP Board of Directors approved plans for the development of a GEDA

TABLE 56.1 ■ GED Guidelines

#	
1.	A guideline to define criteria for access to geriatric care from ED triage
2.	A standardized delirium screening guideline with appropriate follow-up
3.	A standardized dementia screening process
4.	A guideline for the standardized assessment of function/functional decline with follow-up
5.	Standardized fall-assessment guidelines with appropriate follow-up
6.	A guideline for the identification of elder abuse with appropriate follow-up
7.	A guideline for medication reconciliation in conjunction with a pharmacist
8.	A guideline to minimize the use of potentially inappropriate medications
9.	A guideline for pain control in elderly patients
10.	A guideline for accessing palliative care consultations in the ED
11.	A guideline for accessing geriatric psychiatry consultations in the ED
12.	At least three order sets for common geriatric ED presentations developed with attention to geriatric-appropriate medications, dosing, and management plans
13.	A guideline to standardize and minimize urinary catheter use
14.	A guideline to minimize NPO designation and promote access to appropriate food and drink
15.	A guideline to promote mobility
16.	A protocol to guide the use of volunteer engagement
17.	A standardized discharge guideline that addresses age-specific communication needs (e.g., large font, lay person's language, clear follow-up plan, evidence of patient communication)
18.	A guideline for notifying the patient's primary care provider
19.	A guideline to address transitions to residential care
20.	A guideline to minimize the use of physical restraints
21.	Standardized access to geriatric-specific outpatient clinics
22.	A guideline for postdischarge follow-up
23.	Access to transportation services for return to residence
24.	A pathway program providing easy access to short- or long-term rehabilitation services
25.	Access to an outreach program providing home assessments of function and safety
26.	An active relationship with community paramedicine follow-up services
27.	A program that provides outreach to residential care homes

program in 2017 with a goal of standardizing the care being delivered to older adults throughout the nation (**Table 56.2**). The GEDA criteria are based on the GED guidelines, which are subsequently divided into three different levels of accreditation based on several important factors.[10,11]

Level 3 GED

Level 3 signifies excellence in geriatric care as represented by one or more geriatric-specific initiatives that are reasonably expected to elevate the level of care of older adults in one or more areas. Additionally, staff are identified and trained to implement and manage these efforts.

Level 2 GED

Level 2 identifies sites that have integrated and sustained geriatric initiatives into their daily operations. They demonstrate interdisciplinary cooperation for the delivery of services targeted to older adults and have an established supervisor that directs the staff.

TABLE 56.2 ■ GED Outcome Measures

#	
1.	Percentage of eligible patients who receive available intervention(s)
2.	Number of patients who screen positively for applicable intervention(s)
3.	Designation of a referral pathway for positively screened patients
4.	Percentage of eligible positively screened patients who are referred as designated
5.	Percentage of eligible positively screened patients who complete the referral
6.	Outcomes of all completed referrals for positively screened patients
7.	Number of older adults admitted to the hospital, including the primary admitting diagnosis and chief complaint
8.	Number of older adults discharged, including the primary ED diagnosis and chief complaint
9.	Number of older adults with repeat ED visits and the percentage of all geriatric visits this represents
10.	Number of older adults with repeat ED admissions and the percentage of all geriatric visits this represents
11.	Number of older adults staying >8 hours in the ED and the percentage of all geriatric visits this represents

Level 1 GED

Level 1 defines EDs with policies, guidelines, procedures, and staff that provide a coherent system of care targeting and measuring specific outcomes for older adults and elevating operations and transitions of care both to and from the ED. This includes physical plant enhancements designed to improve the care of geriatric patients.

Key Components of a GED

With the expansion of GEM, the GED guidelines formed the foundation for the accreditation criteria, which were expanded to focus on seven key areas.[11]

Staffing

A specially trained staff is a requirement to have an accredited GED. While staffing arrangements will vary across sites, all GEDs operate with an interdisciplinary team. At a minimum, a GED should have at least one doctor and one nurse on staff with geriatric-focused emergency medicine training; this is the requirement for ACEP level 3 GED accreditation. An ACEP-designated level 1 or level 2 GED offers a more comprehensive set of services and referrals and may have additional specially trained ED staff to support operations. These facilities should also provide access to a broad range of hospital staff from other departments (e.g., physical therapy, psychiatry) and offer coordination services that connect the patient to community resources outside of the hospital.

Education

Education is a key element for all GEDs. It is essential that all GEDs provide specialized staff education with a focus on best practices for the acute care of older adults. Appropriate documentation of that training is required for GED accreditation. The field of GEM emphasizes learning in eight principal domains[12]:

- Atypical presentations of disease
- Trauma including falls

- Cognitive and behavioral disorders
- Emergency intervention modifications
- Medication management/polypharmacy
- Transitions of care
- Effect of comorbid conditions
- End-of-life care

Education and training opportunities include but are not limited to in-house lectures, conferences, continuing medical education work, and self-guided learning. As interest in GEM has grown, so too have the educational resources available on the topic. Among the many offerings are on-site GED "boot camps" (provided by GEM experts with preconference sessions), online lecture series, review courses, and learning modules. Several programs are tailored to clinicians in the GED. Details and links to many of these resources are available in the GED guidelines and GEDA criteria.[13,14]

Policies and Procedures

Policies and protocols, guidelines, and procedures are an important part of accreditation because they document, guide, and reflect the GED's commitment to the care of older adults. Many GEDs begin by incorporating geriatric-specific content into the department's existing policies and procedures. Developing and establishing new protocols to address the needs of older adults in the ED requires significant attention and time.

The GED guidelines and GEDA criteria require a specific number of policies for each level of accreditation. However, each GED may choose which protocols to incorporate into its program. For instance, a level 3 unit only requires one policy or guideline, whereas a level 2 requires 10; a level 3 GED requires 20 policies from the list in **Table 56.1**.[15]

Quality Improvement

A GED's quality-improvement program should include mechanisms(s) to track, report on, and ensure implementation of the policies they enact. Institutions undertaking a quality-improvement plan may choose to focus on one area first (e.g., falls, medication safety, etc.) and then expand to other areas as resources allow. Ideally, this plan would include monitoring and evaluating a range of relevant process and outcome metrics.

Outcome Measures

The GEDA criteria focus on 11 possible outcome measurements, including the number of patients screened, the number of revisits for the same complaint, and other metrics frequently tracked by emergency medical directors and chairs (**Table 56.2**). Of note, these requirements are based on the desired level of accreditation. A level 3 GED does not have any specific requirement for outcomes measures, while a level 2 requires three outcome measures, and a level 1 requires five outcome measures.

Equipment and Supplies

Geriatric emergency departments may incorporate specialized equipment and supplies to better accommodate older patients. At a minimum, these supplies should include mobility aids (e.g., walkers, canes) for use in the ED. Other, resource-dependent supplies include nonslip socks, pressure ulcer-reducing mattresses and pillows, blanket warmers, hearing-assist devices, and reading glasses to improve the patient experience. Bedside commodes, condom catheters, low beds, and reclining lounge chairs are designed to improve the quality of care and provide comfort. Other considerations include enhanced signage, large wall clocks, and additional chairs for family members and caregivers.

Although the GEDA criteria do not mandate a separate physical space, they do require attention to aspects of the physical environment, including:

- Safety amenities like adequate hand rails and nonslip floors
- Comfort amenities, such as raised toilet seats and access to food and drink
- Other amenities, including enhanced lighting and acoustic noise-reduction

Transitions of Care

A protocol for improving transitions of care is one of the 27 options listed in the GEDA criteria and is also a component of the GED guidelines. Geriatric emergency departments strive to reduce avoidable return visits and hospital admissions. Well-developed transitions of care can help facilitate appropriate follow-up and build connections to community resources.

Resources

Most communities across the United States, regardless of size, can provide resources that may be beneficial to the older adult population, including church groups, senior daycare centers, visiting nurses, and homecare programs. A list of community resources can easily be developed by the hospital's case managers and community leaders.

Department leaders should discuss the goals of improving care for older adult patients and identifying geriatric care initiatives. In particular, it may be helpful to ask these stakeholders how they can help both at the time of a patient's discharge and during admission. Some of these resources may be covered by insurance, others may require payment by the patient, and some may be free. A continually updated list provides the patient and ED team with invaluable discharge options.

ED LEADERSHIP DECISIONS

When creating a GED, department leaders must focus first on the primary goal of delivering high-quality, comprehensive care to older adults. Experience reveals the existence of common operational opportunities and pitfalls. These challenges include bed utilization, triage variations, flow strategies for geriatric beds, and effective utilization of existing resources—both in the hospital and community.

When designing a GED, departmental bed use should be an early consideration. Many ED leaders have used the formula of 1,000 geriatric ED patients per bed to calculate these needs. A unique feature of geriatric patients is that their arrival times can easily be predicted. Unless it is a life-threatening problem, most older adults present to the ED during daylight hours.[16] These patients may wait until morning to call their family doctors, only to be told to go to the ED. Other older patients may wait until morning before they venture out.

When planning a GED, it is also important to determine which patients will be seen. Space limitations may influence the chosen inclusion categories based on chief complaint, condition on arrival, or living arrangements (nursing home vs independent living) to name a few. Ultimately, the goal is to identify patients who will benefit most from specialized care, regardless of age, acuity level, or living situation.

Number of GED Beds

Department leaders must determine the actual number of beds required. Generally, most GEDs plan on one bed for every 1,000 geriatric ED patients.[17] For example, if the ED sees

10,000 geriatric patients per year, it would be appropriate to plan for 10 geriatric beds. Alternatively, if the space will only allow five geriatric beds, it may be helpful to more narrowly define the patients who can be managed in the unit (e.g., adults aged >75 years, excluding nursing home patients, etc.). It is wise to focus on a specific subset of the geriatric population first, based on what the GED can accommodate, and then expand the inclusion criteria as bed capacity allows.

Triage Strategies

In one very busy ED, the door-to-doctor time for GED patients is less than 15 minutes. This is achieved by immediately placing appropriate patients into GED beds. In many GEDs, geriatric patients bypass triage and are immediately put in the first available bed; this approach prioritizes the patient, minimizes door-to-doctor time, and improves the clinical experience. In this scenario, geriatric patients are quickly assessed by a member of the interdisciplinary GED team, who orders appropriate disposition and/or referrals. While this flow process is an efficient use of time, it also raises the challenge of how to best utilize open GED beds for patients who do not meet geriatric criteria.

If there are open GED beds but no patients who meet the GED criteria, the space can be used for nongeriatric patients who have minor complaints that can be managed rapidly. This expansion of utilization criteria is often based on objective tools, such as the emergency severity index (ESI); ideal patients might be vertical 3, 4, or 5s. For example:

A 25-year-old woman who presents to the ED with right lower-quadrant pain may require an extensive workup that would tie up a geriatric bed for an extended period, making it unavailable to the next geriatric patient. Alternatively, a 45-year-old with an ankle injury could be placed in a GED bed. The patient could be managed rapidly and easily moved if a geriatric patient arrives and requires the bed.

Separate GED Space

Certain beds in the ED are more desirable than others; in some EDs, these beds are selectively given to VIP patients, such as physicians and staff, board members, patrons, and so on. These beds may be in quieter locations, away from uncooperative and noisy patients, and possibly close to a nurses' station, with greater privacy and additional amenities. These same characteristics are ideal for geriatric patients.

While older adult-specific care can be improved without undertaking physical changes to the ED space, there are several modifications that can reduce the risk of in-hospital falls and create a calming environment through the use of soothing colors and soft background music. The GED guidelines detail the ideal specifications for these enhancements.

Although it is ideal to reserve a separate area of the ED for older adults, it is important to note that few GEDs have the money or resources required. If establishing a separate unit is not an option, enhancing existing space is the next best strategy. This approach entails ensuring that appropriate equipment and supplies are readily available.

Online Resources

Online resources and expert consultations can be used to enhance the team's education and understanding of successful GEDs. Among the available online programs are Geri-EM.com modules and NICHE modules from the ENA. Other free online resources specifically address staffing and training, notably the Portal of Geriatrics Online Education, Geri-EM.com, and GEMCAST.[18,19] Furthermore, the Geriatrics Emergency

Department Collaborative is an excellent resource for designing and sharing best practices in GEM.[20]

IMPLEMENTATION SCENARIOS

The following three cases illustrate GED implementation in different circumstances.

Case One: Mid-Sized ED With Available Space

Hospital A has 30,000 annual ED visits; one-third of the hospital's patients are aged 65 years and older. Based on these numbers, the team has determined that a GED would be an ideal addition. A six-bed area that was formerly an observation unit has become available. When envisioning the GED, several questions should be answered, including:

- Does this space work for the GED?
- How many patients can be managed in the space?
- Will reconfiguration of this space meet the geriatric volume needs?
- Can the GED be effectively operationalized (e.g., staffing, equipment, protocols)?

These and other questions must be addressed to determine how to operationalize the department. There are 10,000 patients aged 65 and older who could potentially use this GED every year. Approximately 40% (4,000) are from the large nursing home served by Hospital A, most of whom are older than 75. What is the best use of the six GED beds?

Option 1 entails excluding nursing home patients from the GED. These patients benefit less from the geriatric initiative and can still be managed in the regular ED by the GEM team if available. The six-bed GED space can be utilized for patients who will receive the greatest benefit — those who are functionally independent. By excluding nursing home patients, at the utilization rate of 1,000 patients/bed, the six-bed unit is a perfect for the 6,000 (non-nursing home) older adult patients per year.

Option 2 might be to exclude patients between the ages of 65 and 74 and develop GED criteria that are focused on patients aged 75 and older. Based on the numbers, the six-bed unit might be a good fit for any patient aged 75 and older.

Case Two: Large Inner-City ED With Limited Resources

Hospital B has a 100,000 volume inner-city ED that treats 22,000 geriatric patients annually. Since a lack of resources cannot support the addition of new beds, the focus will be on redistricting the department's current beds. One area of the ED is a 17-bed unit that is used for general medical care, typically patients with ESI scores of 2 or (horizontal) 3. The ED leaders determine that this is the perfect place for a GED. How can the unit be operationalized in this space?

Based on the ratio of 1,000 geriatric patients per GED bed, the ED would require a 22-bed unit to provide care to all adult patients aged 65 and older. By limiting the criteria to patients 70 years and older, the GED might more closely meet the ideal patient-to-bed ratio. Taking into account that some of these patients will not go to the GED because of high acuity (e.g., requiring resuscitation), this 17-bed unit might be a perfect fit.

Case Three: Low-Volume ED Developing Level 2 GED

Hospital C has a 20,000-volume ED and wants to create a geriatric program. Since the department leaders do not want to create a separate space for older adults, they focus on achieving a level 2 GED accreditation. Reviewing the geriatric guidelines and accreditation standards, they confirm that a separate space is unnecessary. Instead, they decide to concentrate on critical issues like transitions of care and medical screenings. To help achieve their goal, the ED leaders establish an interdisciplinary GED team, including physician and nurse champions and members of multiple hospital services.

To earn level 2 accreditation, the ED opts to implement policies addressing cognitive impairment, falls, and medication safety (employing resources already being utilized in the inpatient setting). Relying on existing resources ensures that the screening and assessment tools are familiar to hospital staff. It further simplifies the documentation process by using existing fields within the health record. Specific protocols (e.g., urinary catheter use) can be modified from existing hospital policies, making them applicable for older adults in the ED.

ADDITIONAL CONSIDERATIONS

Several additional considerations include managing budgeting constraints by starting small, treating patients who require resuscitation, establishing hours of operation, determining ED length of stay (LOS), and naming or branding the GED.

GED on a Shoestring Budget

It is not uncommon to go through the early stages of GED development only to find that the human (staff) and financial resources are unobtainable. However, it is vital to understand that the most important component of any GED is unrelated to its physical space. First and foremost, a GED has a culture of care designed to address the needs of older adults. This cultural transformation comes in many different forms, not all of which are resource-intensive. If resource constraints limit the full implementation of a desired GED, department leaders should consider starting small. For example, using the level 3 accreditation criteria as a starting point, a dedicated physician and nurse can initiate a program with a subset of geriatric patients by restricting care to those who are aged 75 years or older, not residing in a nursing home, and functionally independent. Starting small builds momentum by achieving incremental success and expanding as appropriate.

One ED was able to make minor GED structural improvements for less than $2,000 per room, including soundproofing, enhanced lighting, refinished floors, and dense foam pressure-reducing mattresses. Both the hospital and community will have existing resources and equipment that the ED leaders should access as appropriate. Creating a multistakeholder group when planning the GED will make it possible to maximize its capabilities.

When developing policies and procedures, ED leaders may find that many of the risk-screening tools being utilized in GEDs around the country are publicly available. It is also recommended that programs employ screening tools that are already being leveraged at the hospital, notably within the inpatient setting. This will prevent the duplication of existing resources and create consistency with other hospital departments.

Consider using free access to expert consultants with a vested interest. Invite some of the ED staff's parents or grandparents in to share what is important to them in a GED. A department designed by older members of the community focuses on the priorities of those most likely to benefit from a high-quality service.

Patients Requiring Resuscitation

Another consideration when planning a GED is whether to include patients who are actively being resuscitated or have a high risk of decompensation. Given the limited number of beds in most GEDs, the medical director must decide whether to include these patients or treat them in the standard ED. One triage approach is to place deteriorating patients in the main ED and allow anyone who is decompensating while in the GED to remain there.

Hours of Operation

Geriatric emergency departments may operate under capacity during certain hours based on need and resources. Most EDs tier the openings of specific bed types during slow (early morning) hours by closing certain areas like the fast track. In developing the GED, a demand-capacity study can assess patient arrival times to determine the appropriate hours of operation. Many GEDs find that their volume peaks between 8 AM and 8 PM. Generally, the workup for older adults averages approximately 4 hours, and most will have dispositions by midnight. Therefore, consider the appropriate hours of operation described in Case Study One, which highlights an ED with 6,000 functionally independent geriatric patients. Based on the average workup, the appropriate hours of operation would be 8 AM to midnight, enabling the final disposition of all patients in the GED.

Length of Stay

Emergency department leaders are appropriately concerned about the LOS of patients in the ED. Studies show that the longer a patient stays in the ED, the greater the risk of bad outcomes.[4] This is especially true of older patients, who frequently have comorbidities and may require long, complicated workups that include lab tests, diagnostic imaging, and consultations. The waiting period between testing and results is the perfect time to complete geriatric assessments and screenings.

By incorporating GED assessments into "downtimes," a complete workup can be performed without any increase in LOS. The admission rates of geriatric patients can be reduced by providing more comprehensive transition-of-care strategies and increasing the use of visiting nurses and observation units. Since admission requires additional time to acquire an inpatient bed, fewer admissions decreases the average LOS of geriatric patients.

Naming the GED

While it may seem insignificant, the name of a GED makes a difference by conveying the services provided to hospital and community stakeholders. The challenge is to ensure that the public understands that *general* emergency care is also provided. The unit does not need to be called a "GED." Common terms include "senior emergency care" and "older adult ED." Most people accept the label "older adult" as part of their age bracket. While the term "geriatric" is frequently used within medical circles, it may not be as commonly recognized by members of the general public. It is appropriate to canvas select members of the community who would use the GED to determine the most appropriate name.

CONCLUSION

The GED is designed to decrease risk and improve care transitions, making each clinical encounter safer and more productive for older patients. As the geriatric population continues to grow, so does the number of geriatric patients who present to the ED.[21] For many older adults, the ED remains the only option for addressing their health-care needs, regardless of clinical, social, or insurance status. Given this reality, it is necessary to build a service that ensures that the medical requirements of older adults are addressed during each ED encounter—the raison d'etre of GEDs.

REFERENCES

1. Rui P, Kang K. *National Hospital Ambulatory Medical Care Survey: 2015 Emergency Department Summary Tables*. Centers for Disease Control National Center for Health Statistics; 2016.
2. Mather M, Jacobsen LA, Pollard KM. Aging in the United States. *Population Bulletin (Population Reference Bureau)*. 2015;70(2).
3. Inouye S, Studenski S, Tinetti M, et al. Geriatric syndromes: clinical, research, and policy implications of a core geriatric concept. *J Am Geriatr Soc*. 2007;55(5):780-791.
4. Ackroyd-Stolarz S, Read Guernsey J, MacKinnon NJ, et al. The association between a prolonged stay in the emergency department and adverse events in older patients admitted to hospital: a retrospective cohort study. *BMJ Qual Saf*. 2011;20(7):564-569.
5. Carpenter C, Shelton E, Fowler S, et al. Risk factors and screening instruments to predict adverse outcomes for undifferentiated older emergency department patients: a systematic review and meta-analysis. *Acad Emerg Med*. 2015;22(1):1-21.
6. Earl-Royal E, Kaufman E, Hanlon A, et al. Factors associated with hospital admission after an emergency department treat and release visit for older adults with injuries. *Am J Emerg Med*. 2017;35(9):1252-1257.
7. Cousins G, Bennett Z, Dillon G, et al. Adverse outcomes in older adults attending emergency department: systematic review and meta-analysis of the Triage Risk Stratification Tool. *Eur J Emerg Med*. 2013;20:230-239.
8. Deschodt M, Devriendt E, Sabbe M, et al. Characteristics of older adults admitted to the emergency department (ED) and their risk factors for ED readmission based on comprehensive geriatric assessment: a prospective cohort study. *BMC Geriatrics*. 2015;14:54-63.
9. Galvin R, Gilleit Y, Wallace E, et al. Adverse outcomes in older adults attending emergency departments: a systematic review and meta-analysis of the Identification of Seniors At Risk (ISAR) screening tool. *Age Ageing*. 2017;46:179-186.
10. American College of Emergency Physicians. Geriatric emergency department guidelines. *ACEP*. Available at: http://www.acep.org/by-medical-focus/geriatrics/geriatric-emergency-department-guidelines/#sm.0001seyt10126qfpasec16kbx134u. Accessed August 20, 2018.
11. Geriatric Emergency Department Accreditation Program, American College of Emergency Physicians. 2020. Available at: https://www.acep.org/geda. Accessed July 19, 2020.
12. Hogan T, Losman E, Carpenter C, et al. Development of geriatric competencies for emergency medicine residents using an expert consensus process. *Acad Emerg Med*. 2010;17:316-324.
13. Geriatric Emergency Department Guidelines. *Ann Emerg Med*. 2014;63(5):e7-e25.
14. American College of Emergency Physicians. Geriatric emergency department accreditation criteria for levels 1, 2, & 3. Available at: https://www.acep.org/geda/. Accessed March 3, 2020.
15. Criteria for Levels 1, 2, & 3 – ACEP Geriatric Emergency Department Accreditation. American College of Emergency Physicians. 2019. Available at: https://www.acep.org/geda/. Accessed July 19, 2020.
16. Lo A, Flood K, Biese K, et al. Factors associated with hospital admission for older adults receiving care in U.S. emergency departments. *J Gerontol A Biol Sci Med Sci*. 2017;72:1105-1109.
17. Fayyaz J, Khursheed M, Umer M, et al. Pattern of emergency department visits by elderly patients: study from a tertiary care hospital, Karachi. *BMC Geriatr*. 2013;13:83.
18. POGOe. The portals of geriatrics online education. Available at: https://www.pogoe.org. Accessed August 20, 2018.
19. GEMCAST. Available at: https://gempodcast.com. Accessed August 20, 2018.
20. Geriatrics Healthcare Professionals. Geriatrics emergency department collaborative. *AGS*. Available at: https://www.americangeriatrics.org/programs/geriatrics-emergency-department-collaborative. Accessed June 30, 2019.
21. Moore B, Stocks C, Owens P. Trends in emergency department visits, 2006-2014. Available at: https://www.hcup-us.ahrq.gov/reports/statbriefs/sb227-Emergency-Department-Visit-Trends.pdf. Accessed August 20, 2018.

CHAPTER 57

PRACTICE DIVERSIFICATION IN EMERGENCY MEDICAL SERVICES

Thomas Blackwell, Thom A. Mayer, Ed Racht, Kathy Robinson

Emergency nurses and physicians consistently work with emergency medical services (EMS) systems and providers, so fostering collegial relationships with these organizations and their employees is essential for emergency department (ED) professionals. Thus, practice diversification in EMS is one of the most common and logical strategies for emergency care providers. A substantial percentage of ED patients arrive by EMS (10%-30%, depending on location, acuity, access to care, and other factors), so interaction with prehospital care providers is a daily occurrence and a necessity for the practice of emergency medicine.[1] In addition to the providers, developing a solid working relationship with the EMS system's medical director, the physician who has specialized interest in and knowledge of patient care activities and who provides clinical oversight for care provision, is equally important.[2]

Often referred to as the operational medical director (OMD), the medical director is legislatively mandated in all 50 states when advanced life support (ALS) is the designated scope of practice of an EMS system. In the past, EMS physicians came from many different specialties, but the vast majority of them today are now emergency physicians.[3] Since the OMD will have an important impact on care delivery, directly and indirectly, many physician groups wisely choose to pursue diversification of their practice so that one or more of their members serve as EMS physicians. **Box 57.1** lists several reasons why diversification in EMS is an attractive option (each of which is discussed next).

ROLE OF EMS MEDICAL DIRECTOR

The oversight provided by the OMD extends through all phases of prehospital care, from selection and training of providers, through communications, to all components of field care. Depending on the state, EMS personnel are either licensed or certified to practice in that

---

BOX 57.1 ■ REASONS TO PURSUE EMS PRACTICE

- EMS medical director/OMD issues
- Medical protocol integration with ED care
- Integration with emergency nursing and nursing directors
- Quality and process improvement
- Destination decisions
- Skills maintenance
- Contract retention
- Community support

state, and each provider is credentialed, competencies verified, and ultimately supervised by the local system's OMD. The OMD is also responsible for determining the limits of each provider's scope of practice, approving care protocols, and ensuring that the quality of that care is appropriate and considered the community standard. The OMD should have the authority to restrict, suspend, or terminate a provider's credentials if local standards are not achieved. Guidelines describing the performance, qualifications, and activities of the OMD have been developed by the American College of Emergency Physicians, the National Association of EMS Physicians, the National Highway Traffic Safety Administration, and for pediatric patients, the Health Resources and Services Administration.[4-6]

Medical direction comprises both indirect (off-line) and direct (online) oversight. Indirect medical direction includes the development of patient care protocols, dissemination of the protocols to the ED and medical community, education of field providers, and identification of key performance indicators for prospective and retrospective quality improvement (QI) processes. Quality improvement should include patient care information from the ED and inpatient admissions to continuously update and improve field care. Direct medical oversight refers to concurrent interactions between the OMD or their designees and the field provider, whether through direct observation or through radio or telephone communication.

In most cases, the OMD has a contractual arrangement with the EMS agency detailing the authority to develop, implement, and monitor protocols, participate in QI programs, and when necessary, remove a provider from further practice if the medical care provided deviates consistently from protocol or requisite skills are not maintained. Typically, the EMS agency compensates the medical director for time depending upon the resources of the jurisdiction. In some cases, the emergency physician group may choose to supplement this stipend when funding from the agency is insufficient because of the importance of the medical director to the overall group strategy for community engagement.

For those ED groups that pursue EMS diversification as a strategy, the group member who is selected must be carefully chosen. First, the OMD must have a deep and abiding interest in and passion for the provision of care in the prehospital setting. The work of being an OMD is too taxing and requires too much commitment to be performed by anyone who is not fully invested. While formal fellowship training in EMS is now offered at many emergency medicine residency training programs, completion of a fellowship, while desired, is not required to become an OMD. The American Board of Emergency Medicine now recognizes EMS as a subspecialty (EMS Medicine), a core content has been published, and examinations are offered every other year to those meeting eligibility requirements.[7,8] Note that sitting for the Certificate of Added Qualifications examination requires completion of a 1-year, Accreditation Council for Graduate Medical Education-approved EMS fellowship since the practice pathway ended on July 1, 2019.

In addition to an interest and passion in EMS-related issues, the OMD should possess or have an active plan to acquire significant leadership and political skills, since the role requires, by its very nature, the ability to work across numerous boundaries and with many different stakeholders (see Chapter 12).

Medical Protocol Integration with ED Care

The most important off-line responsibility of the OMD is to develop and implement patient care protocols for field providers. Those protocols must always be developed with the intent of integrating prehospital care with ED and, in some cases, inpatient care. Collegial input from the emergency physicians and nurses who continue the care provided in the field is essential to an effective relationship between EMS and ED staff. While participation can occur even when the OMD is not a member of the ED group, it is much easier and more effective when they are working together and interpersonal relationships already exist. Further, coordination with inpatient care protocols is easier when the OMD has access to the physicians and nurses providing that care.

The provision of prehospital care is subject to a great deal of change and, occasionally, controversy regarding the most effective methods of providing quality patient care. Airway management, cardiopulmonary resuscitation, field resuscitation of trauma victims (including spinal stabilization), and pediatric care are only a few of the areas where major changes in field management have been implemented and where even more changes can be anticipated as the application of outcomes research to EMS becomes more prevalent (**Box 57.2**).

Coordination of patient care protocols with the physicians and nurses providing continuing care in the ED and inpatient settings, along with alignment of evidence-based medicine, ensure that patients receive quality care in the prehospital setting.

Integration with ED Nursing

Diversification into EMS is also an important issue for ED nursing, since close cooperation between EMS providers and ED nurses is an essential aspect of the transfer of care.[9] In many systems, the initial radio communication with the ED is handled by nurses, with physicians being available for backup consultation when needed. Typically, the first person to greet the EMS providers following arrival is the ED nurse, and formal transfer of care and patient reporting is always provided to the nurse. Each of these functions is facilitated and enhanced when nursing staff are familiar with EMS providers and their patient care protocols.

As mentioned previously, educational opportunities and relationships with providers are often easier to attain when the OMD is also a practicing physician and affiliated with the local hospital or practice. As with physicians, ED nurses should always be encouraged to provide positive or negative feedback to the EMS providers. In some cases, a hospital may select a nurse to serve as a liaison with EMS to communicate issues or concerns including

---

BOX 57.2 ■ AREAS OF EMERGING CONTROVERSY AND CHANGE IN EMS CARE

Clinical Area	Emerging Changes
Airway management	• Intubation vs supraglottic airway vs bag-valve mask ventilation
Trauma resuscitation	• Limited use of fluid boluses
	• Use of extremity tourniquets and pelvic binders
	• Use of spinal motion restriction
Cardiovascular	• Public use of automatic external defibrillators
	• Minimally interrupted chest compressions
	• Post-arrest induced hypothermia
	• Outcomes research on medications
Pediatrics	• Bag-valve-mask ventilations vs intubation
Destination decisions	• Alternative options for care
	• Trauma, stroke, cardiac centers

participating in "ride-along" programs. In verified trauma centers, the connections among ED and trauma nursing staff and EMS are even more important, since trauma registry, QI, mechanism of injury and scoring in trauma patients, destination decisions, and other factors are integral to a fully functioning trauma program.[9] This is also true of specialty care centers that treat primary and comprehensive stroke, chest pain, and ST-elevation myocardial infarction (STEMI), where time from symptom onset to presentation is a determining factor in selecting appropriate treatment options.[10]

QUALITY AND PERFORMANCE IMPROVEMENT

Similar to ED and inpatient settings, effective QI programs lead to performance improvement and are essential for effective care delivery. These initiatives must be an integrated component of any EMS system. Robust programs should monitor compliance with field protocols, system operations that may impact care, coordination with ED and inpatient care and outcomes, and be integrated with provider continuing education programs to ensure compliance.[11]

Perhaps the best example of QI may be the care of the trauma patient, particularly in a verified or designated trauma center. The diagnosis and treatment of trauma patients has always been subject to a high degree of evidence-based, standardized protocols.[12,13] The trend toward controlling hemorrhage with limited fluid resuscitation (permissive hypotension) is clearly an area where coordination of EMS field care, ED resuscitation, and inpatient trauma care must be carefully managed. The OMD must be familiar with the protocols of both the ED and trauma team to ensure that EMS protocols reflect the community standard of care and that the reasons for those protocols are clearly and consistently communicated.

Another example of QI is in the care of pediatrics. While the actual number of children requiring ALS care is relatively small compared to adults, effective pediatric evaluation and treatment skills are critical for all EMS providers. Indeed, this area is one in which field, ED, and inpatient protocols must be seamless and guided by evidence. For example, Gausche and her colleagues demonstrated that bag-valve-mask ventilation in the field setting is the preferred method of oxygenation and ventilation of pediatric patients, and this study changed EMS airway management.[14]

In summary, since the care of many ED clinical entities is changing as new evidence emerges, an open, collegial approach to QI activities is a fundamental part of an effective EMS system. Further, outcomes research and evidence-based protocols are a major thrust for progressive EMS systems, and these activities are easier to implement and coordinate if EMS diversification for emergency physicians and nurses is included.

EMS DESTINATION DECISIONS

In rural and some suburban EMS systems, destination decisions are fairly straightforward: only one hospital serves as the primary destination facility. However, even in these settings, destination decisions must be made for patients requiring tertiary or subspecialty care. The choice of whether a patient should go to the local hospital ED by ambulance versus helicopter transport from the scene to a specialized-care facility is an ongoing debate. Such decisions will be more effective when the OMD is a practicing emergency physician who understands the factors that impact these decisions. The guiding force should always be the quality of care that the patient receives, with all other factors being strictly secondary.

Destination decisions in suburban and urban EMS systems can also be challenging. The closest hospital may not be the most appropriate for a specific patient, unless their medical condition requires immediate stabilization. For example, a patient who recently had surgery at hospital A but lives closer to hospital B may be best served by being transported to the facility where their surgeon and medical records reside. Understandably, this may be inconvenient to the EMS system since distant or even out-of-county transports result in fewer available resources for potential incoming calls. If the patient is stable and does not require regionalized tertiary care, most patients would likely prefer to be transported to their local facility or one closer to their residence.

Destination decisions for EMS can almost always be best coordinated when the OMD has a strong working relationship with the EDs, tertiary care centers, and specialty facilities in the community. However, under no circumstances should the OMD appear to have made destination decisions based on financial incentives. This can be complicated and contentious for the OMD, especially when two competing hospitals are in proximate locations and both are capable of providing the same services. Patient preference should always be the guiding parameter on destination decisions as long as the facility is appropriate for the care needed and the patient is deemed stable for transport.

It is in cases where the patient who has no destination preference where issues may surface. Fortunately, mapping programs now exist that can assist EMS crews in determining the closest facility prior to scene departure. More sophisticated programs base distance on additional data, including traffic-flow patterns, weather, and alternate routes using side streets. Thus, objective data can be presented when questions arise about which facility was actually closer. In summary, destination decisions are perhaps one of the most political and controversial aspects of prehospital care. Best practices include honoring a patient's request unless the patient needs a specialty level of care. Even with the latter, a patient's request may still be honored, those without a preference should be transported to the closest appropriate facility.

SKILLS MAINTENANCE

Emergency medical services providers must maintain an adequate level of skill competency, particularly with regard to invasive procedures, including the stabilization of critically ill or injured patients. In urban systems, these skills are routinely used; however, in rural or suburban systems, maintaining skill proficiency is challenging since providers have fewer opportunities to practice these skills, especially those that are rare, such as pediatric intubation. Interestingly, at least one non-peer-reviewed report in the lay press asserts that, as the number of ALS providers in a community increases, the survival rate from cardiac arrest decreases.[15] As implausible as this may seem, it is possible that the number of patient encounters per paramedic and the level of technical skills performed might decline if a community has an abundance of paramedics. Establishing rotations for field providers in the ED and inpatient units can be an effective way of ensuring that skill maintenance is addressed. For example, in those systems in which field rapid-sequence intubation is used for specified patients, rotations through the operating room or ED under the supervision of physicians can be extremely helpful in ensuring that providers remain competent in this vital skill.[16]

Contract Retention

The more the emergency physician group is integrated into the fabric of the community, the more likely it is that the group will be able to maintain contract longevity. There are few, if any, other initiatives that support the community more than EMS. Since EMS is such a fundamental part of ED practice, it is a logical area for diversification; however, the most important aspect for this diversification is, and should always be, the ability to provide optimal patient care.

FUTURE HORIZONS

The rise of value-based purchasing, accountable care organizations, and population health has made the integration of EMS and inpatient care even more important than it has been in the past. Hospital ED surge, length of stay, satisfaction scores, and readmission rates are but a few of the issues that the health-care system faces in which the emerging role of EMS may be critical (**Box 57.3**). For example, establishing a nurse referral line as part of the communications system where 911 calls triaged as low acuity are connected to a nurse who can determine resources required and arrange appropriate care at a clinic or other facility instead of an ED may be useful. Similarly, many systems have implemented community paramedicine or mobile-integrated health programs that follow up with patients who have chronic conditions.

In terms of interoperable communications, the US Department of Commerce has created the First Responder Network Authority (FirstNet), which has the capability to broadcast live audio and video feeds to hospitals while on the scene or during transport.[17] This system allows a secure method of transmitting sensitive patient data, providing improved situational awareness at incidents, and augmenting on-scene reports with images, videos, geolocation, weather updates, and traffic data. It also features patient tracking and bed management software for real-time monitoring of hospital status. With this advance in telecommunications, nursing directors and physicians will be integral to designing systems that meet the needs of the ED to ensure continued quality care.

Finally, another growing trend is having field providers work alongside ED nurses and physicians in the clinical setting. Depending on the provider's scope of practice, responsibilities may be at the level of an ED technician or extend beyond this to include direct patient care, triage, medication administration, and monitoring. Individual states may also have rules or regulations that govern such practices. For example, a state office of EMS may not allow a paramedic to work in a clinical setting under that designation because paramedic certification is for patient care provision in the field under OMD oversight. Further, a state's board of nursing may not sanction paramedics practicing their skills in the ED. Therefore, in such cases, the provider would likely be referred to by another title and work under the physician group. Regardless, such programs require physician and nurse collaboration and support and a solid understanding of state and board requirements.

With the landscape of health care changing rapidly, EMS systems and agencies will be wise to incorporate these changing needs, often in ways that are fundamentally different from traditional views of EMS.

BOX 57.3 ■ INTEGRATION OF EMS WITH INPATIENT AND OUTPATIENT HEALTH CARE

Value-Based Purchasing Issue	Possible EMS Response
Hospital length of stay	• More effective transport to home • Medical home EMS transport
Readmission rates	• EMS coordination with home health services • Community paramedics rounding on patients recently discharged
Inpatient satisfaction scores	• "Leading up" between EMS-ED-inpatient

CONCLUSION

Practice diversification in EMS is one of the oldest and most fundamentally sound investments that emergency physicians and nurses can pursue. While there are many business and system reasons to pursue this strategy, most important is the ability to provide better health care that improves patient outcomes. Creative innovation in this area is important not only as health care systems change but also as the measures that validate the success of health care and EMS systems change as well.

REFERENCES

1. Williams DM, Ragone M. 2009 JEMS 200-city survey. Zeroing in on what matters. *JEMS*. 2010;35:38–45.
2. Blackwell T. Emergency medical services: overview and ground transport. In: Marx J, ed. *Rosen's Emergency Medicine: Concepts and Clinical Practice*. 9th ed. Philadelphia, PA: Elsevier; 2018.
3. Institute of Medicine. *Committee of the Future of Emergency Care in the U.S. Health System: Hospital Based Emergency Care at the Breaking Point*. Washington, DC: National Academy Press; 2006.
4. National Association of EMS Physicians. Physician oversight of emergency medical services. *Prehosp Emerg Care*. 2017;21(2): 281–282.
5. American College of Emergency Physicians. The role of the physician medical director in emergency medical services leadership. *Ann Emerg Med*. 2018;71(3):E39-E40.
6. Federal Emergency Management Agency. *Handbook for EMS Medical Directors*. 2012. Available at: http://pehsc.org/wp-content/uploads/2014/10/USFA-Medical-Directors-Handbook-2012.pdf. Accessed September 2, 2020.
7. Perina DG, Pons PT, Blackwell T, et al. The 2019 core content of emergency medical services medicine. *Prehosp Emerg Care*. 2012;16(3):309–322.
8. Delbridge TR, Dyer S, Goodloe JM, et al. The 2019 core content of emergency medical services medicine. *Prehosp Emerg Care*. 2020;24(1). Available at: https://www.tandfonline.com/doi/full/10.1080/10903127.2019.1603560?scroll=top&needAccess=true. Accessed September 2, 2020.
9. American College of Surgeons Committee on Trauma. *Resources for the Optimal Care of the Injured Patient*. 6th ed. Chicago, Ill: American College of Surgeons; 2014.
10. Acker JE, Pancioli A, Crocco TJ, et al. Implementation strategies for emergency medical services within stroke systems of care. *Stroke*. 2007;38:3097.
11. Lerner EB, Pirrallo RC, Swor R, et al. *Evaluating and Improving Quality in EMS*. Lenexa, Kan: National Association of EMS Physicians; 2011.
12. Blackwell TH, Kline JA, Willis JJ, et al. Lack of association between prehospital response times and patient outcomes. *Prehosp Emerg Care*. 2009;13:444.
13. Newgard CD, Schmicker RH, Hedges JR, et al; Resuscitation Outcomes Consortium Investigators. Emergency medical services intervals and survival in trauma: assessment of the "golden hour" in a North American prospective cohort. *Ann Emerg Med*. 2010;57:235.
14. Gausche M, Lewis RJ, Stratton SJ, et al. Effect of out-of-hospital pediatric endotracheal intubation on survival and neurological outcome: a controlled clinical trial. *JAMA*. 2000;283:783.
15. Davis R. Many lives are lost across USA because emergency services fail. *USA Today*. May 20, 2005. Available at: http://www.usatoday.com/news/nation/ems-day1-cover.htm.
16. Davis DP. Prehospital intubation of brain-injured patients. *Curr Opin Crit Care*. 2008;14:142.
17. Careless J. How FirstNet will broaden communications. The wireless broadband network will connect police, fire, and EMS through mobile devices. *EMS World*. 2015;44:36.

CHAPTER 58

AIR MEDICAL SERVICES AND INTERFACILITY GROUND TRANSPORT

Thom A. Mayer, James Augustine, Luis F. Eljaiek Jr, Thomas Judge, Renee Holleran

One of the earliest areas of subspecialty diversification in emergency medicine was emergency medical services (EMS), which is addressed in detail in Chapter 57. The EMS subspecialty is recognized by the American Board of Emergency Medicine, the American Osteopathic Board of Emergency Medicine, and the American Board of Medical Specialties as a Certificate of Added Qualification.[1] Air medical transport, interfacility ground transport, and tactical EMS are discrete areas within EMS, providing opportunities for diversification for emergency physicians, nurses, and paramedics with the passion for caring for patients in these unique environments.

DEFINING TRANSPORT MEDICINE

Transport medicine has been a common component of emergency department (ED) practice for over a half century. Just as the ED is the "front door of the hospital" to the local community, air medical and interfacility ground transport are the front doors to the regional community for critically ill or injured patients.[2] It is also increasingly a part of the healthcare systems' efforts to "brand" and promote their tertiary and quaternary services to the region.[3] Utilizing air transport, approximately 85% of the US population lives within 1 hour of a level I or level II trauma center, but that figure drops to 56% without it.[4]

Interfacility inpatient transports have grown in importance because there are an increasing number of patients who are transferred out of one ED for admission to another hospital. The data from 2019 show about 2.1% of patients initially seen in one ED were transferred to another hospital for admission.[5] That amounts to about 3 million patient transfers per year. The transfer rate in small-volume EDs is higher and has grown to about 5.4% of the patients who are seen in those facilities.

Rural community hospitals seldom have the resources to keep and manage complex patients. These hospitals have had to close service lines and have been unsuccessful recruiting specialty clinicians. Rural facilities also can't afford to absorb the costs of inpatients with prolonged lengths of stay, resulting in decreased reimbursement. This financial penalty also encourages higher ED transfer rates.

Some of this increasing use of transport services relates to the regionalization of specialty care and the evolution of tertiary care and trauma centers to encompass neonatal intensive care units (NICUs), pediatric specialty centers, acute cardiac interventional centers, stroke centers, high-risk obstetrical care, and others.

Interhospital transports, whether by ground or air, may involve highly specialized technology, including intra-aortic balloon pumps (IABPs), left ventricular assist devices

(LVADs), resuscitative endovascular balloon occlusion of the aorta (REBOA), and extracorporeal membrane oxygenation (ECMO). At the other end of the hospitalization, as health care grows more complex and evolved, the need for coordinated transporting of patients from hospitals to rehabilitation centers, skilled nursing homes, home care, and other facilities is changing out-of-hospital care. Indeed, proper health-care resource utilization, cost-appropriate care, and profitability require effective and efficient movement of patients within the medical system to meet the "Quadruple Aims" of:[6]

- Improving the health of the general population
- Improving patient experience of care (including quality and satisfaction)
- Reducing the cost of care
- Improving the work life of clinicians

Historical Perspective

Out-of-hospital transport services are areas of practice diversification that have a rich history for emergency physicians, nurses, and paramedics. They provide substantial opportunities for ED groups and the physicians comprising them. The mid- to late 1980s saw a tremendous growth in the number of transport programs, primarily in rotor-wing aircraft, but also including fixed-wing transports.[7]

This growth was due to the regional expansion of trauma center and tertiary care programs with corresponding funding mechanisms to offset their operating costs. As more hospitals incorporated trauma and acute care, there was expansion of the:

- Trauma systems infrastructure
- Need for a rapid and reliable method of transport
- Requirement for critical care capabilities during transport (in the aircraft)

The medevac model from the Korean and Vietnam wars was adapted to civilian practice. Further, hospital-based medevac programs included highly trained critical care crews capable of substantial interventions far beyond that available in the military model, which at that time focused largely on speed of transport.[8] (See Chapter 53 for current concepts in military medicine and sophisticated transport teams over long distances.)

More recently, both peer-reviewed literature and the lay press have questioned the safety and the need for the number of air medical programs in operation.[9,10] However, a careful and dispassionate review indicates that regionalization of trauma, critical care, and neonatal–pediatric critical care centers is best supported and sustained by air medical critical care transport capabilities.[11] The American College of Emergency Physicians (ACEP) and National Association of EMS Physicians (NAEMSP) have issued a joint statement on guidelines for air medical dispatch.[12]

As the number of air transports grew, the inherent limitations of weather, appropriateness of air transport, risks to the patient and air crew, costs, and utilization of the most appropriate transport vehicle contributed to the growth of interfacility ground transport. Integration of the transport models was necessary and led to a systems approach for the delivery of care to patients, hospitals, and communities (**Figure 58.1**).

Current Status

Air medical transport includes rotor-wing (helicopter) and fixed-wing transports. Air medical helicopters generally fly using a single-pilot plus two-crew-member configuration, instrument flight rating (IFR), and travel between 100 and 175 miles per hour, depending on the aircraft model, number of engines, wind speeds, weight loads, and altitude. Because helicopters travel without regard to road configuration and traffic conditions, they are

FIGURE 58.1 ■ Coordinated Rescue Effort

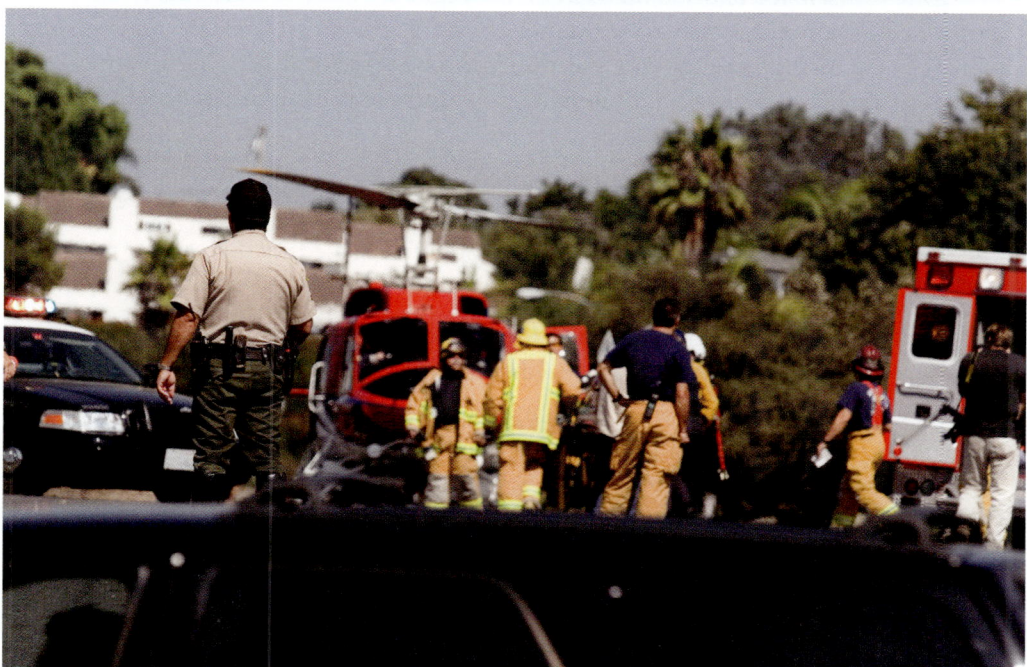

extremely efficient at arriving on scene rapidly. Most aircraft operate under rules that require visual ground reference throughout the flight, although some have IFR capability. Due to changes in the Centers for Medicare and Medicaid Services reimbursement protocols, the number of rotor-wing aircraft flying medevac missions has tripled in the last two decades.

Fixed-wing aircraft are significantly faster, with speeds between 250 and 600 miles per hour. Most aircraft fly a two-pilot crew and many aircraft flying in the 150 to 1,000-mile range are twin-engine turboprops, capable of short take-off and landing flights. For many air transport systems, the "break point" between rotor and fixed-wing transport is 150 to 200 miles.[13,14] Helicopters do not have pressurized cabins and typically operate at less than 3,000 feet above base altitude, with some exceptions for mountain rescue.

Ground transport systems initially focused on the critically ill. However, it soon became clear that the efficient, safe transport of patients along the acuity spectrum was a necessity. Currently, many ground transport services offer multiple levels of care, including wheelchair, basic life support, advanced life support, adult and pediatric critical care, and even bariatric transports.[15] The goals for medevac and critical care ground programs are to:

- Provide a rapid and safe method of medical transportation
- Maintain stability until the patient receives definitive care and, when necessary, initiate resuscitation
- Provide a balance between the need for immediate care, quality outcomes, and the cost and risk of transport

For over 40 years, it has been shown that the time it takes to get the patient to the regional critical care center is less important than the time it takes to get expert resources to the patient.[16] This process requires oversight and leadership using ongoing quality-improvement efforts and collegial outreach education. These goals and care methodologies are strikingly similar to those of emergency medicine and nursing. Emergency physicians and nurses are, by virtue of their training and experience, ideally suited to lead transport medical services. In addition, emergency physician groups are always available to provide online medical direction and support for both air and ground medical crews.

To varying degrees, patients transported by air and advanced-level ground medical services are resuscitated and stabilized in ED settings both prior to and at the conclusion of the transport (before admission to the trauma service or critical care units). Not surprisingly, most clinicians involved in the medical direction of air medical services are emergency physicians.[17] Emergency physicians pursuing the subspecialty of air medical and/or ground transport services have several options:

- Participation as a full- or part-time operational medical director (OMD)
- Involvement as a member of the flight or ground crew itself
- Participation as a member of the ED group providing medical direction to the air medical and/or ground transport service

In many cases, these roles overlap substantially, and some programs have elements of all three. The role of the OMD provides the emergency physician with many opportunities for career expansion.

Emergency nurses often choose to become flight nurses or members of ground critical care teams, particularly with trauma and adult critical care transport teams. (Neonatal transport teams use NICU nurses and physicians. Pediatric ICU teams typically use pediatric ICU nurses and physicians.) While there are many configurations for air and critical care ground transport teams, the most common is flight nurse–paramedic crews.

QUALIFICATIONS AND EXPERIENCE

Involvement in air medical and ground transport services requires a high degree of clinical expertise because most of these programs manage a medically diverse patient population. Residency training and board certification in emergency medicine provides the basic clinical background required (**Box 58.1**). Leadership involvement requires emergency physicians to meet the regulatory requirements for training and education and continuing medical education for OMDs within their state. Emergency physicians should also be aware of the overall strategic mission and operating goals of their particular service. which may be hospital based, a consortium model, private enterprise, or a combination. It is also important for physicians involved in medical transport services to have a working knowledge of hospital operations beyond the ED, including:

- Operations of the receiving critical care units
- Hospital leadership goals for service to the community and region (tertiary care)
- Financial contribution of the transport patients to the hospital's bottom line
- Scientific understanding of the value and risks of air transport services

---

BOX 58.1 ■ AIR MEDICAL PHYSICIAN QUALIFICATIONS

- Residency training and/or board certification by ABEM or AOBEM
- Meet the requirements of state regulatory agencies for operational medical directors of EMS services
- Awareness of the strategic mission and operating goals of the flight program
- Working knowledge of the ED, critical care, and operative capabilities of the hospital
- Basic understanding of the financial and reimbursement aspects of the program
- Scientific foundation in aeronautics and air medicine
- Professional society participation

There is substantial literature addressing these areas.[18,19] In addition, emergency medicine residency programs established at institutions that provide air and/or ground medical transport services can offer the residents insight into this subspecialty and the opportunity to fly as a medical team member. Fellowships in air medical or transport services will continue to grow in number, just as EMS fellowships have.[20] Several professional organizations also provide the foundation necessary to be involved in air medical services. They include:

- Air Medical Physician Association (www.ampa.org)
- Association of Air Medical Services (www.aams.org)
- NAEMSP (www.naemsp.org)
- ACEP (www.acep.org)
- Air and Surface Transport Nurses Association (www.astna.org)
- International Association of Flight and Critical Care Paramedics (www.iafccp.org)
- Commission on Accreditation of Medical Transport Systems (www.camts.org)

PRACTICE DIVERSIFICATION

Why should an individual physician or an ED group consider diversification into air medical and/or ground transport services (**Box 58.2**)?

Supporting the Hospital's Mission

Most hospitals enter air medical or ground transport services with a clear understanding of the strategic importance of extending the market of the hospital far beyond its existing boundaries. Emergency medicine participation allows the group—and the medical director specifically—to support and drive the hospital's strategic needs in a critical area of service. Because critical care air and ground medical transport services extend the hospital's service area, the ED group can provide immense support to an important strategy within the overall mission, profitability, and long-term plan of the hospital.

Health-Care Integration

The transport systems of large health-care systems, both air and ground, cut across the boundaries of all critical care functions, including trauma, cardiac, stroke, high-risk obstetrics, neonatal, pediatric, and bariatric services. This gives the OMD, the transport nurses and paramedics, and the entire staff a chance to represent these services and assist in not only transporting their patients but also in outreach to the region they serve. It

---

BOX 58.2 ■ ADVANTAGES OF DIVERSIFICATION

- Allows the medical director to participate in the hospital's strategic mission at a high level
- Allows the ED to integrate within the hospital's broader mission
- Allows for higher visibility of emergency physicians and nurses as members of the critical care team
- Allows the medical director and other emergency physicians a path into physician leadership and management at the hospital or health-care system level

affords a unique opportunity to cut across "the seams of the teams," meaning all aspects of the care of the patients who are cared for by the various specialty teams in the hospital or the system.

Protocols for transport will be integrated carefully with each of the services provided, which should be closely coordinated between the medical and nursing directors of those services and the transport team. Similarly, the flight or transport crew are quintessential representatives of the system when they arrive at the referring hospital, so they serve a substantial branding and customer service function by the way they interact with staff at the referring hospital. The same representation applies to their interaction with ground EMS crews when transporting trauma patients.

A Path to Institutional Leadership

Air and ground medical services are high-visibility symbols of the hospital's presence within the community. They are regularly featured in media accounts of the hospital's service. Emergency physician and nurse involvement further elevates the stature of the ED and its providers. Involvement in these programs also provides emergency physicians and nurses with additional expertise in financial management and analysis. Similarly, this experience ensures the medical and nursing directors of the service participate more broadly in the field of health-care management. Finally, because the emergency physicians usually provide online medical direction for the critical care patients transported by air or ground, the clinical skills and abilities of the entire physician group are broadened.

Potential Disadvantages

Although there are substantial benefits to diversifying air medical or ground transport services, there are also some potential disadvantages (**Box 58.3**). If the program is organized and managed, the physician and group will benefit from affiliation with a program that has an excellent reputation and record of service. However, if proper program support and leadership are not in place and there is no definite plan to build those elements, it may be best to pass on the opportunity.

There are typically competitive factors in place in the regional health-care market. Affiliation with one air medical or ground transport service will usually prevent a

---

BOX 58.3 ■ DISADVANTAGES OF DIVERSIFICATION

- Roles and responsibilities of the medical director need to be integrated into the emergency physician group.
- Administrative time needs to be compensated (usually by the flight program or hospital).
- Critically ill and injured patients who will be flown to the ED can demand resources that disrupt the flow of other ED patients.
- Medical direction for online control can place greater demands on emergency physicians during their clinical duties.
- Unsafe or poorly managed services may have negative effects on the medical directors who are affiliated with it.
- Regional competitive transport and emergency care programs and their employees may not forget who served their competitor system.

significant relationship with a competitive program. If the potentially competing program has a superior group of services, employs many influential members of the regional EMS community, or has better long-term viability, affiliation with the less-viable program may have long-term negative effects on the physicians and their practice.

A program that does not compensate the medical director for the substantial time, energy, liability, and effort necessary to provide medical direction does not recognize the significant importance of the program or the medical leader's time. If the emergency medical director expends administrative time to participate in or lead the service, those hours must be factored into the ED group structure and appropriately compensated. This compensation is usually an administrative stipend, particularly if the system is hospital based. If the transport system entails a fee-for-service model, the stipend is typically a line item in the budget.

The critical care transport service brings critically ill patients to the ED. Many of these cases require the immediate attention of ED providers, staff, and other non-ED resources. Some require immediate and prolonged resuscitative efforts. All emergency physicians and nurses recognize that trauma and other critically ill patients are disruptive to emergency medicine services and can pull human, clinical, and other essential resources away from existing ED patients. Unless these contingencies are addressed in advance, the ED team will inevitably be disappointed by its inability to deliver organized care.[21]

Online, real-time medical direction of helicopters or critical care ambulances requires time and effort by the emergency physician on duty at the time of the transport. Despite these potential difficulties, one final fact should be kept in mind. If the hospital is already providing (or intending to provide) air medical or ground transport services, the emergency physician group and the ED staff will be required to work with this service anyway. It is far preferable to ensure that prospective controlling guidance is provided by the emergency physician group rather than by physicians and/or staff from other areas of the hospital. For multiple reasons, the ED group will find it beneficial to provide medical direction for non-EMS out-of-hospital transport services.[22]

EMERGENCY PHYSICIANS AS OMDs

The medical director of any out-of-hospital service (private or public, for-profit or not-for-profit, air or ground or both) must assume many new roles and responsibilities and further develop the skills of the physician manager. These skills include leadership, motivational theory, development and implementation of mission statements, conflict resolution, complaint management, personnel management, departmental budgets, financial analysis, administrative policy creation and implementation, and negotiation proficiency. In addition, the competencies listed in **Box 58.4** are specific for optimal clinical and administrative achievement.[23,24]

Protected time to meet the various obligations of supervision and management is required. The medical director should carefully assess the level of involvement within the transport program and the many tasks that will be demanded by outside organizations. Ensuring this protected time requires adequate reimbursement for this valuable position. The time spent on nonclinical or administrative processes requires the involvement of the emergency medicine group and its director, the transport entity, and to some extent, the hospital. This position is a 24-hour, on-call job. Additional funds should be set aside for the director to attend relevant meetings, continuing medical education, and other special circumstances that may be pertinent to the program operation. Professional liability insurance also must be addressed, often in the form of a "rider" on the physicians' existing

> **BOX 58.4 ■ COMPETENCIES OF THE MEDICAL DIRECTOR**
>
> - Clinical and administrative supervision of the medical crew
> - Integration of legal, regulatory, and bureaucratic elements of the program
> - Integration with the hospital, municipality, or corporate administrative structure, whichever is the case
> - Establishment of relationships with tertiary care specialists within the accepting facilities
> - Establishment of relationships with air and ground emergency medical services within the hospital's and the non-EMS transport provider's service area
> - Establishment of relationships with outlying physicians and hospitals
> - Involvement in community relations
> - Marketing
> - Knowledge of air physiology, prolonged out-of-hospital patient care, and crew stressors
> - Knowledge of aircraft capabilities, aeronautical principles, and regulations for ground-based programs-traffic patterns, vehicle regulations, resource management
> - Management of relations between the emergency and transport programs

policy. Alternatively, the hospital (if hospital based) could indemnify the physician for providing medical direction, oversight of other caregivers, and clinical supervision.

The transport crew and medical director should collaboratively write the medical guidelines to achieve a comfort level and balance of medical and clinical skills. It is particularly important that these protocols are "field-tested" to reflect the realities of the often-taxing conditions in which air medical crews operate (**Figures 58.2** and **58.3**).

Protocol development is a labor-intensive but critical aspect of any program. As medical care advances, so does the external regulatory environment in which transport medicine is practiced. As such, these guidelines require periodic revisions. Cooperative

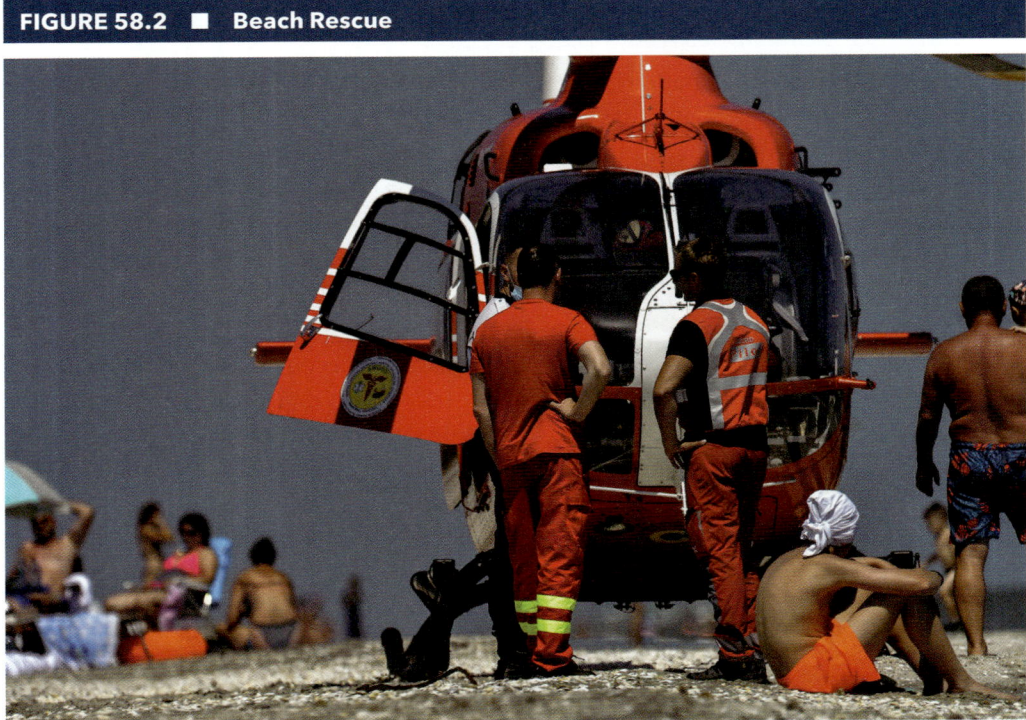

FIGURE 58.2 ■ Beach Rescue

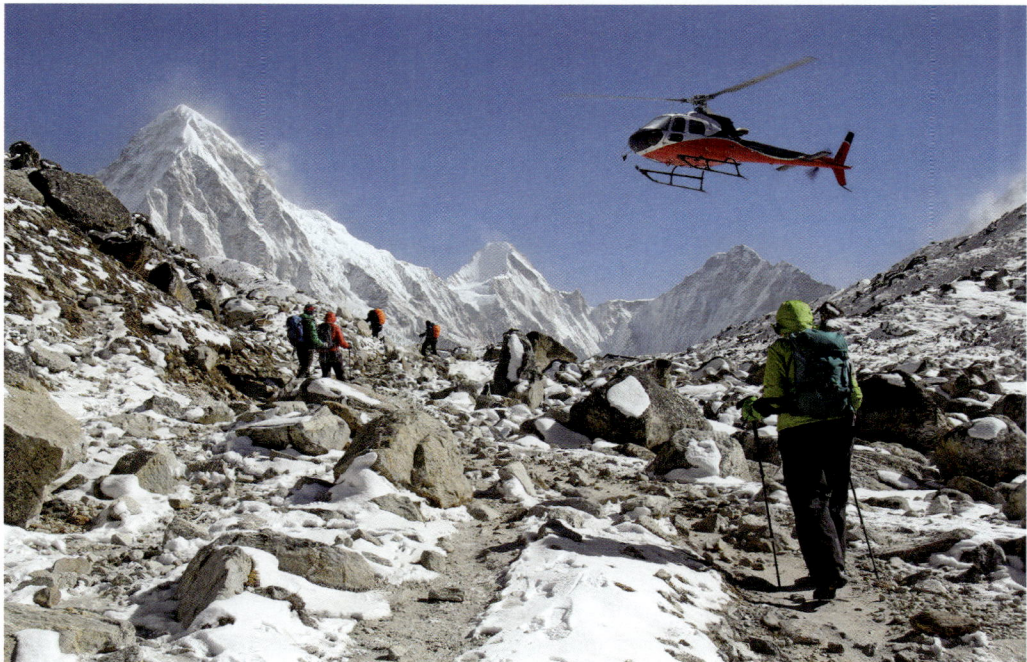

FIGURE 58.3 ■ Winter Rescue in Nepal

operational protocols should also be developed by the transport medical crew, communications specialists, drivers, and pilots. This collaborative approach results in optimum patient care.

Administrative Skills and Integration

Responsibility for the didactic and skills training of the transport medical crew rests with the medical director. Some of these skills, including specialty training that is beyond the usual scope of the medical director, may be delegated to others.

The way in which the medical director interacts with the rest of the ED group is also important. There are many effective ways to communicate and promote the activities and operations of the transport program back to the ED. These include regularly scheduled department meetings, newsletters, and memos.

Consistent communication helps to integrate the program into the hospital's administrative structure. The medical director should continually demonstrate to the administrative team how vital the transport medical program is to the overall success of the institution. This integration places the medical director in the role of a physician leader–manager (see Chapter 18).

The medical director must always maintain the best interest of the patient while skillfully balancing the goals and interests of the transport program and the various institutions involved. A successful medical director is capable of merging two different roles:

- *Clinical leader*: The clinical model addresses the care of the patient and the relationship between the patient and the physician.
- *Manager*: The managerial model deals with the overall goals of the department, transport entity, or institution and is not established on a personal level.

Adept medical directors address the concerns of the primary care and specialty or tertiary care physicians who use the transport program. The key to success in this realm is being flexible enough to meet the expectations of those who depend on these services.

One way to ensure communication is to establish a medical advisory committee for the transport program. The members should include key representatives and other stakeholders who may be vital to its success. Ideally, this committee becomes a forum for the collaborative exchange of ideas and knowledge, including the review and revision of medical guidelines. It is also one of many opportunities to ensure that the medical director is informed of any clinical or administrative problems. This approach reinforces the perception that management is interested in hearing any feedback that can improve the service.

Community Relations and Outreach

The primary focuses of the transport program are the referring ground EMS and the referring physicians and hospitals. Each of these areas is unique and consequently must be dealt with differently. The ground emergency medical transport system provides a doorway unique to that community's particular tertiary medical needs. The medical director must understand and work collaboratively within the existing structure. The contact established also provides the referring community with a glimpse into the role that a transport program plays in the continuum of out-of-hospital care.

Health-care providers appreciate access to ongoing medical education, case reviews, instructive and timely feedback, and focused emergency training. The medical director's relationships with referring physicians and hospitals are essential to the program's continuing success. There should be clear and regular communication among all involved parties. The medical director may wish to meet with referring services to discuss several specific topics, including:

- Medical necessity of transfers (i.e., criteria)
- Medical guidelines for transfer of patients, such as patient preparation and pretransfer communications
- Program goals and updates
- Quality issues from the point of view of the transferring facility and agencies
- Financial issues, including the costs involved with both air and ground medical transports

The goal is to ensure that the level and process of transport matches the level of care required for the patients' safe and efficient transport while remaining cost efficient.[8]

EMERGENCY PHYSICIANS AS TRANSPORT CREW MEMBERS

Most transport programs in this country do not routinely utilize physicians as crew members. This is quite different from the European models in which a physician is frequently utilized in that role.[25,26] The majority of US air medical programs use a flight nurse–paramedic configuration. Some crews operate with either two flight nurses or two paramedics. Occasionally, a respiratory therapist replaces either the flight nurse or paramedic. Rarely, programs fly with a single paramedic.

In contrast, ground transport programs typically utilize paramedic configurations based on the level of care required. As an example, a critical care ground team may consist of two EMT-Paramedics (EMT-Ps), at least one critical care trained, and often an additional EMT at either the EMT-P level or lower. Advanced life support transport teams use two or three crew members with training and certification commensurate with the care required.

Although there is a federally recognized level of certification, many states mandate different levels of training and certification. As the acuity of critical care ground transport patients has risen, many programs have assembled critical care nurse–paramedic teams, which may be augmented by a respiratory therapist or cardiac technician to operate IABPs, LVADs, ECMO, or REBOAs.

An emergency physician may be involved as a transport crew member on an as-needed basis for the most critically ill or injured patients. Emergency physicians who are directly involved with patient care during the transport process are part of the medical transport crew, providing real-time orders and/or supervision.

The medical director may also need to consider, design, and implement programs that include physicians with particular areas of expertise. This would include programs where specialty physicians are transported to initiate IABPs, LVADs, ECMO, neonatal, or high-risk maternity services, especially in long-distance transports that are performed in fixed-wing programs. There are also times when a surgical emergency response team must be activated to perform field amputations or similar surgical crisis services. In some of these encounters, a ground unit may be involved in transporting the patient, specialist, and care team back to the specialty center.

When a physician is a member of the transport team, routine medical protocols can be exceeded, based on the physician's judgment. Transport physicians should be members of, or intimately familiar with, the receiving facility as well as the transporting team and its operations.

Flight medicine is a special area of knowledge, particularly for programs that have a long-distance fixed-wing element. It is particularly important that transporting physicians on air transports are familiar with flight programs, the stresses of flight, and the physiological changes associated with this subspecialty. Flight medicine is not simply an extension of the ED or ground transport vehicle. Many transport crews have had the experience of physicians unfamiliar with the aircraft (or transporting vehicles) becoming a hindrance rather than a complement to the delivery of quality patient care. To avoid this problem, physicians must know the limitations of patient care within the aircraft or vehicle and have in-depth familiarity with the respective operation. In all transport vehicles, but particularly in flight programs, safety features are paramount. Physicians must employ all of the standard precautions used routinely by the flight crew, which includes wearing flame-retardant material and helmets (**Figure 58.4**).

Physicians contracted as medical directors and routine members of the transport team must address several key issues. The most problematic one may be conflicting schedules. Most flight programs require eight hours of rest before starting flight duty. This schedule requirement must be followed. It is extremely difficult to maintain appropriate discipline and adherence to standard operating procedures if "all rules are off" when an emergency physician is flying. Malpractice, disability, and life insurance must also be negotiated and rated for this line of work.

PHYSICIAN GROUP INTEGRATION

Participation in transport medicine, either air or ground, is usually advantageous to the entire physician group. The medical directors of these programs often have protected administrative time and provide fewer clinical services than other emergency physicians. To prevent resentment about the lower clinical load of the physicians participating in the flight program, the advantages to the entire group should be discussed early, openly, and

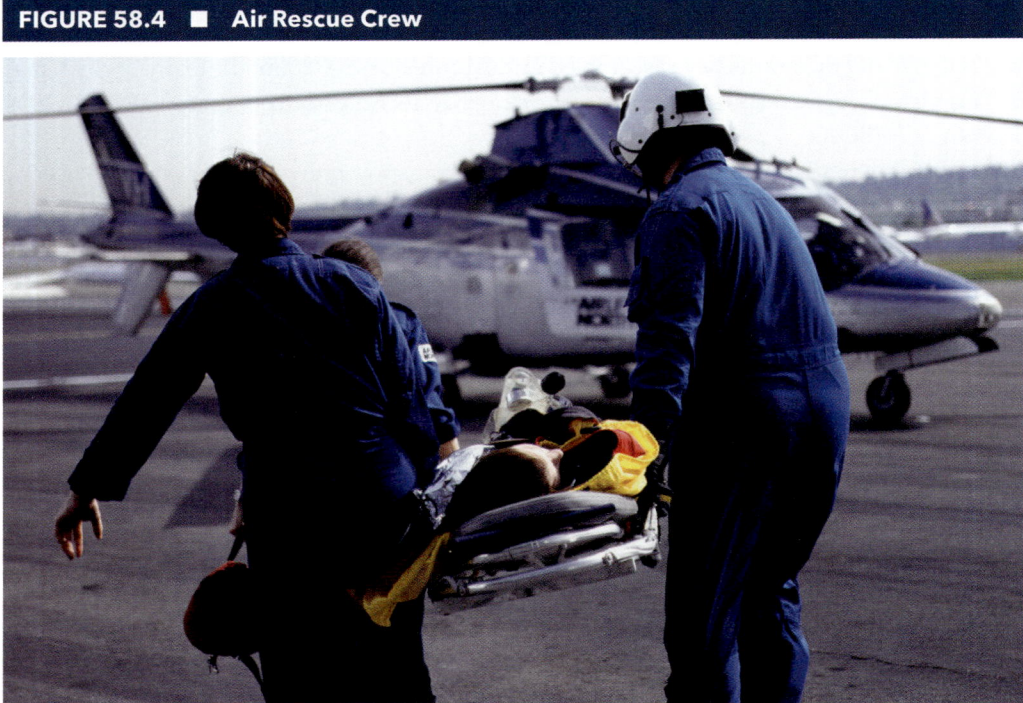

FIGURE 58.4 ■ Air Rescue Crew

clearly. The emergency physician group should be provided with routine information about the progress of the transport program and its role in advancing the strategic goals and objectives of the entire team.

TACTICAL EMERGENCY MEDICINE

Tactical emergency medicine and EMS comprise training, care, and support to ensure the safety, physical and mental health, and overall well-being of military and law enforcement special operations teams during training and incident deployments (see Chapter 53). There are many emergency physicians, paramedics, and some nurses who provide support to law enforcement teams and serve through special operations, high-threat deployments, and medevac operations. They may act as civilians or, in rare cases, as sworn officers. Tactical medicine, which requires the ability to function in stressful or austere conditions, also demands proficiency in weapons and marksmanship, aircraft operations, environmental medicine, and wilderness and urban search and rescue.[27] ACEP's Tactical Emergency Medicine Section is an excellent source for information on this topic.[28]

CONCLUSION

As transport programs and the expertise in this area of medicine continue to mature, emergency physicians and nurses will find multiple opportunities for diversification. Air medical and critical care ground transport is an exciting, high-profile subspecialty. For the medical director, there is ample opportunity to branch out into management and administration. This merging of skills and disciplines provides clinical leaders with the opportunity to work collaboratively with many customers in differing roles and functions.

REFERENCES

1. American Board of Emergency Medicine. Emergency medical services. Available at: https://www.abem.org/public/become-certified/subspecialties/emergency-medical-services. Accessed November 24, 2020.
2. Werman HA, Falcone RE. Indications for air medical transport: practical applications. In: Blumen IR, Lemkin DL, eds. *Principles and Direction of Air Medical Transport*. Air Medical Physicians Association; 2006:13–14.
3. Kemp E, Jillipalli R, Becerra E. Healthcare branding: developing emotionally based consumer brand relationships. *J Serv Marketing*. 2014;28:126–137.
4. Branas CC, MacKenzie EJ, Williams JC, et al. Access to trauma centers in the United States. *JAMA*. 2005;293(21):2626–2633.
5. US Government Accounting Office. Air Ambulance: available data show privately-insured patients are at financial risk. 2019. Available at: https://www.gao.gov/products/GAO-19-292. Accessed November 23, 2020.
6. Bodenheimer T, Sinksy C. From triple to quadruple aim: care of the patient requires care of the provider. *Ann Fam Med*. 2014;12(6):573–576.
7. Wedige-Stecher T. In-flight cardiac support: aeromedical transport of IABP and LVAD patients. *AeroMedical J*. 1988;3(6):16–19.
8. Benson NH, Low RB, Chisholm CD, et al. Air medical transport: an annotated bibliography of the recent literature. *Am J Emerg Med*. 1991;9(5):510–519.
9. Baker SP, Grabowski JG, Dodd RS, et al. EMS helicopter crashes: what influences fatal outcome? *Ann Emerg Med*. 2006;47(4):351–356.
10. Khoury SI, Moorer L, Stone CK, et al. Air vs ground transport and outcome in trauma patients requiring urgent operative interventions. *Prehosp Emerg Care*. 1998;2(4):289–292.
11. Stewart KE, Cowan LD, Thompson DM, et al. Association of direct helicopter vs ground transport and in-hospital mortality in trauma patients: a propensity score analysis. *Acad Emerg Med*. 2011;18(11):1208–1216.
12. Thompson DP, Thomas SH. Guidelines for air medical dispatch. *Prehosp Emerg Care*. 2003;7(2):265-271. Available at: http://aams.org/wp-content/uploads/2014/01/GuidelinesAirMedDispatch.pdf.pdf. Accessed November 24, 2020.
13. Guyette F. Controversies in air medical care. Paper presented at: the National Association of EMS Physicians Annual Meeting; January 7-12, 2019; Austin, Tex.
14. Norton EG. Model curriculum in air medical transport for emergency medicine residencies. *Ann Emerg Med*. 1991;20(4):431–432.
15. National Highway Traffic Safety Administration. Guidelines for interfacility patient transfer. 2020. Available at: https://www.ems.gov/pdf/advancing-ems-systems/Provider-Resources/Interfacility_Transfers.pdf. Accessed November 23, 2020.
16. Black RE, Mayer T, Walker ML, et al. Air transport of pediatric emergency patients. *N Eng J Med*. 1982;307:1465–1486.
17. Thomas SH, Williams KA Claypool DW. Medical director for air medical transport programs. *Prehosp Emerg Care*. 2002;6(4):455–457.
18. McGinnis K, Hutton K. *Air Medical Services: Critical Component of Modern Healthcare Systems* MedEvac Foundation International; 2011. Available at: http://aams.org/wp-content/uploads/2014/01/Public-Education-Paper.pdf. Accessed July 1, 2020.
19. Walker RA. Qualification and training of the air medical director. In: Blumen IR, Lemkin DL, eds. *Principles and Direction of Air Medical Transport*. Air Medical Physicians Association; 2006:121.
20. National Association of Emergency Medical Services Physicians (NAEMSP). Table: EMS fellowships. Available at: https://naemsp.org/NAEMSP/media/NAEMSP-Documents/0-Fellowship-Programs-for-website.pdf. Accessed July 1, 2020.
21. Kelly M. Sky High Air Ambulance Prices. *Ann Emerg Med*. 2020;76:17A–20A.
22. American College of Emergency Physicians Interfacility Transportation of the Critical Care Patient and Its Medical Direction. 1999. Available at: http://www.acep.org/webportal/PracticeResources/ PolicyStatements/. Accessed November 23, 2020.
23. Fitch JJ, Gerard WC. Qualification and training of the air medical director. In: Blumen IR, Lemkin DL, eds. *Principles and Direction of Air Medical Transport*. Air Medical Physicians Association; 2006:137–141.
24. Carrubba C. Role of the medical director in air medical transport. In: Blumen IR, Lemkin DL, eds. *Principles and Direction of Air Medical Transport*. Air Medical Physicians Association; 2006:114.
25. Coenen FH, Micheels J, Muller N. Air medical transport in Belgium. In: Blumen IR, Lemkin DL, eds. *Principles and Direction of Air Medical Transport*. Air Medical Physicians Association; 2006:614.
26. Reichert A. Air medical transport in Germany. In: Blumen IR, Lemkin DL, eds. *Principles and Direction of Air Medical Transport*. Air Medical Physicians Association; 2006:631.
27. Schwartz RB, McManus Jr JG, Swienton RE. *Tactical Emergency Medicine*. Lippincott, Williams, and Wilkins; 2008.
28. American College of Emergency Physicians (ACEP). Tactical emergency medicine. Available at: https://www.acep.org/how-we-serve/sections/tactical-emergency-medicine/. Accessed July 1, 2020.

CHAPTER 59

END-OF-LIFE ISSUES

Kenneth V. Iserson

Emergency department (ED) deaths represent a significant management concern as well as a major clinical issue. Practitioners and managers often see patient deaths as time-consuming and stressful interruptions in the normal workflow, whether they occur in the prehospital or ED setting. There are multiple reasons that patients requiring end-of-life (EOL) care come to the ED, including symptom management such as pain, nausea, vomiting, diarrhea, and shortness of breath. Caregiver stress may cause a family to "give up" and come to the ED for assistance. Finally, the fear of what to do when a patient is actively dying may drive a family to send a patient to the ED.[1,2,3]

Death will always be an integral part of the ED milieu. By proactively establishing appropriate policies, implementing targeted education, using protocols, and partnering with other stakeholders such as local hospice agencies, ED managers can improve staff morale, decrease unnecessary and unproductive work, and generate patient, family, and survivor gratitude. The tools exist; management's responsibility is to make them readily available to their staff. As with any challenging issue in the ED, a team approach is required.

END-OF-LIFE AND PALLIATIVE CARE

End-of-life care describes multidisciplinary medical and community services to care for and support people with only months (or less) to live. It includes a variety of services, including palliative care and perimortem care for the patient and their caregivers. Palliative care is the provision of pain and symptom relief and spiritual and psychosocial support for those who face life-threatening illness, whether it is curable or not (**Figure 59.1**).[4] Because EOL

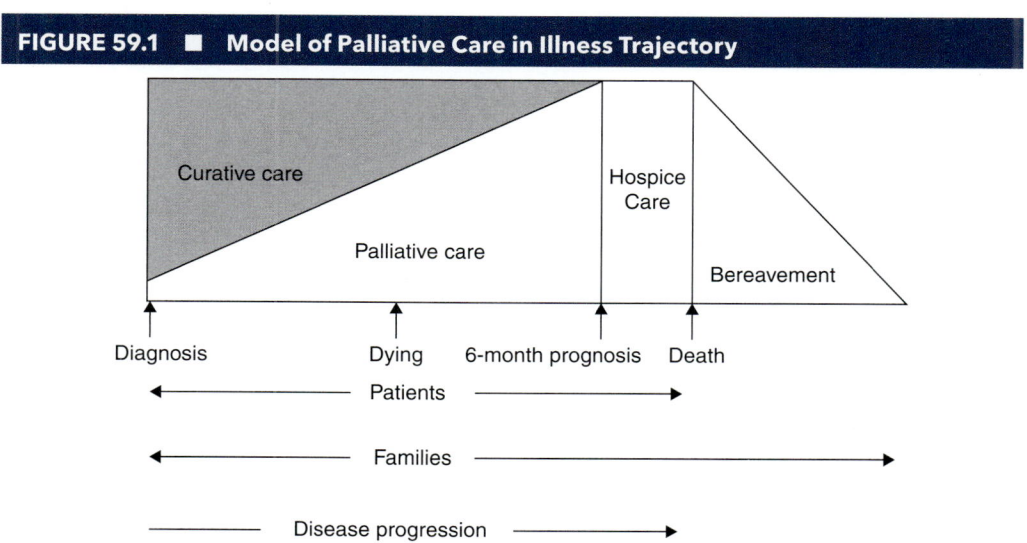

FIGURE 59.1 ■ Model of Palliative Care in Illness Trajectory

Adapted from "The Integrated Model of Care" proposed by World Health Organization [WHO]. 1990.

TABLE 59.1 ■ Treatable Reasons for Cancer Patients' Emergency Department Visits During Their Final Six Months of Life[5]		
1.	Abdominal pain	4.75
2.	Pneumonia	3.57
3.	Dyspnea	3.18
4.	Malaise/fatigue	2.56
5.	Chest pain	2.30
Less common (1%-2% of patients)		
6.	Pleural effusion	1.89
7.	Nausea/vomiting	1.82
8.	Anemia	1.81
9.	Back pain	1.78
10.	Constipation	1.75
11.	Fever	1.64
12.	Dehydration	1.62
13.	Chronic obstructive pulmonary disease	1.58
14.	Urinary tract infection	1.55
15.	Intestinal obstruction	1.48
16.	Altered consciousness	1.48
17.	Congestive heart failure	1.23
18.	Gastrointestinal hemorrhage	1.06
Least common (<1% of patients)		
19.	Chemotherapy	0.91
20	Neutropenia	0.88
21.	Ascites	0.88
22.	Urinary retention	0.83
23.	Phlebitis/thrombophlebitis	0.83
24.	Hematuria	0.79
25.	Convulsions	0.70

patients frequently present to the ED with treatable symptoms (**Table 59.1**), emergency clinicians routinely provide palliative care in the form of symptom relief, pain management, and discussions of critical decisions with patients and their families.[6] These palliative care interventions improve outcomes, reduce hospital lengths of stay and ICU use, provide hospice referrals, generate improved patient and family satisfaction, and lead to more timely care and reduced costs.[6]

> **BOX 59.1 ■ BARRIERS TO PALLIATIVE CARE[6,7]**
>
> - ED crowding
> - Chaotic environment
> - Long wait times
> - Physician attitudes/perceptions
> - Lack of good patient prognostic models
> - Lack of knowledge about:
>   - Palliative care
>   - Patient condition/status/wishes
>   - Available resources
>   - Communicating prognosis
>   - Medical legal issues
>   - Ethical issues (e.g., withholding and withdrawing treatment)
>   - Culturally appropriate spiritual issues
> - Availability/response time of in-house palliative care team
> - Financial constraints/reimbursement issues

There are several potential barriers to optimizing palliative care in the ED (**Box 59.1**). Some of these can be overcome by developing ED-specific protocols for various aspects of the process (**Box 59.2**). Both the American College of Emergency Physicians (ACEP) and the Emergency Nurses Association (ENA) offer resources to assist in the develop of protocols for EOL care in the ED.[6,7]

Managers have the opportunity to positively affect how their staff deal with death by (1) helping to change prehospital practice standards, (2) changing how their staff deal with patients who are dying in the ED, (3) establishing better methods to interact with survivors of patients who die in the ED, and (4) working on other management and educational issues that overlay the clinical setting.

DEAD AND DYING PATIENTS

Emergency department staff care for dying patients and manage the deaths of patients who are receiving palliative care in connection with three main settings: prehospital, at-home, and skilled nursing facilities (SNFs).

Prehospital Setting

Emergency department staff may spend significant time managing deaths in the prehospital setting via the provision of direct medical oversight to emergency medical service (EMS) units and the personnel they supervise. The patients (or surrogate decision-makers) frequently do not want resuscitative efforts or further acute medical interventions, yet standard practice in many locations is to proceed with resuscitative efforts and, in most

> **BOX 59.2 ■ ED PALLIATIVE CARE PROTOCOLS TO DEVELOP[6]**
>
> - Identify ED patients who may benefit from palliative interventions
> - Pain management
> - Non-pain symptom management (i.e., nausea, constipation, pruritis)
> - Comfort care
> - Coordination of in-house palliative care team

cases, to transport the patient to the ED. This is particularly true when no durable advanced directives are immediately available for review. While this may be unavoidable in situations where the death occurs in public, ED leadership has several methods to lessen this problem with expected deaths that occur in homes and SNFs.

At-Home Deaths

Expected deaths at home may be associated with patients who are enrolled in home hospice or receiving other EOL treatment. In these cases, neither patients nor their caregivers desire additional, often expensive and intrusive medical interventions other than palliative care. Yet EMS and police protocols often require that ambulances respond, and crews provide treatment and then transportation to the ED. This "last rite" from emergency medical providers is neither welcome nor viewed positively by the public.

To remedy this situation, managers should consider implementing an easily used, readily available prehospital advance directive (PHAD). This protocol allows EMS to forgo resuscitative measures in appropriate situations and permits them to pronounce death on the scene, rather than transporting the deceased patient's body to an ED where death is then pronounced. Many PHAD examples exist, with Arizona's statute being a clear and simple model that has been successfully used for nearly 20 years.[8,9] Written by an emergency physician, the law's passage demonstrates the type of coordination and collaboration needed to successfully change existing systems.[10,11] The Arizona coalition included the state's medical, nursing, and bar associations; the AARP; and some elder-care groups. There are three unique elements of the statute: it requires only an adult witness, rather than a health-care provider's agreement; it is available online; and only a "good faith effort" is needed to identify the patient. The term good faith effort "includes all health-care decisions, acts, and refusals to act based on a health care provider's reasonable belief of a patient's desires, a patient's best interest, or the directives of a patient's surrogate if these decisions, acts, or refusals to act are not contrary to the patient's express written directions in a valid health care directive." For EDs in other states, an alternative to working through legislature is the implementation of PHADs through state health departments or regional EMS councils.

Emergency department staff must also be familiar with other forms patients or their family members may complete that declare what care they may or may not want at the end of life. An example of one such form is the Physician Orders for Life-Sustaining Treatment (POLST) form.[12] The POLST form can assist ED team members, especially when a patient suffering cardiopulmonary arrest is brought in (**Figure 59.2**). States accept different versions of POLSTs as demonstrated by the National POLST Paradigm Map.[13] A POLST form addresses whether resuscitation should be attempted, as well as what mode of resuscitation (CPR, intubation, etc.) should be utilized, which is helpful in this situation. Some POLST forms allow advance directives, such as the inclusion of such procedures as bilevel positive airway pressure or other resuscitation procedures.[14] Note that Arizona's PHAD explicitly omits these options, since they were found to often conflict with each other and with appropriate resuscitation and palliative care measures. Ideally, fillable copies of EOL forms are readily available in the prehospital and hospital environments.

Skilled Nursing Facilities

Death frequently occurs in SNFs. Many patients with dementia reside in SNFs at the end of their lives, and many of them, along with their surrogate decision makers, have no desire to receive acute medical treatment other than necessary palliation. Yet frequent ED visits are the norm,

FIGURE 59.2 ■ **Sample POLST Form (First Page)**[12]

HIPAA PERMITS DISCLOSURE OF POLST TO OTHER HEALTH CARE PROVIDERS AS NECESSARY

Physician Orders for Life-Sustaining Treatment

Last Name - First Name - Middle Initial

Date of Birth   Last 4 #SSN   Gender M F

FIRST follow these orders, THEN contact physician, nurse practitioner or PA-C. The POLST is a set of medical orders intended to guide emergency medical treatment for persons with advanced life limiting illness based on their current medical condition and goals. Any section not completed implies full treatment for that section. Everyone shall be treated with dignity and respect.

Medical Conditions/Patient Goals:

Agency Info/Sticker

A | **CARDIOPULMONARY RESUSCITATION (CPR):** Person has no pulse and is not breathing.
Check One
☐ CPR/Attempt Resuscitation   ☐ DNAR/Do Not Attempt Resuscitation (Allow Natural Death)
Choosing DNAR will include appropriate comfort measures and may still include the range of treatments below. When not in cardiopulmonary arrest, go to part B.

B | **MEDICAL INTERVENTIONS:** Person has pulse and/or is breathing.
Check One
☐ **COMFORT MEASURES ONLY** Use medication by any route, positioning, wound care and other measures to relieve pain and suffering. Use oxygen, oral suction and manual treatment of airway obstruction as needed for comfort. **Patient prefers no hospital transfer:** EMS contact medical control to determine if transport indicated to provide adequate comfort.

☐ **LIMITED ADDITIONAL INTERVENTIONS** Includes care described above. Use medical treatment, IV fluids and cardiac monitor as indicated. Do not use intubation or mechanical ventilation. May use less invasive airway support (e.g. CPAP, BiPAP). **Transfer** to hospital if indicated. Avoid intensive care if possible.

☐ **FULL TREATMENT** Includes care described above. Use intubation, advanced airway interventions, mechanical ventilation, and cardioversion as indicated. **Transfer** to hospital if indicated. Includes intensive care.

Additional Orders: (e.g. dialysis, etc.) _____

C | **SIGNATURES:** The signatures below verify that these orders are consistent with the patient's medical condition, known preferences and best known information. If signed by a surrogate, the patient must be decisionally incapacitated and the person signing is the legal surrogate.

Discussed with:
☐ Patient   ☐ Parent of Minor
☐ Legal Guardian   ☐ Health Care Agent (DPOAHC)
☐ Spouse/Other: _____

PRINT — Physician/ARNP/PA-C Name | Phone Number
✗ Physician/ARNP/PA-C Signature (mandatory) | Date

PRINT — Patient or Legal Surrogate Name | Phone Number
✗ Patient or Legal Surrogate Signature (mandatory) | Date

Person has: ☐ Health Care Directive (living will)   ☐ Living Will Registry
☐ Durable Power of Attorney for Health Care
Encourage all advance care planning documents to accompany POLST

SEND ORIGINAL FORM WITH PERSON WHENEVER TRANSFERRED OR DISCHARGED

Revised 2/2011   Photocopies and FAXes of signed POLST forms are legal and valid. May make copies for records

Washington State Medical Association — Physician Driven Patient Focused   WSMA   Washington State Department of Health

OVER ▶

---

rather than the exception for patients with dementia. Patients, surrogates, EMS personnel, and ED staff wonder about the benefit of these visits. The ultimate misapplication of planned care results when patients who are dying an expected and natural death are sent to the ED "for resuscitation." Everyone involved understands that this unplanned and inappropriate care contravenes the duty to first do no harm, but most feel powerless to prevent it. Emergency department leadership can change the situation by working with SNFs and EMS systems to implement a process whereby SNF providers can write do-not-hospitalize (DNH) orders **(Figure 59.3)**. Successfully used for decades, DNH documents spare everyone the misfortune of participating in the futile exercise of trying to resuscitate the "truly dead."[11,15,16,17]

FIGURE 59.3 ■ Do-Not-Hospitalize Order (Sample)

I,_____,
being over the legal age required by law and of sound mind do voluntarily and intentionally make known my desire and will that a Do Not Hospitalize Order be placed in my medical records. I direct that (1) I not be hospitalized (as provided by state law) for any condition for which I may receive the same type medical treatment in my own residence (home or care facility); (2) I not be subjected to diagnostic testing of possible illnesses or diseases for which treatment would not be expected to positively contribute to my quality of physical and mental life; (3) I am hospitalized only after the attending physician and I, or the attending physician and my health care surrogate, deem hospitalization to be absolutely necessary for my comfort and/or pain control.

In the event I have a hopeless (not necessarily terminal in the legal sense) condition as determined by at least two licensed medical physicians (more if required by state law) who have personally examined me and determined there is no reasonable medical probability of my recovery from said condition to a meaningful quality of physical and mental life, I direct that my treatment be one of comfort measures only and that treatment be limited to pain management and comfort.

I fully understand I will only be hospitalized after the attending physician and I, or the attending physician and my health care surrogate, have determined hospitalization to be absolutely necessary for my comfort and/or pain management. I fully understand that I may revoke this directive at any time. I understand the importance of this decision; I am competent to make this decision; and I voluntarily and freely sign this on (**date**) in the presence of witnesses refuse resuscitative efforts—unless it is done via surrogate decision makers or the discovery of a previously completed advance directive.

Patient or Legal Surrogate's Signature _____

Print Full Name: _____

Address: _____

City / State / Zip: _____

Witness Signature: _____

Print Full Name: _____

Address: _____

City / State / Zip: _____

Acknowledgment: (Notarize if required by State Law)

State of: _____

County of: _____

On this date _____ before me personally appeared _____ to me, known to be the person described in and who executed the foregoing instrument, and acknowledged to me that (she/he) executed the same as (her/his) _____ free act and deed.

(Notary Public): _____

My commission expires: _____

CARE DURING RESUSCITATION

Patients requiring resuscitation constitute most of those who die, or are near death, in the ED.[10] Providing care for a patient who is dying or dies in the ED requires the involvement of providers, family members, and, at times, the patient. Several issues frequently encountered include providing timely information, allowing family members to witness resuscitation, preparing or notifying the family of the patient's death, and caring for the caregivers.

Those awaiting news of their loved one often complain that they lack adequate and timely information. Further, the room in which they are sequestered—if they are not relegated to the waiting room—is often at some distance from where the resuscitation is occurring.[11] Finding and providing a private area for a patient's family and significant others should be a priority when possible. A team member, generally a nurse, social worker, or chaplain, should be assigned to the family or significant others. This allows for the development of an interpersonal relationship between the family and team member that has been viewed by those experiencing loss as providing death with dignity.[16-21]

Another way to assist families during this difficult time is to allow key relatives to witness the resuscitation attempts. This has been found to significantly decrease anxiety and demonstrate that the ED staff is doing all that can be done at the patient's end of life.[16-21] Witnessed resuscitation was pioneered decades ago in pediatric ICUs and in some EDs. In 1992, Hanson and Stranser published a paper that described the results of 9 years of allowing family presence during resuscitation in the ED.[20] This description and other papers began a discussion about how to meet family needs during a difficult situation. This is a practice that emergency and critical care nurses have supported and implemented for many years. In 1993, the ENA published *Clinical Practice Guideline: Family Presence During Invasive Procedures and Resuscitation*, which has been revised several times and includes evidence-based recommendations for family presence during resuscitation.[22]

The process of witnessed resuscitation involves asking one or two family members or significant other individuals if they wish to observe the resuscitation in the company of an experienced clinician (nurse, social worker, chaplain) who can answer their questions. The family participants are instructed ahead of time that they must not interfere with the medical team and that they may leave whenever they want. For departments who have initiated family presence during resuscitation, this has rarely been a problem.

The resuscitation team is told that "family is in the room," so they are not surprised. During witnessed resuscitations, the resuscitation team shares only vital communications and, in addition to occasionally providing explanations to the family, the staff concentrates on what they are doing.

For resuscitations involving only the ED staff, management can make family attendance during resuscitaitons a department policy, encouraging the physician and nursing staff to "buy in" to the practice. It helps to also have the chaplains and social work staff agree to support and facilitate the effort. Family presence during resuscitation and other invasive procedures has become an expectation over the past years.[16-21]

The presence of these survivors generally does not hinder the resuscitative efforts and often leads to quieter, more effective team efforts. Experience has shown that survivors who witness ED resuscitative attempts never question whether the team "tried hard enough," do not ask whether the person is "really dead," and spend less time in the ED trying to come to terms with the death. In addition, survivors may thank the ED team for their efforts, a situation that rarely occurs under other circumstances, and the ED staff never has to "notify" survivors of the death.

In summary, the general procedure for including family presence during resuscitative attempts is as follows:

1. Ask survivors if they want to view resuscitative efforts.
2. If they do, give them a quick briefing about what they will see and have a knowledgeable staff member, usually a chaplain, social worker, or ED nurse who can answer their questions, accompany them.
3. Give them a chair, particularly if they are older adults, and allow them to leave and re-enter as they wish.
4. Staff should attempt to cover as much of the patient as is compatible with effective resuscitative efforts.
5. Team members should be advised that family is in the room.
6. The survivors should be encouraged to talk to and touch the patient during the resuscitation.
7. The decision to pronounce the patient dead, while often discussed with the family, is generally in the format of advising them that "we must stop now." Witnesses should never be asked whether to stop the resuscitative effort; this is a medical decision.
8. Experience shows that the process of having key survivors view resuscitations often works best if EMS personnel notify the receiving hospital in advance of this request.[22]

For resuscitations involving others, such as a trauma team or pediatric intensivists, it is important to involve all team members in the discussions regarding possible implementation. To gain support, care providers must participate in discussions about implementing this protocol. Experience shows that, while there may be initial reluctance from the ED staff to initiate this policy, they become enthusiastic supporters once they have some experience with it—especially when they find they are being thanked for their efforts.

Deadcare of the Decedent in the ED?

Emergency department deaths may occur after a resuscitation attempt or when patients are brought in and officially declared dead. Death, especially when it is sudden and unexpected—as often happens in the ED—shocks and devastates patients' families and friends. For them, it is a seminal, life-changing event, with every nuance burned into their memories. Furthermore, although they may not consciously acknowledge it, ED personnel may also be deeply affected by such losses, despite their almost constant exposure to life's disasters. This emotional component makes death notifications and dealing with the survivors both vitally important and very difficult.[21]

Even though notifying survivors of a sudden, unexpected death is one of the most difficult parts of emergency clinicians' jobs, they are rarely taught the skills necessary to perform this task. Whether in-person or via telephone (**Box 59.3**), notifying survivors is emotionally draining: 70% of emergency physicians find death notifications to be personally difficult. Perhaps this is because only one-half of physicians received any type of death notification education in medical school, and only one-third received any such training during residency.[21,23] Moreover, there are a variety of significant barriers to successful death notification in EDs (**Box 59.4**).

Death notification protocols can assist ED staff when they must notify survivors, either via telephone or in-person.[22,24,25,26] It is true that no protocol can anticipate every eventuality; every notification will differ in some way, and no protocol can enable notifiers to break bad news painlessly. Death notification protocols can, however, help notifiers prepare for their task and understand what to expect. Protocols combined with staff education have had a significant effect on how survivors perceive and respond to sudden death notifications.[22,26]

BOX 59.3 ■ TELEPHONE NOTIFICATIONS[18]

The first step after a sudden, unexpected death is to contact survivors. This must often be done via telephone. Yet, telephone contact, let alone notification, can be problematic because there is no ongoing relationship between the ED staff and the survivors. The person designated to call the survivors should identify him- or herself and establish the identity of the person with whom he or she is speaking. Always talk to an adult, and try to determine whether someone is present to provide emotional or physical support.

The question constantly arises: should ED personnel notify someone of the death by telephone? Most Americans, especially if they live locally, prefer to be told that the patient is "critical" and then to be told of the death when they arrive at the hospital. The majority of those who wish to be told immediately are men.

For relatives in the local area, the caller should initially say that the patient is in critical condition and that their presence is requested. Be certain that the recipient writes down all necessary contact information; have them repeat it back. If they demand to know whether the person is dead, you must tell them.

When calling relatives outside the local area, tell them of the death. They should never be put in a position of rushing to the side of a "critical" or "dying" relative when the person is already dead.

The only information appropriate to leave on a telephone message system is that a specific person, identified by name or position (e.g., son of George White), should return the call as soon as possible. Leave the name and telephone number of someone with information about the death who will be available for the following 24 hours. This may require providing a pager number or a number for the hospital chaplain or social worker. There should also be a system for each shift to pass on relevant information to the next shift. Protocols and other materials are available to teach and to aid ED telephone notifiers.

Obviously, optimal survivor notification, especially in cases of sudden unexpected deaths, includes the staffs' emotional commitment to and personal investment in the process. There must also be a way to begin learning this difficult task and to measure the quality of notifications. Protocols fulfill these two goals.

For many in the healing professions, as well as other professionals tasked with notifying survivors of sudden, unexpected deaths, protocols have become a standard method of learning complex material. Certainly, as they become more experienced, these professionals will deviate from the protocols to meet the needs of individual situations. Protocols provide both notifiers and death educators a framework on which to build. Emergency department management should ensure that such protocols are readily available, use educational sessions to practice using them in simulations, and openly discuss resulting staff anxiety when performing this difficult task. Possibly even more difficult than death notification is asking survivors for organ and tissue donations, but here, protocols can also be useful.[24] (The process is so difficult that specially trained personnel now often assume this task.)

BOX 59.4 ■ BARRIERS TO EFFECTIVE ED NOTIFICATION[19]

- **No preexisting relationship** with medical staff
- **Survivor stress:** fear, grief, remorse, anxiety, panic
- **Time:** staff has limited time, needs to treat other patients/crises, and may be interrupted to make other decisions
- **Strange environment:** surroundings, noises, smells, lack of privacy
- **Survivor status/behavior:** anger, inebriation, disbelief, not available, cultural or language differences
- **Medical staff stress:** must deliver bad news, ask for autopsy (or notify about medical examiner requirements), ask for organ/tissue donation, and allow time in the midst of other patients' emergencies

> **BOX 59.5 ■ VIEWING THE DECEDENT**[19]
>
> - Ask survivors if they wish to view (use the decedent's name).
> - Prepare them for what they will see. Explain the condition of the body (usually with tubes in place and, if post trauma, some disfigurement).
> - Address common questions before entering the room (Why aren't the eyes closed? Will those marks go away? Why is the mouth open?)
> - If the viewing is in the resuscitation room, clean the floor and cover the body. Leave a hand or foot exposed so that survivors can touch the decedent if they wish.
> - Stay with the survivors while they view the body. Touch the decedent's hand, head, or foot to show them that it is permissible to do so. (Wearing standard precautions for survivors is usually optional.)
> - Leave most of the resuscitation equipment in place; this shows that the decedent received medical interventions.
> - If the decedent is a child, the parent or caregiver may wish to hold the body.

Emergency department managers should involve EMS personnel, chaplains, and social workers in these educational sessions, since separate death notification protocols exist for these groups.[16-22,27] Also, the experiences and comments of these different professionals during the sessions provide substantial validation to the importance of learning this material.

Two other changes may also help lessen stress after ED deaths. One is to develop a protocol based around survivors viewing the decedent (**Box 59.5**), and training personnel to assist in this process. While this practice may seem morbid, it prevents survivors from having the common experience of wondering if their loved one is "still alive." The other practice is to identify media-trained personnel, often on-call, from the hospital's public affairs office who can effectively deal with media inquiries and requests for interviews after the deaths of high-profile patients or those whose deaths are likely to generate media attention.[23-26,28]

One of the most difficult issues, since it involves financial investment (or a lot of inventiveness), is to establish family rooms for death notifications and for relatives awaiting news during resuscitation attempts. These rooms should be near the resuscitation areas, close to restrooms, and contain telephones, tissues, toys for young children, and a door for privacy. It is important to remember that the management of death, whether sudden or expected, requires a team effort. It is also imperative to consider the needs of the team and make resources available to support and comfort them.

EDUCATION AND MANAGEMENT ISSUES

ED management will find that some issues surrounding ED deaths will need time, effort, and patience to resolve. It is worth the time spent. In addition to supporting the decedent's survivors' needs, it is necessary to support the needs of the staff who have provided care. As noted previously, any death can place strain on the ED. However, some are more stressful than others. A "critical incident" has been described as any event that has a stressful impact sufficient enough to overwhelm the usually effective coping skills of an individual. Critical incidents are abrupt, powerful events that fall outside the range of ordinary human experiences. In particular, the sudden death of a child, coworker, law enforcement officer, or EMS personnel may trigger a critical incident.[26,28,29]

A useful tool that should be added to the ED toolbox is a critical incident stress management (CISM) team. A CISM team can assist the ED staff, as well as the EMS, fire, and police personnel involved in the incident to accept the loss of the patient. The leaders of such sessions should briefly and nonjudgmentally review the events involved in the patient's death and allow each staff member to air his or her feelings about the situation. Information about CISM can be found at the National CISM website.[30]

Emergency department staff members should be taught to recognize their peers' symptoms of abnormal stress adaptation. Symptoms may include confusion, poorer concentration, denial, guilt, depression, anger, changes in interactions with others, unusual behavior, increased anxiety, and problems with sleep. Department policy should mandate that the resuscitation leader provides a short debrief for the resuscitation team.

CONCLUSION

Death's frequent appearance is inherent in ED practice. It has been called our society's "last taboo," and even experienced clinicians often avoid speaking about it openly and honestly. The ED management's task is to reduce the stress for staff and survivors while making the process of a patient's dying and death as compassionate as possible for everyone involved.

REFERENCES

1. Solberg L, Hincapie-Echeverri J. Palliative care in the emergency department. *Crit Care Nurs Clin N Am.* 2015;27(3):355–368.
2. McEwan A, Silverberg JZ. Palliative care in the emergency department. *Emerg Med Clin North Am.* 2016;34(3):667–685.
3. Forero R, McDonnell G, Gallego B, et al. A literature review on care at the end-of-life in the emergency department. *Emerg Med Int.* 2012;2012:486516. Available at: https://www.researchgate.net/publication/224006717_A_Literature_Review_on_Care_at_the_End-of-Life_in_the_Emergency_Department. Accessed April 8, 2018.
4. World Health Organization. Definition of palliative care. 2020. Available at: http://www.who.int/cancer/palliative/definition/en/. Accessed July 23, 2020.
5. Barbera L, Taylor C, Dudgeon D. Why do patients with cancer visit the emergency department near the end of life? *CMAJ.* 2010;182(6):563–568.
6. American College of Emergency Physicians. Emergency department palliative care: information paper. 2012. Available at: https://www.acep.org/globalassets/uploads/uploaded-files/acep/clinical-and-practice-management/resources/administration/palliative_care_ip_final_june2012_edited.pdf. Accessed July 23, 2020.
7. Emergency Nurses Association. Palliative and end-of-life care in the emergency department. 2019. Available at: https://www.ena.org/docs/default-source/resource-library/practice-resources/position-statements/palliativeendoflifecare.pdf?sfvrsn=1777bb45_8. Accessed July 25, 2020.
8. ARS. Sample health care power of attorney. 36-3224. Available at: www.galenpress.com/extras/extra1.htm. Accessed June 4, 2018.
9. Arizona Revised Statutes Title 36. Public Health and Safety § 36-3205. Health care providers; immunity from liability; conditions. Available at: https://codes.findlaw.com/az/title-36-public-health-and-safety/az-rev-st-sect-36-3205.html. Accessed June 4, 2018.
10. Iserson KV. A simplified prehospital advance directive law: Arizona's approach. *Ann Emerg Med.* 1993;22(11):1703–1710.
11. Iserson KV. *Death to Dust: What Happens to Dead Bodies?* 2nd ed. Tucson, Ariz: Galen Press, Ltd; 2001:33.
12. National POLST Form. 2019. Available at: https://polst.org/wp-content/uploads/2020/05/2020.05.11-National-POLST-Form-with-Instructions.pdf. Accessed July 26, 2020.
13. National POLST Paradigm Map. 2020. Available at: https://polst.org/programs-in-your-state/. Accessed July 26, 2020.
14. POLST and Advance Directives. The National POLST Paradigm. 2020. Available at: https://polst.org/polst-and-advance-directives/. Accessed July 26, 2020.
15. Dobalian A. Nursing facility compliance with do-not-hospitalize orders. *Gerontologist.* 2004;44(2):159–165.
16. Pekmezaris R, Breuer L, Zaballero A, et al. Predictors of site of death of end-of-life patients: the importance of specificity in advance directives. *J Palliat Med.* 2004;7:9–17.
17. Mitchell SL, Teno JM, Intrator O, et al. Decisions to forgo hospitalization in advanced dementia: a nationwide study. *J Am Geriatr Soc.* 2007;55(3):432–438.
18. Beckstarn, RL, Rasmussen, RJ, Luthy KE, et al. Emergency nurses' perception of of department design as an obstacle to providing end-of-life care. *J Emerg Nurs.* 2012;38:e27–e32.
19. Del Mar Diaz-Cotes M, Granero-Molina J, Hernandez-Padilla JM, et al. Promoting dignified end-of-life care in the emergency department: a qualitative study. *Int Emerg Nurs.* 2018;37:23–28.
20. Hanson C, Stranser D. Family presence during cardiopulmonary resuscitation: Foote hospital emergency department's nine-year perspective. *J Emerg Nurs.* 1992;18:104–106.
21. Iserson K. Bereavement and grief reactions. In: Wolfson AB, Hendey GW, Henry PL, et al, eds. *Harwood-Nuss' Clinical Practice of Emergency Medicine.* 5th ed. Philadelphia, Pa: Lippincott Williams & Wilkins; 2009:817–820.
22. Iserson KV. *Grave Words: Notifying Survivors About Unexpected Deaths.* Tucson, Ariz: Galen Press, Ltd; 1999.
23. Olsen JC, Buenefe ML, Falco WD. Death in the emergency department. *Ann Emerg Med.* 1998;31(6):758–765.
24. Iserson KV. *Pocket Protocols: Notifying Survivors About Sudden Unexpected Deaths.* Tucson, Ariz: Galen Press, Ltd; 1999.
25. Wolfram RW, Timmel DJ, Doyle CR, et al. Incorporation of a "Coping With the Death of a Child" module into Pediatric Advanced Life Support (PALS) curriculum. *Acad Emerg Med.*1998;5(3):242–246.

26. Adamowski K, Dickinson G, Weitzman B, et al. Sudden unexpected death in the emergency department: caring for the survivors. *CMAJ*. 1993;149(10):1445–1451.

27. ENA Emergency Nursing Resources Development Committee, Clinical Practice Guideline: Family Presence during Invasive Procedures and Resuscitation. 2009. Available at: https://www.ena.org/docs/default-source/resource-library/practice-resources/cpg/familypresencecpg3eaabb7cf0414584ac2291feba3be481.pdf?sfvrsn=9c167fc6_12. Accessed May 20, 2018.

28. Emergency Nurses Association, American Academy of Pediatrics, American College of Emergency Physicians. Death of child in the emergency department. 2013. Available at: https://www.ena.org/docs/default-source/resource-library/practice-resources/white-papers/deathofachildined-jointtechnicalreport.pdf?sfvrsn=b78f4ea3_4. Accessed May 20, 2018.

29. Decker K, Lee S, Morphet J. The experience of emergency nurses in providing end-of-life care to patients in the emergency department. *Aus Emerg Nurs J*. 2015;18(2):68–74.

30. US Department of Health and Human Services. Critical incident stress management. 2020. Available at: https://foh.psc.gov/NYCU/CISMInfo.asp. Accessed July 26, 2020.

CHAPTER 60
PRACTICAL IMPLEMENTATION OF OPIOID-REDUCTION INITIATIVES

Alexis M. LaPietra, Donald E. Stader, Sergey Motov, Lewis Nelson

The opioid epidemic is among the greatest public health crises the United States has faced in recent years, affecting people of all socioeconomic classes, geographical locations, and ethnicities.[1] The opioid epidemic encompasses several long-term use disorders, including addiction, dependence, hyperalgesia, and abuse, and patients often suffer from overlapping disorders. The crisis can be traced back to the mid-1990s, when a steady increase in opioid prescribing began, ultimately resulting in a quadrupling of opioid prescriptions by 2010.[2-4] In 2016 alone, approximately 42,000 Americans died from a drug overdose involving an opioid, amounting to more than 115 deaths each day. Drug overdose is now the most common cause of preventable death in Americans under the age of 50.[5,6] Currently, there are an estimated 2 million Americans who report misusing or abusing prescription opioids.[7] Recently, the number of deaths from illicit opioids, such as heroin and fentanyl analogs, has exceeded those from prescription opioids, although the latter remain responsible for an increasing number of annual fatalities.[5,6]

Although the most common reason patients present to the emergency department (ED) is pain, emergency physicians are responsible for writing less than 5% of opioid prescriptions nationally.[8] However, in an effort to improve the practice of pain management, ED-specific nonopioid algorithms as well as agency- and state-endorsed best practice guidelines have been developed.[9-15] The increased focus on nonopioid therapies has opened the door for providers to use and combine medications and techniques not traditionally used for the acute management of patients with pain.[16,17] The concept of a multimodal, evidence-based, and systematic approach to pain management empowers emergency physicians to utilize alternatives first in an effort to decrease unnecessary exposure to prescription opioids in both opioid-naïve and opioid-tolerant patients presenting with pain.

Similarly, the role of emergency physicians in the management of patients with long-term opioid use is evolving, requiring a greater understanding of the complex spectrum of this disease. For example, there is increasing evidence to support the use of medications like buprenorphine for the management of acute severe opioid withdrawal.[18,19] Additionally, EDs can integrate harm reduction into clinical practice by implementing a naloxone dispensing program or via collaboration with local needle-exchange programs. Harm-reduction initiatives can provide important and potentially lifesaving resources and information that may otherwise be unavailable to patients with opioid use disorder (OUD).

PRESCRIPTION OPIOID-REDUCTION STRATEGIES

A tenet of assessing opioid risk is understanding that there are few telltale signs that a person is likely to develop an adverse consequence from opioid analgesics, particularly addiction. More importantly, it appears that many patients without risk factors suffer long-term consequences, making it unlikely that we will ever adequately define baseline risk. Since absolute opioid avoidance is an unrealistic option, especially for acute pain management, the goal is to use the principles and tools available to reduce the likelihood of long-term dependency.

Long-term use often starts with a medically provided opioid. Since risk-factor assessment is very limited, opioids must be prescribing cautiously.[20,21] Opioid-naïve patients obviously have an undefined risk, highlighting the need to use these agents conservatively when managing this population. Paradoxically, the only patients with defined risk are those with a history of OUD. Assistance determining prior opioid use, nonuse, and potentially aberrant use can be obtained by querying the state's prescription drug monitoring program (PDMP).[22] These longitudinal online databases track the individual dispensing of controlled substances over years, and provide valuable information about the patient's history of opioid use.[23] Many states require providers to consult the PDMP prior to prescribing a controlled substance. It is also important to check surrounding states' databases if they are accessible.

Although this theory is unproven, most believe that opioids used for acute severe pain are less likely to trigger long-term use; a parenteral opioid remains the initial treatment of choice for most patients with severe pain. This may be followed by oral opioids or alternative analgesics as the pain becomes more tolerable, a process that generally takes 3 to 5 days.[24] Opioids are generally not indicated for nonsevere pain, such as pain from an ankle spain.[25] Most ED and postoperative opioid guidelines focus on exposure minimization through appropriate patient selection, dosing, and treatment duration.

After observing the failure of the health-care system to reduce opioid use, however, many states have implemented restrictive prescribing limitations for patients with acute pain. In New York, no more than 7 days may be prescribed, and in New Jersey, the limit is 5 days.[26] Although, most guidelines call for using the lowest effective dose for the shortest necessary duration, the subjectivity this introduces allows aberrant prescribing opportunities (e.g., how many pills are appropriate for a 5-day prescription?). These guidelines have proven valuable in reducing opioid use, are useful to prescribers, and do not appear to adversely affect patient outcomes.[27,28]

Reducing the default prescribing amount in the electronic health record (EHR) can reduce the quantity (in pill count) prescribed and does not appear to adversely affect outcomes.[29] Interestingly, removing defaults altogether appears to slightly increase the amount of opioids prescribed.[30] Effective decision support may allow specific opioids to be ordered by default or recommend alternative pain management strategies through the use of best practice alerts. Furthermore, prescriber feedback contextualizing an individual within a group can normalize prescribing behavior.[31] However, some clinicians may be unwilling to change their practices given fixed beliefs about the role of opioids in pain management.[32]

Although long-term opioid use for chronic pain generally includes the use of a patient–provider agreement that lists risks, benefits, goals, and exit strategies, this information also should be communicated with patients prior to prescribing opioids even for short-term use. Unintended consequences include abuse, addiction, dependence, and hyperalgesia, each of which limits the individual's ability to readily discontinue use. The benefits of short-term opioid use are widely accepted but often overrated, but the data to support these medications for chronic painful conditions are limited and generally negative. More educated patients often decline opioid analgesia when provided an explanation of the risk–benefit balance.[33]

For patients with current long-term use (or an OUD, as described in the *Diagnostic and Statistical Manual of Mental Disorders, 5th Edition*), a clear distinction must be drawn between

TABLE 60.1 ■ One Concept of an Opioid Stewardship Committee

Patient-centered strategies

- Involvement in shared decision-making about:
  - The opioid type, dose, route, and alternatives
  - Short- and long-term adverse effects
  - Potential for development of abuse, dependence, hyperalgesia, and addiction
- Counseling about proper opioid storage and disposal
- Counseling about an existing OUD and referral for treatment

Physician-centered strategies

- Consideration for combination of nonopioid and opioid analgesics in the ED
- Utilization of immediate-release (short-acting) oral opioids only in the ED and at discharge for mild-to-moderate pain
- Utilization of morphine sulfate as a first-line opioid for parenteral and oral administration in the ED
- Prescription of the shortest effective course with minimal effective dose at discharge—usually 3 days of immediate-release opioids
- Elimination of ED administration and prescribing of hydromorphone, oxycodone, hydrocodone, codeine, and tramadol
- Querying prescription drug monitoring program for identification of excessive dosages and dangerous drug combinations
- Identification of patients with long-term use disorder and consideration of medication-assisted treatment in the ED with suboxone

Department-centered strategies

- Creation of syndrome-specific pain management protocols by combining nonpharmacological, nonopioid, and opioid analgesics
- Conversion of opioid analgesics into morphine milligram equivalents
- Use of defaults in EHR
- Review of monthly faculty opioid prescribing data
- Creation of departmental pain management protocols

a legitimate need for additional opioid analgesia and diversion for nonanalgesic reasons (e.g., abuse to get high, withdrawal due to dependence). Patients with a history of OUD who are currently in recovery should be offered opioids with extreme caution and only when absolutely necessary.

The 2018 Joint Commission regulations favor the development of a leadership group to create safe opioid practices.[34] Well intended as this is, a refocusing from safe opioid use to opioid alternatives may better serve public health. Many health systems are configuring these leadership groups as multidisciplinary opioid stewardship programs, in which the initiation of opioids, alternative (nonopioid, nonpharmacological) options, harm-reduction strategies, and addiction treatment coexist along a continuum (**Table 60.1**).

ALTERNATIVES TO OPIOIDS

Increasing interest in opioid-sparing pain management has led to the development of innovative ED treatment models. Many approaches have been developed, most notably the Channels-Enzymes-Receptors-Targeted Analgesia (CERTA) principles and the Alternatives to Opioids (ALTO) program. The details of these are presented in **Tables 60.2** and **60.3**. The CERTA concept is based on an improved understanding of the neurobiological aspects of

TABLE 60.2 ■ Acute Pain Management Protocols

Headache/migraine	• Metoclopramide, ketorolac
	  ◦ If <50% relief:
	    — Magnesium 1 g
	    — Valproic acid 500 mg IV
	    — Dexamethasone 4-8 mg IV
	  ◦ If <50% relief:
	    — Haloperidol 2.5-5 mg IV
	  ◦ If <50% relief:
	    — Observation with neurology consultation

Extremity fracture or dislocation	• Nitrous oxide + intranasal ketamine
	  ◦ Set up for block:
	    — Ultrasound-guided regional anesthesia

Musculoskeletal pain	• Ibuprofen + acetaminophen • Lidocaine 5% or diclofenac patch • Cyclobenzaprine or diazepam • Trigger-point or other soft-tissue injection
Lumbar radiculopathy	• Ibuprofen + acetaminophen • Cyclobenzaprine or diazepam • Gabapentin • Lidocaine 5% patch • Ketamine
Renal colic	• Ketorolac, acetaminophen + intravenous fluids • Cardiac lidocaine 1.5 mg/kg IV, max 200 mg

pain. This targeted patient-focused analgesic method utilizes combinations of nonopioid analgesics and the judicious use of opioids. By mixing classes of analgesics that act on different target sites, greater pain relief can be obtained than with individual agents alone. This approach also reduces the dose of each individual medication, potentially leading to fewer side effects, shorter length of stay, and improved ED throughput.[14,35,36] The ALTO program provides practitioners with innovative syndrome-specific opioid-sparing algorithms to assist in the management of acutely painful conditions commonly seen in the ED (**Tables 60.2** and **60.3**)[15] The use of opioid alternatives has been rapidly adopted in EDs across the nation, reserving these drugs as second-line or rescue agents.[37] The ultimate goal of these programs is to broaden the analgesic armamentarium of ED clinicians while promoting patient-specific, pain syndrome-targeted analgesia.

Program Development

New treatment strategies must be implemented in collaboration with other clinicians and staff outside of the ED. For example, pharmacy leadership may be able to assist clinicians in building appropriate algorithms regarding formulary considerations, medication stocking, and dose appropriateness. Furthermore, they can offer clinical decision support and education for staff. The pharmacy is a cornerstone of this strategy, since the ease of use is an extremely important part of practical implementation.

TABLE 60.3 ■ CERTA Concept

Target site	Medications	Pain syndromes
Sodium channel-blocking agents	Local anesthetics: • Articaine: 4% • Bupivacaine without epi: 0.25%-0.5%, bupivacaine with epi: 0.25%-0.5% • Chloroprocaine 2%-3% • Lidocaine without epi: 0.5%-2% • Lidocaine with epi: 0.5%-2% • Mepivacaine: 1%-2% • Prilocaine: 4% • Procaine: 0.25%-0.5% • Ropivacaine: 0.2%-1% • Tetracaine: 0.5% eye drops Antidepressants: • Nortriptyline • Amitriptyline	Acute musculoskeletal pain (fractures, dislocations, subluxations, muscle sprains, strains, spasms [triggers]) Acute soft-tissue pain (laceration, abscess, foreign bodies) Acute visceral pain (renal colic) Acute neuropathic pain (acute herpetic neuralgia) Acute corneal abrasion (tetracaine) Chronic Musculoskeletal pain (flare of rheumatoid arthritis, osteoarthritis) Chronic neuropathic pain (post-herpetic neuralgia, trigeminal neuralgia)
Calcium channel-(central) blocking agents Cox-1, Cox-2 enzyme inhibitors	• Gabapentin, pregabalin NSAIDs: • Ibuprofen • Naproxen • Diclofenac • Ketoprofen • Ketorolac • Acetaminophen (possible Cox-3 inhibition)	Acute postoperative pain Acute neuropathic pain Chronic neuropathic pain (nerve palsies, neuralgias, diabetic neuropathy, post-herpetic neuropathy, sciatica, fibromyalgia) Acute musculoskeletal pain (sprains, strains, contusions, fractures, dislocations, subluxations, tendinopathies, arthralgias, back pain) Acute visceral pain (renal and biliary colic, abdominal pain) Acute soft-tissue pain (lacerations, contusions, foreign bodies, abscesses) Acute headache Chronic musculoskeletal pain (osteoarthritis, rheumatoid arthritis, gout)
Central alpha-1, -2 receptor agonists	• Clonidine • Dexmedetomidine	Acute pain (neuropathic) Chronic pain (neuropathic pain, vaso-occlusive sickle cell painful crisis)
D1 and D2 receptor antagonists	• Haloperidol • Droperidol • Metoclopramide • Prochlorperazine • Chlorpromazine	Acute pain (migraine headache) Chronic abdominal pain Cyclic vomiting syndrome

(Continued)

TABLE 60.3 ■ (Continued)

GABA receptors agonist/ NMDA antagonist	• Propofol	Intractable migraine headache
5HT-2, 5HT-3 receptor antagonists	• Metoclopramide • Haldol • Droperidol	Acute pain (migraine headache) Chronic abdominal pain Cyclic vomiting syndrome
5HT-1 agonists	• Sumatriptan	Acute pain (migraine headache, cluster headache)
NMDA/glutamate receptor antagonists	• Ketamine • Magnesium	Acute traumatic/nontraumatic pain: abdominal/flank/back pain, musculoskeletal pain (sprains, strains, contusions, fractures, dislocations, subluxations, tendinopathies, arthralgias, back pain) soft-tissue pain (lacerations, contusions, abscesses) Abdominal migraine Acute/chronic neuropathic pain Refractory migraine headache Vaso-occlusive painful crisis of sickle cell disease Opioid-tolerant painful conditions Opioid-induced hyperalgesic states Cancer-related pain
Opioid receptor agonists (Mu-receptors)	• Morphine • Hydromorphone • Fentanyl	Acute traumatic musculoskeletal pain (fractures, dislocations, subluxations) Acute visceral pain (Abdominal pain: biliary colic, pancreatitis, diverticulitis), renal colic, acute traumatic pain Sickle cell vaso-occlusive pain Cancer-related pain
TRPV1 receptor agonists	• Acetaminophen • Capsaicin	Musculoskeletal pain (sprains, strains, contusions, fractures, dislocations, subluxations, tendinopathies, arthralgias, back pain) Soft tissue pain (lacerations, contusions, abscesses) Musculoskeletal pain (sprains, strains, contusions) Herpetic//postherpetic neuralgia
Volatile anesthetic (endogenous opioid receptor agonist)	• Nitrous oxide	Acute musculoskeletal pain (traumatic/nontraumatic): fractures, dislocations Acute traumatic/nontraumatic soft-tissue painful conditions (lacerations, contusions, abscesses)

Implementing an ALTO approach requires preparation, education, and commitment from the ED team. As with any disruptive innovation, it may be advisable to assign champions with a passion for this change, both in the emergency physician and nurse realms. In some cases, EDs have tasked specific individuals with such change efforts, naming them as assistant or associate medical/nursing directors.

Physician Education

To be effective, an ALTO program must represent a consensus approach that is uniformly (or near-uniformly) adopted and practiced by every emergency physician and advanced practice provider on the team. This requires educating all clinicians on CERTA and ALTO principles. This step may take some time. The American College of Emergency Physicians (ACEP) has recently developed an evidence-based approach to these topics, which may be of benefit.

An extremely important perimeter of developing ALTO is the education and input of medical staff referral physicians, particularly those taking ED call. For example, if sphenopalatine ganglion blocks will be used for migraine headaches, it is essential to ensure that primary care physicians and neurologists understand this analgesic approach. Similarly, if ultrasound-guided femoral nerve blocks will be used for eligible patients with femoral fractures, orthopedic surgeons who take ED calls should be made aware.

Nursing Education

Education is particularly paramount for nurses, who traditionally play a pivotal role in the administration of medication. Nurse educators should identify and work with nurse champions who have an interest in driving change. There may be regulatory barriers regarding the administration of certain medications. One of the more common problematic drugs is subdissociative ketamine (SDK).[38,39] As stated in the ACEP policy, "SDK is effective and safe for use in the emergency setting, though many hospitals and state regulators are slow to ease restrictions on its use in this setting. It may be safely administered by nursing under the same provisions and protocols as other typical emergency analgesics such as opioids and tends to receive positive feedback from both patients and providers."[39] Although there may be required regulatory changes in some states before SDK can be implemented, discussion around the agent's efficacy and safety should continue.

Information Technology

The information technology (IT) team within the ED or health-care system can contribute greatly to the success of a new program. Support from the IT team, with the implementation of refined pain management order sets in the EHR, can facilitate the use of opioid alternatives. The physician and nursing champions should be involved in building and testing new order sets and developing decision support "cheat sheets" that include, for example, indications, contraindications, and dosing information.

Collaboration With the Health-Care System

Collaboration within the health-care system will improve transitions of care and ensure the appropriate follow-up of patients who are discharged or admitted. By involving primary care services, ED clinicians will be able to transition patients comfortably to a specific treatment regimen. The physician champion may even extend training to different departments as a means of justifying novel treatment strategies.

Additionally, a focus on physical therapy, acupuncture, or other nonpharmacological modalities plays an important role in targeted, focused pain treatment. By developing a relationship preimplementation with physical medicine and rehabilitation, ED practitioners may discover new or improved referral patterns and faster follow-up. The goal of the opioid alternatives program should be to explore novel strategies in an effort to reduce the potential harms associated with opioid exposure.

Public Relations

Finally, the public relations team can serve as a liaison to the community by educating the public and debunking the myths surrounding the new program. Some ALTO programs have been deemed *opioid free* when, in fact, most are not. The public relations department should work with local media outlets to properly summarize the importance of ALTO programs in promoting patient safety and public health. The message should focus on quality and effective pain management as opposed to a reduction in opioid use. A patient whose only experience with pain medication is an opioid may be concerned about visiting an ED that doesn't provide them.

Barriers to Implementation

Specialties outside of the ED have traditionally "owned" certain interventions and may not agree with the necessity of their use in the ED. Some common examples of drugs with administrative barriers include inhaled nitrous oxide, SDK, and ultrasound-guided regional anesthesia (USRA). Because of the need for interdisciplinary cooperation, the support of department leaders is important when evaluating the feasibility of these alternatives. Department leadership must be well educated on the evidence, indications, contraindications, complications, and appropriate use of each modality, as they will be negotiating with the hospital and extradepartmental leadership on most of the key issues.

The use of nitrous oxide as an analgesic for procedural pain (e.g., incision and drainage or foreign body removal) in the ED is much different than its use in combination with anesthetic gases by anesthesiology. Increasing evidence to support the use of nitrous oxide as an anxiolytic and analgesic in the out-of-hospital, pediatric ED, and adult ED settings makes it an attractive option for the management of acute pain.[40-43] Nitrous oxide use does not require fasting, IV access, or cardiac monitoring. The patient's oxygen saturation should be evaluated before, during, and after the procedure, although delivery units are metered to limit the concentration of the drug and avoid hypoxia. Upon completion of the procedure, patients are ready for discharge and can leave without restriction.[44,45]

Since 2007, URSA has become an ideal modality for the management of pain associated with extremity fractures and joint dislocations. This approach provides superior pain relief for patients with extremity trauma, as it can reduce opioid requirements, improve pain with transfer and transport, potentially reduce length of stay, and decrease the risk of adverse events compared to procedural sedation.[47] However, it is important to collaborate with anesthesiology and other relevant services, such as orthopedics, who will ultimately be responsible for providing operative inpatient care. A multidisciplinary meeting should take place to discuss training, quality assurance, and good transitions of care. A physician champion, ideally with formal USRA training, can be enlisted to provide ED staff education and support.

HARM REDUCTION

In 2011, it was estimated that approximately 6.6 million Americans had used IV drugs in their lifetimes, and 774,434 Americans admitted to using them within the past year.[48]

According to the Centers for Disease Control and Prevention, heroin overdoses have increased from 300% since 2011, and heroin use has risen by more than 62%.[49,50] IV drug use is now the number one cause of new hepatitis C infections and the second leading cause of HIV. Moreover, patients who inject drugs have a 16-fold greater incidence of invasive MRSA infections, including endocarditis, epidural abscess, cellulitis, and septic emboli.[51] We are in an era of unprecedented morbidity and mortality from illicit drug use, but there is a proven way for emergency clinicians to intervene.

Harm reduction is a set of practical strategies and ideas aimed at reducing the negative consequences associated with drug use. The approach is predicated on respecting patients and their choices, removing stigma, and meeting them where they are and not where we believe they should be. The goal is not to motivate patients to abstain from drugs but to provide counseling and interventions that decrease the dangers of drug use. Harm reduction acknowledges that most patients with OUD will continue to misuse opioids upon discharge, despite physician counseling. In many cases, counseling that is too simplistic (e.g., "stop using because you may die") is ineffective and often deleterious to the physician–patient relationship.

Initially developed in response to the AIDS epidemic, the harm-reduction philosophy primarily applies to people who inject drugs (PWIDs); however, its principles are broadly applicable to most substance-using patients. Adopting harm reduction in the ED should involve educating physicians and nurses on IV drug use, increasing their knowledge of unsafe injection practices, and understanding how to counsel patients on using drugs safely. Clinicians should attempt to lean into this difficult and taboo topic and embrace discussions about safe drug use.

Educating Patients and Staff

Table 60.4 serves as a quick guide to several harm-reduction organizations, but more can be found through a variety of other resources. A pertinent introduction for emergency physicians and staff is presented in guidelines written by the Colorado chapter of ACEP, available at https://coacep.org/docs/COACEP_Opioid_Guidelines-Final.pdf.

In many communities, syringe exchange programs (SEPs) serve as a resource for patients struggling with IV drug use. Establishing a relationship between the ED and these institutions can help provide seamless referrals for appropriate patients. In many cases, harm-reduction agencies can serve as educators for the ED when implementing harm-reduction initiatives. In communities without SEPs, the health department will often be involved with harm reduction.

Naloxone is a potentially lifesaving drug with no abuse potential.[52] Most states permit the antidote to be prescribed to a person with whom the prescriber does not have a clinical relationship, and they permit naloxone to be dispensed via a non-patient-specific mechanism, such as a standing order.[53] Take-home naloxone programs decrease the barrier of patients needing to fill a prescription and may reduce mortality in high-risk populations.[54,55] In 2018, the US Surgeon General issued an advisory encouraging the availability of naloxone for patients with OUD and the friends, family members, and medical professionals with whom they interact. The creation of a take-home naloxone program includes training for staff and patients, stocking of medication kits, and billing considerations. For more information, consult Prescribe to Prevent: http://prescribetoprevent.org/prescribers/emergency-medicine/. If the ED does not have a program to discharge patients with take-home naloxone, physicians should be encouraged to prescribe the antidote to high-risk individuals (**Table 60.5**).

TABLE 60.4 ■ Key Harm-Reduction Interventions

Preventing drug overdose	Counsel patients to do the following: • Never use alone; use in a witness environment or with a sober friend. • Try a tester shot if using a new product. • Utilize fentanyl test strips. • Do not mix drugs. Provide naloxone, and encourage its use: • Best practice: Dispense naloxone take-home kit to high-risk individuals. • Prescribe naloxone if unable to dispense from the ED.
Preventing invasive bacterial infections	Counsel patients to do the following: • Always use new sterile equipment. • Use a sterile water supply. Do not use a water bottle that you have drank from. • Encourage patients to cook their product as it will help sterilize the infused drug. Assure them they will not be cooking off their heroin (boiling point of heroin is 273°C). • Ask about, and discourage, practice of licking needles before insertion into skin. • Use alcohol pads to cleanse injection site or wash injection site with soap and water prior to injection. • Try to avoid injecting in high-risk areas (groin, neck, back of hands). Critical intervention: • Refer patient to syringe exchange program.
Preventing viral infections (hepatitis B, hepatitis C, HIV)	Counsel patients to do the following: • Always use new sterile equipment. • Never, never share equipment, including needles, syringes, cookers, cottons. • Get tested for HIV, hepatitis C, hepatitis B, and know your status. • If positive, seek treatment. Critical intervention: • Refer patient to syringe exchange program.

Strongly consider creating new discharge instructions that contain the above materials; **Appendix 60.1** provides a sample of harm-reduction discharge paperwork.

Good discharge instructions and teaching following an ED visit for an opioid-related problem (e.g., overdose) can help prevent repeated complications and serve as a valuable resource for patients. These educational materials can be integrated into EHR discharge instructions and should be tailored to local resources, such as syringe exchange or free HIV and hepatitis testing programs. When combined with bedside education, these serve as powerful interventions for at-risk patients.

TABLE 60.5 ■ 2015 ACEP Policy on Who Should Be Prescribed Naloxone
Discharged from the ED following opioid intoxication or poisoning
Taking high doses of opioids or undergoing chronic pain management
Receiving rotating opioid medication regimens
Having legitimate need for analgesia combined with history of substance abuse
Using extended-release/long-acting opioid preparations
Completing mandatory opioid detoxification or abstinence programs
Recent release from incarceration and a history of opioid abuse

MEDICATION-ASSISTED THERAPY

Emergency departments have begun partnering directly with institutional and regional treatment centers to provide what is often called a *warm handoff*. Using this cost-effective model, the ED provides a direct link to an addiction provider and, in some cases, the provider can engage with the patient in the ED prior to discharge.[56]

Regardless of whether and how the warm handoff is performed, a short course of medication-assisted therapy (MAT) will provide the best opportunity for successful engagement.[18,19] Buprenorphine and methadone are widely utilized in MAT and have historically been provided only through long-term care venues, such as addiction treatment centers. The initiation of MAT reduces cravings and withdrawal symptoms following discharge. Buprenorphine is regulated less intensively, safer to administer to unfamiliar patients, and easier to use in the ED.

At its simplest, an appropriately titrated dose of buprenorphine for a patient who is in moderate opioid withdrawal, as assessed by the Clinical Opioid Withdrawal Scale, can reduce signs and symptoms and allow safe discharge. The initial buprenorphine dose is generally 4 to 8 mg, but some patients may require up to 16 mg. Any provider with a Drug Enforcement Administration X-waiver can prescribe a short course of buprenorphine until a follow-up appointment can be arranged, at which point the long-term provider will take over. Buprenorphine often requires preauthorization to dispense from the pharmacy, limiting its availability without extra effort by the prescriber. In these situations, or for prescribers without an X-waiver, the patient may return to the ED for up to 72 hours to receive a daily dose of buprenorphine.[57]

Community Outreach and Communication

As programs centered on safe opioid use, harm reduction, and the treatment of OUD have proliferated, communicating about new services and policy changes has become a challenge to administrators and clinicians alike. With the intense focus that the opioid epidemic has received from press, the community, and legislators, it behooves ED administrators to develop a solid communication plan.

Internally, new treatment paradigms, such as ALTO, CERTA, and MAT, have obvious downstream effects on consultants who may be admitting patients and are unfamiliar with the new ED procedures. For instance, an orthopedist who examines a patient after a fascia iliaca compartment block may wonder what is going on in the ED! This highlights the need to communicate effectively with other clinicians so that the good care implemented in the ED is carried forward when patients are admitted to the hospital.

Externally, ED directors should coordinate with their hospital public relations team, administrators, and legal counsel when promoting new programs. It is important to remain sensitive to state and federal regulations, hospital policies, and patient expectations.

CONCLUSION

The ED is uniquely positioned to address the prevention and treatment of OUD. Emergency physicians have an abundance of tools for preventing opioid exposure—and hopefully long-term use—via multimodal protocols for managing acute and chronic pain. Additionally, EDs can treat patients with acute opioid withdrawal effectively and engage them in a comprehensive recovery process in collaboration with a local addiction center or outpatient practice. Lastly, harm-reduction strategies like naloxone prescribing, education on safe injection, and referral to needle-exchange facilities can reduce the morbidity and mortality associated with IV opioid abuse. The aforementioned approaches can empower emergency physicians to successfully address key issues specific to the nation's opioid epidemic. Emergency clinicians can help prevent dependency, treat long-term use disorders, and mitigate the harm associated with opioid use—and, in doing so, can potentially change the course of many lives, families, and communities.

APPENDIX 60.1: SAMPLE DISCHARGE INSTRUCTIONS FOR HARM REDUCTION IN PWID

Reproduced with permission from Swedish Medical Center in Englewood, Colorado.

Harm Reduction for Heroin Users and PWIDs

Addiction is a true medical disease. Our team cares about you and wants to protect your health. Heroin and IV drugs are particularly addictive, difficult to quit, and dangerous. IV drug use has high rates of overdose, skin and blood infections, hepatitis C, and HIV. We encourage you to seek help for your addiction to heroin and/or IV drugs as soon as possible. However, we understand that entering into recovery and seeking help can be a difficult process. We care about you and want you to be healthier and safer. We also understand that you may continue to use IV drugs, but we want to be sure that you don't suffer an infection, overdose, or complication.

How to Inject Safely

To Avoid an Overdose

1. *Never use alone.* Injecting with another person can help avoid an accidental overdose. Colorado's Good Samaritan Law protects individuals who call 911 to report an overdose. This law will exempt arrest and charges for small amounts of drugs on the patient or caller.
2. *Always carry naloxone.* Naloxone can reverse the effects of a heroin overdose and saves lives. It is available at most syringe access programs and Colorado pharmacies. Medicaid and other insurances will pay for it.

3. ***Try tester shots.*** When trying a new product or after any period of abstinence, patients should use a small test dose (i.e., tester shot) to gauge the drug's potency. Heroin purity in Denver is between 2% and 37%, so you never know what's in the product you've bought.
4. ***Do not mix drugs.*** Mixing heroin or opioids, especially benzodiazepines (e.g., Xanax, Valium, or Ativan), alcohol, or barbiturates, substantially increases your risk of overdose! If you *do* mix, decrease the amount of each drug you are using.
5. ***Use fentanyl test strips.*** These are available for purchase online and are provided through many harm-reduction centers. They can detect if your heroin contains fentanyl.

To Avoid Hepatitis and HIV

Avoid sharing equipment. Although HIV can survive only minutes outside the body, the virus can live for days to weeks inside hollow-bore needles. The risk of transmission is highest when drug paraphernalia is shared between multiple people within a short period of time. Hepatitis B and C are particularly hardy viruses that can survive between 1 and 3 weeks outside of the body. Hepatitis can be spread in every piece of injection equipment, including needles, syringes, cookers, water (lives in injection water for 62 days), and cottons. **AVOID SHARING OR BORROWING ANY INJECTION ITEMS!**

To Avoid Skin and Soft-Tissue Infections

1. ***Practice good hygiene.*** Always wash your hands and clean the injection site. Use an alcohol pad to sterilize the skin immediately prior to injecting. You can buy 100 alcohol pads for under $2 at most pharmacies, and syringe access programs provide them for free.
2. ***Use sterile water to prepare the product.*** Many infections stem from unsafe water supplies. Try not to use river water, toilet water, or saliva to dissolve product into an injectable form. Never lick a needle before putting it into your skin! **Bottled water is safer than standing water, but it is NOT sterile! Do not use a bottle of water that has already been opened and used; it may be contaminated by mouth bacteria, which can cause serious infections!** The safest water comes from single-use containers, which are available through most syringe-access and needle-exchange programs. If single-use containers are unavailable, water should be sterilized by heating it at rolling boil for 10 minutes then letting it cool down.
3. ***Use sterile equipment.*** Try not to reuse equipment on yourself, as reused equipment is often colonized with bacteria. If you must reuse equipment please clean it by soaking it in bleach for 2 minutes and completely flushing all components with clean, cold water. This step should be repeated multiple times.
4. ***Cook your product.*** The boiling point of water is 100°C. The boiling point of heroin is over 270°C! So you will not boil off your heroin, but you will kill bacteria that can cause infections. Boiling your product can help prevent infection, but be sure to let it cool for adequate time before injecting.

To Protect Your Veins

Use the smallest needle possible, and try to rotate between injection sites. Do not inject in the neck, groin, or foot veins, as these areas pose a higher risk of infection. You should also avoid injecting the wrist, as there are arteries and nerves that can be accidentally hit. Staying well hydrated by drinking plenty of water can make it easier to locate your veins. Never use lime juice or lemon juice if you need to dissolve a product. These fluids can cause infections and are very damaging to veins. Use a citric acid solution if your product is very hard to dissolve.

Local syringe access programs are available in Colorado that can help provide clean supplies, as well as provide additional assistance and medical referral.

2016 Colorado Syringe Access Locations

1. Harm Reduction Action Center
231 E. Colfax Avenue
Denver, CO 80203
(303) 572-7800

2. Denver Colorado AIDS Project
2480 W 26th Avenue, Suite B-26
Denver, CO 80211
(303) 837-0166

3. Jefferson County Public Health Clinic
645 Parfet Street in Lakewood, CO 80215
(303) 271-5700

4. Access Point Pueblo
Available Fridays Only
505 West 8th Street
Pueblo, CO 81003
(719) 621-1105

5. Aurora Syringe Access Services
1475 Lima Street
Aurora, CO 80010

6. The Works
3450 Broadway
Boulder, CO 80304
(303) 413-7533

7. Northern Colorado AIDS Project
400 Remington, Suite 100
Ft Collins, CO 80524
(970) 484-4469

8. Rocky Mountain Morpheus Project
414 Taos Street, #B
Georgetown, CO 80444
720-401-6569
(Syringe services not currently offered at this site.)

9. West Colorado Aids Project
805 Main Street
Grand Junction, CO 81501
(970) 243-2437

National Help Line

SAMHSA's National Helpline provides free confidential information to individuals and family members who are facing substance use disorders; it is available 24 hours a day, 365 days a year in English and Spanish. For more information about recovery options and treatment opportunities near you, we encourage you to call SAMHSA's National Helpline (Substance Abuse and Mental Health Services Administration) at 1-800-662-HELP (4357).

REFERENCES

1. Bosman J. Inside a killer drug epidemic: a look at America's opioid crisis. 2017. Available at: https://www.nytimes.com/2017/01/06/us/opioid-crisis-epidemic.html. Accessed July 18, 2018.

2. Kolodny A, Courtwright DT, Hwang CS, et al. The prescription opioid and heroin crisis: a public health approach to an epidemic of addiction. *Ann Rev Public Health.* 2015;36:559–574.

3. US Department of Justice. *Automation of Reports and Consolidated Orders System (ARCOS).* Springfield, VA: US Department of Justice, Drug Enforcement Administration (DEA); 2011.

4. Paulozzi LJ, Jones CM, Mack KA, et al. Vital signs: overdoses of prescription opioid pain relievers—United States, 1999–2008. *MMWR.* 2011;60(43):1487–1492.

5. Centers for Disease Control and Prevention. Understanding the epidemic. Available at: https://www.cdc.gov/drugoverdose/epidemic/index.html. Accessed July 18, 2018.

6. Centers for Disease Control and Prevention. Prescription opioid overdose data. Available at: https://www.cdc.gov/drugoverdose/data/overdose.html. Accessed July 18, 2018.

7. Substance Abuse Center for Behavioral Health Statistics and Quality. Results from the 2016 National Survey on Drug Use and Health: Detailed Tables. SAMHSA. 2017. Available at: https://www.samhsa.gov/data/sites/default/files/NSDUH-DetTabs-2016/NSDUH-DetTabs-2016.htm. Accessed July 18, 2018.

8. Axeen S, Seabury SA, Mechine M. Emergency department contribution to the prescription opioids epidemic. *Ann Emerg Med.* 2018;71:659–667.e3.

9. Washington State Chapter of American College of Emergency Physicians. Washington emergency department opioid prescribing guidelines. Available at: http://www.washingtonacep.org/postings/edopioidabuseguidelinesfinal.pdf

10. Oregon Chapter of American College of Emergency Physicians. Oregon emergency department (ED) opioid prescribing guidelines. Available at: https://www.oregon.gov/oha/PH/PREVENTIONWELLNESS/SUBSTANCEUSE/OPIOIDS/Documents/oracep-ed-opioid-prescribing-guidelines.pdf

11. American College of Emergency Physicians Opioid Guidelines Writing Panel. Clinical policy: critical issues in the prescribing of opioids for adult patients in the emergency department. *Ann Emerg Med.* 2012;60:499–525.

12. Colorado Department of Regulatory Agencies. Policy for prescribing and dispensing opioids. Available at: http://www.painpolicy.wisc.edu/sites/www.painpolicy. (wisc.edu/files/Colorado_Joint%20Bd_Policy%20for%20Prescribing%20and%20Dispensing%20Opioids.pdf).

13. Centers for Disease Control and Prevention. Guideline for prescribing opioids for chronic pain. Available at: www.cdc.gov/drugoverdose/prescribing/guideline.html

14. Cohen V, Motov S, Rockoff B, et al. Development of an opioid reduction protocol in an emergency department. *Am J Health Syst Pharm.* 2015;72(23):2080–2086.

15. St. Joseph's Health. Reducing opioid addiction & overdose. An innovative solution to the epidemic. Available at: http://stjosephsalto.org. Accessed July 18, 2018.

16. LaPietra AM, Motov SM, Rosenberg MS. Alternatives to opioids for acute pain management in the emergency department: Part I. AHC Media. 2016. Available at: https://www.ahcmedia.com/articles/138799-alternatives-to-opioids-for-acute-pain-management-in-the-emergency-department-part-i. Accessed July 30, 2018.

17. LaPietra AM, Motov SM, Rosenberg MS. Alternatives to opioids for acute pain management in the emergency department: Part II. *AHC Media.* 2016. Available at: https://www.ahcmedia.com/articles/138951-alternatives-to-opioids-for-acute-pain-management-in-the-emergency-department-part-ii. Accessed July 30, 2018.

18. D'onofrio G, O'connor PG, Pantalon MV, et al. Emergency department-initiated buprenorphine/naloxone treatment for opioid dependence: a randomized clinical trial. *JAMA.* 2015;313(16):1636–1644.

19. D'onofrio G, Chawarski MC, O'connor PG, et al. Emergency department-initiated buprenorphine for opioid dependence with continuation in primary care: outcomes during and after intervention. *J Gen Intern Med.* 2017;32(6):660–666.

20. Cicero TJ, Ellis MS, Surratt HL, et al. The changing face of heroin use in the United States: a retrospective analysis of the past 50 years. *JAMA Psychiatry.* 2014;71(7):821–826.

21. Iwanicki JL, Severtson SG, McDaniel H, et al. Abuse and diversion of immediate release opioid analgesics as compared to extended release formulations in the United States. Landau R, ed. *PLoS One.* 2016;11(12):e0167499.

22. Weiner SG, Griggs CA, Langlois BK, et al. Characteristics of emergency department "doctor shoppers". *J Emerg Med.* 2015;48(4):424–431.e1.

23. Cheatle MD. The Impact of prescription drug monitoring programs and prescribing guidelines on opioid prescribing behaviors: a time for institutional and regulatory changes. *Pain Med.* 2017;18(5):823–824.

24. Rodgers J, Cunningham K, Fitzgerald K, et al. Opioid consumption following outpatient upper extremity surgery. *J Hand Surg Am.* 2012;37(4):645–650.

25. Delgado MK, Huang Y, Meisel Z, et al. National variation in opioid prescribing and risk of prolonged use for opioid-naive patients treated in the emergency department for ankle sprains. *Ann Emerg Med.* 2018.

26. Affirm Health. Opioid prescribing guidelines: a state-by-state overview. Available at: www.affirmhealth.com/blog/opioid-prescribing-guidelines-a-state-by-state-overview

27. Howard R, Brummett C, Englesbe M, et al. Reduction in opioid prescribing through evidence-based prescribing guidelines. *JAMA Surg.* 2018;153(3):285–287.

28. Nagel FW, Kattan JA, Mantha S, et al. Promoting health department opioid-prescribing guidelines for New York City emergency departments: a qualitative evaluation. *J Public Health Manag Pract.* 2018;24(4):306–309.

29. Delgado MK, Shofer FS, Patel MS, et al. Association between electronic medical record implementation of default opioid prescription quantities and prescribing behavior in two emergency departments. *J Gen Intern Med.* 2018;33(4):409–411.

30. Zwank MD, Kennedy SM, Stuck LH, et al. Removing default dispense quantity from opioid prescriptions in the electronic medical record. *Am J Emerg Med.* April 2017.

31. Michael SS, Babu KM, Androski C, et al. Effect of a data-driven intervention on opioid prescribing intensity among emergency department providers: a randomized controlled trial. *Acad Emerg Med.* March 2018.

32. Pomerleau AC, Perrone J, Hoppe JA, et al. Impact of prior therapeutic opioid use by emergency department providers on opioid prescribing decisions. *West J Emerg Med.* 2016;17(6):791–797.

33. Platts-Mills TF, Hunold KM, Bortsov AV, et al. More educated emergency department patients are less likely to receive opioids for acute pain. *Pain.* 2012;153(5):967–973.

34. The Joint Commission. Pain Management. Available at: www.jointcommission.org/topics/pain_management.aspx. Accessed August 17, 2018.

35. Ducharme J. Non-opioid pain medications to consider for emergency department patients. 2015. Available at: http://www.acepnow.com/article/non-opioid-pain-medications-consider-emergency-department-patients/.

36. Motov S. Lyness D. CERTA Concept of Analgesia. Available at: http://www.propofology.com/infographs/certa-concept-of-analgesia. Accessed July 31, 2018.

37. Duncan RW, Smith KL, Maguire M, et al. Alternatives to opioids for pain management in the emergency department decreases opioid usage and maintains patient satisfaction. *Am J Emerg Med.* 2018.

38. American College of Emergency Physicians Sub-Dissociative Ketamine for Analgesia Policy Resource and Education Paper. 2017. Available at: https://www.acep.org/patient-care/policy-statements/sub-dissociative-dose-ketamine-for-analgesia/. Accessed July 30, 2018.

39. Bowers KJ, Mcallister KB, Ray M, et al. Ketamine as an adjunct to opioids for acute pain in the emergency department: a randomized controlled trial. *Acad Emerg Med.* 2017;24(6):676–685.

40. Lee JH, Kim K, Kim TY, et al. A randomized comparison of nitrous oxide versus intravenous ketamine for laceration repair in children. *Pediatr Emerg Care.* 2012;28(12):1297–1301.

41. Herres J, Chudnofsky CR, Manur R, et al. The use of inhaled nitrous oxide for analgesia in adult ED patients: a pilot study. *Am J Emerg Med.* 2016;34(2):269–273.

42. Kariman H, Majidi A, Amini A, et al. Nitrous oxide/oxygen compared with fentanyl in reducing pain among adults with isolated extremity trauma: a randomized trial. *Emerg Med Australas.* 2011;23(6):761–768.

43. Ducassé JL, Siksik G, Durand-béchu M, et al. Nitrous oxide for early analgesia in the emergency setting: a randomized, double-blind multicenter prehospital trial. *Acad Emerg Med.* 2013;20(2):178–84.

44. Pasarón R, Burnweit C, Zerpa J, et al. Nitrous oxide procedural sedation in non-fasting pediatric patients undergoing minor surgery: a 12-year experience with 1,058 patients. *Pediatr Surg Int.* 2015;31(2):173–180.

45. Gozal D, Mason KP. Pediatric sedation: a global challenge. *Int J Pediatr.* 2010;2010:701257.

46. Liebmann O, Price D, Mills C, et al. Feasibility of forearm ultrasonography-guided nerve blocks of the radial, ulnar, and median nerves for hand procedures in the emergency department. *Ann Emerg Med*. 2006;48(5):558–62.

47. Gadsden J, Warlick A. Regional anesthesia for the trauma patient: improving patient outcomes. *Local Reg Anesth*. 2015;8:45–55.

48. Lansky A. Estimating the number of persons who inject drugs in the United States by meta-analysis to calculate national rates of HIV and hepatitis C virus infections. *PLoS One*. 2014;9(5):e97596.

49. CDC. Annual surveillance report of drug-related risks and outcomes—United States, 2017. Atlanta, GA: US Department of Health and Human Services, CDC. 2017. Available at: https://www.cdc.gov/drugoverdose/pdf/pubs/2017-cdc-drug-surveillance-report.pdf

50. Jones CM, Logan J, Gladden RM, et al. Vital signs: demographic and substance use trends among heroin users—United States, 2002–2013. *MMWR Morb Mortal Wkly Rep*. 2015;64:719–725.

51. Jackson KA, Bohm MK, Brooks JT, et al. Invasive methicillin-resistant Staphylococcus aureus infections among persons who inject drugs—six sites, 2005–2016. *MMWR Morb Mortal Wkly Rep*. 2018;67:625–628.

52. Maxwell S. Prescribing naloxone to actively injecting heroin users: a program to reduce heroin overdose deaths. *J Addict Dis*. 2006;25(3):89–96.

53. Davis C. State legal innovations to encourage naloxone dispensing. *J Am Pharm Assoc*. 2017;57(2):S180-S184.

54. Enteen L. Overdose prevention and naloxone prescription for opioid users in San Francisco. *J Urban Health*. 2010;87(6):931–941.

55. McDonald R. Are take-home naloxone programmes effective? Systematic review utilizing application of the Bradford Hill criteria. *Addiction*. 2016;111(7):1177–1187.

56. Busch SH, Fiellin DA, Chawarski MC, et al. Cost-effectiveness of emergency department-initiated treatment for opioid dependence. *Addiction*. 2017;112(11):2002–2010.

57. Substance Abuse and Mental Health Services Administration. Special circumstances for providing buprenorphine. Available at: https://www.samhsa.gov/medication-assisted-treatment/statutes-regulations-guidelines/special-circumstances

CHAPTER 61

DEVELOPING AND IMPLEMENTING EMERGENCY DEPARTMENT ULTRASOUND

Thompson Kehrl, Robert Jones, Mark Collin

Point-of-care ultrasound (POCUS) has become a fundamental component in the evaluation and management of patients presenting with a wide variety of conditions to the emergency department (ED). As the number of emergency physicians (EPs) skilled in POCUS has grown, issues regarding management of these important programs have become more complex.

HISTORY AND POLITICS OF POCUS

The road to recognition for POCUS has not been smooth or easy. Traditional users of ultrasound (US) have long frowned on its use by nontraditional point-of-care users and, in some cases, have resisted bringing it to the bedside. One of the major victories for POCUS was the passage of American Medical Association (AMA) House of Delegates Resolution (HR) 802 in 1999. This resolution affirmed that US is not "owned" by any one specialty and that US privileges should be granted at the level of hospital medical staff based on specialty-specific educational standards.[1] In 2001, the Agency for Healthcare Research and Quality included US guidance for central venous catheter placement as one of its top patient safety measures.[2] This, in conjunction with the growing use of the Focused Assessment with Sonography for Trauma (FAST) exam in United States trauma centers, sowed the seeds for significant growth in the numbers and types of US users and applications in EDs. In 2001, the American College of Emergency Physicians (ACEP) released comprehensive guidelines on the many issues that POCUS programs faced.[3]

The emergency US community has been and continues to be the leader in the advancement of POCUS. The US community continues to move forward and has obtained focused practice designation from the American Board of Emergency Medicine (ABEM).[4] Despite the progress that has been made, more barriers must be overcome to advance the proliferation of POCUS, including:

- Training of the various different providers who care for emergency patients
- Uniform methods of quality assurance (QA)
- Credentialing pathways
- Integrating handheld devices into workflow

DEPARTMENTAL ORGANIZATION

The development, growth, and maintenance of a POCUS program depends largely on the efforts of a number of key stakeholders. Support from administration, both within the department and at a hospital level, is paramount. Understanding the importance of POCUS, including its impact on clinical care, patient flow, and even patient satisfaction, is required.[5-7] The most important individual role within a POCUS program is the director. When recruiting for this position, the hiring committee should consider individuals who have completed a clinical US fellowship or have prior experience as a POCUS director. More than 100 clinical US fellowships and fellowship-trained EPs exist in both academic and community EDs. Completion of a fellowship provides focused, dedicated training in all aspects of POCUS. While it may be difficult to recruit a fellowship-trained physician to some locations, finding the right person for the position is key to any POCUS program's longterm success.

The depth of commitment and the amount of work required of a POCUS director are substantial and should be recognized by all involved parties. Protected time for management, development, and supervision is frequently a point of discussion among POCUS directors and medical directors or chairs. The leader(s) must have adequate time to address the following considerations:

- Program size
- Training aspects
- Quality assurance and performance improvement
- Hardware and software requirements

A new leader must understand the program's current status. The work needed to develop a POCUS program at an institution where prior groundwork has been laid is different than the work required at an organization without an existing POCUS program. Easing the burden on the POCUS director by aligning the department's priorities with the hospital's goals can help significantly.

A growing number of medical institutions are creating a system-wide POCUS director role. This position provides many benefits, including the standardization of processes, uniform education, and economies of scale. It also enhances the reputation of the ED and its POCUS program.

EDUCATION

No internationally recognized guidelines address POCUS training programs.[8-10] Current national guidelines support a competence-based approach, and ACEP has identified the following 11 core competencies: trauma, intrauterine pregnancy, abdominal aortic aneurysm, cardiac, biliary, urinary tract, deep venous thrombosis, soft-tissue/musculoskeletal, thoracic, ocular, and procedural guidance.[11,12]

Both didactics and hands-on scanning are necessary aspects of training that should be followed by an objective demonstration of competency. According to ACEP, EDs are individually entitled to determine and assess competencies for their US programs. Evidence supports the use of a task-specific checklist (unique to each application) and a global rating scale in the evaluation of trainees.[10,13] Training varies based on the practitioners' prior education and is typically divided into residency versus practice-based pathways. Either pathway can be broken into three parts: knowledge acquisition, practical scanning, and proficiency assessment.

Residency-Based

POCUS skills are critical to the clinical development of an EP, and a minimum skill set should be mandatory for all graduating emergency medicine trainees.[14,15] In 2013, ED leaders determined that POCUS is a skill integral to emergency medicine practice and therefore incorporated goal-directed focused US into the Accreditation Council for Graduate Medical Education (ACGME) EM Milestones project.[16] Requirements to graduate from residency include didactics and completion of at least 150 to 300 proctored, high-quality US scans, as well as demonstrated competency in POCUS.[17] Skill in image acquisition is sometimes assumed when the trainee performs a certain number of practice scans. This skill acquisition number may range from 25 to 300 depending on the exam type.[8,18] There is evidence that competency is better assessed through observation by an expert reviewer and a checklist of specific exam functions.[19,20] Department leadership should look for competence-based assessment of POCUS skills when recruiting recent emergency medicine residency graduates.

Practice-Based

The ACEP lays out specific elements for practice-based POCUS training in the ED. These guidelines address practicing clinicians who have not undergone formalized clinical US education. The recommendations include an introductory course, 25 to 50 documented and reviewed cases in each core area, non-core POCUS application, and a QA program to ensure quality, facilitate education, and satisfy credentialing pathways.[8] Some of the practice-based pathways can mirror the residency-based pathways, but this will be dependent on local resources and the capacity of available trainers. Dissemination of information and skills can occur via lectures, demonstrations, hands-on skills sessions with human models, simulations, web-based learning and assessment, and practical scanning on patients.

Continuing Medical Education

Regular clinical utilization of POCUS is necessary in order to prevent erosion of skills.[21] Peer QA and continuing medical education (CME) are important to maintain skills as well as to keep knowledge up to date. Continuing medical education can include conference attendance, online educational activities, preceptorships, research, teaching, QA, and image review. Five to 10 hours of CME related to US activities per year are recommended for POCUS directors, and 2 1/2 to 5 hours or 5% of total CME time are recommended for individually credentialed physicians.[3]

Advanced Practice Providers

Recommendations for advance practice provider (APP) education mirrors the medical school model of education.[22] A fund of medical knowledge is obtained via a didactic phase and clinical skills follow with clerkships and rotations in multiple specialties. Clinical US education should be incorporated into APP educational programs similar to the way it is being adopted in medical schools (discussion follows). Advance practice providers who have not had integrated POCUS teaching as a part of their initial coursework or training can follow the practice-based pathway to achieve competency with a focus on the anticipated practice patterns. Of note, a number of 1-year clinical US fellowships now accept APPs into their programs.

Nursing

Development of a training program for POCUS use by nursing staff has many advantages, including both improving patient care and nursing job satisfaction. Program needs include focused training with lectures followed by proctored practical scanning centered on desired applications such as US-guided peripheral intravenous (IV) line insertion. Clear supervisory, documentation, and scope of practice protocols are imperative.

Undergraduate Education

The AMA supports the integration of US throughout the continuum of medical education.[23] Supplementation of anatomy, physiology, pathophysiology, and physical examination classes as well as integrated longitudinal exposure, problem-based learning, and exposure on clinical rotations and US electives are some of the methods whereby medical students are gaining exposure to US. A longitudinal approach promises the greatest opportunity for progression of skills.[24] There is, however, significant variability in the quality and quantity of US teaching in medical schools.

CREDENTIALING AND PRIVILEGING

Credentialing is the process of obtaining, assessing, and verifying the qualifications of a medical practitioner to provide services or care for a health-care organization. Privileging is the process whereby the scope or content of the patient care services are authorized by a health-care organization or hospital based on the individual's credentials, training, and performance. Credentialing and privileging of practitioners within a medical organization or hospital are essential to ensure accountability and competence. At the heart of the credentialing and privileging processes is the issue of competence.

Ultrasound as an Extension of the Physical Examination

The evolution of US technology has led to the development of smaller machines, including handheld units. Clinicians now have the ability to easily bring POCUS to the bedside and rapidly evaluate patients for a wide variety of conditions that physical examination alone might not be able to detect. Many view US as the stethoscope of the 21st century and consider it to be an extension of the physical examination, not a clinical service requiring specific privileging. This stance, however, is not supported by ACEP.[25]

Decision-Making in Clinical Privileging

Pertaining to POCUS, both ACEP and the AMA recommend hospitals' credentialing committees follow specialty-specific guidelines for hospital credentialing decisions related to US use by clinicians.[1,3] The AMA HR 802 provides clear support for hospital credentialing committees to grant clinical US privileging based on the specialty-specific guidelines without requiring approval from other departments, and it affirmed that the use of clinical US is within the scope of practice of appropriately trained physician specialists. Furthermore, AMA HR. 802 states that opposition to POCUS that is clearly based on financial motivation meets criteria to file an ethical complaint to the AMA.

Unfortunately, a perception exists within the medical community that medical or surgical specialties that are first to perform a specific clinical service own the procedure and can prevent other specialties from adopting it into their practices. Point-of-care ultrasound has been a common cause of privileging disputes for EPs despite appropriate clinical training and the overwhelmingly supportive literature. Therefore, it is essential that these issues not be taken lightly when approaching the privileging process and that the specialty-specific guidelines set forth in the current ACEP guidelines be followed.[3]

Privileging Structure

Practitioners within a group will have different levels of POCUS competency. ACEP recommends that EDs create a credentialing system that gathers data on individual physicians.

That information should be communicated in an organized fashion (at predetermined thresholds) to the institution-wide credentialing committee. Emergency departments should list POCUS within their core privileges as a single separate privilege and add them directly to the core privileges. Department leaders should monitor the core applications being used and track the practitioners in each of them. As new core applications are adopted, privileging in them should be granted by an internal credentialing/privileging system.

The providers eligible for privileging in POCUS should include appropriately trained EPs as well as other providers who complete the necessary training set forth in the current ACEP Ultrasound Guidelines (attained through residency or practice-based training). Advance practice providers have been integrating POCUS into their practices in recent years; however, there is a paucity of data available regarding the training and evaluation of APPs in the area of POCUS.[26] As such, an APP supervision policy that is tailored to the local circumstance should be in place.

Registered nurses and emergency medical technicians are also integrating POCUS into their practices. Within the hospital setting, this is usually limited to performance of US-guided peripheral IV line insertion and requires that practitioners go through the appropriate level of training and supervision.

Maintenance of Competency

The Joint Commission (TJC) mandates a detailed evaluation of the practitioner's professional performance.[27,28] This standard has been part of the process of granting and maintaining practice privileges since 2008. Ongoing Professional Practice Evaluation (OPPE) and Focused Professional Practice Evaluation (FPPE) are the two evaluation processes that TJC is now using. The Ongoing Professional Practice Evaluation is used to assess professional performance on a continual basis. Specifically, OPPE monitors professional competency and provides data for determining continuance of practice privileges. These evaluations must be done more frequently than annually. The Focused Professional Practice Evaluation involves more specific and time-limited monitoring of a practitioner's performance and is utilized when:

- A provider is initially granted practice privileges
- Performance nonconformance involving an already privileged provider is identified
- New privileges are requested for an already privileged provider

The period of monitoring for these evaluations varies depending on how commonly the procedure is performed. For commonly performed procedures, a 3- to 6-month period might be reasonable, while a longer period of monitoring, such as 6 to 12 months, might be required for infrequently performed procedures.

ACCREDITATION

Accreditation is a process of review that allows hospitals and health-care organizations to demonstrate their ability to meet regulatory standards and requirements established by a recognized accreditation organization. Pertaining to US, the American Institute of Ultrasound in Medicine, the American College of Radiology, and the Intersocietal Accreditation Commission already accredit maternal–fetal medicine, radiology, and cardiology/vascular medicine practices, respectively. Due to the lack of a nationally accepted formal accreditation program in clinical US, the ACEP Accreditation Subcommittee of the Ultrasound Section developed the Clinical Ultrasound Accreditation Program (CUAP) in 2015.[29] The CUAP is an ACEP-governed national accreditation organization with the purpose of establishing a system of review for departments performing POCUS examinations. The goal of the accreditation system is to promote the goals of patient safety, quality, communication, responsibility, and clarity pertaining to the use of POCUS. This program includes standards in several areas:

- Administration of US programs
- Training and education of health-care providers
- Equipment management
- Image acquisition and retention
- Transducer disinfection
- Performing and interpreting US examinations
- Confidentiality/privacy

The accreditation process evaluates group practice and not an individual's practice. Achieving accreditation demonstrates a health-care organization's commitment to maintaining quality, improving patient outcomes and safety, and driving continuous improvement. It is possible that programs that do not achieve certification in clinical US may eventually have more difficulty billing for POCUS.

CERTIFICATION

No nationally accepted formal recognition exists for EPs with significant expertise in clinical US. In recent years, ACEP has been working with ABEM to create a path for specialty certification. Two options for certification currently exist. The first is subspecialty certification by ABEM through the American Board of Medical Specialties (ABMS), which represents the highest standard and level of recognition. To qualify for this level of certification, physicians must complete an ACGME-accredited fellowship training program. The second is the FPD, which is a new type of recognition that was approved by ABMS in 2017. The FPD offers providers an opportunity to set standards for, assess, and recognize areas of additional expertise acquired through practice in a particular area of a specialty and/or subspecialty. This designation serves as an additional indication of a provider's commitment to delivering high-quality care for patients' specific health needs.

ABEM offers a FPD for clinical US. The application was supported by an ABEM survey of EP members of the ACEP Ultrasound Section, the Society of Academic Emergency Medicine Academy of Emergency Ultrasound, and the Society of Clinical Ultrasound Fellowships. Physicians who achieve certification or FPD in clinical US will likely experience greater recognition of their expertise; formal recognition could accelerate the use of clinical US in EDs, with common high standards, quality control procedures, and protocols, fostering widespread improvement in patient care. Once approved by ABEM and ABMS, physicians who meet the criteria for certification should move forward with the certification process.

ULTRASOUND MACHINES

When selecting a US system, it is necessary to consider the intended applications, size and weight, screen size, image quality, number and types of transducers, and budget.

Hardware

When purchasing US hardware, it is necessary to strike a balance between the needs of the operators and the overall cost. The two ways to procure US equipment include purchasing a fully outfitted US machine or incrementally. The cost of the probes comprises a significant percentage of the total cost of a machine.

A number of US companies provide point-of-care platforms. Each offers US machines that can meet the needs of the POCUS user. Selection is largely a matter of personal and institutional preference. As each practice location and physician group requirements are different, it is reasonable to obtain quotes from a number of different vendors. Much like buying a car, it helps to test drive the machine with an onsite demonstration or, more preferably, a short-term loaner that can be put to use in its possible future environment. All of this can be done with help of the vendor sales representative.

The hospital purchasing the equipment may belong to a group purchasing organization, which can help drive the cost of the US machine down. If a hospital's biomedical engineering department has extensive experience and a strong relationship with a specific vendor, this will make servicing machines smoother in the long run.

Among the nonprice considerations, the most important is the selection of a machine that everyone in the group feels comfortable using, balancing the needs of different skill sets. A platform that is too advanced and imposing for novice users will hamper the development of skill sets. Another important purchase consideration is the number and type of probes. If the needs of a facility/group are purely to perform vascular access, then purchasing a small, easy to maneuver, and economical machine can be an attractive choice; however, this approach can limit options if there is a future desire to perform a wider variety of studies.

Limiting the number of probes, while decreasing cost, can compromise patient care as providers may be required to perform scans with suboptimal probes. An example of suboptimal purchasing might occur if providers were required to use a phased array probe to perform an array of abdominal examinations. While the phased array probe might be acceptable, a curvilinear probe is the preferred probe for many of these examinations.

In addition to the number of probes, there are other considerations related to purchasing an US machine. For example, the images taken by the US machine must be reviewed for credentialing and QA purposes as well as archived for billing purposes. If a digital solution is desired, the machine will require a Digital Imaging and Communication in Medicine platform. If images are to be printed, it will be necessary to purchase an image printer. Further considerations include the purchase of various types of Doppler modes. Most machines come standard with color and pulse-wave Doppler. Some include tissue and continuous wave Doppler, while others do not. Most point-of-care platforms do not include more advanced adjuncts such as elastography or speckle tracking.

Middleware and Image Archival

Optimizing workflow for both front- and back-end users is key when designing and managing a POCUS program. Poorly planned processes create the potential for substantial waste. Improper workflow will lead to on-shift mistakes and delays. Scans must be reviewed for both quality and credentialing purposes. If the program includes trainees, it will be necessary to track numbers of appropriately performed scans for graduation and credentialing. Using middleware is a potential solution for how to handle this tracking. Middleware is software that, in addition to other capabilities, receives US studies, permitting review, QA, and collation of images by user. The major barrier to using middleware is the upfront costs of both the software/hardware and the information technology resources needed for its installation and support. Images must be stored digitally, and server space can cost tens of thousands of dollars. However, if installed and utilized properly, middleware can significantly ease the administrative burden placed on US program staff.[30]

There are a number of reasons to archive images, including billing, medicolegal, and QA purposes. The most common archival method is a picture archival and communication system (PACS), which allows archiving of images for the two main reasons noted previously.

The Centers for Medicare & Medicaid Services (CMS) requires images to be archived for five years.[31] In case of an audit, images must be retrievable.

The PACS systems are generally kept on system servers and have redundant backup capabilities, ensuring the security of billed images. The PACS systems also permit consulting services access to images for medical decision-making. The downside of using PACS is that POCUS programs must abide by system information technology rules and regulations, adherence to some of which can be difficult. Other image storage methods include scanning thermal images into medical records and maintaining images on middleware servers.

Infection Control

Developing and maintaining strict POCUS infection control policies are critical to any POCUS program. Point-of-care ultrasound examinations and procedures carry a risk of transmittable infection based on the exposure of the equipment to normal patient microflora and bodily fluids and the degree of the procedure's invasiveness. Practitioners should follow general principles of infection prevention. These include:

- Hand hygiene before and after patient contact
- Decontamination of transducers and other equipment before and after each case
- Regular deep cleaning of the entire US equipment
- Use of protective transducer covers when appropriate
- Use of sterile US gel when appropriate
- Suitable waste disposal

Cracks, abrasions, or tears in US transducers may act as safe havens for infectious organisms or harbor chemical contaminants, and such transducers should not be used.[32] Single-use items (e.g., needle guides) are recommended when possible.

In noninvasive POCUS exams, the general consensus is that low-level disinfection (LLD) is sufficient. Gel removal with soap and water or detergent wipes is essential to remove invisible gel remnants that may harbor pathogens. The transducer should then be dried prior to using the LLD agent to avoid diluting it. Approved LLD agents with antibacterial, antiviral, and antifungal properties in the form of wipes, foams, or sprays can clean surfaces and should be used in accordance with manufacturers' recommendations. The transducer should then be allowed to dry to allow time for the disinfectant to achieve optimal results.

When performing invasive POCUS exams (including US-guided procedures, contact with mucous membranes or bodily fluids), the general consensus is that high-level disinfection (HLD) is required. A single-use protective cover should be used over the transducer (except in the use of a transesophageal echocardiography probe). After the examination is complete, the protective cover should be removed to avoid additionally contaminating the transducer. Even with transducer covers, the rate of perforation or contamination is high, and sterile gel should be used both inside and outside of the sterile transducer cover.[33-37] Gel removal with soap and water or detergent wipes is essential. Approved multistep disinfectant wipes validated for HLD, standardized automated systems employing hydrogen peroxide or UV light, or other HLD validated and approved techniques such as immersion bath are appropriate. To allow time for the disinfectant to achieve the best results, the transducer should then be allowed to dry. A mechanism to ensure that decontamination of probes between patient contact occurs, such as a log, should be in place. After HLD, transducers should be stored in such a way as to avoid accidental contamination before reuse.

Ultrasound gels may allow bacterial survival and multiplication. Outbreaks related to gel use have been reported.[38-40] Single-use bottles of gel are recommended when possible. The user should avoid patient contact of the gel dispensing tip. Opened gel should be used within a short period of time. Warmed gels may increase pathogen reproduction and should only be for immediate use.[41] Decontamination of gel warmers should be performed regularly.

BILLING AND CODING

Setting up a compliant (regulatory) billing schedule can help a POCUS program prosper, allowing reinvestment in both hardware and manpower. Billing for POCUS is outlined by the AMA's annual Current Procedural Terminology (CPT) publication.[42] The CPT codes are set by the AMA's Specialty Society Relative Value Scale Update Committee and published by the CMS. Appropriately trained clinicians privileged and credentialed by his or her institution to perform POCUS may bill accordingly.

It is important to note the difference in the billing specifics for diagnostic versus procedural CPT codes.[42] Most procedural guidance codes are used in addition to the surgical code for the procedure itself. As an example, when central venous catheter placement in a patient older than 5 years (CPT code 36556) is performed under US guidance, the US guidance can be billed separately under CPT code 76937. However, there are CPT codes that combine both the surgical procedure and US guidance (e.g., CPT code 20604).[43]

An understanding of CPT modifiers is important to maintain compliance and optimize billing. As POCUS combines the image generation and interpretation, EDs (both free-standing and hospital-based) generally utilize a combination of technical (-TC) and professional (–26) CPT modifiers. The technical fee is used to cover machine and infrastructure maintenance and is billed by the owner of the machine, which generally is the facility. The technical fee cannot be billed without a professional component. Some insurers prohibit the payment of the technical fee to practitioners. The professional fee is generated by the interpretation of the images. There are a number of other CPT modifiers. Notably, the technical fee can be substantially greater than the professional fee.

Limited codes are generally used by POCUS users when assessing a single organ, anatomic area, or clinical problem. Comprehensive codes are used for the evaluation of multiple organs and require detailed interpretations. For example, a comprehensive abdominal US requires imaging and detailed descriptions of all abdominal organs, whereas a limited examination focuses on a specific organ. EPs can perform and bill for comprehensive US exams and, when doing so, are expected to meet the comprehensive standards. Some US examinations do not have a limited CPT code (e.g., transvaginal US) and require a –52 service reduction modifier if a comprehensive study is not completed. Other CPT codes include modifiers for repeat examinations for a change in clinical condition (–76) or planned serial examinations (–77).

To adhere to billing requirements, certain standards must be met (**Box 61.1**).[42] Importantly, there is no specification regarding the type or number of images required or method utilized to archive images. A number of different processes can be used to accomplish this, including

---

BOX 61.1 ■ REQUIREMENTS FOR ULTRASOUND BILLING[42]

1. Order placed in medical record
2. Documentation of medical necessity
3. Maintenance of archived image
4. Written interpretation
5. Performing and interpreting attending physician's signature

use of the electronic medical record and various middleware solutions. Medical necessity is illustrated via *International Statistical Classification of Diseases and Related Health Problems (ICD-10)* codes. Reimbursement for POCUS is largely governed by Medicare Administrative Contractors (MACs) who determine local coverage determinants. Understanding these rules, including which *ICD-10* codes will support medical necessity, is important, as there is variation between the various MACs.

QUALITY ASSURANCE

Quality assurance and improvement components are vital to maintaining and improving POCUS standards and are necessary at sites performing POCUS. Quality assurance helps to ensure quality, foster ongoing education, and satisfy credentialing pathways. As noted previously, using a middleware program can improve the QA workflow and allow for timely feedback. Highlighting both QA cases where POCUS made an immediate clinical impact as well as those where pitfalls were encountered is important to foster ongoing education. The use of a PACS program has many benefits, including the ability to share POCUS images with consulting services; however, POCUS QA should be kept within the confines of the ED.

Quality assurance should focus on both image acquisition and interpretation. This process includes assessing individual studies for such features as image resolution, gain, depth, orientation, focus, and appropriate labeling. Impressions should be compared with radiology-performed US and/or other imaging modalities as well as pathology reports, surgical procedure notes, and clinical outcomes when available. When discrepancies between the interpretation of images by the acquiring practitioner and the over-read by the QA processors are identified, a mechanism should exist to inform the patient and update the medical record, much like other discrepancy workflows. Quality assurance should also provide timely feedback to providers about the quality of their POCUS studies; however, this must be balanced with a sufficient QA/QI review. The percentage of scans to be reviewed by a QA process should be determined at each site. This number may vary based on factors like the complexity of the POCUS program, including the type of US application in question and provider experience.[3]

CONCLUSION

As EPs have increasingly incorporated US into their daily practices, the complexity of managing a POCUS program has grown substantially. This chapter reviews many of the key components of a successful program, including education, credentialing and privileging, accreditation, certification, hardware, billing and coding, and QA.

REFERENCES

1. AMA Policy Finder. Available at: https://policysearch.ama-assn.org/policyfinder/detail/Ultrasound%20imaging?uri=%2FAMADoc%2FHOD.xml-0-1591.xml. Accessed July 2018.

2. Shojania KG, Duncan BW, McDonald KM, et al, eds. *Making Health Care Safer: A Critical Analysis of Patient Safety Practices*. Rockville, Md: Agency for Healthcare Research and Quality; 2001. AHRQ Publication No. 01-E058.

3. American College of Emergency Physicians. ACEP emergency ultrasound guidelines–2001. *Ann Emerg Med*. 2001;38(4):470-481.

4. American Board of Emergency Medicine Recognition for Clinical Ultrasonography Expertise. Available at: https://www.abem.org/public/docs/default-source/default-document-library/clinical-ultrasonography-fact-sheet.pdf?sfvrsn=8. Accessed August 2018.

5. Blaivas M, Harwood RA, Lambert MJ. Decreasing length of stay with emergency ultrasound examination of the gallbladder. *Acad Emerg Med*. 1999;6(10):1020-1023.

6. Moore CL, Copel JA. Point-of-care ultrasonography. *N Engl J Med*. 2011;364(8): 749-757.

7. Howard ZD, Noble VE, Marill KA, et al. Bedside ultrasound maximizes patient satisfaction. *J Emerg Med*. 2014;46(1):46-53.

8. American College of Emergency Physicians. ACEP emergency ultrasound guidelines—2008. *Ann Emerg Med*. 2009;53:550-570.

9. Henneberry RJ, Hanson A, Healy A, et al. Use of point of care sonography by emergency physicians. Canadian Association of Emergency Physicians Position Statement. *CJEM*. 2012;14(2):106-112.

10. College of Emergency Medicine Ultrasound Subcommittee: Emergency medicine ultrasound, level 1 training. Available at: https://secure.rcem.ac.uk/code/document.asp? ID=3570. Accessed July 2018.

11. European Federation of Societies for Ultrasound in Medicine and Biology: Minimum training requirements for the practice of medical ultrasound. *Ultraschall Med*. 2006;27(1):79-105.

12. Neri L, Storti E, Lichtenstein D. Toward an ultrasound curriculum for critical care. *Crit Care Med*. 2007;35(5):S290-S304.

13. Sisley AC, Johnson SB, Erickson W, et al. Use of an Objective Structured Clinical Examination (OSCE) for the assessment of physician performance in the ultrasound evaluation of trauma. *J Trauma*. 1999;47(4):627-631.

14. Heller M, Mandavia D, Tayal V, et al. Residency training in emergency ultrasound: fulfilling the mandate. *Acad Emerg Med*. 2002;9(8):835-839.

15. Reardon R, Heegaard B, Plummer D, et al. Ultrasound is a necessary skill for emergency physicians. *Acad Emerg Med*. 2006;13(3):334-336.

16. ACGME EM Milestone Project. Available at: https://www.acgme.org/Portals/0/PDFs/Milestones/EmergencyMedicineMilestones.pdf. Accessed August 2018.

17. Lanoix R, Leak LV, Gaeta T, et al. A preliminary evaluation of emergency ultrasound in the setting of an emergency medicine training program. *Am J Emerg Med*. 2000;18(1):41-45.

18. Cheitlin MD, Alpert JS, Armstrong WF, et al. ACC/AHA guidelines for the clinical application of echocardiography: a report of the American College of Cardiology/American Heart Association Task Force on Practice Guidelines (Committee on clinical Application of Echocardiography). *Circulation*. 1997;95(6):1686-744.

19. Jang TB, Ruggeri W, Dyne P, et al. The learning curve of resident physicians using emergency ultrasonography for cholelithiasis and cholecystitis. *Acad Emerg Med*. 2010;17(11):1247-1252.

20. Hertzberg BS, Kliewer MA, Bowie JD, et al. Physician training requirements in sonography: how many cases are needed for competence? *AJR Am J Roentgenol*. 2000;174(5):1221-1227.

21. Kimura BJ, Sliman SM, Waalen J, et al. Retention of ultrasound skills and training in "point-of-care" cardiac ultrasound. *J Am Soc Echocardiogr*. 2016;29(10):992-997.

22. Jones PE. Physician assistant education in the United States. *Acad Med*. 2007;82(9):882-887.

23. AMA Policy Finder. Available at: https://policysearch.ama-assn.org/policyfinder/detail/Ultrasound%20imaging?uri=%2FAMADoc%2FHOD.xml-0-4351.xml. Accessed July 2018.

24. Royer DF. The role of ultrasound in graduate anatomy education: current state of integration in the United States and faculty perceptions. *Anat Sci Educ*. 2016;9(5):453-467.

25. American College of Emergency Physicians. Ultrasound guidelines: emergency, point-of-care, and clinical ultrasound guidelines in medicine. *Ann Emerg Med*. 2017;69:e27-e54.

26. Daymude ML, Sumeru M, Gruppo L. Use of emergency bedside ultrasound by emergency medicine physician assistants: a new training concept. *J Physician Assist Educ*. 2007;18(1):29-33.

27. The Joint Commission. Focused Professional Practice Evaluation (FPPE)—Understanding the requirements. 2020. Available at: https://www.jointcommission.org/standards/standard-faqs/critical-access-hospital/medical-staff-ms/000001485/. Accessed October 17, 2020.

28. The Joint Commission. Ongoing Professional Practice Evaluation (FPPE)—Understanding the requirements. 2020. Available at: https://www.jointcommission.org/standards/standard-faqs/critical-access-hospital/medical-staff-ms/000001500/. Accessed October 17, 2020.

29. ACEP Emergency Ultrasound Section, Clinical Ultrasound Accreditation. 2015. Available at: https://www.acep.org/how-we-serve/sections/emergency-ultrasound/news/june-2015/acep-launches-clinical-ultrasound-accreditation-program/. Accessed October 17, 2020.

30. Tayal VS, Weekes A, Tassone H, et al. Early impact on workflow and administrative costs of a web-based ultrasound data management network on a large volume emergency ultrasonography program. *Ann Emerg Med*. 2010;56(3):S243-S244.

31. MLN Matters Number: SE1022. Medical Record Retention and Media Formats for Medical Records. Available at: https://www.cms.gov/Outreach-and-Education/Medicare-Learning-Network-MLN/MLNMattersArticles/downloads/SE1022.pdf. Accessed October 18, 2020.

32. Seki M, Machida H, Yamagishi Y, et al. Nosocomial outbreak of multidrug-resistant *Pseudomonas aeruginosa* caused by damaged transesophageal echocardiogram probe used in cardiovascular surgical operations. *J Infect Chemother*. 2013;19(4):677-681.

33. Ma ST, Yeung AC, Chan FK, et al. Transvaginal ultrasound probe contamination by the human papillomavirus in the emergency department. *Emerg Med J*. 2013;30(6):472-475.

34. Casalegno JS, Le Bail CK, Eibach D, et al. High risk HPV contamination of endocavity vaginal ultrasound probes: an underestimated route of nosocomial infection? *PLoS One*. 2012;7(10):e48137.

35. Kac G, Podglajen I, Si-Mohamed A, et al. Evaluation of ultraviolet C for disinfection of endocavitary ultrasound transducers persistently contaminated despite probe covers. *Infect Control Hosp Epidemiol*. 2010;31(2):165-170.

36. Storment JM, Monga M, Blanco JD. Ineffectiveness of latex condoms in preventing contamination of the transvaginal ultrasound transducer head. *South Med J*. 1997;90(2):206-208.

37. Milki AA, Fisch JD. Vaginal ultrasound probe cover leakage: implications for patient care. *Fertil Steril*. 1998;69(3):409-411.

38. Muradali D, GoldWL PA, Wilson S. Can ultrasound probes and coupling gel be a source of nosocomial infection in patients undergoing sonography? An in vivo and in vitro study. *Am J Roentgenol*. 1995;164:1521-1524.

39. Oleszkowicz SC, Chittick P, Russo V, et al. Infections associated with use of ultrasound transmission gel. Proposed guidelines to minimize risk. *Infect Control Hosp Epidemiol*. 2012;33(12):1235-1237.

40. Olshtain-Pops K, Block C, Temper V, et al. An outbreak of *Achromobacter xylosoxidans* associated with ultrasound gel used during transracial ultrasound guided prostate biopsy. *J Urol*. 2011;185(1):144-147.

41. Westerway S, Basseal JM, Brockway A, et al. Potential risks associated with an ultrasound examination—a bacterial perspective. *J Ultrasound Med Biol*. 2016;43(2):421-426.

42. Ultrasound coding and reimbursement document 2009. Emergency Ultrasound Section, American College of Emergency Physicians. Available at: https://www.acep.org/globalassets/uploads/uploaded-files/acep/membership/sections-of-membership/ultra/running-a-program/coding.pdf. Accessed July 2018.

43. Goldstein JR, Wu S. Point of care ultrasound reimbursement and coding. In: Tayal VS, Blaivas M, Foster TR, eds. *Ultrasound Program Management*. 2018:353-354.

CHAPTER 62

RURAL EMERGENCY DEPARTMENTS

Autumn M. Brogan, Stephen J. Jameson, Alex J. Beuning, Scott W. Rodi

In the United States, physicians of various specialties had been working as *emergency doctors* for years when, in 1979, a vote by the American Board of Medical Specialties approved emergency medicine (EM) as a recognized specialty. The movement toward specializing EM started with the American College of Emergency Physicians (ACEP), which formed in 1968. And, in 1972, the American Medical Association (AMA) started residency training programs. These efforts attempted to fill the growing need for hospitals to manage emergencies with organized care teams rather than by individual moonlighting physicians.[1,2] As medical care became more complex and specialized, the old model was unable to provide the necessary sophisticated system of care, and EM filled the void.

Rural emergency care continued in a more traditional manner. While residency-trained emergency physicians were increasing the number of staff in urban and suburban settings, general practitioners continued to manage most emergencies in rural hospitals, filling a critical need in the health care of rural populations.[3,4] Even today, rural family physicians have a much broader scope of practice than urban family physicians and are more likely to deliver emergency care.[5]

DEFINING RURAL EM

ACEP developed a definition of rural EM in June 2017:

> *Rural EM is urgent or emergent medicine practiced in geographical areas with low population densities and resource constraints, including ready access to more specialized care facilities. Rural emergency departments (EDs) provide critical services for their communities, including facilitating earlier evaluation and entry into the health-care system, stabilization and initiation of treatment, and coordinated transfer to a tertiary care facility.*[6]

This statement makes clear the critical importance of rural EDs as a safety net for rural populations. But the exact population density to define an area as rural is unclear. While a variety of definitions of population *rurality* are available, the following are derived from rural-urban continuum codes as used by the Rural and Underserved Health Research Center:

- Frontier (<2,500)
- Small rural (2,500–19,999)
- Large rural (20,000–250,000)
- Metropolitan (>250,000)[7]

From an ED-specific mindset, annual volumes may be used as a surrogate for broader population size. The ED Benchmarking Alliance (EDBA) defines ED size based on annual volume as below 20,000, 20,000 to 40,000, 40,000 to 60,000, 60,000 to 80,000, and above 80,000.[7] For the purposes of discussion related to rural ED staffing and operations, it may be beneficial to add two additional ED annual volume categories: below 5,000 (frontier ED) and 5,000 to 10,000 (very small rural ED).[8]

Large Rural Facilities

As of 2014, 69% of emergency physicians practicing in rural EDs were American Board of Emergency Medicine (ABEM) or American Osteopathic Board of Emergency Medicine (AOBEM) board certified or EM residency-trained. Emergency physician density decreases from 10.3 per 100,000 in urban areas to 5.3 for large urban areas.[9] The annual ED volumes in these areas may be above 20,000, and both the volume and acuity of patients seen in these departments are often similar per physician to that seen in an urban ED.[9]

> *Dr. Bruce Burns is an American Board of Internal Medicine-certified physician who has been practicing EM in Alabama since 1995. His staffing agency runs multiple rural Alabama EDs in cities ranging in size from 15,000 to over 50,000 residents. He is the program director for a network of post-graduate training programs for family medicine and internal medicine physicians. He comments, "We want to hire EM residency graduates, but it is hard to get them to move to the rural Alabama communities that we serve."*

Dr. Burns and others have seen the limitations of family medicine and internal medicine physicians covering EDs directly out of their residency training. These clinicians often have inadequate experience with trauma care, including procedural skills and pediatric EM, while having a sufficient base in most other areas of emergency management. Dr. Burns' agency requires a one-year EM training program, focusing on acquiring emergency skills and experience under the watchful eye of program faculty. He believes his program of EM didactics and simulation is superior to old-fashioned on-the-job training, where physicians are often required to figure out the practice of EM without guidance or supervision. His program's graduates have helped to staff numerous hospitals in Alabama, alleviating the EM workforce shortage.

Small Rural Facilities

In small rural EDs with annual volumes between 10,000 and 20,000, EM residency-trained and ABEM- and AOBEM-board certified physicians can be difficult to attract. Non-EM residency trained physicians are often required to meet staffing needs.[9]

Dr. Guy Nuki has practiced rural EM since 1995, when he graduated from his family medicine residency program in Ventura, California and started his first job in rural Washington state. In addition to ED coverage, he did broad-spectrum family medicine, including obstetrics and cesarean sections. In 2001, he moved to Maine and, after a few years, started practicing full time in a rural ED because he was passionate about improving rural emergency care. He states, "The mindset that we should accept less quality emergency care in rural locations is unacceptable."

Dr. Nuki is the chief medical officer of his EM staffing agency that staffs four EDs in Maine, Vermont, and Massachusetts with annual volumes ranging from 10,000 to 16,000. His group hires both physicians and advanced practice providers (APPs), that is, nurse practitioners (NPs) and physician assistants (PAs). The physician group comprises approximately 70% ABEM and AOBEM and 30% family medicine and internal medicine physicians, some of whom have alternative board certification. While non-EM residency-trained physicians have less trauma and intensive care unit (ICU) experience than EM residents, he finds that some EM residents initially struggle in rural EDs. He states:

> Rural EM should be its own specialty. It requires all of the skill sets for high-risk, low-frequency procedures, but also a deep understanding of resource limited system constraints and the differing goals of care and expectations of rural populations that you serve.

Very Small Rural Facilities

In very small rural EDs, critically ill and injured patients arrive at all hours, just like in the largest EDs in the country. While that happens with less frequency, the stakes are just as high, and ED providers must be prepared. In a 2016 survey, 31% of all EDs in the US had annual patient volumes below 10,000.[10] Given the low volumes, hospitals have a difficult time attracting and affording the salary expected by board-certified EM physicians.

Furthermore, reimbursement rates have plummeted throughout the country, leaving hospitals struggling with difficult decisions about how to safely staff their departments while also balancing their budgets.[11] Those who work in rural EDs often recognize the following benefits to this unique practice: opportunity to spend more time with the patients, greater esteem in the community, opportunity for early leadership positions, lower burn out rate, and lower cost of living, among others.

Both Dr. Nuki's and Dr. Burns' EDs utilize APPs to assist the physicians during high volume times. Near Dr. Nuki's hospital in Vermont, Lee Morissette, a Certified PA, independently covers a rural Vermont emergency department. As a former Navy Corpsman, with 25 years of active service, he was often the only medical provider on a Navy vessel serving hundreds of sailors and Marine Corp units deployed overseas. Lee states, "Covering a rural ED feels about the same. I still need to be comfortable making critical decisions, doing critical procedures, and knowing when to ask for help to optimize the care of my patients."

Lee is a former president of the Society of Emergency Medicine Physician Assistants (SEMPA) and has been involved in many discussions about the role of PAs in the ED, both with ACEP leadership and as the SEMPA liaison to the ACEP Rural Section. Humorously, he says, "Covering an ED shift can be easier than some of those conversations." He has great relationships with the emergency physicians he consults with at the nearby tertiary center. "They don't want to cover the ED where I work, but they do appreciate the stabilization care I give to critical rural patients before transferring them."

Frontier Facilities

Frontier EDs are distinguished by both their low volumes and their distance from tertiary care.[10] They also struggle to attract EM residency-trained physicians; in some cases, they would prefer family physicians, who have the flexibility to both cover the ED and manage patients in the hospital and clinics.[5]

Dr. Scott Owens did his EM residency in Fresno, California but moved to Alaska in 2017 to complete a fellowship in Global Emergency Medicine and Rural Health through the University of Washington. This program is a two-year fellowship based in the Alaska Native Tribal Health Consortium that also involves clinical work in South Sudan, Uganda, and Malawi. His wife, Dr. Erica Delsman, is a family physician with fellowship training in obstetrics and cesarean section training who shared his interest in working in Alaska. Scott covers most of his shifts at the Level 2 trauma center in Anchorage but works regularly in Bethel, Alaska. Bethel is a town of 6,493 but serves an area the size of

Nebraska, despite having no roads leaving town. Patients are transported to the ED in Bethel by plane, boat, all-terrain vehicle, or by snow machines and dogsleds.

Often patients are unable to get to Bethel easily, so Scott gives radio advice to local community health aides about basic care to give before the patient can be evacuated. Even after patients arrive in Bethel, it may take days to transport them to Anchorage so his critical care knowledge and skills are important. He says, "I've had an intubated patient in Bethel, taken care of them on the ventilator throughout my shift and then extubated them once they improve. Our ED sometimes has to be a mini-ICU."

Sometimes patients make it into the Bethel hospital late for their clinic appointment but have a plane flight home before the clinic reopens in the morning. In some instances, the most reasonable thing is to prescribe their diabetic medication, blood pressure pills, or give other primary care in the ED. Based on lack of exposure to management of chronic illness, Scott was initially uncomfortable in these situations. His wife, Erica also covers ED shifts in Bethel, as well as Seward, Alaska, which is an even smaller community, with a population of 2,729, where she covers the ED, hospital, and even obstetrics with cesarean section coverage when she works in these rural hospitals. They support each other to help improve the care they give to the rural populations they serve. The cooperation between EM and family medicine within the Owens-Delsman family may be a useful model to consider when exploring ways to improve rural EM in the US.

Critical Access Hospitals

Many of the rural EDs discussed above, in addition to the size niche they fill, are also an integral part of their critical access hospitals (CAHs). These facilities have higher reimbursement from government payers such as Medicare.[11,12] Critical access hospitals receive 99% of reasonable costs for most inpatient and outpatient services, which is a significant difference from urban and suburban hospitals.[13-14] Critical access hospitals must provide 24/7 emergency care services. Failure to staff a rural ED continually is a risk for a rural hospital to lose CAH status, which often is required to make the hospital financially viable.[11-13] This will be discussed further in this chapter.

Physician and APP Relationships

The relationship between rural EM APPs and the physicians who collaborate with them is highly variable in these very small rural EDs, ranging from almost complete independence to close oversight. The training and experience level of these APPs upon entering EM practice, even solo practice, are widely variable. One Mayo Clinic CAH, based in a northwestern Wisconsin town of 3,400 residents and with an ED annual volume of 8,000, has a model that combines physician oversight with significant but progressive APP autonomy. This rural ED partners with a larger, tertiary care ED 50 miles south.

In this system, APPs start their practice, initially shadowing board-certified emergency physicians. Once the APP graduates from this period of orientation and oversight, the APP moves to independently run a pod in the larger ED, with slightly lower patient acuity while also assisting in resuscitations, procedures, and complex patients. Eventually, the APP runs these cases as a team leader, with EM physician oversight. After several years in this system, and an experiential and didactic educational program, these APPs start to bridge to solo practice where they begin covering shifts with experienced APPs in the smaller CAH.

Unlike Dr. Nuki's ED, the busy part of the day in this rural ED is covered by a board-certified EM physician from the hub site practice who, along with the experienced APP, can assess how new providers are acclimating to work in a rural ED. Dr. Aaron Triplett is an EM residency-trained ABEM-certified physician and is the medical director of this hospital.

He grew up in this rural Wisconsin county and was happy to come home to work here but enjoys his ability to work many of his shifts at the larger the American College of Surgeons (ACS) level 2 trauma center where he feels he can better maintain his critical care skills. Today, Dr. Triplett is working with Jon Farm, PA-C, who has worked in this ED for almost 20 years and (Farm) supervises the other local APPs.

Some of the APPs Jon supervises gained their skills through traditional on-the-job training, as he did. Others have gone through a structured Mayo Clinic onboarding program, which has been in place since 2006. Still others are graduates of the Mayo Clinic's formal 18-month EM NP/PA Fellowship program. Over the last 20 years, multiple pathways have been created to both recruit and train providers for rural EDs.

RURAL VS URBAN

Emergency care is not identical in all locations. Approximately half of the nation's EDs are located in rural hospitals.[15,16] Institutions vary greatly in terms of the patient population, staffing, and the available resources by which hospitals can care for patients. Key differences exist between rural and urban EDs.

Patient Population

Rural EDs have often been referred to as a safety net to provide initial time-sensitive care to those living far from urban settings. The population shifts have led to fewer people living in rural settings, due to a movement of industries from community settings. The rural patient population demographics have also shifted to a more elderly and poorer population than urban settings.[17] These patients tend to have several comorbid diseases and require more prescriptions, causing their care to be more complex.[18] Despite falling populations, rural EDs have seen a 50% rise in utilization in the last 12 years.[19] Patients presenting to rural facilities also tend to have a higher proportion of payments from Medicare, Medicaid, and self-pay, which have led to further financial instability for these hospitals and providers.[20]

Training

As mentioned, it is challenging to staff rural EDs with boarded EM physicians. Many creative staffing and training models have developed to meet these challenges, including the use of APP providers and non-ABEM/ABOEM boarded physicians. In rural EM, many physicians and APPs have not participated in a formalized training program in EM. Instead, many rely on skills obtained in their non-EM residencies or through experience working in the field.[21]

Scheduling

Scheduling can also be difficult in rural EDs. Many rural hospitals use contracted staff or locum tenens providers to fill gaps in scheduling. Some have questioned the quality of care and risk associated with bringing in staff on a nonpermanent basis to fill gaps in provider coverage. In addition, organizations contracting to supply these providers may charge a 25% commission, which adds to the hourly ED coverage expense. Literature specific to EM practice and the use of locum physicians is quite limited. Some smaller studies have suggested locum providers could have a detrimental impact on safety due to a lack of familiarity with local policies.[22-23]

The duration of shifts may also be quite different in rural EDs. The length of shifts varies greatly from 8 hours, to 24 to 48 hours of care delivered by providers depending on the volume and acuity of patients. Multiple studies have shown that productivity decreases significantly on an hourly basis for physicians as the shift length grows longer.[24] Additionally, the risk of sentinel events grows with shift length. Both communication errors and the risk of missing important information required to safely care for patients increase with each hour worked.[24,25]

These facts as well as concern for clinician well-being have led the Accreditation Council for Graduate Medical Education (ACGME) to mandate scheduling changes for physicians in training. Many hospital systems have adopted similar provider scheduling changes to enhance wellness, optimize productivity, and reduce risk.[26] However, these models are not always practical in many rural EDs which struggle to provide adequate staffing.

Nursing and Ancillary Staff

The educational background of emergency nurses varies. Some complete a two-year associate degrees (ADNs) by accredited institutions. Others pursue a four-year bachelor's degree (BSN). Once formal education is completed, nurses completing either degree are required to pass the National Council Licensure Exam (NCLEX-RN).[27] After working in an ED for a minimum of two years, an additional certification, certified emergency nurse, can be earned. Many academic and urban centers have shifted toward hiring those who have completed a BSN or requiring the completion of a BSN within a specified amount of time once employed. This requirement is not always feasible or practical in rural areas where it can be more difficult to recruit nurses.[27,28]

Skills, Technology, and Resources

In 2018, there were 139 million ED visits in the US. Forty million were injury related, and 2 million resulted in ICU admissions.[29] Both of these types of patients frequently require procedural skills for stabilization. Over the years, EM has continued to add skills to the specialty training in order to better care for these patients.

From video laryngoscopes for airway management and intubations to point-of-care ultrasound exams, emergency providers must master numerous procedural skills in order to effectively care for patients.[30-32] These procedures require specialized equipment. Additionally, providers practicing in hospitals with low acuity and volume may require refresher training programs to ensure that staff retain knowledge in the use of this equipment. These devices, while sometimes costly, can provide the ED with the capability to perform high income-generating procedures.[31,32]

Technological advances have also led to a decline in the need for specialists to come to the ED to see patients (see Chapter 71). Video laryngoscopies can help less skilled providers successfully intubate patients and improve first time success for all providers.[30] Nasopharyngeal scopes now aid emergency providers in airway management skills, such as awake intubations, and help them assess for infection and foreign objects. Finally, through the use of ultrasound, emergency providers can make quicker and more accurate diagnoses when caring for a variety of patients. From trauma to surgical abdomen pathology, retinal detachments to the drainage of abscesses, and even the placement of intravenous lines has been improved by this one machine.[33,34]

Additionally, the decreasing availability of specialists in rural hospitals has also paved the way for new procedural skills to develop in EM leading to an increase in the number of critical procedures performed in EDs. The ability of ED providers to perform more skills is an advantage to rural hospitals.[32] As skilled rural emergency physicians perform a wealth of procedures, more patients are able to avoid transfer and remain in a local facility when receiving care. For example, with the advent of various novel nasal packings, patients with epistaxis should rarely require transfer to tertiary centers for otolaryngologic care.[35,36]

While there have been many advances in rural care, emergency providers still may face challenges interpreting subtle diagnostic tests without the assistance of cardiology and radiology. The lack of consultants has placed increasing responsibility on rural providers, whose scope of practice can be quite extensive.

Telemedicine

Telemedicine, or telehealth, has been a pivotal change in the care of rural emergency patients. Founded in 1998, telehealth was slow to take off in EDs.[37] Telehealth providers allow patients to be seen virtually, often with the assistance of a nurse or technician. Various telehealth machines exist, but some allow for auscultation of the patient and have zooming features to allow a near full physical exam. Telehealth was designed to provide consultant services and to advise physicians and APPs in the management of critically ill or complex patients, such as those with an acute stroke or trauma.[38] Through telehealth, patients can now access specialty services such as neurology, trauma surgery, cardiology, and psychiatry, for example. Patients and their clinicians can access specialty care from rural EDs and save the time and expense of a transfer to a tertiary center.[37,38]

Staffing and Supervision

Telehealth has since grown and some systems, such as Mayo Clinic, use this service to augment staffing in rural EDs. When a provider is overwhelmed with a sudden rise in volume, telemedicine physicians are able to see patients virtually in triage or exam rooms. Use of this technology allows patients to receive care in an expedited manner. Additionally, telehealth physicians can provide supervision of APPs for the management of critically ill patients and for those patients whom the APP feels uncomfortable managing independently. These telehealth physicians often work in tertiary centers and may even continue to care for the patient if the patient transfers to that tertiary facility.[38]

The COVID-19 pandemic created a widespread push for digital providers who could care for patients while minimizing the risk of exposure. In rural communities, where staffing is more difficult and the number of cross-covering providers is limited, telehealth allows quarantined providers to continue to see patients. These providers, with proper licensing, can work remotely from another state or even another country.[39]

Drawbacks

Drawbacks to telemedicine include payment, speed of data, and reliability. Until recently, reimbursement for telemedicine has been limited. State laws regulating private payer reimbursement are inconsistent.[40] Furthermore, some locations in rural America do not have the consistent bandwidth and internet connectivity necessary to reliably take full advantage of telemedicine.[38,40]

Transportation of Patients

As specialty services become increasingly unavailable at rural medical facilities, more patients are obtaining their care in tertiary centers. This shift has also led to an increase in volume of EMS ground and air transports.[41] Most patients would prefer to stay in their communities for their medical care. Transferring a patient to a tertiary center can be costly, time-consuming, and inconvenient to the patients and their families and friends, who are often involved in care decisions and patient transport upon discharge. Furthermore, areas with extreme weather conditions may not be able to consistently transfer patients to tertiary centers in a timely manner, leaving local providers to manage these critical patients for prolonged periods of time. These issues pose unique challenges to clinicians working in rural communities. In certain situations, these emergency providers must also serve as intensivists until the transfer conditions improve.

ECONOMICS OF CAHs/RURAL FACILITIES

According to the 2018 American Hospital Association Annual Survey, approximately 30% of hospitals in the US (1,821/6,146) are rural.[42] Most of these facilities, or 61%, are designated as CAHs. The remainder are sole community hospitals (17%), Medicare-dependent hospitals (8%), or prospective payment system (PPS) hospitals (14%).[13] It is beyond the scope of this chapter to discuss the relative merits of each model, but a brief overview of the financial benefits of CAHs is helpful to understand the financial challenges facing many small, rural hospitals and to consider how these challenges may impact services offered and strategies employed.

Cost-Based Reimbursement

In 1983, Medicare changed its hospital payment methodology from cost-based reimbursement to a PPS.[13] In this system, all inpatient clinical diagnoses are classified into diagnosis-related groups (DRGs) and hospitals are paid according to the DRG assigned to each patient upon admission, regardless of the actual cost associated with caring for that patient.[13]

A rise in closures of small, rural hospitals following this change led to the creation of the Medicare Rural Hospital Flexibility Program (Flex Program) in 1997, which allowed a return to cost-based reimbursement of CAHs for care rendered to Medicare patients.[13] Unlike the PPS, the Flex Program was originally designed so that Medicare would pay CAHs 101% of the reported costs for most hospital-based and outpatient services provided to Medicare beneficiaries. The intention of this cost-based model was to help low-volume hospitals survive financially, and its impact was magnified in rural areas where a disproportionate number of elderly, Medicare-eligible patients reside (in 2010 21% of Medicare beneficiaries lived in rural areas, though they represented just 15% of the total US population).[13]

In 2011, the Budget Control Act imposed a penalty on Medicare known as sequestration that required Medicare providers, including CAHs, to reduce costs by 2%.[13,43] This Act has resulted in current cost-based reimbursement for CAHs at 99% of cost rather than the 101% originally implemented. Thus, what had commonly been regarded as a "cost plus 1" plan was changed to a "cost minus 1" plan. The result is that even under ideal circumstances CAHs lose money on patients covered by Medicare and Medicaid—a majority of patients at most rural facilities.[42,43]

The CAH reimbursement from Medicare under the Flex Program is determined based on the cost of providing care to covered beneficiaries according to the hospital's annual Medicare cost report. The cost report is a document submitted annually by CAHs that records their total costs and charges associated with providing services to all patients and the proportion of those costs allocated to Medicare, as well as all Medicare payments received. Over the course of the year, Medicare provides interim payments to cover the allowable costs, as determined by Medicare, associated with caring for that population. This methodology means that commercial (nongovernmental) insurance profitability, which still applies to non-Medicare beneficiaries, is enhanced by cost-based reimbursement for Medicare patients.

As an example, if a CAH with a 40% Medicare population purchases a computerized tomography (CT) scanner for $1 million, the hospital will receive $400,000 (40% × $1,000,000) in cost reimbursement over the life of the scanner from Medicare cost reporting. The remaining $600,000 would then be offset by the non-Medicare population through negotiated nongovernmental (commercial) payments.[44]

Another important advantage of CAH designation is that most CAH beds can be used as swing beds. The swing bed program allows hospitals with 100 beds or fewer to change a patient's designation (or *swing* the patient) from acute care to skilled nursing without physically changing beds.[43] In the case of CAHs, these beds are also paid at 99% of cost by Medicare, rather than by the patient-driven payment model used to pay PPS hospitals. Swing beds help stabilize a CAH's census and allow the facility greater flexibility to meet unpredictable demand for acute care and skilled nursing facility (SNF) care. These beds can also be used for long-term care of Medicaid patients in some states and offer an alternative to stand-alone SNFs, which do not exist in many rural communities.[44,45]

Implications for ED Management

Although most hospital-based services are allowable (i.e., can be included on the cost report), there are important exclusions, such as for hospitalist and EM provider salaries, which generally cannot be included in the cost report. There is an exception to this exclusion for EM providers (but not for hospitalists) because CAH designation requires that the ED be staffed around the clock. Specifically, if a hospital can demonstrate that during a portion of each day, there are no patients being managed in their ED, the EM providers' salaries during those standby hours can be included in the cost report.

Another important consideration for ED management in a CAH setting is that a portion of many nonclinical, overhead expenses attributed to the ED can also be included in the cost report. For example, a proportion of human resources, environmental services, and administrative expenses can be stepped down or attributed to the ED and included in the cost report. Similarly, administrative expenses such as an ED medical director's stipend can also be included on the cost report.[46]

Ultimately, cost-based reimbursement under the CAH model provides better financial support for small EDs than a traditional PPS model. However, the fact that emergency physician salaries are generally excluded from cost-reporting creates a continuing financial challenge for low-volume, rural EDs to pay the going rates for residency-trained EM physicians who are also being recruited by high-volume, urban departments. This challenge is of course exacerbated by traditional, nonfinancial considerations that have made it hard to recruit highly trained professionals to rural areas, such as the community's quality of schools, proximity to airports, and availability of arts and entertainment resources.

Financial Challenges

The CAH designation could add millions of dollars annually to a hospital's bottom line. Within five years, the program was so popular that nearly one-third of rural hospitals had become CAHs. By 2019, almost 30% of all hospitals in the country were identified as CAH.[45] A recent study by the North Carolina Rural Health Research Program found that critical access status should be a better fit than PPS for many small, rural hospitals.[46] Using a predictive algorithm, the Office of Financial Research Financial Distress Index found that the percentage of CAHs predicted to be at high risk for financial distress remained essentially stable during the period 2015 to 2019 (6.8%-7.3%) but increased significantly for rural PPS hospitals (from 12.1% to 19.3%).[46,48]

Despite the advantages associated with critical access status, statistics regarding the financial health of rural facilities remain sobering. In 2016, urban hospitals were twice as profitable as rural hospitals, and nearly 50% of rural hospitals were unprofitable as compared with roughly 10% of urban hospitals.[48] According to the National Rural Health Association,

121 rural hospitals have closed in the last decade, and 19 closed in 2019 alone, the greatest single-year total in at least 15 years.[48] The causes of rural hospital closures have generally been divided into internal and external factors.

Internal (hospital-based) factors include poor financial health, aging facilities, low occupancy, staff recruitment and retention difficulties, and fewer medical services. External (market-based) factors include socioeconomic factors such as payer mix and poverty rates, and market share. Protective features include higher outpatient and surgical volumes.[49] A more recent review of rural hospital closures by the Sheps Center for Health Services Research at the University of North Carolina identified the following causes of closure:

- Demographics (as rural populations decline the market for hospitals and other business declines)
- Bypass (tendency of residents to not seek care at the closest hospital)
- Changes in health-care delivery (mergers which result in referral systems that may exclude rural hospitals)
- State and federal policy (e.g., whether states expanded Medicaid under the Affordable Care Act)
- Technology and health care (e.g., services that previously required an inpatient stay can now be done on an outpatient basis)
- Mismanagement (quality concerns or fraud have led to legal interventions resulting in restrictions or closure)[49]

Today's demographic trends, which demonstrate a declining, older and more impoverished rural population, combined with health system consolidations that concentrate medical services in larger tertiary centers and drive referral patterns away from small, rural hospitals, will inevitably add significantly to the financial strain already facing most small, rural facilities.[48] Even with favorable CMS reimbursement models such as CAH designation, unless demographic trends are reversed or health systems thoughtfully and intentionally integrate these hospitals into their systems, rural hospitals will continue to be forced to pursue nontraditional ED staffing (e.g., PAs and NPs) and other care delivery models (e.g., telemedicine) to simply survive.

THE EXPANSION OF EM PROVIDERS

Despite over 50 years since the specialization of EM and advances in emergency care, rural EDs continue to struggle to find EM-trained and board-certified physicians.

Physicians

The backbone of coverage for rural EDs had fallen on local primary care physicians for many years since the 1960s, but in 1986, the Emergency Medicine Treatment and Active Labor Act required hospitals participating in Medicare to staff EDs with onsite (or limited response time) qualified medical personnel.[50] Local physician interest in staffing EDs waned greatly, and primary care shortages began to take its toll on rural ED coverage. A rural health study from 1992 revealed that 86% of rural EDs contracted for physician coverage, and the majority of those physicians were not living locally.[51] For decades, the Association of American Medical Colleges and the AMA have recognized the lack of numbers of primary care physicians and continue to advocate for more of these providers in order to fill the gap in coverage in rural America.[52]

In 1988, ABEM closed the practice track for non-residency-trained physicians as was required by the ABMS.[53,54] The American Academy of Emergency Medicine was established in 1993, created out of concern that non-EM trained physicians were providing substandard care for emergency patients in addition to the concern that unfair practices exploited emergency physicians.[54] Out of this turmoil, another alternative board, the American Board of Physician Specialties (ABPS), created another means for non-EM residency-trained physicians to become boarded in EM with the Board Certification in Emergency Medicine (BCEM). This track does require doctor of medicine (MD) or doctor of osteopathic medicine (DO) degrees, completion of a primary care residency, a minimum of five years (and 7,000 hours) of EM clinical practice, and passage of an exam in order to earn BCEM.[55,56] These physicians help to fill the provider gap needed in rural EDs.

Despite this increase in the EM workforce, there has not been a substantial rise in ABEM/AOBEM-certified physicians working in the rural setting. Rural hospitals represent about 24% of all emergency patient visits and 53% of all hospitals in the US.[57,58] This has led some emergency physicians to question whether there should be active efforts to decrease the expansion of the number of EM programs, particularly since the expanded number of graduates has not met the demand in rural America, including CAHs.[59]

The Role of APPs

One of the responses to this call for emergency provider coverage in rural EDs has been that of APPs. Both NPs and PAs have a long history of working collaboratively with physicians for more than 50 years. The past two decades, however, have seen a dramatic increase in the number of APPs and an increasing move toward independent practice. From 2003 to 2013, there was a 119% increase in the number of PAs, reaching 43,500 in the US. By 2018, there were 123,000 practicing PAs, nearly a 300% increase in just five years.[60]

In 2007, there were about 120,000 NPs, and by 2018, that number grew to over 240,000, a 100% increase in 11 years.[61] The NP programs (467 in the US as of 2017) graduate nearly as many NPs annually as medical schools graduate physicians. By 2030, there will be two NPs for every five physicians, compared to less than one NP per five physicians in 2016.[62] Roughly 13% of PAs and 3% of NPs work in EDs, and they help care for patients across the entire spectrum of EM, from large urban trauma centers down to the smallest of CAHs.[63,64]

In the 1980s, Alaska, New Hampshire, Oregon, and Washington were the first states to broaden NP licensing authority and move toward medical practice independent of a collaborative physician agreement. This was largely a move to provide greater access to care in the vast rural areas of these states. Many more states joined this movement over the next 20 years, but with the passage of the ACA in 2010 and an anticipated surge of patients requiring a primary provider, the following five populous states granted independent practice to NPs: California, Massachusetts, Michigan, Pennsylvania, and New Jersey.[65]

As of December 2019, 28 states allow full independent practice authority to NPs; half of the states allow this immediately after graduation from a NP program, and half allow independent practice after a specified time period of practicing with a physician.[65,66] With the momentum of NPs gaining independent practice, it was inevitable that PAs would seek similar independence. Over the past decade, there have been many political efforts federally and in multiple states to advance independent practice for PAs, and this is beginning to come to fruition.[67] In time, there is little doubt that PAs will achieve the same independent practice as NPs, despite efforts by the AMA and other major physician organizations to halt this trend.

Assistant Physicians

Another trend that has developed regarding the care of the underserved rural EM population is the creation of the assistant physician. With the expansion of US medical schools outpacing the availability of residency positions, an increasing number of medical students are graduating without being able to match to a US residency. Many of these graduates are from international medical schools. These physicians cannot obtain a state license until they have completed at least one year of residency and, in some states, two or more years of residency training.

The assistant physician concept was first trialed in Missouri, where clinicians can practice in the ED under a delegation agreement within 50 miles of their supervising physician upon graduating from medical school, passing the US Medical Licensing Examination (USMLE) and working with a supervising physician for a fixed period of time (e.g., one month).[68] Many other states are considering adding assistant physician licensure.[69]

RURAL EM PROCESS AND QUALITY IMPROVEMENTS

The EDBA has effectively defined best practices in EDs of various sizes. The EDBA compares EDs based on multiple metrics like ED volume, admission rate, flow statistics, boarding, and so on.[70] This approach promotes quality comparisons of like EDs based on volume and acuity, for example. In some rural locations that are distant from tertiary care centers, the acuity is high and admission rates may be high enough that many of these rural patients will obtain their definitive care at these rural hospitals despite the absence of many of the specialty services present at larger urban hospitals.

Rural EDs should develop infrastructure to improve the care they give when problems are identified. In many rural hospitals, even with CAH funding, margins are thin and support for quality improvement time for physicians and nurses is limited. An ED nursing director and/or medical director may be in charge of quality for all aspects of EM care in addition to daily operations, whereas the work will often be divided in higher volume urban EDs. When staffing or other operational needs divert the leaders, quality improvement or peer review may suffer. To address the lack of resources, many rural ED leaders have found that partnering with a larger ED is a benefit to both organizations.

The larger ED may make recommendations that improve the quality of care given to patients transferred from the rural ED and simultaneously gain perspective on the resource limitations of the smaller hospital. The rural ED may benefit from the administrative resources and expertise available at their tertiary referral center. Just as telemedicine can help support care for rural EDs in real time, teleconferencing quality meetings may assist offline care improvement. Many systems that have both urban and rural EDs currently have regular regional system meetings, and this trend is likely to increase as more rural hospitals become affiliated with health systems.

When tertiary care hospitals support the quality improvement of rural hospitals, it is important that their quality leadership understands the resource limitations and geography of the rural hospital. For example, an ST-elevation myocardial infarction improvement process for a rural hospital may include timely administration of thrombolytics, rather than timely transfer to the cardiac catheterization lab, given the realities of transfer distances and times from the rural facility.

CMS quality initiatives are also affected by a lack of specialists or providers. For instance, rural hospitals may not have a radiologist to interpret a stroke patient's CT scan within the recommended 45-minute time frame, resulting in some facilities reprocessing images and sending them electronically to a radiology service for interpretation. This delays the patient's care. In solo-provider sites, an influx of arrivals can lead a higher number of patients who leave without being seen. The inequality in providers and resources between large and rural hospitals can make quality comparisons difficult, if not impossible.

THE FUTURE OF RURAL EM

When it comes to emergency medical care, all patients should have a basic consistent standard. Residency training is the gold standard for practicing EM.

Workforce: Staffing Rural EDs

Currently, staffing all rural EDs with EM-trained physicians is not possible. However, EM leaders can and should work with all EM providers to develop practical and sustainable workforce solutions. While some observers express concerns regarding non-EM trained providers working in EDs, this practice already exists, and it is unlikely to significantly change in the foreseeable future. It is therefore important to consider how to improve the EM training and support of this workforce.

Ideally, multiple organizations with an interest in continuous workforce improvement could form a collaboration on behalf of all EM providers to establish guidelines for ED competency levels. It is suboptimal to have non-EM-trained physicians, assistant physicians, PAs, and NPs working without support or guidance. Emergency care should be a collaborative process with a system that allows for comprehensive review with consistent standards. Leaders in EM have begun to lead this effort, but there is still much work to do.[71]

The following recommendations are aimed at reducing some of the critical gaps in training that exist for different providers.

Residency-Trained Physicians

- *Increase health system expansion into rural hospitals.* More EM residency-trained physicians would presumably enter the rural EM workforce as the health-care systems or physician groups that employ them manage rural hospital EDs.
- *Increase EM resident exposure to rural practice settings.* EM residency training programs can help prepare their graduates for these employment opportunities by increasing rural rotations for EM residents.[72]
- *Improve EM telemedicine outreach.* In most urban EDs with more than one physician working at a time, a physician with a complex case will ask a nearby colleague for advice. Two clinicians may meet at the bedside for challenging airways or difficult procedures. Yet, often less well-trained clinicians in a solo-covered rural ED are expected to manage these situations with minimal support staff and no additional assistance. While a telemedicine EM physician cannot literally lend a hand, the real-time support can enhance care during the management of complex cases or procedures. The EM telemedicine physician can also assist with transport, improve communication with the receiving facility, obtain specialty video or telephonic consultation (telestroke, teleneonatology, etc.), and even place orders when done with shared electronic medical record platforms, all while the rural EM provider is working at the bedside. This support reduces the cognitive load of the local EM provider and has the potential to improve the efficiency and quality of care provided to the patient.[73,74]

Non-Residency-Trained Physicians

- *Improve EM exposure in primary care residency programs.* The majority of rural emergency care provided by non-EM residency-trained physicians is provided by family physicians, and occasionally by internal medicine, surgical, and other physicians. The American Academy of Family Medicine published a set of core curriculum guidelines for family medicine residents addressing acute and emergency care designed to ensure adequate preparedness for its graduates.[75]

- *Ensure continuing education in EM for non-EM residency-trained physicians.* Non-EM residency-trained physicians practicing rural EM often maintain their primary care board certification for state licensing requirements. However, many do not have requirements to make an effort to complete EM-based training or competency education. To improve the ongoing training of these providers, ABMS and other certification boards could coordinate efforts to ensure that every EM provider has continuing emergency medical education requirements.
- *Move from on-the-job training to more formalized EM education.* As noted, family physicians get basic EM training during their residencies, but they need additional experience in critical care, trauma, and procedural medicine if they intend to practice in an ED. The College of Family Physicians of Canada offers a two-year residency training program in family medicine with the option of an additional year of training in EM to obtain the Canadian College of Family Physicians–Emergency Medicine (CCFP-EM) certification.[14] In the United States, post-primary care residency graduate training programs in EM have developed to fill this training void and should be encouraged for non-EM residency-trained clinicians practicing EM.
- *Train in trauma care.* The ACS has recognized the need to improve rural trauma care and has advised that all providers working in rural EDs take advanced trauma life support (ATLS).[76] The ACS has also developed a course for teaching a fluid team response to trauma for resource-limited rural EDs: Rural Trauma Team Development Course (RTTDC).[77] Some states have allowed a more comprehensive rural EM course, Comprehensive Advanced Life Support (CALS), as a replacement of ATLS for level 3 and 4 trauma centers. Comprehensive Advanced Life Support has the core components of ATLS in regard to trauma care but has more extensive coverage of other critical emergencies (airway, medical, obstetric) and how to manage them in a rural ED. For non-EM boarded physicians covering rural EDs, it is important that they take one or both of these courses.

Advanced Practice Providers

- *Encourage development and support of EM fellowship programs.* Basic APP training does not sufficiently prepare APPs for rural EM practice. Additionally, there are no standardized requirements for APPs choosing to practice EM. Experience with EM board-certified physicians can minimize mistakes made from gaps in knowledge. Advanced practice providers EM fellowship programs offer experience through additional training and education, including procedural skills, ultrasound, and rotations in orthopedics, pediatrics, critical care, and other subspecialties. Fellowship programs are intended to provide a portion of EM physician training. In 2020, the Accreditation Review Commission on Education for the Physician Assistant began accrediting EM fellowship programs. Accreditation provides a standard for the educational requirements of APP specialization in EM, similar to the ACGME requirements for physician residency programs.[78]
- *Encourage extended on-the-job training or apprenticeship with formalized didactics when EM fellowship experience is not available.* The demand for EM APPs currently exceeds the number of EM APP fellowship programs. When EM APPs require on-the-job training, it is important to ensure adequate orientation with EM board-certified physician oversight. Even when EM APPs are managing patients in lower acuity areas, knowledge, training, and experience can significantly improve quality of care and lower patient risk. Orientation should include both clinical supervision and a comprehensive didactic program in EM and simulation skills.

- **Train in trauma care.** For reasons noted previously, APPs should take both ATLS and a course such as CALS to prepare them to work in the rural setting. Taking the ACS-developed RTTDC or CALS course can also teach team response to trauma.

Future directions in the improvement of rural EM should be made with the input and leadership all organizations concerned about the future of this critical subspecialty. Of these, ACEP, through the work of its Rural Section, is in an excellent position to advocate for and participate in the recommendation of standards and education for rural EDs.

Other organizations, such as the American Academy of Family Medicine, the ABPS Board of Certification in Emergency Medicine, SEMPA, and AAENP, should actively participate in this discussion of standards. As an example, ACEP is collaborating with SEMPA to create guidelines for the EM APP workforce, which is an excellent first step toward developing national standards for rural EM practice.[79,80]

CONCLUSION

Practitioners of rural EM face many challenges. Partnerships between emergency physician and other provider groups continue to work toward standards of excellence while elevating care for rural communities. Through innovative solutions and new training programs, rural EDs are meeting scheduling and financial challenges to keep their EDs afloat. These steps offer support to rural hospitals who provide life-saving care to our rural communities.

REFERENCES

1. American College of Emergency Physicians. About ACEP. Available at: https://www.acep.org/who-we-are/about-us/. Accessed November 5, 2020.
2. American Academy of Emergency Medicine website. History. Available at: https://www.aaem.org/about-us/our-values/history. Accessed November 5, 2020.
3. Peterson LE, Fang B. *Rural Family Physicians Have a Broader Scope of Practice Than Urban Family Physicians*. Lexington, KY: Rural and Underserved Health Research Center; 2018.
4. Gerald C Banks et al. Family physicians play integral role in emergency medicine. *Ann Fam Med*. 2017;15(1):84–86.
5. American Academy of Family Physicians Position Paper. Family Physicians Delivering Emergency Medical Care—Critical Challenges and Opportunities. 2020.
6. ACEP webpage. Available at: https://www.acep.org/patient-care/policy-statements/definition-of-rural-emergency-medicine/. Accessed November 5, 2020.
7. Welch SJ, Augustine JJ, Dong L, et al. Volume-related differences in emergency department performance. *Jt Comm J Qual Patient Saf*. 2012;38(9):395–401.
8. Rodi S, Carpenter C, Hirsch S. Defining "rural"—what's in a name? *J Rural Emerg Med*. 2015;2(1).
9. Macht M, MacKenzie A, Ginde AA. The rural emergency physician workforce. *J Rural Emerg Med*. 2014;1(1).
10. Emergency Medicine Network, 2016 National Emergency Department Inventory—USA. 2016 National and State-Specific ED Data. Available at: https://www.emnet-usa.org/research/studies/nedi/nedi2016/. Updated 2020. Accessed August 15, 2020.
11. Medpac. Payment basics—Critical Access Hospitals Payment System. Available at: www.medpac.gov. Accessed November 5, 2020.
12. Rural Health Information Hub. Critical Access Hospitals—Introduction. 2018. Available at: https://www.ruralhealthinfo.org/topics/critical-access-hospitals.
13. National Rural Health Resource Center. Critical Access Hospital Finance 101. Updated June 2017.
14. American College of Emergency Physicians Position Paper: The Impact of Unreimbursed Care on the Emergency Physician.
15. Urban K. Patient visits higher at rural emergency departments. University of Michigan, "M" Health Lab. 2019. Available at: https://labblog.uofmhealth.org/industry-dx/patient-visits-higher-at-rural-emergency-departments. Accessed November 5, 2020.
16. Health Resources & Services Administration. Rural Hospital Programs. Available at: https://www.hrsa.gov/rural-health/rural-hospitals/index.html. Accessed November 5, 2020.
17. United States Department of Agriculture Economic Research Service. Population & Migration. Available at: https://www.ers.usda.gov/topics/rural-economy/population/population-migration/. Updated February 25, 2020. Accessed November 5, 2020.
18. ACEP. Delivery of Emergency Care in Rural Settings: An Information Paper. Available at: https://www.acep.org/globalassets/sites/acep/blocks/section-blocks/rural/delivery-of-emergency-care-in-rural--settings.pdf. Last reviewed August 2017. Accessed November 5, 2020.
19. Greenwood-Ericksen MB, Kocher K. Trends in emergency department use by rural and urban populations in the United States. *JAMA Netw Open*. 2019;2(4):e191919.
20. ACEP. The Impact of Unreimbursed Care on the Emergency Physician. Available at: https://www.acep.org/administration/reimbursement/the-impact-of-unreimbursed-care-on-the-emergency-physician/. Accessed November 5, 2020.
21. Groth H, House H, Overton R, Deroo E. Board-certified emergency physicians comprise a minority of the emergency department workforce in Iowa. *West J Emerg Med*. 2013;14(2):186–190.

22. Upper Midwest Rural Health Research Center: Policy Brief. Rural Emergency Department Staffing: Potential Implications for the Quality of Emergency Care Provided in Rural Areas. 2007. Available at: http://rhrc.umn.edu/wp-content/files_mf/caseyedstaffing.pdf. Accessed November 5, 2020.

23. Ferguson J, Walshe K. The quality and safety of locum doctors: a narrative review. *J R Soc Med.* 2019;112(11):462–471.

24. Joseph JW, Davis S, Wilker EH, et al. Modelling attending physician productivity in the emergency department: a multicentre study. *Emerg Med J.* 2018;35:317–322.

25. Wagner M, Wolf S, Promes S, et al. Duty hours in emergency medicine: balancing patient safety, resident wellness, and the resident training experience: a consensus response to the 2008 Institute of Medicine Resident Duty Hours Recommendations. *Acad Emerg Med.* 2010;17(9):1004–1011.

26. Shanafelt, T., Noseworthy, J. Executive leadership and physician well-being: nine organizational strategies to promote engagement and reduce burnout. *Mayo Clin Proc.* Special Article. 2017;92(1):129–146.

27. RegisteredNursing.Org. What is an ER nurse. Available at: https://www.registerednursing.org/specialty/emergency-room-nurse/. Accessed November 5, 2020.

28. ED Nurse Salary and Career. Available at: https://nurse.org/articles/emergency-room-er-nurse-salary/. 2020. Accessed November 5, 2020.

29. Center for Disease Control and Prevention: National Center for Health Statistics. Emergency Department Visits. Available at: https://www.cdc.gov/nchs/fastats/emergency-department.htm. 2017. Accessed November 5, 2020.

30. Gao YX, Song YB, Gu ZJ, et al. Video versus direct laryngoscopy on successful first-pass endotracheal intubation in ICU patients. *World J Emerg Med.* 2018;9(2):99–104.

31. Burke LG, Wild RC, Orav EJ, Hsia RY. Are trends in billing for high-intensity emergency care explained by changes in services provided in the emergency department? An observational study among US Medicare beneficiaries. *BMJ Open.* 2018;8(1): e019357.

32. Rosenblatt RA, Hart LG. Physicians and rural America. *West J Med.* 2000;173(5):348–351.

33. Whitson MR, Mayo PH. Ultrasonography in the emergency department. *Crit Care.* 2016;20(1):227.

34. Hall M, Omer T, Moore C, et al. Cost effectiveness of the cardiac component of the focused assessment of sonography in trauma examination in blunt trauma. *Acad Emerg Med.* 2016; 23(4): 371–513.

35. Singer AJ, Blanda M, Cronin K. Comparison of nasal tampons for the treatment of epistaxis in the emergency department: a randomized controlled trial. *Ann Emerg Med.* 2005;45(2):134–139.

36. Mathiasen R, Cruz R. Prospective, randomized controlled clinical trial of a novel matrix hemostatic sealant in patients with acute anterior epistaxis. *Laryngoscope.* 2005;115:899–902.

37. ACEP: How-We-Serve: Sections: Telemedicine. Telemedicine in Emergency Medicine: A Primer. Available at: https://www.acep.org/how-we-serve/sections/telehealth/. Accessed November 5, 2020.

38. ACEP Emergency Telemedicine Section: Telemedicine Primer. Available at: https://www.acep.org/globalassets/uploads/uploaded-files/acep/membership/sections-of-membership/telemd/acep-telemedicine-primer.pdf. Accessed November 5, 2020.

39. Hollander J, Carr B. Perspective: virtually perfect? Telemedicine for COVID-19. *N Engl J Med.* 2020;382:1679–1681.

40. Fanburg J, Walzman J. Telehealth and the law: the challenge of reimbursement. *Medical Economics.* 2018.

41. Miller K, Hailey J, Holmes G, et al. The effect of rural hospital closures on emergency medical service response and transport times. *Health Serv Res.* 2020;55(2):288–300.

42. AHA Hospital Statistics, 2018 Ed. Health Forum LLC. 201813.

43. Rural Health Information Hub. Critical Access Hospitals—Introduction. Available at: https://www.ruralhealthinfo.org/topics/critical-access-hospitals. Accessed June 8, 2018.

44. National Rural Health Resource Center. Critical Access Hospital Finance 101. Updated June 2017.

45. Dalton K, Slifkin R, Poley S, Fruhbeis M. Choosing to convert to critical access hospital status. *Health Care Financ Rev.* 25(1):115–132. 2003. PMID: 1499769.

46. Thomas S, Pink G, Reiter K. Trends in financial distress among rural hospitals from 2015–2019. The Cecil G. Sheps Center for Health Services Research. The University of North Carolina. 2019. Available at: www.shepcenter.unc.edu/programs-projects/rural-health. Accessed November 5, 2020.

47. Pink G, Thompson K, Howard H, Holmes M. Geographic variation in the 2016 profitability of urban and rural hospitals. NC Rural Health Research Program. The Cecil G. Sheps Center for Health Services Research. The University of North Carolina. 2018. Available at: www.shepcenter.unc.edu/programs-projects/rural-health. Accessed November 5, 2020.

48. Kaufman B, Thomas S, Pink G, et al. The rising rate of rural hospital closures. *J Rural Health.* 2015;32(1).

49. 170 Rural Hospital Closures: January 2005-Present. More Information—Sheps Center. 2020. Available at: https://www.shepscenter.unc.edu/programs-projects/rural-health/rural-hospital-closures/rural-hospital-closures/. Accessed November 5, 2020.

50. Zibulewsky J. The Emergency Medical Treatment and Active Labor Act (EMTALA): what it is and what it means for physicians. *Proc (Bayl Univ Med Cent).* 2001;14(4):339–346.

51. Williamson HA, Rosenblatt RA, Hart LG. Physician staffing of small rural hospital emergency departments: rapid change and escalating cost. *J Rural Health.* 1992;8(3):171–177.

52. AMA Resolutions: July 2019. International Medical Graduates Section 2019 Annual Meeting Summary of Actions. Available at: https://www.ama-assn.org/system/files/2019-07/a19-imgs-summary-actions.pdf. Accessed November 5, 2020.

53. American Board of Emergency Medicine. ABEM History. Available at: https://www.abem.org/public/about-abem/abem-history. Accessed November 5, 2020.

54. American Academy of Emergency Medicine. History. Available at: https://www.aaem.org/about-us/our-values/history. Accessed November 5, 2020.

55. American Board of Physician Specialties. Board Certification in Emergency Medicine. Available at: https://www.abpsus.org/emergency-medicine. Accessed November 5, 2020.

56. EMRA match data. 2020. Available at: https://www.emra.org/students/newsletter-articles/em-match-2020-by-the-numbers/. Accessed November 5, 2020.

57. Urban K. Patient Visits Higher at Rural Emergency Departments. University of Michigan, "M" Health Lab. 2019. Available at: https://labblog.uofmhealth.org/industry-dx/patient-visits-higher-at-rural-emergency-departments. Accessed November 5, 2020.

58. Health Resources & Services Administration. Rural Hospital Programs. Available at: https://www.hrsa.gov/rural-health/rural-hospitals/index.html. Accessed November 5, 2020.

59. Blazer E. Viewpoint: emergency medicine doesn't need more residencies. *Emerg Med News.* 2019;41(2):6–7.

60. NCCPA 2013 Statistical Profile of Certified Physician Assistants. An Annual Report of the National Commission on Certification of Physician Assistant. Available at: https://prodcmsstoragesa.blob.core.windows.net/uploads/files/2013StatisticalProfileofCertifiedPhysicianAssistants-AnAnnualReportoftheNCCPA.pdf.

61. AANP. Number of Nurse Practitioners Hits New Record High. 2018. Available at: https://www.aanp.org/news-feed/number-of-nurse-practitioners-hits-new-record-high.

62. Kacik A. Nurse practitioner workforce doubles amid primary-care push. *Modern Healthcare*. 2020. Available at: https://www.modernhealthcare.com/providers/nurse-practitioner-workforce-doubles-amid-primary-care-push. Accessed November 5, 2020.

63. NCCPA 2017 Statistical Profile of Certified Physician Assistants PA's. Available at: https://prodcmsstoragesa.blob.core.windows.net/uploads/files/2017StatisticalProfileofCertifiedPhysicianAssistants%206.27.pdf. Accessed November 5, 2020.

64. AANP. Nurse Practitioner Role Grows to More Than 270,000. 2019. Available at: https://www.aanp.org/news-feed/nurse-practitioner-role-continues-to-grow-to-meet-primary-care-provider-shortages-and-patient-demands. Accessed November 5, 2020.

65. Vestal C. Nurse practitioners slowly gain autonomy. *Kaiser Health News*. July 19, 2013. Available at: https://khn.org/news/stateline-nurse-practitioners-scope-of-practice/. Accessed November 5, 2020.

66. Rappleye E. 28 States with full practice authority for NP's. *Becker's Hospital Review*. December 23, 2019. Available at: https://www.beckershospitalreview.com/hospital-physician-relationships/28-states-with-full-practice-authority-for-nps.html. Accessed November 5, 2020.

67. Cheney C. More states pushing for autonomy in scope-of-practice battle. *HealthLeaders*. 2019. Available at: https://www.healthleadersmedia.com/clinical-care/more-states-pushing-autonomy-scope-practice-battle. Accessed November 5, 2020.

68. Porter S. Study Reveals Troubling Test Scores of Assistant Physicians, Data Show Low First-time USMLE Pass Rates for Holders of New Missouri License. *AAFP*. November 9, 2018. https://www.aafp.org/news/practice-professional-issues/20181109asstphys.html. Accessed November 5, 2020.

69. Association of Medical Doctor Assistant Physicians. SB718, The 2017 Assistant Physician Modified Provisions. 2019. Available at: https://assistantphysicianassociation.com/news. Accessed November 5, 2020.

70. Welch C, Augustine J, Camargo CA Jr, Reese C. Emergency department performance measures and benchmarking summit: the consensus statement. *Acad Emerg Med*. 2006;13(10):1074–1080.

71. Freess D. ACEP Task Force Examining Collaboration with Advanced Practice Providers, American College of Emergency Physicians. *ACEPNow*. July 17, 2019. Available at: https://www.acepnow.com/article/acep-task-force-examining-collaboration-with-advanced-practice-providers/. Accessed November 5, 2020.

72. Wadman MC, Clark TR, Kupas DF, et al. Rural Clinical experiences for emergency medicine residents curriculum template. *Acad Emerg Med*. 2012;19(11):1287–1293.

73. Wiborg A, Widder B. Teleneurology to improve stroke care in rural areas. *Stroke*. 2003;34:2951–2956.

74. Dharmar M, Romano PS, Kuppermann N, et al. Impact of critical care telemedicine consultations on children in rural emergency departments. *Crit Care Med*. 2013;41(10):2388–2395.

75. American Academy of Family Physicians. Recommended Curriculum Guidelines for Family Medicine Residents. Urgent and Emergent Care. Available at: http://www.aafp.org/dam/AAFP/documents/medical_education_residency/program_directors/Reprint285_Urgent.pdf. Accessed November 5, 2020.

76. American College of Surgeons, Committee on Trauma. *Resources for Optimal Care of the Injured Patient*. Chicago, IL: American College of Surgeons; 2014.

77. American College of Surgeons. Inspiring Quality: Highest Standards. 7. Available at: https://www.facs.org/quality-programs/trauma/education/rttdc. Accessed November 5, 2020.

78. ARC-PA. Accreditation Review Commission on Education for the Physician Assistant, Inc. Available at: http://www.arc-pa.org/accreditation/postgraduate-programs/accreditation-process/. Accessed November 5, 2020.

79. American College of Emergency Physician Board of Directors Information Paper: Advanced Practice Providers (Physician Assistant and Nurse Practitioner) Medical-Legal Issues. 2016.

80. Society of Emergency Medicine Physician Assistants, Standards for Postgraduate Training of Emergency Medicine Physician Assistants. 2012.

81. Freess D. ACEP Task Force Examining Collaboration with Advanced Practice Providers, American College of Emergency Physicians. *ACEPNow*. 2019. Available at: https://www.acepnow.com/article/acep-task-force-examining-collaboration-with-advanced-practice-providers/. Accessed May 20, 2020.

INFORMATICS

SECTION 5

CHAPTER 63

INTRODUCTION TO CLINICAL INFORMATICS

Ali S. Raja

Technology, in the form of comprehensive electronic health record (EHR) systems, has transformed processes and practices in emergency departments (EDs). It is critical that nurse and physician directors are knowledgeable about clinical informatics and EHR regulations. They must have the requisite knowledge and skills to understand the clinical context of EHR design, implementation, and maintenance. Section 5, Informatics provides ED leaders with the resources and skills necessary to understand, operationalize, and measure the success of ED information technology implementation.

A DYNAMICALLY CHANGING ENVIRONMENT

The American Recovery and Reinvestment Act of 2009, and more specifically the Health Information Technology for Economic and Clinical Health (HITECH) Act, created the economic and policy challenge to medicine to implement EHRs. Since then, the rapid implementation of EHRs by hospitals has dramatically changed the ED, and the positive and negative consequences of these systems continue to present challenges and opportunities for ED clinical leadership. Hospital executives expect physicians to participate in the successful implementation of EHRs and to be responsible for governance of clinical content, order sets, and decision support rules.

An EHR brings many new tools and techniques into the ED. The old white board becomes an electronic tracking board, visible to anyone with a display device (e.g., personal computer [PC], laptop, mobile phone). Information about processes of care is presented in real time. The pen and paper of a documentation system give way to electronic templates, keyboards, and voice recognition software. Computerized provider order entry systems link physicians directly to lab, imaging, and nursing, eliminating the need for a paper chart and unit secretary to enter orders. The benefits of clinical decision support are balanced by a myriad of potential unintended consequences on both workflow and physician burnout. A new set of skills is required to manage the impact of EHR on processes, productivity, patient and clinician satisfaction, and quality measures.

The complexity and brevity of the ED encounter elevates the importance of communicating the patient's health status and the overall plan to all parties quickly and effectively. It is difficult, if not impossible, to fully and effectively communicate with other clinicians (e.g., inpatient teams, primary care physicians, and specialists) when patients' electronic records are inaccessible to them. Interoperability has become an essential aspect of an organization's informatics strategy and key to the EHR. Department leaders must balance the desire to have efficient systems (best-of-breed) with the enterprise requirements for achieving the overall goals and organizational mission.

CLINICAL INFORMATICS

I am fain to sum up with an urgent appeal for adopting . . . Some uniform system of publishing records of hospitals. There is a growing conviction that in all hospitals, even in those which are best conducted, there is a great and unnecessary waste of life . . . In attempting to arrive at the truth, I have applied everywhere for information, but in scarcely an instance have I been able to obtain hospital records fit for any purposes of comparison . . . If wisely used, these improved statistics would tell us more of the relative values of particular operations and modes of treatment than we have means of ascertaining at present.

—Florence Nightingale, 1863[1]

Despite Florence Nightingale's lament in 1863, the state of hospital information management scarcely changed until the end of the 20th century. Two major circumstances influenced a new perspective. The first was technology; after the 1940s, computer technology evolved at an astonishing rate, from mainframes in the 1950s and 1960s to PCs in the 1970s, to the cell phones and tablets we use today. The Internet dates back to only the 1990s, and it spearheaded a technology revolution that paralleled an information revolution.

Second, health-care systems became increasingly expected to provide better outcomes, better service, and improved patient safety. Governments, payers, and patients expected higher accountability and transparency, and improved information management through a transformed medical record was considered key to meeting those goals. As physician and nurse leaders, we cannot ignore this key dimension of our specialties, and we must become skilled at navigating the complexity of technology in order to integrate it into our practice.

EMERGENCY MEDICINE CLINICAL INFORMATICS

Emergency medicine has been at the forefront of clinical informatics. In 1992, the American College of Emergency Physicians (ACEP) Board of Directors approved the creation of the section for computers in emergency medicine evolving into the Section of Emergency Medicine Informatics. The American Academy of Emergency Medicine Board approved an informatics subcommittee in 2006. Subsequently, the Society for Academic Emergency Medicine (SAEM) created an Academic Informatics Section. All three serve as fora for their members to share, discuss, and advocate for informatics issues impacting emergency medicine.

The importance of informatics in emergency medicine was reaffirmed during a 2004 SAEM Consensus Conference: Developing Consensus in Emergency Medicine Information Technology. Attendees from a number of emergency medicine organizations jointly published 10 recommendations that year; key among them was the recognition of the need for informatics leadership.

In keeping with this recommendation, a modern full-service ED should identify nurse and physician leaders from within the department to guide its informatics efforts. These leaders should be closely tied to clinical patient care to fully experience the impact that informatics has on their frontline teams. Acute awareness of the operational and clinical needs allows these leaders to support usability and efficiency, while simultaneously focusing on data collection.

CLINICAL INFORMATICS RESOURCES

Practicing emergency physicians interested in clinical informatics have a number of educational and professional resources available to them. These resources provide a variety of opportunities to enhance skills and knowledge; they include:

- *American Medical Informatics Association (AMIA)*: A national organization with regular meetings and a monthly journal—*The Journal of the American Medical Informatics Association*.
- *ACEP Emergency Medicine Informatics Section*: Membership benefits of the section include access to an informatics listserv for posting of questions and topics of interest to informaticians.
- *SAEM Academic Informatics Section*: For academic emergency physicians, membership benefits of this section include a listserv, mentorship, and the opportunity to participate in position papers for the Society.
- *ACEP/AMIA/Oregon Health and Science University 10 × 10 Informatics Education Program*: A 16-week online course culminating in an optional on-site session during the ACEP Scientific Assembly.
- *Accreditation Council for Graduate Medical Education (ACGME) Fellowships*: At the time of this publication, there were more than 40 ACGME-approved fellowship programs. These informatic fellowships are formal 2-year programs sponsored by nine specialties, with most willing to consider fellows with any primary specialty training. All ACGME-approved programs can lead to subspecialty certification in clinical informatics.
- *Other informatics education resources*: A number of universities and medical schools have developed graduate programs in informatics leading to a master's or doctor of philosophy (PhD) degree.

SECTION FOCUS

The authors of the subsequent chapters within this section focus on the key areas of informatics impacting emergency medicine. Each chapter written by experts in the field defines why each topic is important to supporting ED operations.

- *Electronic Health Records*: Todd B. Taylor, MD, FACEP and James C. McClay, MD, MS, FACEP, FAMIA, describe electronic EHR systems and ED-specific components, explore ways to enhance EHR utility, reflect on the implications of the HITECH Act, and emphasize the importance of continued support and evolution of EDIS.
- *EHR Tracking Systems*: Zachary Jarou, MD, and Thomas Spiegel, MD, MBA, MS, evaluate tracking systems (e.g., patient, equipment, staff), their role in supporting daily ED operations, and the collection of key data to support process flow metrics.
- *EHR Documentation Systems*: John Brown, MD, and Zachary Jarou, MD, describe the current state of EHR clinical documentation tools. They define the keys for success, the impact on processes and productivity, and how they create credible documents for communication, reimbursement, and risk management.
- *Computerized Provider Order Entry and Clinical Decision Support*: Brian Fengler, MD; Nicholas Genes, MD, PhD; and I describe the benefits and risks of these systems as they are deployed in the ED.

- ***Data Acquisition and Analysis:*** Sean Michael, MD, MBA, FACEP, and Jennifer Wiler, MD, MBA, FACEP, discuss data sources, quality, collection, analysis, and presentation as well as the infrastructure necessary to support this work.
- ***Essential Support Technologies:*** Sujal Mandavia, MD, and Phillip F. Gruber, MD, review other technologies that impact successful ED management, from mobile devices and voice recognition to patient kiosks and portals.
- ***Social Media in Medicine:*** Matthew Richard Klein, MD; Ryan Stanton, MD; and Michael Gottlieb, MD, take a look at the hot topic of social media in medicine, including its use in education, wellness, and career advancement as well as its inherent potential risks.
- ***New Technologies and Applications in Emergency Medicine:*** Timothy Boardman, MD, and Gita Pensa, MD, describe cutting-edge advances in mobile applications and diagnostic technologies as well as reference and productivity tools used to advance the care of patients in the ED.
- ***Telemedicine in Emergency Medicine:*** Judd Hollander, MD, and Rahul Sharma, MD, MBA, describe digital health and telemedicine, including a proven framework for the establishment of a telemedicine program from the ground-up and use cases for its success.

REFERENCE

1. Nightingale F. *Notes on Hospitals*. London: Longman, Green, Longman, Roberts, and Green; 1863:175.

CHAPTER 64

ELECTRONIC HEALTH RECORDS

Todd B. Taylor, James C. McClay

Emergency care is complex, information intensive, and technology driven. In fact, the necessary body of knowledge for patient care in the emergency department (ED) far exceeds the ability of individual practitioners to manage without multiple electronic devices.[1] This is further complicated in the context of managing patients without aggregated, organized, and well-presented data—otherwise known as relevant "information."[2] Health information technology (HIT) has been touted to increase efficiency, enhance quality, and reduce costs (**Box 64.1**). However, since much focus has been centered on the development of the electronic health record (EHR), the promise remains largely unrealized.[3-5] This prompts the question, what can be done to finally realize benefits from the huge investment of time, effort, and funding for HIT?[6]

This chapter explores the history of EHRs, with a focus on ED information systems (EDISs); current EHR state-of-the-art technologies, with a focus on enhancement and utilization; and emerging technologies that promise to deliver on the HIT investment (**Box 64.2**).

HEALTH INFORMATION TECHNOLOGY

For historical context, it is worth briefly exploring how we arrived at the current state of HIT. As early as 2001, an Institute of Medicine report outlined concerns of decreased quality, excess costs, and avoidable errors, calling for new tools and methods to manage health-care processes and knowledge.[10] This led some to recommend universal adoption of HIT, particularly EHR systems.[11] Advanced interconnected EHRs promised streamlined care coordination, personalized health care, and improved processes.

With the passage of the American Recovery and Reinvestment Act of 2009, Congress made a $49 billion "bet" that increased the implementation of HIT (including computers, software, and network connections throughout the health-care system) would improve quality and efficiency of health care in the United States.[12] This effort became known as the Health Information Technology for Economic and Clinical Health (HITECH) Act, with an express purpose to accelerate the adoption of HIT as a method of improving the quality, safety, and efficiency of health care.[13]

HITECH Methodology

HITECH started with monetary incentives via enhanced Medicare and Medicaid payments, then, in 2016, it began levying penalties for noncompliance. It required the use of EHRs that were certified to meet requirements put forth by the Office of the National Coordinator (ONC) and certified by an ONC-authorized testing and certification body via a testing process defined by the National Institute of Standards and Technology. Further, the certified EHR technology had to be used in a "meaningful way," extensively spelled out in published regulations called "meaningful use."

> **BOX 64.1 ■ HEALTH INFORMATION TECHNOLOGY DEFINED**
>
> Health information technology is defined as "the application of information processing involving both computer hardware and software that deals with the storage, retrieval, sharing, and use of health care information, data, and knowledge for communication and decision-making."[7]

> **BOX 64.2 ■ EHR, EMR, AND EDIS**
>
> Although often used interchangeably, these terms have distinct meanings.[8]
>
> An EDIS may be a subset of an EHR (i.e., a module of an enterprise hospital-wide electronic medical record [EMR]) or a standalone application (aka "Best-in-Breed") with or without an interface to the hospital EMR. In short, EDIS refers to electronic record functions relevant to the ED, which may rely upon systems from many other departments.
>
> Early EMRs were the first to begin to integrate various segregated departmental information systems into a single system used mostly for clinical purposes. In time, they became more highly integrated, subsuming more and more functions and even expanding outside of the hospital environment.
>
> To better reflect the increasing breadth of features and functions, the term EHR came to mean everything the EMR is, plus a broader view of patient care, administrative and workflow functions, and a secure platform to share data across the entire health care ecosystem, including patients and entities external to the hospital.[9]

Under HITECH, emergency physicians were not listed as "eligible providers." As such, the ED had little direct involvement with the program and only minimally contributed to the hospital's compliance efforts with Meaningful Use. While the legislation may have accelerated the development and implementation of some key HIT functions, it inhibited others (**Box 64.3**).[14]

In a cruel twist of fate, while not directly focused on EDISs, HITECH negatively impacted nearly every ED in the United States. In the effort to meet Meaningful Use criteria, many hospitals were forced to update or replace their EHRs. In most instances, that meant the loss of time-tested, stand-alone "best-in-breed" systems, which were rapidly replaced by certified enterprise EMR/EHR "ED modules."[15] In addition, virtually all the new modules had much less functionality than the "best-in-breed" EDISs that EDs had come to rely upon.[16] From an HIT functionality and efficiency standpoint, this set progress back at least 10 years.

> **BOX 64.3 ■ HITECH IMPACT ON EDs**
>
> 1. Displacement of a functional, well-established EDIS toward enterprise EHR ED modules with substantially less functionality
> 2. Diversion of hospital IT and vendor resources toward meeting meaningful use criteria
> 3. Substantial consolidation in the EDIS and enterprise EHR industry (resulting in fewer vendors to choose from)
> 4. Minimal to no input from emergency physicians as to the selection of the EHR they are destined to use

> **BOX 64.4 ■ EMERGENCY PHYSICIANS UNDER MACRA**
>
> 1. Elimination of the longstanding, counterproductive sustainable growth rate formula that would have resulted in major Medicare rate cuts for clinicians
> 2. Emergency physicians are now eligible for MIPS but also subject to penalties
> 3. Advancing Care Information Performance Category is worth 25% of MIPS final score
> 4. Performance measures must still be submitted via certified EHR technology
> 5. Emergency physicians now find themselves struggling to acquire sufficient data to meet MIPS reporting requirements, and many are forced to largely rely on a Quality Clinical Data Registry to submit quality measures to avoid MIPS penalties

Enter MACRA

By 2015, a decade of the HITECH program had led to the adoption of at least a basic EHR by 84% of nonfederal acute-care hospitals.[17] However, a substantial number of institutions failed to meet the deadline for Stage 2 Meaningful Use criteria.[18] Ongoing criticism of the program led to replacement of Meaningful Use with the Advancing Care Information performance category in the Medicare Access and CHIP Reauthorization Act of 2015 (MACRA) as part of the Merit-based Incentive Payment System (MIPS).[19]

Ongoing legislative updates continue to impact EHR requirements, often adding incrementally to user burden. Suffice to say, hospitals and EDs must be prepared to adjust as policymakers seek to drive health care in a direction often intended to suit evolving political ideology (**Box 64.4**).

Electronic Health Record Systems

Despite technical differences, for the purposes of this chapter, we will consider EMR and EHR to be analogous with respect to the ED. Further, we will refer to the specific ED functions of the EHR or a "best-in-breed" system as the EDIS. Electronic health record systems include a collection of historical patient data, information-management tools, data linkages, and knowledge sources to organize, interpret, and respond to the data.[20] Because the ED is a unique care setting, specialized tools to manage these data have evolved into a subset of functions called EDISs.

BRIEF HISTORY OF THE EDIS

Emergency departments have traditionally relied upon the hospital's main information system for basic administrative functions like registration (demographic/billing data), computer provider order entry (CPOE), results reporting, and visit tracking. Similar to most health-care environments in the past, EDs were otherwise largely paper-based. One early exception was a manual electronic "whiteboard" (grease board) for patient tracking in the ED.[22,23] Subsequently, several of the early EDISs were merely computer-based electronic tracking boards, some of which became quite sophisticated. Of note, virtually all of the early EDISs were created by zealous emergency physicians. Over time, some of these stand-alone systems included additional functionality that allowed them to serve as comprehensive ED management tools; a few achieved modest commercial success. There have been multiple commercially available EDISs, although relatively few had more than a handful of installations. These became known as the "best in breed." As noted, the HITECH Act signaled a death knell for stand-alone EDISs, and by 2019, there were only two best-in-breed EDIS vendors clinging to life, representing less than 1% of the EDIS market share combined. As noted, this phenomenon had a dramatic negative impact on EDIS usability and functionality.

Two notable activities contributed to the early advancement of EDISs. In 1992, ACEP formed a special interest group, originally called the Computer Section, dedicated to the advancement and promotion of HIT. Renamed the Section for Emergency Medicine Informatics (SEMI), the group now boasts more than 400 emergency physician members. SEMI's landmark inaugural project, *A View of the Emergency Department of the Future*, remains as relevant today as it was 25 years ago.[24]

From 1995 to 2010, the Pennsylvania ACEP chapter held an annual EDIS symposium that brought together experts in HIT, vendors, and emergency physicians hungry for IT solutions. As the EDIS/EMR market consolidated due to HITECH, the need for this meeting waned. Reality had set in; for the most part, ED physicians would no longer have significant input regarding the selection of the IT tools they would now be forced to use.

Consolidation has also been significant for the enterprise EMR market. As of April 2020, three vendors (EPIC = 29%, Cerner = 26% and MediTech = 17%) control 72% of the entire hospital EMR market. For large hospitals (>500 beds), EPIC (58%) and Cerner (27%) own 85% of the market.[25]

What Is a Modern EDIS?

In 2005, the HL7 Emergency Care Work Group (ECWG) developed the EDIS Functional Profile.[26] It described the EDIS as "an extended EHR system used to manage data in support of ED patient care and operations. The functions of an EDIS may be provided by a single application or multiple applications" (**Box 64.5**).[27]

In 2010, the EDIS was "designed specifically to manage data and workflow in support of ED patient care and operations."[28] The ECWG recognized that an EDIS may be assembled from components by different vendors or even homegrown software. However, in order to realize the full benefit of an EDIS, "all components, modules, and applications within an EDIS should respond to users in a well-integrated fashion."[29] This interoperability should extend to integration with the host EHR system at the local hospital or health system.

Therefore, the EDIS should be viewed as a set of features and functions operating on a common set of patient and departmental data. These functions can be subdivided into

---

BOX 64.5 ■ FUNCTIONAL DESCRIPTION OF EHRS[11]

1. Longitudinal collection of electronic health information for and about persons, where health information is defined as information pertaining to the health of an individual or health care provided to an individual
2. Immediate electronic access to person- and population-level information by authorized, and only authorized, users
3. Provision of knowledge and decision-support that enhance the quality, safety, and efficiency of patient care
4. Support of efficient processes for health-care delivery

TABLE 64.1 ■ EDIS Functions

Core Functions[29]	Administrative Functions[21]
Patient entry and triage	Hospital/departmental statistical metrics
Clinical documentation (physician, nurse, ancillary)	Coding/billing
Results reporting	Integration with public health and other registries
Document management	Disaster management
Order entry	Disease surveillance
Decision support and risk management	Integration of patient satisfaction data
Patient and resource tracking	
Discharge management	

direct patient care requirements, departmental operations, and administrative functions (**Table 64.1**). No current EHR software excels in all of these areas, so certain compromises are inherent in any system. Nevertheless, the purpose of an EDIS is to support all users and all features of an EHR, which is important for a complete application package. As such, careful consideration of the local environment is necessary to balance the local needs with the particular system offerings.

Various stakeholders may place different weight on various functions depending on their points of view. Departmental operations and direct patient care support should be considered primary uses. Direct-care providers are most affected by their ability to utilize the system to support workflow as patients are moved through the care process.

Providers must maintain a contextual awareness of the overall department activities. They must keep track of patients, respond to urgent needs, and generally maintain the departmental flow. As such, providers depend on the unique departmental functions embodied in the EDIS tracking component. Traditionally, the remaining uses of the EDIS have been considered secondary (**Table 64.2**). However, this may be changing due to the integration of clinical decision support systems (CDSS) and the emergence of artificial intelligence (AI).[30,31] As these new technologies develop, they will become primary functions, indispensable to patient care and departmental efficiency.

In addition, administrators must be able to analyze staffing and resource requirements; researchers need to retrieve data across multiple patients; and external (regulatory) and affiliated (billing) agencies must obtain data organized into reports. These administrative functions may be met by the EDIS and/or the larger hospital EHR system. There are also additional core functions, such as data analysis, and uses that share characteristics with enterprise EHR systems.

TABLE 64.2 ■ EDIS Uses[20]

Primary Uses	Secondary Uses
Patient care delivery	Education
Patient care management	Regulation
Patient care support processes	Research
Financial and other administrative processes	Public health and disease surveillance
Patient self-management	Policy support

EDIS INTEGRATION AND INTEROPERABILITY

As part of the larger hospital environment, patient-care activities in the ED require coordination and integration with the rest of the health-care system, even beyond the walls of the hospital (**Figure 64.1**).[32] Up to 55% of hospital inpatients begin their stays in the ED, making the ability to share data between the EDIS and the hospital-wide EHR system critically important.[33]

For these reasons, hospital chief information officers tend to value integration, interoperability, and cost over ease of use or functionality. All EHRs have strengths and weaknesses, but physicians "report less intuitive interfaces and less efficient clinical functionality" in many enterprise products.[21] The problem is that these programs are not being developed for the end users (i.e., physicians). They are being developed for IT departments in hospitals so they can say they are using technology to get their Meaningful Use money.

In the current EHR market environment, ED physicians are typically not involved in choosing their EDIS. As such, it is important for physicians to optimize the systems they do have. There have been very reasonable successes and unmitigated disasters with exactly the same EDIS vendors. The differentiator is often in the implementation process and, subsequently, how the new system is maintained and optimized.

An EDIS must be customized to the local hospital and unique ED workflow environment, hospital preferences (e.g., pharmaceuticals), physician and staff preferences, and so on. Failing to do so means a very unsatisfactory EDIS experience. Yet, many EDs fail to do even the most basic customization in advance of an implementation or upgrade, instead leaving it to individual providers or IT "champions." In addition, very useful features are often either not purchased or fail to be implemented by IT for cost or expediency reasons. As a result, many EDs never achieve the full benefits of even a modest EDIS. Over time, resentment tends to grow, staff satisfaction declines, and productivity suffers.

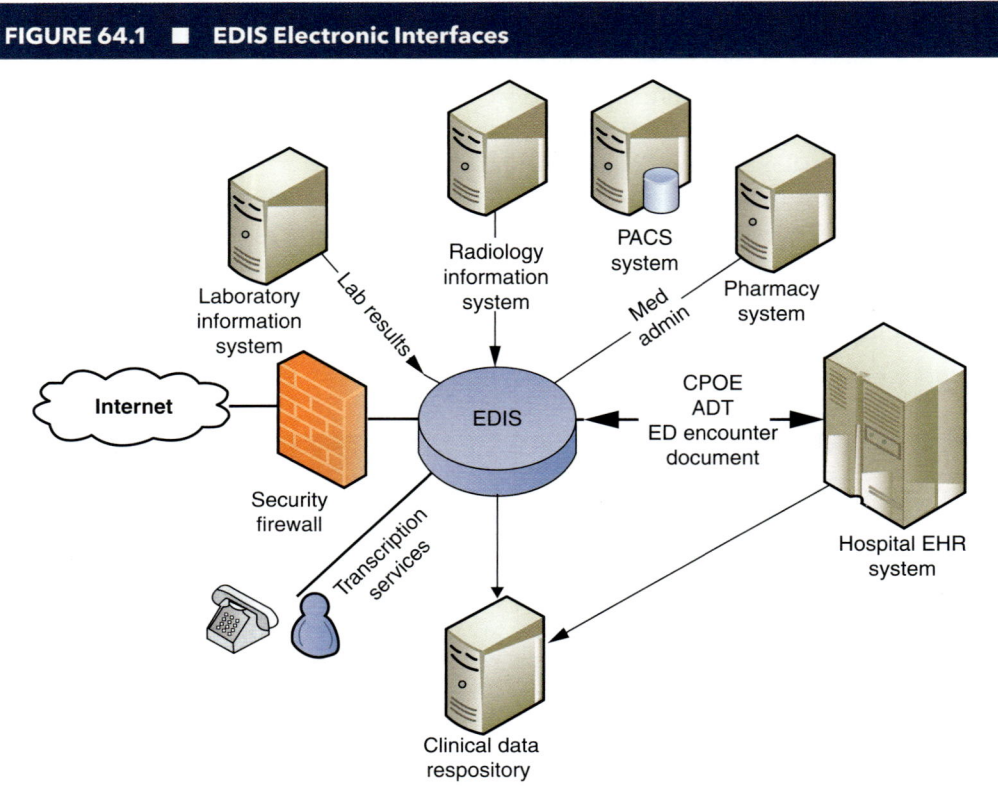

FIGURE 64.1 ■ EDIS Electronic Interfaces

> **BOX 64.6 ■ FAST HEALTHCARE INTEROPERABILITY RESOURCES**
>
> Fast Healthcare Interoperability Resources (FHIR), pronounced "fire," is a standard describing data formats and elements (known as resources) and an API for exchanging EHRs.

While the issue of EDIS interoperability has largely been eliminated by the transition to enterprise EHRs, it remains an issue for a host of third-party productivity solutions that are not native to the EHR. This often leads to frustration by clinicians who feel thwarted by hospital IT departments any time a new useful software gadget comes along but is felt to be too costly to integrate.

In recent years, EHR data export has become fairly straightforward due to adoption of standards. However, there are multiple types of HIT standards, which are a related challenge in addition to cost. An emerging standard, Fast Healthcare Interoperability Resources (FHIR) has the potential to reduce cost by employing application programming interface (API) technology, opening a door into the EHR at low cost (**Box 64.6**).[34] But this specification relies on EHR vendors making APIs available. So, while promising, implementation of FHIR has been delayed by resistance from the vendor community. The recently enacted 21st Century Cures Act, signed into law in December 2016, specifically requires EHR vendors to support APIs "without special effort."[35] However, like all standards, FHIR has limitations, and its success remains to be demonstrated.

Bidirectional interoperability with third-party external systems, such as the import of (especially clinical) discrete data, remains problematic. For example, it may not make sense to have a digital blood pressure monitor, only to have a nurse manually enter the values into the EHR. But automating the input of this type of data can cause a variety of untoward consequences, including patient misidentification, spurious values, and data corruption. Often seemingly simple transactions are actually quite complex in the current world of HIT.

In summary, "Hospitals have a duty to patients, staff, and the community to provide HIT that is suitable for use in the ED. Health information technology should facilitate the delivery of patient care, conform to relevant standards, and comply with applicable privacy and security constructs to ensure the secure availability of relevant health-care information."[36]

Direct Patient Care, Medical Records, and Workflow Functions

The direct-care functions of an EDIS support the workflow of individual patients throughout the ED encounter and even prior to arrival (**Box 64.7**). Discreet functions include prehospital documentation, structured triage, nursing/physician documentation, order entry, results

> **BOX 64.7 ■ POTENTIAL BENEFITS OF AN EHR[37]**
>
> - Coordinate care
> - Improve communication between providers
> - Error checking/adverse drug event elimination
> - Quality improvement through CDSS
> - Monitor compliance
> - Facilitate patient education
> - Improve patients' access to their physicians

reporting, care planning, electronic prescribing, disposition planning, and patient education. Multiple providers are involved in transitioning patients from an ambulance provider, to intake/triage, to a room for assessment/treatment, to disposition. Yet, because every patient is different (simple to complex), this workflow must be flexible. Therein lies the challenge for the EDIS development and implementation. The workflow must provide support for documentation of findings across a large variety of conditions and circumstances. The EDIS must also ultimately collect numerous sources of data into a comprehensive ED record. These direct-care functions are very sensitive to good design and usability. Unfortunately, the current state-of-the-art in this respect is often poor and leads to the need for workarounds.

The EHR should support the maintenance of a longitudinal description of each individual patient's health status including, but not limited to, basic demographics, a problem list, past medical history, allergies, prescriptions, and prior diagnostic results. Ideally, this record is shared across the enterprise and community (e.g., via health information exchange) through integration and interoperability.

Nevertheless, the EDIS is organized around an individual ED encounter rather than the longitudinal patient record. While acute findings are recorded during the ED encounter, the EHR ideally should support access to longitudinal patient data. Information about the ED visit should include elements the chief complaint, history of present illness (HPI), physical examination findings, medical decision-making, and disposition plan. Relevant EHR longitudinal data may include a visit history, problem list, allergies, medications, prior diagnostic results, and so on. Integration of these two functions is fundamentally important.

CLINICAL DOCUMENTATION

With respect to the EDIS, nothing is more important nor more challenging than clinical documentation. The promise of EHR technology to enhance efficiency, reduce workload, improve patient care and safety, and reduce cost is yet to be realized. It has been estimated that the transition from paper templates or dictation to electronic documentation results in a sustained 10% to 20% decrease in physician productivity.[38] In fact, this overhead burden has increased to the point that Congress has tasked the US Department of Health and Human Services "to articulate a plan of action to reduce regulatory and administrative burden relating to the use of health IT and EHRs."[39]

Nevertheless, clinical documentation by physicians, nurses, and other ED staff is an essential EDIS function. It should permit quick, accurate, and complete documentation of observations and medical decision-making, reflecting exactly what the user wishes to convey without requiring redundancy. The key to documentation is the clinician's ability to leverage previous documentation; review, harmonize, or incorporate existing data related to the current visit; and finally, provide a summary of pertinent findings and medical decision-making.

While documentation is ideally completed contemporaneously, physicians often wait until the end of their shift to fully complete records. However, nurses and other personnel must document in tandem with patient care, since these data are utilized throughout the ED encounter. Therefore, it is important to view the state of completion for each chart by role while in use.

The documentation process should move seamlessly from patient to patient and be abandoned quickly if necessary without loss of work. Unfinished items should be plainly seen with a hard stop for critical missing items. The EDIS must support multiple authors, as two or more providers may need to document patient data at the same time.

Finally, although considered a secondary function, the correlation between documentation and coding/billing is unavoidable. Yet, the desire to achieve the maximal coded level of service often leads to overdocumentation that pollutes the medical record with useless verbiage. Nevertheless, a failure to achieve an appropriate coding level as supported by documentation has serious financial consequences.

Mitigating Electronic Documentation Overhead

Electronic documentation, with all of its promise, has its negative aspects, including decreasing the efficiency of the clinician and requiring more time in front of a computer and less time with the patient. Multiple programs and work-arounds have been developed to mitigate these inefficiencies.

Computer Template (Checkbox)

The computer template (checkbox) is the most common, yet most inefficient, type of documentation. It has the advantage of creating discrete data that can be checked against a variety of parameters (e.g., coded level of service, risk assessment, etc) and may also enhance research or quality measures. More sophisticated systems feature cascading menus to prompt consideration of subordinate details. But the biggest challenge of this method is that templates may force the provider into a linear path that does not follow ED workflow. The use of bedside tablets and electronic templates has been successful for some third-party documentation systems. An example is T-System EV™, which still enjoys significant EDIS market share as a stand-alone and third-party add-on documentation tool. Finally, while perhaps ideal for billing, the final output of more typical electronic templates tends to be inadequate for communicating patient care, often to the point of being almost useless.

Scribes

To address the challenge of template documentation, some have employed scribes to "check the boxes" while clinicians focus on patient care. Some clinicians even use two scribes: the first person remains behind to complete the chart, while the clinician moves on to the next patient with a second scribe. The term "scribe" is actually a misnomer. While they certainly document, they also serve as assistants, helping to organize data, track results, or even get the patient a pillow. The return on investment (ROI) for the use of scribes varies widely depending on ED characteristics, patient demographics, and how they are utilized. However, the typical ROI for a busy ED with a good scribe program is 100% or more. Improved provider satisfaction and decreased burnout are secondary, albeit very important, factors as well.[40]

Typed Free Text

Most EDISs offer the user the ability to enter typed free text for at least partial documentation. Adding comments can improve communication, albeit at the cost of efficiency (unless using a scribe). But for virtually all providers, typing an entire note is impractical. A technique from the early EDIS years was to utilize macros that would paste standard text in the record or create an entirely new one. The provider would then modify the text to match the actual clinical details. This was sometimes referred to as "charting by deletion." As one might imagine, it was fraught with opportunity for error and has largely been abandoned.

Speech Recognition and Natural Language Processing

Often inaccurately called voice recognition, speech recognition and natural language-processing technology leverages the ability of a machine to identify spoken words and phrases and then convert them to machine-readable format (text or commands). Often touted as an alternative to typing or transcription, this technology is hampered by error rates of 5%

to 10%, with virtually no document without at least one error.[41] This forces the provider to carefully edit the text. This may not be an issue for short passages; however, as an alternative for full documentation, this technology's time has not yet come. As with typed text, there are no discrete data unless the information is being used to complete an electronic template.

Dictation and Transcription

Cost notwithstanding, the tried-and-true method of dictation and transcription is the second-most efficient and by far the best method for communication. Unfortunately, due to cost, delay in availability, and lack of discrete data, it has largely fallen out of favor, at least for EDs.

Scanned Paper Template

Perhaps not surprising, scanned paper templates remain the most efficient method for documentation, although they suffer from poor (often illegible) communication. Yet, this method is one of the more popular ED documentation methods in use today. Various techniques have aimed to get the best of both worlds. For example, a special type of machine-readable coded paper with a preprinted template is able to translate checkmarks into a discrete machine-readable format; however, the cost of the paper and inaccuracy rate made this unworkable.

Blended Documentation Methodologies

Emergency departments tend to use a broad variety of ways to collect data. Certain data are only amenable to scanning (e.g., paper EMS report); other data types are suitable for templates (e.g., allergies, medications, review of systems, physical exam); still others use some sort of free text (HPI, medical decision-making, disposition). In such cases, perhaps the best option might be to use templates where they make sense and use free text for the remainder.

Visit Abstract

A prose (free text) visit summary of pertinent details can be the most useful part of the record, perhaps aside from coding/billing. Leveraging the blended data collection methods mentioned previously for the bulk of the record and then leveraging dictation/transcription, speech recognition, or typed text to create a brief, albeit meaningful bullet (i.e., what the next provider needs to know) might be conducive for optimal communication.

Patient-Provided Documentation

Finally, we often miss the opportunity to leverage tech-savvy patients by having them enter data via a well-designed app for a mobile device. Perhaps 50% of necessary data could be obtained in this way, including various required screenings (e.g., HPI, social history, and family medical history). For the most part, patients have nothing but time, which might pass a bit faster if they were engaged in this activity. This and other automated data-collection methods can help to significantly reduce the documentation burden that even modern EDISs impose.

CLINICAL DECISION SUPPORT SYSTEMS

A major promise of EHR use is to provide automated tools to help avoid errors and optimize care, with AI suggesting the best choices for the patient's management. Unfortunately, these objectives remain largely unrealized, as EHRs accumulate more data than anyone has time to review and in a format that cannot be efficiently processed.

One solution to this data glut is the broad application of CDSS, enabled by robust data aggregation/transformation and automated background analysis that produces near real-time information. As an analogy, consider autonomous vehicles (self-driving cars). The human occupant merely provides the destination, then the vehicle's decision-support system collects ambient data, analyzes the best route, monitors/reacts to changes along the way, and only alerts the occupant of any variances the system cannot handle.

To help better understand CDSS in the ED, it is helpful to consider the Society of Automotive Engineers automation levels (**Box 64.8**). Current EMR CDSSs are at or below level 0 and, at best, partial level 1. Level 0 examples might include allergy and adverse drug event (ADE) alerts, which have become fairly standard, but often suffer from alert fatigue due to poor implementation and reliance upon drug databases that are not well-designed for this purpose. Various other checklist-type CDSSs have been deployed but are hardly automated.

Emerging level 1 examples include third-party solutions that garner basic data from the EMR and help direct care by employing integrated clinical pathways. For example, the CDSS monitors various clinical parameters and warns of possible sepsis, then suggests further diagnostics and even treatment recommendations. More sophisticated systems can be integrated with the EDIS order entry system to avoid redundant steps.

In comparison, fully automatous vehicle (level 5) systems are actually much more complex than many ED care pathways. Consider a laceration: there are a finite number of variables that must be remembered and addressed multiple times a day. Yet how many times is a patient's tetanus status still not addressed? An automated system does not miss such details and further allows clinicians to focus on more important tasks.

Clinical knowledge management refers to the process and tools for encoding knowledge, such as order sets, protocols, and guideline components, into a CDSS system.[43] The CDSS is typically a rules-based process dependent on input of discrete patient data that offers user actions by the display of alerts, results, reminders, and workflow for the end user. The knowledge layer in an EDIS contains structures such as preconfigured order sets, structured vocabulary, documentation forms, and patient instructions. Modern EMRs typically have the ability to employ these components, but they are rarely preconfigured, and the task of customizing them for individual providers can be daunting. Some example CDSS tools allow individual- or departmental-configured alerts for out-of-range results, time events, and reminders of missed documentation components. A more sophisticated CDSS may

BOX 64.8 ■ LEVELS OF DRIVING AUTOMATION[42]

Level 0: Warnings—no sustained vehicle control

Level 1: Hands on—shared control of the vehicle, e.g., adaptive cruise control

Level 2: Hands off—fully automated control with driver monitoring and taking actions when necessary (i.e., not truly "hands off")

Level 3: Eyes off—fully automated control with driver ability to divert attention (watch a movie while in driver's seat); however, must still be prepared to intervene within a limited time when called upon

Level 4: Mind off—fully automated control with driver ability to completely divert attention (sleep); vehicle may abort the trip (pull over) if driver intervention necessary

Level 5: Steering wheel optional—no human intervention required at all

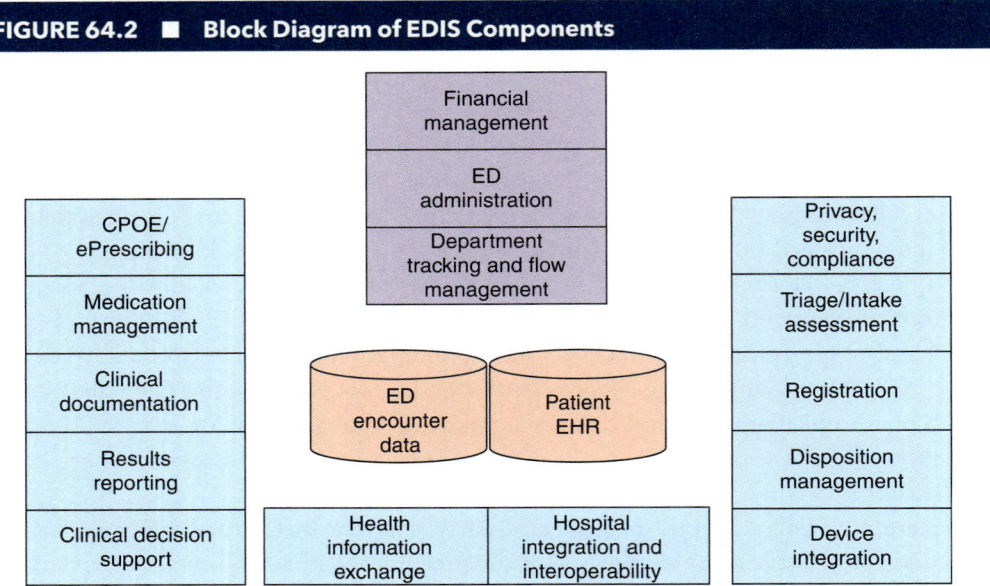

FIGURE 64.2 ■ Block Diagram of EDIS Components

recommend order sets, documentation forms, and discharge instructions. As noted, this is immature technology, and careful consideration must be given to the EDIS's ability to meet the department's needs (**Figure 64.2**).

Workflow changes may be necessary to support an efficient CDSS. For example, ADE functions are ineffective until both of the patient's allergies and medication lists have been entered, and such alerts are typically not retrospective. Other historical factors are also important, such as pregnancy status or diabetes, that may impact diagnostic tests or medication administration. These functions must be entered as early as possible in the ED workflow and delayed/post hoc entry must be avoided.

Ongoing CDSS maintenance and updates require special attention and resources that may not be available from the hospital IT department. Failing to apply appropriate resources to these activities is often the cause of EDIS inefficiency and user dissatisfaction. Further complicating CDSS is the fact that certain components are supplied by third-party vendors, such as drug databases used for drug–drug and drug–allergy interaction checking. These are updated regularly and require maintenance in and of themselves.

Administrative Functions

The EDIS must provide tools to manage ED resources and patient flow. Additionally, these tools must provide measurements, alerts, and reports to various stakeholders—both internal and external—and generate coding and billing information. The ED is a unique, unscheduled care setting without the ability to control external events. As a result, this complex, sometimes-chaotic environment requires robust tools to track multiple patients (often placed in hallways) and allocate resources. An effective system is necessary for providers and team leaders to monitor department status, constantly reprioritize and adjust workflow, and redeploy resources to acute needs (**Box 64.9**).

Analytics

Department dashboards are administrative views of key performance indicators derived from various tracking metrics. These typically include the number of patients in the waiting

> **BOX 64.9 ■ EDIS ADMINISTRATIVE FUNCTIONS**[44]
>
> 1. Patient flow management
> 2. Resource allocation (e.g., provider assignment)
> 3. Process metrics measurement and analysis
> 4. Regulatory compliance
> 5. Revenue cycle support
> 6. Maintain patient records, internal/external clinical documents and notes
> 7. Manage patient demographics, problem lists, medication lists, history
> 8. Present/manage care plans, guidelines forms, and protocols
> 9. Generate/record patient-specific instructions

room, awaiting an inpatient bed assignment, and so on. Relevant dashboards should be viewable on the main EDIS screen to communicate the status of patient flow. The dashboard may be configured to change colors to indicate changes in a patient's status. Department status should also be available to hospital administration as a means of anticipating increased inpatient occupancy and subsequent overcrowding. Some dashboards have become fairly sophisticated and evidenced-based, such as the National Emergency Department Overcrowding Score and Community Emergency Department Overcrowding Score.[45]

Administrative functions typically involve a post-hoc data analysis, with the ability to do patient- or complaint-specific reviews. Most vendors include standard reports, which may or may not meet a specific ED's needs. Billing and financial management is a key administrative use of clinical data, and standard vendor reports tend to focus on these. The EDIS may facilitate coding by providing feedback at the point-of-care for clinical documentation. The EDIS should transmit an accurate representation of the care delivered in the ED, so that billing can be done expeditiously. Mandated public health disease reporting may be an additional supported function; others include reporting for hospital administration, clinician profiling, staffing projections, and patient satisfaction. Disaster management and community-wide resource management can also be enhanced with an EDIS.

Security and Privacy

Security and privacy are closely related in health care and largely regulated by the Health Insurance Portability and Accountability Act of 1996 (HIPAA).[46] Security refers to how personal information is protected. Privacy relates to the rights individuals have to control their information and how it is used.

The HIPAA Security Rule requires appropriate administrative, physical, and technical safeguards to ensure the confidentiality, integrity, and security of electronic protected health information. The HIPAA Privacy Rule requires appropriate safeguards to protect the privacy of personal health information and sets limits and conditions on its uses and disclosures without patient authorization. It also gives patients rights regarding their health information (including rights to examine and obtain a copy of their health records) and to request corrections. These regulatory initiatives have now become a movement, championed by the OpenNotes philosophy that "urges doctors, nurses, therapists, and others to invite patients to read the notes they write to describe a visit."[47]

An extension of the traditional medical record, patient portals offer important benefits to patients and provider organizations. These technologies, particularly when integrated with an EHR, have the potential to improve both quality and access to care through features that enable patients to communicate electronically and securely with their provider; access their medical records; schedule appointments; pay bills; and refill prescriptions. By providing these tools as well as easy access to online resources, portals have the potential to benefit providers by increasing care efficiency, improving the management of chronic illness, and actively engaging patients and families in care.[48]

While ED managers and personnel might not be expected to know the technical aspects of maintaining data privacy and security, they are accountable for ensuring functional HIPAA compliance, especially related to the EDIS. Typical activities include username/password management, role/rights access levels, control of data copying (e.g., texting, e-mail, and cell phone photo of computer screen), and unauthorized access to unrelated patient charts. Ensuring computer screens are not visible to unauthorized personnel and patients is another privacy issue affecting EDIS deployment. More obscure aspects include education of personnel to the fact that EHR systems log virtually every action with a timestamp, whether or not it is finalized, visible on screen, or visible in the published record.

Mobile devices used in the ED environment add additional challenges, even if they are not connected to the EDIS. Careful consideration of HIPAA is a must if such devices are to be allowed for use in the ED.

CONCLUSION

Basic functions of EDISs include registration (ADT), patient tracking, order entry, results reporting, and discharge planning. Due to requirements in the HITECH Act, most EDISs now also include a number of advanced functions, such as electronic documentation, CPOE, and ADE prevention as integrated tools to support ED workflow. More advanced features continue to emerge, such as CDSS, positioning and automated tracking (automated wireless tracking), AI predictive modeling, and many others.

An unfortunate reality is that there is often little incentive for hospital IT departments to address concerns and enhancements of the EDIS due to competing interests, distance, and complexity. IT may take advantage of the ED leadership's lack of IT knowledge and experience by simply saying, "It can't be done." Therefore, it is imperative that every ED have a designated IT advocate liaison who stays abreast of emerging technologies to assure they are considered for implementation at an appropriate stage: neither too soon nor too late in their evolution.

Despite setbacks, EHR vendors are closing the functionality gap, approaching the "best-in-breed" EDIS functionality of the past while retaining the advantage of full integration with the hospital enterprise EHR.[49] The market dominance of EPIC and Cerner is good news for their customers, who can now leverage other users' experiences and content, as well as band together to apply pressure on these companies to enhance their products.

Finally, after years of resistance, EMR vendors are beginning to embrace third-party solutions by allowing bidirectional integration. This may signify a coming age of renewed best-in-breed third-party feature vendors, such as CDSS and integrated evidenced-based treatment care plans.

APPENDIX 64.1

The following section has been retained for the few that may experience a transition to a new EMR/EDIS. As new third-party enhancement solutions emerge, you may have a role to play in evaluating and selecting them. These ACEP Policy Statement excerpts may serve you well in such circumstances (**Box 64A.1**).

> **BOX 64A.1 ■ ACEP POLICY STATEMENT: HIT[38]**
>
> 1. Evaluation, selection, implementation, and ongoing assessment of HIT that impacts emergency care is best accomplished with active involvement of emergency physicians, nurses, and other emergency care providers. Emergency physicians should have a role in the selection and approval of any HIT that impacts the ED or the local emergency medicine community.
> 2. EDISs include best-in-breed (stand-alone) and ED modules of larger enterprise EMR systems, specifically designed to manage data in support of ED patient care and operations. EDISs should be properly implemented, sufficiently integrated, and well maintained.
> 3. Emergency physicians must have a role in the selection and configuration of an EDIS. Clinical functionality, usability, efficiency, and interoperability should be the primary criteria by which systems are evaluated. Preference should be given to systems that ensure support for ED workflow, clinical accuracy, patient safety, and operational support. System costs and assessment of ROI should take into account the impact on physician and staff productivity.

IMPLEMENTING AN EDIS EMR MODULE

Installation Disruption

Installation or replacement of an EDIS is universally disruptive to any ED and should be done carefully to avoid pushing the ED past its breaking point.[32,50] There are numerous aspects of implementation to focus on, but the overriding principle is active involvement of ED staff. This includes identifying a physician and nurse champion with protected time to actively participate with the implementation team. Ideally, one or both should have expertise in clinical informatics, or else you may wish to consider an emergency physician clinical informaticist consultant to assist with the process. Your hospital IT department may have competing interests in both time and objectives, so it is critical that you have your own representative to advocate on your behalf.

Due to the inevitable initial disruption in workflow and efficiency, success of an EDIS implementation is more often a result of good planning and support during/after go-live than it is the product itself. Some hospitals phase-in individual components of the EDIS by starting with the tracking board and then adding results reporting, nursing/physician documentation, and order entry, followed by other components (**Table 64A.1**). An alternative is to simply choose a date to transition all at once. This "Big Bang" approach is often necessary due to the nature of an enterprise EMR in which services are highly integrated

TABLE 64A.1 ■ Phased EDIS Implementation Example	
Phase 1	Patient tracking with hospital registration interface
Phase 2	Triage
Phase 3	Discharge planning and instructions
Phase 4	Laboratory and radiology results reporting
Phase 5	Nursing care documentation and device integration for vital sign capture
Phase 6	Physician documentation and charge capture
Phase 7	Computerized physician order entry and electronic prescribing
Phase 8	Closed-loop medication administration with bar code medications

> **BOX 64A.2 ■ TYPICAL EDIS IMPLEMENTATION CHALLENGES**
>
> - Major alterations to workflow and increased IT overhead
> - Unanticipated unfavorable or unworkable workflow
> - Ad-hoc workarounds, including reverting to paper
> - Incomplete system configuration
> - Changes in communication practices
> - Negative feelings toward the new system
> - Enabling new kinds of errors
> - Changes in power structure and loss of professional autonomy
> - Focus on technology rather than patient care

and interdependent. Nevertheless, the risk and consequences of failure are significantly increased with this approach. You may find it necessary to have twice the usual staff for the first several days, just to survive the go-live.

Regardless of approach, close attention to preparing, testing, and training is essential.[51] Multiple pitfalls can be avoided by anticipating commonly known challenges with new system installation. An analysis of multiple CPOE implementations demonstrated numerous problems that required some form of mitigation.[52] The issues clustered around the categories are listed in **Box 64A.2**.

Successful Implementation

Successful implementations are as much about change management (staff and workflow) as technology. In other words, success has been shown to be more about the people and processes than the technology.[53] In addition, detailed attention must be paid to the way the system works and how the staff interacts with it.[54] Early involvement of nurses, physicians, and ancillary staff provides an opportunity for champions to emerge as leaders (**Table 64A.2**). These special people help build enthusiasm while demonstrating proper usage to their peers. When these champions are identified, they should be supported and allowed to determine the best way to configure and use the system while defining new workflows within the department.

Workflow Analysis

A new EDIS may require major changes to departmental operations, so preimplementation is the appropriate time to analyze existing processes and communication patterns.[55] Overlaying technology onto poor existing workflow processes will inevitably make things

TABLE 64A.2 ■ Keys to Implementation Success

Technical details	Provide access to workstations, including wiring and power, wireless configuration, and security setup.
Workflow	Plan for and implement workflow changes to best use the system's capabilities.
Training	Provide comprehensive training, including just-in-time training.
Scheduling and staffing	Provide additional staff coverage, as patient care and documentation will likely take much longer initially.
Ongoing support	Support users through the performance impact while learning new workflows and integrating the system into daily work. Monitor for workarounds and continue to optimize the user experience.

> **BOX 64A.3 ■ BILL GATES ON TECHNOLOGY**
>
> *"The first rule of any technology used in a business is that automation applied to an efficient operation will magnify the efficiency. The second is that automation applied to an inefficient operation will magnify the inefficiency."*

worse (**Box 64A.3**). A comprehensive workflow analysis provides a starting point for defining how work gets done once the new system is installed. For example, if a CDSS is to be successful, much of the data collection must be done as early as possible in the workflow process. Such systems cannot check against things that are not as yet known. Worse, bad habits of completing charts after patients have been discharged or at the end of shift can have severe untoward consequences.

Creating flowcharts that depict steps involved in common workflow scenarios allows staff to step through and consider how work will get done with the new system. This allows both the workflow and the system to be adapted to best meet users' and patients' needs. Defining workflow and necessary configuration of the system in advance of go-live also provides an opportunity to create training materials and educate users.

It is always difficult, due to shift-work demands and limited resources, to find the time to train ED physicians, nurses, and staff, but failing to do adequate training all but guarantees failure. In addition to orientation of system features, significant time should be spent walking through common patient-care scenarios, from routine ankle sprain to female abdominal pain to cardiac arrest. Doing this in teams (physician, nurse, technician) also allows an opportunity to see how everything fits together.

System usability and features may require changes to workspace. The new system may feature mobile options that require new tablet hardware, or a more highly intensive documentation system may require dedicated workstations, for example. The vendor may provide guidance on many of these details, but do not assume it will be conveyed directly to end users. Hospital IT departments may try to save money by purchasing the bare minimum of hardware and training resources. Equipment redundancy is a must for a department that never stops.

Conferring with outside colleagues who have been using the same system for a while is important in identifying pitfalls. Another option is conferring with the ACEP Section of Emergency Medicine Informatics.[56]

Technical Considerations

Common technical issues center on the ability to easily access the system. Issues such as multiple username/passwords that change frequently, lack of adequate number or nonfunctional workstations, screen size, nonstandard keyboard/mouse, and convenient printer location must all be identified and addressed long before go-live (**Box 64A.4**). Further, the notion that all the new hardware can be installed and never maintained is a common misconception. Twenty-four access to redundant plug-and-play swappable hardware is a must.

Go-Live Support

Choosing the best day and time for go-live should be carefully considered. Ideally, it might be a traditionally "slow" time of year on an anticipated "slow" day during business hours.

Numerous strategies exist to mitigate disruption, and they all involve additional resources to provide help during the transition. Clinicians who have been well-trained on

> **BOX 64A.4 ■ PHYSICAL WORKSPACES TO CONSIDER**
>
> - Proper and convenient location and configuration of workstations
> - Appropriate installation of wiring and power
> - Effective placement of wireless access
> - Convenient printer access
> - Workstation-on-wheels (WOW) location and charging
> - Mobile device charging, maintenance, antitheft, damage
> - Secure wireless access

the system can provide support to others as needed. As noted, scribes can have a significant impact, and some have used the implementation of a new EMR as the impetus to begin using them. Regardless, virtually all EMR go-lives include additional personnel for several days to weeks. Typical return to baseline productivity ranges from 4 to 8 weeks post-go-live.[57] Transition from a paper-based system to an EMR typically results in a sustained loss in physician productivity of 10% to 20%.[20] However, merely shifting from one EMR to another is unlikely to have a sustained negative impact, and in most instances, a positive one in the long term due to improved technology.

While focusing on the technology, it is important to recognize the human process regarding major changes in the high-stress environment of the ED. There is often significant resistance and anxiety around the change. Physicians, nurses, and staff who have developed their expertise over many years may feel a loss of autonomy, a shift in power structures, and loss of control.[58] Support from leadership and peers are critical to the successful incorporation of the new EDIS into the users' workflow.

ED personnel are much more willing to adopt new technology if it enhances productivity; however, a lack of responsiveness, irritating software behavior, and increased burden on the staff will result in anger and frustration. Continued support, troubleshooting, and fast turnaround for configuration changes are all key to improving user satisfaction.

Ongoing Education and Support

ED staff turnover, locum tenens physicians, part-time help, and ED nurse vacancy rates place an increased premium on the ability to rapidly bring new users up to speed with the EDIS. Careful attention to well-defined procedures and effective training materials provide critical support for new staff long after the intensive go-live training process. Vendors and current users from other hospitals can often help with the best techniques, but local customization processes require at least some locally developed training materials. Nevertheless, with the EMR market consolidation, vendor-supplied training materials, and a more technology-savvy workforce, this is much less an issue today than even a few years ago.

APPENDIX CONCLUSION

A physician and/or nurse EDIS champion should be allotted dedicated time and receive advanced training on the system and, ideally, have advanced expertise in informatics.[59]

Department administrators and staff must continue to optimize EDIS use while implementing additional advanced functionality. Increasingly, ED personnel select work environments where the EDIS is well integrated, well supported, and familiar. They may even choose where to work based on a particular EDIS vendor product.

Planning for changes and obtaining the necessary trained personnel is a major consideration for health-care administrators. Hospital IT departments must provide around-the-clock support resources to ensure system stability outside normal business hours. Further, sufficient IT resources must be available to provide ongoing maintenance for system upgrades and constantly refine the system to meet ongoing needs. It is ACEP's position that hospitals have an obligation to use an EDIS that is "properly implemented, sufficiently integrated, and well maintained."[46]

An often-overlooked detail after EDIS purchase is ongoing vendor support, since any system will require continued software updates. Therefore, software maintenance should be included in the initial contracting process and fully utilized after go-live. Vendors have been known to alter and even disable functionality either intentionally or as a consequence of an unrelated upgrade. Without careful monitoring and advanced testing, routine upgrades may disrupt existing features and workflow. Continuing EHR development requires the active involvement of a dedicated team of informatics-savvy providers, including physician and nursing staff. Either a consultant or a staff member should be engaged to keep up with changing regulations and features.

Material for this chapter is drawn in part from prior work by:

- ACEP Section of Emergency Medicine Informatics, including ACEP policy statements, information papers, and newsletter submissions.
- Former ED Certification Commission for Health Information Technology (CCHIT) Committee
- HL7 Emergency Care Work Group
- Friends, colleagues, vendors, and HIT innovators

REFERENCES

1. Mickan S, Tilson JK, Atherton H, et al. Evidence of effectiveness of health care professionals using handheld computers; a scoping review of systematic reviews. *J Med Internet Res*. 2013;15(10):e212.
2. Lee CH, Yoon H-J. Medical big data: promise and challenges. *Kidney Res Clin Pract*. 2017;36:3–11.
3. Agha L. The effects of health information technology on the costs and quality of medical care. *J Health Econ*. 2014;34:19–30.
4. Gold M, McLaughlin C. Assessing HITECH implementation and lessons: 5 years later. *Milbank Q*. 2016;94(3):654–687.
5. Soumerai SB, Mahjumdar SR. A Bad $50 Billion Bet. *The Washington Post*. Published 2009.
6. Kellermann AL, Jones SS. What it will take to achieve the as-yet-unfulfilled promises of health information technology. *Health Aff*. 2013;32(1):63–68.
7. Thompson T, Brailer D. *Health IT Strategic Framework*. Washington, DC: US Department of Health and Human Services; 2004.
8. Garrett P, Seidman J. EMR vs EHR—what is the difference? Office of the National Coordinator for Health Information Technology (ONC). Published 2011. https://www.healthit.gov/buzz-blog/electronic-health-and-medical-records/emr-vs-ehr-difference. Accessed August 20, 2020.
9. What is an electronic health record (EHR)? Office of the National Coordinator for Health Information Technology (ONC). https://www.healthit.gov/faq/what-electronic-health-record-ehr. Accessed August 20, 2020.
10. Committee on Quality of Health Care in America. *Crossing the Quality Chasm: A New Health System for the 21st Century*. Washington, DC: National Academy Press; 2001.
11. Tang PC. Key capabilities of an electronic health record system: a letter report. Committee on Data Standards for Patient Safety: Institute of Medicine Committee on Data Standards for Patient Safety. Washington, DC: Institute of Medicine; 2003.
12. Burke T. The health information technology provisions in the American Recovery and Reinvestment Act of 2009: implications for public health policy and practice. *Public Health Rep*. 2010;125(1):141–145.
13. Blumenthal D. Stimulating the adoption of health information technology. *N Engl J Med*. 2009 Apr 9;360(15)1477–1479.
14. Botta MD, Cutler DM. Meaningful use: floor or ceiling? *Healthc (Amst)*. 2014;2(1):48–52.
15. *KLAS: Emergency Department Information Systems Is Best of Breed Still the Best Approach?* Orem, UT: KLAS Research; 2009.
16. *KLAS Performance Report: EDIS 2013: Revealing the Physicians' Voice*. Orem, UT: KLAS Research; 2013.
17. US Hospital EMR Market Share 2019 Report. KLAS. 2019.
18. Adler-Milstein J, DesRoches C, Furukawa M, et al. More than half of US hospitals have at least a basic EHR but stage 2 criteria remain challenging for most. *Health Aff (Millwood)*. 2014;33(9):1664-1671.
19. MIPS overview. Quality Payment Program website. https://qpp.cms.gov/mips/overview. Accessed August 20, 2020.
20. Dick RS, Steen EB, Detmer D. *The Computer-Based Patient Records: An Essential Technology for Health Care*. Washington, DC: National Academy Press; 1997.
21. Rothenhaus T, McClay JC, Taylor TB, et al. Emergency department information systems: primer for emergency physicians, nurses and IT professionals. ACEP. 2009.
22. Aronsky D, Jones I, Lanaghar K, et al. Supporting patient care in the emergency department with a computerized whiteboard system. *J Am Med Inform Assoc*. 2008;15(2):184-194.
23. Groner GF, Rockwell MA. Computer-based Information Systems for a Hospital Emergency Department. Santa Monica, Calif: Rand Corporation; 1977:R-2240-RC.

24. Taylor TB. *A View of the Emergency Department of the Future (Monograph), Millennial Addition.* Dallas, Tex: ACEP Section for Emergency Medical Informatics; 2000.
25. Roth M. Epic dominates EMR market share wars; Cerner Loses Ground. 2020. Available at: https://www.healthleadersmedia.com/innovation/epic-dominates-emr-market-share-wars-cerner-loses-ground. Accessed July 26, 2020.
26. HL7 Emergency Care Work Group. *Emergency Department Information Systems Functional Profile.* Vol. 2011. Ann Arbor, Mich: Health Level 7; 2007.
27. VanWagenen S. *Emergency Department Information Systems: Is Best of Breed Still the Best Approach.* Oren, UT: KLAS; 2009.
28. Baumlin KM, Shapiro JS, Weiner C, et al. Clinical information system and process redesign improves emergency department efficiency. *Jt Comm J Qual Patient Saf.* 2010;36(4):179–185.
29. Health Level 7 Emergency Care Special Interest Group: Emergency Department Information Systems Functional Profile. Health Level 7. 2007. Available at: https://www.hl7.org/documentcenter/public/wg/emergencycare/EDIS%20FP%20R1.pdf. Accessed August 29, 2020.
30. Tcheng JE, Bakken S, Bates DW, et al, eds. *Optimizing Strategies for Clinical Decision Support: Summary of a Meeting Series.* Washington, DC: National Academy of Medicine; 2017.
31. Jiang F, Jiang Y, Zhi H, et al. Artificial intelligence in healthcare: past, present and future. *Stroke Vasc Neurol.* 2017;2:e000101.
32. Taylor TB. Information management in the emergency department. *Emerg Med Clin North Am.* 2004;22:241–257.
33. Owens P, Elizhauser A. *Hospital Admissions That Began in the Emergency Department* 2003. Rockville, MD: Agency for Healthcare Research and Quality; 2006. Statistical Brief #1.
34. ONC Fact Sheet. "What Is FHIR®?" Office of the National Coordinator for HIT Website. Available at: https://www.healthit.gov/sites/default/files/2019-08/ONCFHIRFSWhatIsFHIR.pdf. Accessed May 5, 2020.
35. Mandl KD, Kohane IS. A 21st-century health IT system-creating a real-world information economy. *N Engl J Med.* 2017;376(20):1905–1907.
36. ACEP Policy Statement: *Health Information Technology.* 2015. ACEP Website: Available at: https://www.acep.org/patient-care/policy-statements/health-information-technology/. Accessed May 5, 2020.
37. Handel DA, Hackman JL. Implementing electronic health records in the emergency department. *J Emerg Med.* 2010;38(2):257–263.
38. EDIS: Primer for Emergency Physicians, Nurses, and II Professionals—Information Paper. 2009. ACEP Website. Available at: https://www.acep.org/patient-care/policy-statements/. Accessed May 5, 2020.
39. Section 4001 of the 21st Century Cures Act: Public Law No: 114–255 (12/13/2016).
40. Use of Scribes an Information Paper. 2011. ACEP Website. Available at: https://www.acep.org/patient-care/policy-statements/. Accessed May 5, 2020.
41. Goss F, Meteer M, Bates D. NLP to Improve Accuracy and Quality of Dictated Medical Documents. Brigham and Women's Hospital. AHRQ funded research: 09/30/2015-09/30/2019.
42. "Levels of Driving Automation" Standard J3016. 2018. SAE International Website. Available at: https://www.sae.org/news/press-room/2018/12/sae-international-releases-updated-visual-chart-for-its-%E2%80%9Clevels-of-driving-automation%E2%80%9D-standard-for-self-driving-vehicles. Accessed May 5, 2020.
43. Sittig DF, Wright A, Meltzer S, et al. Comparison of clinical knowledge management capabilities of commercially-available and leading internally-developed electronic health records. *BMC Med Inform Decis Mak.* 2011;11:13.
44. Health Level 7 Basic EHR Functions. AAFP Website. Available at: https://www.aafp.org/practice-management/health-it/product/features-functions.html. Accessed May 5, 2020.
45. Hoot N, Aronsky D. AMIA an early warning system for overcrowding in the emergency department. *AMIA Annu Symp Proc.* 2006; 2006:339–343.
46. The Health Insurance Portability and Accountability Act of 1996 (HIPAA); Privacy & Security Rules: 45 CFR Part 160 and Subparts A, C & E of Part 164.
47. OpenNotes Website. Available at: https://www.opennotes.org/. Accessed May 5, 2020.
48. Emonc S. Measuring the impact of patient portals: what the literature tells us. 2011. California Healthcare Foundation Website. Available at: https://www.chcf.org/. Accessed May 5, 2020.
49. Miliard M. EHRs in 2019: still a source of frustration, but getting better bit by bit. 2019. Healthcare IT News Website. Available at: https://www.healthcareitnews.com/news/ehrs-2019-still-source-frustration-getting-better-bit-bit. Accessed May 5, 2020.
50. Institute of Medicine 2007. *Hospital-Based Emergency Care: At the Breaking Point.* Washington, DC: The National Academies Press. Available at https://doi.org/10.17226/11621. Accessed May 5, 2020.
51. Longhurst C, Davis T, Maneke A, et. al. Local investment in training drives electronic health record user satisfaction. *Appl Clin Inform.* 2019;10(2):331.
52. Campbell EM, Sittig DF, Ash JS, et al. Types of unintended consequences related to computerized provider order entry. *J Am Med Inform Assoc.* 2006;13(5):547–556.
53. Ash JS, Stavri PZ, Dykstra R, et al. Implementing computerized physician order entry: the importance of special people. *Int J Med Inf.* 2003;69(2-3):235–250.
54. Bates DW, Kuperman GJ, Wang S, et al. Ten commandments for effective clinical decision support: making the practice of evidence-based medicine a reality. *J Am Med Inform Assoc.* 2003;10(6):523–530.
55. Linder JA, Schnipper JL, Tsurikova R, et al. Barriers to electronic health record use during patient visits. In: *Proceedings for AMIA Annual Symposium.* AMIA Symposium; 2006:499–503.
56. Section of Emergency Medicine Informatics. ACEP Website. Available at: https://www.acep.org/how-we-serve/sections/emergency-medicine-informatics/. Accessed May 5, 2020.
57. Ward MJ, Froehle CM, Hart KW, et al. Transient and sustained changes in operational performance, patient evaluation, and medication administration during electronic health record implementation in the emergency department. *Ann Emerg Med.* 2014;63(3):320–328.
58. Zhou L, Soran CS, Jenter CA, et al. The relationship between electronic health record use and quality of care over time. *J Am Med Inform Assoc.* 2009;16(4):457–464.
59. Clinical Informatics Certification. American Board of Preventive Medicine Website. Available at: https://www.theabpm.org/become-certified/subspecialties/clinical-informatics/. Accessed May 5, 2020.

ELECTRONIC HEALTH RECORD TRACKING SYSTEMS

CHAPTER 65

Zachary J. Jarou, Thomas Spiegel

The "whiteboard" was the primary way of organizing and tracking patients in the emergency department (ED) for decades. These large dry-erase boards were typically placed in high-visibility areas, allowing staff to see the locations of all patients being treated. Department staff typically used markers or symbols to help communicate and coordinate care among doctors, nurses, and other team members. Unfortunately, whiteboards were cumbersome to maintain, requiring staff to walk to a central location to see or make updates; the data contained were not robust; and frequent phone calls were still required between team members. Additionally, they did not contain important information like length of stay (LOS) and were not integrated with other information systems within the hospital.[1] Today, ED whiteboards are a relic unknown to most new physicians, aside from experiences during electronic health record (EHR) downtime or disaster planning.

EVOLVING FROM PHYSICAL TO DIGITAL

Electronic whiteboards, or "trackboards," eventually replaced dry-erase boards, although many of these early innovations were implemented as part of a nonintegrated (stand-alone) ED information system.[2,3] For example, in the era of paper charting, after writing orders for medications, imaging, or blood or urine tests, a physician or other staff member had to log into the electronic trackboard to flag each individual task that needed to be performed. Failure to manually flag these actions may have led to significant delays in patient care. Similarly, early trackboards were not linked to the hospital medical records and lacked access to notes, lab, or imaging results from patients' prior visits.

Today, ED trackboards are included as a standardized module within a comprehensive EHR system. The trackboard, which is accessible throughout the ED from any computer workstation, displays detailed, real-time information about a patient's chief complaint, LOS, care team members, vital signs, test results and imaging status, and more. Systems have also evolved to track equipment, staff, and patients prior to hospital arrival. It has been estimated that between 10% and 15% of an emergency physician's time is spent viewing or interacting with the ED trackboard, a shift that may reduce face-to-face interruptions, increase situational awareness, and improve collaboration among team members (**Table 65.1**).[4,5]

Electronic systems have several advantages over dry-erase boards. They can be accessed throughout the ED, and information entered into one system can be automatically used to populate information in another. With dry-erase boards, information is not automatically replicated and cannot be recovered once removed. Staff were able to easily change the structure of dry-erase whiteboards by adding new columns and could make notations or use symbols that may not be as easily implemented in an electronic format. This more spontaneous formatting process led to increased variability of information.

TABLE 65.1 ■ Advantages of Patient Tracking Systems[6]	
Task management	Synchronous and asynchronous communication
Team attention management	Multidisciplinary problem-solving and negotiation
Task status tracking	Socialization and team building
Task articulation	Resource planning and tracking

PURPOSE AND DESIGN OF THE ED TRACKBOARD

While the graphical user interfaces (GUIs) of ED trackboards will continue to evolve as new features and functionality are developed, a few basic principles must be considered. First, the ED trackboard should provide a high-level, summary overview of the ED's entire operation (including emergency medical services (EMS) diversion status and number of patients in the waiting room or awaiting admission), while also providing physicians and staff with fast and easy access to more detailed information about individual patients. The trackboard can be customized to track patients within each of many designated zones or care areas of the department, as well as patients with certain statuses, such as patients whose workups have been completed and are awaiting a final disposition.

Second, the trackboard should support collaboration between all members of the patient care team as well as hospital bed control and environmental services. Recoordination between team members is a continuous activity in the ED. Trackboards function as transitional elements, filling the gap between the work that needs to be performed and formal documentation that the work has been completed.[7]

Third, the trackboard functions as a real-time, interactive data display along three axes (**Figure 65.1**). The vertical axis contains a row for tracking the location of each patient in the department. The horizontal axis contains columns for patient-specific data elements such as name, chief complaint, acuity level, LOS, vital signs, and comments. A third axis represents the temporal aspect of the patient moving through the ED, including indicators like whether they are waiting for nursing triage, a particular ED clinician, a consult, or laboratory or imaging results.

Patient-Level Information

The specific patient information columns on the trackboard are dependent upon the capabilities of the EHR software vendor and the way the software has been locally

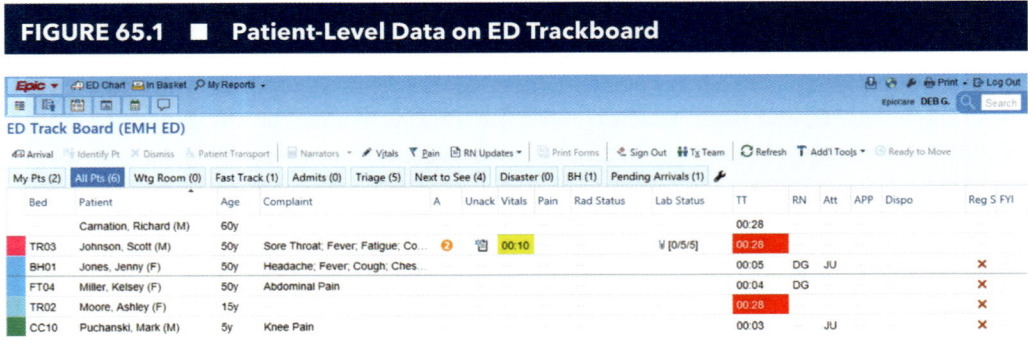

FIGURE 65.1 ■ Patient-Level Data on ED Trackboard

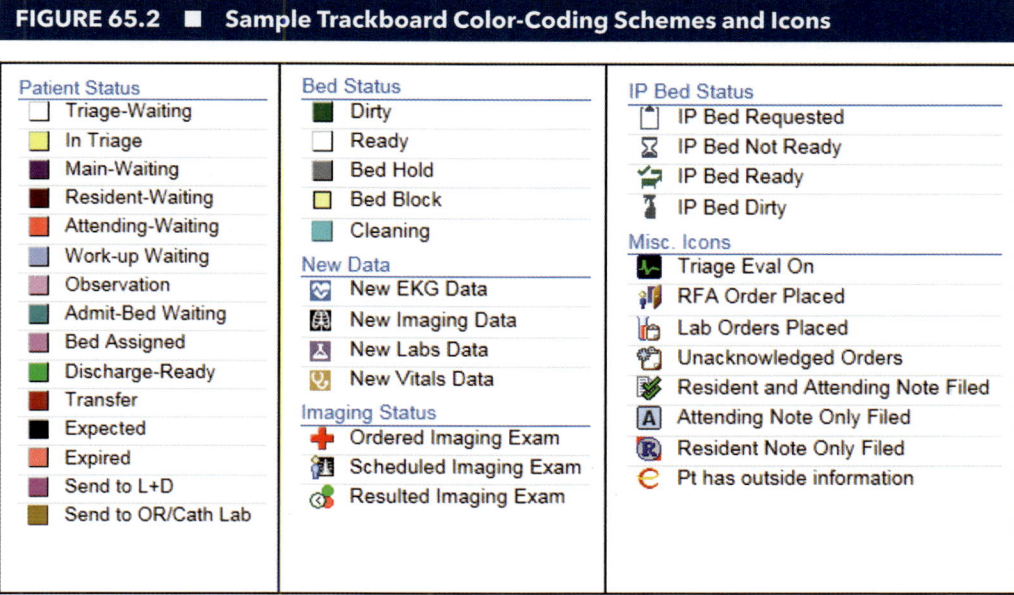

FIGURE 65.2 ■ Sample Trackboard Color-Coding Schemes and Icons

implemented. A large variety of information can be represented using text, icons, or color-coding schemes (**Figure 65.2**).

Examples of Information Represented Using Text

- Bed number
- Acuity (emergency severity index) level
- Patient name
- Age/gender
- Chief complaint
- Total LOS
- Time since last status update (e.g., roomed, admission order placed)
- Names (and phone numbers) of care team members
- Vital signs (blood pressure, pulse, temperature, respiratory rate)
- Comments (to communicate between team members)
- Disposition

Examples of Information Represented Using Icons

- Unacknowledged orders or other "action needed" flags (e.g., needing to reorder patient restraints)
- Electrocardiogram (ECG) status
- Lab status (icon displays if labs ordered, status summarized using [# resulted/#anticipated to return during ED visit/#total labs ordered])
- Imaging status (icon updates to represent each step of the process; may also include numerical summary similar to lab status)
- Recent admission or ED visit
- Status of provider notes
- Level of service completed
- Out-of-network insurance status
- Availability of data via health information exchange (HIE)
- Critical result flag
- Triage status
- Contact precautions or history of multidrug-resistant organism

- Incarceration or restraints
- Mental health hold
- Registration status
- Primary care physician status

Examples of Information Represented by Color Coding (i.e., Patient Status)

- Patient expected (or room holds)
- Waiting for triage
- In triage
- Awaiting resident
- Awaiting attending
- In process
- In process (attending only)
- Results returned/reevaluation needed
- ED observation status
- Anticipated admission
- Inpatient bed requested
- Inpatient bed assigned
- Ready for discharge (for use by residents to asynchronously communicate to attending for final approval)
- Discharge (approved by attending MD)
- Discharge when orders complete

It is crucial that trackboards are configured to clearly represent important clinical information, allowing caregivers to have a shared understanding of the patient's status. By doing so, ED trackboards function as communication tools with the potential to minimize interruptions that may pose a threat to patient safety and delay throughput. Any member of the clinical team should be able to glance at the ED trackboard and quickly answer "What is this patient waiting for?" This is accomplished by advancing a patient's color-coded status as they move through each step of their ED visit using icons that show the status of diagnostic studies.

While some clinicians may believe that updating the trackboard is equivalent to directly communicating with other members of the care team, for communications that require urgent or emergent actions, it is best to not rely upon updating the trackboard alone.[8]

Optimizing Functionality

Information technology staff often take the lead in implementing ED trackboards based upon interoperability, cost, and other factors. However, clinicians should also be involved in implementation since they have a better understanding of what configuration will best assist them with patient care. Those responsible for trackboard customization should respect the delicate balance between providing enough data to enhance patient care while avoiding information overload. It is important to follow the visualization mantra "overview first, zoom and filter, then details-on-demand."[9] For example, including too many columns, especially those containing information that may not routinely affect care, may clutter the trackboard or, in the extreme, force column sizes to be extremely narrow, making their contents unreadable.

Advanced Trackboard Features

Current trackboards allow clinicians to access substantial patient information without ever leaving the trackboard, saving users time—and clicks. ED trackboards provide multiple ways to view detailed patient data without opening the chart. A "report viewer" maintains the list

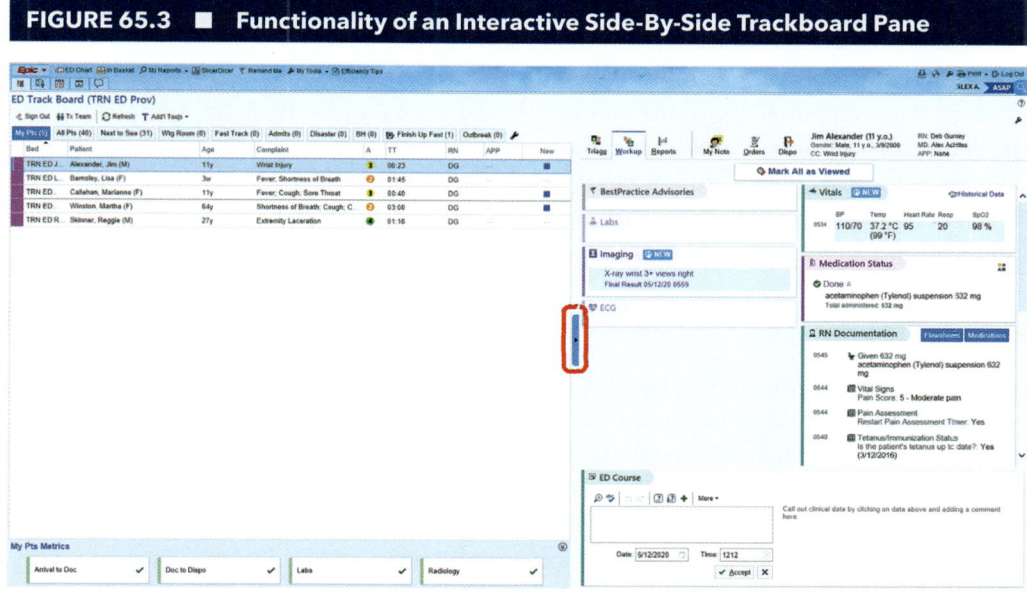

FIGURE 65.3 ■ Functionality of an Interactive Side-By-Side Trackboard Pane

of patients across the full width of the screen with the full set of information columns, while allowing navigation between different static "report types" at the bottom portion of the screen.

A "side-by-side" track board view is an enhanced viewing option, which displays an abbreviated list of columns alongside an interactive pane. This option allows users to view time-stamped updates that auto-populated an "ED Course" SmartLink in the patient's note. The ED Course SmartLink can also be used to provide real-time interpretation of lab results, ECGs, and imaging with single-click access to historical lab records, picture archiving and communication system images, or ECG tracings (**Figure 65.3**).

Advanced ED trackboards allow clinicians to create notifications for a recently resulted lab or imaging test, enabling them to reduce their data-to-disposition decision time. The notifications avoid wasted time and frustration attributable to the necessity of regularly opening screens or constantly scanning the trackboard to determine if the result is available (**Figure 65.4**). As one example use case of this functionality, it has recently been demonstrated

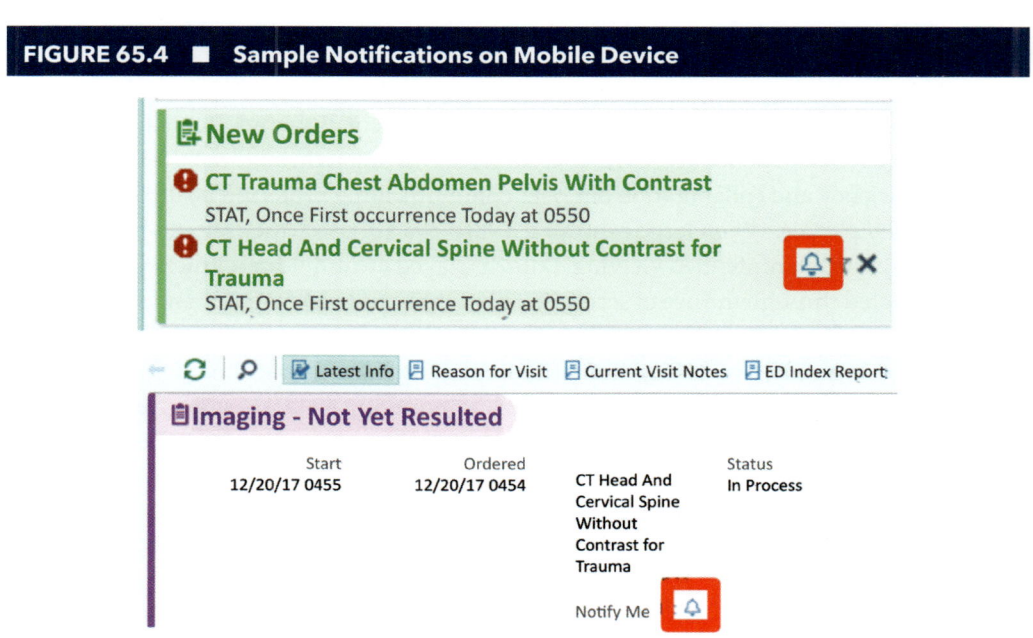

FIGURE 65.4 ■ Sample Notifications on Mobile Device

that creating push-alert notifications of troponin results to smart phones enabled emergency physicians to discharge patients 25.8 minutes sooner.[10]

While EHR software vendors currently allow limited screen customization, it is possible that individual clinicians will be allowed to customize their trackboards beyond the departmental default view or experience functionality that allows orders to be placed without having to open a patient chart. Trackboards could also be linked to patient call lights for specific requests, such as bathroom assistance, food, water, or blankets, displaying unique icons regarding a request to help make completing each task more efficient.

Patient Safety

Electronic trackboards are ideally positioned to maximize patient safety by highlighting critical information about patients as well as leveraging information within the EHR. For example, most electronic ED trackboards are equipped to flag patients with the same or similar last names. Displaying these names in a different font or color alerts staff that the potential for error exists, signaling to physicians and nurses to exercise additional caution when placing or acknowledging orders for these patients.

Trackboards also enhance patient safety by enabling shared situational awareness and teamwork among clinical staff and preserving critical information across shift changes. Trackboards can be used to display icons that inform clinicians about the availability of records from outside hospitals that have not been reconciled with the patient's local health record and to remind team members about unacknowledged orders or the need to reassess a patient or update vital signs at a specified time interval.

Trackboards can also alert providers to abnormal vital signs, critically abnormal laboratory results, returned diagnostic results, and the need for patient reassessments. High-risk patients (either recently discharged from the hospital or recently treated in the ED) can be highlighted. This alert allows care teams to appropriately research prior treatment plans and possibly contact prior providers for additional information. Finally, trackboards can be equipped with flags/colors to highlight institutional patient safety priorities. For example, such priorities might include documentation regarding procedural sedation requirements, restraint reassessments/reorders, or any other compliance/patient safety priorities.

Privacy Concerns

Jeopardizing patient privacy is always a significant risk when dealing with health-care information. This concern also applies to ED trackboards of any kind. Publicly displaying information about a patient's age, chief complaint, and location throughout the ED may help improve efficiency and collaboration but risks communicating protected health information to unintended parties. When large centralized displays are used, they should be located in areas that minimize unintended viewing. Data displayed on individual clinical workstations can be protected through the use of screen savers, automatic timed logoffs, and screen filters that prevent viewing unless directly in front of the monitor.

However, imposing too many limitations to accessing the trackboard may result in unintended consequences. There is a need to continually balance safety, privacy, and operational efficiency. In their 2004 article, Feied et al argue that "clinician access to clinical data should not be unnecessarily restricted" and that "one of the most important causes of clinical error is lack of awareness of existing information; thus, security measures that impede access to clinical data may increase error rates. The liability (malpractice and otherwise) resulting from clinical errors is real, immediate, and substantial, while the liability associated with breaches of privacy and security remains poorly defined. When clinical information needs are in conflict with privacy or security rules, the best possible clinical outcomes should be supported even at the expense of security and privacy."[2]

MANAGING DEPARTMENT FLOW

Trackboards function as the command center of the ED and have many uses in addition to representing patient-specific information.

Bed Management

Department-centered tracking allows users to understand many aspects of ED flow at one time. This real-time tracking is accomplished by displaying views that answer crucial questions, such as:

- How many patients are waiting for ED beds?
- How many patients are waiting for inpatient beds?
- How long have patients been here?

In addition to indicating bed occupancy and patient location, the ED trackboard can designate a location or bed being held for specific purposes. For instance, a nurse may hold a bed for a patient's return from another location in the department (e.g., X-ray), the hospital (e.g., magnetic resonance imaging), or reserve a room for a patient arriving from the prehospital setting (e.g., from EMS or an outside clinic). Staff can also designate rooms and beds requiring special services such as housekeeping, isolation, or pest control.

Prehospital Patient Tracking

When critically ill patients arrive in the ED, it is crucial that they are registered and placed on the trackboard as soon as possible so that physicians may begin entering orders and reviewing prior records without delay. In the event that critically ill patients are arriving by ambulance, a temporary patient record can be created and assigned to a room prior to patient arrival to eliminate delays in orders and charting.

In most cases, EMS will radio ahead to inform the ED that they are en route with a patient. Charge nurses are able to place "room holds" to ensure that the patient will have a bed upon arrival. Many times, the ambulance bay entrance will have a display informing EMS to which room their patient has been assigned. Critically ill patients will be preregistered as a "John Doe," and in cases of trauma, stroke, heart attack, or other chief complaints requiring multiple care teams, an estimated time of arrival can be provided so the ED team can be mobilized.

When transport times are long or inaccurate, this unreliability may result in inefficient use of clinician time that could be spent seeing other patients in the ED or reviewing the past medical history of the patient who is en route. Several technologies are currently being developed to address these issues, including systems that streamline workflows between EMS and the ED by eliminating the need for a phone call. The EMS providers are able to send photos of patient IDs, insurance cards, ECGs, clinical images, vital signs, and critical alerts in real time. This technology enables patients to be preregistered under their previous medical

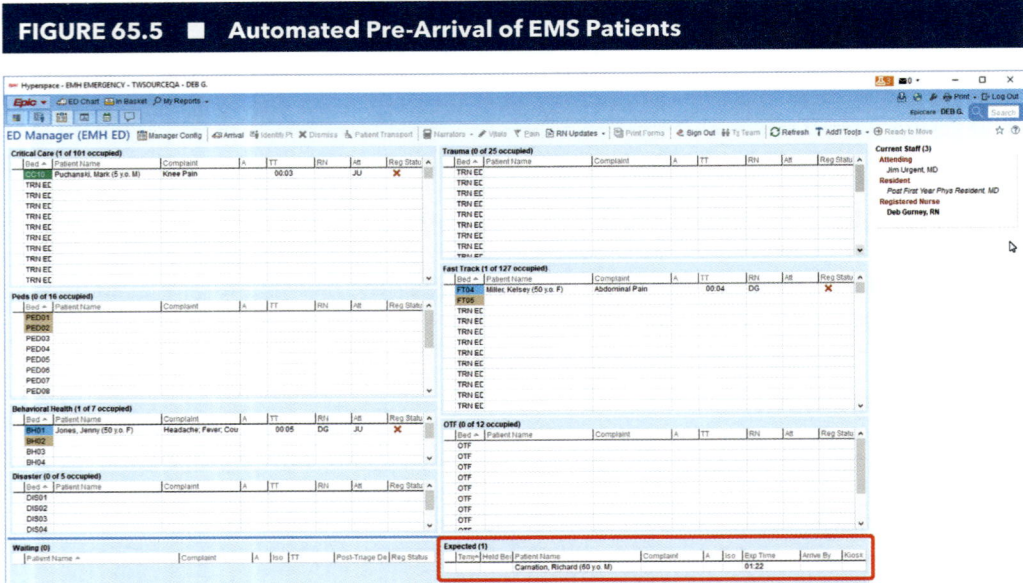

FIGURE 65.5 ■ Automated Pre-Arrival of EMS Patients

record numbers. Important clinical information can be reviewed by emergency physicians and consultants prior to patient arrival (**Figure 65.5**).

To provide more accurate arrival times, these systems also provide GPS-based estimated time of arrivals, which are often more reliable than traditionally reported time estimates. Staff can continue to provide care to patients who are actually in the ED, rather than waiting while anticipating the new arrival.

Fewer phone calls save time for ED nurses. Emergency medical services providers also reported faster throughput after implementing this technology.[11] Similar programs have been independently developed at academic medical centers such as the University of California San Diego (UCSD), where EMS systems have become integrated with the local HIE. The UCSD program allows EMS to query the HIE upon arrival to the scene to match the patient with the hospital's HIE record. This program eliminates the need to perform redundant data entry and leverages the patient information available within the HIE. Early results of the UCSD program have demonstrated:

- Reduced data entry time for paramedics
- Patient reports of having a better chance of being taken to "their" ED
- ECGs and EMS-run reports automatically transfer into the EHR
- EMS personnel are more easily able to obtain information on patient outcomes[12]

REAL-TIME LOCATION TRACKING

Some trackboards have GUIs in addition to those already presented such as maps of the ED that indicate room location, bed occupancy, and patient status (**Figure 65.6**).

Patient Tracking

Updating the location of patients on the trackboard to match their real-world location within the ED is crucial. Patients are often identified by the bed that they occupy in the ED. If patients are moved and the trackboard is not updated, significant errors may arise, including incorrect medication dosing, treatments, or tests. Wristbands, barcodes,

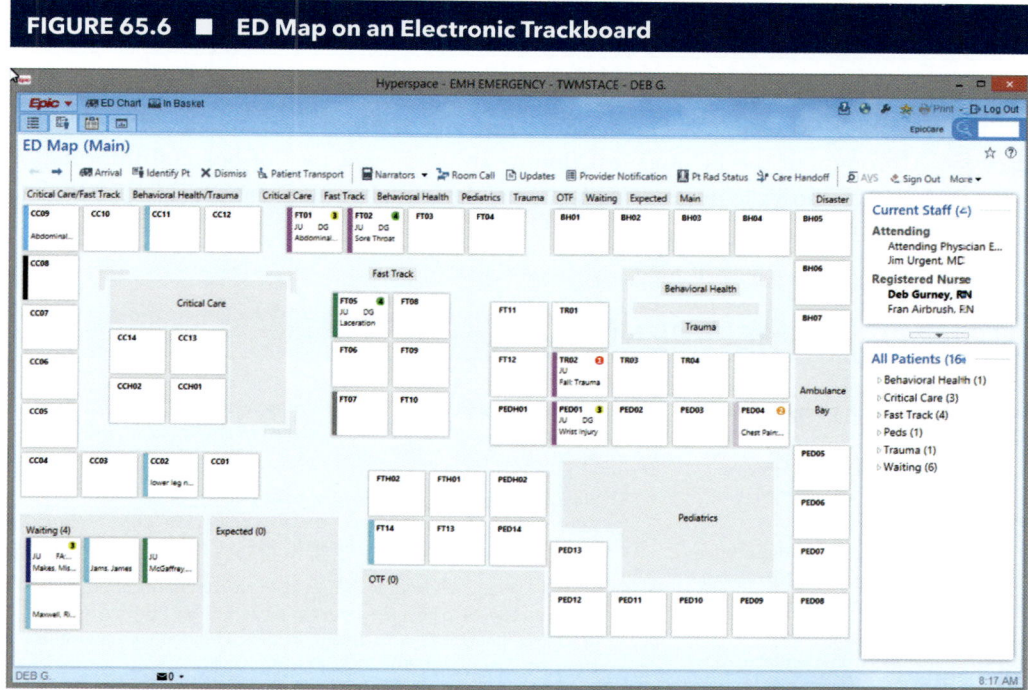

FIGURE 65.6 ■ ED Map on an Electronic Trackboard

and other methods of two-factor authentication are now required steps for medication administration in most EDs. In the future, hospitals may make use of radiofrequency identification (RFID) or Bluetooth Low Energy (BLE) systems capable of automatically updating patients' locations in real time as they move through the ED or hospital. Tracking patient movements is an important element in performance-improvement efforts, particularly related to ED patient flow.[13]

Equipment and Staff Tracking

In addition to facilitating enhanced patient tracking, RFID and BLE could allow tracking of equipment such as infusion pumps, ultrasound machines, video laryngoscopes, Wood's lamps, Tonopens, procedure carts, and other items that need to be located quickly. This process would decrease time searching for equipment and increase time caring for patients.

Similar technologies can be used to track the movements of individual team members. Studying the step patterns of clinicians throughout their shifts might allow for optimization of inefficient workflow processes and create a safer and more secure environment for staff. In a critical emergency, a staff member in a room with a closed door could be found immediately. Obtaining and reviewing a tracking history would also be helpful in cases of occupational exposure to pathogens and for quantifying the intensity of caring for individual patients to ensure that workloads are fairly distributed among staff.

In the future, the physical resources in the ED may be tracked as objects in an "Internet of Health-Care Things" that interact with one another. For instance, as a computer on wheels or ultrasound machine is rolled into a patient's room, wireless transponders will automatically recommend a task according to the patient's physical location, opening the chart or ultrasound acquisition series for the patient within closest proximity. Perhaps one day, physicians will wear location-aware devices with a display that would allow them to quickly review patient data, document encounters using natural language-processing tools, and facilitate hands-free order entry.

CONCLUSION

Accurate patient tracking is an essential element of ED operations. The evolution from solitary, centrally located dry-erase whiteboards to sophisticated trackboards that are accessible throughout the ED and function as an integrated part of hospital information systems has been shown to improve patient care, staff collaboration, patient satisfaction, and ED operations.

REFERENCES

1. Boger E. Electronic tracking board reduces ED patient length of stay at Indiana hospital. *J Emerg Nurs.* 2003;29:39–43.
2. Feied CF, Handler JA, Smith MS, et al. Clinical information systems: instant ubiquitous clinical data for error reduction and improved clinical outcomes. *Acad Emerg Med.* 2004;11(11):1162–1169.
3. American College of Emergency Physicians. "Emergency department information systems": Primer for Emergency Physicians, Nurses, and IT Professionals. Resolution 22(07) Task Force White Paper. 2009.
4. France DJ, Levin S, Hemphill R, et al. Emergency physicians' behaviors and workload in the presence of an electronic whiteboard. *Int J Med Inform.* 2005;74(10):827–837.
5. Xiao Y, Schenkel S, Faraj S, et al. What whiteboards in a trauma center operating suite can teach us about emergency department communication. *Ann Emerg Med.* 2007;50:387–395.
6. Bisantz AM, Pennathur PR, Guarrera TK, et al. Emergency department status boards: a case study in information systems transition. *J Cogn Eng Dec Mak.* 2010;4(1):39–68.
7. Chen Y. Documenting transitional information in EMR. In: *Proceedings of the CHI2010 Conference on Human Factors in Computing Systems.* ACM Press; 2010:1787–1796.
8. Hertzum M, Simonsen J. Visual overview, oral detail: the use of an emergency-department whiteboard. *Int J Hum-Comput St.* 2015;82:21–30.
9. Shneiderman B. The eyes have it: a task by data type taxonomy for information visualizations. In *Proceedings of the 1996 IEEE Conference on Visual Languages.* IEEE Press; 1996:336–343.
10. Verma A, Wang AS, Feldman MJ, et al. Push-alert notification of troponin results to physician smartphones reduces the time to discharge emergency department patients: a randomized controlled trial. *Ann Emerg Med.* 2017;70(3):348–356.
11. Twiage. Available at: http://www.twiagemed.com/. Accessed October 15, 2018.
12. Killeen J, Branning M. "SAFR" care coordination between paramedics and ED. HIMSS18 Conference, Las Vegas, NV, March 9, 2018. Available at: http://365.himss.org/sites/himss365/files/365/handouts/550235671/handout-287.pdf. Accessed October 15, 2018.
13. Taylor TB. Information management in the emergency department. *Emerg Med Clin North Am.* 2004;22(1):241–257.

ELECTRONIC HEALTH RECORD DOCUMENTATION SYSTEMS

CHAPTER 66

John C. Brown, Zachary J. Jarou

> *As clinicians, we are historians, not transcriptionists. Use the EHR to your advantage to paint a unique picture of the patient!*
>
> —Michael Weinstock, author of the *Bounceback!* series

Of all the components in an electronic health record (EHR), the adoption and optimization of the documentation tools can be the most challenging. Adequate preparation with strong executive support and accountability at the highest level are essential for success. Physician and/or nurse managers must be committed to driving the process from conception through implementation to the continuous upgrading of clinical content, features, and functionality.

A BRIEF HISTORY OF EHRs

The primary purpose of physician documentation has always been to communicate a concise clinical summary of the patient's evaluation and treatment. The ideal document is a brief, well-organized narrative that focuses on positive and pertinent negative signs and symptoms, clinically significant test results, and the medical decision-making (MDM) thought process.[1] Historically, physicians were free to write anything they felt was relevant and omit what they felt was not pertinent. Diagnoses could be written using the physician's personal choice of words.

Medicare Documentation Requirements for Reimbursement

Physician documentation changed in 1995, when the US Medicare program published evaluation and management (E/M) documentation guidelines for reimbursement.[2] The guidelines specify the number of elements that must be documented in each part of a history and physical (H&P) examination in order to receive compensation for patient E/M. Failure to include all elements, even if the physician does not consider them to be pertinent, results in less compensation. Submitting claims with extensive documentation to justify an inappropriately higher level of service constitutes fraud subject to possible penalties and fines. While these guidelines were initially intended for Medicare patients, they were subsequently embraced by commercial insurance companies as well.

International Classification of Disease, 10th Version

On October 1, 2015, the US Department of Health and Human Services (DHHS) mandated the use of over 70,000 International Classification of Disease, 10th version Clinical Modification (ICD-10-CM) diagnosis codes, or ICD-10-CM, further increasing the documentation burden on physicians.[3] Physicians are no longer free to use their personal choice of wording for a diagnosis. They must search for and select a coded diagnosis that most closely matches what they would have written. Multiple other stakeholders continue to add and change physician documentation requirements for purposes other than what is needed for direct patient care.[4]

The rising rate of medical litigation in the United States has prompted a more extensive ordering of tests, further increasing the amount of documentation based on a "not documented, not done" mentality.[5]

From Handwriting to Electronic Documentation

Handwriting and dictation produce a document in the physician's own words with complete flexibility to accommodate any workflow. But handwriting is time-consuming and often illegible. Dictation is costly and not available immediately.

Prior to the development of EHR documentation systems, the majority of emergency departments (EDs) transitioned from filling in the blank space documentation systems to paper templates. A collection of just 50 or so complaint-based paper templates allowed a nurse or a physician to record a complete patient encounter by making marks on a single sheet of paper. Well-designed templates included prompts for reimbursement requirements, key data elements required for regulatory compliance, and reminders of high-risk considerations. Users reported that making marks on a template was more efficient than writing or typing prose and even faster than traditional dictation. Paper templates have been proven to improve reimbursement levels.[6] The cost for paper templates is a fraction of that for dictation.

The Mandate for Electronic Documentation

In April 2004, President George W. Bush issued an executive order calling for the widespread use of EHRs for most Americans by 2014. The challenge was intended to accelerate the adoption of health-care information technology (HIT) by medical providers. In September 2005, DHHS awarded the Certification Commission for Healthcare Information Technology (CCHIT), a three-year contract that provided hospitals and clinicians with a single independent certification for implementing HIT products that included a minimum set of features and functionality. The CCHIT would not establish standards for HIT products but would select standards established by other organizations.

However, certifying functionality was not enough. A product could be capable of performing a desired function, but if it took 20 keystrokes to do so, that product was essentially useless. It became clear that HIT usability and interoperability must also to be considered. In February 2009, President Barack Obama signed the Health Information Technology for Economic and Clinical Health Act as part of the American Recovery and Reinvestment Act. This introduced "Meaningful Use," a concept backed by $19.5 billion in incentives for health-care providers to adopt the technology over an aggressive four-year time line.[7] Eight years later, data from HIMMS Analytics Logic indicated that 73.1% of US hospitals were using electronic physician documentation templates by the end of 2017.

UNDERSTANDING ED WORKFLOW

A fully functional EHR documentation system can achieve a number of objectives that are not typically possible with other methods (**Table 66.1**).

Access to Prior Records

Key components of a longitudinal patient record that supports quality documentation and patient care include up-to-date information on patient allergies and home medications, an active problem list, prior test results, and prior surgeries.

> *Example:* A hemoglobin value of 10.0 g/dL can indicate significant anemia requiring hospitalization if the value was 15.0 g/dL a few days ago or it can indicate significant improvement in a patient with renal failure whose hemoglobin was 8.0 g/dL last month.

Electronic health record interoperability has evolved to provide users with access to this information from different records within the same health system, as well as EHRs used by other health-care institutions. Users must consider the integrity of data from other systems before using or adding that information to their EHR. Users must also know if their EHR is

TABLE 66.1 ■ Objectives of an EHR Documentation System

Objective	Description
Concise clinical summary	An EHR documentation system should never lose sight of the primary purpose of documentation: to provide a concise clinical summary of the patient evaluation.
Rapid access to recent test results	Efficient physician documentation relies on rapid access to recent test results.
Timely access to prior records	Timely access to key elements of the patient's longitudinal record, including: • Allergies and medications • Active problem lists • Prior test results • Prior surgeries
Point-of-care feedback	Well-designed point-of-care feedback can: • Optimize reimbursement • Ensure regulatory compliance • Assist in risk management • Enhance diagnostic accuracy • Promote evidence-based best practice
Avoid alert fatigue	Excessive pop-ups can lead to "alert fatigue" in which all prompts are ignored.
Provide clinical decision support	Medication interactions and allergy checking are examples of clinical decision support.
Maintain or improve efficiency	Adequate preparation, physician training, and physician support are the key to maintaining or improving efficiency.
Meaningful reports	Standardized data structure is required for effective point-of-care and retrospective reporting.

able to store the data from other systems in the same format that it is being stored in their own system. For example, medication data from other systems may come across as a string of text rather than as discrete data fields for medication strength, dose, route, and frequency. This can create problems during the admission medication reconciliation process.

In addition to accessing these data, the health-care provider must be able to edit and update the allergies, medications, and problem lists. Ideally, a single entry should update the information every place that it is stored. The need to reenter the same data in another place within the EHR or in another system has a detrimental impact on efficiency and user acceptance while increasing the potential for errors.

While both physicians and nurses need to access prior records, the EHR documentation system must also accommodate workflows that differ between physicians and nurses.

Physician Documentation

Emergency physicians care for and document information about multiple patients at the same time with many interruptions. They need to be able to start by recording their initial H&P, then return later to document their interpretation of test results; the patient's response to treatments; their thought process on how they arrived at their clinical impression; any consultations with other physicians; and finally, the plan for the patient's post-ED treatment. Clinicians must be able to jump from one patient's documentation to another patient's documentation, each of which are at different stages of completion. They also need to be able to review various portions of the patient's record as they document.

Nurse Documentation

Emergency department nurses also care for and document on multiple patients at the same time with many interruptions. However, the content of their documentation is very different than that of the emergency physician. Nurses create time-stamped logs of the care they provide and any changes in the patient's condition. They are also tasked with documenting multiple different types of patient screening assessments. Unlike physician documents that have one author, the nursing documentation for a patient may have many authors.

DATA ENTRY

Physician charting has been recognized as one of the most challenging aspects of EHR adoption. In 2005, the Healthcare Information and Management Systems Society (HIMSS) created an Electronic Medical Record (EMR) Adoption Model to compare progress in utilization of HIT by individual hospitals and integrated delivery systems. The model (**Figure 66.1**) is based on seven stages of progressively higher levels of HIT adoption. In this model, physician charting is ranked as fifth out of the seven stages of a fully functioning EMR. In 2017, the HIMSS Analytics Database reported that two-thirds of US hospitals still had not implemented physician documentation using structured templates and discrete data in at least 50% of the facility and had not installed a security system to prevent unauthorized intrusions into the hospital network.[8,9]

There are multiple modes of data entry to consider when evaluating and implementing an EHR system. What works best for one person may be very inefficient for another. Optimal documentation often incorporates multiple modes of data entry for a single document. Forcing the user to employ a single mode of data entry can have a negative impact on end-user satisfaction, efficiency, and adoption of the technology. Any requirement to document the same information in more than one place should be avoided unless the duplication can be achieved automatically.

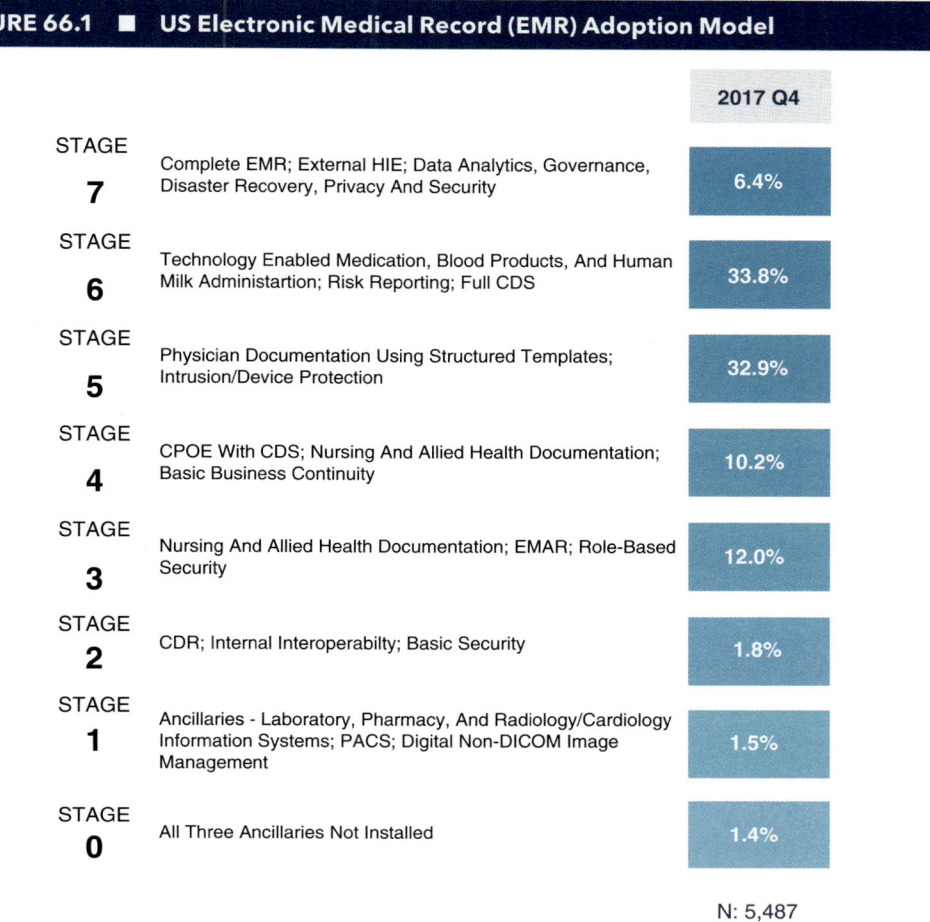

FIGURE 66.1 ■ US Electronic Medical Record (EMR) Adoption Model

Scanned Documents

The ability to scan a paper document into the EHR can be essential when documents come from outside sources or are created during scheduled or unscheduled EHR downtimes. The ability to scan and store each document in a specific location within the EHR increases the probability that subsequent users will find it. However, the information is stored as a computer image, not as text, and certainly not as structured data. The usefulness of this form of "computerization" is extremely limited. For instance, lab results on a scanned document will not appear in a display of prior values unless the EHR includes the capability to convert the picture of the value to a discrete numeric value.

Templates

Every EHR documentation system provides a way for the user to type a document. While this is very efficient for those with good typing skills, it can be the pathway to retirement for others. Documentation templates provide a method of capturing standardized data elements in a structured format instead of storing the information as sentences and paragraphs. These templates can prompt the user to include elements considered essential for quality care and appropriate reimbursement.[10] The structured data can feed computer logic that drives real-time addition or elimination of documentation elements based on patient-specific data that have already been entered.

Standardization, Customization, and Personalization

Maintaining eye-to-eye contact when talking to a patient and others in the room can greatly enhance the experience for everyone involved while improving the quality of the information obtained by both parties. The computer should not get in the way.

Optimal use of computer templates requires familiarity with the content and layout of a template beforehand. This can decrease the need to look at the computer for prompts, allowing for more eye contact with the patient and family. Success is often greater when the end users are involved in the design of the template. Some EHR templates can only be modified by the vendor. Others can be customized by the hospital's HIT team. Adoption can be greatest when each user is able to create a personalized version of the template. Personalization can involve changing titles or the wording surrounding data entry fields to better match that clinician's workflow and thought process without changing the standardized data entry field. Personalization may also include the ability for users to add their own data fields to capture elements that the user finds helpful but are not required.

Point-and-Click Templates

A common method for documenting in the EHR involves moving the computer mouse over an item and clicking the mouse to include the item in the document or to toggle between a positive and pertinent negative. Only a limited number of options can be reasonably displayed on the computer screen. This creates a tendency for point-and-click documentation to contain similar or identical content. Therefore, use of point-and-click templates tends to work best for portions of a note that consist of established, predefined data elements. One example might be the 14 body systems recognized by the Centers for Medicare and Medicaid Services (CMS) that make up a medical review of systems (ROS).[11] Another example could be the well-established components of a physical exam (PE).

Electronic Forms and Flow Sheets

An EHR that provides a means to convert paper forms into electronic forms eliminates legibility issues and the need to scan a paper document into the computer. However, these forms often include information that is documented in other places within the medical record. A well-designed EHR will automatically populate fields on the electronic form if the information has already been documented elsewhere in the patient's record. Likewise, if the first time those data elements are entered is on the electronic form, the information should automatically populate the other areas of the patient's record where it is needed. Examples include past medical history obtained by the nurse that can then be verified by the physician as needed as well as medications, vital signs, and test results.

Electronic flow sheets typically list data elements in rows, with different values for each element entered chronologically in date/time columns. The discrete data can be used to display the information as a time line or as a graph of values over time. Nurses rely heavily on the use of flow sheets for their documentation.

Text-Block Templates

Predefined phrases, sentences, paragraphs, or entire documents can be the foundation for a text-block template. An effective EHR documentation system will allow users to easily create and name their own personal text blocks. This gives them the ability to quickly insert a block of text using words that they use consistently for specific situations either when documenting in the patient's EHR or entering patient instructions.

Although useful, text-block templates can also significantly increase the risk of "cloning" where every note looks essentially identical. When text blocks are used in areas of the record that are not expected to be identical for all patients, the risk of cloning can be reduced if portions of the text are created from a list of predefined phrases or the ability to manually type these portions. Some lists permit the selection of a single phrase, while others enable the selection of multiple phrases. The computer replaces the list with the phrase or phrases that were chosen.

Advanced EHR documentation systems also allow portions of the text block to be automatically filled with specific information that has already been documented elsewhere in the patient's record. The use of this functionality should be limited to include only pertinent information used by the physician to determine the clinical impression and treatment plan.

Macros, Copy/Paste, and Copy Forward

Macros are computer commands available in some EHR documentation systems that allow the user to generate predetermined text or a series of operations with a single keystroke. They are typically used with point-and-click templates. When available, users can make a set of selections on the template for future use with names like "Normal Complete ROS," "Normal Medical PE," or "Normal Trauma PE." The CMS has recognized macros and has approved their use by teaching physicians.[12] Copy/paste functionality allows the user to copy something in one part of the record and paste it into their note. Copy forward functionality provides a means to copy the contents of a prior note into the current note.

These tools can be tremendous time savers, but they must be used with caution. It is very easy to inadvertently include unwanted information, which can have significant adverse financial and/or medical–legal consequences. For example, it is very easy to generate a "normal" physical examination with a single keystroke. The acronym PERRLA (pupils equal, round, reactive to light and accommodation) is often included as part of a normal physical examination. If that phrase is part of the normal examination on a patient with a glass eye, accommodation is not actually assessed, then the medical record is inaccurate with no defense in a billing dispute or a malpractice lawsuit.

A 2017 study of inpatient progress notes found that only 18% of information was manually entered, while 46% was copied, and 36% was imported.[13] Copying and importing 82% of a note significantly increases the chance of unintentionally, including information that is not currently accurate; The False Claims Act specifies that "it is illegal to submit claims for payment to Medicare or Medicaid that you know or should know are false or fraudulent."[14] These cases can result in fines in excess of $150,000.[15]

Dictation

Dictation can be used to create an entire document. It can also be used to insert information into an electronic template by positioning the cursor and dictating instead of typing. It can be one of the most effective means of "telling the patient's story" or explaining one's thought process. For emergency physicians, this is typically the history of present illness (HPI) or MDM portion of the document.

Traditional Dictation

Those who choose traditional dictation typically use a separate dictation device, a microphone connected to the computer, or a cell phone app to record their dictation. When using a separate dictation device, the person dictating must manually enter data identifying the patient, the location, and the identity of the person dictating. Using a microphone or cell phone app that connects to the EHR documentation system allows the user to place an electronic bookmark that gets replaced by the text created by a trained medical transcriptionist.

Most providers have developed a high level of efficiency in dictating. One of the major disadvantages of traditional dictation is the time it takes for the transcriptionist to produce the document before the clinician can proofread it, make changes as necessary, and sign it, making it available for others to read. A second major disadvantage is the cost of the transcriptionist's services. Also, unlike templates, the data are typically stored as text strings and are not available as discrete data.

Voice-to-Text Dictation

Commercially available speech recognition solutions for ED documentation have progressed significantly since their early use in the 1990s.[16,17] Today, voice-to-text solutions are much more widely used than speech recognition in health care. Voice-to-text dictation is done using a microphone connected to a computer or a cell phone app with a wireless connection to the computer. There is no need to manually enter data to identify the patient, the location, or the person dictating since the computer already has that information. The cost of a trained transcriptionist is eliminated. The user watches the computer-generated text based on what they are saying, often at a very fast rate. Any editing is done immediately, eliminating a delay in the ability of others to read what was dictated.

Physicians using voice-to-text dictation software should take care to ensure the accuracy of the text that is generated prior to signing their notes. A published study of a random sample of 100 emergency medicine notes dictated between January and June 2012 and reviewed independently by two board-certified emergency physicians found a total of 128 errors or 1.3 errors per note.[18] These two physicians concluded that 15% of the notes contained one or more critical errors that had the potential to impact patient care.

The term "discrete-reportable transcription" was introduced in 2009 by Mark Anderson, CEO of AC Group, Inc.[19] The concept involves software that converts dictation into discrete data that can be used for reporting and analysis. This conversion can occur during dictation or afterward. Conversion to discrete data after dictation involves the application of natural language processing technology to "read" text, "understand" its context, and map the concepts to established coding systems (e.g., *ICD*, Current Procedural Terminology, Systematized Nomenclature of Medicine–Clinical Terms, Logical Observation Identifiers Names and Codes, etc.). Use of this technology to provide real-time clinical documentation assistance is just beginning to be available at the time of this writing.

Mobile Technology

Smartphones and computer tablets offer a dizzying array of apps that many emergency physicians find useful as they care for patients in the ED. But use of mobile applications for documenting the patient encounter remains limited. The primary reason rests in the fact that while cell phones and computer tablets excel in providing a convenient means of consuming data, they are not as good for data entry. Another issue is that EHR vendors have been slow to offer their products on mobile platforms.

While typing on a cell phone or tablet is cumbersome, many physicians have used the camera on their smartphones to capture clinical images that provide visual documentation of findings that are difficult to fully describe in words. This can be a very efficient way to share images with consultants, insert data obtained from another facility into the EHR, and add visual images to the documentation that demonstrate clinical progression. Vendors offer apps that allow the physician to transmit the information directly into the EHR without storing any patient information or images on the mobile device. Mobile technology also provides a means to dictate notes that are transmitted directly into the EHR without any of the text being stored on the mobile device.

Scribes

Some emergency physicians have found that using a scribe to do their documentation increases their ability to see more patients. In one adult ED, there was an increase in both the number of patients treated per hour and in the relative value units generated per hour by emergency physicians using scribes.[20] In another academic medical center, scribes increased the average charge for ED visits by 15%.[21] Caution must be taken to ensure that this increase in ED charges does not result from inappropriate up-coding of the ED visits.

In many cases, scribes are college students who are very facile with technology and aspire to attend medical school.[22] In 2011, The Joint Commission published their "stand that the scribe does not and may not act independently" based on the understanding that scribes were unlicensed individuals.[23] More recently, The Joint Commission has recognized that "there are individuals with the official title of 'scribe' for whom documentation assistance is their only role, and there are individuals who perform dual roles that include clinical responsibilities as well as documentation assistance."[24] While The Joint Commission has always made it clear that they do not support or prohibit the use of scribes, they do specify the need for:

- Minimal training requirements
    - Medical terminology
    - Health Insurance Portability and Accountability Act of 1996 (HIPAA)
    - Principles of billing, coding, and reimbursement
    - EHR navigation and functionality
    - Computerized provider order entry (CPOE) and clinical decision support
- Organizational policy and procedure requirements
- Job description that includes minimal qualifications
- Authorization to enter orders based on the individual's certification and scope of licensure or practice in accordance with organizational policy as well as local and federal laws and regulations[24]

The emergence of skilled remote scribe services that are available 24 hours a day has also increased the use of scribes in the ED (see Chapter 25).[25]

POINT-OF-CARE DOCUMENTATION SUPPORT

Most hospitals and physician groups have clinical documentation improvement (CDI) specialists who help physicians understand how their choices of words or omissions of certain elements can impact the level of reimbursement for hospital and professional services. Performing well on quality initiatives, participating in registries, and partnering in research projects all require accurate documentation of key elements in specific places of the EMR. Documenting discussions with the patient, family, and consultants can mitigate medical risks and help track patient satisfaction efforts.

An EHR documentation system can use several methods to supplement the efforts of CDI specialists and prompt the physician to include documentation of key data elements in the appropriate places.

Push vs Pull vs Neither

In some cases, the user can click a link to *pull* up information that is not visible. This method is frequently used to access context-specific reference material. While this method does not directly interfere with the user's workflow, it does require to user to:

- Decide whether to interrupt workflow to view the information.
- Take the necessary action.
- Filter through the information to find what might be useful.

At other times, context-specific information is automatically *pushed* to the user. The effectiveness depends on what triggered the push, the accuracy and appropriateness of that trigger, the time in the physician's workflow when the information appears, and how the information is delivered. For example, if the user enters a diagnosis of a humerus fracture, they could be prompted to specify whether it is the left or right humerus. The accuracy and appropriateness of this prompt would be extremely high; the best time in the workflow to display the prompt would be at the moment the user enters the diagnosis instead of waiting until the next time the user accesses the patient's record.

Pop-ups that interrupt the physician's workflow are usually not well received and can lead to *alert fatigue*, a condition where users ignore messages because there are too many of them.[26] Systems that update a to-do list to the side of the physician's documentation location can push information in a way that is less disruptive and less likely to cause alert fatigue. The effectiveness of information push versus information pull has been studied in marketing and learning environments with varying conclusions.[27,28] An ideal solution would blend both methods to maximize effectiveness.

Some EHRs include an electronic rules engine that monitors data elements as they are entered, applies encoded rules when specific conditions are met, and delivers the key information to the user at the specified time in the specified manner. In some cases, only the vendor is able to code the rules. In other cases, the hospital's information technology specialists create rules that are customized for the particular hospital. These engines determine the triggers for when information is pushed to the user. The information that is pushed can prompt for clarification needed for billing, data needed for quality metrics, or provide suggestions to help the user comply with policies and regulations. They can also be used to create *dynamic templates* with portions that are added or deleted based on these rules. For example, the computer can remove a portion of a template that is only appropriate for females if the patient is a male, or it can display age-specific templates for documentation on pediatric patients depending on the patient's age.

One form of clinical documentation support that is very well received involves neither push nor pull. The clinical content of documentation templates can be strategically designed to prompt the user for items that might be overlooked when dictating or typing. Examples mentioned previously include listing the 14 body systems recognized by CMS in a ROS or listing well-established components of a PE. Another example would be a template chosen to document a particular chief complaint that includes a list of elements in the patient's history section that are known to be useful in differentiating the various diagnostic possibilities associated with that chief complaint. This list can reduce the chance of the physician forgetting to ask a key question that could help confirm or rule out a particular diagnosis. Diagnostic errors are among the most common errors made in medicine, outnumbering both medication and surgical errors as causes of outpatient malpractice claims and settlements.[29]

Imagine documenting an ED encounter for a burn patient:

- A good EHR documentation system would include a template designed to document the encounter and a link to a current summary reference.
- A better EHR documentation system would display an age-appropriate pediatric template if the patient is a child and a different template if the patient is an adult with a link to a current summary reference for pediatric versus adult care.
- The best EHR documentation system would also include a tool to calculate percentage of body burned and recommended fluid volumes. In addition, documentation of the ROS and the PE would be done using templates saved by the user with their personal choice of defaulted terms.

ACCOMMODATING OTHER USERS

As the physician enters information in an EHR, it is important to consider how others will use that information. The sequence in which data are acquired does not match the priority of information needed by readers of the document. Others caring for the patient are most interested in the author's clinical impression and plan that are traditionally located at the end of the document. One way to facilitate the reader's priorities is to place the clinical impression and plan at the top of the document. Some EHRs include an option to display the note with portions of the document collapsed into a single line which reduces or eliminates the need to scroll to the bottom to see the clinical impression and plan.

The real value of EHR systems over other documentation methods is their ability to access data for various purposes besides just looking at a single chart for a single patient. Meaningful reports include information about multiple patients or multiple visits for a single patient. The shift from volume-based to value-based payment has significantly increased the need for data to be documented in specified data fields for quality reporting, transfer of data to registries, and to feed electronic rules engines. As natural language processing has evolved into natural language understanding, the technology is better able to determine context and can reduce the need for specific data fields, as the technology is able to extract the information from strings of text regardless of how the information was entered in the system.

Sharing Notes With Patients

In addition to their use for patient care, patient safety, billing, quality improvement, and medicolegal purposes, physician documentation can also be shared directly with patients. In 1996, HIPAA gave patients the right to access their medical records,[30] and in 2001, the Institute of Medicine's *Crossing the Quality Chasm* report encouraged notes to be viewed as interactive documents between patients and providers.[31] However, it was not until the OpenNotes demonstration project in 2010 that this practice was evaluated by more than 100 primary care physicians and 25,000 patients in Massachusetts, Pennsylvania, and Washington.[32] Potential advantages of OpenNotes include improved patient understanding, adherence with treatment plans, and accuracy and completeness of notes as well as patient insight into MDM, better patient preparation for clinic visits, and ability of patients to share notes with others.

Potential disadvantages of OpenNotes include increased clinical time spent addressing patient concerns about the note, changes in documentation that would prohibit candid observations or reasoning, patient confusion or misunderstanding medical terminology, patients taking offense by what was documented, potential for security breaches, and perceived pressure for patients to read notes.[33]

After the 12 months of the OpenNotes demonstration at three large medical centers, greater than 80% of patients opened at least one note, and two-thirds reported understanding their conditions better, increasing their medication adherence, taking better care of themselves, and feeling more in control of their care. Very few patients reported confusion, worry, or offense about what they read in their notes (1%-8% across sites). Two out of 10 patients shared their notes with others, and greater than 85% said that ability to access notes would influence their choice about future providers.

From the physician's perspective, only 3% of doctors reported spending more time answering patient questions between visits, 11% reported spending more time writing or editing notes, and there was no significant increase in the number of e-mails between physicians and patients.[34]

Based upon the success of the initial pilot, OpenNotes have expanded beyond the primary care setting, around the world, and may include notes from the inpatient or ED settings.[35] As of March 2020, there were multiple organizations successfully participating in the US OpenNotes movement.

DOCUMENTATION CONCERNS

While the unintended consequences of EHRs in terms of patient safety have been widely reported, these cases have involved issues with CPOE, not EHR documentation.[36-38] One of the primary concerns specific to EHR documentation is the potential for decreased efficiency. Recent published experience has been mixed. One institution was able to measure the isolated impact of implementing provider documentation software designed by that institution to replace paper documentation in the setting of existing patient tracking and CPOE. Analysis of 1 year of data that included roughly 60,000 patient visits demonstrated a slight increase in patient length of stay (less than 12 minutes) without the use of scribes or voice-to-text dictation.[39] Another study at a different institution found no significant difference in the productivity of 31 emergency physicians 6 months after transitioning from paper documentation to electronic charting.[40]

Too Much Information

The problem of too much information has been recognized in almost every industry, and medicine is no exception. The concerns regarding how much information must be entered and how to filter through all the noise of information overload are more a reflection of new requirements than of the EHR documentation system itself.

The ability to automatically pull information from other places in medical record into the physician's note can make the document very long. This is often referred to as "note bloat" and requires readers to filter through the note to find the information they need. The problem can be avoided by judicious use of links and limiting imported information to data that are essential to the medical decision process.

SOAP to APSO

Electronic notes can also be made more easily navigated by considering alternative ways of presenting information. For instance, the SOAP (subjective, objective, assessment, plan) note format that was developed during an era of paper charting translates into having to scroll considerably before arriving to the assessment and plan portion of the note that best conveys the MDM that occurred during the interaction. Some health systems have implemented APSO (assessment, plan, subjective, objective) note formats to make the assessment and plan readily available and easy to find at the top of each note. In one study, this resulted in 70.6% clinicians reporting that it was (much) easier to find clinically relevant data, 76.3% reporting that it was (much) faster to browse multiple EHR notes, and 67.6% reporting that it was (much) easier to follow clinical reasoning.[41]

Liability Risk

Concern about liability risk is also reported. Inappropriate use of macros and copy/paste functionality without necessary editing has already been mentioned. Suffice it to say that prudent users of EHR documentation systems should avoid known common pitfalls, such as cloning, adding single-click default values without careful review, and failing to document key facts because options could not be found.[42,43]

Physicians should be cautious about modifying notes after care has been provided. Minor corrections that are made in close proximity to the time that care was rendered will most likely not be problematic, while major changes that occur long after the patient has been seen, especially if there was a subsequent unexpected poor outcome, may be viewed as deceptive or fraudulent. Printed versions of addended electronic notes will show the updated time the note has been addended, and forensic analysis of EHRs makes it possible to track exactly which information in the note was modified and at what time. Despite all these medical–legal concerns, there is actually evidence that physicians who use EHR documentation systems are less likely to pay malpractice claims.[44]

Usability

Electronic health record usability has been a concern for some physicians. Evaluation of usability is a significant challenge due to the fact that usability is far more subjective than features or functions. The literature is full of strategies for use of color, numbers, graphs, and visualizations in other industries.[45-48] Researchers have published extensive discussions of multiple approaches for improved cognitive design for health information technology.[49-51]

A document titled "Electronic Health Record Usability: Interface Design Constraints" prepared in 2009 for the Agency for Healthcare Research and Quality, a division of the US DHHS, describes a significant void in any comprehensive standards or guidelines.[52] This lack of usability standards continues to be an issue. Consequently, usability and information design are more a product of each vendor's unique style and design constraints. Until standards are established for health-care technology usability and cognitive design, evaluation of the user interface will rely on the subjective opinions of HIT physician champions. These opinions are based on vendor demonstrations, direct observation of successful installations, and hands-on use in a simulated environment.

THE FUTURE OF EHR DOCUMENTATION SYSTEMS

While current EHR systems produce documents that tend to reflect the paper records they replaced, future developments may include a more layered representation that allows the user to drill down into diagnosis-specific portions of the patient's history to rapidly assemble a working knowledge of the clinical course regarding a specific diagnosis or surgery.[53]

Nuance Communications, Inc is currently demonstrating utilization of their ambient listening and natural language processing technology to capture key portions of the doctor–patient conversation, distinguish between the voice of the physician and that of the patient, and automatically construct a document that includes the HPI. It also includes the physician's verbal description when performing the PE, their clinical impressions and plan as conveyed to the patient, and any test results. Microsoft is also developing a similar product, the EmpowerMD Intelligent Scribe, which transcribes conversations between physicians and their patients. Suggestions are mapped to the subjective, objective, assessment, and plan sections of the note and ranked with a confidence level from high to low. Physicians can map each suggestion back to the transcript for more context and can decide whether to accept or reject each suggestion.

Future documentation systems may allow for text-based notes to be enhanced with multimedia formats beyond images, such as audio or video recordings, or more easily facilitate the inclusion of images to multimedia involved in MDM, such as radiology images or electrocardiography/telemetry tracings. Multimedia-enhanced radiology reports with hyperlinks to annotated images and tables and graphs that quickly display trends over time have recently been implemented in some health systems.[54] It is easy to imagine that provider notes may include similar functionality in the future or that unequivocal radiology impressions or diagnoses based upon laboratory results might automatically suggest visit diagnoses, discharge instructions, orders, and more.

Machine learning and predictive analytics are expected to work alongside the physician, processing information about the patient and integrating it with health surveillance data to provide insights that would otherwise require active data gathering and assimilation.

Finally, as clinician reimbursement becomes increasingly dependent upon adherence to quality measures, delivery of value, and effective documentation, automated feedback systems will likely identify deficiencies and alert the provider to address them prior to signing a note.

Keys to Successful EHR Implementation and Optimization

Successful implementation of an electronic documentation system is more about process and preparation than it is about the specific solution that is selected. Factors to consider include:

1. **Strong leadership team**
   - Executive leadership and accountability is essential.
   - Early creation of multidisciplinary teams is also essential.
   - Physician champions should be identified and involved from the very beginning.
   - Appropriate compensation for physician time will need to be a part of the budget.

2. **Highly reliable infrastructure**
   - A fast connection is required.
   - Reliable wireless connectivity must be tested in every corner of the ED.
   - Redundancy to minimize downtime should be considered.
   - Simple single sign-on with sharing of patient data across applications is important.
   - User preferences for the location and type of workstations and mobile devices must be considered. (Since workflows can change significantly with implementation of an electronic solution, the final purchase of devices may be delayed until after implementation once physicians and clinicians understand their new workflows.)

3. **Equate planning**
   - Realistic time lines need to be established anticipating the need for adjustments.
   - The physician champions must insist on adequate physician training by all physicians prior to going live. (Successful implementation can involve anywhere from 6 to 24 hours of physician training. Most successful programs involve individual web-based training, one-on-one training, and/or training in small groups of four or fewer physicians.)

4. **Metrics for success**
   - Users should be involved in establishing meaningful metrics for success prior to going live.
   - Metric values should be measured before implementation as well as at 30 days, 90 days, and 1 year after implementation.

5. **Caveats**
   - When signing a vendor contract, the prudent institution will not allow the vendor to include a clause that holds the vendor harmless for all medicolegal liability.[26]
   - It is essential to maintain transparency for everyone affected throughout all aspects of preparation, implementation, and evaluation of the success of an electronic documentation system.

Beyond Implementation

One of the more common oversights that can threaten successful adoption of an EHR documentation system is the failure to recognize that implementation is not the end. Three more steps are essential:

1. *Stabilization:* Users must be given time to get used to the system, feel more comfortable with it, and adapt to new workflows. Different workflows for different users will surface and will need to be accommodated. Support systems may need to be adjusted.

2. **Optimization:** Motivated users will identify opportunities to improve the system, but allowing time for stabilization before implementing changes can be very helpful. A system of governance should be established and communicated so that opportunities to improve the system are prioritized in an orderly manner.
3. **Realization:** Realization of the full benefits of "going electronic" comes only after allowing adequate time for stabilization and successful optimization. Moving resources to other projects before completing the stabilization and realization processes can increase the risk of failure.

CONCLUSION

There are many purposes and audiences of medical documentation, including recording information used for direct patient care, billing, ensuring quality/improvement, maintaining patient safety, communicating among care team members, and communicating with patients themselves. Medical documentation has transformed over time, from paper charting to EHRs. The ways in which information is recorded in health records has evolved from handwritten notes to scanned documents, from paper templates to electronic forms, and from asynchronous dictation to natural language processing and scribes. The burden of note writing can be mitigated by efforts to develop documentation support systems that suggest templates based upon age, chief complaint, and other data contained within the EHR.

REFERENCES

1. Bickley MD, Lynn S. *Bates' Pocket Guide to Physical Examination and History Taking.* 6th ed. Philadelphia, Pa: Wolters Kluwer Health/Lippincott Williams & Wilkins; 2009:1–14
2. Centers for Medicare and Medicaid Services (CMS). *Documentation Guidelines for Evaluation and Management Services.* 1995.
3. Department of Health and Human Services (DHHS). *International Classification of Diseases (ICD-10-CM/PCS) Transition.* 2015.
4. Kuhn T, Basch P, Barr M, et al. Clinical documentation in the 21st century: executive summary of a policy position paper from the American College of Physicians. *Ann Intern Med.* 2015;162(4):301–303.
5. Mandell M. Not documented, not done. *Nursing.* 1994;24(8):62–63.
6. Mulvehill S, Schneider G, Cullen CM, et al. Template-guided versus undirected written medical documentation: a prospective, randomized trial in a family medicine residency clinic. *J Am Board Fam Pract.* 2005;18(6):464–469.
7. Health Information Technology for Economic and Clinical Health (HITECH) Act. Title XIII of Division A & Title IV of Division B of the American Recovery and Reinvestment Act of 2009. ARRA; Pub. L. no 111-5: 2009.
8. Cohen JK, How many hospitals are on each stage of HIMSS Analytics' EMR Adoption Model? Becker's Health IT. 2018. Available at: https://www.beckershospitalreview.com/ehrs/how-many-hospitals-are-on-each-stage-of-himss-analytics-emr-adoption-model.html. Accessed September 19, 2020.
9. U.S. EMR adoption model: HIMSS Analytics. 2017. Available at: https://www.himssanalytics.org/emram. Accessed August 1, 2020.
10. Kohn D. Patient engagement and the legal electronic health record. Presented at: the American Health Information Management Association Legal Electronic Health Record Summit, August 15, 2011; Chicago, Ill.
11. Centers for Medicare and Medicaid Services (CMS). Evaluation and Management Services Guide. Available at: https://www.cms.gov/Outreach-and-Education/Medicare-Learning-Network-MLN/MLNProducts/Downloads/eval-mgmt-serv-guide-ICN006764.pdf. Accessed October 14, 2018. Updated August 2017.
12. Centers for Medicare and Medicaid Services (CMS). Pub 100-04 Medicare claims processing. Transmittal 881. Change request 3928. 2006.
13. Wang K, Najafi N. Characterizing the source of text in electronic health record progress notes. *JAMA Intern Med.* 2017;177(8):1212–1213.
14. Office of the Inspector General, U.S. Department of Health and Human Services. A roadmap for new physicians, avoiding Medicare and Medicaid fraud and abuse. Available at: https://oig.hhs.gov/compliance/physician-education/roadmap_web_version.pdf. Accessed October 14, 2018.
15. Levinson S, Grider D, Linker R, et al. The perfect storm. *Med Eco.* 2009;86(7):18–20, 22, 24.
16. Zick RG, Olsen J. Voice recognition software versus a traditional transcription service for physician charting in the ED. *Am J Emerg Med.* 2001;19(4):295–298.
17. Hoyt R, Yoshihashi A. Lessons learned from implementation of voice recognition for documentation in the military electronic health record system. *Perspect Health Inf Manag.* 2010;7:1e.
18. Gross FR, Zhou L, Weiner SG. Incidence of speech recognition errors in the emergency department. *Int J Med Inform.* 2016;93:70–73.
19. Anderson MR. DRT-enabled EHRs Healthcare Information and Management Systems Society (HIMSS) 2009. Paper presented at: HIMSS Europe Digital Conference, February 3, 2009.
20. Arya R, Salovich DM, Ohman-Strickland P, et al. Impact of scribes on performance indicators in the emergency department. *Acad Emerg Med.* 2010;17(5):490–494.

21. Terry C, O'Conner R, Cardella K, et al. The use of a medical scribe program to improve emergency medicine resident documentation at an academic medical center. *Acad Emerg Med*. 2008;15(supp s1):216.

22. Scheck A. The next big thing: medical scribes: scribes push emergency medicine closer to adoption of electronic medical records. *Emerg Med News*. 2009;31(2):13–16.

23. The Joint Commission. Use of unlicensed persons acting as scribes. 2011. Available at: http://www.jointcommission.org/mobile/standards_information/jcfaqdetails.aspx?StandardsFAQId=345&StandardsFAQChapterId=66. Accessed April 3, 2014.

24. The Joint Commission. Documentation assistance provided by scribes: what guidelines should be followed when physicians or other licensed independent practitioners use scribes to assist with documentation? *Perspectives Newsletter*. 2018;38(8). The Official Newsletter of the Joint Commission. Available at: https://www.jointcommission.org/standards_information/jcfaqdetails.aspx?StandardsFAQId=1809. Accessed October 14, 2018.

25. Gellert G, Ramirez R, Webster SL. The rise of the medical scribe industry: implications for the advancement of electronic health records. *JAMA*. 2015;313(13):1315–1316.

26. Lo H, Matheny M, Seger D, et al. Impact of non-interruptive medication laboratory monitoring alerts in ambulatory care. *J Am Med Inform Assoc*. 2009;16(1):66–71.

27. Unni R, H R. Perceived effectiveness of push vs. pull mobile location-based advertising. *J Interact Adv*. 2007;7(2):28–40.

28. Tehrani A, Lee H, Matthews S, et al. 25-Year summary of US malpractice claims for diagnostic errors 1986-2010: an analysis form the National Practitioner Data Bank. *BMJ Qual Saf*. 2013;22(8):672–680.

29. Santos A, Powell JA. Effectiveness of push and pull learning strategies in construction management. *J Workplace Learn*. 2001;13(2):47–56.

30. Solove DJ. HIPAA turns 10: analyzing the past, present and future impact. *J AHIMA*. 2013;84(4):22–28.

31. Committee on Quality of Health Care in America, Institute of Medicine. *Crossing the Quality Chasm: A New Health System for the 21st Century*. Washington, DC: National Academy Press; 2001.

32. OpenNotes. Available at: https://www.opennotes.org/. Accessed July 7, 2020.

33. Delbanco T, Walker J, Darer JD, et al. Open notes: doctors and patients signing on. *Ann Intern Med*. 2010;153(2):121–125.

34. Delbanco T, Walker J, Bell SK, et al. Inviting patients to read their doctors' notes: a quasi-experimental study and a look ahead. *Ann Intern Med*. 2012;157(7):461–470.

35. DesRoches CM, Leveille S, Bell SK, et al. The views and experience of clinicians sharing medical record notes with patients. *JAMA Network Open*. 2020:3(3). Available at: https://jamanetwork.com/journals/jamanetworkopen/fullarticle/2763607. Accessed August 1, 2020.

36. Walsh KE, Adams WG, Bauchner H, et al. Medication errors related to computerized order entry for children. *Pediatrics*. 2006;118(5):1872–1879.

37. Koppel R, Metlay JP, Cohen A, et al. Role of computerized physician order entry systems in facilitating medication errors. *JAMA*. 2005;293(10):1197–1203.

38. Han YY, Carcillo JA, Venkataraman ST, et al. Unexpected increased mortality after implementation of a commercially sold computerized physician order entry system. *Pediatrics*. 2005;116(6):1506–1512.

39. Feblowitz J, Takhar S, Ward M, et al. The operational effects of implementing electronic provider documentation in the emergency department. *Ann Emerg Med*. 2015;66(4):S99.

40. Sarangarm D, Lamb G, Weiss S, et al. Implementation of electronic charting is not associated with significant change in physician productivity in an academic emergency department. *JAMIA Open*. 2018;1(2):227–232.

41. Sieja A, Pell J, Markley K, et al. Successful implementation of APSO notes across a major health system. *Am J Account Care*. 2017;5(1):29–34.

42. Dimick C. Documentation bad habits: shortcuts in electronic records pose risk. *JAHIMA*. 2008;79(6):40–43.

43. Hammond KW, Helbig ST, Benson CC, et al. Are electronic medical records trustworthy? Observations on copying, pasting and duplication. *Proceedings from Annual Symposium of American Medical Informatics Association (AMIA)*. 2008;269–273.

44. Virapongse A, Bates D, Shi P, et al. Electronic health records and malpractice claims in office practice. *Arch Intern Med*. 2008;168(21):2362–2367.

45. Tufte ER. *The Visual Display of Quantitative Information*. 2nd ed. Cheshire, Conn: Graphics Press; 2006.

46. Few S. *Information Dashboard Design: The Effective Visual Communication of Data*. Sebastopol, Calif: O'Reilly Media; 2008.

47. Few S. *Show Me the Numbers: Designing Tables and Graphs to Enlighten*. El Dorado Hills, Calif: Analytics Press: 2004.

48. Wickens CD, Lee JD, Gordon-Becker S. *An Introduction to Human Factors Engineering*. 2nd ed. Upper Saddle River, NJ: Prentice Hall; 1998.

49. Patel VL, Kushniruk AW. Interface design for health care environments: the role of cognitive science. *Proceedings from the Journal of American Medical Informatics Association (JAMIA) Symposium*. 1998;29–37.

50. Patel VL, Kushniruk AW, Yang S, et al. Impact of a computer-based patient record system on data collection, knowledge organization, and reasoning. *J Am Med Inform Assoc*. 2000;7(6):569–585.

51. Cimino JJ. An integrated approach to computer-based decision support at the point of care. *Trans Am Clin Climat Assn*. 2007;118:273–288.

52. Armijo D, McDonnell C, Werner K. *Electronic Health Record Usability: Interface Design Considerations*. James Bell Associates and the Altarum Institute; 2009.

53. Dunagan W. quoted in "The Future of Electronic Health Records: 6 Predictions." Institute of Informatics (I²) website, Washington University School of Medicine. Available at: https://informatics.wustl.edu/2017/04/04/the-future-of-electronic-health-records-6-predictions/. Accessed October 15, 2018.

54. Folio LR, Machado LB, Dwyer AJ. Multimedia-enhanced radiology reports: concept, components, and challenges. *RadioGraphics*. 2018;38(2):462–482.

COMPUTERIZED PROVIDER ORDER ENTRY AND CLINICAL DECISION SUPPORT

Brian Fengler, Nicholas Genes, Ali Raja

Computerized provider order entry (CPOE) has crossed the threshold from a function used in daily practice by only a small number of clinicians to a general work expectation; it was mandated as part of the "Meaningful Use" expectations of the 2009 HITECH Act.[1] While CPOE and clinical decision support (CDS) can exist independently of one another, in most electronic health records (EHRs), CPOE is associated with the implementation of CDS. From a physician-leader standpoint, the methods for managing the implementation of CPOE and CDS within the emergency department (ED) are quite similar. For nurse leaders, attention to the order sets, order entry approval functionality, and reporting of performance metrics and quality outcome measures are essential.

The adoption of CPOE changes provider workflows. When utilizing a well-designed CPOE system and an EHR that has been integrated into provider workflow with an excellent user interface, the end result can be quite beneficial to both patients and providers.[2] In the absence of this synergy, however, the institution of CPOE and CDS has been demonstrated to adversely impact patient safety and provider efficiency.[3-8]

With a regulatory emphasis on the reporting of quality measures, CDS has become a tool to improve organizational performance, reduce errors, and improve patient safety. As such, it is anticipated that CDS deployment will evolve and expand over time, increasing its impact upon clinical users within the department. For a CPOE and CDS project to be successful, emergency physicians and nurses must thoughtfully advocate throughout the development, implementation, and deployment cycles. However, inadequate leadership and resources or a failure to understand the potential clinical and organizational impact of CPOE and CDS can lead to profound consequences. Preventable decrements in core ED throughput metrics, clinician satisfaction, patient safety, and provider reimbursement may all follow if CPOE and CDS implementations are characterized by insufficient clinical leadership, governance, or participation.

ELECTRONIC HEALTH RECORDS

As clinicians spend more of their time in front of a computer, the usability of the ED's EHR is an essential factor when contemplating new CPOE and CDS processes. The Healthcare Information and Management Systems Society defines EHR usability as "the effectiveness, efficiency, and satisfaction with which specific users can achieve a specific set of tasks in a particular environment." Usability isn't simply about a pleasant user experience; poor EHR usability contributes to errors associated with patient harm. It also results in clinicians spending extra time using EHRs and can lead to frustration, which can jeopardize patient safety.[9] In the ED, efficient interactions are particularly important. The acute, unscheduled care provided in the ED makes it an interruption-driven environment.[10,11] One early study

> **BOX 67.1 ■ EHR USABILITY CRITERIA[12]**
>
> 1. Simplicity
> 2. Naturalness
> 3. Consistency
> 4. Forgiveness and feedback
> 5. Effective use of language
> 6. Efficient interactions
> 7. Effective information presentation
> 8. Preservation of context
> 9. Minimize cognitive load

showed that emergency physicians are interrupted an average of 10.3 times per hour.[11] While computers can multitask and reliably return to disrupted processes, human beings often find themselves distracted and unable to concentrate when they return to tasks.[7] Thus, minimizing interruptions generated by the EHR should be a leadership priority. The "usability" of a particular system can be assessed against criteria in nine key categories (**Box 67.1**).[12]

Relatively basic usability enhancements to the EHR system are associated with better physician cognitive workload and performance. A recent review of 557 clinician-submitted reports identified seven safety and usability challenges of which physicians must be aware (**Table 67.1**).[13]

TABLE 67.1 ■ Safety and Usability Challenges of EHRs[13]

Type	Challenge	Example
Data entry	A clinician's work process may make it hard or impossible to appropriately enter the desired EHR data.	A clinician chose the wrong frequency for a drug to be administered because he didn't realize that the order in which the options were populated in the EHR had changed.
Alerting	EHR alerts or other feedback from the system may be absent, incorrect, or ambiguous.	Although a patient's gelatin allergy was listed in the EHR, a clinician wasn't alerted to the allergy while prescribing a medicine containing gelatin.
Interoperability	Communication of information in an EHR may be hindered because interoperability is inadequate within components of the same EHR or from the EHR to other systems.	Clinicians were unable to access laboratory results for a patient from records held in a different part of the hospital.
Visual display	Clinically relevant information is hindered because it is entered or stored in the wrong location or is otherwise inaccessible in the EHR.	A clinician attempted to order 3.125 mg of a medication, but the EHR listed a 6.25 mg prescription, with a 3.125 mg dose listed in small print, confusing the clinician.
Availability of information	The EHR automates or defaults to information that is unexpected, unpredictable, or not transparent to the clinician.	A hospital lab employee was unable to access a section of a patient's EHR in which the clinician ordered diagnostic tests; consequently, the tests were not performed.
Workflow support	The EHR workflow is not supported due to a mismatch between the EHR and the end user's intent.	A physician ordered diagnostic tests and included instructions for the lab in a special field. However, laboratory staff could not see that information, and the tests were not conducted.

COMPUTERIZED PROVIDER ORDER ENTRY

CPOE is becoming standard; since 2016, these systems have been used in 96% of US hospitals.[14] Frequently upheld as a means to improve patient safety, CPOE can provide important safety features, such as allergy alerts and drug–drug, drug–food, and drug–disease interaction checks; it can also suggest safe medication dose ranges and intervals. However, it has been challenging to assess whether the profound improvements in patient care that were anticipated by transitioning to CPOE have, in fact, been realized. The majority of studies related to CPOE implementation have been conducted in tertiary care centers with large informatics and information technology support structures, and CPOE benefits have not been well demonstrated in scenarios outside of large academic facilities.[15] Also, many studies of the effects of CPOE have included bundled CDS tools, making it difficult to assess the isolated outcomes of CPOE implementation.

While there have been some reports of reductions in medication errors based upon isolated CPOE implementations, increased errors related to CPOE have also been reported.[3–8,15,16] Sometimes this effect can be attributed to "shining a light on a dirty room," as CPOE and its associated reporting tools allow mistakes to be easily captured, while older paper-based workflows may result in underreported errors. Within the ED, CPOE also enables parallel processing (i.e., allowing for nursing, radiology, and other orders to be placed and acted upon simultaneously) without requiring a physical chart.

A body of literature regarding the unintended and adverse consequences of CPOE is developing.[4–8,17] Notable examples include the perception of more or new work for physicians, mismatches between the CPOE system and current workflow, changes in the hospital's power structure due to reduced physician autonomy, and an overdependence on technology.[5] CPOE systems are accepted or rejected by clinical providers based upon their user interface and capabilities. A system that is labor intensive, not integrated with current workflow, or hampered by a poor user interface will meet resistance.[18]

Selecting and Implementing a CPOE System

As enterprise EHR implementations have predominated, ED leaders are no longer likely to be involved in the selection of a CPOE provider. Furthermore, few institutions are developing custom-built CPOE systems. Selection decisions are typically made at an institutional level, with the expectation that all providers within the hospital will be using one vendor's product across many different practice environments. Emergency physician leaders should ensure that they are involved in the implementation and governance of CPOE, as well as the integration of CDS at a departmental and institutional level, with the ability to tailor the EHR to the ED staff's specific needs. The absence of interested clinicians in CPOE decisions may lead to negative workflow-related consequences.[19–21]

Understanding the capabilities and limitations of the chosen CPOE product is instrumental to its success within the ED. By being a leader on the hospital's governance committee and a champion of CPOE within the organization, the physician leader will help ensure the implementation of a clinically driven product (as opposed to an information technology project). The development of order sets and order functionality for a CPOE system can be time and labor intensive, and the contents of those sets are predicated upon the capabilities of the product itself. The CPOE and CDS capabilities of EHR applications vary widely, impacting the functionalities that are available within the system as well as the resources needed to curate and maintain this knowledge base.[22–25]

Medication-specific considerations when selecting a CPOE system include whether to default the priority on most ED medications to STAT x1, as opposed to scheduled and recurring times. STAT dosing orders can lead to a nursing management dilemma: If every medication is given STAT, are all medications overdue the moment they are ordered? Can a STAT order also include a grace period, so that nurses are not automatically penalized? Similarly, some EDs do not allow as needed (PRN) medication dosing. Can the CPOE vendor accommodate this policy, or can ED drugs be listed without the PRN option?

Being present, visible, and committed to the success of CPOE deployment and maintenance will help ensure that adequate hospital resources are committed to meet the needs of the department. After the initial creation of a CPOE system, nursing and physician involvement will be an ongoing requirement in the maintenance, upkeep, and adjustment of the system to support ED workflow. Clinicians need to be identified, trained, and made available to support departmental requirements.

CLINICAL DECISION SUPPORT

In this chapter, CDS is defined as a series of tools designed to inform and influence clinical decision-making. Ideally, CDS systems may be described in terms of doing five *right* things: They "provide the right information, to the right person, in the right format, through the right channel, at the right point in workflow to improve health and health care decisions and outcomes."[26] While appearing simple at the onset, the design, implementation, and use of CDS can have a significant impact on provider practice and workflow.

As EHRs have grown in functionality and complexity, the ability to provide CDS at different stages of the provider workflow and decision support that extends beyond passive means has become possible. As an example, CDS extends the range of feedback to clinical providers, providing information at new locations within their workflow. While it may be associated with CPOE implementation, CDS within the ED can provide many forms of support that extend well beyond the CPOE system itself (**Table 67.2**).

The goal of CDS is to provide contextual, real-time decision support at the point of care. This ability exists due to the presence of discrete patient-specific data, including demographics, chief complaints, past medical history, vital signs, laboratory values, charting elements, orders, and phases of ED care. Based upon the complexity of the EHR and the resources available to provide the programming, set up, and maintenance of CDS, the decision support can include simple tasks like color-coding abnormal laboratory values or providing icons to identify new, actionable information regarding a patient. Links to supporting literature and references may be embedded into the workflow based upon diagnoses, medications, or other discrete data elements. "Hard stops" can be implemented to confirm high-risk orders. More complex rules and engine-based workflows, present within some EHRs, allow for branching order sets, suggested order sets, and automated alerts based upon a mixture of demographics, laboratory values, orders, and documentation elements within the chart.

CDS Adoption

David W. Bates—the medical director of clinical and quality analysis and information systems at Partners HealthCare System, Inc.—identified 10 "commandments" for the adoption and effective use of CDS.[27] They emphasize that the presentation of CDS influences provider acceptance and overall functionality of the system. Eight of the ten requirements for implementation and maintenance revolve around the provider experience (**Box 67.2**).

TABLE 67.2 ■ Potential CDS Support in the ED

Type	Examples and Considerations
Medication-allergy checking	CDS can alert the ordering provider to a potential medication allergy at the time an order is placed. However, not all previous symptoms may represent a true allergy. For example, if a patient vomited once after taking codeine, should all future IV opioid orders trigger an alert?
Medication-medication interaction checking	Medication interactions can also be flagged at the time of order entry, although some interactions are potential rather than actual. For example, should a doctor ordering a statin refill see a warning for a theoretical interaction with the patient's SSRI, even though the patient has been taking both medications for years without incident?
Weight-based and renal dosing recommendations	CDS recommendations to adjust a medication dose for a patient's weight and creatinine clearance facilitate good practice. However, if these values are not readily available, drug ordering should not be delayed.
Antibiotic selection and stewardship	Guidelines for initiating treatment, results from prior cultures, and the ED's local antibiogram should be available to the clinician at the time of prescribing.
Opioid prescribing	One-click, single sign-on access to a state prescription drug monitoring program should be available, or ideally, prior scheduled drugs should be automatically imported into the chart, and clinicians should be alerted to similar existing prescriptions.
Suggesting appropriate clinical calculators and decision rules	Linking to a website that facilitates calculation of a PERC rule upon ordering a D-dimer may encourage appropriate usage; exporting relevant patient values (heart rate, O_2 saturation) and importing the calculated results into a note can improve efficiency and documentation. However, requiring calculations before orders can be placed encourages workarounds.
Appropriate use criteria for imaging	When an ED clinician ordering a radiology study clicks an indication from a predefined list, recommendations for the most appropriate test can appear. But, if the list does not include ED-specific indications or suggests unavailable tests, the utility of the CDS is limited.
Bed status determination	Access to clinical criteria to determine the appropriate level of care or bed status (observation, inpatient, ICU) can accelerate ED patient throughput. However, providers may not have the time to expend on case management.
"Coupled" order suggestions and panels	When ordering a *Clostridium difficile* toxin study, the ED clinician may appreciate a suggested order for contact isolation. But if the isolation order is required, it may inappropriately cut down on testing in crowded EDs.
Prompts/reminders to complete one aspect of a workup before embarking on another	Highlighting an opportunity to enter pharmacy information before e-prescribing can save clicks and time for a clinician, but requiring pharmacy details may discourage some prescribing. Similarly, some radiology tests can prompt for pregnancy testing, but requiring a test for a woman with a hysterectomy or in an emergent situation can lead to workarounds or delays in care.
Reminders to meet quality-reporting goals	Status indicators on trackboards may include features like timers to meet throughput goals or improve sepsis metrics. While these indicators can highlight patients who have been waiting too long for a study or inpatient bed, too many indicators can make track boards overwhelming.

> **BOX 67.2 ■ EIGHT REQUIREMENTS FOR EFFECTIVE CDS[27]**
>
> 1. Speediness
> 2. Anticipation of a clinician's need
> 3. Fitting into a clinician workflow
> 4. Clinician usability
> 5. Not interrupting or stopping a clinician workflow, if possible
> 6. Redirection of clinicians within their intended task
> 7. Simple interventions
> 8. Only asking for information when truly necessary

A recent survey on clinical preferences highlighted four beneficial features for CDS systems:[29]

1. Providing actionable CDS alerts that minimized disruption to clinical workflow
2. Letting providers make the CDS smarter by informing it when to alert, rather than interruptive CDS alerts for all clinicians in the same way for all patients (also called cooperative decision support)
3. Programming CDS alerts to include patient-specific information to inform clinical decisions, such as pertinent laboratory results, vital signs, and drug allergies
4. Adhering to CDS recommendations with the "least amount of clicks" and having the EHR populate text in their clinical documentation or patient instructions to reflect decision-making

Investigators in Norway recently created a comprehensive checklist to support health-care teams in considering the factors that affect the success of CDS interventions.[30] The GUIDES checklist includes 16 factors across several domains (**Table 67.3**).

Types of CDS

Both an advantage and disadvantage of modern EHRs is their ability to incorporate CDS in multiple locations in a provider's workflow and with various degrees of visibility and interactivity. Types of CDS systems have been described in various ways to reflect their method of interactivity with the user. Common descriptors related to CDS systems are active and passive, although that methodology has been criticized.[31] By this definition, *passive* CDS is something that occurs "behind the scenes" from the provider's standpoint and, in general, is something that does not force an action upon the provider. *Active* CDS, in contrast, requires some action on the part of the provider, though the appearance of an alert may not be a direct consequence of a provider's action.

Passive CDS

Passive CDS systems seek to inform and suggest, with the goal that end users exploit the provided resources to make better decisions. Real-world analogies might be "on-sale" tags placed on items in a store or a social media notification on a cell phone. These kinds of alerts may be driven by sophisticated algorithms or simple if/then logic. Users can act on the information or choose to ignore it and proceed with other tasks. An early form of passive decision support was Microsoft Clippy, a cartoon paper clip that tried to infer a Microsoft Office user's goals and offer help with certain tasks. Clippy was persistent, and some found its efforts unnecessary and annoying; ultimately, however, it could be ignored. Examples of passive CDS in an EHR include adding specific checkboxes for fever and incontinence

TABLE 67.3 ■ GUIDES Checklist

Domain	Domain Factors	Evaluation of Domain Factors
Context	The circumstances in which CDS can be potentially successful	• CDS can achieve the defined quality objectives. • The quality of the patient data is adequate. • Stakeholders and users accept CDS. • CDS can be added to the existing workload, workflows, and systems.
Content	The factors shaping the success of the advice produced by the CDS system	• The content provides trustworthy evidence-based information. • The decision support is relevant and accurate. • The decision support provides an appropriate call to action. • The amount of decision support is manageable for the target user.
System	Features belonging to the CDS tool	• The system is easy to use. • The decision support is well delivered. • The system delivers the decision support to the right target person. • The decision support is available at the right time.
Implementation	Factors affecting the integration of CDS into practice settings	• Information about the CDS system and its functions is appropriate. • Other barriers and facilitators to compliance with the decision support advice are assessed/addressed. • Implementation is stepwise, and the improvements in the CDS system are continuous. • Governance of the CDS implementation is appropriate.

to improve documentation for back pain complaints, providing a link to departmental guidelines and protocols in the EHR main menu, having a Wells score calculator appear when a CT chest angiogram is ordered, and surfacing a patient's older laboratory data when new results come in. Many emergency physicians are already familiar with passive CDS through the use of an electronic trackboard with colors or icons representing a patient's status, such as "ready to be seen" or "orders pending." Passive CDS may also be embedded within CPOE systems, for example, restricting a list of medications that can be ordered to those currently on-hand within the ED's medication-dispensing system.

Many forms of passive decision support are contextual and based upon patient-specific data. They may automatically appear to the provider, preferably at appropriate points within their workflow. A shortcoming of passive CDS is that the provider must be using the EHR during the time of patient care. Documenting the case after the fact (e.g., at the end of the shift) will make any of the passive guidance within the documentation system irrelevant. Similarly, if the CDS system is triggered by specific patient data that are not yet available, the provider will not benefit. In addition, the use of a scribe to overcome a slow or poor user interface will have a deleterious effect on a CDS system designed to improve documentation. An advantage of passive CDS is that, because it does not interrupt or redirect providers away from the task at hand, it is minimally intrusive to the clinician's workflow.

Administrators and others may ask: Why not prompt a clinician to acknowledge every alert? For documentation purposes and when reconstructing events, wouldn't it be better to know when an alert was seen and how the provider responded? While the ability to ignore passive CDS may seem suboptimal, in some circumstances, this can be advantageous. Engineering a process with barriers to quickly reading a patient's chart or placing orders carries its own risks, particularly in emergent situations.

Active CDS

Active CDS requires the provider's acknowledgment or forces the provider to stop within their current workflow. In some circumstances, these could be classified as "hard stops." Intuitively, this form of CDS is more intrusive and less likely to be well tolerated by clinicians.[27] An example of active CDS in the ED is the identification of a potential allergy to a prescribed medication, which then requires the clinician to manually indicate a desire to continue with or cancel the order. The challenge with alerts that require active intervention is that they are disruptive. The development and implementation of effective CDS requires an extremely gentle hand with active decision support. It has been demonstrated that clinicians often ignore drug safety alerts in CPOE systems.[32-36] Reasons cited include "alert fatigue," resulting from inappropriate alerts and lack of specificity.[34]

In response to injudicious use of alerts and the resulting alert fatigue, it may seem tempting to implement even "harder" stops for truly dangerous drug interactions. Under limited circumstances, active CDS can cause behavior changes more effectively than passive support; however, clinicians may not tolerate this type of CDS and may work to subvert it.[7] For instance, one study documented an inpatient unit where the CPOE design made it impossible to order trimethoprim/sulfamethoxazole and warfarin for the same patient without a phone call to an inpatient pharmacist.[6] The study had to be terminated early, as several participants ended up without antibiotic coverage or anticoagulation for days. Hard stops to prevent patient discharge without complete documentation can also lead to abbreviated notes.

There is no universal recommendation regarding the most appropriate timing of active CDS or hard stops; it varies by application and appropriateness. In a study of clinician preferences, roughly equal numbers of providers preferred the CDS to alert at different times, such as 1) the first opening of an encounter, 2) when ordering a medication or reviewing medications, 3) entering the patient's visit diagnosis, or 4) at the end of the encounter.[19] In a comprehensive review of the literature on the topic of active CDS and hard stops, several design characteristics that appear to be associated with positive outcomes were identified.[37] These included integrating important clinical decision-making aids, such as recent relevant lab results and specific score or risk calculators; triggering the alert at a natural and relevant place in the physician's workflow; enabling a third-party override; and having a comprehensive implementation plan involving user engagement, multiple iterations, and a rapid response to feedback.

Outcomes of CDS

Despite the promises of improvement in patient safety and clinical outcomes from CDS, results have been mixed. A review of 42 studies found that 83% of institutions reported a positive effect, although only a few actually addressed patient-centered clinical outcomes.[38] Many of the outcomes studied were process measures immediately downstream from implemented interventions, including documenting, prescribing, and the ordering of tests. While these studies are useful and provide evidence that CDS can modify clinician behavior, they do not make a strong case for its utility in improving patient outcomes.

In studies that have reported an improvement in patient-centered outcomes, benefits have been seen in improved rates of screening tests and immunizations; improved antibiotic stewardship; and (with more comprehensive CDS) improvement in the detection and care of patients with pneumonia, syncope, sepsis, asthma, and appendicitis.[39-47]

Results from the application of CDS for making diagnostic imaging decisions are especially interesting in light of the upcoming mandate from the Centers for Medicare and Medicaid Services, which requires that advanced imaging tests be accompanied by a qualified CDS mechanism.[48] Multiple studies have shown that the application of CDS modestly reduces imaging orders while improving the documentation of appropriateness scores.[49-52]

CDS Governance

Any institution hoping to change provider behavior via CDS will need to commit significant resources to the process. The two non-provider-based commandments cited by Bates revolve around the implementation, tracking, and maintenance of CDS.[27] Their recommendations include monitoring the impact of CDS, getting and responding to feedback from providers, and managing and maintaining the CDS knowledge base. Additionally, **Table 67.4** identifies 18 activities that are part of the institutional commitment to CDS effectiveness.[53]

Support and Maintenance

Ongoing support and maintenance of a CDS system can be labor intensive. Best practices regarding tools and techniques to develop and maintain a knowledge base for CDS have been suggested.[54,55] The resource and time commitments involved in implementing and maintaining effective CDS highlight the importance of tying organizational goals and metrics to the system while setting expectations to exceed specified thresholds.

TABLE 67.4 ■ Activities to Support CDS Effectiveness[52]

Areas	Activities
Fostering relationships across the organization	• Training and support • Visibility/presence on the floor • Liaising between people • Administration and leadership • Project management • Cheerleading/buy-in/sponsorship • Preparing for CDS implementation
Assembling the system	• Providing technical support • CDS content development • Purchasing products from vendors • Knowledge management • System integration
Using CDS to achieve the organization's goals	• Reporting • Requirements: gathering/specifications • Monitoring CDS • Linking CDS to goals • Managing data
Participation in policy and standards activities	• Internal governance • Engagement with medical societies and authors of clinical guidelines

If CDS is frequently overridden or the organization is not achieving its goals, then something about the current system is unhelpful or poorly designed. The work effort to monitor alerts, overrides, and address potential problems is significant; yet in its absence, CDS will likely not achieve its intended goal (and is likely generating alert fatigue, workarounds, burnout, and other unintended consequences).

Tracking Metrics

Ideally, an organization should be committed to defining and tracking ED metrics related to CDS. A lack of adherence or a system that elicits frequent provider complaints due to its intrusiveness or restrictiveness must prompt department leaders to consider a change. This requires physician leaders to have a strong representation within the CDS governance process, as well as an investment of time by both clinicians and IT resources to build, restructure, and readdress CDS within the EHR.[53] Inherent in this discussion is having an EHR that allows for changes to the provided CDS; this ability varies by vendor.[22]

In addition to measuring CDS performance based upon safety and compliance measures, it is also critical to evaluate the system's effect on clinician and nursing performance. Little published literature exists regarding the impact of CDS systems on nursing or physician performance in the ED. It is intuitive, however, that poorly implemented systems will succeed in reducing acceptance of the CDS and EHR and make the ED run less efficiently.

False-Positive Alerts

The impact of CDS upon providers and nurses cannot be effectively determined by gross measures like the average patient length of stay. More effective measures to calculate its effects are likely to come from provider feedback and the number of false-positive alerts. An example of a false-positive alert is one that fires every time a patient who had a previous reaction to codeine has an order for fentanyl placed in the ED. While drug-allergy checking can be effective, if the database does not have the granularity to distinguish between different categories of medications, there will be a number of inaccurate alerts presented to providers.[32] In addition, if the system is acting on incorrect data (such as drug intolerances listed as allergies) or outdated data (such as a drug-drug interaction regarding a medication the patient is no longer taking), providers will develop a skepticism related to these alerts. In one outpatient study, physicians found that 36.5% of medication alerts provided by their CDS were inappropriate.[36]

CDS Feedback

A formal feedback process from end users to a multidisciplinary team managing CDS for the ED is important.[53] Using submitted comments and exploring, understanding, and minimizing workflow limitations and constraints related to CDS will allow the organization to maximize the system's benefits while limiting potential adverse experiences. Once EHRs are implemented, the application of a CDS system (or its failure) must become a standard consideration during root-cause analyses and workflow mapping. Lessons learned can allow for the thoughtful implementation of CDS to prevent future adverse outcomes; however, CDS can also be a cause for errors or delays in treatment.[16]

Alternatives to CDS

Not all efforts to improve clinician adherence to guidelines and patient safety need to be implemented as point-of-care CDS. As the capabilities of EHRs to record provider behavior and decision-making have grown, peer-comparison feedback (also called social norm feedback) has emerged as a powerful new tool to drive physician behavior. Giving feedback to individual providers by showing their individual guideline adherence compared to the distribution of a group has been shown to reduce practice variation and achieve clinical goals, such as antibiotic stewardship and reduced opioid prescription.[56,57] This method of feedback cannot be given at the point of care and requires adequate data collection and administrative review; however, the process is less intrusive than EHR-based CDS for some clinical scenarios, and perhaps more effective.

Challenges of CDS Implementation

When implementing CDS functionality within the ED or transitioning to a new EHR system, many operational and clinician workflow challenges must be considered. The implementation of an enterprise-wide EHR with CDS, where the ED previously had a stand-alone ("best-in-breed") system, can also lead to unanticipated and undesired consequences. Enterprise-wide decisions related to CDS interactivity and alerts can be implemented with little consideration of department-specific workflow. Some enterprise EHR systems allow the regulation of CDS at a departmental level; however, this is not always possible.

The operational goals of hospital organizations often influence the application of CDS. **Box 67.3** contains a list of CDS goals that can be used to educate and inspire researchers, developers, finders, and policymakers.[58] In a 25-year retrospective on CDS, researchers laid out the following factors that contribute to the current dissatisfaction with CDS:

First, the difficulty in aligning the CDS with the clinician user's mental model of the patient and potential diagnostic or therapeutic interventions. Second, the difficulty in developing, maintaining, and integrating the clinical logic required to generate accurate, patient-specific, clinical suggestions. Third, the difficulty in gathering and assessing the quality of the data upon which this logic acts. Last, the rapid evolution of technology platforms — clinician end-users now may be accessing patient records via a desktop application, a hand-held application, or via a web-interface on a variety of devices, which implies significant technology and implementation challenges.[59]

As the ED transitions from one EHR to another, or from a paper system to an electronic one, it is imperative that the leadership maps current physician and nursing workflows. By going through these workflows in their entirety, the ED can effectively itemize currently used CDS (whether computerized or not) and ensure an equivalent level of support with the new EHR. This process will also allow physician and nursing leadership to prioritize new CDS requirements and clearly define expectations about where and how the system will be used. The implementation of a new EHR may provide significant opportunities for

---

BOX 67.3 ■ GOALS FOR CDS IMPLEMENTATION[58]

- Improve the human-computer interface.
- Disseminate best practices in CDS design, development, and implementation.
- Summarize patient-level information.
- Prioritize and filter recommendations to the user.
- Create an architecture for sharing executable CDS modules and services.
- Combine recommendations for patients with comorbidities.
- Prioritize CDS content development and implementation.
- Create internet-accessible CDS repositories.
- Use free-text information to drive CDS.
- Mine large clinical databases to create new CDS.

improved workflow and communication within the department that were lacking based upon prior system capabilities, but only if clinical leaders are aware of the new system's abilities and advocate for their appropriate use.

The lack of active participation by ED leadership, especially when transitioning to an enterprise-wide EHR, can result in new processes that are neither effective nor efficient and can potentially have adverse consequences for patient care and safety.

Next-Generation CDS

Among the many challenges of CDS adoption is the fact that the system must provide guidance in a consistent manner, while also being coherent with the individual user's mental model of the patient, processes, and context of care and decision-making. Recently, it was suggested that as CDS becomes more complex, the service-oriented integration of these systems will become more prevalent, allowing for the separation of knowledge and inference from the presenting EHR while still permitting deep workflow integration.[59] This fully modular approach may allow more innovation to occur in and around EHRs. Indeed, many of the EHR vendors are now moving toward an "app store" model to create a more scalable approach to CDS.

One desired but largely unattained aim of clinical informatics has been enabling CDS across multiple EHR systems. Although many factors limit the adoption of CDS, one main reason is that CDS capabilities are typically tightly coupled to custom modules within specific EHRs, making it difficult to share information across multiple platforms and care settings. A potential opportunity to enable scalable CDS systems is to leverage EHR-supported, web-based development platforms along with standard application programming interfaces (APIs), including Fast Healthcare Interoperability Resources.

One notable study proposed a staged approach, enabling a scalable web-based CDS platform to facilitate interoperability, with the CDS web tool displaying within the EHR's native user interface instead of a separate web browser.[60] This would allow the CDS tool to be coupled to a specific patient's chart and provide patient-specific recommendations. For example, while documenting an ED patient with chest pain, a standardized HEART score calculator would appear, importing the chart elements that facilitate the score calculation (comorbidities, troponin levels) and allowing users to enter or edit other values. Upon completion of the HEART score calculation, text would be generated in the note to reflect the score and subsequent decision-making. To the user, the HEART score calculator and tools would appear to be part of the EHR. In reality, however, this data would be independent of it and work with multiple EHR vendors.

As computing power and available patient data continue to grow, increasingly sophisticated algorithms become possible. Algorithms trained on outcomes from pre-existing patient data sets (machine learning) can be deployed in the EHR to forecast possible outcomes in new patients (predictive analytics). In the ED, predictive analytics for sepsis, clinical deterioration, and the likelihood of inpatient admission have been studied. These predictions can be based on demographic data, vital signs, lab results, comorbidities, and other factors, such as the time of day or words that appear in triage notes. With so many factors, it can be difficult or impossible for clinicians to review what triggered the alert. While the hope is that these algorithms lead to improved, timelier patient care, inevitable false-positives could drive unnecessary resource utilization, and false-negatives could lead to misdiagnosis or delays in care. As the triggers for the alerts are hard to evaluate, they may prompt clinician second-guessing and "erring on the side of caution" and agreement. Further, as these alerts prompt interventions and change clinician behavior, they could lead to "concept drift," a known machine-learning phenomenon in which predictions become less accurate over time.

Today's CDS systems have something in common with the first "expert systems" of the 1970s, an early approach to artificial intelligence. For example, MYCIN delivered predictions about the likely causes of bacteremia and meningitis based on inputted history, exam, and lab findings, and incorporated unknowns and degrees of certainty well before cultures were resulted. MYCIN also worked better than doctors—blinded infectious disease faculty evaluators rated MYCIN's choices for antibiotics as correct 65% of the time, beating the human specialist ratings of 42.5% to 62.5%.[61]

The expert systems had the advantages of memory and a methodical nature, but these advantages were also shortcomings. The knowledge base and hundreds of rules took a long time to develop and were hard to maintain; each diagnosis also required asking the user many dozens of questions. These were time-consuming solutions that didn't scale well. Also, critics lamented the "Greek oracle" proclamations of these systems, which relegated the physician to the role of passive data-entry clerk. But the arrival of machine learning and predictive analytics to CDS, more than 40 years later, may herald the return of inscrutable "Greek oracle" proclamations in medicine.

CONCLUSION

CPOE and CDS systems have been touted for years as revolutionary solutions to complex patient safety issues within health care. It is clear that we are riding a wave of new CDS functionalities that will soon permeate our working environment.

Accustomed to working in a complex, high-risk environment, emergency physicians and nurses have already established processes and procedures to reduce risk and improve throughput. The greatest potential for new CDS tools is their ability to provide decision support at the time of need based upon discrete information within the patient's record. The new risk for ED practice with the deployment of CDS is the ability to create active decision support. This is a powerful tool that can also be intrusive, limiting, and obstructive. It must be used thoughtfully, cautiously, and with objective goals and expectations in mind.

Per earlier analogies, an "on-sale" tag generally works well as a passive alert to shoppers, and a smartphone notification works well for social media users. But if a barrier existed with every notification, requiring acknowledgment and giving an option to reply, workflow rules would be necessary to use the phone emergently without reacting to pending notifications. Active alerts that demand a response can be powerful tools to prompt reflection and limit severe errors in judgment, but they are inherently disruptive and can lead to their own problems and errors. The implementation of active CDS within the ED requires aggressive clinical participation during the development, implementation, maintenance, and revision processes.

There is a clear take-home point for the emergency physician leader: Successful CPOE and CDS systems require active involvement in the hospital organization's IT governance and leadership. It is necessary for individuals to bridge the gap between clinical medicine and information technology for CPOE to work.[20] That requirement only increases with the implementation of complete, and frequently enterprise-based, EHRs within the department.

CDS and CPOE have the potential to decrease errors and improve patient safety, access to information, efficiency, and workflow. Just like any other tool, however, they can be used poorly. If CPOE and CDS are implemented improperly, employed without clinical participation, and applied without an understanding of their relationship to the clinical workflow, they will have unexpected consequences and possibly counterproductive results.

REFERENCES

1. Goldstein MM, Thorpe JH. The First Anniversary of the Health Information Technology for Economic and Clinical Health (HITECH) Act: the regulatory outlook for implementation. *Perspect Health Inf Manag.* 2010;7(Summer):1c.

2. Terrell KM, Perkins AJ, Hui SL, et al. Computerized decision support for medication dosing in renal insufficiency: a randomized, controlled trial. *Ann Emerg Med.* 2010;56(6):623–629.

3. Barron WM, Reed RL, Forsythe S, et al. Implementing computerized provider order entry with an existing clinical information system. The Joint Commission. *J Qual Patient Safety/Jt Comm Res.* 2006;32(9):506–516.

4. Koppel R, Metlay JP, Cohen A, et al. Role of computerized physician order entry systems in facilitating medication errors. *JAMA.* 2005;293(10):1197–1203.

5. Ash JS, Sittig DF, Dykstra R, et al. The unintended consequences of computerized provider order entry: findings from a mixed methods exploration. *Int J Med Inform.* 2009;78(Suppl 1):S69-S76.

6. Nebeker JR, Hoffman JM, Weir CR, et al. High rates of adverse drug events in a highly computerized hospital. *Arch Intern Med.* 2005;165(10):1111.

7. Han YY, Carcillo JA, Venkataraman ST, et al. Unexpected increased mortality after implementation of a commercially sold computerized physician order entry system. *Pediatrics.* 2005;116(6):1506.

8. Sittig DF, Ash JS, Zhang J, et al. Lessons from "Unexpected increased mortality after implementation of a commercially sold computerized physician order entry system." *Pediatrics.* 2006;118(2):797.

9. Ratwani RM, Savage E, Will A, et al. Identifying electronic health record usability and safety challenges in pediatric settings. *Health Aff (Millwood).* 2018;37(11):1752–1759.

10. Chisholm CD, Collison EK, Nelson DR, et al. Emergency department workplace interruptions: are emergency physicians "interrupt-driven" and "multitasking?" *Acad Emerg Med.* 2000;7(11):1239–1243.

11. Chisholm CD, Dornfeld AM, Nelson DR, et al. Work interrupted: a comparison of workplace interruptions in emergency departments and primary care offices. *Ann Emerg Med.* 2001;38(2):146–151.

12. Schoeffel R. The concept of product usability. *ISO Bulletin.* 2003;34:6–7.

13. Howe JL, Adams KT, Hettinger AZ, et al. Electronic health record usability issues and potential contribution to patient harm. *JAMA.* 2018;319(12):1276–1278.

14. Pedersen CA, Schneider PJ, Scheckelhoff DJ. ASHP national survey of pharmacy practice in hospital settings: prescribing and transcribing-2016. *Am J Health Syst Pharm.* 2017;74(17):1336–1352.

15. Shojania KG, Jennings A, Mayhew A, et al. The effects of on-screen, point of care computer reminders on processes and outcomes of care. *Cochrane Database Syst Rev.* 2009;(3):CD001096.

16. Strom BL, Schinnar R, Aberra F, et al. Unintended effects of a computerized physician order entry nearly hard-stop alert to prevent a drug interaction: a randomized controlled trial. *Arch Intern Med.* 2010;170(17):1578.

17. Ash JS, Sittig DF, Dykstra RH, et al. Categorizing the unintended sociotechnical consequences of computerized provider order entry. *Int J Med Inform.* 2007;76(Suppl 1):S21-S27.

18. Campbell EM, Guappone KP, Sittig DF, et al. Computerized provider order entry adoption: implications for clinical workflow. *J Gen Intern Med.* 2009;24(1):21–26.

19. Sittig DF, Ash JS, Guappone KP, et al. Assessing the anticipated consequences of computer-based provider order entry at three community hospitals using an open-ended, semi-structured survey instrument. *Int J Med Inform.* 2008;77(7):440–447.

20. Ash JS, Stavri PZ, Dykstra R, et al. Implementing computerized physician order entry: the importance of special people. *Int J Med Inform.* 2003;69(2–3):235–250.

21. Aarts J, Ash J, Berg M. Extending the understanding of computerized physician order entry: implications for professional collaboration, workflow and quality of care. *Int J Med Inform.* 2007;76(suppl 1):S4-S13.

22. Wright A, Sittig DF, Ash JS, et al. Clinical decision support capabilities of commercially-available clinical information systems. *J Am Med Inform Assoc.* 2009;16(5):637–644.

23. Sittig DF, Wright A, Meltzer S, et al. Comparison of clinical knowledge management capabilities of commercially-available and leading internally-developed electronic health records. *BMC Med Inform Decis Mak.* 2011;11:13.

24. Mccoy AB, Wright A, Sittig DF. Cross-vendor evaluation of key user-defined clinical decision support capabilities: a scenario-based assessment of certified electronic health records with guidelines for future development. *J Am Med Inform Assoc.* 2015;22(5):1081–1088.

25. Ash JS, Sittig DF, Mcmullen CK, et al. Multiple perspectives on clinical decision support: a qualitative study of fifteen clinical and vendor organizations. *BMC Med Inform Decis Mak.* 2015;15:35.

26. Osheroff JA, Pifer EA, Sittig DF, et al. *Clinical Decision Support Implementers' Workbook.* Chicago, Ill: HIMSS; 2004.

27. Bates DW. Ten commandments for effective clinical decision support: making the practice of evidence-based medicine a reality. *J Am Med Inform Assoc.* 2003;10(6):523–530.

28. Kawamoto K, Houlihan CA, Balas EA, et al. Improving clinical practice using clinical decision support systems: a systematic review of trials to identify features critical to success. *BMJ.* 2005;330(7494):765.

29. Trinkley KE, Blakeslee WW, Matlock DD, et al. Clinician preferences for computerised clinical decision support for medications in primary care: a focus group study. *BMJ Health Care Inform.* 2019;26(1).

30. Van de velde S, Kunnamo I, Roshanov P, et al. The GUIDES checklist: development of a tool to improve the successful use of guideline-based computerised clinical decision support. *Implement Sci.* 2018;13(1):86.

31. Carter JH. *Electronic Health Records.* 2nd ed. Philadelphia, PA: ACP Press; 2008.

32. Abookire SA, Teich JM, Sandige H, et al. Improving allergy alerting in a computerized physician order entry system. *Proc AMIA Symp.* 2000;2–6.

33. Hsieh TC. Characteristics and consequences of drug allergy alert overrides in a computerized physician order entry system. *J Am Med Inform Assoc.* 2004;11(6):482–491.

34. van der Sijs H, Aarts J, Vulto A, et al. Overriding of drug safety alerts in computerized physician order entry. *J Am Med Inform Assoc.* 2006;13(2):138–147.

35. Cavuto NJ, Woosley RL, Sale M. Pharmacies and prevention of potentially fatal drug interactions. *JAMA.* 1996;275(14):1086–1087.

36. Weingart SN, Toth M, Sands DZ, et al. Physicians' decisions to override computerized drug alerts in primary care. *Arch Intern Med.* 2003;163(21):2625–2631.

37. Powers EM, Shiffman RN, Melnick ER, et al. Efficacy and unintended consequences of hard-stop alerts in electronic health record systems: a systematic review. *J Am Med Inform Assoc.* 2018;25(11):1556–1566.

38. Patterson BW, Pulia MS, Ravi S, et al. Scope and influence of electronic health record-integrated clinical decision support in the emergency department: a systematic review. *Ann Emerg Med.* 2019;74(2):285–296.

39. Dean NC, Jones BE, Jones JP, et al. Impact of an electronic clinical decision support tool for emergency department patients with pneumonia. *Ann Emerg Med.* 2015;66(5):511–520.

40. McGuire R, Moore E. Using a configurable EMR and decision support tools to promote process integration for routine HIV screening in the emergency department. *J Am Med Inform Assoc.* 2016;23(2): 396-401.

41. Venkat A, Chan-Tompkins NH, Hegde GG, et al. Feasibility of integrating a clinical decision support tool into an existing computerized physician order entry system to increase seasonal influenza vaccination in the emergency department. *Vaccine.* 2010;28(37):6058-6064.

42. Sharp AL, Hu YR, Shen E, et al. Improving antibiotic stewardship: a stepped-wedge cluster randomized trial. *Am J Manag Care.* 2017;23(11):e360-e365.

43. Melnick ER, Genes NG, Chawla NK, et al. Knowledge translation of the American College of Emergency Physicians' clinical policy on syncope using computerized clinical decision support. *Int J Emerg Med.* 2010;3:97-104.

44. Nelson JL, Smith BL, Jared JD, et al. Prospective trial of real-time electronic surveillance to expedite early care of severe sepsis. *Ann Emerg Med.* 2011;57(5):500-504.

45. Dexheimer JW, Abramo TJ, Arnold DH, et al. Implementation and evaluation of an integrated computerized asthma management system in a pediatric emergency department: a randomized clinical trial. *Int J Med Inform.* 2014;83(11):805-813.

46. Kharbanda AB, Madhok M, Krause E, et al. Implementation of electronic clinical decision support for pediatric appendicitis. *Pediatrics.* 2016;137(5). pii: e20151745.

47. Hendrickson MA, Wey AR, Gaillard PR, et al. Implementation of an electronic clinical decision support tool for pediatric appendicitis within a hospital network. *Pediatr Emerg Care.* 2018;34(1):10-16.

48. Centers for Medicare & Medicaid Services. Medicare Program; Revisions to Payment Policies Under the Physician Fee Schedule and Other Revisions to Part B. 2020. Available at: https://www.cms.gov/Medicare/Medicare-Fee-for-Service-Payment/PhysicianFeeSched. Accessed August 1, 2020.

49. Medicare Program; Revisions to Payment Policies Under the Physician Fee Schedule and Other Revisions to Part B for CY 2018; Medicare Shared Savings Program Requirements; and Medicare Diabetes Prevention Program. Rules and regulations. *Fed Regist.* 2017;82(219):52976-53371.

50. Raja AS, Gupta A, Ip IK, et al. The use of decision support to measure documented adherence to a national imaging quality measure. *Acad Radiol.* 2014;21(3):378-383.

51. Huber TC, Krishnaraj A, Patrie J, et al. Impact of a commercially available clinical decision support program on provider ordering habits. *J Am Coll Radiol.* 2018;15(7):951-957.

52. Doyle J, Abraham S, Feeney L, et al. Clinical decision support for high-cost imaging: a randomized clinical trial. *PLoS One.* 2019;14(3):e0213373.

53. Wright A, Ash JS, Erickson JL, et al. A qualitative study of the activities performed by people involved in clinical decision support: recommended practices for success. *J Am Med Inform Assoc.* 2014;21(3):464-472.

54. Wright A, Sittig DF, Ash JS, et al. Governance for clinical decision support: case studies and recommended practices from leading institutions. *J Am Med Inform Assoc.* 2011.

55. Sittig DF, Wright A, Simonaitis L, et al. The state of the art in clinical knowledge management: an inventory of tools and techniques. *Int J Med Inform.* 2010;79(1):44-57

56. Hallsworth M, Chadborn T, Sallis A. Provision of social norm feedback to high prescribers of antibiotics in general practice: a pragmatic national randomised controlled trial. *Lancet.* 2016;387(10029):1743-1752.

57. Witt TJ, Deyo-Svendsen ME, Mason ER. A model for improving adherence to prescribing guidelines for chronic opioid therapy in rural primary care. *Mayo Clin Proc Innov Qual Outcomes.* 2018;2(4):317-323.

58. Sittig DF, Wright A, Osheroff JA, et al. Grand challenges in clinical decision support v10. *J BioMed Inform.* 2008;41(2):387-392.

59. Middleton B, Sittig DF, Wright A. Clinical decision support: a 25 year retrospective and a 25 year vision. *Yearb Med Inform.* 2016;(Suppl 1):S103-S116.

60. Zhang M, Velasco FT, Musser RC, et al. Enabling cross-platform clinical decision support through Web-based decision support in commercial electronic health record systems: proposal and evaluation of initial prototype implementations. *AMIA Annu Symp Proc.* 2013;2013: 1558-1567.

61. Shortliffe EH, Davis R, Axline SG, et al. Computer-based consultations in clinical therapeutics: explanation and rule acquisition capabilities of the MYCIN system. *Comput Biomed Res.* 1975;8(4):303-320.

CHAPTER 68

DATA ACQUISITION AND ANALYSIS

Sean Michael, Jennifer Wiler

Pray, Mr. Babbage, if you put into the machine wrong figures, will the right answers come out?

—Charles Babbage, *Passages from the Life of a Philosopher* (1864)

Entire books and business school courses have been written and taught on the topic of business intelligence and analytics. Given the apparent technical complexity of the subject, many clinical leaders feel more comfortable delegating analytic tasks to information technology/information services (IT/IS) professionals, hospital analysts, or external consultants. Perceiving that they lack the time or interest to master aspects of data acquisition and analysis themselves, these well-meaning leaders cede control to stakeholders outside the emergency department (ED), many of whom have exceptional technical skills but may lack expertise on the core operations of an ED.

Consequently, ED leaders lose the ability to tell stories using data, shape the narrative of their departmental successes and challenges, and maintain awareness of their processes and people. They may also find themselves feeling defensive or blindsided when operational data is taken out of context by hospital administrators, policymakers, partners, or payers. When confronted with an interesting question or opportunity, they may spend months of back-and-forth with IT, finally settling on a report that is "close enough" and several months out of date. Sound familiar? In contrast, the ED leader who has both a command of operational principles and a strong grasp on data analytics is well positioned to understand, manage, communicate, and improve clinical, operational, financial, quality, educational, and satisfaction outcomes for the department.

USES AND OUTPUTS OF ED DATA

On a walk through any ED these days, you cannot go more than a few feet without seeing a nurse, technician, or physician interacting with some kind of an electronic device. Computer, telemetry monitoring, and departmental tracking screens are everywhere. Patients sometimes see push notifications with their lab results on their smartphones before their clinicians do. As hospitals continue to invest heavily in technology (even after Meaningful Use incentives have been sunset), the data entry of clinical and administrative information has become a normal part of ED culture.[1] This cultural evolution has resulted in an exponential increase in the availability, volume, and richness of the information captured.

Hospital administrators, especially those in the C-suite, are being told by their chief information officer and IT/IS departments that all data required to validate staffing, evaluate quality, monitor productivity, track patient satisfaction, and prove return on investment on requests made by ED leaders can be obtained from currently installed computer systems. Electronic health record (EHR) vendors purport that all of the required information is

> **BOX 68.1 ■ COMMON USES OF ED DATA**
>
> **Regulatory reporting:**
>
> Prioritizes precise adherence to data definitions with integrity monitoring/audit trails but may have significant time lags
>
> **Quality and process improvement:**
>
> Prioritizes minimal time lag and patient-centered outcomes but may be difficult to capture exact clinical workflows of interest
>
> **Business development:**
>
> Prioritizes high-level summaries of long time periods but may oversimplify clinical nuances as rough estimates are often "good enough"
>
> **Research:**
>
> Prioritizes high-resolution detail with precise definitions but encumbered by regulatory requirements and may be poorly generalizable to larger ED population
>
> **Daily operations:**
>
> Prioritizes high refresh rate and minimal time lag, but the most easily measured daily metrics may be the most difficult to convert to actionable intervention

available at the push of a button, either through built-in reporting or ad-hoc reporting tools. The reality, unfortunately, is slightly more nuanced because the list of use cases for ED data is diverse and long, and different applications have different tradeoffs and requirements (**Box 68.1**).

Regulatory Reporting

The bulk of investment in standard reports tends to address domains that have regulatory requirements for data reporting, which apply broadly to most health-care organizations. For example, the National Committee for Quality Assurance, Joint Commission, and Centers for Medicare and Medicaid Services all require quality metrics to be reported in predefined formats.[2-4] Historically, requirements of the Affordable Care Act, Meaningful Use, the Health Information Technology for Economic and Clinical Health Act of 2009, and other regulatory obligations have incrementally increased the need for data reporting.[1,5,6] The transition to the Quality Payment Program under the Medicare Access and CHIP Reauthorization Act of 2015 only adds complexity and data requirements.[7]

Many states and payers have an additional list of mandatory metrics for reporting, and hospitals and health systems may require ED groups to independently self-report additional operational and financial data, as well.

Quality and Process Improvement

Internally, ED leaders are faced with increasing competition among hospital departments for dwindling dollars. They are simultaneously challenged to improve their department's clinical, financial, operational, and patient experience outcomes. These responsibilities include coordinating and supporting a number of parallel quality-improvement initiatives, both internal to the ED and in collaboration with other hospital stakeholders. The Lean Six Sigma process-improvement methods are notably data-centric and require clean data, often captured in high resolution (such as time-stamp events down to the second, or clinical data attributable to individual patients). Department leaders are expected to know how to produce and obtain robust information to support these activities, including repeated measurements over time to evaluate improvement efforts.

Business Development

Almost all future planning for major ED investments (e.g., asking for a new CT scanner, hiring another doctor or nurse, investing in a new ultrasound machine) are—at their core—data-driven decisions. For ED groups structured as hospital contractors, the periodic dance to renegotiate agreements with hospital administrators or boards may feel like an annual (or less frequent, if you are lucky) pitch to keep the contract, often relying heavily on quality, financial, and operational performance data from the prior contract period. Exploration of new services, partnerships, and endeavors (e.g., adding virtual care, expanding observation services, implementing substance abuse treatment services) also requires the careful development of a business plan, typically based on recent historical data and projected benefits.

Research

Even nonacademic EDs are increasingly involved in clinical research and implementation studies. Academic centers often have an even higher expectation of such involvement. In both cases, obtaining research-grade patient data—complete with safeguards for protected health information, missing value tracking, audit trails, and partitioned billing—can present unique challenges. Fortunately, investigators typically expect to provide both financial and technical support, but using ED data for research may still be a major undertaking, and the ED leader may be the primary data-point-of-contact for interested researchers, especially in community settings.

Daily Operations

The most common (and perhaps most exciting) use of ED analytics is to support daily operations. Real-time reporting helps ED leaders identify operational trouble spots, allocate resources more effectively, tweak departmental and hospital patient flow, and follow trends of core operational importance. In practical terms, analytics may range from rather straightforward to quite complex. Many operational leaders rely on static daily reports of the previous day's "numbers" e-mailed each morning. Larger, more sophisticated teams may hold robust multidisciplinary daily huddles and weekly data-dives or employ real-time predictive intelligence with automatic mobile alerts pushed to key leaders when operations go awry.

COMMON DATA SOURCES

Every computer system used in the clinical environment to care for patients (and every behind-the-scenes supporting system used to bill them) stores information from which analytics can be produced. A standard set of reports and reporting tools are often built into these systems, but more advanced analyses may require custom logic and report development (discussed later in this chapter).

As most ED leaders don't exercise direct control over the information systems integral to department operations, leaders may choose to assign an administrative assistant or physician member with interest and expertise to be responsible for generating standard reports. The leader may also opt to work with someone in the hospital analytics or IT/IS departments to run the reports needed. Depending on the availability and responsiveness of IT/IS, additional assistance may be required, such as consultants, who have already mastered vendor-reporting tools, and business intelligence professionals, who offer products and services capable of extracting the data from the ED's systems.

Enterprise EHRs

Increasingly, EHRs (also called electronic medical records, or EMRs) are fully integrated systems spanning outpatient, inpatient, ED, perioperative, obstetrical, and other care in a single system. Emergency departments are typically integrated by virtue of a module within the larger enterprise-wide hospital information system. Alternatively, several "best-of-breed" ED information systems (EDIS) interface with enterprise-wide hospital information systems, allowing the ED to use purpose-built systems that have bidirectional information flow with the other hospital systems. **Box 68.2** provides examples of key metrics obtainable from EHRs, including common methods of stratifying or summarizing data. Implications for ED leaders include:

- The EHR is often the richest source of clinical and operational data for the ED.
- In order to effectively exploit the data that reside within the EHR, ED leaders or their delegates must become familiar with the data methodologies, including what data is entered, by whom, and at what point in the workflow. Individual staff members deviating from the prescribed workflows may introduce data discrepancies.
- Department leaders must develop an understanding of how data is entered and stored.
- Most EHR data are tied to a specific patient or encounter. This is beneficial in that it provides drill-down capability, but it adds complexity because aggregation functions are often required to obtain meaningful "big-picture" analytics.

BOX 68.2 ■ KEY METRICS OF EHR SYSTEMS

- Time stamp events in the context of each patient's visit (used to calculate performance metrics, such as LOS, arrival-to-disposition decision time)
- Chief complaint
- Mode of arrival to the ED
- Patient demographics
- Prior visit history
- The Joint Commission and other publicly reported quality measures
- Patient-level resource utilization statistics (e.g., room, imaging, lab, consults, medications)
- Clinical data (e.g., lab results, vital signs)
- Billing codes
- Diagnosis codes and dispositions

Data are often summarized or stratified by:

- Date/time
- ED area/zone/treatment team
- Triage acuity
- Chief complaint groupings
- Clinician or staff member
- Time increment groupings (e.g., day shift, night shift)
- Patient final disposition
- When and what labs are ordered
- When and what diagnostic tests have been ordered
- Payer status
- Patient demographics
- Behavioral health patients
- Accountable care organization patients

Metrics that may be calculated from EHR source data using more advanced logic:

- ED census at a given time (Because individual patient arrival and discharge times are readily captured, an "ED moment-in-time" can be computationally reconstructed.)
- Returns to the ED within a specified number of hours (Because individual patients are linked by a unique identifier across encounters, a "look-back function" can identify prior visits within a specified time range.)

Legacy Health Information Systems

Before the advent of the enterprise-integrated EHR, hospitals used a hodgepodge of purpose-built systems networked together through interfaces and data-communication channels. Many hospitals still use a collection of legacy systems, where multiple data sets may reside in different locations.

The "admission, discharge, transfer" (ADT) system collects information on every patient who registers for ED services, and it is usually the same system used for demographic and registration details. Lab, cardiology, and imaging systems may house information for supporting services; document image captures may archive old paper records; and ED patient tracking, orders, and documentation may reside in one or more other systems. While the practicing clinician may see these data stores as integrated, the ED leader or analyst may need to search multiple systems, linking a unique encounter or medical record identification number to other records across systems.

Implication for ED Leaders

- Information may be available only for registered patients.
- The implementation of "quick" or "early" registration processes will be necessary to collect complete data on patients who have left prior to receiving a medical screening examination, as well as record accurate patient arrival times.
- Disparate systems may have different data storage structures or even wildly contradictory data that must be reconciled. (For example, the patient's disposition may be "discharged" in the EDIS but "against medical advice" in the ADT record.)

Billing Systems

Even with a modern EHR, some hospitals and practice groups may store financial and billing for each patient visit in a separate system, sometimes managed by a separate billing company (often, in the case of professional fee billing). **Box 68.3** gives examples of key metrics often obtainable from billing systems.

BOX 68.3 ■ KEY METRICS OF ADMINISTRATIVE SYSTEMS

Billing systems:

- Documentation of the specific physician under whom each patient encounter is billed (More than one physician may care for a patient during their entire ED visit.)
- Each patient's charges, CPT, and ICD codes billed, including breakdowns of evaluation and management codes and modifiers
- Patient insurance and demographics
- Account billed date and accounts receivables
- Down-codes
- Payments, adjustments, refunds, and total charges
  - Total RVUs (when linked to an RVU look-up table)
  - RVUs per patient billed
  - Procedure counts
  - Diagnostic counts by ICD code
  - Payer mix
  - Payments per billed visit

Schedule, payroll, and human resource systems:

- Start and end times and overlapping times
- Specific "area" or location with the ED
- Hours worked, total and by provider
- Type of provider worked
- Productivity by type of provider
- Sick calls, swaps, and schedule changes

Implication for ED Leaders

- Billing and coding professionals may be the only data source for numeric current procedural terminology (CPT) and International Classification of Diseases (ICD) values, which have been reviewed and validated.
- It is important that ED leaders understand the procession and time lines of data flow from a hospital computer system into a billing system (if separate). Billing systems often operate on batch jobs that move large swaths of data periodically, and billing data may be many months behind real time. Delays in the billing process may also be caused by the untimely signing of patient charts, coder queries, manual coding reviews, and slow data-exchange processes.
- The development of a productivity-incentive program is often dependent on data obtained by the billing process, and there are likely important nuances and idiosyncrasies to understand, especially pertaining to provider attribution (who saw the patient versus who the billed provider is), the number of relative value units (RVUs) generated, and so on.
- Questions that the ED leader may wish to ask the billing department/vendor include:
    - What is the time lag between patient disposition (discharged, admitted, transferred) and time of data entry into the billing system?
    - By what process is a signed chart submitted?
    - Does the coder revise any CPT or ICD information submitted by the physician if that data is already available within an EHR?
    - Does the billing computer system maintain a stored record of all patient visits, billed and unbilled, or can reports only be produced from billed accounts?
    - If the group monitors RVUs and physician productivity statistics, when does the billing company close the "month of service" records? (For example, the total patients seen in January were 2,000, of which 1,800 were billed in January, 150 billed in February, 25 billed in March, etc).

Schedule, Payroll, and Human Resource Systems

Various systems may store work-hour information for physicians, advance practice providers, nurses, ED staff, and others outside of the EHR. This may include scheduling systems, time-clock systems, or hospital practice payroll systems. **Box 68.3** gives examples of key metrics often obtainable from these administrative systems.

Implications for ED Leaders

- As EDs segment flow into separate units (fast track, urgent care, observation), leaders may be able to evaluate staffing and productivity and perform demand–capacity matching by drilling down into each separate subunit.
- A number of scheduling tools exist that ED leaders may use to manage physician, nursing, and other staff. Best practice is to conduct a thorough evaluation of these tools. Some additional questions that may be considered when evaluating a scheduling tool or vendor include:
    - How are schedule changes logged when someone calls in sick or takes a day off?
    - How is shift sharing/splitting handled?
    - How are final work hours verified?
    - What is the process of moving scheduled hours to payroll?

- To assess the true cost of staff services provided to the different patients, ED leaders must obtain accurate data from the available scheduling tool.
- Analyzing scheduling information in association with visit and acuity information allows leaders to identify when different providers should be scheduled and which patients (by acuity and diagnosis) may need different provider types.
- Drilling down into productivity by area may also help leaders find creative ways to reduce the "provider cost" of care delivered in the ED.

Patient Experience Data Providers

Providers of internal or external patient experience/satisfaction surveys often store data apart from the medical record. Ideally, the information is available at the individual practitioner and patient level (by including a patient identifier that links the satisfaction results to the patient).

Implications for ED Leaders

- Hospital leaders often care very much about satisfaction survey scores and results.
- It is important to resist the temptation to dismiss satisfaction results due to poor sampling, low response rates, or invalid survey methodology. Instead, learn how to dissect the results to create usable feedback for providers and measure improvement over time.
- If the hospital only samples a few patients each month or quarter, best practice may be to implement a callback system. Callback systems provide early feedback about problems, accomplish some element of clinical follow-up and quality assurance, and have been shown to increase patient satisfaction.[8]
- Qualitative free text data often require special textual analysis and processing to be aggregated.

Special Operational Systems

This catch-all category includes hospital transport and environment-services tracking systems, phone and communication systems, patient call-light systems, medical device integration, remote monitoring, security and premise monitoring systems, and so on. Depending on the application and specific vendor, reporting may be quite useful for specific operational analyses. However, sometimes these systems are not linked to the context of a particular patient.

THE INFORMATION PIPELINE

The management of information requires a formal systematic process of creation, collection, processing, interpretation, distribution, and distribution. To ensure the information is operationally useful, those for whom it is intended should have a thorough understanding of its component processes.

Raw data are often too granular to be useful; a complex pipeline of processing techniques is typically required to transform it into actionable information and intelligence. As the old adage "garbage in, garbage out" suggests, the integrity of the entered data determines the usefulness of the results. Therefore, data quality and source workflows should become obsessions of ED leaders. The definition of "quality data" varies depending on the metric being analyzed.

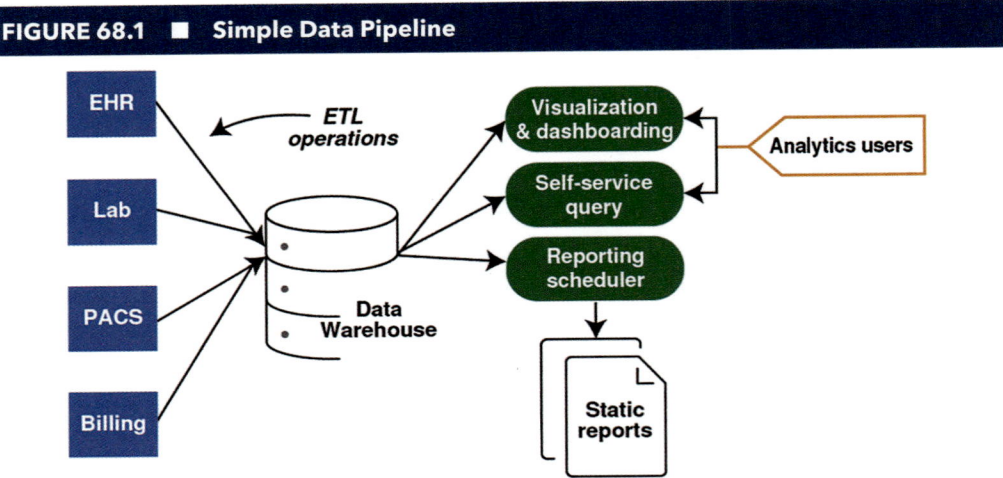

FIGURE 68.1 ■ Simple Data Pipeline

Functional Layers

Figure 68.1 shows an overview of the data pipeline generally applied to moderately complex health-care data sources.

Source Systems

Source systems are the initial locations of data storage. This may be the system for a lab-component result (such as a WBC count, the EHR for a patient-roomed time stamp, or the billing system for a coder-verified CPT evaluation and management code). While many source systems have built-in reporting capabilities, they often lack any integration with other sources. For example, the WBC in the lab system may not be linked to the patient in a way that is traversable to the analyst. Source systems are the most reliable input for later reporting operations because, by definition, they are not summarized, aggregated, filtered, modified, or otherwise contaminated by logic and assumptions that may occur later in the processes.

Extract, Transform, Load Operations

Extract, transform, and load (ETL) operations take data from source systems, modify it as needed and then load the "cleaned" data into another system (often a data warehouse). Clean data refer to a set with parts (specific rows or columns of data) that are devoid of invalid or inaccurate information. Invalid and inaccurate data can be a result of poor computer system design, incorrect computer system usage, recent workflow changes, or an information architecture that allows frequent missing fields as a matter of course. A partnership between clinical and technical staff is critical to determine why data are not clean; unclean data can produce invalid results and may promote inaccurate conclusions and poor decision-making.

Examples of data-cleaning and metric-filtering rules implicit in ETL operations include:

- Eliminate all:
  - Patients directly admitted to labor and delivery who are not seen in the ED
  - Time stamps when the event is after the documented arrival time (creating impossible intervals, such as a negative arrival-to-rooming time)
  - Patients with a disposition of "entered in error"
  - Patients with a medical record number of 0000000 or 9999999

- Calculate intervals, such as:
  - Door-to-room times—excluding patients who arrive by ambulance, who have a different flow and are registered while already in their room
  - Room-to-first-provider times—excluding all detail for patients whose room-to-first-provider metric is <0 where patients did not arrive by ambulance. Providers probably aren't seeing these patients before they are roomed.
  - Door-to-discharge times—excluding all patients who leave without completing treatment
- Summarization and aggregation

Once key metrics and data-cleaning rules have been defined, ETL operations may also define segmentation and classification dimensions. Examples of such dimensions are given in **Box 68.2**. After extraction and transformation, loading data into the next system may happen periodically or continuously, according the specific needs of a given ED or hospital. Frequently, the ETL operation from the EHR to a data warehouse may run as a daily batch job, sometimes overnight or in the early morning. Consequently, analytics may be a day old. Streaming (real-time) ETL is possible as well, but it is often more technically complex and computationally intensive, so it may be reserved for specific-use cases requiring true real-time data.

Data Warehousing

Many questions are only answerable when data are combined from multiple sources into a centralized repository, where their relationships can be traversed and exploited for reporting. The terms "centralized database," "separate reporting database," and "data warehouse" typically refer to the same general concept of using a system optimized to combine data from multiple sources, usually loaded via ETL jobs.

Other industries, including banking, insurance, travel, and retail, have been moving data out of operational systems into centralized data repositories, and then reporting from that system for years. Similarly, EHR systems are often designed for transactional data, which is to say they are optimized for the millisecond-to-millisecond recording and retrieval of information used to directly support operations.

Summarization and reporting have different computational and data-structure requirements and are best accomplished in a data warehouse. Domain experts—in this case ED leadership/management, billing, and process improvement experts—are necessary to drive these management strategies and development efforts. Some benefits of moving operational data into a separate technical infrastructure include the ability to:

- Clean operational data in the exact way that fits the defined needs, and verify accuracy before the information is used for real-time or retrospective reports.
- Dissect data independently from source computer systems in ways that are currently unavailable from the vendors.
- Use advanced visuals for data presentation.
- Incorporate statistical programs capable of better analyzing specific data types with higher performance. (This is particularly applicable to the analysis of large data sets of time stamp, genomic, or discrete sensor data.)
- Combine all data into one location, creating a "single source of truth."

By combining data from multiple systems into a centralized warehouse, it becomes feasible to evaluate questions like the financial benefits of operational changes (e.g., split flow, observation units, point-of-care testing) or tie patient satisfaction data to diagnosis groupings, particular time intervals, census, payer class, and so on.

Visualization and Dashboards

The data-presentation layer (i.e., the software that actually displays a dashboard, chart, or interactive report to a user) is often distinct from the data warehouse itself. A visualization engine may sit on top of the warehouse, accessing data and stored procedures but transforming data further, segmenting it visually, and rendering tables, charts, and graphics. Because they usually do not store data on their own and instead link to a warehouse to pull information in real time, this layer enables the creation of dynamic dashboards, reports, and visuals that are refreshable. Popular current products include Tableau and Microsoft PowerBI. While the end user may view these systems as "the dashboard," they are only one layer in the reporting architecture.

Reporting Services

Many static reports are built in behind-the-scenes subsystems, which may include instructions for computing and displaying tables and charts, complete with a distribution list of e-mail addresses and a scheduler to automatically run and e-mail the report at a prespecified time. Crystal Reports is one popular application utilized in many organizations.

Ad Hoc and Self-Service Query

Finally, another layer may allow authorized users to run custom queries and exports from the data warehouse without building a report. Examples include SAP/Business Objects and Microsoft Power Query. These systems are often reserved for a few "power users" with both technical and domain knowledge, and IT professionals often perceive these systems as posing a higher security risk and performance penalty. However, record-level and field-level safeguards are common in such systems, as are performance limits that prevent authorized users from accessing inappropriate information. Two examples are efforts to obtain social security numbers and large queries, which could crash the system when attempting to download the entire text of all notes for all patients for the last decade.

THE ANALYSIS PROCESS

To guide initial data analysis efforts, the ED team should define and apply departmental and institutional management goals as guides for key performance indicator (KPI) identification. The ED team should also determine the dashboards, reports, and metrics that are currently and easily available from the built-in reporting tools.

Measure Development and Metadata

Department leaders may find previous information (retrospective analytics) to be quite helpful when developing department goals and translating them into KPIs, dashboards, or reports. The retrospective analytics may offer insight into the longitudinal state of KPIs, allowing the identification of trends and longer-term interventions necessary to support management goals. However, real-time analytics are the most meaningful way to recognize and redirect poor performance and outcomes. When translating a goal into a KPI, the ED leader should consider the following:

- What are the obvious "pain points" in the ED? What processes do the team members describe as requiring improvement?
- Are the "pain points" measurable?

- In what computer system (e.g., EHR, billing) does this measurable data exist, and what is the best method for obtaining it?
- Can vendor standard reports provide needed data on these KPIs?
- Are the data on these standard reports clean?

What KPIs Are Already Used

When developing departmental KPIs, it is best practice to take an inventory of standard reports available in each system. This information helps the ED leaders quickly understand what is currently being measured. The more valuable reports provide actionable evidence for giving feedback to staff and recommending process improvements.

While taking a standard report inventory to support KPI production and monitoring, it is important to develop an understanding of the underlying data and imperfections of the information used to generate the aggregated statistics (mean, sum, median values, etc). Too often, the information provided does not measure the requested information.

A common example is found when comparing volume metrics obtained through billing, EHR, and clerical data (overall volume, admissions, patients leaving AMA, etc). Yet many leaders rely on this contradictory information to make critical judgments.

Department leaders should scrutinize the reported information carefully and work closely with technical partners to clarify the logic and ETL processes underlying the metrics. It is helpful to specifically note data exclusions and filters and make this information available to those viewing and interpreting KPIs. **Box 68.4** gives examples of questions to ask during this process.

Common Pitfall

The translation of management goals into KPIs and then into data may reflect a variable degree of inaccuracy due to human error. While these inaccuracies may be discouraging at first, they are routine and, in fact, afford an opportunity to fine-tune the system. High-performance ED leaders should educate staff so that they understand the importance of accurate data; it will allow the team to assess their performance and continually improve.

BOX 68.4 ■ EXAMINING "UNCLEAN" DATA

Regarding patient volume metrics:

- Have voided patients (those registered in error or for testing purposes) been removed from the total count?
- Have duplicate entries been removed? (Duplicate patients are those with the same data listed twice.)
- Have direct admits been removed? (These patients may not have been provided ED services. Or maybe they have.)
- Are patients who register and leave prior to medical screening examination included in total count statistics?

Regarding door-to-provider time interval:

- How are arrival times being obtained? What exact human action triggers the time stamp, and where does that fit in the workflow? What interaction (triage nurse, greeter, kiosk, sign-in sheet, etc.) in what computer system creates the time stamp being used?
- How is a "provider" defined (physician, APP, resident)?
- What exact event triggers the ending time stamp?
- What happens when the time interval is calculated as a negative number?

Defining KPIs

Best practice is to define each KPI's primary objective: from what system and/or report the KPI is produced, and all related data-logic inclusions and exclusions. Data management experts refer to data definition as a type of metadata. During this exercise, problems with source systems are often identified. Data management best practice includes:

- Addressing what information is collected and why
- Determining how data should be collected and stored as well as its attributes, its desired behavior, and its relationship to other data
- Defining dimensional information (items that can be dissected and diced into various components)
- Defining calculated metric information (items that can be used in mathematical equations)

Use a precise and unambiguous vocabulary to refer to operations, metrics, and measurements. Always use standardized terminology whenever applicable terms and definitions exist in national consensus documents.[9-11] For terms, metrics, and measurements that do not have a standard definition, document the agreed-upon institutional or departmental definition in an accessible dictionary that includes, at minimum, the elements in **Box 68.5**.

Data Aggregation

Summary statistics (e.g., mean, median) pose a number of problems when reported as a KPI or used as an outcome measure. While it seems more straightforward to report summary statistics (mean length of stay [LOS], median door-to-provider, etc), this approach is information-poor and removes much of the actionable information obtained from the entire distribution of patients. In other words, when only the mean or median LOS for a patient is obtained, rather than a distribution of outliers by time of day, shift, clinician, and so on, valuable improvement opportunities are lost. The entire distribution—including the minimum, maximum, central tendencies, shape of the distribution, outliers, measures of dispersion—is far more valuable.

Summary statistics are like any other statistical method: assumptions must be understood, and valid use cases must be met. The majority of metrics used in ED operations violate the assumptions of most parametric methods (normal probability models). Even simple questions ("What was the average LOS?") imply that the LOS follows a normal distribution curve, which it rarely does.

BOX 68.5 ■ MINIMUM DATA DICTIONARY ELEMENTS

- Label name (including abbreviations that may appear in tables and graphs) and textual descriptive definition
- Data type (categorical, numeric ordinal, continuous, etc)
- Units
- Numerator, denominator, or calculation formula, if applicable
- Inclusion and exclusion criteria, if applicable
- Intervals defined by start and end time stamps for events
- Source (including source for numerator and denominator terms, if applicable)
- Target/threshold values, including desired directionality (e.g., "fewer than 2% left without being seen is desirable," not "target: 2%")

Furthermore, most commonly used summary statistics are mean or median measures. Managing the middle LOS is not inherently desirable or actionable. A corollary and common pitfall occurs when the ED leader creates a staffing plan for a median department census. The department will be understaffed 50% of the time. The central tendency is too information-poor for operational decision-making, let alone research.

A more patient-centered KPI definition sets a desirable target from the patient's perspective (e.g., goal LOS <120 minutes for a discharged patient) and reports the proportion of patients who met the goal, or how many minutes in excess were cumulatively accrued by patients with a long LOS on a given day. Knowing that the middle patient was discharged within 120 minutes is a blunter instrument and makes management more difficult.

Trends and Time Series

Department leaders are interested in trends, rather than a single point in time. A table of summarized data for consecutive time intervals (such as months, days, hours) creates a time series. Time series exhibit autocorrelation, which recognizes that measurements may be affected by prior observations. In other words, each consecutive observation (e.g., hourly ED census) is not an independent observation and can be predicted as some function of the prior values.

Take, for example, consecutive measurements of monthly median LOS depicted in **Figure 68.2**. The ED leader would be unable to discern if the LOS were going up or down over time related to natural variation, operational interventions, or changes in patient volumes. Further, if the system is unstable with significant baseline variation, the leader could not determine if the next month's LOS increase or decrease is just random noise. The details of time-series methods are beyond the scope of this chapter, but a discerning ED leader may choose to learn more about statistical process control and will be a healthy skeptic of any "normal" statistical test, table, or graph that involves consecutively collected time series data.[12]

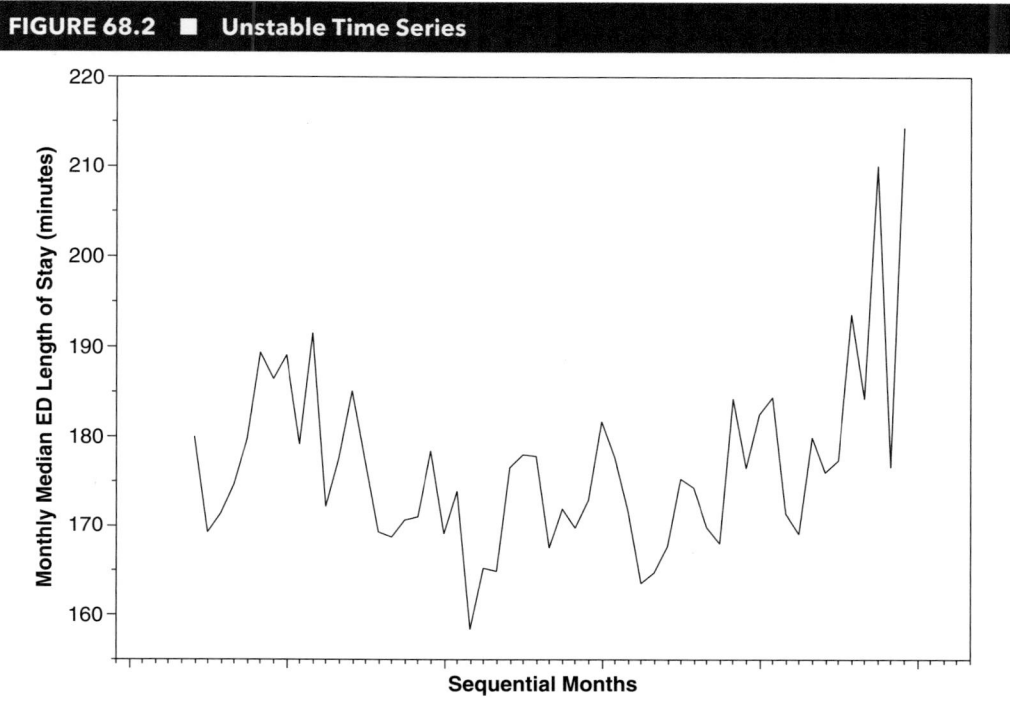

FIGURE 68.2 ■ Unstable Time Series

Before/After Special Case

The case for measuring changes in a KPI before and after an operational intervention warrants special mention. Like time series analysis, this is a common-use case of ED analytics. For example, suppose that the ED LOS before trialing a front-end intake model was "X" minutes. The ED leadership team intentionally changes a feature of the operations and measures the results. Suppose that change works by reducing LOS for the "exposed" postintervention patients. Simultaneously, however (and unbeknownst to the leaders), patients with psychiatric needs were not exposed to the intervention and subsequently experienced prolonged boarding times. These boarded patients offset the gains made in the successful intervention, and the overall ED mean/median LOS increases postintervention. The team might inappropriately conclude that the intake pilot was unsuccessful. This example exposes one common pitfall of before/after designs that have numerous uncontrolled variables.

Second, consider an intake trial that provides a benefit for many patients but does not change the overall ED LOS. Perhaps at baseline, an occasional patient had a door-to-provider time of 150 minutes, while many others had a time of only 10 minutes. The mean at baseline in the whole population was 20 minutes, but the dispersion was large. What if the intervention narrowed the variation such that all of the patients had door-to-doctor times between 15 and 25 minutes, but the mean did not change? The ED leaders would have no way to see that effect in the summary statistics chosen.

It is difficult to know what else changed between the before-and-after time periods. There are almost always unmeasured confounders in these designs. Furthermore, condensing and summarizing performance before and after an intervention may mask its true effects, falsely attributing unrelated outcomes to the intervention and oversimplifying the analysis. A proper before/after analytical design requires careful thought and probably advanced methods, such as interrupted time-series analyses.[13]

Data Presentation

Many books are available that provide a comprehensive discussion and guidance on best practices for data visualization.[14] A few key best practices are shown in **Boxes 68.6 to 68.9**.

The timely presentation of actionable metrics has the greatest potential to produce a desired change in behavior. As described earlier, it is necessary to determine how frequently

---

BOX 68.6 ■ BEST PRACTICES FOR DATA VISUALIZATION

- Use consistent, meaningful, and legible fonts, colors, and text effects (e.g., capitals, bold, italics, underlines) throughout the document, and tailor these choices to the audience and display medium.
- When possible, rather than reporting summary statistics or central tendency (such as mean or median), report the frequency with which a particular patient-centered outcome is met (or report how closely the observed value matches the expected).
- Whenever summary data are reported, always clearly label the summary operation used, such as mean or median.
- Avoid insinuating or assuming that random variation in unstable systems or seasonality in time-series data constitutes meaningful trends.

BOX 68.7 ■ BEST PRACTICES FOR TABLES

- People perceive quantitative information much more effectively via spatial and visual relationships than tabular displays of numbers. Display data in a table only when the tabular format adds value over an alternative visualization, such as when:
  - The reader must be able to look up or compare individual values with a great deal of precision.
  - The data must be reported with high precision (for example, when the difference between 2.487 and 2.459 is important, rather than reporting 2.5).
  - It is important to know the raw values of a measurement over time, as opposed to the trend (for example, when the values 2.487 and 2.459 are themselves more important than simply reporting a 1.1% or 0.028 unit decrease).
  - Values with multiple units of measure with different scales must be displayed together and cannot be separated into different visualizations.
- If a table is used to present trends over time, it should have embedded sparklines to visually depict each trend, rather than relying on the reader to infer trends from the numeric data.
- Groups of related rows or columns, as well as summary cells, should be visually distinguished by the meaningful and consistent use of text effects, lines, borders, and/or shading.
- Whenever possible, simple tabular data should be sorted in numeric order.
- Except when displayed with the numeric data itself (such as the percent sign in "30%"), table headers should include units.

BOX 68.8 ■ BEST PRACTICES FOR GRAPHS AND CHARTS

- Consider the intended purpose, audience, and display medium before creating any visualization. Select a technique that is optimized for the goal and type of data, and take into account whether the purpose is primarily exploratory or explanatory.
- In general, select the visualization type that is most information-rich and minimizes the need to summarize or remove valuable data.
- Avoid insinuation of relationships in the data that do not exist in reality or are illogical.
- Design visualizations intentionally to minimize the cognitive load required to interpret them and to take maximal advantage of natural human visual processing.
- Maximize the "data-to-ink ratio." In general, the default graph settings in Microsoft Excel result in a lot of non-value-added "chart junk," where excessive lines, shading, shadows, colors, and text add zero additional information and inhibit visual information processing.
- Format chart axes with integrity and transparency:
  - All axes should be labeled, and axis labels should include units.
  - Set axis minimum and maximum values to create meaningful comparisons that neither exaggerate nor understate relationships.
  - Avoid using an interrupted axis without a clear and compelling reason. If it is mandatory, make it visually obvious that the axis is interrupted.
  - Avoid displaying data with different units, scales, or meanings on the same chart, even if separate axes are used for each series. If it is mandatory, make it visually obvious that the display is nonstandard.
  - When values on a chart have a desired directionality, clearly indicate that direction visually on the chart.
- 3D charts almost never adhere to these best practices. If you are considering a 3D chart, reconsider the intended purpose.

> **BOX 68.9 ■ BEST PRACTICES FOR SUMMARIES AND STATISTICS**
>
> - Before reporting the central tendency of a population (e.g., mean or median), consider whether there may be an alternative measure that is more information-rich or patient-centered (such as the frequency with which a particular goal is met).
> - When measures of central tendency are appropriate, use the summary statistic most suited to the distribution of the data, and consider including a measure of dispersion.
> - The analyst must verify all prerequisite assumptions of a given statistical test prior to employing that test or reporting the results.
>   - Do not assume that a relationship between variables is linear without verifying that assumption. Most complex systems in real life are nonlinear.
>   - Be wary of any variables involving time. Time series are naturally ordered, nonindependent, and frequently autocorrelated and heteroscedastic, which violates the assumptions of many statistical tests.

the information can and should be available for reporting. For example, EHR data may be available in real time, while other data regarding billing, physician hours, and satisfaction may not be available or complete until after the end of each month.

For data that are not available on a real-time basis, the ED leader may create a management-level visualization layer (i.e., a scorecard or dashboard) with 10 to 12 KPIs. These KPIs should be metrics that can be directly impacted by ED staff through a modification of process or other behaviors. If selected KPIs placed on this dashboard can be improved by ED staff, they are more likely to use the reports to effect change.

When designing this dashboard, consider a balance of at least one KPI specific to each subject matter grouping—finance, operations, clinical care, satisfaction, and so on. Once top-level visualizations have been developed, drill-down paths from the associated KPIs may be established to determine ways to improve those metrics. For example, a department's top-level metric might be their walkout percentage. Below that might be the "left without being seen" percentage by time of day and day of week, further segmented by triage acuity, physician on duty, or even triage nurse.

The focus of the report often depends on the audience—physicians, physicians and nurses, other clinical staff, hospital administrators, and others. Regardless of the audience, the focus should generally be on a metric that is actionable.

ANALYTIC INFRASTRUCTURE

The ED leadership team does not control the actual hardware and software running any of the source systems, especially the EHR. Thus, a strong partnership with IT and IS professionals is crucial. Equally valuable is a partnership with other departments that share an interest in developing sophisticated analytic capabilities.

Technical Systems

The technical investments and maintenance required to set up a system to extract, transform, and load ETL information into the data-warehousing program are large and require collaboration. Subject-matter expertise will invariably be required, but core technical installations should be managed by technical staff who serve more than just the ED.

Human Systems

Similarly, hospitals and health systems may already have an analytics team on which ED leaders can rely. However, a capable IT team with little understanding of ED operations can develop timely and accurate reporting with the help of a small number of ED analytic specialists. Some groups without substantial internal support hire and embed an ED-specific expert, who can become familiar with the data structures specific to emergency care. The ED analysts can provide direction and expertise while working closely with IT/IS, who additionally maintain the servers, code, and databases. In some organizations, the ED also has its own technical infrastructure.

CONCLUSION

Successful data acquisition and analysis require a partnership between clinical and technical ED and hospital resources. Department leaders can and should call on technical professionals for help with actual coding, implementation, and IT operations. However, effective ED leaders know these systems in detail, ensuring clear and actionable goals, accurate data input, and the regular analysis of results. A credible ED leader must understand operations data science and implement systems to improve the care of their patients.

Special thanks to Jeff A. Finkelstein and Jonathan Rothman, who participated in a previous edition of this chapter.

REFERENCES

1. Centers for Medicare and Medicaid Services (CMS). Medicare and Medicaid programs; electronic health record incentive program-stage 3 and modifications to meaningful use in 2015 through 2017. *Fed Regist.* 2016;80(200):62761–62955.
2. National Committee for Quality Assurance (NCQA). HEDIS Measures and Technical Resources. Available at: https://www.ncqa.org/hedis/measures/. Accessed October 20, 2018.
3. The Joint Commission. Core Measure Sets. 2020. Available at: https://www.jointcommission.org/measurement/measures/. Accessed August 4, 2020.
4. Centers for Medicare and Medicaid Services (CMS). Quality Measures. 2020. Available at: https://www.cms.gov/Medicare/Quality-Initiatives-Patient-Assessment-Instruments/QualityMeasures. Accessed August 4, 2020.
5. Patient Protection and Affordable Care Act, 42 USC § 18001 et seq. (2010).
6. US Department of Health and Human Services. The Health Information Technology for Economic and Clinical Health (HITECH) Act. *Fed Regist.* 2009;74(209):56123–56131.
7. Centers for Medicare and Medicaid Services (CMS). MACRA. 2019. Available at: https://www.cms.gov/Medicare/Quality-Initiatives-Patient-Assessment-Instruments/Value-Based-Programs/MACRA-MIPS-and-APMs/MACRA-MIPS-and-APMs.html. Accessed August 3, 2020.
8. Guss DA, Gray S, Castillo EM. The impact of patient telephone call after discharge on likelihood to recommend in an academic emergency department. *J Emerg Med.* 2014;46(4):560–566.
9. Wiler JL, Welch S, Pines J, et al. Emergency department performance measures updates: proceedings of the 2014 emergency department benchmarking alliance consensus summit. Zink B, ed. *Acad Emerg Med.* 2015;22(5):542–553.
10. Welch SJ, Asplin BR, Stone-Griffith S, et al. Emergency Department Benchmarking Alliance. Emergency department operational metrics, measures, and definitions: results of the second performance measures and benchmarking summit. *Ann Emerg Med.* 2011;58(1):33–40.
11. Welch SJ, Stone-Griffith S, Asplin B, et al. Emergency department operations dictionary: results of the second performance measures and benchmarking summit. *Acad Emerg Med.* 2011;18(5):539–544.
12. Benneyan J, Lloyd R, Plsek P. Statistical process control as a tool for research and healthcare improvement. *Qual Saf Health Care.* 2003;12(6):458–464.
13. Kontopantelis E, Doran T, Springate DA, et al. Regression based quasi-experimental approach when randomisation is not an option: interrupted time series analysis. *BMJ.* 2015;350:h2750.
14. Tufte ER. *The Visual Display of Quantitative Information.* 2nd ed. Graphics Press; 2001.

ESSENTIAL SUPPORT TOOLS AND TECHNOLOGIES

Sujal Mandavia, Phillip F. Gruber

CHAPTER 69

The science of today is the technology of tomorrow.

—Edward Teller,
Hungarian-American Theoretical Physicist, 1908–2003[1]

One of the effects of the Health Information Technology for Economic and Clinical Health Act was the widespread implementation of enterprise-wide electronic health records (EHRs). While these software packages are usually touted as comprehensive solutions, significant institutional variability remains. Modern emergency departments (EDs) are more interconnected than ever before, and while large EHR vendors are racing to incorporate additional features into their software, most EDs rely on multiple add-on systems and technologies that serve a variety of ancillary functions, from augmenting communication to realizing unmet potential from core systems (**Table 69.1**).

TABLE 69.1 ■ Overview of ED Support Technologies					
Application	**Institutional Support Needed**	**Initial Cost/Investment**	**Ongoing Costs**	**Pros**	**Cons/Other Notes**
Front-end speech recognition	High	Moderate	Moderate	Improves provider experience, faster documentation turnaround compared to traditional dictation	Not for everyone, significant error rate, ongoing licensing costs, does not always improve overall provider efficiency
Scribes	Moderate	Low	High	Improves provider experience and efficiency	Significant ongoing costs, significant turnover, not as easily scalable as software implementation
E-prescribing of controlled substances	Moderate	Low	Low	Improved opioid prescribing documentation and decision support, regulatory compliance	Operational challenges (e.g., troubleshooting of issues after discharge, preferred pharmacy selection, insurance issues, etc), provider adoption

(Continued)

TABLE 69.1 ■ Continued

Internet marketing/ communication	Low	Low	Low	Inexpensive, enables communication with potential patients/staff	Limited utility, requires ongoing content management
Clinical reference tools	Low	Low	Moderate	Can enhance clinical decision-making, requires very little ongoing administrative effort	Ongoing paid subscription/ licensing costs
Residency management software	Moderate	Moderate	Moderate	Increasingly critical for ensuring regulatory compliance in academic environments	Requires significant ongoing administrative commitment
Real-time location services	High	High	High	Unparalleled security and data accuracy in large departments	Requires extensive infrastructure and support
Scheduling systems	Low	Low	Moderate	Simplifies what may be an otherwise impossibly difficult task	Still requires human oversight and involvement
Patient kiosks	High	High	High	Many potential benefits including patient experience and throughput	Expensive, requires implementation planning and ongoing administrative oversight
Patient portals	High	Moderate	Moderate	Improved patient engagement and experience	Intimately tied to hospital system's EHR and patient experience efforts

COMMON THEMES

Although the support technologies discussed in this chapter may require a fraction of the budget and resources of an EHR, their implementation should receive the same thoughtful attention from administrators and other interested stakeholders. As with EHRs, the success or failure of these technologies often depends much more on planning and preparation than on intrinsic technological considerations.

Information Technology Collaboration

With rare exception, the implementation of any of the technologies discussed here requires the full support and involvement of the facility's information technology (IT) department. Access to high-quality, secure, and well-maintained network resources is required for any connected tool or application. Hardware devices need stable (nonvarying) power and robust maintenance and repair resources. No matter how simple or trivial it may seem, software requires accessible and responsive support. In some cases, the role of the ED director may be to draw attention to the needs of the ED in facility-wide IT decision-making.

Practicality and Simplicity

It is critical to envision the actual application of a given technology, not the vendor's promised uses. Clinical end-user needs are frequently simpler and more practical than those envisioned by the engineers who design devices and the software they run. Individuals who represent the ED in IT decision-making should be familiar with real-world, frontline operations and ensure that this perspective is incorporated into procurement and implementation plans.

Adequate Resources and Ongoing Attention

A frequent pitfall—from the biggest enterprise-wide project to the smallest niche product—is underestimating the resources that are needed for adequate implementation and ongoing maintenance. Incremental costs can add up to an unanticipated financial commitment.[2] Even the smallest projects require:

- Ongoing education for new users
- Occasional maintenance or updating
- Customization to accommodate department operational changes
- Reassessment of value

MOBILE DEVICES AND APPS

Clinicians and other end users are now accustomed to the excellent user interfaces and extensive capabilities of their personal mobile devices, including voice recognition, virtual assistants, and automatic personalization through machine learning. Many health-care software systems have complex foundations and user interfaces that lag far behind modern mobile operating systems and apps. This is a reality that will be slow to change and that administrators and leaders should be aware of when managing change and expectations with their clinical staff.

The ED and hospital or health system should have a clear mobile device strategy that balances the needs of clinical operations, data safety, and usability. This strategy may rely on personal devices with secure apps, mobile-device management software (also known as BYOD—bring your own device), or corporate-issued devices (**Table 69.2**).

For all of the apps available for use in the ED, it is critical that patient and staff data are segregated and protected from each other and from malicious attack and unintended disclosure. This is an area that is especially reliant on collaboration and consultation with larger organizations, many of which now mandate enterprise management solutions for BYOD mobile devices. These solutions allow for corporate control of certain security settings and business/patient data on the enrolled mobile device (including remote-wipe capability in case of loss or theft), without affecting the user's personal data. All end-user access to protected health information must be logged and audited. If a device is able to access patient data from networks (e.g., cellular) that are not under facility control, two-factor authentication must be used, and data must be encrypted during transmission.

Facility IT/IS participation is critical for the successful implementation and maintenance of any mobile device in the ED, even when relying on BYOD devices. Well-maintained and secure network access, ongoing support for end-user questions and problems, and repair and replacement service (if applicable) must all be considered.

TABLE 69.2 ■ Overview of Mobile Devices

Factor	Smartphone/PDA	Tablet Computers	COW or WOW	Enterprise Communication Devices
Cost	Good—especially if user owned	Moderate	Poor—often last resort when physical space inadequate for workstations	Moderate
Usability	Moderate—data entry can be difficult	Good—larger screens ease data manipulation	Excellent—functions as a workstation	Moderate—usually limited and dedicated functions that are well integrated
Portability	Good—usually holstered or in pocket	Poor—difficult to hold in hand or pocket	Poor—large art that may trail an extension cord	Good
Durability	Good—with case or holster	Moderate—not as easily protected as small devices	Good—COW carts are ruggedized and designed for hospital use	Good—designed for health care environment
Battery	Good—but device dependent	Good—but device dependent	Poor—frequently have large batteries that fatigue quickly	Good—but device dependent
Infection control risk	Poor	Poor	Moderate	Poor
Physical security	Poor	Poor	Good	Poor
Data security	Poor	Moderate—device and application dependent	Good	Excellent—anchored to local network infrastructure
Ownership	Usually user owned	Variable	Facility owned	Facility owned

SPEECH RECOGNITION

Along with the ubiquity of EHRs has come widespread clinician dissatisfaction. Doctors and nurses now feel like they are spending more time doing clerical tasks on the computer and less time with their patients. Simultaneously, the widespread use of speech recognition (SR) tools has led to a sense of inevitability that SR software will become standard in all areas of our lives—including the medical environment. Many users feel that dictating instead of typing would improve their speed and efficiency.

Speech recognition is already very well established in certain health-care settings. Computer-aided medical transcription and front-end speech recognition (FESR) reduce costs and improve turnaround times in radiology, anatomic pathology, and any environment where traditional medical transcription was previously utilized. As with many technologies in medicine, the published literature regarding SR is inconclusive and of mixed quality, especially in the ED setting. Potential industry sponsorship and publication bias must be considered, just as with the literature around other profitable endeavors in medicine.

However, some general themes can be drawn from the higher-quality studies and reviews on the topic:

- FESR is associated with a faster turnaround time for report generation as compared to traditional medical transcription.[2]
- FESR requires providers to spend more time correcting the document.
- Documents generated by FESR have higher error rates than those generated by traditional medical transcription.[3,4]
- Providers report satisfaction with FESR usage despite time spent correcting errors.[5-7]
- One 2017 study showed that FESR documentation in EHR using real-world ED tasks was slower and more error prone; however, this study used a product that is already out of date compared to today's technology.[8]

Front-end SR is a particularly dynamic area of technology, where the quality of algorithms, sophistication of background noise cancellation and accent recognition, and convenience of cloud-based solutions make it a moving target for evaluation in any given scenario. Perhaps the most important principle to keep in mind when involved in FESR procurement and implementation is to realize that not everyone will use it. This variability has significant implications for the cost effectiveness of software licensing and should be accounted for in the purchasing evaluation.

Ultimately, FESR will most likely become a routine tool that is available per user preference; anywhere you can click and type, you should be able to click and talk instead.

SCRIBES

Another response to the poor usability of EHRs has been the hiring of scribes (in-person on-site transcribers) or virtual scribe services (scribes who observe the patient visit via telepresence technology). Some data show that scribes improve physician efficiency and experience enough to justify their ongoing cost.[9-12] However, this benefit is dependent on the reimbursement environment of each particular practice, and revenue may be diminished in academic institutions.[9] In many cases, scribes are premed students. This can result in the administrative burden of high turnover, including training and orientation, as scribes move on to attend medical school or other professional training.[13]

In theory, scribes should transcribe the physician's verbal interactions with the patient in real time; they should never have the authority to act independently. However, in practice, scribes frequently become unofficial "EHR wranglers," which makes them even more popular with physicians with suboptimal computer skills. This becomes especially problematic if physicians are tempted to have scribes enter orders on their behalf. One of the core promises of the EHR is the decision support that accompanies computerized physician order entry. Nonclinicians who enter orders on behalf of providers receive decision-support cues that they do not have the background and training to properly interpret. For this reason, regulatory agencies strictly forbid scribes from entering orders in the EHR; this practice is also an area of risk for ED medical directors contemplating the implementation of a scribe program.

DIGITAL RESOURCES

Electronic Prescribing

The opioid crisis has captured the attention of the medical community, creating a nationwide push to reduce the illegal diversion of controlled substances and encourage lower-risk prescribing patterns. However, effective monitoring, decision support, and ED policies and procedures are all hampered by incomplete data sources and paper prescriptions that are not recorded electronically. In response, many organizations are implementing electronic prescribing of controlled substances (EPCS), which allows for better decision support and more complete prescribing data. Additionally, eliminating paper-controlled prescription pads removes an avenue for illegal diversion.

The US Drug Enforcement Administration (DEA) requires significant security precautions, both around initial provider enrollment in EPCS and at the time of prescribing.[14] Although these precautions may initially seem daunting, they are achievable and already mandatory in many states. Enrollment requires in-person verification of the prescriber's identity with a government-issued photo ID, proof of medical credentials (e.g., license, DEA registration), and enrollment in "two-factor authentication." For successful implementation, appropriate expectations must be communicated to providers around the enrollment process.

Currently, the ability to transfer, change, and cancel prescriptions via electronic transactions is not yet widely available, so it is also important to account for new operational challenges. For example:

- Who will record the patient's preferred pharmacy?
- Will that staff member understand the implications of the patient's insurance on acceptable pharmacy options?
- Who will respond to after-hours or post-shift issues with prescriptions or pharmacies?
- What is the expected action and operational response if there is a prescribing irregularity or suspected security breach?

Internet Marketing and Communication

With increased competition among hospitals to attract a payer mix compatible with financial success, institutions are more focused on creating a positive and robust web presence. There are new opportunities to communicate individually or as a group with patients and potential patients, enhance business, and improve customer satisfaction. A department's web presence can also be used as an ancillary physician-recruitment tool.

One of the first issues to address when updating or creating a virtual presence is ownership and maintenance. In other words, who hosts and maintains the site, and who is responsible for its content? If the hospital already has a website of sufficient quality, this is an opportunity for the ED to piggyback onto the resources of the facility. Ideally, hosting and content management would be taken care of by IS/IT, while the ED maintains control over content. Departmental involvement provides an opportunity for the medical and nursing directors to sell the benefits of an effective web presence to the hospital's administration. If the facility's online presence is of low quality or absent, a multitude of commercial web design and hosting resources are available.

Before developing content for a department's website, it is helpful to carefully consider the intended audience and communication goals, which may include the following:

- *Physician recruitment*: Data from academic programs indicate that residency searches are frequently geography-based.[3] It is likely that similar considerations guide all job searches. While it is not a substitute for traditional methods, basic information about the characteristics of a department and contact information can augment recruitment for independent groups.
- *Patient recruitment*: Although published evidence is lacking, some believe that an online marketing presence can have a beneficial effect on payer mix. The theory is that those patients with the resources to check available services are more likely

to be insured. This correlation, if it exists, may diminish as Internet access and familiarity become more ubiquitous.
- *Patient satisfaction*: Many EDs now broadcast real-time wait times, quality data, and appointment scheduling. This web-based information attracts well-informed, proactive patients and allows them to avoid high-volume times (wait times) or wait in a location other than the waiting room (appointments). The intent is to redistribute volume spikes and increase patient satisfaction. Appointment systems expect patients to exercise good judgment about what constitutes an emergency.

When the goals of web-based communication are clearly defined, logical information will follow. The best and most useful content is accessible to users and search engines (search engine optimization). The details of these principles are beyond the scope of this text but should be an integral part of web design and hosting services, whether obtained in-house or outsourced.

Clinical Reference Tools

Emergency providers constantly look up clinical knowledge, perhaps forgotten or rarely encountered, to assist with patient care and decision-making. A plethora of medical references are available—some free, some subscription-based. Since references are constantly changing and updating, this discussion focuses on the pros and cons of these two broad categories—free versus paid.

- *Free content*: Free medical content on the web is of highly variable quality.[4] Without an obligation to paid subscribers, even advertising-supported publishers do not have the same incentive to maintain and update information. If used, free- or advertising-supported content requires a curator (either in-house or from a trusted source) to evaluate its quality and reliability—or significant and ongoing personal effort and education. Advertising-supported search engines are ubiquitous and familiar; they are easy to use but require a discerning approach when interpreting the information.
- *Subscription-based content*: Subscription-based online references are expensive but have the advantage of being curated. Ideally, access to these resources is purchased through coordination with a larger institution, that is, the hospital or affiliated academic institution. Although EDs may not be individually considered when a large institution obtains access to online medical references, many publishers include emergency medicine-focused content as part of their institutional packages.

There is minimal research to recommend one resource over another. One study supports the reliability and speed of using both paid subscription services and search engines over traditional MEDLINE literature searches.[5] In any case, practitioner familiarity and preference should be considered when evaluating any resource. Users must know what is available and how to use it, regardless of the brand name. As with the implementation of any technology, user education and training, ongoing maintenance, and downtime and backup procedures must be addressed. Basic hard-copy texts and resources should be available for disaster scenarios and the occasional technophobe.

Real-Time Location Systems

Real-time location systems (RTLS) have been used extensively in multiple industries, including health care. The two most frequent use cases involve tracking the movement of people (including doctors, nurses, and patients) and equipment. Real-time location systems capable of tagging people and equipment each have their own pros and cons, but they all require extensive infrastructure and ongoing support. Real-time location systems are ideally suited for large departments or facilities that are already making the investment for other purposes (e.g., for tracking costly and mobile capital equipment, such as hemodialysis machines).

RTLS can provide unparalleled data on the movement of people and equipment, especially in departments with multiple points of entry and large numbers of providers and patients. These systems can be especially useful for security purposes, particularly when managing special populations like neonatal, pediatric, or psychiatric patients. They can also improve the accuracy of data that is challenging when relying on human entry and recall, including encounter and transport times, and can inform operational analysis and decisions in ways that are impossible without them.

Scheduling Systems

From the smallest groups to the largest organizations, provider shift scheduling is a mundane yet important task that can become an enormous problem if managed inappropriately. A number of commercially available scheduling software packages exist. Many go beyond simple shift placement and schedule printing with the most full-featured packages, including:

- Remote access
- Vacation requests
- Shift swaps
- Secure communication among group members and administrators
- Automatic shift reminders
- Calendar software interface
- Payroll interface

For maximum staff satisfaction, online access to scheduling tools is a must have. Some scheduling solutions are enterprise-wide, providing another reason to coordinate with facility IT/IS to avoid the duplication of effort and/or costs. Although scheduling software packages permit complex rulemaking when assigning shifts, it is prudent to maintain oversight, as the ultimate responsibility for staff work assignments lies with the person running the software, not the program.

PATIENT KIOSKS AND PORTALS

Customer kiosks have become widely used in other industries (e.g., airline and hotel) and are quickly finding a place in the ED setting. Kiosks for patient-care purposes typically involve a custom hardware solution with a touchscreen interface that can be installed in waiting areas, patient rooms, and other departments. Most kiosks are designed to augment rather than replace nursing or registration staff. The utilization of kiosks has permitted other industries to decrease their number of "live" personnel.

As applied in the ED, a typical flow process might point incoming patients to a kiosk whenever triage or registration personnel are not immediately available. The clinician then directly reviews the patient-entered information as it becomes available. One advantage of this approach is that in the interim, the entire team can access the electronic data and escalate the patient's priority if necessary. This approach also eliminates a server (i.e., triage) queue when the flow process is delayed by crowding. Patient flow for lower-acuity conditions may be enhanced as well. Patients requesting prescription refills or suture removals can be automatically directed to a fast-track waiting area or intake department.

Exit interviews offer another opportunity to put the patient kiosk into service. At the conclusion of their visits, patients and families can be directed to a kiosk, where they can complete a survey on their experience. Feedback is then sent to key stakeholders while giving frontline staff the opportunity for "real-time" service recovery. This application can also help identify potential risk/quality events.

As standalone products or used in conjunction with an enterprise EHR, kiosks are technologically simple to execute and require a relatively small investment. They are particularly efficacious in departments with queuing issues and large variations in arrival patterns. They have the potential to offer greater privacy, more accurate data, and increased patient satisfaction by reducing wait times and improving the responsiveness of the department.

Sophisticated health-care systems are implementing portals to enhance efficiency and improve the patient experience. Accessed from the web, a mobile device, a kiosk, or a terminal in the patient's room, portals allow patients and families to participate in their care. The portals commonly provide access to demographic information, some parts of the health record, lab, imaging, and other ancillary test results. Many organizations are now moving forward with OpenNotes, which allows patients to access clinical information from the patient portal.[15] The effective use of portals may reduce unnecessary or marginally productive office visits.

Historically, non-face-to-face visits were associated with reduced reimbursement. However, as telemedicine is becoming more ubiquitous and reimbursement shifts away from fee-for-service to value-based models, additional opportunities to leverage nontraditional access to care will become available. As an example, patients can e-mail questions, concerns, or requests for prescription refills, eliminating an office visit. However, some states require insurers to cover and reimburse for phone, online, and telemedicine efforts by the physician. Portals can also "push" after-care instructions and disease-specific educational materials to patients.

AVOIDING PITFALLS

In addition to the pitfalls mentioned regarding security and devices, some pitfalls are unique to the implementation of new technology. By keeping these in mind, the chances of success are enhanced.

- *Misspecification*: It is important to define as clearly as possible the "problem" that the new support technology is intended to solve. When this critical step is missed, there is inevitably an expectation gap between the implementation team and users.
- *Examine the process(es) surrounding the problem(s)*: Too often, new technology is purchased to solve rather than understand and address a dysfunctional process, which may still exist after the purchase of the new technology. By defining the problem, engaging the pertinent stakeholders, and examining the process, this misstep can be avoided.
- *Lack of dedicated resources for implementation and training*: It is necessary to budget proper resources to both train and support new users. Otherwise, the technology may not be utilized, or the users may become cynical and resist further attempts, making reimplementation very challenging.
- *Lack of leadership support*: As with any new change, participation begins at the top. If the technology is important enough to purchase and implement, the support of the leaders is essential.
- *IT department collaboration*: Related to allocating resources, it is paramount to get buy-in and support from the IT department, whose business processes are designed to support new technologies.

CONCLUSION

While support technologies may not be essential to daily operations, when chosen and implemented well, they have the ability to dramatically enhance staff satisfaction, operational efficiency, communication, and patient safety. As IT becomes more integrated within health care, a convergence of these technologies will occur. Users will be able to access these essential resources in a convenient form at the point of care. While the user interface of these technologies may change, the principles of their use will not.

REFERENCES

1. Today in Science History. Technology Quotes. 2020. Available at: https://todayinsci.com/QuotationsCategories/T_Cat/Technology-Quotations.htm. Accessed October 26, 2020.
2. Zick RG, Olsen J. Voice recognition software versus a traditional transcription service for physician charting in the ED. *Am J Emerg Med.* 2001;19(4):295–298.
3. Goss FR, Zhou L, Weiner SG. Incidence of speech recognition errors in the emergency department. *Int J Med Inform.* 2016;93:70–73.
4. Blackley SV, Huynh J, Wang L, et al. Speech recognition for clinical documentation from 1990 to 2018: a systematic review. *J Am Med Inform Assoc.* 2019;26(4):324–338.
5. Vogel M, Kaisers W, Wassmuth R, et al. Analysis of documentation speed using web-based medical speech recognition technology: randomized controlled trial. *J Med Internet Res.* 2015;17(11):e247.
6. Lyons JP, Sanders SA, Fredrick Cesene D, et al. Speech recognition acceptance by physicians: A temporal replication of a survey of expectations and experiences. *Health Informatics J.* 2016;22(3):768–778.
7. Clarke MA, King JL, Kim MS. Toward successful implementation of speech recognition technology: a survey of SRT utilization issues in healthcare settings. *South Med J.* 2015;108(7):445–451.
8. Hodgson T, Magrabi F, Coiera E. Efficiency and safety of speech recognition for documentation in the electronic health record. *J Am Med Inform Assoc.* 2017;24(6):1127–1133.
9. Heaton HA, Nestler DM, Jones DD, et al. Impact of scribes on patient throughput in adult and pediatric academic EDs. *Am J Emerg Med.* 2016;34(10):1982–1985.
10. Heaton HA, Nestler DM, Lohse CM, et al. Impact of scribes on emergency department patient throughput one year after implementation. *Am J Emerg Med.* 2017;35(2):311–314.
11. Shuaib W, Hilmi J, Caballero J, et al. Impact of a scribe program on patient throughput, physician productivity, and patient satisfaction in a community-based emergency department. *Health Inform J.* 2019;25(1):216–224.
12. Addesso LC, Nimmer M, Visotcky A, et al. Impact of medical scribes on provider efficiency in the pediatric emergency department. *Acad Emerg Med.* 2019;26(2):174–182.
13. DeWitt D, Harrison LE. The potential impact of scribes on medical school applicants and medical students with the new clinical documentation guidelines. *J Gen Intern Med.* 2018;33(11):2002–2004.
14. EPCS Approved Certification Processes. Available at: https://www.deadiversion.usdoj.gov/ecomm/e_rx/thirdparty.htm. Accessed October 11, 2020.
15. Open Notes. Available at: https://www.opennotes.org. Accessed October 11, 2020.

CHAPTER 70

SOCIAL MEDIA IN MEDICINE

Matthew Richard Klein, Ryan Stanton, Michael Gottlieb

Social media is defined as a form of electronic communication through which users share information, ideas, personal messages, and other content.[1] These sites allow people to communicate with acquaintances and strangers, often with a focus on common interests. Technology has revolutionized the ways in which we gather information, communicate, learn, and play. For hundreds of years, medical education and learning took place through books, libraries, and in-person teaching. However, in the last 20 years, the entire paradigm has changed. The breadth of human medical knowledge is now at our fingertips, and information that once took hours or days to locate can be accessed in seconds.

The unfolding digital revolution creates a dramatic increase in the pace of knowledge dissemination and discussion. Social media continues to disrupt the ways in which we create and consume medical information, so it is critical to understand the strengths and limitations of these novel resources.

TECHNOLOGY REVOLUTION

Computers have been around for nearly a century and a half; the original "punched cards" (precursors of the first "computers") were developed in 1750 for the control of textile looms.[2] In 1890, Herman Hollerith designed a punch card-based system to assist with the 1880 US Census.[2] The US population had grown to a point that it took seven years to tabulate the results. This new system was able to perform the task in three years, however, saving the government an estimated $5 million. Hollerith created a company that would later become International Business Machines.

The personal computer (PC) is a relatively new term first published in a 1962 *New York Times* article.[3] Although the idea had been around since the 1940s, it took significant advancements to get the size and cost in a range that made these machines practical for the general public. Prototypes and resemblances to the PC existed prior to 1981; the Datapoint 2200 was released in 1970 and was the first to resemble what we would recognize as a PC.

The rapid advancement of technology that we've experienced in the last 30 years started in the 1980s with increasing processing speeds, memory space, and gaming platforms. During this pivotal period, personal computing became a reality as technology advanced and costs decreased. In the 1990s, the development of the internet allowed the public to directly communicate with others. The decade also ushered in the early use of online services like Prodigy and America Online. PCs transitioned from advanced word-processing devices and basic gaming platforms to global communication tools.

The 2000s featured advanced computers with a rapidly growing capacity to store data in a shrinking footprint. With the advent of smartphones, computing power that once required rooms of machinery could fit in the palm of a hand. Advancements in access, connectivity, and speed allowed medical knowledge that was once confined to journals and textbooks to become digitized and instantly searchable. These advancements also allowed the medical community to move to paperless systems for medical records, sharing of information, and real-time access to integral patient data.

In recent years, our online connectivity has allowed clinicians to establish interest groups, share information, and create movements like Free Open Access Medical Education (FOAMed or FOAM), which revolutionized the distribution of education and research.[4]

The Evolution of Social Media

Social media initially emerged in the 1990s for recreational purposes to connect friends and strangers via chat rooms. Initial dial-up internet connections and limited computer capabilities gave way to improved technology, access, and speed. The first big social media "success story" launched in 2003 with Myspace, a large-scale platform that provided individuals with the opportunity to create a social media presence. Myspace had over 72 million users at its peak in 2008, the same year it was overtaken by Facebook, a rival social networking site founded in 2004.[5] Twitter was founded in 2006, allowing users to share short, 140-character messages. As of 2020, there were over 2.6 billion monthly Facebook users with 1.75 billion daily users and 330 million monthly Twitter users with 145 million daily users.[6,7]

According to the Pew Research Center, roughly 70% of Americans use some form of social media, and a majority of Americans use the internet to gather health information.[8,9] Mirroring the general population, physicians also utilize social media as consumers and creators of medical content.[10] One example is EMDocs, a private Facebook group of several thousand international emergency physicians who share information related to and outside of medicine. Twitter represents an open-source information exchange in which conversations and comments are public and visible to anyone who "follows" a particular person or group. Twitter's design promotes rapid information exchange, debate, and conversations.

SOCIAL MEDIA AND LEARNING

The impact of social media on emergency medicine education cannot be overstated. Textbooks, lectures, and bedside teaching were the predominant educational tools available to previous generations of medical trainees. Today's learners, on the other hand, can augment these traditional modalities with blogs, podcasts, streaming video, infographics, and discussion boards. Although these innovative resources offer novel opportunities to engage learners, they also present new challenges. The evolution of online resources has allowed for the more rapid dissemination and translation of medical information, but it has also called into question the methods by which data is reviewed and vetted.

The early 21st century has seen an exponential growth in the number of digital education resources in emergency medicine.[11] Although these tools are predominantly utilized in high-income countries, emergency medicine and critical care websites reach a global audience.[12] Unsurprisingly, trainees use these resources more frequently than their program directors.[13] In one survey of emergency medicine residents, listening to podcasts was more popular and believed to be more beneficial than reading textbooks.[14]

FOAMed

FOAMed is a constantly evolving collection of interactive and free medical education resources, including blogs, podcasts, tweets, online videos, text documents, photographs, Facebook groups, and so on. Many of these resources exist under the umbrella of FOAM or FOAMed. Advocates of FOAMed cite inspiration from the Hippocratic Oath's urging to teach the art of medicine "without fee and covenant."[15] Some proponents of social media argue that these novel digital resources have the advantage of disseminating knowledge more rapidly than traditional publication models.[16] As emergency medicine pioneer Joe Lex explains:[17]

If you want to know how we practiced medicine five years ago, read a textbook. If you want to know how we practiced medicine two years ago, read a journal. If you want to know how we practice medicine now, go to a (good) conference. If you want to know how we will practice medicine in the future, listen in the hallways and use FOAMed.

Some digital resources, such as Emergency Medicine Reviews and Perspectives (EM: RAP. org), employ a paid subscription model. Other sites are truly FOAMed. In recent years, hybrid models have emerged, particularly among academic journals. Although these publications often require subscriptions and host articles behind paywalls, many publish open-access papers for a limited time and disseminate them using blogs and podcasts.

Common Critiques

Although digital educational resources continue to proliferate, concerns about quality have arisen. Some social media conversations may help drive practice changes but may also come at the expense of covering more "bread and butter" topics. One analysis found that FOAMed resources produce imbalanced and incomplete coverage of core emergency medicine content.[18] This imbalance requires continued attention as trainees increasingly turn to social media for their educational needs. Another common critique of FOAMed is that the peer-review process that accompanies textbooks and journals affords higher-quality content than the latest blog post or tweet. While there is undoubtedly value in content that is curated by experts, proponents of FOAMed suggest that immediate, open-source feedback provides a unique opportunity to address incorrect information.

In the online world, there is a challenge in clearly distinguishing strict evidenced-based medical information from opinions, bad data, and misinterpreted research. As this digital revolution continues to unfold, efforts to assess quality in social media education continue to evolve. For example, the popular website Academic Life in Emergency Medicine (ALiEM.com) created instructional resources that are curated by an editorial board.[19] Operating in parallel, an international group of emergency medicine educators is working to develop an instrument called the *Social Media Index* to measure the quality of online resources.[20]

RISKS OF SOCIAL MEDIA

As with any aspect of medicine, the benefits of social media must be weighed against its risks, both to patients and providers. The adage "the internet is forever" serves as a reminder that once a social media post is shared, it should be considered permanently available to patients, colleagues, and employers. Inappropriate online behavior can jeopardize patient relationships, professional reputations, and physicians' licenses.

Regulatory Mandates

Violations of patient privacy and confidentiality are primary concerns with the use of social media in medicine.[21] In the United States, patient health information is protected by the Health Insurance Portability and Accountability Act (HIPAA).[22] All clinicians should familiarize themselves with the requirements of HIPAA to prevent violations of this federal mandate, including those related to social media. Patient identifiers (e.g., name and date of birth) are obviously illegal to share on social media, as are videos or photographs that could be used to identify patients. Posting other information that could be used to identify a patient—such as details of a rare presentation or the date of a specific encounter—may be less commonly recognized as violations but are equally inappropriate.

Ethical Considerations

The use of social media by health-care professionals should also be governed by ethical considerations. In 2011, the American Medical Association Council on Ethical and Judicial Affairs published recommendations on the use of social media by physicians and students.[23] In addition to raising concerns regarding patient privacy, these guidelines call for maintaining appropriate boundaries with patients, reporting unprofessional posts by colleagues, and recognizing that inappropriate social media behavior can undermine public trust in the medical profession. The Council of Residency Directors in Emergency Medicine has also published guidelines for the use of social media by residency programs.[24]

State medical boards have engaged in disciplinary actions against physicians for violations of online professionalism.[25] This is particularly germane since emergency physicians underestimate the likelihood of official investigations related to social media behavior involving alcohol or derogatory speech.[26] The importance of maintaining patient privacy and professional behavior is not limited to the online environment. By adhering to the same standards that govern interpersonal interactions, physicians can mitigate the hazards of using social media and avail themselves of its merits.

SOCIAL MEDIA AND CAREER ADVANCEMENT

Social media can be a valuable tool for career advancement because it can increase the potential for collaboration and help develop a virtual community of practice.[27-31] This can be an invaluable tool for health-care professionals with limited local mentorship by enabling them to expand their network of potential collaborators.[28] Additionally, there is an increasing recognition of the scholarly value of social media content. Sherbino and colleagues have suggested that four criteria are necessary to qualify as scholarship (**Box 70.1**); ensuring adherence to these criteria may enhance the utility of social media-based study for career enhancement.[32] Increasingly, social media-based scholarship is also recognized by promotion and tenure committees.[30,33,34] Finally, social media can be utilized to expand research influence. Research findings can be shared via social media platforms and blog posts.[30] A number of journals are incorporating infographics to improve the visibility of research papers.[35] As an added benefit, this exposure can also increase the visibility of the researcher, leading to potential collaborations or speaking opportunities. In fact, some authors have even utilized these infographics to recruit study participants.[36]

SOCIAL MEDIA AND PHYSICIAN WELLNESS

Social media is a double-edged sword with the potential to reduce or exacerbate physician burnout. As stated previously, virtual communities of practice allow users to connect with colleagues and collaborators, irrespective of geographic boundaries,

---

BOX 70.1 ■ SOCIAL MEDIA-BASED SCHOLARSHIP[27]

Social media-based scholarship must:
- Be original
- Advance the field of medical education by building on theory, research, or best practice
- Be archived and disseminated
- Provide the medical education community with the ability to comment on and provide feedback in a transparent fashion that informs wider discussion.

> **BOX 70.2 ■ TAKE-HOME POINTS**
>
> 1. Social media provides opportunities to connect with colleagues, advance education, and support others. Take advantage of peer support, wellness, and potential connections that can be built.
> 2. Social media is public information; even "private" posts can be easily shared.
> 3. The internet is forever... relatively. Posts and information live on for long periods of time and may come back up in the future.
> 4. Social media is held to the same HIPAA and other privacy standards as any level of health-care communication.
> 5. The First Amendment may protect speech from government regulation, but it does not offer the same protection from employers, lawyers, or the public.
> 6. Choose social media platform(s) based on individual interests and goals.
> 7. Be respectful. Similar to holiday meals with the extended family, certain topics (e.g., politics, religion, gun control) can lead to discord on social media.
> 8. Check facts and confirm data for practice-changing posts. Not all opinions are consistent with evidence.
> 9. Assume statements could appear in court. The legal system uses social media posts during litigation, including medical malpractice cases.
> 10. Do not be afraid to take a break or suspend social media activities. Social media can enhance lives, but time spent online must be balanced.

to facilitate projects and even debrief on stressful situations.[27] This expanded network can provide greater opportunities to connect with others who have shared similar experiences and to discuss coping strategies for challenging situations. However, social media also has the potential to diminish wellness by adding to the workload as users try to keep up with the massive amount of information released daily. Additionally, developing a social media presence requires consistent effort, which may detract from time for work or family.

Limiting Intrusion

Several strategies are helpful for maintaining engagement on social media while avoiding burnout. First, determine boundaries and prioritize social media use accordingly. Set aside dedicated time for social media, and avoid keeping up with every post that is released. This can be facilitated by limiting notifications to only those that directly reference the user, halting notifications entirely, or establishing a specific start and end time for notifications.

Rich Site Summary (RSS) feeds can be used to deliver regularly changing web content and identify topics of interest. Create electronic alerts (e.g., Google Scholar) to notify the user when new citations or papers on topics of interest are published. However, it is also important to avoid excessive notifications and emails, so RSS feeds should be continuously reassessed and refined.

CONCLUSION

Social media is a rapidly evolving tool available to health-care professionals to greatly expand access to expertise, colleagues, and collaboration. However, these powerful platforms carry a number of potential risks. All clinicians must strictly adhere to laws and standards related to patient privacy when using social media. It is also important to understand that much of the information provided via social media is limited and may not include adequate context. Therefore, the user remains responsible for gathering appropriate evidence (**Box 70.2**).

REFERENCES

1. Social media. Merriam-Webster.com. 2019. Available at: https://www.merriam-webster.com/dictionary/social%20media.
2. da Cruz F. Early Card Punch Machines—Columbi University Computing History. 2019. Available at: http://www.columbia.edu/cu/computinghistory/oldpunch.html#:~: Accessed October 24, 2020.
3. Wikipedia. History of personal computers. 2020. Available at: https://en.wikipedia.org/wiki/History_of_personal_computers. Accessed October 24, 2020.
4. Chan TM, Stehman C, Gottlieb M, et al. A short history of free open access medical education. the past, present, and future. 2020. Available at: https://www.atsjournals.org/doi/full/10.34197/ats-scholar.2020-0014PS. Accessed October 24, 2020.
5. Arrington M. Facebook no longer the second largest social network. Tech Crunch. 2008. Available at: https://techcrunch.com/2008/06/12/facebook-no-longer-the-second-largest-social-network/.
6. Statista. Number of daily active Facebook users worldwide as of 1st quarter 2020. 2020. Available at: https://www.statista.com/statistics/346167/facebook-global-dau/#:~: Accessed August 1, 2020.
7. Lin Y. 10 Twitter statistics every marketer should know in 2020. 2020. Available at: https://www.oberlo.com/blog/twitter-statistics#:~: Accessed October 24, 2020.
8. Pew Research Center. Social Media Fact Sheet. 2018. Available at: www.pewinternet.org/fact-sheet/social-media.
9. Fox S. Chronic Disease and the Internet. Pew Research Center. 2010. Available at: https://www.pewresearch.org/internet/2010/03/24/chronic-disease-and-the-internet/.
10. Pershad Y, Hangge P, Albadawi H, et al. Social medicine: Twitter in healthcare. *J Clin Med.* 2018;7(6):E121.
11. Cadogan M, Thoma B, Chan TM, et al. Free Open Access Meducation (FOAM): the rise of emergency medicine and critical care blogs and podcasts (2002–2013). *Emerg Med J.* 2013;31(e1):e76–e77.
12. Burkholder T, Bellows J, King R. Free Open Access Medical Education (FOAM) in emergency medicine: the global distribution in 2016. *West J Emerg Med.* 2018;19(3):600–605.
13. Purdy E, Thoma B, Bednarczyk J, et al. The use of free online educational resources by Canadian emergency medicine residents and program directors. *Canad J Emerg Med.* 2015;17(2):101–106.
14. Malin M, Schlein S, Doctor S, et al. A survey of the current utilization of asynchronous education among emergency medicine residents in the United States. *Acad Med.* 2014;89(4):598–601.
15. Nickson C, Cadogan M. Free Open Access Medical Education (FOAM) for the emergency physician. *Emerg Med Australas.* 2014;26(1):76–83.
16. Thoma B, Mohindra R, Artz J, et al. CHM and the changing landscape of medical education knowledge translation. *CJEM.* 2015;17(2):184–187.
17. Cadogan M. FOAM. 2020. Available at: https://litfl.com/foam-free-open-access-medical-education/. Accessed October 24, 2020.
18. Stuntz R, Clontz R. An evaluation of emergency medicine core content covered by free open access medical education resources. *Ann Emerg Med.* 2016;67(5):649–653.
19. Lin M, Joshi N, Grock A, et al. Approved instructional resources series: a national initiative to identify quality emergency medicine blog and podcast content for resident education. *J Grad Med Educ* 2016;8(2):219–25.
20. Thoma B, Chan T, Kapur P, et al. The social media index as an indicator of quality for emergency medicine blogs: a METRIQ study. *Ann Emerg Med* 2018;72(6):696–702.
21. Lambert K, Barry P, Stokes G. Risk management and legal issues with the use of social media in the healthcare setting. *J Healthc Risk Manag* 2012;31(4):41–7.
22. Health information privacy. HHS.gov. Available at: https://www.hhs.gov/hipaa/index.html. Accessed February 4, 2018.
23. Shore R, Halsey J, Shah K, et al. Report of the AMA council on ethical and judicial affairs: professionalism in the use of social media. *J Clin Ethics.* 2011;22(2):165–172.
24. Pillow M, Hopson L, Bond M, et al. Social media guidelines and best practices: recommendations from the Council of Residency Directors Social Media Task Force. *West J Emerg Med.* 2014;15(1):26–30.
25. Greysen S, Chretien K, Kind T, et al. Physician violations of online professionalism and disciplinary actions: a national survey of state medical boards. *JAMA.* 2012;307(11):1141–1142.
26. Soares W, Shenvi C, Waller N, et al. Perceptions of unprofessional social media behavior among emergency medicine physicians. *J Grad Med Educ.* 2017;9(1):85–89.
27. Dubé L, Bourhis A, Jacob R. The impact of structuring characteristics on the launching of virtual communities of practice. *J Organ Change Manag.* 2005;18:145–166.
28. Gottlieb M, Fant A, King A, et al. One click away: digital mentorship in the modern era. *Cureus.* 2017;9(11):e1838.
29. Chan TM, Gottlieb M, Sherbino J, et al. The ALiEM Faculty Incubator: a novel online approach to faculty development in education scholarship. *Acad Med.* 2018;93(10):1497–1502.
30. Gerds AT, Chan T. Social media in hematology in 2017: dystopia, utopia, or somewhere in-between? *Curr Hematol Malig Rep.* 2017;12(6):582–591.
31. Yarris LM, Chan TM, Gottlieb M, et al. Finding your people in the digital age: virtual communities of practice to promote education scholarship. *J Grad Med Educ.* 2019;11(1):1–5.
32. Sherbino J, Arora VM, Van Melle E, et al. Criteria for social media-based scholarship in health professions education. *Postgrad Med J.* 2015;91(1080):551–555.
33. Franzen D, Cooney R, Chan T, et al. Scholarship by the clinician-educator in emergency medicine. *AEM Educ Train.* 2018;2(2):115–120.
34. Cabrera D, Vartabedian BS, Spinner RJ, et al. More than likes and Tweets: creating social media portfolios for academic promotion and tenure. *J Grad Med Educ.* 2017;9(4):421–425.
35. Murray IR, Murray AD, Wordie SJ, et al. Maximising the impact of your work using infographics. *Bone Joint Res.* 2017;6(11):619–620.
36. Thoma B, Paddock M, Purdy E, et al. Leveraging a virtual community of practice to participate in a survey-based study: a description of the METRIQ study methodology. *AEM Educ Train.* 2017;1(2):110–113.

CHAPTER 71

NEW TECHNOLOGIES AND APPLICATIONS IN EMERGENCY MEDICINE

Timothy Boardman, Gita Pensa

Advances in medical technology are typically borne out of perceived need. In 1816, the stethoscope was invented by French physician Rene Laennec, who was having difficulty hearing the heartbeat of a young woman suffering from a cardiac disorder.[1] From this sentinel event, a symbol of medicine was created; it is now almost inconceivable to see a health-care provider without this essential piece of medical equipment.

While the stethoscope was considered a technological advancement in the 1800s, the term "technology" is now commonly associated with electronic devices and digital applications. Historically, the first push for computerized health solutions is attributed to Medicare and Medicaid in 1965, as the United States developed a need for more efficient and accurate health-care information systems.[2]

The demand for better and more efficient systems, which led to the introduction of multiple new technologies, increased significantly in 1999 with publication of the Institute of Medicine report *To Err is Human: Building a Safer Health System*. Given estimations that between 44,000 and 98,000 people were dying in hospitals each year as a result of preventable medical errors, the report called for a new "culture of safety."[3] As a direct response to this report, the US government mandated the development of new technologies directed at reducing medical errors, including computerized provider order entry systems and more efficient ways to track and report safety events. Subsequently, President George W. Bush called for the full implementation of computerized health records in his 2004 State of the Union address.[4] This initiative was later mandated by President Barack Obama in 2009 with the signing of the Health Information Technology for Economic and Clinical Health Act, which established "meaningful use" and the full adoption of electronic health records (EHRs) by 2014.[2]

Over the past decade, the growth of mobile health-care technology has been exponential; the potential for new advances almost seems infinite.[5] The specific devices and applications discussed in this chapter represent new technologies designed to increase safety, productivity, and efficiency in the emergency department (ED). Their inclusion is not meant as endorsement over other similar products, nor is this list exhaustive; these examples are provided simply as illustrations of the myriad ways in which technology is changing the practice of modern emergency care.

MOBILE APPLICATIONS: POINT-OF-CARE/BEDSIDE

Mobile applications may be used away from a fixed "computer station," allowing providers to utilize point-of-care, bedside, and other remote technologies. Among other advantages, mobile applications give ED providers quicker access to the patients' EHR without the need to log into a desktop computer and offer additional resources to efficiently manage patients and demonstrate visual diagnosis and treatment options.

Electronic Health Record Companion Applications

A patient presents to the ED with complaints of fevers and increased redness around and drainage from a surgical incision. The emergency physician evaluating the patient opens the EHR companion application on their tablet and takes a photo of the wound, which is immediately and securely added to the patient's EHR. Additionally, the physician orders an infectious workup, imaging, and a surgical consult directly from the application. While leaving the room, the physician dictates a note directly into the tablet and moves on to evaluate the next patient.

Several years ago, this scenario may have seemed like science fiction, but with the newest companion applications for EHRs, it is now a reality. Most of the major EHR companies have created mobile applications that not only give the user access to medical records from virtually any location but also allow for data entry and mobile ordering.

As the EHR continues to become more user-friendly, so should the associated companion applications. These applications have the potential to significantly reduce the amount of time emergency physicians are confined to a desktop computer, allowing them to spend more time at the bedside with their patients. Their use will also allow for timely order entry and can help minimize the occurrence of "verbal orders," a common source of medical errors.[6]

Epic Haiku and Canto

Epic Systems Corporation (Epic), one of the most widely used medical record software companies in the US, offers a set of mobile companion applications. Epic Haiku is a smartphone application that allows access to patient records without having to log onto a computer. This application also allows users to take clinical photographs with their smartphones that are uploaded directly to the EHR without being stored locally on the device.[7] Epic Canto is an application created specifically for tablet computers. In addition to the functionality included in the Haiku application, Canto allows the user to dictate notes directly into the EHR through a Nuance dictation system.[8] The application also has a whiteboard-like function that allows the provider to write down observations and details that are only viewable by the user who created them and are not made part of the patient's EHR. Lastly, Canto offers mobile physician order entry with access to the user's order preferences.

Patient Communication

Patient satisfaction is linked to the quality of communication between provider and patient and to how well patients understand their care.[9-11] This poses a challenge for emergency providers, as the fast-paced and demanding environment of the ED often leaves little time for patient interaction and even less time for thorough explanations of diagnoses and treatment plans. Unfortunately, health-care providers often speak *at* their patients, who may retain very little of the conversation. The use of bedside visual tools can improve communication and may help emergency clinicians better explain diagnoses and treatments to patients and help obtain informed consent for procedures.[12,13]

drawMD

drawMD is a free mobile application designed specifically for use in the health-care setting. It includes premade anatomical templates that allow providers to add "stamps,"

FIGURE 71.1 ■ drawMD Application

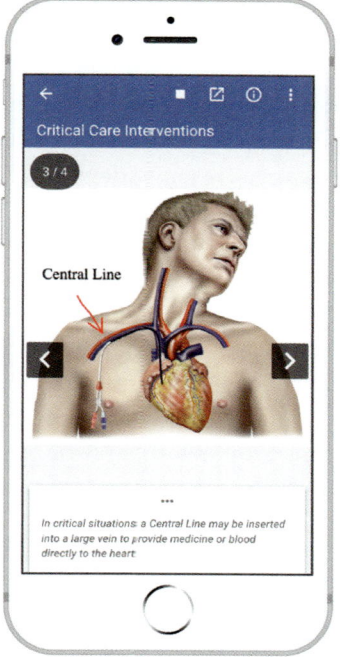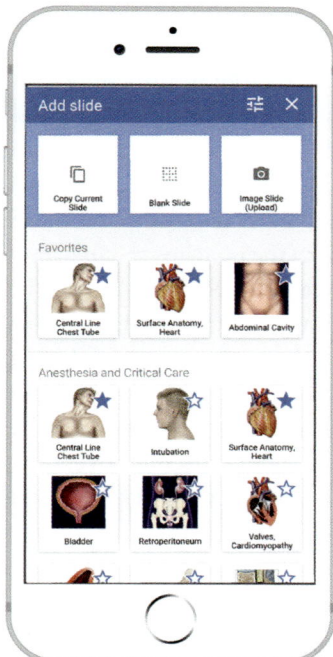

Image © Copyright Visible Health, Inc.

such as a triple-lumen catheter, or to draw directly onto the templates in order to facilitate conversations with patients. The application can be used for a real-time explanation and annotation or to create presentations used for recurring discussions, such as obtaining consent for a central line (**Figure 71.1**). The application can also use custom images, such as the patient's own radiograph, to aid in explaining a diagnosis. With account registration, drawMD can be used in a cloud-based format, allowing presentations created on one device to be accessed with a separate device registered on the same account.

CardioVisual

CardioVisual is a video-based mobile application that helps to explain various cardiovascular disorders. The basic form of the application is available for free download; a purchased professional version includes additional features. The educational resource contains over 100 videos that can help emergency providers explain conditions like atrial fibrillation, deep vein thrombosis, acute coronary syndrome, or heart failure. The application also includes videos regarding therapies and can help prepare a patient and their family for cardiac catheterization or other treatments that are often poorly explained in emergent situations.[13-15]

Whiteboard Applications

A number of whiteboard applications are available for download, each with similar functions. These applications are ideal for the provider who does not want to rely on premade videos or templates and would rather be able to draw and write without constraint. Many of these applications also allow for image upload for annotation; some are cloud-based and allow for real-time collaboration between peers. Examples of these applications include Explain Everything, BaiBoard, and Whiteboard.

Ultrasound

The use of point-of-care ultrasonography is becoming increasingly popular among emergency physicians, and with this, bedside ultrasound is quickly becoming the standard of care.[16] With this surge in utilization, there is a potential for increased revenue for EDs when emergency providers are able to submit their point-of-care ultrasound studies for reimbursement.[17] However, many departments, especially those not in urban or academic settings, have limited access to adequate point-of-care ultrasound devices. This is partly due to the high cost of purchasing and maintaining ultrasound equipment.[18]

However, with the push for reliable mobile technology, handheld ultrasound devices are starting to provide reliable, high-quality imaging comparable to the traditional ultrasound machines at a fraction of the cost. Handheld ultrasound devices have the potential to be a solution for EDs that struggle to purchase and maintain traditional ultrasound equipment, as multiple devices can be purchased for the price of one new ultrasound machine.[18,19] This would enable these EDs to provide high-quality bedside imaging and faster diagnosis and could potentially generate higher revenue by means of billable diagnostic procedures. At the same time, costs to patients could be decreased by reducing the need for resource-intensive studies by radiology departments.[20]

Butterfly iQ

The Butterfly iQ is a handheld ultrasound device that is currently compatible with iPhone (Apple iOS 12.0 or newer) and Android devices (Android OS 9 for Samsung devices and Android OS 10 for Google and OnePlus devices). Unlike other handheld ultrasound devices, it uses a single transducer that can emulate linear, curved, or phased array exams. This is possible through the use of a 2-D array of 9,000 microsensors that replaces the piezoelectric crystal technology found in traditional ultrasound transducers. To address patient privacy and data security concerns, the information obtained with the Butterfly iQ (**Figure 71.2**) can

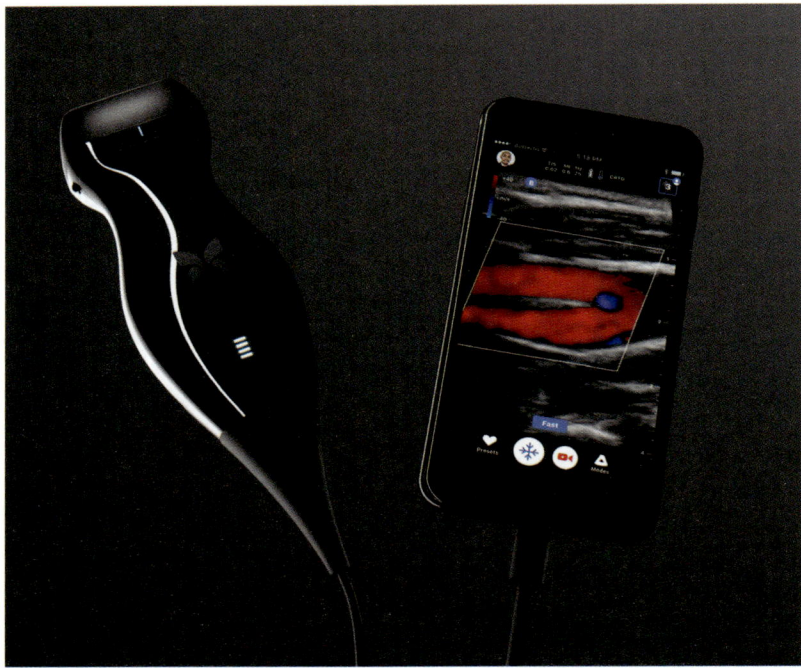

FIGURE 71.2 ■ Butterfly IQ Ultrasound Device

Image courtesy of Butterfly Network, Inc.

be stored locally on the device with 256-bit advanced encryption standard security, or it can be sent to the Butterfly Cloud or to colleagues or patients using secure 1.2 encryption.

Philips Lumify

Philips Lumify is an Android-based handheld ultrasound machine. It utilizes three separate transducers (linear, curved, and phased array) that rely on the piezoelectric effect generated by crystals similar to that of traditional ultrasound machines. These transducers connect directly to Android devices using universal serial bus-type C technology and are captured using the Lumify mobile application. The Lumify application and cloud allows for image interpretation and processing similar to a traditional ultrasound machine. All images and videos are stored in the application or cloud in compliance with the Health Insurance Portability and Accountability Act (HIPAA) and can be shared with colleagues or sent to a picture archive and communication system. The application also includes an integrated barcode reader than can be configured to read most patient identification systems for easy data input.

Ophthalmoscope

Fundoscopy is a core physical exam skill that, despite its high utility in the ED, is challenging for many medical providers.[21,22] The introduction of the Welch Allyn PanOptic ophthalmoscope has helped to increase the accuracy and ease of this exam, but it is still often difficult to convey findings accurately to consultants.[23] This poses a clear challenge for emergency providers who do not have an ophthalmology consultation readily available or who must make the decision to either transfer patients to a referral center or send them home with outpatient ophthalmology follow-up.

A potential solution to this problem is the use of a mobile smartphone device to capture high-quality images of the eye exam that can be easily shared with ophthalmology consultants. Through use of this technology, management decisions can be made with consultants based on their direct visualization of the eye exam images instead of relying on descriptions that may not be complete or fully accurate. Several devices exist that are designed for this purpose. All require the use of a smartphone camera and are either used in conjunction with a separate ophthalmoscope or have built-in magnification technology.

Welch Allyn

The Welch Allyn iEXAMINER consists of an adapter that fits onto an iPhone device and then attaches to a PanOptic ophthalmoscope. The system is then used through the iEXAMINER mobile application and allows the user to capture several images of the fundus in a field-of-view that is up to 25°. Stored locally on the mobile device, these images can be printed or sent as e-mail attachments to any desired consultants.

D-EYE

The D-EYE Digital Retina imaging system does not require the use of a separate ophthalmoscope. The technology uses the built-in light-emitting diode (LED) source and smartphone camera to capture images or videos of the patient's retina. The device is able to capture a field-of-view up to 20°. The images can then be sent securely via local area networks or directly from the D-EYE mobile application through e-mail or other messaging services.

oDocs Eye Care

oDocs Eye Care offers several eye examination products. The visoScope connects directly to an iPhone device and uses its LED source and camera. Using the companion application, the visoScope can obtain images up to a 50° field-of-view with eye dilation.

The oDocs Fundus is similar to the visoScope in its operation and functionality but is designed to fit a wider range of smartphones. The device itself follows a "do-it-yourself" concept. It can be purchased either as an assembly kit or preassembled; it is also available through an open-source platform, and the digital specifications for the device can be obtained for self-3D printing.

The oDocs Nun is a handheld device with built-in optics, light source, and focusing capabilities that can be used as a standalone device. Images and video can be obtained through the use of a mobile smartphone via a built-in mount that can accept a range of iPhone and Android devices. The Nun can be used on nondilated pupils as small as 2 mm. With pupils at 4 mm, the device can obtain images at a 30° field-of-view.

Stethoscope

The stethoscope has been evolving since 1816.[1] Traditionally, a discussion of a patient's cardiac and pulmonary exams with a remote consultant required a verbal description of the physical exam findings. Now, through the use of digital stethoscopes, cardiac and pulmonary exam findings can be amplified and recorded and then subsequently shared with consultants, posing a great opportunity in telemedicine.[24] The audio exam findings can also be stored in the patient's medical record for further medical decision-making. Several digital stethoscope products are available.

3M Littmann

3M Litmann's initial concept for a digital stethoscope revolved around pure sound amplification. More recent iterations have incorporated ambient noise reduction to mitigate the amount of interference from movement and breath sounds while listening to the heart. Additionally, their most recent model includes the capability to record sound clips and transmit them wirelessly to a nearby computer for inclusion in the medical record and direct visualization of the generated sound waves using companion software. The use of an additional web-based platform enables the secure transmission of auscultated heart sounds to a remote consultant for real-time listening. This poses an opportunity for those providers involved with telemedicine or who do not have access to cardiology consultants.

Eko Devices

Eko Devices produces multiple stethoscopes, including attachments for a currently owned nondigital device and a combination digital stethoscope and electrocardiogram (ECG). The digital stethoscope attachment can be switched from digital mode to the more traditional analog mode if necessary. It includes noise reduction and amplification technology and can transmit sounds via Bluetooth to nearby computers and mobile devices. Using companion software and applications, the sounds can be directly visualized with the software to help aid in the rapid diagnosis of hard-to-hear murmurs. This software also allows real-time streaming of the exam for remote consultation and telemedicine purposes.

The combination digital stethoscope adds a built-in 1-lead ECG, which allows the simultaneous bedside auscultation of heart sounds and visualization of ECG tracing using the companion software. This stethoscope can also transmit real-time data to other providers and consultants. This product is not an attachment and does not adapt to an existing stethoscope, but it uses a 3.5-mm audio jack that can be connected to an earpiece or headphones.

Eko Devices can stream recorded heart sounds to Bluetooth-enabled hearing aids. This addresses an accessibility concern in medicine for those providers who are hard of hearing and utilize hearing aids or capable cochlear implants.

FIGURE 71.3 ■ **Wireless, Bluetooth-Capable Digital Stethoscope**

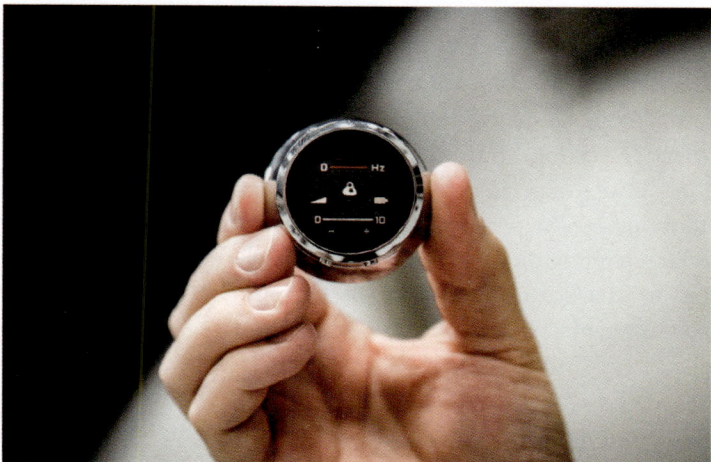

Thinklabs

The Thinklabs One digital stethoscope does not rely on traditional binaural tubes but rather transmits sound through a 3.5-mm audio jack that can be used with compatible headphones (**Figure 71.3**). It does not transmit wirelessly but can be attached to a Bluetooth transmitter to send signals to any Bluetooth-capable device (e.g., computers, mobile devices, and capable hearing aids and cochlear implants). The One also comes with an inline linking adapter that can plug directly into a computer or mobile device for the immediate recording or streaming of captured audio. Much like the other digital stethoscopes discussed, this allows for remote listening by other providers.

REFERENCE AND DECISION-MAKING APPLICATIONS

Most clinicians are familiar with several of the increasing number of applications available to access information, support immediate patient management, and enhance productivity.

Reference Applications

An ever-expanding number of mobile health-care applications are available, and with the increasing adoption of mobile technology, current and evidence-based information is readily available to aid in critical decision-making.[25,26] This easy access to information can increase the efficiency of health care providers, helping them make clinical decisions and providing them with real-time refreshers on less-familiar topics. It is impossible to cover the thousands of available medical reference applications in detail. There is also a range of preferences for mobile applications, and opinions on their utility vary.[27]

UpToDate

The UpToDate mobile application is a companion to the web-based UpToDate reference repository. The application is available with a subscription to the UpToDate service and may be installed on two mobile devices per account. Subscriptions can be obtained on an individual or institutional level. This application accesses over 11,000 clinical topics that are updated as evidence changes. It also provides access to over 175 medical calculators and information regarding over 6,000 drugs. A small positive association has been reported between the use of UpToDate and reduced length of stay, lower risk-adjusted mortality rates, and better quality performance in smaller, nonteaching hospitals.[28]

Epocrates

Epocrates is a web-based reference tool that primarily focuses on pharmacology. The mobile application is available as a free download and gives access to information regarding medication dosing, indications, contraindications, adverse reactions, potential drug interactions, and safety information. Additionally, the application features a pill identification tool that can help providers identify unknown medications quickly, without having to sift through many pictures of similar-looking tablets. A paid version of Epocrates provides access to disease information, including decision-support tools, treatment strategies, and common history and physical exam findings.[29]

PediSTAT

Medication dosing and equipment selection for pediatric patients is based heavily on the child's size and weight. This variability makes the selection of appropriate treatment more prone to error in the pediatric population, particularly in stressful and emergent situations.[30] PediSTAT is a mobile application that provides quick access to weight-based and age-specific medication dosing and equipment sizes. Information can be accessed by entering the patient's age, weight, length, or Broselow category. Once the data has been entered, the application provides information on appropriate equipment selection, resuscitation formulas (e.g., Parkland formula), and medication selection.

The Emergency Medicine Residents' Association

The Emergency Medicine Residents' Association (EMRA) Antibiotic Guide mobile application is a quick reference for the treatment of infectious disease. This popular handbook is organized by diagnosis and provides primary and alternative treatment strategies for each condition. Additionally, many diseases come with a list of common causative organisms, additional "pearls," and isolation recommendations.

The EMRA Peds Meds focuses on the treatment and care of pediatric patients. The mobile application provides access to a Centers for Disease Control and Prevention-based clinical weight estimator and guides the user in appropriate drug dosing. Additionally, the application includes video tutorials specific to pediatric patients and aids in the selection of equipment, including endotracheal tubes and laryngoscope blades.

The primary focus of EMRA's PressorDex is the many infusions, pressors, and vasoactive drugs used to treat critically ill patients. The application can be organized by diagnosis, system, or medication and provides treatment algorithms and clinical decision support. The application also provides critical care reference information, such as blood pressure goals for spontaneous subarachnoid hemorrhage and criteria for massive versus submassive pulmonary emboli.

Clinical Decision Tools

Clinical decision tools and scores are an everyday part of practicing medicine. Validated tools, including the Wells criteria for pulmonary embolism or deep venous thrombosis and the Pediatric Emergency Applied Research Network pediatric health injury/trauma algorithm, help providers make clinical choices based on scientific evidence. These tools are not intended to replace clinical gestalt but are designed to guide physicians and improve patient care. Research suggests that instant access to these clinical decision tools by way of mobile devices may improve clinical decision-making and efficiency.[31]

MDCalc

MDCalc provides easy access to evidence-based equations, medical calculators, and clinical decision rules. The mobile application is free and, once registered, the user can search for the desired clinical tool based on name or keyword (e.g., "bleeding" or "stroke"), or use a list of tools filtered by their own medical specialty. For most of the clinical tools, the application provides suggested next steps on what to do with the information obtained, advice on how to use the tool correctly, and links to supporting evidence.

HIPAA-Compliant Messaging

Emergency department directors are tasked with managing complex organizations and overseeing an array of providers, staff, and initiatives unique to their departments. Traditionally, organizations use frequent e-mails and meetings in an attempt to keep staff members "on the same page," but e-mail chains can become cumbersome, and meetings are often unproductive and time-wasting. Using HIPAA-compliant communications and effective collaboration applications, organization members can give and receive real-time updates on projects and assign tasks easily without the use of in-person meetings or e-mails.

The widespread use of mobile devices makes it easier than ever to communicate with colleagues. On a busy shift in the ED, it may be preferable to send a text or image to a consultant rather than wait on hold or wait for the consultant to reach a computer to view an image in the medical record. However, communication via conventional messaging software is not secure and is considered a violation of patient privacy laws.

Several available solutions exist for messaging that comply with HIPPA requirements. They all provide the common service of secure text messaging and image sharing. Some are standalone messaging services, while others are based through larger EHRs or management platforms. These applications all attempt to reduce the time clinicians spend engaging in administrative duties and streamline the discussion of cases with consultants. Some examples of HIPAA-compliant messaging applications are:

- OhMD
- TigerConnect TigerText
- Imprivata Cortext
- Epic Haiku or Canto built-in messaging
- PerfectServe
- Spok Mobile

Slack

Slack is a web- and application-based software that allows for group collaboration organized by channels. Members of an organization can be given access to various channels that can be customized and created to reflect various work groups, organization divisions, or projects. Members can use a text-based chat to engage the team or use voice and video chat for face-to-face conversations. Additionally, members can utilize screen sharing to further aid in collaboration. Slack has the ability to integrate with commonly used productivity tools like Google Drive and Dropbox, which enables easy file sharing without the need to upload data into a separate cloud platform. Slack also offers a HIPAA-compliant version.

Basecamp

Basecamp is another example of organizational software that is web- and application-based. This software organizes members into teams and projects. Each team and project group have a built-in message board, to-do list, schedule, and file-sharing section. Tasks and deadlines can be assigned to members through the to-do list and updated in real-time as they are completed; this makes the entire team aware of a project's status without the need for in-person check-ins. Basecamp also provides a central location for files and schedules so that these items are no longer lost in e-mail chains. Basecamp uses robust encryption for data transfer and storage but is not considered HIPAA-compliant.

FUTURE DIRECTIONS

With more and more patients seeking care at EDs, there is growing need for technology that will aid in the efficiency and accuracy of emergency providers. Right now, innovators are tapping into mobile technology to fulfill this purpose, and the market is replete with well-developed mobile applications and portable, cost-effective devices.

The field of toxicology provides an example of the future of technology for emergency providers. With the widespread adoption of wearable biosensors, such as the Fitbit, toxicologists are studying how to use these biosensors to rapidly and accurately diagnose toxic exposures. Through the use of real-time biometric data, including heart rate, respiratory rate, skin temperature, and electrodermal activity, toxicologists may be able to recognize toxidromes or changes in a patient's condition at the bedside or remotely.[32]

The development of noncontact vital signs also has the potential to advance patient monitoring and detect sudden changes in patient stability. Several types of technology for noncontact vital signs exist and are being refined. One example involves placing a sensor underneath the patient's mattress, and other forms are even more remote, using cameras or microwave Doppler signals.[33] It is proposed that with advancement of this technology, changes in patient status may be detected earlier than with conventional monitoring, allowing for faster interventions.[34]

Biosensing devices and remote patient monitoring represent only a small fraction of the many potential innovations in emergency medicine technology. Many other areas are currently being developed and include advancements in telemedicine, real-time sharing of data between providers, computerized decision-making, and even the prevention of emergency visits using at-home patient monitoring.[35,36]

CONCLUSION

Current advances in technology have the potential to positively impact emergency health care. The use of portable, cost-effective mobile devices is increasing the quality of care for patients, as well as the efficiency of health-care providers. Machines that pose a significant expense for EDs are becoming more affordable, and with the advances in digital communication, bedside findings can now be shared remotely with consulting providers. The growing number of mobile health-care applications, which is expanding from the bedside to evidence-based research, may be linked to improved patient care and error reduction.

REFERENCES

1. David L, Dumitrascu DL. The bicentennial of the stethoscope: a reappraisal. *Clujul Med*. 2017;90(3):361–363.
2. The history of healthcare technology and the evolution of EHR. Vertitech IT. 2017. Available at: https://www.vertitechit.com/history-healthcare-technology/. Accessed September 5, 2018.
3. Institute of Medicine. *To Err is Human: Building a Safer Health System*. Washington, DC: The National Academies Press; 2000.
4. Thielst CB. The future of healthcare technology. *J Healthc Manag*. 2007;52(1):7–9.

5. Steinhubl SR, Muse ED, Topol EJ. The emerging field of mobile health. *Sci Transl Med*. 2015;7(283):283rv3.

6. Wakefield DS, Wakefield BJ. Are verbal orders a threat to patient safety? *Qual Saf Health Care*. 2009;18:165–168.

7. Husain I. MD tech tips: use Epic's Haiku app to instantly upload medical documents to a patient's chart. iMedical Apps. 2017. Available at: https://www.imedicalapps.com/2017/03/epic-haiku-upload-medical-documents-patients-chart/. Accessed September 15, 2018.

8. Dolan B. Nuance voice-enables Epic Haiku, Canto apps for clinical info input. *Mobi Health News*. October 12, 2012. Available at: https://www.mobihealthnews.com/18740/nuance-voice-enables-epic-haiku-canto-apps-for-clinical-info-input#:~:text=Nuance%20voice%2Denables%20Epic%20Haiku%2C%20Canto%20apps%20for%20clinical%20info%20input,-By%20Brian%20Dolan&text=Just%20one%20week%20after%20Nuance,a%20similar%20deal%20with%20Epic. Accessed September 15, 2018.

9. Locke R, Stefano M, Koster A, et al. Optimizing patient/caregiver satisfaction through quality of communication in the pediatric emergency department. *Pediatr Emerg Care*. 2011;27(11):1016–1021.

10. Rutherford KA, Pitetti RD, Zuckerbraun NS, et al. Adolescents' perceptions of interpersonal communication, respect, and concern for privacy in an urban tertiary-care pediatric emergency department. *Pediatr Emerg Care*. 2010;26:257–273.

11. Simmons SA, Sharp B, Fowler J, et al. Implementation of a novel communication tool and its effect on patient comprehension of care and satisfaction. *Emerg Med J*. 2013;30:363–370.

12. Goyal AA, Tur K, Mann J, et al. Do bedside visual tools improve patient and caregiver satisfaction? A systematic review of the literature. *J Hosp Med*. 2017;12:930–936.

13. Schenker Y, Fernandez A, Sudore R, et al. Interventions to improve patient comprehension in informed consent for medical and surgical procedures: a systematic review. *Med Decis Making*. 2011;31:151–173.

14. Dathatri S, Gruberg L, Anand J, et al. Informed consent for cardiac procedures: deficiencies in patient comprehension with current methods. *Ann Thorac Surg*. 2014;97:1505–1511.

15. Leclercq WK, Keulers BJ, Scheltinga MR, et al. A review of surgical informed consent: past, present, and future. A quest to help patients make better decisions. *World J Surg*. 2010;34:1406–1415.

16. American College of Emergency Physicians Policy. Emergency ultrasound guidelines. *Ann Emerg Med*. 2009;53(4):550–570.

17. Hall MD, Hall J, Harish NJ, et al. Use of point-of-care ultrasound in the emergency department: insights from the 2012 Medicare national payment data set. *J Ultras Med*. 2016;35(11):2467–2474.

18. How much does an ultrasound machine cost? LBN Medical. 2017. Available at: https://lbnmedical.com/ultrasound-price-guide/. Accessed September 15, 2018.

19. Landon J. The butterfly effect. EPM. 2018. Available at: https://epmonthly.com/article/the-butterfly-effect/. Accessed September 15, 2018.

20. Moore C, Copel J. Point-of-care ultrasonography. *NE J Med*. 2011;364:749–757.

21. Cordeiro MF, Jolly BC, Dacre JE. The effect of formal instruction in ophthalmoscopy on medical student performance. *Med Teach*. 1993;15:321–325.

22. Wu EH, Fagan MJ, Reinert SE, et al. Self-confidence in and perceived utility of the physical examination: a comparison of medical students, residents, and faculty internists. *J Gen Intern Med*. 2007;22:1725–1730.

23. Petrushkin H, Barsam A, Mavrakakis M, et al. Optic disc assessment in the emergency department: a comparative study between the PanOptic and direct ophthalmoscopes. *Emerg Med J*. 2012;29(12):1007–1008.

24. Swarup S, Makaryus A. Digital stethoscope: technology update. *Med Devices*. 2018;11:29–36.

25. Ventola CL. Mobile devices and apps for health care professionals: uses and benefits. *Pharm Ther*. 2014;39(5):356–364.

26. Wiechmann W, Kwan D, Bokarius A, et al. There's an app for that? Highlighting the difficulty in finding clinically relevant smartphone applications. *West J Emerg Med*. 2016;17(2):191–194.

27. Kaine J, Ranney M. Mobile applications for the ED provider. Brown EM Blog. 2018. Available at: http://brownemblog.com/blog-1/2018/1/28/mobile-applications-for-the-ed-provider. Accessed September 21, 2018.

28. Isaac T, Zheng J, Jha A. Use of UpToDate and outcomes in US Hospitals. *J Hosp Med*. 2012;7(2):85–90.

29. Bhanot S, Sharma A. App review series: Epocrates. *J Digit Imaging*. 2017;30(5):534–536.

30. Stucky ER. American Academy of Pediatrics Policy. Prevention of medication errors in the pediatric inpatient setting. *Pediatrics*. 2003;112(2):431–436.

31. Mickan S, Tilson J, Atherton H, et al. Evidence of effectiveness of health care professionals using handheld computers: a scoping review of systematic reviews. *J Med Internet Res*. 2013;15(10):e212.

32. Chai P. Wearable devices and biosensing: future frontiers. *J Med Toxicol*. 2016;12(4):332–334.

33. Hall T, Lie DYC, Nguyen TQ, et al. Non-contact sensor for long-term continuous vital signs monitoring: a review on intelligent phased-array Doppler sensor design. *Sensors (Basel)*. 2017;17(11):2632.

34. Zhao F, Li M, Jiang Z, et al. Camera-based, non-contact, vital-signs monitoring technology may provide a way for the early prevention of SIDS in infants. *Front Neurol*. 2016;7:236.

35. Bhavnani SP, Narula J, Sengupta PP. Mobile technology and the digitization of healthcare. *Eur Heart J*. 2016;37:1428–1438.

36. Carley S, Laing S. How can emergency physicians harness the power of new technologies in clinical practice and education? *Emerg Med J*. 2018;35:156–158.

CHAPTER 72

TELEMEDICINE IN EMERGENCY MEDICINE

Judd E. Hollander, Rahul Sharma

While policymakers debate ways to reduce medical expenditures and industry searches for ways to increase profit, patients maintain that the most important aspect of health care is easy, affordable access to treatment.[1,2] Emergency department (ED) visits continue to rise nationally. A shortage of primary care providers (PCPs), coupled with an expansion of the percentage of Americans with health insurance, makes it difficult for many people to obtain timely medical care for routine conditions. Rural hospitals face a shortage of qualified providers; urban areas face a shortage of appointments. While primary care visits are falling, patients now make over 130 million ED and 160 million urgent care visits, retail pharmacies have entered the health care space, and telemedicine is projected to grow to a $30 billion industry by 2020.[3]

Telemedicine addresses some of the issues surrounding access, patient experience, cost, and effectiveness. By 2017, 71% of hospitals had adopted some version of telemedicine, up from 54% in 2014.[4] Nearly half of physicians surveyed in 2017 reported using some version of telemedicine in the outpatient setting.[5] In addition, 92% of health-care executives surveyed in 2014 ranked telemedicine services as important or very important to their institutions.[6]

Telehealth and telemedicine are means to an end. Telemedicine is not about the technology; it is about access. It helps to bring care to the patient when and where they need it. Framing the user experience as important in health care is also a part of a bigger societal shift. Patient-centered care, patient satisfaction, and a buyer's market have created forces that reward not just high-quality care but highly convenient care.

Emergency physicians may provide remote services in a variety of settings, including EDs, urgent care clinics, observation medicine units, out-of-hospital clinics, and disaster sites. Technical requirements and digital health care outside the realm of telemedicine are beyond the scope of this chapter.

UNDERSTANDING TELEMEDICINE

Telehealth and telemedicine represent two-way communication between parties who are at a distance from one another (**Figure 72.1**). Although subject to some debate, the terms telemedicine and telehealth are typically used interchangeably.

Case One: Frances is a 63-year-old retired teacher with mild-to-moderate heart failure. One morning, she feels a little more winded than usual and texts her doctor's office. The office responds with a text link to 10 different time slots for a video visit later that day. She selects one and later completes a 10-minute video chat with her doctor, who suggests some alterations to her medications. Feeling reassured, she goes to bed but awakens in the middle of the night with shortness of breath. Frightened, she touches the JeffConnect app (described further below) on her phone, and is connected with an emergency physician within minutes. The emergency physician takes a history and performs a "virtual examination." As they speak, the emergency physician is reassured by the patient's respiratory rate, and the patient is reassured by being assessed by a physician. She takes an additional dose of diuretic, and the emergency physician schedules an early morning visit by the community paramedicine team. They check her blood pressure, heart rate, oxygenation, and weight, and conduct a 5-minute check-in to review the medication plan with her PCP. They leave her a Bluetooth scale that communicates with her PCP's office and discuss a plan for diuresis to achieve a 5-pound weight loss over the next few days.

Although different types of telemedicine can be discussed based on specialty (e.g., telestroke, telecardiology, teledermatology), we prefer a categorization that spans specialties. The simplest framework is the following:

- *Synchronous versus asynchronous.* Synchronous communication is a live interaction between two parties (e.g., a real-time audio–video medical visit). Asynchronous communication is the transmission of recorded information that can be interpreted later (e.g., forwarding an image of a rash to a physician to review tomorrow).
- *Patient-to-provider versus provider-to-provider.* This distinction identifies the two parties who are involved. Direct-to-consumer care is typically patient-to-provider. A neuro-stroke network, where an emergency physician in a rural hospital receives a consult from a specialist at a remote hospital, is classified as provider-to-provider care.
- *Remote monitoring.* This is the real-time transmission a patient's vital signs or other clinical findings to continuously track the data and proactively alert the monitor or provider to an aberration. An example includes when the paramedic leaves Frances a Bluetooth scale that communicates with her PCP's office.
- Other relevant telemedicine terms:
  - *Originating site.* This is a term relevant to payment for telemedicine services. Although one can imagine more options, originating sites are most often the patient's home or office, the hospital, a dialysis center, or a nursing home. Insurance providers may only reimburse telemedicine visits that originate from a particular location. In some cases, the patient may have to travel to a less-convenient, costlier venue like a physician's office, hospital, rural health clinic, or skilled nursing facility to conduct a reimbursable visit.
  - *Store and forward.* This term is used when videos and images are digitally transmitted to a provider who then reviews the data to render a service in an asynchronous manner.

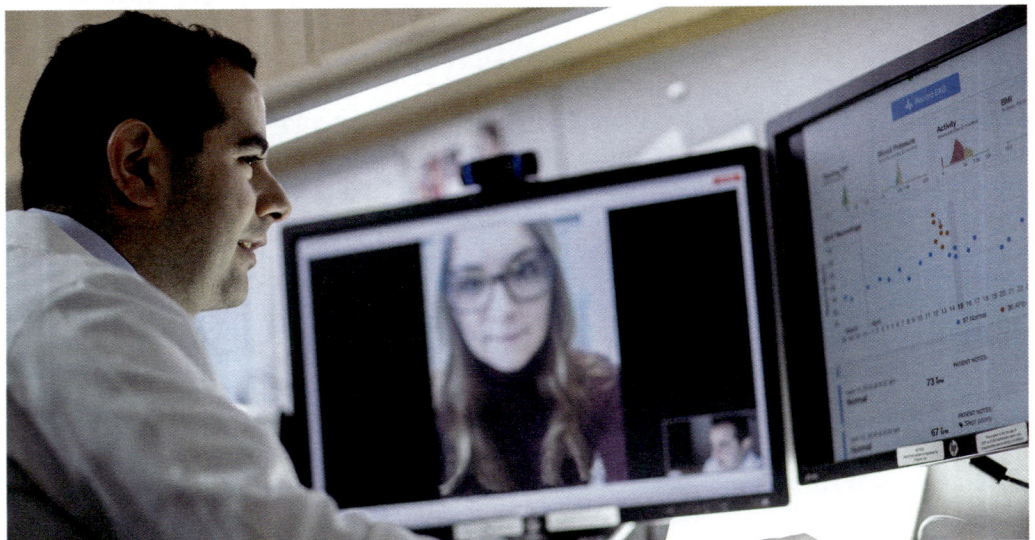

FIGURE 72.1 ■ Physician at the Cleveland Clinic Demonstrates a Virtual Consultation

EMERGENCY TELEMEDICINE USE CASES

Telemedicine encompasses a wide range of ways to provide remote health care.[7] Acute and urgent care providers can use telemedicine across a broad continuum, depending on where the needs are greatest in their community.

Direct-to-Consumer (or On-Demand) Care

Case Two: Anthony is home alone on Sunday evening when he notices a linear pruritic rash on his lower leg, just above his sock line, as well as multiple other patches of redness on sun-exposed areas, including his face. He spent a lot of time gardening last week. He uses his smartphone app and conducts a video visit with a physician from his health system. The physician diagnoses poison ivy, calls in a prescription for steroids, and gives instructions for topical symptom control. The physician documents the visit in the institution's electronic medical record and sends a copy to the patient's PCP.

Patients seek care both when they need it and when they want it. As a result, many patients cared for in the ED do not require a time-sensitive critical intervention, yet they feel they have nowhere else to go to get care *now*.

The most common type of urgent or emergency telemedicine involves a synchronous audio–video visit between a patient and a clinician. Although some health systems provide these services directly, the most common scenario involves a for-profit provider network, such as Teladoc Health or MDLive, through which care is rendered by subcontracted clinicians who take the calls. These providers may be contracting on behalf of a specific health system, caring for patients under an employer subscription model, or providing care to patients directly from the community. On the patient-facing side, visits with most providers can be conducted using smartphone apps, tablets, or webcam-enabled computers. The provider side has the same variety of options across vendors, but some vendors may not have all options.

On-demand, direct-to-consumer telemedicine programs are not, in and of themselves, likely to generate a positive return on investment (ROI). The ROI for an on-demand program comes from indirect sources, such as:

- The competitive advantage of an established program
- Ability to redirect patients from higher-cost to lower-cost venues
- New patient acquisition and retention
- Improving patient and provider experience
  - Convenience
  - Overall satisfaction
- Cost effectiveness from patient and payer perspective[6]
- Adherence with clinical guidelines

The most common chief complaints of patients who use these urgent care services include coughs, upper respiratory symptoms, urinary tract infections, and rashes.

ED Teletriage

Telemedicine can easily be integrated into the ED triage process to expedite intake evaluations, decrease walkout rates, and improve operational efficiency. The initial evaluation includes an assessment of the patient's vital signs and chief complaint by a technician, medical assistant, or nurse followed by a virtual history and physical examination completed by the provider. This type of telemedicine encounter can help replace some traditional "provider in triage" models. In one model, patients are still seen by an on-site provider, thus the teletriage provider is not ultimately responsible for the care rendered. In another model, the teletriage provider can facilitate the discharge of low-acuity patients after the initial medical screening exam is performed in the ED.[8] ROI for ED teletriage comes from:

- Reduced left-without-being-seen rates (enhancing revenue)
- Improved throughput and efficiency of bed turnover
- Reduced front-end staffing, especially in programs that have providers in triage
- Synergies with one provider being able to triage at multiple facilities

At the present time, it is unclear whether teletriage visits meet the requirements of the Emergency Medical Treatment and Labor Act (EMTALA) and can be categorized as medical screening exams. Although different Medicare regional offices have given disparate opinions regarding EMTALA compliance, none have prohibited telemedicine visits.

Specialty Consultation

Case Three: Bill presents hypotensive and febrile to a community ED, where he is met by an emergency physician who recognizes that he is septic. The emergency physician sends a panel of lab tests, orders a chest x-ray, establishes large-bore IV access, orders a fluid bolus and antibiotics, and engages the virtual resuscitation consult service. After about an hour, Bill has worsened despite aggressive resuscitation and is started on pressors by the resuscitation service. The two physicians agree on a plan to intubate Bill and transfer him to a referral center. The onsite emergency physician performs the intubation, and the resuscitation expert transitions his care to the ICU at the receiving hospital by giving a virtual video report to the receiving team.

A number of specialties and subspecialties currently provide telemedicine in a hub-and-spoke model. For example, institutions have implemented telestroke programs to connect regional hospitals with a neurologist and reduce the time to treatment and improve patient outcomes.[8] Telestroke programs represent one form of synchronous provider-to-provider telemedicine that is commonly employed in emergency medicine. They connect regional and critical access hospitals with a neurologist who can consult with the emergency physician, review the CT scan, and provide specialty video consultation. This method of telemedicine was adopted early in the ED setting to assess stroke patients for tPA administration and involve trauma specialists in the evaluation of crash victims in rural EDs.[9,10] Telestroke programs have been shown to reduce door-to-treatment times and improve patient outcomes.[11]

Moreover, the launch of hospital-based mobile stroke units is growing. A mobile stroke treatment unit is an ambulance that can provide acute stroke care; it contains a CT scan, point-of-care laboratory testing, and the capability to facilitate a telemedicine encounter between the patient, ambulance personnel, and hospital. Preliminary data from these mobile stroke units show that they speed treatment and may improve outcomes.[11] This approach may offer major advantages in congested urban areas or rural areas, where transport times cannot compete with telestroke networks.[12]

Established provider-to-provider networks with mature telestroke programs may be leveraged to expand critical care services to regional hospitals. Sepsis, cardiac arrest, and other critical conditions requiring emergency interventions represent additional opportunities.[13] Behavioral health and dermatology are also common specialty consultation requests by hospitals. ROI for a telemedicine specialty consultation comes from:

- Building the brand with patients and families
- Creating goodwill with providers and regional health-care systems
- Tertiary care transfer of patients who can benefit from the higher level of care
- Enabling patients who will not benefit from tertiary services to receive care closer to home

Family Engagement

"Virtual rounds" connect caregivers and family members with the patient's providers in real time while the patient is in the ED or hospital inpatient unit.[14] Common uses of bedside telehealth to engage family members in virtual rounds are:

- When the patient is present without family, but there is an interest in having the family join the conversation
- Enhancing the quality of resident-attending communication and education
- To revisit patients who were off the floor (e.g., on observation units) during initial rounds or who had important test results come back later in the day
- To convene a multiparty meeting, including physicians(s), the patient, family members, care managers, and home-care personnel

ROI for virtual rounds comes from:

- Improved patient satisfaction and Hospital Consumer Assessment of Healthcare Providers and Systems (HCAHP) scores
- Improved physician efficiency
- Expedited patient care, with issues more readily addressed by the team outside of normal rounds
- Improved resident supervision and decreased malpractice risk

Post-Discharge Transitions in Care

Case Four: David was evaluated in the ED and is being discharged on an oral antibiotic for a 10-cm area of cellulitis. He is offered placement in the observation unit, but his daughter is getting married the next day. He asks whether he could be treated via a video call instead. The physician agrees, marks the area of cellulitis, and helps him download the app. A nurse shows the patient how to use the app and conducts a practice visit with him. David is then discharged home. The next morning, he has a video visit with the "follow-up provider," who is able to visualize his leg and compare it to previous pictures in the chart. The rash is improving, and David is instructed to follow up for any further concerns. He is able to participate in his daughter's wedding.

Following discharge from the ED, patients can better participate in their transition-of-care planning through the use of telemedicine.[15] This enhances adherence to discharge recommendations and provides patients and caregivers the opportunity to re-engage and better understand follow-up recommendations. ROI for post-discharge telemedicine can come from:

- Reduced length of stay
- Improved transitions of care during a time that patients cannot be seen in an outpatient setting
- Improved patient satisfaction and HCAHP scores
- Decreased return visits
- Decreased readmissions

Community Paramedicine

Case Five: Mrs. Smith is being discharged from the hospital later today after an exacerbation of heart failure. She is relatively immobile and does not have access to a car. She lives 1.5 miles from her pharmacy in a two-story walk-up. Prior to discharge, she is visited by a paramedic who promises to periodically check on her at home over the next 30 days. During the first visit, the paramedic notices that Mrs. Smith has not filled her new beta-blocker prescription and is taking both an older Lasix and newer furosemide prescription of the same dose. The paramedic makes arrangements for the new medication to be delivered and educates Mrs. Smith that the Lasix and furosemide are the same medication. They agree that she will take the older pills first and save the new pills for later. At the 3-week visit, Mrs. Smith has gained 6 pounds and is slightly short of breath. The paramedic and Mrs. Smith schedule a telemedicine visit with her doctor, which she completes later that day. Once her medications are adjusted, she gradually loses weight, and her shortness of breath resolves.

Community paramedicine allows paramedics and EMTs to operate in expanded roles by assisting with public health, primary health care, and preventive services for underserved populations. The goal is to improve access to care and avoid duplicating existing services. Equipped with audiovisual capabilities, paramedics can deliver a wide variety of services. The community paramedicine model can benefit EMS agencies and health systems by:

- Reducing nonurgent transport services
- Using down time between transport calls, exercising medical skills, and improving access to providers to meet the community's primary care needs
- Increasing revenue by billing patients or third-party payers for services provided, when appropriate
- Decreasing readmissions
- Helping to coordinate transition-of-care services

The Virtual ED

Creation of a virtual ED will allow emergency physicians to provide enhanced care to patients when they want it, where they want it, and in a lower-cost environment. For some patients, this may be through a smartphone app, and they may not require further diagnostic testing. Other patients may require a telemedicine assessment with expedited diagnostic testing in an outpatient facility, urgent care center, or hospital. Processes should enable patients to walk in and receive testing, then walk out and receive their follow-up recommendations virtually. For others, a referral to a PCP or specialist may be appropriate. A virtual ED can provide:

- Direct-to-consumer care for low-acuity conditions that do not require any further testing
- Direct-to-consumer care for moderate acuity conditions that may require rapid diagnostic testing with a time-appropriate referral to a PCP, specialist, or the ED following results of testing
- Direct-to-consumer care for patients with more time-sensitive conditions who need expedited testing, referrals, or intervention
- Physician-to-physician consultation/backup for patients in urgent care centers who are treated by physician assistants or nurse practitioners

Patients using the virtual ED could be directed from home, urgent care centers, or even the ED waiting room to the location with the most capacity for the care they need.

Disaster Response Support

Case Six: Following Hurricane Maria in Puerto Rico in 2017, there was a shortage of local medical care. New York-Presbyterian used telemedicine to provide provider-to-provider specialty consultation that was not otherwise available at some relief sites. This allowed hurricane victims access to dermatology, endocrinology, psychiatry, and otolaryngology.[16]

Telemedicine can be used in disaster-response scenarios. The growing ability to provide care virtually can be mobilized and scaled to reach people when traditional means of in-person disaster relief are not available. When done well, telemedicine in disaster relief has the potential to provide individually tailored medical care where and when the patient determines it is necessary.[16,17] However, it is critical to note that telemedicine can only be scaled for deployment in disaster settings if the program pre-exists and can be maintained during normal daily operations.

DEVELOPING A TELEMEDICINE STRATEGY

The business case for telehealth can be made on the basis of these factors:

- The Institute for Healthcare Improvement has developed a framework to describe the optimization of health system performance based around the "Triple Aim" of 1) improving how the patient experiences care (including quality and satisfaction), 2) improving the health of populations (outcomes), and 3) reducing the cost of health care.[18] As providers move to a more patient-centric model, they are looking for ways to deliver care to patients when they want it, how they want it, where they want it.
- The Affordable Care Act and Comprehensive Primary Care Plus programs have moved payment models from fee-for-service toward value-based care. There is a growing recognition that, for their own success and sustainability, PCPs have to find cost-effective ways of engaging patients.[19] Telehealth is one possible method.
- The payer market continues to consolidate. The remaining companies have increased size and bargaining power. It is incumbent on providers to be more efficient and cost-effective, and telemedicine is believed to be one way to accomplish those goals.
- Telehealth may create new entry points into the health-care system in a cost-effective, accessible manner. Early entrants into telehealth have the opportunity to service their existing patients and attract new ones from providers who do not offer telehealth. This is critical in local markets, which will continue to consolidate as patients seek out patient-centric providers.

Developing the Strategy

Case Seven: You are approached and asked to begin a telemedicine program for your group or institution. You are given no further direction.

Several approaches to developing a business plan for telemedicine are possible, but all include at least some component of each of the following:

- Define the problem you are trying to solve.
    - Payment models are changing from fee-for-service to value-based care.
    - Patients now consider cost and convenience a higher priority than the ability to see their own PCP. There is discordance between when patients want care and when most providers want to deliver care.

- It is critical to recognize that telemedicine is a care-delivery model. Anyone developing a program must decide what kind of care they need to deliver.
- Meet with key stakeholders, including patients, to identify unmet needs and program goals.
- Group unmet needs into domains that can be addressed with a common approach. For example, Thomas Jefferson University Healthcare Center in Philadelphia developed the strategy shown in **Figure 72.2**, where the approach to outpatient care, transitions of care, and inpatient care are similar across service lines.

■ Conduct a market assessment.
- Market forces favor emergency care-delivery models. Emergency physicians now have a unique opportunity created by the shift in patient priorities and payment reform. Emergency physicians should be available where the patients desire, which is increasingly likely to be in their backyard (urgent care or retail clinic) or over the phone (telehealth).

■ Prioritize your initiatives.
- Prioritize financially lowest-risk, lowest-cost opportunities.
  o If self-insured, explore programs for your employees.
  o Focus on conditions that carry high readmission penalties.

■ Understand the financial consequences of your programs.
■ Develop an implementation strategy (discussed in the next section).

It is critical to recognize that, when a telehealth program is implemented, there is not going to be an immediate ROI. Rather, it should be considered as an enterprise-wide strategy preparing for the move from fee-for-service to value-based care. Viewed through this lens, telehealth is a necessary loss leader during this time of transition. Ultimately, the value of the program will be measured by changes in health-care use and the transformation of care delivery. This will include inpatient admissions, outpatient visits, home visits, readmissions, and downstream growth in volume. The concept of developing patient "stickiness," convenience, shorter hospital length of stay, less time lost from work, redistribution of care to less-costly environments, patient and employer satisfaction, and improved care coordination should also be considered. Even in the absence of any remuneration, there are types of care that will still be cost-effective. Bundled care, post-procedure care, and interventions that decrease uncompensated (readmissions) are three examples.

FIGURE 72.2 ■ Classification of Original Telemedicine Programs at Jefferson Health

	LEAST Transformative		MOST Transformative
	←		→
Outpatient	Covered employees		Virtual ED and urgent care
	On-demand care signature services		
Transitions of Care	Pre-admission testing		
	Virtually augmented discharge processes		
Inpatient	Post-discharge care		Expanded critical care network
	Teleconsultation		
	Virtual rounds		
Academic	Research grants		Live CME
		Certificate program	Research training programs

IMPLEMENTING A TELEMEDICINE PROGRAM

An important consideration in implementing a new telemedicine program is to understand that providers do not always embrace change and may not believe that patients want them to change. Therefore, implementation is about change management, which begins with a clear mission statement, organization, staffing, and alignment of incentives.

At Thomas Jefferson University Healthcare Center, the mission statement is clear: "JeffConnect" is medical care without walls. The aim is to deliver comprehensive, high-quality, *coordinated* care to patients when they want it, where they want it. The JeffConnect program was built to enhance the care coordination of patients regardless of where they receive treatment.[20]

Patients who fall off their baseline and become a "little sick" can be treated by their own provider through scheduled e-visits or by an on-demand emergency physician who is available around the clock. In the acute setting, ED teletriage allows a physician to begin care immediately on arrival, even before patients are roomed. Jefferson Expert Teleconsulting allows Jefferson providers to collaborate with partnering hospitals and participate in provider-to-provider remote consults for neuro-stroke care. Virtual rounds further connect caregivers and family members with patients and their providers in real time, increasing patient and family engagement as well as coordination and communication. Following discharge, patients have the option of participating in their transition-of-care planning and post-discharge visits virtually.

New York-Presbyterian provides another example of an academic medical center program (**Figure 72.3**). The hospital launched a comprehensive, enterprise-wide digital health program, which includes the first mobile stroke unit on the East Coast and the first ED-based telehealth Express Care Service in the nation. New York-Presbyterian has expanded its ED-based suite of services to include ED Express Care, NYP OnDemand kiosks at Walgreens, specialty consults, chronic heart failure patient follow-up, and telemedicine medical screening exams. The suite expands access by not only providing care during the initial patient encounter but also post visit, when the patient is home and needs follow-up care.

FIGURE 72.3 ■ New York-Presbyterian OnDemand Services

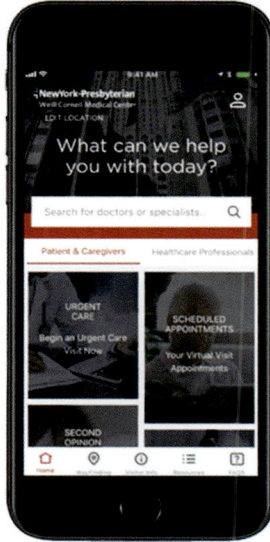
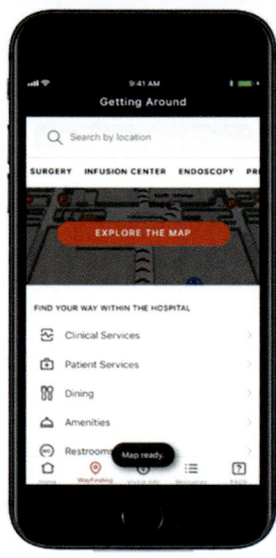
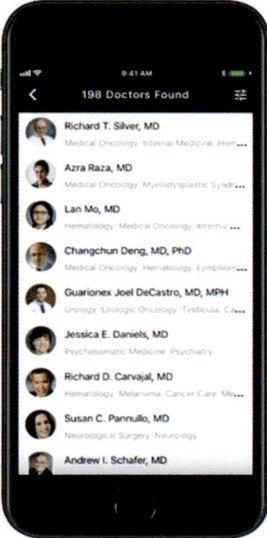

Key takeaways learned from implementing these types of programs: Be sure to align proposals with the strategic goals of the institution, disseminate data, and use patient stories to highlight the benefits of telehealth. Managing change requires the development of telehealth champions at all staff levels and uses career development opportunities and rewards to incentivize them to take on that role. To enroll a heterogeneous population of patients in telehealth programs, teams should use multiple methods of education to accommodate different learning styles. We recommend that teams develop telehealth-specific outcome measures and repeatedly use them to drive improvement.[18]

Leadership Structure

Telemedicine programs with a leadership structure that empowers decision-making have an advantage. We recommend that there be a "guiding team" or "governing council" that meets monthly. Telemedicine should maintain an enterprise-wide structure to enhance synergies and leverage the experience of the team. Recommended membership for a telehealth guiding team include:

- Clinical lead
- Chief medical officers of relevant practices (hospital- and ambulatory-based)
- Chief medical information officers of relevant practices
- Legal
- Compliance
- Billing and payer contracts
- Marketing and public relations
- Finance
- Academic representation if at academic medical center
- Telehealth operations team

Staffing

The number and qualifications of the telehealth staff depend on the size the program. Generally, positions to be considered include a director, program and project managers, and telehealth coordinators. We recommend staffing with people dedicated to telehealth alone; expecting staff to balance telehealth with other job responsibilities could inhibit the growth of your telehealth program.

Operational Challenges

There are a number of challenges to implementing telehealth services.

Legal Compliance and Regulatory Challenges

Current legal and regulatory challenges in telehealth largely stem from the fact that these rules are not well codified. As a result, department leaders should work with their attorneys to determine the legal risks of these programs and the best way to move forward. The organization's legal and compliance experts should be involved in reviewing materials (e.g., terms of use, privacy statements, and public-facing websites) to help minimize risk.

The largest challenge at present is for groups with providers who cover multiple states. The provider must be licensed in the state where the patient is located at the time care is rendered. The appropriate business entities, tax forms, DEA certificates, and malpractice coverage must be obtained. For ED teletriage programs, the team will need to decide how to approach medical screening exams and ED discharges until federal guidance determines whether teletriage can count as a medical screening exam.

The National Consortium of Telehealth Resource Centers and the American Telehealth Association (ATA) have up-to-date information that can help address rapidly changing federal and state policies.

Reimbursement

Concerns about reimbursement, for both private insurers and public programs such as Medicaid, continue to limit the implementation and use of telehealth services. When certain telehealth services are not reimbursed or are reimbursed at lower levels than in-person services, the incentives to provide telehealth services decrease.

Accessibility challenges exist in both urban and rural settings. Much federal legislation has focused on expanding telemedicine in rural areas; however, although there may be a provider shortage in rural areas, there is an appointment shortage in urban areas.[11] This has been shown to be true in primary care practices and specialty practices such as orthopedics and dermatology.[11] Current Medicare payment policies target geography and therefore do not focus on the real problem: *accessibility*. The ability to utilize health care resources via telemedicine would allow for improved access to care in the same way that virtual connectivity has decreased access barriers in other industries, such as banking and commerce. The best way to care for patients in rural environments is to build programs that synchronize rural and urban care. Hospitals, patients, and providers are all poised to interact with the health-care system differently; aligning payment structures to focus on the availability of timely care, rather than historic geographic constructs, is essential.

More than 30 states now provide for coverage parity—which essentially means that, if the service is covered in person, it should be covered if delivered via telemedicine; however, it leaves the rates to be negotiated by the provider and payer. Only three states have parity whereupon payment is the same regardless of whether the care is delivered in person or via telemedicine. Details regarding your own state's laws can be found on the National Consortium of Telehealth Resource Centers and the ATA websites.

Incentive Programs

It is critical to align incentives with strategy. If your existing strategy is still aligned with fee-for-service reimbursement—for example, relative value units (RVUs)—it will be difficult to grow value-based programs like telemedicine. One successful incentive strategy requires providers to participate in a minimal number of telehealth calls to qualify for their RVU-based incentive bonus.

Provider Engagement and Change Management

This requires a complex strategy that includes integrating telehealth into pre-existing provider workflows. Items to address regarding provider engagement include:

- Align compensation with strategy.
- Make training as painless as possible.
  - Legal and regulatory
  - Platform use
  - How to do video visits
- Don't make your future strategy penalize today's provider. Recognize the lack of fee-for-service compensation, but pay the provider for aligning with strategy.
- Dispel myths.
  - "Patients don't want it." Surveys show they do.
  - "It is not as good as an in-person visit." Most of the time, it is; and it is always better than no visit, which is many patient's alternative.
  - "You cannot examine the patient." You can do everything but listen to heart and lungs. In return, you see them at home.

☐ "It is too hard." You have been doing this with your family for years.
☐ "I work in an urban area, where patients do not want or need this." Telemedicine still saves patients time, travel, and parking expenses and may fit better into other competing priorities in their life.

Defining Metrics

As with every clinical care program, it is important to establish metrics and track the success of any telemedicine initiative. New programs will typically focus on measures of adoption. Depending on the particular use case, data will vary. Most commonly assessed metrics include:

- Number of app downloads
- Number of patient registrations
- Patient experience (satisfaction) reports or scores
- Number or proportion of providers trained
- Provider utilization
- Provider experience/satisfaction, as assessed by formal surveys
- Platform performance (audio–video connectivity rates)
- Number of telemedicine encounters
- Number of repeat visits
- New customer acquisition

As telemedicine programs expand, metrics can often be tied to specific-use cases like the time from the patient's first contact to visit completion, readmission avoidance, and decreased cost of care. More mature programs will align their metrics to national quality standards. In response to a request from the US Department of Health and Human Services, the National Quality Forum (NQF) recently convened a multistakeholder Telehealth Committee that was charged with identifying a foundation for the development of new measures to assess the quality of telehealth care. Their final report, *Creating a Framework to Support Measure Development for Telehealth*, provides a framework for telehealth measurement organized into four main domains: 1) access to care, 2) financial impact/cost, 3) experience, and 4) effectiveness (**Table 72.1**).[19] Quality of care crosses all of these domains.

TABLE 72.1 ■ NQF Telehealth Measurement Framework

Domain	Subdomain(s)
Access to care	• Access for patient, family, and/or caregiver • Access for care team • Access to information
Financial impact/cost	• Financial impact to patient, family, and/or caregiver • Financial impact to care team • Financial impact to health system or payer • Financial impact to society
Experience	• Patient, family, and/or caregiver experience • Care team member experience • Community experience
Effectiveness	• System effectiveness • Clinical effectiveness • Operational effectiveness • Technical effectiveness

The NQF report recommends measuring whether sufficient information was obtained during a telemedicine encounter to make clinical decisions regarding intervention. Obtaining the appropriate actionable information is more important than measuring diagnostic accuracy. The committee recognized that, just like in the ED, sometimes more information is needed to make a diagnosis. Thus, not knowing the diagnosis is not critical, but failing to issue a referral to obtain the important information would be problematic.

Outcome measures should depend on the specific application of telemedicine. Some examples are mortality, frequency of prescriptions such as antibiotics, testing ordered, or frequency of clinical worsening requiring an in-person visit or hospitalization.

Patient and provider experience (rather than just satisfaction) are important quality components that require special attention in telemedicine, where direct in-person patient–provider contact is lacking. Satisfaction with the technological aspects of the interaction should be separated from that of the provider. Since seeing a patient over telemedicine requires some differences in interaction, such as eye contact, environment, and audio–video quality, these aspects should be monitored.

The NQF measures are likely to be universally adopted; therefore, mature programs should be encouraged to measure and report quality outcomes in alignment with these recommendations. The four domains in the NQF report have already been incorporated into program metrics in the fields of primary care and internal medicine, urology, general surgery, otolaryngology, preadmission testing, and oncology.[20-26]

EDUCATION AND TRAINING

As the medical landscape continues to evolve, educational strategies will need to be adapted to prepare the clinical workforce for these new telemedicine approaches. New models of care delivery will require new skill sets to effectively diagnose and treat health conditions.[27,28] Training programs should meet the needs of all learners and foster interprofessional education and collaboration (e.g., physicians, nurses, allied health professionals, and patients). In fact, the American Medical Association recommends including telemedicine as a core competency in training programs.[29-31]

Participants in the First National Academic Consortium of Telehealth universally agreed that the gold standard is to embed telemedicine training into the nascent stages of health providers' professional development.[31] Rather than serving as an independent elective, telemedicine education should be integrated into the management of patients with stroke, asthma, rashes, and so on. Several medical institutions, such as Thomas Jefferson University and Weill Cornell Medicine, are already providing training and education in telemedicine and digital health care, and we expect this trend to spread throughout the industry.[32,33]

Telehealth Facilitator Certificate Programs

Telehealth facilitator certificate programs are designed for affiliates of health-related fields who are interested in further developing their careers. These training programs teach how to improve health-care access, efficiency, and safety, as well as patient outcomes. This entails acquiring an arsenal of telehealth skills that enable learners to successfully facilitate, evaluate, and advocate for telehealth within their respective organizations.

Students are immersed in modules that promote the skills needed to support clinical telehealth encounters, including but not limited to using the approach in both inpatient and outpatient settings and providing technical assistance when needed. Some programs provide a hands-on practicum module through which students have the opportunity to practice skills covered in previous modules. In these modules, trainees can learn how to avoid commonly encountered problems and/or how to troubleshoot common issues faced during typical telehealth encounters.[33] Education for telehealth staff can be found online through the telehealth resource centers or some academic medical centers.

Telehealth Fellowships

A few programs offer telehealth fellowships that are not approved by the Accreditation Council for Graduate Medical Education; they are usually specific to the provider's specialty. They tend to tailor the curriculum to the fellow's personal interests, allowing for individualized concentrations of research and knowledge application as well as the option to complete an advanced degree or certificate.

Resident Physicians and Medical Student Electives

Several institutions now offer telehealth electives for residents and medical students wanting to explore all aspects of novel care delivery systems. Electives generally include a base educational curriculum with an opportunity for learners to further pursue interests appropriate for their degree of training. Ideally, in addition to basic readings and an interactive curriculum specifically tailored for their level of education, all learners get to participate in the conception, development, and implementation of various telehealth use cases throughout the health system, regional accountable care organizations, and large community groups.

A telehealth elective was developed at Thomas Jefferson University, where residents performed telehealth follow-up visits on post ED-discharged patients.[16] After discharge, the patients had scheduled televisits with the physicians, who were able to reassess their clinical conditions, confirm that follow-up appointments were scheduled, and perform medication reconciliation. Both patients and providers found this an effective and positive experience.[16]

VENDOR SELECTION CAUTIONS

Ideally, telemedicine programs are vendor agnostic, customer focused, and cost effective. All too often, unfortunately, institutions begin a telemedicine program before determining their strategy. We caution against evaluating any vendors' new technological "toys" before developing a roadmap. Rather, we recommend an approach that first answers the following questions:

- What problem am I trying to solve?
- Do we already have something that can solve this problem?
- If not, do we want to buy or build a solution to the problem?
- What are the specifications that we need?

Only then should you begin a search for the right product. Here are some tips to consider as you develop a program and look for the right vendor:

- Remember that most start-ups are in it for the exit strategy. They are building a product to sell and are less concerned with customer retention and more concerned with selling the company. More stable public companies may be better long-term bets.
- Test drive the product behind your own firewall before the sale to ensure that your vendor and your IT department don't eventually run into a problem each says is caused by the other.
- Assess compatibility with all common devices (e.g., smart phones, tablets, computers).

- Test functionality with all common browsers.
- If you plan to see new patients, make sure they can register for the program without first being enrolled by someone else.
- If you plan to conduct scheduled visits, make sure you can do this in the same system that allows on-demand calls.
- Multiparty capabilities that allow you to link providers, patients, families, and consultants, if needed, should be possible without requiring anyone to download an app or register (or there will be excessive delays).
- Assess the ability to easily transfer a call to another provider without the patient needing to call back to speak to someone else.
- Ensure the ability to upload data during the interaction. No one wants to disconnect and reconnect before or after uploading a picture.
- Require EMR integration with the capability to transfer more than just pdf documents into the EMR.
- Assess the ability to communicate with both patients and other providers and coordinate care.
- Require the ability to send prescriptions electronically to the pharmacy.
- Determine the system's capability to know who and how many people are waiting.
- Require unlimited publication rights (other than the vendor's intellectual property).

Vendors should provide a solution to your problems. If you don't make them develop that solution before purchasing the product, it is unlikely they ever will.

CONCLUSION

Telemedicine represents a new health-care delivery mechanism with many possible uses in EDs, urgent care centers, and outpatient settings. Although emergency physicians should embrace the change and continue to be available to patients 24/7, they may no longer need to provide care from within a bricks-and-mortar hospital setting.

REFERENCES

1. Daughtery A. What do consumers want from primary care? Advisory.com. 2014. Available at: https://www.advisory.com/Research/Market-Innovation-Center/expert-insights/2014/get-the-primary-care-consumer-choice-survey-results?WT.ac=4member_MPLC_LB_PrimaryCare. Accessed February 6, 2019.
2. Bhatt J, Bathija P, Ensuring Access to Quality Health Care in Vulnerable Communities. Acad Med. 93:9 (1271–1275) Sep 2018. Available at: https://journals.lww.com/academicmedicine/Fulltext/2018/09000/Ensuring_Access_to_Quality_Health_Care_in.13.aspx?WT.mc_id=HPxADx20100319xMP. Accessed September 19, 2020.
3. Hollander J, Ranney M, Carr B. No patient left behind: patient-centered healthcare reform. *Healthcare Transformation*. 2016;1(2):114–119.
4. 2017 Inpatient Telemedicine Study. HIMSS Analytics. 2017. Available at: https://www.himssanalytics.org/sites/himssanalytics/files/HIMSS%20Analytics%202017%20Inpatient%20Telemedicine%20Essentials%20Brief%20Snapshot%20Report.pdf. Accessed September 4, 2018.
5. 2017 Outpatient Telemedicine Study. HIMSS Analytics. 2017. Available at: https://www.himssanalytics.org/sites/himssanalytics/files/HIMSS%20Analytics%202017%20Outpatient%20Telemedicine%20Essentials%20Brief%20Snapshot%20Report_0.pdf. Accessed September 4, 2018.
6. Lacktman N, Vernaglia L. 2014 Telemedicine Survey Executive Summary. Foley and Lardner LLP. Available at: https://www.foley.com/2014-telemedicine-survey-executive-summary/. Published 2018. Accessed September 4, 2018.
7. Telehealth basics. American Telemedicine Association. 2018. Available at: https://www.americantelemed.org/resource/why-telemedicine/. Accessed August 2018, 2020.
8. Sharma R, Fleischut P, Barchi D. Telemedicine and its transformation of emergency care: a case study of one of the largest US integrated healthcare delivery systems. *Int J Emerg Med*. 2017;10(1):21.
9. Sharma R, Gordon J, Greenwald P, et al. Telehealth express care service: revolutionizing care for ED patients. *NEJM Catalyst*. 2017. Available at: https://catalyst.nejm.org/telehealth-express-care-service-revolutionizing-ed-care/. Accessed September 4, 2018.
10. Itrat A, Taqui A, Cerejo R, et al; Cleveland Pre-Hospital Acute Stroke Treatment Group. Telemedicine in prehospital stroke evaluation and thrombolysis: taking stroke treatment to the doorstep. *JAMA Neurol*. 2016;73(2):162–168.
11. Patient-Centered Outcomes Research Institute Comparing Mobile Stroke Treatment with Emergency Room care—the BEST-MSU Study. 2018. Available at: https://www.pcori.org/research-results/2016/benefits-stroke-treatment-delivered-using-mobile-stroke-unit-compared-standard). Accessed September 4, 2018.

12. Huigol, YS, Joshi AU, Carr BG, et al. Giving urban health care access issues the attention they deserve in telemedicine reimbursement policies. *Health Affairs Blog*. 2017. Available at: https://www.healthaffairs.org/do/10.1377/hblog20171022.713615/full/. Accessed September 4, 2018.

13. Agarwal AK, Gaieski DF, Perman SM, et al. Telemedicine REsuscitation and Arrest Trial (TREAT): a feasibility study of real-time provider-to-provider telemedicine for the care of critically ill patients. *Heliyon*. 2016;2(4):e00099.

14. Rising KL, Ricco JC, Printz AD, et al. Virtual rounds: observational study of a new service connecting family members remotely to inpatient rounds. *Gen Int Med Clin Innov*. 2016;1(3):50–53.

15. Papanagnou D, Stone D, Chandra S, et al. Integrating telehealth emergency department follow up visits into residency training. *Cureus*. 2018;10(4):e2433.

16. How NewYork-Presbyterian Used Telemedicine to Expand Care in Puerto Rico. NewYork: Presbyterian Health Matters Blox. 2018. Available at: https://healthmatters.nyp.org/newyork-presbyterian-used-telemedicine-to-expand-care-in-puerto-rico/. Accessed September 4, 2018.

17. Uscher-Pines L, Fischer S, Tong I, et al. Virtual first responders: the role of direct-to-consumer telemedicine in caring for people impacted by natural disasters. *J Gen Intern Med*. 2018;33(8):1242–1244.

18. The IHI Triple Aim. Ihi.org. Available at: http://www.ihi.org/Engage/Initiatives/TripleAim/Pages/default.aspx. Accessed February 11, 2019.

19. Comprehensive primary care initiative. Center for Medicare & Medicaid Innovation. Innovation.cms.gov. Available at: https://innovation.cms.gov/initiatives/comprehensive-primary-care-initiative/. Accessed February 11, 2019.

20. Ellimoottil C, An L, Moyer M, et al. Challenges and opportunities faced by large health systems implementing telehealth. *Health Affairs*. 2018;37(12):1955–1959.

21. NQF: creating a framework to support measure development for telehealth. Qualityforum.org. 2017. Available at: https://www.qualityforum.org/Publications/2017/08/Creating_a_Framework_to_Support_Measure_Development_for_Telehealth.aspx. Accessed September 4, 2018.

22. Powell RE, Henstenburg JM, Cooper G, et al. Patient perceptions of telehealth primary care video visits. *Ann Fam Med*. 2017;15(3):225–229.

23. Powell RE, Stone D. Hollander JE. Patient and health system experience with implementation of an enterprise wide telehealth scheduled video visit program: mixed methods study. *JMIR Med Inform*. 2018;6(1):e10.p1–7.

24. Rimer RA, Christopher V, Falck A, et al. Telemedicine in otolaryngology outpatient setting—single center head and neck surgery experience. *Laryngoscope*. 2018;128(9):2072–2075.

25. Mullen-Fortino M, Rising KL, Duckworth J, et al. Presurgical assessment using telemedicine technology: impact on efficiency, effectiveness and patient experience of care. *Telemed and e-Health*. 2018. Available at: https://doi.org/10.1089/tmj.2017.0133. Accessed August 27, 2020.

26. Rising KL, Ward MM, Goldwater JC, et al. Framework to advance oncology related telehealth. *JCO Clinical Cancer Informatics*. 2018. Available at: http://ascopubs.org/doi/pdfdirect/10.1200/CCI.17.00156. Accessed August 27, 2020.

27. Papanagnou D, Sicks S, Hollander JE. Training the next generation of care providers: focus on telehealth. *Healthcare Transformation*. 2015;1(1):52–63.

28. West DC, Robins L, Gruppen LD. Workforce, learners, competencies, and the learning environment: Research in Medical Education 2014 and the way forward. *Acad Med*. 2014;89(11):1432–1435.

29. Warsaw R. *From Bedside to Webside: Future Doctors Learn How to Practice Remotely*. Association of American Medical Colleges. 2018. Available at: https://news.aamc.org/medical-education/article/future-doctors-learn-practice-remotely/. Accessed September 5, 2018.

30. *AMA Encourages Telemedicine Training for Medical Students, Residents*. American Medical Association. 2016. Available at: https://www.ama-assn.org/ama-encourages-telemedicine-training-medical-students-residents. Accessed July 27, 2017.

31. Hollander JE, Davis TM, Doarn C, et al. Recommendations from the First National Academic Consortium of Telehealth. *Pop Health Management*. 2018;21(4):271–277.

32. Khullar D. Telemedicine is getting trendy, but doctors may not be keeping up. *The Washington Post*. April 22, 2018. Available at: https://www.washingtonpost.com/national/health-science/telemedicine-is-getting-trendy-but-doctors-may-not-be-keeping-up/2018/04/20/681e1644-2178-11e8-badd-7c9f29a55815_story.html?utm_term=.e24362f82c2f. Accessed September 5, 2018.

33. Telehealth Facilitator Certificate—Philadelphia University + Thomas Jefferson University. *Jefferson.edu*. Available at: https://www.jefferson.edu/university/emerging-health-professions/programs/telehealth-facilitator-certificate.html. Accessed September 4, 2018.

ACEPStore

acep.org/store

PEERprep
For Physicians

PEERcert+
Train. Test. Thrive.

The ONLY EM Board Prep You Need

ACEP Online Learning COLLABORATIVE

200 Courses, 750 Hours of Online Education

The American College of Emergency Physicians is accredited by the Accreditation Council for Continuing Medical Education to provide continuing medical education for physicians.

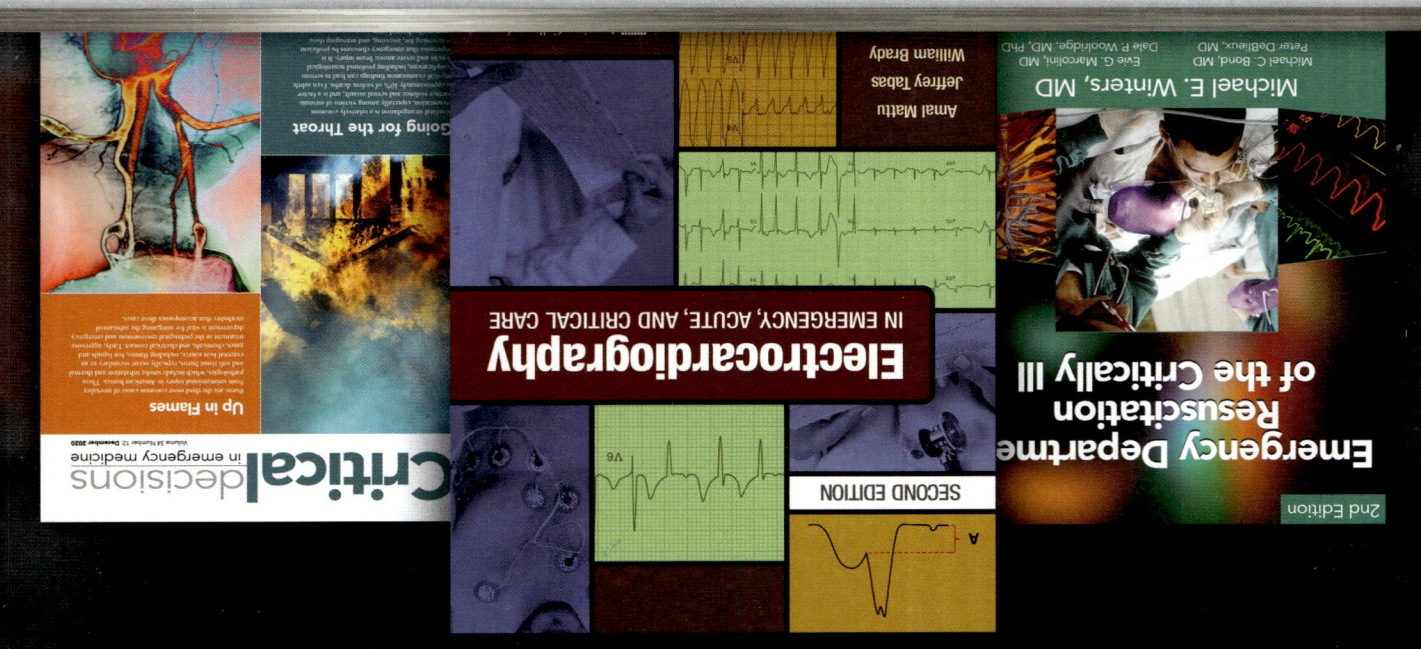

VISIT THE ACEP STORE
FOR MORE EDUCATIONAL PRODUCTS

Dedications

To my wonderful wife, Phyllis Bossin, who views life with astonishing clarity and passion and enriches mine every day; to my children, Bo Strauss and Shelby Strauss Demody, for whom I have the utmost love and admiration; to my sisters Susan Stark, my friend and confidant, and Nancy Dale, for always providing insight and perspective; to my late parents Bob and Aileen, for their remarkable intellects and emotional intelligence; and to Aaron and Lauren Bossin Kull, I am grateful that you are part of my family.

Robert W. Strauss

To my brilliant, beautiful, and forever-inspiring wife, Maureen; to our three kind, generous, and thoughtful sons, Greg, Kevin, and Josh; to Josh's wife, Valerie, and their incredible children, Eve, Audra, Clara, and Ryan; to Kevin's fiancée, Nicola, and to the memory of my parents, Bette and "Grandpa Jim" Mayer, and to the memory of Maureen's wonderful parents, Georgette and Dr. John B. Henry.

Thom A. Mayer

Contents

Contributors   *xi*
Preface   *xxiii*
Acknowledgments   *xxv*

VOLUME 1

SECTION 1	**LEADERSHIP PRINCIPLES**	**1**
Chapter 1	**Leadership, Management, and Motivation**	**3**
Chapter 2	**Vision, Mission, Values, Strategy, and Tactics**	**21**
Chapter 3	**Change and Project Management: A Practical Approach**	**43**
Chapter 4	**Power vs Influence**	**59**
Chapter 5	**Interaction With Hospital Governance**	**73**
Chapter 6	**Managing Professionals in Organizations: The Role of Physician and Nurse Leaders**	**89**
Chapter 7	**Mentoring and Coaching**	**103**
Chapter 8	**Conflict Management**	**113**
Chapter 9	**Conducting High-Impact Meetings**	**133**
Chapter 10	**Patient Safety: Error Reduction**	**155**
Chapter 11	**Defining Patient Experience and Leading Change**	**173**
Chapter 12	**The Discipline of Teams and Teamwork**	**191**
Chapter 13	**Maintaining Personal and Professional Balance**	**219**
Chapter 14	**Ethical Issues in the Emergency Department**	**237**
Chapter 15	**Practice Management Leadership: The Role of the Site Medical Director**	**249**
Chapter 16	**Women in Emergency Medicine Leadership**	**267**
Chapter 17	**Leadership in Times of Crisis**	**285**
SECTION 2	**OPERATIONS: GENERAL**	**301**
Chapter 18	**Medical Director Leadership**	**303**
Chapter 19	**Nursing Director Leadership**	**335**
Chapter 20	**The Medical Director–Nurse Director Relationship**	**345**
Chapter 21	**Emergency Department Provider Staffing**	**359**
Chapter 22	**Nurse Staffing**	**373**
Chapter 23	**Physician and Nurse Productivity Assessments**	**385**

Chapter 24	**Physician Assistants and Nurse Practitioners**	**397**
Chapter 25	**Scribes**	**413**
Chapter 26	**Violence in the Emergency Department**	**433**
Chapter 27	**Emergency Department Facility Design**	**449**
Chapter 28	**Effective Marketing of the Emergency Department**	**473**
Chapter 29	**Multicultural Approach to Emergency Department Patients**	**489**
Chapter 30	**Emergency Department Management Essentials**	**501**
Chapter 31	**The View from the C-Suite**	**517**
Chapter 32	**Emergency Management of Drug and Supply Shortages**	**533**
SECTION 3	**OPERATIONS: FLOW**	**543**
Chapter 33	**Patient Throughput: Why It Matters, How It Is Done**	**545**
Chapter 34	**Patient Flow Principles**	**559**
Chapter 35	**Improving the Front-End Process to Add Value**	**573**
Chapter 36	**Front-Loading Flow**	**585**
Chapter 37	**The Role of Emergency Department Fast Tracks**	**599**
Chapter 38	**Optimizing Patient Throughput**	**613**
Chapter 39	**Role of Observation Units/Rapid Treatment**	**629**
Chapter 40	**Expediting Admissions**	**641**
Chapter 41	**Decision to Discharge: Finishing Strong**	**653**
Chapter 42	**Managing Waits: The Psychology of Waiting**	**669**
Chapter 43	**Hospital-Wide Patient Flow**	**681**
Chapter 44	**Effective Response to Full Capacity**	**699**
Chapter 45	**Defeating Bounce Backs: Managing High-Utilizer Patients**	**707**
Chapter 46	**Innovative Strategies to Enhance Flow**	**721**
SECTION 4	**OPERATIONS: EMERGENCY DEPARTMENT DIVERSIFICATION**	**735**
Chapter 47	**Poison Centers and Medical Toxicology**	**737**
Chapter 48	**Pediatric Emergency Medicine: Improving Quality and Readiness**	**749**
Chapter 49	**Undersea and Hyperbaric Medicine**	**763**
Chapter 50	**Behavioral Health in Emergency Care**	**773**
Chapter 51	**Hospital Medicine**	**785**
Chapter 52	**Disaster Planning and Response**	**805**
Chapter 53	**Military Emergency Medicine**	**823**

Chapter 54	**Freestanding Emergency Departments**	**841**
Chapter 55	**Sports Medicine**	**861**
Chapter 56	**Geriatric Emergency Departments**	**871**
Chapter 57	**Practice Diversification in Emergency Medical Services**	**883**
Chapter 58	**Air Medical Services and Interfacility Ground Transport**	**891**
Chapter 59	**End-of-Life Issues**	**905**
Chapter 60	**Practical Implementation of Opioid-Reduction Initiatives**	**917**
Chapter 61	**Developing and Implementing Emergency Department Ultrasound**	**933**
Chapter 62	**Rural Emergency Departments**	**945**
SECTION 5	**INFORMATICS**	**963**
Chapter 63	**Introduction to Clinical Informatics**	**965**
Chapter 64	**Electronic Health Records**	**969**
Chapter 65	**Electronic Health Record Tracking Systems**	**989**
Chapter 66	**Electronic Health Record Documentation Systems**	**999**
Chapter 67	**Computerized Provider Order Entry and Clinical Decision Support**	**1015**
Chapter 68	**Data Acquisition and Analysis**	**1031**
Chapter 69	**Essential Support Tools and Technologies**	**1049**
Chapter 70	**Social Media in Medicine**	**1059**
Chapter 71	**New Technologies and Applications**	**1065**
Chapter 72	**Telemedicine in Emergency Medicine**	**1077**

VOLUME 2

SECTION 6	**QUALITY AND SERVICE**	**1093**
Chapter 73	**Patient Experience: The Survival Skills Approach**	**1095**
Chapter 74	**Scripts: Using Evidence-Based Language to Improve Service**	**1113**
Chapter 75	**The A-Team Toolkit**	**1129**
Chapter 76	**Complaint Management**	**1143**
Chapter 77	**Effective Medical Staff Relationships: A Case-Based Discussion**	**1175**
Chapter 78	**Improving Performance Through Mutual Accountability**	**1193**
Chapter 79	**Patient Safety and Error Reduction**	**1209**

Chapter 80	**Promoting Rational Thinking: An Ethical Imperative**	**1223**
Chapter 81	**Debiasing Strategies: Cognitive Pills for Cognitive Ills**	**1237**
Chapter 82	**The Revolving Door of Readmissions**	**1251**

SECTION 7   FINANCE   1269

Chapter 83	**Developing a Business Plan**	**1271**
Chapter 84	**Resource Utilization**	**1289**
Chapter 85	**The Financially Successful Emergency Department**	**1303**
Chapter 86	**Optimizing Physician Performance Through Incentives**	**1313**
Chapter 87	**Optimizing Nursing Performance Through Incentives**	**1339**
Chapter 88	**Financially Successful Private Physician Groups**	**1351**
Chapter 89	**Financial Success in Academic Emergency Medicine**	**1361**
Chapter 90	**Financial Planning for Individuals**	**1371**

SECTION 8   REIMBURSEMENT   1389

Chapter 91	**Reimbursement Issues**	**1391**
Chapter 92	**Introduction to Coding**	**1411**
Chapter 93	**Advanced Billing and Coding**	**1437**
Chapter 94	**Facility Revenue Considerations**	**1461**
Chapter 95	**Billing and Collecting**	**1483**
Chapter 96	**Creating a Culture of Compliance**	**1499**
Chapter 97	**Quality and Reporting in the Era of Payment Reform**	**1517**
Chapter 98	**Alternative Payment Models**	**1539**

SECTION 9   CONTRACTS   1553

Chapter 99	**Negotiation Skills**	**1555**
Chapter 100	**Contracts With Physicians**	**1583**
Chapter 101	**Contracting With Hospitals**	**1603**
Chapter 102	**Employee vs Independent Contractor**	**1615**
Chapter 103	**Equity, Parity, and Group Structure**	**1631**

SECTION 10   LEGAL AND REGULATORY ISSUES   1651

Chapter 104	**EMTALA for Emergency Department Leaders**	**1653**
Chapter 105	**Consent to and Refusal of Medical Treatment**	**1673**
Chapter 106	**Emergency Department Documentation**	**1685**
Chapter 107	**Reporting Requirements: Confidentiality, Data Breaches, and HIPAA**	**1697**
Chapter 108	**Disposition, Discharge, and Follow-Up**	**1709**

SECTION 11   MALPRACTICE   1733

Chapter 109	**Risk Management: Challenges and Opportunities**	1735
Chapter 110	**Risk Management in Practice**	1749
Chapter 111	**Medical Malpractice Insurance**	1761
Chapter 112	**Malpractice: The Personal Toll**	1777
Chapter 113	**Medical Malpractice**	1783
Chapter 114	**Anatomy of a Lawsuit**	1805
Chapter 115	**Being an Expert Witness: Telling the Story of the Case**	1815
Chapter 116	**Medical Defense Experts: A Defense Attorney's Perspective**	1829

SECTION 12   HUMAN RESOURCES   1835

Chapter 117	**Human Resources Management: Basic Principles**	1837
Chapter 118	**Physician Recruitment, Credentialing, and Orientation**	1847
Chapter 119	**Physician Retention and Professional Development**	1863
Chapter 120	**Nurse Recruitment, Orientation, and Credentialing**	1881
Chapter 121	**Nurse Retention**	1897
Chapter 122	**Managing Impaired Professionals**	1911
Chapter 123	**Generational Differences in Emergency Medicine**	1927
Chapter 124	**Gender Balance**	1945
Chapter 125	**Burnout: Diagnosis, Treatment, and Prevention**	1975
Chapter 126	**Compassion Fatigue Resiliency**	2001
Chapter 127	**Late Career Toolkit**	2021

SECTION 13   HEALTH-CARE POLICY   2031

Chapter 128	**Inclusion, Equity, and Diversity**	2033
Chapter 129	**Health Policy and Advocacy**	2047
Chapter 130	**Mechanics of Advocacy**	2053
Chapter 131	**Federal Advocacy**	2071
Chapter 132	**State Advocacy**	2089
Chapter 133	**Private Sector Engagement**	2105

Contributors

Gallane D. Abraham, MD
Assistant Professor Emergency Medicine
Icahn School of Medicine at Mount Sinai

Paul Allegretti, DO, FACOEP, FACOI
Clinical Professor of Emergency Medicine
Midwestern University/Chicago College of Osteopathic Medicine
Medical Director, Emergency Medicine
Provident Hospital of Cook County

W. Clayton Alexander IV, MBA
Vice President, Geesbreght Group

Andrew Amaranto, MD
Department of Medicine, Division of Cardiology
NewYork-Presbyterian/Columbia University Irving Medical Center
Department of Emergency Medicine
NewYork-Presbyterian Brooklyn Methodist Hospital

Kimberly Anderson, MHA
Performance Integration Director
The Permanente Medical Group, Inc.
Kaiser Permanente South Sacramento Medical Center

Francisco Javier Andrade Jr, MD
Ultrasound Fellow and Clinical Instructor
University of Arizona College of Medicine | Banner Health

Knox Andress, RN, BA, FAEN
Designated Regional Coordinator, Louisiana Region 7 Hospital/Healthcare Coalition
Assistant Director, Louisiana Poison Center
Department of Emergency Medicine
Louisiana State University Health-Shreveport

Louise B. Andrew, MD, JD, FACEP
Former Office and Chair, ACEP Wellness Committee
Senior Member, ACEP Medical-Legal Committee

Jonathan D. Apfelbaum, MD, FACEP, FAAEM
EMS Medical Director, Parker Adventist Hospital
Medical Director, Weber State University Paramedic Program

Tim W. Attebery, DSc, MBA, FACHE
President and CEO, Attebery & Associates
Adjunct Professor
College of Public Health, East Tennessee State University

Andrea Austin, MD, FACEP, FAAEM, CHSE
Associate Physician Diplomate of Emergency Medicine
University of California San Diego

Brooks Babcock, MBA
Senior Vice President, PSR LLC

Stephanie N. Bailey, MD
Emergency Medicine and Primary Care Sports Medicine
Greenville Health Systems
Clinical Assistant Professor
University of South Carolina School of Medicine, Greenville

Erik D. Barton, MD, MS, MBA, FACEP, FAAEM
Chief of Emergency Medicine
Samaritan Pacific Communities Hospital

Denise Bayer, MS, RN, FAEN
Independent Emergency Nursing Consultant
Past President, Emergency Nurses Association

Gigi Baniqued, MHA, MSN, RN, CHC
Director, Supportive Care Services, Continuing Care, and Complex Needs
South Sacramento Service Area
The Permanente Medical Group

Vikhyat S. Bebarta, MD
Director, CU Anschutz Center for COMBAT Research
Director, CU TRIAD Research Colorado
Vice Chair, Strategy and Growth
Professor (tenured), Emergency Medicine and Medical Toxicology, Pharmacology
Department of Emergency Medicine, University of Colorado School of Medicine, Aurora

Kevin H. Beier, MD, FAAEM
Associate Program Director, Emergency Medicine Residency
University of Tennessee

Elijah Berg, MD, FACEP
Chief Executive Officer, LogixHealth

Jeffrey Bettinger, MD, FACEP
Managing Member, BSA Healthcare

Alex Beuning, MD
Emergency Medicine, Mayo Clinic Health Systems

Graham Billingham, MD, FACEP, FAAEM
Chief Medical Officer, MedPro Group and Princeton Insurance Company
Founder, The Center for Emergency Medicine Education

Kevin Biese, MD, MAT, FACEP
Associate Professor, University of North Carolina
Consultant, West Health

Tom Blackwell, MD, FACEP, FAEMS
Assistant Dean, Longitudinal Clinical Education
University of South Carolina School of Medicine, Greenville
Professor of Emergency Medicine, Prisma Health
Executive Director, Greenville County EMS

Kay Bleecher, CRNP
EMS-Nursing Educator, Harrisburg Area Community College
Wellspan Health

Timothy J. Boardman, MD
Assistant Professor and Clinician Educator
Department of Emergency Medicine
Warren Alpert Medical School of Brown University

J. Stephen Bohan, SM, MD
Associate Physician, Brigham and Women's Hospital
Corresponding Member of the Faculty of Emergency Medicine, Harvard Medical School

Ed Boudreau, DO, FACEP, FAAEM, CPPS
CEO, Emergency Physicians Insurance Exchange RRG
Value Stream Managers LLC

Robert M. Bramante, MD, FACEP
Chairman, Department of Emergency Medicine
Catholic Health Mercy Hospital
Progressive Emergency Physicians
Clinical Associate Professor of Emergency Medicine
NYIT College of Osteopathic Medicine
Clinical Assistant Professor of Emergency Medicine
Stony Brook University School of Medicine

Autumn M. Brogan, MD, MPH
Department of Emergency Medicine, Mayo Clinic

John C. Brown, MD, FACEP
Medical Director, San Francisco Emergency Medical Services Agency
Associate Clinical Professor of Emergency Medicine; EMS and Disaster Medicine
Associate Fellowship Director, University of California San Francisco Medical School
Medical Officer, Disaster Medical Team CA-6

Diane Calello, MD, FAAP, FACMT, FAACT
Executive and Medical Director
New Jersey Poison Information and Education System
Associate Professor of Emergency Medicine
Rutgers-New Jersey Medical School

Janet Carr, MBA
Vice President of Operations, Emergency Medicine
Sound Physicians

L. Anthony Cirillo, MD, FACEP
Board of Directors, American College of Emergency Physicians
Director of Government Affairs, US Acute Care Solutions LLC
Past Chair, Emergency Medicine Policy Institute
Senior Medical Advisor, Graphene Composites - USA
Clinical Adjunct Associate Professor, University of Rhode Island College of Nursing

Mark Collin, MD
Director, Division of Point-of-Care Ultrasound
Director, Emergency Medicine Ultrasound Fellowship
Department of Emergency Medicine
Wellspan York Hospital

Stephen Colucciello, MD, FACEP
Professor and Vice Chair, Department of Emergency Medicine,
Carolinas Medical Center and Atrium Health

Norma Cooney, MD, FACEP, UHM/ABEM
Clinical Assistant Professor of Emergency Medicine
SUNY Upstate University Hospital
Chief Operating Officer, MedSpa Solutions LLC

Michael Corvini, MD, MBA, FACEP, FACP
President, Southeast Group
TeamHealth

Pat Croskerry, BSc, MD, PhD, CCFP, FRCP
Professor of Emergency Medicine. Division of Medical Education
Dalhousie University
Professor
Canadian Patient Safety Institute

Randal L. Dabbs, MD, FACEP, FAAFP
Co-Founder and President, Practice Development
TeamHealth

Keith DellaGrotta, MD, MBA
Assistant Medical Director, Department of Emergency Medicine
West Hills Hospital and Medical Center

Christina Dempsey, DNP, MBA, RN, CNOR, CENP, FAAN
Chief Nursing Officer Emerita, Press Ganey Associates Inc.
Adjunct Faculty
Missouri State University School of Nursing

Colleen Desai, RN
Chief Nurse Officer, Holyoke Medical Center

Joseph P. Dervay, MD, MPH, MMS, FACEP, FAsMA
Flight Surgeon, Space Medicine Operations Division
NASA Johnson Space Center
Clinical Instructor, Division of Emergency Medicine, Dept. of Surgery
Clinical Assistant Professor, Dept. of Preventive Medicine & Community Health
The University of Texas Medical Branch

Taylor T. DesRosiers, MD
Lieutenant, Medical Corps, United States Navy
Naval Medical Center Portsmouth

Jeffrey "Jim" Dietz, MD
Chair, Department of Emergency Medicine (retired)
Coordinator, Vitality Professional Resilience Project (retired)

Sue Dill Calloway, RN, AD, BA, BSN, MSN, JD, CPHRM, CCMSCP
President, Patient Safety and Healthcare Education & Consulting

Valerie Dobiesz, MD, MPH, FACEP
Director of Internal Programs, STRATUS Center for Medical Simulation
Brigham & Women's Hospital
Department of Emergency Medicine, Harvard Medical School

Jeff Druck, MD
Co-Director, Office of Professional Excellence
Assistant Dean for Student Affairs, Office of Student Life
Professor of Emergency Medicine
University of Colorado

Pamela L. Dyne, MD
Professor of Clinical Emergency Medicine
UCLA David Geffen School of Medicine
Designated Institutional Official, Department of Emergency Medicine
Olive View-UCLA Medical Center

Caral Edelberg, CPC, CPMA, CAC, CCS-P, CHC
Honorary Member, American College of Emergency Physicians
Founder and Chairman, Edelberg + Associates

Jim Ellis, MD, FACEP
Emergency Preparedness Consultant, NFL
President, Prisma Health Medical Group-Midlands
Clinical Associate Professor of Emergency Medicine
University of South Carolina School of Medicine-Greenville

Luis F. Eljaiek Jr, MD, FACEP, FAAEM
Medical Director, Physicians Transport Service

Jeffrey Eye, RN, MSN
Vice President, Patient Care Services
Chief Nursing Officer
Murray-Calloway County Hospital

Ugo A. Ezenkwele, MD, MPH, FACEP
Chief, Mount Sinai Queens Emergency Department
Associate Professor of Emergency Medicine
Icahn Mount Sinai School of Medicine

Brian Fengler, MD
Co-Founder and CEO, EvidenceCare

Kathleen Flarity, DNP, PhD, CEN, CFRN, FAEN
Deputy Director, CU Anschutz Center for COMBAT Research
Associate Professor and Research Nurse Scientist, Department of Emergency Medicine
University of Colorado School of Medicine, Aurora
Brigadier General, US Air Force

Cyndy Flores, PA-C
Senior Director, Advanced Providers, Vituity

Edward R. Gaines III, JD, CCP
Chief Compliance Officer, EM Division, Zotec Partners LLC

Gus M. Garmel, MD, FACEP, FAAEM
Clinical Professor (Affiliate) of Emergency Medicine
Stanford University
Senior Staff Emergency Physician, TPMG, Kaiser Santa Clara
Senior Editor, *The Permanente Journal*, KWFCO

Chelsey Geiger, MS
President, CareThrough

Nicholas Genes, MD, PhD, FACEP
Associate CMIO, Mount Sinai Health System
Associate Professor of Emergency Medicine
Icahn School of Medicine at Mount Sinai

J. Eric Gentry, PhD, LMHC, DAAETS, FAAETS
President, FORWARD-FACING INSTITUTE

Aaron George, DO
Chief Medical Officer, Meritus Health

James E. George, MD, FACEP
Co-Founder and Strategic Advisor to the President and CEO, TeamHealth

Michael Gottlieb, MD, RDMS, FAAEM, FACEP
Associate Professor of Emergency Medicine
Director, Emergency Ultrasound Division
Program Director, Clinical Ultrasound Fellowship
Department of Emergency Medicine
Rush University Medical Center

Pawan Goyal, MD, MHA, FAMIA, FHIMSS, FAHIMA
Associate Executive Director, Quality
American College of Emergency Physicians

Louis Graff IV, MD, FACEP, FACP, FACC
Physician Advisor, Hartford Healthcare Corporation
Professor of Surgery and Emergency Medicine, Clinical Professor of Medicine
University of Connecticut School of Medicine

Charles Grassie, MD, JD, FACEP
Retired CEO, Emergency Physicians Medical Group
Emeritus Physician, St. Joseph Mercy Health System

Andrea L. Green, MD, FACEP
Chair, ACEP Diversity, Inclusion, and Health Equity Section
Vituity Healthcare Partner
Department of Emergency Medicine
UMC Medical Center Northeast

Phillip Gruber, MD
Chief Medical Information Officer
LAC+USC Medical Center

Alison Haddock, MD, FACEP
Assistant Professor of Emergency Medicine, Baylor College of Medicine
Vice President, American College of Emergency Physicians

Blaine Hannafin, MD, MBD, RDMS
Chief of Cost Performance, Northern California Clinical Lead for Medi-Cal Operations
Medical Director, Kaiser Geographic Managed Care (Kaiser GMC Medi-Cal)

Gregory L. Henry, MD, FACEP
Clinical Professor of Emergency Medicine
University of Michigan Medical School
Former President, American College of Emergency Physicians
Risk Consultant, Emergency Physicians Medical Group

Judd E. Hollander, MD
Senior Vice President for Healthcare Delivery Innovation, Jefferson Health
Associate Dean for Strategic Health Initiatives, Sidney Kimmel Medical College
Vice Chair for Finance and Healthcare Enterprises, Department of Emergency Medicine
Thomas Jefferson University

Michelle Hoppes, RN, MS, DFASHRM
President/CEO, Michigan Professional Insurance Exchange
Adjunct Faculty, Loyola School of Law

Kenneth V. Iserson, MD, MBA, FACEP, FAAEM, FIFEM
Professor Emeritus, Department of Emergency Medicine
University of Arizona
Visiting Professor, Emergency Medicine Residency
Georgetown Public Hospital, Guyana

Sujit S. Iyer, MD
Director, Pediatric ED Outreach
Associate Fellowship Director
Assistant Medical Director, Pediatric Emergency Medicine
Associate Professor of Pediatrics, UT Austin Dell Medical School
Dell Children's Medical Center of Central Texas

Stephen J. Jameson, MD, FACEP
Chair, ACEP Rural Section
Co-Editor, Emergency Medicine Core Training
Emergency Trauma Center
St. Cloud Hospital

Zachary J. Jarou, MD, MBA
Clinical Associate, Section of Emergency Medicine
Department of Medicine, University of Chicago
Fellow in Administration, Quality, Informatics, and Policy
American College of Emergency Physicians
Immediate Past President, Emergency Medicine Residents' Association

Mark M. Jones, JD, MEd
Retired Partner, Wilson, Elser, Moskowitz, Edelman, and Dicker LLP

Robert Jones, DO, FACEP
Systemwide Clinical Ultrasound Co-Chair, MetroHealth System
Assistant Dean for Clerkship Education
Block 7 Leader, Clinical Ultrasound and Professor of Emergency Medicine
Case Western Reserve University School of Medicine

Thomas Judge
Paramedic/Critical Care
Executive Director, LifeFlight of Maine/LifeFlight Foundation

Jay Kaplan, MD, FACEP
Medical Director of Care Transformation, LCMC Health
Clinical Associate Professor of Medicine, LSU Health Sciences Center
Attending Physician and Academic Faculty, LSU Emergency Medicine Residency, University Medical Center New Orleans
Past President, American College of Emergency Physicians

Mark Kauffman, BSN, MBA
Director, Strategic Initiatives
Kaiser Permanente South California

Thompson Kehrl, MD, RDMS, FACEP
Chair, Department of Emergency Medicine
WellSpan York Hospital

A. Michael Kelen, CFA, CFP
Director of Financial Services, Sortino Financial Group

Marylou Killian, DNP, RN, FNP-bc, ENP-c, FAEN
Emergency Medicine, TeamHealth

Matthew R. Klein, MD, MPH
Assistant Professor of Emergency Medicine
Northwestern University Feinberg School of Medicine

Kevin M. Klauer, DO, EJD, FACEP, FACOEP
CEO, American Osteopathic Association
Assistant Clinical Professor, Michigan State University College of Osteopathic Medicine
Clinical Assistant Professor, University of Tennessee Health Science Center
Assistant Clinical Professor, Ohio University College of Osteopathic Medicine

Kirk R. Klemme, MD
Addiction Medicine, Aspirus Keweenaw Hospital

Kelly J. Ko, MS, PhD
Director of Clinical Research
West Health Institute, La Jolla, CA

Kathy Kopka, RN, MHSA
Administrative Director Clinical Operations
Skyline Medical Center, HCA TriStar Division, Nashville, TN

Linda Lawrence, MD, CPE, FACEP
Col (ret) USAF, MC
Associate Dean for Clinical Affairs and Clinical Associate Professor of Emergency Medicine
Northeast Ohio Medical University
Adjunct Associate Professor of Military & Emergency Medicine
Uniformed Services University of the Health Sciences

Alexis M. LaPietra, DO, FACEP
Chief, Pain Management and Addiction Medicine
Assistant Professor of Clinical Emergency Medicine
Rowan University School of Osteopathic Medicine

Adriane Lesser, MS
Associate Director, Clinical Research
West Health Institute, La Jolla, CA

Resa E. Lewiss, MD
Director, Point-of-Care Ultrasound
Professor of Emergency Medicine and Radiology
Thomas Jefferson University

Ori Litvak, MBA
Executive Director, Innovation and Process Improvement
LogixHealth

Bernard L. Lopez, MD, MS, CPE, FACEP, FAAEM
Associate Provost for Diversity and Inclusion
Associate Dean for Diversity and Community Engagement
Professor and Executive Vice Chair, Department of Emergency Medicine
Sidney Kimmel Medical College, Thomas Jefferson University

Sujal Mandavia, MD, FRCP(C), FACEP
Clinical Assistant Professor of Emergency Medicine
LAC/USC Medical Center, Keck School of Medicine
Senior Board Examiner, American Board of Emergency Medicine

Nancy Mannion, DNP, RN, CEN, FAEN
President, NMB Global Leadership LLC
Senior Nursing Consultant
Brigham and Women's Hospital

Ricardo Martinez, MD, FACEP
Chief Medical Officer, Adeptus Health
Assistant Professor of Emergency Medicine
Emory School of Medicine

Catherine A. Marco, MD, FACEP
Professor of Emergency Medicine
Wright State University Boonshoft School of Medicine

Donna Mason, RN, BS, MS, CEN, FAEN
Retired Nurse, Emergency Medicine

James C. McClay, MD, MS, FACEP, FAMIA
Chair, Biomedical Informatics Graduate Program
Professor of Emergency Medicine and Informatics
University of Nebraska Medical Center

David A. McKenzie, CAE
Reimbursement Director, American College of Emergency Physicians

Abhi Mehrotra, MD, MBA, FACEP
Vice Chair, Strategic Initiatives & Operations
Professor of Emergency Medicine
University of North Carolina

Sean Michael, MD, MBA, FACEP
Medical Director
Physician Informaticist and Pathways Lead
Department of Emergency Medicine
University of Colorado School of Medicine

Angela M. Mills, MD
J. E. Beaumont Professor and Chair
Department of Emergency Medicine
Columbia University College of Physicians and Surgeons
Chief of Emergency Medicine Services, NewYork-Presbyterian | Columbia

Nicholas M. Mohr, MD
Associate Professor of Emergency Medicine and Anesthesia Critical Care
University of Iowa Carver College of Medicine

William Montei, CPA
Chief Medical Officer, Meglodon Insurance Systems

Michael D. Moon, PhD, MSN, RN, CNS-CC, CEN, FAEN
Former President, Texas Emergency Nurses Association
Professor of Nursing
University of the Incarnate Word
Ila Faye Miller School of Nursing and Health Professions

Lisa A. Moreno-Walton, MD, MS, MSCR, FAAEM, FACEP, FIFEM
President, American Academy of Emergency Medicine
Professor of Emergency Medicine
Director, Latino Health Scholars Program
Louisiana University Health Sciences Center, New Orleans

Rhonda M. Morgan, RN, DNP, CNS, APRN
Professor, King University
Director, Doctor of Nursing Practice Program

Eric J. Morley, MD, MHA, MS
Associate Professor, Vice Chair for Clinical Affairs, and Clinical Director
Department of Emergency Medicine
Deputy CMIO
Renaissance School of Medicine at Stony Brook University

Sergey M. Motov, MD, FAAEM
Research Director, Department of Emergency Medicine
Maimonides Medical Center
Professor of Emergency Medicine
SUNY Downstate Medical College

Karen Murrell, MD, MBA, FACEP
Medical Director, Lodi Memorial Hospital
Performance & Innovation Consultant, TeamHealth
Clinical Consultant, Qventus Inc.

Anthony Nader
Chairman, Inova Health Systems

Joanne Navarroli, MSN, RN, CEN
Chandler Regional Medical Center

Susan Nedza, MD, MBA
Adjunct Assistant Professor of Emergency Medicine
Feinberg School of Medicine
Northwestern University

Lewis S. Nelson, MD
Professor and Chair, Department of Emergency Medicine
Director, Division of Medical Toxicology
Rutgers New Jersey Medical School
Chief of Service, Emergency Department, University Hospital of Newark
Senior Consultant, New Jersey Poison Information & Education System

Diana Nordlund, DO, JD, FACEP
Corporate Compliance Officer, Emergency Care Specialists
Attorney/Partner, Nordlund | Hulverson PLLC
Board of Directors, Michigan College of Emergency Physicians

Marlaina Norris, MD, MBA
Director of Utilization Review and Care Coordination
Vituity Emergency Department
Presence Mercy Medical Center

Charles Noon, PhD, MEng
Professor, Physician Executive MBA Program
Haslam College of Business, University of Tennessee
Faculty, Institute for Healthcare Improvement
Co-Founder/Consultant, X32 Healthcare

Ashley Booth Norse, MD, FACEP
Associate Chair of Operations, Medical Director, and Associate Professor of Emergency Medicine
University of Florida College of Medicine - Jacksonville

Sara Nourazari, PhD
Assistant Professor
California State University - Long Beach

India Owens, MSN, RN, CEN, NE-BC, FAEN
India T Owens Consulting
Adjunct Faculty, Indiana University School of Nursing
Adjunct Faculty, University of Indianapolis

Rebecca Bollinger Parker, MD, FACEP
Chief Coding Officer, Health Care Financial Services of TeamHealth, Knoxville TN
President, Team Parker LLC, Tucson, AZ

Gita Pensa, MD
Clinical Assistant Professor, Department of Emergency Medicine
Warren Alpert School of Medicine of Brown University

Ava E. Pierce, MD, FACEP
Associate Professor and Associate Chair of Diversity and Inclusion
Director of Texas Emergency Medicine Research Associates Program
Department of Emergency Medicine
UT Southwestern Medical Center

Susan B. Promes, MD, FACEP
Professor and Chair of Emergency Medicine
Penn State Milton S. Hershey Medical Center

Ed Racht
Chief Medical Officer, American Medical Response

Mark Reiter, MD, MBA, MAAEM, FAAEM
CEO, Emergency Excellence
Professor and Residency Director, Department of Emergency Medicine
University of Tennessee-Murfreesboro/Nashville
Chair, American Academy of Emergency Medicine Physician Group

Katherine Remick, MD, FAAP, FACEP, FAEMS
Medical Director, San Marcos Hays County EMS System
Executive Lead, National EMS for Children Innovation and Improvement Center
Associate Medical Director, Austin-Travis County EMS System
Assistant Professor of Pediatrics, Dell Medical School at the University of Texas at Austin

Matthew Rice, MD, JD, FACEP
Emergency Medicine Physician
Gig Harbor

Lynne D. Richardson, MD, FACEP
Professor of Emergency Medicine and Health Evidence and Policy
Vice Chair for Academic Research and Community Programs, Department of Emergency Medicine
The Icahn School of Medicine, Mount Sinai

Hammad Rizvi, DO, MBA, CPE, FHM
Senior Vice President, TeamHealth

Kathy Robinson, RN, BSHA, FAEN
Strategic Partnerships Director, National Association of State EMS Officials
Past President, Emergency Nurses Association

Scott W. Rodi, MD, MPH
Inaugural Chair, Department of Emergency Medicine, Dartmouth-Hitchcock Medical Center
Director, Regional Emergency Medicine, Dartmouth-Hitchcock Health
Associate Professor of Emergency Medicine, The Geisel School of Medicine at Dartmouth

Adam Rodos, MD, FACEP
Program Director, Internal Medicine/Emergency Medicine Residency
Director of Quality, Department of Emergency Medicine
Assistant Professor of Clinical Emergency Medicine and Medicine
University of Illinois at Chicago

Marie-Laure Romney, MD, MBA
Vice President of Operations
NewYork-Presbyterian Hospital
Columbia University Irving Medical Center

Mark Rosenberg, DO, MBA, FACEP, FAAHPM
President, American College of Emergency Physicians
Associate Professor and Chairman Emeritus of Emergency Medicine
St Joseph's University Medical Center

Alexander M. Rosenau, DO, CPE, FACEP
Chief, Division of Emergency Medicine, Department of Emergency and Hospital Medicine, Lehigh Valley Health Network
Professor, Morsani College of Medicine, University of South Florida
Former President, American College of Emergency Medicine

William F. Rutherford, MD
Associate Medical Director, IU Health Revenue Cycle Services
Physician Lead, Denial Management

Tracy G. Sanson, MD, FACEP
Founder, TracySansonMD
Emergency Physician, Consultant, Educator

James J. Scheulen, PA, MBA
Chief Administrative Officer, Emergency Medicine and Capacity Management
Johns Hopkins Medicine

Gillian R. Schmitz, MD, FACEP
Associate Professor, Department of Military and Emergency Medicine
Uniformed Services University
Vice Chair of Education
Brooke Army Medical Center

Bill Schueler, MSN, RN, CEN, CPPS, WVTS, FAEN
Patient Safety Specialist, Providence Health - Oregon Region
Owner, WJS Services LLC

Jean Scofi, MD, MBA, MS
Director of Informatics & Analytics
Assistant Director, Healthcare Leadership and Management Fellowship
Assistant Professor of Emergency Medicine
New York Presbyterian Weill-Cornell Medical Center

Aviva Segal, PhD
Faculty, Department of Education, Concordia University
Postdoctoral Fellow, Centre for Research on Children and Families
McGill University, Concordia University

Rahul Sharma, MD, MBA, FACEP
Professor and Chairman, Emergency Physician-in-Chief
New York Presbyterian-Weill Cornell Medicine
Executive Director, Center for Virtual Care
Weill Cornell Medicine

David Singley Jr, MHA
Chief Executive Officer, PSR LLC

Mary Kay Silverman, DNP, RN, CEN, NEA-BC
Director of Pediatric Emergency Services and Pedi/Neo Transport Team
Golisano Children's Hospital of SW Florida

Michael A Silverman, MD, FACEP
Chairman, Department of Emergency Medicine
Virginia Hospital Center

Rebecca Smith-Coggins, MD
Professor (Teaching) of Emergency Medicine
Stanford Hospital and Clinic

Jeff Solheim, MSN, RN, CEN, TCRN, CFRN, FAEN, FAAN,
President, Solheim Enterprises
Past President, Emergency Nurses Association
Past President, Nursing Organizational Alliance

Thomas Spiegel, MD, MBA, MS, FACEP
Assistant Professor of Medicine and Administrative Fellowship Director
Emergency Department Medical Director, Center for Care and Discovery
Section of Emergency Medicine, Department of Medicine, University of Chicago

Donald E. Stader III, MD, FACEP
Emergency Physician, Swedish Medical Center
Founder and President, Stader Opioid Consulting LLC
President, Triage Films LLC

Jennifer L'Hommedieu Stankus, MD, JD, FACEP
Physician, Department of Emergency Medicine
Madigan Army Medical Center
Co-Founder, Comprehensive Medical Legal Consultants LLC

Ryan A. Stanton, MD, FACEP
Central Emergency Physicians
Member, American College of Emergency Physicians Board of Directors
Medical Director, Lexington Fire/EMS
AMR/NASCAR Safety Team

Charles (Chuck) D. Stokes, BSN, MHA, FACHE
Founding Partner, Relia Healthcare Advisors
Former CEO, Memorial Hermann Healthcare System, Houston
Past President, American College of Healthcare Executives

Suzanne Stone-Griffith, RN, MSN, CNAA
Affiliate Faculty, Regis University

Cary J. Stratford, PA-C, DFAAPA
President, Emergency Services of New England Inc.

William Sullivan, DO, JD, FACEP
Emergency Physician, St. Margaret's Hospital
Clinical Assistant Professor of Emergency Medicine
Midwestern University
Law Office of William Sullivan
Co-Founder, BAM Medical Staffing
Senior Editor, *EP Monthly Magazine*

John Sverha, MD
Vice Chair, Department of Emergency Medicine
Virginia Hospital Center
Alteon Health

Abbie G. Tapp-Pearson, RN, MSN, MBA
Director of Clinical Education
Director, TeamHealth Patient Safety Organization

Theresa Tavernero, RN, PhD, MBA
Senior Vice President
Performance & Innovation Consultants

Todd B. Taylor, MD, FACEP
Health Information Technology Consultant
Vice-Chair, ACEP Health Innovation & Technology Committee

Aisha T. Terry, MD, MPH, FACEP
Associate Professor of Emergency Medicine and Health Policy
George Washington University School of Medicine and Hospital
Member, American College of Emergency Physicians Board of Directors

Sarah Todt, RN, CPC, CPMA, CEDC
Senior Director, Revenue Integrity
LogixHealth

Vaishal Tolia, MD, MPH, FACEP
Department of Emergency Medicine
University of California San Diego

Jeremy D. Tucker, DO, FACEP, FACOEP, FACOI
Chief Medical Officer, New Frontier Aerospace
Co-Founder, Drone Delivery Systems Corporation
Chief Medical Officer/Co-Founder, Medssenger
US Acute Care Solutions

Pam Turner, RN, MBA
Independent Healthcare Consultant, Clarksville, TN
Senior Consultant, Quality Matters, Salt Lake City, UT

Joseph Twanmoh, MD, MBA, FACEP, FAAEM
President and Founder, Queue Management LLC

Brad Uren, MD
Associate Professor of Emergency Medicine
University of Michigan

Arjun Venkatesh, MD, MBA, MHS, FACEP
Chief, Section of Administration
Associate Professor, Department of Emergency Medicine
Yale University School of Medicine
Scientist, Center for Outcomes Research & Evaluation
Yale New Haven Hospital

(Asa) Peter Viccellio, MD, FACEP
Professor, Vice Chairman, and Associate Chief Medical Officer
Department of Emergency Medicine
Stony Brook School of Medicine

Barbara Weintraub, RN, MSN, MPH, APN, CEN, CPEN, FAEN
Trauma/EMS Coordinator
Gottlieb Memorial Hospital, Melrose Park, IL

Winnie T. Whitaker, MD, FAAP, FACEP
Assistant Professor of Pediatrics
University of Texas at Austin Dell Medical School
Assistant Medical Director, Pediatric Emergency Medicine
Dell Children's Medical Center of Central Texas
Medical Director, Camp Longhorn

Dennis C. Whitehead, MD, FACEP
Emergency Physician, UP Health System - Portage
Associate Professor of Emergency Medicine
Michigan State University
Past Chair, ACEP Wellness Committee
Past Speaker, ACEP Council

Winnie T. Whitaker, MD
Pediatric Emergency Medicine, Dell Children's Medical Center of Central Texas
Assistant Medical Director and Director of Advance Practice Providers
Clinical Assistant Professor or Emergency Medicine
UT Austin-Dell Medical School

Jennifer Wiler, MD, MBA, FACEP
Chief Quality Officer Denver Metro | UCHealth
Co-Founder CARE Innovation Center | UCHealth
Professor of Emergency Medicine
University of Colorado School of Medicine

Jeannette Wolfe, MD, FACEP
Professor of Emergency Medicine
UMass-Baystate

Christopher M. Ziebell, MD, FACEP
Assistant Professor and Division Chief, Dell Medical School
Emergency Department Medical Director, Dell SETON Medical Center at the University of Texas

Frank Zilm, DArch, FAIA, FACHA emeritus
Chester Dean Director of the Institute for Health-Wellness Design
University of Kansas

Brian J. Zink, MD, FACEP
Senior Associate Dean for Faculty and Faculty Development
Professor of Emergency Medicine
University of Michigan Medical School

Leslie Zun, MD, MBA, FAAEM, FACEP
Professor and Chair, Department of Emergency Medicine
Chicago Medical School
Medical Director, Lake County Health Department and Community Health

Preface

*Be not afraid of greatness. Some are born great, some achieve
greatness, and others have greatness thrust upon them.*

William Shakespeare, *Twelfth Night*

Deep political divides, emerging infectious diseases, inconsistent mandates, recognition of and response to systemic racism, overwhelming burnout and increased risk of suicide, and the safety risks to our team members and families all put inordinate pressure on leaders to get it right.

The health-care sector is undergoing dramatic and disruptive change. National leaders and marketplace pressures are mandating the provision of higher-quality, lower-cost care to an aging population. And so, like the quote from Shakespeare, survival and success during these uncertain times require greatness, strong leadership, and collaboration. Emergency department (ED) leaders must approach these transformative changes with a steady nerve, sustained ingenuity, and a willingness to creatively embrace the ever-shifting landscape.

Approximately, 150 million patients are seen in EDs annually (411,000 patients per day), with 27 million patient admissions from the ED (74,000 patients per day). Furthermore, ED admissions account for 70% of all hospital admissions.[1,2] With such staggering data, it's vital that ED leadership and management continuously assess, adapt, and redesign their approach to patient care. One constant is that EDs continue to be both the critical safety net for their patients, communities, hospitals, and the entire health-care system, *and* a central cog in health-care coordination.

A RAND Corporation research report acknowledged the value of the ED in the health-care system.[3] Though ED care is sometimes referred to pejoratively as "the most expensive care there is," this overly simplistic view "ignores the many roles that EDs fill, and the statutory obligation of hospital EDs to provide care to all in need without regard to their ability to pay." As fewer patients are directly admitted from primary care physician (PCP) practices, PCPs increasingly rely on EDs to perform "complex diagnostic workups and [handle] overflow, after-hours, and weekend demand for care." The report goes on to recognize that the physicians and nurses staffing the EDs "are increasingly serving as the major decision-maker[s] for [the majority of] hospital admissions in the United States."

With approximately one-third of US health-care dollars currently spent on hospital patients, it is no surprise that emergency care providers are under increasing scrutiny.[4-6] On the current growth path, some would argue that health-care costs might "bankrupt America."[7,8] All ED leaders are obligated to actively engage in the health-care debate, and in so doing analyze their services, ensure increasing value, institute evidence-based best practices, provide a caring environment, build transparent and meaningful information systems, and inspire teams of caregivers. Department leaders must go beyond meeting critical metrics; rather, they must create a team that consistently delivers "acts of kindness . . . the highest level of compassion . . . one patient at a time."[9-11]

The purpose of this book is to help leaders respond to the complex and evolving ED environment by organizing the contained information into a unified body of knowledge. The intent is to provide both broad philosophic concepts and granular tools and techniques for delivering best and evidence-based practices. The book is organized into 13 sections, which cover the broad array of ED logistics and operations:

- Leadership Principles
- Operations: General
- Operations: Flow
- Operations: Emergency Department Specialization
- Operations: Informatics
- Quality and Service
- Finance
- Reimbursement
- Contracts
- Legal and Regulatory Issues
- Malpractice
- Human Resources
- Health Care Policy

The mission of this book is to develop and enhance the skills of those leading and managing ED services. It is designed to support the ED and its caregivers—emergency physicians, nurses, department directors, administrators, and other staff members—in the provision of those services. It is our privilege as editors to provide a resource to support that endeavor.

Robert W. Strauss and *Thom A. Mayer*

REFERENCES

1. CDC.gov, "National Center for Health Statistics: Emergency Department Visits." Updated February 21, 2020. Accessed October 31, 2020. https://www.cdc.gov/nchs/fastats/emergency-department.htm

2. Augustine JJ. Latest Data Reveal the ED's Role as Hospital Admission Gatekeeper. Published December 20, 2019. Accessed October 31, 2020. https://www.acepnow.com/article/latest-data-reveal-the-eds-role-as-hospital-admission-gatekeeper/#:~:text=Every%20day%2C%20emergency%20physicians%20in,admitted%20to%20hospitals%-20each%20day.

3. Morganti KG, Bauhoff S, Blanchard JC, et al. The Evolving Role of Emergency Departments in the United States. Santa Monica, CA: Rand Corporation, 2013. http://www.rand.org/pubs/research_reports/RR280.html. Accessed May 23, 2013.

4. Abelson R. "ER's Account for Half of Hospital Admissions, Study Says." http://www.nytimes.com/2013/05/21/business/half-of-hospital-admissions-from-emergency-rooms.html?_r=0. Accessed May 21, 2013.

5. Kavilanz P. "6 Reasons Health Care Costs Keep Going Up." http://money.cnn.com/2012/07/12/news/economy/health-care-costs/index.htm. Accessed July 15, 2012.

6. Gee E. "The High Price of Hospital Care." From Center for American Progress: Healthcare. Published June 26, 2019. Accessed November 22, 2020. https://www.americanprogress.org/issues/healthcare/reports/2019/06/26/471464/high-price-hospital-care/

7. Tikkanen R, Abrams MK. "U.S. Healthcare from a Global Perspective, 2019: Higher Spending, Work Outcomes? Published by The Commonwealth Fund, January 30, 2020. Accessed November 23, 2020. https://www.commonwealthfund.org/publications/issue-briefs/2020/jan/us-health-care-global-perspective-2019?gclid=CjwKCAiAtej9BRAvEiwA0UAWXqXw8XC-a4gihZyf-6PkDhtLhsR8LHsxfGePXrcWu9x31MfgO_jbcxoC7BYQAvD_BwE

8. Brockman K. "The expense nearly half of Americans think can bankrupt them." Published in USA Today, May 31, 2019, Accessed November 21, 2020. https://www.usatoday.com/story/money/2019/05/31/45-american-worried-healthcare-expenses-could-bankrupt-them/1292919001/

9. Feinberg D. CEO UCLA Hospital System in a speech delivered to TEDx uploaded to youtube.com August 2, 2011. http://www.youtube.com/watch?v=cZ5u7p-ZNuE. Accessed November 11, 2011.

10. Michelli JA. *Prescription for Excellence: Leadership Lessons for Creating a World-Class Customer Experience from UCLA Health System.* Co-published by McGraw-Hill Companies and Second River Healthcare Press, Bozeman, MT; 2011.

11. Brenner J, Rosenblatt M. "Transforming Healthcare One Patient at a Time." Published in thehill.com, December 8, 2014. Accessed November 20, 2020. https://thehill.com/blogs/congress-blog/healthcare/226165-transforming-healthcare-one-patient-at-a-time

Acknowledgements

The overwhelmingly positive reaction to the 1st edition of this book was extremely gratifying and deeply appreciated. When the American College of Emergency Physicians approached us about updating the book, we both took several deep breaths but quickly agreed to do so, owing primarily to the dramatic, even cataclysmic changes health care *writ large* and emergency departments, in particular, were undergoing. This meant that leadership and management must adapt and react quickly to those changes while finding innovative and creative ways to change systems and processes. The only reason this work has a chance of being successful is because of the amazing work of our friends, who happen to be among the most talented leaders in the specialty of emergency medicine.

To our senior associate editor, Kirk Jensen, and our associate editors Jim Augustine, Jeanne Proehl, and Sandy Schneider, thank you for your incredible insights, unflagging energy, and pure hard work. The same goes for our section editors, who were the "tactical commanders" responsible for ensuring that the content was consistent, accurate, and timely. Finally, to our authors, all highly respected and busy emergency department leaders: Thank you for your dedication and for sharing your invaluable insights, which will make patient care better and the jobs of those who provide that care easier.

Finally, Linda Sokhor Cooper was our editorial assistant throughout this process, and her contributions to the work permeate every page. Her intelligence is exceeded only by her unflagging positive and proactive spirit, which kept us working when it wasn't always easy to see through to the end. As Shakespeare said of Hermia in *A Midsummer Night's Dream*, "Though she be but little, she is fierce."

DR. MAYER'S ACKNOWLEDGMENTS

Henry Adams once wrote, "A teacher affects eternity. He can never tell where his influence ends." In co-editing this book, I have felt the influence of many teachers who materially contributed to its development, even if they were not explicitly aware of it.

I have had the honor of working with many of the brightest lights of health-care leadership, whose thoughts have deeply influenced my work, including Chuck Stokes, Quint Studer, Dr. Don Berwick, Charles Barnett, Steve Brown, Toni Ardabell, Nicholas Beamon, Candace Saunders, and Drs. Tom Jenike and John Brennan. I am grateful to all of them. My friend Tom Peters is a legend in the field of leadership and management, whose praise for the work I have done is both fulsome and excessive. I simply try to live up to it in large or small ways.

My clinical home at the Inova Health System has exposed me to some of the finest leaders in health care, including its CEO, Dr. Stephen Jones, the chief of clinical enterprise, Dr. Steven Motew, and the president of the Inova Fairfax Medical Campus, Dr. Steve Narang, whose definition of culture as "coming straight from the airway of the organization" is as lyrical and succinct as it is pragmatic. I continue to learn from them and from my emergency medicine colleagues, including Drs. Glenn Druckenbrod, Rick Place, Bob Cates, and Dan Hanfling. Exceeding me in intelligence and wit, they collectively form a leadership brain trust without peer.

While he is mentioned above, Dr. Kirk Jensen has been a sage and gimlet-eyed friend and mentor, whose insights have influenced almost every area of my thinking. The memory of three friends and major contributors to the field of emergency department leadership is always with me: Joan Kyes, Martin Gottlieb, and Dr. Stephen Dresnick.

As the medical director of the NFL Players Association, I have benefited from the wisdom of two executive directors, Gene Upshaw (who gave me the job in 2001) and Demaurice "De" Smith, who is as wise and articulate as he is kind and generous. Sean Sansiveri has been my principal partner in health and safety work, as well as Tom DePaso, Ira Fishman, Dr. Don Davis, Ernie Conwell, Tom Carter, and Mark Verstegen.

Finally, words alone fail to express my respect, esteem, and affection for Dr. Rob Strauss, who has been a friend, mentor, and constant source of wisdom for my entire career. There is no one for whom I have more gratitude, and admiration. He is truly a national treasure to all of those who are fortunate enough to lead emergency departments.

DR. STRAUSS'S ACKNOWLEDGMENTS

I would like to thank several individuals who have helped launch and nurture my professional career. Harvey Meislin introduced me to emergency medicine and helped me discover my professional passion. John Lumpkin, Bob Hockberger, and Frank Baker at the University of Chicago provided both rigorous training and invaluable mentoring. Involvement in emergency medicine organizations has been professionally enriching and has also given me great satisfaction. I am grateful late Hal Jayne for introducing me to the realm of national EM education, both program leadership and teaching. I would like to express my deep gratitude to Greg Henry, both for opening doors that allowed me to attain positions of leadership and for being an inspiration to enhance my skills as an educator.

A special thanks to my friends and colleagues at TeamHealth, who have demonstrated astonishing leadership during good and difficult times. I have the honor to work among people with a steadfast focus on improving health care and supporting the well-being of the clinicians providing that care. Among the exemplary leaders, colleagues, role models, mentors, and friends on this "dream team" are Jody Crane, Lynn Massingale, Michael Wiechart, Leif Murphy, Jim George, Theresa Tavernero, Stan Thompson, Randal Dabbs, David Hogan, Abbie Tapp-Pearson, and John Haeberli.

I am fortunate to have been affiliated with institutions that are deeply committed to providing patient care at the highest levels, including the University of Chicago, which provided my foundation in EM and leadership; St. Francis Hospital in Poughkeepsie, which gave me the opportunity to lead and grow for more than 20 years; and the Christ Hospital in Cincinnati for its consistent commitment to excellence.

And finally, my enormous appreciation to Dr. Thom Mayer, my partner in this endeavor; Thom is brilliant and an inspiration to me and all who have the good fortune to work with him. He has great vision, deep passion, and a profound positive regard for others. Thom is a "level 5 leader" possessing great will and humility. I am one of Thom's innumerable fans, whose life he has indelibly enriched.

QUALITY AND SERVICE
SECTION 6

PATIENT EXPERIENCE: THE SURVIVAL SKILLS APPROACH

CHAPTER 73

Thom A. Mayer, Joan Kyes, Robert J. Cates

Far too often, patient experience has been viewed as the "softer," less-scientific aspect of medical care. However, there are considerable data born out of extensive clinical experience that support both the utility and effectiveness of an evidence-based approach to this area.[1-8] More than 25 years ago, the increasing emphasis on patient experience led to the development of the "Survival Skills" approach summarized in this chapter.[4-8]

Chapter 11 defined patient experience and addressed the importance of getting the "why" of intrinsic motivation right before the "how" of detailed implementation. This chapter summarizes those messages and provides a detailed approach to implementing a plan for making the teams' jobs easier while improving the patient experience (**Figure 73.1**). This brief summary is important, after which the details of the "how" are delineated.

FIGURE 73.1 ■ Evidence-Based Disciplines for Patient Experience

01	Making the patient part of the team; providing precise, personalized care	06	Three Survival Skills core competencies
02	Intrinsic motivation: accentuate the A-Team, eliminate the B-Team	07	Taxi, takeoff, flight plans, landing, and Druckenbrod's details
03	The open-book test approach to surveys	08	Dispelling the myths of impossibility and autonomy
04	ED team as performance artists and chief storytellers	09	Shadow shifting and focused coaching
05	Three A-Team behaviors	10	The A-Team toolkit

GETTING THE "WHY" BEFORE THE "HOW"

- Patient experience is the difference between what the patient expected and what the patient actually experienced during their ED visit.[5-8]
- Complaints occur when the team fails to meet the patient's expectations.
- Compliments come from loyal patients whose expectations have been exceeded.
- Unhappy patients tell 16 to 20 people about their bad experience, but happy patients tell 40 to 50 people, which explains the power of creating loyal "customers."[9,10]
- Making the patient a part of the team is critical to success.
- This important question should be asked of each patient: "What's the most important thing we can do to make this an *excellent* ED experience?"[5-8]
- Getting the "why" right before the "how" is made up of these elements[3-7]:
  - ☐ The number one reason to get patient experience right is it makes your job easier!
  - ☐ The entire move to patient experience as an evidence-based discipline is based on intrinsic, not extrinsic motivation.
  - ☐ This is demonstrated by comparing A-Team and B-Team behaviors.[10-13]

Will understanding the "why" of service excellence assist in raising and sustaining patient satisfaction scores? Unequivocally, the answer is a resounding and consistent "Yes!" However—and this is a critically important distinction—the focus should not primarily be on the scores themselves but rather on the A-Team behaviors that make their job easier and the patients' experience better. Wise ED leaders will ask themselves this question every day: "What have I done *today* that makes life easier for the ED staff for whom I am responsible?" By doing so, those leaders will have unleashed a powerful, pervasive, and sustainable force—intrinsic motivation to constantly and consistently be an A-Team member.

The "Open-Book Test"

Every survey is an "open-book test." Department leaders need to help the staff recognize and acknowledge that the questions on the survey are or should be well known well in advance of the survey itself.[5-8] The current most common surveys are the Press Ganey Survey (or variations of it) and the recently completed CMS–Rand Survey adopted by the Agency for Healthcare Research and Quality and the Consumer Assessment of Healthcare Providers and Systems survey team and called the Emergency Department Consumer Assessment of Healthcare Providers and Systems (ED CAHPS) survey.[13] Emergency nurse and physician leaders should ensure that the entire team is aware of the elements that make up the surveys and treat them as open-book tests.

Once everyone knows the composition of the surveys, the "Huddle Up" approach should be used to guide the initial service excellence efforts.[8] "Huddle Up–1st Down" means that the respective groups of the ED team (physicians, nurses, registration, laboratory, radiology—all the elements of the team that is being assessed) should examine the questions about their service and identify A-Team behaviors and processes that help ensure patients and their families are best served in this area. Once this is completed, move on to "Huddle up–2nd Down," where the responses of the physicians are shared with nurses and vice versa across the elements of the team.

If an ED medical director wants to identify the best A-Team physicians, should they ask their fellow emergency physicians? Or should they ask the ED nurses who work most closely with those physicians? Without question, leaders would ask the nurses, who can best identify the A-Team doctors. "Huddle Up–2nd Down" recognizes both this insight and the fundamental team nature of ED care.

"Huddle Up–3rd Down" emphasizes the critical importance of hardwiring patient flow (see Chapters 33 through 46) into the patient experience and the tools and techniques necessary to accentuate A-Team processes and eliminate B-Team processes, which stand in the way of meeting or exceeding patients' expectations. "Huddle Up–4th Down" stresses the use of coaching and mentoring.

ED TEAM MEMBERS AS PERFORMANCE ARTISTS

In the ED, every member of the team is always on stage, creating a performance that makes sense of the patients' symptoms and telling the story of what is done and why (**Figure 73.2**).[15] It is sometimes helpful to remind the team that patients don't just wake up and say, "It's a great day. I think I'll go to the ED!" Instead, they have some symptom, problem, or pain that causes them to seek care. Understanding the concepts of performance artists acting as chief storytellers and sensemakers helps clinicians move from the "problem side" to the "solution side" as quickly as possible.[1-8]

A key lesson from the Disney theme park experience is the concept of *expectation creation*. Signs at each of the rides tell the customers how long they can expect to wait. However, Disney creates an expectation that the park is capable of exceeding; if the wait sign says 30 minutes, Disney knows from statistical analysis that the wait is usually 22 minutes or less. When park visitors are able to board the ride in under 30 minutes, they usually feel they have gotten special treatment.[14]

Expectation creation can also be used in the ED to help manage waits and delays by systematically increasing the estimate of how long a test or treatment might take. For example, if a chest radiograph takes 20 minutes to complete based on analysis of data, team members might be trained to say, "A chest x-ray usually takes 45 minutes, but we will do our best to beat that." Once the radiograph is completed, perhaps in 30 minutes, patients are typically happy, since it appears to them that the target was beaten.[5-8]

A-TEAM BEHAVIORS

Putting these concepts to practical use is the job of each of the members of the ED team. It starts with three fundamental, yet often neglected behaviors that everyone should use consistently as a discipline to be followed with each ED patient.

FIGURE 73.2 ■ Clinicians as Performance Artists

You are a Performance Artist!

- You are the chief storyteller of the ED!
- Patients don't wake up and say, "Great day! Off to the ED!"
- The faster and more effective you are at making yourself a "solution" instead of a part of the bad experience, the easier the job.
- It's the perception of flow that matters!
- It's not just how much time you spend, it's how you spend the time
- Onstage — off stage
- Expectation creation

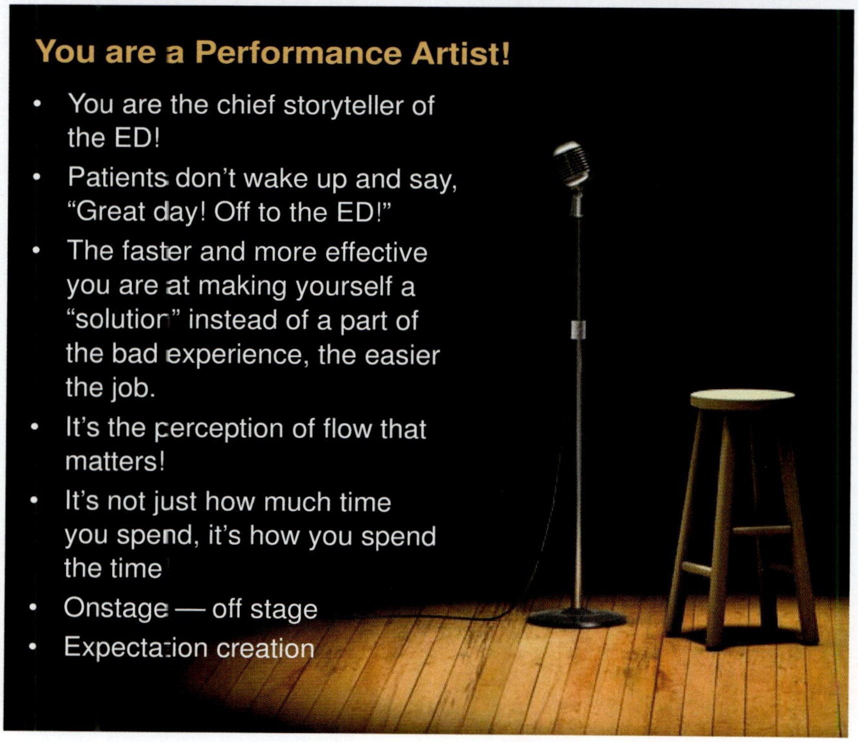

Body Language

While it may seem obvious, taking the time to speak to the patient and family is extremely powerful. It not only shows that the provider is taking the time to really listen, it "changes the plane" by moving the provider nearer to the eye level of the patient. Open communication takes the ED team member from an unintentionally intimidating figure in a white coat or scrubs to a compassionate professional. Studies indicate that patients and families estimate that clinicians who sit during the encounter spend three to five times longer in the room than those who stand.[5,17,18] To be sure, having the ability and a place to sit is paramount, as many EDs do not have stools or chairs. In addition, there should be hangers in each room, so the patient can hang up their clothes; otherwise, the stool or chair will have clothes on it.

Sitting face to face with the patient also makes it more likely that the provider will smile at the patient. The power of a smile is exerted both for the benefit of the patient and for the ED team members. (Research indicates that when endorphins are measured, a smile is worth 200 chocolate bars![19]) Smiling makes it much more likely that others will smile in response, generating a sort of endorphin cascade.

When sitting, it is much easier to approach the patient with open body language than when standing. Standing tends to encourage most people to fold their arms across their chest. This gives the patient and family a defensive message, which unintentionally communicates that the provider has a negative image of the encounter.[20,21] Finally, sitting at the bedside makes it easier to touch the patient by holding a hand or simply taking a pulse. The art of healing is often perceived to begin with the "healing touch." The earlier that healing touch occurs, the better will be the patient's experience, particularly if the physician or nurse says something like, "Your pulse is nice and strong. That's always a good sign."

Active Listening

Active listening is an evidence-based approach that results in co-creation (with the patient) of optimal outcomes in clinical and patient experience through interactive communication.[5,6] The importance of active listening is perhaps best demonstrated by data that indicate that the average amount of time a provider interrupts a patient after asking a question is 48 seconds for a nurse and 12 seconds for a doctor.[22] Health-care providers generally have not been taught to listen well or patiently.[20] **Box 73.1** illustrates ways in which active listening can be put to use.[23] Regardless of which specific techniques are utilized, active listening should be

---

BOX 73.1 ■ ACTIVE LISTENING EXAMPLES

- "Discharge instructions are very important to us. In fact, they are so important, I am going to ask you to repeat them back to me when I finish."
- "You have pain in your right upper quadrant, which we call 'guarding'; however, you don't have rebound, which is good. You also have some 'crackles' in your right lung base, which I think is due to the pain, not pneumonia. The nurse will give you some pain medication and something to help the nausea and then she will draw some blood at the same time she starts the IV. The blood work will look for infection, check your blood count, and look at your liver and gall bladder function. We'll also bounce some sound waves off your gall bladder to check out and a chest x-ray, just to make sure there isn't any pneumonia. To make sure you understand, please repeat what I just told you; we want to keep you well-informed."
- "So, if I understand correctly, this chest pain is sharper, more sudden, and doesn't feel like the heart attack you had two years ago—is that right?"

a fundamental discipline that all ED team members exhibit in their daily care of patients. Its effectiveness has repeatedly been shown in multiple studies.[3,7-9]

Blameless, Effective Apologies

Parents teach their children that the two most powerful words in the English language are "I'm sorry." This is particularly true in the health-care environment, where so much of what is done seems cold and impersonal—from the delays patients encounter to the frankly dehumanizing gowns they are forced to wear, to the fact that they are sometimes referred to as numbers instead of persons. The apology should be blameless in that it doesn't assign or accept fault; instead, it should simply emphasize that an apology is in order.

These aren't scientific or technical ways of speaking; they are personal ones. For most people, it gets the relationship back on track. There are many excellent resources on apology and its power in human communication.[5-8,24] Recent work has also accentuated the role of compassionate language in health care. Indeed, the term *compassionomics* proposes that empathy has a clear financial value.[24]

THE THREE SURVIVAL SKILLS

Patient Experience Diagnosis and Treatment

The first ED service excellence core competency is making the patient experience diagnosis and providing the right treatment. When this concept is initially presented, many experienced ED clinicians legitimately ask: "Are you saying the patient experience diagnosis is more important than the clinical diagnosis?" The answer is—and always should be—a resounding, "No, of course not!" To be clear, the patient experience diagnosis is never more important than the clinical diagnosis. However, as noted earlier, this insight is equally true: The clinical diagnosis and the patient experience diagnosis cannot ever be separated one from the other. They are inextricably and unavoidably linked.[5-8]

A simple exercise called the Patient-CustoMeter illustrates this shows a simple meter that will point either toward "patient" or toward "customer," depending upon the reaction of those hearing three simple case scenarios. There are no right or wrong answers—only the honest answers of the clinicians hearing the scenarios.

> *Scenario one:* A 65-year-old woman with "crushing" substernal chest pain arrives via ambulance with an ECG that shows dramatic ST-segment elevation. She is clearly having a major anterior myocardial infarction. Is this more a patient or more a customer?
>
> *Scenario two:* A 3-year-old boy is brought to the ED at 3 a.m. by his parents, having been seen by the child's pediatrician at 3 p.m. the same day. The pediatrician diagnosed otitis media, gave the child a dose of antibiotic, a prescription for the antibiotic, and fever-control instructions. He has a temperature of 99.2°F and the parents say they "can't get the fever down." Is this more of a patient or more of a customer?
>
> *Scenario three:* Scenario three is precisely the same as scenario two, with this difference — this time it is your child. Now is this a patient or a customer?

Having conducted this experiment with tens of thousands of health-care providers, without exception, scenario one is listed as a patient and scenario two is listed as a customer. (For scenario three, the needle wavers a bit.) Consistently, the reasoning is the woman in scenario one is considered a patient because she is severely ill and needs immediate care. The child in scenario two is rated as a customer because the gestalt feeling is that he is not acutely ill and only needs reassurance and fever-control instructions for his parents. The point is simple: Each time ED clinicians enter a room to evaluate and treat those served, a tacit, silent question arises: "Is this a patient, or is this a customer?"

This resonates with ED providers because they understand that rule means "patients," when horizontal, are clearly ill or injured; require more immediate stabilization, evaluation, and treatment; tend to be brought in by ambulance; require a room or stretcher quickly; and need our technical skills, often immediately. In contrast, "customers" are perceived as not as acutely ill or injured, are usually ambulatory, can afford to wait, and need our service skills to a higher degree than our purely technical skills (or so the ED staff believes). Of considerable interest is the response to this question:

Who has higher expectations: the woman (patient) or the child with the fever (whose parents are considered customers)?

Having asked this question of thousands of ED providers, without exception, the answer has been that the parents of the child have higher expectations than the woman with the heart attack. As curious as this may seem at first, for trained critical care emergency physicians and nurses, this makes a curious sort of sense, in that what the woman expects—lifesaving care, expertly and immediately provided—is precisely what those nurses and doctors *love* to provide. After all, it is largely what drew them to the ED in the first place. What the parents need—education and reassurance (so they can confidently go to sleep!)—is not all that difficult, but it is also not something discretely taught in medical and nursing schools. *Make the patient experience diagnosis in addition to, not to the exclusion of, the clinical diagnosis—and offer the right treatment for both.*

Making the customer service diagnosis and offering the right treatment involve a number of specific skills (**Table 73.1**). The first is to provide a clear, concise, and disciplined introduction to the patient, which can be done in many ways but needs to be consistent. As Spinoza wisely notes, "Excellence is what we strive for, but consistency is what we demand."[25] One way to do that is to use the mnemonic developed by Huron Consulting, AIDET (**a**cknowledge, **i**ntroduce, **d**uration, **e**xplanation, and **t**ime estimate).[10]

Regardless of the specific system, all ED staff must understand first the importance of disciplined communication, starting with the introduction. Second, ensure that family members and visitors are acknowledged professionally. It is equally important to ensure that the patient is asked what information they want to share with family members and visitors, as well as whether they want them to be present for the examination, treatment, and other phases of care.

Patients and families should be given a preview of what the ED clinical team is thinking and the reason each test or procedure is being done and what information will be gained. Because patients consistently rate health-care providers as not providing an adequate amount of explanation and information, letting patients know, in detail, what they can expect is a key part of exceeding expectations.[17,18,22] In providing previews, active

TABLE 73.1 ■ Making the Customer Service Diagnosis

CLINICAL Diagnosis	CUSTOMER SERVICE Diagnosis
Pediatric fever	Meningitis
Chest pain	Myocardial infarction
Abdominal pain	Appendicitis
Abdominal >50 years old	Cancer

> **BOX 73.2 ■ COMMUNICATE REASONABLE EXPECTATIONS**
>
> 1. Introduce yourself in a professional fashion. Consider AIDET.
> 2. Address family members and bring them into the encounter, guided by the patient.
> 3. Provide "previews" of what to expect, and use expectation creation.
> 4. Provide information as soon as it becomes available to reduce fear and anxiety.
> 5. Establish a high level of professionalism—on stage, always.
> 6. Check the patient's progress multiple times.
> 7. Never underestimate creature comforts: pillows, warm blankets, water, juice, and information.

listening (discussed later in this chapter) is valuable in ensuring patients and families have understood the information provided. In making time estimates, it is wise to create expectations that the team could reasonably exceed.[15] For example, if a chest radiograph is expected to be complete within 45 minutes, the staff might be encouraged to say, "The chest x-ray may take as long as an hour to an hour and a half to complete. Once the results are back, you will know as quickly as we do." **Box 73.2** gives examples of scripts that emphasize previews and expectation creation.

In the ED clinical encounter, knowledge is power, so the staff must be taught to provide information to the patient as soon as possible after receiving it. For example, for a patient older than 50 years with abdominal pain, cancer is a major part of the patient's fear or customer service diagnosis. If a CT scan is obtained, the patient and family intuitively know that this study has the answer to the question of whether cancer has been detected or not. Once the patient returns from the CT scan, the results of the scan should be made available to the patient as quickly as possible to allay fear and anxiety. This helps exceed expectations by quickly and efficiently addressing what is known is to be a concern.

Checking the patient's progress multiple times through the course of their ED stay—particularly if they will be there more than an hour—is an important way to make sure the patient and family know the staff members are checking in. Research has consistently shown that patients value multiple evaluations to a single, even longer encounter.[16-18]

Finally, all staff members should be encouraged to identify and address the "creature comforts," including pillows, warm blankets, water, and food (unless the patient is to have nothing by mouth). Who should address these needs? Simply stated, whoever identifies the need should address the need. As an experienced emergency physician once said, "It actually takes me less time to get the blanket out of the warmer and give it to the patient than it does to find a technician to do it." All of these small measures are ways of enhancing the ED patient's sense of dignity, which is extremely important in that many EDs appear as if they were systematically designed to strip patients of their dignity.

All of these steps constitute a strategy designed to ensure that the staff consciously puts forth an effort to make both the clinical diagnosis and the customer service diagnosis. The first is treated with technical skills and the latter with effective communication skills.[18]

Negotiating Agreement and Resolution of Expectations

The second service excellence core competency is *negotiating agreement and resolution of expectations*. As indicated in the beginning of this chapter, it is essential to recognize that patients and families bring their own discrete set of expectations to the ED clinical encounter. Perhaps less well known is that each ED staff member brings a set of expectations to the

> **BOX 73.3 ■ DISCOVERING OUR EXPECTATIONS**
>
> **The first step in negotiating expectations is for the staff to discover their own, which can be done by addressing these questions:**
>
> - Am I well-rested?
> - Where is my stress tolerance level?
> - How many hours/patients are left in the shift?
> - How stressful has the shift been so far?
> - What are my specific expectations for this patient?
> - Am I ready to be open-minded, unstressed, and at the top of my game with this patient?

encounter as well. Discovering the expectations of the ED staff begins even before they go to work and requires an introspective look at the several issues listed in **Box 73.3**.

Perhaps the most important question is what the individual staff member's specific expectations are for the specific patient being treated. Once that is known, it is essential to determine the patient's expectations for his or her ED care. How can this be done? Simply use the Precision Patient Care question: "What's the most important thing we can do to make this an *excellent* ED visit?"

Once the patient's or parents' expectations are known, they should be verbalized back to confirm their expectations. (This process, known as *active listening*, is discussed in more detail later in the chapter.) To the extent that there are differences between the providers' and the patients' expectations, those differences must be negotiated, so there is a common understanding of what the staff can do to meet or exceed expectations. While the ED staff negotiates on various issues in health care throughout the course of a clinical shift (**Box 73.4**), very few providers have been through a formal course on negotiation skills.

Chapter 99 provides an excellent and in-depth treatment of negotiation skills. One of the best treatises available on negotiation is the book *Getting to Yes* by Fisher, Ury, and Patton, which presents a key concept: inventing options for mutual gain.[26] Too often, negotiation is viewed as "splitting the difference," but inventing options for mutual gain is a far more pragmatic way of dealing with negotiations around differences in patient and staff expectations.

Building Moments of Truth Into the Clinical Encounter

The third service excellence core competency is creating moments of truth in the clinical encounter. The concept of moments of truth was first described by Jan Carlzon, then the CEO of Scandinavian Airlines.[27] Upon undertaking the difficult role of guiding an airline that

> **BOX 73.4 ■ COMMON ED NEGOTIATIONS**
>
> - Can this patient be moved out of the room?
> - Can I get a critical care bed for my patient?
> - Shall I admit this patient to your service or to the cardiologist?
> - We are two nurses down; how shall we cover the patients we have?
> - There are 10 hospital boarders in our rooms and hallways; how can we get beds upstairs?

was fraught with problems and near bankruptcy, Carlzon wisely addressed huge gatherings of the employees of Scandinavian in this (paraphrased) way:

> As employees of Scandinavian Airways, you have been defining the success of the airlines as a certain number of planes taking off and landing on time, getting there safely, with specified revenue and load capacities, assuring the appropriate fuel burn rates, and getting the bags to the right place at the right time. All of this is certainly important, but it is not actually how the airline is defined. The airline is defined by 50,000 moments of truth a day. Those moments of truth occur when you, the employees of the airline, have contact with the 50,000 customers who fly our airline each and every day. That's how the airline is defined — not by metrics alone or even by the CEO or the board of directors — but by you, the frontline employees who take care of the customer.

Each member of the ED team has a chance, each day and with each patient, to define the department. It is the care and concern of those evaluating and treating the patient that is remembered far more than the technical skills needed to deliver that care. Indeed, most experienced emergency nurses and physicians have learned, many times over, that the kindness and compassion shown to patients and their families not only outlives the clinical encounter, it sometimes outlives the patient.

TAXI, TAKEOFF, FLIGHT PLANS, LANDING

When Karl Weick and Katherine Sutcliffe presented their landmark work on high-reliability organizations, two of the entities they studied were naval aircraft carriers and EDs.[29] Stimulated by their insights, Mayer undertook site visits to Nimitz-class aircraft carriers to examine similarities between naval aircraft and ED operations.[4-8] Among many insights, one of the most important is the analogy of launching aircraft from the carrier to the patient encounter: "taxi, takeoff, flight plans, and landing."

Taxi

The amount of preparation it takes to move aircraft into position to takeoff is staggering. The aircraft is brought to the flight deck by massive elevators. With incredible precision, they are positioned on the flight line while being monitored from the tower. So detailed and precise are these operations that a review of naval operations indicates there is only one "crunch" (an aircraft touching another aircraft) in every 2 million aircraft movements. The aircraft is weighed, rechecked, and complete taxiing to the flight line. In health care, the team members also "taxi" as they prepare each time to enter the patients' rooms.

Takeoff

The "takeoff" is the most dramatic aspect of carrier flight, but it has a strong correlation with ED patient care as well—rapid, heart-racing for the patient and the caregiver and even a bit dangerous, if not handled well.

Parents often tell their children: "You never get a second chance to make a first impression!" Simple, yet true in so many ways. The patient and their family will take a distinct and lasting impression from each team member's first entry and their first words. Make these interactions count. Enter with a flourish—whether as the doctor or the nurse—they are the ones who the patients have come to see. They will be the chief storytellers, the sense makers, of their journey. Knock on the door if possible and say who you are, what you are there for, and that you are a part of team. If appropriate, ask "May we come in?" All of these are ways of showing courtesy and respect.

Make sure the first words to the patient are carefully thought through, rehearsed, and designed to make the maximum impact.[31] Make sure you know what your script will be when you enter the room. Think it through. To be sure, it will be somewhat different, depending upon the clinical situation. But don't leave it to chance. Prepare. Everyone will handle this aspect of the "takeoff" differently, but it should never be left to chance.

> ***Example:*** *Good morning Mrs. Smith. I'm Dr. Thom Mayer, and I am working with the entire team to take care of you in our emergency department today. I'm sorry you're not feeling well, but I am very happy to be your doctor today. Here's what I know so far regarding your symptoms based on my conversation with your nurse, Caroline, and Dr. Jones, the emergency medicine resident on your team. Is that information correct?*

That language may not work for everyone, but find language that *does* work, seems comfortable, and reflects both professionalism and personal commitment. The last line is an example of using active listening to make sure the information obtained is correct and pulls the patient into their care at the outset—the takeoff! Patients will definitely have questions. Acknowledge this by asking, "What questions do you have?" This is more effective than simply asking, "Do you have any questions?" Make sure they know that you and the team will listen carefully and answer them.

Use the A-Team behavior of sitting down at the bedside to meet the patient's eye level. Remember, patients will estimate that you spent considerably more time with them if you do. Establish physical contact. There is nothing stronger than the ancient ritual of "laying on of hands" by doctors and nurses, and it should never be neglected.

The Flight Plan

Just as pilots file a different flight plan for each trip, depending on their destination and existing conditions, physicians and nurses need to understand that the flight plan for each patient is different, depending upon their clinical presentation. Use evidence-based language and expectation creation (estimating the time needed for tests and treatment, increasing the amount to ensure we meet our goals, and communicating this to the patient and family) to help them understand the flight plan for their clinical presentation. Make sure the patient and family are told: "These tests will tell us . . .," "This medicine is for . . .," and "This medicine has the following side effects . . ."

All of this is part of the role as chief storyteller, a role that helps patients and families make sense of their journey by explaining the details of what is being done and why. Not only does this take an "open-book test" approach by addressing the specifics of the patient experience they will be asked about on the survey, it also shows courtesy and respect. It also serves the fundamental purpose of making a patient and family an important part of the team, changing them from recipients of care into participants in their care.

Below is an important verbal technique developed by Ralph Badenowski, an emergency physician at St. Vincent's in Jacksonville, Florida. Consider the following conversation between a fictional physician and patient with abdominal pain. Keep in mind that patients with this common presentation must typically remain in the ED for several hours.[32]

> *Ma'am, my experience with evaluating and treating patients like you with abdominal pain, which is actually the most common type of complaint we see, is that it will take us about 4 hours to complete your workup since we will be getting lab work, giving you IV fluids, medication, and a CT scan.* **But during those 4 hours, we'll be getting about 10 days' worth of work done!**

It's a brilliant way to handle expectation creation, negotiate expectations, and help the patient understand the distinct bargain that an ED visit represents. It also lets the family know how long the patient is expected to be there, in case they have to pick up the kids from the bus or they have a call they need to make. It is a fundamental sign of respect.

Patients present to the ED confused, concerned, and often in pain. Part of the "flight plan" should be to tell them: "We knew you were coming. We just didn't know your name!" All good emergency nurses and physicians know from experience the types of patients they see in a typical day and even the times of day they see them. To be sure, statistical analysis can be used to verify this, but the gestalt of an experienced clinician is more than adequate to predict the type of cases that will present in a given day. Letting the patient know that the team "expected" them helps them understand that, while their symptoms may be new or more severe to them, an experienced team who handles cases like theirs every day is on the job.

Abdominal Pain

What is the most common clinical presentation in the ED? A careful statistical analysis of ED visits makes clear what instincts have already suggested: It is abdominal pain. A carefully thought out and rehearsed abdominal pain "flight plan" should include several essential elements. First, remember that the patient always has both a clinical diagnosis and a customer service diagnosis. Most patients under 50 years of age are concerned they have appendicitis, while those over 50 often are concerned they might have cancer. Of course, if they have chronic conditions, that will change the customer service diagnosis. Evidence-based scripts should be used to communicate:

It must be scary to have so much pain. We'll be giving you some medication for that.

I am so sorry you are so nauseated, but we have a great medication called ondansetron that will shut that down. Fortunately, it doesn't have any significant side effects.

All this vomiting has made you dehydrated, which can make the nausea worse, so we'll be giving you IV fluids to correct that. When the nurse starts your IV, he'll also draw your blood at the same time so we don't have to stick you twice.

Make sure to tell them why each test is being done and what it is expected to help in making their diagnosis. Give them a preview and use expectation creation with the patient and the family.

Example: I'm concerned your symptoms may represent inflammation of your gall bladder. We will be bouncing some sound waves off your abdomen to check that out. You also have some "crackles" in your right lung base, so we'll get a chest x-ray to check that as well. I don't think that it is pneumonia. I think the pain is keeping you from breathing deeply, which can keep your lungs from expanding.

Be sure to explain the lab tests as well.

Example: We're going to run a CBC. It will tell us if your white blood cells are elevated, which can be a sign of inflammation or infection, and how your red blood cells are as well. A chemistry panel will tell us a lot of information, including if your bilirubin is elevated, which we often see with gallbladder disease and which could explain your dark urine and the change in skin color.

Chest Pain

The second most common clinical presentation in the ED is chest pain. While the vast majority of these patients do not have myocardial infarctions, their biggest fear (the customer service diagnosis) is that they are having a heart attack. A consistent and highly evidence-based clinical approach for all of these patients is taken in the ED. But many could improve on the language used to communicate what that approach means to the patient.

Intuitively, ED team members know that patients with acute chest pain are having the worst day of their lives and are terribly afraid their heart health is in jeopardy. If the initial ECG and troponin are normal, the ED staff knows the patients will be monitored for a few hours, with a repeat troponin and ECG in 2 to 4 hours (depending upon the particular protocol for acute chest syndrome). Evidence-based language to let the patient and the family know what will be done, why, and when is highly effective.

Example: We know that chest pain can be really scary and you've told us your biggest fear is that this could be a heart attack. The good news is that your initial ECG is totally normal.

Take the time to actually show the ECG to them, explaining what areas would be different if there were signs of an MI.

Example: And the troponin level, which is an enzyme that leaks out into the blood if there is damage to the heart muscle, is also completely normal, so that's good.

Now move into previews and expectation creation.

Example: While that's all great, we have a detailed approach to patients with chest pain, so we'll be putting you in this protocol. First, we have you on cardiac monitoring, which the team is constantly watching. We do that because the number one threat if a heart attack were to develop is an abnormal cardiac rhythm, so we'll we monitoring your heart for that. So, even when we're not in the room, we're still monitoring your heart.

If you develop any chest pain, let us know immediately and we'll repeat the ECG, so you are a critical part of our team. If you don't have any further pain, in 2 hours we'll recheck both your ECG and your troponin level. All of that should take about 4 hours. If those tests are normal, our protocol is to have you monitored in our cardiac chest pain unit, where they usually do a cardiac stress test to fully evaluate your potential for cardiac risk. I'll let your doctor know you are here and what the tests show. What questions do you have?

The Pain Flight

One of the most difficult challenges faced in the ED is dealing with patients with chronic pain. While a review of ED statistics actually shows that these patients rarely account for more than 7% to 10% of total cases, most clinicians say it is one of the areas with which they most need help. It is essential that each emergency physician and nurse carefully thinks through what their pain "flight plan" will be, since this clearly is an area of major concern in our society writ large.[33,34]

It is almost always a mistake to refer to patients as "pain patients" or, even worse, as "chronic pain patients" when speaking to them. This will invariably be taken as pejorative at best and judgmental and demeaning at worst. The terms *patients with pain* and *patients with chronic pain* serve better. A discussion among the team regarding this issue is an important and worthwhile approach. Words matter, and these words matter *a lot* to this group of patients. Further, the entire ED team should have open discussions on how, as a department, the team will approach caring for these patients in an evidence-based manner. Some institutions have created "opioid-lite EDs," which focus on managing acute pain with fentanyl and other less-addictive agents.[34]

At its core, our interaction with patients with pain requires us to be highly effective at negotiation, an essential Survival Skills core competency.

Example: Sir, I understand that your current pain level is 8 out of 10. What pain level would you consider successful in managing your pain?

Some patients will say "0," which goes to the point of doing everything we can to reduce their pain. However, "0" is not attainable in most cases. But this question establishes what their expectations are. The majority of patients are reasonable and often say that "2 to 4" is an acceptable level of pain. Once the ED has at least a broad plan for the management of pain patients, each clinician should consider their experience with and approach to pain patients and adopt scripts-evidence-based language. AIDET can be a good start to teeing up such conversations.[34]

Example: My experience with helping thousands of patients with pain is that, while we may not be able to completely eliminate your pain, we can make you much more comfortable. Is that your experience as well?

Example: I'm sorry you are in so much pain.

Example: What medications have worked for you in the past when you've had this level of pain? (Note: The logic of this question may be counterintuitive, but it is a way of directly assessing what the patient's expectations are in a direct and straightforward manner. It brings the issue to the forefront, so it can be dealt with through negotiation.)

Example: How is that medication working? We started out at a pain level of 8 with a goal of cutting it in half to a 4. Have we gotten there?

While it is obvious that multiple nonpharmacologic methods can be used to reduce pain, they may not be as apparent to the patient. Be sure to explain the role of ice, elevation, compression, anti-emetics, and so on. Many EDs (particularly pediatric EDs) have used headphones, music, biofeedback, and other mechanisms to decrease the perception of pain.

Patients With Chronic Pain

Patients with chronic pain clearly warrant special thought and specific actions, representing as they do a group of patients for whom there has traditionally been no easy answer. As ED clinicians, caring for major trauma and acutely ill patients can be challenging, and to care for them is guided by well-known evidence-based guidelines. But far too little literature exists on approaches for chronic pain.

For clinical reasons, always ensure that acute etiologies and sequelae are considered. For example, patients with chronic abdominal pain who are on opiates have extremely thin bowel walls, so perforation needs to be considered and ruled out clinically. Once the "science" side is completed, we need to address the "service" side as well. First, take time to sit down at the bedside. As noted previously, any difficult conversation needs to be done eye to eye, so change the plane and sit at the bedside, preferably establishing some appropriate physical contact (taking the pulse or a hand on the arm or shoulder are good examples). Second, think the conversation through ahead of time. This is a crucial conversation and a script that you will use often.

Example: Ma'am, as I've said before, I am so sorry that you are suffering from this chronic pain. I'm also sorry that no one seems to have figured out a plan to help you reduce this pain to a level that's more tolerable.

We have done tests that have ruled out the most common causes of acute issues that might be contributing to your pain, but those have fortunately all come back negative.

Our team here is really good at dealing with acute pain, and we've tried to do that for you. But, unfortunately, EDs are neither designed nor equipped to deal with chronic pain like yours, I'm sorry to say.

But I have contacted our Pain Management Service, which is a team of specialists who will coordinate your care with your doctor to help in every way they can.

Sometimes nothing works and the patient demands specific medications or doses with which the team is not comfortable. In that case, be clear, concise, and specific.

Example: Sir, I'm very sorry, but I am simply not comfortable prescribing that medication dose because it could ultimately be harmful to do so. I understand you don't agree with me on that, but my experience is that it's not the right thing to do, based on your best interests.

When all else fails, give them someone else to talk with by referring them to the ED medical director or nursing director's voice or email.

Example: I'm sorry we couldn't agree on this, but our emergency department team cares about your experience, so with your permission, I'll let our medical director know about your concerns so she can follow up with you. Is that acceptable?

Landing

As aviators attest, the landing is the most dangerous part of aircraft carrier operations. It also is in many ways the most critical part of the ED experience. Even if the taxi, takeoff, and flight plan phases have gone well, they won't help if the landing is missed.

Discharged Patients

As the chief storytellers of the ED, summarizing the patients' journey for them, pulling aspects of their care together in way that explains their symptoms, their treatment, their diagnostic workup, their presumptive diagnosis, and the treatment plan (another "flight plan"!) they will follow at home are all essential but often-neglected aspects of care. This is an opportunity to tie the entire visit into a summary that gives the patient closure and a chance to ask final questions. Use this opportunity to tie their symptoms to the tests and treatment done, as well as to their follow-up plan.

- Remind them of the previews and expectation creation you gave them during "takeoff."
    - "These tests showed . . ."
    - "These medications are for . . ."
    - "The medication has these possible side effects . . ."
    - "Did you experience any of those side effects?"
- Use ECGs, lab results, and radiographic findings as "tools and toys" by bringing them to the bedside to show the patient.
    - "Have we met your expectations?"
    - "What other questions do you have? We want to answer all your questions."
- Finally, ask them Druckenbrod's details, named for Glenn Druckenbrod, the medical director at Inova Fairfax Medical Campus in Annandale, Virginia[35]:
    - "Have we met your expectations?"
    - "What questions do you have?"
    - "How did we do?"

Other language that can help seal the deal effectively with patients:

- "Are you comfortable with what we've discussed?"
- "Is there anything we can explain better?"
- "I'm sorry this happened to you, but it has been a privilege being your emergency physician/nurse today."
- "Thanks for coming to see us!"

Here's some simple language that works well for ankle sprains:

When I first examined your ankle after you twisted it playing basketball, I was concerned that you had a second-degree ankle sprain since you have pain over your anterior and posterior talo-fibular ligaments here. (Gently touch the ligaments to demonstrate.)

We put ice on it and kept it elevated to help reduce the swelling and gave you ibuprofen for the pain and inflammation as well. As I told you, medicine can cause some slight burning in the abdomen if taken on an empty stomach, but you haven't had that, correct?

As I suspected, your x-ray did show swelling here and here (point to the x-ray), but fortunately there are no signs of fracture, so our diagnosis of a second-degree ankle sprain is confirmed.

Do you remember me saying that if it was a sprain, we would plan to have you rest, ice, wear a compression dressing, and keep this ankle elevated whenever possible, which we call the "RICE" treatment? (Because you gave him a preview and used expectation creation, he was expecting to hear the diagnosis confirmed and has any questions ready.)

This is Jim, a great ED technician with a lot of experience (managing/leading up). He's going to put on a compression dressing and show you how to walk with the crutches he will give you. In the RICE treatment, these are the letters R for rest and C for compression. What questions do you have?

To make sure you understand your discharge instructions, could you please repeat them back to me when I finish? That way we can be sure we understood each other. (Active listening at work.)

Have we met your expectations? How did we do? Here's my card.

Like the "flight plans," it is a good idea to proactively think about the different ways you will handle each of the clinical "landings." You also should discuss with your colleagues what works and what doesn't.

Admitted Patients

The transition from the ED to inpatient care deserves clear, thoughtful closure, incorporating previews, expectation creation, managing/leading up, and the other tools.

Example: *Mrs. Smith, as you recall when you came to us with pain in the upper right side of your abdomen and the terrible vomiting, we suspected that it might be your gallbladder acting up and causing all these problems.*

We started you on IV fluids for dehydration and gave you medication for your pain and your nausea, which seems to have resolved. Is that right?

As we predicted, the gallbladder ultrasound did show thickening of the wall, which means inflammation and gallstones, which are producing the change in your skin color and the dark urine.

Your blood tests showed an elevated white blood cell count and a high bilirubin, which means those stones are creating an obstruction. All of this means you have acute cholecystitis, which means an inflamed gall bladder.

As I promised, I discussed this with your doctor and she agreed you should come into the hospital so we can treat you with antibiotics, which we have already started, and continue to manage your pain and nausea.

> *I called Dr. Rodriguez, who is a specialist in hospital medicine your doctor and I know very well, and he'll take great care of you. I also called Dr. Moynihan, who is an excellent general surgeon, in case it becomes necessary to remove your gallbladder, which is a very common and safe operation he has done hundreds of times. (Managing up and previews)*
>
> *I called the bed control nurse and she tells me they have a bed ready for you and will move you up in the next hour to hour-and-a-half. (Expectation creation)*
>
> *I'm sorry this happened to you, but I am very pleased I could be your doctor here in the ED. Have I met your expectations? How did we do? What questions do you have? Here's my card if you need it.*

THE MYTHS OF IMPOSSIBILITY AND AUTONOMY

Dealing with low scores, sometimes as low as single digits, can be extremely frustrating for members of the ED team. To them, it seems that it just can't be done, at least not here. It's common to hear that "Our patients are different; you can't get high scores with them!" The frustration is understandable, and a search for the reasons often ends by blaming the patient. The *myth of impossibility* rests on the belief that it can't be done here!

Department leaders must disabuse their teams of that notion if progress is to be made. First, remember to focus on the intrinsic motivation of making their jobs easier and not on the scores per se. Use the scores as a tool to accentuate A-Team behaviors, language, and processes, not a club. Second, use individual scores for physicians or shift scores for nurses and the rest of the team to identify higher performers. To be clear, these may not be at the highest levels attainable but are simply those whose scores are higher than others. For example, if the mean scores for the ED or any component group (e.g., physicians, nurses, etc.) are in the single digits, but one or more of the emergency physicians has scores in the 30th percentile, that is significantly higher than the rest of the group, even if they aren't in the 90th percentile. Make the point to the team that, despite the myth of impossibility, high scores are already being achieved by certain members of the team.

A related but distinct concept is the *myth of autonomy*, in which those who have low performance scores say, "I am an autonomous physician/nurse, professionally trained, and I do not practice in the way you are describing." However, in the increasingly evidence-based environment of an ED, autonomy is largely a myth in many clinical areas. Cardiac resuscitation, trauma care, pediatric care, and strokes are but a few examples of highly evidence-based, protocol-driven care in which consistency is valued over autonomy. As has been emphasized, the science of patient experience is simply an extension of the disciplined, evidence-driven manner in which the job can be made easier.

A way to deal with the myth of autonomy is by accentuating the team concept of mutual accountability, meaning all team members hold each other accountable for adherence to "patient first" and "excellence always," if those are the values of the team. For ED leaders, this means having frank conversations.

> **Example:** We respect your desire for autonomy in how you practice, but emergency medicine is always a "team sport," where everyone's practice affects others. You are free to ignore the excellent results that others are getting, but *only if you are able to attain similar or better results. If not, we as a team will coach and mentor you with specific habits, language, and behaviors from those whose scores have been consistently better. And we think you'll find it also helps you to enjoy your job more.*

Disabusing team members of the myths of impossibility and autonomy is best handled through coaching, mentoring, and "shadow shifting."

COACHING, MENTORING, AND SHADOW SHIFTING

It is important to emphasize the critical role that using the effective and highly specific experience of the A-Team members to guide improvement among the B-Team members (as well as to sustain improvement in themselves) requires using the tools of coaching and mentoring. "Shadow shifting" is a concept whereby A-Team members, whose habits have produced predictably high results, work with B-Team members to help coach and mentor them toward best-practices language and behaviors that would help make their jobs easier and their patients' lives better. This tool is highly successful in delivering specific guidance, based on the A-Team members' experience and their demonstrated results on the "how" habits resulting in excellent performance. Shadow shifting typically is done for only 3 to 4 hours per session, in which the A-Team member shadows the other physician or nurse, after which a discussion occurs in a positive and collegial fashion.

Example: *I noticed that you only sat down with a few patients. My experience has been that I had to develop sitting down as a habit, which helps my communication.*

It seems to me that you have a tendency at times to stand with your arms crossed over your chest. I've found that if I sit, it sort of forces me to use more open body language, which helps me communicate with the patient better.

One habit I've developed is giving the patient their lab and radiology results as soon as I get them, which my patients seem to like, as opposed to giving them all the results at the end, when they are all back.

CONCLUSION

Achieving and sustaining excellence in patient experience requires a disciplined, evidence-based approach that entails 10 discrete yet related skills that use intrinsic motivation to make the job easier while improving the patient experience.

REFERENCES

1. Mayer T. Putting it all together: education and the right tools to create a culture of service. *Healthc Exec.* 2011;26(1):56–59.
2. Mayer T. Patient experience and ED team engagement. Paper presented at: American College of Emergency Physicians (ACEP) Emergency Department Directors Academy (EDDA); November 12, 2018; Dallas, TX.
3. Mayer T. Leadership for great customer service: getting the "why" right before the "how." *Healthc Exec.* 2010;25(3):66,68–69.
4. Mayer T. Drive service excellence to the next level. *Healthc Exec.* 2010;25(6):54,56.
5. Mayer T, Cates RJ. *Leadership for Great Customer Service: Satisfied Employees, Satisfied Patients.* 2nd ed. Health Administration Press; 2014.
6. Mayer T, Cates RJ. *Leadership for Great Customer Service: Satisfied Patients, Satisfied Employees.* Health Administration Press; 2004.
7. Mayer T. Drive service excellence to the next level. *Healthc Exec.* 2010;25(6):54–56.
8. Studer Q. *Results That Last: Hardwiring Behaviors That Will Take Your Company to the Top.* Hoboken, NJ: John Wiley and Sons; 2008.
9. Studer Q. *Hardwiring Excellence: Purpose, Worthwhile Work, Making a Difference.* Pensacola, Fla: Fire Starter Publishing; 2003.
10. Delbanco T, Berwick DM, Boufford JI, et al. Healthcare in a land called PeoplePower: nothing about me without me. *Health Expect.* 2001;4(3):144–150.
11. Barry MJ, Edgman-Levitan S. Shared decision making—the pinnacle of patient-centered care. *N Engl J Med.* 2012;366(9):780–781.
12. Harlow H. Motivation as a factor in the acquisition of new responses. In: Brown OH, Judson S, Harlow H, et al, eds. *Current Theory and Research on Motivation—A Symposium.* Lincoln, Neb: University of Nebraska Press; 1953.
13. Emergency department consumer assessment of healthcare providers and systems (ED CAHPS) survey. Available at: https://www.cms.gov/Research-Statistics-Data-and-Systems/Research/CAHPS/ED. Accessed February 1, 2020.
14. Lee F. *If Disney Ran Your Hospital: 9 ½ Things You Would Do Differently.* Bozeman, Mont: Second River Healthcare Press; 2004.
15. Mayer T. Dealing with the B Team members: holding the mirror up can have a positive effect on them and the organization. *Healthc Exec.* 2010:52–54.
16. Spinoza B. *Ethics.* Curley E, ed. New York, NY: Penguin; 1994.
17. Lee F. *If Disney Ran Your Hospital: 9 ½ Things You Would Do Differently.* Bozeman, Mont: Second River Healthcare Press; 2004.

18. Aristotle. *Nichomachean Ethics*. Ross D, trans. Oxford: Oxford University Press; 2009.
19. Baker SK. *Managing Patient Expectations: The Art of Finding and Keeping Loyal Patients*. San Francisco, Calif: Jossey-Bass; 1998.
20. Baker SJ. Hourly rounding in the emergency department: how to accelerate results. *J Emerg Nurs*. 2012;38(1):69–72.
21. Grossman A, Sutton JR. Endorphins: what are they? how are they measured? what is their role in exercise? *Med Sci Sports Exerc*. 1985;17(1):74–81.
22. Swayden KJ, Anderson KK, Connelly LM, et al. Effect of sitting vs standing on perception of provider time at bedside: a pilot study. *Patient Educ Couns*. 2012;86(2):166–171.
23. Chen PW. What doctors are telling us even when they're not talking. *Well* (blog). Available at: http://well.blogs.nytimes.com/2012/02/09/what-doctors-are-telling-us-even-when-theyre-not-talking/. Accessed April 15, 2019.
24. Groopman J. *How Doctors Think*. Boston, Mass: Houghton Mifflin; 2009.
25. Reichheld FF. *The Loyalty Effect: The Hidden Force Behind Growth, Profits, and Lasting Value*. Brighton, Mass: Harvard Business Press; 1996
26. Trzeciak S, Mazzarelli A. *Compassionomics: The Revolutionary Scientific Evidence That Caring Makes a Difference*. Pensacola, Fla: Studer Group; 2019.
27. Spinoza B. *Ethics*. Curley E, ed. New York, NY: Penguin; 1994.
28. Fisher R, Ury WL, Patton B. *Getting to Yes: Negotiating Agreement Without Giving In*. New York, NY: Penguin; 2004.
29. Carlzon J. *Moments of Truth: New Strategies for Today's Customer-Driven Economy*. Pensacola, Fla: Ballinger; 1987.
30. Angelou M. Personal communication to the author (TM), September 1, 2012.
31. Weick KE, Sutcliffe KM. *Managing the Unexpected: Sustaining Performance in a Complex World*. 3rd ed. Hoboken, NJ: Wiley and Sons; 2015.
32. Scheider R, as Bob Fosse. In: *All That Jazz*. Bob Fosse, Director. 20th Century Fox Columbia Pictures; 1979.
33. Peters T. *The Brand You 50: Or Fifty Ways to Transform Yourself From an "Employee" Into a Brand That Shouts Distinction, Commitment, and Passion*. New York, NY: Knopf; 1999.
34. Badenowski R. Personal communication to the author, August 18, 2000.
35. Tefera L, Lehrman WG, Conway P. Measurement of the patient experience: clarifying facts, myths, and approaches. *JAMA*. 2016;315(20):2167–2168.
36. Salam M. The opioid epidemic: a crisis years in the making. *The New York Times*. October 26, 2017. Available at: https://www.nytimes.com/2017/10/26/us/opioid-crisis-public-health-emergency.html. Accessed November 20, 2019.

CHAPTER 74

SCRIPTS: USING EVIDENCE-BASED LANGUAGE TO IMPROVE SERVICE

Robert W. Strauss, Thom A. Mayer

What we say and the words we choose has a tremendous impact on our patients. The right words can calm, comfort, and reassure. The wrong words can produce anxiety and create confusion in a situation that is likely already stressful.[1]

—Regina Shupe

Every patient's journey through the emergency department involves a series of service transitions from one area and person to another, involving predictable interactions among patients and staff. The concept of using powerful communication tools to plan for and script the interaction with the patient simply anticipates these communications. Further, it supports providers by empowering them with specific words or phrases to effectively address patient issues and improve the interaction with the patients and their families. Scripting is evidence-based because it relies on verbal skills that reliably and predictably manage the service transitions and interactions in a positive fashion. These communication tools enhance the patient and family perceptions of care. Just as an evidence-based approach is widely used in clinical settings, scripts allow clinicians to benefit from decades of experience with patients to guide our language skills.

—Paraphrased from Mayer and Cates[2]

Our patients and their families come to us at a time of desperation—often confused and in pain. They have the sincere hope that we will provide comfort and relief and that our words will help to alleviate, and not exacerbate, their fear and anxiety. Yet some health-care personnel don't even introduce themselves or describe what is going to happen. Excuses like "I'm too busy," or "My job is to make you better, not be nice," ignore the well-understood healing power of warmth, sympathy, and understanding as described in the modern version of the Hippocratic Oath[3]:

> *I will remember that there is art to medicine as well as science, and that warmth, sympathy, and understanding may outweigh the surgeon's knife or the chemist's drug.*

The American Association of Medical Colleges (AAMC) is responsible for designing and administering the Medical College Admissions Test (MCAT). In an effort to better prepare physicians to work in a reformed health-care system in which patient satisfaction is highly valued, an entire section on the social and behavioral aspects of care was added to the MCAT in 2015. The AAMC recognizes the importance of sociocultural and behavioral determinants, including communications skills, in the successful practice of medicine. As of 2016, all medical students have been educated in a system in which communication skills are highly valued.[4]

RESISTANCE

Staff members may initially resist the concept of "scripting" patient interactions. Some resistance stems from the perception that it is demeaning for a professional to be told what to say. These clinicians may assert that a sophisticated health-care worker is not an actor who just "parrots" words in response to certain cues. Rather, they claim, clinicians must address every situation differently without preconceived phrases or lines.

Scripts Are a Cultural Necessity

While many may initially state that scripts are objectionable, all will admit that the dictates of culture lead everyone to use scripts on a daily basis and even teach these scripts to children. These routine phrases conform to societal expectations and allow communications to occur easily and habitually. **Table 74.1** provides several examples of typical key phrases that people learn as children and use throughout life.

Another form of resistance occurs when professionals are encouraged to take responsibility for their patients and then are told to perform certain functions in a particular way, as is exemplified by the statement:

> *First you tell us we are empowered to do whatever is best for the patient, then you try to control what we say and exactly how we say it.*

Staff members can be simultaneously empowered and encouraged to use time-tested, evidence-based approaches when communicating. This concept is similar to using proven clinical protocols, such as advanced trauma life support for trauma patients, advanced cardiac life support for cardiac patients, and advanced pediatric life support for pediatric patients. By practicing and implementing these known protocols, clinicians produce consistent results. In a similar way, evidence-based language can be used daily to consistently and effectively guide communications with patients in the emergency department (ED).

The ED "Why"

The concept of using key phrases to enhance patient interactions simply recognizes the frequency of patients' concerns and provides specific "previously considered" words or

TABLE 74.1 ■ Common "Scripts" Used Every Day	
In Response to a . . .	**Admitted Version A**
Kind gesture	Thank you.
Accidental intrusion	Excuse me.
Typical greeting	Fine thank you, how are you?
Recognizing a person in need	May I help you?
Introduction	Hello, I'm Rob. What's your name?
When you need some time	I'll be with you in a moment.

phrases to effectively address them. When clinicians are stressed, spontaneous responses seldom lead to resolution and sometimes exacerbate the situation. It is generally accepted that patient satisfaction surveys reflect how a patient (or family member) feels about the care they received. Because patient concerns are common and familiar, well-formulated phrases can be used to successfully address them. Beyond this intuitive concept, patients who like and trust their providers are much more likely to follow their advice and be more compliant with the instructions they receive.

Adaptive Scripts

> *As a leader, it is OK to tell people what to do, but not exactly how to do it.*
>
> —David C. Leach, MD, Executive Director, Accreditation Council for Graduate Medical Education (ACGME) (1997-2007)[5]

The goal is to help others understand:

- *Why* it is important to communicate effectively with patients, their families, and other ED stakeholders who may be experiencing extreme stress
- *What* type of communication is most likely to decrease that stress

The goal is *not* to tell them:

- Exactly *how* to say the words
- Precisely *which* words to use

The concept of adaptive scripts permits staff, within reason, to create variations on the phrases that allow them to comfortably use their own words to address patient needs. It is certainly acceptable for staff members to adapt, modify, and improve on scripts. However, avoiding communications that can effectively address a patient's anxiety, fears, or requests for information is not an acceptable solution. As discussed in detail later in this chapter, well-formulated patient satisfaction phrases accomplish several goals. They are easy to use, provide consistent approaches to sometimes-difficult situations, and address concepts that enhance the patient's experience of care.

PATIENT EXPERIENCE SURVEYS

Since most patients are incapable of determining the clinical quality of the care they receive (e.g., whether the x-ray was correctly read or the best antibiotic chosen), they typically evaluate the quality of their visit based on the quality of the "caring" they experienced. In general, health-care providers (with the possible exception of Dr. House from the TV series "House" [2004-2012]) prefer that patients perceive both the care and the caring to be excellent. The effective use of scripts or, as the Studer Group refers to them, "key words at key times," allows the intent of high-quality care and caring to be simultaneously demonstrated and perceived.[6]

Multiple companies assess the patient experience.[7] More than 20 of these firms responded to Modern Healthcare's recent survey. Payments to clinicians are increasingly affected by results of these surveys. Medicare utilizes Consumer Assessment of Healthcare Providers and Systems (CAHPS) principles and has developed hospital-specific "HCAHPS" surveys. The Centers for Medicare and Medicaid Services now uses Emergency Department Patient Experience of Care (EDPEC) surveys for assessing the experiences of patients discharged to the community and those admitted from the

TABLE 74.2 ■ Number of Questions Relating to Various Aspects of ED Care

Questions Relating to:	Admitted Version A	Admitted Version B	Discharged
Going to ED	3	4	4
During ED visit	5	8	12
ED staff	3	2	8
Leaving ED	1	2	6
ED experience	1	2	2
Total	13	18	32

ED.[8] These surveys recognize that the ED is a unique area of care within the health-care environment that:

- Bridges outpatient and inpatient care
- Provides short-term care, distinct from hospitalization or a primary care physician's ongoing care
- Provides a "safety net" and resources for patients who may have no other access to care

For these reasons, ED surveys require a distinct set of questions (**Table 74.2**) relating to patient arrival, care, and transition (discharge or admission). The EDPECS survey was implemented in 2020, initially as an elective choice for hospital EDs. The increased detail in these questions may enable nurses and emergency physicians to better improve the patient experience. As the results of these surveys are increasingly tied to reimbursement, their outcomes will be accepted by the health-care industry and our hospital C-suites as an accurate reflection of the patient experience.

If one accepts that these survey questions (**Box 74.1**) adequately reflect how patients feel about the service they received, well-formulated scripts can be used to successfully address any important concerns. Regardless of which survey is used, all ED team members should be familiar with the questions being asked by their institution.[2] The survey should be

BOX 74.1 ■ TYPICAL PATIENT SATISFACTION QUESTIONS

- Staff cared about you as a person?
- Kept you informed about delays?
- Medical care worth the money charged?
- Reasonable length of stay?
- Physician and nurses informative about treatments?
- Adequacy of information provided to family/friends?
- Physician and nurses' attention shown to you?
- Courtesy shown to family/friends?
- Nurses took problem seriously?
- Courtesy of nurses?
- Nurses' concern for privacy?
- Physician and nurses addressed pain effectively?

treated as an "open book test."[9] In other words, knowledge of what is essential to patients and their families gives providers and staff the ability to address these important issues through the use of scripts.

Expectation Management

If the satisfaction of customers (patients) is defined as the degree to which their expectations are met or exceeded, then it is necessary to first understand their expectations.[10-13] In emergency medicine, patients expect:

- Quality care
- Rapid and efficient care
- Caring care

Expectation management is simply a matter of anticipating and addressing the patient's assumptions:

> To create patient satisfaction, it is necessary to meet, to exceed, and sometimes to negotiate *lower* expectations.[14]

Although it may seem counterintuitive, in order to meet expectations, the expectations must first be lowered. Many consumers have developed an expectation that products and services (especially "emergency" care) will be immediate. Patients and their families may be familiar with any of several ED television series, such as "ER," in which multiple lives are saved in 42 minutes of programming. This poor understanding of the exigencies of a real ED may prompt unrealistic assumptions. Negotiating lower, more realistic expectations by describing what will actually happen may create the only opportunity to subsequently meet or exceed (now-lowered) expectations.

The authors of this chapter suggest providing patients with a slightly exaggerated estimate of the duration of their visit. There are two reasons for this. First, when describing duration, most providers convey, in hopeful tones, the "best-case" time frame. In fact, the actual procedures, tests, and reports, often take longer than estimated. Second, if the process takes less time than described, then the provider can actually *exceed* the patients' (new and lowered) expectations.

WELL-FORMULATED SCRIPTS

A well-formulated scripted response (**Table 74.3**) is designed to simultaneously accomplish several goals. All scripts should:

- Be easy to use
- Provide consistent approaches to sometimes-difficult situations
- Utilize words that appear in subsequent patient experience surveys
- Communicate what patients want to hear (empathy, concern) in words that are comfortable to use
- Incorporate feedback and input from ED team members to hone or improve the scripts

Effective communicators share what is important to them. Providers who use "I" statements or use the words "to me" or "by me" create a personal connection while taking responsibility for the intention described. Similarly, when personalizing the action by including "you" or "your," the patients know that the actions and efforts that the providers are taking are about them, their comfort, their privacy, and so on. Using the words "important to me" or "care about your . . ." lets the other person know that the issue has significance

TABLE 74.3 ■ Four Components of the Ideal Script	
Component	Words
Personalizing the provider	I, me, we
Personalizing the patient	You, your
Importance to (sincerity of) the speaker	"... important to ..." "... care about ..."
Issue addressed	"Privacy, comfort, inform ..."

to the speaker. This is an additional way of personalizing care and demonstrating that the provider is an empathetic individual whose intent is to provide excellent care.

The fourth component of effective scripts is "naming the issue." Consider the action of closing the door (or curtain) to ensure the patient's privacy:

- Closing the door will not be remembered two weeks later as an act of ensuring privacy.
- Stating, "I'm closing your curtain" only describes the action but not the intent.
- Declaring, "I'm closing the door so that we can have *privacy*," lets the patients know why and allows them to recognize the specific way the provider is meeting their needs. Further, when the survey asks about "privacy," it is likely that the patients will answer positively.

Phrases like, "I care about your ..." and "Your ... is important to me," all add to the patient's perception that the provider cares about them as a person.

Patient Privacy and Comfort

Every provider recognizes the need for patient privacy and discreet communication. The Health Insurance Portability and Accountability Act (HIPAA) and institutional compliance programs regularly emphasize this requirement.[15] To address patient privacy, providers typically close curtains/doors and, when appropriate, lower their voices. While providers understand what *they* are doing to ensure patient privacy, the patients themselves are often unaware of this important process, and the sincere effort goes unrecognized. Surprisingly, patients may give low scores even when their privacy was effectively addressed. To ensure that patients recognize the steps being taken to guard their privacy, clinicians may want to verbally describe their actions:

I am closing the curtain because your privacy is important to me.

I am closing the door to give you privacy.

I am very sorry you are in the hallway, but we will get you into a more private setting as quickly as possible.

When I leave, would you like me to close the door for your privacy?

Lack of privacy can be very disturbing to patients, especially those who must initially remain in hallways and other open treatment areas. These people, who often feel vulnerable and exposed, may be subjected to multiple conversations, laughter, and drama that are totally unrelated to their current situation. It is critical to use language that puts these patients at ease and explains the advantages of addressing their complaints now, rather than keeping them in the waiting room:

> *I'm sorry that we do not have a room for you at this moment. I felt it was important to take care of you now, rather than make you wait in the waiting room. We'll do whatever we can to give you some privacy until we get you in a room. I will start your treatment now. Is that OK?*

Emergency departments are uncomfortable. Patients, who are ill and often in pain, are put in rooms that are small and too cold (or warm), placed on gurneys that are awkward and uncomfortable, and given food that is tasteless. And, of course, much of what providers do causes additional discomfort. Thus, every effort staff members take to address comfort can change the entire patient experience. Rather than feeling like a "number," comfortable patients recognize that the staff actually cares about them. There are many phrases that can be adapted to demonstrate concern for comfort:

> *I am concerned about your comfort. May I get you a warm blanket?*
>
> *What can I do to make you more comfortable?*
>
> *You look uncomfortable. May I raise (lower) the back of your bed?*
>
> *You look like you're in pain. May I order something to make you more comfortable?*

Delays in Care

Preprocess waits feel longer and create more anxiety than in-process waits.[16] In other words, the time patients spend waiting to see the provider is generally more difficult than the time they spend in the ED after being seen. Simply acknowledging the patient's wait can have an appeasing effect:

> *I'm sorry that you've had to wait . . . I'm here to take care of you now.*
>
> *It's difficult to wait when you're ill . . . I will take care of you now.*

It's really no surprise that patients who are forced to wait become frustrated. After all, how many readers have become angry when simply waiting "too long" for someone to respond to a fast-food order? Frustrated people often look for someone to blame. The examples above offer a "blameless apology/acknowledgment." The provider acknowledges but does not take specific responsibility for the patient's wait. Further, the provider has followed the blameless apology by giving the patient exactly what he or she wanted—the provider's care and attention.

Generally, ED patients don't know what to expect during their visit, which increases their anxiety and, correspondingly, their perception of pain. Even the most minor ED visits involve some degree of anxiety and disruption, and it is wise to address this prospectively by acknowledging and then reassuring:

Initial acknowledgment

> *I'm sorry this happened to you . . .*
>
> *It sounds like what happened to you was very scary . . .*

Followed by a reassuring statement

> *We handle cases like yours all the time and we will give you the best possible care.*
>
> *I am glad I'm here to take care of you. You will get excellent care by our team.*

> **BOX 74.2 ■ A-I-D-E-T**
>
> **A** = Acknowledge
> **I** = Introduce
> **D** = Duration
> **E** = Explanation
> **T** = Thank you

Despite the best efforts of ED providers, the multitude of processes involved in patient management often simply take longer to complete than desirable. Patients often don't understand the details of these operational processes and perceive them as "delays." It is advisable to provide patients with an explanation of what is to occur and an estimate of the time it will take: the "D" and "E" of "A-I-D-E-T" (**Box 74.2**).[6]

Because perceived delays in care are often the most frustrating part of an ED visit, most surveys ask if patients were informed about delays. Using the same theories described above, it is important to not only keep patients abreast of any delays but also to let them know that they are being informed about those holdups. It is acceptable, but not ideal to say:

We're still waiting for your laboratory test. Do you have any questions?

The above or similar words that come across like an excuse demonstrate that the providers and staff do not control their own environment. It is substantially more effective to say:

*It's **important** to **me** that **you** are kept **informed** (about delays). We're expecting your laboratory test results. What questions do you have?*

Patients mind waiting less if the providers are courteous and show concern about the wait, and the promise of excellent care make patients believe the wait was worthwhile.

*Hello, I'm _____. I'm the physician (nurse, technician, phlebotomist, nurse practitioner, or other) who will be taking care of you. I'm sorry that you've had to wait. **I intend** to give **you** excellent care.*

There is a three-phased approach to keeping patients informed that, if adopted, almost always leads to an excellent satisfaction score:

1. *Initial interaction*: After the exam and explanation of next steps: "It is **important** to **me** that **you** are kept **informed**. Do you have any questions?"
2. *After updating the patient during the visit*: "Keeping **you informed** is **important** to **me**. Do you have any questions?"
3. *At close*: After explaining the diagnosis and providing discharge instructions: "As I've mentioned, it is **important** to **me** that **you** have been kept **informed**. Do you feel like all your questions have been answered?"

If they answer "yes" to this final question, it is highly likely that they will answer the survey question with a "5" (the highest score).

It is important to remind the staff that blaming other members of the team is both unacceptable *and* unhelpful. Statements like the one below make everyone look bad and encourage the patient to think that the provider does not have control over the care being provided, a sobering thought:

I don't know what's wrong with the lab today. Sometimes they are just so slow!

Encouraging Patient Involvement

Far too often, patients are passive recipients of care rather than active participants who are encouraged to become involved in their health-care decisions. The following examples show ways in which patients can be made a part of the team:

> Mrs. Jones, we have a team of dedicated people who are here to serve you, but you are the most important member of our team. We want to keep you fully informed of every aspect of your care. If you have any questions, please ask them at any time.
>
> As the key team member, we want you to participate in the diagnostic and treatment decisions and understand them completely.
>
> I'd like to perform a physical exam – is this a good time to do that? Would you be more comfortable if your family stayed or stepped out?
>
> Based on what we know so far, here's what we think our plan should be . . . Does that all make sense? Do you agree with the plan?

Addressing Pain

The vast majority of patients who come to an ED have a complaint that involves pain or discomfort.[17-19] Patients have an expectation that their complaint will be addressed.[20] While emergency providers should be experts at managing the clinical aspects of pain as well as addressing patients' expectations of pain, unfortunately, many are not. Even worse, some providers take offense when patients have specific requests regarding pain management. While it may be unrealistic to entirely meet the patients' expectations, it is always appropriate to address them.

To avoid the negative consequences of denying a patient's request, a provider may simply respond: *Yes, it is important to me that your pain is addressed. Let's discuss it.* This acknowledgment neither implies that the provider will acquiesce to any demand nor does it create an unrealistic promise that the pain will be completely eliminated. It simply recognizes the concerns of the patient and expresses the provider's willingness to engage in a discussion about them.

A common and difficult ED problem relates to the care of patients with chronic pain. While there are actually relatively few of these patients, ED staff members may believe that there are many more. When queried about the number of patients inappropriately seeking medication for chronic pain, it is common for groups of ED providers to offhandedly state between 30% and 50%. This exaggerated number reflects the difficulty providers have when managing these cases. To deal with such cases, scripts like the following can be very helpful:

> I am sorry you have chronic pain. It must feel terrible. It's unfortunate that your doctors haven't been able to manage your pain. In the emergency department, we deal with acute pain every day, but we are neither experts at nor qualified to manage chronic pain on an ongoing basis. I'm happy to speak with and coordinate your care with your doctor. That is the person who is best qualified to care for your chronic pain needs.

Provider Courtesy and Effective Listening

It is an absolute expectation that providers will be courteous to patients. In 2008, the American Board of Medical Specialties performed a consumer survey.[21] The highest response was reported this way:

95 percent of participants surveyed said that bedside manner or communication skills are very important or important as a key factor when choosing a doctor.

Consider the alternative approach, sometimes sarcastically described as "I'm here to save your life, not fluff your pillow." Patients arrive fearful, in pain, and vulnerable. Then their clothes are taken away, and they are placed in an uncomfortable room where multiple personnel may come and go with no regard for their privacy. Worse, patients may undergo painful procedures. If, in addition, the patient's dignity is taken away by rude, sarcastic, and uncaring staff, the providers are literally "adding insult to injury." It is no wonder that surveys ask about the courteousness of the providers.

There are many treatises on active listening skills that may be accessed by interested readers.[22-24] For the purposes of this discussion, effective listening enhances the trust between patients and their providers because it:

- Improves relationships
- Demonstrates sincerity
- Enhances understanding
- Decreases misunderstanding
- Promotes cooperation

There are several skills that can improve the perception that the provider is listening, including sitting in a chair at eye level, maintaining active eye contact, avoiding interruptions, paraphrasing, speaking in a soft tone, and exhibiting open body language. Depending on the situation, specific scripts may be used to improve patient perceptions of provider listening, including:

I'm going to sit here so that I can listen carefully to you.

It's important to me that I listen to what you have to say.

If I heard you correctly, you said that . . .

Initially: Concisely repeat the patient's complaint and then ask, "Have I heard you correctly?"
During care or at the end: "It is important to me that I address your needs and answer your questions. Have I?"

Managing Up

All too often, well-meaning ED team members express their own frustration by blaming others, most often related to delays; for example, "The lab is slow," or "You'll have to wait because the nurse/doctor is busy with a sick patient." This approach does not accomplish the likely intention of shifting the blame, as patients do not differentiate one part of the hospital's care from another. In fact, patients and their families assume that we are all a part of the same health-care team.

A more appropriate approach is to instead "manage up". Consider the positive perception of the patient when told that all of the team members (doctors, nurses, technicians, advanced practice providers, phlebotomists, and others) are working together to take care of them. It instills confidence when a doctor or nurse says:

- *I see that Tiffany (Dr. Jones) is your nurse (doctor) today. That's great! She's a great nurse (doctor).*
- *Tiffany (Dr. Jones) and I work really well as a team. If you need anything while your tests are being processed, you can ask her or me and we'll make sure you get what you need.*

TABLE 74.4 ■ Scripts Designed to Address Patient Concerns

Patient Experience Principle	Reason	Script
Privacy	Doors and curtains are closed for privacy, but patients are usually unaware of this intent.	"I am closing your curtain because I care about your privacy." Or ask permission, "When I leave, would you like me to close the door for privacy?"
Comfort	Comfort measures are provided without patient awareness.	"Your comfort is important to me. May I get you a blanket?"
Anxiety	ED patients are often anxious, in pain, and uncertain about what will transpire.	"I'm sorry you're having (symptoms). We treat this all the time and will take excellent care of you."
Informing about treatment delays	Patients and families wait without understanding the reason. Sharing the reason and describing concern dramatically improves the patients' perceptions of the providers' caring.	"It's important to me that you are kept informed (about delays). We're expecting your laboratory test results. What questions do you have?" See "three-phased approach" in the chapter text and Table 74.8.
Patients as members of the team	Encouraging active patient participation in decision-making likely leads to better outcomes.	"Based on what we know so far, here's our plan... Does that all make sense? Do you agree?"
Pain	While eliminating pain is not always possible or appropriate, addressing it always is.	"It is important to me that your pain is addressed. Let's discuss the most appropriate way."
Chronic pain	A few patients have chronic pain syndromes that are difficult to fully address in the ED.	"I'm sorry that you have this pain. While providing your care, I will communicate with your doctor to ensure that your treatment is consistent with your pain management program."
Courtesy	Patients and their families expect courtesy and concern.	See "A-I-D-E-T" in Box 74.2. "Your comfort is important to me, may I get you a warm blanket?"
Taking time to listen and address needs	Throughout the interaction, it is critical to patients that their needs are addressed.	Initially: Concisely repeat the patient's complaint and then ask, "Have I heard you correctly?" During care or at the end: "It is important to me that I address your needs and answer your questions. Have I?"
Safety	Avoid unsafe events by ensuring right patient, right procedure.	"For your safety, let me check your armband and your chart to make sure everything is accurate."
Managing up	Patients and families want to know that the health-care personnel are part of an effective team.	"I see that Tiffany (Dr. Jones) is your nurse (doctor) today. That's great! She's a great nurse (doctor)."

It is even better to say this in front of your counterpart (team member) to let her know that you are proud to work with her, to clarify your recognition of the importance of the team, and just to let her know what you've said about her to the patient. **Table 74.4** demonstrates actual scripts that can be used to improve patients' perceptions of care and, therefore, their satisfaction. These scripts may be reformulated into phrases that are comfortable for the health-care worker and yet still contain the key content concepts and words. Note that many of these scripts include patient questions to determine if a particular need is being met. When actively engaged in the conversation, the patient is more likely to remember that the issue has been addressed. Consider the example regarding "informing about delays." If the patients affirm that they have been kept informed during the time of care, it is highly likely that they will give the provider a 5 when later queried during the patient care survey. In other words, the provider will have been successful at "driving a 5."

Scripts and Electronic Medical Records

The nearly universal use of electronic medical records (EMRs) creates the need for additional scripts. Without helping patients to develop an understanding, they might often wonder why the doctor or nurse is spending so much time in front of the computer instead of with them. (Experience has shown that, without scripts, patients may even incorrectly believe that the clinician is on the computer for completely nonclinical reasons.)

A particularly effective method of addressing the additional demands created by implementation of the EMR is through the use of scribes. These team members accompany the emergency physician and document the pertinent history, physical examination, and preliminary order sets on the computer (for the physician to then complete the computerized order entry.) Examples of scripts to use when addressing the use of the EMR, either with or without scribes, are provided below:

> **With scribes:** *This is Valerie, who is one of our scribes. She is working with me to ensure that we accurately document all your pertinent information on your computerized medical record. This process is both for accuracy and for your safety.*

> **Without scribes:** *Now that I have all of your initial information, I will be spending some time on the computer to make sure that I document this information in the medical record. This process is both for accuracy and for your safety.*

Other Scripts

There are many examples of scripts that have been devised by others, all with the goal of improving the communication between and perceptions of the patients/families and caregivers.

Creating Previews and Expectations

Two areas in which scripts can be particularly helpful (**Box 74.3**) are:

- Creating previews for the patients (a sense of what will happen to them during their ED visit)
- Creating expectations (creating time expectations that can be exceeded)

BOX 74.3 ■ SCRIPTS THAT CREATE PREVIEWS AND EXPECTATIONS[6,25,26]

- "Do you have any questions? I have plenty of time."
- "I'm Dr. _____. <Name>, your nurse, and I are leading an excellent team that will be caring for you."
- "Even when we're not in the room, we're still guiding your care."
- "I'm sorry this happened to you."
- "Come back any time! We never close."
- "Thank you for allowing us to take care of you."
- "I must leave to respond to a call, but I will try to be back in 5 (actual expected time is 5 minutes, but instead states . . .) 20 minutes."

Note that in the final example described in **Box 74.3**, the provider may have believed that he or she would be back to the patient in 5 minutes. Using the theory of (exaggerated) expectation setting, the provider set an expectation of returning in 20 minutes but actually took 15 minutes. By creating an exaggerated time expectation, though the provider returned later than he or she expected, it was less time than the patient expected, and therefore, the provider exceeded the patient's expectation.

The best scripts are those the team members devise themselves. They are most likely to put them into practice on a daily basis in the course of their work. **Box 74.4** shows scripts used by emergency medicine leader Denis Pauzé, who devised them to help communicate more effectively with his night-shift patients. Emergency medicine specialist Constandino Tsagaratos devised the statements in **Table 74.5** when he was a senior resident. Emergency physician Daniel Getz adapted a "go-to" question (**Table 74.6**)

BOX 74.4 ■ PAUZE'S PEARLS

- "I'm going to be here all night. If you have any questions, give me a call."
- "I'll be on duty Tuesday and Wednesday nights. If you need to see me, come back then."
- "You've already had to wait tonight. If you come back Tuesday or Wednesday, give this card to the triage nurse, and I'll see you in the triage area as soon as I can."

BOX 74.5 ■ MIANO'S ACKNOWLEDGMENT

Acknowledge what you already know about the patient, and then give the patient 1 minute to tell his/her story *uninterrupted*:

"I read Val's triage note. It sounds like you started having pain early today and have thrown up two times. Tell me more about what's going on today."

TABLE 74.5 ■ Tsagaratos's Statements

Issue	Goal	Statement
Closing	Close well (everyone wants to leave on a "good note").	"Thank you. It has been an honor taking care of (you/your . . .)"
End-of-life care	Improve the family's comfort with a difficult decision.	"Any decision that you make out of love is a good decision."

TABLE 74.6 ■ Getz's Go-to Question

Complaint	"I wanted to let you know that your chaplain visited with me and said a very beautiful prayer. I just wish he would have asked me what I wanted to pray about."
Resolution	Ask every patient, "Is there anything that you would like me to know about you personally that can help me to provide you with the best possible care?"

TABLE 74.7 ■ Sternberg's Suggestions

Accompanying Family Member	Issue	Suggestion/Result
Child	Fearful child	First, introduce yourself to the child, and then address the parents. "Hello, Mr./Ms. Smith. It's an honor to meet you, sir/madam!"
Elderly patient	Upset family member	When the family member of a senior citizen is upset about the quality of the patient's care, first address the immediate concern and then express an understanding of their anger. "Thank you so much for bringing this issue to my attention. I can't tell you how much I appreciate your being here with your mother. Too often I have patients who have nobody to support them and the fact that you are here with her really warms my heart and helps us care for her more effectively." This clarifies that the family member and I are on a team, working toward the same goal: the patient's well-being.

after learning of a patient complaint. Medical director Marlea Miano in her statement to patients (**Box 74.5**) demonstrates both team cohesiveness and the desire to avoid wasting the patient's time by asking the same question again. Emergency physician Daniel Sternberg (**Table 74.7**) focuses on the concerns of family members accompanying the young and the old.

CONCLUSION

Neuro-linguistic programming teaches that the words one uses reflect one's perceptions and beliefs. Further, what people say repeatedly, they believe.[27] This has direct implications for developing and using key phrases or scripts in the ED. Although adopting a new script may initially feel awkward, the process becomes increasingly comfortable over time. With continued use, providers come to believe the phrases and words that they use consistently.

TABLE 74.8 ■ The Three Phases and Effects of Adopting New Scripts

Phase I	Discomfort	Using new words feels somewhat awkward the first few times.
Phase II	Comfort	Because of positive feedback from patients demonstrating their appreciation, it becomes increasingly comfortable to use scripts.
Phase III	Belief	Through the process of repetition (neuro-linguistic programming), the practitioner using the script increasingly believes in the importance of patient privacy.
Effect	Positive patient perception	The patients (families) recognize the concern of the practitioner and answer positively on subsequent surveys.

BOX 74.6 ■ PROCESS FOR CREATING SCRIPTS

- **Goal:** Provide the best care in the most caring manner.
- **Patient satisfaction survey:** Review questions asked of patients who receive emergency department services.
- **Current patient perceptions:** Use actual patient satisfaction scores (individualized by practitioner if available).
- **Scripts:** Describe proven successful scripts.
- **Personalized scripts:** Modify scripts to both contain critical words and ensure the comfort of the provider using the script.
- **Commitment:** Ensure a commitment to using scripts.
- **Follow-up:** Monitor the use of scripts, and review ongoing results on surveys.

As an example, a practitioner who decides to use the phrase "I am closing the curtain because your privacy is important to me," will go through the three phases described in **Table 74.8**. Patients and family members will increasingly recognize the concern that is being conveyed. This expression of care will be reflected on subsequent patient surveys by high scores.

Staff meetings are an excellent place for the ED team discussions on the development and use of scripts. The leader(s) should go through a process that always focuses on the primary goal of addressing patient needs first (**Box 74.6**). It is important to continue to monitor the use of scripts, particularly through the patient compliments and complaints and the feedback in staff meetings. Department leaders should continue to show individuals their scores and use this feedback to improve and motivate the members of the team.

REFERENCES

1. Shupe R. The power of our words. 2012. Available at: https://www.studergroup.com/resources/articles-and-industry-updates/insights/february-2012/the-power-of-our-words. Accessed October 22, 2018.
2. Mayer T, Cates RJ. *Leadership for Great Customer Service: Satisfied Patients, Satisfied Employees*. Chicago, Ill: Health Administration Press; 2004.
3. Lasagna L. Hippocratic Oath. Modern Version. 2014. Available at: https://www.pbs.org/wgbh/nova/article/hippocratic-oath-today/. Accessed October 14, 2018.
4. Robeznieks A. New rounds for med students. Revised admissions test, changing focus for essential skills will bring a fresh look to the next generation of physicians. *Mod Healthc*. 2012;42(9):6-7.

5. Leach DC. *In an Address to the Chairs of the Residency Review Committees.* Chicago, Ill; 2001.

6. Studer Q. *Hardwiring Excellence.* Gulf Breeze, Fla: Fire Starter Publishing; 2003.

7. Largest patient-satisfaction measurement firms. *Modern Healthcare.* October 25, 2017.

8. Centers for Medicare & Medicaid Services. Available at: https://www.cms.gov/Research-Statistics-Data-and-Systems/Research/CAHPS/ed.html. Accessed September 30, 2018.

9. Mayer T. Customer relations and patient satisfaction. Presented at: The ACEP Emergency Department Directors Academy; 2014-2018.

10. Miriam Webster. 2019. Available at: https://www.merriam-webster.com/dictionary/customer. Accessed December 14, 2019.

11. Business Dictionary. 2019. Available at: http://www.businessdictionary.com/definition/customer.html. Accessed December 14, 2019.

12. Cambridge Dictionary (American). 2018. Available at: https://dictionary.cambridge.org/dictionary/english/satisfaction#dataset-cacd. Accessed October 18, 2018.

13. Wikipedia. 2018. Available at: https://en.wikipedia.org/wiki/Customer_satisfaction. Accessed October 25, 2018.

14. Strauss RW. Complaint management system. In: Salluzzo R, Strauss RW, Mayer T, et al., eds. *Emergency Department Management: Principles and Applications.* Philadelphia, Pa: Mosby; 1997.

15. U.S. Department of Health and Human Services, Health Information Privacy; Available at: http://www.hhs.gov/ocr/privacy/. Accessed December 14, 2019

16. Jensen K, Kaplan J, Dempsey C. The psychology of waiting: managing waits. In: Strauss RW, Mayer T. *Strauss and Mayer's Emergency Department Management.* Philadelphia, Pa: McGraw-Hill; 2013.

17. Agency for Healthcare Research and Quality, Healthcare 411 Available at: http://healthcare411.ahrq.gov/featureaudio.aspx? id=759. Accessed December 20, 2018.

18. Agency for Healthcare Research and Quality; Chest Pain, a Leading Reason for Hospital Emergency Department Visits. Available at: http://archive.ahrq.gov/news/nn/nn022708.htm. Accessed December 12, 2019.

19. Otto E., List of Common Emergency Cases in the Hospital. Available at: http://www.livestrong.com/article/41781-list-common-emergency-cases-hospital/. Accessed December 20, 2018.

20. Fosnocht DE, Hepas ND, Swanson ER. Patient expectations for pain relief in the ED. *Am J Emerg Med.* 2004;22(4):286-288.

21. American Board of Medical Specialties, Facts About the AMBS Consumer Survey: Lifelong Learning and Other Qualities in Choosing a Doctor. Available at: http://www.abms.org/News_and_Events/Media_Newsroom/pdf/ABMS_Survey_Fact_Sheet.pdf. Accessed, December 16, 2018.

22. Rothwell JD. *In the Company of Others: An Introduction to Communication.* Oxford, England: Oxford University Press; 2012.

23. Goulston M. *Just Listen: Discover the Secret to Getting Through to Absolutely Anyone.* New York, NY: Amacom; 2010.

24. Nichols M. *The Lost Art of Listening.* New York, NY: The Gilford Press; 2009.

25. Mayer T, Jensen K. *Hardwiring Flow.* Gulf Breeze, Fla: Fire Starter Press; 2007.

26. Strauss R. Complaint and Compliment Management. Presented at: the ACEP Emergency Department Directors' Academy. Dallas, Tex; 2004-2019.

27. Dilts R. *Modeling With NLP.* Soquel, Calif: Meta Publications; 1998.

CHAPTER 75

THE A-TEAM TOOLKIT™

Thom A. Mayer, Robert J. Cates

Chapter 11 defines patient experience as the difference or "delta" between patients' expectations and their actual experience of care in the emergency department (ED). If their expectations are not met, they are unhappy and often complain. If they are met, but only *just* met, they are merely satisfied. But if the ED team exceeds patient expectations, they foster patient loyalty, which is the goal of all hospitals and health-care systems.[1-3] Motivating the ED team to provide language, systems, and processes that exceed patient expectations requires using intrinsic motivation and focusing on making the job easier—not extrinsic motivation or focusing on scores. "Do it because the boss says so!" is not and has never been an effective motivation for highly trained and skilled professionals.

Intrinsic motivation is illustrated by the A-Team/B-Team concept, since all ED team members recognize that there are A-Team members, who make the job much easier, but there are also B-Team members, who make the job infinitely more difficult. If ED leaders ask their teams how many B-Team members it takes to destroy an entire shift, the team will shout, "Just one!" The "why" of patient experience is that it makes the job easier, which should always be a central foundation of any patient-experience effort.

Once the definition of patient experience is understood and the importance of getting the "why" right is known, it is important to move to the specifics of "how." This chapter discusses the A-Team Toolkit™, a set of evidence-based disciplines which, if put into action, make the job easier (Box 75.1).

TOOL #1: EMPOWERMENT

"Empowerment" is one of the most overused and least understood terms in health care. Detailed service and health-care research indicate that no service leader has ever succeeded without a deep culture of empowerment.[5,6] Indeed, world-class medical organizations consider it a central tenet of their culture.[7] Empowerment means that those providing the

---

BOX 75.1 ■ THE A-TEAM TOOLKIT™

The 10 elements of the A-Team Toolkit assist clinicians and leaders in exceeding patients' expectations.

1. Empowerment
2. Dealing with B-Team patients and B-Team members
3. Focused patient-experience coaching, mentoring, and shadow shifting
4. Rounding—yours, next, sign-outs, and post-discharge phone calls
5. Scripts—using evidence-based language to improve service
6. Hire right—screen for the service gene
7. Taking 4s to 5s—going from "usually" to "always"
8. Hardwiring flow and the psychology of waiting
9. Reward the champions—harvesting compliments
10. Leave a legacy

service have the ability to change or improve their processes to better meet the needs and expectations of their patients.

At a large, prestigious health-care system with a reputation for having progressive programs, the question was posed, "Are you empowered?" The silence, frankly, was a bit disquieting, until a small voice from the back of the auditorium said, "They *tell* us we are . . ." If the team is told they are empowered, but the reality of that empowerment is not clear, it's time to start over.

Thick-Rulebook vs Thin-Rulebook Organizations

Emergency departments that deliver excellent patient care understand that service doesn't reside in a thick manual that explains every detail of what to do; true empowerment comes from "think" rulebooks, not thick ones. Thick-rulebook organizations delineate every way in which patient care is to be delivered, and they demand specific compliance with the policies. Thin-rulebook organizations outline their broad values, mission, and vision but rely on leaders and managers to act as catalysts to help the team uncover the best ways to deliver excellence. It is better to have one person practicing empowered patient experience than a hundred posted mission statements proclaiming it.

Narrow Corridors vs Wide Corridors

Excellent patient experiences occur in EDs that not only have thin rulebooks but also have wide corridors on the path to success. There are many ways to succeed, not just "the boss' way" or "the company way." Hire right (discussed below), train your employees well, give them servant leaders who exemplify the organization's values, and then turn them loose. Both the literature and practical experience show that staff will create more and better details on "how to do it" than any leadership team could because they have been given values and are empowered.

Point of Impact Intervention™

The first tool in empowerment is the Point of Impact Intervention™, which combines the concepts of empowerment and negotiation. It begins with the insight from patients who registered a complaint about their care: When their caregivers were asked if they had any notion that the patient was unhappy at the time, 92% of the time, the answer was "yes." In other words, usually when complaints occur, the ED staff already knows that there is a problem.[3-4] Point of Impact Intervention simply recognizes this fact and puts a tool in the hands of the caregiver to resolve the problem at the patient's bedside, the "point of impact."

The eight steps of this technique (**Box 75.2**) simply represent a disciplined approach to avoid making the incident report bigger than the incident itself by addressing the patient's

---

BOX 75.2 ■ POINT OF IMPACT INTERVENTION™

Point of Impact Interventions help ensure that problems are identified and addressed at the bedside, before the patient leaves the ED.

1. Identify the problem and address it immediately.
2. Establish the fact you know there has been a breakdown.
3. Wipe the slate clean.
4. Establish their expectations: what's the "delta" between their expectations and their experience?
5. Negotiate and resolve issues.
6. If possible, meet their expectations.
7. Offer reasonable alternatives.
8. When all else fails, offer an alternative person to talk to.

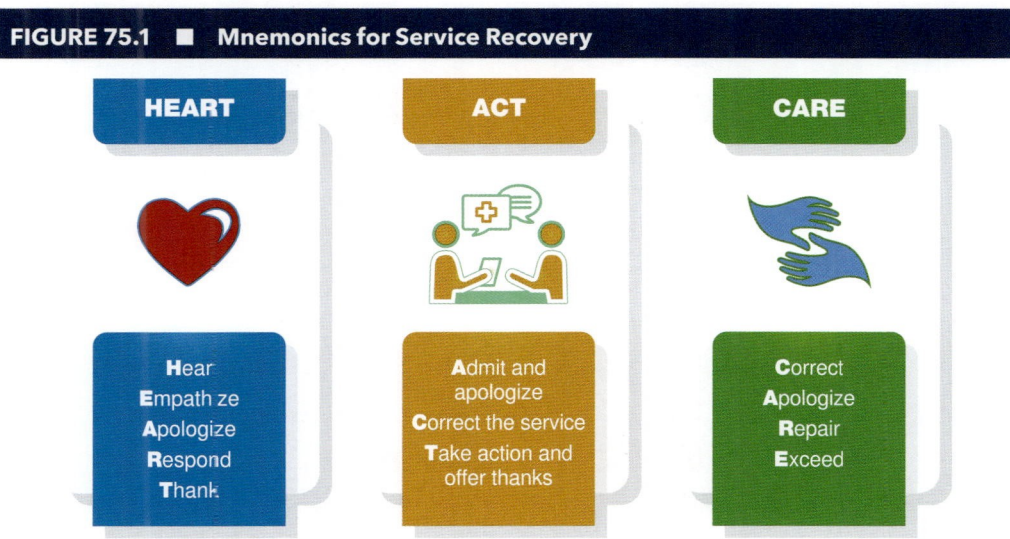

FIGURE 75.1 ■ Mnemonics for Service Recovery

expectations in real time. Step four is of particular significance because patients often feel the staff has not met their expectations. Ensuring that the team goes back to the patient to re-establish their expectations is key to the Point of Impact Intervention, which dramatically reduces complaints by addressing them at the bedside.[4,8]

Service Recovery

The second tool in the empowerment category is service recovery. While the Point of Impact Intervention is a form of complaint *prevention*, service recovery is a form of complaint *management*. There are many formulations for service recovery, many of which are associated with a mnemonic (**Figure 75.1**). Most hospitals and health-care systems have developed their own processes, mnemonics, or forms to use in service recovery, so these efforts should be coordinated with existing systems.[9] All such programs recognize the fact that once a service failure occurs, the sooner it is recognized and addressed, the higher the magnitude of the recovery and the more loyal the patient (**Box 75.3; Figure 75.2**).

Regardless of the system chosen, it is imperative that service recovery be treated using a focused, disciplined approach that requires careful monitoring to ensure the source of patient complaints is carefully tracked and that appropriate follow-up is provided.

Harvesting Compliments, Cultivating Complaints

A-Team behaviors lead to compliments, and B-Team behaviors cause complaints. With this simple yet effective insight, ED leaders and managers must "harvest compliments" to discover which A-Team behaviors exceed expectations and create a positive patient

---

BOX 75.3 ■ SERVICE RECOVERY PROGRAM BEST PRACTICES

- Listen actively.
- Apologize: "What can I do to make this right?"
- Fix it.
- Follow up and follow through.
- Give something extra.

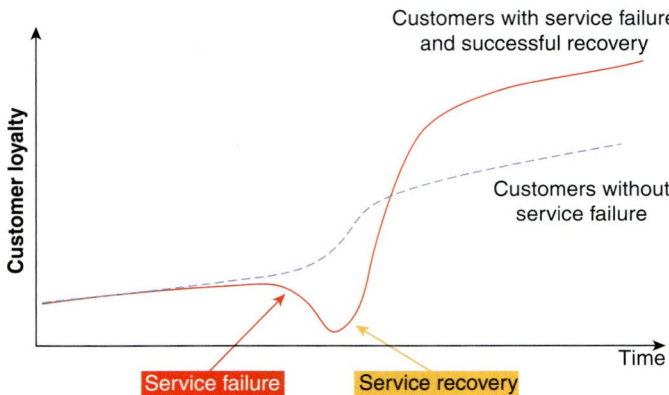

FIGURE 75.2 ■ Service Recovery Paradoxon

experience. Likewise, leaders must "cultivate complaints" to understand the source of B-Team behaviors and processes, which fail to meet patient expectations. For this reason, all compliments and complaints should be discussed openly at ED staff meetings to foster group learning. The ninth element of the A-Team Toolkit discusses harvesting compliments in more detail.

The third empowerment tool is a concept known as either "leading up," or as the Studer Group refers to it, "managing up".[10] This technique refers to empowering others by using verbal service transitions to ensure patients are led to expect excellence from those taking over their care (**Box 75.4**). While the primary benefit of leading or managing up is that it prepares the way for a smooth service transition from one person and one service to another, it also serves to "lead up" the person to whom care will be transferred. In other words, it helps them understand that a great deal will be expected of them, given their superb introduction to the patient and family.

BOX 75.4 ■ MANAGING UP

"Leading up" or "managing up" uses verbal tools to transition care to others on the health-care team, which assists in managing expectations and ensuring that teammates know they have been introduced positively.

- "Janet is your nurse; she's the best!"
- "Jim is the ED technician, and he will put your splint on and teach you to walk with your crutches. He's actually better at this than I am!"
- "Let me introduce you to Dr. Strauss, my partner, who will be taking over your care. I have briefed him on your situation, and he will take great care of you."
- "Ma'am, the x-ray shows your bone is fractured, so I spoke with your physician. She recommended I call the orthopedic surgeon, who will be in to take care of you. He is excellent and will do a great job!"
- "As I said earlier, we will need to admit you to the hospital today, so I have called your doctor, who asked that we admit you to one of our specialists in hospital medicine. Dr. Rodriguez will be admitting you today and will keep your doctor informed of your care every step of the way."

TOOL #2: MANAGING THE B-TEAM

The A-Team/B-Team metaphor inevitably gives rise to caregivers asking, "What is the best way to handle both B-Team patients and B-Team members?" It is a perfectly legitimate question. It is one thing to ask our team to exhibit A-Team behaviors, but it is quite another to ask them to deal with the B-Team realities of their patients, families, and teammates.

Dealing With B-Team Patients

Many patients and their families are a joy—appreciative, understanding, and grateful for the care provided to them. Others are, frankly, the bane of our existence. They tax our resources and abilities with expectations that seemingly cannot be met. For these reasons, B-Team patients and members must be handled with a disciplined approach (**Box 75.5**).

The most common and vexing of the B-Team patients might be those with chronic pain. How can their expectations be met or exceeded in a busy ED? Admittedly, it is a difficult problem. However, a disciplined approach allows clinicians to isolate the issue, focus on excluding possible new clinical explanations, and create a solution. Fortunately, many EDs have developed and implemented aggressive alternatives to opioid pain-management practices that are of huge benefit (see Chapter 60). Of particular benefit is shifting the locus of power and control from the ED staff to other areas of the health-care system by:

- Expressing concern for the patient's chronic pain
- Acknowledging the very real nature of the pain
- Explaining that emergency physicians and nurses are trained and credentialed in acute pain management but have no background or expertise in chronic pain
- Addressing any acute pain (new injury or illness) while referring the patient to a chronic pain service
- Effectively shifting the power and control from the ED to the (appropriate) chronic pain management service

Dealing With B-Team Members

It is also critical to understand the best means of dealing with B-Team members, which is a fundamental skill for all health-care providers, particularly in the ED.[1,11] As indicated

---

BOX 75.5 ■ DEALING WITH THE B-TEAM PATIENT

This approach improves the ability of physicians and nurses to deal with difficult (B-Team) patients, many of whom have chronic pain.

- Sit down.
- Use open body language.
- Practice active listening.
- Establish expectations.
- Be proactive.

- Meticulously address the clinical issues:
  - "I am sorry you have chronic pain and the system has failed you . . ."
  - "I don't have what you want, but I can get an appointment for you with those who do."
  - "I'm not trained in chronic pain management!"
  - "But I have 'friends' who have the answer to what you want . . ."

previously, the A-Team members exhibit positive, proactive, and compassionate behaviors in their daily work, which makes our jobs easier. The B-Team members are precisely the opposite. They are negative, reactive, and seemingly constant complainers who devastate the team's morale. In a curious twist to the Pareto principle, which states that 80% of problems come from 20% of causes, leaders and managers spend the majority of their problem-solving efforts cleaning up the messes that the B-Team members create. Everyone knows who the B-Team members are, except the B-Team members themselves. They genuinely don't recognize the havoc they leave in their wake and, indeed, consider themselves bastions of excellence.

Here's a simple exercise that illustrates that idea: Leaders should ask their staff, "When an A-Team member looks in the mirror, what do they see?" It sounds like a bit of a trick question, but on reflection, they will answer, "An A-Team member." The A-Team members are fundamentally self-reflective and usually recognize the behaviors that work for them and their team.

Now follow up with this question: "When a B-Team member looks in the mirror, what do they see?" The answer will come quickly, "An A-Team member!" That is because B-Team members truly do not realize how toxic their words and actions are to the patients, the family, and, most importantly, the rest of the ED team. In this regard, the most fundamental skill in dealing with B-Team members is the ability to hold the "mirror" up to them so they may see the true effect of their actions (**Box 75.6**).

Communication with B-Team members must be specific, clear, and concise. The language used must be focused and staccato in nature. Far too often, the language used by leaders is too vague, as if they were somehow concerned they will hurt the B-Team members' feelings.

> *Example: I've been talking to some of the staff, and we were kind of thinking that things could be going better. We were hoping you could help us make improvements through your actions; when things go better, people feel better. I hope you can help us on this journey. Well, thanks for coming in and giving this some thought.*

What did this manager just say? Nothing! The B-team member comes out of this meeting with no earthly clue as to what they should be doing differently. In fact, if asked what happened in the meeting, they might actually answer, "I think I got a raise."[1-4,10]

It is important for leaders to know what they will say and how they will say it before the meeting ever begins. The message should be clear, concise, and businesslike. Don't exchange pleasantries; this is not a social interaction. Come to the meeting prepared with specific examples in which the employee failed to deliver A-Team words and actions. This begins with ensuring the entire team knows the A-Team/B-Team concept and feels comfortable communicating B-Team incidents to the leadership team. Staff should be encouraged to make their concerns as specific as possible so the

---

BOX 75.6 ■ DEALING WITH B-TEAM MEMBERS

Holding the "mirror" up to B-Team members allows for a focused, disciplined conversation about how their behaviors affect the ED team.

- Be specific, clear, and concise.
- Be timely.
- Be blunt.
- Use the Gordon Method: "When you do X, it makes others feel Y. Try Z instead."
- Give them examples.
- Give them a mentor.

manager can be equally specific. A simple and direct format for holding the mirror up to a B-Team member is the Gordon Method: "When you do X, it makes others feel Y. Try Z instead."[12]

Example: *When you show up late, it makes others feel frustrated and as if you don't have to follow the same rules as the rest of the team. Try leaving 15 minutes earlier than you think you need to.*

The communication is terse, focused, and direct. There is no mention of the leader's position of authority, but the point is clear: This behavior cannot continue and has a negative impact on morale. Once a culture of service and mutual accountability is established, it is common for the staff themselves to have these sort of conversations directly with their B-Team colleagues.

Give the B-Team member a time frame for improving the behavior. If all else fails, give them a mentor. Pair the B-Team members with A-Team colleagues who are admired by the staff for the grace, dignity, and equanimity they bring daily to the ED. Finally, leaders and managers must have the courage of their convictions to replace the B-Team members who can't or won't change.

TOOL #3: PATIENT EXPERIENCE COACHING

All patient experience surveys are "open-book tests" in that the questions are or should be known to the staff (**Box 75.7**). However, focused patient satisfaction coaching takes the results of the scores to design specific improvement strategies. In the case of emergency physicians, Press Ganey scores can be reported by individual providers and used for coaching with specific goals toward improvement.

Shadow Shifting

Taking focused patient experience coaching to the next level involves the concept of "shadow shifting," in which A-Team members spend time working with B-Team members to help improve their scores. Shadow shifting is part of a culture of mutual accountability in which colleagues work together to improve each other's scores, thereby raising the score of the entire team. For example, for a physician or nurse whose scores are low in "took time to listen" or "listened carefully," the coaching might focus on sitting, using active listening, and touching the patient.

The same concept can be used to improve the perception of service in other patient satisfaction surveys. For example, **Figure 75.3** shows how the PRC scores can be used to improve service. For PRC, three "key drivers" are identified on a statistical basis which, for each individual ED, are the main determinants of the overall score. By focusing on these key drivers and coaching to them, the scores can be improved, which is simply another form of focused patient satisfaction coaching.

BOX 75.7 ■ FOCUSED PATIENT SATISFACTION COACHING

Focused coaching based on patient surveys, complaints, and compliments improves both scores and staff satisfaction.

- Open-book test: identify the questions.
- The target score is identified (e.g., 75th percentile).
- Plotting these scores is relatively simple.

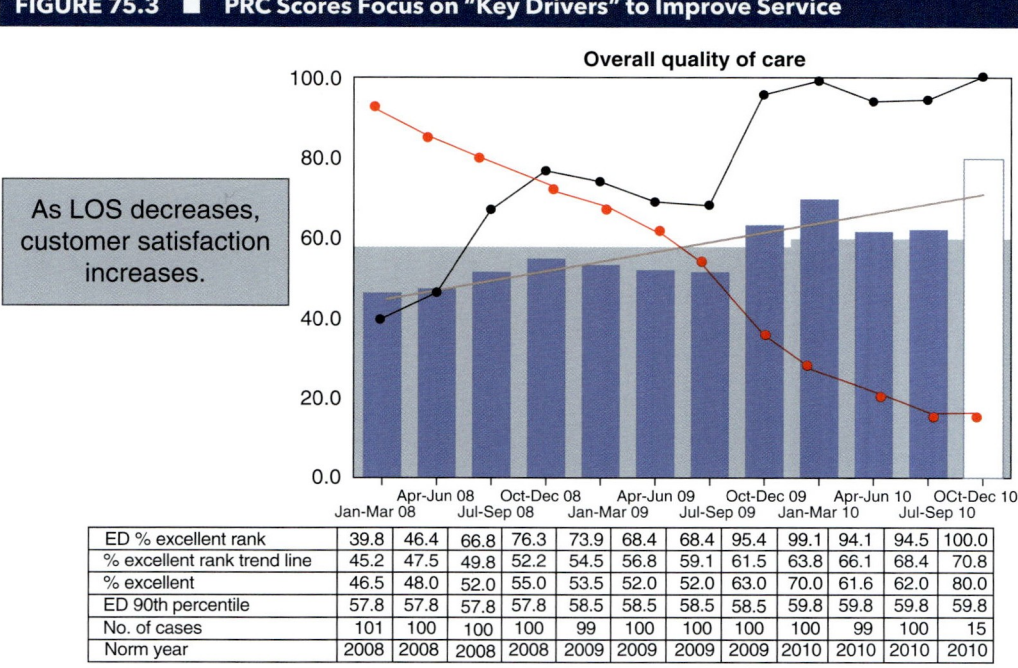

FIGURE 75.3 ■ PRC Scores Focus on "Key Drivers" to Improve Service

As LOS decreases, customer satisfaction increases.

	Jan-Mar 08	Apr-Jun 08	Jul-Sep 08	Oct-Dec 08	Jan-Mar 09	Apr-Jun 09	Jul-Sep 09	Oct-Dec 09	Jan-Mar 10	Apr-Jun 10	Jul-Sep 10	OCt-Dec 10
ED % excellent rank	39.8	46.4	66.8	76.3	73.9	68.4	68.4	95.4	99.1	94.1	94.5	100.0
% excellent rank trend line	45.2	47.5	49.8	52.2	54.5	56.8	59.1	61.5	63.8	66.1	68.4	70.8
% excellent	46.5	48.0	52.0	55.0	53.5	52.0	52.0	63.0	70.0	61.6	62.0	80.0
ED 90th percentile	57.8	57.8	57.8	57.8	58.5	58.5	58.5	58.5	59.8	59.8	59.8	59.8
No. of cases	101	100	100	100	99	100	100	100	100	99	100	15
Norm year	2008	2008	2008	2008	2009	2009	2009	2009	2010	2010	2010	2010

*Ranking are based on PRC norm data.

TOOL #4: ROUNDING AND POST-DISCHARGE FEEDBACK

One of the most powerful tools available to leaders and managers is rounding, which is a systematic way of hearing both the "voice of the patient" and the "voice of the team." There are four fundamental types of rounding: 1) leaders rounding on their own units, 2) leaders, physicians, and nurses rounding on their admitted patients, 3) sign-out rounds, 4) and post-discharge feedback, usually in the form of phone calls. Leader rounding is a core concept of the Studer Group's Evidence-Based Leadership program and has been adopted by many successful health-care systems.[10,13] It requires leaders to round on staff and patients in their unit on a regular basis and systematically record the results. The disciplined use of rounding has shown consistent and dramatic results, including improvements in service scores and length of stay. Focusing on both A-Team and B-Team behaviors, language, and processes is critical.

Rounding on a small group of patients admitted from the ED is an extremely powerful tool, both for patients and the physicians and nurses who care for them. The principle is simple: leaders, doctors, and nurses keep a log of the patients admitted to the hospital. Once a week, physicians and nurses are encouraged to round on these patients, simply to revisit them, check on their progress, and determine how best to improve care. Perhaps the most important benefit of rounding is the genuine respect and gratitude these patients show, almost without exception, when the ED staff visits them. Indeed, in many cases, such patients become gracious friends.

Sign-out rounds are another of the tools that benefit both ED providers and patients. When emergency physicians and nurses are leaving at the end of the shift, they should not only inform the patient they are leaving, they should also go room to room with the provider assuming responsibility for their care. This is an essential service transition and one that dramatically improves patient and staff satisfaction. The Emergency Medicine

Patient Safety Foundation has developed a patient-centered, team-based tool for safe sign-outs (www.safersignouts.com) that is excellent, although it lacks a focus on Precision-Personalized Care™, which would include this aspect: "Mrs. Gonzalez, this is Dr. Chen, my partner, who will be taking over your care. I explained to him that the most important thing we can do to make this an excellent emergency department visit for you is . . ."

Post-discharge follow-up on ED patients should be considered a tool of rounding because it captures the "voice of the patient" with the added perspective of time. The most common and powerful tool is post-discharge telephone calls. Many EDs have nurses, APPs, or other staff perform these calls, but it is most effective to have the emergency physicians, nurses, or APPs who actually provided the clinical care perform the post-discharge follow-up. In general, having a template to guide the calls works better than a "free-form" dialogue.[1-4,10,13-15] There are a number of proprietary formats for these calls, but the essential elements should include:

- *Immediate, succinct introduction*: "Hello, Mr. Smith. This is Dr. Jones. I was the emergency physician who had the pleasure of caring for you in our ED."
- *Courtesy of the call*: "Is this a good time to talk briefly?"
- *Purpose of the call*: "We like to check up on our patients to see how you are doing and to see if there is anything we can do better. This shouldn't take more than 5 minutes. Is that okay with you?"
- *Personalize*:
  - ☐ "How are you feeling?"
  - ☐ "How would you characterize how you are doing?"
  - ☐ "Are you having any symptoms or problems?"
  - ☐ "How is your ___ doing?"
  - ☐ "Were you able to get your prescriptions filled? Are the medications helping?"
  - ☐ "Were our follow-up instructions clear? Any questions?"
  - ☐ "Were you able to schedule your follow-up appointment as we discussed?"
  - ☐ "Is there anyone on our staff you would like to recognize?"
  - ☐ "Is there anything we could have done better?"
- *Positive close*: "Thanks for choosing our emergency department. We are there when you need us. It was my privilege to have been your doctor."

Whatever format is chosen (which should be discussed with the team prior to implementation), the results of the call should be captured in a log, whether on the computer or paper, and the results should be used to compliment team members, correct team problems, and allow trending data to improve clinical care and the patient experience.

TOOL #5: USING SCRIPTS

Because the patients' journey through the ED is a series of service transitions from one area and person to another, there is a high degree of predictability regarding interactions that patients and staff will have. The concept of scripts simply recognizes this predictability and seeks to design specific words or phrases to improve these interactions. Scripts as evidence-based language are addressed in detail in Chapter 74, but the fundamental elements are addressed here. As mentioned previously, two areas where scripts can be particularly helpful are creating *previews* for the patient (a sense of what will happen to him or her during an ED visit) and *expectation creation* (a time expectation that the team should be able to better).[14]

The best scripts are those that A-Team members devise themselves and are seen to practice on a daily basis. Staff meetings are an excellent place for the ED team to discuss such scripts. Patient compliments about the ED team are an excellent resource to help determine which scripts resonate with the patients themselves. Here is an example, received in a handwritten note from an 85-year-old woman cared for in the ED:

> *Doctor Kuhn and Doctor Skibbie have learned at a very young age the true art of medicine — they kept asking me what questions I had and telling me they had plenty of time to answer them. I am an astute observer, and time was the one thing these two gentlemen did not have plenty of! But they were so kind in asking me, and I truly appreciated it. But more than the care I received was the care I saw given to others, of every race, creed, and social stature. I was in a bed in the hallway, so I saw lots of care given, and it was all compassionate and professional. I can't thank you enough for the care I was given.*

Clearly, the script, "What questions do you have? I have plenty of time," meant a great deal to this woman. (By the way, Drs. Kuhn and Skibbie were, at the time of this incident, 41 and 45 years old, respectively; but when you are 85, everyone seems young.) The second comment about observing others is a classic example of the "on stage–off stage" concept that Disney champions, which was previously discussed. It is important to continue to monitor the use of scripts, particularly through patient compliments (and complaints, which identify "B-Team scripts") and the feedback in staff meetings.

TOOL #6: HIRING RIGHT

Creating and sustaining a culture of service excellence makes the following statement abundantly clear: The hiring of a new ED team member is one of the most crucial and expensive decisions an ED leader or manager will ever make.

Because the staff delivering the service define the ED on an ongoing basis, the process of selecting, hiring, orienting, and mentoring those people is a "mission critical" part of the job. In fact, ED physician and nurse leaders are, in effect, the "chief talent officers" because they decide which of the applicants will be a part of the team, as well as structure candidates' exposure to the culture of the department during the interview process. To do this successfully, it is important to check not only applicants' *qualifications* but their *qualities*, as well (**Box 75.8**). When staff are hired, the colleges they attended are checked, but what about the colleagues with whom they studied? Their *curriculum vitae* will tell if they attained honors, but did they

---

BOX 75.8 ■ QUALITIES vs QUALIFICATIONS

Qualities	Qualifications
• Employer	• Employees
• College(s)	• Colleagues
• Honors	• Honor
• Education	• Ethics
• Aptitude	• Attitude
• Degree(s)	• Demeanor
• Credentials	• Integrity
• Intelligence	• Customer service skills
• Computer skills	

comport themselves with honor? Their transcripts and scores will tell about their intelligence, but what about their integrity? Wise leaders and managers realize that it is far easier to educate someone for qualifications than it is to raise their standards on quality.[15,16]

A number of questions can be asked to help delineate those who will be successful in a service culture from those who won't. Two specific questions can be very helpful: "What's the worst thing I am going to hear about you and from whom will I hear it?" and "What's the nurses' facial expression when they see your name on the schedule?" The answers can often help distinguish A-Team members from B-Team members.

Hiring should be a group process, involving members from different parts of the team. Whenever possible, it can be worthwhile to have the applicant observe in the ED for several hours; this not only helps them understand what the ED is really like, it also enables a more casual interview process.

Finally, this rule is almost always true: A-Team members hire A-Team members; B-Team members hire C-Team members. First-rate people always surround themselves with other first-rate people who will challenge them and the entire team. Second-tier people don't want to be challenged and are likely to recommend people who they consider beneath them in talent.

TOOL #7: TAKING FOURS TO FIVES

Driving patient experience to the highest levels requires a fundamental ability to go from "good to great," in the words of James Collins.[17,18] Collins systematically studied companies that were able to attain and sustain excellence in their respective fields, contrasting those near the top of the industry with those that led the way. He also looked carefully at the characteristics of their leaders. This is a strong analogy that can be applied to health-care customer service if one understands the ways in which scores are generated.

Virtually all patient satisfaction scores seek to rank ordinal data of the patient's perception of their care through a Likert scale (named for the Wyoming sociologist, Rensis Likert).[19] The majority of these scales are either five-point Likert scales (Press Ganey and the PRC) or four-point scales (Gallup and NRC+Picker). The Consumer Assessment of Healthcare Providers and Systems (HCAHPS) and EDPECS surveys use a four-point Likert scale with these elements:

- Always
- Usually
- Sometimes
- Never

When scores decline, there is a (natural and reasonable) tendency for physicians to think, "It must be all those people giving us scores of 1, 2, and 3 that are pulling us down. There are some people who just can't be pleased!" But data from Press Ganey, PRC, and HCAHPS indicate this is simply not the case. In fact, it only takes one-quarter to one-third of patients currently scoring a "4" to move to a score of "5" to dramatically change the percentile ranking from the bottom third to the top third. Perhaps equally important is to ensure that the ED staff members with low scores understand this concept and do not despair.

While all of the techniques in the A-Team Toolkit can be used to move scores of "4" to "5," one of the most effective is to ask patients, "What would make this an excellent ED visit for you?" Listening to the voice of the customer is and has always been one of the most powerful ways to go from good to great. Even more important is acting on what the customer says by changing the system to meet the patients' needs.

TOOL #8: HARDWIRING FLOW

The concept of "flow" in ED operations is discussed in detail in Chapters 34 through 48. Interested readers are referred to the work of Mayer and Jensen and Jensen, Mayer, Welch, and Haraden for an in-depth treatment of flow.[20-22] However, "flow" can be briefly defined as "existing to the extent that value is added and waste is eliminated as the patient moves through the service transitions and queues of their care." Further, "value" is defined as a simple ratio of burdens received versus burdens endured in the course of their care. Thus, anything that increases benefit or decreases burden increases value in health care.[20-23] For those familiar with "lean" principles, this is fundamentally a lean definition of flow in that it focuses on value creation and waste elimination.[23]

There are many reasons to use the principles of flow to improve ED operations, but perhaps the most important is this: *Everyone—every patient, every family member, every ED team member—deserves an ED that works!* Effective flow ensures that ED operations are designed to work for everyone involved. Thus, triage bypass when rooms are available, standing orders for certain patient presentations when beds are not available, bedside registration, and front-loading care by placing physicians or midlevel providers in the triage area at peak flow times are all examples of using flow principles to increase value and decrease waste.

Another "flow" concept that can improve patient and staff satisfaction is described by David Maister, an expert on business management practices, as "the psychology of waiting."[24] Maister described the psychological impact of waiting in queues, although he did not focus specifically on health care. Nonetheless, his insights apply to the ED experience; **Box 75.13** illustrate how these principles can be put to use.

TOOL #9: REWARDING THE CHAMPIONS

Because the ED has metrics-based accountability, leaders should recognize when their department is working and aim to sustain those results over time. Length of stay (defined for admitted, nonadmitted, and fast-track patients), left without being seen, patient satisfaction scores, boarder hours, time from admission to bed, use of agency personnel, and fiscal measures are all ways in which ED teams are measured on a regular basis. The concept of rewarding the ED champions simply recognizes the legitimate role that praise has in motivating professionals. "Harvesting compliments" refers to taking an aggressive approach to discovering when, where, and how the ED team members are providing excellent care, which includes:

- Whenever ED staff members receive praise, it should be noted by reading the letter at department meetings or posting them on a board that is visible in the treatment area. A-Team behaviors should be celebrated publicly, not kept in secret.
- All ED staff should be encouraged to acknowledge A-Team behaviors in real time by telling their colleagues how much their help is appreciated. For example: "Randi, you did a great job on this case. It was a tough one, but you made it easier for all of us."
- While success should be made public, failures (B-Team behaviors) should be handled in private and never in front of the patient, the family, or the other members of the team.
- Programs in which ED team members can nominate their fellow teammates for service awards on a monthly, quarterly, and yearly basis can be quite effective in building morale, modeling behaviors, and mentoring the staff.

Chapter 78 discusses this approach in more detail.

TOOL #10: LEAVING A LEGACY

There are many meanings to the term "legacy." In health care, we leave a legacy every time we interact with a patient, the family, or other team members. At the end of a taxing shift, ED staff members should be encouraged to sit in their cars before going home and ask themselves a simple yet powerful question: "What did I leave behind in that ED? What was my legacy today?"

Health care is unique in this regard—the legacy is not something that needs days, months, or years to determine. Clinicians can assess their legacy one patient at a time. A parable inspired by the work of Loren Eiseley, an anthropologist and philosopher, demonstrates this well[25]:

> *A quintessential Type A businessman took his family to the Outer Banks of North Carolina for a vacation, in hopes of relaxing and unwinding from the stress of his high-powered job. The houses on the beach in that area are built on pylons to raise them above the damage that the water and waves would cause from the frequent storms that visit these coastal islands.*
>
> *The businessman and his family checked in on a Saturday afternoon, typical of renters in this area, when the weather was sunny and beautiful. However, that night a sudden storm arose, and he and his family could hear the waves pounding repeatedly against the pylons. The next day he woke early, as was his habit, and looked out to see a gorgeous, sunny morning. But when he walked toward the beach, he discovered that it was nearly covered with starfish, as if the storm had rained them down. He could barely make his way for all the starfish. There seemed to be no one on the beach until he noticed a single person to the north, perhaps 100 yards away. As he stepped carefully up the shore, he became curious and noticed the person repeatedly bending over and standing up. As he grew even nearer, his curiosity grew, until he realized it was a young girl, perhaps 9 years old, who was picking up starfish, one by one, cleaning them off, and then throwing them back into the waves.*
>
> *The businessman couldn't help saying, "Little girl, I don't mean to disappoint you, but what you're doing can't possibly make any difference. I've been watching you throw the starfish back for the past 15 minutes, and you've only been able to clear a small area about 7 feet across. There are thousands of starfish on this beach that we can see – and perhaps millions more that we can't see. So I am sorry to say, what you're doing can't possibly make any difference."*
>
> *The young girl looked at the starfish in her hand and exclaimed, "It does to this one!" And she threw it into the foam.*

What's the point? That's precisely what ED providers do each and every day they go to work. Despite overwhelming demands and even inadequate resources, they "take care of the one in front of them," seemingly oblivious to the surrounding chaos. They do it with style, grace, dignity, and equanimity, and they deserve unending praise for both the job they do and how they do it. They are leaving a legacy, and wise leaders and managers will never forget to praise them for a job well done under the most trying of circumstances.

CONCLUSION

The "why" of improving patient experience is that a disciplined approach makes the job easier for the ED team. The "how" comprises evidence-based approaches gleaned from extensive experience in multiple EDs, whose members delineated what works to improve the patient experience. The A-Team Toolkit™ comprises 10 focused the patient experience and service strategies, which collectively make the job easier, drive mutual accountability, and deliver excellence consistently.

REFERENCES

1. Mayer T, Cates RJ. *Leadership for Great Customer Service: Satisfied Employees, Satisfied Patients*. 2nd ed. Health Administration Press; 2014.
2. Mayer T, Cates RJ. *Leadership for Great Customer Service: Satisfied Patients, Satisfied Employees*. Health Administration Press; 2004.
3. Mayer T. Leadership for great customer service: getting the "why" right before the "how." *Healthc Exec*. 2010;25(3):66,68-69.
4. Mayer T. Putting it all together: education and the right tools to create a culture of service excellence. *Healthc Exec*. 2011;26(1):56,58-59.
5. Peters T. *The Excellence Dividend: Meeting the Tech Tide With Work That Wows and Jobs That Last*. Vintage Books; 2018.
6. Pink DH. *Drive: The Surprising Truth About What Motivates Us*. Riverhead Books; 2009.
7. Berry LL, Seltman K. *Management Lessons from Mayo Clinic: Inside One of the World's Most Admired Service Organizations*. McGraw-Hill; 2008.
8. Mayer T. Drive service excellence to the next level: moving patient satisfaction scores from the 4s to the 5s is key. *Healthc Exec*. 2010;25(6):54-56.
9. Mayer T. Patient experience and ED team engagement. Presented at: The American College of Emergency Physicians (ACEP) Emergency Department Directors Academy (EDDA), November 12, 2018; Dallas, TX.
10. Studer Q. *Hardwiring Excellence*. Fire Starter Publishing; 2004.
11. Mayer T. Dealing with the B team members: holding the mirror up can have a positive effect on them and the organization. *Healthc Exec*. 2010;(Sept-Oct):52-54.
12. Strauss R. Negotiation methods. Presented at: The American College of Emergency Physicians (ACEP) Emergency Department Directors Academy (EDDA), November 14, 2018; Dallas, TX.
13. Studer Q. *Results That Last: Hardwiring Behaviors That Will Take Your Company to the Top*. John Wiley and Sons; 2008.
14. Mayer T. Beyond patient experience. Presented at: The American College of Emergency Physicians (ACEP) Emergency Department Directors Academy (EDDA), May 2, 2018.
15. Studer Q. Four best practices to improve emergency department results. *Becker's Hospital Review*. January 25, 2010.
16. Mayer T. Hire right: the 12-step process for patient experience. Presented at: The American College of Emergency Physicians Scientific Assembly, September 14, 2017; San Francisco.
17. Collins J. *Good to Great: Why Some Companies Make the Leap and Others Don't*. HarperCollins Publishers; 2001.
18. Collins J, Hansen MT. *Great by Choice: Uncertainty, Chaos, and Luck—Why Some Thrive Despite Them All*. HarperCollins Publishers; 2011.
19. Likert R. *New Patterns of Management*. McGraw-Hill; 1999.
20. Mayer T, Jensen K. *Hardwiring Flow: Systems and Processes for Seamless Patient Care*. Fire Starter Publishing; 2009.
21. Jensen K, Mayer T. *The Patient Flow Advantage: How Hardwiring Hospital-Wide Flow Drives Competitive Performance*. Fire Starter Publishing; 2015.
22. Jensen K, Mayer T, Welch SJ, et al. *Leadership for Smooth Patient Flow: Improved Outcomes, Improved Service, Improved Bottom Line*. Health Administration Press; 2007.
23. Studer Q. *Straight a Leadership: Alignment, Action, Accountability*. Fire Starter Publishing; 2009.
24. Maister D. The psychology of waiting lines. *David Maister: Professional Business Professional Life* blog. September 8, 2006. Available at: http://davidmaister.com/blog/201/The-Psychology-of-Waiting-Lines. Accessed November 22, 2018.
25. Eisley L. *The Star Thrower*. Harcourt Brace Jovanovich; 1978.

CHAPTER 76
COMPLAINT MANAGEMENT
Robert W. Strauss

People complain when they are dissatisfied. Add the anxiety, confusion, and potential peril of an emergency, and the number and seriousness of complaints increase. For example, a mother brings her tearful 3-year-old to the emergency department (ED) because of a wrist injury. After waiting for three hours, the child is seen by a hurried nurse, is taken to x-ray, and then is seen once (for 2 minutes) by a physician, who performs a limited examination, barely speaks to either the mother or the child, and mutters something about a fracture. The patient is discharged with a splint and written instructions. Questions are superficially answered. Two days later, the child goes to his family practitioner, who after telling the mother that the child has a broken bone, shares his own complaints about the ED care and then refers the child to an orthopedist. One month later, a very dissatisfied parent receives ED bills totaling $1,050. She is angry and on the phone waiting to speak with you.

Complaint recognition and management are critical components of the successful ED. When handled properly, a dissatisfied and angry person can achieve satisfaction. Alternatively, the improper management of a complaint can lead to a disgruntled person who seeks retribution. The benefits of effective complaint management go far beyond meeting the perceived needs of the individual complainant. Institutions and leaders that recognize the importance of the consumer seek opportunities to improve by taking steps to reduce the root cause of dissatisfaction.

Adding compliment management creates a more comprehensive and balanced system. ED leaders who recognize and publicize compliments celebrate and value the praiseworthy efforts of department members, commonly delivered but uncommonly recognized and appreciated.

THE NATURE OF COMPLAINTS

All EDs receive complaints. Inevitably, some people will voice their dissatisfaction with the quality of care, length of stay, attitude of nurses and physicians, or cost of care. The approach of the department team and the institution distinguishes the organizations seeking improvement and satisfaction from those destined to repeat mistakes. To develop an effective approach, it is necessary to first understand why people complain.

We all experience dissatisfaction with some interactions because "reasonable" expectations go unmet. The ED is particularly prone to create dissatisfaction among those who use its services. Patients, private physicians, emergency medical services providers, and staff all enter the ED with expectations of rapid, quality care by an attentive and kind staff. Unfortunately, it is impossible to always meet these expectations.

The Complainer

Why do people complain?[1,2] Generally, people are dissatisfied when their expectations go unmet. In addition, if they perceive that they have been inconvenienced and treated rudely, they are much more likely to voice their dissatisfaction in the form of a complaint.

Duration of Relationship

Although the reasons for patient dissatisfaction are myriad, certain generalizations can be made. The duration of the relationship between the health-care providers and the patient is positively correlated to patient satisfaction.[3,4] The longer the relationship, the more satisfied the patient. The relationship between emergency care staff members and the patient is measured in minutes rather than years. This brief exposure allows little opportunity to develop the bond that may exist between a patient and a private physician.

Effective Communication

Patient expectations of physicians and nurses go beyond that of clinical competence. Patients expect their practitioners to be friendly, kind, and concerned and to take the time to explain the situation and answer questions.[5,6] As Terry Canale stated in his American Academy of Orthopaedic Surgeons Presidential Address:

> *The patient[s] will never care how much you know, until they know how much you care.*[7]

In the stressful setting of the ED, the ability to develop a rapid rapport with the patient and family enhances patient satisfaction. While many patients complain about delays in care, the greatest number of complaints lodged directly against ED workers relates to attitude and poor communication.[8] It follows that those physicians and nurses who adequately explain the nature of the problem or procedure are found to score higher on patient satisfaction scales than those who do not.[3,9,10] More complete explanations create a better understanding and more realistic expectations of the course and outcome of the illness. In addition, those who are encouraged to and actually do ask questions about their condition are more satisfied.[3,5,10]

The Demographics of Complainers

A substantial amount of literature that reviews the characteristics of the complainer has been published. Considerations of age, sex, and income levels are frequently cited.[4,8,11] The relationship between age and complaint behavior is unclear. Although it has been suggested that the elderly are less likely to voice a complaint, this has not been substantiated in several studies. Women are more likely than men to register complaints, which may relate to the fact that women are more likely to make the family's health-care decisions. And those with higher incomes voice complaints more often and are more likely to choose another provider because they generally have higher expectations, greater resources, and increased options to obtain alternative providers of care.[4]

Reasons for Concern

Successful delivery of emergency care entails recognizing the responsibility to address the needs of those using the service. There are many ramifications of dissatisfied patients, peers, and customers. The ED census may drop, medicolegal cases may increase, and ultimately the ties between the practitioner and the institution may be severed. Dissatisfied patients have three choices: They may voice a complaint, choose another provider ("exit"), or continue to use the service despite being dissatisfied (remain loyal).[12] Interestingly, loyal but dissatisfied consumers are considered passive, seeming to suffer in silence.

Many dissatisfied people do not complain.[8,13-15] They don't express their dissatisfaction because they believe it is not worth their time and effort, they don't know how or where to complain, or they don't believe it will do any good. In fact, fewer than 25% of patients who are dissatisfied voice a complaint to the service provider. Note that many of these "noncomplaining" consumers still may have an impact. Although unwilling to complain to the service provider, they may complain to friends and family, influencing their behavior and creating "negative word of mouth."[16] Further, they may seek satisfaction from third parties, such as governmental agencies or the legal system. Finally, they may choose other providers, as suggested by the following passage:

> *You know me, I'm a nice person. When I get lousy service, I never complain. I never kick. I never criticize, and I wouldn't dream of making a scene. I'm one of those nice customers. And I'll tell you what else I am. I'm the customer who doesn't come back. I take whatever you hand out because I know I'm not coming back. I could tell you off and feel better, but in the long run, it's better to just leave quietly. You see, a nice customer like me, multiplied by others like me, can bring a business to its knees. There are plenty of us. When we get pushed far enough, we go to one of your competitors.*[17]

Census Impact

Changing providers ("exiting") once a relationship is well established seems difficult and requires substantial effort.[15,18] However, literature reveals that up to 63% of patients change physicians when dissatisfied, a number that is much higher than previously believed.[15,19] Those with medical (quality of care) complaints are twice as likely to seek alternative providers as those with nonmedical complaints.[4] A nonmedical study on dissatisfaction among aging consumers shows that they are more than 12 times more likely to report an intention to switch providers than satisfied consumers.[20]

As the environment becomes increasingly competitive, patients may find the option of changing providers and institutions more attractive. This is particularly true in an ED setting, where:

- The caregiver–consumer relationship is superficial.
- Interactions occur unpredictably.
- The consumer's absence will go unnoticed.
- Many alternatives are available.

In the ED, a contraction of census will decrease the need for service, nurses, physicians, and support staff. For an emergency physician group that exists within a fee-for-service environment, a dwindling census may be devastating. For employed emergency physicians and emergency nurses, fewer patients may obviate the need for their positions.

Medicolegal Implications

Aggrieved patients frequently turn to the legal system to seek redress.[21] Multiple agencies exist to receive and respond to consumer complaints. These include the Office of Consumer Affairs, Better Business Bureau, Centers for Medicare and Medicaid Services (CMS), Office of the Inspector General, and quality-improvement organizations, medical societies, medical boards, departments of health, and so on.

Consumers have a greater tendency to seek third-party redress when they perceive that more direct interaction, such as voicing a complaint to the hospital's consumer advocate, is unlikely to lead to resolution. There is evidence that consumers perceive medical providers to be among the least responsive to complaint resolution among the service industries.[18] Only about one-third of the consumers who voiced complaints believed their problems were satisfactorily addressed.[13] By ignoring or inadequately handling complaints, ED leaders may unwittingly encourage third-party actions.

Contract/Job Security

If there is a perception of ineffective problem management, the nurse's or practitioner's (group's) relationship with the institution may become tenuous. Effective consumer-oriented administrators expect problems to be identified and solved with the subsequent development of procedures to ensure that the problem does not recur. Department leaders are expected to supervise this improvement. Leadership nonparticipation (avoidance) is perceived as an "I don't care" attitude, which is often the reason for the complaint in the first place. Hospital administrators and medical staff leadership may react decisively against unresponsive individuals and organizations by looking for alternative contractual relationships.

The Regulatory Imperative

Regulatory agencies look at problems, the systems used to handle those problems, and the methods to prevent their recurrence. The presumption is if there is an effective system, future problems will be prevented through early recognition and resolution. The Joint Commission looks specifically at the institution's complaint-management process. Reviewers often ask for evidence of a comprehensive system. The Joint Commission requires complaint-management guidelines to be incorporated into the organization' procedures. The 2010 Joint Commission standards require that:

> *The Elements of Performance Standard RI 01.07.01 address the resolution of patients' complaints. The standards require a complaint resolution process and informing individuals about the process. The standards also require response by the organization and the organization informing patients about their right to file complaints with the state authority.*[22]

Other regulatory bodies further define the process necessary for institutional complaint management. For example, the New York State Department of Health, Code 405.7.23, states:

> *[The hospital shall ensure that all patients . . . are afforded their rights [to]]: . . . express complaints about the care and services provided and to have the hospital investigate such complaints. The hospital shall provide the patient or his/her designee with a written response indicating the findings of the investigation. The hospital shall notify the patient or his/her designee if the patient is not satisfied with the hospital's oral or written response, the patient may complain to the New York State Department of Health's Office of Health Systems Management. The hospital shall provide the telephone number of the local area office of the Health Department to the patient.*[23]

Hospitals and their leaders are responsible for developing and implementing mechanisms to promptly receive and respond to patient and family complaints. All hospitals provide their patients with a "bill of rights." Most agencies refer to a constructive complaint resolution process. The organizations must thoroughly analyze the complaints and when indicated take appropriate corrective actions. And the patients or family members making the complaint must receive responses that substantively address their complaints.[18]

Providing Patient Satisfaction

The job of leaders entails providing high-quality care while satisfying the perceived needs of those around them. It is helpful to look at patients, colleagues, staff, and others who use and interact with the ED and its services as customers. This business philosophy enables ED leadership to look closely at what patients and others want. To do this, it is necessary to first define customer service:

> *Customer service is a series of activities designed to enhance the level of customer satisfaction – that is, the feeling that a product or service has met the customer expectation.*[24]

> **BOX 76.1 ■ THE 4 Cs OF PATIENT SATISFACTION**
>
> - Convenience
> - Caring
> - Care (quality)
> - Cost

Therefore, satisfaction can only occur by meeting, surpassing, or modifying expectations. And yet, so often, caregivers thoughtlessly create dissatisfaction by raising expectations. Consider:

- An emergency physician who says, "The nurse will discharge you in *a minute*."
- The emergency nurse who says, "I'll be *right back*."
- A private physician who says, "Just go to the ED and get an x-ray." The inexperienced patient may believe this will be a 20-minute excursion. If it takes 2 hours and the patient did not plan for it, every little additional delay creates frustration.

Patients are customers, and the ED offers a service. If it is not delivered properly, EDs will lose their customers.

The Definition of a Customer

Merriam-Webster defines a customer as "one that purchases a commodity or service." Unfortunately, some practitioners who work in the ED reject the concept of patients as customers. This disregard is a form of arrogance that essentially communicates, "If the patients don't like what I say or how I say it, they can go somewhere else." Patients are not fundamentally different from people who buy computers, gas, or food. The basic expectations of a person who comes for treatment of a broken bone and one who orders food in a restaurant have several similarities. While a patient will likely have a greater sense of urgency, both want what "customers" universally expect—service delivered quickly, courteously, with quality, and at a fair cost.

Patient Expectations

Patients want the same things that all customers want: the Four Cs, or **c**onvenience, **c**aring, **c**are (quality), and **c**ost (**Box 76.1**).[23]

- ***Convenience:*** When patients have a choice about emergency care, they tend to choose the institution that will get them in and out most quickly. Interestingly, health-care professionals rarely have the patience to wait in the waiting room of their own EDs when they or their family members are ill. In fact, most will bypass the typical front-end triage process and go straight to the care area to get their medical problems addressed immediately.
- ***Caring:*** Emergency professionals must develop rapport quickly. The success of the treatment approach once the patient is discharged depends on the trust developed. Patients judge caregivers most often based on the level of caring rather than the level of care.[8,13,13] Caring goes beyond giving a high standard of care. The classic response, "I did everything correctly; just look at the chart," just isn't good enough. When dealing with people and complaints, the complaint manager (CM) initially must focus on how the process did not work for the patient ("complainer") rather than trying to "educate" the patient and defend the process.

- ***Care:*** Generally, the lay public cannot judge the quality of care provided. Consider how difficult it is for an unsophisticated consumer to assess whether the examination was complete, the testing was appropriate, or the antibiotic was correct. It is only when the outcome is poor and unexpected that questions arise, perhaps even leading to questions of competence. Therefore, it is critical to recognize the patients' expectations and meet, surpass, or modify them. It is often prudent to both say and document some form of the following: "You should improve with this treatment. If you are not better in _____ days or you get worse, I would like you to immediately see your doctor or come back here and see me or one of my partners."
- ***Cost:*** Value is an increasingly important issue for those who use the ED. If a patient waited for hours, was treated rudely, or had a condition that got worse in spite of treatment, the cost of care may seem inappropriate no matter how inexpensive. Conversely, patients who perceive that they received value—treated quickly, courteously, and correctly—are much more willing to accept a reasonable bill.

Complaint Prevention

Though it is not always possible to meet patients' initial expectations, ED nurses and physicians have many opportunities to modify or reset patients' expectations. In other words, unrealistically high expectations can be lowered and then met or surpassed (**Box 76.2**).

Realistic Triage

The initial interaction with the ED, which is often triage, provides the first opportunity to recognize and influence the patient's expectations. One of the most common patient complaints is related to duration of stay, perhaps based on patients' unrealistic expectations or a poor understanding of the process. The triage clinician may positively modify the patient's expectations by spending a few extra seconds to explain the process:

- Describe what will happen.
- Share (with slight exaggeration) the anticipated duration of the clinical process, perhaps lowering preconceived expectations.
- Answer questions.
- Provide satisfaction by surpassing the now lowered expectations.

For example, to a patient requiring an x-ray in a busy traditional ED, the triaging staff member could explain like this:

From here you will be taken to an examination room. I'll order an x-ray now, and once you're in the examining room, you will receive a more in-depth evaluation by both the nurse and the physician who will review your x-ray. The physician will determine your treatment and follow-up, and then your nurse will give you discharge instructions. Generally, the entire process takes 90 minutes. Do you have any questions?

BOX 76.2 ■ COMPLAINT-PREVENTION TECHNIQUES

- Realistic triage
- Triage ordering
- Reset expectations
- Theory of "Yes"
- Questionably necessary test
- Closing questions

While the care might be expected to only take an hour or less, it is appropriate to add a few minutes to the estimate of the patient's duration of stay to allow for the interruptions that typically occur in an ED. If the evaluation is completed sooner, the patient is thrilled because the lowered expectation will have been surpassed.

Operational protocols that empower the nursing staff to order necessary tests and begin treatments on patients can dramatically reduce the duration of stay. As in the example above, an x-ray or lab test that has been completed by the time the patient arrives in the examining room will reduce unnecessary waits.

Resetting Expectations

While patients expect rapid care, it is not always possible to meet this expectation. There are several appropriate opportunities to modify patient expectations during the wait. After a particularly busy time, such as a resuscitation, the nurse or physician can go out to the waiting room with two or three charts in hand. An apology for and explanation of the delay, displaying respect, and providing a legitimate reason are usually very much appreciated. Then bringing two or three patients into the ED proper will confirm that the situation is improving. Once a patient is in an examining room, the same outcome can be achieved on an individual basis:

Hello, Mrs. Jones. I am Dr. Smith. I am sorry that you have had to wait. I am taking care of a very unstable patient and expect to be back with you in about 20 minutes. In the meantime, I will ask the nurse to make sure we get your evaluation started and to keep me informed.

The caveat is that if providing a specific time resets the expectation, the promising health-care professional must be there at or before the promised time. If the professional gets "tied up," he or she must send someone in to say it will be a little longer.

Just Say "YES"

It is often helpful to begin the response to a request or inquiry with a form of "YES!" The "yes" in this situation is only meant to acknowledge the point of view of the other person, not to agree to the request. Consider the following responses to a patient who asks for something unreasonable:

- "No, you don't need that." The message is "I am the trained specialist, and I know what you need better than you do." Once the response begins with "No," the communication and therapeutic relationship may deteriorate.
- Alternatively, according to the "yes" theory, one might respond by saying, "Yes (sure), I can see that this is bothering you. Let me take a closer look so that we can figure out exactly what is wrong." The communication now is one of acceptance—affirmation that the patient has a reasonable perspective. The practitioner has agreed to work with the patient to further elucidate the problem without actually agreeing to meet the unreasonable request.

The Questionably Necessary Test

The patient requests a questionably necessary test, convinced that the test is essential. When practical, a successful strategy is to involve the trusted private practitioner in the discussion. On other occasions, it may be appropriate to provide the desired test. The patient will leave satisfied and believing that the practitioner cared enough to make sure that he or she is okay. This is not substantially different from the practice of most practitioners who obtain x-rays or provide antibiotics that are of questionable necessity. Alternatively, if the practitioner successfully convinces the patient not to get the test and eventually pathology is found, the vindicated patient may be very resentful.

> **BOX 76.3 ■ CLOSING QUESTIONS**
>
> - Is there anything else that I can do for you?
> - Have I fully addressed your medical problem?
> - Have you and your family been kept fully informed?
> - Have we provided you with excellent care?

Closing Questions

It is a good practice for each practitioner who participates in the discharge of the patient to routinely ask the "closing question" to ensure that nothing has been overlooked from the patient's perspective (**Box 76.3**). When given the opportunity, occasionally patients divulge their true concern only at the end of the visit, such as "Will I be okay?" or "Is it cancer?" Without that final opportunity to ask the question, the patient may leave dissatisfied. Other patients may notice or describe an additional complaint, such as "What about my...?," which may have been previously overlooked. Most often, the patient will respond with a "No, but thanks." Some practitioners ask a closing question to obtain feedback on their own and the staff's performance. The closing question allows the patient and the practitioner to come to a definitive closure.

Satisfying Other Stakeholders

The appropriate management of complaints, including trend analysis, cannot be overemphasized as one of the key tasks of ED leadership. When an effective emergency complaint-management system exists, the process of handling a complaint proceeds down a consistent pathway:

- An administrator or other hospital representative receives a complaint about the ED.
- The complaint is immediately and confidently forwarded to the ED leader/CM for rapid resolution.
- The complaint is resolved quickly and effectively.
- The ED leader/CM communicates the resolution to the administrator (in writing).
- The root cause is identified and processes are put in place—and ED personnel are immediately informed of them—to limit the occurence of similar complaints.
- The resolution of the complaint is communicated to appropriate stakeholders.

Administration

The hospital administration runs a service business. To be effective, they must listen to their customers and user groups. Included among the most influential are the patients and their insurers, who use the service and pay the bills; the primary care physicians (PCPs) and proceduralists, who control which of the paying patients will use the hospital's service; and the hospital board of trustees, the institution's governing body, which directly oversees the administrator. Note that emergency care professionals are not among the most influential groups. Administrators typically want ED staffs who:

- Are problem solvers
- Do not generate a lot of complaints
- Keep the influential customers—the patients, physicians, and the board—happy

ED Staff

The emergency staff requires leadership that solves problems. For instance, if a nurse or physician comes to the ED leader and states that there is a problem with another person or a process, it is incumbent upon the leader to investigate, attempt to resolve the problem (when appropriate), and communicate back to the person raising the issue. Staff issues generally do not go away and, if ignored, erode the confidence of the staff in the department leaders. Leaders who don't address the problem become part of the problem.

Medical Staff Members

Emergency department complaints from non-ED medical staff generally involve effectiveness of communication and quality of care.[25] Department leaders should actively seek out those complaints and the people who make them. Once made aware of a complaint, the CM should rapidly investigate it and communicate the results of the investigation. By moving quickly to resolve the concerns of the medical staff, ED leaders demonstrate that the greatest interest of the ED staff is to provide the best care possible. To achieve success, the ED leaders should articulate and promote a philosophy of partnership with the members of the medical staff.

THE COMPLAINT-MANAGEMENT SYSTEM

A positive approach to the sometimes-unpleasant task of complaint management can be the first step in improving others' perceptions of your services. People who complain are looking for something they did not get during their first interaction with the system—*satisfaction*. By calling, the complainer is providing a challenge and an opportunity to transform the previously dissatisfying interaction into a favorable one. A response that conveys the sentiment, "Oh, no, not another complaint!" will confirm the complainer's misgivings. Alternatively, an open and sincere approach that conveys the sentiment "I want to understand and address the problem" will demonstrate the caring and concern that may have been absent during the earlier encounter.

Real-Time Management

Ultimately, it is best to rectify a situation while it is occurring to achieve immediate resolution. Five minutes spent getting an acutely developing situation back on track may obviate hours of investigation and embarrassment later.

In fact, most practitioners recognize when a patient is frustrated and dissatisfied. Leaders may wish to teach team members real-time service recovery; that is, to recognize and effectively respond to escalating problems. For instance, the simple key phrase—"You seem upset. How can I help?"—may lead to a definition of the problem and the potential for resolution. As an alternative approach, the primary provider can ask a colleague to investigate the perceptions of an unhappy patient. A problem uncovered may be then resolved as it is occurring. An undisclosed and therefore unresolved problem may leave the patient dissatisfied and frustrated, which in turn can result in a complaint voiced directly to an institutional leader and to multiple friends and acquaintances.

Tripping the System

Determining which complaints require a formal process of resolution is individual to each institution. This is one of the primary reasons that it is difficult to objectively compare ("benchmark") the volume of complaints among institutions. As examples, the following complaints are considered minor in some institutions and significant and worthy of full investigation in others:

- "My patient Mrs. Smith says that she had to wait to be discharged because your emergency doctor/nurse was on the phone ordering dinner!"
- A "repeater" who often comes to the ED to get warm and sober describes being ignored and then treated rudely.
- The patient complains no one called her primary care practitioner.

How each leader differentiates legitimate from "bogus" (groundless) complaints is telling. It is similar to asking, "What is a true emergency?" Is it the leader's definition, or is it the patient's? The same dilemma exists for defining true complaints. From the perspective of the complainer, they are all legitimate. It is the contention of this author that more rather than fewer complaints should be included in the formal system of complaint management.

Handling the Complaint

Unfortunately, the staffs and leaders of many organizations react adversely to complaints, ignoring them, which in turn perpetuates the problem. Complaints are most appropriately viewed as an "asset." On one hand, complaints create additional and sometimes difficult work for the CM. On the other hand, the person who calls and lets the organization know that the service or system didn't work cares enough to let the leaders know about the failings. Only by seriously considering the complaint does that person have the potential to be satisfied and does that problem have the potential to be resolved, now and in the future.

The CM should demonstrate concern, sincerity, and empathy, conveying the feeling that the perceived problem is important to the manager. In one sense, all emergency practitioners are experts at handling complaints, because it is part of the ED routine when trying to assess and respond to the patient's medical problem. It is simply a matter of putting the same effort into managing the service complaint. The CM may be able to rapidly change the complainer's perception by starting with a positive and empathetic attitude. The message should be some form of:

Thanks for letting me know. Your experience is a real concern to me. I'm going to investigate it now and get back to you.

Complaint managers who are continually trying to improve their systems may say with sincerity:

Your call comes at an opportune time. I am looking at ways to improve our service. What happened? How is the patient doing now?

This type of attitude displayed to a complainant may actually transform the complainer's self-perception from a slighted, depersonalized object into a valued consultant. Thus, the first step in resolving the complaint has been taken.

Determining the Issue

The second step is to find out what the complainer really wants, which can be accomplished only by hearing it from the complainant's perspective. The goal is to allow the person to

> **BOX 76.4 ■ COMPLAINERS WANT RESOLUTION**
>
> - Respect and understanding
> - Immediate investigation and follow-up
> - Censure
> - Assurance of nonrecurrence
> - Compensation or reduction of the bill

leave the conversation thinking "I'm glad I called. I've made a difference." People who have complaints want one or a combination of the following (**Box 76.4**):

- *Respect and understanding*: It is necessary for complainers to believe that the CM sincerely wants to hear about and resolve the issue, that it *is* important. Empathetic listening may itself provide the caring and compassion that were missing from the initial interaction, which in many cases is all the complainer wants.
- *Immediate investigation and follow-up*: The genuine desire to address the issue can be demonstrated by simply agreeing to perform an immediate and thorough investigation and promising rapid follow-up. The powerful message conveyed by this sincere approach lets the complainer know: "You are so important that I will promptly address your issues and report back to you." A neglected person who has been frustrated by the system is now able to establish some control and a promise of action.
- *Censure*: Some complainers have been so slighted by the process that they believe satisfaction can best be achieved by some form of punishment, reprimand, or censure. These people want to know that the responsible person "will pay the penalty." This most often occurs as the result of uncaring, inattentive, or rude behavior exhibited by a caregiver. While the CM cannot share specific actions related to a clinician, he or she can describe the general quality procedure, including investigation and action based on the results of that investigation, without describing the specific results. If convinced of the CM's sincerity, this explanation usually satisfies those looking for "censure."
- *Assurance that the problem will not recur*: It is very satisfying to conclude an interaction knowing "I've made a difference." If the CM is able to transform the complaint into a system or a behavior change, the complainer can walk away with the feeling that he or she has improved the system and the care rendered to others who follow. Though these complainants may not themselves achieve a change in the care they personally received, they can achieve the satisfaction of their "altruistic" action: "My experience will improve the experience of others."
- *Reduction of the bill*: Many complaints occur at the time the bill is received. For a variety of reasons, the patient may not believe the service rendered justifies the bill received. These patients will want reconsideration of the charge. Patients with a complaint about the bill may be satisfied with a negotiated reduction of the bill. Some will ask for complete elimination of the bill, and a few may even request compensation.

The Complaint Manager

To achieve the greatest success and effect the greatest system improvements, it is necessary to formalize the complaint-management process. A formal approach requires hardwiring

> **BOX 76.5 ■ COMPONENTS OF A COMPLAINT SYSTEM**
>
> - Complaint manager
> - Situation assessment form and process
> - Systematic tracking process—Log
> - Follow-up and reporting mechanism

several integrated processes (**Box 76.5**). To ensure consistency, a CM should be identified to assume responsibility for the overall management of complaints. This CM should be a person with leadership skills, integrity, and the authority to effect change. By creating the position and title, the potential other recipients of a complaint (administrator, chief of staff, etc.) are prompted to immediately forward the complaint to the identified complaint handler.

Preferably, the CM will be the nursing or physician director or associate director of the department—a person with the imprimatur of leadership and authority. If a complaint is received involving the person who typically handles the complaint, then it is appropriate for another person to manage the process.

The Situation Assessment

A sample situation assessment form is provided in **Figure 76.1**. (Note: The form is presented as a single page for the convenience of the reader. An actual completed situation assessment form might be longer because specific sections require expansion to thoroughly document all aspects of the complaint.)

Identifying Information

Using this form, the patient name and medical record number are placed on the top of the sheet, as well as a unique identifying number particular to the tracking system ("log"). Practitioners may also be identified by a number, rather than by name, when referring to them in the body of the situation assessment. For instance, in the example that follows, Dr. Smith is referred to as "emergency physician #107," and Nurses Jones and Peters are referred to as "emergency nurses #2214 and #1020," respectively.

Dates

Delineating the dates of service, complaint, and resolution is valuable because it gives an indication of the type of complaint, as well as helps to track the responsiveness of the system. A complaint expressed immediately after care is rendered implies a problem with the care or caring. A complaint articulated weeks later may be related to the receipt of the bill. A review of the average time between date of complaint and date of resolution will measure the efficiency of the system. It might be appropriate to have an additional line for "date complaint received," particularly in institutions that do not immediately forward complaints to the ED CM.

Types of Complaints

Differentiating the type of complaint into various subtypes, such as quality, attitude, and length of stay, allows data trending. The trends may then be used to create a focus of individual or system improvement and monitor the success of those efforts. A single complaint may involve more than one subtype.

Sources (Initiated By)

Anyone can be the source of a complaint, so access to the system should be easy. The complaint can arise from a patient (oral or written), physician (directly or by word of mouth),

FIGURE 76.1 ■ Situation Assessment Form

ABC Hospital Emergency Department
Performance Improvement program
Situation Assessment

Patient _____ ID# _____ LOG# _____

Type of Complaint

Date of Service _____   ____ Attitude   ____ Cost of Care
Date of Complaint _____   ____ Documentation   ____ Follow-Up Instruction
Date of Receipt _____   ____ Length of Stay   ____ Other (Specify)
Date of Resolution _____   ____ Quality of Care   _____

Initiated by: NAME   DATE
____ Chart Review
____ Hospital Administration
____ Nurse
____ Patient
____ Physician
____ Billing Rep
____ Other

Sources of Information: _____

Issue: _____

Investigation: _____

Assessment: _____

Discussed with: NAME   DATE
____ Emergency Nurse
____ Emergency Physician
____ Patient (Family)
____ Private Physician
____ Hospital Representative
____ Billing Representative

Rating: Standard of Care Met   ____ Yes   ____ +/-   ____ No

Adverse Patient Outcome   ___0   ___1   ___2   ___3   ___4   ___5

Investigated By: Signature   Date:
_____   _____   _____

Practitioner:
_____   _____   _____

or a staff member. Other sources include legal inquiries and routine chart reviews, such as 72-hour return visits, that may uncover possible problems of care and become an entry point into the system.

Assessment

The actual assessment generally contains three components: the issue, the investigation, and the resolution. The assessment may at times require in-depth documentation of the information gathered.

The issue: The issue is ascertained by discussion with the complainant and review of the records. The perspective of the complainant should be documented in an objective manner. For instance, a patient might state, "The doctor was a jerk and treated us like animals!" This could be documented as: "The patient was angry and felt emergency physician #107 was rude and uncaring." The issue section should be brief, concisely describing enough detail to understand why the complaint is being lodged and to direct the subsequent investigation. Occasionally, the complainant describes several issues. Each should be delineated in this section and then addressed in the subsequent process of investigation and resolution.

The investigation: This investigation section of the form should begin with a description of the sources of the investigation and end with the results of it; for example, "The following sources were used to investigate this case: the patient, the medical record, emergency physician #107, emergency nurses #2214 and #1020, and *The ABC Textbook of Emergency Medicine*."

The investigation is driven by the desire to objectively determine what actually occurred. To be effective, the CM must gather information without preconceived notions of right or wrong. It is normal to empathize with the point of view of the complainant; however, the complainant, no matter how compelling, represents one side of the story. It is inappropriate to adopt any point of view that would cloud objectivity during the investigative portion of the complaint-management process. Investigation is not meant to assess blame but rather to clarify perceptions and performance. In other words, when approaching the practitioner, the query should be without reproach or criticism; for example, "It was Mrs. Smith's perception that her care was . . . What happened?" Each person implicated or with substantive information to add should get an opportunity to describe the occurrence from his or her own perspective.

The resolution: The resolution must address each concern raised in the previous sections of the form. The goal is to educate, improve performance, and correct inappropriate behaviors, faulty perceptions, and misinformation. Follow-up and feedback are critical to the complaint-management and behavioral modification process. It is incumbent on the CM to communicate to both the complainant and to the complaint recipient that the process has been completed. Complaint-specific resolutions are presented in detail later in this chapter. **Table 76.1** lists problems with typical resolutions. Complaints may require specific actions to effect a change in behavior, fill a knowledge gap, etc.

However, the CM will also determine that many complaints, after investigation, do not require any change in the system or individual behavior. Follow-up and feedback from positive

TABLE 76.1 ■ Potential Problems and Solutions	
Problem	**Example Resolution**
Misread x-ray	Review x-ray; if trend or significant misread, read chapter and spend time with radiologist
Misunderstood process (i.e., referral)	Perform in-service (by complaining practitioner)
Delay in care	Improve lab reporting system
	Decrease door to doctor time
	Shorten triage process
	Implement staffing change
Perceived but not actual incorrect care	Explanation to patient, supportive feedback to practitioner
Behavioral issue	Coaching practitioner with expected standards of behavior

TABLE 76.2 ■ Standard of Care Assessment

Symbol	Standard of Care
+	Met
+/−	Questionable
−	Deficient

assessments are particularly valuable. The CM not only satisfies the complainer by a thorough investigation and follow-up but also supports the caregivers by a positive conclusion.

Signature

The final sections of the form identify the individual caregivers, rate the care, and provide an opportunity for feedback by the caregiver. It may be judicious to complete these sections on a subsequent page to avoid having ratings visible to all who might read the complaint and its investigation. The CM or person investigating the complaint determines a rating and then signs the form. The involved physician or nurse reads, signs, and may make a comment on the form. This process ensures that the practitioner has knowledge of the complaint, investigation, and conclusions. Occasionally, the CM may draw a conclusion that is erroneous or lacks complete information. In these cases, the review by the practitioner allows appropriate modification.

Full disclosure is another reason for practitioner review. Since the complaint file resides in the practitioner's file, it is inappropriate to hold this information without knowledge of the involved person. Concealing the information limits the opportunity to change and improve. Further, if the information only surfaces subsequently when the practitioner is applying for another position, the CM might be subjected to legal scrutiny.

Rating

The rating system describes the final appraisal of the issue's significance. The rating should incorporate two elements. First, the CM must judge whether the standard of care has been met (**Table 76.2**). If the standard of care has not been met, there must then be a determination of whether an adverse patient outcome (APO) occurred as a direct result of the deficiency (**Figure 76.2**). If the standard of care was met and the patient has a poor outcome unrelated to the standard of care, the rating will not reflect an adverse outcome. (Examples are illustrated in **Table 76.3**.)

FIGURE 76.2 ■ Adverse Patient Outcome Grid

Symbol Type	Change in Patient Outcome/ Management	Examples (management changes directly attributable to a deficiency in standard of care)
0	None	
1	Minor-temporary	Additional visit, splint antibiotics
2	Minor-permanent	Facial scar, decreased function fifth digit
3	Major-temporary	Ruptured appendix, pneumothorax, ICU care
4	Major-permanent	Loss of functional use of limb, cardiac cripple
5	Death	

TABLE 76.3 ■ Rating System Demonstrating Relationship of Standard of Care (SoC) and Adverse Patient Outcome (APO)

Issue	SoC	APO	Explanation
Iatrogenic pneumothorax	– (deficient)	3 (major, temporary)	Deficient SOC caused APO
ªPatient death	+ (met)	0 (no negative outcome related to SOC deficiency)	SOC met, even though patient did not survive resuscitation
Poor documentation requiring re-evaluation	– (deficient)	1 (minor, temporary)	Deficient SOC caused APO, leading to additional patient care
ªRude practitioner	– (deficient)	0 (no change in outcome)	No resultant adverse outcome

ª In these cases, there was either no APO or the APO was unrelated to a deficient SoC (The previously published example).

The Tracking Log

The log is a tracking mechanism used to document in a single and consistent manner the essential data and status of all complaints (**Figure 76.3**). Information entered directly into the log correlates with information on the situation assessment form. At minimum, the log should be used as a tracking system to identify the patient, nature of the complaint, its current status, and resolution.

A more sophisticated log can be used to trend data and extract a variety of information about the caregivers and the provision of care in the institution. For instance, a comprehensive log can be used to determine the number of complaints, types of complaints, and outcome data. The number and types of complaints broken down by individual can be used to create comparative data. When comparing individual caregivers, it is important to factor in the variations in practice, that is:

- Number of patients cared for and hours worked by each health-care professional—the denominator
- Types of shifts worked (days, nights, swing, fast track)
- Complaint type, severity, and patient outcome

FIGURE 76.3 ■ Example of a Complaint-Management Log

Name	Date of service	Date of complaint	Date of resolution	Type	Investigator	Provider number	Assessment complete	+/- 0-5	Comment
R Jones	6/6/12	6/8/12	6/11/12	Attitude	RS	27	✔	-/0	Provider counseled
W Clinton	5/4/12	6/13/12	6/15/12	Quality	GN	19	✔	-/1	CME required
A Einstein	5/11/12	6/19/12	6/19/12	Cost	RS	36	✔	+/0	No action required
M Jordan	6/18/12	6/25/12	6/28/12	Quality	RS	44	✔	+/0	Follow up with orthopedist (complainant) – in service
M Ghandi	7/1/12	7/1/12		Attitude	GN	27	✔		

Over time, an effective tracking mechanism can expose or confirm system and individual problems such as delays, attitude, quality, and cost-of-care issues. Attention to the outcome data may quickly identify individuals whose care is associated with poor outcomes or a "particular type" of poor outcome. For example, a caregiver with several complaints and an APO of 0 may be delivering high-quality care but low-quality caring. Alternatively, a professional who has more than one case per year with an APO of 2 or greater is likely to have significant quality of care problems.

Follow-Up and Reporting

The complaint-management process is not concluded until the appropriate stakeholders are notified of a resolution and the completion of the investigation is documented in the institution's quality management system.

When possible, the CM should contact each complaint source. While not all persons registering a complaint will achieve complete satisfaction, it is usually possible to provide them with the gratification of knowing that their issue was reviewed and addressed quickly and with respect and sincerity.

Further, it may be appropriate to send a letter to the complaining party thanking him or her for sharing the issue with you. An example of such a letter:

> *Dear Mr. Jones:*
>
> *Thank you for taking the time to let us know how we can better serve you. Your direct feedback about our services is vital to us. Though we closely monitor the medical care in our department, evaluating the perceptions of the patients and their families is more difficult to assess. Letters (feedback) such as yours are the best means we have of determining how well we are achieving our goal of providing excellent medical care in a caring manner. I am encouraged that part of your experience was positive. I hope that should you or your family need emergency care in the future that you again consider _____ Hospital.*
>
> *Sincerely,*
>
> *_____*
>
> *Director, Department of Emergency Medicine*
>
> Joseph E. F. Shanahan, MD, personal communication,
ED Medical Director, Chicago, IL

Caregiver Follow-Up (Monitoring Performance)

Comparisons of performance against individual benchmarks and within the group are measured and trended over time. Initially, it may be necessary to compare practitioners with their cohorts to persuade them to change. Some practices openly share this information. In the long run, it is more important for practitioners to be made aware of their own strengths and weaknesses so that they can recognize and address individual areas for improvement. Regular feedback can also demonstrate progress and provide positive reinforcement.

An effective monitoring system identifies practitioners with particular types of deficiencies. When a trend is noted, the CM should provide direct feedback to the individual caregiver and, when appropriate, develop a plan of corrective action. This should be communicated and agreed to in both orally and in writing.

Reporting and Confidentiality

The complaint-management process is an essential part of the overall performance improvement program. Practitioner complaint data can be incorporated into the credentialing and reappointment process. When discussing, documenting, and reporting situation assessments, it is imperative to avoid specifically referring to the practitioner. Names should not appear on any circulated data. Many systems use coded numbers to identify staff members. To maintain the tightest security, some EDs have their own coding system separate from the hospital's system, which can only be decoded by quality management personnel in the institution.

As with all performance improvement materials, situation assessments should never be circulated except on a limited "need-to-know" basis. If these materials are widely available, they lose the protection of confidentiality usually afforded to peer-review activities. Situation assessments should not appear in e-mails, either by reference or attachment, unless part of a secure intrafacility system. In some institutions, situation assessments are distributed for discussion during departmental performance improvement meetings and collected at the conclusion of the meeting. Participants in the process, including the support personnel who gather the materials and enter data, must be made aware of the significance, sensitivity, and confidential nature of these documents and processes.

The Four Phases of Implementation

When first implementing a complaint-management system, the CM should be prepared for the four typical phases, including preimplementation (planning and communication) and testing.

Preimplementation

The CM should promote the new, improved, and perhaps, more comprehensive system. Explaining the "enhanced" program at executive committee and the nursing directors' meeting has the potential to positively change the clinical leaders' perceptions of the ED. Beyond the general announcement, it is beneficial for the CM to meet individually the chief medical officer, chief nursing officer, chief of staff, department chairs, and other institutional leaders to accomplish two goals:

- Share information about how to use and activate the program (trip the system).
- Gain commitment from the leader to both utilize the system and encourage others who complain to communicate their issues directly to the CM. Rather than sympathize with the colleague, they can say, for example, that the doctor or nursing director is looking for ways to improve the ED services and "why don't you share your experience with her."

Once a new complaint-management system is implemented, the CM should be prepared for three typical phases of utilization: testing, high utilization, and steady state.

Testing Phase

Some older complaints that were previously ignored or unrecognized will be sent. Complainants who may have had particularly difficult encounters may angrily share their negative experiences, even though some are remote, perhaps occurring months or even years ago. They will be testing the sincerity of the CM and the effectiveness of the system.

High Utilization

A moderate increase in the number of complaints may follow the first phase. Positive experiences will encourage clinical colleagues to express their concerns about how they or their patients were handled. While this phase might seem burdensome, system users are giving the ED the chance to address their issues and improve the services.

Steady State

If the complaints are managed effectively and the "root causes" of the complaints are addressed, CMs will enter a low-utilization steady-state phase.

CHANGING PERCEPTION AND BEHAVIOR

This section provides examples of and reviews the most common ED complaints and then describes the basic techniques for resolving these complaints. After defining the issue, the resolutions will be examined from two perspectives. The "retrospective solution" will deal with the complaint that has already been voiced. This process focuses on damage control and satisfying a dissatisfied person. The "prospective solution" will describe prevention strategies, specifically examining the behavior or the system that has been identified as a problem.

The common complaints that will be reviewed in this final section of this chapter are listed in **Table 76.4**. Every CM will confront these issues.

Managing Actual Complaints

When possible, the CM should collect relevant information before talking with the complainant. Responding to a complaint without information is like walking in a minefield. If an assistant answers the phone, that person should make arrangements for the CM to return the call. Prior to the call back, the CM should obtain the chart and critically review the records with an eye for the appropriateness of the medical care. If it is not possible to prepare for the complaint in advance with a copy of the chart, the following approach will create the necessary time to review and respond to the complaint:

- Take all of the information.
- Empathize: "Given what you are describing, I can understand why you might be upset."
- Promise to call back after an investigation.

Dr. Zippy: He only saw me for 30 seconds!

"He never touched me" or "He only saw me for 30 seconds and his bill was $400. That means he's making $48,000 per hour! No wonder health care is so expensive!"

TABLE 76.4 ■ Typical Complaints Received by ED Leaders

Focus of Blame	Perceived Issue
Dr. Zippy	"He only saw me for 30 seconds…"
Molasses General Hospital	"I waited so long…"
Mercedes Medical Center	"Your charge was way too much…"
Dr. Frankenstein	"But he was dead when he got there…"
Nurse Jerkyl	"The nurse yelled at me for coming to the ED…"
Dr. Vesuvius	"He blew his stack at the nursing station again."
Dr. Terry Bradshaw	"The Monday morning quarterback"
Dr. Blunder	"He missed my child's broken bone…"

At Issue

This patient is expressing concern about one of three problems:

- Lack of caring and thoroughness
- Possible missed problem
- Expense of the bill.

To respond effectively to the actual concern, the CM must listen carefully and ask questions to determine the true nature of the patient's complaint. If the review demonstrates a consistent pattern of complaints related to a particular practitioner, a clinician-specific problem may exist.

"Dr. Zippy" appears in a variety of forms (**Figure 76.4**). He or she may be lazy, unconcerned, or simply lack an understanding of what patients want. Some practitioners are good "openers"; they evaluate the patient near the beginning of their emergency visit but don't provide closure. They do not tell the patient the results of test, summarize, or provide the opportunity for the patient to ask questions. Instead, these physicians send in another professional (such as a discharging nurse) to act as a designee.

Other physicians may be good "closers," only arriving to meet the patient for the first time after the decisions have been made. Such a doctor may believe the patient has come to the ED for a simple answer to a simple question, "Is it broken?" or "Do I need to be admitted?"

Patients want more than an answer. They want time and touching. They want caring, compassion, and consideration.

Retrospective Solution

Once the specific nature of this complaint is determined, the CM can address the issue. Perceived poor caring during the initial visit can be addressed by demonstrating compassion and concern during the current conversation. Additionally, the CM can ensure appropriate aftercare by offering to have the patient return or helping to arrange an appointment with the patient's PCP. Addressing the patient's concern may help:

- Satisfy the patient.
- Resolve any ongoing medical issue.
- Address a missed problem.

Prospective Solution

If the system identifies multiple practitioners with complaints of too little patient communication, then the staffing pattern might require review. However, an individual caregiver who regularly gets a complaint of not enough time or caring requires retraining. Education for this clinician entails teaching him or her how to provide the patient with early contact, middle contact, and late closure. With only a single visit, the patient may believe that the caregiver has only a fleeting awareness of the patient's presence. Evaluating the patient at the beginning of the visit, updating in the middle, and providing a conclusion at the end create in the patient the belief that the practitioner is aware of and concerned about the patient during the entire visit.

There are several simple techniques that this practitioner can utilize. Sitting with good eye contact will increase the perception of time spent without necessarily increasing the actual time spent. Multiple short visits to keep the patient informed will increase the perception of caring. Scripting or using a "key phrase" may be helpful (see Chapter 74). The perceptions of the patient, who might otherwise feel ignored, will improve if "Dr. Zippy" simply states, "It's important to me that I spend enough time with you to address your medical problems and answer your questions."

Molasses General Hospital

"I waited forever!" or "Those party animals! I kept waiting in pain and nothing was done. The staff was just sitting around laughing and figuring out what they were going to have on their pizza!"

At Issue

The two most important issues for patients who have a choice of where they get their emergency care are convenience and caring. Convenience means easy access and parking, efficient systems, and being evaluated and treated quickly so that they can return to their routine. However, even ED leadership and hospital administration that continually work toward implementing effective means of improving turnaround times cannot always provide efficiency.

When unable to deliver convenience and efficiency, providing a caring environment becomes even more important to patients and their families. While the quality of care is essential to those delivering it, most patients lack the sophistication to scrutinize the actual quality of care provided, and so: Emergency caregivers are usually judged more for the level of caring than for the quality of care.

Retrospective Solution

When confronted by a patient who complains about lack of caring, it is necessary to demonstrate empathy with an expression of understanding. People who complain that they were not taken care of in a timely and caring way when first seen are asking to be taken care of in a timely and caring way now. It is often enough to acknowledge and validate the concern: "Yes, it is frustrating to wait when your child is in pain. How is he doing now?" There is very little to offer other than empathy and a promise that you will investigate the delay and get back to them.

Prospective Solution

Particularly during the periods of time that the ED is unable to provide rapid and efficient care, it is necessary to provide "caring" care. Methods include the following:

- ***The sit-down approach.*** Whenever possible, when obtaining a history, practitioners should sit with the patient. Sitting often results in a more efficient communication, because patients may be more trusting and specific when the practitioner sits at eye level and appears unrushed. This approach demonstrates a willingness to spend the time necessary to complete the evaluation.
- ***The frequent touch.*** Some practitioners walk by patients as if wearing blinders. Clinicians state they are worried that if they make eye contact, the patient may try to pull the practitioner away from the important matters at hand. In fact, a comment such as "Mrs. Jones, we are waiting for your lab tests to come back. Is there anything I can do for you?" or "Are you okay?" will usually not result in a demand but rather demonstrate that the practitioner is concerned and caring. Most patients respond with a smile and a "Thanks, I'm okay." Some may request for something to make them more comfortable. Occasionally, patients may describe a change in their condition. And always they are appreciative. Patients' perceptions of caring and satisfaction are higher when multiple clinicians regularly check on them.
- ***Provide realistic expectations.*** When providing care in a busy setting, patients particularly appreciate a realistic appraisal of what to expect the duration of their visit. Many patients in an ED do not have an appreciation of the many steps

involved in rendering care. Describing the steps in the evaluation, estimating (perhaps even slightly exaggerating) the time, and providing occasional updates will both keep the patient informed and decrease the anxiety associated with not knowing what to expect.

Mercedes Medical Center

"I can't believe they charged me this much money! All they did was . . .."

At Issue

For many CMs, the majority of the complaints come at the time the patient receives the bill. However, it is a mistake to assume that this is simply a patient trying to get out of paying for service. The CM must listen carefully to discern the patient's concern. The three most common reasons for a billing complaint are limited ability to pay, perception of inappropriate bill, and dissatisfaction with care.

Retrospective Solution

When addressing these concerns, reason should prevail. If a bill is decreased or eliminated, it is important to clarify that the change in the patient charge is related to enhancing patient satisfaction rather than addressing poor quality care. The appearance of the latter could be perceived as an admission of guilt.

- *No money*: Some patients may voice dissatisfaction with the care, the lack of care, or the cost of care because of their inability to pay the typically expensive bill generated by a visit to the ED. An uninsured or underinsured patient may have great difficulty paying a charge of $1,000. When cost is recognized as the issue, a patient may be satisfied to develop a payment plan and avoid being sent to collection. On occasion, it may be appropriate to write-off part or all of a bill. However, write-offs should be carefully considered to avoid developing a reputation as the "no charge ED" in the community. Usually, patients are willing to pay part or most of the bill, and it is reasonable after the discussion to say, "I understand that it is difficult to pay this bill, would you be able to pay . . .?" or, although somewhat more risky, "What do you think would be fair?"
- *Inappropriate bill*: Occasionally, the bill is incorrect. Removal of a superficial tick may get coded mistakenly as a removal of a deeply embedded foreign body. When an incorrect bill is brought to the attention of the CM, it is appropriate to apologize, correct the bill, and make an immediate change in the billing process. With acknowledgment of this last step, the patient will feel like he or she made a difference. Without it, the patient may believe that the ED is trying to gouge the public and trying to get away with it.

Explanation of Charge Reduction

When a bill is decreased or eliminated for either of the two reasons above, it is appropriate to send an explanatory letter to the patient. There should be no reference to having done anything wrong in the provision of care. Instead, describe the reason for the change as a means of satisfying the patient and maintaining the patient's patronage, such as:

> *I understand that you are not satisfied with the bill you received as a result of your visit to the ED. Your satisfaction and patronage are important to us at XYZ Hospital and for that reason we have decreased your bill to $_____. Thank you for the opportunity to discuss this matter. I hope that in the event you require emergency services in the future, you will again give us the opportunity to serve you.*

Dissatisfaction With Care

The third reason a person may complain about the bill is because of dissatisfaction with the care—a quality issue that should be addressed directly. The CM should find out in what way the patient's expectations weren't met, investigate the situation, and get back to the patient quickly.

A variation on this theme arises when follow-up reveals a poor outcome, and upon review, the quality of care is questioned. Because an expensive bill may be perceived as adding "insult to injury," some CMs advocate not sending a bill in this situation. However, this practice is potentially dangerous. If it is discovered that the bill was intentionally eliminated, a plaintiff's attorney will argue that the decision not to bill is "evidence of guilt." It might be wise to obtain counsel when deciding whether or not to reduce a bill in this circumstance.

Prospective Solution

The best prospective solutions for managing the bill are to ensure compliance (accuracy and appropriateness) and deliver high-quality care and caring. An organization that effectively provides the first three of the four "Cs" **(Box 76.1)**—convenience, caring, and care—gets fewer complaints about the fourth—cost. Nonetheless, it is inevitable that an ED will receive some complaints about the cost of care. ED care is very expensive. With increasing scrutiny by various payors, each facility should review its charge structure to be certain that it remains competitive.

It is judicious for ED and administrative leaders to coordinate charge reductions both for individual patients and in general. It is unfair for the hospital administration to ask the ED to decrease its bill while continuing to charge a full facility fee. Alternatively, the ED leaders might ask the hospital to reduce its bill. The strategies for bill reduction should be well thought out and organized.

Dr. Frankenstein: But He Was Dead When He Got There

The ambulance arrived and I overhead them say there was no chance . . . but they kept working on him. I'm not sure why. And now I've got this huge bill. Why are you charging me so much? He was dead!

At Issue

This is a particularly poignant variation of "too much money." (See "Mercedes Medical Center" earlier in chapter.) Clearly, the anguish and suffering associated with the grieving process are only compounded by the receipt of the very large bill that typically follows a resuscitative effort. This situation becomes particularly distressful when the grieving party believes that "there was no chance" or that "you were working on the dead body of my loved one." Arguing with the grieving person or trying to explain how the billing process works will only reinforce the belief that the institution and its representatives are uncaring and only interested in money.

Retrospective Solution

The grieving person may be distraught and dealing with many unresolved issues. It is important to empathize, acknowledge, and validate the concern, for example, "I'm very sorry your husband died. It is difficult to deal with money at a time like this." If the CM is a good and patient listener, the grieving relative may soon be ready to listen. It then may be appropriate to explain the situation in a way that demonstrates compassion and caring.

The resuscitation team was called. We really thought that there was good reason to try our hardest to resuscitate your husband. We performed x, y, and z just as the American Heart Association recommends, but unfortunately he didn't survive. We did the best that we could. However, I understand that what you're going through is difficult, and it is a lot of money. Let's work something out.

Prospective Solution

Some EDs and hospitals, by policy, do not bill for care rendered to patients who are dead on arrival (DOA). Though the definition of DOA may vary broadly, the intent is usually the same—to avoid the additional burden of an expensive bill to an already grief-stricken family. In this situation, it may be appropriate to send a letter of condolence describing your concern for the grieving spouse and your resulting determination to eliminate the bill. This practice allows the department to give solace and get credit for the good deed. The process of forgiving a bill should be done in a way that does not imply that something went wrong. (See "Mercedes Medical Center: Too Much Money" earlier in chapter.)

Nurse/Doctor Jerkyl

"She yelled at me because I came in last week for the same thing. Well, it wasn't better," or *"He said that this is an ED, and that my case was not an emergency. Well, it was to me and to my own doctor, who admitted me the next day!"*

At Issue

It is difficult for some practitioners to understand that everyone has his or her own definition of an emergency. Instead these practitioners are often intent on explaining how the ED works rather than listening to the patient's issue. The pedantic attitude is humiliating to the patient. Worse still, the reprimand may be dangerous if, as a result, the patient is reticent to seek appropriate care in the future.

The caregiver may justify the lecture stating that he or she is just educating the patient. The patient, on the other hand, may believe that the practitioner is arrogant, lazy, and unwilling to spend the appropriate time with the patient. There is an expression: "Jerks who are right are jerks; jerks who are wrong are defendants." When insulted, the patient may get angry. When things go wrong, the patient may seek retribution.

Retrospective Solution

Once it is determined that the complaint is about practitioner rudeness or inappropriate behavior, the CM should empathize and agree to quickly investigate and get back to the complainant. If the patient believes that the practitioner was disrespectful, the CM has the opportunity to give the patient the caring and compassion that was initially lacking. The CM may wish to describe the expected standards of behavior, including respect and courtesy. It is acceptable to admit guilt about caring, but not about care.

"It seems that you've been treated rudely, and we did not meet either your or our expectations. This type of attitude is unacceptable. Thank you for letting me know. I will investigate it and get back to you on Tuesday."

During the follow-up conversation, the CM will, ideally, apologize on behalf of the practitioner: "Nurse/Dr. Jones is sorry that you perceived him as rude. It was not intended. In fact, he was very upset that you left dissatisfied. We both appreciate that you brought this to our attention."

Prospective Solution

If this is a consistent problem of a particular practitioner, it is necessary to create a behavior change. (Changing the behavior of an individual is beyond the scope of this chapter. However, this issue is addressed more fully in Chapters 78, 103, and 119.)

Dr. Vesuvius

A private physician on staff charges up to the nursing station and blows his stack again, screaming: "I can't stand to have my patients come to this ED! You never get anything right around here!"

At Issue

Following this type of outburst, there is consistent discomfort and embarrassment among those within hearing range, including the patients. Worse, if this criticism is directed at a particular person, that person may be humiliated.

Some medical staff members had their only significant ED experience during their residency. The memory of the ED may be a wild, uncaring, chaotic environment with nobody responsible or particularly interested. The ED rotation may have been brief and distasteful, with the only intent of providing exposure or meeting a service obligation.

Further, the non-ED medical staff members may be accustomed to a supportive private office staff that responds immediately to their needs (see Chapter 77). Arriving in the more clamorous, confusing, and seemingly disorganized ED environment may be very stressful. Unfortunately, some practitioners handle high-stress situations by becoming aggressive and blaming.

Retrospective Solution

Success with this type of physician requires maintaining a respectful countenance and then creating the understanding that the ED is the emergency physician's office that is in many ways similar to his or her office. As the ED leader, it is important that the ED staff members are treated with the same courtesy and respect that his or her own staff members deserve. It might even be helpful to make an appointment and go to the physician's office, which simultaneously demonstrates respect for the physician and the seriousness of the issue. Then the ED leader can:

- *Define the issue creating the physician's ED outburst and address it*: Once the nature of the problem that caused the frustration is determined, it can be acknowledged, explored, and, if appropriate, rectified. The disgruntled physician's issue must be heard with a commitment to investigation and resolution before he or she will listen and address the ED leader's concern.
- *Describe your complaint-management process*: The ED leader should encourage the complaining physician to raise concerns immediately and directly to the leader any and every time that there is a problem with the ED or the care being rendered there. The complainant should know the importance of the ED being perceived as a user-friendly environment and that ED leadership takes very seriously any concerns about the care provided there. Once the practitioner is convinced that the problem is a concern and will be addressed, the practitioner will then be in a position to help solve the ED leader's problem.
- *Describe the ED as the office of its providers*: The ED leader may share that he or she:
  - ☐ Assumes responsibility for the patients and staff in the ED, just as the private practitioner does in his or her office

- Wants to create the most positive and caring environment for those who use the facility, just as the private practitioner does in his or her office
- Would go directly and privately to the private practitioner's staff member if a problem surfaced, just as ED leaders would expect the practitioner to do
- Would never go to private practitioner's office and complain publicly and would expect similar behavior from the private practitioner;
- *Gain commitment to communicate directly when problems arise.*

Prospective Solution

The person expressing his or her discontent may not recognize the inappropriateness of the behavior. If a disruptive and inappropriate expression of emotion in this public arena is occurring, the ED leader may be able to intervene by doing the following (also see Chapter 8):

- When possible, the ED leader should walk up to, stand in front of, establish eye contact with, and get the attention of the dissatisfied person.
- Once the dissatisfied person is engaged, the ED leader may quietly and firmly say, "I can see you are upset. I want to find out more about the issue, over here, in private." Then the leader should walk the other person to a more private space. Once the practitioner is engaged with the ED leader and the leader is in a position of authority, it is likely that the practitioner will follow.
- It is important to address the practitioner's issue first and then follow the steps listed in the previous section, "Retrospective Solution."

Dr. Terry Bradshaw

"My doctor said that I had a ruptured appendix and that your doctor screwed up!"

At Issue

This patient is angry and wants satisfaction. It is important to recognize that by calling, the patient may be offering the only opportunity to resolve a high-risk situation. Ignoring the issue at this point is fanning the fire. It is essential to determine what the patient wants. However, in the long run, it may be even more important to ascertain if and why the physician criticized the ED care. The private physician may be upset with the care and inadvertently have planted a seed of discontent; may be angry with the ED, an emergency physician, or the hospital; or may be implicating another for his or her own protection.

Retrospective Solution

This case requires communicating directly with both the patient for damage control and the private physician to discourage future inappropriate and inflammatory remarks to patients.

The patient: When talking with the patient, the CM should immediately demonstrate concern by listening carefully to the story and seek to understand what the patient wants as a result of this discussion. Even ask: "What would you like to see happen?" (**See Box 76.4.**) Perhaps it is to make sure that this mistake does not happen again. The patient may want the practitioner to be punished ("his head on a platter!"). The CM should agree to look into the situation and get back to the patient quickly.

If the care rendered was within the acceptable standard, then the CM must address the patient's perception and expectations. It is important to avoid further complicating the situation by impugning "Dr. Bradshaw" because this criticism may lead to a battle that the

ED is likely to lose. At the very least, it is important for the CM to empathize with the patient and try to provide a satisfactory answer. One response is the following:

Yes, I've talked with Dr. Bradshaw [private physician] and understand his concern There are several ways to evaluate and treat abdominal pain. Dr. Jones [emergency physician] was very concerned about you and your pain. He performed the correct tests and encouraged you to see your doctor or return to the ED immediately if the pain got worse. He is sorry that you continued to be ill but is very glad to hear that you did follow-up with Dr. Bradshaw as he recommended.

If the care did not meet the standard, the CM must still address the patient's perception and help to meet his or her expectations. The CM must carefully avoid making statements that the patient might subsequently use against the ED, its practitioners, or the hospital. A statement to the patient that implies that poor care was rendered is equivalent to becoming the plaintiff's witness.

Dr. Bradshaw should discuss the situation with the private physician. The CM should make an appointment to meet with the physician in his or her own office. It demonstrates a level of deference that may help while trying to enlist the support of the private physician. It is important to ascertain why the physician denounced the patient's care. This should be done in a nonaccusatory manner, such as: "It was the patient's perception that you were not happy with his care in the ED and that you thought that the emergency physician provided poor care. How might we have done better?"

Usually when directly confronted with this type of situation, the private physician will recognize the gravity and implications of his or her conversation with the patient. As with "Dr. Vesuvius" earlier in this chapter, the CM should familiarize the complaining physician with the ED's complaint-management program and further emphasize your team's desire to provide excellent care. An effort should be made to gain a commitment to call directly when a perceived problem occurs. "Dr. Bradshaw" may be drafted by a request to participate the advancement of the department. Methods include designing a clinical protocol, giving a lecture, participating in a journal club, selecting upgraded equipment, and so forth.

Some private physicians when confronted with "the patient's perception" will deny that they had criticized the ED or the care provided. You can then state that you thought it was unlikely that he or she had disparaged the ED. After all, your team sees many of the private physician's patients and you would never allow your staff to voice concerns about the care that had led to the ED visit. You can be sure you have made a point that is likely to prevent future inappropriate remarks to patients.

Prospective Solution

The only prospective solutions to this problem involve techniques of prevention. The ED leaders should seek out physicians or groups of physicians who are unhappy with the care of their patients in the ED. As their issues are ascertained, the ED leaders can work with them to seek solutions, demonstrating eagerness to continuously improve ED care for the patients and those who care for the patients, the medical staff members (see Chapter 77). They may be drafted into the development of clinical guidelines. Above all, the leaders must assure them that providing the best care to their patients is of paramount importance.

Dr. Blunder

"The doctor told me my x-ray was okay, and now you tell me that my son has a broken bone!"

At Issue

Patients expect high-quality care and accurate diagnoses. They are sometimes intolerant of what they perceive to be mistakes. As in other complaints, this is a second opportunity to provide the correct care and caring.

Retrospective Solution

There are two important strategies in the resolution of this problem. First, it is necessary to ensure that the patient has gotten or gets the necessary care for the injury. If appropriate, the CM may demonstrate concern by bringing the patient back to the ED for further care. "How is your child now? Would you like to come in now, and I'll take care of him myself?" Alternatively, the CM may take the initiative to secure definitive care for the patient by making all the necessary arrangements with the PCP, orthopedist, and so on.

The second important strategy is to assure the patient that the system "worked." The CM may admit that, though not often, the first interpretation of the diagnostic image is not always correct. That is exactly why the ED developed a sophisticated system of overreads in cooperation with the radiologists. The system ensures that a second expert, a radiologist, reviews every diagnostic image taken in the ED. The CM should be in a position to say, "I'm pleased that the system works so well."

Depending on what the patient expects, such as that it won't happen again, it may also be appropriate to add, "Our system also requires that Dr. Jones (emergency physician) review the x-ray to become an even better physician."

Prospective Solution

The prospective solution involves three components: an overread system, patient education, and performance improvement.

- *Overread system*: Develop an effective protocol for overreading diagnostic images. Elements include those listed in **Box 76.6**.
- *Patient education*: Patients evaluated in the ED should always get a thorough and caring explanation of the continued management of the injury. As part of the discharge process, it is appropriate to advise the patient that, "Though I don't see anything wrong with your x-ray, we always have the radiologist review the films in the morning." By informing the patient of the overread system before discharge, subsequent misunderstanding and anger may be averted.

BOX 76.6 ■ ELEMENTS OF AN EFFECTIVE RADIOLOGY OVERREAD SYSTEM

- Rapid identification of misread radiographs
- Immediate notification of emergency personnel
- Determination of significance, and when appropriate
- Patient and physician notification
- Arrangements for follow-up care
- Documentation
- Emergency physician review of radiograph
- Emergency physician trending, and when appropriate
- Physician education

- *Performance improvement:* The performance improvement system must identify members of the department who misread radiographs, particularly those that lead to a subsequent change in patient management. (See adverse patient outcome [APO] 1 or higher in **Figure 76.2**.) Depending on the type, frequency, and seriousness of the misread radiographs, the practitioner may require further education.

COMPLIMENT MANAGEMENT

An approach based on responding to complaints alone is only part of a complete system. Most systems concentrate so heavily on complaints and "what went wrong" that the opportunity to recognize and share "what went right" is squandered. A comprehensive approach to performance improvement includes the management and promotion of compliments. Implementing a thoughtful "compliment management system" creates balance in the process of reviewing the clinicians' quality of care and caring.

The Logistics of Sharing Compliments

The comprehensive system should look for opportunities to praise, and even celebrate, success. A compliment tracking system demonstrates to all who participate in the quality system—practitioners, administrators, and even regulatory personnel—that the system is balanced and that excellence regularly occurs in the ED. The CM should look for, document, and incorporate compliments in the practitioners' performance appraisals.

Documented compliments, such as cards, letters, and e-mails, should be gathered and sent to the CM, department director, or administrative assistant for inclusion into the system. Department members who personally receive a compliment letter should also be strongly encouraged to submit the letter for processing through the compliment management system. Explain to those who are reticent, citing humility, that these letters provide balance to staff and institutional leaders, who usually only hear about what went wrong.

Processing of the Compliment

Once a compliment letter is received, copies should be made. A copy should be:

- Placed in the caregiver's file.
- Sent directly to the practitioner with a letter of congratulations. As an example, a card could be replicated onto one of several predesigned memos that begins with a congratulation, such as: "Lauren, congratulations and thank you for once again being recognized for your stellar care and upholding the "Crest of Values" of _____ Hospital." Or "James, we are proud that you are a member of our department." The copy of the compliment letter plus the card are then sent to "Lauren" (or "James") and prominently displayed in the ED for other department members to see and to have the opportunity to personally recognize the recipient.
- Sent to each member of a predetermined distribution list. Consider who would like to receive a letter demonstrating a job well done at the hospital. The CEO is constantly addressing problems, complaints, and unhappy customers, some of which are related to the ED. Imagine the pleasant surprise of seeing a note from the ED, expecting a problem, and being delighted to see the praise of a clinician who was appreciated for a job well done. The list of those copied can be determined by ascertaining who has a stakeholder interest in the ED and its success.
- Some leaders close the loop by sending a "thank you" letter back to the person who wrote the original compliment letter.

Example Compliment Letters

The following are the contents of two actual compliment letters received by a practitioner:

Dear Dr. ____,

We know that you were instrumental in saving our son ____'s life. We can't even begin to imagine our lives without him and are so grateful that he is healing. You are a very special person, and we would like to commend you and your staff for excellence in every area. We have a long road but are progressing. You will never ever be forgotten, and we will remember you in our prayers always. Thank God you were there.

God Bless You

Our Love,

The ____'s

Dear Dr. ____,

I've never met you, but I feel a great deal of gratitude for the kind of man you are. Nearly two weeks ago, my dear father-in-law, ____ ____, was admitted to the ____ ER following a massive stroke. You admitted him in the morning and pronounced him dead in the evening. In the meantime, according to our family who were present with him, you were a clear, strong, honest, compassionate presence.

____ was a bright light for those of us in his world. He was a deep thinker, a professor of East Asian religion, a lover of poetry and music and beauty. We thank you for your help in allowing his safe and peaceful passage from this world.

With gratitude,

____ ____

These written compliments were sent to the provider with a cover letter of congratulations for a job well done. The congratulatory notes and letters were then distributed widely throughout the institution. They had an incredibly positive effect on the hospital's chief medical officer, who often deals with physician problems; the CEO, who expects the vast majority of written material to create more work; and all the others who share responsibility for the institution's success.

CONCLUSION

The management of complaints is a critical function of ED leadership that performed properly can transform angry or disappointed patients, staff members, and other important stakeholders into satisfied customers. Going further and seeking and resolving the root causes of the complaints can smooth operational inefficiencies, improve behaviors, and substantially reduce the number of complaints. Adding a robust compliment management system encourages best practices and boosts morale by recognizing and promoting the exceptional work routinely performed in the ED.

APPENDIX 76.1: SCHWAB CASE RATING SYSTEM

Richard M. Schwab, MD, personal communication, Previous ED Medical Director, Holy Name Medical Center, Teaneck, NJ

0 **No clinical issue identified:** Includes events that may be related to cost, utilization, or other factors not specific to patient outcome. Tracking data from this category may provide opportunity to identify trends useful to department or hospital-wide management.

1 **Not practitioner-related:** Includes events causally related to factors intrinsic to the patient (i.e., underlying disease, biologic/anatomic variation, hypersensitivity reaction in absence of history of allergy), institutional support (i.e., delayed turn around for lab/x-ray studies, unavailability of scans), or care provided outside of hospital. Trending data from this category may demonstrate trends useful for departmental or hospital-wide management.

2 **Practitioner-related:** The following subcategories should include those events that either individually or collectively are related to specific practitioner. Data from these categories are trended and will allow department chairpersons and practitioners to identify opportunities to enhance practice in terms of quality, effectiveness, or efficiency.

2a* **Predictable Event Within Standard of Care:** Refers to events that are widely reported in literature, may be anticipated, and are relatively frequent. "Within Standard of Care" indicates care was provided in accordance with contemporary standards of the specialty and departmental staff.

2b* **Unpredictable Event Within the Standard of Care:** Refers to events that are infrequent and not anticipated but have been described in literature to occur in cases where the standard of care is met.

2c **Marginal Deviation from the Standard of Care:** Refers to care that is "minimally" outside the contemporary standards of the specialty or expected standards of the department.

2d **Moderate Deviation from the Standard of Care:** Refers to care that is "moderately" outside the contemporary standards of the specialty or expected standards of the department.

2e **Significant Deviation from the Standard of Care:** Refers to care that is gross departure from the expected standards of the department.

*Both category 2a and 2b meet accepted standards of care.

REFERENCES

1. Reader TW, Gillespie A, Roberts J. Patient complaints in healthcare systems: a systematic review and coding taxonomy. *BMJ Qual Saf*. 2014;23(8):678–689.

2. Taylor DM, Wolfe R, Cameron PA. Complaints from emergency department patients largely result from treatment and communication problems. *Emerg Med*. 2002;14(1):43–49.

3. Adamson TE, Tschann JM, Gullion DS, et al. Physician communication skills and malpractice claims: a complex relationship. *West J Med*. 1989;150(3):356–360.

4. Solnick SJ, Hemenway D. Complaints and disenrollment at a health maintenance organization. *J Consumer Affairs*. 1992;26(1):90–103.

5. Korsch BM, Gozzi EK, Francis V. Gaps in doctor-patient communication. *Pediatr*. 1968;42(5):855–871.

6. Lateef F, Patient expectations and the paradigm shift of care in emergency medicine. *J Emerg Trauma Shock*. 2011;4(2):163–167.

7. O'Dowd J. How to improve doctor-patient communication. AOSpine Newsletter. 2015. Available at: http://xfiles.aospine.org/users/publications/community_newsletter/2015_01/doctor-patient-communication.html. Accessed October 3, 2020.

8. Schwartz LR, Overton DT. Emergency department complaints: a one year analysis. *Ann Emerg Med*. 1987;16(8):857–861.

9. Buller MK, Buller DB. Physicians' communication style and patient satisfaction. *J Health Soc Behav*. 1987;28(4):375–388.

10. Evans BJ, Kiellerup FD, Stanley RO, et al. A communication skills programme for increasing patients' satisfaction with general practice consultations. *Br J Med Psychol*. 1987;60(4):373–378.

11. Dennis B, Overton DT, Schwartz LR, et al. Emergency department complaint frequency: variation by patient median household income. *Ann Emerg Med*. 1992;21(6):746–748.

12. Hirschman AO. *Exit, Voice, and Loyalty: Responses to Decline in Firms, Organizations, and States*. Harvard University Press; 1970.

13. Best A, Andreasen AR. Consumer responses to unsatisfactory purchases: a survey of perceiving defects, voicing complaints, and obtaining redress. *Law Society Rev.* 1977;11(4):701–742.

14. Ley P. Complaints made by hospital staff and patients—review of the literature. *Bull Br Psychol Soc.* 1972;25:115–120.

15. Schneiderman N. Patient complaints. In: Henry GL, ed. *Emergency Medicine Risk Management.* American College of Emergency Physicians; 1991.

16. Day RL, Gabicke K, Schaetzle T, et al. The hidden agenda of consumer complaining. *J Retailing.* 1981;57(3):86–106.

17. *Bits and Pieces.* Vol. 3. Pamphlet. The Economic Press; 1991.

18. Singh H. Industry characteristics and consumer dissatisfaction. *J Consumer Affairs.* 1990;25:19–56.

19. Andreasen AR. Consumer responses to dissatisfaction in loose monopolies. *J Consumer Res.* 1985;12(2):135–141.

20. Cameron MP, Richardson M, Siameja S. Customer dissatisfaction among older consumers: a mixed-methods approach. *Ageing Soc.* 2016;36(2):420–441.

21. Malpractice risks in communication failures. 2015 CRICO Strategies National Comparative Benchmarking System (CBS) Report. Available at: https://www.rmf.harvard.edu/Malpractice-Data/Annual-Benchmark-Reports/Risks-in-Communication-Failures. Accessed March 23, 2018.

22. The Joint Commission International. Complaint Management/Quality Monitoring. 2015. Available at: https://www.jointcommissioninternational.org/-/media/deprecated-unorganized/imported-assets/jci/default-folders/documents/18-complaint-management-and-quality-monitoringpdf.pdf?db=web&hash=25F11FAAC50A3E9CCD811324D72A80AC https://www.jointcommissioninternational.org/assets/3/7/18-Complaint-Management-and-Quality-Monitoring.pdf. Accessed October 11, 2020.

23. *Comprehensive Accreditation Manual for Hospitals.* The Joint Commission; 1996.

24. Title: section 405.7–patients' rights. New York Codes, Rules, and Regulations. Available at: https://regs.health.ny.gov/content/section-4057-patients-rights. Accessed April 27, 2018.

25. Griffey RT, Bohan JS. Healthcare provider complaints to the emergency department: a preliminary report on a new quality improvement instrument. *Qual Saf Health Care.* 2006;15(5):344–346.

CHAPTER 77

EFFECTIVE MEDICAL STAFF RELATIONSHIPS: A CASE-BASED DISCUSSION

Robert W. Strauss

Emergency medicine has undergone several transitions. In the 1970s and 1980s, the emergency department (ED) was perceived as "mission required"—perhaps a necessary evil. The ideal ED was one that did not cause any problems for the administration. In the 1990s, with the prominence of managed care and capitation, the ED began to shrink in importance and became "mission unnecessary," as fewer patients were likely to use its services. This was a time when many EDs were afforded very limited resources.

More recently, the ED has become "mission critical." Hospital boards and administrations, as well as national regulatory agencies, scrutinize the ED, its services, and the satisfaction of all who interact with it. To succeed, department leaders must do more than simply cover the schedule with highly qualified practitioners. They must address the demands of multiple stakeholders, most of whom insist that both the patient's needs and their own are fully addressed.

The key relationship between ED medical staff and non-ED medical staff (referred to in this chapter as "medical staff") must be thoughtfully and intentionally nurtured. While developing and maintaining effective working relationships with the medical staff can be challenging, there are multiple daily opportunities to successfully collaborate with them to provide quality care to patients. Effective relationships are built on a foundation of mutual respect and appreciation for each other's roles.

BUILDING RELATIONSHIPS

From the ED's limited vantage point, it is difficult to recognize that medical staffs comprise large numbers of individuals, each potentially overwhelmed with the intricacies of the changing health-care environment, increasing patient demands, decreasing reimbursement, contradictory regulatory interventions, government oversight, and so on. Department leaders have a choice: Either allow the ED to become another burden and the source of complaints, or become friends, colleagues, supporters, and facilitators of the medical staff. The primary advantages of the latter approach are both improved relations and, more importantly, *improved patient care*.

The consequences of the inability to integrate with the medical staff are quite serious and all too often lead to a physician's or group's departure from an institution. A pattern of inattention to staff issues and reactively (rather than proactively) addressing them will ultimately create frustration, anger, and a reputation of neglect and disregard. Can a pattern of poor relationships and medical staff dissatisfaction with the group be turned around? It can, but it's like turning the Titanic; it takes enormous effort and may be too late anyway. Titanic-like disasters can be avoided with:

- Advance planning
- A thorough understanding of the environment
- Constant attention to changing tides and new obstacles
- An alert team
- A well-orchestrated, proactive problem-prevention program

The continued presence of the ED group often depends on maintaining the good will of the medical staff. Establishing peer relationships is critical to this alliance. Though not common, a particularly strong relationship with a medical staff may help to turn the tide of an administrative decision to change ED groups.

Conversely, it is common for a poor relationship with the medical staff to be the cause of the loss of a contractual relationship. Perceived poor quality or inadequate care leading to complaints quickly erodes the position of the ED group. Even positive relationships will not overcome substandard performance.

Hierarchy of Emergency Physician Success

Success among the medical staff may be compared to a modified version of Maslow's hierarchy of needs, which describes attaining self-actualization by moving through several stages.[1] One can move only sequentially up the hierarchy and cannot realize a higher level without first successfully achieving all of the levels below. A parallel model can describe the hierarchy of ED (leadership) needs (**Table 77.1**).[2]

Level 1: Survival

The basic *sine qua non* of achieving ED success requires filling the schedule with safe and reliable providers. This fundamental need is equivalent to Maslow's first level: the basic requirements of survival. So, the first job of the new medical director is ensuring that this basic need is rapidly fulfilled. It is only after establishing consistent quality providers that the ED can begin to demonstrate success in Level 2: providing safe, quality care. Conversely, the inability to consistently provide practitioners in whom the medical staff has confidence will significantly limit integration and progression.

Level 2: Safe, Quality Care (Maslow's "Safety, Protection")

The medical staff will not recognize the care in the ED as safe until they experience a consistent presence of high-quality, reliable, and familiar emergency physicians—in

TABLE 77.1 ■ Maslow's Hierarchy of Needs		
Ascending Need	**Hierarchy**	**Strauss ED Hierarchy**
Level 1	Basic survival	Schedule covered by excellent practitioners
Level 2	Safety	Safe, quality care
Level 3	Belonging	Effective member of medical staff—committees
Level 4	Esteem, status	Leader of medical staff
Self-actualization	Personal growth and fulfillment	

other words, practitioners they can trust. Only then, with the ED leadership's hard work and "demonstration" of an effective quality program, including responsive complaint management, will the medical staff perceive that the ED functions well.

Level 3: Effective Members of the Medical Staff (Maslow's "Belonging")

When the group has successfully demonstrated consistent safe, quality care, emergency physicians have the potential to be perceived as true colleagues and effective members of the larger team. Membership requires participation in the committee structure to improve the hospital and medical staff processes.

The early emergency medicine entrepreneur and leader Karl Mangold once said, "If you think your only responsibility is to practice high quality medicine, you will lose your contract in a minute." He simply meant that emergency physicians exist in a community (of providers and other stakeholders) and must help in both the provision and the coordination of care. It is more than the patient who must be satisfied.

Successful membership also requires involvement in social and professional events.

Level 4: Leadership (Maslow's "Esteem, Status, Responsibility, Reputation")

When ED directors are perceived as active members of the medical staff with effective programs in place, they have the potential to assume the mantle of leadership. This advancement requires subjugating parochial needs for the larger good of all patients (not just those of the ED).

Self-Actualization: Personal Growth and Fulfillment

The ED group and its leaders can achieve success (self-actualization) through continuous attention to the:

- Needs of the patients (first), staff, clinicians, and the institutional leadership
- Consistent provision of quality providers in the ED
- Integration into the medical staff and organizational structures and leadership

Becoming Clinically Indispensable

No matter what else is accomplished, no matter how extraordinary the administrative effort, the foundation of the relationship with the Medical Staff always exists within the role of providing clinical expertise. Because of the frequent interactions with a large number of clinicians (primary care physicians [PCPs], surgeons, hospitalists, radiologists, etc.), emergency physicians more than other staff members have the opportunity to develop or squander a clinical partnership (**Box 77.1**).

BOX 77.1 ■ TIPS FOR SUCCESS WITH THE MEDICAL STAFF

- Know the clinicians by their first names
- Quickly meet and orient new staff members to the ED
- Hardwire the process by active membership on the credentials committee
- Welcome opportunities to see manage (consult on) medical staff patients in the ED

Emergency Physicians as Medical Staff Consultants

Some emergency physicians moan when a medical staff member sends a patient to the ED for evaluation. Is such a referral inherently good or bad? *It is wonderful!* Why? Emergency physicians have an opportunity to be perceived as consultants. And what do good consultants do? They:

- Evaluate the patient.
- Call the referring physician.
- Recommend a course of action.
- Earn appreciation for facilitating the care of the patient.

Unfortunately, some emergency physicians neglect the opportunity to communicate their findings to the referring physician. Or they may call and act like interns presenting to a senior resident. Part of the ED director's orientation to the providers should include a description (perhaps including role playing) of these crucial conversations (**Box 77.2**).

CASE STUDIES

The following five cases demonstrate stereotypical problems that clinicians will confront over the course of a practice—and sometimes over the course of a day! Each case (**Table 77.2**.) contains the fact pattern, a description of the issue, potential solutions, and a discussion. The first three cases address issues in the lower end of the hierarchy (providing safe, quality care). The final two cases demonstrate the importance of emergency physician involvement in the staff structure. On the hierarchical scale, these final cases are Level 3 (participation among the larger group, or belonging) and Level 4 (leadership and respect, or esteem). *Please note: These cases are exaggerated for purposes of illustration.*

Case One: Creating Consistent Protocols for Medstaff Notification

After completing a lengthy workup, the emergency physician calls an irritated PCP, who claims, "You should have called much earlier . . . I know the patient, and I could have prevented the lengthy and unnecessary workup. *I was in the hospital!*" The chastened emergency physician calls "Dr. Lose-Lose" a few hours later (at 3 am) after performing an initial evaluation of a patient. Dr. Lose–Lose is furious that he was called prior to obtaining the results of the lab tests and computed tomography (CT). He complains, "Now you're going

---

BOX 77.2 ■ DO'S AND DON'TS OF SPEAKING WITH STAFF

Avoid:
- Meandering presentations
- Appearing stupid: "What should I do?"
- Being rude: "You know you could have admitted the patient directly!"

Do:
- Obtain relevant information.
- Describe the patient concisely.
- Know in advance what you want the outcome of the conversation to be.
- Thank the referring physicians for the opportunity to "consult" on their cases.
- Refer perfectly and notify the PCP when his/her patient is being admitted.

TABLE 77.2 ■ Common Problems Between EDs and Medical Staff

Case	Hierarchy	Clinician Name	Issue
1	Level 1-2	Dr. Lose–Lose	Notifying medical staff about their patients in the ED
2	Level 1-2	Dr. Vesuvius	Addressing medical staff needs when in the ED
3	Level 1-2	Dr. Vesuvius	Going beyond the "call of duty"
4	Level 3-4	Dr. Casper/Dr. Backstabber	Addressing the "invisible" director
5	Level 3-4	Dr. Terry Bradshaw	Addressing the "monday morning quarterback"

to have to call and wake me up a second time to give me the information that I needed to hear the first time."

At Issue

Nonhospitalist medical staff members with mature practices do not want or need the ED to fill their clinical practices, and they find the requirement to take ED calls a frustrating irritant. Responding to calls from emergency physicians usually interrupts some other preferred activity, such as managing office patients, spending time with family, or sleeping. There is simply no best time to call, and the emergency physician will continue to fall into the trap of never communicating at the right time.

Solution

The ideal solution requires developing an agreeable communication system in advance. Can everyone's needs be met? Probably not. As an example, consider the particularly difficult consultant who wants to be called between 8 am and 10 am or between 4 pm and 6 pm, but not during office hours or surgery time and never at night, at which point the emergency physician becomes, in his or her mind, a practitioner with newfound surgical expertise.

Discussion

A solution to this perplexing issue is to create a limited list of options, and encourage all medical staff to choose one for communication that will be consistently used (and annually updated). The list of options should cover the majority of communication requests (**Box 77.3**). Provide this list to each member of the medical staff for completion and careful review.

BOX 77.3 ■ MEDICAL STAFF NOTIFICATION PREFERENCE LIST

The emergency care provider will contact the PCP:

- After the initial evaluation
- After a complete evaluation
- Only if the patient requires admission/urgent follow-up

_____ _____ ___/___/___

Signature   Print Name   Date

While this system may not work for every situation, it does work for most and encourages each PCP to select and accept a consistent standard. Minor modifications may be required for practitioners with limited service requirements or special circumstances. For instance, general surgeons may wish to be notified prior to or following the completion of an abdominal CT on a stable patient. Of course, unstable or deteriorating patients warrant immediate consultation. It is appropriate to build support for a consistent standard by having a discussion with the executive committee in advance of the program rollout.

Case Two: Addressing Medical Staff Needs

"Dr. Vesuvius," an irritated hot-headed medical staff member charges up to the ED staff (nursing) station and blows his stack *again*, loudly proclaiming, "My patients get lousy care! Why is it that this place never gets anything right? Where is the chart?"

At Issue

Following this type of outburst, there is consistent discomfort and embarrassment. Worse, if directed toward an individual, that person may feel humiliated. This behavior may happen for a variety of reasons. Many medical staff members had their only significant ED experience during their residencies. For some, their memory of the ED is of a wild, uncaring, chaotic environment in which no one is responsible or particularly interested. The experience may have been part of a brief and distasteful assignment, the purpose of which was to provide exposure or meet a service obligation. Further, most practitioners are accustomed to a supportive private office, where they are like Star Trek captains, sitting at the bridge and calling out orders to people who respond immediately. Arriving in the more clamorous and confusing ED environment may be very stressful, disruptive, and frustrating.

Solution

Generally, medical staff members want the ED to provide them with exactly the same environmental qualities that lead to patient satisfaction. They want a pleasant experience in a professional environment; in other words, the three Cs (**Box 77.4**).

Medical staff members in the ED want to get in and out quickly so they can resume their other responsibilities. They prefer a consistent, comfortable, quiet, well-organized area to sit, with all documents, information systems, communication systems, and so on, immediately available. The effective ED provides its team with:

- A simple way to communicate and leave orders.
- Easy phone access into and out of the ED.
- A simple visual method to determine where their patients are located.
- Ready access to the caregivers managing the patient.

BOX 77.4 ■ THE THREE Cs FOR MEDICAL STAFF SATISFACTION

- **Convenience:** Provide a consistent, fully functional, quiet area.
- **Caring:** Demonstrate concern and appreciation for the medical staff.
- **Care:** Ensure that quality care is provided to the patients.

Arriving medical staff members should be recognized and warmly greeted. It is appropriate for the ED staff, including emergency physicians, to ask: "Is there anything that you need or that I can do for you?" Medical staff members are and should be treated as guests. The effective ED consistently demonstrates quality patient care to the medical staff members who evaluate patients:

- The quality of care provided by the ED staff must be unassailable.
- Medical staff must have easy access to the tools and equipment necessary to access and provide care to their patients.

Discussion

Effective ED leaders recognize that quality patient care can only be ensured by listening to and solving medical staff members' problems. These ED leaders work diligently to address the predicament that caused the physician's frustration. An effective response can be hard-wired through a three-step process: demonstrate concern, describe the intended environment, and follow-up (**Box 77.5**). (See Chapter 76 for more information.)

Demonstrate concern: Once an inefficient process or problem is brought to the attention of the ED leadership, it is incumbent upon them to determine the nature of the issue in an open and nondefensive manner. This follows Stephen Covey's fifth principle as described in *The Seven Habits of Highly Effective People*:

Seek first to understand, then to be understood.[4]

The complaining physician should be encouraged to come to the ED leader each and every time that there is a problem. This encouragement should be directly communicated to the disgruntled party by an ED leader who believes and communicates that the ED should be a user-friendly environment and that all concerns of the practitioners and their patients will be taken seriously. This approach creates the foundation of trust that allows the ED to be described in positive terms.

Describe the intended environment: Describe the similarities between the medical staff and ED practices. Explain the importance of creating a positive and caring environment for patients and those who care for them. While the medical staff member's office and the ED have several similarities, it is appropriate to emphasize the unpredictable nature of patient arrivals and acuities. It may be appropriate to remind the medical staff member that the emergency physicians see all patients who present to the ED. In particular, when the medical staff member's outpatient care does not go as intended, many of these patients wind up in the ED. As a member of the patient care team, the ED leader would never speak negatively to the patient about the care provided by the medical staff or walk into the practitioner's office and loudly proclaim that care was inadequate.

BOX 77.5 ■ THE THREE-STEP PROCESS OF PROBLEM RESOLUTION

1. Demonstrate concern by listening effectively, working to resolve problems, and encouraging regular feedback.
2. Describe the goal of a highly professional environment.
    a. Describe the ED as the emergency physician's office.
    b. Assume responsibility for the ED practice environment.
3. Follow up: call to check for problems.

Rather, the ED leader would always be supportive in front of the patient and respectful toward the medical staff member by "privately" calling or making an appointment to discuss any concerns.

Follow up: Hardwire the process by intermittently calling to check for problems. This step is critical to achieve success and demonstrate a sincere commitment to attaining operational effectiveness and promoting an open relationship. One week after the problem, the emergency physician should call to determine if the practitioner had patients in the ED and, if so, what were the patients' and practitioner's experiences. The practitioner should be reminded to call any time that a problem arises. The physician should follow up with a second call several weeks later. The follow-up process demonstrates that the ED leadership is serious about problem identification and resolution and further creates an expectation to follow the appropriate communication pathway.

Case Three: Going Beyond the Call of Duty

"Dr. Please–Please" calls from home to ask you for a favor (**Box 77.6**). After all, you're right there!

At Issue

While the specific nature of these requests may vary, the dilemma created is similar in each situation. The emergency physician might wish to help a colleague in need when the performance of this duty is substantially more convenient for the emergency physician. However, by addressing the medical staff member's need, the emergency physician risks setting a precedent that might lead down a very slippery slope.

Solution

These issues require a thorough discussion by the emergency physician group to clarify in advance and script the responses to each of these requests. There has been a great deal of discussion on these issues by our national organizations, including the American College of Emergency Physicians.[5]

Discussion

Admitting and transition orders: Extending the care provided by the emergency physician to inpatient care, including writing orders and responding to situations outside of the ED, is fraught with many subtle and complex risks. The legal theory that creates the greatest risk relates to the assumption by courts, juries, and other physicians that the emergency physician who writes inpatient orders has accepted responsibility for the patient's care until the medical staff member evaluates the patient. If the patient's condition deteriorates prior to

---

BOX 77.6 ■ STEREOTYPICAL MEDICAL STAFF REQUESTS

- Write admitting orders (I don't have time, you know the patient).
- Run up to the floor to evaluate a sick patient (you're already there).
- Sign the death certificate (you're there).
- Evaluate the patient postprocedure.
- I want to use your rooms to see my patients.

that evaluation, even if it occurs long after the emergency physician has left the hospital, the "admitting" medical staff member may:

- Perceive the emergency physician to be at fault.
- Choose to deny any responsibility.
- Directly implicate the emergency physician by implying that the full liability rests with the practitioner who saw the patient last and wrote the most recent orders—the emergency physician.

On the other hand, *bridging orders* written by the emergency physician can create greater efficiency of patient care. These transition orders may expedite patient flow from the ED to the inpatient units, while only minimally increasing the emergency physician's risk. These orders should include essential treatment and assessment parameters required before preparation of suitable admission orders. In addition, hospital and ED policies should clearly delineate who is responsible for writing bridge, transition, and admission orders and should further clarify the period of time that those orders remain active (the maximum time for the admitting physician to see the patient and prepare full admission orders). Alternatives to writing inpatient orders include:

- *Phone orders*: After the emergency physician provides a thorough explanation of the patient's condition, the call can be transferred to the nurse managing the patient to obtain admission orders from the admitting medical staff member.
- *Time-limited orders or a policy related to the timely re-evaluation of admitted patients*: Working through the medical staff committee structure (i.e., medical executive, quality and safety, bylaws, etc.), the ED leader can make a compelling case for the creation of a policy that ensures a rapid transition of care. This may include a statement on the order set, such as, "These orders will automatically expire within 1 hour of the patient's admission to the unit. The unit nurse will call the primary admitting physician to obtain orders within 30 minutes of the patient's admission to the unit." These policies should include specific times for reassessment by the medical staff member based on the acuity of the patient.
- *Predefined order sets*: The ED leaders may work with the medical staff to create evidence-based order sets (basic admitting, coronary care unit, pneumonia, transient ischemic attack, etc.) that simplify the process for the medical staff to admit the patient. If the medical staff member requests that the emergency physician implements a particular order set, then the emergency physician should act as a "scribe with a license" and perform and document the same safe "read-back process" for verbal/phone orders mandated throughout the hospital.
- *Development of a contractual preclusion*: When initially contracting with the hospital, emergency physicians may suggest avoiding "competition and interference" by inserting contractual language, such as: "The patient's attending shall be responsible for writing all admitting orders."

Managing Patients Outside of the ED

No matter how compelling the reasons to respond to patient management outside of the ED, emergency physicians have a primary responsibility to be immediately available to patients with urgent, emergent, and critical needs in the ED. Nonetheless, arguments can be made for responding to non-ED patient care needs.

Resuscitations outside of the ED: There is no more critical need than the management of patients with acute deterioration of their cardiopulmonary status (i.e., cardiac or respiratory arrest). If there is no other clinician in the hospital available to respond, it may be incumbent upon the emergency physician to respond. But what if he or she is simultaneously managing a critically ill patient in the ED? To address this complex situation, it is reasonable to stipulate in the contract that:

> *The emergency physician on duty will assist the hospital and its staff with calls involving life-threatening emergency situations — defined as cardiac and respiratory arrests — occurring on hospital premises provided that such services shall only be provided when, in the sole discretion of the emergency physician on duty, the condition of the patients within the ED permits such emergency physician to respond to such calls. The hospital is responsible for providing "trained first responders" to respond to and initiate the resuscitation of deteriorating patients.*[6]

In-house nonemergencies (out-of-ed requests): When is it appropriate for the emergency physician to go to the floor to manage a nonemergency? There are several common requests of the emergency physicians by the medical staff (**Box 77.7**). But even in the quietest of EDs, the agreement or obligation to manage non-ED patients creates a clinical risk for the remaining patients and a liability risk for the emergency physician. Though there are exceptions, nonemergent, non-ED requests generally should be avoided.

Alternatively, the pre- or post-shift visit to patients admitted to patient care units from the ED has several advantages[7]:

- The patients may not recognize these visits as unusual. However, they very much appreciate and remember the physician who cares enough just to see how they are doing.
- Emergency physicians can get follow-up on their patients' course and condition. This clinical feedback may improve practice.
- The medical staff perception of the emergency physicians improves when they recognize that emergency physicians are interested in the ongoing care, concern, and responsibility for admitted patients. The occasional visit to the floor favorably changes the opinion of medical staff members.

Requests to Assess a Patient

Perhaps a nurse from an inpatient unit calls and states that the medical staff member would like a patient to be evaluated or reevaluated. While the increasing accessibility of electronic information has decreased the frequency of these requests, it has not eliminated them. If it is the determination of the emergency physician group that this service will be provided, the emergency physician should perform it as a consultation. When a nonphysician calls to pass on a request by a clinician, politely require a direct physician-to-physician request. This approach is the best way to get appropriate clinical background, while compelling the medical staff member to give the same respect given to any consultant of whom a favor is asked. After the interpretation, the emergency physician should document the interpretation and call the requesting medical staff member with the result.

BOX 77.7 ■ LIST OF COMMON NON-ED REQUESTS

- Declaration and documentation of death
- Evaluation of a patient fall
- Management of a laceration
- Oversight of patient restraints
- Assessment of a nonemergency airway

Case Four: Showing Up Is More Than Half of the Battle

It is common for people to complain about those who are not present to defend themselves. Since medical staff committees and the medical executive committee, in particular, comprise members who are passionate and vested, the ED leader (or designee) should always be present to share information and provide perspective.

A medical staff department chair comes to executive committee to complain about the "lousy care in the ED." Then another member of the executive committee asks, "Just who is in charge in the ED? They referred my patient to another group!" This discussion gains steam, and several criticisms are directed at the ED. There is nobody present as an ED advocate because the department director has been very busy with personal and professional responsibilities and attendance at the medical executive committee has become a low priority. Subsequent to the meeting, the CEO calls the ED director in to discuss this lack of involvement and apparently poor-quality care. What can be done?

At Issue

The medical director wasn't present at a meeting of the medical staff leadership. There is a much greater tendency to complain about a person or process when the individual responsible for the process is not present. The Cowardly Lion from *The Wizard of Oz* manifested similar behavior.[8] He was willing to growl threateningly, but only when there was no opposition in sight.

Solution

The medical executive committee is a critical gathering of medical staff leaders, and the ED director should actively participate. Even if the ED director is not an official voting member, he or she should attend, as most executive committees are open to the medical staff. Attending and participating eliminates many of the complaints that might have been voiced against a defenseless group and further provides the department leader with a voice among other medical staff leaders.

Retrospectively, the ED leader should go immediately to "Dr. Backstabber" and in an open and nondefensive manner, determine the nature of the complaint, investigate it, resolve it, and communicate back. The complaining physician should be assertively asked to address concerns more directly for all future problems. (Refer to the three-step process described in **Box 77.5**.)

Discussion

Refer perfectly. Ensuring proper referrals deserves great emphasis within the emergency physician group. In an environment that includes physicians who do not like taking calls, the frustration is compounded when:

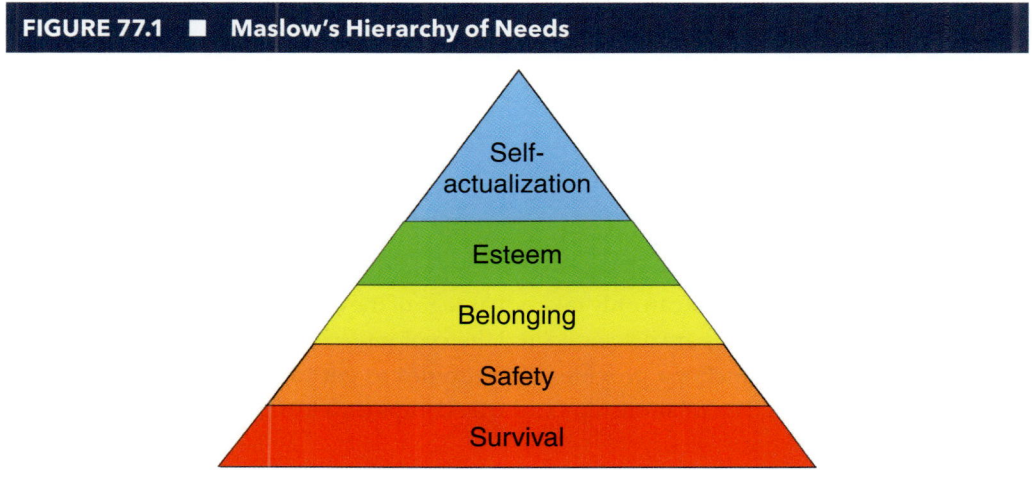

FIGURE 77.1 ■ Maslow's Hierarchy of Needs

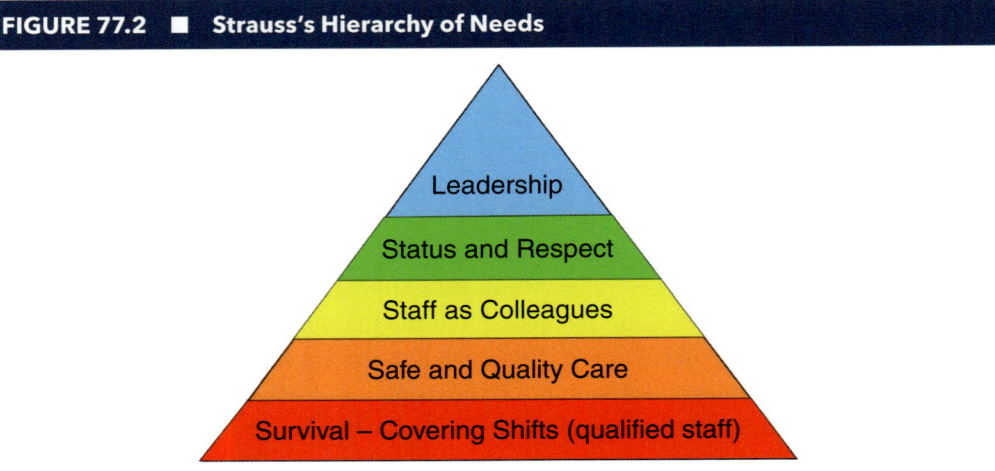

FIGURE 77.2 ■ Strauss's Hierarchy of Needs

- One physician is pressed to admit or follow a patient who should have been the responsibility of another clinician;
- The appropriate physician loses the opportunity to admit or follow his or her own patient.

A patient admitted to the wrong physician, particularly early in a group's tenure, can create enmity, perceptions of favoritism, and paranoia. All incorrect referrals must be addressed immediately.

Medical Staff Integration

Administrative effectiveness (Level 3 on the hierarchy described in **Table 77.1** and **Figure 77.2**) can only occur after establishing clinical effectiveness and demonstrating quality care. Then the process of becoming more fully assimilated into the medical staff occurs by actively participating in the committee system to improve care in the hospital.

Participating requires more than just showing up for a committee. Emergency physicians have the opportunity to sit at the table with their colleagues to work on common problems and develop new strategies.[10] The broad perspective of emergency physicians makes them ideal problem-solvers in the realm of difficult operational processes. Active involvement creates high visibility within the hospital community. The opportunities to participate abound, including working with the medical staff and administration to develop or expand a variety of programs, as described in **Table 77.3.**

Contemporary emergency medicine has expanded the role and visibility of emergency physicians in system leadership, including medical staff leadership and hospital strategic planning and governance. Once emergency physicians are recognized as "team players" by their consistent involvement, they may have the opportunity to become "team captains" by chairing and leading the committees (Level 4 in **Table 77.1**). Effective ED leaders have reputations as problem-solvers. The administration of the hospital will appreciate that, while other specialties are increasingly competing with the hospital (orthopedists and neurologists with their own magnetic resonance imagings and community surgeons with a surgical center), emergency physicians may be among the administrator's few remaining friends. Emergency physicians can only take advantage of the opportunities by being present when these critical initiatives are discussed and then volunteering to be part of the solutions.

Professional social functions provide opportunities to get to know hospital members in a nonclinical setting. The relationships and friendships developed can create substantial support.

TABLE 77.3 ■ Key Initiatives for Emergency Physician Involvement

Initiative	Examples
Clinical programs	Develop stroke-designation programs, sepsis protocols, orders sets, LEAN programs, and guidelines for door-balloon time efficiency.
Outreach programs	Participate in EMS, community, and school programs. Develop referral center programs and telemedicine protocols.
Safety and quality	Address core measures, medication reconciliation, safety standards, risk management, and patient satisfaction.
Medical staff committees	Get involved in committees geared toward hospital executives, performance improvement, safety, credentials, clinical practice, etc.

Hardwiring visibility: There are many ways of developing and maintaining a high profile among the medical staff (**Table 77.4**). While some may question the effort versus value of medical staff cultivation and social integration, there are several potential positive outcomes. The most important result is that strong relationships with other care providers lead to better patient care and, as a second benefit, greater longevity of the emergency group.

Medical staff members who know and trust the emergency physicians are more likely to agree with and respond positively to specific patient management requests. There will be fewer challenges and retrospective criticisms. Additionally, practicing in an environment of collegiality creates a more nurturing and enjoyable workplace. To maintain trust, ED leaders must respond promptly and decisively to clinical complaints by investigating all problems, issues, and rumors and providing rapid follow-up to the complainant (see Chapter 76).

Additionally, there is a substantial financial incentive for the emergency group to become integrated with their colleagues. Assume the emergency group consists of eight physicians,

TABLE 77.4 ■ Methods to "Hard-Wire" Medical Staff Visibility

Chairs of divisions/departments	Meet and communicate on a regularly scheduled basis in a neutral environment.
	Use the "servant leadership" approach, determine their expectations for the ED.
	Provide contact information.
	Share initiatives and garner support.
Meetings of divisions/departments	Occasionally go to the division/department meeting.
	Describe willingness to address all complaints and issues.
	Provide contact information.
	Share initiatives and garner support.
Physician outreach program	Assign specific medical staff members to individual emergency physicians.
	Emergency physicians call monthly to check for satisfaction, uncover problems, and share initiatives (may be scripted).
	Leadership follows up on problems.

each making $250,000 a year. Isn't it worth $2 million a year to figure out how to "play well in the sandbox"?

Physician outreach program: Creating a physician outreach or "ambassador program" helps to ensure continuing communication with critical medical staff members (**Box 77.8**). Assigned emergency providers regularly reach out to and document communications with medical staff members. The departmental administrative assistant tracks the frequency and results of the calls. As a result of this type of program, medical staff change their old perceptions of the ED and emergency physicians from uncaring to attentive and concerned about delivering high-quality care. This program is particularly effective at addressing cynical medical staff members who might bear a grudge years after an incident occurred. During these regular calls, emergency physicians can:

- Reemphasize the goal of high-quality patient care.
- Uncover patient care problems.
- Share initiatives.
- Further develop positive relationships.

Case Five: Addressing Indirect Criticisms by Medical Staff Members

The Monday morning quarterback, "Dr. Terry Bradshaw," tells the patient that the care provided in the ED was malpractice: "You should have immediately called me first! I could

---

BOX 77.8 ■ STRAUSS, YAMAGUCHI, HAYES POP FORM

Medical staff member name _____ Date _____ Phone number _____

Talking points at your discretion:

- We appreciate that you send your patients to us and I would like to make sure that we are meeting their needs. So I'm calling to talk with you about your patient's and your perception of the care in the ED.
- Have you or your patients had any recent issues that you could share with me? (If yes—what, i.e., communication, care, delays)
- Have you heard any compliments about the care received by your patients?
- What is your perception of the ED and the care given?
- I'd like to continue to follow up every once in a while to get further feedback.
- Please call me with any issues, because we can't address what we don't know about. Here is my phone number and my email . . .
- What is your level of satisfaction with our service (5 = very satisfied, 1 = very dissatisfied)? (If less than 5, what can we do better?)

Specific Issues, complaints, compliments:

_____

_____

_____

Physician making call (print) _____ ☐ Needs call back

have provided the proper care." The patient calls the ED and leaves the following message, "Dr. Bradshaw said that I had appendicitis and that your doctor screwed up!"

At Issue

The phrase "Hindsight is 20/20" is applicable to clinicians who were not present during when emergency care was provided to their patients. Since it's easy to criticize from afar, it is appropriate to communicate an effective complaint process to all medical staff members. This patient is angry and wants satisfaction, but this interaction provides the ED leader with a valuable opportunity to resolve the issue directly. (To address the patient aspect of this case, see Chapter 76.) The issue here relates to the medical staff member; in the long run, it is critical to ascertain if and why their criticism was voiced in front of the patient. The medical staff member may be:

- Upset with the care and inadvertently (or not) planted a seed of discontent
- Angry with the ED, an emergency physician, or the hospital
- Purposely implicating another physician simply for self-protection or self-aggrandizement

Solution

Immediately call the medical staff member with whom the patient followed up. Ideally make an appointment to meet with the physician in their own office. Going to the physician's office has two potential advantages: It can demonstrate a level of respect that will be helpful when trying to enlist the support of the medical staff member. Often, it also can change the medical staff member's attitude because most will treat a visiting physician as a guest.

When meeting with the medical staff member, the ED leader should directly describe the statement that was alleged to have been made. Using the three-step process (**Box 77.5**), determine if and why the physician denounced the patient's care. This must be done in a nonaccusatory manner, such as "It was the patient's perception that you were not happy with his care in the ED. [Pause.] How might we have done better?"

Usually, when confronted, the medical staff member will recognize the gravity and implications of the conversation with the patient. Even if denying the allegation, the staff member will be chastened by the direct confrontation and less likely to make such a statement in the future. The ED leader may solicit further support by asking the disgruntled physician to participate in the advancement of care in the ED. Methods include designing a clinical protocol, giving a lecture, participating in a journal club, selecting upgraded equipment, and so on. A participating medical staff member, whose issues have been heard and addressed and who then contributes to the improvement of the ED, is much more likely to be supportive.

Prospectively, effective leaders seek to find and address problems while in the early stages. These leaders meet with medical staff members as soon as dissatisfaction comes to their attention. This proactive approach demonstrates an easily recognized commitment to continuously improve the level of care in the ED. The emergency physician must regularly reach out to and follow up with the medical staff member to demonstrate a sincere interest in improving both patient care and the relationship.

WORKING WITH HOSPITALISTS

Born of the quest for quality and efficiency, hospital medicine has proven to be a transformative influence, improving both performance and satisfaction in a large segment of hospital-based health-care delivery. Hospitalists simultaneously improve the patient experience, clinical outcomes, and the use of hospital resources.

> **BOX 77.9 ■ ADVANTAGES OF HOSPITALIST PROGRAMS**
>
> - Reduced length of stay
> - Decreased cost per case
> - Reduced readmission rates
> - Fewer patient tests
> - Higher patient/family satisfaction
> - Patient-physician access 24/7
> - Improved quality measures
> - Core measure compliance
> - Improved HCAHPS scores

Inpatient Care Coordination

The hospitalist's role starts with the patient's evaluation after being informed (usually) by the emergency physician that inpatient management is required. The hospitalist then works to admit the patient, provide appropriate treatment, monitor patient progress, provide real-time care supervision, plan for postdischarge management and follow-up, and ultimately discharge the patient to the next stage of care. The advantages of a properly managed hospitalist program can include all of the advantages noted in **Box 77.9.**

The opportunities for improving service to the patient as well as enhancing operational efficiency are substantial. Hospitalists are positioned to efficiently manage admissions, quickly getting the patient from the point of entry to a bed on the inpatient floor. Based on their roles, hospitalists can potentially benefit multiple stakeholders (**Table 77.5**).

Quest for the Ideal Hospitalist-ED Relationship

The hospitalist program has a significant and direct impact on the performance of the ED, often generating more than 50% of a hospital's admissions.[11] A positive respectful working relationship between the ED providers and hospitalists enhances the ability of both to provide best care to patients, with several specific advantages to the ED and its providers. Working collaboratively, the two departments can have a significant impact on the hospital's and each other's performance. Efficient transfer of patients to the inpatient setting reduces the likelihood of hospital boarders in the ED by opening the "back door" of the ED so the "front door" can remain open."[7]

TABLE 77.5 ■ Hospitalists Benefit Multiple Stakeholders

Beneficiary	Hospitalists
Patients	Are in-hospital care experts, shorten LOS, provide frequent communication
Families	Are nearby when the family is present to explain and answer questions
PCP	Allow PCPs to focus on office patients and avoid onerous call obligations
Emergency provider	Facilitate throughput, provide consultations, reduce ED backlogs
Surgeons	Manage complex surgical patients allowing surgeons to concentrate on surgery
Nurses	Provide improved access and coordination of patient care
Hospital	Improve efficiency, decrease LOS, perform with evidence-based care

Ideally, the relationship between hospitalists and emergency physicians is the best relationship in the hospital because the functions of the two groups are so intertwined. These clinicians spend their professional practices within the walls of the hospital and become uniquely and intimately familiar with all of the existing processes (both effective and ineffective).

Unfortunately, in some hospitals, there is little trust between the ED providers and hospitalists, creating a strained, or worse, an adversarial and competitive relationship. This conflict is more likely to occur when the incentives and goals of the groups are divergent and result in delays, inefficiencies, and provider frustration. Furthermore, this strife may compromise clinical care; studies have shown that the longer a patient "boards" in the ED, the worse the outcome.[12]

Case Six: A Patient Requiring Admission

The emergency physician calls to admit a patient. He realizes that the hospitalist on duty today is generally irritable, always questioning whether patients "really" need to be admitted and then demanding more tests to be completed in the ED. The hospitalist seems to delay the process until the next hospitalist takes over. The hospitalist is about to call the ED but realizes that it is that doctor who usually calls with several patients at the end of the shift. The patients are inadequately worked up, and it is often impossible to determine into which bed (unit) the patient should be placed. In some cases, the patient hasn't required admission at all.

At Issue

Poor relationships and inconsistent processes result in deteriorating trust, inadequate transitions, and suboptimal patient care. The differences in the driving forces and incentives lead to unclear communication, slower throughput, poor service to the patient, increased frustration and dissatisfaction, poorer performance, and increased liability. Inevitably, time and resources are wasted for evrreyone involved. The patient suffers most and is caught in the middle of the conflict between the two departments.

Solution

Emergency providers are driven by speed. Since length of stay is measured in minutes, they move fast and make critical decisions quickly. Hospital medicine physicians, on the other hand, are driven by careful and thorough analyses. Because length of stay is measured in days, they make slower, well-thought-out decisions. It is not easy to change these mindsets. This transformation must start with leadership. The leaders of each group must meet and come to a common understanding of the *raison d'être* of their programs—"service to the patients." Once agreed upon, several effective programmatic changes can occur (discussed in detail in Chapter 51). Inevitably, success requires the development of trust based on communication and regular meetings to discuss improvements:

- Commitment to goal of most efficient patient care
- Development of protocols acceptable to both groups
- Definition of combined (aligned) and separate metrics to be reviewed by both groups
- Review of cases and behaviors that fall outside agreed-upon protocols
- Establishment of regular formal meetings to discuss progress and issues
- Social interactions outside of the routine medical setting

Once the ED providers and hospitalist are all rowing in the same direction, efficiency, patient care, and interdepartmental relationships will all improve.

CONCLUSION

Above all, it is important that medical staff members recognize that the greatest interest of the ED staff is to provide the best possible care to theie patients and those who care for them. To achieve success, an ED group must articulate a philosophy of partnership between the emergency physicians and the rest of the medical staff. It is necessary to deliver and be recognized for providing high-quality patient care. After establishing a foundation of clinical excellence, effective groups become integrated in the medical staff structure. Emergency physicians can then become leaders in the medical staff process and gain the esteem afforded to those who hold these pivotal roles.

REFERENCES

1. Maslow AH, revised by Frager R, Fadiman J, McReynolds C, Cox R. *Motivation and Personality.* New York, NY: Harper and Row;1987.
2. Strauss RW. Effective medical staff relationships. Strauss RW, Mayer T, eds. *Strauss and Mayer's Emergency Department Management.* Philadelphia, PA: McGraw Hill; 2013.
3. Mayer T. Customer service. Presented at: the American College of Emergency Physicians (ACEP) Emergency Department Directors Academy (EDDA), April 18, 2004, Dallas, Tex.
4. Covey SR. *The Seven Habits of Highly Effective People.* Free Press; 2004.
5. Policy statements. American College of Emergency Physicians (ACEP). Available at: https://www.acep.org/policystatements/. Accessed November 20, 2020.
6. Zun L, Strauss RW, Kalifon D. Contracts with physicians. In: Salluzzo RF, Mayer TA, Strauss RW, Kidd P, eds. *Emergency Management: Principles and Applications.* Mosby; 1997.
7. Mayer T, Jensen K. *The Patient Flow Advantage: How Hardwiring Hospital-Wide Flow Drives Competitive Performance.* Pensacola, FL: Firestarter Publishing; 2015.
8. *The Wizard of Oz.* Metro-Goldwyn-Mayer; 1939.
9. Tom Peters Blog. 2006. Available at: https://tompeters.com/2008/06/eighty-percent-of-success-is-showing-up/. Accessed September 30, 2020.
10. Greenleaf RK. *Servant Leadership: A Journey Into the Nature of Legitimate Power and Greatness.* Paulist Press; 2002.
11. Owens P, Elixhauser A. Hospital admissions that began in the emergency department, 2003. *Healthcare Cost and Utilization Project (H-CUP) Statistical Brief #1.* 2006. Available at: https://www.hcup-us.ahrq.gov/reports/statbriefs/sb1.pdf. Accessed October 5, 2020
12. Singer AJ, Thode HC, Viccellio P, Pines JM. The association between length of emergency department boarding and mortality. *Acad Emerg Med.* 2011;18(12):1324–1329.

CHAPTER 78

IMPROVING PERFORMANCE THROUGH MUTUAL ACCOUNTABILITY

Thom A. Mayer, Robert W. Strauss, Jay Kaplan

Excellence is what we strive for, but consistency is what we demand.

—Baruch Spinoza[1]

Rewarding champions and corralling the stragglers requires holding members of the emergency department (ED) team mutually accountable for aligned strategic incentives and metrics-based results—good for the patient and good for the team taking care of the patient.[2] This process is sometimes difficult, but it should never be *complicated*, as this chapter will show. It requires an understanding of human motivation combined with an approach that is transparent, direct, data-driven, and effective. Elements of leadership as well as "followership"—the ability of team members to come together—produce measurable results for mutual benefit. Plans that are team generated align strategic incentives to produce the best results.[3] Department leaders must embrace the concepts of rewarding champions and corralling the stragglers (and their behaviors) in a culture in which success is not only possible but likely.

Emergency departments are complex, adaptive systems that involve individuals with varying backgrounds and levels of education and training. All ED staff members come together as a team to deliver the best possible care for their patients, the vast majority of whom they have never seen before. Department leaders must engage and align the providers to work in an accountable fashion with the common goal of serving these patients, their families, the medical staff, hospital leadership, and, of course, each other.

A CULTURE OF MUTUAL ACCOUNTABILITY

Rewarding champions and corralling stragglers assumes that there is a "right way" to do things, guided by a culture of excellence with a clear definition of what success comprises. Each ED must come to a team-based understanding of how it defines success. However, all effective teams have at their core some variation of the way Best Practices, Inc defines success:

- The **Science** of Clinical Excellence
- The **Art** of Patient Experience
- The **Business** of Execution

Rewarding ED champions simply recognizes the adage, "What gets rewarded gets repeated." While intrinsic motivation is the key to meaningful and lasting change (as discussed in detail in Chapter 1), most people respond positively to the genuine expression of appreciation for a job well done under difficult circumstances. In addition, a culture of appreciation accelerates the development of additional champions.

"Corralling the stragglers" requires leaders to temporarily separate poor performers from the group and meaningfully motivate them. The leader must directly help the straggler(s) address the goals of providing higher levels of care and caring through specific programs and mentoring. The most important of these processes is the development of a culture of mutual accountability.

Mutual accountability is a system in which personal responsibility is intertwined with a culture that prizes team engagement.[4] Leader accountability ("top down") certainly has a place, but so does team accountability ("bottom up"), wherein team members are empowered to hold each other responsible for the processes and behaviors to which they have mutually agreed. Generally, leader accountability should work in tandem with team accountability. Whenever team accountability fails, leaders must aggressively step in to ensure that all team members are aligned, engaged, and held responsible for the choices inherent in their actions.

If the stragglers cannot be motivated or refuse to change, they must be removed from the team. While this mandate may seem harsh, failure to hold people accountable for behaviors that are counterproductive to the team's goals exhibits poor leadership. Further, it is fundamentally deceptive and dishonest. Telling team members, "It's OK" when it is decidedly and transparently "not OK" will eventually bring the team down. Team members quickly recognize leaders who are both inconsistent and insincere about their expectations. In fact, lack of mutual accountability usually will cost some of the team members their jobs . . . and it may cost the leader theirs as well.

Lack of accountability creates a culture in which there are two sets of rules—one for the champions who follow and embody them and another for the stragglers who get away with disregarding them. That is a recipe for mediocrity fueled by the "inertia of anonymity."[5]

DEFINING SUCCESS IN THE ED

The first task is to ensure there is a clear, concise, actionable, and team-generated definition of success. Part of this wisdom is recognizing that all positive things are created twice: first in the mind or vision and then in the action taken to achieve the vision. Without a clear definition of success, it is impossible to attain it. Aligning strategic incentives around a clear, proactively stated definition of success creates a culture where excellence is not only attainable but also sustainable. Both Peter Drucker and Ed Schein, each in his own voice, note that "Culture eats strategy for breakfast."[6-8]

Culture is the oil that makes the ED team able to create success in as frictionless an environment as possible.

Aligning strategic incentives should begin with the hiring and onboarding process, and both the culture and the alignment of "why" and "how" should be communicated clearly to the new team members at the outset. During the onboarding process, newcomers should be encouraged to verbalize their understanding of the mission, vision, values, and strategies across the team, as well as their role in attaining them.[9]

Once the "why" is clear, there are many ways to set and measure progress, including Pillar Management, balanced scorecards (**Figure 78.3**), dashboards displaying real-time metrics, and more formal 360-degree approaches to evaluation.[10-13] The specific approach used is less important than ensuring a clear statement of the vision, mission, values, strategies, and measurements by which success will be judged (Chapters 1 and 2 discuss these concepts in more detail).

This chapter focuses on how both individual and team behaviors contribute to the delivery of success, elaborating on the attributes of:

- *Great* emergency physicians
- *Great* emergency nurses
- *Great* ED technicians
- *Great* ED unit administrative assistants
- *Great* essential services personnel (imaging, laboratory, bed board, and so on)

The answers begin with an understanding of the ED as a complex adaptive system, in which multiple aspects of success must be integrated into a meaningful whole.

Creating Mutual Accountability

In his excellent book *The Fifth Discipline: The Art and Science of Learning Organizations*, Peter Senge emphasizes the concept of "shared mental models," defined as:

> . . . deeply ingrained assumptions, generalizations, or even pictures or images that influence how we understand the world and how we take action.[14]

One of the most important shared mental models for health-care leaders and managers is the concept of "connecting the gears." The patient is at the center of all we do in health care, and each of the "gears" (clinical effectiveness, patient safety, hardwiring flow, patient experience, and all others) is connected through its relationship to the patient. In other words, each discipline has value only inasmuch as it has an impact on the patient.[15]

Talented leaders and managers ensure that all new processes not only have a direct effect on the patient but also are clearly connected to the other gears. It is necessary to consider this concept in every change effort or innovation. Equally important, mutual accountability requires leaders to help all team members connect these gears—all day, every day, and for every patient.

Defining A-Team Behaviors

To hire those who are or aspire to be champions, it is imperative to know the attributes ingrained in those who are capable of hardwiring excellence into their practices. Generally speaking, search for team members with:

- ***Clinical knowledge and technical skills***: They know what to do and how to do it across a wide range of clinical entities. (The Science of Clinical Excellence)
- ***Demonstrated productivity and efficiency***: They can multitask (task-switch) in the most difficult and trying of circumstances. (The Business of Execution)
- ***Excellent bedside manners***: They have a goal of high patient, family, and team member satisfaction. (The Art of Patient Experience)
- ***Team-player attitudes***: They work across boundaries for the good of the patient and those who care for the patient.
- ***Humility, dignity, and grace***: They are able to maintain the perspective that it is not about them but rather about achieving the team goals on behalf of the patient. As C.S. Lewis wrote, "Humility is not thinking less of yourself, but thinking of yourself less".[16]

As noted in the patient experience chapters in this book, one of the simplest ways to view staff attitudes and behaviors is through the A-team/B-team concept. All ED staff members recognize that there are certain days when they go to work, see their (A-team) colleagues, and think, "Great! Bring it on—this team can make things happen!" But there are other days they go to work, see those with whom they are working (B-team members) and think, "Get me out of here!—I can't work with these people!" If the staff is asked, "How many B-team members does it take to destroy an entire shift?" it should be no surprise if the answer is "One!"

The A-team members are the champions, consistently making a difficult job much easier through their disciplined use of the talents and skills requisite to deliver great patient care, defined in the broadest possible sense. (That discipline is detailed in Chapter 12.) The B-team members (or worse, the C- or D- team members) are the stragglers, the ones who just cannot seem to focus adequately on taking care of the patients and their families, let alone their fellow team members.

Passion, Engagement, and Burnout

The psychological relationship between people and their jobs can be conceptualized as a continuum, from the positive experience of engagement to the negative experience of burnout.[17] Viewed in this way, the three interrelated aspects of the continuum are *energy*, *involvement*, and *efficacy*—all of which can lead to burnout if not properly managed and supported by leadership and the entire team:

Engagement	↔	Burnout
Energy	↔	Exhaustion
Involvement	↔	Cynicism
Efficacy	↔	Inefficacy

Engagement is defined as a positive, energetic state of job involvement that enhances one's sense of professional accomplishment or efficacy. To what extent is the ED (and the entire hospital) committed to meaningful, demonstrable ways of promoting the three core qualities necessary for success: high energy, committed involvement, and maximum effectiveness? A commitment to engagement is a commitment to change the job and its effect on the team . . . rather than focusing on burnout alone, which leads to strategies that change the *person*.[17]

While engagement is an important concept to consider in health care, passion is really the element that drives those in highly stressful environments, although that aspect is admittedly less easy to capture in surveys. As Wilbur Wright said about the invention of man-powered sustainable flight:

> *Orville and I were having so much fun, we couldn't wait to get up in the morning.*[18]

That is precisely the type of passion needed to work well in an ED—where mere engagement may be just a step from the joy of passion to the tragedy of burnout:

Passion	→	Engagement	→	Burnout

The solution to burnout is restoring passion, not just attaining engagement. *Passionate engagement* as opposed to engagement alone is a helpful construct in which to consider the prevention of health-care burnout.[19] One effective way to confirm that engagement exists is to present the vision of success and simply ask, "Is there anyone here who can't commit to this? If you cannot, tell us now."

B-team members predictably consume 80% to 90% of their ED leaders' time (Pareto's paradox) and detract from the A-team members' ability to effectively do their jobs. If allowed to continue, they fundamentally destroy the culture of excellence by proving that there are two sets of rules in their ED: one for the A-team and a completely different set for the B- and C-teams. A culture of excellence requires mutual accountability. Emergency department leaders must be fundamentally committed to this concept if they are to create and sustain high-performing teams.[20]

REWARDING THE CHAMPIONS

In his book *Inside the Magic Kingdom*, Tom Connellan notes the curious but wise fact that people are subject to a "compliment-to-criticism ratio," which describes the necessity of using praise over criticism as a motivating strategy.[21]

Harvesting Compliments

Connellan points out that the negative effect of a criticism has double the power of a compliment, so that if you balance one criticism with one compliment, the effect is negative. One criticism with two compliments has a neutral effect, and after one criticism, three compliments are needed to produce a positive effect (**Table 78.1**).

The implication of Connellan's work for ED leaders is clear—they must have both a commitment to and a system for capturing compliments. Health-care systems that have transformed their culture have found effective ways to "harvest" compliments, a method that has two important functions. First, once the compliments have been harvested, they can be fed back to the champions who created them, with a preference for a system that celebrates these successes publicly. Second, by celebrating the success, both the champion and the rest of the team have practical examples of how compliments were created. This system becomes a treasure hunt for successful behaviors.[22] There are number of effective ways of doing this, including:

- Direct observation in the clinical areas
- Leader rounding (ask, "With whom do you most enjoy working and why?" "Whose name do you *love* seeing on the schedule?")
- Patient experience surveys (free-form compliments)
- Patient thank-you letters, notes, verbal comments, e-mails
- Leader rounding on patients and families
- Boards or panels posted either in the treatment area (for patients, families, and staff) or in the staff lounge (for staff)

One very effective model for promoting compliments publicly is the "Caught Caring" program at Inova Health System and the "Catch-a-Star" program at Best Practices. Both use boards with notepads and pens in which any one can compliment A-team members for the kindness, thoughtfulness, or professionalism of their actions. These notes are then collected and kept in the files of the staff, after the champion and staff members have been made aware of the compliment.

Regardless of the system used (and using multiple mechanisms to catch compliments characterizes the highest-performing systems), it is essential to feed the results back to the caregivers in real time (see Chapter 76). The closer the compliment to the action, the more powerful the reinforcement. (The same applies to stragglers and complaints.) Other

TABLE 78.1 ■ Connellan's Praise Over Criticism

Compliment-to-criticism ratio	Effect on employee
1 compliment/1 criticism	Negative
2 compliments/1 criticism	Neutral
3 compliments/1 criticism	Positive

essential elements of programs that reward champions by capturing compliments are that they:

- Must reflect genuine admiration for the work done
- Should be as specific as possible
- State the outcome of the action (how it made the patient, family, or other staff feel)
- Should be encouraged whenever and wherever a kindness occurs

Many successful EDs use these compliments as the basis for monthly, quarterly, and yearly awards for high-performing team members. Plaques, prizes, gift certificates, parking spaces, and other incentives have all been used successfully to tangibly acknowledge excellent work.[23] While leaders need to drive these recognition efforts, it is important that staff members have a role in designing and implementing them as well.

While these programs can be good motivators, none should replace the primacy of communicating directly to the champions with heartfelt and genuine appreciation, preferably tied directly to specific actions. All leaders should use this method of communication widely, keeping in mind the 3:1 compliment-to-criticism ratio necessary for success. In many physician groups, patient, family, or staff satisfaction is actually a part of the financial incentive program. Some programs emphasize team-based scores, while others use individual scores or compliment-to-complaint ratios.

A common question for EDs is whether to maintain a separate rewards program or to integrate these efforts into the hospital's recognition program. Former Speaker of the House of Representatives Tip O'Neill famously said, "All politics is local." This wisdom certainly applies to the ED and suggests that having a separate system ensures the timely and robust recognition of A-team behavior. However, if the hospital also has a program, it is usually wise to participate in it as well to ensure that the ED is viewed as a part of the hospital team.

CORRALLING THE STRAGGLERS

One of the great failures of many EDs is their often-inexplicable reluctance to call to task those who are, at best, distracting and, at worst, disruptive. These "C-team" members can create intense frustration among their colleagues, as they consistently (and perhaps consciously) behave in ways that thwart the already-difficult task of providing patient care.

These "stragglers" exhibit behaviors that pull them away from the majority of well-meaning and hardworking providers—the "herd" to use one metaphor. The stragglers' behaviors must be brought into a constrained space, in which consistently acceptable parameters are followed. Both leaders and staff ("top down" and "bottom up") must help corral the B-team behaviors, which distract the team from achieving their purpose. To extend the metaphor, the "fences" of the corral are the parameters of alignment and expectations of the team. In some cases, stragglers who refuse to stay within the fences must be "cut from the herd" by finding other places in which they might be successful.

These stragglers:

- Occupy 80% to 90% of leadership's time
- Create constant distractions from the team's efforts to provide quality care
- Demoralize the rest of the team, who wonder why no one holds them accountable
- Create an environment where patients and their families feel the ED fell below their expectations
- Make the job much more difficult for the A-team members.

Worse, having more than one B-team member on the same shift can be exponential in its negative effects. It has been wryly noted that poor performers are, "space-occupying lesions that suck the life out of those with whom they work."[23] Leaders must deal with low performers in a disciplined, aggressive, but fair fashion. Otherwise, the continuous improvement of the other team members will be severely limited. The stragglers may be identified by simply asking these questions:

- Who occupies the majority of the problem-solving ("putting the fires out") time of the ED leadership?
- Which team members are viewed as distractors versus enhancers during a difficult ED shift?
- Who takes coaching and mentoring well? Who does not?
- Whose name(s) does the staff dread to see on the schedule?
- Whose personnel files have the most complaints?
- Whose files have the same types of complaints over and over?

Although low performers are usually well known to the leadership team, going through these questions does occasionally identify an unknown straggler, and it certainly clarifies the poor level of their performance. In addition, listen for these phrases, which are often key clues to B- and C-team members:

- "That's not my job."
- "That's not my responsibility."
- "I see there was a problem, but I didn't do anything wrong."
- "That's not a legitimate complaint."
- "That's a problem for the next shift."
- "That's not a nurse/doc/ED problem, it's someone else's problem."
- "What do you want me to do about it?"

Each of the above responses is an attempt to avoid and redirect responsibility. Alternatively, A-team members respond to complaints by recognizing that poor performance reflects on the entire team; rather than making excuses, these high performers engage in finding solutions. The good news for ED leaders is that there are highly specific and effective tools that can be used to corral the stragglers and pull the B-team members back onto the A-team (**Figure 78.1**).

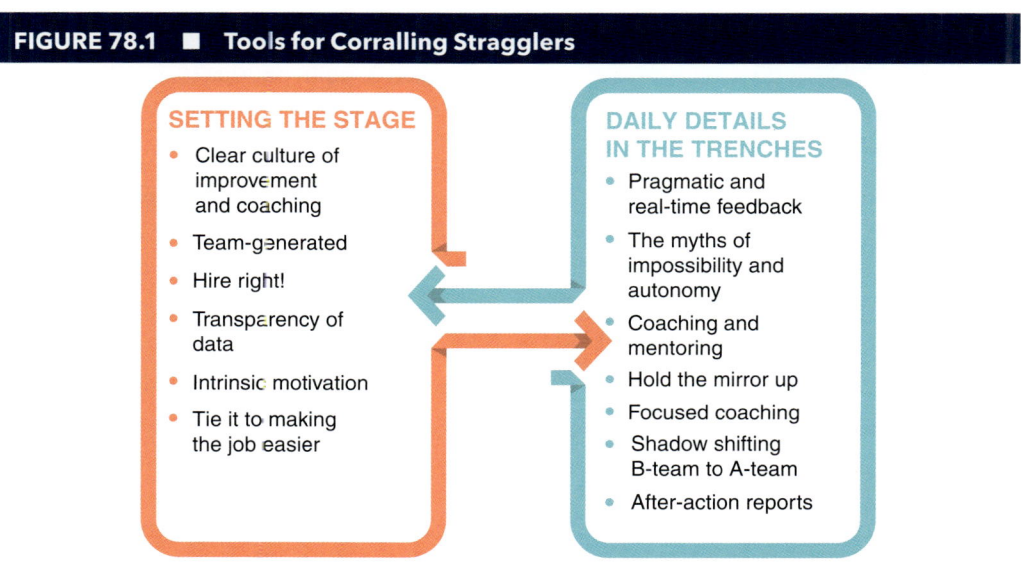

FIGURE 78.1 ■ Tools for Corralling Stragglers

SETTING THE STAGE
- Clear culture of improvement and coaching
- Team-generated
- Hire right!
- Transparency of data
- Intrinsic motivation
- Tie it to making the job easier

DAILY DETAILS IN THE TRENCHES
- Pragmatic and real-time feedback
- The myths of impossibility and autonomy
- Coaching and mentoring
- Hold the mirror up
- Focused coaching
- Shadow shifting B-team to A-team
- After-action reports

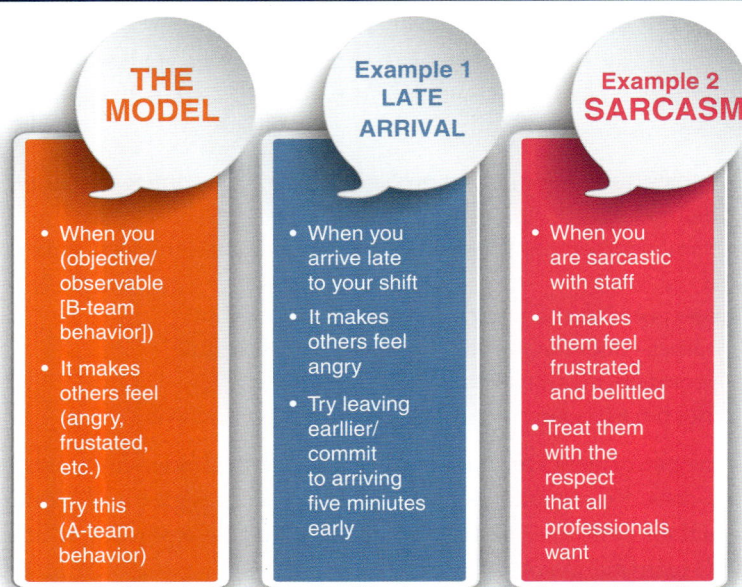

FIGURE 78.2 ■ Gordon's Model for Handling B-Team Members

Pragmatic and real-time feedback is essential to tying behavior to results. The closer and more practical the feedback, the greater the impact. Use specific information regarding what happened, what the negative effects were, and how to move to being a champion. The Gordon Method (**Figure 78.2**) is a practical and powerful way to ensure the message is delivered. This effectively holds a mirror up to the B-team members to show them what effect their behavior has, not only on patients, but on their colleagues.

Debunking Myths

Two stubborn myths can impede success in the ED: *the myth of impossibility* and the *myth of autonomy*.

The Myth of Impossibility

Stragglers always have a reason why things "can't be done here." Expect this reaction because it will occur. When it does, it is imperative to use the data to point out that it actually *is* being done here; after all, *others* on the team have been able to do it. The following evidence-based script may be helpful:

> *I understand that the march to metrics we have agreed to as a team requires change, and change can be frustrating. You mentioned, "It can't be done here." But, in fact, it is being done here, since Dr. Ortega has been able to produce 90th percentile scores. So, it can be done, it just isn't being done by you — yet . . . I'd suggest we have you work with her to see what she is doing differently to attain those scores.*

The myth of impossibility is one of the most common issues in dealing with stragglers, but these tactics can easily overcome it.

The Myth of Autonomy

This myth is a related concept, in which professionals maintain that they have an autonomous practice, and nobody should interfere with it. First, ED care is a "team sport" by its very nature, and autonomy is not a necessary or desirable component. Every member of the team must realize the impact their work has on their colleagues. When leaders hear some variation of, "I'm a professional with 20 years of experience—you can't tell me how to practice!" they are hearing some variation of the autonomy myth. The following are examples of language that can be helpful for addressing such attitudes:

> *As I'm sure you recall, when you went through the process of joining our ED, we stressed that we practice in a team environment, where everyone's work affects that of the other team members. Do you remember that conversation?*
>
> *I respect your professional qualifications, but you must respect the fact that we have shared goals, which require that every team member coordinate their care with the other team members, including the use of evidence-based clinical, quality, safety, and patient experience protocols. Your autonomy, and that of every team member, cannot be counter to attaining those goals.*
>
> *However, what we have noticed is that your results on XYZ metrics are excellent. Would you be willing to work with some of your colleagues who are lagging behind on those measures . . . and they can work with you on improving your ABC metrics?*

To corral the stragglers, the myths of impossibility and accountability must be met head on.

CREATING A CULTURE OF CHAMPIONS

The culture of the ED should be one in which alignment, engagement, and accountability are part of the recruitment, orientation, and re-recruitment processes. During recruitment, leaders should clarify the expectations to everyone on the team and encourage them to continuously elevate the "level of their game." There will be a series of crucial conversations directed around these questions:

- "What do we want to see more of?"
- "What do we want to see less of?"
- "What is going well?"
- "What is not going well?"
- "What are your suggestions to improve?"
- "When might we expect improvement to occur?"
- "Are you committed to doing what is necessary to meet expectations?"

Highly successful organizations encourage a culture in which any team member at any level can raise what they perceive to be a problem, with one provision—they have to have thought through the problem in enough depth to provide at least one possible solution.

Data, Delta, Decision

Conversations concerning the specific changes required to improve team and individual performance are a necessary, if sometimes uncomfortable, part of leadership. To simplify these interactions, the three "Ds" should frame every conversation regarding performance improvement:

- ***What are the Data?*** The "data" focus on specifics of an effective metrics-based approach on which the team can agree (see Chapter 2).
- ***What is the Delta?*** The "delta" is simply the difference between current results and the target. How far is the team or the individual from the established target, and why have we failed to achieve it? If we have achieved or exceeded our metrics targets, why

and how did that occur? It is important to know the reasons for success (so they can be shared) and for failure (so they can be eliminated).
- ***What is the Decision?*** The "decision" is the specific plan for sustaining success or eliminating the reasons for failure. What will be done differently, and why will these changes result in better performance?

Coaching and Mentoring

While culture is critical to effective leadership, it is no less essential for the team to be willing to be coached and mentored. What is the best way to ensure that team members are open to coaching? It is simple . . . ask them. During the recruiting and orientation process, leadership should tell potential team members that coaching and mentoring are a fundamental part of the fabric of the organization and that they will be formally evaluated on a regular basis. Practical experience has shown that quarterly or semiannual reviews, at a minimum, are beneficial to B-team members.[24] However, the closer the coaching and mentoring are to suboptimal performance, the greater and faster the improvement. With C-team members (who may require formal counseling), monthly or even weekly coaching and mentoring sessions may be necessary, and the sessions should be documented.

While the formal process of counseling is often governed by hospital or system policy (at least for hospital employees), physician groups often craft their own independent processes. Nurses and physicians, at a minimum, should be assigned a mentor when they are hired. This mentoring process can range from highly informal (helping with orientation, catching up on a periodic basis for a "reality check") to extremely structured (weekly session during the first 3 to 6 months to discuss successes, failures, problem areas, and other issues).

Redesigning Performance Assessments

In many hospitals and health-care institutions (including EDs), the performance assessment process contains far too much hierarchical and authoritarian interaction and far too few opportunities to compare the demands of the job with the resources needed to complete the tasks. As management experts Peter Block, Tom Peters, and Peter Drucker note, the sessions often have almost a neocolonial feel, where professionals feel they are fundamentally being told:[25-27]

- "Here are your deficiencies."
- "Here are the data supporting your deficiencies (which you had no voice in generating . . .)"
- "Here's the timeline for reassessing your deficient performance."
- "Fix it!"
- ("Oh, by the way, I basically own you . . .")

It is far more productive to use these assessments as a means of coaching and mentoring team members. An effect process includes ways the individual can augment their capacity to deal with job stressors and also ways in which the job itself can be changed to make it more manageable. (This revolutionary concept utilizes a performance assessment that takes into consideration both how the person is performing in the job and also *how the job is performing for the person!*) Leaders should ensure that the performance assessment process reflects both concepts.

FIGURE 78.3 ■ Focused Coaching (CTs per 100 Patients)

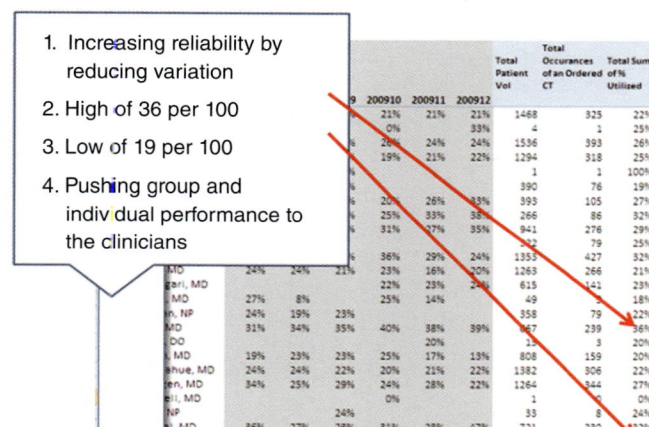

Focused Coaching

For many of the metrics approaches (pillar management, balanced scorecard, 360-degree feedback, etc.), data can show how an individual compares with others on the team. Using these data to focus on highly-specific areas improves performance. After all, physicians and nurses are scientists, and scientists love data. And, of course, no one wants to be in the bottom third!

Use these insights to drive the crucial (data, delta, decision) conversation. The "decision" should focus on ways that the individual (or team) can outline a strategy for achieving specific performance goals. For example, most hospitals can obtain flow, patient safety, clinical effectiveness, and patient experience scores for specific physicians (**Figure 78.3**). Focused coaching allows leaders to help individual team members improve these metrics in meaningful and actionable ways.

Focused coaching can also be effective for improving patient experience scores. The Press Ganey scores for physicians are calculated based on a Likert scale in four categories:

- Courtesy
- Took time to listen
- Informed regarding treatment
- Concern for comfort

For nurses, the same Likert scale is used to measure performance in five categories:

- Courtesy
- Took time to listen
- Informed regarding treatment
- Attention to your needs
- Concern for privacy

FIGURE 78.4 ■ Focused Patient Satisfaction Coaching (Doctor A)

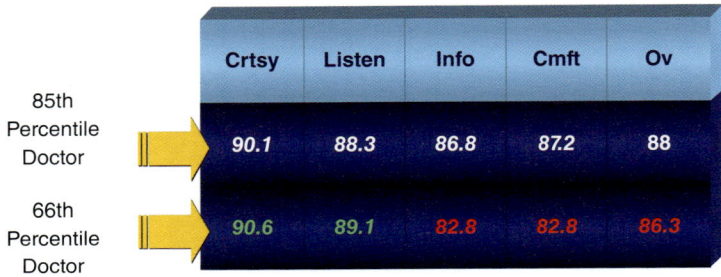

This doctor has scores that are above target (green) as well as scores that are below target (red), with an overall 66th percentile placement in contrast to the target 85th percentile.

Compare two physicians whose overall scores were subpar:

- **Doctor A:** This physician has an overall score in the 66th percentile, well below the 85th percentile target (**Figure 78.4**). He has *above target* scores for "Courtesy" and "Took time to listen." However, the low scores for "Informed regarding treatment" and "Concern for comfort" have pulled his overall score down. Note that his A-team behaviors on "Courtesy" and "Took time to listen" should be celebrated and accentuated while he is encouraged to improve the other two areas.
- **Doctor B:** The second doctor at the same facility during the same measurement period has a higher overall score in the 77th percentile (**Figure 78.5**). However, her scores are the opposite of the first physician's. Her scores are higher than the target for "Informed regarding treatment" and "Concern for comfort," but her scores for "Courtesy" and "Took time to listen" need improvement.

Instead of exhorting both physicians to improve their scores, focused coaching allows the clinicians to emphasize specific behaviors in specific categories. In this example, both physicians were made aware of their scores and discussed their approaches together, after which they worked several shifts together so each could learn from the other. The result was that the scores for both doctors rose to above the 90th percentile.

Shadow Shifting

One of the most powerful tools to drive improvement is often initially resisted. *Shadow shifting* pairs B-team members with A-team members, allowing lower-performing providers

FIGURE 78.5 ■ Focused Patient Satisfaction Coaching (Doctor B)

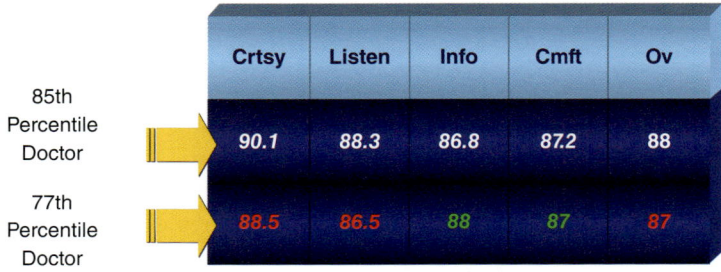

In contrast to the doctor in Figure 67.4, this doctor has the reverse of scores that need improvement (red) and those that are above target (green), with an overall 77th percentile placement (in contrast to the target 85th percentile).

to see how great results occur. Shadow shifting is most commonly used to improve patient experience scores through specific behaviors and language, but it can be helpful in other dimensions as well. Shadow shifting can occur in two directions, with B-team members shadowing A-team members during their shifts or vice versa.

The Method

Start by having the A-team member shadow the B-team member for 4 to 6 hours. The B-team member can simply tell the patient, "I am working with Dr. Smith today, who is one of my partners." The champion can coach and mentor the straggler outside the patients' rooms, beginning with a gentle, "Here's what's worked for me in the past . . ." or "I noticed you don't sit down when you come in the room—that works really well with patients and families."

Overcoming Resistance

Shadow shifting may be resisted by both B-team and A-team members. The stragglers do not readily accept the perceived "punishment" of having someone watch them practice. The champions, on the other hand, often find it difficult to assume the role of coach and mentor.

Focused coaching and shadow shifting are highly effective. Inevitably, both require and represent a fundamental cultural change by all team members. To use a sports analogy, what highly competitive team would refuse coaching from high performers? None would—they welcome any advice that improves their chances of winning. That analogy can be very helpful when transitioning to a culture of coaching. In addition, it should be clarified that the poor results simply cannot continue.

After-Action Reviews

An after-action review (AAR) is a method of understanding a suboptimal outcome, as well as critiquing ways in which all efforts can be improved, even if the outcome was acceptable. After-action reviews were developed by the US Army and Marine Corps to better enable their war fighters to assess combat encounters. They can be used to define how an average or good outcome could have been turned into an even better one. An AAR analyzes the factors listed in **Figure 78.6.**

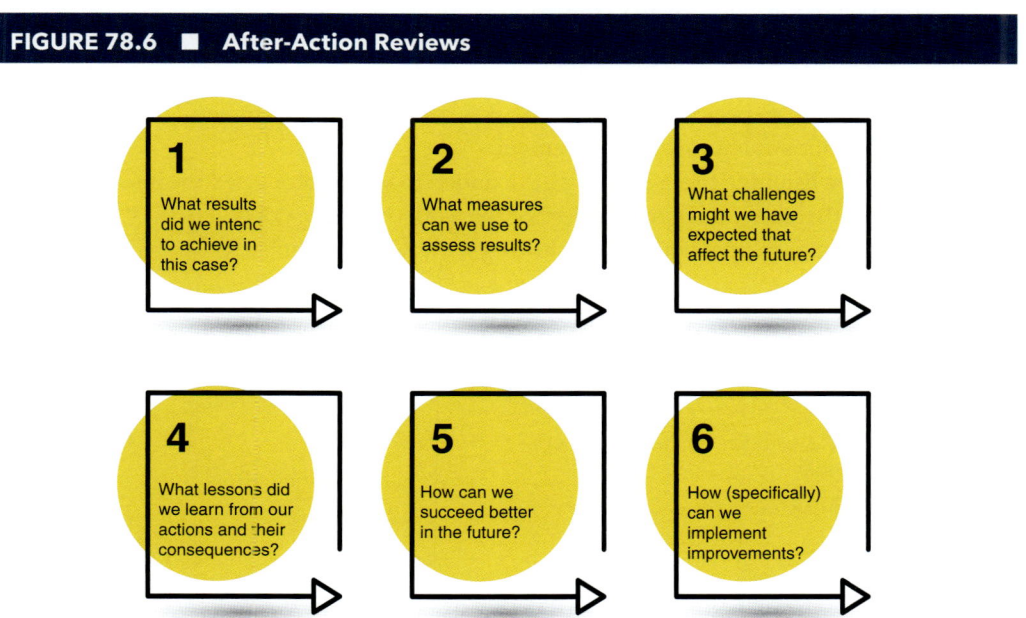

FIGURE 78.6 ■ After-Action Reviews

1. What results did we intend to achieve in this case?
2. What measures can we use to assess results?
3. What challenges might we have expected that affect the future?
4. What lessons did we learn from our actions and their consequences?
5. How can we succeed better in the future?
6. How (specifically) can we implement improvements?

This approach can be applied at the bedside or used for deeper dives into performance improvement and error reduction. After-action reviews can also be used to leverage change in stragglers by introducing the entire team to this improvement concept. They are particularly effective when introduced in high-acuity, high-risk cases like trauma or cardiac resuscitations and extended to other ED patients. Learning why and how errors occur involves an iterative set of discussions, investigations, and analyses.

When performing an AAR, it is important for leaders to take the time to talk to the people involved in the case and then, after the review, return to those people with a clarification (armed with the acquired knowledge about the events surrounding the case). Making simple assumptions about why an error occurred and settling for the first set of conclusions is seldom sufficient to hardwire improved processes and outcomes. Conversely, AARs also should be used to highlight where excellence was attained and accentuate A-team behaviors, which should be celebrated and shared with the entire staff.

A-, B-, and C-Team Members

Effective communications with various types of team members include the following.

A-Team Members

- Reiterate alignment, engagement, and accountability, taking time to note the current direction of the department's strategic objectives.
- Continuously re-recruit them to the team:
  - Thank them for their role in moving the team forward toward its goals.
  - Whenever possible, provide specific examples to reinforce their A-team behaviors.
  - Let them know how important they are to the team and how much they are personally and professionally appreciated.
- Ask them if they would be willing to mentor B-/C-team members, that is, focused coaching and shadow shifting.
- Ask what can be done to help them.
- Reward champions (**Box 78.1**)

B-Team Members

- Reiterate alignment, engagement, and accountability, taking time to note the current direction of the department's strategic objectives.
- Let them know the specific positive attributes that the team has noticed.
- Let them know if there has been improvement noted since the last review.
- Inform them of specific areas where work is needed—give examples.
- Give specific strategies for improvement.
- Use active listening to ensure they have understood and processed the information.
- Close with thanks and appreciation for the work they have done.
- Have them participate in shadow shifting with A-team members.

BOX 78.1 ■ WAYS TO REWARD CHAMPIONS

- "Patient-first" award certificate and pin on a monthly basis
- Catch of the day (real-time each day)
- Treasure grams
- Beads for deeds
- Star cards
- WOW grams
- Wheel of recognition
- E-mail "trophies"
- Handwritten notes
- Earn an extra day off

C-Team Members

- Reiterate alignment, engagement, and accountability, taking time to note the current direction of the department's strategic objectives.
- Make clear in which areas their work has fallen below accountability standards.
- Create and share plans for corrective action.

CONCLUSION

In order to build and sustain a high-performing ED team, there must be a culture in which alignment, engagement, and accountability are at the core. All staff, particularly nurses and physicians, should be recruited, oriented, and continuously re-recruited with the understanding that coaching and mentoring are fundamental and valued aspects of team membership. Rewarding the champions and corralling the stragglers is not a motto—it is a disciplined, formal, carefully considered approach to delivering the results that matter to our patients and our colleagues.

REFERENCES

1. Spinoza B. In: Curley E, ed. *Ethics*. New York, NY: Penguin; 1994.
2. Mayer T. Leadership for great customer service: getting the "why" right before the "how". *Healthc Exec*. 2010;25(3):66-69.
3. Jensen K, Mayer T, Welch S, Haraden C. *Leadership for Smooth Patient Flow: Improved, Outcomes, Improved Service, Improved Bottomline*. Chicago, Ill: Health Administration Press; 2007.
4. Mayer T. Leadership, management, and motivation. In: *Strauss and Mayer's Emergency Department Management*. Dallas, Tex: American College of Emergency Physicians; 2019.
5. Mayer T. Rewarding the champions, corralling the stragglers. Presented at: the American College of Emergency Physicians Leadership and Advocacy Conference; Washington, DC; May 18, 2018.
6. Drucker P. *Adventures of a Bystander*. Hoboken, NJ: John Wiley and Sons; 1994.
7. Schein E. *Organizational Culture and Leadership*. Hoboken, NJ: John Wiley and Sons; 2017.
8. Cave A. *Culture Eats Strategy for Breakfast. So What's for Lunch?* Jersey City, NJ: Forbes; 2017.
9. Mayer T, *Active Listening*, Presented at: the American College of Emergency Physicians Emergency Department Directors Academy, Dallas, Tex, February 5, 2019.
10. Studer Q. *Hardwiring Excellence: Purpose, Worthwhile Work, Making a Difference*. Gulf Breeze, Fla: Fires Tarter Press; 2008.
11. Kaplan RS, Norton DP. The balanced scorecard: measures that drive performance. *Harv Bus Rev*. 1992;70(1):71-79.
12. Mayer T. Drive service excellence to the next level. *Healthc Exec*. 2010;25(6):54,56.
13. Bracken DW, Dalton MA, Jako RA, McCauley CD, Pollman VA. *Should 360-Degree Feedback be Used Only for Developmental Purposes?* Greensboro, NC: Center for Creative Leadership; 1997.
14. Senge P. *The Fifth Discipline: The Art and Science of the Learning Organization*. New York, NY: Doubleday; 2006.
15. Mayer T. Dealing with the 3 team members: holding the mirror up can have a positive effect on them and the organization. *Healthc Exec*. 2010;25(5):52-54.
16. Lewis CS. *Mere Christianity*. New York, NY: Harper One; 1952.
17. Mayer T, Maslach C. Burnout in emergency departments, In: *Strauss and Mayer's Emergency Department Management*. Dallas, Tex: American College of Emergency Physicians; 2019.
18. Kelly FC. *The Wright Brothers*. New York, NY: Dover; 1989.
19. Mayer T. Putting it all together: education and the right tools establish a culture of service. *Healthc Exec*. 2011;26(1):56-59.
20. Studer Q. *Results That Last*. Hoboken, NJ: John Wiley and Sons; 2008.
21. Connellan T. *Inside the Magic Kingdom: 7 Keys to Disney's Success*. New York, NY: Bard Press; 1997.
22. Mayer T, Cates RJ. *Leadership for Great Customer Service: Satisfied Patients, Satisfied Employees*. Chicago, Ill: Health Administration Press; 2004.
23. Mayer T. *Teams and Teamwork*. Dallas, Tex: American College of Emergency Physicians Emergency Department Directors' Academy; 2018.
24. Mayer T, Jensen K. *Hardwiring Flow: Systems and Processes for Seamless Patient Care*. Gulf Breeze, Fla: Fire-Starter Publishing; 2009.
25. Block P. *Stewardship: Choosing Service Over Self-Interest*. 2nd ed. San Francisco, Calif: Berrett-Kohler; 2013.
26. Peters T. *The Excellence Dividend: Meeting the Tech Tide With Work That Wows and Jobs That Last*. New York, NY: Vintage; 2018.
27. Drucker P. *Managing Oneself and What Makes an Effective Executive*, Boston, Mass: HBR Press; 2004.

CHAPTER 79
PATIENT SAFETY AND ERROR REDUCTION

Kirk Jensen, Thom A. Mayer, With John Howell, Leslie M. Flament

Every system is perfectly designed to generate precisely the results it produces.

—Paul Batalden[1]

When clinicians are repeatedly interrupted while delivering patient care, it is because the system is designed to deliver this outcome. When a radiograph or lab test is not resulted for several hours, it is because certain systems are designed to deliver that outcome. When a patient cannot get through triage in under an hour, it is because the system is designed to deliver that result. The effects of these kinds of patient safety issues are measured in human cost, malpractice risk, and contractual instability. If emergency department (ED) leaders are delighted with their results, they should be delighted with the system that produces them. For far too many EDs, less-than-acceptable results mean the system is designed poorly and requires redesign.

Providing a safer environment prevents harm and improves care. In 2000, the Institute of Medicine (IOM) conservatively estimated that 44,000 deaths in the United States could be attributed to medical errors every year—more people than died from motor vehicle accidents.[2] Errors, patient harm, and malpractice all take a significant toll on everyone involved. The high costs of malpractice litigation (and correspondingly high premiums from malpractice insurance) also provide motivation for reducing errors and improving safety. Group practices in emergency medicine typically allocate 5% to 10% of their budget for malpractice premiums—their third largest expense. Improving patient safety not only affects the lives of patients and their caregivers, it also affects the bottom line.

The toll on the ED team is considerable—it produces burnout, a syndrome of exhaustion, cynicism, and inefficiency that is derived from a failure to adapt to work–life stressors.[3] Several health-care systems have developed and implemented changes to help alleviate stress, noting a substantial return on investment.

Organizations become highly reliable, in part, by developing efficient and effective processes. The triage process is changed to direct bedding during the hours when ED beds are available. The patient with cardiac chest pain rapidly receives an ECG. The patient with stroke symptoms is fast-tracked to a clinical evaluation and head CT scan. These types of process changes mostly benefit patient care. Broader benefits accrue in terms of global satisfaction, clinical metrics, and market position.

While process improvement and operations management underpin effective risk reduction, other strategies can make major contributions to patient safety: risk surveillance, outcome measurement, human resource strategies, decision support, education, and development of a culture of excellence.

CONCEPTS AND DEFINITIONS

High-Reliability Organizations

Karl Weick and Katherine Sutcliffe coined the term "High-Reliability Organizations" (HROs) following their study of high-risk, high-pressure organizations, including nuclear power plants, naval aircraft operations, and . . . emergency departments.[4] High-reliability organizations have fewer accidents or bad outcomes than other systems. Organizations are viewed as a complex summation of inter-related processes. Errors occur when processes fail. As a practical example, consider **Table 79.1**.

The vertical axis of this table is the number of elements in an event, encounter, or decision. The horizontal axis is the probability of successfully performing a given action. Looking at the .95 (95%) column—if an ED cares for 100 patients in a day, the odds of success for all 100 patients is less than 1% (.006). Alternatively, consider an ED that cares for 200 patients each day. Imagine each patient encounter involving an average of five decisions or actions, for a total of 1,000 such elements per day. The probability of being 100% successful in this scenario becomes infinitely small.

High-reliability EDs attack risk reduction from this perspective by addressing the following issues:

Anticipation: "Staying out of trouble"

1. Preoccupation with failure
2. Sensitivity to operations
3. Reluctance to simplify

Containment: "Getting out of trouble"

4. Commitment to resilience
5. Deference to expertise

Preoccupation with failure reflects a culture that not only recognizes the potential for failure but the likelihood (near-inevitability) it will occur in complex, adaptive systems, such as EDs populated by fallible human clinicians. Errors should be viewed as consequences, not causes, whose origins are more frequently systemic than arising from an individual's failure.

"Swiss Cheese" Model of Organizational Errors

When performing a focused review of a case with a suboptimal outcome, reviewers frequently note a series of errors. Each identified error requires analysis and understanding; HROs do not settle for simple explanations or superficial interpretations.

TABLE 79.1 ■ Probability of Performing Perfectly

Number of Elements	Probability of Success (Each Element)			
1	0.95	0.990	0.999	0.999999
25	0.28	0.78	0.98	0.998
50	0.08	0.61	0.95	0.995
100	0.006	0.37	0.90	0.99

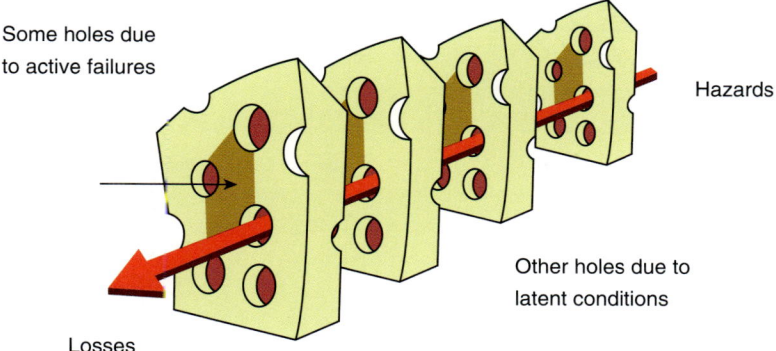

FIGURE 79.1 ■ "Swiss Cheese" Model of Organizational Accidents

This concept is graphically represented in **Figure 79.1**. This "Swiss cheese" model illustrates how errors and harm only occur when the "holes" in the system are aligned perfectly to allow the vector of error to occur, which reemphasizes the systemic nature of organizations.[5] Notably, these "holes" are constantly opening, closing, and shifting, making error management even more complex. Reliability is a "dynamic nonevent" that can be achieved with a series of timely adjustments that result in safe, successful outcomes that rarely call attention to themselves.[5]

A Culture of Safety

As highlighted in a report by the IOM, *Keeping Patients Safe*, when leadership overtly embraces a culture of safety, it becomes just as important as finance and productivity.[6] A culture of safety is a culture of trust in which patient well-being and quality are promoted without fear of retaliation or the clashing of egos. A nurse who is concerned about a specific dosage or volume of medication should be free to question the ordering physician before administering the drug. If a workflow process has the potential to compromise patient safety, any staff member has permission to question it and suggest improvements.

STRATEGIES FOR RISK REDUCTION

Strategies that minimize risk and promote safety include hiring and keeping the right people, focusing on operations, and instituting after-action reviews (AARs) as well as Failure Mode and Effects Analysis (FMEA) reviews (discussed in detail later in the chapter).

Human Resources: "A" Team Versus "B" Team

One of the most important strategies to optimize safety is hiring, training, and retaining the right staff. Competent and effective team members are essential partners when building a high-reliability ED. Hire "A-team members," as originally described by Mayer and Cates:[7]

> A-team members get things done efficiently and effectively. They come to work on time and with energy to spare. A-team members are committed to working with the team and doing what is right for the patient.

TABLE 79.2 ■ A-Team and B-Team Attributes	
A-Team Members	**B-Team Members**
Positive	Negative
Proactive	Reactive
Confident	Constant complainers
Competent	Late
Compassionate	Lazy
Team players	Poor communicators

Avoid hiring B-team members whose behaviors are often the opposite of A-team behaviors (see **Table 79.2**). It may take months of working side by side before differences in team members become apparent. One substantial challenge is a B-team member who lacks self-awareness. This is the B-team member who looks in the mirror and sees an A-team member. Measuring outcomes is an effective strategy for modifying B-team behavior. Measuring clinical metrics (by provider) and feeding them back to everyone allows B-team members without self-awareness to compare themselves to peers. Mentoring and coaching, in selected cases, effectively improves performance. Measuring performance outcomes, aligning incentives, and requiring professional accountability are critical to maintain these performance gains.

Establish and candidly communicate performance expectations when a staff member's citizenship performance (e.g., participation in department meetings, medical staff committees, or community affairs) is unacceptable. Alternatively, having fellow team members evaluate each provider during performance reviews (i.e., 360° evaluation) is a powerful method of improving B-team citizenship issues. When used as a mirror, these type of performance reviews allow B-team members to see how their work is perceived by others. Shadow-shifting, where A-team members work alongside B-team members to offer coaching and mentoring, is also an effective strategy.[8] Ultimately, deciding that a B-team member does not (and most likely is never going to) fit into the system is just as important as hiring correctly.

Focus on Operations

Increased ED volume and diminished hospital capacity lead to overcrowding. Increasingly, patients are older, more medically complex, and often chronically ill. Caring for a chronically ill elderly patient with acute sepsis in a crowded ED is difficult. Caring for that same patient in an ED with fragmented and unreliable systems consistently produces errors and bad outcomes.

Studies show that HROs have found ways to avoid disasters in complex environments where the risk of disaster is inherently high. These HROs focus on developing and consistently using systems that prevent the risk of failures. Strategies to improve processes to ensure success include:

- *Using the Lean approach to process improvement*: Lean uses a variety of analytical tools to preserve value with less work. It identifies and removes steps that do not add value. This set of tools is particularly effective in complex processes like triage and admission.
- *Measuring outcomes*: Clinical metrics and risk outcomes should be measured by each individual provider. Having providers review their individual outcomes allows them to participate in the process of improving patient care, which in turn helps reduce risk.
- *Managing outliers*: Identifying and analyzing outliers identifies opportunities for system- and risk-related improvement. For example, outliers for length of stay frequently encounter multiple delays and process errors (**Figure 79.1**). This approach typically requires persistence and attention to detail.

> **BOX 79.1 ■ QUESTIONS TO ANSWER IN AFTER-ACTION REVIEWS**
>
> 1. What results did we intend to achieve in this case?
> 2. What measures can we use to assess results?
> 3. What challenges might we have anticipated that affect the future?
> 4. What lessons did we learn from our actions and their consequences?
> 5. How can we succeed better in the future?
> 6. What specific measures can we implement and how?

After-Action Reviews

The AAR is a method of understanding what has led to a suboptimal or bad outcome.[9] Developed by the US Army and Marine Corps to better enable their war fighters to assess combat encounters, an AAR can also be used to define how an average outcome could have been turned into a better outcome. An AAR analyzes the questions listed in **Box 79.1**.

This approach can be applied at the bedside or used for deeper dives into performance improvement and error reduction. It is important to point out that in the organizational accident/industrial safety experience, 70% to 80% of errors are blamed on the last person involved in the situation. Following investigation, less than 20% of errors are attributed to the last person involved.[10] Learning why and how errors occur involves an iterative set of discussions, investigation, and analysis. When performing an AAR, it is important for leaders to take the time to talk to the people involved in the case and then, after the review, return to those people with clarification (armed with the acquired knowledge about the events surrounding the case). Making simple assumptions about why an error occurred and settling for the first set of conclusions is seldom enough to hardwire improved processes and outcomes.

Failure Modes and Effects Analysis

Another strategy for risk reduction is FMEA, a proactive risk-assessment strategy required by the Joint Commission. Hospitals and other health-care organizations are mandated to analyze one high-risk procedure every 18 months, identify failures that have occurred during the process, and dissect steps that led to the failure. In the context of the ED, FMEA provides an incisive analysis of the situation, failure points, and suggested improvements.

FMEA assessments can reduce staff stress about proposed changes and also pinpoint and prevent unnecessary interruptions in patient flow that could result from new processes. Without a meaningful FMEA review, organizations can inadvertently add counterproductive regulations, constraints, and complexity that may add waste and act as barriers to the provision of safe, effective service.

TEAMWORK AND COMMUNICATION

An F/A-18 pilot in a plane above the vast shining waters of the Pacific Ocean must find a steel postage stamp (also known as an aircraft carrier) bobbing in the waves and land on its limited surface area deck. The wind is blowing, and the waves are choppy. The landing crew is new, and success depends largely on communication and synchronized interactions among crew members. Few errors in action or communication can be tolerated. (This is an excellent example of why it is the military that has developed highly effective disaster avoidance systems for many high-risk military procedures.)

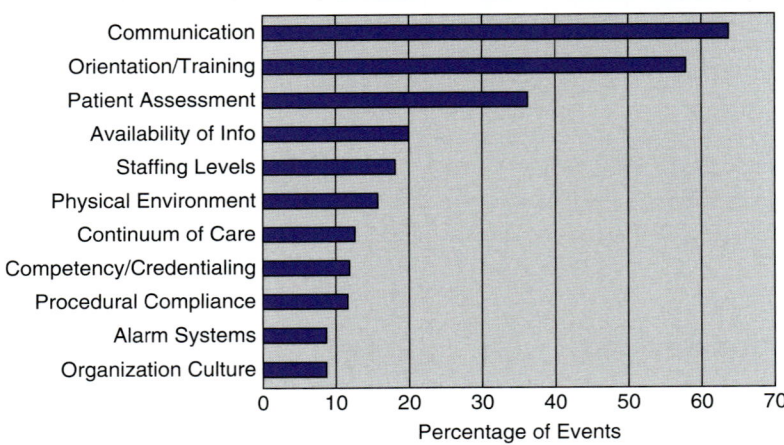

FIGURE 79.2 ■ Root Causes of Sentinel Events (1995-2002)

Equivalent scenarios occur daily in EDs across the country. While many are perhaps less dramatic than landing a plane on the deck of an aircraft carrier, they are still fraught with the potential for teamwork errors and miscommunication (**Box 79.2**). Consider results from The Joint Commission's study of root causes of sentinel events, graphically illustrated in **Figure 79.2**. The top reason for these events was not careless doctors and nurses. The top reason was *communication*. A study by Dynamic Research Corporation that analyzed 50 closed ED malpractice cases over a 10-year period identified 8.8 teamwork errors per case and determined that 50% of the actual harm could have been avoided (see Chapter 12).

Teamwork behavior and skills are teachable. Superb individual clinical skills do not guarantee effective team performance or perfect outcomes. Even though teamwork does not replace clinical skills, it should be embraced because it establishes a safety net for patients and providers. Even the best practitioners anchor and prematurely close on a diagnosis when tired or overworked. Teamwork, along with effective processes and communication, buffers patients from these errors.

The IOM safety report recommends that a dedicated plan should ensure adequate education and training so that every individual working in the ED has the resources to stay current in the latest evidence-based practices.[12] The educational provisions of the ED should reflect the constant advances of medicine as well as the ongoing recommendations of regulatory bodies. All ED staff members need access to educational materials and course offerings, such as journals, seminars, and classes. In addition, both new and experienced staff members need to review infrequently used skills, equipment, and supplies.

SBAR: A Teamwork and Change Communication Tool

SBAR stands for Situation, Background, Assessment, and Recommendations. This tool fosters teamwork and effective communication by standardizing patient reporting and

---

BOX 79.2 ■ REQUIREMENTS FOR EFFECTIVE TEAMWORK

- Collegial teams must be developed with an intention of catching one another's mistakes.
- These collegial teams must work together, demonstrating respect and kindness.
- Barrier-less communication allows subordinates to speak up for patient-safety measures.

TABLE 79.3 ■ SBAR Functions	
SBAR Component	Definition
Situation	Describe the situation with clear facts and data (e.g., pulse rate, respiratory rate, and concerns).
Background	Describe the patient's background clinical information.
Assessment	Give a clear assessment of the problem.
Recommendations	Follow up with recommendations to manage the case or situation.

discussion and establishing communication protocols to build a culture of safety at all practice levels (**Table 79.3**).

Establish Clinical Red Rules and Pathways

"Red rules" describe behaviors that require compliance all of the time. One easily recognizable example of this are the red rules designed to avoid patient misidentification. Analogous clinical red rules, varying in length and complexity, can be developed to preclude diagnostic and therapeutic misadventures. These protocols should be based on high-frequency and high (closed-claim) dollar-loss chief complaints and diagnoses.

To illustrate, one such red rule is designed to prevent the misidentification of testicular torsion. The red rule states that a Doppler ultrasound will be performed for all patients with acute testicular pain. The rule recognizes a patient's history and physical examination are inaccurate when attempting to diagnose testicular torsion. Doppler use is a measurable outcome that can be tracked by individual provider and built into performance reviews and incentive programs.

Red rules like this can be broadened to limit risk across a system. Similarly, pathways can be developed to standardize approaches to clinical presentations based on evidence-based information and expert review. Pathways (**Figure 79.3**) can be developed using process-flow mapping techniques to analyze decision points and value-added steps.[11,12] Once a consensus pathway is developed, a simple representation of the pathway can be made available to providers, either as part of an electronic medical record (EMR) or as a physical document. Outcomes can be tracked by health-care personnel.

Use Decision Support Tools

In the case of testicular torsion, practitioners may need clinical information or reminders about this topic. The support may be provided as evidence-based synopses of disease processes available in the ED. More advanced decision support may take the form of focused reminders (embedded into an EMR), such as:

- Perform a Doppler ultrasound when evaluating suspected testicular torsion.
- Consider a spinal epidural abscess in patients with acute back pain.

When establishing or updating an EMR, one must be careful to balance the number of automated decision support reminders with the risk of "alert fatigue"—an excessive number of warnings that may cause desensitization and result in alerts being ignored or avoided.

Monitor the System for Misses and Near Misses

Leaders should monitor the practice for misses and near misses and use the information to improve processes and performance. Such assessments may include reviews of unexpected

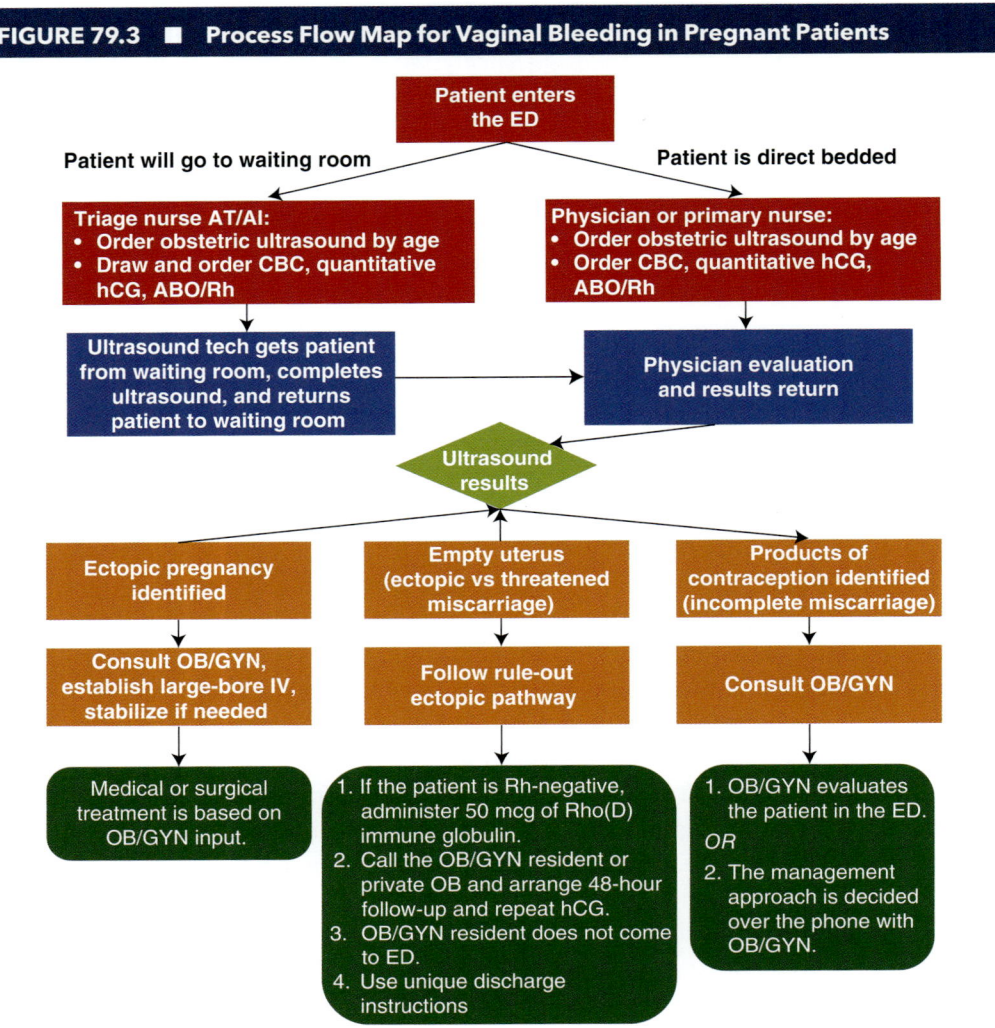

FIGURE 79.3 ■ Process Flow Map for Vaginal Bleeding in Pregnant Patients

returns to (or deaths in) the ED. At the system level, consider monitoring for near misses as well as unfavorable outcomes. Providers may be encouraged to anonymously or discreetly report these cases by establishing an online link to a survey instrument. To be effective, providers must feel secure that reporting will not lead to action against any individual.

Acquiring information about near misses allows a health-care system or unit to learn from its experiences. Trends are identified. Do providers anchor and prematurely close in on certain diagnoses at night? Is a heavy clinical schedule associated with misses and near misses? This information can be used to develop provider feedback and leverage process improvements. The system continuously monitors itself, learns, and uses that knowledge to improve. Example of pathways to avoid an OB/GYN miss or near miss:

Goal: To rapidly evaluate and treat pregnant patients with vaginal bleeding.

Exclusion: This pathway does not pertain to unstable patients.[13]

Consulting in-house OB/GYN: Call the in-house OB/GYN attending (see daily call sheet). The attending will decide if a resident should be involved and, if so, who.

Timing around diagnostic studies: If a serum hCG is to be sent with a pelvic ultrasound, the blood test must be drawn and sent before the patient undergoes imaging. However, do not wait for the hCG result to send the patient for ultrasound.

> **BOX 79.3 ■ PATIENT SAFETY WALK-ROUNDS QUESTIONS**
>
> - Were there any recent events that resulted in prolonged stays for a patient?
> - Have there been any near misses?
> - Have there been any incidents recently that concern you or your team members about patient safety?
> - What can be done to recognize and prevent an adverse event?
> - What is working well from a patient safety perspective?

Conduct Patient Safety Walk-Rounds

Clinical leaders should tour the ED on a regular basis with a focus on patient safety to garner value-added information from providers and staff. Asking the questions listed in **Box 79.3** is a good framework. Patient safety walk-rounds help identify strengths and weaknesses and provide opportunities for improvement.

IMPROVING RELIABILITY

Like the notion of improving safety, the concept of high reliability may seem obvious: service and outcomes one can count on every time they are delivered. However, in the context of organizational dynamics, the concept has been given a specific meaning: an organization that operates in a field where conditions are stressful and challenging that nonetheless operates with a low rate of mistakes.[4]

For example, consider older ATM machines, which took the customer's card and ejected money. To get the ATM card back, the customer was required to press a button. There were many incidents of forgotten and lost cards. A low-reliability approach to solve this problem

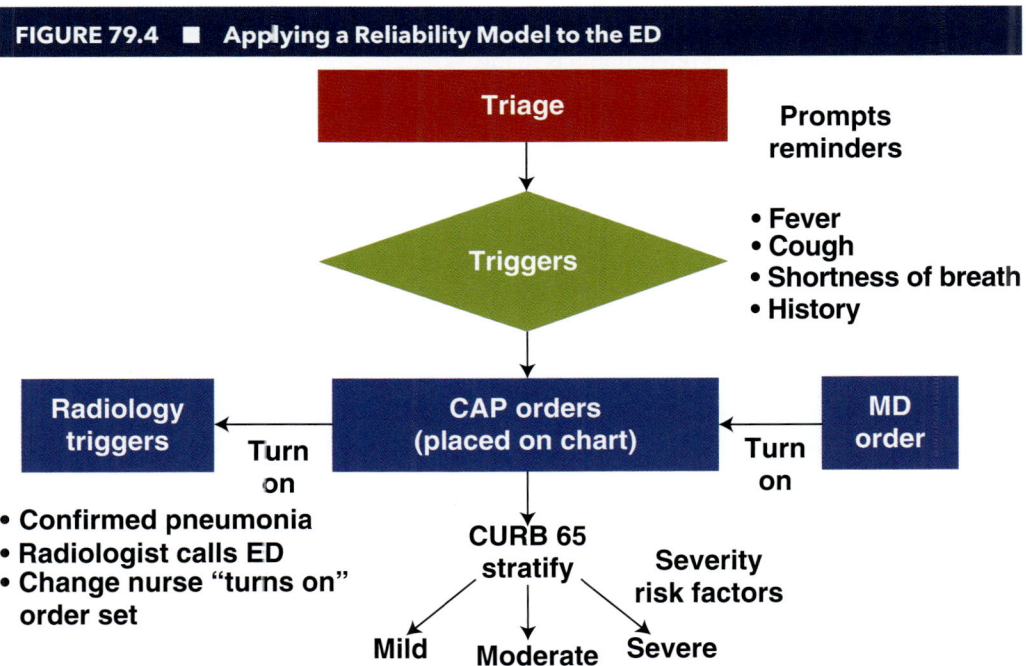

FIGURE 79.4 ■ Applying a Reliability Model to the ED

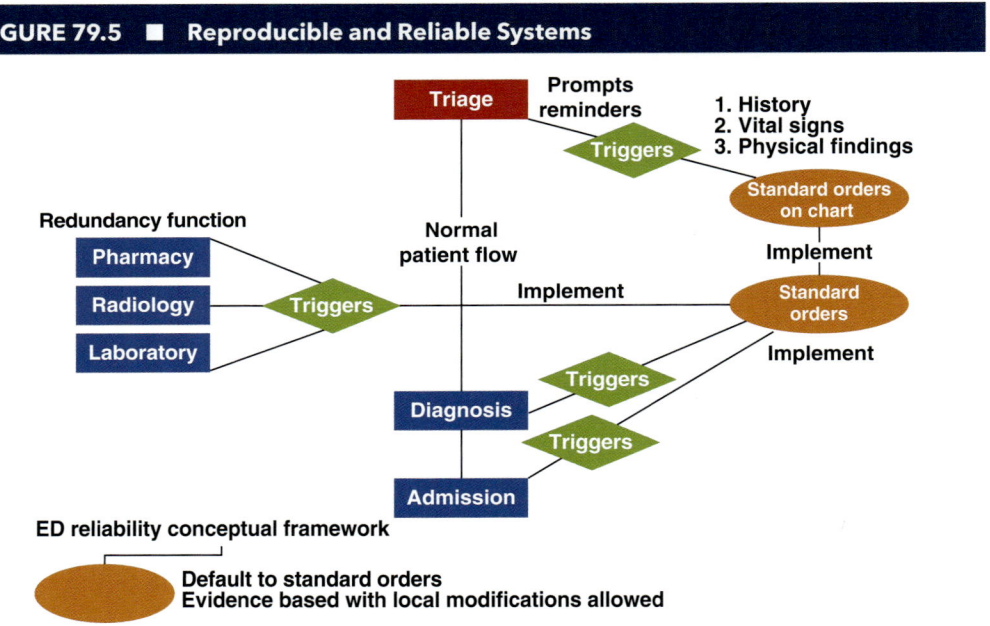

FIGURE 79.5 ■ Reproducible and Reliable Systems

could have been "blame, shame, and train"—penalties, reminders, or perhaps educational seminars. Instead, the machines were redesigned to eject the card before money is dispensed (a high-reliability approach—engaging an appropriate forcing function). Newer ATMs simply allow swiping the card, so there is no possibility for the card to be retained in the machine. These process redesigns have built safety and reliability into the ATM system. These same principles can be applied to any system, including medicine (**Figure 79.4**).

To illustrate, this concept can be applied to the management of community-acquired pneumonia. Rather than applying the standard triage model, consider the advantages of using "triggers" for certain helpful or critical actions. For instance, flag patients for a chest x-ray if they are older than 50 years and present with a productive cough, high temperature, or symptoms suggestive of pneumonia.

Let's say the diagnosis of pneumonia is made, What if:

- The pharmacy, after receiving a request for antibiotics, automatically sent a message back to the ED asking, "Is this patient on the pneumonia pathway?"
- Radiology, when pneumonia is noticed on the chest x-ray or CT, triggered a cue in their system that flagged the ED and asked, "Is this patient being treated for pneumonia?"

Mandating actions like this can mitigate risk occurrences by fostering a reproducible and reliable system (**Figure 79.5**) to avoid errors or failures.

CREATE AND SUSTAIN A SAFE ED

How does an ED undertake and sustain safe and effective health care in a climate of constant change? Addressing safety concerns already identified by reputable sources (e.g., American College of Emergency Physicians, Emergency Nurses Association, National Academy of Medicine, Agency for Healthcare Research and Quality, Institute for Healthcare Improvement, and National Patient Safety Foundation) provides a quick and easy start. Recognize that errors occurring in different departments or other hospitals also have the potential to occur in the ED; much can be learned from the experience of others. Leaders should query staff about concerns and barriers to safety while allowing these staff members to recommend solutions for

> **BOX 79.4 ■ FAMILY-FOCUSED TASKS**
>
> - Compile and maintain an accurate list of medicines and known allergies.
> - Wear a medical bracelet. Some medical alert devices come with USB port capabilities which may be useful for those with complicated medical histories.
> - Provide copies of power of attorney and do-not-resuscitate (DNR) forms.
> - Maintain a ready-to-go emergency bag with appropriately sized equipment (e.g., tracheostomy tubes) and an updated standardized medical information form. The American Academy of Pediatrics and American College of Physicians have developed an emergency information form for children with special needs.
> - Provide copies of various indwelling devices with the manufacturer's contact numbers.

problems identified. Explore opportunities to improve in the ED by conducting retrospective chart audits or hands-on simulations using high-risk scenarios (e.g., resuscitation).

Engaging patients and families as advocates is another avenue to elicit safety suggestions and build reliability. Encourage families to participate in safe behaviors at the bedside (e.g., fall precautions) or even across the health-care continuum. A family-centered approach is an underutilized tactic for engaging families in actions that support patient safety and eliminate harm. Specific steps for families to take when promoting patient safety are largely dependent on the patient's overall status (e.g., age, development, decisional capacity, dependence on technology, language barriers, special health-care needs). Family-focused tasks may include some of the activities listed in **Box 79.4**.

The National Academy of Medicine's Keeping Patients Safe program offers an abundance of advice for rectifying safety problems that can be useful in a busy ED:[6]

- Interruptions should be limited so that staff can focus on direct hands-on activities (e.g., assessment, medication administration, and bedside procedures).
- Nurses should spend more time on direct clinical activities and less time on indirect clinical activities (e.g., finding supplies, redundant charting, and specimen transports).
- Current staffing practices should be continually evaluated by departmental leadership to assess current workflow processes and to facilitate ample direct hands-on patient care.

Design a Safe Environment

When designing the work environment, ED leadership should solicit the involvement of physicians and nurses in order to help identify opportunities for reducing errors. Many solutions recommended by the IOM and others can offer a big impact, and several are as simple as assigning accessible locations for hand soaps and foams, which can assist in decreasing nosocomial infections.[6] With numerous handoffs occurring in an ED, it is important to determine the most essential and concise amount of information that should be relayed. Knowing which steps to reduce or eliminate in order to avoid unnecessary or redundant documentation potentially increases the amount of direct nursing care at the bedside.

Create a Climate of Trust

Creating a climate of trust with appropriate timing of feedback is essential to foster a prosperous culture of safety work. If patient harm is imminent, immediate intervention and feedback is required to prevent it. If patient harm is *not* imminent, a more thoughtful (nonimmediate) approach will engender trust, particularly if staff can voice their concerns without fear of blame. Explicit mechanisms for staff to report safety issues should be available and include an option for anonymity. Embedding a culture of safety into daily health-care practices can illustrate and reinforce behaviors that prevent patient harm.

Determine Root Causes

Safety strategies should be embraced in order to understand what the root causes of a problem are, how they affect a health-care institution, and how to hardwire reasonable fail-safe solutions. All safety strategies are not created equal; what works in one institution may not in another. Despite the many variables that influence EDs, the provision of safe care remains a basic and universal expectation.

CONCLUSION

To achieve safe and effective emergency care, it is essential to establish a multidisciplinary health-care team that is committed to safety and quality. Collaborating with other departments may leverage a powerful partnership for promoting patient safety. Working with other facilities to share the tools of evidence-based practice, including patient safety assessments, training, equipment, and supplies, may be a cost-effective strategy when contemplating an ED's capabilities to improve care. Most importantly, current emergency care practices must be constantly reviewed with an eye on safety, effectiveness, and reliability to ensure the desired outcomes for both our patients and our health-care teams.

Pitfalls to avoid:

- Failing to understand that an efficient ED is a major driver of risk reduction
- Being timid in human resources strategies and team building
- Failing to develop a robust performance review process
- Failing to appreciate that effective risk reduction takes time and sustained effort; there is plenty of opportunity, but there is no silver bullet.

REFERENCES

1. Batalden P. Like Magic (Every system is perfectly…). Institute for Healthcare Improvement. Available at: http://www.ihi.org/communities/blogs/origin-of-every-system-is-perfectly-designed-quote. Accessed September 14, 2020.
2. Kohn LT, Corrigan JM, Donaldson MS, eds. *To Err Is Human: Building a Safer Health System*. Washington, DC: National Academy Press; 1999.
3. Mayer TA, Maslach C. Burnout in emergency departments: diagnosis, prevention, and treatment. In Strauss RJ, Mayer TA, eds. *Strauss and Mayer's Emergency Department Management*. 2nd ed. Dallas, Tex: American College of Emergency Physicians; 2019.
4. Weick KE, Sutcliffe KM. *Managing the Unexpected: Assuring High Performance in an Age of Complexity*. San Francisco, Calif: Jossey-Bass; 2001.
5. Reason J. Human error: models and management. *BMJ*. 2000:320(7237);768-770.
6. Page A, ed. *Keeping Patients Safe: Transforming the Work Environment of Nurses*. Washington, DC: National Academies Press; 2003.
7. Mayer TA, Cates RJ. *Leadership for Great Customer Service: Satisfied Employees, Satisfied Patients*. 2nd ed. Chicago, Ill: Health Administration Press; 2014.
8. Mayer TA, Beyond Patient Experience. Paper presented at: the ACEP Emergency Department Directors Academy; November 10, 2018; Dallas, Tex.
9. Darling M, Perry C, Moore J. Learning in the thick of it. *Harv Bus Rev*. 2005;83(7):84-92.
10. Reason J. *Managing the Risks of Organizational Accidents*. Burlington, Vt: Ashgate; 1997.
11. Nance JJ. *Why Hospitals Should Fly: The Ultimate Flight Plan to Patient Safety and Quality Care*. Bozeman, Mont: Second River Healthcare Press; 2008.
12. Haig KM, Sutton S, Whittington J. SBAR: a shared mental model for improving communication between clinicians. *Jt Comm J Qual Patient Saf*. 2006;32(3):167-175.
13. BestPractices. *Process Flow Map for Vaginal Bleeding in Pregnant Patients*. Fairfax, Va: BestPractices; 2012.

ADDITIONAL READINGS

- ACEP. Croskerry P, Cosby KS, Schenkel SM, Wears RL, eds. *Patient Safety in Emergency Medicine*. 2008.[AQ7: Please insert publisher name and location for "ACEP. P. Croskerry, K. S. Cosby, S. M. Schenkel, R. L. Wears, eds…"]

- ACEP Patient Safety Task Force. *Patient Safety in the Emergency Department*. Dallas, Tex: American College of Emergency Physicians; 2001.

- American Academy of Pediatrics. Emergency Information Form for Children with Special Needs. www2.aap.org/advocacy/eif.doc. Accessed July 9, 2013.

- Bogner M. *Human Error in Medicine*. Hillsdale, NJ: Lawrence Erlbaum Associates; 1994.

- Bosk C. *Forgive and Remember: Managing Medical Failure*. Chicago, Ill: University of Chicago Press; 1984.

- Brennan TA, Leape LL, Laird NM. Incidence of adverse events and negligence in hospitalized patients. *N Engl J Med*. 1991; 324:370-376.

- Cheung DS, Kelly JJ, et al. Improving handoffs in the emergency department. *Ann Emerg Med*. 2010;55(2):171-80. 10.1016/j.annemergmed.2009.07.016.

- Croskerry P. Critical thinking and decision making: avoiding the perils of thin-slicing. *Ann Emerg Med*. 2006;48:720-722.

- Dynamics outcomes management: a short history of CRM. Collierville, Tenn; 2003. http://www.saferpatients.com.

- Helmreich R. On error management: lessons from aviation. *BMJ*. 2000; 320:781-785.

- Kachalia A, Gandhi Tk, Puopolo AL, et al. Missed and delayed diagnoses in the emergency department: a study of closed malpractice claims from 4 liability insurers. *Ann Emerg Med*. 2007; 49:196-205.

- Kohn LT, Corrigan JM, Donaldson MS, eds. *To Err Is Human: Building a Safer Health System*. Washington, DC: National Academy Press; 1999.

- Leape LL. Error in medicine. *JAMA*. 1994;272:1851-1857.

- Morey JC, Simon R, Jay GD, et al. Error reduction and performance improvement in the emergency department through formal teamwork training: evaluation results of the MedTeams project. *Health Serv Res*. 2002;37(6):1553-1581.

- Perry S. Transitions in care: studying safety in emergency department signovers. *Focus Patient Safety*. 2004;7:1-3.

- Risser DT, Rice MM, Salisbury MM, et al. The potential for improved teamwork to reduce errors in the emergency department. *Ann Emerg Med*. 1999;34(3):373-383.

- Sexton JB, Thomas EJ, Helmreich RL. Error, stress, and teamwork in medicine and aviation: cross sectional surveys. *BMJ*. 2000; 20:745-749.

- Spear SJ. Fixing healthcare from the inside, today. *Harv Bus Rev*. 2005;83:78-91.

- Spear SJ, Schmidhofer M. Ambiguity and workarounds as contributors to medical error. *Ann Intern Med*. 2005;142(8) 627-630.

- Uhlig P, Haan CK, Nason AK, et al. Improving patient care by the application of theory and practice from the aviation safety community. Presented at: 11th annual Ohio State Symposium Aviation Psychology; Columbus, Ohio; March 6, 2001.

- Virshup BB, Oppenberg AA, Coleman MM. Strategic risk management: reducing malpractice claims through more effective patient-doctor communication. *Am J Med Qual*. 1999;14(4):153-159.

- Wears R, Leape L. Human error in emergency medicine. *Ann Emerg Med*. 1999;34:370-372.

PROMOTING RATIONAL THINKING: AN ETHICAL IMPERATIVE

CHAPTER 80

Thom A. Mayer, Pat Croskerry

Teaching critical thinking to emergency physicians, emergency nurses, and the entire emergency department (ED) team will improve diagnostic reasoning, which, in turn, improves patient safety. The outcomes of effective clinical decision-making are correct diagnoses and appropriate treatment plans. If the first is correct, the second has a significantly greater chance of being correct as well.[1]

Improved critical thinking must be a priority, as early estimates imply that 40,000 to 80,000 patients die each year from preventable diagnostic failures, defined as an incorrect or delayed diagnosis.[2] Given that the annual death rate from all medical errors is now estimated to be about 250,000, the early figures undoubtedly underestimated the magnitude of the problem.[3] While diagnostic error is associated with significant morbidity and mortality (including out-of-hospital care), the precise rate is not known. As the tools of patient safety continue to expand, more precise data on morbidity and mortality associated with medical mistakes will become available.

DEFINING DIAGNOSTIC ERROR

Misdiagnoses occur for two reasons: system failures and individual failures. Generally, individual failures account for 75% of diagnostic errors, while system failures account for about 25%.[4] This chapter primarily focuses on ameliorating individual errors. Three broad categories define what causes clinicians to make diagnostic errors:

- *Cognitive laziness*: They don't try hard enough.
- *Knowledge deficits*: They don't know enough.
- *Cognitive errors*: They don't think correctly.

While cognitive laziness and knowledge deficits clearly occur, most diagnostic errors result from the third category, incorrect thinking. Rare, esoteric diagnoses are sometimes missed; however, very common illnesses are frequently misdiagnosed. For example, the presenting signs and symptoms as well as the pathophysiology of pulmonary embolism (PE) are well known by most clinicians. Yet because those signs and symptoms are highly variable and are similar to those of numerous other diseases, this critical presentation was misdiagnosed a surprising 55% of the time in a series of fatal cases.[5]

> **BOX 80.1 ■ COGNITIVE FACTORS IN DIAGNOSTIC FAILURE**
>
> - Knowledge deficits
> - Reasoning
> - Problem-solving
> - Logical competence
> - Vulnerability to bias

A 35-year study of autopsies of nearly 6,000 intensive care unit (ICU) patients published in the *British Medical Journal* supports this concept. At least 28% of patients had at least one misdiagnosis, 8% of which caused or significantly contributed to death, with the following four diagnoses accounting for 75% of the diagnostic errors[6]:

- PE
- Myocardial infarction (MI)
- Pneumonia
- Aspergillosis

Given that these diagnoses are relatively common, the findings lend support to the notion that clinician thinking is a primary cause of diagnostic errors, many of which result in preventable deaths. Winters and his colleagues estimated from this study that "as many as 40,500 adult patients in an ICU in the United States may die with an ICU misdiagnosis annually." Research from Harvard and the Netherlands also supports the view that diagnostic errors are not due to esoteric diagnoses but rather occur most frequently with common diagnoses such as MI, PE, sepsis, and appendicitis.[7,8] In addition, these studies bear out the rate of system errors at 25% versus individual diagnostic errors at 75%.

The cognitive factors that appear to be most responsible for diagnostic failures include knowledge deficits, a failure to reason effectively, imperfect problem-solving, logical incompetence, and vulnerability to bias (**Box 80.1**).[9] The two main factors most critical to patient safety are the clinician's ability to make a correct, timely diagnosis and provide the right treatment, with the former driving the ability to deliver the latter.[1]

Diagnostic acumen . . . is every doctor's measure of his own abilities: it is the most important ingredient in his professional self-image.

—Nuland, 1994[10]

Despite this wisdom, it is surprising how long it has taken for diagnostic error and the role of clinician thinking to be emphasized in the conversation about patient safety and high reliability. Succinctly stated, 75% of the time it is not what the clinician doesn't know (a knowledge deficit) but rather the incorrect thinking of the clinician (cognitive error) that must be improved.

CURRENT ESTIMATES OF DIAGNOSTIC ERROR

Applying the science of patient safety to various specialties leads to diagnostic error rates as low as 2% to 3% in specialties like general radiology, anatomic pathology, and dermatology; however, the rates in emergency medicine are similar to those in internal and family medicine (approximately 15%).[1,11-13] While a 15% diagnostic error rate clearly calls for improvement, it is perhaps unsurprising, given the fact that ED clinicians rarely know their patients and, therefore, have no context in which to place the patients' current complaints. Famed psychologist James Reason cites Shakespeare's *Henry V*, "We are but warriors for the working day," and then states:

> *Emergency physicians and nurses stand on the front line between the hospital (the rear echelons) and the hostile world of injury, infections, acute illness. The nature and extent of these enemies are not really known until the moment of the encounter. And the encounter itself is brief, singular, hugely critical, largely unplanned and full of surprises and uncertainties. These skirmishes offer an almost unlimited number of opportunities for going wrong.*[14]

These lines accurately reflect the challenges faced in EDs each day. Nonetheless, leaders must be resolute in their efforts to reduce medical mistakes.

DEFINING CRITICAL THINKING

Critical thinking is the ability to be in control of one's thoughts while in the process of reflection. It includes the ability to consciously examine the elements of one's reasoning, or that of another, and evaluate that reasoning against universal intellectual standards, including:

- Clarity
- Accuracy
- Precision
- Relevance
- Depth
- Breadth
- Logic

A structured examination of information is an important part of critical thinking, as is the ability to consider the applicability and reliability of that information in a clinical setting. Finally, critical thinking integrates the intellectual traits of humility, autonomy, integrity, courage, perseverance, confidence, empathy, and fair-mindedness (**Figure 80.1**).[15]

Critical Thinking Guidelines

Several elements of critical thinking guidelines deserve emphasis. In the ED, critical thinkers should define the purpose of their inquiry. In other words:

- Choose significant and realistic purposes.
- State the purpose clearly.
- Distinguish the purpose from related (less significant) purposes.
- Periodically check that the purpose is still valid.

The *question or problem must be stated with precision* and reformulated in several ways to clarify its meaning and scope. Identify if the question being asked has one right answer, is a matter of opinion, or requires reasoning from more than one point of view. *Assumptions* must be identified and determined to be justifiable. Consider how the assumptions are changing and shaping the point of view, while checking for bias at each step. Much of the functioning of the human brain is subject to numerous biases, which influence decision-making and behavior.

As an example, a "frequent flyer" alcoholic patient is brought into the ED on a routine Saturday night. The emergency physician performs a brief assessment and recognizes the patient's typical presentation, including slurred speech, alcohol on breath, confusion, and agitation. Blood is drawn, and the patient is placed in a room to "sober up." Two hours

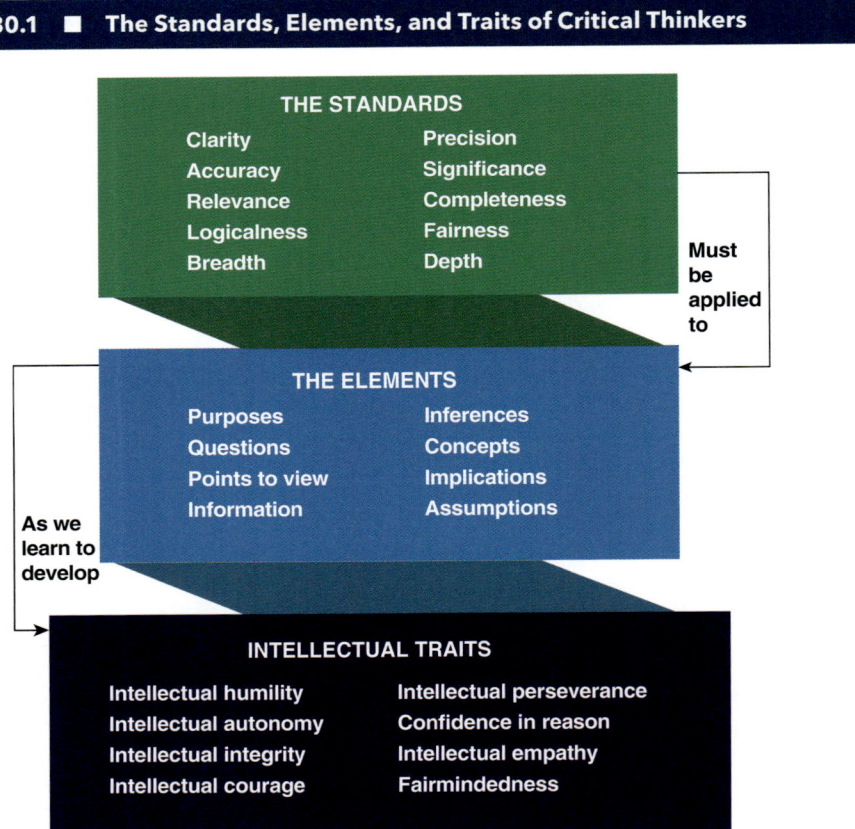

FIGURE 80.1 ■ The Standards, Elements, and Traits of Critical Thinkers

later, when the physician has caught up, he reviews the laboratory tests, and notes that the patient's alcohol level is actually quite low. The patient is reevaluated and responds only to painful stimuli with decorticate posturing. A computed tomography of the head shows a subdural hematoma.

Since critical thinking requires reflection, the *practitioner's point of view* should be clearly identified. The strengths and weaknesses of other ideas should be considered; it is important to keep an open mind when evaluating all reasonable perspectives, while simultaneously checking for biased reasoning. All assertions should be restricted to factual *data, information,* and *evidence* that support the conclusions. Critical thinkers search for evidence that both supports and opposes their positions. In addition, they ensure that all information is clear, accurate, unbiased, and relevant to the question at hand. In short:

- Concepts and ideas should be identified, explained, and used with care and precision.
- Alternative concepts, inferences, and conclusions should go as far as the evidence supports them.
- Inferences should be checked for consistency, identifying assumptions that lead to these inferences and determining if they are evidence based.
- Finally, the implications and consequences must follow from the reasoning. The critical thinker searches for negative as well as positive implications, achieving a balanced position that includes both the pros and the cons. All possible consequences should be considered, especially those related to a "confirmation bias"—the tendency to accept information that supports the conclusion and to ignore or rationalize information that does not.

The Stages of Critical Thinking

The Foundation for Critical Thinking defines six stages of critical thinking development (**Box 80.2**) that are relevant to medical and nursing staff.[16]

Several points deserve emphasis:

- None of these six stages of critical thinking development represent innate skills or abilities. Instead, these are stages for which the skills can be learned.
- Moving through the stages does not necessarily occur at an even pace; with effective training, thinkers can advance rapidly once the early skills are mastered.
- Most medical people reside in stage 3 (beginning thinker), as there has been little emphasis placed on critical thinking in their medical training.

While nursing schools are better than medical schools at training students in this area, the limited knowledge of critical thinking skills among health-care personnel in general suggests that few are reaching their potential to become "practicing," "advanced," or "accomplished" thinkers. Greater emphasis should be placed on this set of skills during training, since given the right education and a commitment from leadership, most can advance.

Accomplished Critical Thinkers

Enhanced critical thinking decreases errors and produces more consistent and appropriate care. Stage 6 (accomplished) thinkers understand the standards of clarity, accuracy, and relevance. They also have the capacity to actively reflect on their own thinking processes. This is known as *metacognition*—the ability to detach oneself from what is immediately occurring and evaluate how one is thinking. A component of metacognition is the ability to recognize distracting stimuli, propaganda, and irrelevant items and set them aside. Another fundamental skill of an accomplished critical thinker is intellectual humility, including the:

- Ability to identify their own cognitive and affective biases
- Discipline to identify, analyze, and challenge assumptions
- Capability of assessing the credibility of information
- Ability to define alternatives
- Capacity to work through problems in an organized fashion to make effective decisions
- Awareness of the value of practice and training in critical thinking skills throughout their professional and personal life

---

BOX 80.2 ■ THE STAGES OF CRITICAL THINKING

- **Stage 1:** The unreflective thinker
- **Stage 2:** The challenged thinker
- **Stage 3:** The beginning thinker
- **Stage 4:** The practicing thinker
- **Stage 5:** The advanced thinker
- **Stage 6:** The accomplished thinker

The attributes of enhancing critical thinking skills, ideally to the stage 6 level, are essential to improving patient safety in EDs and health care *writ large*. Unfortunately, the literature demonstrates that too few medical schools, residencies, and health-care systems encourage or provide critical thinking training.[17-19] In 1998, Scott noted:

> *The development of critical thinking—the ability to solve problems by assessing evidence using valid inferences, abstractions, and generalizations—is one of the global goals advanced by most medical schools.*[18]

Progress in this area has been slow. Therefore, reducing diagnostic errors and improving patient safety will require health-care leaders and managers, specifically in the ED, to develop and implement critical thinking training.

DUAL-PROCESS THEORY

In 2011, Daniel Kahneman, a Nobel Prize-winning psychologist from Princeton, wrote a best-selling book, *Thinking Fast and Slow,* which describes the dual-process system of human thinking.[20] This theory proposes that human decision-making is divided into two basic patterns: system 1 (intuitive thinking) and system 2 (rational or analytical thinking) (**Figure 80.2**). The dual-process system is consistent with the two known neural processes involving separate cortical mechanisms, each with associated neuroanatomical and neurophysiologic substrates. Functional magnetic resonance imaging scans display changes in neuronal activity as processes move (or "toggle") between the two systems.[21]

System 1–Intuitive Thinking

System 1, or intuitive, thinking is extremely fast, occurring in hundredths of seconds. Most humans use this thinking process 95% or more of the time. It is also largely autonomous, meaning that the brain "automatically" utilizes this process (leading to decisions) without involving the higher cognitive centers of the cerebral cortex. System 1 thinking is context dependent and qualitative in nature (less objective/data driven), making it more error

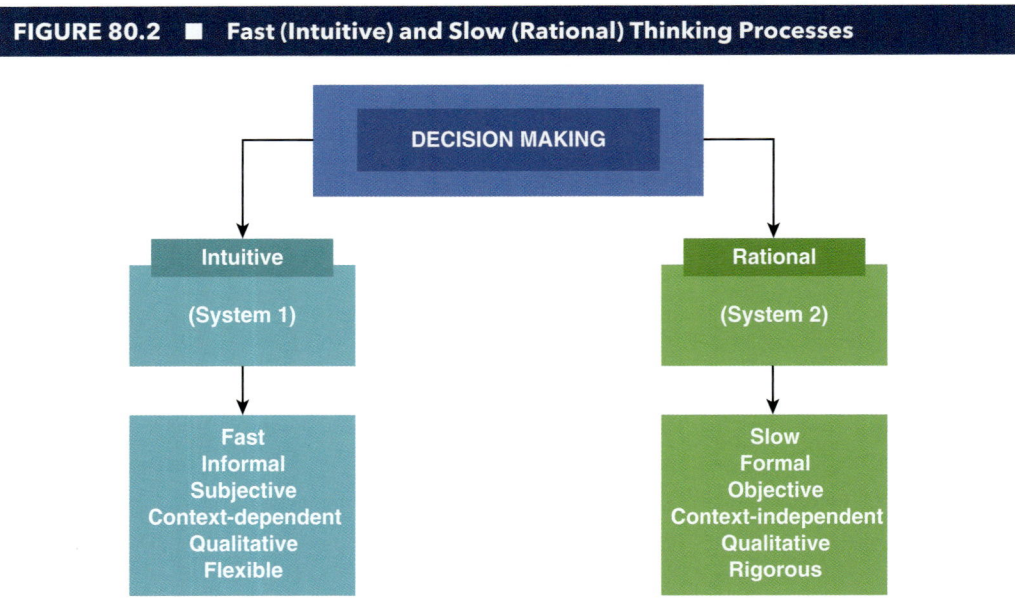

FIGURE 80.2 ■ Fast (Intuitive) and Slow (Rational) Thinking Processes

prone. Although there is a tendency to characterize system 1 thinking as more primitive and simplistic, it is often entirely appropriate and highly effective.

For example, asystole on a cardiac monitor in an unconscious patient prompts an immediate reaction from the emergency physician and nurse. No time is lost deciding what the etiology might be. A quick, definitive, and decisive intervention based on evidence-based approaches must be made to reestablish circulation. However, asystole on the cardiac monitor in a patient who is awake and conversing drives the team to conclude that one or more cardiac leads are off the patient. Both are examples of how intuitive or system 1 thinking is used.

System 2–Rational Thinking

System 2, or rational, thinking is a reflective, deliberate, thoughtful process that is objective, has scientific reference points and, if done correctly, results in very few errors. It is what comes to mind when a "thinker" is pictured—one who can detach himself or herself from the immediate pull of the situation and through careful, reasoned, and logical thought, arrive at a well-calibrated decision. The downsides of rational thinking are:

- More extensive and costly use of resources
- Longer decision-making process
- More extensive evaluations take more time, often an undesirable option in the ED

The average clinician spends most of his or her time in the intuitive mode, with relatively little time in the rational mode, usually 5% or less. Early in the course of training, physicians and nurses spend more time in system 2. But as their knowledge and experiential base increases, and pattern recognition develops, they move to more system 1 thinking. Repeated presentations of a particular illness or injury processed in system 2 can eventually result in its being relegated to system 1.[13] The risk of bias (e.g., confirmation bias—interpreting new evidence as confirming existing assumptions) and subsequent error are much greater when clinicians unconsciously rely on intuitive thinking.

For example, when patients present with the rash of herpes zoster, clinicians who see the rash for the first few times approach the patient in system 2, analytically describing it as a collection of oval or round intensely painful vesicles superimposed on patchy redness in a dermatomal distribution. After seeing this pattern several times, the recognition and diagnosis is virtually automatic and is processed intuitively in system 1.

This process applies to many diagnoses, particularly those with pathognomonic features, such as Colles fractures, anterior shoulder dislocations, renal colic, and even highly acute diagnoses such as tension pneumothorax or hypovolemic shock. Under certain circumstances, it can be highly efficient to relegate a problem previously processed in system 2 to an unconscious system 1 process. With the unavoidable challenges and pressures inherent in all ED practices, it can be difficult to balance the speed of system 1 thinking with the time required to perform a more reflective analysis, even when system 2 thinking might help avoid potential misdiagnoses and errors.[22]

Dual-Process Theory in Diagnosis

Figure 80.3 presents a universal model of reasoning that may be used when making a clinical diagnosis. When evaluating a patient, the clinician's brain uses a pattern recognition process common to all animal brains, which will either discern the pattern or not. If the pattern is distinctly familiar, the thought process becomes intuitive. This occurs extremely fast, leading the clinician to a diagnosis quickly, possibly without reflection.

FIGURE 80.3 ■ A Universal Model of Reasoning

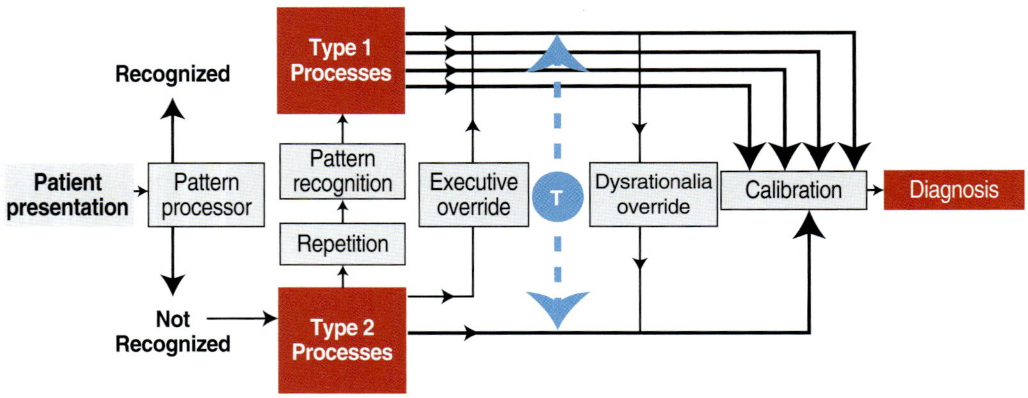

If the pattern is not recognized, the brain enters into rational thinking patterns: a slower, more deliberate process. The clinician takes additional time to provide a much more reflective and balanced response. After repeated exposures, the brain eventually begins to recognize the pattern, making it more likely that the clinician will use system 1 when assessing similar presentations in the future.

The first-time driver finds himself surrounded by levers, buttons, switches, wheels, and other features with which he is unfamiliar. Learning to drive requires substantial rational effort with the well-known tendency in the novice driver to overcorrect. Over time, through repetition, the driver develops psychomotor and haptic (sense of touch) skills and eventually can drive a car in system 1. In fact, it is not uncommon for an experienced driver to have no conscious memory of a particular drive at all; the process becomes automatic once the driver moves from system 2 to system 1 thinking.

A patient is brought in from triage in a wheelchair with a vomit basin, looking ill and gray, writhing in pain, and holding his flank. The triage nurse is holding a urine sample and says it is positive for blood. The clinician's brain is presented with this pattern of flank pain, nausea, vomiting, hematuria, and an inability to find a position of comfort, leading to an immediate diagnosis of renal colic. This decision is made within milliseconds to seconds in system 1. Without reflection and consideration (system 2), other possible diagnoses and associated treatments might be missed or at least delayed.

An autonomous (immediate and intuitive) process made in system 1 can be superseded, a process known as *executive override*.[23] This is accomplished through intentional reflection, which slows and monitors the intuitive system. The "T" in **Figure 80.3** represents a toggle function. In other words, clinicians can move back and forth between the intuitive and the analytical systems.

In the aforementioned example, if the patient with presumed renal colic is found to be hypotensive with diminished femoral pulses and a history of cardiovascular disease, the clinician's executive override should switch to system 2, and considerations of other diagnoses, such as abdominal aortic aneurysm, will be considered.

In the example of the rash of herpes zoster, a master learner exhibiting a high level of critical thinking (i.e., stage 6) should be able to toggle back and forth based on the results of thoughtful inquiry. For example, the rash was noted to be in a cervical dermatome (an unusual distribution for zoster), and on closer examination, the rash clearly crosses the midline. While system 1 indicates the probability of herpes zoster, these unusual features should cause the thinker to pause and revert to system 2. In this case, a more detailed history might reveal that the patient is an arborist with an affinity for oak trees; as such, a more analytical approach would lead to the correct diagnosis: a poison oak rash.

A related irrational thinking process is known as *dysrationalia override*, in which rapid intuitive thinking is followed without question despite the realization that a better approach requires slow system 2 thinking.[24] The tendency to ignore information that is counter to one's initial impression is dysrationalia override: system 1 intuition overrides system 2 analytical thinking. Road rage is an example of irrational override, but so is immediately making judgmental assumptions regarding the intent of patients with chronic pain. In addition, having an angry, visceral reaction to a patient with a borderline personality disorder is an example of dysrationalia override that might well lead to inappropriate treatment. Similarly, making an immediate assumption that a patient's chest pain does not have a cardiac etiology can be driven by dysrationalia override based on immediate gestalt assumptions, particularly in female patients.

In all of these cases, the rational approach entails avoiding the tendency to react quickly; rather, the clinician should build in a moment of reflection (system 2) to circumvent dysrationalia override. Thus, inserting higher thinking (stages 4-6) or calibration should occur to prevent an intuitive response from interfering with a correct diagnosis and treatment.

The Development of Expertise

Figure 80.4 illustrates what is currently known about the percentage of time a person spends in system 1 (intuitive) versus system 2 (rational) thinking, as well as the role of "rule-based" reasoning (e.g., evidence-based clinical guidelines). As seen on the right side of the figure, novices spend about 75% of their time in system 2 and about 5% in system 1. The remainder of time is spent in the rule-based area, where clinical decision rules are essentially developed and implemented in system 2.

Do critical thinkers make better decisions? And can these skills be taught? The answer to both questions is a definitive "yes." A major meta-analysis by the United Kingdom Thinking Schools Review Group (TSRG) evaluated more than 6,000 papers and sources focused on thinking interventions in children between the ages of 5 and 16 years.[25] The results revealed that interventions designed to improve critical thinking had a significant positive impact. In addition, the effect of thinking interventions exceeded those of all

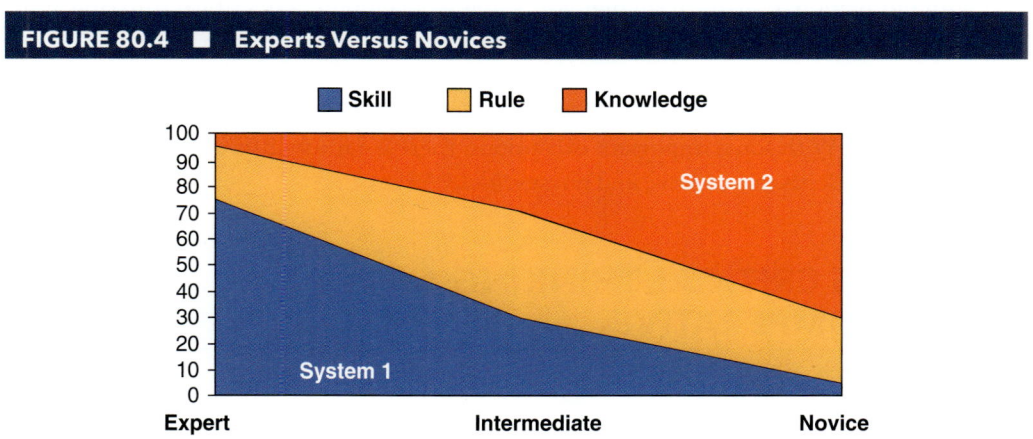

FIGURE 80.4 ■ Experts Versus Novices

other interventions. The effect on improving performance on tests of cognitive measures such as Raven's matrices was 0.62, which is staggering. This is the equivalent of having a class that began at the 50th percentile move up 26 percentile points to the 76th percentile as a result of applying these interventions. This analysis provides convincing evidence that thinking interventions can be taught and lead to dramatic performance improvement.

Teaching Critical Thinking to Medical Students, Residents, Physicians, and Nurses

The TSRG study and others that have reached similar conclusions clearly indicate that teaching thinking skills improves performance in the age-group tested, up to and including the age of 17. Since these studies address young learners, several questions arise:

- Has the opportunity to teach and learn critical thinking skills been lost by the time students get to medical or nursing school?
- Have older thinkers lost brain plasticity?
- Is the critical period for acquiring these thinking skills (using similar interventions) absent in mature students?
- Is it possible that these studies simply show some corrective effect of pulling outliers in, which increases the average?

The data do not support any of these hypotheses; in fact, research shows the opposite.[26,27] There are four major categories of brain function: *memory, reasoning, spatial visualization*, and *speed*. Early studies show that people experience a general decline in all of these areas from the time they are in their early 20s until they reach their late 50s.[28,29] However, more recent data show a clear flattening of the lines of decline, if indeed there is one at all. The question then becomes: *How dramatically does aging affect critical thinking? And what interventions work to improve critical thinking in mature learners?* There is good evidence that adults can improve their thinking and educational skills throughout their lives. Several international studies demonstrate that specific interventions can enhance these skills, even when brief. Psychology students showed a 15% gain in critical thinking after only 10 hours of generic critical thinking training, and a Korean study using comparable 10-hour sessions revealed similar improvements.

Without specific training in critical thinking, however, progress is slow, even in fields that depend on this vital skill. One study of medical students over a 4-year period showed a yield of improved critical thinking skills between 2% and 3%.[30] Despite their intelligence and high motivation, they have smaller gains in the development of critical thinking skills during medical school than those who undergo more focused training. In fact, some people have said that traditional medical school curricula actually *suppress* critical thinking, since so much emphasis is placed on the acquisition of knowledge at the expense of other cognitive skills.[1] With some important exceptions, there is far too little emphasis placed on how medical students, physicians, and nurses *think*.[13-15,23]

TEACHING CRITICAL THINKING AS A MORAL IMPERATIVE

When proposing additions to the training content (in medical schools, nursing schools, residency training programs, orientation to hospitals, and continuing medical and nursing education), it is common to hear the plaintive response: "But we already have substantial constraints on the time available we have to teach our learners. If we include critical thinking, we will have to leave something critical out—just what critical information would you have us *not* teach?" While the time limitations of professional education are well known, a diagnostic error rate approaching 15% is simply not tolerable. Patient safety and high-reliability organizations are an essential part of the fabric of health care. Stark and Finns address this in the *Cambridge Quarterly of Healthcare Ethics*:

> *While the medical ethics literature has well explored the harm to patients' families and the integrity of the profession in failing to disclose medical errors once they occur, less often addressed are the moral and professional obligations that take all available steps to prevent errors and harm in the first instance. As an expanding body of scholarship further elucidates the causes of medical error, insufficient progress in systematically evaluating and implementing suggested strategies for improving critical thinking skills and medical judgment is of mounting concern.*
>
> *Continued failure to address pervasive thinking errors in medical decision making imperils patients' safety and professionalism, as well as beneficence and non-maleficence, fairness, and justice. We maintain that self-reflective and metacognitive refinements of critical thinking should not be construed as optional, but rather be considered an integral part of medical education, a codified tenet of professionalism and by extension a moral and professional duty.*[31]

No more forceful nor succinct argument can be made for the inclusion of critical thinking, which is not only an effective strategy for reducing diagnostic errors, but also is an ethical imperative for the good of all patients and the clinicians who care for them. As T. S. Eliot notes in *The Hollow Men*:

> *Between the idea*
> *And the reality*
> *Between the motion*
> *And the act*
> *Falls the shadow.*[32]

Extrapolating from Eliot, between the *idea* of professing the importance of critical thinking in health care and the *reality* of formally addressing this knowledge deficit, "the shadow" is far too long. Ethics compels implementation of an explicit solution to narrow it.

CONCLUSION

Critical thinking is an integral part of clinical reasoning, which is marked by the ability to observe, ask questions, analyze, synthesize, evaluate, make valid conclusions, assess the strength and validity of arguments, and demonstrate skill in understanding differing perspectives. Substantial evidence shows that interventions to augment cognitive skills significantly improve problem-solving and, therefore, would be expected to improve diagnostic performance. Of the interventions, critical thinking is a discrete skill that can be taught without a major time commitment. However, these interventions must be explicit. Simply expressing support is insufficient; rather a formal, written plan with content must be implemented.

Does current medical training suppress critical thinking because of its primary emphasis on memorization and knowledge acquisition? Probably, but it's not too late to address these shortcomings in undergraduate, postgraduate, and continuing medical education. Furthermore, it is an ethical imperative to teach critical thinking because there is good evidence that the current diagnostic process fails at a 15% rate, and the tools to improve people's thinking, reasoning, problem-solving, and diagnostic abilities are readily available.

Among the medical and nursing schools that have developed substantial courses and resources for teaching critical thinking is Dalhousie University. This program includes an online course for faculty known by the acronym TACT (Teaching and Assessing Critical Thinking). In addition, the Society to Improve Diagnosis in Medicine has multiple resources available on its website: improvediagnosis.org.

In 2015, the AAMC (American Association of Medical Colleges), the organization that develops and administers the Medical College Admission Test, began to include questions that assess critical thinking abilities in prospective medical students. Some medical schools have also developed structured personal interviews to evaluate these vital skills. Medical educators and ED leaders and managers should promote processes to improve critical thinking and reasoning in order to reduce cognitive errors. The training should include a review of the major cognitive and affective biases and the manner in which they affect thinking. In addition, hospital leaders should encourage the appropriate use of intuitive system 1 and reflective system 2 thinking to enhance the clinician's reasoning process.

Socrates wrote, "The unexamined life is not worth living." To paraphrase Socrates and apply the concept to the need for critical thinking and reasoning skills among health-care professionals, the unexamined thought is not worth *thinking*.[1]

REFERENCES

1. Croskerry P. From mindless to mindful practice—cognitive bias and clinical decision making. *N Engl J Med*. 2013;368:2445-2448.

2. Leape L, Berwick D, Bates D. Counting deaths from medical errors. *JAMA*. 2002;288:2404-2405.

3. Makary M, Daniel M. Medical error—the third leading cause of death in the UC. *BMJ*. 2016;353:i2139.

4. National Academies of Science, Engineering, and Medicine. *Improving Diagnosis in Healthcare*. Washington, DC: National Academies Press; 2015.

5. Abrami PC, Bernard RM, Borokhovski E, et al. Instructional interventions affecting critical thinking skills and disposition: a stage 1 meta-analysis. *Rev Educ Res*. 2008;78:1102-1134.

6. Winters B, Custer J, Galvagno SM Jr, et al. Diagnostic errors in the intensive care unit: a systematic review of autopsy studies. *BMJ Qual Saf*. 2012;21:894-902.

7. Schiff GD, Hasan O, Kim S, et al. Diagnostic error in medicine: analysis of 583 physician-reported errors. *Arch Int Med*. 2009;169:1881-1887.

8. Zwann L, de Brujine M, Wagner C, et al. Patient record review of the incidence, consequences, and causes of diagnostic adverse events. *Arch Int Med*. 2010;170:1015-1021.

9. Graber ML, Trowbridge R, Myers JS, et al. The next organizational challenge: finding and addressing diagnostic error. *Jt Comm J Qual Patient Saf*. 2014;40:102-110.

10. Nuland SB. *How We Die: Reflections on Life's Final Chapter*. New York, NY: Alfred A. Knopf; 1994.

11. Berner ES, Graber ML. Overconfidence as a cause of diagnostic error in medicine. *Am J Med*. 2008;121(5 suppl):S2-S23.

12. Berlin L. Radiologic errors past, present, and future. *Diagnosis*. 2014;89:79-84.

13. Croskerry P. Critical thinking and reasoning in emergency medicine. In: Croskerry P, Cosby KS, Schenkel SM, et al., eds. *Patient Safety in Emergency Medicine*. Philadelphia, Pa: Wolter Kluwer; 2009:39, 219.

14. Reason J. Foreward. In: Croskerry P, Cosby KS, Schenkel SM, et al., eds. *Patient Safety in Emergency Medicine*. Philadelphia, Pa: Wolter Kluwer; 2009:xi.

15. Croskerry P. A universal model of diagnostic reasoning. *Acad Med*. 2009;84:1022-1028.

16. Paul R, Elder L. *Critical Thinking: Tools for Taking Charge of Your Personal and Professional Lives*. 2nd ed. Upper Saddle River, NJ: Pearson Publishing; 2014.

17. Sharples JM, Oxman AD, Mahtani KR, et al. Critical thinking in healthcare and education. *BMJ*. 2017;357:j2234.

18. Scott JN, Markert RJ, Dunn MM. Critical thinking: change during medical school and relationships to performance in clinical clerkships. *Med Educ*. 1998;32:14-18.

19. Croskerry P. The importance of cognitive errors in diagnosis and strategies to prevent them. *Acad Med*. 2003:78:775-780.

20. Kahneman D. *Thinking Fast and Slow*. New York, NY: Farrar, Straus, and Giroux; 2011.

21. Ivanoff J, Branning P, Marois R. fMRI evidence for a dual-process account of the speed-accuracy tradeoff in decision making. *PlosOne*, Available at: https://journals.plos.org/plosone/article?id=10.1371/journal.pone.0002635. Accessed January 31, 2019.

22. Croskerry P, Singhal G, Mamede S. Cognitive debiasing 1: origins of bias and debiasing. *BMJ Qual Saf*. 2013;22(suppl 2):ii58-ii64.

23. Stanovich KE. Dysrationalia: a new specific learning disability. *J Learn Disabil*. 1993;26:501-515.
24. Higgins S, Baumfield V, Lin M, et al. Thinking skills approaches to effective teaching and learning: what is the evidence for impact on learners. In: *Research Evidence in Education Library*. London, United Kingdom: EPPI-Centre, Social Science Research Unit, Institute of Education, University of London; 2004.
25. Twardy CR. Argument maps improve critical thinking. *Teach Philos*. 2003;27:1-19.
26. Seesholtz M, Polk B. Two professors, one valuable lesson: how to respectfully disagree. *Chronicle of Higher Education*. Available at: http://chronicle.com/article/Two-Professors-One-Valuable/48901/. Accessed October 10, 2009.
27. Salthouse TA. When does age-related cognitive decline begin? *Neurobiol Aging*. 2009;30:507-514.
28. Denney NW. Critical thinking during the adult years: has the developmental function changed over the last four decades? *Exp Aging Res*. 2007;21:191-207.
29. Maudsley G, Strivens J. Promoting professional knowledge, experiential learning, and critical thinking for medical students. *Med Educ*. 2000;34:535-544.
30. Stark M, Fins JJ. The ethical imperative to think about thinking: diagnostics, metacognition, and medical professionalism. *Camb Q Med Ethics*. 2014:23:386-396.
31. Eliot TS. The hollow men. In: *Selected Poems*. New York, NY: Faber and Faber; 1964.

CHAPTER 81

DEBIASING STRATEGIES: COGNITIVE PILLS FOR COGNITIVE ILLS

Thom A. Mayer, Robert W. Strauss, Kirk Jensen, Pat Croskerry

> *We cannot change the human condition, but we can change the conditions under which humans work.*
>
> —James Reason[1]

> *Our judgments are erroneous because we attend to variables that we should ignore and ignore variables to which we should attend.*
>
> —Jonathan Baron[2]

Decision density and clinical complexity are higher in emergency departments (EDs) than in any other environment in health care.[3] Decision-making is the most common activity emergency physicians and nurses undertake in their daily work, since decisions necessarily precede every deliberate and purposeful action taken in the ED. It is also the most important activity because it guides all actions undertaken on behalf of the patient. Almost all ED patients are previously unknown to the physician and nurse and are seen in small windows of focused time. The imperative to move patients through the ED in an expeditious manner places even more pressure on decision-makers by adding the "need for speed."

The process has been likened to the plate-spinning acts previously seen on television variety shows, where multiple plates balanced on sticks must be kept in constant motion to keep them from falling. When one plate comes off, another instantly replaces it, and the performer of necessity leaps from plate to plate, doing whatever is needed to keep everything spinning. The difference for emergency physicians and nurses is that instead of being a 5-minute "act," managing multiple patients with varying needs and acuities is a 10-hour "reality." How can this decision-density dilemma be managed?

WHY CHANGE MATTERS

In order for effective change to occur, humans generally and professionals specifically need to understand *why* change is necessary to move from one way of thinking to another. One of the most important distinctions of critical thinkers is their ability to recognize cognitive and affective bias in both themselves and others. While traditional undergraduate and medical education typically cover the characteristics and reliability of diagnostic tests (e.g., pretest probabilities, positive- and negative-predictive values), principles of evidence-based medicine (EBM), and often some elements of Bayesian analysis, these lessons are focused only on the "what" of the thinking and reasoning done in EDs. Clearly, the "what" of thinking is important because it is a *necessary* condition for a successful ED practice. But it is not a *sufficient* condition and does not reliably ensure success. (One of the major constraints of both morbidity and mortality conferences and case reviews is their inherent inability to recreate the ambient conditions, context, time of day or night, staffing situation, and so on that have an important impact on outcomes.)

"How" thinking involves the role of biases and heuristics and is an essential part of effective critical thinking in complex adaptive systems such as the ED. "What were you thinking?" focuses on the selection of diagnostic tests (and the exclusion of others), the applicability and use of evidence-based guidelines, and the patient's response to therapeutic interventions. "How were you thinking?" adds the role that bias plays in this analysis, which is too often ignored or subliminal. It adds the unique effect in which the context and way decision-making is made.

An additional factor informing the "how" of medical and nursing thinking is *heuristics*, which are "rules of thumb, maxims, and other mental shortcuts." Heuristics form a "cognitive process that simplifies decision-making operations, describing the everyday intuitive decisions that emergency physicians make without resorting to formal decision analysis."[4] Heuristics allow ED professionals to make multiple decisions and avoid "paralysis by analysis" by providing information processing rules. However, when heuristics fail, they are often called *cognitive biases*.

Heuristics are an abbreviated form of decision-making that results in a shortened route to a reasonable conclusion. Most heuristics and biases are unconscious, type 1, reflexive processes that skip the laborious process of deductive reasoning and system 2 thinking.[4] While heuristics are neither bad nor good, it is necessary to recognize heuristics at work and understand the effect they have on decision-making. Examples of heuristics include:

- Be careful in treating elderly patients who "don't quite look right."
- The younger (and older) the patient, the less "typical" the presentation of acute appendicitis.
- Determine quickly if the patient is stable, unstable, or potentially unstable.
- Assume the worst, hope for the best, and settle often for something in between.

Recognizing Bias

Definitions should not simply provide a clear taxonomy and understanding of terms; they should also contain pathways toward solutions.[5] The origin of bias comes from a desire to use past experience to predict future behavior. However, the term *bias* unavoidably carries negative connotations and results in attributions of judgment, neither of which are helpful for improving patient care, outcomes, and professional fulfillment for those involved in that care. For example, *bias* is often associated with highly charged terms like "racial bias," "gender bias," or "age bias," which suggest some unjustified and unfair predilection resulting in patients being treated unfairly.

Nonetheless, for advanced critical thinkers and cognitive psychologists, whose role it is to study how thinking occurs, *bias has no intrinsic moral value*, and as such, no stigma should be attached to it. For example, consider these definitions of *cognitive bias,* all of which carry negative connotations:

- "Flaws or distortions in judgment and decision-making"[6]
- "Predictable deviations from rationality"[7]
- "Mental contamination"[8]

For these and many other reasons, *disposition to respond* is a far more appropriate way to describe bias, both because it destigmatizes the term and results in less resistance when attempting to identify, examine, and improve those very dispositions.[9] Dispositions to respond are factors leading health care professionals to respond to specific situations in predictable ways, which may be positive or negative. A cognitive disposition to respond (CDR) is a predictable, understandable, and analyzable deviation from purely objective rationality. Consider the following example:

> A 56-year-old woman presents with vague symptoms, including indigestion, bloating, anxiety, and a sense of fullness in the epigastric area. She denies chest pain, pain on exertion, shortness of breath, and a cardiac history. Her initial electrocardiogram is normal.

The emergency physician may think, "This can't be an acute coronary syndrome (ACS) because she doesn't have any of the 'classic' symptoms. She looks great and just seems anxious." This thinking is a form of *anchoring bias* in that the physician has anchored early to the belief that this is not ACS. It is a CDR that is dangerous and ignores evidence (as well as practical experience) that women with cardiac disease often present with a much different clinical picture than men.

However, an experienced clinician does precisely the opposite and uses a heuristic (rule of thumb or shortcut) that women with vague symptoms should be evaluated for cardiac disease. Other positive effects of heuristics and bias include what the US Marine Corps refers to as "a bias toward action," which is an innate cultural tendency toward action versus inaction. For ED professionals, this is a positive characteristic in most circumstances, given the decision-density dilemma they face. Removing the stigma of bias clears the way for the capriciousness of decision-making and alerts us to strategies that improve the likelihood of responding in a more positive and predictable fashion.

Because definitions drive solutions, the definitions of bias CDRs and heuristics should form the basis of debiasing strategies, which can also be used to recognize existing CDRs and affective dispositions to respond (ADRs) and find strategies to improve their effect on the quality and speed of decision-making.[10] The first step in that process is understanding the taxonomy of bias.

TAXONOMY OF BIAS

In *The Fifth Discipline*, Peter Senge describes the importance of "shared mental models" to understand complex adaptive systems. Shared mental models are defined as:

> . . . deeply held internal images of how the world works, images that limit us to familiar ways of thinking and acting. Very often, we are not consciously aware of our mental models or the effects they have on our behavior.[11]

Cognitive Dispositions to Respond

> With disease, injury, or illness, the diagnosis is often obvious and may involve no more than simple pattern recognition. Where there is uncertainty, however, there is a need for clinical reasoning and decision-making; both of these processes show considerable vulnerability to error."[12]

In and of themselves, CDRs are neither positive nor negative; it is their application in practice that produces outcomes that may be desirable or undesirable. **Table 81.1** describes six general CDRs that result in 35 discrete classifications often seen in the ED. Some of the factors that might influence these dispositions are described in **Figure 81.1**.

When the diagnosis and appropriate response are uncertain, the way in which the caregivers think about and organize the information—in the context of the determining

TABLE 81.1 ■ Classification Scheme for Cognitive Dispositions to Respond

Errors can be due to:

- Overattachment to particular diagnosis
- Anchoring
- Confirmation bias
- Premature closure
- Sunk costs

- Failure to consider alternative diagnoses
- Multiple alternative bias
- Representativeness restraint
- Search satisficing
- Unpacking principle

- Inheriting someone else's thinking
- Diagnosing effect
- Framing effect
- Bandwagon effect

- Patient characteristics or presentation context
- Fundamental attribution error
- Affective bias
- In-group bias
- Triage cueing
- Contrast effect
- Yin-yang out

- Prevalence perception
- Availability bias
- Ambiguity effect
- Base-rate neglect
- Gambler's fallacy
- Hot-hand fallacy
- Hindsight bias
- Playing the odds
- Posterior probability error
- Order effects

- Physician affect, personality, or decision style
- Commission bias
- Omission bias
- Outcome bias
- Visceral bias
- Overconfidence
- Belief bias
- Ego bias
- Sunk costs
- Zebra retreat

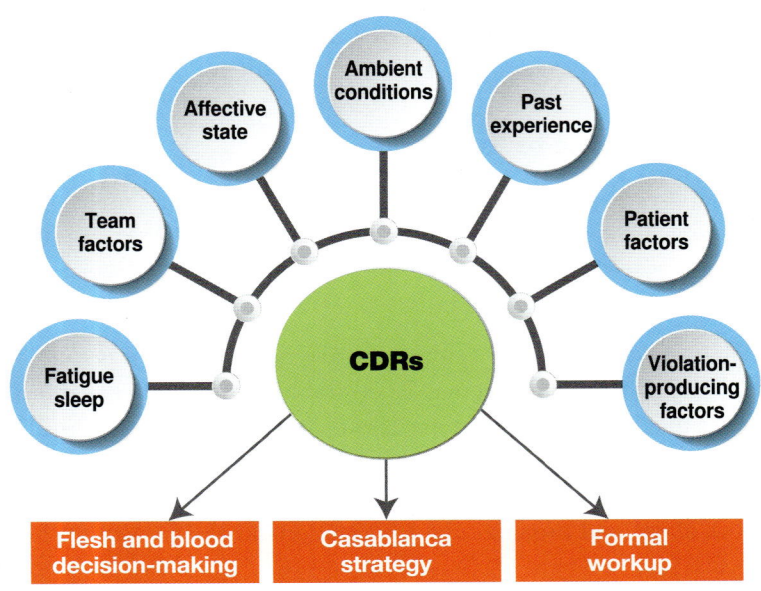

FIGURE 81.1 ■ CDR Determining Factors and Actions

factors combined with the heuristics (mental shortcuts)—may lead to a correct or incorrect outcome. These biases, or tendencies, are generally unconscious and, when flawed, may have significant negative consequences. For example:

> *A patient with a history of multiple visits for alcoholic stupor arrives with alcohol on his breath and delirium. Based on multiple previous similar presentations, the patient's examination is deferred until a more convenient time and leads to a delayed diagnosis of a traumatic intracerebral hemorrhage.*

Affective Dispositions to Respond

Affective, perhaps oversimply stated as "emotional," dispositions to respond may also positively or negatively influence the caregivers approach to care and patient outcomes. For example:

> *Patient A is likeable, young, and attractive. The caregiver establishes a strong rapport with the patient and takes extra time to understand the complaint, symptoms, and signs. Through an exhaustive process, a previously undiscovered obscure diagnosis is made and leads to resolution.*

> *Patient B presents with a long history of multiple changing symptoms and a diagnosis of "fibromyalgia." The somewhat histrionic patient is irritating to the provider. The result is a superficial evaluation and a diagnosis based on a feeling that "there is nothing seriously wrong with this patient, or at least nothing I can treat in the ED."*

Although a distinction is often made between cognitive and affective factors in decision-making, affect (emotion) forms a perimeter for most cognitive decisions, especially in the ED. Though many health-care professionals minimize or deny the role of emotion, affect should not be discounted in ED reasoning and decision-making, because taking ADRs into account can lead to debiasing strategies and improve outcomes. Recently, it has become more widely accepted that emotions are inseparable from cognition, and a classification has begun to develop for ADRs (**Box 81.1**).[10] In this sense, all ADRs should be considered CDRs.

COGNITIVE DEBIASING STRATEGIES

Can the path to clinical expertise be shortened, straightened, or otherwise improved by specific training to recognize, eliminate, or at least blunt the effect of bias? Are there, in fact, "cognitive pills for cognitive ills?"[10] At its most elemental level, the debiasing process starts when clinicians begin to understand and override their intuition and fundamentally restructure their decision-making processes with more objectivity. The fundamental premise is that if thinking in the ED can be debiased, clinicians will think more clearly and become better diagnosticians, which will improve treatment and outcomes.[12]

BOX 81.1 ■ SOURCES OF AFFECTIVE DISPOSITIONS TO RESPOND

- Ambient, chronobiological, and other influences
- Endogenous affective status of the physician/nurse
- Depressive disorders
- Anxiety disorders
- Burnout
- Manic disorders
- Emotional dysregulation of professionals
- Unconscious defenses, avoidance, anxiety
- Excessive emotional involvement or detachment
- Specific affective biases in decision-making

TABLE 81.2 ■ Debiasing Strategies	
Educational	Training to recognize and address biases through development of critical thinking, mentoring, educational interventions, etc
Workplace	Implementing highly efficient systems to improve safe flow and accurate information
Forcing Functions	Developing evidence-based rules that enable broader consideration

One of the biggest obstacles to developing and implementing debiasing strategies is a specific type of bias CDR, called "blind-side bias," a belief that an individual is less susceptible to bias CDRs than others. The thought process goes something like this: "Fortunately, based on my experience and objectivity, I am not as subject to bias as others are."

Table 81.2 describes the three fundamental categories of debiasing strategies: *educational, workplace,* and *forcing functions*.[13]

Educational Strategies

Educational strategies proactively make physicians and nurses aware of the existing CDRs, the risks of ignoring them, and the context and importance of improved decision-making, including real-time recognition of CDRs in clinical care. These strategies include training in critical thinking, theories of reasoning and decision-making, specific educational

TABLE 81.3 ■ Educational Strategies for Cognitive Debiasing		
Strategy	**Comment**	**Examples**
Educational training on reasoning and medical decision-making	Achieving improved diagnostic reasoning requires an understanding of cognitive theories about decision-making and the impact of cognitive biases.	Educational curricula can cover theories of decision-making, major cognitive and affective biases, and their application to diagnostic reasoning.
Bias inoculation	A key recommendation is to teach about cognitive and affective biases and develop specific tools to test and mitigate them.	A "consider-the-opposite" procedure marginally reduced anchoring in judgments of personality traits. Cognitive forcing strategies to counteract cognitive bias showed minor effects.
Specific educational interventions	Teaching specific skills may mitigate bias by providing basic knowledge that leads to greater insight.	People trained in inferential rules committed fewer bias rate errors. Combining a nonanalytical with an analytical approach for reading ECGs improved diagnostic accuracy.
Cognitive tutoring systems	Computer-based systems can be used to construct a learner's decision-making profile and provide feedback on specific biases and strategies to mitigate them.	Decision-monitoring software of virtual slide cases detected cognitive biases according to preset criteria.
Simulation training	Simulation may be a venue for teaching about, identifying, and remediating cognitive errors.	Residents experienced a simulation involving a difficult diagnosis with a cognitive error trap.

interventions, cognitive tutoring/mentoring systems, and simulation training (widely available, particularly in regional health-care systems).

Educational strategies need to "start early" and "stay late." "Start early" means ensuring that the curricula for medical students, nursing students, residents, and fellows include critical thinking and debiasing strategies. As important as this approach is, it will take several years to ensure the entire next generation of clinicians—the future of EDs—will be exposed to these educational strategies (**Table 81.3**).

"Stay late" refers to educating the current clinicians, many of whom have not been systematically exposed to these principles and precepts. This approach includes:

- Making training widely and easily accessible, including technology-based access
- Making training mandatory for all emergency nurses and physicians
- Making decision-making a part of monthly clinical meetings
- Increasing the number of team-based, evidence-based forcing functions
- Creating "communities committed to change" by sharing learnings across boundaries and sites, using ListServ and other information technologies
- Using simulation labs to educate cognitive error traps

All educational strategies primarily aim to increase the ability of clinicians to identify and effectively debias CDRs in the future. Emphasis must also be placed on strategies that can be implemented at the time of decision-making. This requires effective workplace strategies and forcing functions.

Workplace Strategies

Workplace strategies (**Table 81.4**) focus on cognitive processes and the settings and processes through which decisions are made. Ensuring that the maximum amount of information can be attained and interpreted in the shortest amount of time helps ensure that the maximum necessary information (attributes) can be identified and considered. Electronic medical record systems can be designed to assist in this workplace strategy by using larger or multiple screens to show data, allowing past medical records, imaging studies, and laboratory results to be displayed simultaneously. Slowing strategies using "time-outs" when managing critical cases can improve patient outcomes by helping clinicians actively consider alternate diagnoses. Similarly, group decision-making can also enhance the clinical judgment of individual providers.

Forcing Functions

Cognitive forcing functions are evidence-based rules that "force" clinicians to consider alternative possibilities, specific diagnostic or therapeutic measures, or some combination of both. They form a perimeter or "bumper" outside of which the clinician cannot traverse except with a conscious, deliberate override. Properly developed and implemented, these cognitive forcing functions should be viewed as *enabling* functions. The use of clinical prediction rules, evidence-based protocols, checklists, and other strategies are all examples of cognitive forcing functions designed to improve decision-making and outcomes.

For example, Mayer and Jensen developed a highly evidence-based set of clinical protocols for the most high-risk entities presenting to the ED.[14] These best practices were a requirement for all emergency physicians prior to working their first day **(Table 81.5)**. The course material was followed by a brief test, which was monitored via a survey instrument. A similar course was developed and implemented for emergency nurses.

TABLE 81.4 ■ Workplace Strategies for Cognitive Debiasing

Strategy	Comment	Examples
Gathering more information	Heuristics and biases often arise in the context of insufficient information. Diagnostic accuracy is related to the thoroughness of cue acquisition.	The more attributes of a problem can be identified, the greater the likelihood of selecting the best alternative.
Structured data acquisition	Forcing deliberate data acquisition may avoid "spot diagnoses" by ensuring that less-obvious symptoms are considered.	Traditionally, data acquisition has been pursued by establishing a differential diagnosis list or, more recently, a differential checklist tool.
Affective debiasing	Virtually all decision-making involves some degree of affective influence. Many affective biases are hardwired. Decision-makers often are unaware of these influences.	An overview of affective biases and recommendations for debiasing are available.
Metacognition, decoupling, reflection, mindfulness	Deliberately disengage from intuitive judgments, and engage in analytical processes to verify initial impressions.	Deliberately reflecting upon an initial diagnosis led to better diagnoses in difficult cases and counteracted availability bias.
Slow-down strategies	Accuracy suffers when diagnoses are made too hastily, but it improves when decisions are slowed down.	A planned time-out in the operating room
Skepticism	A tendency in human thinking is to believe rather than disbelieve. Type 1 processing occurs by viewing something as more predictable and coherent than it really is.	No published examples
Recalibration	When the decision-maker anticipates additional risks, recalibration may reduce error.	When bias is anticipated (e.g., medical comorbidities in psychiatric patients), the decision-maker may recalibrate.
Group decision strategy	Seeking others' opinions in complex situations may be valuable. Crowd wisdom can be more powerful than the opinions of a single decision-maker.	Group rationality exceeded individual rationality in studies with experimental games in other domains.
Personal accountability	When people know their decisions will be scrutinized, their performance may improve.	Participants who knew they had to justify their responses performed better than those whose responses were anonymous.
Supportive environments	Friendly and supportive environments improve the quality of decision-making.	Avoid cognitive overload, fatigue, and sleep deprivation. The ready availability of protocols, clinical guidelines, and patient-care pathways can reduce variance.
Exposure control	Limit exposure to information that might influence judgment before an impression is formed.	Although there are no published examples, some clinicians avoid reading nurse's notes until after they have assessed the patient. Similarly, clinicians can discourage patients and colleagues from providing a presumed diagnosis until they have formed their own impressions.
Sparklines	Informational mini-graphics can be embedded in clinical data and have the potential to mitigate specific biases.	A graphic outlining pediatric respiratory virus prevalence provided immediate and accurate estimates of respective base rates and trends.
Decision support systems	Support systems are available for clinical use.	A reminder system reduced diagnostic errors of omission and improved quality scores.

TABLE 81.5 ■ Forcing Function Strategies for Cognitive Debiasing

Forcing Function	Comment	Examples
Statistical and clinical prediction rules (SPRs and CPRs)	Explicit SPRs and CPRs typically equal or exceed the reliability of expert "intuitive" judgment. Easy to use, they address significant issues.	The superiority of SPRs and CPRs over clinical judgment has been shown. Physicians demonstrate pretest probability variability in specific diagnoses.
Cognitive forcing strategies (CFSs)	CFSs require clinicians to internalize and apply them deliberately. They represent a systematic change in clinical practice. CFSs may range from universal to generic to specific.	Training might help identify situations that promote the use of heuristics and biases. Clinical scenarios can be identified in which particular biases are likely to occur, and explicit CFSs can be taught to mitigate them.
Standing rules	May be used when a given diagnosis should be avoided until other pathologies have been ruled out	No published examples
General diagnostic rules in clinical practice	Diagnostic "rules" intended to prevent medical errors	Specific tips to avoid diagnostic error
Rule out worst-case scenario (ROWS)	A simple but useful general strategy to avoid missing important diagnoses	No published examples
Checklists	A standard in aviation that is now incorporated into medical practice	Catheter-related bloodstream infections were sustainably reduced when clinicians adopted five evidence-based procedures and used reminders such as reinforcing strategies. The implementation of a surgical safety checklist reduced deaths and surgical (noncardiac) complications in a multicenter study.
Stopping rules	An important forcing function to determine when enough information has been gathered to make an optimal decision.	No published examples
Consider the opposite	Seeking evidence to support a decision that contradicts your initial impression	Experimental psychological studies show that by considering the opposite viewpoint, participants could counteract their biased judgments of personality traits.
Consider the control	Causal claims are often made without an appropriate control group.	No published examples

Called "Creating the Risk-Free ED," the initiative reduced professional liability loss runs, loss reserves, and insurance rates by 70% and was recognized by the Robert Woods Johnson Urgent Matters Program as the "Innovation of the Year Runner-Up."[14] **Figure 81.2** shows an example of a "Risk-Free ED" best practice. These forcing functions can vary from mandated efforts (removal of all concentrated potassium solutions, mandated EBM protocols) to simple encouragement. However, as experience with these strategies expands, the less optional (and more successful) they become.

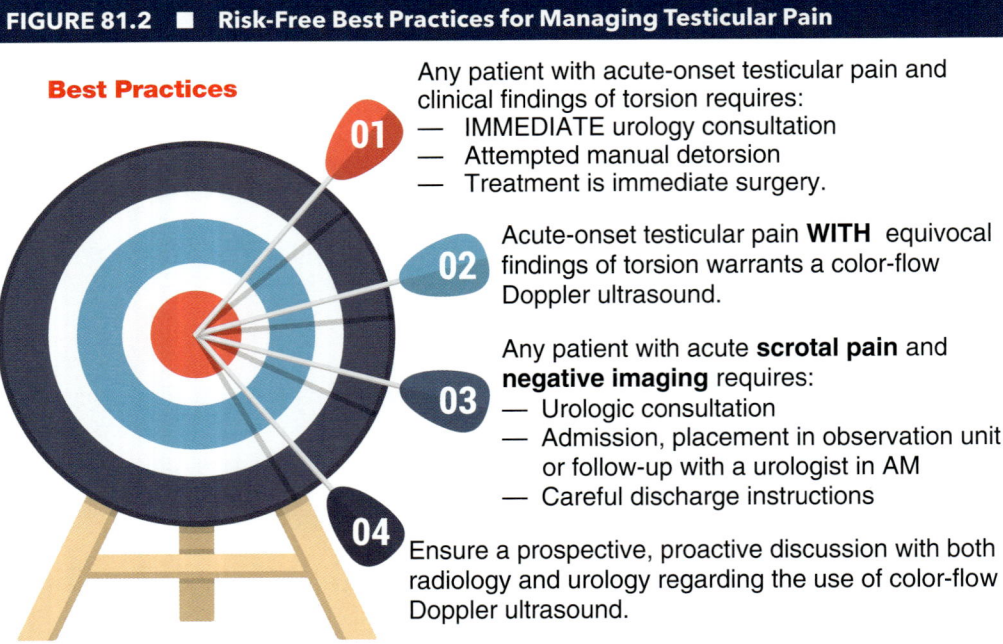

FIGURE 81.2 ■ Risk-Free Best Practices for Managing Testicular Pain

Best Practices

01 Any patient with acute-onset testicular pain and clinical findings of torsion requires:
— IMMEDIATE urology consultation
— Attempted manual detorsion
— Treatment is immediate surgery.

02 Acute-onset testicular pain **WITH** equivocal findings of torsion warrants a color-flow Doppler ultrasound.

03 Any patient with acute **scrotal pain** and **negative imaging** requires:
— Urologic consultation
— Admission, placement in observation unit, or follow-up with a urologist in AM
— Careful discharge instructions

04 Ensure a prospective, proactive discussion with both radiology and urology regarding the use of color-flow Doppler ultrasound.

BRINGING IT TO THE BEDSIDE

How can one practically utilize the debiasing strategies to move from the dilemma of decision density to effective decision-making? What are the "cognitive pills for cognitive ills" that can be used every day?[15] The following debiasing strategies were chosen because they are common and represent the classification system noted previously.

Anchoring–Confirmation Bias

Anchoring occurs when the clinician locks onto a diagnosis at the exclusion of other considerations too early in the course of the patient's care, focusing on initial impressions instead of staying open to a broader range of possibilities. (It is often associated with confirmation bias, looking for confirming data and avoiding nonconfirming data, as well as premature closure). For example:

> *A patient with a known seizure disorder presents to the ED with a seizure. The emergency physician and nurse anchor onto this previous diagnosis and fail to note that the ECG shows an arrhythmia.*

The debiasing strategy includes asking questions such as "What if it's not . . .?" "What are three other possibilities?" and "What if this were the patient's first seizure?" Slow down early in the course of care and expand the differential diagnosis list.

Premature Closure

Premature closure (overattachment to a diagnosis) is a common CDR that causes a high proportion of missed diagnoses. Caregivers apply premature closure prior to assembling and interpreting the pertinent facts. It leads to the maxim: "Once the diagnosis is made, the work is done—and the thinking stops." For example:

> *A patient with a history of alcohol abuse presents with intoxication and altered mental status. The ED team prematurely closes in on a diagnosis of ethanol intoxication and*

discharges him. The patient is found dead at home the next day. An autopsy shows an epidural hematoma.

The debiasing strategy is to expand divergent thinking and restrict convergent thinking in the early stages of care. Consider alternate diagnoses. Despite the previous encounters of alcohol intoxication, perform a detailed neurologic exam and document it carefully. Repeat the previous step. Consider, "Ensure that this presentation is not acute head trauma, metabolic disease, space-occupying mass, and so on, because . . ." Create a list of specific reasons why the alternative etiologies are not the final diagnoses.

Search Satisficing

Search satisficing (the failure to consider alternative diagnoses) is the universal, understandable yet dangerous tendency to call off a search once an initial explanation is found. The maxim that applies is: "Call in the dogs and put out the fire because the 'hunt' is over." For example:

A patient presents with acute pain that began after she stepped on a piece of glass. A glass foreign body is found and removed, the wound is irrigated, and the patient is discharged. She returns 2 days later with a swollen foot, cellulitis extending to the lower leg. After a careful wound exploration, several additional pieces of glass are found. (The same applies to multiple fractures, drug poisonings, and additional comorbidities.)

The debiasing strategy to keeping looking, keep searching. Ask: "What else is in there?" "What else is going on?" Spend twice as much time looking for additional foreign bodies as it took to find the first.

Unpacking Principle

The *unpacking principle* is the failure to elicit pertinent information (unpacking) before establishing a differential diagnosis, resulting in significant possibilities being missed. For example:

A patient presents with a temperature of 39°C, dysphagia, cervical lymphadenopathy, and previous bouts of "strep throat." The throat cannot easily be visualized. A diagnosis of pharyngitis is made, and the patient is presumptively started on antibiotics. The patient returns 2 days later with respiratory distress, drooling, and complete inability to swallow, including fluid. An indirect laryngoscopy shows epiglottitis.

The debiasing strategy is to pause and consider alternative information sources; persist in completing a history, past history, and a physical examination; and "pull up" instead of "pulling out."

Diagnosing Effect–Diagnostic Momentum

Diagnosing effect–diagnostic momentum (inheriting other's thinking) refers to diagnostic labels that, once attached to a patient, become difficult to dislodge and lead clinicians to ignore other possibilities. These labels can come from emergency medical services, physicians, nurses, the medical record, the family, and even the patient. With repetition, these labels gather increasing momentum, blocking consideration of alternate diagnoses. For example:

During "sign-out rounds," a patient is handed off with a presumptive diagnosis of gastroenteritis and instructions to "check the electrolytes and then send him home." The emergency physician does just that, but the nurse asks that a repeat examination be performed, explaining, "The patient seems sicker to me." The repeat exam shows increasing right lower quadrant tenderness with rebound, and a diagnosis of acute appendicitis is correctly made.

The debiasing strategy is to start fresh and avoid assumptions when assuming care of a patient, regardless of colleagues' diagnostic impressions. Specifically, when taking over care of a patient, reverify the history and physical exam findings and review laboratory and imaging findings independently.

Bandwagon Effect

The *bandwagon effect* (inheriting other's thinking) is similar in some respects to diagnostic momentum. It is the tendency for people to believe and do what others are doing, virtually guaranteeing the same outcome. Bandwagon effects can have a disastrous effect on team decision-making. For example:

> *A patient with a stated and documented history of fibromyalgia arrives with pain in a new location. Because the pain is somewhat similar in nature to previous pains and the patient states, "I think it's my fibromyalgia," other causes are not considered.*

The debiasing strategy is similar to solutions to other CDRs, that is, the bandwagon effect can be overcome by eliminating preconceived notions and thoroughly evaluating each new presentation.

Gender Bias

Gender bias (sex discrimination) is the (nonevidence-based) tendency to see the patient's gender as a significant determining factor in the probability of a particular diagnosis. Gender bias results in both over- and underdiagnosis. For example:

> *A woman presents with anxiety, fatigue, difficulty sleeping, and mild tachycardia. The clinician's evaluation results in a diagnosis of "anxiety disorder" (overdiagnosis) and does not investigate or consider the actual diagnosis: hyperthyroidism (underdiagnosis).*

The debiasing strategy is to recognize that gender bias is common (review data) and has been subtly incorporated into caregiver training. Then maintain awareness of the possibility in all patient encounters; rely on evidence-based information rather than "gut instinct," and when training others, ensure that this bias is brought to light and discussed.

Availability Bias

Availability bias (errors in prevalence perception) occurs when what most readily comes to mind is considered most likely and relevant. What is most available to memory drives decision-making instead of a careful assessment of alternatives. "When you hear hoofbeats, think 'horses,' not 'zebras' " is the applicable maxim. For example:

> *In the midst of an influenza outburst, a child presents with flu-like symptoms and is the seventh patient that day with those symptoms. A diagnosis of influenza is made, but the nurse notes that the child has significantly more respiratory distress and is much more anxious than previous patients. A more in-depth reconsideration reveals the patient has a lobar pneumonia; he is admitted under a pneumonia-sepsis clinical pathway.*

The debiasing strategy is to recall that what is most common is not necessarily most likely. When assessing an individual patient, it is important to consider:

- "Those patients had common, mild findings, but *this one* is sicker and/or has a presentation variation. Does this presentation suggest other possible etiologies?"
- "Sometimes zebras come to this ED, even if they have the same hoofbeats as horses."

- "Though this patient may have a common and benign explanation for the symptoms, what else is consistent with this presentation?"

Gambler's Fallacy

Gambler's fallacy (errors in prevalence perception) is the belief that past events affect the probability of future events. A gambler may reason that, since a coin has turned up heads 10 times in a row, the odds are that the 11th toss will be tails, whereas the real odds are always 50:50. For example:

> An emergency physician evaluates four patients in succession, each of whom are diagnosed with acute chest syndrome and are admitted to the short-stay cardiac unit. When the fifth chest pain patient presents, the physician assumes that the diagnosis is less likely to be ACS and discharges the patient.

The debiasing strategy is to recognize this CDR early and remember that each patient is different, with discrete findings and needs. Ask: "Why am I assuming that this can't be . . .? What specific data leads me to that conclusion versus alternate diagnoses?" and "Would it be helpful to seek a colleagues' input for a fresh viewpoint?"

Yin-Yang Out

Yin-yang out (an error of patient characteristics or presentation context) is a CDR that occurs when patients have received extensive or repeated clinical workups, creating the impression that everything that can be done has already been done. In other words, the patient has been "worked up out the 'yin-yang.'" For example:

> A patient with chronic abdominal pain of unknown etiology presents to the ED with another bout of pain. He has already had multiple CT scans and upper and lower endoscopy (including an endoscopic retrograde cannulation of the pancreas), all of which are negative. The patient is discharged but returns 1 day later with mesenteric ischemia.

There are a number of debiasing strategies for this CDR:

- Review the patient's history and diagnostic studies (including the images themselves and the radiology readings).
- Examine the patient thoroughly and repeatedly with a focus on new findings.
- Make a list of alternate diagnoses that have not been considered.
- Separately, consider new changes that might herald the onset of acute, chronic abdominal pain.
- Seek an opinion from ED colleagues.

Visceral Bias

Visceral bias (an error of affect, personality, or decision style) is a form of "hot button" bias. Representing the strong pull of affective factors on CDRs, it is a bias that is widely underestimated. Both positive and negative visceral responses can result in countertransference. For example:

> A clinician with a family history of abusive behavior is evaluating a patient/family with a presentation suggestive of similar abuse. Unintentionally, the clinician is hostile to the potentially abusive member, making care and discussion more difficult.

The debiasing strategy should start before the encounter begins: Recognize the potential for visceral bias; "disconnect" hot buttons so they do not have an impact on the encounter; and regularly reflect on what types of patients and interactions cause positive or negative involuntary reactions.

CONCLUSION

Emergency clinicians face an unprecedented level of decision-making. Forcing the use of heuristics, which are formulated to improve the speed, if not the accuracy, of this process. Effectively used, heuristics provide information-processing rules and allow ED professionals to more efficiently manage patient care and avoid "paralysis by analysis." Diagnostic and therapeutic errors often result from biases, of which there are at least 35 discrete types common in emergency medicine. Heuristics and biases are almost always unconscious, type 1, reflexive processes that skip the laborious process of deductive reasoning.

While the terms "bias" and "heuristics" are neither positive or negative, they often are associated with negative connotations. The more objective, alternative term "cognitive disposition to respond" is more useful. In fact, using this positive, analytical term helps clinicians not only consider "What were you thinking?" but also "How were you thinking?"

Cognitive debiasing strategies may be considered "cognitive pills for cognitive ills" in that they can improve decision-making by highlighting biases/CDRs and helping clinicians implement strategies to blunt the negative and accentuate their positive effects.[10] These debiasing techniques may be grouped as educational, workplace, and cognitive forcing/enabling strategies.

REFERENCES

1. Reason J. Human error: models and management. *BJM.* 2000;320(7237):768–770.
2. Baron J. *Thinking and Deciding.* New York, NY: Cambridge University Press; 2008.
3. Croskerry P. Cognitive and affective dispositions to respond. In: Croskerry P, Cosby KS, Schenkel SM, et al, eds. *Patient Safety in Emergency Medicine.* Walters Kluwer; 2009.
4. Mayer T. Burnout, rustout, resilience, and engagement: learning to love the job you have while creating the job you love. Presented at: the American College of Healthcare Executives Congress, 2019; Chicago, IL.
5. The Joint Commission. Cognitive biases in healthcare. *Quick Safety.* Issue October 28, 2016. Available at: https://www.jointcommission.org/assets/1/23/Quick_Safety_Issue_28_Oct_2016.pdf. Accessed July 30, 2020.
6. Arnott D. Cognitive bias and decision support systems development: a design science approach. *Info Syst J.* 2006;16(1):55–78.
7. Wilson TD, Brekke N. Mental contamination and mental correction: unwanted influences on judgments and evaluations. *Psychol Bull.* 1994;116(1):117–142.
8. Croskerry P. Cognitive forcing strategies in clinical decision-making. *Ann Emerg Med.* 2003;41(1):110–120.
9. Croskerry P, Abbass AA, Wu AW. How doctors feel: affective issues in patients' safety. *Lancet.* 2008;372(9645):1205–1206.
10. Senge PM. *The Fifth Discipline: The Art and Practice of the Learning Organization.* Doubleday; 2006.
11. Croskerry P. Achieving quality in decision making: cognitive strategies and detection of bias. *Acad Emerg Med.* 2002;9(11):1184–1204.
12. Croskerry P. Diagnostic failure: a cognitive and affective approach. In: Henriksen K, Battles JB, Marks ES, et al, eds. *Advances in Patient Safety: From Research to Implementation, Volume 2: Concepts and Methodology.* Agency for Health Research and Quality; 2005.
13. Croskerry P, Singhal G, Mamede S. Cognitive debiasing 1: origins of bias and theory of debiasing. *BMJ Qual Saf.* 2013;22:ii58–ii64.
14. Mayer T, Jensen K. Creating the risk free ED. *Robert Woods Johnson Urgent Matters Innovation of the Year.* Available at: https://smhs.gwu.edu/urgentmatters/news/innovations-risk-free-ed. Accessed July 30, 2020.
15. Kerken G. Cognitive aids and debiasing methods: can cognitive pills cure cognitive ills? *Adv Psychol.* 1990;68:486–498.

CHAPTER 82

THE REVOLVING DOOR OF READMISSIONS

Jean Scofi, Arjun Venkatesh

Nearly one in five Medicare beneficiaries discharged from the hospital is readmitted within 30 days at a cost of approximately $26 billion per year.[1] In addition to increasing medical costs, high readmission rates can negatively impact patient outcomes, burden providers and caregivers, and contribute to emergency department (ED) and hospital overcrowding. Notably, patients who were readmitted to the hospital are susceptible to "posthospitalization syndrome," which includes infections, gastrointestinal conditions, mental illness, metabolic derangements, and trauma unrelated to the original admitting diagnosis.[2]

Significant efforts have been made over the past decade to improve hospital admission policies. These efforts include the creation of readmission benchmarks, financial penalties under the Hospital Readmissions Reduction Program (HRRP), patient and community education programs, new hospital admission and observation protocols, and improved discharge planning and care coordination processes.[3] As a result, readmission rates have declined from 17.7% in 2010 to 15.8% in 2016 (for all-cause national readmissions reported by the Centers for Medicare and Medicaid Services [CMS]).[4] However, there is still opportunity to further improve ED readmissions.

The ED is the largest source of unscheduled hospitalizations in the United States. A large national study in 2016 found that the ED is responsible for over 40% of adult admissions and over 50% of elderly admissions.[5] Traditionally, hospital administrators and policymakers viewed the ED simply as a contributor to the readmission problem. However, recent evidence has shown that ED interventions and policies can have a significant impact on readmission rates.

DEFINING READMISSIONS

Although general readmission terms are agreed upon by the medical community, the specific definition of "readmission" can vary based on the purpose of measurement and the policy lens applied. A hospital readmission occurs when a patient is discharged and admitted again within a specified time interval. The first admission is commonly referred to as the "index admission," and the subsequent admission is called the "readmission." The CMS defines "readmission" as:

> ... an admission to an acute care hospital within 30 days of discharge from the same or another acute care hospital [regardless of the cause for readmission].[6]

Index admissions are excluded if the patient was transferred between hospitals, discharged against medical advice, or admitted for cancer treatment, rehabilitation, or a primary psychiatric diagnosis. The CMS also focuses on specific clinical cohorts like congestive heart failure (CHF), pneumonia, and so on. By contrast, researchers may choose to define "readmission" using much longer time intervals (60 days, 90 days, or a year from hospital discharge) and include other acute care admissions, such as observation stays.[7] They may also focus on different clinical cohorts outside of national quality measures, including vulnerable or niche patient populations.

Planned vs Unplanned Readmissions

In 2015, CMS added an addendum to its definition to account for "planned" versus "unplanned" readmissions.[6] "Planned" readmissions are those that are anticipated and controlled and therefore do not reflect gaps in quality of care. "Unplanned" readmissions are those that arise from unanticipated clinical events (**Figure 82.1**). According to national data from 2008 to 2016, CMS found that only approximately 5% of all readmissions are planned.[4]

Furthermore, studies have shown that some fraction of these unplanned readmissions are potentially preventable. Exactly how many is somewhat controversial and varies by institution, patient population, and the definition of "preventability." One systematic review

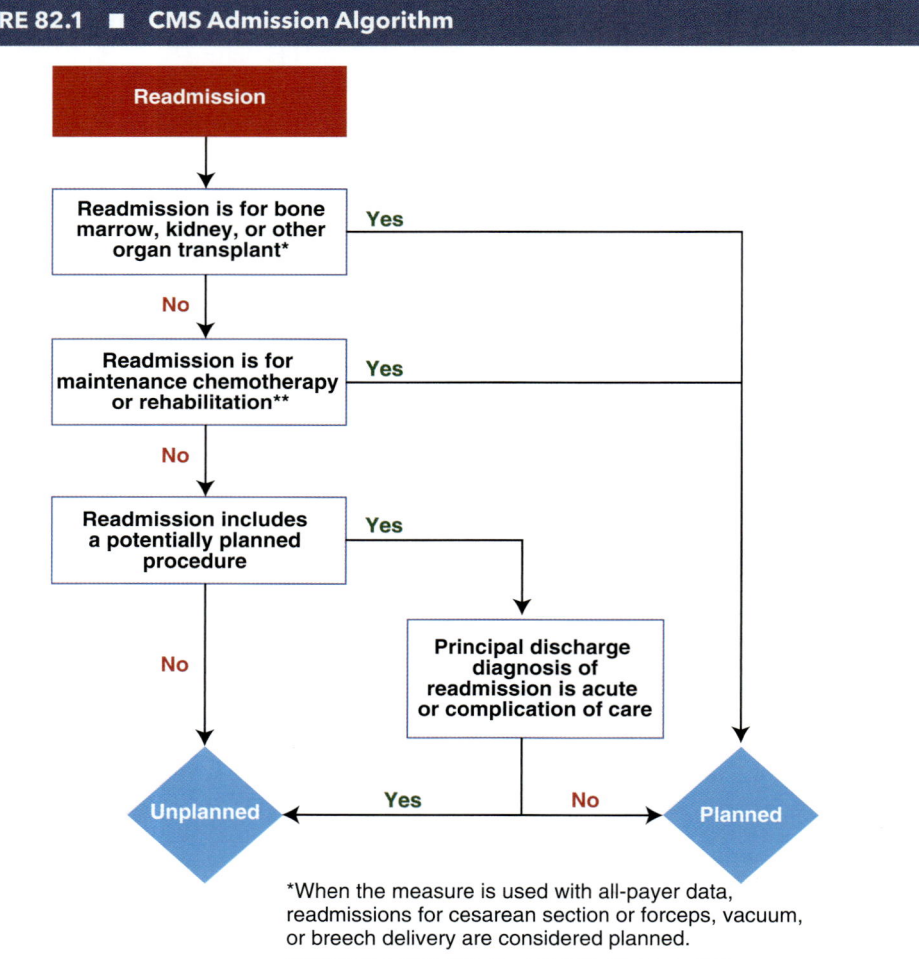

FIGURE 82.1 ■ CMS Admission Algorithm

*When the measure is used with all-payer data, readmissions for cesarean section or forceps, vacuum, or breech delivery are considered planned.

**When the measure is used with all-payer data, readmissions for forceps or normal delivery are considered planned.

of 34 institutional studies indicates that the fraction of all readmissions that are potentially preventable may range from as little as 5% to as many as 79% across different hospitals.[8] Most national studies in the past decade agree that the median fraction of potentially preventable readmissions (PPRs) for all conditions and US hospitals is somewhere between 20% and 30%.[9-11]

Potentially Preventable or Avoidable Readmissions

Potentially preventable readmissions are the main focus of policy efforts because this special subset can be directly influenced by hospital-level interventions (**Figure 82.2**).[12] However, the "preventability" of readmissions remains understudied, and the degree to which acute events are truly preventable is contested in the literature. For instance, one study of chronic obstructive pulmonary disease (COPD) patients at the Mayo Clinic in 2017 found that a commonly used reporting algorithm classified 78% of all COPD 30-day readmissions as potentially preventable, while a group of practicing physicians found that only 53% were potentially preventable. Studies like this have led to the critique that administrative data without clinical review may inflate PPR rates.[13]

A systematic review of risk-prediction models for hospital readmission also found that most models perform poorly, and few account for social determinants and functional status.[14] Nonetheless, significant efforts are being made to identify risk factors for PPRs and predict which are causal and actionable.[15]

This issue is further complicated by terms such as "inappropriate hospitalizations," which may be mistakenly used interchangeably with "PPRs." The latter refers to quality gaps during the index admission (e.g., undertreatment of hyperglycemia that leads to readmission for diabetic ketoacidosis), whereas "inappropriate hospitalization" refers to a problem with initiating the index admission (e.g., admitting a patient for hyperglycemia amenable to outpatient management).[16]

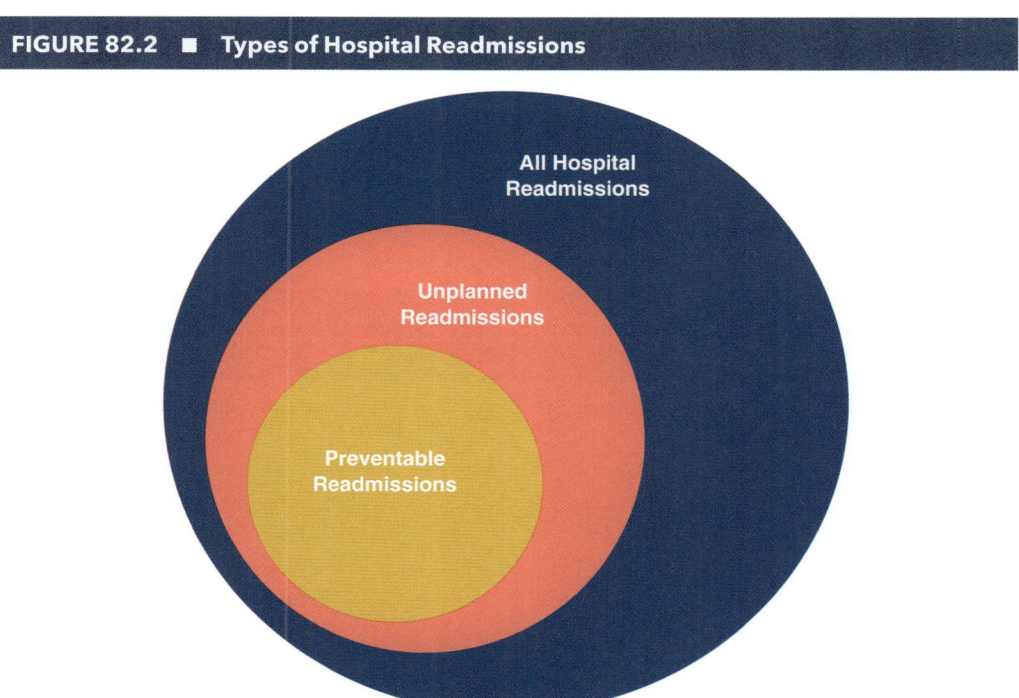

FIGURE 82.2 ■ Types of Hospital Readmissions

Commonly Reported Readmission Measures

Currently, a total of six inpatient readmission measures are publicly reported by CMS on its Hospital Compare website and can be used to calculate payment penalties in the HRRP (**Table 82.1**). These include excess readmission rates for acute myocardial infarction, coronary artery bypass graft surgery, COPD, heart failure, hip/knee replacement, and pneumonia.[6]

In addition, several readmission measures apply to ambulatory surgical centers, cancer hospitals, and other settings where patients are likely to incur emergency care. For these measures, CMS calculates a risk-standardized readmission rate (RSRR) for each hospital that used administrative claims data to account for differences in the hospital case mix.[17] The CMS also reports an excess readmission ratio (ERR) for specific conditions.[18] Unlike the RSRR, which is a measure of absolute performance, the ERR is a measure of a hospital's relative performance. It is the ratio of a hospital's predicted or measured readmission rate to the expected readmission rate among hospitals in the same peer group. Because the ERR controls for differences among hospitals and patient populations, it is considered a fairer measure than the RSRR. More recently, CMS has also begun to evaluate and publicly report excess days in acute care.[19] These are condition-specific readmission measures that capture the risk-adjusted number of days patients are in hospital settings (ED, observation, or inpatient) out of the 30 days following hospital discharge.

In addition to CMS measures, another notable readmission metric is the 3M Health Information Systems measure of "PPR," which is used by large hospital groups for public reporting, payment incentives, and quality-improvement strategies.[20,21] A PPR is defined as a readmission within a specified time interval that is clinically related to the index admission. Therefore, a PPR rate that is higher than expected suggests that the readmission could have been reasonably prevented by providing quality care at the index admission, adequate discharge planning, or adequate care coordination.

While both the CMS-reported "unplanned readmission rate" and the 3M-defined "PPR rate" are commonly used, only the CMS-reported measures are tied to hospital payment incentives. In addition, while all these metrics capture overall hospital readmission rates, none of them directly quantify emergency care. However, EDs have become an integral partner in hospital strategies to reduce readmissions and improve patient care transitions.

TABLE 82.1 ■ List of Commonly Reported Readmission Measures

	Measure Name	Source	Use
HRRP	Hospital readmissions reduction program	CMS	Used to calculate payment penalties
RSRR	Risk-standardized readmission rate	CMS	Applies to ambulatory surgical centers, cancer hospitals, etc. to address case-mix differences
ERR	Excess readmission ratio	CMS	Compares readmission rates to similar (peer group) hospitals
PPR	Potentially preventable readmission	3M	Focuses on readmissions that could have been prevented by attention to quality, discharge planning, or care coordination

Factors Affecting Readmission Rates

Hospital readmission is the result of complex and multifactorial processes that can fail at multiple decision points, including:

- *Care delivery*: diagnostic and therapeutic errors or quality gaps during the index admission
- *Care coordination*: failed handoffs, premature discharge, lack of patient education or communication, or inadequate follow-up or patient support after discharge
- *Care complications*: iatrogenic infections and adverse events incurred during the index admission
- *Patient risk factors*: include but are not limited to) comorbid conditions, progression of diseases, and social determinants such as low income or poor housing[22-26]

Which of these factors are potentially preventable? Studies and prediction models have cited many candidates over the past decade. For instance, a landmark report by the Dartmouth Atlas Project in 2011 found that more than half of discharged Medicare patients do not see a primary care clinician or specialist within 2 weeks of leaving the hospital.[27] More recently, a 2016 study found that ED decision-making was most strongly associated with preventability at US academic medical centers (adjusted odds ratio: 9.13), followed by a failure to relay important information to outpatient providers (adjusted odds ratio: 4.19), and lack of discussion about goals of care (adjusted odds ratio: 3.84).[9]

However, not all drivers of readmissions are modifiable or within the individual provider's control. The optimal readmission rate is therefore unknown. However, the broad variation in readmission rates among hospitals and evidence of successful interventions suggests that ED administrators have significant opportunities to reduce unnecessary readmissions and improve patient outcomes.

NATIONAL READMISSIONS DATA AND TRENDS

As part of a national policy effort to track and reduce hospital readmissions, CMS began publicly reporting hospital readmission rates for myocardial infarction, heart failure, and pneumonia in 2010. This information is published on Hospital Compare, a CMS website that houses public information for 4,000+ Medicare-certified hospitals in the United States.[28] Since 2010, CMS has added hospital readmission rates for COPD, hip/knee replacement, and coronary artery bypass graft surgery; surgical readmission rates for lower extremity bypass, colon surgery, and surgeries in patients 65 years of age or older; and the Hospital Wise Readmission measure to its publicly reported data.[29]

Figure 82.3 shows the all-cause, unplanned, and PPR rates reported by CMS between 2008 and 2016. All-cause and unplanned readmissions are defined using CMS criteria, whereas PPRs are defined using 3M criteria (see the "Defining Readmissions" section above). The trends for all three rates are similar, with relatively flat rates from 2008 to 2010, followed by a steady decline from 2010 to 2016 (17.7%-15.8% for all-cause, 16.7%-15.0% for unplanned, 11.2%-9.7% for potentially preventable).[4]

There is little variation in readmission rates among all hospitals, with approximately half of US hospitals reporting RSRR within 1% of the median and the full range of RSRRs varying from 11.0% to 21.4% in 2010 to 2013.[30] However, some studies show that there is actually much greater variability among hospitals of similar type (urban vs rural, academic vs nonacademic, etc.) compared to all hospitals of different types (aggregate data).[31]

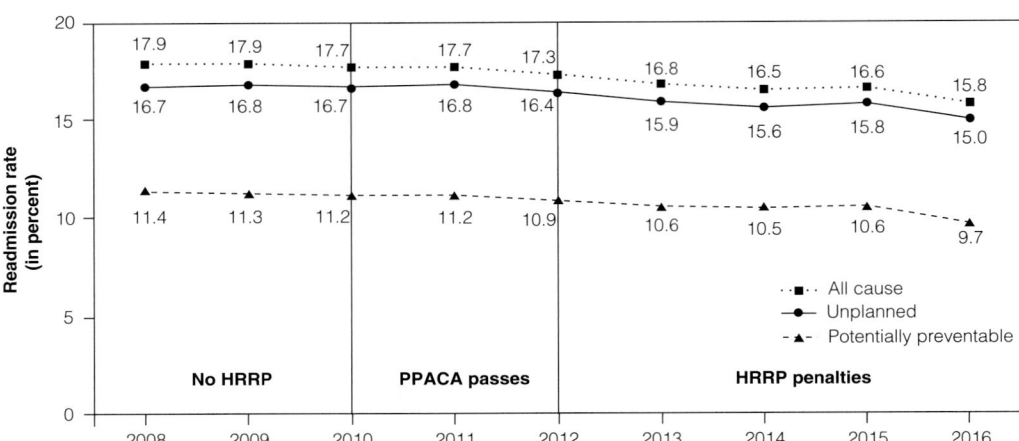

FIGURE 82.3 ■ CMS-Reported All-Cause, Unplanned, and Potentially Preventable Readmission Rates Across All Conditions

Decline in Unplanned Readmission Rates

Notably, readmission rates in 2010 to 2016 declined not only for Medicare patients but also for patients with Medicaid or private insurance and those with non-HRRP conditions.[32] **Figure 82.4** shows that unplanned readmission rates for non-HRRP-covered conditions decreased by 2.6% between 2010 and 2016. The decline in unplanned readmission rates for HRRP-covered conditions was even greater (3.9% for heart failure, 3.7% for acute myocardial infarction, 3.0% for pneumonia, and 1.4% for hip and knee replacements).

What caused this decline in readmission rates? In general, the literature credits the large wave of national and local quality-improvement efforts that started between 2011 and 2012. These efforts were initiated in response to the HRRP, the Community-Based Care Transitions Program, and the Independence at Home Demonstration Program. **Figure 82.4** demonstrates that the average unplanned readmission rate was flat prior to the HRRP (16.7% in 2008 and 2010) but declined by an average of 0.15% to 0.35% per year

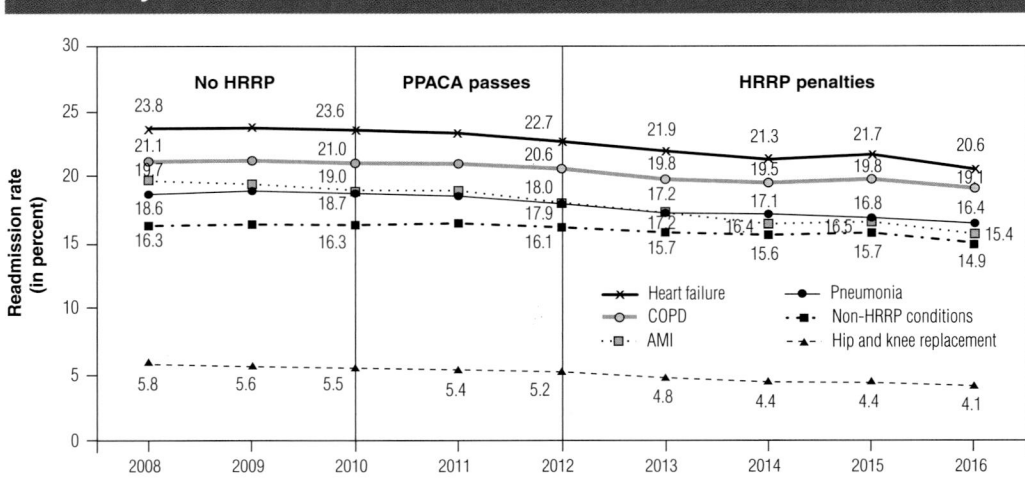

FIGURE 82.4 ■ CMS-Reported Unplanned Readmission Rates for Conditions Covered by the HRRP

after the HRRP was implemented.[4] While these findings do not demonstrate causation, they do suggest that the decline in is associated with national policy efforts. However, the data also showed concurrent increases in observation stays and ED return visits as readmission rates declined.

Analysts were initially concerned that patients were simply being shifted from inpatient to observation status with no significant change in health-care utilization overall.[33,34] However, the growth in both ED visits and observation stays was not unique to admitted patients and reflected a global phenomenon of increased ED and observation use for all patients nationwide over the past decade.

WHY READMISSIONS MATTER

High readmission rates can negatively impact patient outcomes, contribute to ED and hospital overcrowding, and increase health-care costs.

Impact on Patient Outcomes

Repeat admissions can negatively impact patients in three major ways. First, inpatient stays are not benign. They expose patients to risks and complications unique to the hospital setting, including medical errors, hospital-acquired infections, delirium, and deconditioning. These risks disproportionately affect the chronically ill, medically complex, and/or elderly and can compound with repeat admissions.[2,35,36]

Second, repeat admissions increase the risk of poor patient compliance, inadequate follow-up, and communication errors. Studies have shown that patients and caregivers are particularly vulnerable when discharged from inpatient care, compared to other types of care transitions.[37] They may not know who to contact for follow-up, how to obtain and deliver adequate home care services, or how to navigate myriad outpatient visits. This confusion can result in inadequate treatment, care errors, or missed appointments that worsen the patient's condition and increase their morbidity or mortality. Similarly, repeat admissions to different inpatient teams and specialty services complicate the medical record, increase the risk of miscommunication, and can result in poor longitudinal care.

Finally, repeat admissions have been shown to take a toll on the emotional well-being of both patients and families. Hospital admissions are disruptive and stressful events, and repeat admissions can prolong this disruption. Most elderly and chronically ill patients show higher satisfaction with home care services compared to repeat inpatient stays.[38,39]

Operational Impact

High readmission rates can create two major operational inefficiencies: overutilization of inpatient resources and high patient turnover. Overutilization of inpatient resources results in high occupancy rates that have a trickle-down effect to the ED and other points of entry to the health-care system. If inpatient beds are constantly occupied, fewer new patients can be admitted. Current occupants with unnecessary reasons for admission therefore take up precious hospital resources that could be better utilized for others awaiting inpatient beds. As ED resources become overwhelmed, patients are at greater risk for quality gaps, medical errors, and worse outcomes.[40] High patient turnover has been shown to increase adverse events, including medication errors, faulty handoffs, fragmentation of care, and patient mortality, particularly when combined with understaffed or overcrowded conditions.[41,42]

Financial Impact

In 2007, the Medicare Payment Advisory Commission (MedPAC) estimated that 30-day Medicare readmissions cost approximately $26 billion per year, of which $12 billion was attributable to potentially preventable admissions (an average of $7,200 per PPR based on 2005 dollars).[27,43] In 2013, MedPAC suggested that reducing avoidable readmissions by 10% could achieve a savings of $1 billion per year or more.[44]

Ever since readmissions received the policy spotlight in 2007, researchers have struggled to parse this financial impact in greater (and more actionable) detail. One major area of concern is whether higher readmission rates translate to worse financial performance for individual hospitals. While there are no studies that can definitively demonstrate causality, there is certainly a strong correlation between safety net hospitals (with low margins) and higher readmission rates (among disadvantaged or vulnerable populations).[45] This suggests that some hospitals are serving patients with special conditions that are consistently costlier than others to readmit.[46,47]

For instance, one study found that sepsis is both more prevalent and costlier than other conditions penalized by the HRRP, and another found that unplanned readmissions for knee replacement are strongly correlated with reduced hospital profits.[48,49] There is debate as to whether certain conditions should be penalized disproportionately, given their higher financial impact, or if this will disproportionately punish safety net hospitals.[50]

Another concern is whether the financial impact of readmissions extends beyond the simple cost of the second hospital stay. In particular, high hospital readmission rates can have downstream effects, including increased overcrowding and ED boarding. A preventable readmission can also result in costly complications, including hospital-acquired infections. Since readmission is a complex event that causes ripple effects along the entire health-care delivery chain, the true financial impact to the medical system may actually be understated.

Policy Measures

Due to the negative clinical, operational, and financial impact of PPRs, this topic has become a high priority for policymakers and administrators. In 2007, CMS published a report to Congress, "Promoting Greater Efficiency in Medicare," which made a case for reducing hospital readmissions.[43] In 2009, CMS began tracking and publicly reporting hospital readmission rates nationwide to increase awareness of this issue. As a result, the 2010 Affordable Care Act required CMS to penalize hospitals for "excess" readmissions when compared to "expected" levels of readmissions in an effort to reduce health-care costs.[51] The CMS responded by creating the Hospital Readmission Reduction Program (HRRP) in 2010, which tied payment incentives to publicly reported hospital readmission rates for certain conditions.

Initially, the HRRP reduced Medicare payments by up to 1% for hospitals with above-average readmission rates for three conditions: acute myocardial infarction, heart failure, and pneumonia. By 2018, the HRRP had increased the readmission penalty to a maximum of 3% and expanded the list of conditions to include COPD, pneumonia, coronary artery bypass graft surgery, and elective primary total hip arthroplasty and/or total knee arthroplasty. This list will likely continue to be expanded in the future. For a full timeline of the implementation and evolution of the CMS HRRP policy, see **Figure 82.5.**

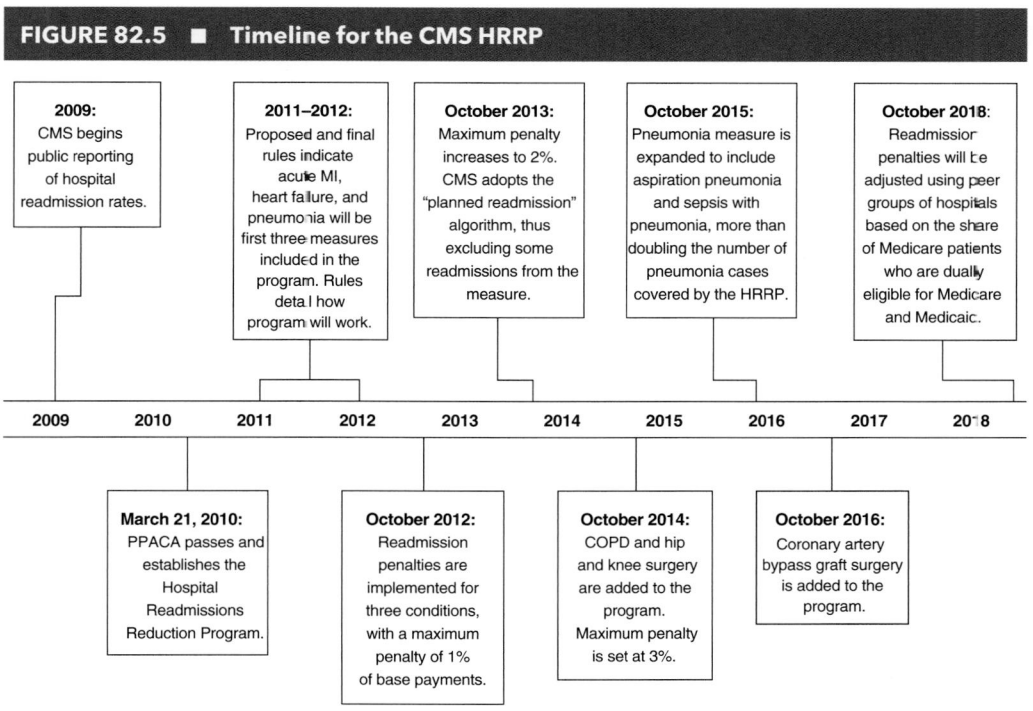

FIGURE 82.5 ■ Timeline for the CMS HRRP

Since implementation of the HRRP, hospitals have incurred over $1.9 billion in penalties.[51] As a result, local and national efforts to reduce hospital admissions have surged since 2010. These efforts were initially highly varied and scattered, ranging from clinical protocols to community partnerships to patient engagement. They were also siloed among disciplines, likely due to HRRP penalties that focused on specific conditions rather than global care delivery or coordination across health systems. Finally, since the HRRP emphasized a financial penalty, initial efforts focused heavily on cost savings rather than mortality or other outcome measures.

For instance, a large 2016 systematic review of 123 primary studies over the past decade found that quick diagnostic units, observation units (OUs), and hospital-at-home all showed near-universal cost savings when implemented as alternatives to inpatient hospitalization.[52] A 2017 systematic review of 50 studies related to the economic impact of quality-improvement strategies to prevent hospital readmissions also found net savings, with the greatest savings associated with interventions that engaged patients and caregivers.[53] More recently, studies have shifted away from pure cost savings toward quality, strategy, and coordination. For instance, numerous studies have confirmed that hospitals that utilize multiple strategies have significantly greater reductions in 30-day hospital readmissions compared to those that utilize only one or two.[3,54,55]

Hospital Factors That Affect Readmission Rates

In addition to national CMS-reported data, numerous studies have examined readmission rates for specific conditions and patient populations, characterized hospitals with low versus high readmission rates, and evaluated the impact of national and local efforts to reduce hospital readmissions. For instance, studies have consistently shown that large hospitals, teaching hospitals, and safety net hospitals tend to have higher readmission rates and are therefore more likely to be penalized under the HRRP.[45] In particular, safety net hospitals have an average RSRR that is 0.21% higher than non-safety net hospitals and are more likely to be penalized (odds ratio: 2.38).[31,33] However, one study found that readmission rates for safety net hospitals decreased more rapidly than those of non-safety net hospitals (mean RSRR declined from 18.0% in 2008 to 13.6% in 2015 for safety net hospitals versus 15.4% to 12.7% for non-safety net hospitals).[12]

To address the implication that the HRRP may have the unintended consequence of worsening outcomes for socially disadvantaged patients, CMS enacted a policy in 2018 that defines hospitals with similar low-income shares as peers for determining readmission penalties.[4] Efforts to accurately account for sociodemographic factors, index hospital admission rates, and implement equitable, risk-adjusted penalties and incentives for readmissions are ongoing.

THE ROLE OF THE ED IN READMISSIONS

The ED is a primary entry point for both index hospital admissions and readmissions.[56-58] A 2016 study of 216 million hospitalizations found that the ED was the source of admission for 57.3% of elderly patients (age 65 and older) and 44% of adult patients (age 64 and younger), making it the primary source of hospitalizations in the United States.[5] As described earlier in this chapter, CMS measures focus on unplanned readmissions only, omitting elective or planned readmissions. Since the vast majority of ED visits resulting in admission are unplanned, the ED plays a critical role in influencing readmission rates under CMS guidelines.

Over the past decade, researchers and policymakers have identified several evidence-based strategies in which the ED plays a prominent role in reducing readmissions. Departments with lower preventable readmission rates tend to follow the same broad principles, which include robust reporting and monitoring practices, continuous performance assessments to provide feedback and identify evolving targets for improvement, and the utilization of multiple strategies across disciplines.[54,59]

Administrative Levers

Seven strategies are described that EDs can use to deliver value to the hospital and play a strategic role in readmissions. Keep in mind that these strategies require continuous measurement and feedback to be successful. Further, multiple coordinated strategies tend to be more successful than singular interventions.

Decrease Index Hospital Admissions

Efforts to reduce hospital readmissions tend to focus on transitions of care. However, multiple studies have shown that overall admission rates strongly predict readmission rates. For instance, a major study of Medicare data in 2011 found that all-cause admission rates accounted for the highest proportion of variation in readmission rates for heart failure (27.5% at 30 days) and pneumonia (22.8% at 30 days).[60] Reducing index hospital admission rates is therefore a key strategy for reducing hospital readmissions.

The ED can decrease index hospital admissions in different ways. One way is the ED can utilize validated clinical decision support tools such as the CURB-65 tool for pneumonia or the HEART score for low-risk chest pain to reduce admissions for certain conditions. These tools can have a large impact by decreasing the significant practice variation in ED admissions across institutions. For instance, a large national study in 2016 found that risk-standardized admission rates varied drastically across EDs, especially for mood disorders (coefficient of variation: 0.81), nonspecific chest pain (0.66), skin and soft-tissue infections (0.51), urinary tract infections (0.43), and COPD (0.33).[61] This information suggests that some admissions may not be necessary, and using decision support tools or ED admission guidelines for these conditions may result in improved efficiency and cost savings.

Another way for the ED to decrease index hospital admissions is to collaborate with coordinators and consultants to plan high-quality alternatives to admission during the index ED visit.[56] This strategy is most successful when the ED has formal partnerships with other disciplines, such as a practice of routinely contacting primary care providers to arrange next-day follow-up as an alternative to admission. This strategy also requires a robust infrastructure of hospital care managers, navigators, and social workers. For example, having 24-hour care coordination available to ED providers at the index visit can minimize preventable "social" admissions during off-hours and weekends.[62] Access to ED pharmacists who can perform medication reconciliation and patient education at the index ED visit has also been shown to decrease both readmissions and repeat ED visits.[63]

Finally, note that decreasing index hospital admissions does not mean the ED should simply shift to a different type of hospitalization (i.e., from inpatient status to observation status). There was some initial concern that EDs would rely on this strategy to avoid readmission penalties under the HRRP, but this did not turn out to be the case. The CMS data from 2008 to 2016 showed that, while readmission rates decreased, there was no correlated increase in observation status.[64]

Engage With Community Partners

The "community setting" refers to the collection of clinical and nonclinical services outside the hospital and ED. These services include outpatient providers, community paramedic programs, primary care clinics and medical homes, social service agencies, nursing homes or skilled nursing facilities, and home-based care. Studies have shown that care coordination programs can decrease inefficiencies in transitional care and reduce hospital readmissions.[40,62] However, due to the large number of stakeholders involved, it can be overwhelming for providers and policymakers to decide where best to spend resources in order to maximize gains. This inconsistency has led to the mixed success of hospital- and ED-based transitional care programs overall, with some resulting in markedly improved outcomes and cost savings, while others had no effect.[14,65-68]

Nonetheless, some tried-and-true strategies have been shown to effectively reduce PPRs.[40,69,70] A 2014 meta-analysis of 47 trials regarding care coordination strategies for heart failure readmissions found that home care programs and multidisciplinary clinic interventions were most effective for reducing all-cause readmission rates and producing a mortality benefit.[71]

Home care programs have also been shown to be particularly effective at reducing readmissions for elderly patients.[72] Other large studies have found high-intensity strategies that bundle multiple interventions are most effective for patients with chronic illnesses.[73] These include structured ED-to-primary-care communications, scheduled home visits shortly after ED discharge, and ED-based care coordination by designated nurses or care managers. Emergency department discharge planning and follow-up have also been shown to be particularly effective at reducing hospital readmission rates.[74,75] Rapid referral clinics are a notable and successful ED-based intervention in this area.[76]

Health information technology plays a critical role in transitional care efforts by supporting the robust exchange of medical information.[62,77] For instance, EMS information should be immediately available upon ED arrival with standardized fields for EMS vital signs, interventions, and reason for transport. Similarly, ED and community providers should have access to the same integrated information regarding medications from pharmacies, prescription drug monitoring programs, and local clinics. When appropriate, outpatient providers should be alerted when patients arrive or depart the ED, and ED providers should receive call-in and transfer information in a standardized format.[78]

Due to the large number of possible transitional care interventions available to the ED, it is critical to approach this problem strategically before deploying resources. In particular, ED managers should differentiate between system-level interventions that target all ED patients and specific interventions that target the much smaller subset of patients at high risk for chronic readmissions. For instance, not every patient will need automatic alerts to outpatient providers and social services upon ED arrival, but patients managed by numerous specialists for complex medical conditions may benefit greatly from this intervention. ED managers should also pay particular attention to the special needs and capabilities of high-risk patients that may aid or hinder care coordination efforts. As an example, older adults may not benefit from ED follow-up interventions due to underrecognized cognitive impairments.[79]

Educate Patients and Caregivers

Emergency department levers for this strategy—educating patients and caregivers—fall into several broad categories:

- Educating patients about their condition and anticipated treatment and recovery process
- Making shared decisions with patients when appropriate
- Providing robust discharge and follow-up instructions
- Ensuring that community resources are available to both patients and caregivers

Shared-decision making (SDM) between patients and ED providers has been shown to be a particularly successful means of reducing hospital readmissions and resource utilization for a variety of different conditions.[80,81] Shared-decision making is a process in which clinicians and patients make clinical decisions together by balancing evidence-based risks and benefits with patient preferences and values.[82] This approach is typically used for preference-sensitive conditions for which there is evidence of more than one medically acceptable diagnosis or treatment option, such as imaging for low-back pain. A 2016 randomized trial found that a shared decision aid for low-risk chest pain decreased ED admission rates by 15% with no major associated adverse cardiac events.[80] A 2013 randomized study examined SDM more broadly across all conditions by utilizing trained health coaches with decision-support aids. They found that patients who received enhanced support SDM had 12.5% fewer hospital admissions and 5.3% lower overall medical costs compared to patients receiving usual care.[83] In the context of current nationally reported readmission measures, SDM may serve as an important tool in reducing index admissions or subsequent readmissions for patients with mild or moderate illness severity suitable for either inpatient or outpatient management, such as CHF exacerbations.

Develop and Implement ED Protocols for Admissions

Department administrators can screen for patients who are at high risk for ED hospital readmissions and develop specific care pathways for these patients. Numerous risk-prediction models have been developed by researchers to assist with the screening process. These include models originally developed for inpatients that have been adapted to the ED setting, including screening for high- versus low-risk heart failure, hypertension, pneumonia, and other specific disease processes.[83-85] They incorporate variables like comorbidity and illness severity indexes, overall functional status, prior use of medical services, and social determinants of health (e.g., insurance status, education, etc.), among many others.[14,86,87]

Are there certain risk prediction models that have been proven to be consistently accurate? Unfortunately, not yet. Most systematic reviews agree that readmission risk prediction is still poorly understood, with unreliable performance and poor predictive ability.[14] One large review of 60 studies and 73 predictive models from 2011 to 2015 found that only 11 models had modest discrimination ability, and only two assessed PPRs.[86] This is likely due to the fact that numerous systemic, cultural, and sociodemographic factors contribute significantly to risk but are notoriously difficult to quantify. Models are also limited by their heavy reliance on administrative data to predict human behaviors. Nonetheless, the highest and lowest risk scores were associated with clinically meaningful variation in readmission rates, suggesting that the highest-risk patients could benefit from interventions.[14]

The use of risk models alone is insufficient and should be paired with "clinical care pathways" that operationalize patient care plans. With or without a structured risk prediction model, ED care pathways can be developed for patients with different characteristics, conditions, or available community resources. They can also be oriented by stakeholder or intervention type. For instance, care management pathways can transfer elderly patients with poor baseline functional status directly to rehabilitation or skilled nursing facilities. They can also be used to provide home care services for patients with medically intensive chronic conditions, such as cancer or end-stage renal failure.

Overall, evidence-based clinical care pathways have been shown to decrease ED admission rates without increasing return revisits.[88] Successful care pathways share a few common characteristics:

- An interdisciplinary or multidisciplinary approach
- A development process that accounts for barriers and enablers at multiple levels, including individual providers, ED teams, and broader departmental and hospital leadership
- Robust monitoring and feedback mechanisms to address evolving areas for improvement[89]

Utilize ED Observation Units

An OU is a dedicated unit in the ED or hospital that provides protocol-based short-term observational care for patients with well-defined diagnoses before decisions about admission or discharge are made.[90] Rather than directly admitting patients with chest pain, asthma, pyelonephritis, or other specific conditions, ED providers can choose to send them to the OU instead. Observation units have become increasingly popular in the United States over the last few decades (see Chapter 39).[91] However, these units have only been shown to successfully reduce hospital admissions, return ED visits, and medical costs under specific circumstances for certain conditions.[92,93] Department managers should therefore approach this particular strategy with caution. Simply creating an OU does not automatically translate to fewer index admissions or readmissions. In general, OUs have only been shown to decrease ED hospital readmissions if two conditions are met: the unit has high patient volumes and provides high-acuity care.

For example, a 2013 study of statewide data in Georgia showed that patients in OUs with defined protocols had a 17% to 44% lower probability of subsequent inpatient admission and $950 million in potential cost savings each year.[94] Similarly, the Mayo Clinic successfully reduced hospital admission rates by 20% for atrial fibrillation (AF) patients after implementing an ED OU algorithm in 2014. There was no associated increase in return ED visits or adverse cardiac events.[95] Several lessons can be learned from this case:

- The algorithm utilized a high-intensity strategy that bundled multiple interventions including standardized rate control protocols, discharge prescribing criteria, patient education, and prompt outpatient follow-up.
- The Mayo Clinic saw a high volume of high-acuity AF patients with a baseline admission rate of 45%. This represented a significant opportunity for cost savings and improved care coordination.
- The AF patients could receive the same high acuity care in the OU as they could in the ED, including cardioversion, diltiazem drips, and direct access to cardiologists.

Utilize ED Telehealth

Numerous studies have shown that telehealth or telemedicine is associated with fewer unplanned health-care encounters, improved monitoring, and increased patient compliance with therapy across a variety of conditions.[96-98] While the evidence linking telemedicine to reduced readmissions is weaker, this emerging intervention is still promising, particularly in low-resource or rural ED environments. For instance, a 2015 study of pediatric patients at eight rural EDs found that the patients with access to telemedicine had significantly fewer hospital admissions compared to patients who only used traditional telephone communications (59.5% vs 87.5%).[99]

In terms of quality, telemedicine has been found to have similar patient outcomes as in-person nursing visits for elderly patients.[100] Although this evidence is promising, ED managers do have to consider the significant upfront costs in equipment, infrastructure, and training required to develop an in-house ED telemedicine program. However, as these services continue to expand nationwide, they are becoming increasingly more accessible and cost-effective.

Support Alternative Payment Models

Support alternative payment models to incentivize care coordination. For instance, hospitals can move toward global budgets that provide multidisciplinary rewards for care coordination, offer direct payments for coordination activities like ED-based outpatient referrals, or directly invest in transitions-of-care or disposition-planning programs (e.g., initiatives to reduce unplanned ED return visits).[101] Policymakers could also develop new reimbursement codes for OUs or referral clinics that provide intensive care coordination services or for primary care physicians who coordinate follow-up with ED providers.[102] In addition, new payment models could be linked to accreditation programs that include recommended standards for transitions of care, such as electronic health records with the ability to communicate across all health-care settings.[103]

CONTROVERSIES AND LIMITATIONS

National measurement and improvement efforts focused on readmissions have advanced significantly over the past decade. However, several controversies have come to light, particularly regarding potential unintended consequences.

Overly Narrow Focus

Focusing on a single measure related to "readmissions" may cause hospitals to ignore other related measures or systemic factors for a complex medical problem.[27] Some experts have argued that hospital readmission rates are more accurately a measure of utilization than a measure of quality. Under this definition, it may be counterproductive to conserve resources for admissions by spending excess resources in other areas. Similarly, the resources spent by EDs and hospitals to avoid the HRRP penalty may create significant opportunity costs for other important but unmeasured activities.[104] Using "30-days" as the standard time interval may also be shortsighted and ignore long-term downstream effects at 90 days, 1 year, and beyond.

Decreasing Admissions

Reducing readmission rates does not automatically translate to improved quality or better patient outcomes. As noted by a 2013 Robert Wood Johnson Foundation report, "keeping patients healthy after hospitalization is without question a good patient outcome. This does not mean, however, that reducing readmission rates necessarily means that patients are generally doing better."[27] In fact, declining readmission rates may be associated with increased mortality for some conditions. A 2018 study of 8.3 million hospitalizations found that the implementation of the HRRP readmissions penalty was associated with increased mortality rates within 30 days of discharge for patients with heart failure and pneumonia (0.52% and 0.44% increase, respectively).[105] A separate research group in 2018 found similar results for longer-term outcomes in heart failure patients. While the 1-year risk-adjusted readmission rate declined from 57.2% to 56.3% after HRRP implementation, the 1-year risk-adjusted mortality rate increased significantly from 31.3% to 36.3%.[106]

Limited Incentive Structure

Payment incentives tied to a single measure may result in disproportionate penalties to some hospitals. This is a particular concern for academic medical centers and safety net hospitals, which have higher readmission rates.[107] As with all single measures, it is important to be aware of the limitations and useful application of hospital readmission rates when creating ED policies. Overreliance on the measure rather than the bigger clinical or operational picture can result in unintended consequences and negative outcomes.

CONCLUSION

A "hospital readmission" occurs when a patient is discharged from the hospital and admitted again within a specified time interval. High readmission rates can contribute to health-care costs, negatively impact patient outcomes, burden providers and caregivers, and exacerbate ED and hospital crowding. Significant efforts have been made over the past decade to improve hospital admission policies. These include the creation of readmission benchmarks, financial penalties under the HRRP, patient and community education programs, new hospital admission and observation protocols, and improved discharge planning and care coordination processes. As a result, readmission rates have declined since 2010.

However, there is still room for further improvement. The ED is the biggest source of unscheduled hospitalizations in the United States, and ED leaders play a critical role in reducing readmissions and improving performance on related national metrics. The administrative levers available to emergency physicians include:

- Decreasing initial or "index" hospital admissions by using clinical decision support tools and collaborating with consultants and care coordinators
- Engaging with community resources, including outpatient providers, community paramedics, social service agencies, and home-based care

- Educating patients and caregivers by using SDM tools and providing robust ED discharge resources and follow-up instructions
- Developing ED admission protocols for patients at high-risk for readmissions
- Utilizing ED OUs
- Utilizing ED telehealth
- Supporting alternative payment models that incentivize care coordination and quality of care

Going forward, ED leaders should be prepared to tackle challenges regarding new federal quality measures, the scope of readmissions policies, the incentive structure surrounding readmission rates, and the long-term impact of reducing readmissions on patient outcomes.

REFERENCES

1. Jencks SF, Williams MV, Coleman EA. Rehospitalizations among patients in the Medicare fee-for-service program. *N Engl J Med.* 2009;360(14):1418–1428.
2. Krumholz HM. Post-hospital syndrome–an acquired, transient condition of generalized risk. *N Engl J Med.* 2013;368(2):100–102.
3. Kripalani S, Theobald CN, Anctil B, et al. Reducing hospital readmission rates: current strategies and future directions. *Annu Rev Med.* 2014;65:471–485.
4. Medicare Payment Advisory Commission (MedPAC). Report to the Congress: Medicare and the Health Care Delivery System. 2018. Available at: http://www.medpac.gov/docs/default-source/reports/jun18_medpacreporttocongress_rev_nov2019_note_sec.pdf?sfvrsn=0. Accessed August 2, 2020.
5. Greenwald PW, Estevez RM, Clark S, et al. The ED as the primary source of hospital admission for older (but not younger) adults. *Am J Emerg Med.* 2016;34(6):943–947.
6. Hospital Readmissions Reduction Program (HRRP) Archives. Centers for Medicare & Medicaid Services (CMS). Available at: https://www.cms.gov/Medicare/Medicare-Fee-for-Service-Payment/AcuteInpatientPPS/HRRP-Archives.html. Accessed May 29, 2019.
7. Sabbatini AK, Wright B. Excluding observation stays from readmission rates—what quality measures are missing. *N Engl J Med.* 2018;378(22):2062–2065.
8. van Walraven C, Bennett C, Jennings A, et al. Proportion of hospital readmissions deemed avoidable: a systematic review. *CMAJ.* 2011;183(7):E391–E402.
9. Auerbach AD, Kripalani S, Vasilevskis EE, et al. Preventability and causes of readmissions in a national cohort of general medicine patients. *JAMA Intern Med.* 2016;176(4):484–493.
10. van Walraven C, Jennings A, Forster AJ. A meta-analysis of hospital 30-day avoidable readmission rates. *J Eval Clin Pract.* 2012;18(6):1211–1218.
11. Donzé J, Aujesky D, Williams D, et al. Potentially avoidable 30-day hospital readmissions in medical patients: derivation and validation of a prediction model. *JAMA Intern Med.* 2013;173(8):632–638.
12. Salerno AM, Horwitz LI, Kwon JY, et al. Trends in readmission rates for safety net hospitals and non-safety net hospitals in the era of the US Hospital Readmission Reduction Program: a retrospective time series analysis using Medicare administrative claims data from 2008 to 2015. *BMJ Open.* 2017;7(7):e016149.
13. Dulohery M, Lim K, Peterson S, et al. COPD hospital readmissions: what should be considered potentially preventable? In: *D13 The Revolving Door: COPD Hospitalization and Readmission.* Abstract presented at: American Thoracic Society 2017 International Conference, May 10-24, 2017; Washington, DC. Available at: https://www.atsjournals.org/doi/book/10.1164/ajrccm-conference.2017.D13
14. Kansagara D, Englander H, Salanitro A, et al. Risk prediction models for hospital readmission: a systematic review. *JAMA.* 2011;306(15):1688–1698.
15. Lindquist LA, Baker DW. Understanding preventable hospital readmissions: masqueraders, markers, and true causal factors. *J Hosp Med.* 2011;6(2).
16. Klein, S. In focus: preventing unnecessary hospital readmissions. The Commonwealth Fund. https://www.commonwealthfund.org/publications/newsletter-article/focus-preventing-unnecessary-hospital-readmissions. Accessed August 2, 2020.
17. Yale New Haven Health Services Corporation/Center for Outcomes Research & Evaluation (YNHHSC/CORE). 2014 measure updates and specifications report: hospital-wide all-cause unplanned readmission–version 3.0. 2014. Available at: https://altarum.org/sites/default/files/uploaded-publication-files/Rdmsn_Msr_Updts_HWR_0714_0.pdf. Accessed September 11, 2020.
18. Hospital Readmissions Reduction Program (HRRP). Centers for Medicare & Medicaid Services (CMS). 2018. Available at: https://www.cms.gov/medicare/quality-initiatives-patient-assessment-instruments/value-based-programs/hrrp/hospital-readmission-reduction-program.html. Accessed May 29, 2019.
19. CMS Measures Inventory Tool: Excess days in acute care (EDAC) after hospitalization for heart failure. Centers for Medicare & Medicaid Services (CMS). 2019. Available at: https://cmit.cms.gov/CMIT_public/ViewMeasure?MeasureId=2708. Accessed Aug 2, 2020.
20. 3M Heath Information Systems. Potentially Preventable Readmissions Classification System: Methodology Overview. 2012. Available at: http://multimedia.3m.com/mws/media/849903O/3m-ppr-grouping-software-fact-sheet.pdf. Accessed August 2, 2020.
21. 3M Heath Information Systems. 3M Potentially Preventable Readmissions (PPR) Grouping Software. Available at: http://multimedia.3m.com/mws/media/1042610O/resources-and-references-his-2015.pdf. Accessed August 2, 2020.
22. Feigenbaum P, Neuwirth E, Trowbridge L, et al. Factors contributing to all-cause 30-day readmissions: a structured case series across 18 hospitals. *Med Care.* 2012;50(7):599–605.
23. Rico F, Liu Y, Martinez DA, et al. Preventable readmission risk factors for patients with chronic conditions. *J Healthc Qual.* 2016;38(3):127–142.
24. Jiang HJ, Andrews R, Stryer D, et al. Racial/ethnic disparities in potentially preventable readmissions: the case of diabetes. *Am J Public Health.* 2005;95(9):1561–1567.
25. Proctor EK, Morrow-Howell N, Li H, et al. Adequacy of home care and hospital readmission for elderly congestive heart failure patients. *Health Soc Work.* 2000;25(2):87-96.

26. Goldfield NI, McCullough EC, Hughes JS, et al. Identifying potentially preventable readmissions. *Health Care Financ Rev.* 2008;30(1):75–91.
27. The Robert Wood Johnson Foundation. The revolving door: a report on US hospital readmissions. An analysis of Medicare data by the Dartmouth Atlas Project. 2013. Available at: https://www.rwjf.org/content/dam/farm/reports/reports/2013/rwjf404178. Accessed August 2, 2020.
28. Centers for Medicare & Medicaid Services (CMS). Hospital Compare: The Official US Government Site for Medicare. Available at: https://www.medicare.gov/hospitalcompare/search.html?. Accessed August 2, 2020.
29. Centers for Medicare & Medicaid Services (CMS). Quality Initiatives Patient Assessment Instruments: Hospital Compare. Available at: https://www.cms.gov/Medicare/Quality-Initiatives-Patient-Assessment-Instruments/HospitalQualityInits/HospitalCompare.html. Accessed August 2, 2020
30. Centers for Medicare & Medicaid Services (CMS). Medicare Hospital Quality Chartbook: Performance Report on Outcome Measures. 2014. Available at: https://www.cms.gov/medicare/quality-initiatives-patient-assessment-instruments/hospitalqualityinits/downloads/medicare-hospital-quality-chartbook-2014.pdf. Accessed August 2, 2020.
31. Horwitz LI, Bernheim SM, Ross JS, et al. Hospital characteristics associated with risk-standardized readmission rates. *Med Care.* 2017;55(5):528–534.
32. Angraal S, Khera R, Zhou S, et al. Trends in 30-day readmission rates for Medicare and non-Medicare patients in the era of the Affordable Care Act. *Am J Med.* 2018;131(11):1324–1331.e14.
33. Joynt KE, Jha AK. Characteristics of hospitals receiving penalties under the Hospital Readmissions Reduction Program. *JAMA.* 2013;309(4):342–343.
34. Himmelstein D, Woolhandler S. Quality improvement: become good at cheating and you never need to become good at anything else. *Health Affairs* blog. 2015.
35. Sacks GD, Lawson EH, Dawes AJ, et al. Which patients require more care after hospital discharge? An analysis of post-acute care use among elderly patients undergoing elective surgery. *J Am Coll Surg.* 2015;220(6):1113–1121.e2.
36. Bjorvatn A. Hospital readmission among elderly patients. *Eur J Health Econ.* 2013;14(5):809–820.
37. Fuji KT, Abbott AA, Norris JF. Exploring care transitions from patient, caregiver, and health-care provider perspectives. *Clin Nurs Res.* 2013;22(3):258–274.
38. Farber N, Shinkle D, Lynott J, et al. Aging in place: a state survey of livability policies and practices. National Conference of State Legislatures (NCSL) and the AARP Public Policy Institute. 2011. Available at: https://www.ncsl.org/documents/transportation/Aging-in-Place-2011.pdf. Accessed August 2, 2020.
39. Covinsky KE, Pierluissi E, Johnston CB. Hospitalization-associated disability: "She was probably able to ambulate, but I'm not sure." *JAMA.* 2011;306(16):1782–1793.
40. Wallace E, Smith SM, Fahey T, et al. Reducing emergency admissions through community based interventions. *BMJ.* 2016;352:h6817.
41. Needleman J, Buerhaus P, Pankratz VS, et al. Nurse staffing and inpatient hospital mortality. *N Engl J Med.* 2011;364(11):1037–1045.
42. Weissman JS, Rothschild JM, Bendavid E, et al. Hospital workload and adverse events. *Med Care.* 2007;45(5):448–455.
43. Report to the Congress: Promoting Greater Efficiency in Medicare. Medicare Payment Advisory Commission (MEDPAC). 2007. Available at: http://www.medpac.gov/docs/default-source/reports/Jun07_EntireReport.pdf. Accessed September 11, 2020.
44. Report to the Congress: Medicare and the Health Care Delivery System. Medicare Payment Advisory Commission (MEDPAC). 2013. Available at: http://medpac.gov/docs/default-source/reports/jun19_medpac_reporttocongress_sec.pdf. Accessed September 11, 2020.
45. Figueroa JF, Joynt KE, Zhou X, et al. Safety-net hospitals face more barriers yet use fewer strategies to reduce readmissions. *Med Care.* 2017;55(3):229–235.
46. Hong Y, Zheng C, Hechenbleikner E, et al. Vulnerable hospitals and cancer surgery readmissions: insights into the unintended consequences of the Patient Protection and Affordable Care Act. *J Am Coll Surg.* 2016;223(1):142–151.
47. Sheingold SH, Zuckerman R, Shartzer A. Understanding Medicare hospital readmission rates and differing penalties between safety-net and other hospitals. *Health Aff.* 2016;35(1):124–131.
48. Mayr FB, Talisa VB, Balakumar V, et al. Proportion and cost of unplanned 30-day readmissions after sepsis compared with other medical conditions. *JAMA.* 2017;317(5):530–531.
49. Clement RC, Kheir MM, Derman PB, et al. What are the economic consequences of unplanned readmissions after TKA? *Clin Orthop Relat Res.* 2014;472(10):3134–3141.
50. Berenson J, Shih A. Higher readmissions at safety-net hospitals and potential policy solutions. *Issue Brief (Commonw Fund).* 2012;34:1–16.
51. The American Hospital Association (AHA). *Fact Sheet: Hospital Readmissions Reduction Program.* 2016. Available at: https://www.aha.org/system/files/2018-01/fs-readmissions.pdf. Accessed August 2, 2020.
52. Conley J, O'Brien CW, Leff BA, et al. Alternative strategies to inpatient hospitalization for acute medical conditions: a systematic review. *JAMA Intern Med.* 2016;176(11):1693–1702.
53. Nuckols TK, Keeler E, Morton S, et al. Economic evaluation of quality improvement interventions designed to prevent hospital readmission: a systematic review and meta-analysis. *JAMA Intern Med.* 2017;177(7):975–985.
54. Bradley EH, Sipsma H, Horwitz LI, et al. Hospital strategy uptake and reductions in unplanned readmission rates for patients with heart failure: a prospective study. *J Gen Intern Med.* 2015;30(5):605–611.
55. Bradley EH, Curry L, Horwitz LI, et al. Contemporary evidence about hospital strategies for reducing 30-day readmissions: a national study. *J Am Coll Cardiol.* 2012;60(7):607–614.
56. Schuur JD, Venkatesh AK. The growing role of emergency departments in hospital admissions. *N Engl J Med.* 2012;367(5):391–393.
57. Singh S, Lin Y-L, Nattinger AB, et al. Variation in readmission rates by emergency departments and emergency department providers caring for patients after discharge. *J Hosp Med.* 2015;10(11):705–710.
58. Kocher RP, Adashi EY. Hospital readmissions and the Affordable Care Act: paying for coordinated quality care. *JAMA.* 2011;306(16):1794–1795.
59. Silow-Carroll S, Edwards JN, Lashbrook A. *Reducing Hospital Readmissions: Lessons from Top-Performing Hospitals.* The Commonwealth Fund. 2011. https://www.althfund.org/publications/case-study/2011/apr/reducing-hospital-readmissions-lessons-top-performing-hospitals. Published April 6, 2011, Accessed October 9, 2020.
60. Epstein AM, Jha AK, Orav EJ. The relationship between hospital admission rates and rehospitalizations. *N Engl J Med.* 2011;365(24):2287–2295.
61. Venkatesh AK, Dai Y, Ross JS, et al. Variation in US hospital emergency department admission rates by clinical condition. *Med Care.* 2015;53(3):237–244.
62. National Quality Forum. *Emergency Department Transitions of Care: A Quality Measurement Framework Final Report.* National Quality Forum. 2017. https://www.qualityforum.org/Publications/2017/08/Emergency_Department_Transitions_of_Care_-_A_Quality_Measurement_Framework_Final_Report.aspx. Published August 2017, Accessed October 9, 2020.
63. Phatak A, Prusi R, Ward B, et al. Impact of pharmacist involvement in the transitional care of high-risk patients through medication reconciliation, medication education, and postdischarge call-backs (IPITCH Study). *J Hosp Med.* 2016;11(1):39–44.
64. Zuckerman RB, Sheingold SH, Orav EJ, et al. Readmissions, observation, and the Hospital Readmissions Reduction Program. *N Engl J Med.* 2016;374(16):1543–1551.

65. Joint Commission Resources. Project RED. Available at: https://www.jointcommissionjournal.com/article/S1553-7250(17)30481-6/abstract Accessed May 29, 2019.
66. Hansen LO, Greenwald JL, Budnitz T, et al. Project BOOST: effectiveness of a multihospital effort to reduce rehospitalization. *J Hosp Med*. 2013;8(8):421–427.
67. Crocker JB, Crocker JT, Greenwald JL. Telephone follow-up as a primary care intervention for postdischarge outcomes improvement: a systematic review. *Am J Med*. 2012;125(9):915–921.
68. Kwan JL, Lo L, Sampson M, et al. Medication reconciliation during transitions of care as a patient safety strategy: a systematic review. *Ann Intern Med*. 2013;158(5 Pt 2):397–403.
69. Vigod SN, Kurdyak PA, Dennis CL, et al. Transitional interventions to reduce early psychiatric readmissions in adults: systematic review. *Br J Psychiatry*. 2013;202(3):187–194.
70. Hickman LD, Phillips JL, Newton PJ, et al. Multidisciplinary team interventions to optimise health outcomes for older people in acute care settings: a systematic review. *Arch Gerontol Geriatr*. 2015;61(3):322–329.
71. Feltner C, Jones CD, Cene CW, et al. Transitional care interventions to prevent readmissions for persons with heart failure: a systematic review and meta-analysis. *Ann Intern Med*. 2014;160(11):774–784.
72. Linertová R, García-Pérez L, Vázquez-Díaz JR, et al. Interventions to reduce hospital readmissions in the elderly: in-hospital or home care. A systematic review. *J Eval Clin Pract*. 2011;17(6):1167–1175.
73. Verhaegh KJ, MacNeil-Vroomen JL, Eslami S, et al. Transitional care interventions prevent hospital readmissions for adults with chronic illnesses. *Health Aff*. 2014;33(9):1531–1539.
74. Hansen LO, Young RS, Hinami K, et al. Interventions to reduce 30-day rehospitalization: a systematic review. *Ann Intern Med*. 2011;155(8):520–528.
75. Hesselink G, Schoonhoven L, Barach P, et al. Improving patient handovers from hospital to primary care: a systematic review. *Ann Intern Med*. 2012;157(6):417–428.
76. Slaughter GRD, Shadowitz S. Reducing hospital admissions from the emergency department. *Harvard Business Rev*. October 15, 2013.
77. Rider AC, Kessler CS, Schwarz WW, et al. Transition of care from the emergency department to the outpatient setting: a mixed-methods analysis. *West J Emerg Med*. 2018;19(2):245–253.
78. Ben-Assuli O. Electronic health records, adoption, quality of care, legal and privacy issues and their implementation in emergency departments. *Health Policy*. 2015;119(3):287–297.
79. Marengoni A, Winblad B, Karp A, et al. Prevalence of chronic diseases and multimorbidity among the elderly population in Sweden. *Am J Public Health*. 2008;98(7):1198–1200.
80. Hess EP, Hollander JE, Schaffer JT, et al. Shared decision making in patients with low risk chest pain: prospective randomized pragmatic trial. *BMJ*. 2016;355:i6165.
81. Flynn D, Knoedler MA, Hess EP, et al. Engaging patients in health care decisions in the emergency department through shared decision-making: a systematic review. *Acad Emerg Med*. 2012;19(8):959–967.
82. Veroff D, Marr A, Wennberg, DE. Enhanced support for shared decision making reduced costs of care for patients with preference-sensitive conditions. *Health Aff*. 2013;32(2):285–293.
83. Wallace E, Stuart E, Vaughan N, et al. Risk prediction models to predict emergency hospital admission in community-dwelling adults. *Med Care*. 2014;52(8):751–765.
84. Rahimi K, Bennett D, Conrad N, et al. Risk prediction in patients with heart failure: a systematic review and analysis. *JACC Heart Fail*. 2014;2(5):440–446.
85. Amarasingham R, Moore BJ, Tabak YP, et al. An automated model to identify heart failure patients at risk for 30-day readmission or death using electronic medical record data. *Med Care*. 2010;48(11):981–988.
86. Zhou H, Della PR, Roberts P, et al. Utility of models to predict 28-day or 30-day unplanned hospital readmissions: an updated systematic review. *BMJ Open*. 2016;6(6):e011060.
87. Billings J, Blunt I, Steventon A, et al. Development of a predictive model to identify inpatients at risk of re-admission within 30 days of discharge (PARR-30). *BMJ Open*. 2012;2(4):e001667.
88. Norton SP, Pusic MV, Taha F, et al. Effect of a clinical pathway on the hospitalisation rates of children with asthma: a prospective study. *Arch Dis Child*. 2007;92(1):60–66.
89. Allegri MD, Schwarzbach M, Loerbroks A, et al. Which factors are important for the successful development and implementation of clinical pathways? A qualitative study. *BMJ Qual Saf*. 2011;20(3):203–208.
90. Napolitano JD, Saini I. Observation units: definition, history, data, financial considerations, and metrics. *Curr Emerg Hosp Med Rep*. 2014;2(1):1–8.
91. Huffman A. Use of observation units growing: but variable billing practices sometimes leave patients on the financial hook. *Ann Emerg Med*. 2013;61(2):A21–A23.
92. Schrock JW, Reznikova S, Weller S. The effect of an observation unit on the rate of ED admission and discharge for pyelonephritis. *Am J Emerg Med*. 2010;28(6):682–688.
93. Rydman RJ, Isola ML, Roberts RR, et al. Emergency department observation unit versus hospital inpatient care for a chronic asthmatic population: a randomized trial of health status outcome and cost. *Med Care*. 1998;36(4):599–609.
94. Ross MA, Hockenberry JM, Mutter R, et al. Protocol-driven emergency department observation units offer savings, shorter stays, and reduced admissions. *Health Aff*. 2013;32(12):2149–2156.
95. Bellew SD, Bremer ML, Kopeky SL, et al. Impact of an emergency department observation unit management algorithm for atrial fibrillation. *J Am Heart Assoc*. 2016;5(2):e002984.
96. Hwang U, Shah MN, Han JH, et al. Transforming emergency care for older adults. *Health Aff*. 2013:32(12):2116–2121.
97. Raaber N, Botker MT, Riddervold IS, et al. Telemedicine-based physician consultation results in more patients treated and released by ambulance personnel. *Eur J Emer Med*. 2018;25.
98. Langabeer JR, Champagne-Langabeer T, Alqusairi D, et al. Cost-benefit analysis of telehealth in pre-hospital care. *J Telemed Telecare*. 2017;23(8):747–751.
99. Yang NH, Dharmar M, Kuppermann N, et al. Appropriateness of disposition following telemedicine consultations in rural emergency departments. *Pediatr Crit Care Med*. 2015;16(3):e59.
100. Antonicelli R, Testarmata P, Spazzafumo L, et al. Impact of telemonitoring at home on the management of elderly patients with congestive heart failure. *J Telemed Telecare*. 2008;14(6):300–305.
101. Selevan J, Kindermann D, Pines JM, et al. What accountable care organizations can learn from Kaiser Permanente California's acute care strategy. *Popul Health Manag*. 2015;18(4):233–236.
102. Blecker S, Gavin NP, Park H, et al. Observation units as substitutes for hospitalization or home discharge. *Ann Emerg Med*. 2016;67(6):706–713.e2.
103. Pines JM, McStay F, George M, et al. Aligning payment reform and delivery innovation in emergency care. *Am J Manag Care*. 2016;22(8):515–518.
104. Joynt KE, Jha AK. Thirty-day readmissions-truth and consequences. *N Engl J Med*. 2012;366(15):1366–1369.
105. Wadhera RK, Joynt Maddox KE, Wasfy JH, et al. Association of the Hospital Readmissions Reduction Program with mortality among Medicare beneficiaries hospitalized for heart failure, acute myocardial infarction, and pneumonia. *JAMA*. 2018;320(24):2542–2552.
106. Gupta A, Allen LA, Bhatt DL, et al. Association of the Hospital Readmissions Reduction Program implementation with readmission and mortality outcomes in heart failure. *JAMA Cardiol*. 2018;3(1):44–53.
107. Fonarow GC, Yancy CW. Consequences of reductions in hospital readmissions. *JAMA*. 2017;318(19):1933–1934.

FINANCE

SECTION 7

CHAPTER 83

DEVELOPING A BUSINESS PLAN

Brooks Babcock, Robert W. Strauss, Thom A. Mayer

Failing to plan is planning to fail.

John Wooden, 10-time NCAA Men's Basketball Division I coach at UCLA[1]

An uninformed clinician might ask, "Why is a business plan necessary? The solution is obvious and doesn't require all that work!" A business plan is a matter of effective communication. It is necessary to speak the language of those who must be convinced of the importance and necessity of the proposed solution to a problem. The necessary steps for progress may be obvious among emergency department (ED) leaders. However, an effectively crafted business plan clearly describes both the opportunity and the desired outcomes to the ED's administrative business partners, who are responsible for implementing institutional programs and may not initially recognize their value.

It is perhaps easier for clinicians to recognize the importance of speaking "their language" when communicating with other clinicians (**Table 83.1**). Similar to a clinical description, the business plan communicates the *vision* of the intended program (medical care) and persuades the listener to support the described goals (desired patient care). It enlightens the listener by giving enough detailed information to concisely address most questions that might arise and, in the case of the business plan, also describes the scope of the project, time lines, costs, profitability, and metrics by which progress can be measured.

TABLE 83.1 ■ Examples of Effective Communication		
Specialist	**Poor Request**	**More Effective Request**
Orthopedist	"I've got a guy with a busted wrist."	"... trans scaphoid peri-lunate fracture dislocation."
Psychiatrist	"I need you to take care of this crazy person!"	"... agitated, paranoid with active delusions and command hallucinations, requiring chemical sedation. The patient is medically clear."
Cardiologist	"A 63-year-old whom I just don't feel comfortable discharging."	"... a significant family history, three risk factors, including a highly suspicious story, a nonspecific repolarization abnormality, and a heart score of 6."
Oncologist	"Her WBC is low and she's sick!"	"She has a neutropenic fever."

While this chapter focuses on a business plan for a private, fee-for-service emergency physician group, the same principles apply to all groups. Regardless of the entity compiling the plan, the following key principles must be considered:

- Seek input, using the principle that, "If they aren't with you on the *take-off*, they won't be with you on the *landing*."
- Integrate the perspectives of the:
  - Entire ED team, especially taking advantage of the critical relationship with the nursing staff
  - Key stakeholders among the medical staff
  - Administrative leadership team
- Ensure that there is a chance for the stakeholders to give their opinions, even—or especially—if there are areas of disagreement.
- Anticipate the resistance that accompanies all change.
- Write the plan in clear, declarative sentences, using the active voice. Edit and then reedit the document. Clarity comes from thoughtful revisions.
- Be succinct, remembering Churchill's statement: "This document, by its very length, ensures that it will never be read."[2]

The 7 Ws

In its simplest expression, a business plan is a document detailing seven Ws: **w**hy, **w**hat, **w**here, **w**ho, **w**hen, ho**w** much, and **w**hat next? A business plan represents the summation and quantification of critical components, assumptions, and projections used to support the organization's goals and objectives. A well-functioning strategy is an essential component of an organization's operations. *Initially, a business plan is a tool that helps to evaluate and summarize a business opportunity.* Assuming an organization pursues the opportunity, the plan allows postimplementation monitoring and reporting. The development and implementation of a business plan follows the old adage, "plan the work and work the plan."

What a Business Plan Is and What It Is Not

There are several approaches to and uses for a business plan. For example, a business plan may be used to evaluate potential investment opportunities, that is, a *prospectus* for an external audience. These investment-oriented business plans typically describe the opportunity to a currently noninvested audience. The intended consumer of this type of business plan may or may not be familiar with the type of venture described and may or may not take an active and ongoing role in the management of the venture proposed.

While the investment-oriented business plan just described may conjure up images of Wall Street, venture capitalists, and initial public offerings, a business plan focused on the ED will likely be more utilitarian in nature. This type of plan serves as a guide to ED financial operations, as well as to future growth and profitability.

An ED business plan typically represents how the organization will pursue and manage the business of the department. The business plan is typically a written document developed by the practice manager(s) and ED leaders, with appropriate input by competent, professional business managers including accounting and legal professionals. Because of the hectic and sometimes unpredictable pace of the ED, the concept of planning might sound like wishful thinking. To the contrary, a well thought-out approach is essential to the successful management of the ED or of some specific program within it, for example, pediatrics, geriatrics, EMS, alternatives to opioids, and so on.

A good business plan can be characterized as a potential set of directions for the business to follow; this implies that the organization's leaders actually know where they want it to go and why they want it to go there. As management consultant Peter Drucker says, "Management by objectives works if you first think through your objectives. Ninety percent of the time you haven't."[3] An effective business plan is like a set of guardrails which do not *restrict* but rather *guide* the best direction for the effort.

THE "WHY"

The Drucker statement highlights the need for planning that supports the creation of a business plan. When creating a business plan, it is important to initially address the first W: the *why*. In the planning continuum, this basic consideration is commonly referred to as a strategic planning approach. Strategic plans are perhaps more philosophical in nature and certainly address more long-range issues than the average business plan. Strategic planning deals with the big picture and helps to define and reinforce the reason(s) for an organization's existence, that is, the organization's mission. In most corporate cultures, any discussion of mission also includes a discussion of vision and values, or mission, vision, and values (MVV; see Chapter 2).

Vision Statement

Vision and mission statements are distinct yet highly interrelated parts of a business. The vision statement answers why the group exists, while the mission statement answers what the organization is attempting to do. The vision statement should be a succinct and easily understood statement outlining the group's purpose, answering the questions:

- Why are we here—what is our purpose?
- Who are we?
- How do we define ourselves to others?

Vision and mission statements should be reviewed and reaffirmed frequently. Many successful groups include a reading of the vision and mission statements as a key element of each business meeting.

Organizations can and frequently do spend hours and days defining their vision and mission statements. It is not uncommon to see an organization's mission statement prominently displayed in offices and on websites as a way of telling others who they are while also reminding themselves of who they want to be. The vision and mission statements should be included in the business plan, usually either as the frontispiece or in the executive summary.

Mission Statement

The mission statement defines what a group envisions accomplishing and answers the following three questions:

1. What is the group attempting to do?
2. What steps need to be taken to be successful?
3. What goals will be set to aid in measuring success?

In other words, the mission provides the foundation for the strategic direction that will allow the group to accomplish the vision. Refer to the following example.

"We will:

- organize a highly talented emergency medicine team into a model business of owners and leaders empowered to provide high-quality, patient-focused emergency care,
- develop and implement clinical and administrative practices for excellence, efficiency, and growth, and
- partner with others to deliver exceptional emergency services."

Values Statement

The values statement serves as the touchstone for decision-making that keeps an organization true to itself by answering the questions:

- Which core and fundamental beliefs guide the organization?
- What do we value about the team members?
- Do the deeds and actions support how the vision and mission?

The values statement embodies the corporate *moral compass*. While properly chosen values should be revisited and sharpened, they are typically deeply held core concepts that do not fundamentally change. Below is an example of an ED values statement.

"Emergency Doctor Associates (EDA) is committed to:

- Functioning in partnership with our nursing and essential services staff as a world-class, high-performing team,
- Treating each other with dignity, compassion, and respect, and
- Bringing the same excellence and integrity to the business practice that the team brings to patient care."

Successful organizations frequently hold dedicated strategic planning retreats. Young organizations may have ongoing sessions during their start-up phases, while more mature enterprises may hold these sessions on an annual or semiannual basis. A strategic plan may encompass, but is not the same as, a business plan. The strategic plan supports the vision and mission; the business plan supports the strategic plan. If the strategic plan sets the roadmap to the horizon, the business plan will identify the waypoints. The business plan acts as the global positioning system for an organization, asking and answering the question:

Are we on track and if not, how do we get back on course?

Some detours may occur along the way, but the final destination remains the same. Thus, frequent review of the strategic plan, and the strategies and tactics selected for accomplishing its objectives, is key. Finally:

- The strategic plan is more *strategic*. (Are the right choices being made?)
- The business plan is more *tactical*. (How specifically will it be accomplished?)

DEVELOPING THE PLAN

The process of holding a successful meeting provides a good analogy for a business plan (see Chapter 9). Most productive meetings have a written agenda, providing a roadmap for the intended accomplishments. That agenda is circulated in advance so the team can give it appropriate consideration. The elements of a refined agenda contain all the elements of a business plan:

- Objective(s)/key considerations
- Actions items
- Potential barriers to success
- Accountability
- Quantification (measures by which success or failure can be measured)
- Regular progress reviews and follow-up

Accordingly, an effective business plan can be described as the business management agenda. The business plan of a fictitious group, EDA, serves as an illustration. This example is internally focused and operational in nature. The plan—addressing a business expansion opportunity—will demonstrate the group's comprehensive analysis and decision-making as well as future review and performance monitoring. The following is the background information:

- EDA has been in business for the past 10 years as a multiowner, democratic group partnership.
- EDA is the exclusive provider of emergency services for the Local Hospital Corporation of Cold Springs, North Carolina (LHC).
- EDA's current contract with LHC is subject to renewal in two years.
- EDA has been approached by the hospital CEO regarding the group's interest in covering LHC's newest facility in Jackson Junction, which LHC considers a key strategic opportunity.
- LHC has informed EDA that for planning purposes, EDA should anticipate the same payer mix and managed care reimbursement rates that they have at Cold Springs.
- In order to properly respond, EDA's management committee has established a committee, whose role is to develop a business plan relating to this opportunity and present it to the owners for a vote.
- EDA's working committee has compiled what they believe to be the salient facts to be included in their review.

EDA's committee worked closely with a financial advisor to compile a business plan (**Appendix 83.1**).

The Business Plan Document

A typical business plan document of this type is relatively short. For an internally oriented plan, a document of five to 10 concisely worded pages with supporting information (i.e., financial and demographic data) is usually sufficient. The document should clearly indicate and explain sources of information as well as the basis for any assumptions and define or avoid uncommon acronyms or insider terms. It is appropriate to present the information as if it is written for someone unfamiliar with the topics and with enough detail to provide a general understanding of the intended meaning.

Above all, the plan must be scrupulously and brutally honest. Flowery language and overly optimistic projections create false impressions that may be misleading and later become the subject of intense scrutiny. One of the key elements of the plan is accountability. Included information must be vetted and accurate. Inaccurate data or assumptions will invalidate the conclusions, or as the expression goes, "Garbage in, garbage out." As an example, if the fastest provider is able to see 2.25 patients per hour, then a plan based on all providers managing 2.75 patients per hour doesn't pass the "sniff test."

The business plan should include financial and operational projections on worst-case, base-case, and best-case scenarios.

Title Page

The title page should use straightforward words describing what the document represents and avoid overly officious descriptions, such as:

- Poor examples:
  - "Analysis of the Select Committee on Proposed Operational Extension of Business Opportunities to Include a Service Model for Delivery of Professional Component Emergency Services at Jackson Junction"
  - "Growing Our Business, Knocking It Out of the Park"
- Good examples:
  - "Service Expansion Business Plan for Jackson Junction"
  - "Business Expansion through Enhanced Community Services"
  - "Horizontal Integration through Development of Pediatric Emergency Capability"
  - "Vertical Integration through Development of Hospital Medicine Services"

All internal and external reviewers can understand the intent of the second, more straightforward titles.

Executive Summary

While the executive summary appears first in the document, it is most effective when written last, creating a "front-end" summary of what the plan will describe in more detail. It is sometimes referred to as an "elevator memo," implying that the reader can digest the summary and obtain a relevant understanding of the plan in a short period of time, that is, an elevator ride. Ideally, the purpose and desired outcome of the business plan is clearly described in a single page, unless the plan covers multiple organizational growth programs.

As the executive summary is a compilation of the entire plan, it actually summarizes the critical information in the document, requiring its completion as a late or last step in the plan development. If the plan requires outside funding, this fact and the amount of support required should be described in the executive summary, as well as possible sources for financing, duration of the credit line, interest rates, amortization of those costs, and so on. The executive summary should conclude with a definitive statement in favor of moving forward (assuming that the analysis has resulted in a positive projection). Putting that declarative statement in writing can help to crystallize the support for the plan.

The executive summary should simply clarify the intended outcomes in a way that allows the reader to recognize what initial and ongoing successes look like. The executive summary may incorporate the MVV statements as a means of confirming that the plan is organizationally aligned. Alternately, the MVV statements may exist as a stand-alone section immediately following the executive summary. A well-written executive summary should be a narrative that pulls the reader in to explore the document in more detail. It is a brief summary of what will be required, by whom, and when.

Table of Contents

The table of contents (TOC) allows the reader to quickly discern what is in the plan, the order in which it is presented, and where specific information may be found. The TOC may be used as a checklist to ensure that the plan includes all critical components. This checklist concept is particularly important if the document is created over a period of time with input from multiple individuals. The TOC helps the writers keep track of the progress and who is responsible for which components. As such, the TOC also serves the additional purpose of establishing early accountability. The case example in **Appendix 83.1** lists the key topics of analysis appropriate for this type of review.

The Business Opportunity

The business opportunity section presents a summary of the opportunity, for example, service expansion. It includes:

- "What" is the opportunity that the group has gathered to discuss?
- "Where" will this opportunity occur?
- "When" will this will happen? Is the opportunity right now, time dependent, or is a date certain, or dependent on other factors? Will there be loss of advantage or opportunity based on delay?

The timing is a critical component of planning and aids greatly in the appraisal of the plan (e.g., Can the group recruit three new BCEM providers in 45, 90, 180 days?).

Performance Indicators

The summary of the business opportunity also provides an early opportunity to introduce the project's performance indicators, such as "how" the success of the new opportunity will be determined. The case example in **Appendix 83.1** defines the physician group's success as the collection of sufficient professional fees to pay its practicing physicians, meet its modest overhead, and manage any start-up capital debt repayment. Simply put, when revenue exceeds expenses, the project will be considered a success. While this definition of success seems intuitive, it may not always be the case.

- *Example 1:* Expansion into a new location at an acceptable level of loss might be preferable to allowing a competitor to encroach on the group's system (area of influence). Also, the group might take on a modest loss, if the primary contract is quite profitable and the value of the relationship with the hospital is great. If so, how much of a loss would be acceptable? The group may wish to further develop the plan to improve marketing, enhance reimbursement, or reduce operational costs?
- *Example 2:* Expansion into a new location at a loss might be unacceptable, even if a profit is certain. Some of the reasons might include:
    - The group's administration is overwhelmed.
- The members of the group prefer the current small size of the group.
    - Recruitment is difficult.
- The expected profit is not worth the effort.
- There are other better and easier opportunities.

Key Assumptions of the Business

This section lists all of the key variables influencing the decision-making. A review of the underlying assumptions provides the reader with another opportunity to consider the plan's validity, including its integration with the overall strategy. For instance, consider a group whose mission includes maintaining all board-certified emergency physician owners. Because of inability to attract necessary clinicians/partners, they must adjust their ownership policy to offer equity partnership tracks to nonboarded providers.

Divergence from the principal mission could require specific actions, such as unanimous or super majority shareholder approval. At a minimum, new business plan assumptions that entail changes in the organizational structure or culture require candid dialogue and subsequent consensus. Potentially, this type of discussion could lead to the creation of a new and separate entity.

History of the Enterprise

This section will sometimes be called "About the Company" if the business plan is intended for an external audience. It provides an opportunity to define the organization and its principals, their respective roles, and its evolutionary history. If the MVV was not included in the executive summary, it should be added here.

Description of the Business

This section describes what, where, and how services are to be provided and what needs are to be addressed. Distinct competitive advantages relative to the proposed venture should be introduced here. The description also explains the organization's general function and how it accomplishes its mission. Some of the more quantitative aspects of the business plan may be presented here, and as such, it is often appropriate to introduce measurable standards (e.g., performance metrics). In this context of expanded ED services, the data might include metrics like productivity and patient satisfaction scores.

Structural aspects of the organization, such as the legal structure of the company (e.g., a limited liability company) are generally depicted in this section. These and other administrative components are generally developed in consultation with financial, tax, and legal professionals since there can be subtle advantages and disadvantages to various configurations.

If the plan requires outside funding, this section should discuss overall projected profitability and financial performance. In addition, lenders will request a comprehensive set of financial statements for review. These documents, sometimes called bankers' financials, are generally attached as an appendix to the plan and include a substantial level of detail, analysis, and comment. Such documents are compiled in conjunction with the business management team, certified public accountant, or banking partners. The financial analysis is a core component of the business plan.

Market Analysis

The market analysis formalizes the where and who. For instance, the *where* (in what specific location) is the ED at Fibula Junction. The *who* is "who will utilize the service?" By completing an in-depth market analysis, these questions can be easily answered in the necessary detail.

> *One of the best explanations for performing a market analysis comes from the* The Music Man *by Meredith Wilson. A salesman on a train opines, "You can talk . . . you can bicker . . . you can talk all you want, but you gotta know the territory."*[4]

With all of the statistical and analytical reference tools available today, "knowing the territory" is a more easily accomplished task and should take advantage of the views of the entire team.

Market Definition

To begin with, it is critical to define the market. Specifically, "Who are the potential customers?" since projected volume is the first variable. In the case example, the organization has determined that there are at least 36,500 opportunities for the delivery of that care in Fibula Junction. Beyond raw volume, it is important to know the demographic profile/analysis of the customer base. Sources for this information can include the US Bureau of Labor Statistics, the US Census Bureau, local or regional chambers of commerce, state employment commissions, hospital marketing departments, and even word of mouth. The market analysis evaluates and answers questions about:

- What is the service area? Is it a neighborhood, a city, or a county? US census data are available through metropolitan statistical areas and can provide an indicator of contiguous or potential customer populations. In an existing facility, historical patient data can detail exactly from where the patients are, and are not, coming.
- Who is the competition? In the case example, LHC operates the only hospital ED in the county. Generally, competitors could include a hospital, freestanding ED, urgent care center, extended-hours primary care practice, and so on.
- Is the population aging? Census data can be queried to ascertain this information. Generally, an aging population can indicate higher acuity potential but may also mean reimbursement at fixed Medicare rates. Will patient ages create a future opportunity for geriatric services or pediatric services?
- Is the population growing or declining? Is there potential to grow the volume through new business growth or housing developments or to lose volume because of an economic downturn or decreasing community census?
- What are the socioeconomic factors related to the proposed service area? Is unemployment high? This can mean a higher percentage of self-pay patients leading to lower reimbursement. Are there a large percentage of manufacturing or industrial jobs in the community? Is the underlying business community shrinking or growing? Is there new industry on the horizon?
- What is the expected payer mix? Is managed care reimbursement going to be a significant percentage of the revenue? Will there be an opportunity to negotiate favorable rates, or must the group "go along with" or "participate in" the existing hospital contracted or regional rates?
- What are the worst-case, base-case, and best-case scenarios for all of these variables?

The examples are by no means exhaustive. Each plan will have its own unique set of characteristics. The sample plan has detailed the critical components related to EDA's proposed service expansion.

Risk Factors

There are other external aspects of the market, such as the following business risk factors that are relevant to this analysis:

- What will be the impact of health-care reform?
- Will there be reimbursement reductions due to unresolved issues with the sustained growth rate?
- What is the local malpractice environment and what is the status of tort reform in the state?
- What is the effect of experiencing the worst-case scenario?

Partners

EDA's silent partner must be considered. Though the hospital may not have any direct management involvement with the group's internal affairs, it certainly will have day-to-day involvement in the management of the ED. Further, the entities may enter into a financial arrangement, such as a subsidy from the hospital, in order for the group to operate and cover the costs of providing services.

The ED business plan should include a candid assessment of the hospital as a stakeholder in the venture. One of the unique aspects of the business of emergency medicine is that the physical space, nurses and ancillary staffing, and supplies are all provided and paid for by the hospital. Accordingly, it would be important to have a good appreciation for any hospital instability. Critical questions include:

- Is the hospital profitable?
- Is the administrative team stable and experienced?
- Does the group participate at the administrative level through committee involvement or medical staff representation?
- Does the hospital plan on any physical plant or service line expansions?

These issues are relevant to the key assumptions and they have been included in the case example.

Strengths, Weaknesses, Opportunities, Threats Analysis

A strengths, weaknesses, opportunities, threats (SWOT) analysis is a critical component of a market analysis. It is valuable to review related questions, such as:

- Does the opportunity match the organization's strengths?
- Is the opportunity likely to succeed?
- Are there significant competitors?
- Is there substantial trust between the ED group and the hospital?
- Does the opportunity depend on the flawless execution in a part of the organization that has previously been defined as a weak?

Marketing Plan

Once the market, including its various risks, rewards, liabilities and opportunities, is analyzed, a plan utilizing that information for market growth is created. With a thorough understanding of the environment, a plan can be formulated to promote the program to the prospective customers. A successful ED requires far more than an "if you build it, they will come" mentality. Some ED leaders may not automatically associate the concept of sales with the provision of EM services, but promoting the product as well as the business is integral to the success of the venture.

4Ps of Marketing

A useful framework for a marketing plan is the 4Ps of marketing:

Product: What is being sold? In this case, the primary service offered by EDA is comprehensive ED medical care. The description of the product should be simple and as always consistent with the mission. It may sound impressive to suggest that, "EDA delivers care like you are a member of our family." However, in reality that might prove difficult to quantify and deliver.

Price: How much should it cost? The price of the services could be evaluated at the patient, provider, and the hospital level. Patient charges are primarily a function of reimbursement and market-driven rates. There are several services available to assist in the development and indexing of the fee schedule, that is, the prevailing rates are easily obtainable. A standard rule of thumb is that charges are approximately 350% of collections. If a hospital subsidy is required, the hospital will consider that subsidy in its cost-price calculation. Evaluation of this metric includes a discussion about fair market value and the requirement to have open books, and so on (see Chapter 101).

Place: Unless the organization is considering an independent free-standing ED or urgent care center, emergency services are provided under the auspices of a hospital. The specific location is important, and traffic patterns, parking access, ease of entry into the ED, distances from competitors, access to EMS, and so on, help to define the pros and cons of the location.

Promotion: Promotion of the ED is an increasingly significant focus for most groups. It is not uncommon to have billboards throughout the community promoting the hospital and ED. Wait times may be posted on these same billboards or online through various apps that patients can access. Hospitals are zealous about reporting such numbers, including patient satisfaction scores. Government websites such as Hospital Compare (https://www.cms.gov/Medicare/Quality-Initiatives-Patient-Assessment-Instruments/HospitalQualityInits/HospitalCompare) provide consumers with detailed information about the facility. Groups can take advantage of health fairs, community service articles, radio spots, or high school athletic physicals as further examples of promotional opportunities.

Financial Plan

The financial plan is the "how much." This section of the business plan provides realistic financial projections over a definable time period, at a minimum of 1 year and up to 5 years. The financial projections contained in the business plan provide the framework for the project budget and can be used to monitor performance.

The Income Statement

A detailed discussion of the accounting principles relevant to emergency medicine is beyond the scope of this chapter. However, the income statement, the most commonly used reporting tool in EM finance, is of critical importance. This document measures and reports financial performance over defined periods of time, usually months, quarters, and years. It is the backbone of the budget In this case, the *projected* income statement measures anticipated activity in both units of service (patient visits) and units of time (typically months).

The revenues and expenses of the provided services over the designated time period are summarized to show profit or loss. Simply stated, the revenues are the collections associated with patient visits plus any subsidies, and the expenses are the costs required to care for those patients plus the business costs of the group. These general terms (i.e., units of service, revenue generation, etc.) are common to every business. After taking into account (validating) the key assumptions, the business plan's potential for profitability can be evaluated.

Budget Projections

Generally, the ED financial plan or budget is driven by patient visits. Therefore, the first financial projection step is to accurately forecast the patient census, which is known as demand forecasting. In this business plan, demand forecasting involves planning how many and what types of visits will be generated during a given time period. The information provides important factors to the equation of expected revenue generation and anticipated expenses. As an example, it may be common in certain locations to experience varying volumes by season. The seasonal variation will be important when evaluating appropriate staffing as well as the cash flow necessary to pay back loans, meet payroll, fund employee retirement funds, and so on.

Changing regulatory requirements, decreasing government payments, and emerging public health urgencies, such as an influenza epidemic, can impact demand forecasting as well. Budgets can be updated and revised as necessary. The forecast should be based upon the best data at the time of the plan creation.

Acuity is an additional factor that influences both revenues and expenses. More acutely ill and complicated patients have higher charges and accounts receivables and associated expenses. The assessment of acuity, provider documentation, and coding trends are useful to identify opportunities to improve revenue.

Budgets are organized by line item. Generally, the first line item is the expected overall revenue generated from the patient visits for the defined measurement period, typically a month. In the case example, it is estimated that there will be 3,667 visits per month at an average collection per visit of $120.

Cash and accrual are budgetary items that require explanation. Cash is the money collected and deposited in the group's account during a defined time period. The accrual method is common in emergency medicine, since payment for services rarely occurs in the same month that the service was provided. In accrual accounting, the money is applied to the budget as if it were received today. By utilizing an accurate accrual methodology, more realistic projections across periods of time can be made.

Cash Flow

Once a patient is seen in the ED, the process of generating a bill, submitting that bill to the payer, and collecting the money may take months. During the first month of service, while the group will accrue money, it will collect very little cash. It is likely that there will be a several month lag between the inception of service and the achievement of steady state collections. Depending on external factors such as payer type, enrollment, and claim processing, the lag period to achieve steady state is usually between three and six months. However, practitioners and business partners, such as malpractice carriers, secretaries, billing companies, and attorneys, expect to be paid on a timelier basis. Accordingly, evaluating the lag in collections is a critical component of determining if, or how much, money may need to be borrowed to support the group's start-up costs.

In the case of service expansion of a mature business, it may be possible to defer borrowing by using profits from the existing business. It is also common for owners to accept reduced compensation during a start-up to avoid or reduce borrowing. Occasionally, the hospital partner may provide access to funds during transition periods. In the example provided, the group has sufficient access to internal capital to bring on the second location without having to secure a loan. Nevertheless, borrowing costs should be considered as part of the budget analysis in order to evaluate all potential scenarios.

The time value of money should always be considered, including current interest rates, the return on investment, and perhaps some financial measures such as internal rate of return.

Practice Expenses

Expenses must also be considered. The primary (largest) component of expense is the professional services component, compensation of the providers. For service expansion, compensation expenses are known. The next largest expense is likely to be billing costs. In the case example, billing costs are shown as a negative adjustment to revenue rather than as a direct expense (either methodology can be used). In addition to clinical costs, EDA provides a budgeted administrative stipend to the Fibula Junction Medical Director. EDA providers are all employees, and the cost of benefits and payroll taxes have also been included. Group expenses will include:

- Provider compensation
- Billing costs
- Director's stipend

- Payroll taxes
- Malpractice insurance payments
- Overhead—operating expenses
- Practice administration—legal, accounting payroll processing, management support
- Interest payments on borrowed money

Once assembled, the budget becomes the financial plan. Many additional related topics are discussed elsewhere in this book.

Goals and Objectives

A summary description of how the business is expected to operate should begin with the intended outcomes. In the case of EDA, a concise statement accomplishes this goal:

"The primary objectives of this plan are to:

- Expand the EDA physician group to the Jackson Junction campus
- Finalize the ED staffing and management contract with the new hospital
- Obtain capital funding, as necessary
- Commence operations
- Stabilize the cash flow within 6 to 9 months."

The business plan is a tool for future management and accountability. The key measures of performance should be outlined, comparing the financial projections to actual performance, that is, the variance analysis. Negative and positive variances are evaluated monthly and, if possible, negative variances are rectified. In addition to the anticipated monthly review, the plan provides a critical opportunity to develop performance benchmarks with the intention of minimizing or avoiding negative variances. These benchmarks should be developed for short-, mid-, and long-range bases, moving the group's thinking from a primarily tactical approach (e.g., covering shifts) to a more strategic approach (e.g., expanding the business).

CONCLUSION

Finally, the last W: **W**hat next? EDA proceeds with the service expansion based upon their analysis and a well thought-out business plan. The creation of the plan allows them to reduce risk by reviewing and comparing the proposal to the group's current operations. EDA is able to obtain unanimous buy-in from all current owners based on an approach that is consistent with the group's mission, vision, and values.

The plan must still be implemented with the same care and attention that was used to create it; even a perfect plan that is poorly implemented is likely to fail. In order to maintain a vested sense of participation, it is wise to delegate key aspects of the plan development, implementation, and monitoring to champions within the group. Even in a sole proprietorship model, there will likely be opportunities to share responsibilities with key participants. By distributing responsibility and accountability, the likelihood of achieving the desired outcomes is enhanced.

APPENDIX 83.1: EXAMPLE BUSINESS PLAN

Emergency Doctor Associates (EDA)

1234 Medical Road, Cold Springs, North Carolina

Executive Summary

This business plan evaluates the business opportunity of EDA, LLC to provide emergency physician staffing and medical direction to the Local Hospital Corporation (LHC), Cold Springs, North Carolina ED. EDA has been the exclusive provider of emergency services to LHC for the past 15 years. The LHC acquired the facility in Cold Springs six months ago.

A new emergency medical practice requires experience and expertise to provide effective leadership, clinical care, collaboration, and growth. The relationship between the hospital and EDA reveals a long history of alignment and success. The hospital intends to provide the physical space, the nurses and ancillary staffing, the supplies, and so on. EDA will provide expert clinical and administrative services and utilize these facilities, evaluate and treat patients, bill professional fees for their services, and pay its providers.

Among EDA's core competencies are provider recruiting, credentialing, scheduling, managing provider performance, demonstrated quality, customer service, physician–nurse collaboration, medical staff leadership, ED operations, billing and collecting for the providers' services, and maintaining the books and records of the corporate entity. EDA possesses, or has contracted to obtain, all of the resources necessary for conducting its business. The business plan addresses the key assumptions of the new practice opportunity and incorporates these into a financial plan that is attached as Appendix A.

Table of Contents

1. Title Page
2. Executive Summary
3. Table of Contents
4. The Business Opportunity
5. Key Assumptions of the Business
6. History of the Enterprise
7. Definition of the Business
8. Services Offered by EDA and Practice Philosophy
9. Market Analysis (with SWOT)
10. Ownership and Management Structure
11. EDA Goals and Objectives

The Business Opportunity

Emergency Doctor Associates has the opportunity to contract with the new LHC to provide the emergency physician staffing and emergency medical direction for the Cold Springs ED. EDA was founded in 1993 and currently contracts with LHC at the main campus, a 49,000-visit ED. To be successful, the new practice must generate sufficient professional fees to pay its employees, meet its modest overhead, and service its start-up capital loan.

Key Assumptions of the Business

The attached financial analysis is based on the following key assumptions of the medical practice:

- 36,500 annual billable ED visits
- Annual growth estimated at 4%
- An average patient charge of ~$320 per visit
- An average net collection of ~$150 per visit
- Billing cost of 8.0% of net collections
- Physician compensation of $175 per hour as employees of EDA
- Benefits (physician) approximately 20% of direct provider compensation

- EDA obtains the malpractice liability insurance
- Medical malpractice expense ~$5.50 per visit for the first year
- 36 hours of physician staffing per day, 7 days per week
- 16 hours of advanced practice provider (APP) coverage per day at $85 per hour
- APPs will be employees of EDA
- Benefits (MLPs) approximately 22.25% of compensation
- Medical Director stipend $10,000 per month
- Practice management expense 6% of practice collections
- Working capital interest rate and terms assumptions: 4%, 1-year interest only, 5-year amortization after first year

History of the Enterprise

EDA was founded in August 2008 for the purpose of providing exclusive emergency management services to the LHC, Cold Springs Medical Center (CSMC). EDA operates at CSMC through an agreement with the hospital with automatically renewals every three years. The group president, Dr. Foster, is board certified in emergency medicine and has been affiliated with EDA since its inception.

Collectively, the group has more than 150 years experience in the practice of emergency medicine. All EDA physician providers are board certified, or board prepared, in emergency medicine. In addition, the organization employs 3.5 full-time equivalent physician assistants. Five of the company's clinicians are natives of Brown County, NC. Since its inception, EDA has treated in excess of 500,000 Cold Springs patients.

[*Note: MVV can be included here as well—especially if it was not included in the executive summary.]

Definition of the Business of EDA

The clinicians of EDA are engaged in the full-time practice of emergency medicine in a hospital-based setting. The term "full-time" implies that the physicians of EDA have limited or no outside practice obligations. The term "hospital-based" signifies that the practice is conducted within the hospital setting where the physical space, equipment, supplies, staff, and so on, of the practice are provided and paid for by the hospital and not EDA.

Services Offered by EDA and Practice Philosophy

The primary services offered by EDA are comprehensive emergency medical care. There are currently approximately 36,500 annual patient visits for services. The ED patient volume at this location is averaging a 4% annual growth rate. Additional product lines for future consideration include:

- ED fast track/convenience care
- Occupational medical services
- ED observation/critical decision unit
- EDA affiliated hospitalist program

Various forms of community-based advertising and promotion in conjunction with the hospital are necessary to develop these product lines. The physicians of EDA adhere to the philosophy that the ED exists to serve the needs of the community. This broad definition of the scope of emergency medical services includes:

- Primary urgent and emergency care for all patients, including those who lack access to primary care services

- Critical medical emergency and trauma care
- Convenience, episodic, and occupational care

This definition of the scope of emergency medical services is consistent with the "prudent layperson" definition of an emergency medical care need.

Given the requirement for organized physician staffing of the ED 24 hours per day, the practice of emergency medicine must, by definition, comprise a group practice. For that reason, the physicians have formed a limited liability corporation with physician ownership.

EDA does not anticipate the introduction of additional product lines that would be scheduled to come online during the first year of the new practice start-up. The focused attention to this program permits the basic business unit to become stabilized.

Market Analysis

The next county over and the surrounding counties are currently a single-hospital metropolitan area with a population of approximately 145,000 as of the 2020 census. With no other ED in the county and very limited drop-in and after-hours care availability, the Brown County marketplace has about 52,000 potential ED and urgent care visits available per year. There is significant growth predicted due to a recently passed casino law allowing casinos in the southern part of Brown County.

- *Strengths*: EDA is a mature organization with boarded emergency physicians who live in the community. The group has demonstrated consistent leadership aligned with and integrated into the hospital and its leadership. EDA remains financially sound.
- *Weaknesses*: EDA will require supporting financial resources to manage a start-up. However, it is anticipated based on sound financial evaluation that the resource requirement will be of short duration. While EDA does not currently have enough clinicians to staff the new institution, the organization has begun speaking with clinicians who are interested in joining the group and will have adequate staffing to expand services to LHC.
- *Opportunities*: LHC is an underserved market, and this collaboration with EDA presents a natural growth opportunity for all parties. With community growth in the LHC service area, there is increasing need for high-quality emergency care.
- *Threats*: There are no current competitors. However, it is possible that a nonaffiliated facility that is structurally separate and distinct or an urgent care center could establish local services. Future pandemics similar to COVID-19 could limit ED volume.

Ownership and Management Structure

Emergency Doctor Associates is a limited liability corporation. Ownership in the corporation is held equally among the six founding principles of EDA. EDA will offer new ownership opportunities as at least three of the current EDA owners are planning to retire within the next three to five years.

Goals and Objectives

The primary goals and objectives for EDA are to:

- Expand the EDA physician group to the Fibula Springs campus.
- Finalize the ED staffing and management contract with the new hospital.

- Obtain start-up capital funding, as necessary.
- Commence operations.
- Stabilize the cash flow, estimated to require 6 months to 9 months.

The practice revenue and expense budgetary goals are set forth in the financial proforma attached as Appendix A. The short-term operational goals are to:

- Hire all necessary staff within 90 days: two full-time and two part-time physicians.
- Manage credentialing and scheduling to ensure the ED staffing coverage.
- Ensure medical records completion and flow of data to the billing company to achieve optimum collections in the shortest possible time frame.
- Establish coding procedure controls.
- Manage charges/coding to their optimum levels.
- Establish cash control procedures.
- Establish the accounting system and books.
- Closely monitor billing company performance.
- Establish a process to address hospital issues with patient quality and satisfaction.

Intermediate term goals are to:

- Establish an ongoing recruiting program to meet future, anticipated physician recruiting needs.
- Establish a compliance program.
- Conduct regular management team meetings.
- Develop medical staff relationships by becoming members of committees, performing outreach, and determining communication preferences.
- Create an ED nurse–physician shared governance program.

Long-term goals are to:

- Develop a long-term stable group of emergency physicians practicing exclusively at the LHC, Cold Springs campus.
- Fully repay the start-up capital debt.
- Become leaders of the medical staff.
- Expand the product line to generate other revenue streams to the practice.

REFERENCES

1. Wooden J, Jamison S. *Wooden on Leadership: How to Create a Winning Organization*. New York, NY: McGraw-Hill; 2005.
2. Churchill W. *Quoted in Roberts A. Churchill: Walking With Destiny*. New York, NY: Penguin Random House; 2018.
3. Drucker P. *The Effective Executive: The Definitive Guide to Getting It Right*. New York, NY: HarperCollins; 2006.
4. Wilson M. *The Music Man*. New York, NY: Fireside Theatre Book Club; 1958.

CHAPTER 84

RESOURCE UTILIZATION

John Sverha

Optimal utilization of resources is an essential concern for all practitioners of medicine. Emergency departments (EDs) are uniquely positioned to identify and address issues of value and efficiency in the application of resources.

For many years, health-care costs in the United States have been growing faster than other sectors of the economy. In 1970, total health-care costs were estimated to be $75 billion and represented 6.9% of gross domestic product (GDP). In 2018, health-care costs were estimated at more than $3.6 trillion (or $11,172 per person) and comprised 17.7% of GDP.[1] This steady increase is universally considered unsustainable.

The percentage of health-care costs that can be directly attributed to the ED is small but significant. These costs have been variably estimated at 2% to 10% of total health-care expenditures.[2] However, the unique position of the ED at the interface of inpatient and outpatient care allows it to have an even greater impact on total health-care costs. The ED has been estimated to be the source of 66% of hospital admissions, and hospital-based care currently comprises 33% of all health-care expenditures.[1,3] Emergency physicians often serve as the gatekeepers of these hospital admissions, and opportunities exist to impact the downstream medical expenses of patients discharged from the ED.

PAYMENT MODEL REFORM

Multiple organizations and agencies are making a determined effort to transform the health-care delivery system by expanding insurance coverage, improving quality, and reducing cost. The Patient Protection and Affordable Care Act (PPACA), signed into law in 2010, was designed specifically to address those three aims. More recently, the Medicare Access and CHIP Reauthorization Act (MACRA) was enacted in 2015 with the goals of controlling physician costs and improving quality. Both programs contain incentives that will impact ED resource utilization in coming years.

Patient Protection and the Affordable Care Act

One of the goals of the PPACA is to ensure that Medicare payments to hospitals are based on quality performance. In order to do this, the Centers for Medicare and Medicaid Services (CMS) has created a long list of quality measures that are revised annually.[4,5] Several of the current CMS quality measures are partly determined by the appropriateness of ED imaging utilization (**Table 84.1**). Medicare fee-for-service beneficiaries are included if they had the relevant imaging study performed as a hospital outpatient. Emergency department patients are considered outpatients and are potentially included in these measures if they are discharged or admitted to observation status.

TABLE 84.1 ■ CMS Quality Measures Impacted by ED Imaging Utilization (2020)[6]

Measure	Description
OP-8 MRI Lumbar spine for low back pain	This measure calculates the percentage of MRIs of the lumbar spine studies with a diagnosis of low-back pain on the imaging claim and for which the patient did not have prior claims-based evidence of antecedent conservative therapy. Patients are excluded if an *ICD-10* diagnosis is listed related to one of the accepted indications for emergency imaging.
OP-10 Abdomen CT, use of contrast material	This measure calculates the percentage of CT abdomen studies performed with and without contrast out of all CT abdomen studies performed (those with contrast, those without contrast, and those with both). Patients are excluded if an *ICD-10* diagnosis is listed related to one of the accepted indications for obtaining separate CT scans with and without contrast.
OP-11 Thorax CT, use of contrast material	This measure calculates the percentage of CT thorax studies that are performed with and without contrast out of all CT thorax studies performed (those with contrast, those without contrast, and those with both). Patients are excluded if an *ICD-10* diagnosis is listed related to one of the accepted indications for obtaining separate CT scans with and without contrast.
OP-14 Simultaneous use of brain CT and sinus CT	This measure calculates the percentage of brain CT studies with a simultaneous sinus CT. Patients are excluded if an *ICD-10* diagnosis is listed related to one of the accepted indications for obtaining simultaneous brain and CT scans.

Other CMS quality measures are designed to measure ED throughput (**Table 84.2**). While many factors contribute to ED throughput times, the elimination of unnecessary testing is one strategy that can be used to improve performance on these metrics. Adherence to CMS quality measures is listed publicly, which provides an incentive for hospital leaders to improve performance. In addition, some of these public metrics are included in the CMS quality star program, which assigns between one and five stars to hospitals based on their performance on selected quality, safety, and patient experience measures and provides additional motivation for hospitals to perform well on utilization-related quality measures.[7]

Besides publicly posting performance, PPACA also provides financial incentives for hospitals utilizing quality and utilization data. There are three "pay for performance" programs that were created by the PPACA: the Value-Based Purchasing (VBP) program, the Hospital Readmissions Reduction Program (HRRP), and the Hospital-Acquired Conditions (HAC) program.[8]

TABLE 84.2 ■ CMS Quality Measures Related to ED Throughput (2020)

Measure	Description
OP-18a	Median time from ED arrival to ED departure for discharged patients: overall rate
OP-18b	Median time from ED arrival to ED departure for discharged patients: reporting measure (does not include patients from OP-18c or OP-18d)
OP-18c	Median time from ED arrival to ED departure for discharged patients: psychiatric/mental health patients (does not include most psychiatric/mental health patient transfers)
OP-18d	Median time from ED arrival to ED departure for discharged patients: transfer patients (does not include psychiatric/mental health patients)
OP-22	Percentage of patients who left without being seen

Value-Based Purchasing Program

The VBP program evaluates a hospital's performance in the domains of clinical outcomes, patient experience, patient safety, and "efficiency and cost reduction" to create a "total composite score." Hospitals have 2% of their Medicare reimbursement placed at risk and can be either "winners" or "losers" depending on how well they perform relative to other hospitals. The efficiency and cost reduction domain score is determined by the Medicare spending per beneficiary (MSPB-1) metric. This complex measure, defined as total spending on Medicare patients 3 days prior to and 30 days after a hospital admission, comprises 25% of a hospital's VBP program score. Given that the majority of Medicare admissions begin in the ED, department utilization patterns can have a significant impact on MSPB-1 performance.

Hospital Readmissions Reduction Program

The HRRP creates strong admission disincentives among certain patient groups. In this program, a hospital's 30-day readmission rates for patients whose index admission was for one of several selected conditions (myocardial infarction [MI], congestive heart failure, pneumonia, chronic obstructive pulmonary disease [COPD], total knee or hip replacement, or coronary artery bypass graft) are compared to that of other hospitals. Hospitals are penalized (a "lose-only" measure) if their readmission rates are above average compared to other hospitals for any of the conditions. Three percent of their Medicare reimbursement is at risk.

Hospital-Acquired Conditions Program

The HAC program assigns a score to a hospital based on the rate of hospital-acquired conditions, including central line-associated bloodstream infections and catheter-associated urinary tract infections. The inclusion of hospital-acquired conditions creates incentives for EDs to reduce utilization of certain procedures to avoid complications. This is another "lose-only" measure for hospitals; if their performance is in the bottom quartile, hospitals lose 1% of their Medicare reimbursement.

Global Payment Models

Also created by the PPACA, global payment models permit hospitals and/or providers to receive predetermined payments for the care of populations of patients and specific conditions. Two types of global payment models legislated by PPACA are "accountable care organizations" (ACOs) and "bundled payments." Both of these programs were designed by CMS for Medicare patients and provided waivers against "fraud and abuse" laws (such as the Stark Law and Anti-Kickback Statute).[9] Without the waivers, these programs would have been considered illegal.

Accountable Care Organizations

The Medicare Shared Savings Program (MSSP) established the ACO model.[10] Accountable care organizations are networks of providers and facilities that are financially accountable for all the health-care costs incurred by a defined population of patients over a period of time. If an ACO is successful in reducing the costs associated with these patients (while still meeting specified quality metric standards), then the ACO is eligible to share in the savings. As of July 2019, there were 559 Medicare ACOs serving over 12 million Medicare patients.[11] Accountable care organizations can also contract with commercial payers and Medicaid. In

2017, over 20 million commercially insured or Medicaid patients were members of ACOs.[12] In 2017, approximately 10% of Americans were members of ACOs, although the penetrance varied between 2% and 30% depending on the state.[12]

Health systems and physician groups that participate in ACOs are strongly incentivized to reduce all utilization—including preventing ED visits—for patients who are members of their ACO. When an ACO patient does present to the ED, providers are typically encouraged to avoid unnecessary testing and admission. Accountable care organizations sometimes provide resources (e.g., case manager assistance or IT infrastructure) that may result in decreased hospital utilization. Thus far, direct participation by emergency physician groups as members of ACOs with financial risk sharing is rare but may become more common in the future.[13,14]

Bundled Payments for Care Improvement Initiative

The Bundled Payments for Care Improvement Initiative (BPCI) provides additional incentives to decrease ED utilization. In this voluntary program (recently relaunched as BPCI Advanced), participating hospitals or physician groups are guaranteed a "bundled payment" for the total cost of a given episode of care lasting 90 days.[15] Participants in the program may choose from one of 32 medical and surgical clinical episodes (e.g., chest pain, cellulitis, joint replacement), with most of the eligible clinical episodes initiated by an inpatient hospitalization. Participants in a bundled-care program benefit financially if the total costs are less than projected for the risk-adjusted episode of care; however, they incur a financial penalty if the costs are higher than projected or if they fail to meet specified quality metric standards.

Hospitals and physicians participating in a bundled-payment program are incentivized to avoid ED visits and readmissions within the 90-day payment window. Commercial payers have also started experimenting with bundled payments, typically for surgical procedures.[16] Similar to ACOs, direct participation of emergency physicians with financial risk sharing for bundled payments is rare at this time. However, the American College of Emergency Physicians (ACEP) has proposed an ED-specific bundled payment methodology to CMS called the Acute Unscheduled Care Model. This voluntary program would focus on specific episodes of care for Medicare patients and bundle the costs associated with the ED visit with the costs incurred in the subsequent 30 days. It would provide incentives to reduce inpatient admissions and observation stays when appropriate through enhanced care coordination.[17]

The Medicare Access and CHIP Reauthorization Act

The MACRA was enacted in 2015, five years after PPACA, with a similar goal of improving the value of care delivered to patients. And similar to PPACA, MACRA provides incentives for emergency physicians to optimize utilization. The MACRA established the Quality Payment Program (QPP), which provides financial incentives for individual providers or provider groups for quality and utilization performance.[18] Under the QPP, nonexempt providers must participate in either an Advanced Alternative Payment Model (APM) or the Merit-Based Incentive Program System (MIPS) to avoid a significant financial penalty. Examples of Advanced APMs include participation in an ACO or the BCPI Advanced program. Given that very few emergency providers are direct participants in an Advanced APM at this time, the vast majority will be participating in the MIPS program.

Merit-Based Incentive Program System

The MIPS program continues provider reimbursement through a fee-for-service model with a value modifier applied to all Medicare provider payments. The MIPS program began in January 2017, placing 4% of Medicare payments at risk in 2019 (two years later). The amount of money at risk increases to a maximum of 9% of Medicare reimbursement by 2022. A MIPS score for a provider or provider group is calculated using:

- Quality measure performance
- Cost performance
- Advancing care information performance
- Participation in specified clinical practice improvement activities

These four categories contribute to the total score, although their percentage contribution may change each year. The quality measures that a physician group reports can be chosen by the provider or provider group (six total) from either a list of approved measures from CMS or a qualified data registry. Several of the quality measures provided by CMS for emergency physicians are related to appropriate utilization (e.g., head computed tomography [CT] utilization in pediatric head trauma).

Optimizing Resource Utilization

Beyond the incentives provided by payment model reforms, there are several other approaches that encourage ED providers to eliminate unnecessary utilization. First, unnecessary utilization (especially blood tests and radiology studies) increases a patient's length of stay (LOS).[19] Besides being a publicly reported quality metric, ED LOS also determines an ED's effective capacity, impacts patient safety if it results in increased wait times, and is strongly associated with patient experience scores. Second, unnecessary radiology studies expose patients to radiation risks and subject them to workups for insignificant incidental findings. Lastly, unnecessary utilization may expose patients to increased health-care costs, especially if they are uninsured or carry a high deductible.

There are multiple strategies available to optimize resource utilization and thereby create value within the ED. Some strategies discourage procedures that provide little value (e.g., CT scans that are not indicated per validated clinical decision rules). Other strategies recommend providing the same resource at lower cost (e.g., using the optimal mix of staff to care for patients). Still other strategies suggest that, by investing in new resources (e.g., case management for frequent users or palliative care services), significant value may be achieved.

Utilization Metrics

An essential first step is developing the capacity to measure utilization. Electronic health records permit easier access to utilization data, resulting in reports that demonstrate the department's use of laboratory, radiology, and pharmacy resources. Data related to CT utilization should typically be obtained by both study type and overall rate. Data related to hospital admissions, consultations, and transfers should also be tracked. It is important to utilize accepted definitions for the various metrics when reviewing and comparing data.

TABLE 84.3 ■ Utilization Metrics Definitions

Area of Utilization	Metric
Radiology	Plain radiograph studies per 100 visits
	CT studies per 100 visits
	MRI studies per 100 visits
	Ultrasonographic studies per 100 visits
Laboratory	Number of patients per 100 ED visits who had any laboratory testing performed
Pharmacy	Number of medication doses administered by any route per 100 patients
Admission/Transfer	Percentage of patients admitted to inpatient status
	Percentage of patients admitted to ICU
	Percentage of patients admitted to observation status
	Percentage of patients transferred
Consultations	Behavioral health consultations per 100 visits
	Case management and/or social work consultations per 100 visits
	Specialty consultations per 100 visits
	Palliative care consultations per 100 visits

Standard definitions for various ED metrics were most recently revised at the Third ED Performance Measures and Benchmarking Summit held in 2014 (**Table 84.3**).[20]

Obtaining consistent throughput data is similarly important. Typical throughput metrics include median times for arrival to provider, total LOS, and time from discharge order to actual patient ED exit. The latter two metrics should be separately reported for admitted, observation, behavioral health, and discharged patients. Data related to the percentage of patients who leave prior to a medical screening examination, as well as those who leave before being seen by a provider (LBS or elopement), should also be tracked.

Utilization metrics should be collected for both the department and the individual provider. When analyzing provider data, measurements should control for patient variability among the various providers. For example, providers who predominantly work fast-track or night shifts typically manage patients of different acuity, as defined by measures like the Emergency Severity Index. Another proxy for acuity may be the percentage of patients seen by that provider who arrive via emergency medical services.

Provider Variability

Resource utilization variation among emergency providers is common, with significant disparities reported in the utilization of emergency diagnostic imaging, laboratory testing, and admission resources.[21-24] It is not unusual to observe as much as a threefold difference in utilization between low- and high-utilization providers.[22,25] The drivers of provider utilization variability are not well understood. It has been suggested that these patterns might be correlated with the provider's age, level of experience, training location, and risk tolerance, although this has not been consistently validated.[26] Providers can have limited insight into how their utilization patterns compare to their peers' until they are provided comparative utilization data.[27]

Simply bringing awareness to how the outliers' practices compare to those of their peers may be enough to significantly reduce variation. For other providers, a concerted effort promoting evidence-based guidelines with clinical decision support and chart audits may be necessary to reduce variability among providers.

Diagnostic Testing

Reduction of "low-value" testing helps optimize resource utilization in the ED. "Choosing Wisely" is a joint initiative founded in 2012 by the American Board of Internal Medicine and *Consumer Reports*. More than 75 specialty societies each identified low-value or potentially harmful tests and treatments that should typically be avoided.[28] ACEP joined Choosing Wisely in 2013 and has developed 10 recommendations to improve the quality and value of emergency care.[29] More recently, an effort was made to identify Choosing Wisely recommendations by other specialties that are relevant and actionable to emergency medicine (**Table 84.4**).[30]

CT utilization is an area of special importance given its cost and associated radiation risks. The ED Benchmarking Alliance reports a CT utilization rate of 23 studies per 100 patients seen in 2018. This rate has been relatively stable over the past 10 years.[3,31] The ED should promote evidence-based guidance for CT utilization whenever possible. Evidence-based guidance is available for the evaluation of mild traumatic brain injury, headache, cervical spine trauma, pulmonary embolism, atraumatic low-back pain, and renal colic.[32-40]

In the future, emergency medicine providers may need to comply with the Protecting Access to Medicare Act of 2014. This program requires providers to use clinical decision support tools containing "appropriate use criteria" when ordering advanced imaging studies, which include CT scans, MRIs, and nuclear medicine scans, but exclude plain radiographs and ultrasound imaging.[41]

Hospital Admissions

The most costly resource for any ED is a hospital admission. For this reason, it has been argued that the most effective strategy for optimizing resource utilization in the ED is to focus on patients currently being admitted who could be effectively treated in other, less-costly settings.[42,43] Nationally, ED admission rates are reported as between 11.1% and 15.3%, depending on the data source.[44,45] Significant variability in admission rates has been found between hospitals, even when controlling for socioeconomic and clinical characteristics.[46] Risk-standardized admission rates have also been shown to vary according to the clinical condition, with some of the least variability associated with sepsis and acute MI and the largest variability associated with chest pain, skin and soft-tissue infections, COPD, urinary tract infections, and mood disorders.[47,48]

Evidence-Based Guidelines

There is evidence-based admission guidance for several ED conditions, including pneumonia, asthma, low-risk chest pain, and deep vein thrombosis.[49-57] Prioritizing awareness and implementation of admission clinical pathways may have the greatest impact on overall utilization of health-care resources. Payers have also created admission-related protocols for gauging the appropriateness of an admission and authorizing reimbursement (e.g., McKesson's Interqual Decision Support and the MCG Health guidelines). Unfortunately, these guidelines have practical limitations because of their complexity and variability. In

TABLE 84.4 ■ Choosing Wisely Recommendations Related to Low-Value ED Testing

Organization	Recommendation
American College of Emergency Physicians	Avoid ordering CT of the abdomen and pelvis in young, otherwise healthy ED patients (age <50) with known histories of kidney stones, or ureterolithiasis, presenting with symptoms consistent with uncomplicated renal colic.
American College of Emergency Physicians	Avoid lumbar spine imaging in the ED for adults with nontraumatic back pain, unless the patient has severe or progressive neurologic deficits or is suspected of having a serious underlying condition (such as vertebral infection, cauda equina syndrome, or cancer with bony metastasis).
American College of Emergency Physicians	Avoid CT pulmonary angiography in ED patients with a low pretest probability of pulmonary embolism and either a negative Pulmonary Embolism Rule-Out Criteria (PERC) or a negative D-dimer.
American College of Emergency Physicians	Avoid CT of the head in asymptomatic adult patients in the ED with syncope, insignificant trauma, and a normal neurological evaluation
American College of Emergency Physicians	Avoid CT scans of the head in ED patients with minor head injury who are at low risk based on validated decision rules.
American Gastroenterological Association	For a patient with functional abdominal pain syndrome (as per Rome III criteria), CT scans should not be repeated unless there is a major change in clinical findings or symptoms.
American Academy of Pediatrics	Neuroimaging (CT, MRI) is not necessary for a child with simple febrile seizure.
American College of Radiology	Do not conduct CT for the evaluation of suspected appendicitis in children until after ultrasonography has been considered as an option.
Society of Cardiovascular Computed Tomography	Do not use coronary CT angiography for high-risk ED patients presenting with acute chest pain.
American Society of Nuclear Cardiology	Do not perform cardiac imaging for patients who are at low risk.
American College of Radiology	Do not conduct imaging for uncomplicated headache.
American Society of Plastic Surgeons	Avoid obtaining radiographs in instances of facial trauma.
Society of Nuclear Medicine and Molecular Imaging	Avoid using a CT angiogram to diagnose pulmonary embolism in young women with a normal chest radiograph result; consider a radionuclide lung study ("V/Q study") instead.
Infectious Diseases Society of America	Avoid testing for a *Clostridium difficile* infection in the absence of diarrhea.

addition, the "evidence" on which these guidelines are based is not readily available to providers, leading to the perception of arbitrary application.

Case Managers

Emergency department case managers have been shown to effectively reduce hospital admissions by identifying the most appropriate level of care for a patient and making the necessary placement arrangements.[58-60] As an example, a hospital admission may not be necessary if home care and equipment can be provided or the patient can be directly transferred to a nursing home, rehabilitation center, or subacute care facility. Alternatively, some patients can be safely discharged home if a follow-up appointment or test (e.g., stress test) can be scheduled expeditiously. Case managers can also help coordinate care.

Observation Units

For those patients who cannot be discharged directly from the ED, there are still opportunities for emergency medicine to assist in the delivery of high-quality, cost-efficient care. Observation units have been shown to significantly reduce the costs associated with the care provided for selected clinical conditions.[61-65] Placing appropriate patients in observation units can result in an estimated savings of greater than $1,500 per patient.[66] While the number of hospitals with dedicated observation units continues to increase, less than half currently place their observation patients in a dedicated unit.[67,68]

A well-designed observation unit decreases costs through a variety of mechanisms. The patients selected for the unit must be considered to have a high probability (80%-90%) of discharge within 24 hours, a single acute problem, and a well-defined plan of care. This organized approach typically results in the "observation" of a limited number of clinical conditions. Protocols that include scheduled diagnostic and therapeutic interventions are available for each of these conditions. Ideally, the observation beds are geographically segregated from the primary ED and not dispersed throughout the hospital. Placing appropriate patients in well-organized observation units can reduce LOS by almost half when compared to care delivered on traditional inpatient units.[62-65] This is thought to be a significant contributor to the decreased costs associated with observation care.

More recently, CMS changed its payment model for observation care so that the facility fee is provided in a bundled payment, whereas previous charges were paid separately (e.g., diagnostic imaging, stress testing, and medication infusions).[69] This change provides additional incentives for hospitals to eliminate unnecessary testing and treatments for observation status patients.

Palliative Care

Early palliative care consultations have been shown to decrease hospital LOS, ICU utilization, and hospital deaths.[70-75] A recent meta-analysis estimated that early palliative interventions decreased hospital inpatient costs by 10% to 30%.[76] Unfortunately, most of these consultations occur after the patient has been admitted.[77] The potential impact of early palliative services on the value of care provided is reflected in one of ACEP's ten recommendations for the Choosing Wisely initiative: "Don't delay engaging available palliative care and hospice care services."[29]

Palliative care principles should ideally be adopted by all frontline providers, including emergency physicians. This requires developing more expertise in symptom alleviation and gaining greater comfort and skill with goals-of-care conversations. The availability of palliative care resources is variable in hospitals but is becoming more common; as of 2016, 75% of hospitals with over 50 beds offer palliative care services.[78] A variety of screening tools have been developed to assist ED providers in identifying patients who might benefit from an early palliative care consultation.[79]

Several metrics can be used to evaluate the effectiveness of ED palliative care, including the number of palliative care consultations requested by ED providers, direct placement of patients into hospice care from the ED, and averted admissions. Additional metrics include hospital LOS and the satisfaction of patients who received an early palliative care consultation. Barriers to ED palliative care integration include the relative paucity of palliative care resources at some hospitals as well as the cultural resistance of emergency providers.

Frequent Users

Patients who regularly visit the ED consume a disproportionate number of resources. "Frequent" users have been defined variably in the literature, although these patients are often considered to have at least four visits over one year (accounting for 21%-28% of all ED visits).[78,80] Frequent users comprise between 4.5% and 8% of all ED patients, although higher percentages have been reported with the advent of health information exchanges, which allow access to regional patient data.[80,81]

The uninsured represent only 15% of frequent users and are no more likely to visit the ED than the insured.[82] However, patients with Medicare or Medicaid insurance are more likely to be frequent users, with 60% of frequent users publicly insured, whereas 36% of "occasional" ED users are publicly insured. The acuity of frequent users is on average higher than that of occasional ED users, although the very frequent users (more than 20 ED visits per year) typically present with lower-acuity complaints.[83,84]

The most common reasons frequent users visit the ED include chronic pain, mental illness, and chronic medical illness. The proportion of frequent users that fall into each category varies significantly among EDs.[80] Patients with the highest level of ED use are more likely to have substance abuse and mental health diagnoses.[85]

The most common strategy described to address ED frequent users is the "case management" approach.[86,87] In this model, a multidisciplinary team composed of physicians, nurses, social workers, and case managers reviews each case and determines what resources are needed to most appropriately manage the patient. A "care plan" is created, allowing ED providers to implement informed, consistent treatment. The case management approach is successful according to most reviews.[87,88] Ideally, if resources are available, efforts should address the social determinants of the health of ED frequent users and engage these patients with primary care resources.[89]

Low-Acuity Patients

Low-acuity patients provide an additional opportunity to optimize ED resources. Charges for low-acuity visits are significantly higher in the ED than in other locations of care, such as a physician's office or clinic. With the increasing prevalence of global payment models, financial incentives broadly exist to prevent low-acuity ED visits or to "triage out" low-acuity patients after a medical screening exam (MSE). An MSE is required by the Emergency Medical Treatment and Labor Act (EMTALA) and is typically performed after triage.

If developing a "triage out" program, be aware that some patients will require additional testing as part of the MSE, even those identified as low acuity by the triage nurse. Lastly, the program should consider the "triaged out" patients' access to the referral centers and the related potential financial or geographic barriers.

Staffing

Staffing costs are a significant component of overall ED costs. There are several factors that should be considered when working to optimize the utilization of the ED team.

Staffing Mix

As a general principle, a provider or other member of the staff should not regularly perform work that can be done effectively by a less-costly provider. This means finding the appropriate mix of secretaries, technicians, scribes, nurses, advanced practice providers (APPs), and physicians to efficiently perform the work of an ED. The use of APPs in the ED deserves special mention because it has steadily increased in recent years. According to the National Ambulatory Care Survey, the percentage of ED visits that involved care provided by an APP increased from 17.4% in 2010 to 28.9% in 2016. The percentage of ED visits in which the patient was treated only by an APP (not seen by a physician) increased from 7.5% in 2010 to 12.1% in 2016.[45,90]

Using ED scribes to enhance provider efficiency has become commonplace in recent years, although concerns exist related to their cost and possible decreased utility as improvements are made in EMR usability and voice-recognition technology.

Telemedicine may allow more cost-effective and efficient access to specialty consultations in EDs. A recent survey showed that 58% of US EDs utilized telemedicine services, most commonly neurology/stroke care, psychiatric care, pediatric care, and trauma care.[91] Telemedicine has also been reported to allow a more efficient initial evaluation of a patient by a physician or APP at triage.[92] Some EDs are also using telemedicine to provide care for the entire encounter for very low-acuity patients.[93]

Demand-Capacity Matching

Patient arrivals vary by hour of day and day of the week in all EDs. It is important to schedule staff in response to the variations in the demand for care. It is common to find variations that require changes in shift start and end times (or even extra shifts) during different days of the week and months of the year.

Throughput Times

Many experienced physician and nursing ED leaders consider discharge patient LOS to be the "secret sauce" in running a successful department. While not easy to achieve, reducing the LOS increases the effective capacity of the department, improves the patient experience, and requires less staffing. On the other hand, if your department is routinely boarding admitted patients, staff should be scheduled to care for the overflow.

PITFALLS TO RESOURCE UTILIZATION

Several pitfalls may arise when addressing resource utilization in the ED:

- Decreased utilization does not necessarily lead to increased value. It is tempting to presume that the ED or the provider using the least resources is providing the "best" care. However, in many cases, the "right" amount of resource utilization is unknown. For instance, should a provider order a head CT scan for 5% or 15% of patients with confusion? Efforts to decrease utilization should be determined by evidence-based medicine, and all efforts to decrease utilization must be paired with a watchful eye on quality.
- Reductions of utilization in the ED may increase utilization elsewhere in the healthcare system. For instance, reducing CT utilization for abdominal pain is a laudable goal; however, it may result in a greater percentage of patients being admitted for observation. Given changes in payment models, it is increasingly important to consider costs when making decisions related to utilization.
- Efforts to reduce utilization must comply with legal and regulatory requirements. An initiative to "triage out" low-acuity patients must comply with EMTALA. Any decreased utilization leading to financial sharing by ED providers must occur within the confines of CMS-sponsored programs such as the MSSP or the BPCI Advanced program and be compliant with federal laws and regulations related to gainsharing.

CONCLUSION

The rate of growth in health-care spending in the United States is unsustainable. While direct costs attributed to emergency care are relatively small, care decisions made in the ED can greatly affect the trajectory of resource utilization by patients. The PPACA and MACRA create financial incentives for both hospitals and individual providers to reduce the cost and improve the quality of ED care.

Efforts to address utilization in the ED require access to standard ED utilization metrics. Evidence-based guidance should be promoted to encourage appropriate diagnostic testing, especially related to CT scanning. A special effort should be made to ensure the appropriateness of inpatient admissions, the costliest resource used by the ED.

Additional opportunities to optimize ED resource utilization are provided by observation units, the integration of palliative care, and efficient staffing. Populations that may benefit from efforts to optimize utilization include frequent users and low-acuity patients. When addressing utilization in the ED, it is important to avoid pitfalls, which include equating decreased utilization with increased value, decreasing ED utilization at the expense of increasing total health-care utilization, and violating legal and regulatory requirements.

The incentives to provide high-value care in the ED, while currently significant, are anticipated to strengthen considerably in coming years. The ability to deliver quality care will increasingly be viewed as a "core competency" of ED directors. Directors should expect to work continuously on issues related to driving value while increasingly prioritizing efforts to optimize ED resource utilization.

REFERENCES

1. Centers for Medicare and Medicaid Services. National Health Expenditure Data: NHE Fact Sheet. Available at: https://www.cms.gov/research-statistics-data-and-systems/statistics-trends-and-reports/nationalhealthexpenddata/nhe-fact-sheet.html. Accessed December 16, 2019.
2. Lee M, Schurr J, Zink B. Owning the cost of emergency medicine: beyond 2%. *Ann Emerg Med*. 2013;62(5):498–505.
3. Emergency Department Benchmarking Alliance (EDBA) Operational Resources. 2019. Available at: https://www.edbenchmarking.org/operational-resources. Accessed July 31, 2020.
4. Hospital Inpatient Quality Reporting (IQR) Program: Overview. Centers for Medicare & Medicaid Services. Available at: https://www.qualitynet.org/inpatient/iqr. Accessed December 16, 2019.
5. Hospital Outpatient Quality Reporting Program: Overview. Centers for Medicare & Medicaid Services. Available at: https://www.qualitynet.org/outpatient/oqr. Accessed December 16, 2019.
6. Centers for Medicare and Medicaid Services. Hospital Outpatient Quality Reporting Program. 2020. Available at: https://www.cms.gov/Medicare/Quality-Initiatives-Patient-Assessment-Instruments/HospitalQualityInits/HospitalOutpatientQualityReportingProgram. Accessed August 1, 2020.
7. Five-Star Quality Rating System. Centers for Medicare & Medicaid Services. 2019. Available at: https://www.cms.gov/Medicare/Provider-Enrollment-and-Certification/CertificationandComplianc/FSQRS. Accessed December 16, 2019.
8. Centers for Medicare and Medicaid Services. Hospital Readmissions Reduction Program. 2020. Available at: https://www.cms.gov/Medicare/Quality-Initiatives-Patient-Assessment-Instruments/Value-Based-Programs/HRRP/Hospital-Readmission-Reduction-Program. Accessed August 1, 2020.
9. 42 U.S. Code § 1395nn—Limitation on certain physician referrals. 2020. Available at: https://www.law.cornell.edu/uscode/text/42/1395nn. Accessed July 29, 2020.
10. Medicare Shared Savings Program. Centers for Medicare & Medicaid Services. Available at: https://www.cms.gov/Medicare/Medicare-Fee-for-Service-Payment/sharedsavingsprogram/index. Accessed December 16, 2019.
11. National Association of ACOs. Available at: https://www.naacos.com. Accessed December 16, 2019.
12. Muhlestein D, Saunders RS, McClellan MB. Growth of ACOs and alternative payment models in 2017. *Health Affairs* blog. 2017. Available at: https://www.healthaffairs.org/do/10.1377/hblog20170628.060719/full/. Accessed August 26, 2020.
13. Ali NJ, McWilliams JM, Epstein SK, et al. Emergency department involvement in accountable care organizations in Massachusetts: a survey study. *Ann Emerg Med*. 2017;70(5):615–620.
14. Lin M, Richardson LD, Carr B, et al. Acute care redesign and alternative payment for emergency medicine within accountable care organizations: a qualitative study. *Ann Emerg Med*. 2017;70(4):S81–S82.
15. BPCI Advanced. Centers for Medicare & Medicaid Services. Available at: https://innovation.cms.gov/initiatives/bpci-advanced. Accessed September 27, 2018.
16. Murray R, Caballero A, Delbanco SF. The state of evidence on payment reform. *NEJM Catalyst*. 2018. Available at: https://catalyst.nejm.org/state-evidence-payment-reform-shared-savings/. Accessed August 26, 2020.

17. ACEP develops an FAQ to explain its alternative payment model. *ACEP Now*. November 24, 2019.
18. MACRA. Centers for Medicare & Medicaid Services. Available at: https://www.cms.gov/Medicare/Quality-Initiatives-Patient-Assessment-Instruments/Value-Based-Programs/MACRA-MIPS-and-APMs/MACRA-MIPS-and-APMs. Accessed December 16, 2019.
19. Kocher KE, Meurer WJ, Desmond JS, et al. Effect of testing and treatment on emergency department length of stay using a national database. *Acad Emerg Med*. 2012;19(5):525–534.
20. Wiler JL, Welch S, Pines J, et al. Emergency department performance measures updates: proceedings of the 2014 emergency department benchmarking alliance consensus summit. *Acad Emerg Med*. 2015;22(5):542–553.
21. Dean NC, Jones JP, Aronsky D, et al. Hospital admission decision for patients with community-acquired pneumonia: variability among physicians in an emergency department. *Ann Emerg Med*. 2012;59(1):35–41.
22. Levine MB, Moore AB, Kuehl DR, et al. Variation in use of all types of computed tomography by emergency physicians. *Ann Emerg Med*. 2012;60(4):104S-105S.
23. Mahler SA, Goff DC, Hoekstra JW, et al. Variability of emergency physicians utilization of chest pain units for "very low risk" chest pain patients. *Ann Emerg Med*. 2011;58(4):190S.
24. Jain S, Elon LK, Johnson BA, et al. Physician practice variation in the pediatric emergency department and its impact on resource use and quality of care. *Ped Emerg Care*. 2010;26(12):902–908.
25. Chen YA, Gray BG, Bandiera G, et al. Variation in the utilization and positivity rates of CT pulmonary angiography among emergency physicians at a tertiary academic emergency department. *Emerg Radiol*. 2015;22(3):221–229.
26. Andruchow JE, Raja AS, Prevedello LM, et al. Physician risk tolerance and diagnostic yield of CT pulmonary angiography: are they related? *Ann Emerg Med*. 2012;60(4):S4.
27. Kadhim-Saleh A, Worrall J, Taljaard M, et al. Self-awareness of computed tomography ordering in the emergency department. *CJEM*. 2018;20(2):275–283.
28. Choosing Wisely. Available at: http://www.choosingwisely.org. Accessed September 27, 2018.
29. Clinician lists: American College of Emergency Physicians. Choosing Wisely. Available at: http://www.choosingwisely.org/clinician-lists/#parentSociety=American_College_of_Emergency_Physicians. Accessed September 27, 2018.
30. Maughan BC, Rabin E, Cantrill SV; ACEP Quality and Patient Safety Committee Workgroup on Choosing Wisely. A broader view of quality: Choosing Wisely recommendations from other specialties with relevance to emergency care. *Ann Emerg Med*. 2018;72(3):246–253.
31. Augustine, JJ. Diagnostic testing in the ED supports development of new metrics as quality indicators. *ACEP Now*. May 15, 2017.
32. Kuppermann N, Holmes JF, Dayan PS, et al. Identification of children at very low risk of clinically-important brain injuries after head trauma: a prospective cohort study. *Lancet* 2009;374(9696):1160–1170.
33. Jagoda A, Bazarian JJ, Bruns JJ, et al. Clinical policy: neuroimaging and decision-making in adult mild traumatic brain injury in the acute setting. *Ann Emerg Med*. 2008;52(5):714–748.
34. Edlow JA, Panagos PD, Godwin SA, et al. Clinical policy: critical issues in the evaluation and management of adult patients presenting to the emergency department with acute headache. *Ann Emerg Med*. 2008;52(4);407–436.
35. Stiell IG, Wells GA, Vandemheen KL, et al. The Canadian c-spine rule for radiography in alert and stable trauma patients. *JAMA*. 2001;286(15):1841–1848.
36. Stiell, IG, Clement CM, McKnight RD. The Canadian c-spine rule versus the NEXUS low-risk criteria in patients with trauma. *N Engl J Med*. 2003;349(26):2510–2518.
37. Hoffman JR, Mower WR, Wolfson AB, et al. Validity of a set of clinical criteria to rule out injury to the cervical spine in patients with blunt trauma. *N Engl J Med*. 2000;343(2):94–99.
38. Raja AS, Greenberg JO, Qaseem A, et al. Evaluation of patients with suspected acute pulmonary embolism: best practice advice from the Clinical Guidelines Committee of the American College of Physicians. *Ann Intern Med*. 2015:163(9):701–711.
39. Chou R, Qaseem A, Owens DK, et al. Diagnostic imaging for low back pain: advice for high-value health care from the American College of Physicians. *Ann Intern Med*. 2011;154(3):181–189.
40. Smith-Bindman R, Aubin C, Bailitz J, et al. Ultrasonography versus computed tomography for suspected nephrolithiasis. *N Engl J Med*. 2014;371(12):1100–1110.
41. Kaplan J, Tomar B. Appropriate use criteria: another hoop for emergency physicians to jump through? *ACEP Now*. August 1, 2017.
42. Smulowitz PB, Hongman L, Landon BE. A novel approach to identifying targets for cost reduction in the emergency department. *Ann Emerg Med*. 2013;61(3):293–300.
43. Venkatesh AK, Schuur JD. A top-five list for emergency medicine: a policy and research agenda for stewardship to improve the value of emergency care. *Am J Emerg Med*. 2013;31(10):1520–1524.
44. Owens PL, Barrett ML, Gibson TB, et al. Emergency department care in the United States: a profile of national data sources. *Ann Emerg Med*. 2010;56(2):150–165.
45. Rui P, Kang K, Ashmann JJ. National Hospital Ambulatory Medical Care Survey: 2016 Emergency Department Summary Tables. 2016. Available at: https://www.cdc.gov/nchs/data/nhamcs/web_tables/2016_ed_web_tables.pdf. Accessed December 16, 2019.
46. Capp R, Ross JS, Fox JP, et al. Hospital variation in risk-standardized hospital admission rates from US EDs among adults. *Am J Emerg Med*. 2014;32(8):837–843.
47. Venkatesh AK, Dai Y, Ross JS, et al. Variation in US hospital emergency department admission rates by clinical condition. *Med Care*. 2015;53(3):237–244.
48. Sabbatini AK, Nallamothu BK, Kocher KE. Reducing variation in hospital admissions from the emergency department for low-mortality conditions may produce savings. *Health Aff*. 2014;33(9):1655–1663.
49. Fine MJ, Auble TE, Yealy DM, et al. A prediction rule to identify low-risk patients with community-acquired pneumonia. *N Engl J Med*. 1997;336(4):243–250.
50. Lim W, van der Eerden MM, Laing R, et al. Defining community acquired pneumonia severity on presentation to hospital: an international derivation and validation study. *Thorax*. 2003;58(5): 377–382.
51. Camargo CA, Rachelefsky G, Schatz M. Managing asthma exacerbations in the emergency department: summary of the National Asthma Education and Prevention Program Expert Panel Report 3 guidelines for the management of asthma exacerbations. *Proc Am Thorac Soc*. 2009;6(4):357–366.
52. Chalut DS, Ducharme FM, Davis GM. The Preschool Respiratory Assessment Measure (PRAM): a responsive index of acute asthma severity. *J Pediatr*. 2000;137(6): 762–768.
53. Gorelick MH, Stevens MW, Schultz TR, et al. Performance of a novel clinical score, the Pediatric Asthma Severity Score (PASS), in the evaluation of acute asthma. *Acad Emerg Med*. 2004;11(1):10–18.
54. Backus BE, Six AJ, Kelder JC, et al. A prospective validation of the HEART score for chest pain patients at the emergency department. *Int J Cardiol*. 2013;168(3):2153–2158

55. Mahler SA, Riley RF, Hiestand BC, et al. The HEART Pathway randomized trial: identifying emergency department patients with acute chest pain for early discharge. *Circ Cardiovasc Qual Outcomes*. 2015;8(2):195–203.

56. Poldervaart JM, Langedijk M, Backus BE, et al. Comparison of the GRACE, HEART, and TIMI score to predict adverse cardiac events in chest pain patients at the emergency department. *Int J Cardiol*. 2017;227:656–661.

57. Kearon C, Akl EA, Ornelas J, et al. Antithrombotic therapy for VTE disease: CHEST guideline and expert panel report. *Chest*. 2016;149(2):315–352.

58. Gautney LJ, Stanton MP, Crowe C, et al. The emergency department case manager: effect on selected outcomes. *Lippincotts Case Manag*. 2004;9(3):121–129.

59. Bristow DP, Herrick CA. Emergency department case management: the dyad team of nurse case manager and social worker improve discharge planning and patient and staff satisfaction while decreasing inappropriate admissions and costs: a literature review. *Lippincotts Case Manag*. 2002;7(3):121–128.

60. Kulkarni R, Pell F, Agocs-Holler EJ, et al. Care coordination in the emergency department: avoiding inappropriate hospital admissions. *Ann Emerg Med*. 2007;50(3):S71-S72.

61. Ross MA, Aurora T, Graff L, et al. State of the art: emergency department observation units. *Crit Pathw Cardiol*. 2012;11(3):128–138.

62. Sun BC, McCreath H, Liang L-J, et al. Randomized clinical trial of an emergency department observation syncope protocol versus routine inpatient admission. *Ann Emerg Med*. 2014;64(2):167–175.

63. Decker WW, Smars PA, Vaidyanathan L, et al. A prospective, randomized trial of an emergency department observation unit for acute onset atrial fibrillation. *Ann Emerg Med*. 2008;52(4):322–328.

64. Peacock WF, Remer EE, Aponte J, et al. Effective observation unit treatment of decompensated heart failure. *Congest Heart Fail*. 2002;8(2):68–73.

65. Rydman RJ, Isola ML, Roberts RR, et al. Emergency department observation unit versus hospital inpatient care for a chronic asthmatic population: a randomized trial of health status outcome and cost. *Med Care*. 1998;36(4):599–609.

66. Baugh CW, Venkatesh AK, Hilton JA, et al. Making greater use of dedicated hospital observation units for many short-stay patients could save $3.1 billion a year. *Health Aff*. 2012;31(10):2314–2323.

67. Wiler JL, Ross MA, Ginde AA. National study of emergency department observation services. *Acad Emerg Med*. 2011;18(9):959–965.

68. Baugh CW, Pines J. Observation status: the new treatment, payment paradigm. *Emergency Physicians Monthly*. August 15, 2017.

69. Baugh D, Granovsky M. New CMS rules introduce bundled payments for observation care. *ACEP Now*. March 16, 2016.

70. Meier DE. Increased access to palliative care and hospice services: opportunities to improve value in health care. *Milbank Q*. 2011;89(3):343–380.

71. Grudzen CR, Stone SC, Morrison RS. The palliative care model for emergency department patients with advanced illness. *J Palliat Care Med*. 2011;14(8):945–950.

72. Morrison RS, Penrod JD, Cassel JB, et al. Cost savings associated with US hospital palliative care consultation programs. *Arch Intern Med*. 2008;168(16):1783–1790.

73. Morrison RS, Dietrich J, Ladwig S, et al. Palliative care consultation teams cut hospital costs for Medicaid beneficiaries. *Health Aff*. 2011;30(3):454–463.

74. Waselewsky D, Zalenski R, Burn J, Hong Y. Palliative care consultation initiated in ED is associated with significant reductions in hospital length of stay. Presented at: 2009 *Society of Academic Emergency Medicine* Annual Meeting. May 14–17, 2009; New Orleans, LA.

75. Wu FM, Newman JM, Lasher A, et al. Effects of initiating palliative care consultation in the emergency department on inpatient length of stay. *J Palliat Med*. 2013;16(11):1362–1367.

76. May P, Normand C, Morrison RS. Economic impact of hospital inpatient palliative care consultation: review of current evidence and directions for future research. *J Palliat Med*. 2014;17(9):1054–1063.

77. Osta BE, Palmer JL, Paraskevopoulos T, et al. Interval between first palliative care consult an death in patients diagnosed with advanced cancer at a comprehensive cancer center. *J Palliat Med*. 2008;11(1):51–57.

78. National Palliative Care Registry. Annual Survey Summary: Results of the 2016 National Palliative Care Registry Survey. Center to Advance Palliative Care (CAPC). Available at: https://www.capc.org/national-palliative-care-registry/. Accessed on September 27, 2018.

79. George N, Phillips E, Zaurova M, et al. Palliative care screening and assessment in the emergency department: a systemic review. *J Pain Symptom Manage*. 2016;51(1):108–119.e2.

80. LaCalle E, Rabin E. Frequent users of emergency departments: the myths, the data, and the policy implications. *Ann Emerg Med*. 2010;56(1):42–48.

81. Han X, Lowry TY, Loo GT, et al. Expanding health information exchange improves identification of frequent emergency department users. *Ann Emerg Med*. 2019;73(2):172–179.

82. Sandoval E, Smith S, Walter J, et al. A comparison of frequent and infrequent visitors to an urban emergency department. *J Emerg Med*. 2010;38(2):115–121.

83. Ruger JP, Richter CJ, Spitznagel EL, et al. Analysis of costs, length of stay, and utilization of emergency department services by frequent users: implications for health policy. *Acad Emerg Med*. 2004;11(12):1311–1317.

84. Peabody C, Gruber P, Lam CN, et al. Medical necessity and resource use among frequent emergency department users. *Ann of Emerg*. 2014;64(4S):S10.

85. Doupe MB, Palatnick W, Day S, et al. Frequent users of emergency departments: developing standard definitions and defining prominent risk factors. *Ann Emerg Med*. 2012;60(1):24–32.

86. Althuas F, Paroz S, Hugli O, et al. Effectiveness of interventions targeting frequent users of emergency departments: a systemic review. *Ann Emerg Med*. 2011;58(1):41–52.

87. Moe J, Kirkland SW, Rawe E, et al. Effectiveness of interventions to decrease emergency department visits by adult frequent users: a systemic review. *Acad Emerg Med*. 2017;24(1):40–52.

88. Soril LJJ, Leggett LE, Lorenzetti DL, et al. Reducing frequent visits to the emergency department: a systemic review of interventions. *PLoS One*. 2015;10(4):e0123660. https://doi.org/10.1371/journal.pone.0123660

89. Capp R, Misky GJ, Lindrooth RC, et al. Coordination program reduced acute care use and increased primary care visits among frequent emergency care users. *Health Aff*. 2017;36(10):1705–1711.

90. National Ambulatory Care Medical Care Survey: 2010 Emergency Department Summary Tables. Available at: https://www.cdc.gov/nchs/data/ahcd/nhamcs_emergency/2010_ed_web_tables.pdf. Accessed August 26, 2020.

91. Zachrison KS, Boggs KM, Hayden EM, et al. A national survey of telemedicine use by US emergency departments. *J Telemed Telecare*. 2020;26(5):278–284.

92. Watson J, Bhat R, Izzo J, et al. Telemedicine model of physician intake decreases door-to-provider time. *Ann Emerg Med*. 2017;72(4):S128–S129.

93. Sharma R, Clark S, Torres-Lavoro J, Dhaded A, Hsu H, Greenwald P. Telemedicine in the emergency department: a novel, academic approach to optimizing operational metrics and patient experience. *Ann Emerg Med*. 2018;70(4S):Supplement 128. Available at: https://www.annemergmed.com/article/S0196-6644(17)31295-7/abstract. Accessed July 31, 2020.

CHAPTER 85

THE FINANCIALLY SUCCESSFUL EMERGENCY DEPARTMENT

Michael A. Granovsky, Ori Litvak, Sara Nourazari

The most significant determinant of a financially successful emergency department (ED) is its payer mix. With sufficient revenue, even the most poorly led and managed department can be financially successful. Alternatively, even the most efficiently run ED will struggle to achieve financial success if it has high levels of self-pay and underinsured government entitlement program patients.[1] It takes resources to attract and support the best leaders and clinicians while updating and maintaining the physical plant. In an era when "making do with less" is the rule, financial success is measured by an ED's ability to delivery quality care without increased subsidies.

This chapter primarily focuses on those EDs in which there are enough revenues to fund the activities required for success and a strong commitment by leadership, physicians, and nurses. The financially successful ED requires a superior leadership team with the ability to operationalize critical workflow programs and billing processes.

KEYS TO SUCCESS

The success of an ED can be measured in many different ways—economically, the quality of the care, community reputation, patient safety, patient satisfaction, and so on. EDs do not achieve success by doing a few big things right but, rather, by paying attention to detail and actively managing hundreds of smaller issues. These details might be as big as the average number of billable relative value units (RVUs) per hour of provider staffing cost or as small as the color of the cap on the urine sample that tells the lab technician that this is a stat test.

No two EDs have the same collections per visit, provider RVUs per hour, or nurse staffing ratios, but all successful EDs share a set of common attributes characterized by standardized processes, close attention to detail, and leaders capable of developing and retaining a well-trained and motivated team with a clear mission and vision.

Superior Leadership

Aside from payer mix, an ED's financial success depends more on its leadership than anything else. A department's leaders must be aligned in their problem-solving approach, know how to balance criticism with praise, and demonstrate respect for each other. The leaders must be committed to crafting and maintaining a departmental culture where the staff feels safe and encouraged to share ideas and voice concerns without fear of reprisal. Simultaneously, leaders should not tolerate chronic poor performance; rather, they must inspire and mobilize the entire ED team while anticipating and adapting to change. The leadership role does not, as some might assert, revolve around continuous process improvements. Department leaders must instead focus on removing barriers, supporting their staff, and coordinating the work of their respective teams.

A Trained Team

Leaders of financially successful EDs make time to step out of the whirlwind that is their typical day to provide their team members with the relationship, communication, and project management skills needed to achieve success. Cultural barriers and complex or long-standing problems are harder to solve and require a plan and a team. Since the basic unit of organizational accomplishment may be considered the "project" or undertaking, ED personnel should receive, at minimum, basic project management training. Mobilizing and engaging staff members on project teams enables the department to achieve much more than it can when only the leaders address problems. Serving on a project team or as a project team leader is a great place to start spreading problem-solving capacity and building the next generation of leaders. Examples of internal ED projects include creating triage protocols to lessen wait time and streamlining the arrival-to-provider time. Interdepartmental ED projects include expediting patient admissions and reducing the time between ordering imaging or lab tests and getting the results.

A Clear Vision of the Future

Great leadership "begins with the end in mind," the second habit of Stephen Covey's *The 7 Habits of Highly Effective People*.[2] Highly successful organizations begin the journey toward excellence with a mission, vision, and values exercise that engages the entire department. That chosen direction should align with the greater organization's strategic vision and mission. When everyone participates, the members of the department are more invested in "owning" the vision than when these goals are merely dictated to them. The result of such an exercise is a written statement that addresses all three of the elements.

- *Mission* is the answer to the question "Why does the team exist?"
- *Vision* describes what the team aspires to become.
- *Values* include how the team members will treat each other on the journey to achieve the vision.

It is difficult, if not impossible, to hold ED team members accountable for goals they had no role in establishing. Alternatively, universal participation in crafting an organization's vision helps create a safe atmosphere in which both leaders and members are encouraged to recommend improvements and are expected to be held accountable. An outside facilitator may help avoid the appearance, or the reality, that leadership is dominating the process. As many members of the department as possible should be involved in the creation of the vision statement and the strategic planning session that typically follows it.

Successful leaders also know that money is only one motivator; the desire for autonomy and being part of a larger purpose are key drivers for staff engagement and satisfaction. It is the leader's job to encourage autonomy and continually reinforce the vision statement, which embodies the kind of higher purpose that makes team members want to go to work each day.

Once the department mission, vision, and values are articulated and embraced, it's time to create the projects that improve the department. Projects aimed at decreasing length of stay, wait time, or turnaround time for key labs or images; increasing patient satisfaction; and delivering better service levels benefit from a scientific approach to problem-solving. The problem-solving cycle can involve a repetitive process of planning, implementation, testing, and measurement. A team can be formed to craft a fitting problem statement and write a charter (either with the help of an outside facilitator or trained project manager) that defines the obstacle, identifies wastes in the process that yield errors and extra work, outlines common goals, and addresses the gap between the current and ideal states. A robust communication plan is also key, especially in an ED that operates with many staff across all hours of the day.

MANAGING CHANGE

Nothing in emergency medicine stays the same for long. The ability to anticipate and lead change is extremely important for any financially successful ED. The American health-care "system" of the 21st century appears to prize the acceleration of change. Addressing these near-constant shifts requires the continual development of high-yield projects designed to improve service. The vision statement itself should be regularly reviewed to ensure that it is consistent with the organization's direction.

A critical component of the change process includes staff and leadership training on communications and project management. Typically, health-care organizations spend very little time training staff on effective ways to provide input, make and implement positive change, communicate clearly, and hold each other accountable. This change process is an ideal opportunity for the medical and nurse directors to develop and practice their delegation skills. Leader expertise in these areas helps all of the team members become more proficient in participating in or leading a project team. The delegation process also allows nontraditional leaders to become involved in project management; such opportunities can groom new leaders, who can be valuable assets for succession planning. By learning how to manage a project, team members learn the basic skills of leadership and change management. In order to keep the team engaged and motivated, it is important to chart progress, provide feedback to staff, and celebrate when goals are reached.

Matching Staff to Patient Needs

Personnel cost is by far the largest ED operational cost. Efficient and cost-effective resource allocation in the ED is only possible if ED leaders become experts at managing staffing levels. The ED is inherently always either over- or understaffed and may rapidly switch from one to the other with the arrival of multiple critically ill patients. The management objective is to identify staffing levels that balance cost and patients' wait times. While total cost is predictable based on the number and mix of the providers working, patient wait times can vary significantly based on the number of arrivals, the needs of these patients, the number of providers working, the rate that each of these providers can see patients, and their respective practice patterns. Modeling the complete ED system is a complex task. However, actionable information can be created by using queuing theory and a few simplified assumptions.

Utilizing queueing theory, ED leaders can perform a mathematical study of how customers wait in service systems. Using information about patient arrivals, servers

FIGURE 85.1 ■ Staffing Related to Patient Length of Stay

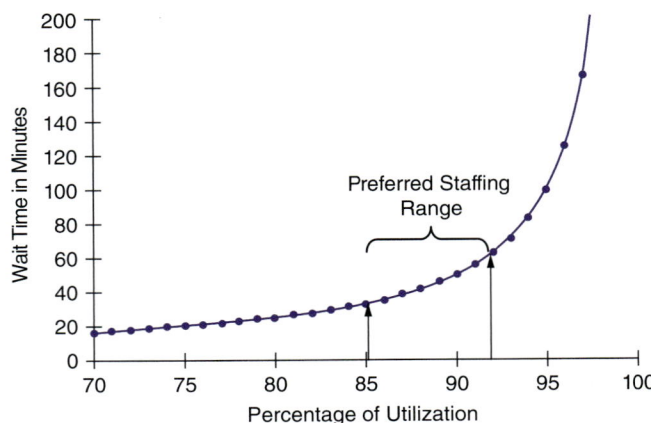

(providers and beds), and the rate that providers can see patients, queueing theory can be used to model flow and predict wait times and the number of patients waiting to see a provider (**Figure 85.1**).

A useful queueing equation called Little's Law can be used to relate arrivals, average length of stay, and census. Little's Law states that the average number of patients in the facility (L) is the product of the patient arrival rate (λ) and the average time to meet each patient's need (W), which in this case is the ED's length of stay (**Box 85.1**).

Little's Law demonstrates that reducing length of stay can reduce bed census and the likelihood of a server deficiency (bed or clinician). As length of stay increases, both server constraints and the waiting room patient lengths of stay grow, further increasing unnecessary wait times. Thus, process improvements that reduce the length of stay can significantly reduce bed census, relieve space and staffing constraints, and diminish wait times without adding costly provider coverage. Additional benefits will result from waiting room patients having shorter "door-to-provider" times, reducing the number of patients leaving prior to medical screening examination and increasing revenue. By improving efficiency and flow, the financially successfully ED reduces nonprovider constraints and increases revenue opportunities.

Financial success is partially determined by the EM group matching its human resources servers (emergency physician, advanced practice provider, or allied health professional) with the patient need while maintaining high-quality care. In order to ensure cost-effective matching of providers (the right level of training in the right area of the ED), providers must have optimal nursing and ancillary support. Similarly, facility-side success requires attention to its servers—"right" staffing and beds. Staffing levels are set most often by staff full-time equivalent (FTE) to patient-visit ratios using various benchmarking tools from the Emergency Nurse's Association or private benchmark providers such as Premier.[3] Other approaches

BOX 85.1 ■ LITTLE'S LAW

$$L = \lambda \times W$$

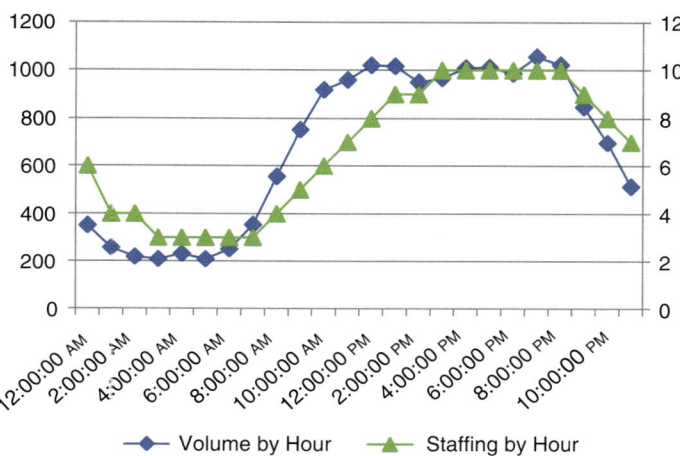

FIGURE 85.2 ■ Patient Volume and Staffing by Hour of Arrival

include staffing by hour of arrival, hour of departure, and the use of a dwell time measure to account for ED patient boarding **(Figure 85.2)**.

A rigid hospital budgeting process may unnecessarily complicate the calculation for nurse staffing by counting all FTEs the same regardless of the cost of the FTE rather than focusing on the dollar budget amount. Emergency departments that use all-nurse staffs are inefficient and expensive, compared to those that rely on both registered nurses and technicians. Financially successful EDs eliminate barriers to the use of nurse extenders.

Typical hospitals allow nurse sick call-in shifts to go uncovered, resulting in a fairly constant nurse staffing shortfall. This inadequate staffing may result in the ED regularly exceeding 85%, 90%, or 95% staffing capacity utilization, creating long queues, walkouts, and an unsafe environment. Making matters worse, some facilities do not include boarding patients (admitted patients residing in the ED) in their "count" of ED patients, even though the boarding patients require significant nurse and physician attention to care for the patients. Financially successful EDs provide adequate nursing coverage and find ways to address call-ins, ensuring adequate staffing.

Many state legislatures are discussing and proposing mandatory staffing ratios in the ED and throughout the hospital. The objective is to determine the ideal nursing coverage needs without compromising care or exceeding budget. Again, success requires effective analysis of the arriving patients by:

- Measuring patient arrival times by hour of day and day of week
- Examining the acuity level of patients
- Predicting the resources required to meet that patient demand

The creation of predictive models for appropriate staffing levels will ultimately require a balance between budgets and high-quality, timely patient care and patient satisfaction.

Processes and Flow

ED workflow must change as patient volumes grow. The physical plant layout that is adequate for 20,000 visits must be remodeled to accommodate 40,000 visits. Throughput generally improves when the physical plant changes keep up with the workflow changes.

Nowhere is this more evident than in triage. Some of the most successful EDs completely reconfigure the triage workflow at higher volumes, providing only quick registration—just enough to get essential testing or medications ordered. The rest of the registration is performed at the bedside.

Using this quick registration process, patients bypass triage altogether and go directly to a bed, when available. When there is no bed available, a provider with a dedicated nurse can be placed in triage to evaluate and discharge patients with minor presentations without ever sending them into the ED proper. For other patients, the provider can initiate the workup based on the physician group's consensus order sets, often routing patients to venipuncture or x-ray before sending them to a bed. Patients who have completed their evaluation and no longer need a bed are routed to a "Results Pending" room to await their final interaction with the provider once all the testing is complete.

As volume increases, the financially successful ED stratifies its provider resources by adding nurse practitioners and/or physician assistants to augment physicians as servers and, on the nursing side, by adding nursing technicians, paramedics, and transporters. The goal is to match appropriate provider skills and cost with patient needs.

Electronic medical records (EMRs) have by and large failed to deliver their promised efficiency benefits in the ED. While it is true that the chart may be more complete and additional clinical data become electronically searchable, these benefits are largely offset by serious degradations in provider productivity. From an ED operational perspective, most of the benefits of EMRs accrue to low-cost personnel—medical records, coding, abstracting, and so on—while the greatest productivity losses are experienced by the highest cost resources, the providers. In this situation, scribes and voice recognition dictation become essential resources. Emergency departments are increasingly using scribes to document key pieces of the interaction with the intent of facilitating more timely and accurate chart documentation, allowing the clinicians to work more productively. In addition to documenting key elements of the patient encounter, scribes can assist in managing communication between staff and the ED provider and help track down and organize laboratory, imaging, and other ancillary test results.

Extra-Departmental Resources

The successful ED's output is a satisfied patient treated according to evidence-based guidelines. Achieving this success depends on coordinating and managing many diverse resources, some of which are extra-departmental resources. This management includes, but is not limited to, tracking and eliminating bottlenecks related to:

- Lab turnaround times for common tests (urinalysis, complete blood count, etc)
- X-ray turnaround times for common images
- Respiratory services responsiveness
- Consulting/admitting physician responsiveness
- Timing of disposition decision to patient departure (from the ED)

Operational Metrics

Financially successful EDs are data driven and may spend considerable resources in the pursuit of meaningful and usable data. Regular reporting creates peer pressure on involved stakeholders and helps focus limited management resources on the areas of greatest opportunity. The most useful metrics are listed in **Box 85.2**.

> **BOX 85.2 ■ USEFUL OPERATIONAL METRICS**
>
> - Collected dollars per visit
> - Collected dollars per RVU
> - RVUs per patient, patients per hour, RVUs per hour of staffing cost
> - Door/arrival-to-provider time
> - Initial provider assessment to disposition decision
> - Disposition decision-to-departure
> - LOS for admitted, treated, and released patients
> - Quality measures
> - Patient satisfaction (assuming a statistically valid sample size)

DOCUMENTATION, CHARGES, AND COLLECTIONS

Management of staffing, operations, and resources is irrelevant if documentation, charges, and collections are not managed correctly. The revenue of the ED on both the facility and professional side is highly dependent on adequate physician and nurse documentation, appropriate coding methodology, and fully optimized coding, billing, and collections. A brief overview of the critical steps in the revenue chain and important metrics to consider for best practices and benchmarking is presented here.

Credentialing

Credentialing involves the simple act of filling out forms and completing the necessary paperwork to ensure each physician's National Provider Identifier number and the group's tax ID number are recognized by the insurance carrier. It is imperative that all providers are credentialed with all insurance carriers prior to the providers' placement on the ED schedule. In the past, insurance carriers allowed extended retroactive billing, but that is no longer the norm. Many carriers allow no retroactive grace period, and even Medicare has shortened the retroactive billing window to 30 days.

Physicians who work prior to having active provider numbers pose two potential financial problems for the group. First, if the carrier does allow retroactive billing once the provider number has been assigned, the ED group loses the potential reimbursement and may be put in a difficult cash flow position. Second, although a group may be able to briefly tolerate this cash flow gap, this loss of reimbursement could become financially awkward if it occurred for several physicians or for an extended period of time. This problem is more likely to occur in July and August when groups may have a large number of graduating residents. Typically, allowing 60 to 90 days for provider credentialing in advance of their start dates is advisable to ensure that a new provider is fully credentialed and retroactive billing does not occur (**Box 85.3**).

> **BOX 85.3 ■ REIMBURSEMENT TIP**
>
> Make sure 100% of your physicians are credentialed prior to beginning their clinical work. This is especially true for graduating residents.

> **BOX 85.4 ■ COMMON REGISTRATION SOLUTIONS**
>
> 1. Do not enter "no address or contact information" or put all Xs or identify an address as 999.
> 2. Do not just ask the patient, "Is everything the same?"
> 3. Do not just put the hospital's address when a patient lacks adequate information.
> 4. **Best practice:** Get copies of the insurance card scanned into the hospital IT database. This helps identify the subtypes of insurance the patient may possess. As an example, there are over 50 Aetna PPO products in some metropolitan areas.
> 5. **Best practice:** Registration personnel should be placed directly in the ED with computers on wheels and mobile scanners.
> 6. **Best practice:** The billing agent should interact with and query on an ongoing basis the Hospital Registration Database at a set time (for instance, 3 days) after the visit to determine if registration information has been updated.
> 7. In an effort to create an atmosphere of equality and team building, include the registration staff when ordering food for the ED or when providing holiday gifts.
> 8. State Medicaid eligibility should be checked prospectively through widely available state telephonic systems at the time of the ED visit.
> 9. Calls should be made to gather workers' compensation contact information at the time of treatment while the employer is motivated to assist.
> 10. Every month, your billing agent should monitor the amount of "bad insurance information" and be alert to any changes.

Hospital Registration

The hospital registration system forms the backbone of the ED group's revenue stream. The billing company should monitor inaccurate insurance information and bring it to the attention of the physician leadership as well as the hospital registration department. Best practices include a monthly or quarterly meeting with the registration manager to go through any identified problems (**Box 85.4**).

Documentation

Typical documentation best practices are listed in **Box 85.5**.

> **BOX 85.5 ■ DOCUMENTING BEST PRACTICES**
>
> - Review the chart construct to make sure it supports all aspects of your coding and billing, including ED services (typically 99281-99285 and 99291), procedures, diagnosis coding, and quality reporting.
> - Ensure the billing of electrocardiograms, ED ultrasound interpretations, and plain x-ray interpretations.
> - Provide an ongoing didactic program to the physicians and nurses, including:
>   - Individual chart feedback for educational purposes for underdocumented records.
>   - Monthly or quarterly educational meetings depending on the needs.
>   - Outlier discussions with physicians or nurses who have ongoing deficiencies.
>   - Management-level reports to track down coded and underdocumented records.
>   - A provider-specific documentation opportunity report.
>   - <0.5% of records down-coded.

Chart Reconciliation

Since a lost chart is the equivalent of lost revenue, a robust and redundant system should be in place to minimize lost records. The hospital staff (including the CFO and CIO) and the ED leaders should coordinate efforts to create a log that accurately reflects the "universal denominator" for all ED patients, including some of the more complex categories of admissions, transfers, visits crossing midnight, and patients who leave prior to medical screening or against medical advice. The system should reconcile the records daily, weekly, and quarterly against the ED log and provide an interface with medical records for identifying and securing any and all missing charts, ideally within 60 days.

Coding

Coding methodology is the process by which medical records are scored. Most providers are familiar with the complex "bean-counting" requirements of Medicare's documentation guidelines, which involve recording a specific number of history and exam elements to support the evaluation and management level assigned. In addition, each code requires a specified amount of medical decision-making. These subcomponents are typically identified by the number of diagnosis and management options, the amount and complexity of data, and the patient's level of risk. Only the medical decision-making subcomponent of risk is actually defined in Medicare's 1995 documentation guidelines. ED coding is a sophisticated and nuanced process, and some benchmarks are helpful to ascertain whether a group is coding appropriately. Medicare makes post-claims data available both nationally (**Figure 85.3**) and by state.

Accounting

The management of accounts receivable is the process of turning the coding and gross charges into revenue for the practice. This involves the actual process of submitting the bill, posting of cash, and working of denials.

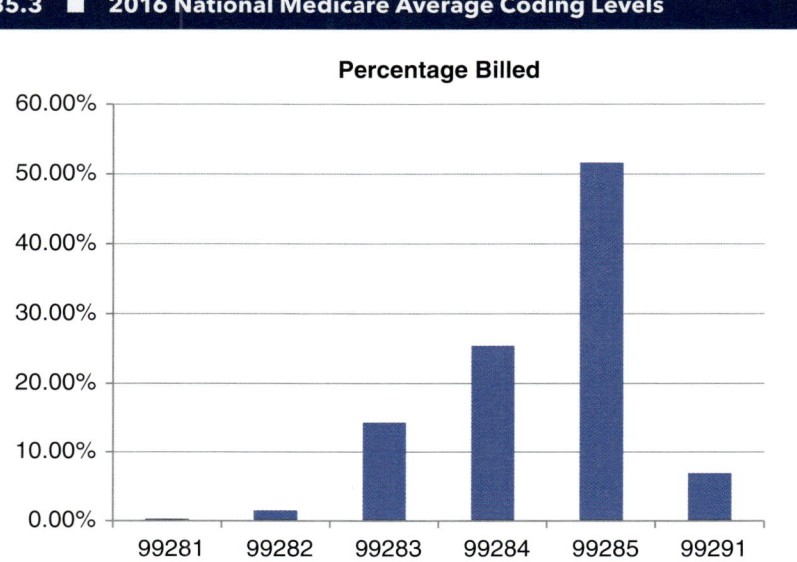

FIGURE 85.3 ■ 2016 National Medicare Average Coding Levels

BOX 85.6 ■ KEY COMPONENTS OF A HEALTHY ED

- A living vision statement
- Consistent staffing with well-trained professionals sufficient to meet the demands for patient flow and quality care
- Operationally intelligent: appropriately equipped, staffed, and designed to support work and flow
- Focused on quality and safety

CONCLUSION

It can be daunting to create a healthy, financially successful ED (**Box 85.6**) in the current economic climate amidst constant, accelerating change. Declining reimbursements, ever-changing payer mixes, and the unknowns presented by health-care reform make "business as usual" a formula for failure. The achievement of financial success requires a dynamic leadership team, a staff committed to excellence, and a departmental willingness to think creatively about the challenges faced by today's EDs. The same dedication to excellence and focus on details that help us provide high-quality, compassionate care to our patients can help us achieve what was once thought of as an oxymoron—a financially successful ED. Outstanding leadership is the most important component of a healthy ED, with the physicians and nursing leaders providing vision and operational direction.

REFERENCES

1. Hsia RY, Kellerman AL, Yu-Chu S. Factors associated with closures of emergency departments in the United States. *JAMA*. 2011;305(19):1978-1985.
2. Covey SR. *The 7 Habits of Highly Effective People*. New York, NY: Simon and Schuster; 2004.
3. Croskerry P, Cosby KS, Schenkel SM, Wears RL. *Patient Safety in Emergency Medicine*. Philadelphia, PA: Lippincott Williams and Wilkins; 2009. Available at: hours_per_unit_of_service.doc. Accessed April 2, 2011.

CHAPTER 86

OPTIMIZING PHYSICIAN PERFORMANCE THROUGH INCENTIVES

Robert W. Strauss, Mark Rosenberg, Erik D. Barton, Thom A. Mayer, Michael Granovsky

There is no medicine like hope, no incentive so great, and no tonic so powerful as expectation of something tomorrow.

—Orison Swett Marden (1850-1924)

How should emergency physicians be paid? This question resonates through emergency medicine and its organizations and publications. There is a plethora of described methodologies, from hourly rate to pure productivity systems. Each has its intended and unintended consequences.

CURRENT PHYSICIAN PAYMENT SYSTEMS

Prior to implementation of the current resource-based relative value scale (RBRVS), there was no widely accepted metric to quantify physician work.[1] Physicians were paid utilizing a fee-for-service system based on the "customary, prevailing, and reasonable" charge structure, established with the creation of the Medicare program in 1965. In an effort to directly measure and attach payments to actual work performed by physicians, Congress required the Health Care Financing Administration (Centers for Medicare and Medicaid Services [CMS]) to develop an RBRVS system in 1992.

The Resource-Based Relative Value Scale System

The American Medical Association (AMA), which maintains the RBRVS program, looks at multiple variables when analyzing reimbursement, including actual work, opportunity cost of training, practice expense, malpractice expense, the geographic location of the practice, and so on. By considering all factors, the program attempts to define the total work expense to see a patient, to provide a service, and to perform a procedure. This process has been standardized and listed for each medical service, both cognitive and procedural medical services.

Over the years, the RBRVS payment reform spread from Medicare to most payors. Currently, practitioners are reimbursed based on the number of relative value units (RVUs) associated with a medical service. The RVU has become the universal metric of physician

BOX 86.1 ■ RVUs ASSIGNED TO EXAMPLE MEDICAL SERVICES

Description	Code	RVUs
ED level 3 evaluation and management service	99283	1.75
Simple abscess	10060	2.79
Endotracheal intubation	31500	4.06
Cardiopulmonary resuscitation	92950	5.34

effort. A number of RVUs are assigned to each reimbursable cognitive service and procedure performed by the medical practitioner (**Box 86.1**).

There are three subcategories of RVUs: *work, practice expense,* and *liability insurance.* Each of the subcategories is then adjusted slightly based on local geographic factors to account for cost differences. Once the number of RVUs for a given service is determined, it is multiplied by the dollar value per RVU (the conversion factor) for that payor to determine the payment amount. The Medicare conversion factor (payment per RVU) has varied over the years between $33 and $39 and is generally the same whether utilized for emergency medicine, neurosurgery, or other specialties. The Centers for Medicare and Medicaid Services and insurance companies modify the conversion factor at least once a year.

Physicians Are Paid for the Work They Do

The RBRVS program is essentially a productivity system—measuring the work done to evaluate and treat a specific patient—that has nothing to do with actual collections from patients or insurers. Physician work is billed on a fee-for-service basis and paid to the physician's employer (hospital, group, or other.) based on the RVU system described earlier. The physician is not necessarily paid based on the money generated by the work and collected by the billing agent (**Box 86.2**). Instead, the physician is paid as determined by his or her contract, which could define an hourly rate, an annual salary, or a productivity model. While there are many variations, most productivity models lead to physician payments that are based in part or entirely on the RVU system (**Table 86.1**). Variations on productivity-based models are discussed in detail later in this chapter.

BOX 86.2 ■ COLLECTION PROCESS STEPS

1. Physician performs a 99283 (level 3) evaluation and management service.
2. Bill is generated with CPT code 99283.
3. Payer (e.g., CMS) calculates payment: 99283 relative value units [RVUs] (1.75) × Medicare payment per RVU ($35.9996).
4. Employer receives a payment of $63.00.

TABLE 86.1 ■ Physician Payment Methodologies

Payment Methodologies	Requirement	Payment
Hourly rate	Work an hour	Hourly
Annual salary	Work a year	Predefined salary
Clinical productivity	Work harder	Relative value units generated
Customer satisfaction	Satisfy patients	A bonus
Citizenship	Get involved	A bonus
Quality care	Comply with standards	A bonus
Differentials	Work undesirable shifts	Increased base

AN INCENTIVE-BASED PRODUCTIVITY PLAN

There are multiple incentive compensation plans, each intended to define and motivate desired behaviors. These plans are created for diverse purposes and with different intended outcomes.

The Concept of Incentives

The essential theory behind an incentive program is that it encourages (rewards) desired behavior. Adam Smith in the *Wealth of Nations* describes the incentives and disincentives for farmers in the sharecropping system.[3] In his landmark text, *Contingencies of Reinforcement*, prominent psychologist B.F. Skinner demonstrates how rewards can control behavior.[4] He found that when a behavior was followed by a valued reward, that behavior was more likely to recur than when there was no reward. Others have found that reward systems may not predictably produce the intended results and may be harmful.[5,6] Nonetheless, incentive pay systems in emergency medicine are extremely common, and many feel they assist in attracting and retaining the best candidates.

Incentives and rewards act somewhat like hypnosis; they will often motivate people to do more than they ordinarily would do. Generally, they will *not* motivate individuals to perform acts they would not normally perform. Very slow practitioners may not know how or be able to manage patients more quickly. Curt (difficult) physicians may be unable or unwilling to learn the skills of good patient experience. Incentives alone (particularly monetary) may not be enough to change the behavior of these clinicians. Focused coaching will help some clinicians to develop the insight needed to change. A physician who believes in and is capable of efficiently moving patients through the system and providing great customer service may, if incentivized to do so, learn additional techniques to be more efficient and to enhance patients' perceptions of the service.

ASMAN Principles

Effective incentive plans are founded on consistent principles that incorporate the participation, understanding, and agreement of the practitioners who will be affected

TABLE 86.2 ■ ASMAN: Tips for Successful Program Development	
Principle	**Strategy**
Agreeable	Create buy-in by involving the group members in the development.
Simple	Keep it simple, resist the "siren song" of fixing everything now.
Measurable	Measure by objective, understandable, and agreed-upon methods.
Achievable	Focus on incremental accomplishable goals.
New value	Create new value rather than simply redistribute current money.

by them (**Table 86.2**). ASMAN is an acronym for the "must" ingredients of an effective incentive plan.[7]

Agreeable: The incentive method must be agreeable to those who are affected by it. If members of the group believe the approach is wrong, even unethical, they will not participate in the program. Well-designed programs involve participants in the development phases. The discussions should establish common goals, identify behaviors to be rewarded, and define the rewards. This method ensures group "buy-in" and agreement. Or, as the saying goes, "If they are not with you on the takeoff, they won't be with you on the landing."[8]

Simple: The program must be simple and understandable to the individuals responsible for carrying out the plan. Some plans try to accomplish too many things and are so complex that, while individual members may understand the components, they are unable to accomplish the plan's goals. New programs should begin with a limited number of components. If appropriate, additional components can be added later. It is important to resist the temptation to modify all behaviors (fix everything) at once. The concept of rapid cycle testing is a useful model for initiating these programs. With cycle testing, discrete, clearly identified, limited-scope changes are made, the results then carefully measured and reported in a timely and transparent manner.

Measurable: The measurement of achievement and success must be based as much as possible on objective and measurable criteria. A poorly defined approach creates confusion. One department chair explained that his approach to incentive payments was based on his subjective evaluation of the individual physician's contributions to the department. Since it is difficult for practitioners to accomplish what cannot be seen, understood, or measured, incentive programs should limit subjectivity, as it will cause those who fall short to believe the decision-maker is arbitrary.

Accomplishable: Goals must be realistic. A program that sets the floor for bonuses at seeing three patients an hour is not achievable if the hospital is constantly on EMS diversion and the ED is crowded with patients waiting to be admitted. "Accomplishable" must be, at least in part, under the control of the provider. An emergency physician can exert some control over his or her time, documentation, politeness, and caring nature. Practitioners will work to achieve accomplishable goals, particularly if they are built in incremental steps. They will not waste their time if they believe the goals are unachievable.

New value: The ideal incentive plan encourages the creation of new value, rather than simply redistributing current value. If the incentive rewards practitioners with money, then an effective program will increase the aggregate amount of money distributable to the practitioners, not simply divide the already-available money differently—more for some practitioners, less for others. Examples of creating new value might include:

- Increased volume of patients—adding revenue to the practice
- Improved documentation—decreasing downcoding and increasing charge capture
- Increased operational efficiency—decreasing the need for additional practitioners
- Improved patient satisfaction—eventually increasing volume by word-of-mouth

How Much Should Be Put at Risk?

Once a decision is made to create a productivity-based incentive program, the leader/group must determine how much money should be placed into the incentive pool. Presumably, a larger incentive pool has greater potential to drive behavior than a smaller pool. Among the many variations of productivity-based incentive plans are those that provide a base compensation rate (percentage of original hourly rate) plus a productivity bonus (based on RVUs). In other words, money is held back from the straight hourly rate and placed into a pool that is distributed based on RVU generation. The tendency, however, is to place too little at risk, which creates minimal incentive to be productive and minimal reward for those who are productive.

As an example, in a hypothetical model, the practitioners are paid $150 an hour. One highly efficient practitioner, physician A, manages 2.4 patients per hour. Working beside physician A is another, much slower practitioner, physician B, who manages 1.6 patients per hour. In other words, physician A manages 60% of the patients, while physician B manages 40% of the patients. (Note that this does not account for the actual work done, as measured by RVUs; it is only the number of patients.)

> **Using the payment formula:**
>
> **Physician A rate = base + 60% of productivity pool**
>
> **Physician B rate = base + 40% of productivity pool**

Table 86.3 demonstrates the hourly differential when holding back X% (10%, 25%, 50%, and 100%) for payment through the productivity pool.

The correct percentage to place in the pool may be a group or practice leader decision. However, if it is only 10% (model 2), physician A, who is working 50% harder than physician B, will only get an additional $3.00 per hour (2% increase) over what he or she was getting in the pre-bonus program (model 1). This distribution might seem quite unfair to physician A. Conversely, if the bonus pool is 100% (model 5), physician B might

TABLE 86.3 ■ Base Plus Productivity Pool Payments

Model	Bonus Pool	Physician A	Physician B
1	No pool	$150.00/hour	$150.00/hour
2	10%	$147.00/hour	$153.00/hour
3	25%	$142.50/hour	$157.50/hour
4	50%	$135.00/hour	$165.00/hour
5	100%	$120.00/hour	$180.00/hour

argue that he or she is getting too little money. What is the correct amount to encourage a change in behavior? There are many opinions on this issue. If too little, very few will make an additional effort. If substantial and some do not hit target, then their payment may substantially decrease.

When developing a program, some members of a group may complain that their friend, Dr. Jones, who is a little slower than other providers, will make less money. Kevin Klauer, MD, FACEP, tells those concerned practitioners, "At the end of the month, [they] are welcome to write a personal check to Dr. Jones out of [their] increased bonus. . . . No one ever does."[9]

How much of the total compensation should be incentive based? It has been said, "The answer to any intelligent question is . . . it depends!"[9] In this case, the answer will depend on whether the individual clinician views himself or herself as a "fast" or "slow" team member and therefore a likely winner or loser under the incentive compensation system. And, do the data generated by the system confirm or refute this view of themselves? The "fast" or efficient providers might feel the entire system should be incentive based, while slower clinicians may want to place little or no money at risk. Experience in dealing with thousands of emergency physicians indicates that an incentive plan must place at least 30% to 40% of total compensation at risk to attain moderate benefit in improving and rewarding performance.[10,11]

100% Productivity Plan

Creating a full-productivity program eliminates the base. In effect, these programs eliminate any guaranteed payments the practitioner earns for working; they are only paid what they earn. This model targets busy EDs with very productive practitioners who are skillful and efficient. Particularly slow (unproductive) physicians would not choose to participate in this type of practice. With a full-productivity plan, the response to shifts that are too slow is to eliminate some of the excess practitioner coverage. 100% productivity models work best in high-volume EDs, in which:

- There is double and triple coverage so the schedule can be adjusted so physicians are generally busy, increasing the earning power of the practitioners.
- Manipulations like a night differential may not be needed if nights are busy through the shift. In fact, night practitioners might be more productive than those working the day shift.

However, 100% productivity plans as described above do not account for patient safety, patient experience, core measures, or teamwork and thus result, at least indirectly, with a definition of value based solely on the speed of seeing patients, not the quality of the care provided.

INCENTIVE PLANS WITH BONUS POOLS

Sophisticated plans set aside money (a "hold back") to create bonus pools to encourage desirable behaviors *beyond productivity*. Incentives can be created for most measurable behaviors. Groups provide incentives for a broad range of activities, including but not limited to customer satisfaction, citizenship, appropriate utilization of established guidelines, meeting core metrics, working undesirable shifts, short door-to-doc times, and so on.

In emergency medicine, the most common incentive bonus systems are based on productivity. Increasingly, incentive compensation plans are broadened to align clinician behaviors with institutional goals and include a blending of additional measurable components such as customer satisfaction, citizenship, and quality.

> *The further the physician's payment methodology is from this reimbursement reality (such as paying by the hour, by the patient, by the charges, etc.), the greater the likelihood of a distortion or misalignment of the relationship between the work performed and the revenue accrued.*
>
> —Ron Hellstern[12]

Patient Experience

The contentment and satisfaction of patients and their families with hospital-based care is a primary focus of health care and is defined as patient experience. This is the sum of the differences between patients' expectations of their care and the actual experience of receiving that care. Patient experience surveys are the most commonly used methodology to assess perceptions of the service recipients. Emergency department–specific surveys have been utilized to provide comparative feedback and demonstrate opportunities for improvement to hospitals, groups, and individual providers.

In 2005, the National Quality Forum formally endorsed the Hospital Consumer Assessment of Healthcare Providers and Systems, leading to adoption of the Inpatient Prospective Payment System.[13,14] More recently, the Emergency Department Patient Experience of Care Survey has been developed and adopted. The clear areas of focus include multiple aspects of effective communication.

Measuring Patient Satisfaction and Providing Feedback

Since patient experience is an increasingly critical feature of hospital–ED alignment, many ED groups choose to include performance on ED surveys as a component of their incentive programs. As payment for services by CMS and other payors is increasingly dependent on successful performance in these and other outcome-based parameters, providers, groups, and health-care institutions will increasingly insist on demonstration of excellence.[15] The bonus pool can be used to motivate practitioners to focus on aspects of caring that are measured by the survey tools.

Surprisingly, many ED staff members are unaware of the specific questions asked on the survey tool. It is illogical to expect high-performance scores on a test in which the questions are unknown. It is imperative to treat all such surveys as an "open-book test" by ensuring that all clinicians know the specific questions asked about them on the surveys.[10] All ED staff members should be completely familiar with the questions. Training in specific skills, such as "scripting" or evidence-based and survey-based language, can significantly improve the understanding and performance of practitioners (see Chapter 74).[9]

There are many complaints about the inconsistencies of the measuring tool: "sample size too small," "only angry patients respond," and so on. Nonetheless, it is widely held that the answers obtained from the surveys accurately represent the subjective experience of those completing the questionnaire. To provide the most effective feedback, the results should be:

- ***Timely.*** Results provided more than a month after a quarter ends are too far removed to change behavior. Feedback provided soon after the behavior occurs is much more likely to lead to change. Consider a practitioner who, upon receiving feedback, tries to modify behavior. One week later, he or she receives additional feedback that the change is or is not working. Contrast that with the practitioner who receives feedback months later and is incapable of determining the effectiveness of a behavior change.
- ***Individualized.*** Ideally, survey results are broken down by individual practitioners. If only group results are available, poorly performing individuals may not recognize the effect of their own behaviors. There is a tendency to believe that "other" members of the group are preventing the team from obtaining high scores. Individuals cannot hide behind the group when results are provided to the individual for his or her specific performance. Even if the results for individual clinicians cannot be obtained, quantifying the type and number of patient complaints and the results of "360-degree" feedback from colleagues and emergency nurses can be effectively utilized.

In programs with residents and advanced practice providers (APPs), it may be difficult to separate the scores of their surveys from those of the supervising attending physicians. This combining of results leads to an inaccurate reflection of the attending physician's patient experience efforts. The inaccuracy can be partially addressed when the attending makes teaching all staff excellent patient-experience behaviors a priority.

Citizenship

The definition of citizenship varies by group, but includes participation in ED departmental, medical staff, and community outreach, as well as educational activities (**Box 86.3**). Some plans create a pool with a point system for bonus distribution. Usually the dollars are small and do not approach the hourly rate for clinical work. Thus, unless the potential distribution is large, an incentive plan that includes citizenship may not have a significant effect on behavior. Rather, this component of the program might simply shift a little of the practice revenue to the practitioners doing more of the "group work," therefore creating less work for the other team members. Rather than bonuses, the keys to having a group populated with good citizens are effective hiring, early and clear expectation setting, and holding individuals accountable.

BOX 86.3 ■ CITIZENSHIP EXAMPLES

- Attendance at meetings
- Teaching residents, medical students, staff
- Participation on hospital committees
- Prehospital care leadership
- Quality management program leadership

Quality

It may be difficult to define payments for "quality." The confusion arises because of the multitude of quality measures and the somewhat arbitrary determination of what merits a bonus payment. Ideally, quality payments will be aligned with group or hospital payments and directly associated with metric-driven outcomes. An example of a successfully employed quality incentive program is provided in Appendix 86.1.

An example of an ED-specific quality measure might involve appropriate utilization of evidence-based guidelines and metrics, such as appropriate computed tomography utilization in patients sustaining head trauma, consistent utilization of a sepsis protocol, or ED length of stay. After developing evidence-based guidelines and metrics, a bonus can be applied to all practitioners who consistently follow the guidelines or document appropriate explanations for management outside of the guidelines. The increasing number and specificity of evidence-based treatment guidelines suggests that compensation based on compliance with such guidelines is likely to increase. Indeed, the "value-based programs" concept is precisely such a measure.[16]

Bonuses

Groups also "hold back" money ($X/hour) to reward practitioners who work full time, a higher percentage of nights and weekends, more holidays, and so on. Distributing the retained money entails creating a formula that fairly measures and rewards valued service:

- *Bonus for working full time*: If the distribution of the bonus is for working full time—an average of "X" or more hours a quarter—then all physicians meeting the full-time standard will get a distribution for each worked hour, paid at the end of each quarter. Additionally, the bonus for other incentive components such as quality, citizenship, and so on, may only apply to full-time clinicians.
- *Bonus for working full-time nights*: If the group finds it appropriate to attract and reward a full-time night practitioner, the most common reward is to pay that night practitioner $X per hour above the base. For instance, in the model used in this chapter, the group might pay a full-time night physician a base of $87.50 per hour ($75.50 plus a $12.50 per night differential). That base is in addition to the RVU-based and other incentives.

CREATING AN INCENTIVE-BASED MODEL

Model 1–Base Model Case (Assumptions)

The preincentive model pays the practitioners $160 an hour (**Table 86.4**). Note that the base model assumes all hours worked are paid at the same rate. The net practice revenue is calculated (billable patients × RVUs/patient × average collection/RVU) less (billing costs). Assumptions about practice expenses in this model include general operational expenses plus director stipend(s) plus malpractice. The difference between these two numbers (practice revenue minus practice expenses) define the distributable pool of revenues. The potential costs for APPs (advanced practice providers: nurse practitioners and physician assistants) are also specified. All further iterations of incentive programs in this chapter will be built using this base model. Actual determinations of revenue and collections per RVU must be based on past collections or a feasibility study of the practice.

TABLE 86.4 ■ Base Model Case (Assumptions)

Practice revenue	
Total patients	36,500
Total billable patients	36,000
Average collection/RVU	$31.50
Average RVUs/patient	3.6
Average collection/billable patient (RVUs × collection)	$113.40
Billing cost (@ $9.00/patient)	$324,000
Annual gross revenue (billable patients × average collection)	$3,758,400
Practice expense	
General operational expenses	$250,000
Director(s)	$135,000
Malpractice	$300,000
Total practice expense	$685,000
Distributable funds (practice revenues − practice expenses)	
Annual	$3,073,400
Daily	$8,420
Advanced practice providers	
Hourly rate including benefits	$55.00
Patients/hour	1.5

Model Variations

Two common variations of the base model are based on physician productivity and adding APPs.

Model Variation 1–Physician Productivity

This model demonstrates variations based solely on differences in physician productivity (**Table 86.5**). The base remains 1.9 patients per provider hour (pph). Less-productive clinicians

TABLE 86.5 ■ Model Variation 1–Physician Productivity

Patients/physician hour	1.7	1.9	2.1	2.3
Base rate	$160	$160	$160	$160
50% RVU	$152	$160	$168	$177
100% RVU	$143	$160	$177	$194

(1.7 pph) are paid less, while more-productive clinicians (2.1 and 2.3 pph) are paid more. Two further variations are:

- The 50/50 model in which physicians are paid a base of $80 (½ of the $160 base) an hour. They would earn the remainder of their payment based on the number of RVUs generated X ½ of the value of the RVUs ($15.75). Both the positive and negative effects of the practitioner's productivity are shared with the group and decreased for the individual practitioner.
- The 100% (full-productivity model) in which practitioners have no base. Their only payment is derived from the RVUs they have generated. In other words, if they are efficient and busy, they will make significantly more money. Less efficient providers will make significantly less money. There is no direct effect on the group.

There are several likely long-term results of physician productivity model.

- *Low-productivity providers*: Less efficient physicians, generating fewer RVUs, will (a) accept lower than average paychecks, (b) learn to be more productive, or (c) leave.
- *Highly productive providers*: More efficient physicians will do well (make more money) with these model variations. Over time, the coverage needs (scheduled physicians' hours) will decrease, ensuring the opportunity for higher physician incomes.
- *The provider group*: Generally, the number of patients to be managed is not a choice but rather is dependent on volume cycles and clinician efficiency. However, the group (management) can fine-tune the schedule to ensure highly productive physicians are able to realize the benefit of their efficiency. These scheduling adjustments will be even more likely if the group itself achieves benefit (value) from higher generation of RVUs. As mentioned, productivity is not the only measure of success. Groups may find it necessary to address other aspects of care through incentive programs.

Model Variation 2—Adding APPs

Groups often reconfigure their staffing patterns to include APPs (nurse practitioners and physician assistants) (**Table 86.6**). Appropriately utilizing these less expensive

TABLE 86.6 ■ Model Variation 2—Adding APPs				
Patients/physician hour	1.7	1.9	2.1	2.3
Base rate	$160	$160	$160	$160
APP hours	12	12	12	12
Rate: 50% RVU	$160	$170	$179	$189
Rate: 100% RVU	$161	$180	$199	$218
APP hours	18	18	18	18
Rate: 50% RVU	$167	$177	$187	$197
Rate: 100% RVU	$173	$193	$214	$234

providers (see Chapter 24) increases the revenue to the physicians. Variation 2 utilizes APPs for 12 and 18 hours, decreasing physician hours of coverage and expense. The model assumes that an APP will:

- Provide care to 1.5 patients per hour
- Generate RVUs like those generated by a physician
- Generate RVUs that are pooled and then divided by the physicians based on the ratio of hours worked
- Cost $55 an hour, including benefits

Note in this model, the use of less expensive APPs can dramatically change the physician incomes. Even the less productive physicians can generate incomes that are approximately the same rate as the base model in which there was no productivity plan. However, the most dramatic changes are seen among the high-productivity physicians. A physician who can see 2.3 patients per hour (~20% over base) can generate $234/hour (~45% over base) in the 100% productivity model: As in model variation 1, this model:

- Will attract high-productivity providers
- Assumes that scheduling will be adjusted over time to allow for the greatest efficiency
- Does not address other aspects of patient care, including customer satisfaction and quality outcomes

Non-RVU Bonus Pool Creation and Payout

The simplest way to create a bonus pool to pay for achievements in quality, citizenship, customer satisfaction, and so on, is to hold back (set aside) an amount of money from the base rate, in this example, $10 per hour. Since there is no base in a 100% productivity plan, a small calculated adjustment to the payment per RVU would create the desired hold back. Payment of the bonus pool would then be based on successful achievement of the desired behaviors/outcomes. There are many variations available to create and adjust a bonus program (**Box 86.4**).

BOX 86.4 ■ VARIATIONS ON BONUS POOL PAYMENT STRUCTURES

- Pay for goal achievement.
    - Payment for full achievement only
    - Partial (pro-rated) payment for partial achievement
    - Redefine success over time
- Pay for multiple goals (citizenship, high patient survey scores, quality).
    - Modify goals based on changing priorities.
    - Pay for group or individual success.
- Enhance the bonus pool by decreasing the base, and pay % or total bonus pool to those who achieve goals.
    - Pay entire bonus to those who achieve goals.
    - Pay a portion of the bonus to those who achieve goals (remainder distributed or used as predetermined by group/director).

As an example, consider a month of 720 hours, with $10/hour withheld, creating a bonus distribution pool of $7,200. The bonus structure is for full-time commitment, defined as 132 or more hours per month. Half the hours are covered by "full-time" clinicians. In this case, full-time practitioners (achieving the goal) could be paid a bonus in one of two ways:

1. Pay all money held back from the full-time individuals for a bonus of $3,600 ($10.00/hour). Group retains $3,600 to address other pending needs.
2. Distribute $7,200 (all money held back) to those earning the bonus. Full-time practitioners would earn a $20.00/hour bonus. No moneys would be retained by the group.

In this simple bonus model, the goal meets the ASMAN principle and a bonus is paid for a desired goal. This bonus program would not work in a system with all full-time clinicians. Note that unforeseen consequences can occur. In the second model, a single full-time practitioner might discourage others from joining the group as full timers, enlarging his or her own bonus. Modifications can be made to the type of bonus and size of the pool by simply modifying the base or RVU payment in a 100% RVU model.

SPECIAL INCENTIVE PLAN CONSIDERATIONS

In the ideal work environment, all health-care providers have aligned incentives. All providers, including APPs and nurses, would work harder and get paid more on a busy day with many sick patients.

APP Incentive Plans

There are two primary variations describing how physicians work with APPs. In one type of practice, the physicians see every patient and perform and document a co-evaluation. In the other, APPs are permitted to primarily evaluate and discharge patients (meeting specified criteria) without requiring involvement of the physician in every case. If physicians co-evaluate patients, the practice may choose to credit the physicians with the RVU's value attributable to those patients.

Some practices attribute all the APP RVUs to the physician responsible for signing off on the case. If the APPs' RVUs are applied to the physicians, the practice must ensure that the value of those RVUs is calculated into the budget, and policies exist to ensure appropriate distribution of RVUs (i.e., discourage physicians from manipulating the system for their own benefit at the expense of their colleagues).

Advanced practice providers can be included in the RVU-based incentive program. However, some APPs are reticent to place their compensation at risk. When employed, RVU systems that include APPs must address several issues, including the recognition that many APPs are averse to accepting a base rate that is less than their current compensation, requiring them to earn the remainder through RVUs. Further, an incentive program for both physicians and APPs may cause them to compete for patients.

An alternative is to allow APPs to earn additional money for each patient managed. Setting the base at 95% of the current compensation and then giving $2 for each patient (or $3 for every patient above two patients per hour) could lead to a bonus of several thousand dollars each year for each APP.

Nursing Incentive Plans

Several forms of ED nurse incentive plans are demonstrated in Chapter 87 and include:

- Traditional incentives merit, performance, and recruitment/retention incentives
- Pay-for-performance–specific metrics
- Career ladders

Very few nurse incentive systems utilize a productivity-based or "fee-for-service" plan. In one practice, a pool of money is created and then divided by the number of the total practice RVUs generated that month. Each nurse is paid a portion of the pool based on the number of RVUs associated with their patients. The details of the program are:

- Monthly census: 2,775 patients
- RVUs per average patient: 3.6
- Nurse bonus pool: $10,000 per month
- Productive nurses earn a bonus of $400 to $500/month
- Nurse bonus per RVU = $1.00
- Monthly bonus pool ($10,000)/(census [2,775] × RVUs/patient [3.6]).

One variation of this model provides a bonus for nurses earning more than "X" RVUs per hour. It is also possible to calculate the bonus based on level of service rather than RVUs.

Academic Faculty Practice Plans/Incentive Programs

Developing incentive-based compensation plans for academic faculty poses an additional layer of complexity. In most academic medical centers (AMCs) and university departments, there are competing "missions" for faculty time and efforts. While *direct patient care* remains a core mission for most academic faculty, teaching staff have the added responsibilities of *education* and *academic productivity*. Also, academic faculty are being asked to assume *administrative roles*, which should also be considered in the compensation plan.

Patient Experience

As mentioned previously, residents may interface with the patient and family to a greater degree than the attending. As such, it may be hard to isolate the results of the patient experience (survey). In this instance, using a group score may be more reasonable, incentivizing the group to improve the interpersonal and communication skills of all residents. Attending staff should be encouraged to observe the interactions between trainees and patients/families, interview patients about their interaction with the trainee, and model appropriate behaviors.

Educational Mission

The trainees educated in emergency medicine may include students, interns, residents, fellows, and other APPs. Teaching requires considerable effort and is usually performed using a variety of approaches and venues, such as didactic lectures, journal clubs, simulation training, "asynchronous" teaching activities (such as online training), procedural skills labs, and bedside teaching. The academic faculty is generally expected to participate in many or all these activities as a condition of employment. Teaching evaluations should be part of the incentive equation.

Academic Mission

The third expectation of faculty members working at AMCs is related to activities that enhance medical evidence and knowledge of the specialty, particularly the development of original research projects and the publication of peer-reviewed articles. Research grants and awards from extramural sources are important pursuits that support the academic mission.

Academic faculty with a primary research focus are evaluated based on the number and types of publications as well as the amount of grant funding awarded on an ongoing basis. Academic productivity, or "original creative activity," is often the primary consideration used for faculty promotion in universities and academic departments.

In addition to original research, academic productivity is evaluated by the publication of case reports, review articles, editorials, chapters, textbooks, and online content. Other forms of productivity include contributions to national medical programs, such as participation in national conferences, specialty societies, ABMS activities, and so on. Academic productivity is important for the success of the department within the institution, but it also has important monetary advantages as it reduces the cost for recruitment, improves retention, and provides opportunities for personal achievements outside the hospital.

Administrative Mission

The success of emergency physician leaders in hospitals across the country has resulted in more academic emergency physicians assuming administrative leadership roles outside the emergency department. A few examples include roles of chief medical officers, associate deans, deans, informatics directors, quality directors, and hospital CEOs. While these roles usually come with reduced clinical hours and/or salary stipend, the consideration of an incentive-based compensation plan should be fairly and transparently applied.

Academic Incentive Plans

The creation of an effective incentive-based compensation plan for academic faculty must consider the competing missions just discussed. Determining the specific prioritization of the incentive plan is a significant challenge. Historically, academic incentive plans relied on academic status and years of service to determine the salaries of its faculty members.[7-29] Now many salary plans are developed with increased emphasis on clinical revenues, patient satisfaction, and most recently, quality and operational throughput quality metrics.[20] Increasingly, AMC emergency departments now employ incentive metrics in their pay plans based on the alignment of the priorities of both the department and the institution. As most academic incentive plans are new, there is lack of uniformity and very little has been written about them in the literature. Transparency and a sense of fairness is as important in academics as in a group practice.

A viable incentive-based compensation plan for academic faculty "balances the priorities" and rewards desirable behaviors unique to each department and institution. Unbalanced or poorly weighted plans may lead to excess attention to certain priorities while not enough to others. Rewards may be financial or include other inducements, such as increased protected time and promotion.

Component-Based Balanced Plan

A balanced academic incentive plan considers the individual components of each mission. For example:

- Clinical mission (30%-50%)
    - Shift base pay/hourly base pay
    - RVU productivity (i.e., average, total, per patient, per shift)
    - Patient satisfaction scores
    - Quality metrics (e.g., pay for performance)
    - Differentials for nights, weekends, holidays, extra shifts
    - Operational metrics (door-to-doc times, admission rates, T utilization, etc)
    - Administrative director stipend

- Education mission (10%-35%)
    - ☐ Attendance/participation (e.g., lectures, meetings, journal clubs, etc.)
    - ☐ Lectures/presentations given
    - ☐ Teaching evaluation scores
    - ☐ Teaching awards/recognitions
    - ☐ Program director stipend

- Academic productivity mission (10%-35%)
    - ☐ Academic base or rank (e.g., professor, associate, assistant)
    - ☐ Publications (i.e., number, type)
    - ☐ Other "creative" activities (online content, podcasts, etc.)
    - ☐ Grant funding (intramural, extramural)
    - ☐ Research director stipend
    - ☐ Contribution to specialty and participation in national activities

The plan components can be individualized to encourage and reward specific behaviors among individual members of the faculty. A good starting point would be to develop consensus on two components from each mission to keep the plans simple and directed toward desired outcomes. More sophisticated plans will weight each element to determine the total compensation. For example, **Table 86.7** presents a structure of an academic incentive plan.

Some academic incentive plans use a "points system" to determine the annual incentive component of salaries, either requiring a minimum number of "points" or providing additional payment for points above a threshold. Specific accomplishments can lead to specific dollar rewards (e.g., "a $1,000 increase in salary for each publication") or incentive payments can be weighted (e.g., "10% more points à 10% more salary").

To effectively encourage and reward behavior, academic incentive plans should include component weightings (point values) that are *meaningful* to faculty members. For example, incentives should have the potential to affect salary by at least a 5% to 10% of the total. To use the current example, if an individual is generating 120% of the average RVU production, that person is rewarded with a 20% increase of that specific clinical mission component (10% of the total compensation; **Table 86.7**) or a net 2% total salary increase. When developing an AMC incentive program, it is wise to begin slowly to avoid excessive incentives in one area that may drive behavior detrimental to other mission components.

TABLE 86.7 ■ Example of an Academic EM-Balanced Faculty Incentive Plan

Mission	Element	Weight %
Patient care (40%)	Contracted annual shifts/hour base pay	20
	Average RVUs per shift compared to group average	10
	Patient satisfaction scores	10
Education (20%)	Teaching evaluation scores compared to group average	10
	Attendance (lectures and meetings)	10
Academic (40%)	Academic base salary (full, associate, or assistant professor)	30
	Publications (number and type)	10

FIGURE 86.1 ■ Simple Blended Scorecard Example

Oct-Dec 2014

	Charges per Shift	WEVU per Shift	Press Ganey-Overall	Median Door-to-Doc	Conference Attendance	Patient per Clinical hour
Faculty X	$ 12,410.22	62.66	85.4	42	5	1.78
Department Avg	$ 13,515.90	$ 70.99	82.2	49	14	2.04

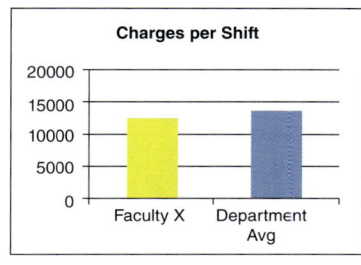
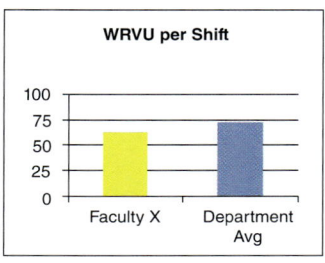
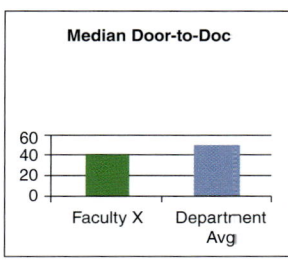
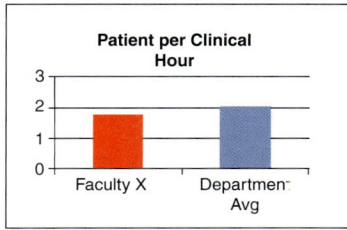
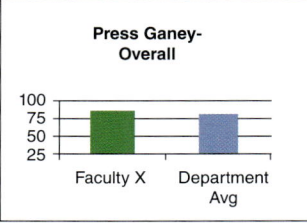
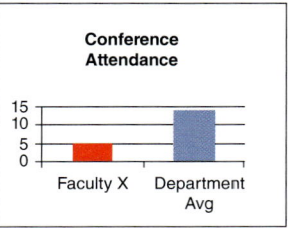

Academic medical center incentive plans require timely bidirectional feedback and periodic adjustments. This is an iterative process that develops over time with "buy-in" from faculty who often see their contributions to the academic department as different from just patient care. Optimally, discussions regarding incentive plan effectiveness and modifications occur both at the faculty retreat and during the annual individual faculty development assessments. Some fine-tuning may occur more frequently as necessary.

Blended Scorecards

In addition, once the annual incentive plan goals are established, regular feedback with the use of blended scorecards given to the faculty on a monthly or quarterly basis are very useful in keeping everyone informed. A good incentive plan should be transparent to the faculty, equitable to all providers, and provide timely feedback so there are no "surprises" when incentive payments are calculated.

When first introducing an AMC incentive program, it is helpful to start with a simple program and scorecard (**Figure 86.1**) so all participants get used to seeing the numbers on an ongoing basis prior to the financial incentives kicking in. The second scorecard (**Figures 86.2a** and **86.2b**) demonstrates a more comprehensive, complex, and nuanced scorecard to track participant activity and provide feedback.

PHASE-IN OF A PRODUCTIVITY INCENTIVE PROGRAM

A phase-in period is advisable when beginning a productivity incentive plan, allowing all parties to observe the plan to ensure it meets defined expectations. The phase-in process can be about 3 months for an established practice and an additional 3 months (6 months total) for

FIGURE 86.2a ■ Comprehensive Blended Scorecard Example

RVU per Hour Worked
Phys versus Dept Mean

V
≥1 Std Dev | ≤1 Std Dev

Phys FY13 YTD	Phys FY12 YTD	Variance	Dept Mean FY13 YTD	Dept Mean FY12 YTD	Phys W, Dept Mean FY13 YTD
6.95	6.60	5%	5.50	5.85	26%

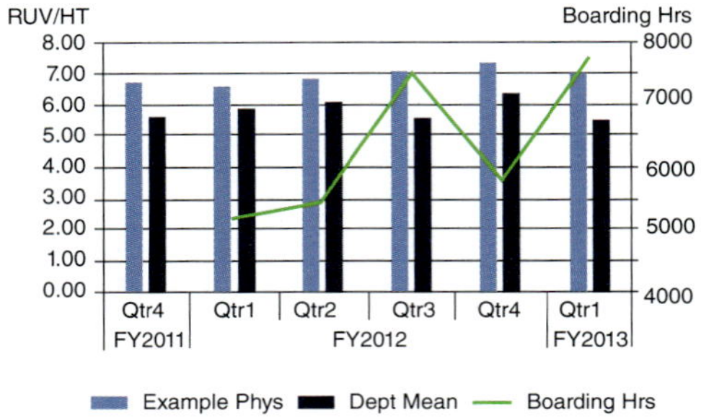

Patients per Hour Worked
Phys versus Dept Mean

V
≥1 Std Dev | ≤1 Std Dev

Phys FY13 YTD	Phys FY12 YTD	Variance	Dept Mean FY13 YTD	Dept Mean FY12 YTD	Phys W, Dept Mean FY13 YTD
3.36	2.39	41%	2.32	2.16	45%

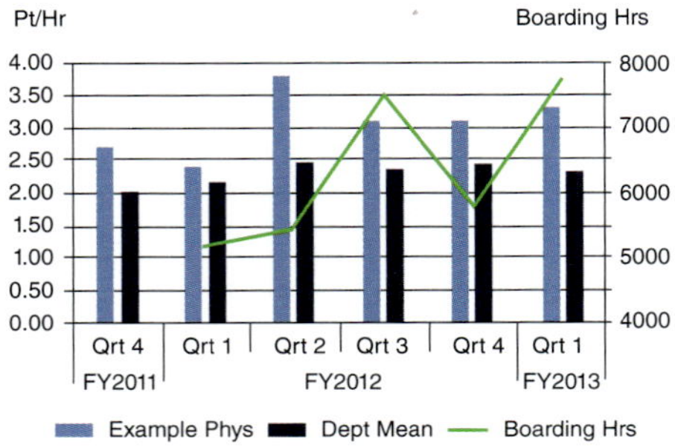

Avg ED LOS - Discharge Patiensts
Phys versus Dept Mean

V
≥1 Std Dev | ≤1 Std Dev

Phys FY13 YTD	Phys FY12 YTD	Variance	Dept Mean FY13 YTD	Dept Mean FY12 YTD	Phys W, Dept Mean FY13 YTD
249	315	−21%	244	295	2%

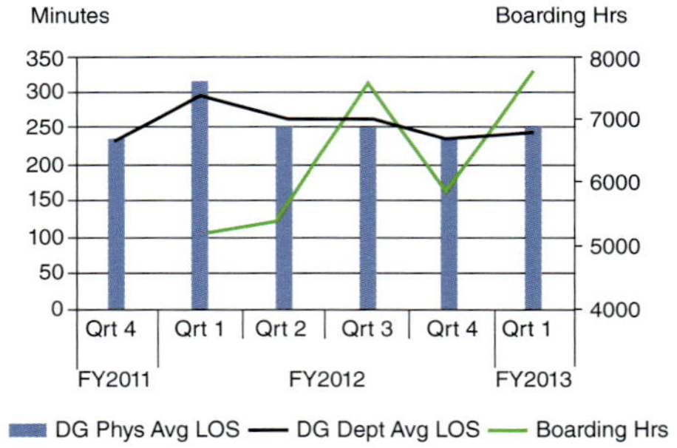

Avg ED LOS - Admit Patients
Phys versus Dept Mean

V
≥1 Std Dev | ≤1 Std Dev

Phys FY13 YTD	Phys FY12 YTD	Variance	Dept Mean FY13 YTD	Dept Mean FY12 YTD	Phys W, Dept Mean FY13 YTD
781	630	24%	795	597	−2%

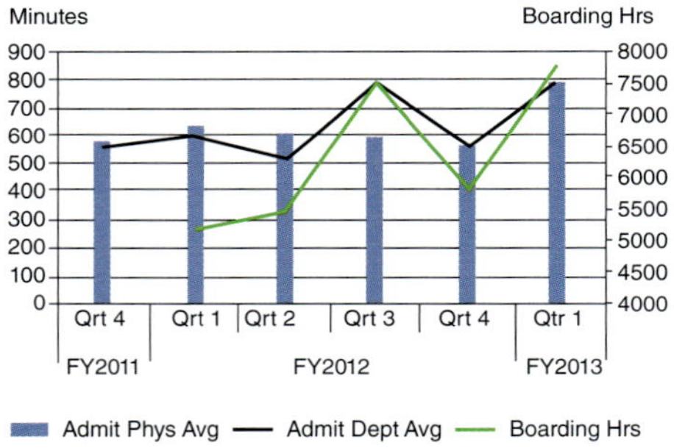

a new practice. (The first three months are necessary to gather the practice data needed to create the plan.) The specific data necessary to develop a *de novo* productivity plan includes information in **Box 86.5.** The goal is to determine (calculate) the correct dollar amount per RVU necessary to implement the plan.

BOX 86.5 ■ DATA FOR A PRODUCTIVITY INCENTIVE PROGRAM

- Billable patient volume
- Patient arrival times/volumes
- Intended practitioner hourly coverage
- Collections per average patient–relative value units (RVUs) × conversion factor
- Calculated RVUs per scheduled hour
- Practice expense operations, stipends, malpractice, etc
- Advanced practice providers expense

FIGURE 86.2b ■ Comprehensive Blended Scorecard Example

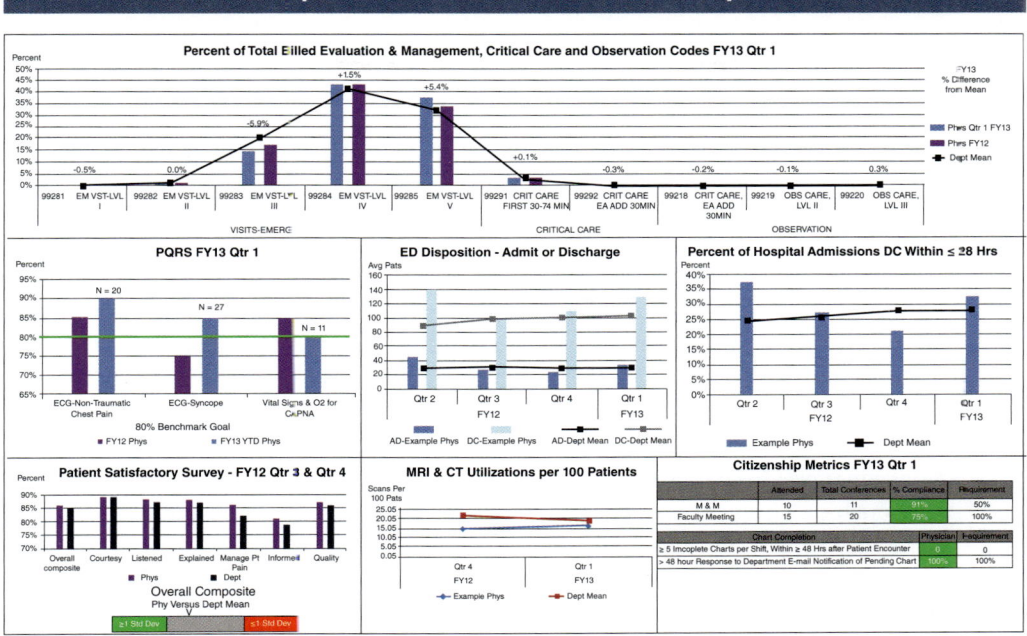

Once the data are gathered, a 3-month, rapid cycle testing phase is advisable. During the testing phase, side-by-side payrolls are compared. For example, payroll 1 can be the actual payroll, the "arbitrary" fixed rate (hourly pay). Payroll 2 is the productivity plan payroll, which demonstrates what the compensation would be using the productivity model. The testing phase allows the group to make necessary adjustments in the amount that will be paid per earned RVU, check the budgetary impact, and test various "what-if" scenarios (**Box 86.6**).

During the phase-in period, each practitioner (including APPs) should be trained to successfully participate in the program. A billing in-service will teach each practitioner how to optimize documentation. An operations analysis (e.g., Lean flow evaluation to add value and eliminate waste) may reveal opportunities to more efficiently provide patient care. Some practitioners may find that using professional scribes substantially increases the number of cases they can manage, improves documentation, and enhances efficiency. Generally, the increased productivity payment is greater than the cost of the scribe.

BOX 86.6 ■ "WHAT-IF" SCENARIOS

What if the practice. . . .

- Experiences volume increase/decrease 5%, 7% . . .
- Changes staffing (increase/decrease hours of coverage)
- Improves documentation increasing relative value units/patient
- Adds advanced practice providers to the practice
- Adds scribes
- Changes the amount of the stipends
- Experiences a malpractice or billing cost increase
- Changes the % of the productivity plan 50%, 75%
- Implements a night shift differential
- Creates a bonus plan for customer service, citizenship, quality

PROS AND CONS OF VARIOUS MODELS

As noted below, the various incentive models have both pros and cons as well as consequences and appropriate mottos.

Hourly Pay

- *Pros*: Simple, no confusion, work an hour, get paid an hour, no matter how busy or quiet.
- *Cons*: The practitioner makes the same amount, no matter what shift is worked (day, night, or holiday) or how busy the ED. Working harder has no personal benefit. The hourly pay system creates an employee mentality. When two physicians are working together and only one is working hard, that practitioner will be frustrated that he or she is carrying the heavy load and does not benefit from this hard work. Busier shifts penalize those who work them.
- *Consequences*: No incentive to perform, provide customer satisfaction, or contribute (citizenship). This practitioner's solution to multiple problems is to add more coverage without consideration of the cost.
- *Motto*: "It's too busy! Let's add more coverage."

100% Productivity: "Eat What You Kill"

- *Pros*: This model provides the greatest incentive to maximize collections (or RVUs). Most practitioners will work very hard in this system. If potential issues (listed in "Cons" below) are addressed, this model can create the greatest efficiency.
- *Cons*: Cherry-picking is a real risk in a double-coverage situation. Most providers will quickly recognize which patient presentations pay the most for time and effort spent. Some may even peruse the list of patients (presentations) to be seen and avoid low-RVU cases. There may be avoidance of low-paying (quiet) shifts requiring manipulation of the base or scheduling equality. It is probably wise to avoid a pure RVU collection-based model, as some practitioners may gravitate toward the better payers and avoid self-pay patients ("wallet biopsies").
- *Consequences*: No patients, no money. Unless quality is emphasized and rewarded, there may be little intrinsic motivation to provide patient satisfaction, participate in "citizenship" programs, and so on. These practitioners may want less coverage than appropriate.
- *Motto*: "I want to be busy."

50% Productivity Plan: "Some for Me, Some for You"

- *Pros*: This model combines a group and an individual focus. Greater productivity inures to the benefit of both the group and the individual. The plan has flexibility and can be combined with bonus pools.
- *Cons*: Slower physicians will earn less money than their more productive colleagues. The system frequently requires adjustments as volume and collections change. This system only addresses productivity. The most productive providers partially support the least productive providers.
- *Consequences*: Hard-working practitioners help the group and themselves (but only partially).
- *Motto*: "We are not all equal, but we are on the same team."

Productivity Plus Bonus: "Quality Is More Than Productivity"

- *Pros*: This model recognizes and values productivity and "quality" by aligning goals through incentives. Incentives can be developed for achievements in patient satisfaction, contributions to the advancement of the group and hospital, and provision of quality improvements.
- *Cons*: Models with multiple components can be overly complex and confusing.
- *Consequences*: When well implemented, this program encourages practitioners to meet the patients' needs and contribute to the group's/hospital's programs while being compensated for their efforts.
- *Motto*: "I work hard, am rewarded for my hard work, and contribute to my community."

UNINTENDED CONSEQUENCES

> *People respond to incentives, although not necessarily in ways that are predictable or manifest. Therefore, one of the most powerful laws in the universe is the law of unintended consequences.*
>
> —Steven D. Levitt and Stephen J. Dubner, *SuperFreakonomics*[21]

Implementation of incentive plans frequently comes with unintended consequences, a concept that was first described in 1936 by Robert Merton.[22] Under the theory of "You get what you pay for (reward)," great care must be exercised in the development and implementation of a productivity plan in order to minimize those unintended consequences. No matter how well intended or thought out in advance, it is not possible to know how all individuals will respond to an incentive program.

Common Causes

The common causes of unintended consequences found when implementing practitioner productivity payment plans are listed in **Box 86.7**. Productivity incentive plans encourage fast doctors to be faster. Practitioners who are paid for productivity may become overly productive, leading to a deterioration in quality, customer satisfaction, and staff/colleague relationships. Quality and compliance monitoring are necessary components of a successful productivity model.

BOX 86.7 ■ CHARGE PHYSICIAN/CHARGE NURSE COMMITMENTS

Primary causes of unintended consequences related to incentive plans:

- Practitioners have negative reactions to the program on "moral" grounds.
- Valued slower practitioners (low producers) leave the practice.
- Practitioners exhibit speed at the expense of accuracy.
- Practitioners exhibit speed without effective communication.
- Current revenue is redistributed—no growth of new revenue.
- Goals are unclear, overly complex, or changing.
- Patients are cherry-picked based on potential revenue.
- Practitioners avoid slow or night shifts.

Two specific examples that are most likely to occur in double- or triple-coverage situations are cherry-picking and overcontrolling the ED:

Cherry-picking: Cherry-picking is preferential selection of "the best people or things from a group and leaving those which are not so good."[23] Practitioners might choose patients who have presentations that allow them to earn "easy" RVUs, that is, chest pain. Conversely, that same practitioner might avoid patients with abdominal pain or a "weak and dizzy" elderly patient as their evaluations are frequently prolonged and difficult.

Overcontrolling: Overcontrolling the ED occurs when practitioners assign themselves to most of or all the patients in the ED. This may occur to the exclusion of other practitioners until eventually the fast practitioner controls most of the beds in the ED. Further, a fast practitioner may avoid providing dispositions for current patients in order to sign up for new patients.

A variation of these two indiscretions occurs when the physician selectively signs up as the supervising physician for patients being managed by APPs or residents. The unattached patients, without resident or APP involvement, are then unfairly left for the other physician(s). The first physician makes more money through this incentive plan, while the other(s) earn less. This problem can be overcome by alternating patients according to their arrival time.

Another troublesome behavior occurs when a clinician signs up for and begins care for a patient but does not complete the care and passes the patient to the next physician at sign-out. This problem is easily addressed by assigning the RVUs to the clinician who completes the work.

A solution to both cherry-picking and overcontrolling the ED is to assign beds, pods, or work areas. Patients can only be placed in open beds/areas, so by assigning areas, each practitioner can only care for another patient when they have beds available, making it more likely that patients will be discharged expeditiously. Another solution is to alternate patient sign-ups. For instance, upon arrival, the new provider accepts the first three unassigned patients and then alternates after that.

Avoiding Pitfalls

Those considering implementation of a productivity plan would do well to avoid critical failure factors that have been observed by the authors (**Box 86.8**). Here are some considerations regarding these failure factors.

Guaranteed minimums: When moving from an hourly rate practice to a productivity-based practice, some practitioners will request a guarantee during a transition period. If it is necessary to provide a guaranteed minimum, the guarantee should be time limited and brief. Extending a guarantee beyond the transition period allows unproductive practitioners—those not meeting the minimum guarantee—to be subsidized by the rest of the practice. In fact, there is little incentive for the low producers to become more efficient or work harder. Even CMS pays physicians on an RVU incentive system and offers no minimums or guarantees. The theory is that a practitioner should get paid only for work performed.

Capping compensation or reducing pay: Should highly productive practitioners have limitations on their compensation? This is in effect a tax on the high producer, taking from the productive (rich) and giving to the less productive (poor).[24] A cap penalizes a practitioner for

---

BOX 86.8 ■ CRITICAL FAILURE FACTORS TO AVOID

- Guaranteed minimums
- Capping compensation
- Incentive plan to reduce pay
- Payment above accrued revenue

efforts beyond that for which he or she is paid (rewarded). If a well-developed incentive plan appropriately modifies behavior, it will pay a person to be more productive. Stopping payment at a certain level of productivity will likely lead the practitioner to stop being productive at that level of productivity. Caps convey a mixed message and create dissatisfaction among the most highly productive practitioners. If a practitioner is earning too much within the current plan design, the practitioner should not be penalized; rather, the plan should be changed. A variation on capping occurs when a plan is designed to decrease revenue to an individual or a group. Enormous practitioner dissatisfaction will ensue in this case.

Payment above the accrued revenue: It is possible to compensate practitioners more than the accrued revenue. This net loss scenario is most likely to occur in a 100%-productivity program (no base) in which expenses are higher, or revenues lower, than anticipated. The "what-if" scenarios must be worked out in advance and the plan, including revenues and expenses, analyzed on a regular basis, and modified as needed. High risk can be avoided if a portion of the accrued revenue is consistently held back and then paid out as a bonus when net revenue has accumulated.

CASE STUDY: THE FAILING PRACTICE

The following case represents an actual ED that was failing.[11]

Background: A 28,000-patient annual volume ED with the following problems:

- Poor staffing–the practice consistently understaffed, recruiting two physicians
- Recruitment efforts unsuccessful
- Poor productivity with an average of 1.6 pph
- Poor documentation that was described by the billing company as "the worst"
- Multiple in-services that did not change performance
- Payment (practitioner) in this hospital ED at 90% of the prevailing rate (compared to surrounding EDs)
- Large retention bonuses paid to keep shifts filled
- Poor clinician morale and camaraderie
- Nurses frustrated by slow, inefficient doctors
- Eight percent of patients leaving prior to medical screening examination
- Practice well over budget

The Goal and Plan Implementation

The goal: Develop and implement a practitioner incentive plan with payment based on RVUs generated through a productivity program. If the physicians increased their productivity to two pph, the practice could be successful.

The implementation: An RVU payment plan was phased in over 90 days. Increased productivity led to higher pay, while those who maintained baseline productivity were paid the baseline rate. The new model:

- Base $75 per hour + $13.50 per RVU
- Bonus $15 per hour for physicians working 12 or more shifts/month
- The model was demonstrated as a "what-if" for the prior 3 months
- One physician was caring for 2.4 patients per hour with an average of 3.6 RVUs per patient. This physician, under the new system, would be paid $191.64 per hour using the following formula:

Patients/hour × RVU × patient × RVU conversion factor + base + bonus
$2.4 \times 3.6 \times \$13.50 + \$75 = \$191.64/\text{hour}$
$206.64/hour (working 12 or more shifts/month)

- Practitioners averaging two patients/hour would make $172.20 ($197.20 if 12 or more shifts/month)

Case Resolution

As the physicians became familiar with the incentive structure, they realized they could be making more money. Managing two patients per hour increased their pay to 15% above the average in surrounding practices. In less than six months, the practice had these results:

- The practice was fully staffed, with a waiting list of physicians who considered themselves highly productive.
- Less than 1% of patients left prior to medical screening examination.
- The physicians felt they were part of a high-performing group.
- Some nurses complained the doctors were working too fast and they could not keep up.
- A nurse incentive was implemented resolving the above complaint.
- Patient volumes increased.

Carefully aligning this incentive program through a well-designed productivity plan accomplished the intended goals.

CONCLUSION

All incentive compensation plans should be developed in a deliberate manner that results in accomplishing the group's goals and avoiding unintended consequences. Plans that follow the ASMAN principles of agreeable, simple, measurable, achievable, and new money (realized) are most likely to endure the often required modifications that result from variations of the reimbursement system and changes in the group's composition or philosophy.

APPENDIX 86.1: QUALITY INCENTIVE PLAN

Created and submitted by Mark Rosenberg

St. Joseph's University Medical Center in Paterson, New Jersey, is the third busiest emergency department in the country with 170,000 visits per year. To ensure quality, we have established a multidisciplinary peer review committee (MDPR) with a comprehensive ED quality plan and an associated quality-incentive plan, described below.

Funds were available to allocate to providers. A pool was created, and each full-time physician given a $10,000 credit that could be earned and distributed at the end of the calendar year. An individual physician's pool could change based on the MDPR assessment of his or her quality of care. The goal is that each physician receives his or her entire bonus.

Cases are identified for MDPR review through preset filters, patient complaints, and referrals from medical staff members, nursing, administration, and so on. The MDPR typically reviews 20 to 30 charts a week and grades each ED physician and nurse using the scoring system below (**Box 86.9**):

Case example: A patient presents to the ED with electrocardiography (ECG) changes consistent with a ST-segment elevation myocardial infarction. The emergency physician does not appreciate the ECG changes and admits the patient to the telemetry unit.

> **BOX 86.9 ■ MDPR SCORING SYSTEM**
>
> ☐ Exemplary nomination
> **0.** No problem with care/documentation
> **1.** Minor process/documentation problem, clinical outcome not affected
> **2.** Problem with process/documentation, disease/symptoms unchanged, adverse consequences possible
> **3a.** Problem with process/documentation, disease/symptoms occurred, made worse, allowed to progress, resolved by chairman
> **3b.** Problem with process/documentation, disease/symptoms occurred, made worse, allowed to progress, referred to MDPR committee
> **4.** Problem with process/documentation, permanent impact/quality of life
> **5.** Death attributable to care provided that is significantly controversial
> **6.** Death attributable to care provided/not provided that should have been provided

Subsequently, the cardiologist identifies a missed intervention opportunity and the patient suffers morbidity. The concern is shared with the ED medical director and referred to the MDPR. After review, a score of 4 is assigned 4,000 is deducted from the physician's potential year-end quality bonus pool. The physician can regain the lost bonus by:

- Participating in acceptable education, for example, a continuing medical education course on ECGs
- Demonstrating excellent future performance

Loss of entire bonus: Any physician who has a score greater than 10, that is, several cases adding up to a score of more than 10, loses his or her entire bonus and is required to submit a work improvement plan to the MDPR.

Exemplary care incentive: At St. Joseph's, a physician can make more than $10,000 based on a bonus plan developed by the medical director. For instance, the physician who most quickly administers thrombolytic therapy in the stroke patient (when appropriate) receives an extra bonus. Other additional incentives can be developed based on budget and department goals.

REFERENCES

1. Hsiao WC, Braun P, Dunn DL, et al. An overview of the development and refinement of the Resource-Based Relative Value Scale: the foundation for reform of U.S. physician payment. *Med Care*. 1992;30 (11 suppl):NS1-NS12.
2. History of Medicare Conversion Factor. Available at: https://www.aap.org/en-us/Documents/Medicare-CF-History-Grid.pdf. Accessed September 4, 2018.
3. Smith A. *An Inquiry into the Nature and Causes of the Wealth of Nations*. Chicago, Ill: The University of Chicago Press; 1976. Book 3, Chapter 2.
4. Skinner BF. *Contingencies of Reinforcement: A Theoretical Analysis*. Englewood Cliffs, NJ: Prentice-Hall; 1969.
5. Kohn A. *Punished by Rewards*. Boston, Mass: Houghton Mifflin; 1999.
6. Herzberg F. One more time: how do you motivate employees? *Harv Bus Rev*. 2003;46:53-62.
7. Strauss RW. Physician compensation plans: show me the money. Presented at: American College of Emergency Physicians Scientific Assembly; San Francisco, Calif; 2011.
8. Mayer TA, Cates RJ. *Leadership for Great Customer Service: Satisfied Patients, Satisfied Employees*. Chicago, Ill: Health Administration Press; 2005.
9. Klauer K. Productivity and compensation: measurement and feedback. Presented at: American College of Emergency Physicians—Emergency Department Directors Academy: Phase I; February 22, 2011; Dallas, Tex.

10. Mayer T. Peer review, physician profiling, and reward systems. Presented at: American College of Emergency Physicians—Emergency Department Directors Academy: Phase 1; February 23, 2011; Dallas, Tex.

11. Strauss R. Physician compensation plans: developing effective incentives. Presented at: American College of Emergency Physician—Scientific Assembly; September 28, 2010; Las Vegas, Nev.

12. Hellstern R. Staffing and scheduling methodologies. Presented at: American College of Emergency Physicians—Emergency Department Directors Academy: Phase I; February 23, 2011; Dallas, Tex.

13. HCAHPS. Available at: http://www.hcahpsonline.org/home.aspx. Accessed June 20, 2013.

14. IPPS final rule. Available at: http://www.aabb.org/programs/reimbursementinitiatives/Pages/11ippsfinalrule.aspx. Accessed June 20, 2013.

15. Available at: https://www.cms.gov/Research-Statistics-Data-and-Systems/Research/CAHPS/ed.html. Accessed September 23, 2018. [Please insert author group/article title for Ref. 15.]

16. Harris R. Value-based purchasing in emergency medicine. Presented at: the Emergency Department Practice Management Association National Meeting; February 2011; Las Vegas, Nev.

17. Guss DA. A simple plan—faculty compensation in an academic department of emergency medicine. *Acad Emerg Med.* 2002;9(6):654-657.

18. Steinwald B. Compensation of hospital-based physicians. *Health Serv Res.* 1983;18(1):17-47.

19. Zun LS, Moss D. Bonus/incentive programs to increase physician productivity in academic emergency medicine. *Am J Emerg Med.* 1996;14(3):334-336.

20. Sikka R. Pay for performance in emergency medicine. *Ann Emerg Med.* 2007;49(6):756-761.

21. Levitt SD, Dubner SJ. *SuperFreakonomics: Global Cooling, Patriotic Prostitutes and Why Suicide Bombers Should Buy Life Insurance.* New York, NY: William Morrow, XIV; 2009.

22. Merton RK. The unanticipated consequences of purposive social action. *Am Sociol Rev.* 1936;1(6):894-904.

23. *Oxford Advanced Learner's Dictionary.* 9th Rev Ed. Oxford University Press; 2014. Available at: https://www.oxfordlearnersdictionaries.com/us/definition/english/cherry-picking?q=cherry+picking. Accessed December 30, 2019.

24. Holt JC. *Robin Hood.* New York, NY: Thames & Hudson; 1982:184.

CHAPTER 87

OPTIMIZING NURSING PERFORMANCE THROUGH INCENTIVES

Jeff Solheim, Fred Neis

Brains, like hearts, go where they are appreciated.

—Robert McNamara, Former US Secretary of State

With an increasing emphasis on improving quality and reducing health-care costs, emergency department (ED) leaders are continually challenged to engage their staff in the process of change. Because the success of their programs rests heavily on the work of others, it is incumbent on leaders to share their vision and motivate their subordinates to strive for the same goals. One way of accomplishing this is through an incentive program, which can be defined as "a formal scheme for inducing someone . . . to do something."[2]

Although there are many varieties, most incentive programs are clustered around four main themes: merit increases, financial compensation, nonmonetary rewards, and career mobility (**Box 87.1**). Nursing leaders must decide which program (or programs) best suits their individual department by analyzing the strengths and weaknesses of each.

CHALLENGES TO NURSING-BASED INCENTIVE PROGRAMS

Regardless of which program is used, leadership must consider impediments to program implementation. One of the major obstacles is the requirement to standardize compensation throughout the institution. Administration and human resources may frown on a financial incentive program that rewards a single department or even a specific job class without providing equal inducements to other employees.

BOX 87.1 ■ COMMON NURSING INCENTIVE PROGRAMS

- Merit increases
- Customary incentives (i.e., recruitment and retention)
- Pay-for-performance evaluation tools
- Career ladders

Programs Limited to a Single Employee Class or Department

A leader may devise a system that rewards registered nurses (RNs) in the ED for obtaining certain goals in patient satisfaction scores. If other departments learn about the program, they may be inclined to complain that RNs within their departments should be equally compensated for patient satisfaction scores. Ancillary departments (e.g., radiology, laboratory) may ask to share in the enhanced compensation program because of the role they play in the satisfaction of ED patients.

Similarly, if only RNs are recognized financially for reaching these goals, it may disincentivize other staff members. ED technicians and other support staff may perceive a lack of fairness because they assist nurses in reaching the goals but do not share in the financial rewards. To avoid the perception of inequality, administration and/or human resources may insist that incentive programs be equally administered and distributed throughout the institution. While this broad program may be laudable, the limitations of the total financial compensation available for the inventive program dilute the reward so much that it does not properly incentivize the majority of staff. Furthermore, if the program includes numerous departments and job classes, it is difficult if not impossible to standardize specific initiatives.

Unions

Unions may create another obstacle to implementation of an incentive program in the ED. A union can be defined as "a grouping of two or more employees aggregated for the assertion of organizational rights or for collective bargaining."[3] While the purpose of the union is to protect and advance the rights of the employees within it, the union must also ensure that its members are treated equitably.[4] The most effective incentive programs reward employees for individual performance, which may result in different rewards for different people. As such, the concept of rewards based on nonstandard evaluations may meet resistance. To further complicate this issue, the bargaining unit may represent employees from both inside and outside the ED, who might initially resist the idea of incentive programs that target the staff of one department only.

OVERCOMING CHALLENGES

Leaders must not let obstacles like single-department inducement plans and unions discourage their attempts to develop incentive programs. ED-specific incentive programs have worked effectively in many organizations. These successes can be shared as part of the background information utilized to propose and implement a program. Generally, unions want what is best for both the members of their bargaining unit and the patients serviced by their members. Therefore, involving the union in the development and implementation of an incentive plan may result in a smoother, more collaborative process.

Incentive Programs

Merit Increases

Perhaps the most widely utilized incentive tool in emergency nursing is the performance-based merit increase. In most institutions, staff is provided with regular pay

> **BOX 87.2 ■ PERFORMANCE QUESTIONS**
>
> - Did the individual meet the personal and professional goals set at the last evaluation period?
> - Did the individual have performance issues requiring discipline since the last evaluation period?
> - How do peers, supervisors, and even the individuals themselves rate their performance (360° evaluations)?

increases. These increases may be automatic raises based on anniversary dates without regard to performance. For example, employees may be given an automatic 2% increase every six months or a cost-of-living increase annually based on the national consumer price index.

To incorporate an incentive into the regular raises in compensation, institutions may choose to provide pay increases based partly or solely on performance. The individual staff member may be "graded" on aspects of performance that can vary between one pay period and another. Questions that might be used to rate performance are listed in **Box 87.2**. An employee's overall score can be used to determine their increase in pay. Because high-achieving employees will earn a better raise than their lower-functioning counterparts, a merit-based system can be a powerful motivator for improved performance.

Numerous factors should be taken into consideration in order to maximize the potential effects of merit-based incentives. The amount of the increase must be substantial enough for the employee to feel that the reward for improved performance is worth the effort. For instance, if the maximum incentive that can be earned is 0.5%, the differential between a low performer and a high performer may be insufficient to encourage improved performance.

Objective Performance Measurements

The ED leader must also use an objective tool when implementing merit increases. If rewards are given based on subjective criteria or standards that are difficult to understand (or achieve), perceptions of inequity may exist, leading to distrust and performance disincentives.[5]

When developing merit increase programs, ED nursing leaders should focus on the priorities of their department stakeholders. For example, if customer service is a focus, then the tool may be primarily based on areas listed in **Box 87.3**. Similarly, if patient

> **BOX 87.3 ■ CUSTOMER SERVICE MEASUREMENT TOOLS**
>
> - Nurse's individual customer service scores
> - Number of episodes of positive patient feedback
> - Negative patient feedback that has been received

> **BOX 87.4 ■ SAMPLE THROUGHPUT MEASUREMENTS**
>
> - Door-to-triage time
> - Triage-to-bed times
> - Left without being seen
> - Door-to-thrombolysis time
> - Disposition decision-to-discharge time

throughput is a focus, then incentives can be based on measurable operational factors (**Box 87.4**).

Recruitment and Retention Incentives

Recruiting and retention incentives are commonly used to engage staff. These programs allow ED leaders to address specific aspects of ED performance. Options include:

- *Specialty certification (e.g., certified emergency nurse, certified trauma registered nurse, sexual assault nurse examiner)*: These types of certifications are becoming increasingly common for hospitals on the journey toward Magnet status.[6] The general costs associated with these programs are listed in **Box 87.5**.
- *Shift differential*: These incentives are intended to provide compensation to ensure coverage (capacity) meets demand. Examples include critical needs, weekend option, and so on. Typically, shift differentials comprise about 3.4% of the total pay for registered nurses.[7]
- *Additional duties (e.g., charge nurse, EMS liaison)*: ED leadership may offer compensation for accepting key duties, some of which may require additional hours to complete outside of assigned shifts.
- *Hospital performance*: Some hospitals set up house-wide plans that reward all employees if larger performance goals are met, such as meeting financial targets, quality care indicators, or service standards. These programs have numerous designations like "contingent or at-risk pay," "profit sharing," and "gain sharing."[8] Hospital performance usually involves staff throughout the institution and is, therefore, not based on a specific unit or job class. To function as an incentive program, the plan requires a high level of visibility and constant communication to maintain organizational awareness. Again, the financial reward must be large enough to be appreciated by the employee.

> **BOX 87.5 ■ SPECIALTY TRAINING/CERTIFICATION COSTS**
>
> - Pay for certification review courses.
> - Compensate for the cost of the certification exam.
> - Provide a stipend or differential in base pay for achieving the certification.
> - Provide funds to assist the staff member obtain enough continuing education hours to maintain certification.

> **BOX 87.6 ■ SAMPLE PAY-FOR-PERFORMANCE METRICS**
>
> - Patient volumes
> - Patient satisfaction scores
> - Unscheduled absenteeism
> - Productivity measures (i.e., hours per patient visit)
> - Left without being seen rates
> - Door-to-bed times
> - Total length of stay
> - Time of disposition to actual discharge
> - Point-of-service cash collections for eligible patients captured
> - Time to clinical intervention (e.g., door to thrombolysis, door to antibiotic administration, etc)

Pay for Performance

As hospital leaders are increasingly focusing on cost and performance, best-in-class organizations are developing innovative department-specific payment programs to reward staff for meeting specific targets. Effective programs align staff performance with the hospital strategies to improve quality, capture market share, and contain cost. As these initiatives are designed, health-care organizations must address metrics, eligibility, measurement and evaluation processes, and returns on investment (ROI).

MEASURING PERFORMANCE

The program's progress and success can be determined by metrics, which are defined as measurements used to gauge/quantify business performance in a pay-for-performance program.[9] The metrics should be **Box 87.6** shows examples of metrics that may be used for pay-for-performance programs.[10,11]

When selecting the specific metrics, it is important to recognize which variables the team controls and which they do not, as described in **Table 87.1**. Performance metrics outside the team's control are difficult or impossible for team members to influence and are, therefore, ineffective components of an incentive program.

Involving the team when determining the metrics fosters a greater sense of team and individual responsibility. Placing the entire responsibility for devising the program on the shoulders of managers decreases team involvement and is less likely to be successful.

TABLE 87.1 ■ Metrics Outside the Control of Team Members

Metric	Reason for Lack of Control
Patient Volume	Not directly controlled by the team
Patient satisfaction	Portions controlled by the team (e.g., keeping patients informed, using keywords)
Employee Absenteeism	Controlled by the individual employee

Determining Eligibility

Determining eligibility for rewards can become a thorny part of the larger plan. While it may seem easy initially, by determining who is included, the leaders must also determine who should be excluded, which may cause divisions among the team members.

A further nuance might include weighting eligibility based on factors like full-time versus part-time classification, job category, cost center, and intradepartmental versus inclusion of all staff affiliated with the ED (e.g., sitters, housekeepers, respiratory therapists). Eligibility decisions may be dictated by the metrics chosen, organizational structure, human resources, payroll process, and the process of ROI.

Evaluating Progress

Once metrics have been defined, targets must be set, related policies must be developed, and the plan must be shared with the staff. In a pay-for-performance initiative, certain targets must be met in order to trigger payment. These goals can come from a variety of internal sources (e.g., board of directors, quality departments) and external sources (e.g., industry norms, published professional protocols). It is important to understand that benchmarks are guidelines rather than absolutes. As such, leaders must consider certain variables when determining how success should be measured. These variables might include overall volumes and census by time of day, time periods measured (by shift, day, hour, or other), patient acuity, physical ED space, hours of operation, and so on. This variability requires the manager to define appropriate targets for comparison.

Goals should also be realistic. If the gap between current performance and target/goals is too wide, staff may become discouraged and view the objective as unattainable. Outlining incremental steps for improvement can help stimulate progress and promote team unity. An effective feedback and evaluation process can also help the ED staff focus on core strategies, understand the importance of the outcome, and obtain rewards for their efforts.

Choosing the measurement frequency (e.g., daily, monthly, quarterly) requires consideration of target adjustments and frequency of payout.

- *Target adjustment*: How frequently should the target goals be modified (updated) or replaced? Adjusting targets that have been met and sustained works well unless the new target is deemed to lead to minimal return for the effort. For example, the manager for an automobile assembly line could be told to increase his daily production of cars from 100 to 120 (i.e., improve throughput). Though the manager might achieve success and meet the stated goal, the unintended consequence could be a higher incidence of cars produced with faulty engines (i.e., clinical quality). Once an acceptable target is reached and maintained, it may be appropriate to go on to an entirely new metric. For example, triage may be a bottleneck to flow. Once the triage process is optimized, rather than further addressing triage issues, which may have little positive return, it might be more appropriate to address another bottleneck.
- *Define metrics*: ED leaders should leave a metric in place long enough to ensure both the process and culture changes achieve sustainability. As a leader, the "art" is knowing when the optimal change in performance has occurred. This definition of "optimum achievable outcomes" should be determined through consensus of leadership and staff before moving to other metrics.

- *Payout frequency*: How often should the rewards for successful achievement of targets be paid? Payouts may occur on paycheck cycles, quarterly, or annually. The payout frequency should be defined when the program is set up. An example of a successful program is provided later with an explanation.

Gauging Return on Investment

Creating the "business case" is another critical aspect of program development and implementation. Hospital administrators, including the chief financial officer, will require an ROI analysis. Successful programs are self-sustaining. In the ED, there are a number of ways to measure ongoing success, including hard returns and soft returns. Hard returns can be directly measured in financial terms and utilized to develop an incentive-based bonus plan as described in **Table 87.2**.

TABLE 87.2 ■ Hard Returns and Incentive Plans

Metric	Definition	Sample Calculation
LPMSE	Left prior to medical screening examination	Annual volume: 60,000 patients LPMSE (current): 1,800 (3%) LPMSE (goal): 300 (0.5%) Average per patient ED facility revenue: $325 Current − goal = Additional revenue 1,800 − 300 = 1,500 × $325 = $487,500 A portion of the additional revenue can be set aside for staff bonuses.
Premium labor spending	Spending on staff overtime, travelers, or agency nursing	Annual expenses based on absenteeism, unfilled slots, etc. Overtime: 12% = $285,000 cost Traveler = $430,000 Total annual expense = $715,000 An 80% reduction of premium labor spending results in savings of $572,000. A portion of the additional revenue can be set aside for staff bonuses with low records of absenteeism.
Staff turnover	Voluntary or involuntary staff turnover, including factor for replacement	Turnover cost per RN = $50,000, annual staff turnover = 12 $400,000 can be saved by a 75% decrease in staff turnover. A portion of the savings can be set aside as a retention bonus.

TABLE 87.3 ■ Soft Returns and Incentive Plans		
Soft Returns	**Description**	**Incentive Bonus Plan**
Patient volume	In the short term, ED providers are only indirectly responsible for volume changes. In the long term, operational efficiency, high patient satisfaction, and word of mouth may directly affect ED reputation and census.	Increased volume requires increased staff- and equipment-related expenditures and limits bonus potential.
Patient satisfaction	Several aspects of patient satisfaction may be outside the control of the ED providers. As an example, inpatient boarding in the ED will create dissatisfaction related to prolonged stays and increased staffing needs.	Plans can be developed around patient satisfaction factors that are under the control of the ED providers. However, patient satisfaction is rarely associated with increased institutional revenue in the short term.
Length of stay	Improving length of stay has several indirect effects on volume. It can decrease staffing needs and improve patient satisfaction.	An incentive plan can be developed related to the direct returns (i.e., higher efficiency requiring lower staffing needs).

Soft returns may be harder to measure objectively in financial terms and are therefore more difficult to use in the development of bonus plans. Some examples of soft returns are listed in **Table 87.3**. **Figure 87.1** provides a sample incentive program.

CAREER LADDERS

Career ladder programs are common in today's health-care organizations and serve to incentivize RNs to become involved in their departments by pursuing further education and becoming vested in their profession.[12] While most hospitals have developed institution-wide career ladder programs, some have created strategies that are focused on the unique goals and needs of the ED.

Defining Goals

Career ladder programs require participants to meet specific standards in order to progress. Each step requires the staff member to complete certain tasks to be successful. When those steps are completed, the staff member can begin to work on the tasks required for the next step. These responsibilities may include:

- *Educational endeavors*: RNs may be required to complete educational courses (e.g., advanced cardiac life support, trauma nursing core courses, etc) in order to either advance or stay at a step in the ladder. Obtaining an advanced degree in nursing, such as a bachelor's or master's degree, may be a minimum requirement for certain steps. Nurses are usually required to provide proof of continuing education hours to be eligible for a specific step in the career ladder.
- *Unit involvement*: Steps in a career ladder may require activities such as:
  - ☐ Participation on department-specific or institution-wide committees
  - ☐ Completing projects for the department, such as an educational session or a poster presentation
  - ☐ Assisting with research on the unit
  - ☐ Advancing the unit through other activities

- ***Unit commitment:*** A certain amount of longevity in the institution or on the unit may be required to reach certain steps on the career ladder. Minimal absenteeism, shift timeliness, and similar factors may also be required.
- ***Performance:*** Directed performance on the annual performance review can be used to accomplish unit-specific goals like customer satisfaction scores or door-to-triage times.

Effective Incentives

Financial Incentives

Career ladders may involve purely financial incentives. Each step in the career ladder may lead to an increase in the nurse's hourly wage or result in a one-time payout. The compensation associated with each step in the career ladder must be sufficient to encourage the desired behavior.

FIGURE 87.1 ■ Sample Incentive Program

Emergency Department Staff Incentive Program

Background: Team members are a key ingredient to the success of the Emergency Department at Main Street Hospital. The ED Incentive Program is designed to increase ED team member involvement, productivity, teamwork, and performance. This program is also intended to enhance patient care and satisfaction and help retain great employees.

Goal: There are three goals to this program:

- Achieve and maintain patient satisfaction scores (% Excellent) above the 80th percentile for three drivers:
  - Triage/registration process
  - Nurses instructions/explanation of treatments/tests (when applicable)
  - Overall quality of care
- Decrease patients who leave prior to medical screening exam (LPMSE) by fostering teamwork and working smarter.
- To be the provider of choice for emergency care in our community.

Structure: For the 24-hour period in which all criteria are met, each nonsalaried staff member involved in direct patient care will receive incentive pay for their hours worked as follows:

- RNs are eligible to receive $2.00/hr.
- ED technicians, unit secretaries, and housekeepers are eligible to receive $1.00/hr.
- To receive the incentive pay, the following criteria must be met:
  - Volume – 20% greater than daily budgeted volume.
  - Hours per patient visit – decrease the hours per patient visit.
  - Patient satisfaction scores for the previously reported quarter must be at or above the 70th percentile.
- **Ineligible:** Any employee who has had an unscheduled absence in the past 90 days (ie, sick call).

Methodology: A daily scorecard will be posted by the ANM at 0700 in the breakroom. It will contain the following metrics:

- Patient volume in the previous 24 hours
- Hours per patient visit
- Previous quarter's patient satisfaction for three drivers.

If all targets are met or exceeded, the staff who worked during that period of time will be eligible for the incentive for the direct hours worked in patient care.

Impact: The program has the opportunity to enhance hospital revenues by $975,000 annually by decreasing the LPMSE rate and increasing volume. Payout to the team members could equal $324,000. Thus, this is a self-funded program.

Career Progress Incentives

Career ladders can also be designed to create eligibility for certain positions within the department. For example, nurses may not be allowed to work in resuscitation rooms or perform the charge nurse role within the ED until they have obtained the minimum competency requirements for that role (**Table 87.4**). Career ladder programs may include a combination of financial and career incentives. In this scenario, the nurse will receive financial compensation and enhanced roles within the department based on the step obtained in the career ladder.

TABLE 87.4 ■ Sample Career Ladder

Level of Achievement	Requirements	Reward
Level 1	• Licensed as an RN	None
Level 2	• Minimum 1-year employment at the hospital, minimum 1-year employment in the ED • 25 contact hours in nursing continuing education within the past year • Serves on at least 1 house-wide or unit-based committee • Has at least 10 points from points list below • Completion of ACLS, TNCC, and ENPC or PALS	$1,500 on anniversary (eligible to work in the resuscitation rooms)
Level 3	• Minimum 5 years of employment at the hospital, with at least 3 years in the ED • 25 contact hours in nursing education within the past year • Serves on at least 1 house-wide or unit-based committee • Has at least 20 points from points list below • Maintenance of ACLS, TNCC, and ENPC or PALS • Completion of "Steps to Leadership" program	$3,000 on anniversary (eligible to serve as permanent charge nurse)
Level 4	• Minimum 10-year employment at the hospital with at least 5 years in the ED • Is currently a certified emergency nurse • 25 contact hours in nursing education within the past year • Serves on at least one house-wide/unit-based committee • Has at least 30 points from point list below • Maintenance of ACLS, TNCC, and ENPC or PALS	$4,500 on anniversary (eligible for scholarship to one national nursing conference)
Points	• Bachelor's degree in nursing (1 point) • Master's degree in nursing (2 points) • Approved national certification (2 points per certification) • Member of a professional nursing organization (1 point) • Member of a hospital or unit-based committee (2 points each)	N/A

Level of Achievement	Requirements	Reward
	- Participation in an evidence-based practice project (1 point each) - Participation in a research project (1 point each) - Participation in a quality initiative project (2 points each) - Leader in a quality initiative project (4 points each) - College credits (1 point for each credit hour in the past year) - Continuing education contact hours (1 point/10 contact hours) - Course instructor (e.g., ACLS, TNCC) (3 points each) - Unit-based poster presentation or presentation at a staff meeting (3 points each) - Involvement as a presenter at competency skills fair (3 points) - Recognition in the "star employee" program (1 point each) - Published in an internal or external publication (3 points) - Preceptor (2 points for every 12 shifts) - Charge nurse role (2 points for every 12 shifts) - Volunteering in a nursing-based activity (1 point/5 hours)	

CONCLUSION

Incentive programs have the potential to dramatically enhance overall performance.[1] If designed well, these programs can partially shift the responsibility of maintaining performance standards from management to members of the staff. Several factors must be considered when designing an incentive plan (**Box 87.7**).

BOX 87.7 ■ INCENTIVE PROGRAM PEARLS

- Ensure the financial incentives are large enough to encourage the desired behavior. Small or insignificant financial incentives may be looked at by the staff as not worth the effort to improve performance.
- Work diligently to implement the incentive plan fairly and objectively. Plans that are perceived as unfair may be counterproductive and disincentivize rather than promote the desired actions.[5]
- Ensure the metrics chosen can be measured easily and the results can be achieved by plan participants. If an incentive plan includes payment for obtaining a desired volume and length of stay in the department's "fast-track" area, but only the nurse assigned to that section can achieve the bonus, others (e.g., triage nurses, charge nurses) may not support the goal.
- Avoid the trap of counterincentives in which star performers are rewarded with more work and low performers do not try yet both receive equal rewards. Effective incentive programs recognize individual performance.[1]

Leaders of a dynamic and professional ED staff can design a compensation program that ensures transparency and equitable administration. There are a number of options that can be used effectively by ED leaders to achieve different goals, including incentives that enhance individual performance, promote greater teamwork, and create accountability.

Plans that align the goals of the ED leaders, the staff, and the hospital promote the ED team's effectiveness. Incentive programs and related policies should be clearly defined and encourage staff alignment with department- and hospital-wide strategic visions and goals. Regardless of changes in health-care payment structures, more innovative ED leaders work to identify programs that drive teamwork, individual and group advancement, institutional market share, quality service, and optimal throughput. Effective programs position the ED and its team members for long-term sustainability and adaptability.

REFERENCES

1. Haim A. *Motivational Management*. New York, NY: Amacom; 2003.
2. Farlex (nd). Incentive program. Available at: http://www.thefreedictionary.com/incentive+program. Accessed August 30, 2011.
3. Sanders LG, McCutcheon AW. Unions in the healthcare industry. *Labor Law J* [serial online]. 2010;61(3):142-151. *Health Business Elite*. Ipswich, Mass. Accessed August 30, 2011.
4. Unions will resist move towards greater regional pay variations. *Nurs Stand* [serial online]. 2006;20(31):9. Academic Search Complete. Ipswich, Mass. Accessed August 30, 2011.
5. Bleich MR. Managing, leading, and following. In: Yoder-Wise PS, ed. *Leading and Managing in Nursing*. 4th ed. St. Louis, Mo: Mosby-Elsevier; 2008:3-26.
6. American Nurses Credentialing Center. (nd). ANCC Magnet Recognition Program. SE4EO 2008 Magnet Manual. Available at: http://www.nursecredentialing.org/Magnet.aspx. Accessed September 16, 2011.
7. United States Department of Labor. Compensation and Working Conditions. 2009. Available at: http://www.bls.gov/opub/cwc/cm20090317ar01p1.htm. Accessed September 16, 2011.
8. American Nurses Association. *RNs and Pay-for-Performance: The Right Prescription*. Silver Spring, Md: American Nurses Association; 1998.
9. SearchCRM.com. Business Metric. 2003. Available at: http://searchcrm.techtarget.com/definition/business-metric. Accessed September 16, 2011.
10. Smiciklas M. Word of Mouth Marketing. 2011. Available at: http://www.socialmediaexplorer.com/social-media-marketing/word-of-mouth-marketing/. Accessed September 16, 2011.
11. Cardello D. Employee and patient satisfaction affects patient flow. *Patient Flow E-Newsletter*. 2007;4(3). Available at: http://urgentmatters.org/346834/318732/318733. Accessed June 19, 2013.
12. Donley R, Flaherty MJ. Promoting professional development: three phases of articulation in nursing education and practice. *Online J Issues Nurs*. 2008;13(8). Available at: http://www.nursingworld.org/MainMenuCategories/ANAMarketplace/ANAPeriodicals/OJIN/TableofContents/vol132008/No3Sept08/PhasesofArticulation.aspx. Accessed June 19, 2013.

CHAPTER 88

FINANCIALLY SUCCESSFUL PRIVATE PHYSICIAN GROUPS

Mark Reiter, Kevin Beier

For a private emergency physician group, a financially successful practice provides increased stability and clinician satisfaction. The group's financial success creates an environment that can provide excellent clinical care within the framework of a positive relationship with the emergency department (ED) staff and hospital administration. As with any other business venture, a financially successful group may reinvest profits in the group to:

- Maintain or increase its revenue stream.
- Recruit and retain quality physicians.
- Improve the practice.

GROUP LEADERSHIP

Effective leadership is a crucial factor for a successful emergency physician group. Prudent group administrators have foresight and are adept at making wise decisions. They additionally possess the personality traits and ability to affirmatively guide, motivate, and mentor the group's physicians. Selection of a group's administrators should also be based on their abilities to communicate and work with the medical and nursing staff and hospital administration. Effective intrahospital relationships help to maintain the contractual relationship that guarantees maintenance of the group revenue stream.

The successful private group should ensure its leadership has the requisite protected administrative time and corresponding financial and administrative support. In many EDs, the amount of time devoted to group leadership is inappropriately low and inadequately supported, leading to poor performance and instability that can place contractual relationships with the hospital at risk. High-volume EDs with active hospital and medical staff leadership should strive to allocate a minimum of 30 to 50 hours a week of combined paid administrative time to their leadership, while low-volume EDs may be successful with a more modest amount of protected time. Paid administrative time should include regular office hours during the daytime. Schedule allowances (particularly fewer overnight shifts) are often required to maximize group leaders' availability for meetings.

The group's physicians should carefully select the most capable leaders. Ideally, the clients of the emergency physician group, including the hospital administration and medical staff, will agree with the selection. Concerns about a potential leader expressed by the hospital or medical staff may hint at discomfort with the individual chosen and eventually lead to friction and discord.

Formal leadership programs may provide the selected leaders with additional skills that propel them and the group forward. These programs, such as the American College of Emergency Physicians (ACEP) ED Directors Academy, the American Academy of Emergency Medicine's (AAEM) ED Management Solutions: Principles and Practice, and the Governance Institute's Leadership Conferences are well worth the time and nominal expense. Additionally, effective groups periodically revisit their leadership decisions. The group may benefit from leadership succession, when:

- Existing leadership becomes less effective, influential, or respected.
- The environment or hospital leadership changes and the current leader(s) is unable to adapt.
- New leaders emerge from within the group.

GROUP STRUCTURE

Selecting a suitable structure is pivotal to the group's formation, stability, and physician professional satisfaction and retention. A properly developed structure maximizes stability, revenue stream, and contractual relations. A poorly conceived or inequitable group structure often results in greater dysfunction, internal friction, and deterioration and may lead to loss of the group's contract with the hospital. The group must also operate within the framework of the relevant state laws and requirements to achieve benefits, such as limited liability, or even a predictable, orderly dissolution.

Political Equity

Political equity (each group member has equitable input in group decision making) aligns and solidifies each emergency physician's short- and long-term goals with those of the hospital and emergency physician group. Smaller groups may offer each individual physician an equal vote for major decisions, and larger groups may elect representatives to make decisions on the behalf of each physician. Individual emergency physicians within a group are more likely to fully support and effect change if they are part of the decision-making process. Further, engaged physicians may have valuable insights about the advantages and disadvantages of a particular proposed change or may offer a more appropriate alternative and thus contribute to better decisions.

Instituting major changes in the ED without participation from the majority of the physicians may lead to poor compliance, poor results, and dissatisfaction within both the physician and the nursing staff. Democratic group models and the benefits associated with their political equality are often viewed as highly desirable by both seasoned emergency physicians and recently graduated and board-certified emergency physicians. Including the hospital administration and nursing staff in major group decisions that directly affect them, such as staffing changes, is also important. An open relationship with internal hospital clients sustains and strengthens contractual relations with the facility and the emergency physician group.

Financial Equity

Financial equity is vital to facilitate alignment of the individual physician's short- and long-term goals with those of the hospital and physician group. Fair business practices are essential for recruitment and retention of high-quality emergency physicians. Fee-splitting is an example of an unfair business practice that is prohibited by both federal and state laws. It occurs when a hospital or physician group receives a portion of physician fees in excess of the market value of services provided.

There are many forms of financial equity, including models that pay clinicians:

- Equally initially, or once they have achieved certain status within the group, that is, partnership
- Based on what each contributes to the group, which may include:
  - Patient billing—relative value units (RVUs) generated
  - Administrative roles—leadership stipends
- Who have met or exceeded certain agreed-upon and desirable performance metrics

CONTRACTS WITH HOSPITALS

A hospital-based physician service contract is complex. As such, obtaining legal advice and counsel is strongly encouraged. While the rare physician may possess the expertise to negotiate a suitable contract with a hospital, most lack the knowledge, substantive experience, resources, and/or skill to ensure that the contractual language precisely meets the intent of the parties without retaining legal counsel. Entering into an unfavorable agreement with the hospital may lead to long-term dissatisfaction. Thus, it may be better to leave a problematic contract on the table than to engage in an onerous and overly restrictive contractual relationship.

Contractual Responsibilities

Preparation for negotiating a contract includes extensive preliminary investigation before expiration of a current contract or bidding on a new contract. A contractual relationship should clearly define the responsibilities of the group and of the hospital. As with any business contract, due diligence and market analysis (the request for proposal [RFP] evaluation) are instrumental. Several other important elements of contract negotiation are listed in **Box 88.1** (see Chapter 101).

The contractual relationship should be clearly, exactly, and unequivocally defined early in the process. This includes defining the scope of patient care services provided by the group that generate revenue, such as ED, observation unit, and in-house code coverage. The contract must also address any unique or facility-specific issues that are potentially nonclinical or nonrevenue generating, such as a mandate for free care of injuries suffered by hospital employees.

BOX 88.1 ■ ELEMENTS OF CONTRACT NEGOTIATION

- Due diligence
- Market analysis
- Exclusivity of the contract
- Contract duration
- Clean sweep and termination provisions
- Due process provisions
- Restrictive covenants
- Noninterference clauses
- Definition of the scope of service
- Limitations on ancillary and uncompensated duties (i.e., providing free care to hospital staff)
- Preservation of the ability to negotiate managed care contracts without hospital approval of fees
- Reasonable staffing structure and expectations
- Admonishment of coercive contracting (disadvantageous contract agreements)

The contract should clearly and expressly state:

- Mechanisms for appointment of the chair of the department, as well as duties and grounds for removal of the chair
- Employment status of the physicians (independent contractor or employees of group)
- A disclaimer for the actions of staff beyond the group and physicians' control
- The hospital's duty to maintain equipment, provide appropriate and adequate nursing and support staff, provide for verification mechanisms of patient insurance, and provide hard equipment for documentation, phones, and so on
- Procedures for sanctioning or terminating physicians, including procedural rights

Financial Assessment

The determination of expected net revenues (i.e., receipts from patient encounters and the estimated costs generated by the contractual obligations) is elemental to the bidding process for an emergency medicine service contract. The RFP process ordinarily allows a period of time to study the payer mix and acuity, survey prior visits for chart demographics and code levels, and provide a period of due diligence to study other factors that affect revenue generation. Although many hospital systems may provide prior data, it is prudent for a group to request a primary chart survey by a reputable billing company to verify payer mix and case mix. Calculations and allowances should be made for different managed care products, frequency of denials, and expected changes in payer mix related to potential regional market changes (i.e., major employers leaving or entering a market). This regional market assessment is particularly important in a locality that is highly dependent on a single large employer.

A knowledgeable billing service can greatly facilitate the study of the anticipated collections and proactively identify problematic fiscal issues. Finally, the contract should specify which entity bills for services and outline the related responsibilities of each entity. If the physician group bills for its own services, the contract should contain provisions mandating timely and prompt access to records, demographic information, and so on. Alternatively, if the hospital bills for physician services, a provision absolving the group for hospital billing errors helps the group avoid a potential "compliance" complaint.

Exclusivity and Clean Sweep Clauses

An exclusivity of services provision is desirable for both the group and the hospital. The exclusivity provision allows the group and its members to be the sole provider(s) of specified services within the hospital. As such, it prevents nongroup physicians from practicing within the designated scope of exclusive services. The hospital benefits from greatly simplified administration of the ED. A broadly exclusive contract ensures that the group is the exclusive provider of all *defined* emergency medical services provided throughout the hospital and its associated facilities. State laws regulate these provisions, and some states have prohibited or imposed limitations on such exclusivity provisions. It is important that the group and hospital agreements are aligned with these laws to avoid potential claims of tortious interference with business relationships.

A *clean sweep* provision frequently accompanies an exclusivity clause. This provision automatically terminates the staff privileges for all physicians in a group upon termination of the group's contract. Such a provision may not be seen as advantageous to an individual emergency physician in the group who may wish to continue practicing in the hospital. However, it does provide significant protection to the group as a whole by preventing the hospital from cherry-picking physicians from the group with whom it would like to renegotiate a contract.

Contract Restrictions

In recent years, contract terms have typically become shorter in duration. While longer-term contracts are preferred by most groups, the duration of contract terms is less relevant, since most contracts contain relatively short *without-cause termination* provisions.

Restrictive Covenants

Hospital and physician groups often request postcontractual restrictive covenants, or noncompete clauses (see Chapter 100) that address:

- Tortious interference—illegally interfering with an existing contract
- Nonhiring—group hiring a hospital employee/hospital hiring a group employee
- Outside practice restriction—working in a competing hospital's ED, urgent care center, and so on
- Noncompete—restricts postcontract practice

Noncompete and Noninterference Clauses

The noncompete form of restrictive covenant provides that upon termination of a professional contract, the physician has certain restrictions placed upon his or her practice, typically related to a defined geographical location and a specific period of time. The American Medical Association, AAEM, and ACEP all discourage the use of the noncompete form of restrictive covenants, arguing that they violate the physicians' professional rights and effectively prevent them from advocating for their patients. Noncompete clauses are unenforceable in many states. In those states in which they are enforceable, "noncompetes" must be reasonable in their duration and geographic limitations.

On the other hand, a *noninterference with contract* (tortious interference) clause is typically considered ethical and enforceable. These clauses prevent physicians from conspiring to seize the ED professional services contract from their colleagues or other parties with whom they have contractual obligations. Similarly, emergency physicians should not conspire with other parties to illegally obtain the ED management contract.

Other Provisions

Third-Party Contracts

Additional economic provisions require close consideration, including the ability of the group to independently and fairly negotiate managed care payer contracts. A group should carefully scrutinize and avoid agreeing to broad provisions that require participation in any and all insurance programs in which the hospital also participates. Such provisions may prevent fair and reasonable compensation for emergency services. Groups may instead wish to either participate with the hospital/physician hospital organization or, perhaps, independently negotiate contracts between the group and third-party payers.

Fraud and Abuse

The close relationship between the physician group and hospital may also increase the risk of fraud allegations against the group or its members. Multiple federal regulations prohibit hospitals from charging more than fair market value for their services and from compensating physicians at a rate under market value.[1,2] There are additional relevant laws that prohibit any hospital incentives to physicians for referring patients or unnecessarily admitting patients. These include the OIG's Special Fraud Alert: Hospital Incentives to Physicians and the Stark Law.[3]

CONTRACT RETENTION

Finally, contract maintenance and retention are critically important to the success of the group and its revenue stream. Of first importance is identification of the principal and secondary clients of the ED and ensuring the long-term satisfaction of these parties. Excellence in patient care and implementation of best practices are as important as they are obvious. However, mistakes are frequently made both identifying and responding to the inherent needs of critical secondary clients. It is essential to recognize the pivotal relationship of the group and its members with the nursing staff, administration, the general medical staff, and other departments. Strong collaborative, patient-care-focused relationships with these groups are the best way to ensure the effective ED care and long-term health of the emergency medicine physician–hospital contract (**Table 88.1**).

While disagreements and friction will periodically occur in each of these relationships, substantial proactive efforts should be undertaken to mitigate discord and quickly resolve conflicts. The importance of a broad, if not universal, perception of the group as a solution and not a problem cannot be overstated. The more adept a physician group is at involving itself in the ongoing administrative operations of the hospital, the more secure the physician hospital contract. Examples of constructive involvement include:

- Membership on hospital committees
- Attendance at hospital and medical staff functions
- Participation in hospital administrative positions (e.g., chief of staff appointments of emergency physicians, chief medical officer, etc.)

The insightful adage "the world is run by those that show up" should be adopted, reiterated, and emphasized to all members of the group. Identification of primary and secondary clients and attending to their needs, striving to integrate the group with the inner workings of the hospital, and working diligently to resolve secondary client conflict ensure long-term retention and success of an emergency medicine physician group.

PERFORMANCE IMPROVEMENT

The successful emergency physician group emphasizes continuous performance improvement. Strict attention to process:

- Facilitates improved patient care and safety (most importantly)
- Maximizes physician and group revenue
- Elevates the primary client (patient) and secondary clients' (hospital, medical staff, and nursing staff) satisfaction

TABLE 88.1 ■ Emergency Physician Group Client Relationships

Primary clients	Patients and their families

Secondary clients	• ED staff (nurses, technicians, unit secretaries, etc.)
	• Medical staff
	• Administration
	• Essential services
	   ○ Imaging services
	   ○ Laboratory services
	• Inpatient units

> **BOX 88.2 ■ CHARACTERISTICS OF KEY PERFORMANCE INDICATORS**
>
> - Meaningful
> - Relevant
> - Measurable
> - Evidence-based (when possible)
> - Lead to performance improvement opportunities

It is essential to identify, update, and incorporate best practices into daily ED operations. A comprehensive assessment of the ED is necessary to fully appreciate its strengths and weaknesses and to identify the most significant opportunities for change.

Proactive Performance Improvement

Waiting for escalation of patient and staff complaints is a poor mechanism to identify problem areas. Routine evaluation of all aspects of patient care, throughput, and primary and secondary client satisfaction improves and strengthens the contractual relationship with the hospital. The ED's performance on a wide variety of metrics, such as time to physician evaluation, time to disposition, lab turnaround, x-ray turnaround, number of inpatient boarding hours, and so on, may be benchmarked against similar EDs and best practices to identify and target areas requiring improvement. Effective groups internally benchmark performance and actively solicit feedback from and provide feedback to key stakeholders (**Box 88.2**).

Successful ED leaders dedicate a substantial amount of their administrative time to development of proactive strategies targeting performance improvement. Performance improvement teams that include key stakeholders and secondary clients provide additional perspectives from outside of the ED leadership. These multidisciplinary teams ensure that performance improvement remains a high priority in the midst of daily operational responsibilities. Performance improvement teams focus on the development of tangible goals with time lines. To be effective, these teams require the resources and power to effect change and successfully achieve the objectives identified.

Political barriers to change can be minimized by creating collegial and institution-wide approaches to solving problems. It is helpful to include and encourage the entire ED staff by seeking their input and keeping them informed about performance improvement initiatives and active measurements, such as via scorecards and dashboards. Champions of successful improvements should be appropriately recognized and celebrated.

It is also essential for the ED medical director to have an excellent working relationship with the department's nursing director. Frequent, effective communication allows department leaders to remain well-informed, align their strategies and priorities, and provide a consistent message to their staff.

STAFFING

Appropriate staffing by both physicians and nonphysician providers is necessary to minimize treatment delays, improve turnaround times, improve patient outcomes, improve patient satisfaction, and maximize staff satisfaction and retention. Understaffing creates a dangerous patient care environment, increases staff turnover, and creates inefficiencies that result in poor primary and secondary client satisfaction. For these reasons, understaffing places the contractual relationship in jeopardy. On the other hand, overstaffing wastes valuable and expensive resources and reduces profitability.

Physician staffing and scheduling are driven by the ED's patient flow. A regular patient volume and acuity analysis is a useful planning aid that can be used to accommodate the fluctuating needs of the department. When initially defining staffing patterns, an evaluation of previous volume and acuity trends is of utmost importance for predicting staffing requirements. Protocols for on-call physician coverage can address a temporary surge in patient volumes and other crises, such as disaster scenarios. Fostering a culture in which group members are potentially available to begin a scheduled shift one to two hours early or to stay a few hours after their scheduled shift ends may be preferable to having on-call coverage. If *flex shift* coverage is frequently needed, additional scheduled coverage should be strongly considered.

Nonphysician Providers

Nonphysician provider staffing, that is, physician assistants and nurse practitioners (collectively advanced practice providers [APPs]), can extend the ability of the physicians to provide cost-effective, efficient, high-quality care for minor care cases and allow concentration of physician attention on high-acuity patients. In general, an APP can extend an emergency physician's productivity by ~50% (additional patients per hour) at a cost that is usually substantially less than half of an emergency physician's cost. Many EDs utilize nonphysician providers to care for low-acuity patients in a dedicated fast track. Dedicated fast tracks improve ED flow and clinician productivity by clustering patients of similar acuity. This approach requires fewer resources and results in less wasted movement by reducing the distractions caused by higher-risk cases.

Many groups consider it a best practice to have the emergency physician review the care provided by the nonphysician provider before the patient has been discharged. This is imperative for all high-acuity patients.

Scribes

Scribes (personal productivity assistants) are extensively used in emergency medicine to improve physician productivity. Emergency physicians typically spend 25% to 50% of their shifts on documentation. Yet, errors in and omissions from medical records are commonplace, which can reduce revenue and increase liability. Implementing a scribe program may improve both professional satisfaction and physician productivity by allowing the physician to dedicate more time to direct patient care and interaction. However, the emergency physician is still responsible for verifying the accuracy of the scribe's documentation.

Typically, a dedicated scribe works one-on-one with a particular physician, documenting the history and physical examination, progress notes, and test results, and preparing discharge instructions. However, physicians and APPs must enter their own patient care orders. In many cases, scribes also perform clerical tasks (e.g., tracking down test results, paging) and assist with nonmedical patient needs (e.g., blanket, beverage). Scribes work best when a long-term working relationship is fostered so that the dedicated scribe understands the specific physician's approach to patient care, flow, and documentation.

A successfully implemented scribe program can easily cover the program costs based on the increased productivity and generated revenues. There are several commercial companies that can help a physician group implement a scribe program (they will typically hire, train, and manage the scribes), or a group can hire, train, and manage its own scribes (most scribes are college students, paramedics, or medical secretarial staff).

INCENTIVES AND REWARD/RECOGNITION PROGRAMS

Productivity-based compensation incentives usually increase physician productivity and are becoming a standard in emergency medicine (see Chapter 86). Typically, physicians see productivity increases of 10% to 30% after implementation of these incentives. Modest incentives (<20% of compensation) have a much smaller impact on performance than more substantial incentives. Utilizing RVUs per hour to calculate physician productivity, rather than patients per hour, more accurately reflects the actual work performed.

Hospitals have strong interest in impacting metrics such as patient satisfaction, clinical/quality measures, turnaround times, and left-without-being-seen rates. When contracting with a physician group, a hospital may insist that rewards and penalties related to these metrics are codified into the hospital-group contract. To ensure alignment between the hospital and physician group, many groups will also include these metrics into performance-based incentive compensation formulas for their individual physicians. However, unlike productivity incentives, these measures typically are much less effective at altering performance, since individual physicians typically has much less control over the associated variables, staffing, boarded patients, and so on.

Rewards and recognition programs are an important method of positive reinforcement and boosting staff morale (see Chapter 78). An effective reward and recognition program can help improve overall ED performance as well as improve staff retention.

CODING/BILLING SERVICES

There are few things more important to a group's financial success than retaining effective and well-matched coding/billing companies. Most groups of small to medium size benefit from outsourcing this function. Large-volume groups (100,000 visits or more per year) may find in-house ownership or management of a billing service financially beneficial but must be aware of the significant complexities of the billing process as well as the substantial penalties for running afoul of regulatory compliance standards (see Chapter 96). Careful selection of the billing company may allow the group to *optimize* patient care revenues while reducing nonclinical, nonessential tasks and lowering the risk of an audit (see Chapter 95). The billing company should have and demonstrate extensive emergency medicine coding/billing experience and possess extensive experience with and knowledge of regional and local payers.

Ongoing, open dialogue between the group and the coding/billing company is essential to maximize profitability. Regular auditing of the billing solution company to ensure that they are providing the best available service for the group is a requisite to financial success. Effective documentation allows the physician group to achieve appropriate reimbursement, decrease liability, and properly communicate clinical information. Incomplete documentation can result in substantial lost revenue. The coding/billing company has the responsibility to provide informative reports that clearly identify any documentation shortfalls and to provide feedback and education to improve performance.

The physician group fee schedule is developed with careful attention to local, regional, and national norms as well as advice from the coding/billing company. Contracts between the physician group and third-party payers require critical data, careful negotiations, and continual monitoring, as well as consideration for the contract implications between the group and the hospital. Effective coding/billing companies must have a clear strategy to ensure that the physician group's services are properly valued.

CONCLUSION

This chapter outlines important components that foster a financially successful emergency physician group. Effective group leadership and structure are the backbone of a successful group. The contract between the hospital and the physician group must be carefully structured. Special attention must be given to continuous, proactive, performance improvement to maximize success. Appropriate staffing keeps the ED running smoothly. Incentive and reward/recognition programs help align behaviors with goals. The coding/billing company is an important partner in the group's success, and ongoing, open dialogue will allow the group's needs to best be served.

REFERENCES

1. Office of Inspector General. Publication of the OIG Compliance Program Guidance for Hospitals. Published in the Federal Register. 1998. Vol 63:35. Available at: https://oig.hhs.gov/authorities/docs/cpghosp.pdf. Accessed October 23, 2020.

2. Office of Inspector General. OIG Advisory Opinion No. 12–15. 2012. Available at: https://oig.hhs.gov/fraud/docs/advisoryopinions/2012/AdvOpn12-15.pdf. Accessed October 23, 2020.

3. Office of Inspector General. OIG Supplemental Compliance Program Guidance for Hospitals. Published in the Federal Register. 2005. Vol 70:19. Available at: https://oig.hhs.gov/fraud/docs/complianceguidance/012705HospSupplementalGuidance.pdf. Accessed October 23, 2020.

ADDITIONAL READINGS

- Camp R. *Benchmarking: The Search for Industry Best Practices That Lead to Superior Performance*. Milwaukee, WI: ASQ Press; 1989.
- Cobb C. *From Quality to Business Excellence: A Systems Approach to Management*. Milwaukee, WI: ASQ Press; 2003.
- Randall BC, Louis SB, Mark WB, et al. Emergency department operations management—an information paper. 2004. Available at: https://www.acep.org/globalassets/uploads/uploaded-files/acep/clinical-and-practice-management/resources/crowding/infoedopermgmt.pdf. Accessed June 21, 2013.
- Salluzzo R, Strauss RW, Mayer T, et al., eds. Emergency Department Management: Principles and Applications. Philadelphia, PA: Mosby (Elsevier); 1997.
- Scaletta T. The business of emergency medicine made easy. 2005. Available at: http://www.aaem.org/education/thebusinessofem.pdf. Accessed June 21, 2013.
- Vega D, Scaletta T. Rules of the Road for Young Emergency Physicians. Milwaukee, WI: American Academy of Emergency Medicine; 2009.

CHAPTER 89

FINANCIAL SUCCESS IN ACADEMIC EMERGENCY MEDICINE

James J. Scheulen, Gabor D. Kelen

A teacher affects eternity. He can never tell where his influence ends.

—Henry Adams[1]

Academic emergency departments (EDs), in addition to providing patient care to the community, are also responsible for training medical students, residents, and nurses—the future providers and leaders of the specialty. The demand for emergency services has continued to grow with few exceptions. The ED is the gateway to the hospital as well as a safety net for the community. Patients expect that their care will be provided by appropriately qualified specialty physicians who have been trained in academic EDs.

While the mission and structure of the academic ED are different in many ways from a private emergency medicine (EM) practice, important similarities exist. Clinical revenue sources are largely the same in both settings. Although the billing and coding elements that drive collections are similar, they are more complicated in the academic environment because of the presence of residents and students.

Revenue from clinical practice generally supports the community/private practice, though occasionally hospital or health-care system subsidies are required. In the academic practice, clinical revenue typically provides a major portion of its income; however, other sources (grants, contracts, institutional support) are more often necessary to subsidize revenue. Thus, the financial management of the academic clinical practice, including staffing, scheduling, recruiting and retaining physicians, and managing the business portion of the academic practice, has similarities to and differences from the private community practice.

The differences between private and academic EDs pose unique challenges. Most private practice EDs are primarily concerned with quality clinical practice and efficient operations and may participate in education, including nursing students, nursing fellowships, in-service education, and clinical rotations for paramedics. In contrast, the academic ED serves a tripartite mission of providing clinical care, educating an expanded group of trainees (medical students, residents, and fellows), and engaging in research and academic scholarship. Each portion of the academic mission requires discrete financial management with a unique set of requirements, revenues, and expenses. The private EM physician practice, with its less-complicated mission(s), must only support clinician practice and the administrative oversight of operations.

Community (private) practice is frequently managed by a physician practice group, contracted for service by individual hospitals. The contracting group may manage a single practice site, a number of regional practices, or even hundreds of practices in multiple states. Some large organizations may operate multiple hospital and out-of-hospital services, including but not limited to hospital medicine, anesthesiology, radiology, urgent care, post-acute care, and telemedicine practices. Larger practices have the ability to spread the fixed costs of operating a physician practice over many patient visits and may have the flexibility to cross-credential providers, permitting shifting providers to different sites on short notice. While some academic practices have engaged in entrepreneurial business ventures by managing community practices, these economies of scale are atypical in an academic practice. Private contract groups occasionally manage academic practices but may find it difficult to manage all aspects of the tripartite mission.

Financial success may vary depending upon institutional expectations and the vision of the department. As in the community practice, emergency practitioners in the academic practice may be incentivized for clinical practice performance. However, participants in the academic ED practice may or may not personally benefit financially from the plan depending on incentives set up by the institution and department administration. In fact, the primary driver in most academic departments is to meet or exceed the institutionally set margins, which support the overall education mission of the organization. The margin includes the "Dean's tax," an assessment applied to professional revenue generated by faculty members for activities like consulting, expert witness testimony, external service agreements, and so on.

Of course, the most fundamental definition of financial success is to optimize revenue from all sources and meet or exceed the expenses required to carry out the departmental mission(s). The successful department generates revenue adequate to cover the costs of the tripartite mission, attracts and retains qualified faculty members, and, if possible, provides some positive financial contribution to the hospital or health system in which it operates. Each academic department mission is not independently self-supportive. Rather, cross-subsidization among the teaching, research, and faculty development, clinical, and other revenue sources is standard, and financial support from the hospital is common. Beyond the mission-driven pursuits, this institutional support is partially in recognition of the service the ED provides to the community and its role as the gateway for hospital admissions.

THE ACADEMIC DEPARTMENT OF EM

The structure of academic EDs varies among institutions. In most academic medical centers and universities, EM has full departmental status and is on equal footing with all other academic disciplines. Autonomous EM departments negotiate directly with the institution for resources much like other academic departments and do not have to rely on the attention and priorities of a parent department.

However, in some centers, EM remains a division within a larger department, typically the department of medicine or surgery. While divisional status can be adequate to support the clinical, educational, and research missions, this lesser status reduces the independence and autonomy with which the ED and its leadership operate.

Departmental Structure

The structure of academic departments generally follows one of two models. The first is a highly centralized structure within limited operational and budgetary control; personnel positions (including academic positions) are centrally managed.

Alternately, decentralized departments operate as a functionally independent financial or business unit, with financial and operational expectations set through a series of budget discussions and negotiations. While some central position control may exist, the department is largely free to manage within its budget. For these independent or decentralized departments, the departmental leadership is responsible for the faculty clinical practice and may also be responsible for hospital ED operations. Hospital responsibilities may include accountability for personnel associated with providing care in the ED (including nurses), managing the operational and nursing budgets, and providing hands-on management of the daily operations of the department. The most decentralized department may also place responsibility for hospital billing and coding in the hands of ED leaders.

Between these two models, partially decentralized departments may still operate with significant independence. Some, including departments in many state universities, operate with the traditional academic activities funded through the home academic institution, while the clinical operation is managed by a separate faculty practice group. For other academic practices, the faculty may be employed by the hospital itself. The structure of the department and its relationship between the institution's medical school and hospital impacts funding and nearly every aspect of how the department operates, including physicians' salary, faculty promotional requirements, and clinical staffing.

Academic Department Budgets

The typical academic ED budget is built around distinct expenses and revenue sources for clinical staffing and operations, academic activities, and research (**Table 89.1**). The largest expense category includes physician and staff salaries and the associated benefits.

In a traditional, nonacademic clinical practice, the financial focus is placed on clinical revenue in order to optimize group profit, while ensuring appropriate staffing, ED efficiency, chart coding, administrative and staff relationships, and billing and collections. The physicians and other providers working in a private practice focus both on the delivery of efficient quality care and the patient experience of that care.

Clinicians (faculty) practicing in academic practices have multiple roles in the department and may be funded through several sources. Academic EM faculty members

TABLE 89.1 ■ Sources of Academic Revenue and Expenses

Revenue	Expense
Clinical billing	Salaries
Research grants	Clinical providers
Contracts	Residents[a]
Institutional support	Administrative support
Clinical effort	Collections
Education effort	Dean's tax
Research effort	Non-salary grant-related expense
Department administration	Office supplies, furniture
Other department managed programs	Overhead (rent, phones, etc.)
Dean's funds[b]	Event costs (retreats, staff events, etc.)
Philanthropy (usually interest only)	
Dowry/grants (initial chair recruitment package)	

[a] Usually a pass through, but some positions may be supported by the department/practice.
[b] Some schools give each department a small amount of funds, usually in recognition of medical school teaching effort.

are more likely to require financial support, particularly early in their careers while they are developing funding streams to support their nonclinical activities. These sources must be carefully calculated when considering the effort dedicated to each mission.

Academic activities (teaching and research) are typically supported by the university (medical school) general funds, a grant negotiated by the chair when offered the position, and/or external sponsors at the "cost" of faculty time; there is essentially no opportunity for profit. Similarly, the teaching mission may be supported through the hospital (for residents) or by the medical school (for medical students). At best nondepartmental support for teaching rarely covers the actual expense of providing and administrating the teaching programs, leaving almost no opportunity for margin. Clinical revenue and other external contracts provide the opportunity to produce a meaningful profit margin and are, therefore, the focus of a great deal of attention.

MAXIMIZING EFFICIENCY AND REVENUE

Appropriate physician recruitment, salary structures that promote advancement and retention, staffing levels that meet demand but limit expense, and a smooth functioning coding and billing operation all contribute to the departmental bottom line. With few exceptions, clinical operations provide the primary revenue stream for the academic ED and may, in part, support its other missions. Therefore, direct revenue from efficient ED operations supports the entire department. Indirect revenue generated by patients admitted to inpatient services and referred to other specialty practices provides significant additional value to the hospital. If this value is not already acknowledged, it is prudent for financial experts in the department to calculate these important contributions and leverage the information when negotiating for resources from the institution.

Staffing Determination

A number of techniques are available to determine appropriate ED staffing (see Chapter 34). Most staffing assessments begin with determining the number of treatment beds that will be needed to meet demand. A reasonable estimate (budget) for the number of patients to be seen in the department in a year is developed. Combining this information with some expectations for bed utilization and dwell time, accounting for bed turnover time (cleaning, restocking, etc.), will lead to an estimate of the appropriate number of treatment spaces needed. It is appropriate to perform analyses with various patient utilization rates. Defining the size and space requirements of the ED is now best accomplished through the use of sophisticated operational modeling techniques.

All EDs experience times of peak and low flow. While there is no consensus about defining peak flow, it is reasonable to design EDs to accommodate a peak flow of 75% to 90% of likely experience (see Chapter 25). Given this information, staffing ratios, and expected levels of productivity, staffing needs may be calculated. It is common practice to assume that a physician in an academic center can see and treat between 1.8 and 2.2 patients per hour (PPH), depending on a number of factors that include patient complexity and the support staff surrounding physician operations. Productivity expectations will also differ for each treatment area; physicians working in a low acuity fast-track area will be expected to see more PPH than a colleague caring for the most complex patients, many of whom might require complex procedures. Staffing demand–capacity modeling will also consider times of peak flow. Inadequate staffing during times of peak demand will result in prolonged waiting and possibly high census throughout the day.

Physician Productivity

Physician productivity is a key metric of clinical practice. Productivity is generally measured as a combination of the number of patients seen by a physician in a period of time (number of PPH) and by the effort required to care for patients in a period of time (relative value units per hour and per patient). Physician productivity in an academic emergency practice is usually negatively impacted by the active teaching of students and resident physicians, a dynamic that decreases the number of patients who can be seen by an attending physician.

Because of the multiple missions served, the salary structure of faculty in an academic practice may be more complex than in a private practice (discussed later in this chapter). While salaries of academic faculty must account for both clinical and academic activity, physician salary should be structured in a way that recognizes strong clinical performance and incentivizes productivity and good patient care. In most practices, clinical performance drives bonus and incentive payments for faculty. Additional components of the academic practice should be considered for faculty performance assessments and related bonuses, typically with a large proportion bonus or incentive payments based upon clinical revenue.

Billing for Clinical Service

Clinical revenue associated with productivity is associated with appropriate documentation of the patient assessment, the complexity of medical decision-making required to come to a conclusion, and the actual care and procedures required to treat the patient. Complete documentation of the clinical encounter captures the required billing elements reflected by the care the patient received. Failure to accurately document care will result in downcoding and submaximal revenue generation (collection for the practice).

The ability to collect the billed revenue for each patient encounter is determined by a number of variables, including:

- Insurance provider policies
- Physician and institutional contracts developed with insurers
- Governmental regulations
- Institutional policies

Rapid processing of bills and minimizing the time to collections (minimize days in accounts receivable) are also central to a successful billing operation.

Many options for coding and billing for services exist. Some academic institutions prefer that all reimbursement-related services are operated internally or through large institution-owned, institution managed/controlled clinical practices. Others allow departments to outsource coding and billing as a way to control expenses. A number of factors should be evaluated when considering the decision to outsource, including the ability to closely monitor and control regulatory compliance and the quality of coding and billing operations. Typically, EM billing requires specific expertise and is often managed more effectively by outsourced organizations specializing in this business area.

It is a commonly held belief that academic practices do not bill and collect revenues efficiently, in part due to the perception that department leadership has little profit motive and is distracted by other department priorities. However, margins in most academic departments are so thin and reliance on clinical revenue so significant that managing the finances of the practice is of equal importance as in the private sector.

Many academic EM practices are unable to fully cover the costs of staffing the clinical operation, typically because the payer mix of academic hospitals existing in urban environments is not favorable. In this case, it is common for hospitals to provide financial support to the ED ensuring the department is adequately staffed. Billing and collections for hospital services are also frequently inadequate to cover all of the hospital-based ED costs. In these situations, financial success is measured by a contribution to margin methodology or by the indirect revenue (hospital admissions) provided by ED operations.

EDUCATION

An additional desirable commitment of academic center faculty is the mission/responsibility for the education of future care providers. The education *jewel* is the EM residency. The academic department may additionally participate in subspecialty fellowships, medical student and nursing education, and advanced practice provider training. Many academic programs also participate in clerkship rotations.

Managing a residency program and providing student education carry significant costs not fully covered by external sources. Residency programs in major teaching hospitals are generally supported by the hospital itself through a federal graduate medical education (GME) program. Each institution negotiates with the Centers for Medicare & Medicaid Services to recover the costs of supporting residents. The total number of residents in a given institution is capped, but in many major teaching hospitals, the resident complement surpasses the GME-negotiated cap. In these cases, the incremental residency positions must be supported by the hospital, departmental funds (clinical margin), or contractual relationships with other affiliated hospitals that utilize the trainees.

Managing an EM residency program is complex and requires significant departmental resources. The Accreditation Council for Graduate Medical Education (ACGME) mandates specific training program requirements, including those related to:

- Program leadership
- Faculty work hours and numbers of support staff
- Institutional support[2]

The hospital may be more inclined to support the administrative costs required to operate a successful residency program if the expenses can be supported by GME funding. Some academic departments may benefit from the philanthropic support of specific educational offerings, fellowships, or even endowed positions.

The responsibility for costs associated with student education is generally borne by the medical school, in contrast to resident training, which is generally seen as a hospital responsibility. Typically, medical schools with a required EM clerkship and elective offerings provide financial support for a portion of one or more EM faculty members. Other faculty, however, are generally required to participate in medical student educational activities outside of the direct clinical environment. These activities are often not funded by the medical school but are considered part of the core faculty responsibilities. Departments may or may not financially recognize such teaching within their compensation plans. If they do, such support would come from clinical margins.

Major academic centers frequently offer fellowship training. The ABEM subspecialty training for EM graduates includes:

- Anesthesiology Critical Care Medicine
- Emergency Medical Servies
- Hospice and Palliative Medicine
- Internal Medicine—Critical Care Medicine
- Medical Toxicology
- Neurocritical Care

- Pain Medicine
- Pediatric EM
- Sports Medicine
- Undersea and Hyperbaric Medicine[3]

Certification for these subspecialties, as well as focused practice designation in advanced EM ultrasonography, is offered through the American Board of Emergency Medicine (ABEM).[4] Graduates of EM programs can also seek training and subsequent subspecialty certification through non-ABEM boards in addiction medicine, brain injury medicine, clinical informatics, and surgical critical care.[3]

In addition, many centers offer non-ACGME-approved fellowship programs, including ultrasound, research, education and global health or international EM, disaster medicine, and administrative fellowships among others. These non-ACGME fellowship programs are generally not supported by GME dollars, and departments typically support them from clinical funds, often offset by revenue generated by having the fellows work as attending physicians.

Academic EDs participate in the clinical training of other health professionals, including PAs and NPs. In most cases, the faculty supervise these students in the clinical setting, often supplemented by other NP/PA trainers, minimizing the role of the EM faculty. However, the high demand for trained EM PAs has led some academic institutions to create and operate PA EM residency programs. Typically, the hospital bears the cost of these programs, including the cost of faculty involvement in PA educational programs. Ideally, a PA residency program would not add un-reimbursed cost to the department, but the general overhead costs of a program (space, support personnel, opportunity cost) are rarely included in budgets.

RESEARCH

While the first two missions are fairly uniformly emphasized in academic EM, research activity is perhaps the most variable among academic departments and is significantly influenced by the institution's mission and expectations, the department chair's vision, and faculty composition. The departmental research enterprise is perhaps the most challenging to develop, maintain, and grow. Compared to clinicians and educators, scholars and researchers are more difficult (and typically more expensive) to recruit and develop. Funding sources and cycles are uncertain; applications for grants and contracts are difficult, time-intensive, and require investment in departmental infrastructure, faculty development, and seed funding. Grant and contract revenue are meant only to cover specific costs and rarely does this funding add to the department's bottom line. And yet, it is the research mission that most clearly differentiates the academic department from all others.

Depending upon the faculty promotional structure, faculty members may be required to perform research or equivalent scholarship and discovery. However, focused, funded research is generally performed by a small subset of a department's faculty, experienced in grant acquisition, program management, and delivering successful output.

A successful research division requires faculty with specific research interests who are able to identify and attract grant funding. Departments can accelerate their research program by recruiting a key senior, established researcher who may come with a full staff and program. Attracting established researchers may be expensive, costing institutions millions of dollars and generally require medical school involvement.

Alternately, a program can develop junior researchers. Junior, less experienced faculty require time to develop their research identities. It is common for faculty members early in their research careers to require partial salary support from clinical revenue before they can

TABLE 89.2 ■ Direct and Indirect Costs of Grants		
	Direct Costs	**Indirect Costs**
Fund	Work performed	Intangibles, e.g., rent, maintenance, administrative, and secretarial support
Paid to	Division performing the work	University (medical school)
Basis	Expense of work = grant	Additional funding (negotiated and variable)

become self-supporting through grants and contracts. Additional incremental costs may be associated with formal training and securing advanced degrees such as a doctorate. Junior faculty may attract career development support grants from external bodies such as the National Institutes of Health (NIH), Society of Academic Emergency Medicine, Emergency Medicine Foundation, and other foundations or from the institution itself. These grants may be encumbered with restrictions that limit clinical and other activities, while not fully covering the faculty member's actual salary. In that circumstance, the department or institution may be required to support the junior faculty member—again in most cases from clinical revenues.

Even for many seasoned researchers, due to capping of NIH and other government grants, the support provided may not cover the related departmental expenses. In the absence of some agreement with the institution, the department bears the incremental salary costs. Some departments have nonphysician researchers on faculty, whose salaries, especially in the early years, do not meet the salary cap. However, when such faculty lose external support, they cannot make up the lost funding by being reassigned to clinical duties. There are additional costs of a research program that cannot be built into the grant award, including:

- Support staff to develop and submit grant applications
- Financial grant specialists to develop budgets with the research faculty
- Individuals maintaining relationships with the institution's office of research administration to manage grant submission
- Additional financial support to monitor budget performance in the post award period

Most grants have two components: direct costs and indirect costs (**Table 89.2**). A department with a small research portfolio is unlikely to have indirect costs returned to the department, though this may be negotiable. When there is no return of indirect costs to the department, the department bears the added expense of the administrative support required to maintain the research programs.

OTHER FINANCIAL CONSIDERATIONS

Many departments generate additional revenue through contracts, external consultation engagements, royalties from discovery or invention, and philanthropy. Commonly, members of the department and faculty contract to provide services outside of the institution. Emergency medicine faculty, for example, may provide medical direction services for local EMS providers or state agencies. The rise of telemedicine provides an avenue for financial growth for academic EDs, which are uniquely positioned to leverage this opportunity. If based on a cost plus basis, the contracted revenue includes the direct cost of the faculty or staff time plus an appropriate operating margin. Before contracting with external agencies, the department should fully understand the cost of each faculty or staff hour to ensure consistency in contracting and adequate financial return.

While a philanthropic revenue stream may be difficult to establish, endowment funding is increasingly common. The most common source of endowments for academic institution is the so-called grateful patient, however, that model may not be a significant source for EM since the relationships are so brief. Resident graduates, corporations, and donations from personal or business relationships are potential additional sources of philanthropic development. Development efforts are frequently supported by a central development office, but all development requires significant, dedicated effort from departmental leaders.

Faculty Composition and Salary Structure

Building a salary structure for academic faculty can be complex. The salary for each faculty member should be developed based upon the effort he or she places in each of the major mission categories: clinical, education, research, or administrative responsibilities. The value of each of those missions can be determined by departmental leaders. Some leaders consider the financial value of each mission to be equal, while others place a higher value on clinical operations.

Faculty compensation plans vary widely for academic EM practices. Compensation plans may be a simple, salary only model, in which the total salary is fixed. Alternatively, plans may include several components: base salary, bonus payments, compensation for extra clinical hours, and stipends (and bonuses) for administrative, educational, and research activities. Even the multifaceted compensation plans typically include a substantial base salary component (e.g., 85% of total salary). Bonus payments are commonly based upon clinical productivity since clinical revenue is the primary source of income.

Budget

The budget is a planning tool that, once developed, provides a way to measure productivity in each of the three areas of the academic practice. Each and every expense added to the operating budget should be carefully reviewed to ensure it meets at least one of the following criteria, and if not, then considered for removal:

- Is it necessary?
- Does it contribute to the mission?
- Does it provide a positive return on investment?

Most of the expenses of a faculty practice are the salary and benefits of faculty and support staff, which might be as much as 80% or more of the operating budget. Usually coding and billing costs are the next largest expenses. Supplies, office management, supplemental staffing, and other overhead expenses are relatively small compared to salary and billing expenses and so optimizing staffing, salary, and billing operations is key to financial success.

CONCLUSION

A successful academic department requires the creation of a thoughtfully considered program that fully addresses the triple mission of clinical service, research, and teaching. Accomplishing these three critical compnents of the academic mission requires a thorough understanding of the budget, both expenses and revenues, and deep involvement in the insitution's leadership.

Planning and implementation entail collaboration at all levels of the institution, including but not limited to the organization's C-suite leaders (CEO, COO, CFO, mission leaders). It is imperative that ED leaders to work closely with other academic leaders to ensure a cooperative educational environment that provides opportunity for all trainees. And finally, funded requires significant investment of human and financial resources and often is significantly enhanced by cross-divisional cooperation and sharing of resources.

REFERENCES

1. Adams H. Chapter 20: Failure. In: *The Education of Henry Adams: An Autobiography*. New York, NY: Modern Library (Random House); 1996.
2. ACGME.com. Common program requirements. Available at: https://www.acgme.org/What-We-Do/Accreditation/Common-Program-Requirements. Updated 2020. Accessed December 12, 2020.
3. ABEM.org. Subspecialties. Available at: https://www.abem.org/public/become-certified/subspecialties. Updated 2020. Accessed December 12, 2020.
4. ABEM.org. Advanced EM ultrasonography. Available at: https://www.abem.org/public/become-certified/focused-practice-designation/advanced-em-ultrasonography. Updated 2020. Accessed December 12, 2020.

CHAPTER 90

FINANCIAL PLANNING FOR INDIVIDUALS

A. Michael B. Kelen, Gabor D. Kelen

Unlike medical practice, which is based on scientific evidence and clinical experience, financial planning is an inexact science at best. While professional education curricula and credentialing standards exist, there are no practice requirements and few restrictions that define who can present themselves as a professional financial planner or advisor.

Financial planning is widely accepted to have been established around 1969. A Certified Financial Planner (CFP) curriculum was first established in 1971, and the first class graduated in 1973.[1] Prior to that time, financial advice was primarily provided by insurance agents, stockbrokers, and sometimes bankers.[2] While these niche professionals continue to provide all-inclusive advice, the authors do not recommend relying on those experts for comprehensive counsel.

Please note that this chapter is not a substitute for competent, compatible professional advice. The authors do not recommend relying solely on "self-help" sources, which would be comparable to relying on web-based materials for health guidance. However, as in medicine, there frequently exists more than one valid approach to financial planning. Further, compared to the general population, financial planning concerns and financial challenges differ for most health-care personnel, particularly physicians.

FINANCIAL PLANNING PROCESS

The following process is considered standard comportment for professionals by the CFP Board of Standards (**Table 90.1**).[3,4]

- *Steps 1 and 2: Identifying detailed qualitative and quantitative information.* Qualitative information includes, for example, current lifestyle, desired lifestyle, risk tolerance, investment and savings philosophy, and cultural and family influences. Quantitative information includes detailed assets and liabilities, contractual and business relationships and obligations, amount and types of insurance, type and reliability employment benefits, and so on.

  While many planners use a template, relying on this process exclusively is of little benefit over the many reasonable templated plans offered by banks and other financial firms. A detailed interview by a financial planner, including a review of the template, is essential. For example, an individual may designate his or her risk tolerance as "moderate" based on the templated definition. However, close questioning may reveal that the quick and sometimes superficially considered answer is inaccurate, and the individual actually prefers riskier or more conservative strategies. If the prospective advisor does not dig deeper into the investor's psychology, short- and long-term goals, and so on, alternate guidance should be sought.

- *Step 3: Setting goals.* A competent advisor assesses a client's stated goals in terms of real-life circumstances. Sometimes the expressed goals are unrealistic or require aggressive risk. A discerning planner should be able to point out potentially important goals not currently considered by the client. An example might be failure to consider disability or long-term care costs. The potential client should be wary of planners that move quickly through this step or offer little coaching in goal development, affirmation, or new considerations.
- *Step 4: Developing the plan.* Plan development is typically hidden from the client, though it is reasonable to inquire about the advisor's methodology during an initial consult. Spontaneous analysis conducted in front of a client is generally considered a red flag. Most planners will use some form of software, some more rigorous and reliable than others, so it is appropriate to discuss the type of software being used. Evasive answers should be suspect. Good planners will also undertake "stress testing" (similar to outcomes sensitivity analysis in medical science) to evaluate the range of possible outcomes of potential recommendations. The planners should be able to describe the limitations of their approach as well as the advantages.
- *Step 5: Presenting the plan.* This is usually the first opportunity to learn the advisor's assessment. Because most clients cannot immediately digest all the information in the plan, written documentation (including an executive summary) should accompany the presentation. The onus is on the client to read the plan fully to ensure that the assumptions as well as current and likely future circumstances have all been accurately addressed. Clients should further consider whether the recommendations are compatible with their expressed goals.

   The client should also ascertain whether the plan is comprehensive or a series of independent suggestions. Strong plans consider the likelihood and impact on the projected results if various conditions are not met, recommendations are not followed, or unexpected circumstances occur. Tax implications should be particularly discussed. Finally, all recommendations should describe possible negative outcomes. A rational assessment of risk should be contained in the plan and possible corrective actions or mitigating strategies outlined.
- *Steps 6 and 7: Implementing and monitoring the plan.* Highly client-dependent, these last two steps are best accomplished with the active assistance of the client.

TABLE 90.1 ■ Developing a Financial Plan	
Step 1	Understand the client's personal and financial circumstances.
Step 2	Determine current circumstances by collecting pertinent data and evaluating potential goals.
Step 3	Analyze the client's current course of action and impact of potential alternative strategies.
Step 4	Develop financial planning recommendations.
Step 5	Present the financial planning recommendations in a manner understandable to the individual client.
Step 6	Help the client implement the financial planning recommendations as may be required and to the degree such assistance is accepted.
Step 7	Monitor progress as defined under the relationship, and update the plan as career and circumstances change.

FINANCIAL ADVISORS

Planners may assist their clients by securing or recommending additional professionals to review and support the plan, including a tax advisor, a chartered public accountant (CPA), an insurance agent, investment specialists, legal advisors, and contracts or real estate planning advisors. Full-service advisors have the capacity to implement or otherwise arrange many, or even all, of the strategies. Some activities (such as drafting of wills) require significant effort and consideration by the client. It should be clear who is responsible for implementation of the various aspects of the plan as well as who is to monitor it and associated fees and commissions. The milestones expected over defined periods of time should also be clear. Agreements and contracts often dictate these terms.

Credentials

The financial advice industry is largely unregulated. According to the Financial Industry Regulatory Authority, there are 190 titled professional designations and several self-designated titles.[5] There are more than 1 million practitioners in the United States.[6] While some categories are highly specialized (e.g., National Social Security Advisor), a title alone does not confer competence and is not an indication of appropriate training.[7] Widely accepted qualifications to provide comprehensive financial planning are:

- Certified Financial Planner
- Chartered Financial Analyst (CFA)
- CPA with additional Personal Financial Specialist (PFS) credential

The CFA credential requires completion of a rigorous curriculum that includes both planning and investment management; it is considered by many to be the premier and most-desired credential. The CFP is the most widely established credential related to financial planning.

Many individuals rely solely on CPAs for all financial advice. CPA is a designation indicating training and proficiency in accounting and taxes. A skilled CPA is important to most physicians and senior administrators for tax planning and preparation. However, without further training and certification, CPAs are generally not recommended for comprehensive financial planning.

For more comprehensive advice, CPAs with PFS credentials could be considered. Personal Financial Specialists are required to possess expertise in estate, retirement, and insurance planning (respectively) in addition to other aspects of financial planning. In addition to CFP, CFA, and PFS, there are other credentials that imply quality training, but it is prudent to seek advice from a professional with one of these three designations. The American Association of Retired Persons has highlighted several credentials geared specifically to the older population; however, these "senior"-oriented designations may often be gratuitous.[8] For most seniors and retired professionals, an advisory with a CFP is appropriate.

Advisors with reputable credentials must abide by standards and codes of ethics.[3,4] They disclose to their clients conflicts of interest, particularly those related to financial products, referrals, and compensation they may receive for various recommendations. Potential clients should avoid any advisor who appears guarded when discussing possible conflicts or associations.

Planner associations may range from employment in a large financial firm to independent sole practitioners. Pros and cons are noted in **Table 90.2.** Many large banks, brokers, insurance companies, and other investment firms have in-house financial planning services. Offerings and fee structures vary significantly.

TABLE 90.2 ■ Pros and Cons of Advisor Organizations		
Firms	**Pros**	**Cons**
Large	Well-resourced with potential for more sophisticated analysis Additional specialist advisors Smooth advisor succession	Potentially higher fee structure Less individual customization May rely on proprietary software In-house investment services or products may create conflicts of interest
Wirehouse **Broker/dealer** **Insurance** **Bank** **Wealth management**	Generally, similar to large firms	Advisors may work for the firm (not client) with possible pressure to steer toward firm investments and products Advisors may be incentivized or bonused based on products/services sold
Small or solo	Likely to cater to individual needs May specialize in niche area (e.g., physicians) Low advisor turnover Advisors less likely to focus on company advancement Seldom tied to specific services/product advice	May not survive major financial downturn or setback Arrangement with products and service may not be apparent (although such relations should be ethically disclosed)

Fee Arrangements

Financial arrangements vary widely within the three most common fee structures.

- Asset-based fees dominate at 58% of industry advisor fees.
- Flat fixed fees are increasing and currently are charged by 36% of industry advisors.[9] However, millennial-aged advisors—those born in the 1980s to 1990s—are more likely to opt for a fixed fee structure.[9]
- Commission-based and hourly fees are charged by a small proportion of advisors.

The advantage to assets-under-management-based fees is the alignment of incentives when the accumulation or preservation of wealth is the goal. However, there is a conflict of interest if the advisor suggests assets are to be managed within the firm, as pressure to include all or most assets will increase the fee. Alternatively, to counter and keep fees lower, the client may be incentivized to hold back assets under management, compromising a comprehensive approach.

Flat-fee arrangements (or even advice charged by the hour) mitigate some of these disadvantages but may dampen the advisor's vested interest in attaining best outcomes. Hourly arrangements have similar disadvantages to flat-fee contracts, with the added issue of the manager working at a less-efficient pace to increase the time charged. While the above arrangements are reasonable for most individuals, the standard commission-based advice is not recommended. Bias is almost unavoidable. It is most important is that the advisor is transparent and openly discloses conflicts of interest.

FINANCIAL PLANNING DOMAINS

Financial planning concerns three related domains: wealth accumulation, wealth protection, and wealth succession. Within those domains, the major issues for consideration include cash flow, budgeting, risk management and insurance, employee (including self-employment) benefit planning, investment/savings planning, tax planning, retirement planning, estate planning, business planning (if applicable), and education planning. Several of these topics are discussed here, though others are beyond the scope of this chapter. There also may be special issues for some (e.g., same-sex partnerships, special-needs dependents). A comprehensive approach must be developed for each individual, as these issues are interrelated and the strength of planning may depend on an otherwise inapparent "weakest link."

Cash Flow

Most planning starts with an understanding of personal cash flow and a current balance sheet. According to a recent American Medical Association survey, 71% of resident physicians have medical school debt; 80% of those have debts of at least $100,000 and 50% of $200,000 or more.[10] Handling debt of this magnitude, while setting realistic future financial goals, can only occur with a full understanding of cash flow.

In its simplest form, cash flow involves defining all income and annual expenses, including current liabilities due (payable in the next 12 months). Cash flow should reflect realized income (inflow) and actual spending (outflow). Notably, cash flow analysis differs from budgeting, which addresses planned inflows and expenditures.

One starts with a current assessment (aggregation) of cash inflow and outflow and then projects that data into the future (*pro forma* cash flows). Expenses can be assessed from bank and credit card statements, paycheck deductions, loan interest statements, and tax returns. One-time large rare expenses are generally not considered unless there are frequent similar expenses. Income and revenues are assessed from W-2 form submissions and other income statements from banks and broker brokerage statements, alimony, trusts, and so on. Utilizing gross earnings and revenues minus related expenses (including taxes) makes it easier to project into the future.

Negative Cash Flow

A negative cash flow is not sustainable for the long term but may be appropriate during training and education, given the potential for very positive margins in future professional years. Nonetheless, even small degrees of negative cash flow during training incur debt or deplete assets. It is appropriate, therefore, to maintain a modest lifestyle during training. Large debt acquired later during high-earning professional years typically does not impact important lifestyle choices, compared to the ability to generate only small positive changes in cash flow during the lean education years.

Assets and Liabilities

Cash-flow analysis paves the way for wealth accumulation. However, there should also be an assessment of *current* wealth (the balance of assets and liabilities). Constructing a balance sheet allows useful insights into potential risks, such as overconcentration in a single investment or clarity regarding degree of debt versus assets. Assets are generally divided into liquid assets and illiquid and hard assets.

- *Liquid assets* are those that can readily be converted to cash. They include checking, savings, stocks, mutual funds, and retirement assets such as 403(b), IRA, and 401(k).
- *Illiquid and hard assets* may have value but are not readily converted to cash. These include assets such as cars, real estate, furniture, and collectibles/art.
- *Liabilities* include debt principal of any kind, such as mortgages, credit cards, and student and other loans.

Useful Planning Formulas

Some useful ratios for planning purposes include liquidity ratio, debt-to-asset ratio, and debt-to-income ratio.

- *Liquidity ratio* is used to help assess capacity to repay debt or support current expenses.

$$\text{Liquidity ratio} = \frac{\text{Liquid assets}}{\text{Current liabilities}}$$

- For example, an individual with $25,000 of liquid assets and debt payments of $75,000 for the upcoming year would have a liquidity ratio of 0.33, implying that current assets-on-hand alone only cover about 4 months of debt expenses. This concept is particularly important if there is potential for job insecurity and/or disability without insurance.
- For those carrying debt, the typical minimally desirable ratio (liquid assets over liabilities) is between 1 and 2.* However, other factors may influence the acceptable ratio—such as training status of potential high earners.[11]
- *Total debt-to-asset ratio* is another useful relationship. Although generally applicable to company balance sheets, it is often useful for individual households. This ratio provides insight into the percent of assets leveraged by debt.

$$\text{Debt-to-asset ratio} = \frac{\text{Short-term debt} + \text{Long-term debt}}{\text{Total assets}}$$

There are different opinions as to what is an acceptable ratio. Obviously, a ratio of debt over assets >1 is generally undesirable unless the future cash flow and liquidity ratio is expected to be high.[12]

- *Debt-to-income ratio* may be more meaningful for professionals who typically start their careers with limited assets. This ratio influences strategies for managing cash flow and paying off liabilities.

$$\text{Debt-to-income ratio} = \frac{\text{Total debt}}{\text{Total (household) income}^\dagger}$$

- Clearly, a high ratio of debt-to-income is undesirable. Yet, the average ratio for medical and surgical residents is 2.5 versus 0.6 for the general public.[12,13] The ideal ratio is unclear. However, in one study, 80% of urology resident trainees with a ratio of 2.38% were significantly concerned about the ability to manage their finances.[13] For resident/fellow trainees who expect to manage current debt burden with future prospects, even small short-term life events could have major ramifications, if current *debt-to-income ratio* (as well as the other ratios) are unfavorable.

---

*Although a complex subject, a ratio well above 2 may imply inefficient asset allocation. However, many individuals psychologically and behaviorally eschew debt altogether and hence the ratio may be factitiously high independent of asset allocation.

†Yearly income.

Debt Management

Once current and prospective cash flow is assessed, debt management becomes an important consideration to improve net cash flow. High debt levels are a major problem for medical professionals, especially early in their careers. While there are many ways to address debt, consideration is complex and necessarily must address each individual's specific situation. As such, specific methodologies are beyond the scope of this chapter.

"Good Debt" and "Bad Debt"

Debt can be considered as "good debt" and "bad debt." A 0% (or minimal) annual percentage rate car loan is considered good debt even though there are monthly obligations. Carrying charges of 18% to 24% or more on credit cards is clearly "bad debt." As a rule, it is a priority for individuals to aggressively dispose of high-interest debt, sometimes by conversion to a lower interest rate debt. Despite being highly illogical, many people focus their debt reduction on the largest monthly payment loans (e.g., student loans or a mortgage) rather than prioritizing their repayments on the highest interest rate debts. It is generally more beneficial to pay off high-interest debt before allocating funds toward lower interest rate savings, even if designated for retirement.

Debt Service Options

Some "debt service" options exist specifically for physicians and new graduates. The Association of American Medical Colleges offers many programs. Loan consolidation to achieve a net lower interest rate may be a helpful strategy. However, if debt is amortized over a longer period of time, it usually results in larger total interest outlays. Nonetheless, lower payments over a longer period may be a good option for those with strong prospects.

Other options include private loans, second mortgages, home equity loans, and even 401(k)/403(b) loans, which may improve overall cash flow position or help mitigate interest charges. Borrowing against the cash value of whole life or universal life insurance policies may be useful only for older policies that have built cash value in the early years.

There are consequences to consolidation or refinancing student debt with private institutions. The refinancing may jeopardize eligibility for public forgiveness programs and income tax benefits. This and each of the listed approaches should be discussed with a dispassionate financial specialist.

Individuals new to medical practice or residency may be eligible for public loan forgiveness after 120 qualifying payments while working full time for a qualified employer (government or nonprofit).[14] Finally, young physicians may also consider income-driven plans that match loan payments to income level and family size.[15] Given that the options are complex, professional consultation is necessary.

RISK MANAGEMENT AND INSURANCE

Risk management and insurance primarily deal with wealth protection. Typical areas of risk include personal property, personal liability, personal illness, sickness or death, financial capital assets, and human capital risks (the latter an intangible asset typically defined as future expected income or economic benefit) such as employment. All of these areas should be thoughtfully considered, even if the decision is inevitably not to insure against a specific risk.

There are four basic approaches to managing risk: avoiding, retaining, controlling/mitigating, and transferring to another party. To determine appropriate action, the individual must understand his or her risk tolerance for loss, the likelihood the loss event will occur, and the duration that the loss is bearable. (The psychology of risk is too complex for a discussion here, but it should be acknowledged that it is an important contributor to risk behavior. Further, many studies have concluded that people violate their own "rational thinking" when confronting risk.[11])

Not every risk is transferable (i.e., insurable), and not all risks should be insured. Individuals typically retain (do not insure for) low-impact financial risks (e.g., extended warrantees on low-cost purchases). Risks with high frequency and significant loss potential should typically be avoided (e.g., owning property in an uninsurable flood plain). Low-frequency risks associated with high losses (e.g., a house fire or malpractice suit) is typically transferred through insurance.[16]

Disability Insurance

Human capital, the economic value of professional skill and experience, is a risk area typically transferred via insurance. It is the projected economic value of one's life, typically defined as future earnings potential. Early in a career, a professional's human capital is quite high. The risk of human capital loss due to disability is typically covered by a disability insurance policy. Ironically, many high-income earners readily insure their lives, homes, cars, and other assets that may be worth a fraction of their human capital but ignore disability insurance. For physicians and senior administrators, this earnings potential may be valued at millions of dollars. For early career doctors and professionals, disability insurance may very well be the most important insurance.

Recent studies indicate that 20-year-old men and women have more than a 25% likelihood of developing at least a year-long disability before age 67. By comparison, the odds of dying without being disabled over that time period is 8.0% for men and 4.2% for women.[17] The likelihood of disability versus death is several-fold higher at all stages of the professional working years. Yet, many people purchase (often an inadequate amount of) life insurance before first considering insuring against disability, despite the significantly lower risk. Interestingly, doctors do disproportionately buy more disability insurance than other professionals; they are also more likely to make a claim.[18]

Group and Private Disability Insurance

Disability insurance products vary. They include two major types: group policies, which are usually offered by an employer or association, and private policies, which are purchased by individuals.

It is important to be aware that the definition of disability varies by insurance carrier. These policies require scrutiny, especially the group products, because they are not designed with the individual in mind. Group policies are typically offered in employee benefits packages. While eligibility is often easier than requirements for private policies, the ability to customize the group policy is highly limited or nonexistent. Group policies are rarely if ever are transportable when changing employers. The later in life a policy change is made, the harder and more expensive it is to acquire a private policy.

In contrast, most private insurance policies are portable. They should be strongly considered even if an employer provides group coverage options.

Short-Term and Long-Term Disability

Disability policies are typically offered in two forms, *short term* and *long term*. Elements of all policies are listed in **Box 90.1**.

Though more expensive, some policies cover "own occupation" rather than "any occupation." The term "any occupation" refers to situations in which the disability inhibits the disabled from working or seeking gainful employment in any occupation. "Own occupation" refers to a disability preventing engagement in the specific regular occupation.[16] For

> **BOX 90.1 ■ COMMON ELEMENTS OF DISABILITY POLICIES**
>
> - Definition of disability
> - Coverage amount (usually percentage of maximum offered)
> - Eligibility period to begin payments
> - Duration of coverage
> - Partial disability coverage (if offered)
> - Premium amounts
> - Riders (amendments under certain circumstances)

professionals such as physicians, it is generally prudent to consider "own occupation" policies, otherwise there is risk the insurers may deny aspects of coverage if they judge the individual could be employed in some other related work (e.g., claims review or even short-order cook). There are further subtleties for "own occupation," particularly relating to specialty care and the clinical practice setting. Because "own occupation" policies generate payments to a clinician who might still be able to earn a significant salary in another occupation, it is not surprising that "own occupation" policies are associated with higher premium costs.

Short-term disability typically covers events of 6 months or less, but some short-term policies may extend benefits up to two years. A short-term policy also may have a much shorter waiting period, sometimes involving one or two weeks or no waiting period at all. In contrast, long-term disability typically begins paying benefits only after a 6-month waiting period and benefit durations can vary from a few years or through retirement age (age 65 or 67 for most policies). Both types of policies typically cover only 60% to 70% of salary. If premiums are paid on a pre-tax basis (like many group plans), then benefits are usually taxable. Premiums paid on an after-tax basis are usually received free of federal income tax.

Partial disability benefits should also be considered. Generally, partial disability benefits will pay a portion of the benefits in the event that not all aspects of the job requirements can be fulfilled.

Life Insurance

Life insurance allows the financial risks associated with death—a low probability but high consequence event—to be transferred to a third party. Life insurance vehicles can be complex, with tax, investment, and savings implications, and cannot be fully covered here. However, because some advisors champion the benefits over the intended purpose, it is important here to focus on actual life insurance needs.

Calculation of Needs Methodologies

Life insurance needs can be considered in two ways. First to consider is "human life value," which is basically the present value of future expected income that dependents would require for support (until those dependents are self-sufficient, if ever). In simple terms, a 35-year-old doctor clearing $175,000 per year in earnings with an expectation of a 30-year career (unadjusted for inflation or promotion) has a projected "life value" of $5.25 million.

The second to consider is a "financial needs analysis," which is a more common way to consider life insurance needs. This calculation computes the requirements of all immediate and ongoing income needs of dependents projected for a given duration. Current family assets and liabilities are also considered. The financial needs approach factors in additional assumptions like investment interest, surviving dependents' life expectancy, and tax and inflation projections.

By taking actual needs into consideration, the financial analysis more closely reflects an individual's actual support requirements. Clearly, the simplistic method of setting a current income target and multiplying it by five years lacks nuance and necessary due diligence. While it is not necessary to buy coverage for the full potential risk, some professionals underinsure by failing to calculate the future value of the insured amount. Further complicating the calculation, life insurance needs may decrease substantially over time as dependents (such as children) become self-sufficient, and retirement and other savings accounts become increasingly accessible.

Term vs Permanent

Life insurance comes in two major forms: term insurance and permanent insurance. There is considerable controversy regarding the best form of insurance for an individual. Some insurance agents may be biased toward which compensates them the best. Competent advice from a dispassionate professional is essential. As with disability insurance, both group and individual policies are available.

Term life insurance provides a defined death benefit during a limited coverage period. It usually requires significantly lower premiums for a given level of coverage. There are many variations, but typically, premiums are fixed for a period (5, 10, or 20 years, and in some cases, longer). Upon expiration, the policyholder may simply allow the policy to terminate or in many cases have the option to renew. Even if the contract has no age limit, premiums tend to increase dramatically at each renewal period eventually rendering the coverage impractical and unaffordable.

Term life insurance has the advantage of being significantly less expensive and is generally advised for a relatively defined period in one's life, ensuring that dependents are adequately covered. Its major drawback relates to potential opportunity costs, such as no cash value or savings (associated with permanent insurance). The premiums are calculated based on actuarial tables that consider age, health, and life expectancy. Once discontinued, it can be difficult and expensive to acquire a new private policy because morbidity and mortality increase as one ages. Some term policies can be converted into permanent life insurance.

Permanent life insurance policies do not expire and are generally offered in two primary forms: whole life and universal life. For simplicity, such policies, once purchased, are in effect for one's entire lifetime. Assuming the policy is properly funded and premiums are fully paid in accordance with a prescribed schedule, the policy remains in effect and cannot be cancelled. Permanent insurance always requires higher premiums than term insurance. The disadvantage is that high upfront costs can be difficult to bear early in one's career. This may be less of an issue for specialties like emergency medicine, in which incomes are at near-peak levels when entering upon graduation.

There are several advantages of permanent over term insurance:

- Permanent insurance is a form of a slow growth (forced) savings account (albeit with some steep initial fees), because the policy has a cash value (premiums paid, less expense charges) that act as deferred tax over time.
- Most new policies allow the owner to access a proportion of the death benefit while alive, which is useful if funds are needed (such as for coverage of illness).
- A policyholder can borrow against the cash value of the policy, essentially as a line of credit on the accrued policy value. Principal and interest are generally paid back by the owner into the policy itself. The death benefit remains even if the cash value is drawn down to the minimum specified by the policy.

Property and Liability

Risks associated with property and liability are also frequently covered by (transferred to) an insurance product. Low-risk but consequential events (a housefire, for example) should be considered for insurance coverage if the impact of the loss is not readily absorbable. Home ownership is the most important component of wealth for most professional Americans. Many homeowners do not fully insure their houses and the contents for "replacement value" or catalog valuable contents and furniture (very easy to do digitally). General policies usually have limits on specific items such as jewelry and art collections.

Homeowner policies should be carefully considered to ensure adequate coverage of property and liability, which are hallmarks of a stable financial plan. In a litigious society, high-wage earner liability coverage related to home events is practically a "must have." It is often offered as an inexpensive policy rider.

Terms and Conditions

The potential policyholder should be aware of several terms and conditions:

- *Perils* relate to the cause of loss in two forms. Named perils cover a specified list of possible covered hazards (fire, storm damage, etc.). Most policies also list specifically excluded perils.
- *Limits* specify the policy's maximum payable for losses. Limits are specified for the entire policy as well as for specific subclassifications, such as jewelry or computers.
- *Loss valuation*, often underappreciated, is either considered as the current cash value of property at the time of the loss or actual replacement cost.
- *Duties of the insured* are often specified to ensure problem-free case settlements. These duties may include keeping receipts of large purchases, recording model and serial numbers, and photo or video evidence of covered possessions—preserved apart from the hazard.

Physicians and other high-income-earning professionals should consider pairing their home and auto insurance in an umbrella liability policy, relatively inexpensive additions. Umbrella policies help cover catastrophic legal claims that stem from personal liability and for which most home and auto policies have inadequate coverage. Typically, policies are issued for a minimum policy limit of $1 million but may be up to $10 million. (These are unrelated to professional malpractice insurance). Such policies are second in line for payouts and are typically relatively inexpensive.

Malpractice-Professional Liability Insurance

Finally, practicing physicians require professional liability (malpractice) insurance (covered in more detail in Chapters 111 and 113). Malpractice insurance is often provided by a hiring entity and, as a result, the provider may have minimal input into the specific coverage. However, this fact does not obviate the need to understand the policy and its ramifications, including the answers to such questions as: Does the policy provide adequate insurance coverage? What are the specific responsibilities of the insured, including reporting? Who is responsible for "tail" coverage, if any? Is there a "consent clause" for settlement?

Claims-Made Policies

Claims-made policies cover claims and incidents only while the policy is in effect (premiums are being paid). Since most claims are made some time after the care is provided, this can become a problem if the claim is filed when the provider is no longer covered by the original policy. The remedy is the purchase of "nose" or "tail" coverage. Nose (prior acts) coverage extends coverage by the new insurer to a claim arising out of care provided while insured by the previous insurer. Tail (extended reporting) coverage essentially continues (extends) the old policy coverage for incidents that occurred during the time premiums were paid and coverage was in place. Tail coverage can be quite costly.

Occurrence Policies

Occurrence policies are generally preferred because they cover all incidents that happen while the policy is in effect, even if the policy no longer covers the provider (e.g., the provider has retired, changed practice, or has a new insurer). Such policies do not require "tails." Of paramount importance to all insurance malpractice policies is the "consent to settle clause." Insurers make decisions based on cost–benefit analysis and may determine that settlement is the best option. It is important to be aware of and understand the various contract clauses.

EMPLOYEE BENEFITS

There is evidence that many employees (if not most) do not appreciate their benefits. Research suggests that fewer than 50% understand their benefits and almost a third do not recognize the value of their benefits. Surprisingly, 80% do not read their benefit materials.[19]

Typical benefit choices include health care, employee retirement options, disability insurance, life insurance, ancillary savings vehicles such as a health savings account (HSA) and a flexible spending account (FSA), and deferred compensation. Some benefit packages include dependent college tuition programs, dental and eye care coverage, tuition remission, and access to legal advice, among others. A few may even offer mortgage assistance and loan repayment programs. Employers may offer or have specific policies concerning sick leave policy, parental leave, dependent care, and in a few cases company stock options, if applicable.

Retirement Plans

Retirement plans are often the cornerstone of effective financial planning. Employer-offered retirement pension benefits fall into two categories: the defined benefit plan (DBP) and the defined contribution plan (DCP). The DBP, or traditional pension plan, is rarely available to practicing physicians and is increasingly disappearing from the employment landscape due to unpredictable costs to the employer.

Deferred Contribution Plans

Due to the short sightedness of a large majority of the working population, the government incentivizes people to save via DCPs. These incentives come largely in the form of tax benefits and forced savings. Defined contribution plan contributions are funded with pre-tax dollars regardless of the source (employer or employee contributions), allowing accrual of positive returns. Defined contribution plans do have deferred tax implications, when funds are withdrawn.

For most employees, employer retirement plans are named 403(b) for nonprofit organizations and 401(k) for-profit enterprises. Some workplaces may also sponsor a 457/457(b) deferred compensation plan in lieu of or in addition to a 401(k)/403(b) plan. The 457/457(b) plans work similarly to 401(k)/403(b) plans but are usually only available to high-wage earners due to the limits imposed on the 401(k)/403(b) plans. In most plans, the employee can make tax-deferred contributions up to an IRS-specified limit ($19,500 in 2020 for both 401(k) and 403(b) plans). If the employee is older than 50, the government permits a catch-up incremental allowance of up to $6,500 (as of 2020). Employers may also contribute either as a percent of salary or a matching contribution up to a certain limit. The employer portion is not considered part of the employee-opted deferral limit. The combined contributions cannot exceed 100% of compensation or $56,000 if under 50 years of age and $62,000 if older than 50.[20]

Unfortunately, many employed physicians do not take advantage of either pre-tax contributions or other tax-deferred advantages. In some cases, individuals wittingly or unwittingly forgo the employer matching contributions as well. It is wise to take advantage of the full individual contribution allowed, unless an individual foresees being in a much higher tax bracket during retirement when (minimum) withdrawals must be taken.

Defined contribution plans are not without risk. The employee usually is given several options of investment vehicles from very safe to highly risky mutual funds. Unless the individual is shrewd at investing (rarely the case), outside professional investment advice as part of the financial planning is advised.

Roth IRAs

Individuals may also be eligible for Roth Individual Retirement Account (IRA) style plans if income does not exceed certain limits. Roth IRA plans are funded with after-tax dollars, but the realized capital gains and interest are tax deferred. Also, for "qualified" withdrawals, neither original contributions nor gains on investments are taxable. Roth 401(k)/403(b) plans exist as well, but unlike Roth IRAs, income limits do not apply, thus making higher income earners eligible if their employer sponsors one of these plans. The Roth IRAs and Roth 401(k) plans have the same contribution limits per year as their traditional counterparts.

A popular misconception is that one type of DCP format (pre-tax vs post-tax funded) is inherently better than the other for accumulating assets. However, the only important factor to consider is the tax rate at the time of contribution versus the likely tax rate when funds are withdrawn. For example:

> *An individual contributes the maximum allowed to either a 401(k)/403(b) or a Roth IRA. Assume a steady growth of assets at 7.2% for 20 years for a given year's contribution. If the top tax rate (or effective tax rate) for the individual is the same at the beginning and end of the 20 years, there is no difference in the actual accrual (**Table 90.3**).*

TABLE 90.3 ■ **Pre-tax 401(k) or 403(b) vs Post-tax (Roth IRA) Plans**

Assumptions		401(k) or 403(b)	Comment	Roth IRA	Comment
Initial available funds for contribution	$18 500	$19,000		$19,000	
Top tax rate at time of contribution	35%	35%		35%	
Initial investment considering tax rate		$19,000	All pre-tax contributions	$12,350	Post-tax contribution at top tax rate
Interest rate	7.2%	7.2%		7.2%	
Term (years)	20	20		20	
Compounding periods (per year)	12	12		12	
Future value after term		$79,849		$51,902	
Tax on accrued value at future projected rate	35%	$27,947		No tax	No tax on accrual
Total post-tax value		$51,902		$51,902	

The federal government set up the Roth IRA to ensure that they (the government) ultimately receive the same taxes in either case. The Roth DCP makes some sense for younger professionals who pay a higher tax rate at the time of retirement. Older professionals would likely prefer the 401(k)/403(b) plan because they are more likely to be at their top tax bracket at the time of contributions versus retirement. Of course, there are many other factors regarding tax rates over a multiple decade period.

Caveats

There are some caveats regarding these retirement plans when compared to no contribution at all. If retirement plan funds are accessed prior to age 59½, a tax penalty usually applies (currently 10% penalty is applied to withdrawals) in addition to the requirement to pay income taxes on the withdrawn money. There are numerous exceptions and exigencies where the penalty is waved, but those details are beyond this chapter's scope.[21]

The vast majority of employer plans have a predetermined lineup of mutual funds and other investment vehicles. The management fees related to these funds can be inherently more expensive than other investment options the individual may have otherwise chosen. Additionally, the retirement plan itself may come with further administrative fees taken from the value of the plan assets. Employees should communicate with the benefit administrator and request a summary plan description including any ancillary expense supplements.

Though a very complicated subject, self-employed individuals (e.g., contract physicians, owners of practices) who garner non-W-2 income are eligible to set up their own DCP. Expert advice should be sought to determine options that fit with the individual's financial plan and to set up these plans properly to avoid running afoul of tax and other regulatory organizations.

Health Insurance

One of the most important employee benefits is health care. The scope of the chapter precludes a detailed discussion and the law. Further, employer-offered plans change frequently and health insurance and related cost reimbursements can be a challenge even for the most well informed. Critical elements of these policies include deductibles, coinsurance and copay schedules, out-of-pocket maximum, covered versus uncovered expenses, and impact of out-of-network care.

Health Savings Accounts

Other possible benefits that may impact an employee's health-care costs are HSA, which have tax benefits both when elected and when used. Capital contributions to these accounts are tax deferred. If used for qualified medical expenses, withdrawals will be tax free. There are contribution limits, however. To be eligible as an HSA, the health insurance vehicle must be a high-deductible plan.[22] Health savings accounts are mobile, which means they are tied to the individual and not to the specific employer. The disadvantage of establishing an HSA is that withdrawals made for a nonqualified expense incur a 20% penalty.[22] However, the penalty may still be less than the top tax rate of the individual.

Flexible Spending Accounts

Flexible spending accounts are similar to HSAs, but generally the entire funded account must be spent in the calendar year, although some plans allow a small amount of unspent funds to be carried forward into the subsequent year, without exceeding the yearly allowed limit. Flexible spending accounts can be established only by an employer. Generally, both HSA and FSA vehicles cannot be simultaneously funded.

Finally, for most individuals, group policies will be less expensive than individually acquired policies, and eligibility requirements tend to be minimal for large group policies. However, a major disadvantage of employer-offered health plans is the lack of portability, which may force some individuals to stay in nonideal employment situations.

Investment/Savings

Although an investment and savings strategy is an important part of any sound financial plan, even the best-laid plans can fail if the topics described in this section go unaddressed. It is widely recommended that individuals develop and maintain a savings plan as early as possible due to the "magic" of compounded returns. Even small sums set aside early may accumulate into large sums over a 30- to 40-year horizon.

The most important part of saving and investing is determining how much readily accessible savings should be set aside for emergencies. Individuals should have the ability to withstand financial setbacks (such as job loss or unanticipated health spending) without liquidating major assets. Many financial planners advise keeping between three and 24 months' worth of cash on hand to cover basic expenses in the event of an unforeseen event.

Risk Tolerance

When emergency savings are considered secured and an investment strategy based on goals and needs is formed, it is necessary for every investor to determine their tolerance for risk.[23] Individuals who invest in portfolios that carry an uncomfortable level of risk will almost certainly abandon their initial strategy, often with highly negative financial results. For example, those heavily invested in US stocks during the 2007 to 2008 downturn likely saw their portfolio values decrease by around 40%. Many such people bailed on their investment strategy and switched to cash or bonds. Because of their aversion to risk, those investors missed the recovery, and their loses were permanent. Other investors, who tolerated the great uncertainty, generally recovered their assets within 18 to 24 months and continued to do quite well in the ensuing "bull market." In fact, virtually all pull-backs, recessions, and collapses recover (**Table 90.4**).[24] Most other recessions last an average of 11 months. Determining and staying with a comfortable strategy will avoid behavior traps that could result in irreparable financial damage.

Some professionals, including many doctors, perceive themselves as highly successful and self-dependent and may be overconfident about their investment acumen. However, most financial novices would do better with the help of a dispassionate professional or, alternatively, by simply keeping their assets in indexed mutual funds for the long term. Having assets managed by professionals is likely to keep psychological demons, overconfidence, and micromanagement at bay.

TABLE 90.4 ■ Time From Collapse to Recovery	
Collapse	**Time to Recovery**
Great Depression	7 years
1970s recession	3 years
Dotcom bubble	5 years
Great recession (recent)	2 years
Other recessions	11 months

Asset Allocation

When choosing a compatible advisor or manager, be aware that the allocation of assets is responsible for 90% of the asset performance.[25] For example, performance of a 60:40 stocks-to-bonds strategy versus an 80:20 strategy is more related to the asset allocation than it is to the manager's ability to pick investments within the strategy.

To determine the appropriate allocation of assets, consider some basic tenets: Stocks are inherently riskier than bonds, but they outperform bonds in the long run. Even relatively "safe" stocks are risker than investment-grade (low-risk) bonds, which can provide some cushion when stocks are stressed. And while international stocks are typically considered riskier than US stocks, many advisors suggest investing some portion of an individual's portfolio in international assets as a means of diversification.

Finally, investment strategies should be reassessed every three to five years to allow adjustment for current circumstances. For example, added risk might be assumed if an investor has a secure high salary, previous dependents are currently independent, and assets have grown significantly. On the other hand, as retirement nears, volatility is less tolerable and investments that pay dividends may be preferable.

CONCLUSION

Financial planning is an essential activity for virtually all individuals, regardless of occupation or station in life. Though it appears complicated, assessment and advice from competent, trained, certified specialists are recommended—for busy professionals, in particular. Financial planning is not a static process and requires cyclical reassessment. A properly drawn plan should match reality and the individual's and household's psychology. Such a plan properly executed will most likely result in realized goals and mitigation of financial challenges throughout one's life and career.

REFERENCES

1. Yeske DA. A concise history of the financial planning profession. *J Financial Planning*. 2016; 29(11):10–13.

2. Walker LJ. The profession of financial planning: past, present, and the next 45 years. *J Financial Planning*. 2018;31(3):20–26.

3. Financial planning practice standards. Certified Financial Planner (CFP) Board: The Standard of Excellence. 2020. Available at: https://www.cfp.net/. Accessed August 5, 2020.

4. Code of ethics and standards conduct. Certified Financial Planner (CFP) Board. 2020. Available at: https://www.cfp.net/ethics/code-of-ethics-and-standards-of-conduct. Accessed August 5, 2020.

5. Professional designations. Financial Industry Regulatory Authority (FINRA). Available at: https://www.finra.org/investors/professional-designations. Accessed January 11, 2020.

6. Raskie S, Martin J, Lemoine C, Cummings BF. The value of financial designations: a consumer perspective. *Social Science Research Network (SSRN)*. 2018.

7. Camarda J. Do designations improve financial advisory quality. *Social Science Research Network*. 2015.

8. Quinn JB. What financial advisor's credential mean: not all designations are the same—or a sign of quality. American Association of Retired Persons (AARP). Available at: https://www.aarp.org/money/investing/info-2014/what-financial-advisers-credentials-mean.html. Accessed January 11, 2020.

9. Britton D. Advisors' use of fixed planning fees on the rise. *Wealthmanagement.com*. 2018. Available at: https://www.wealthmanagement.com/industry/advisors-use-fixed-planning-fees-rise. Accessed January 11, 2020.

10. 2017 Report on U.S. physicians' financial preparedness. AMA Insurance Agency Inc. 2017. Available at: https://www.amainsure.com/research-reports/2017-financial-preparedness-resident-physicians/index.html?page=1. Accessed January 11, 2020.

11. Lemoine C. *Financial Planning Process and Environment*. 6th ed. The American College Press; 2016.

12. Tevis SM, Rodgers AP, Carchman EH, et al. Clinically competent and fiscally at risk: impact of debt and financial parameters on the surgical resident. *J Am Coll Surg*. 2018;227(2):163–171.e7.

13. Teichman JM, Bernheim DB, Espinosa EA, et al. How do urology residents manage personal finances? *Urol*. 2001;57(5):866–871.

14. National Council of Non-Profits, Public Service Loan Forgiveness. 2020. Available at: https://studentaid.gov/manage-loans/forgiveness-cancellation/public-service. Accessed August 3, 2020.

15. *2018–2019 Education Debt Manager for Matriculating and Graduating Medical School Students*. Publication No. 18-077 (07/18). Association of American Medical Colleges (AAMC). 2018. Available at: https://meded.hms.harvard.edu/files/hms-med-ed/files/aamc-2018-2019-education-debt-manager.pdf. Accessed January 11, 2020.

16. Lynch KM. *Fundamentals of Insurance Planning*. 6th ed. The American College Press; 2015.
17. Maleh J, Bosley T. *Disability and Death Probability Tables for Insured Workers Born in 1997*. Publication No. 2017.6. US Social Security Administration. 2017. Available at: https://www.ssa.gov/oact/NOTES/ran6/an2017-6.pdf. Accessed January 11, 2020.
18. Lieber R. The odds of a disability are themselves odd. *New York Times*. February 5, 2010: B1.
19. Employ benefits survey: 2018 survey results. International Foundation of Employee Benefit Plans. Available at: https://www.ifebp.org/store/employee-benefits-survey/Pages/default.aspx. Accessed January 12, 2020.
20. *Retirement Topics – 403(b) Contribution Limits*. US Internal Revenue Service. Available at: https://www.irs.gov/retirement-plans/plan-participant-employee/retirement-topics-403b-contribution-limits. Accessed January 12, 2020.
21. *Retirement Topics – Exceptions to Tax on Early Distributions*. US Internal Revenue Service. 2019. Available at: https://www.irs.gov/retirement-plans/plan-participant-employee/retirement-topics-tax-on-early-distributions. Accessed January 12, 2020.
22. Rosso RJ. *Health Savings Accounts (HSAs)*. Publication No. 7-5700. Congressional Research Service. 2018. Available at: https://fas.org/sgp/crs/misc/R45277.pdf. Accessed January 12, 2020.
23. Behavioral Finance, Individual Investors, and Institutional Investors. Level III, CFA Program Curriculum. Vol. 2. CFA Institute; 2011.
24. Egan M. Worried about a stock market crash? Read this. *CNN Business*. 2015. Available at: https://mcney.cnn.com/2015/02/26/investing/stock-market-crash-bubble-investing/index.html. Accessed January 12, 2020.
25. Ibbotson RG, Kaplan PD. Does asset allocation explain 40, 90, or 100 percent of performance. *Financial Analyst J*. 2000;56(1):26–33.

REIMBURSEMENT

SECTION 8

REIMBURSEMENT ISSUES

Michael A. Granovsky, David McKenzie

CHAPTER 91

Reimbursement describes the general process by which health-care providers are paid for the services they render. The term comes from the practice of rendering care before payment and then subsequently seeking reimbursement from an insurance company or the patients themselves. It is the reimbursement process that identifies the services provided, reports those services, and completes the billing and collection functions necessary to collect revenue. Without fair payment for services, the emergency department (ED) will not have the resources required to provide adequate patient care.

The reimbursement process must be well organized and executed to sustain organizational vitality, thereby ensuring access to quality emergency care for the surrounding community. In addition, payment must be sufficient to attract and retain high-quality physicians who are willing to work nights, weekends, and holidays. Reimbursement and payment must be adequate to attract staff who can sustain a reasonable lifestyle commensurate with their extensive training and must include repayment of the accumulated debt of training. Reimbursement will ultimately be adjusted for local and regional market forces.

The unscheduled, episodic nature of ED care requires a broader understanding of payment rules than most other medical specialties. Layered on top of that are numerous government regulations, not the least of which is the Emergency Medical Treatment and Active Labor Act (EMTALA), which requires EDs to screen and treat—at least until the point of stabilization—all patients who present, regardless of their ability or willingness to pay. Increased audit activity and the evolution of health-care reform further complicate the process. For these reasons, the reimbursement process for emergency medicine is perhaps the most challenging in the industry.

THE NUTS AND BOLTS OF REIMBURSEMENT

Consider the steps in the reimbursement process in detail (**Box 91.1**).

Providing the Medical Service

The reimbursement process begins with the provision of a medical service. All reported services must be medically necessary; performed by providers within the scope of their

---

BOX 91.1 ■ STEPS IN THE REIMBURSEMENT PROCESS

1. Provide the medical service.
2. Document the service.
3. Identify the service.
4. Code the care.
5. Bill (initial claim, appeals, accounts receivable [A/R], collections).
6. Ensure compliance (audits and training).

training and; depending on contractual conditions, a covered service eligible for payment. In the ED, the care usually begins with an evaluation and management (E/M) service to determine the diagnosis and appropriate treatment plan. This E/M service is reported according to the Current Procedural Terminology (CPT) codes 99281-99285 and 99291.

A single E/M code is chosen to represent the intensity of the clinical interaction. The specific history, physical examination, and medical decision-making criteria for each of the ED E/M codes are further discussed in Chapter 92. Separately, procedures (such as laceration repair or lumbar puncture) and diagnostic tests that are required to complete the patient's treatment are also reported as reimbursable events. Providing quality care should be the foremost concern of every emergency physician. However, an understanding of how to bill for and generate revenue for that care is also important.

Documenting the Services Provided

The medical record provides permanent documentation of the care provided, serves as the mechanism to guide future treatment, and justifies the medical necessity required for reimbursement. A well-documented chart may provide protection against potential malpractice claims. This discussion focuses on the requirement to record the medical encounter with a specificity that allows the accurate reporting of services for payment. For example, for reimbursement, laceration repairs require documentation of the anatomical location, length of the repair, mechanism of closure, and the number of layers or extent of undermining involved.

Components of Documentation

The patient's history, physical examination, and related medical decision-making determines the assignment of the ED E/M codes and thus payment for the services provided. Any interpretations of diagnostic tests must have a separately identifiable written report to justify and obtain payment. Documenting the exact nature of treatment for fractures or dislocations is vital. Ultimately, the E/M service, procedures performed, and diagnostic studies are individually listed when submitted for reimbursement.

Centers for Medicare and Medicaid Services

The Centers for Medicare and Medicaid Services (CMS) created the first set of documentation guidelines, which were implemented in 1995. Those guidelines further defined and set numerical thresholds for the components of patient history, physical examination, and medical decision-making. These protocols were determined for most E/M services and are the basis for most payer audit activity. Of note, critical care is a time-based code with its own set of rules and does not have the same documentation requirements as E/M codes. (Critical care is discussed in detail in Chapter 93.)

Traditional documentation systems include electronic health records (EHRs), handwritten notes, dictated records, and the use of templated systems. Most EDs now use EHRs to electronically capture notes and physician orders in a centralized database for system-wide access.

Identifying the Services

Services captured in the documentation process are then extracted by professionally trained coders, who use five-digit CPT codes to identify the appropriate ED E/M codes, procedures, and diagnostic studies. The patient's relevant medical diagnoses are then abstracted to demonstrate the medical necessity for the services provided. This information is submitted using the *International Classification of Diseases, 10th Edition (ICD-10)*.[1] Whereas the CPT codes are reimbursable, ICD-10 codes are not associated with a particular charge; instead, they serve to inform the payer of the medical necessity for the services provided. Modifiers may be appended to CPT codes to identify special circumstances dictated by payer payment policies. These coding systems translate the services documented in the medical record into a language more easily tracked on insurance claim forms and by payer claim-processing software. Physician services are reported on a CMS 1500 form. Hospital services are reported on a distinct billing form, typically a UB-04 (see **Addenda 91.1, 91.2,** and **91.3**).

Billing and Compliance

Once the codes are extracted from the chart, the claim form must be submitted to the appropriate payer. Although many patients have some form of government or private insurance, the ED also sees a significant number of uninsured patients. The billing function identifies the primary payment source (i.e., Medicare, Medicaid, Blue Cross Blue Shield, self-pay) and submits a claim. This important step includes submitting the original list of services to the payment source, all necessary follow-ups, reconciling payments to the services reported, initiating appeals as needed, following up with any secondary insurance, and billing the patient for any remaining balance, up to and including collections if necessary. (For more details, see Chapter 95.)

The billing process must be conducted under the direction of a compliance plan, which is a group- or hospital-created document that governs appropriate billing practices. The compliance plan ensures that all reported claims (including billing codes) are accurate and in accordance with contractual agreements with the various payers. These functions must be closely monitored to avoid overcoding and ensure that the group receives maximum payment for every service to which it is entitled.

THE VALUE OF ED SERVICES

There are two distinct systems at play in the reimbursement process: the CPT system that determines the codes selected and the resource-based relative value system (RBRVS) that determines the value of those codes. More than 80% of all payments are directly or indirectly based on the RBRVS, which was implemented in 1992. The RBRVS changed the traditional payment methodology from one based on usual, customary, or reasonable (UCR) charges to one based on the resources used for the provision of any given service. This is now referred to as the relative value unit (RVU) system.

CPT Coding System

Separate from the RVU system is the governing body that oversees the five-digit CPT codes submitted to the insurance companies. The CPT Editorial Panel is funded by the American Medical Association (AMA) and provides editorial control over the CPT book and its monthly companion piece, *The CPT Assistant*. The panel is made up of 17 physicians representing various medical specialties and payer groups, including CMS, Blue Cross Blue Shield, and the Health Insurance Association of America. Emergency medicine does not have a permanent position on the CPT panel, although it has held one of the rotating seats in the past. The panel is supported by the CPT Advisory Committee, which consists primarily of physicians nominated by national medical societies to serve as content experts and advocate on behalf of their specialties. Meetings have historically been closed to all but members of the panel, the CPT Advisory Committee, and support staff from the AMA and the various medical specialties; however, in recent years, the process has been opened to registered observers. All votes remain secret during the meeting.

The panel is responsible for maintaining the CPT code set and is authorized to revise, update, and modify the content as it deems appropriate. The most common way these revisions are made is for a medical specialty society or a coalition of interested parties to submit a code change proposal (CCP). The rationale for the new or revised code must be presented along with compelling research to justify its need. Interested CPT Advisory Committee members may use a secure website to offer support, make suggestions, or speak out against the proposal. At the scheduled CPT meeting, the presenters will have a few minutes to make an oral argument to the panel before it votes on the proposal or sends it back for refinement. If the CCP is approved, it will appear in the next version of the CPT book.

The two overarching principles of CPT are that 1) a provider must select the code that accurately identifies the service performed and 2) any service or procedure in the CPT book may be used to designate the services rendered by any qualified health-care professional. To illustrate, the ED E/M codes are restricted for use in the ED; however, they are not restricted for use by emergency physicians only. Similarly, radiology or anesthesiology codes are not restricted for use by only those medical specialists.

Category I codes are the five-digit codes that comprise most of the CPT book and are valued through the RBRVS process. A sample category I code may look like this:

92950 Cardiopulmonary resuscitation

Category II codes are for performance measures and are used in value-based purchasing models like Medicare Access and the Children's Health Insurance Program Reauthorization Act of 2015 (MACRA) and the Merit-Based Incentive Payment System (MIPS) initiatives. These codes describe clinical components that may be included in an E/M service or procedure and therefore are not associated with a separate RVU. Not reviewed under RBRVS, these codes appear as five digits with an alpha character "F" in the fifth place, followed by cross references to performance measures associated with the category II. Because these performance measures are created outside the CPT process cycle, they are not published in the CPT book but appear on the AMA website. A category II code looks like this:

1022F Pneumococcus immunization status assessed (CAP, COPD)

Category III codes are assigned for emerging technology services and procedures that, although not currently deemed common enough or otherwise ready for a category I designation, the panel believes could reach that status in time. The category III designation allows the service to be tracked for research purposes. Category III codes are five digits with an alpha character in the fifth place. These codes are considered temporary and will sunset in five years unless they are ready for category I status or the need for a temporary code remains. These codes are not valued by RBRVS and may or may not be covered by payers. A category III code looks like this:

0175T Computer-aided detection (CAD)

According to the Health Insurance Portability and Accountability Act (HIPAA), CPT is the national coding standard for physicians and other health-care professionals. AMA and the CPT editorial panel are careful to make sure the code set meets the needs of providers and payers in order to maintain this important designation.

The RBRVS Process

The fundamental basis of the RBRVS is the RVU, a numeric value that is assigned to a given service based on its relative comparison to other services. For example, a level I ED visit is valued less than a level II ED visit, and so on, within the five available levels of ED E/M codes. Similarly, a 5-cm laceration repair is valued higher than a 2-cm laceration repair because of the

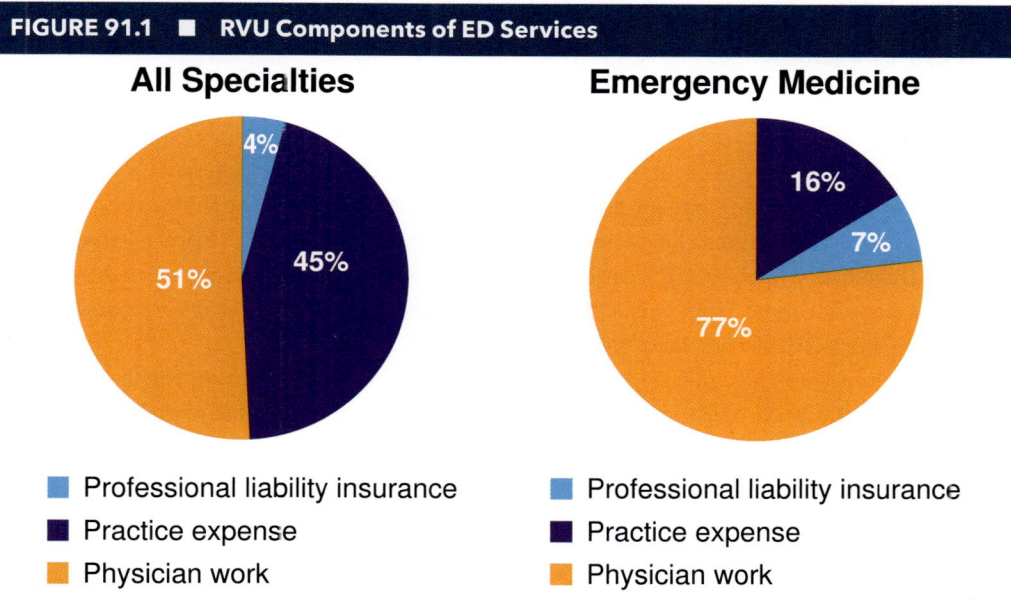

FIGURE 91.1 ■ RVU Components of ED Services

increased resources involved in suturing a longer wound. As presented in **Figure 91.1**, there are three subcategories of RVUs assigned to each code. These are physician work, practice expense (PE), and professional liability insurance (PLI). The three subcategories are not equally considered and are weighted for the ED E/M codes as follows: work 77%, PE 16%, and PLI 7%.

Relative value units for each of those subcategories are adjusted by a geographic practice cost index (GPCI) to account for local variations in costs and then multiplied by a conversion factor to change the resulting numeric value into a dollar amount for payment. The total RVUs for a service are then multiplied by Medicare's conversion factor (the annually determined payment per RVU) to determine the ultimate payment to the provider.

Medicare sets the RVUs for new and revised services based on recommendations from the AMA RBRVS Update Committee (RUC). The RUC is composed of 25 different medical specialties and six assigned positions that represent various organizations or RUC subcommittees, at least two-thirds of which have to agree on the value for any service under consideration. Emergency medicine has a permanent seat on the RUC and has been active in the process since its creation. The RUC considers presentations of compelling evidence, typically based on surveys of those who perform the service in question. The CMS has historically accepted over 90% of the RUC's recommend values.

Physician work is defined as the intensity divided by the time spent providing the service. The RUC survey asks practicing physicians a series of questions that compare a new or revised code to a known reference code familiar to the one under consideration. Respondents are asked to compare the time involved in pre-, intra-, and post-service work for both codes to estimate the total work involved in the provision of both complete services. The survey also compares the physical effort, mental judgment, and psychological stress associated with each service. After carefully considering these comparisons, the survey respondent is asked to suggest a work RVU for the new or revised code.

The PE RVUs are less of a concern to emergency physicians and other hospital-based specialties because they usually do not hire their own nonphysician staff (such as nurses, lab or diagnostic techs) or purchase their own equipment or supplies. Current procedural terminology codes often have two PE RVU values, one for facility and one for nonfacility to account for those differences. Medicare recognizes six categories of PE:

- Nonphysician clinical labor
- Medical equipment

- Medical supplies
- Office overhead
- Administrative labor
- Other

Of note, the specialty of emergency medicine has the highest percentage of work RVUs to total RVUs because of the corresponding lack of direct PE, meaning the first three categories of PE (nonphysician clinical labor, medical equipment, and medical supplies) that can be directly traced to whatever CPT code is performed and reported. As a result, emergency medicine benefits most from any CMS methodological changes that favor increasing or preserving work RVUs over the other two categories.

Fortunately, CMS has adjusted the ED E/M code PE RVUs to account for the nondirect costs associated with providing EMTALA-mandated uncompensated care and standby cost for fully staffing EDs without the ability to efficiently schedule patients. These two costs are included in the "other" category of PE as referenced above.

The PLI component RVUs are not considered by the RUC because they are based on actual claims-made data related to that service. However, the RUC survey does ask the respondent to suggest a PLI crosswalk for a new code from one that is similar in nature. The PLI RVUs are updated periodically based on new available claims made data. The relative value differences assigned by the RUC survey criteria can be used to compare the work, PE, and PLI RVUs for the 20 codes most frequently reported in the ED (**Table 91.1**).

Each year, CMS considers the Medicare fee schedule and often makes adjustments to the assigned RVUs. An ongoing review of work values is conducted to be sure no rank order anomalies have inadvertently occurred with the valuation of all new and revised codes. Periodic adjustments are also made to the PE RVUs based on changes in costs of supplies, as well as to the PLI RVUs based on updated claims data. By statute, CMS must maintain budget neutrality across all codes when new codes are added to the fee schedule or when there are dramatic shifts in payments. For example, in 2007, there were significant increases made in the work RVUs for E/M services, including the ED E/M codes, resulting in an annual shift of about $5 billion from payments for other procedures.

Geographic Practice Cost Index

As described earlier, the GPCIs are factored into the RVU payments and can have a significant impact on regional payments. They are updated at least every three years. A GPCI of 1.000 is considered the national average cost for that RBRVS component. An expensive major metropolitan area will typically have a GPCI weight higher than 1.000; a rural locality's will be lower. Compare the different PE GPCI weights between San Francisco and Puerto Rico in **Table 91.2** to see how significant this impact can be.

Similarly, states with meaningful tort reform laws have significantly lower PLI GPCIs than those that do not. Congress has set a precedent of maintaining an artificial national work GPCI floor of 1.000 in an effort to minimize the pay difference in rural areas and help maintain that workforce. Congress must vote and fund such a threshold each year for it to continue.

These budget-neutrality adjustments are frequently made through changes in the Medicare conversion factor (**Table 91.3**). The formula is complicated, considering a statutory update factor and the budget-neutrality adjustment. After the passage of the Protecting Access to Medicare Act of 2014, Congress stepped in to discontinue the sustainable growth rate (SGR) formula-driven payment cuts.

TABLE 91.1 ■ Top 20 CPT Codes by Frequency of Reporting in the ED as of 2018[2]

Service	CPT Code	Work RVUS	Practice Expense RVUs	PLI RVUs	Total RVUs
Level IV ED exam	99284	2.56	0.53	0.23	3.4032
Level III ED exam	99283	1.34	0.29	0.12	1.75
Level V ED exam	99285	3.80	0.75	0.34	4.89
ECG rhythm interpretation with strip	93042	0.15	0.04	0.01	0.20
Level II ED exam	99282	0.88	0.21	0.08	1.17
Single laceration up to 2.5 cm (scalp, neck, axillae, external genitalia, trunk including hands and feet)	12001	0.84	0.32	0.11	1.27
Single laceration up to 2.5 cm (face, ears, eyelids, nose, lips, and/or mucous membranes)	12011	1.07	0.37	0.14	1.58
Application of short leg splint (calf to foot)	29515	0.73	0.61	0.09	1.43
Critical care first hour	99291	4.50	1.42	0.38	6.30
Single laceration repair 2.6 to 7.5 cm (scalp, neck, axillae, external genitalia, trunk including hands and feet)	12002	1.14	0.39	0.15	1.68
Application of finger splint	29130	0.50	0.26	0.07	0.83
Application of short arm splint (forearm to hand)	29125	0.50	0.57	0.07	1.14
Level I ED exam	99281	0.45	0.11	0.04	0.60
Application of long leg splint (thigh to ankle or toes)	29505	0.69	0.67	0.09	1.45
Treatment of shoulder dislocation	23650	3.53	4.18	0.53	8.24
Spinal puncture: lumbar	62270	1.37	0.69	0.19	2.25
Dressings and/or debridement of partial-thickness burns	16020	0.71	0.76	0.101	1.57
Single laceration 2.6 up to 5.0 cm (face, ears, eyelids, nose, lips) and/or mucous membranes	12013	1.22	0.27	0.17	1.66
Endotracheal intubation	31500	3.00	0.71	0.35	4.06
Incision and drainage of abscess simple/single	10060	1.22	1.44	0.13	2.79

TABLE 91.2 ■ 2018 GPCIs for Select Cities or States

Contractor	Locality	Locality Name	2018 Work GPCI	2018 PE GPCI	2018 PLI GPCI
13202	01	Manhattan, NY	1.052	1.180	1.615
09202	20	Puerto Rico	0.998	1.007	0.990
04412	11	Dallas, TX	1.012	1.014	0.768
03102	00	Arizona	0.980	0.971	0.834
01182	18	Los Angeles, CA	1.046	1.177	0.694
01112	05	San Francisco, CA	1.075	1.325	0.421
01112	75	Rest of California	1.020	1.074	0.562
03602	21	Wyoming	0.983	1.000	0.880

Fee Schedule Determination

As previously mentioned, most payments are based on the RBRVS, so it makes sense to consider the resulting values when determining how to set fees. There is an adage that says, "You will never be paid higher than your asking price." As a result, it is typical for groups (providers) to ensure that their fee schedules adequately cover their costs with a reasonable profit margin. The unfortunate reality is that a considerable portion of ED services are uncompensated. The AMA Patient Care Physician Survey in 2003 estimated that the average EMTALA-mandated debt for each emergency physician was $138,300 annually (the highest of all specialties).[3] For a practice to remain viable, these costs clearly must be considered.

The payer mix is another important factor in setting a fee schedule. The National Hospital Ambulatory Medical Care Survey analyzes ED data each year. The expected sources of payment for the 136 million ED visits are shown in **Table 91.4**.

Most groups set their gross fee schedules based on a multiple of Medicare (e.g., 300%) or a dollar-per-RVU process. Payer contracts consider a group's fee schedule but ultimately base payment on local market forces; this may result in reimbursement as low as 10% to 40% of billed charges. Other groups will use the RBRVS-assigned RVUs and base their fees on their own conversion factor.

Although Medicaid is a shared plan between individual states and the national government, there can be wide variations in the payments for ED E/M services. Some Medicaid payment methodologies include tiers based on patient disposition, while others

TABLE 91.3 ■ Calculation of the Proposed CY 2019 PFS Conversion Factor

CY 2018 conversion factor		35.9996
Statutory update factor	0.25% (1.0025)	
CY 2019 RVU budget neutrality adjustment	−0.12% (0.9988)	
CY 2019 conversion factor		36.0463

TABLE 91.4 ■ Payment Sources for ED Visits[4]

Expected Payment Source	Percentage of Visits
Private insurance	34.3
Medicaid or SCHIP	34.8
Medicare	17.7
Medicare and Medicaid	3.6
Worker's Compensation	0.9
Self-pay	9.0
Charity/no charge	0.9
Other/unknown	14.8

Note: Percentage of visits exceeds 100 because more than one source of payment may be reported per visit.

are based on the specialty and training of the provider (**Table 91.5**). Of note, Medicaid payments are significantly constrained by state budgets and are frequently less than the actual cost of providing the care.

CONTRACTING ISSUES

Social obligation, pressure from hospitals, and the EMTALA mandate to see all presenting patients results in most groups participating in both Medicare and Medicaid programs. Medicare and Medicaid reimbursement schedules are nonnegotiable, whereas private payer contracts can have a wide range of payments depending on the agreement and local market forces. Each

TABLE 91.5 ■ Sample Medicaid Rates By CPT Code (2016)

State	99281	99282	99283	99284	99285	99291	99292	Effective Date
Alabama	13.00	21.00	42.00	66.00	104.00	126.00	63.00	5/23/2016
Arizona	16.89	32.93	49.82	94.06	137.84	176.78	88.78	1/1/2011
Arkansas	22.00	35.00	53.90	71.50	83.75	167.20	83.60	8/24/2009
Colorado	21.25	41.57	61.99	118.21	173.76	275.35	123.40	1/1/2016
Florida	14.80	22.92	42.24	64.69	101.93	151.03	65.98	1/1/2016
Maryland	20.69	40.35	60.30	114.36	168.77	270.16	120.07	1/1/2016
Massachusetts	21.31	41.98	62.65	119.85	175.76	279.71	124.11	6/24/2013
North Carolina	20.71	40.62	60.69	115.63	170.17	219.26	109.76	1/1/2014
Washington	12.11	23.81	35.71	68.08	100.45	162.06	71.84	4/1/2016

Note: Payment amounts for the ED E/M and critical care codes are listed for sample states taken from the respective Medicaid contractor website at the time of publication. Note the variation in payments across the code levels in each state.

emergency physician group negotiates a contractual payment rate and coverage polices with individual private payers. Depending on the circumstances, the group may ultimately decide to refuse the terms, become a nonparticipating provider, and bill the patient directly.

Hospital alliances can greatly influence a group's ability to negotiate a separate arrangement. Health plans will encourage the emergency group to participate in a favorable (for the health plan) arrangement, thereby obtaining the best possible rates and access to care for their covered beneficiaries. The decision to participate depends on how deeply a group is willing to discount its fee schedule and the inconvenience of trying to collect directly from the patient. Many plans further incentivize group participation by refusing to honor the "assignment of benefit" agreements and sending the insurance payments directly to the patients, who may simply keep the money rather than forward it to the providers.

Payers may offer a fee for service, a health maintenance organization (HMO) plan, or a preferred provider organization (PPO) plan to their subscribers. Each of these products has its own reimbursement contractual commitments and must be considered separately. Groups must understand the enrollment and credentialing process, including restrictions and timelines, for every payer plan with which the group intends to contract. For instance, a group may not be eligible for payments and can lose money if it is not fully enrolled by the time the plan's beneficiaries are treated. Medicare and many state Medicaid plans have long credentialing lead times, which can impact a group's cash flow.

Billing Terms and Definitions

The following definitions are helpful in gaining a further understanding of the provider's economic relationship with the insurance carrier.

- *Coinsurance*: A form of medical cost sharing in a health-insurance plan that requires an insured person to pay a stated percentage of medical expenses after the deductible amount, if any, is paid. Once any deductible amount and coinsurance are paid, the insurer is responsible for the rest of the reimbursement for covered benefits up to allowed charges. The insured individual could also be responsible for any charges in excess of the amount the insurer determines to be "UCR." Coinsurance rates my differ if services are received by an approved provider or an out-of-network provider. Rates may also differ for different types of services, such as immunizations or preventive diagnostic screenings.
- *Copayment*: A form of medical cost sharing in a health-insurance plan that requires an insured person to pay a fixed dollar amount when a medical service is received. The insurer is responsible for the rest of the reimbursement. There may be separate copayments for different services. For example, a plan may require a $20 copay for an office visit, $50 for an urgent care visit, and $150 for an ED visit. Some plans require that a deductible first be met for some specific services before a copayment applies.
- *Deductible*: A fixed dollar amount that an insured person pays during the benefit period (usually a year) before the insurer starts to make payments for covered medical services. Plans may have both per-individual and per-family deductibles. Some plans may have separate deductibles for specific services. For example, a plan may have a hospitalization deductible per admission. Deductibles may differ if services are received from providers not on the approved list.
- *HMO*: This is a health-care system that assumes both the financial risks associated with providing comprehensive medical services (insurance and service risk) and the responsibility for health-care delivery in a particular geographic area. The fee is usually prepaid and fixed. The HMO may share the financial risk with its participating providers.

- *Individual practice association*: This is an organization composed of a group of independent practicing physicians who maintain their own offices and band together for the purpose of contracting their services to managed care plans. These plans may include a financial incentive to reduce costs.
- *Managed care plans*: Managed care plans generally provide comprehensive health services to their members and offer financial incentives for using providers who belong to the plan. Examples of managed care plans include:
  - HMOs
  - PPOs
  - Exclusive provider organizations
  - Point of service plans

State Reimbursement Rules

The reimbursement rules governing the physician relationship with the various payers are typically governed at the state level. State laws often address the HMO-related issues of assignment of benefits and balance billing.

- *Assignment of benefits*: The payer may be required to send the monies for a medical service directly to a noncontracted provider, or the payer may refuse to honor the assignment of benefits and send the reimbursement to the patient.
- *Balance billing*: The insurance carrier may not be required to pay the noncontracted (out-of-network) providers their full charges. If a lesser amount is paid, the provider may or may not be permitted to "balance bill" the patient for the difference, depending on local regulations. For example, the ED group's gross charge for 99283 is $200. Hypothetically, the insurance company could pay the physician the out-of-network rate of $150, and the patient would then be responsible for the remaining $50. In some regions, balance billing has been restricted.
- Several years ago, a number of state medical societies entered into a class-action suit against multiple national payers under the Racketeer Influenced and Corrupt Organizations statutes, which were originally developed to fight organized crime. The states claimed that the payers inappropriately bundled their codes and provided misleading explanations of the benefits and the monies owed to their patients. Settlements were eventually reached with the various payers. Providers are cautioned to be vigilant and recognize that once an agreement is signed, the contractual terms must be consistently honored.

Fair Payment and Balance Billing

Private payers, in particular, often scrutinize fee schedules against databases of UCR fees. Several organizations, including the AMA, are building such systems. If they are successful, they may provide practice-blinded comparable fees for a specific region without the resulting antitrust problems if an individual physician or group attempted to collect such data. It is hoped that payers and providers will agree to use the resulting data to set payment rates that are acceptable to both parties. These national fee databases continue to evolve as a possible way to identify "fair payment."

Currently, emergency physician services are often paid by health plans at rates that are substantially below reasonable, customary value. Emergency physicians will not contract if a payer's rates are too low, and the payers will not agree to the physician's fee schedule if they think the rates are too high, thereby creating an impasse. Health plans know that emergency medical care must be provided to their enrollees because of the EMTALA regulations, no matter how poorly the plans pay.

Systematic underpayment of emergency services without a corresponding mechanism of ensuring fair payment has led to the practice of balance billing. Increasingly, state and federal regulations are limiting the collections of out-of-network providers by both eliminating the balance billing of patients and decreasing the obligation of the insurance company to pay the physician's charges. Powerful lobbies in several states are trying to pass laws that would prohibit balance billing. If such laws do pass, there is no incentive for payers to negotiate in good faith, and emergency physicians will have no recourse since they cannot refuse to provide care. This decreasing reimbursement could ultimately result in a future workforce reduction and a corresponding decrease in access to quality emergency medical care.

Payment Policies and Bundling Issues

Fee schedules are typically the primary focus of contract negotiations, but it is also vital to consider payer policies to determine which services are covered. Medicare uses the National Correct Coding Initiative (NCCI) to determine coding combinations that will not be paid when reported together on the same claim. For example, the interpretation and report of chest x-rays are bundled into the code for critical care and not separately payable when reported together. The NCCI does not bundle interpretations of diagnostic tests such as ECGs, x-rays, or ultrasounds into the ED E/M service codes, but many private payers will not reimburse those services separately. In order to obtain reasonable payment for services rendered, it is important to understand the particular contractual language of each payer.

EVOLVING REIMBURSEMENT METHODOLOGIES

One of the stated goals of the current medical reform is to shift reimbursement methodologies away from the traditional fee-for-service models, which reward providers for doing more by paying for every "unit" of medical care produced. Various proposals and government demonstration projects are instead focusing on payment for quality. The underlying concept is that efficient, higher-quality care will ultimately save money for a nation whose medical expenses have increased significantly over the last decade. The aging of the American population and transition of the huge baby boomer generation into Medicare has placed the United States on an unsustainable path of per-capita medical spending (**Figures 91.2** and **91.3**).

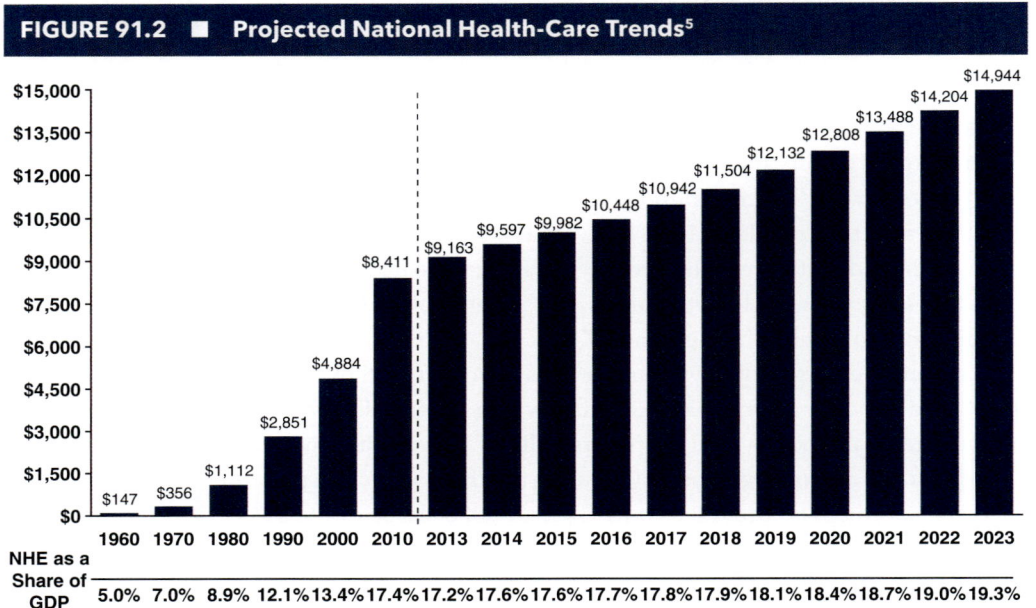

FIGURE 91.2 ■ Projected National Health-Care Trends[5]

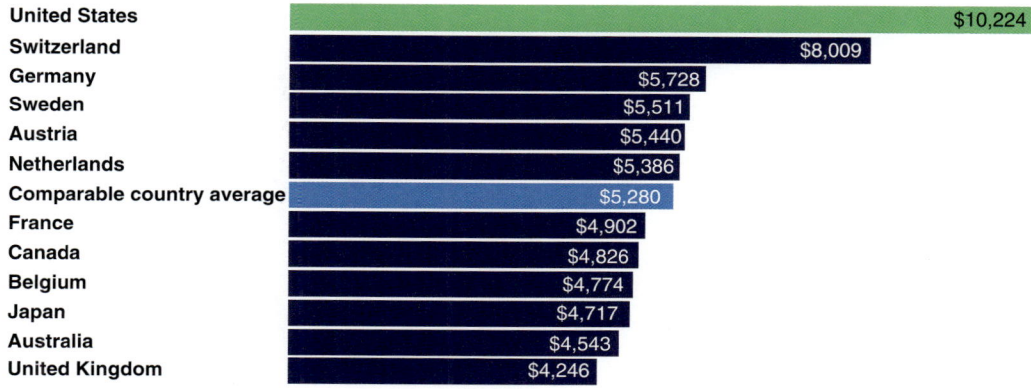

FIGURE 91.3 ■ Total Health Expenditures Per Capita[6]

On average, other wealthy countries spend about half as much per person on health care than the U.S.

- United States: $10,224
- Switzerland: $8,009
- Germany: $5,728
- Sweden: $5,511
- Austria: $5,440
- Netherlands: $5,386
- Comparable country average: $5,280
- France: $4,902
- Canada: $4,826
- Belgium: $4,774
- Japan: $4,717
- Australia: $4,543
- United Kingdom: $4,246

Note: Health consumption does not include investments in structures, equipment, or research.

Pay for Performance

The CMS and some private payers have rolled out a transitional program to reward providers for meeting predetermined clinical performance measures. Medicare's Physician Quality Reporting Initiative (PQRI) and Physician Quality Reporting System (PQRS) programs have given way to MACRA and MIPS reporting.

Congress launched the PQRI program through a provision of the Tax Relief and Health Care Act of 2006. Since its implementation in mid-2007, physicians have been paid a small bonus for reporting on quality measures related to their specialty. The program was initially voluntary and offered an extra bonus payment for participation. The CMS quality program has undergone a rapid evolution. The 2019 conversion factor is not governed by the SGR formula, which mandated continuing annual cuts to physician payments and resulted in years of eleventh-hour congressional short-term fixes. Instead, with the passage of MACRA, 2019 represents the third year of a stabilized conversion factor. In addition to stabilizing the conversion factor, MACRA also combines the quality programs of the PQRS, the "value modifier" process, and "meaningful use" into a single CMS quality payment program: the MIPS.

An overview of the reimbursement impact of the MIPS program is shown in **Table 91.6** with further detail provided in Chapters 97 and 98.

Shared Savings Programs

The implications of shared savings programs continue to evolve. Section 3022 of the Patient Protection and Affordable Care Act (PPACA) required the Secretary of Health and Human Services (HHS) to establish the Medicare Shared Savings Program by January 1, 2012. Three key aims of the program are better care for individuals, better health for the population, and lower per capita costs. Eligible providers, hospitals, and suppliers may participate in the Shared Savings Program by creating or participating in an accountable care organization (ACO).

Incentives have been proposed to align providers with ACOs.[7] In some ways, an ACO greatly expands the idea of a patient-centered medical home. For example, a primary care physician can coordinate care for a select patient population because the ACO encourages multiple providers, including the hospital, to work together to improve quality and reduce costs. The process of aligning primary care physicians and hospital-based systems in developing ACOs has received considerable attention; however, the role of emergency

TABLE 91.6 ■ Evolution of Federal Quality Payment Program

Program	2017	2018	2019	2020	2021	2022	2023	2024	2025	2026+
	0.5%	0.5%	0.5%	0.5%	Base conversion factor update of 0.0 each year					0.25%
HER	Continues under current law		+/-4% MIPS (2017 performance)	+/-5% MIPS (2018 performance)	+/-7% MIPS	+/-9% MIPS				
PQRS	Continues under current law									
VM	Continues under current law									
MIPS	N/A									

physicians (and other hospital-based specialists) has not been fully addressed. The conventional wisdom seems to be that any nontraumatic injury is a failure of the medical system and could be avoided with better preventive care and coordination in other venues.

The CMS began with the Acute Care Episode (ACE) Demonstration Project in 2008. Five sites were selected in five states to participate in a model that made a bundled payment to the hospital for all the costs associated with the provision of care, including all professional and facility charges for select orthopedic and cardiac diagnoses. The sites had the option to reward individual clinicians, teams of clinicians, or other hospital staff who suceeded with measurable clinical quality and efficiency improvements.

An "episode of care" included all services related to an established timeline surrounding a covered service, including a look-back period; any readmissions would not be paid separately (**Figure 91.4**).

Episodes of integrated care programs (e.g., the ACE demonstration projects) require a controlling entity to move forward. Usually, the controlling party is the "player" with the largest slice of the pie. In the ACE project and other pilot programs, the controlling player was the hospital. Eligible entities interested in forming ACOs had to wait for the release of

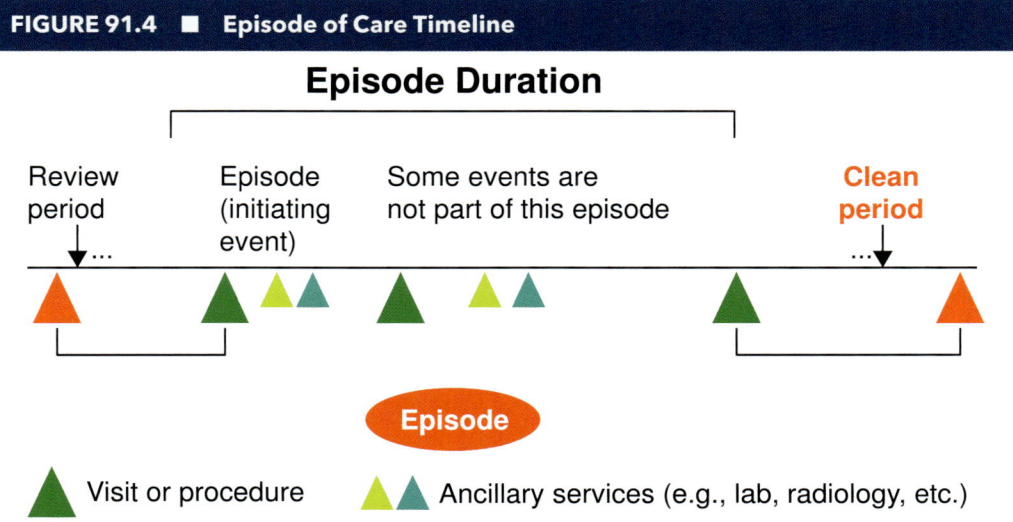

FIGURE 91.4 ■ Episode of Care Timeline

> **BOX 91.2 ■ CMS PRINCIPLES FOR ACOs[8]**
>
> **Eligible organizations must:**
>
> - Be patient centered.
> - Be data rich.
> - Provide seamless care.
> - Include multiple types of providers.
> - Provide better quality than fee for service.
> - Incorporate continuous learning.
> - Have the same value proposition to private payers and Medicare.
> - Allow the beneficiary to choose any provider inside or outside of the ACO.

the CMS ACO rule, which was published in March of 2011. To participate in the voluntary Medicare Shared Savings Program, a potential ACO must file a petition to enter into a three-year agreement with CMS to provide services for a minimum of 5,000 patients in one of two tracks. In both tracks, additional monies are derived from cost "savings."

In the first track, the ACO does not have exposure to losses during the first two years of the agreement but does share in any losses with CMS in the third year. This track is limited to up to 50% of any savings achieved. The second track allows the ACO to assume a share of both savings and losses in all three years and entitles the participating organization to 60% of any savings. CMS determines whether to approve or deny applications from eligible organizations prior to the end of the calendar year in which they are submitted. Additional principles of an ACO appear in **Box 91.2**.[8]

In its release of regulations, CMS estimates the aggregate start-up investments and first-year operating expenditures for ACOs are from $131,643,825 to $263,287,650. A recent study of the CMS Physician Group Practice Demonstration found that after three years in the project, half the participants were still ineligible for any shared savings to offset their initial investment.[9]

There have been significant concerns about the antitrust implications of setting up large regional ACOs, and any potential players must carefully review the guidance outlined in the CMS rule, written in cooperation with the US Office of the Inspector General, US Department of Justice, and others.

A new frontier is now being opened as the American College of Emergency Physicians (ACEP) works with CMS to design alternative payment models that would reward ED groups for demonstrating meaningful reductions in cost (see Chapter 98).

CMS Innovation Center

In an effort to standardize future programs, CMS has brought many of its health-care pilot projects under a single roof, called the CMS Innovation Center. The program was established by Section 3021 of the PPACA. Its mission is to design and rapidly implement innovative methods and models for health-care payment reform. In addition to improving quality, the goal is to "lower the total cost of care." The process is laid out in **Box 91.3**.

> **BOX 91.3 ■ CMS INNOVATION CENTER PILOT PROCESS**
>
> - Solicit ideas for new models.
> - Select the most promising models.
> - Test and evaluate models.
> - Spread successful models.

The CMS Innovation Center is focused on several programs that it believes may yield the greatest change in health-care delivery and cost reduction. Among these approaches are models for seamless, coordinated patient care and community and population health.

Patient Care Models

Clinical care models attempt to match the correct treatments and resources to the patient's medical needs. The goal is to avoid the utilization of too many resources (overspending) and too few resources (undercare). An example that has received significant focus is the ACO model discussed earlier, which initiates payment reform through bundled payments. Providers are incentivized to deliver care more efficiently by minimizing the use of unnecessary resources. Instead of billing using the current fee-for-service process, a single "bundled" payment would be granted for each episode of care.

Seamless and Coordinated Care Models

Seamless care models assist providers working in different settings to provide more coordinated care. Some of the current programs and initiatives that have been launched include state projects to validate and integrate the care of dual-eligibility patients, federally qualified medical centers for the delivery of primary care, and multiple-payer primary care involving bundled payments.

Community and Population Health Model

The community and population health model involves the adoption of payment approaches that are designed to improve public health.

CONCLUSION

The ED reimbursement process continues to be dynamic and challenging. Constant monitoring of current and evolving conditions is vital to remain competitive and profitable. To understand the rules of the game, it is important to be aware of the legislative and regulatory changes that impact ED reimbursement. A time line of relevant changes appears in **Box 91.4**.

Although it is difficult to guess where medical reform will lead, a thorough understanding of the process will create a solid foundation on which to address these changes. The HHS, which is committed to finding more efficient and less costly ways to provide health care, has funded the CMS Innovation Center with $10 billion for testing creative solutions. Emergency physicians must continue to demonstrate value to the health-care continuum in order to achieve and maintain appropriate reimbursement.

BOX 91.4 ■ TIMELINE OF ED REGULATORY CHANGES

1. **Medicare and Medicaid, 1965:** The creation of the Medicare and Medicaid programs provided new sources of funding for ED services and made it possible for hospitals to hire full-time emergency physicians. Medicare was also one of the primary factors in shifting the focus of medical schools from research into training for clinical care.

2. **Introduction of CPT, 1966:** The AMA published the first edition of the CPT, a system of standardized terms for medical procedures used to facilitate documentation.

3. **Tax Equity and Fiscal Responsibility Act (TEFRA), 1982:** Congress passed TEFRA, which disallowed "combined billing" (i.e., physician and hospital charges submitted as one bill) for the governmental payers. This move helped create an entire industry of emergency medicine billing firms.

4. **EMTALA, 1986:** EMTALA became law, which requires the ED to provide assessment and necessary treatment regardless of ability to pay. Further, EMTALA mandates that patient assessment not be delayed by inquiring about ability to pay. The ramifications of this law have a greater impact on the ED than any other site of service and historically have been used as a tool by some payers to significantly reduce or even deny payment based on retrospective review.

5. **OBRA, 1989 and the advent of RBRVS, 1992:** The year 1992 is a watershed mark for reimbursement. Perhaps the most seminal event in reimbursement in the past 40 years was the advent of the RBRVS, used to value physician services based on the actual work, practice expense, and resulting malpractice risk involved with providing that service. Prior to 1992, payments were based on a "usual, customary, and reasonable" standard that arguably was none of those, but rather was based on historic payer data not shared with providers. Moving to the RBRVS gave physicians an active role in valuing their services. ACEP's role in the RUC gives emergency medicine a voice in valuing not only ED-related services but those of all other providers, as well.

6. **Medicare Documentation Guidelines, 1995:** The introduction of the Medicare Documentation Guidelines for E/M services provided a national methodology for assigning a level of service based on numerous criteria related to the medical history, physical examination, and medical decision-making involved in patient care. This revolutionized both the coding and billing industry and also produced standard audit tools for compliance purposes.

7. **The Patient Protection and Affordable Care Act of 2010:** The sweeping healthcare reform legislation is intended to expand insurance to more Americans while controlling costs by moving away from fee-for-service payment methodologies to one based on quality and efficiencies of providing care, including the shared savings plans.

REFERENCES

1. American Medical Association. Current Prrocedural Coding Expert. 2019. Available at: https://www.optum360coding.com/upload/pdf/CE21/CE21.pdf. Accessed August 6, 2020.

2. CMS.Gov. 2020 Medicare Fee Schedule Federal Register. Available at: https://www.cms.gov/Medicare/Medicare-Fee-for-Service-Payment/PhysicianFeeSched/PFS-Federal-Regulation-Notices-Items/CMS-1715-F. Accessed September 25, 2020.

3. Kane CK. *Physician Marketplace Report: The Impact of EMTALA on Physician Practices.* AMA Report #2003-2. American Medical Association Center for Health Policy Research; 2003.

4. Rui P, Kang K, Ashman JJ. *National Hospital Ambulatory Medical Care Survey: 2016 Emergency Department Summary Tables.* See Table 6: Expected source of payment at emergency department visits. National Center for Health Statistics, 2016. Available at: https://www.cdc.gov/nchs/data/nhamcs/web_tables/2016_ed_web_tables.pdf. Accessed August 6, 2020.

5. CMS.Gov. National Health Expenditure data from Centers for Medicare and Medicaid Services, Office of the Actuary, National Health Statistics Group. Updated December 17, 2019. Accessed August 6, 2020. (For 1960-2010 data, see Historical; National Health Expenditures by type of service and source of funds; CY 1960-2012; file nhe2012.zip. For 2013-2023 data, see Projected; NHE Historical and Projections, 1965-2023, file nhe65-23.zip).

6. Sawyer B, Cox C. Peterson-KFF Health System Tracker, How does health spending in the U.S. compare to other countries? 2018. Available at: https://www.healthsystemtracker.org/chart-collection/health-spending-u-s-compare-countries/#item-u-s-increased-public-private-sector-spending-faster-rate-similar-countries. Accessed on August 6, 2020.

7. Haywood TT, Kosel KC. The ACO model—a three-year financial loss? *N Engl J Med.* 2011;364(14):e27.

8. PPACA P.L. 111-148 Sec. 3022 Shared Savings. 2010. Available at: https://www.congress.gov/111/plaws/publ148/PLAW-111publ148.pdf. Accessed August 4, 2020.

9. Damberg CL, Sorbero ME, Lovejoy SL, et al. Measuring success in health care value-based purchasing programs: findings from an environmental scan, literature review, and expert panel discussions. *Rand Health Q.* 2014;4(3):9.

ADDENDUM 91.1: CMS 1500 Form

ADDENDUM 91.2: Reimbursement Tables

Fields on the Reimbursement Form	
Item	**Instructions**
Item 1	Show the type of health insurance coverage applicable to this claim by checking the appropriate box; e.g., if a Medicare claim is being filed, check the Medicare box.
Item 1a	Insured's ID number
Item 2	Patient's name
Item 3	Patient's birth date and sex
Item 4	Insured's name
Item 5	Patient's address and telephone number
Item 6	Patient's relationship to insured
Item 7	Insurance primary to Medicare, insured's address, and telephone number
Item 8	Patient's marital status and whether employed or a student
Item 9	Medigap benefits
Item 9a	Medigap benefits, other insured's policy or group number
Item 9b	Medigap benefits, other insured's date of birth
Item 9c	Medigap benefits, employer/school name
Item 9d	Medigap benefits, insurance plan/program name, payer ID number
Item 10a-c	Condition relationship? Employment, auto liability, or other accident
Item 10d	Use this item exclusively for Medicaid information
Item 11	Insured's policy group or FECA number
Item 11a	Insured's date of birth and sex
Item 11b	Insurance primary to Medicare, employer's name
Item 11c	Insurance plan/program name
Item 11d	Leave blank
Item 12	Patient's or authorized person's signature
Item 13	Medigap benefits, insured's/authorized person's signature
Item 14	Date of current illness/injury/pregnancy
Item 15	Leave blank - not required by Medicare
Item 16	Dates patient unable to work in current occupation
Item 17	Name of the referring or ordering physician
Item 17a	Leave blank

(Continued)

Continued		
Item 17b	NPI of the referring/ordering physician
Item 18	Service furnished as a result of, or subsequent to, a related hospitalization
Item 19	Narrative field
Item 20	Diagnostic and purchased tests
Item 21	Patient's diagnosis/condition
Item 22	Leave blank - not required by Medicare
Item 23	Prior authorization number
Item 24	Service line
Item 24a	Date of service
Item 24b	Place of service
Item 24c	Leave blank - not required by Medicare
Item 24d	Procedures, services, or supplies code
Item 24e	Diagnosis code reference number
Item 24f	Charge amount
Item 24g	Days or units
Item 24h	Leave blank
Item 24i	ID qualifier
Item 24j	PIN/NPI of the rendering provider
Item 25	Provider or supplier federal tax ID (employer identification number)
Item 26	Patient's account number
Item 27	Accept assignment?
Item 28	Total charges for services on claim
Item 29	Total amount the patient paid on the covered services only
Item 30	Leave blank
Item 31	Signature of provider of service or supplier
Item 32	Name and address of facility where services were rendered
Item 32a	NPI of service facility
Item 32b	ID qualifier and PIN
Item 33	Provider/supplier telephone number, billing name, address, and zip code
Item 33a	NPI of billing provider (supplier) or group
Item 33b	ID qualifier and PIN

CHAPTER 92

INTRODUCTION TO CODING

Sarah Todt

The goal of coding is to uniformly describe clinical services. First developed in 1966, *Current Procedural Terminology* (CPT) is published and updated annually by the American Medical Association (AMA). The Healthcare Common Procedure Coding System (HCPCS) is the coding system utilized by Medicare and is based on a combination of CPT codes, regional payer codes, and local payer codes. The HCPCS codes are used by Medicare and monitored by the Centers for Medicare and Medicaid Services (CMS). These codes identify most of the tasks and services provided to a Medicare patient by medical practitioners, including medical, surgical, and diagnostic services. Current Procedural Terminology is a listing of numeric codes. The HCPCS contains both numeric and alphanumeric codes.

Evaluation and management (E/M) services are a subset of codes contained in CPT/HCPCS and are published by the AMA in its annual CPT manual. Evaluation and management services are the most frequently billed emergency department (ED) services. When provided in the ED, these are identified with the ED E/M code levels 99281-99285 and 99291-99292 for critical care. For coding purposes, an ED is defined as "an organized hospital-based facility for the provision of unscheduled episodic services to patients who present for immediate medical attention. The facility must be available 24 hours a day."[1]

The ED E/M codes do not differentiate between new or established patients or initial or subsequent visits, as in the office or inpatient setting. For coding purposes, the level of service is not affected if the patient has been previously seen in the ED. Emergency medicine codes 99281-99285 are based on the documentation of history, exam and medical decision-making (MDM), and do not have referenced standard times like the E/M levels for outpatient office/clinic and inpatient hospital visits.[1] The documentation requirements will be discussed in greater detail later in the chapter.

The CPT/HCPCS codes selected for billing of provider services are entered into a billing form as required by the payer. Claim forms provide a uniform billing format that facilitates payer review and processing of the payment. Whether electronic or paper, claim forms must be completed accurately and signed electronically or personally by the provider. For every claim submitted, the provider assumes full responsibility for the accuracy of the information contained in the claim. It is critically important to ensure that all services are billed accurately.

The level of E/M services is determined by satisfying the listed code descriptor requirements for the key components of history, physical examination, and MDM. The number of key components required to assign an E/M level for emergency medicine requires all three key components to be satisfied. When the ED E/M codes are used, all three key components (history, physical examination, and MDM) must meet or exceed the requirements stated for each level of service. For example, 99284 ED E/M service requires a detailed history, a detailed physical examination, and MDM of moderate complexity.[1]

The only exception to the key element requirement rule for ED visits is 99285. The 99285 code level is uniquely the only level that requires all three key components "within the constraints imposed by the urgency of the patient's clinical condition and/or mental status."[1]

The key element requirements may be waived if the patient's clinical condition or mental status prevent the physician from performing all of the key elements. The E/M exception, commonly known as the emergency medicine "caveat," requires the physician to reference the conditions that prevent completing the required actions. For example, the patient may be intubated, have an altered mental status, be in extreme pain, or experiencing a number of additional problems that may prevent the physician from completing and documenting the required key elements.

Although E/M services are the most commonly performed and are exclusively addressed by Medicare in the documentation guidelines, additional services performed in the ED encompass diagnostic, surgical, and medical treatments. For example, the American College of Emergency Physicians (ACEP) provides a list of the top 20 emergency medicine reimbursement codes on its website (https://www.acep.org).[2]

DOCUMENTATION GUIDELINES

The CMS and the AMA collaborated in creating documentation guidelines to support E/M code choices. The recommendations provide definitions and documentation parameters for the three key components of E/M services. The three key components—history, examination, and MDM—appear in the descriptors for office and other outpatient services, hospital observation services, hospital inpatient services, consultations, ED services, nursing facility services, domiciliary care services, and home services.[1] While the documentation guidelines were not created with an objective "scoring" system to define each E/M level, numerous scoring systems were developed to assist in coding and auditing processes. Although the guidelines contained much of the text from CPT, providers were cautioned to refer to the CPT manual for a complete descriptor for each E/M service level and for more detailed instructions for selecting each level of service. **Table 92.1** illustrates the differences in content for the ED E/M guidelines for CPT and 1995 Medicare documentation guidelines.

Subsequent to the release of the documentation guidelines, the Marshfield Clinic released a scoring system developed to provide a more objective means of assigning each E/M level through use of the guidelines. The Marshfield Clinic scoring system was initially released by Medicare as a suggested method of defining the components of each level, but it was not sanctioned by Medicare for official use. Following publication, however, many Medicare carriers adopted the Marshfield Clinic scoring system for use by their internal audit departments. Over the years since its release, the Marshfield Clinic scoring system has been used and modified by many providers and payers as a documentation and coding/audit tool to add objective elements to each E/M level. For example, National Government Services and First Coast publish an E/M score sheet on their websites.[3,4] Medicare also released an additional version of documentation guidelines. The 1997 version contained a significantly different scoring system that is made up of unique elements for each organ system examination. Because physical examinations in the ED primarily entail multisystem assessments, and Medicare afforded physicians the opportunity to use the version of guidelines that was most beneficial, the 1995 version has become emergency medicine's format of choice.

Currently, the AMA and CMS have not published a revision to the existing documentation guidelines or assigned a nationally recognized scoring mechanism to the existing 1995 guidelines. As a result, there is no clearly recognized standard scoring mechanism or clarification of the more ambiguous terms referenced in the descriptors. There is no single definitive authority dictating how these score sheets are to be used.

TABLE 92.1 ■ Comparison Analysis: E/M Code Content (CMS Guidelines vs AMA/CPT Guidelines)

E/M Level	99281		99282		99283		99284		99285	
	AMA/CPT	HCFA 1995	AMA/CPT	HCFA 1995	AMA/CPT	HCFA 1995	AMA/CPT	HCFA 1995	AMA/CPT	HCFA 1995
Presenting Problem	Self-limiting/ minor severity		Low-to-moderate severity		Moderate severity		High severity, requires urgent evaluation by the physician but does not pose an immediate significant threat to life or physiologic function		High severity and poses an immediate significant threat to life or physiologic function	
History	Problem focused	Problem focused	Expanded problem focused		Expanded problem focused		Detailed		Comprehensive	
HPI (CPT does not recognize "duration" as HPI element)	Brief	One- to three elements	Brief	One to three elements	Brief	One to three elements	Extended	Four or more elements	Extended	Four or more elements
ROS	N/A	N/A	Problem pertinent	Problem pertinent	Problem pertinent	Problem pertinent	Problem pertinent (limited additional systems)	Detailed (two to nine systems)	All body systems	Complete (ten or more systems)
PFSH	N/A	N/A	N/A	N/A	N/A	N/A	Pertinent (directly related to patients' problems)	Pertinent (one of three)	Complete	Complete (two of three)

(Continued)

TABLE 92.1 ■ Continued

Physical examination (CPT does not recognize "constitutional" as an organ system or body area)	Limited examination, affected ba/os	Limited examination, affected ba/os	Limited examination, affected, symptomatic, related ba/os	Limited examination, affected, symptomatic, related ba/os	Limited examination, affected, symptomatic, related ba/os	Limited examination, affected, symptomatic, related ba/os	Extended examination, affected, symptomatic, related ba/os	Detailed examination, extended exam two to seven ba/os	Complete general multisystem examination or complete examination of single system	General multisystem (eight or more OS) or single system complete
Medical decision-making (2 of 3 must meet stated requirements)	Straight-forward	Straight-forward	Low	Low	Moderate	Moderate	Moderate	Moderate	High	High
Amount/complexity of data	Minimal	One point	Limited	Two points	Moderate	Three points	Moderate	Three points	Extensive	Four points
No. Dx./mgmt. options	Minimal	One point	Limited	Two points	Multiple	Three points	Multiple	Three points	Extensive	Four points
Risk (highest level in any one of 3 categories)	Minimal	Minimal	Low	Low	Moderate	Moderate	Moderate	Moderate	High	High
Presenting problem	N/A	Minimal	N/A	Low	N/A	Moderate	N/A	Moderate	N/A	High
Diagnostic procedures	N/A	Minimal	N/A	Low	N/A	Moderate	N/A	Moderate	N/A	High
Management options	N/A	Minimal	N/A	Low	N/A	Moderate	N/A	Moderate	N/A	High

> **BOX 92.1 ■ COMPONENTS TO DEFINE E/M SERVICES[1]**
>
> - History
> - Examination
> - Medical decision making
> - Counseling
> - Coordination of care
> - Nature of presenting problem
> - Time

The descriptors for the levels of E/M services recognize seven components, which are used in defining the levels of E/M services (**Box 92.1**).[1] The first three of these components (i.e., history, examination, and MDM) are the key components in selecting the level of E/M services. An exception to the key element rule is visits that consist predominantly of counseling or coordination of care; for these services, time is the key or controlling factor to qualify for a particular level of E/M service.

For certain groups of patients, the recorded information may vary slightly from that described in CPT. Specifically, the medical records of infants, children, adolescents, and pregnant women may have additional or modified information recorded in each history and examination area. As an example, newborn records may include under history of the present illness (HPI) the details of mother's pregnancy and the infant's status at birth; "social history" will focus on family structure; and "family history" will focus on congenital anomalies and hereditary disorders in the family. In addition, information on growth and development and nutrition will be recorded.

Although not specifically defined in these documentation guidelines, these patient group variations on history and examination are appropriate. The history, physical examination, and MDM components are considered key to selecting a level of E/M services, although the contributory factors may also impact the assignment of an E/M level. The key components are the first components considered when assigning a level of E/M service. Time is not considered a descriptive component for assignment of the ED codes 99281-99285. When scoring an ED record, the MDM level is often determined first, after which the history and physical examination level are scored. If, in reviewing the MDM, it is determined that the ED "caveat" is applicable, the level of history and/or physical examination may necessarily exclude required components as determined by patient's clinical condition and/or mental status.

Determining the accurate level of service requires familiarization with both the CPT manual's instructions for determining a level of service and the Medicare documentation guidelines, which provide more objective definitions of each component. For purposes of accurately identifying the appropriate ED E/M level, the 1995 documentation guidelines are considered significantly more applicable than subsequent versions.

Once all elements are put together, the E/M level is determined by the *lowest* score of the key components (history, physical examination, or MDM) (**Table 92.2**).[5]

Clinical Examples

The importance of the clinical examples in CPT cannot be overlooked. Although the practice of emergency medicine has evolved since creation of these examples, payers often refer to these examples to determine the appropriate level of service for emergency medicine claims. These examples can help define the E/M levels for emergency medicine and provide support for the resources used for each level. However, as they have not been modified in many years,

TABLE 92.2 ■ Determining the E/M Level

CPT Level	History	Physical Examination	MDM
99281	Problem focused	Problem focused	Straightforward
99282	Expanded problem focused	Expanded problem focused	Low
99283	Expanded problem focused	Expanded problem focused	Moderate
99284	Detailed	Detailed	Moderate
99285	Comprehensive	Comprehensive	High

caution should be exercised in using them to illustrate medical necessity for the various E/M levels. The clinical examples can be found in each year's CPT manual in Appendix C.

CONTRIBUTORY FACTORS

Contributory factors are not required to score an E/M service. In the ED, however, the nature of the presenting problem may be a significant factor in determining the E/M level because it is a component of "risk" and thus contributes substantially to the MDM score. Additionally, the nature of the presenting problem will assist in determining the difference between a 99283 and a 99284, because both require moderate MDM. However, the nature of the presenting problem is higher for a 99284.

Nature of Presenting Problem

The presenting problem is the disease, condition, illness, injury, symptom, sign, finding, complaint, or other reason for the visit to the ED with or without a diagnosis being established at the time of the encounter.[1] Although listed as a contributory factor for an ED E/M level, the presenting problem can be a significant indicator of medical necessity and support the need for ED treatment of the condition, the rationale for the ED course, and the medical necessity for diagnostic tests and therapeutic services. As such, it cannot be overlooked as an essential element in determining the level of MDM and confirming medical necessity for the ED visit. As many ED patients do not fully understand the full range of problems that may be represented by their complaint, the emergency physician must develop a history of the complaint and/or present illness, consider contributory factors, and determine the course of treatment during the patient's ED stay. The chief complaint (CC), history, and MDM together present a more accurate picture of the entire problem and the care required during the ED course.

The levels of the presenting problem are shown in **Box 92.2**.[1] The CC/presenting problem may be a significant indicator of risk. It is not uncommon for the patient's presenting problem to be of a very significant nature that extensive testing determines to be less serious. Alternatively, a patient may underestimate the significance of symptoms and may actually have a problem that is more significant once a workup identifies additional concerns. For example, a patient experiencing chest pain presents to the ED and has a full evaluation. The ED workup determines abnormal cardiac enzymes and abnormal electrocardiogram (ECG), and the patient must be admitted to rule out myocardial infarction.

> **BOX 92.2 ■ LEVELS OF PRESENTING PROBLEMS**
>
> **Minimal**
>
> A problem that may not require the presence of the physician, but service is provided under the physician's supervision. This is generally not applicable in the ED.
>
> **Self-limited or minor (99281)**
>
> A problem that runs a definite and prescribed course, is transient, and is not likely to permanently alter the health status or has a good prognosis with management/compliance.
>
> **Low severity (99282)**
>
> A problem where the risk of morbidity without treatment is low; there is little to no risk of mortality without treatment; full recovery without functional impairment is expected.
>
> **Moderate severity (99283)**
>
> A problem where the risk of morbidity without treatment is high to extreme; there is a moderate-to-high risk of mortality without treatment or a high probability of severe, prolonged functional impairment.
>
> **High severity, requires urgent evaluation by the physician but does not pose a threat to life or physiologic function (99284)**
>
> A problem where the risk of morbidity without treatment is high to extreme; there is a moderate-to-high risk of mortality without treatment or high probability of severe, prolonged functional impairment.
>
> **High severity, poses an immediate significant threat to life or physiologic function (99285)**
>
> A problem where the risk of morbidity without treatment is high to extreme; there is a moderate-to-high risk of mortality without treatment or high probability of severe, prolonged functional impairment

Medical necessity can still be supported by the CC/presenting problem even when, after testing, the diagnosis indicates a less significant problem, for example, a patient with chest pain who is diagnosed with indigestion and not a more severe cardiac-related problem after an extensive workup. The presenting problem can misrepresent the true acuity of the patient's problem for an ED service. The accurate judgment of the level of acuity comes after workup, which is indicated by a combination of the CC/presenting problem and the history and physical examination performed to identify the extent of the problem. The MDM is an indication of the physician's judgment of the severity of the patient's injury or illness determined through a review of each of these factors.

Chief Complaint

The CC is a concise statement describing the symptom, problem, condition, diagnosis, or any other factor that is the reason for the encounter, usually stated in the patient's own words.[1] The CC is one or more symptoms or concerns that prompt the patient to seek care in the ED. Symptoms or concerns include:

- Illness
- Injury
- Psychiatric conditions
- Normal bodily process that the patient or family member perceives as abnormal
- Patient's perception of the problem

Elements contained in the CC may also be used to score elements of the history of present illness, review of systems (ROS), and/or past medical, family, and social history (PFSH). The CC may be included in the history statement.[5] The significance of the CC cannot be overlooked when determining the level of MDM. The CC supports the medical necessity for an ED visit when one or more of the problems are urgent in nature, particularly when it supports the differential diagnoses and ED diagnostic tests and interventions.

History

The 1995 documentation guidelines state: The CC, ROS, and PFSH may be listed as separate elements of history, or they may be included in the description of the HPI.[5]

History of the Present Illness

The HPI is one of three components of the history element of an E/M service. The HPI is a chronological description of the development of the patient's present illness from the first sign and/or symptom to the present. It is an elaboration of the CC conducted by the clinician in order to determine the extent of the problem. Problems referenced in the history may also include the status of a chronic condition. The level of HPI is determined by identification of one or more of the following elements: location, quality, severity, timing, context, modifying factors, and associated signs and symptoms (significantly related to the presenting problem).[5]

Review of Systems

Review of systems is the second component of the history and is defined as, "an inventory of body systems obtained through a series of questions seeking to identify signs and/or symptoms that the patient may be experiencing or has experienced."[1] The ROS may be recorded by ancillary staff. To document that the physician reviewed the information, there must be a notation supplementing or confirming the information recorded by the staff. The 1995 Medicare documentation guidelines permit ancillary personnel in the ED to record the ROS and PFSH with physician confirmation. (The physician must personally record the HPI.[5])

The extent of the ROS for 99285 is a review of "at least 10 organ systems," according to Medicare guidelines. Those systems with positive or pertinent negative responses must be individually documented. For the remaining systems, a notation indicating "all other systems are negative" is permissible. In the absence of such a notation, at least 10 systems must be individually documented.[5]

The emergency physician determines the extent of the physical examination required to evaluate the patient from a combination of the elements shown in **Box 92.4**.

Past Medical, Family, and Social History

The three elements of past, family, and social history are grouped under the heading "Past Medical, Family and Social History (PFSH)" and are scored to determine the level of PFSH (**Box 92.3**). The PFSH level contributes to the determination of the overall history level of the E/M. The overall level of history is selected by the level determined as the lowest of the three components (HPI, ROS, and PFSH) as illustrated in **Table 92.3**.

Exception to 99285 Elements

In the ED setting, it is not uncommon for the patient's medical or mental condition to be compromised and prevent the physician from obtaining the required "key" components. Medicare 1995 documentation guidelines state: "If the physician is unable to obtain a history from the patient or other source, the record should describe the patient's condition or other circumstance which precludes obtaining a history."[5] The exception statement applies to any level history and not specifically to the 99285 as is outlined in CPT. Therefore, where the physician was unable to obtain portions of the history due to compromise of the patient's clinical condition and/or mental status and noted the required information was unobtainable, the recording of the patient condition may override the required elements of history.

BOX 92.3 ■ ELEMENTS OF THE PATIENT HISTORY

The *medical history* is defined as a review of the patient's prior experience with illness, injuries, and treatments including significant information about:

- Prior major illnesses and injuries
- Prior operations
- Prior hospitalizations
- Current medications
- Allergies (e.g., drug, food)
- Age-appropriate immunization status
- Age-appropriate feeding/dietary status

Family history is defined in CPT as a review of medical events in the patient's family, including significant information about:

- Health status or cause of death of parents, siblings, and children
- Specific diseases related to problems identified in the chief complaint (CC) or history of the present illness (HPI) and/or system review
- Diseases of family members that may be hereditary (heart disease, cancer, etc.) or that place the patient at risk

The *Social history* is defined in CPT as an age-appropriate review of past and current activities, including significant information about:

- Marital status and/or living arrangement
- Current employment
- Occupational history
- Use of drugs, alcohol, and tobacco
- Level of education
- Sexual history or preference
- Other relevant social factors

Other relevant *social factors* may include references to accommodations such as:

- Living arrangements (e.g., nursing home, homelessness, etc.)
- Social contacts, persons who sent or accompanied patient to ED
- For children the number of siblings, attendance at day care, grade in school, discussion about the child's primary caretaker (e.g., parents, grandparents, foster parents, etc.)
- History of domestic violence or abuse, and so on

Medical Decision-Making

Medical decision-making refers to the complexity of establishing a diagnosis and/or selecting a management option as measured by the elements of MDM (**Box 92.5**)[5]:

In order to determine an overall MDM score, each of the components of MDM that are discussed in this chapter will be scored.[5] To qualify for a given level of MDM, two of the three components (amount/complexity of data, number of diagnoses and management options,

TABLE 92.3 ■ 1995 Documentation Guidelines Scoring

Level of History	HPI	ROS	PFSH
99281	One to three elements	N/A	N/A
99282-99283	One to three elements	One organ system	N/A
99284	Four elements	Two organ systems	One from either past medical, social, or family history
99285	Four elements	Ten organ systems	Two from past medical, social, and/or family history

> **BOX 92.4 ■ ELEMENTS OF THE PHYSICAL EXAMINATION**
>
> **Body areas:**
>
> - Head, including face
> - Neck
> - Chest, including breasts and axillae
> - Abdomen
> - Genitalia, groin, buttocks
> - Back, including spine
> - Each extremity (each counts as one body area)
>
> **Organ systems:**
>
> - Constitutional (e.g., vital signs, general appearance) (Note: The constitutional organ system is not listed in CPT. It is unique to the 1995 documentation guidelines.)
> - Eyes
> - Ears, nose, mouth, and throat
> - Respiratory
> - Cardiovascular
> - Gastrointestinal
> - Genitourinary
> - Musculoskeletal
> - Skin
> - Neurologic
> - Psychiatric
> - Hematologic/lymphatic/immunologic

and risk) must meet or exceed the level of complexity (straightforward, low, moderate, or high) selected for each component.

Medical decision-making is scored by assigning a level to each element of MDM as illustrated in **Tables 92.1 and 92.2** and **Box 92.5**. Individual payer policy may determine the application of the "additional workup planned." However, as the ED provides a wide range of "workups" during the visit, the common interpretation is that less extensive workups are considered "no workup planned," with more extensive workups scored as "additional workup planned."

> **BOX 92.5 ■ ELEMENTS OF MEDICAL DECISION MAKING (MDM)**
>
> 1. The number of possible diagnoses and/or management options that must be considered. The diagnosis/management option element references the number and types of problems addressed during an encounter, the complexity of establishing a diagnosis, and the management decisions made by a physician. It may be illustrated by a differential diagnosis.
> 2. The amount and/or complexity of medical records, diagnostic tests, and/or other information that must be obtained, reviewed, and analyzed. Complexity increases with the decision to obtain and review old medical records and/or obtain history from sources other than the patient; ordering of diagnostic tests and/or the physician's interpretation of tests; discussion of contradictory or unexplained test results with the physician who performed or interpreted the tests; and/or direct visualization and independent interpretation of an image, tracing, or specimen.
> 3. The risk of significant complications, morbidity, and/or mortality as well as comorbidities associated with the patient's presenting problem(s), the diagnostic procedure(s), and/or the possible management options. The ""risk"" element of MDM includes elements often based on risks associated with the presenting problem(s), patient comorbidities, and underlying illnesses; the diagnostic procedure(s) ordered and/or performed, and the options of management of the problem.

Amount and Complexity of Data Reviewed

The level of complexity for each category can be determined by identifying the type of data reviewed during the ED visit. As referenced in CPT, "the actual performance and/or interpretation of diagnostic tests/studies ordered during a patient encounter are not included in the levels of E/M services. Physician performance of diagnostic tests/studies for which specific CPT codes are available may be reported separately, in addition to the appropriate E/M code."[6] The necessity for ordering and/or interpreting diagnostic tests indicates a higher level of acuity. The amount and complexity of data to be reviewed is based on the types of diagnostic testing ordered or reviewed. A decision to obtain and review old medical records and/or obtain history from sources other than the patient increases the amount and complexity of data to be reviewed.

Discussion of contradictory or unexpected test results with the physician who performed or interpreted the test is an indication of the complexity of data being reviewed. On occasion, the physician who ordered a test may personally review the image, tracing, or specimen to supplement information from the physician who prepared the test report or interpretation.

The level of risk is determined by the highest level scored in each of the three MDM risk subcategories. To determine the final MDM level, all components must be reviewed and scored by determining the final score for each of the three components and calculating the final score by the value that meets or exceeds the highest *two* values.

How Payers Determine Payment for ED Services

Payment for services is determined by individual payer policy. Often, the policy is uniformly determined by the type and place of service (Medicare) or may be determined by a fee schedule that assigns a payment amount to each service (Medicare, managed care, private payers). Although the fees that are assigned to each service should be uniformly assigned, payment will vary.

Medicare utilizes the Medicare Physician Fee Schedule, which is calculated and published annually by CMS.[7] The Medicare payment amount is determined by a calculation of the relative value unit (RVU) assigned to each service multiplied by a conversion factor dollar amount and adjusted by economic and regional factors. Medicaid generally assigns a flat rate to each service, which varies from one state to another. Managed care organizations and private payers may utilize contracted amounts that are either calculated independent of the amount charged by the provider or a percentage of the total fee.

Because payers can exercise little control over how subscribers utilize emergency services—and EDs are required by law to provide at minimum a medical screening examination—payers may default to identifying medical necessity to approve or deny payments. Medical necessity is defined differently by individual payers, so it is important for emergency physicians to provide detailed documentation for all of the following:

- Reason the patient came to the ED through the CC and reason for visit
- History and risk factors associated with the presenting problems
- Rationale for ordering and interpreting diagnostic tests, interventions such as intravenous fluids and medications, and disposition

Without providing a rationale for the service provided, emergency physicians may receive denials or reduction for payment of reasonable emergency services.

SURGICAL SERVICES

Current Procedural Terminology has established that certain services are always considered part of the surgery "package," although not always a component of the actual surgical operation. The correct coding initiative (CCI) edits build on the CPT policies to design edits that identify inappropriate code fragmentation in Medicare billing.[7] The purpose of the National Correct Coding Initiative (NCCI) edits is to prevent improper payment when incorrect code combinations are reported. The NCCI contains two tables of edits.

The "Column One/Column Two Correct Coding Edits" table and the "Mutually Exclusive Edits" table include code pairs that should not be reported together for a number of reasons explained in the NCCI Coding Policy Manual. The CCI edits follow CPT policies with a few exceptions while providing detailed information for each service to determine what services are included in each procedure "package." Medicare publishes a booklet that provides instructions for use of the CCI edits for both professional and facility coding.[8]

Emergency physicians provide a wide variety of surgical and diagnostic procedures that are determined by the E/M service and identify an injury and/or illness that requires surgical treatment. Payment for an E/M service with a surgical procedure requires that the physician document both services in detail to avoid packaging of the E/M service into the surgical payment. The "surgical package" concept is defined by the CPT as the services that are included in a given surgical procedure (**Box 92.6**).[1]

Medicare global surgery policy divides surgery into two distinct categories by the number of postoperative follow-up days assigned to each procedure package: 0, 10 days postoperative follow-up for minor procedures and 90 days postoperative follow-up for major surgical procedures. The global surgery concept differs from the CPT "surgical package definition," which applies one uniform package definition to the surgical procedures listed in CPT.[9]

Minor Surgical Procedures

Medicare defines minor surgeries as "000" or "010" postoperative days. Procedures with "000" days do not include postoperative follow-up beyond the day of the procedure. Procedures with "010" postoperative follow-up days include following up starting with the day of the procedure. Intraoperative services are those that are normally a usual and necessary part of the procedure. Visits by the same physician on the same day as minor surgery are included in the payment for the procedure unless a significant, separately identifiable service is also performed (e.g., full neurological examination for the patient with head trauma in addition to suturing a scalp wound).[9]

Billing for an E/M service in addition to the minor surgical procedure would not be appropriate if the physician only identified the need for sutures and confirmed the patient's allergy and immunization status. Services by other physicians are not included in the global fee for minor procedures.[10]

BOX 92.6 ■ SURGICAL PACKAGE CONCEPTS[1]

- Local infiltration, metacarpal/metatarsal/digital block, or topical anesthesia
- Subsequent to the decision for surgery, one related E/M encounter on the day immediately prior to or on the date of procedure (including history and physical) (Note: The ED visit is separate from the procedure as is necessary to determine)
- Immediate postoperative care, including dictating operative notes, talking with the family, and other physicians
- Writing orders (whether or not surgery is required, and if so, the type and extent)
- Evaluating the patient in the post anesthesia recovery area
- Typical postoperative follow-up care (clarified as normal, uncomplicated follow-up care)

Major Surgical Procedures

Medicare defines major surgeries as services requiring "090" postoperative days. For major procedures, the preoperative visit begins the day before the surgery. The intraoperative services are those considered a normal, usual, and necessary part of the procedure. An E/M service on the day before or the day of a major surgical procedure that results in the initial decision to perform the surgery is not included in the global surgery package for a major procedure. For the E/M service that determines the need for surgery, the –57 modifier is applied to E/M service. Medicare clarifies, "If evaluation and management services occur on the day of surgery, the physician bills using modifier –57, not –25."[9]

Medicare Policy on Procedure Codes and Modifiers

The use of modifiers for Medicare global surgery billing applies to major procedures with a 90-day postoperative period and minor procedures with a 10-day postoperative period. The modifier applicable to minor procedures with a "000" day postoperative period is modifier –25. When two physicians within the same practice each provide components of the global surgery package, they may not bill separately for visits or other services included in the global surgery package. For services provided by different physicians in a group practice where both participate in the care, the entire global surgical package is billed as long as the physicians reassign benefits to the group.

Physicians providing part of a global surgery package must agree on transfer of care if the operating surgeon (emergency physician in our case) refers the patient out to another physician for follow-up. The –54 modifier is required to denote that only the surgical care was provided by the physician performing the procedure. The physician providing follow-up care must affix the –55 modifier for postoperative management only. Both bills (surgical care only and postoperative care) must contain the same date of service distinguished by the applicable modifier. Both surgeon and physician providing postoperative care must keep a copy of the written transfer agreement in the beneficiary's medical record. Where a formal transfer of care does not occur, the occasional postdischarge services of a physician other than the surgeon are reported by the appropriate E/M code. No modifiers are necessary.

The emergency physician who performs the minor ED service ("000" or "010" day postoperative period) bills for the surgical procedure without a modifier. The physician who provides the follow-up for a minor procedure performed in the ED bills the appropriate level of office visit code.

When an underlying condition or medical complication requires a service during a postoperative period by a physician other than the surgeon, the physician providing follow-up care is required to report an E/M code without a modifier. Modifiers are not necessary when coding the unrelated follow-up care. The modifier rule for unrelated follow-up applies to both major and minor surgical procedures.

ENSURING ACCURACY WITH MODIFIERS

When a procedure is performed in the ED, modifiers may be required to differentiate the E/M service from the components of the procedure. In addition, if postoperative follow-up is referred outside the ED, additional modifiers may be required by the emergency physician and the physician providing the follow-up and may change depending on how the patient progresses through the follow-up period.

Modifier –25

Modifier –25 was established to identify E/M services on the day of a procedure for which separate payment may be made. Modifier –25 is used on the same day a procedure/service listed in CPT was performed and the patient's condition required a significant, separately identifiable E/M service above and beyond the other service provided or beyond the usual preoperative and postoperative care associated with the procedure. The E/M service may be prompted by the symptom or condition for which procedure and/or service was provided so separate diagnoses are generally not required.[1]

Medicare provides a similar instruction for the use of modifier –25 but instructs that it is not to be used to report the E/M service that results in a decision to perform surgery (see "Modifier –57" next).

Modifier –57

Modifier –57 is required for an E/M service resulting in the initial decision to perform surgery. Medicare guidelines for use of the –57 modifier are complex and the type of procedure (major 10- to 90-day follow-up or minor 0 days follow-up) determines when Modifier –57 is used.

Modifier –54

Modifier –54 is required when postoperative follow-up is referred by the emergency physician to another physician. The –54 modifier is required to be added to the surgical procedure[1]:

- For CPT, application of a modifier is required for ED surgical procedures when follow-up is provided by another physician.
- For Medicare, both the operating physician and follow-up physician must agree on the transfer of care when the -54 modifier is used by the operating surgeon (or, in our case, the emergency physician). The emergency physician would affix the –54 modifier to the code for the surgical procedure.

WOUND REPAIRS

Lacerations and wound repairs are the most common surgical procedures provided to ED patients. Wound repair encompasses three levels of complexity in CPT: simple, intermediate, and complex. Although most are found in the surgical/integumentary section of CPT (10000-19499), additional codes for full-thickness repair of lip, tongue, eyelids, and so on, can be found in the related anatomical sections, for example, lip (CPT codes 40650, 40652, 40654), vestibule of mouth (CPT codes 40830, 40831), and floor of mouth and tongue (CPT codes 41250, 41251, 41252). Wound repairs are classified as simple, intermediate, or complex and include wounds closed with sutures, staples, or tissue adhesives.[1]

Simple Repair

Superficial wounds involve primarily the epidermis, dermis, or subcutaneous tissues without significant involvement of deeper structures. Simple repair involves one-layer closure. Local anesthesia and chemical or electrocauterization of wounds not closed are included in the category of simple repair.

Intermediate Repair

Intermediate repairs are wounds requiring layered closure of one or more deeper layers of subcutaneous tissue and superficial (nonmuscle fascia) in addition to the skin (epidermal and dermal closure). Single-layer closure of heavily contaminated wounds requiring extensive cleaning or removal of particulate matter is also included in the intermediate repair category.

Complex Repair

Complex repairs require more than a layered closure and include scar revision, debridement of traumatic lacerations or avulsions, extensive undermining, stents, or retention sutures. Wounds in the complex repair category may include creation of a defect such as may be necessary for excision of a scar or the debridement of complicated lacerations or avulsions. Complex repair does not include excision of benign or malignant lesions (CPT codes 11400-11446) or malignant lesions (CPT codes 11600-11646), excisional preparation of a wound bed (CPT codes 15002-15005), or debridement of an open fracture or open dislocation.

Wound repair is further subdivided into body areas by classification as shown in **Box 92.7**.

Wounds should be measured and reported in centimeters by the physician. When reported in inches, a coder must convert the length from inches to centimeters, which often results in lost revenue to the practice. For example, Medicare assigns 5.53 RVUs to an intermediate facial laceration under 2.5 cm and 6.63 RVUs to a 2.5 to 5.0 cm intermediate facial laceration. A 1 cm difference equals a difference of 1.10 RVUs; 1 in equals 2.51 cm and 2 in equal 5.08 cm—a dramatic difference in payment if the documentation is not correct.[6]

When determining the length and body area of a wound repair, the coder must add together the lengths of those repairs from the same classification (i.e., intermediate repair of trunk and extremities) and from all anatomic sites that are grouped together into the same code descriptor. When multiple repairs of unrelated groupings are performed (i.e., face and extremities), it is not appropriate to add together the lengths but instead code and report each repair in order of complexity. Code debridement separately only if gross contamination is documented and it is performed as a meaningful and separately identifiable procedure. The

---

BOX 92.7 ■ WOUND REPAIR BODY-AREA SUBDIVISIONS

- Simple repairs of scalp, neck, axillae, external genitalia, trunk, and/or extremities including hands and feet
- Simple repairs of face, ears, eyelids, nose, lips, and/or mucous membranes
- Layered (intermediate) repairs of scalp, axillae, trunk, and/or extremities excluding hands and feet
- Layered (intermediate) repairs of neck, hands, feet, and/or external genitalia
- Layered (intermediate) repairs of face, ears, eyelids, nose, lips, and/or mucous membranes
- Repair complex trunk
- Repair complex scalp, arms, and/or legs
- Repair complex forehead, cheeks, chin, mouth, neck, axillae, genitalia, hands, and/or feet
- Repair complex eyelids, nose, ears, and/or lips

wound repair codes designate closure using sutures, staples, or tissue adhesives. Whether or not the wound is repaired singly or in combination with these repair materials, the repair codes may be used. However, if only adhesive strips are used for wound closure, an E/M level would be coded instead of a wound repair.

MUSCULOSKELETAL INJURIES

Procedures listed in the musculoskeletal section commonly performed in the ED define orthopedic procedures that are determined both by the types of fractures and the type of treatment performed. For the category of fractures, the terms in **Box 92.8** apply.[1]

Fractures

Fracture codes are surgical "global care" procedures and as such include related pre- and postoperative services in addition to the restorative procedure. A key consideration for coding orthopedic treatment in the ED is whether the treatment is similar to that provided by the orthopedist as clarified in CPT assistant, orthopedic "definitive care," or "restorative care." Use of these codes is only appropriate if the emergency physician is providing either restorative care (i.e., manipulating the bones back into place) or definitive care similar to that provided by the orthopedist. The emergency physician's overall management should be comparable to that provided by other physicians performing the same service.[10,11] To determine whether or not the emergency physician provided restorative care, consider the criteria in **Box 92.9**.

Fracture procedures commonly performed by emergency physicians include CPT codes shown in **Box 92.10**.

Dislocation, Subluxation, Strain, Sprain

Dislocation is defined as an injury to a joint causing the adjoining bone to separate. *Subluxation* is defined as a minor dislocation where joint surfaces touch, but not in normal relation to one another. A *strain* is a stretched or torn muscle. A *sprain* is defined as a stretched or

---

BOX 92.8 ■ FRACTURE CATEGORIES

- **Complete:** Bone is completely separated.
- **Incomplete:** ""Greenstick""–bone is not completely separated.
- **Comminuted:** There are mMore than two bone fragments.
- **Open (compound):** Bony fragments have penetrated through the skin.
- **Closed:** Skin has not been violated by the fractured bone.
- **Compression:** Break occurs from extreme pressure on the bone.
- **Impacted:** Broken ends of bone are driven into one another.

- **Avulsion:** Force applied to a strong tendon causes it to pull on and break off a portion of the bone.
- **Pathologic:** A break is caused by a minor injury in bone weakened or destroyed by disease.
- **Stress:** A crack in the bone is caused by repetitive and prolonged pressure.

The type of fracture does not correlate to the type of treatment. The following terms apply:

- **Closed:** The fracture site is not surgically opened.
- **Open:** The fracture site is surgically opened.

> **BOX 92.9 ■ CRITERIA FOR RESTORATIVE FRACTURE CARE**
>
> - Restorative care is treatment to repair, not just stabilize, an injury.
> - If the emergency physician immobilizes the injury and refers the patient to the orthopedist for the definitive/restorative care, the emergency physician has provided immobilization and comfort care and would not bill the orthopedic service. In instances where the emergency physician performs the evaluation and management service and the patient is followed up by another specialist for definitive care of the orthopedic injury, the emergency physician would select the E/M level, append the –25 modifier, and bill for the splint or strap application.
> - If manipulation is required, the treatment would be considered restorative and the emergency physician would bill for the orthopedic service. If the patient is sent to the orthopedist for follow-up, the emergency physician must affix the –54 to the orthopedic code (2XXXX) to indicate that the follow-up is being provided by a physician other than the physician who provided the restorative care.
> - If the fracture does not require manipulation and the emergency physician provides definitive care, which generally includes diagnosis of the fracture, pain management, and immobilization, the emergency physician would add the fracture care code for the service and append the –54 modifier.

torn ligament. Codes for these services are listed throughout the anatomic listing of the musculoskeletal section of CPT.[1] Dislocations commonly treated in the ED are shown in **Box 92.11,** though many other dislocation codes may be used.

Splinting and Strapping

It is appropriate to code for the application of a splint if the service is provided to stabilize, protect, or provide comfort. In the ED, these codes are generally used to define the initial application of the device when a surgical code for the restorative care is *not* billed. When billing for the surgical procedure, the application of a splint or strap is included in the

> **BOX 92.10 ■ CPT CODES FOR FRACTURE TREATMENTS**
>
> - **21310:** Closed treatment of nasal bone fracture; without manipulation
> - **23500:** Closed treatment of clavicular fracture; without manipulation
> - **25600:** Closed treatment of distal radial fracture (e.g., Colles or Smith type) or epiphyseal separation, with or without fracture of ulnar styloid; without manipulation
> - **26600:** Closed treatment of metacarpal fracture, single; without manipulation, each bone
> - **26605:** Closed treatment of metacarpal fracture, single; with manipulation, each bone
> - **26720:** Closed treatment of phalangeal shaft fracture, proximal or middle phalanx, finger, or thumb; without manipulation, each
> - **26750:** Closed treatment of distal phalangeal fracture, finger, or thumb; without manipulation, each
> - **28490:** Closed treatment of great toe fracture, phalanx or phalanges; without manipulation
> - **28510:** Closed treatment of fracture, phalanx or phalanges, other than great toe; without manipulation, each

> **BOX 92.11 ■ CPT CODES FOR DISLOCATION PROCEDURES**
>
> - **23650:** Closed treatment of shoulder dislocation, with manipulation; without anesthesia
> - **24640:** Closed treatment of radial head subluxation in child, nursemaid elbow, with manipulation
> - **26770:** Closed treatment of interphalangeal joint dislocation, single, with manipulation; without anesthesia
> - **21480:** Closed treatment of temporomandibular dislocation; initial or subsequent
> - **24600:** Treatment of closed elbow dislocation; without anesthesia
> - **27250:** Closed treatment of hip dislocation, traumatic; without anesthesia
> - **27265:** Closed treatment of post hip arthroplasty dislocation; without anesthesia
> - **27560:** Closed treatment of patellar dislocation; without anesthesia
> - **27840:** Closed treatment of ankle dislocation; without anesthesia

surgical package if performed by the physician applying the device. Because billing for the splint or strap defines a personal service by the emergency physician, it is necessary that the physician, not the ED nurse, applies the splint or strap. In some cases, the emergency physician only checks the placement of a splint or strap applied by a nurse. If the splint or strap is not personally applied by the emergency physician but the physician examines the placement and circulation in the affected body area, it may also be a billable service.

Local payer rules may place limits on coding for direct supervision of the placement by another clinician. Confirmation of individual payer rules for coding and billing for direct supervision of splint/strap application is advised. As with most additional procedures, the –25 should be applied to the E/M code when also reporting a splint or strapping code. Examples of splint application codes commonly used in the ED are offered in **Box 92.12**.

COMMON PROCEDURES

Incision and Drainage

An abscess is described as a painful, swollen lesion that requires drainage, often by incising the lesion. Treatment also may require the emergency physician to prescribe a course of antibiotics. In all cases, these procedures should be documented with a concise operative note to facilitate correct assignment of the code. CPT recognizes two levels of drainage and several incision procedures (**Box 92.13**).

Nail Procedures

Nail injuries are common to the ED and often result in multiple injuries to the nail and surrounding area. It is important to understand the rules for identification of the surgical

> **BOX 92.12 ■ CPT CODES FOR SPLINT APPLICATION**
>
> - **29105:** Application of long arm splint
> - **29125:** Application of forearm splint
> - **29130:** Application of finger splint
> - **29505:** Application of long leg splint
> - **29515:** Application of lower leg splint

> **BOX 92.13 ■ CPT CODES FOR INCISION AND DRAINAGE**
>
> **CPT recognizes two levels of drainage:**
>
> - Simple—limited treatment;, e.g., incision or minimal irrigation
> - Complicated—beyond limited treatment including debridement, packing, drain placement and/or probing to break loculations, etc.
>
> **Incision and drainage is a common ED service and that includes the following procedures:**
>
> - **10060:** Paronychia or furuncle
> - **10061:** Complex or multiple simple
> - **10080:** Pilonidal cyst simple
> - **10160:** Aspiration of abscess
> - **46050:** Perianal abscess
> - **46040:** Perirectal abscess
> - **42700:** Peritonsillar abscess
> - **56420:** Bartholin's gland abscess

process and the anatomic site treated. These codes are located throughout the CPT coding manual. Coding of nail injuries requires detailed documentation of the type and extent of injury (**Box 92.14**).

Removal of Foreign Body

Codes for the removal of foreign bodies (FBs) can be found in various anatomical sections of CPT, representing the areas of the body from which a FB might be removed. They include FB removal from the eye and skin as well as additional anatomical areas. Coding for the removal requires identification of the type of tissue (skin, muscle) and the type of removal.

> **BOX 92.14 ■ CPT CODES FOR NAIL INJURIES**
>
> - **CPT 11730:** Avulsion of nail plate, partial or complete, simple; single. An *avulsion* is the detachment of the nail from the nail bed. Part or all of the nail plate is removed or avulsed and generally requires local anesthesia. For total nail avulsion, the nail is separated totally from the underlying nail plate and the nail bed. The loosened nail is lifted and removed. For partial nail plate avulsion, the proximal nail fold is freed from the portion of nail to be removed and the portion to be avulsed is separated from the nail bed.
> - **CPT 11732:** Each additional nail plate is listed separately in addition to primary code.
> - **CPT 11740:** Evacuation of subungual hematoma. A *hematoma* results from a blunt injury to the nail. The procedure drains the blood by opening the nail plate. Evacuation usually involves boring a hole with a hot cautery pencil. Blunt injury may also result in damage to the nail matrix, which may include bony fragments.
> - **CPT 11760:** Repair of nail bed. Injury to the nail bed is often the result of blunt trauma and requires removal of the nail to permit suturing of the nail bed.
> - **CPT 10060:** Drainage of paronychia. This involves making an incision along the lateral nail fold to release a build up of purulent material.
> - **CPT 11750:** Excision of nail and nail matrix, partial or complete. Though commonly performed for severely deformed or ingrown nails, it is seldom performed in the ED. The ingrown portion of the nail is removed. The involved germinal matrix is then removed surgically by laser, electrocautery, or chemical techniques, which permanently destroy the portion of the nail.
> - **CPT 11765:** Wedge excision of skin of nail fold identifies removal of tissue from a hypertrophic or ingrown nail.

> **BOX 92.15 ■ CPT CODES FOR FOREIGN BODY REMOVAL**
>
> - **10120:** Subcutaneous simple
> - **10121:** Subcutaneous complex
> - **20520:** Muscle simple
> - **30300:** Intranasal
> - **42809:** Pharyngeal
> - **69200:** Ear auditory canal
> - **28190:** Foot subcutaneous
> - **28192:** Foot deep
> - **46608:** Anoscopy with foreign body removal
>
> Foreign bodies in the eye are differentiated by location, type, and removal method.
>
> - **65205:** Removal of foreign body, external eye, conjunctival superficial
> - **65210:** Conjunctival embedded (includes concretions), subconjunctival, or sclera nonperforating
> - **65220:** Corneal, without slit lamp
> - **65222:** Corneal, with slit lamp

Examples of FB removals performed in the ED are included in anatomical or procedure subsections of CPT. Foreign body removals commonly performed in the ED include the CPT codes in **Box 92.15**.

Nasal Procedures

Nasal procedures in the ED include simple and complex procedures for anterior and posterior nosebleeds (**Box 92.16**).

Digestive System Procedures

Procedures performed on the digestive system range from simple biopsies to the more complex laparoscopy, anoscopy, and tube changes (**Box 92.17**).

Lumbar Puncture

Lumbar punctures are common to the ED and should be coded when performed. When performed and documented appropriately, the following code may be used.

- CPT 62270 spinal puncture, lumbar, diagnostic

> **BOX 92.16 ■ CPT CODES FOR NASAL PROCEDURES**
>
> - **CPT 30300:** Removal of foreign body, intranasal, office type procedure
> - **CPT 30901:** Control nasal hemorrhage, anterior, simple (limited cautery and/or packing), any method
> - **CPT 30903:** Control nasal hemorrhage, anterior, complex (extensive cautery and/or packing), any method
> - **CPT 30905:** Control nasal hemorrhage, posterior, any method

> **BOX 92.17 ■ COMMON DIGESTIVE SYSTEM PROCEDURES**
>
> - **CPT 41250:** Repair of laceration 2.5 cm or less; floor of mouth and/or anterior two-thirds of tongue
> - **CPT 40800:** Drainage of abscess, cyst, hematoma, vestibule of mouth; simple
> - **CPT 42700:** Incision and drainage abscess; peritonsillar
> - **CPT 46050:** Incision of perianal abscess
> - **CPT 40650:** Repair lip full thickness, vermillion only
> - **CPT 46040:** Incision and drainage of ischiorectal and/or perirectal abscess (separate procedure)
> - **CPT 49080:** Peritoneocentesis, abdominal paracentesis, or peritoneal lavage (diagnostic or therapeutic); initial
> - **CPT 41800:** Drainage of abscess, cyst, hematoma from dentoalveolar structures
> - **CPT 43760:** Change of gastrostomy tube
> - **CPT 46600:** Anoscopy; diagnostic, with or without collection of specimen(s) by brushing or washing (separate procedure)
> - **CPT 46608:** Anoscopy; with removal of foreign body

Ear Procedures

Impacted ear wax and ear FBs are common ED problems and can be coded if documented. When wax is truly impacted, its removal should be reported with 69210 if performed by a physician using at minimum an otoscope and instruments such as wax curettes. The following codes may be used.

- CPT 69200: Removal of FB from external auditory canal; without general anesthesia
- CPT 69200: Removal of impacted cerumen using irrigation/ lavage, unilateral
- CPT 69210: Removal impacted cerumen (separate procedure), one or both ears

INTERPRETING DIAGNOSTIC TESTS

Payment for these commonly performed services varies by payer.

ECGs

Medicare will pay for interpretations of ECGs ordered by an emergency MD. The Office of Inspector General memorandum states the payment should be made to the physician on whose interpretation the diagnosis and treatment is based and not to a subsequent interpreter; however, some emergency physicians have chosen not to bill for ECG interpretations.[12] ACEP provides several excellent online resources for interpreting ECGs and x-rays.

There is currently no definitive description of what constitutes a formal interpretation by the emergency physician. It is minimally defined by CMS as a notation in the ED record which addresses the findings, relevant clinical issues, and diagnosis. The documented interpretation should be similar to what a cardiologist would provide. Providers should be aware of practice and individual payer's policy when determining whether to code for an ECG interpretation (**Box 92.18**).

BOX 92.18 ■ CODING FOR ECG INTERPRETATION

When indicated as appropriate to code, the provider should ensure that the emergency physician actually provided an interpretation. To ensure that the interpretation follows objective criteria, the documentation should include two or more of the following:

- Rate
- Rhythm intervals
- Axis
- ST elevation
- T waves
- Acute or chronic changes
- Clinical findings and/or diagnosis as part of the interpretative note

Examples of common interpretation:

- Sinus tachycardia, rate 120, nonspecific ST-T changes; no acute ischemia noted, no ECG available for comparison
- Sinus bradycardia; rate 44, left-axis deviation; no significant changes when compared to prior ECG
- Normal sinus rhythm with rate of 72; PR and QRS intervals within normal limits; elevated T waves in II, III, and aVF. Acute inferior wall myocardial infarction.
- Normal sinus rhythm rate 86 with nonspecific ST changes, normal intervals

Do not code for ECG or rhythm strip interpretation if the physician merely notes, "ECG-normal or negative."

The diagnosis code must establish the medical necessity of an ECG. If diagnosis coding is not precise or if the medical record does not support a diagnosis code, some carriers will consider the ECG "routine" and deny payment for ECG interpretation. It is appropriate to report signs and symptoms (e.g., shortness of breath, fatigue, dizziness, chest pain) to indicate medical necessity when documented in the chart as a patient complaint or problem. Where documented, code a history of cardiac problems.

Coding for ECG interpretations is still a state/payer-specific issue. The issue of "over read payment" (payment to cardiologist) requires research of the individual payer policies to understand the implications for the emergency medicine group and the cardiologists. In addition, specific clients have specific prohibitions about billing for interpretations of ECG and rhythm strips.

X-Rays

Payment for emergency physician interpretation of x-rays is specific to individual payers. The emergency physician must provide an individual, personal interpretation of the x-ray, and it is suggested that documentation includes comments about two or more of the items in **Box 92.19.**

BOX 92.19 ■ ITEMS TO NOTE REGARDING X-RAYS

- Detailed description of findings
- Specific location of imaged organ or area
- Number of views
- Quality of study
- Pertinent positive and negative findings
- Recommendations for other studies or treatment
- Clinical impression or diagnosis as part of the interpretative note

It is not appropriate to code for an interpretation when the physicians merely states, "x-ray negative for fracture." Some examples of acceptable x-ray interpretations are:

- PA and lateral chest, two views, negative for infiltrate with no cardiomegaly or masses noted
- AP and upright abdomen, two views, bowel gas pattern, no ileus obstruction, air-fluid levels, or free air
- Right thumb, two views, fracture of distal tuft with soft-tissue swelling, no FB noted, no other body deformities noted

When coding for x-ray interpretation by the emergency physician, the –26 modifier must be applied to the x-ray procedure code. Application of the –26 modifier denotes the service as a "professional component" only and excludes the technical service of preparing and developing the film for payment purposes. Individual client policy will determine how x-ray interpretations will be identified and billed. Although there is currently no definitive description of what constitutes a formal interpretation by the emergency physician, it is minimally defined by CMS as a notation in the ED record, which addresses the findings, relevant clinical issues, and diagnosis. A simple review of the radiologist's findings by the emergency physician does not constitute a separately billable interpretation (such a review is included in the E/M service). The ED provider should be encouraged to sign or initial the interpretation note to avoid confusion about who actually provided the interpretation. The ACEP addresses emergency interpretations of ECG and x-ray on its website. Also provided is an information packet with historical documents outlining the various clarifications provided by Medicare and other payers.

DIAGNOSIS CODING

Diagnosis coding illustrates the reason and medical necessity for the services performed in the ED. The *International Classification of Diseases, 10th Edition (ICD-10)* is designed to promote international comparability in the collection, processing, classification, and presentation of mortality statistics.[13] The reported conditions are translated into medical codes through use of the classification structure and the selection and modification rules contained in the *ICD-10* code list, which is published by the World Health Organization. These coding rules improve the usefulness of statistics by categorizing condition into categories. The *ICD* has been revised periodically to incorporate changes in the medical field. To date, there have been 10 revisions of the *ICD*.[13]

Application of ICD-10-CM

For diagnosis coding to accurately capture the range of conditions affecting care, the physician must document presenting problems, CC, history, treatment, differential diagnoses, and final diagnosis. These entries are then converted into diagnosis codes through application of the ICD-10 coding policies. As emergency physicians treat acute problems, coding in the ED often prioritizes the presenting problems to underscore medical necessity.

Determining when a symptom, definitive diagnosis, or both should be coded can be challenging for coding professionals. The challenge of coding for symptoms and/or definitive diagnoses is complicated by the varying rules regarding the coding of symptoms versus definitive diagnoses and according to the type of encounter and the particular service rendered. With increased focus/abuse and regulatory compliance, it is especially important for coding professionals to understand and properly apply official coding rules and guidelines.

Conditions Integral to Disease Processes

Conditions that are integral to a disease process should not be assigned as additional codes. For example, nausea and vomiting should not be coded in addition to gastroenteritis; wheezing should not be coded in addition to a diagnosis of asthma. Conditions that may not be associated routinely with a disease process should be assigned additional codes. In the inpatient setting, if a diagnosis documented at the time of discharge is qualified as "probable," "suspected," "likely," "questionable," "possible," or "rule out," the condition should be coded as if it existed or was established. The basis for rule-out guidelines are the diagnostic workup, arrangements for further workup or observation, and initial therapeutic approach that corresponds most closely with the established diagnosis.

In the ED setting, diagnoses documented as "probable," "suspected," "questionable," or "rule out" should not be coded as if they are established. Rather, the conditions should be coded to the highest degree of certainty for that encounter, such as symptoms, signs, abnormal test results, or other reason for the visit. For example, if the physician documents "fever and cough, possible pneumonia" at the conclusion of an ED visit, only the fever and cough should be coded, because those symptoms represent the highest degree of certainty for that encounter. However, if the physician documents "fever and cough, possible pneumonia" on a requisition for an outpatient chest x-ray, and the radiologist's diagnosis on the radiology report is "pneumonia," it is appropriate to code the pneumonia, as a diagnosis of pneumonia represents the highest degree of certainty for the encounter for the x-ray. Based on *Coding Clinic for ICD-10-CM*, it is appropriate to code based on the physician documentation available at the time of code assignment.[14]

With the transition to *ICD-10*, there is a higher need for specificity in diagnosis reporting. Providers should report diagnoses to the highest level of specificity including laterality, chronicity, etiology, specific location, and so on. For example, the diagnosis of "anterior chest pain of unknown etiology" is much better than "unspecified chest pain." Please refer to the Official Guidelines for Coding and Reporting in the current *ICD-10-CM* book for full instructions.

CONCLUSION

Emergency physicians should be aware of the available clarifications on the services they provide to avoid compliance and/or revenue problems. Certainly, the most frequently billed ED services should be documented and reported correctly.

REFERENCES

1. *American Medical Association. CPT 2020: Professional Edition*. Chicago, IL: AMAStore.com; 2019.

2. American College of Emergency Physicians (ACEP). Top 20 reimbursement codes. Available at: https://www.acep.org/administration/reimbursement/top-20-ed-reimbursement-codes/. Updated January 11, 2016. Accessed August 27, 2018.

3. Centers for Medicare and Medicaid Services. Evaluation and management documentation training tool. National Government Services 1074_0317. Accessed October 23, 2020.

4. First Coast Service Options, Inc. E/M interactive worksheet. First Coast. 2017. Available at: https://medicare.fcso.com/SharedTools/faces/EMWorksheet_en.jspx;jsessionid=7oZaYW_Z7sY28UKjMKeE2eQ3BbmnkhLe_MeYeqzvtBPlFDjZ8Mp9!-1701045669?_lob=&_state=. Accessed August October 24, 2020.

5. Centers for Medicare and Medicaid Services. Evaluation and management services guide. Medicare Learning Network. 2017. Available at: https://www.CMS.gov. Accessed November 14, 2020.

6. American Academy of Family Physicians. Coding and Documentation—Answers to Your Questions. Published 2003. Available at: https://www.aafp.org/fpm/2003/0200/p23.html#:~:text=Yes%2C%20as%20long%20as%20the,levels%20of%20E%2FM%20services. Accessed October 23, 2020.

7. Centers for Medicare and Medicaid Services. Medicare physician fee schedule. Available at: https://www.cms.gov/Medicare/Medicare-Fee-for-Service-Payment/PhysicianFeeSched/index.html. Accessed October 24, 2020.
8. Centers for Medicare and Medicaid Services. 2018 National Correct Coding Initiative Coding Policy Manual for Medicare Services (Coding Policy Manual). 2020. Available at: https://www.cms.gov/Medicare/Coding/NationalCorrectCodInitEd. Accessed October 24, 2020.
9. Centers for Medicare and Medicaid Services. 40.1–Definition of a global surgical package. *Medicare Claims Processing Manual*. Chapter 12. Revision 4431. 2019. Available at: https://cms.gov/Regulations-and-Guidance/Guidance/Manuals/Downloads/Clm104c12.pdf. Accessed October 24, 2020.
10. American Medical Association. Application of casts and strapping guidelines broadened. *AMA CPT® Assistant*. 1996;2:3–4.
11. American Medical Association. Reporting fracture and restorative care and dislocations. *AMA CPT® Assistant*. 2018;1:3–5.
12. Health Care Financing Administration. *Medicare Program; Revisions to Payment Policies and Adjustments to the Relative Value Units Under the Physician Fee Schedule for Calendar Year 1996*. Department of Health and Human Services Federal Register. 1995;Vol. 60:236. Available at: https://www.govinfo.gov/content/pkg/FR-1995-12-08/pdf/X95-11208.pdf#page=55. Accessed October 23, 2020.
13. National Center for Health Statistics. *International Classification of Diseases, Tent Revision (ICD-10)*. 2020. Available at: https://www.cdc.gov/nchs/icd/icd10.htm. Accessed October 24, 2020.
14. American Hospital Association. AHA Coding Clinic. 2019. Available at: https://www.codingclinicadvisor.com/about-us#:~:text=Clinic%20for%20HCPCS.-, AHA%20Coding%20Clinic%20for%20ICD%2D10%2DCM%20and%20ICD%2D, NCHS)%20and%20the%20Centers%20for. Accessed October 24, 2020.

CHAPTER 93

ADVANCED BILLING AND CODING

Michael A. Granovsky

> *Reimbursement is a major determinant of how medicine is practiced. When reimbursement changes, so do medical practice and medical education.*
>
> —Dean Ornish[1]

Chapter 92, Introduction to Coding, laid the foundation for the essential items that form the backbone of emergency department (ED) coding—in particular the assignment of the basic 99281 to 99285 evaluation and management (E/M) codes and the Medicare documentation guidelines. Further building on that content, this chapter provides the tools necessary to lead and manage a group successfully in the complex world of coding, compliance, and reimbursement.

DEFINING CRITICAL CARE

Emergency physicians often undervalue their services, failing to adequately document the provision of critical care, which results in lost revenue opportunities. Critical care differs from the 9928x codes discussed in Chapter 92. In contrast to the "bean counting" documentation of the elements of history of the present illness (HPI) and the review of systems (ROS) and the like, critical care is a time-based service.

Critical care is a time-based code that is different than the construct of the more familiar 99281 to 99285 codes covered in Chapter 92. Current Procedural Terminology (CPT) code 99291 describes the first 30 to 74 minutes of critical care.[2] In the last several years, the clinical/coding definition of critical care has been loosened. Initially, patients had to be frankly unstable, and then in later years, they could be potentially unstable. Importantly, the CPT definition for critical care now simply includes the concept that there is a high probability of imminent deterioration in the patient's condition:

> *A critical illness or injury acutely impairs one or more vital organ systems such that there is a high probability of imminent or life-threatening deterioration in the patient's condition....*[3]

The CPT goes on to provide the following detail regarding organ failure:

> *Examples of vital organ system failure include, but are not limited to: central nervous system failure; circulatory failure; shock; renal, hepatic, metabolic, and/or respiratory failure.*[3]

This redefining of critical care allows additional patients to meet the criteria. Now, patients typically qualifying for critical care frequently include:

- Chest pain patients who are at high risk and require sequential nitroglycerin, those with electrocardiogram (ECG) changes, active angina, unstable angina, or acute myocardial infarction (MI)
- Dyspnea patients with concerning vital signs that require aggressive interventions such as multiple nebulizer treatments, high-flow oxygen, and close monitoring, and a clinical condition such as severe asthma, pneumonia, and congestive heart failure
- Severe metabolic derangements like diabetic ketoacidosis or renal failure

Time Requirements

In addition to the patient meeting the definition of "having a critical illness or injury," the physician must deliver a minimum of 30 minutes of critical care outside of separately billable procedures. These sicker patients frequently require 30 minutes of care, including:

- Direct bedside care of the patient
- Review of lab and radiology results
- Gathering a history from family, emergency medical services, and old records
- Discussion of the patient's case with other physicians
- Time spent documenting the record
- Time spent on bundled procedures, such as reading x-rays, interpreting pulse oximetry, ordering blood draws, and inserting peripheral IV catheters

Case Studies

The following case studies illustrate some of the potential critical care patients' emergency physicians care for each and every shift (**Box 93.1**).

Case One

A 30-year-old woman is brought to the ED with supraventricular tachycardia. Her heart rate is 190 beats/minute and blood pressure is 80/60 mm Hg. She is complaining of chest pain and appears in distress. The physician considers electrical cardioversion but feels

---

BOX 93.1 ■ POTENTIAL CRITICAL CARE PRESENTATIONS

- Unstable vital signs
- Arrhythmias requiring urgent treatment (atrial fibrillation [Afib] with rapid ventricular rate [RVR])
- Hypertensive emergencies requiring vasoactive medications
- Severe respiratory distress (chronic obstructive pulmonary disorder [COPD], asthma, congestive heart failure [CHF])—may need bilevel positive airway pressure (BiPAP) or continuous positive airway pressure (CPAP)
- Hemorrhagic stroke
- Sepsis
- Diabetic ketoacidosis
- Severe hyperkalemia
- Acute renal failure
- Multiple trauma
- Pneumothorax
- Anaphylaxis or severe allergic reaction
- Status epilepticus

chemical conversion with adenosine is warranted. After a second dose of adenosine, the patient converts to sinus tachycardia. Her lab results, including thyroid-stimulating hormone and D-dimer tests, are normal. The physician documents several repeat assessments as well as a follow-up ECG, and ultimately, the patient is discharged. The physician states that 30 minutes of critical care were delivered, including time devoted to multiple bedside assessments, review of the labs, a discussion to arrange close follow-up with the primary care physician (PCP), and documentation of the record.

Does this discharged patient qualify for critical care? The physician felt that the patient met the criteria for "imminent danger of deterioration," which is a clinical judgment based on the patient's extremely high heart rate, hypotension, and chest pain.

Case Two

A 55-year-old man presents to the ED complaining of 7/10 chest pain. His history is significant for hypertension, and his blood pressure is 215/117 mm Hg. He has had no previous cardiac evaluation. Initial ECG shows depressed T waves. He is given aspirin, and his chest pain is sequentially relieved after three sublingual nitroglycerin tablets. The physician documents his active presence at the bedside, managing both the chest pain and blood pressure. Cardiac enzymes are normal. Once the chest pain is relieved, the patient receives additional treatment with nitro paste and enoxaparin (Lovenox) and is ultimately admitted to a telemetry bed with a diagnosis of unstable angina.

This patient did not seem to be having an acute MI. Does the clinical presentation described qualify for critical care? Based on the patient's risk factors, severe hypertension, presenting problem, and required treatment, the physician demonstrated that the man was in "imminent danger of deterioration."

Case Three

An 18-month-old child is brought to the ED with a croupy cough, a respiratory rate of 42, and a low-grade temperature. The physician notes moderate-to-severe stridor when the child is crying and residual stridor, significant tachypnea, and retractions at rest. The child is managed with dexamethasone and two racemic epinephrine nebulizer treatments. Following the second nebulizer treatment, the child remains tachypneic but is more comfortable. The physician performs several repeat assessments over the next few hours and also interprets a chest x-ray as normal. The child continues to improve and is discharged several hours later with diagnoses of croup, fever, and tachypnea.

This case demonstrates that the requirements for critical care—a patient in "imminent danger of deterioration" and 30 minutes of physician care—do not necessarily include admission or intravenous medications.

Documentation Requirements

What are the documentation requirements for critical care and are the requirements similar to the documentation rules utilized for the regular ED codes 99281 to 99285? While the standard ED E/M codes 99281 to 99285 have strict bullet-counting documentation requirements, as described in the 1995 documentation guidelines, the same criteria do not apply to critical care.[4] Critical care is the only time-based code used in the ED. The chart should reflect and support that the patient's condition was "critical" and that a minimum of 30 minutes of care was delivered. The typical requirements for HPI, ROS, and other documentation elements do not apply.

> **BOX 93.2 ■ COMMON PROCEDURES TYPICALLY BUNDLED WITH CRITICAL CARE**
>
> - Interpretation of cardiac output measurements: 93561, 93562
> - Chest x-rays: 71045, 71046
> - Pulse oximetry: 94760, 94761, 94762
> - Blood gases and information data stored in computers (e.g., ECGs, blood pressures, hematologic data): 99090
> - Gastric intubation: 43752, 43753
> - Temporary transcutaneous pacing: 92953
> - Ventilatory management: 94002 to 94004, 94660, 94662
> - Vascular access procedures 36000, 36410, 36415, 36591, 36600

Procedures

Certain common procedures are bundled with critical care and may not be reported separately but will count toward the 30-minute requirement (**Box 93.2**). The CPT goes on to state that any additional procedure may be billed: "Any services performed that are not included in this listing should be reported separately" (**Box 93.3**).[3] Providers should remember to subtract the time spent performing separately billed procedures from critical care time. What are the issues governing the reporting of cardiopulmonary resuscitation (CPR) and critical care? CPR may be billed in addition to critical care under certain circumstances. Since CPR (92950) is a separate procedure, the physician must subtract out the time spent overseeing and directing it. If the patient is given CPR the entire time, it will not be possible to meet the 30-minute requirements for 99291.

Clinical presentations that typically qualify for both critical care and CPR include those patients who have resumption of vital signs and end up requiring ongoing care with multiple interventions, vasoactive medications, and admission to a critical care unit for ongoing care.

Additional Time Units

What if substantially more than 30 minutes of critical care is delivered? The CPT allows the reporting of care in various time increments. The first hour runs from 30 to 74 minutes. Additional units of care are reported with the add-on code 99292 (**Table 93.1**).

Most templated documentation formats or electronic documentation systems have either a check box or an area to enter the total critical care time. Physicians should document in the chart the total duration of time spent caring for the critically ill or injured patient, even if the time spent by the physician on that date is not continuous. Best practice includes substantial case-specific detail and several bedside patient assessments.

> **BOX 93.3 ■ COMMON PROCEDURES BILLED IN ADDITION TO CRITICAL CARE**
>
> - Intubation
> - Central venous access
> - Chest tube
> - Pericardiocentesis
> - Transvenous pacemaker placement
> - CPR and ECGs

TABLE 93.1 ■ Time Increments for Critical Care

Total Duration	Codes
<30 min	Appropriate E/M codes
30-74 min (30 min to 1 h 14 min)	99291 X 1
75-104 min (1 h 15 min to 1 h 44 min)	99291 X 1 and 99292 X 1
105-134 min (1 h 45 min to 2 h 14 min)	99291 X 1 and 99292 X 2
135-164 min (2 h 15 min to 2 h 44 min)	99291 X 1 and 99292 X 3
165-194 min (2 h 45 min to 3 h 14 min)	99291 X 1 and 99292 X 4
195 min or longer (3 h 15 min, etc.)	99291 and 99292 as appropriate

BOX 93.4 ■ CRITICAL CARE REIMBURSEMENT PEARL

Increasing your critical care by just 2% yields over $45,000 in collectible money for a 45,000 visit ED.

45,000 × 0.02 = 900 patients/year

Reimbursement gain moving from 99285 to 99291 is ~$50

900 patients × $50/patient = $45,000

Critical Care Benchmarks

What is a good benchmark for the amount of critical care that should be billed? This varies based on the acuity of the practice. Practice parameters, which generally support a higher reporting of critical care services, include tertiary care referral facilities, level 1 trauma centers, higher percent of Medicare patients, and more patients arriving by ambulance. Many highly functioning ED groups average 4% to 6% (**Box 93.4**).

Medicare-published benchmark data are available by state for the reporting of critical care 99291 (**Table 93.2**).[5] One should keep in mind that Medicare patients are more likely to require critical care services than the average patient (**Table 93.3**).

TABLE 93.2 ■ Sample Medicare Critical Care Utilization by State

State	99291
Alabama	6.4%
California (N)	6.7%
California (S)	10.2%
Florida	8.0%
Maryland	7.4%
Texas	7.4%
National average	6.9%

TABLE 93.3 ■ Summary of Observation Coding Scenarios

Level of Care	Care Covers 2 Days	Same-Day Care
1	99218 + 99217	99234
2	99219 + 99217	99235
3	99220 + 99217	99236

OBSERVATION SERVICES

More and more emergency physicians are being asked to evaluate opportunities for involvement in ongoing and longitudinal patient care in the form of providing observation services. This step, outside the traditional role of providing unscheduled episodic care, requires an understanding of the regulatory, documentation, coding, and reimbursement processes that govern how observation care is provided and reimbursed.

These observation codes differ from the more traditional 9928x services. Patients must be designated as being placed in "observation" to use codes from this range. There must be a timed provider order in the chart stating: "Admit to/Place patient in observation." Patients in observation are outpatients because they have not been formally admitted to the hospital. Observation is considered a status, not a location. The hospital does not have to have a separate observation unit to report observation codes.

General Premise and Requirements of Observation Care

The goal of typical observation care is to determine the need for inpatient admission. This is substantiated by the following Centers for Medicare and Medicaid Services (CMS) memoranda:

- "Observation care is a well-defined set of specific, clinically appropriate services, which include ongoing short-term treatment, assessment, and reassessment, that are furnished while a decision is being made regarding whether patients will require further treatment as hospital inpatients or if they are able to be discharged from the hospital."[6]
- "Observation services are those services furnished on a hospital's premises, including use of a bed and periodic monitoring by nursing or other staff, which are reasonable and necessary to evaluate an outpatient's condition or determine the need for a possible admission as an inpatient."[6]

One of the key, and often confounding, requirements involves the need for a prospective order to admit the patient to observation status. As per CMS, "Such services are covered only when provided by order of a physician or another individual authorized by state licensure law and hospital bylaws to admit patients to the hospital or to order outpatient tests..."[6] Based on the premise that observation status is warranted to determine the need for inpatient admission, there are two categories of patients who typically qualify

> **BOX 93.5 ■ POTENTIAL OBSERVATION CANDIDATES**
>
> - Asthma
> - Congestive heart failure
> - Chest pain
> - Abdominal pain
> - Renal calculi
> - Croup
> - Vaginal bleeding
> - Dehydration
> - Syncope
> - Allergic reactions
> - Drug ingestion or overdose
> - Alcohol intoxication

for observation: diagnostic uncertainty and therapeutic intensity. **Box 93.5** lists a more global (though not exclusive) list of potential observation candidates.

Observation Code Sets

The observation codes are broken into two sets: all services that occur on a single calendar day and observation services that cross two calendar days. The same-day admit and discharge codes are defined as follows:

- 99234—low severity
    - Low-complexity medical decision-making (MDM)
- 99235—moderate severity
    - Moderate-complexity MDM
- 99236—high severity
    - High-complexity MDM

If the care takes place on two calendar days, the following codes are utilized:

- Initial day
    - 99218—low severity
        - Low-complexity MDM
    - 99219—moderate severity
        - Moderate-complexity MDM
    - 99220—high severity
        - High-complexity MDM
- Discharge day
    - 99217—observation care discharge

If the patient has an observation stay of greater than two calendar days, the "middle days" (technically referred to as "subsequent days") are reported with the codes listed below:

- 99224—subsequent observation care, per day
    - Low complexity
- 99225—subsequent observation care, per day
    - Moderate complexity
- 99226—subsequent observation care, per day
    - High complexity

TABLE 93.4 ■ Observation Documentation Requirements				
Service	CPT	History	Physical	MDM
Observation discharge	99217	+	+	+
Observation level 1	99218	D or C	D or C	S or L
Observation level 2	99219	C	C	M
Observation level 3	99220	C	C	H
Same-day obs/discharge 1	99234	D or C	D or C	S or L
Same-day obs/discharge 2	99235	C	C	M
Same-day obs/discharge 3	99236	C	C	H

Abbreviations: D, detailed; C, comprehensive; S, straightforward; L, low; M, moderate; H, high.

Observation Documentation Requirements

The observation service codes are governed by the same Medicare (1995 documentation guidelines) and CPT principles (**Table 93.4**) as the previously discussed 9928x codes:

- **D**—Detailed
- **C**—Comprehensive
- **S**—Straightforward
- **L**—Low
- **M**—Moderate
- **H**—High

All but the lowest-level observation codes require a comprehensive history and physical examination (PE).

Documentation Pearl

The higher-level observation codes require a complete past, family, and social history. Stated differently, a comprehensive history for the observation code set requires that all three elements of history are addressed—past, family, and social. That is different from the 9928x ED codes, for which a comprehensive history (e.g., to support 99285) only requires two of the three. Observation codes typically require either a detailed or comprehensive history and PE. Applying the Medicare 1995 Diagnosis-Related Groups yields the following:

- Detailed history and PE for 99218 and 99234
  - HPI: four elements
  - Past family and social history (PFSHx): one area
  - ROS: two systems
  - PE: five to seven organ systems/areas
- Comprehensive history and PE 99219/99220/99235/99236
  - HPI: four elements
  - PFSHx: three areas
  - ROS: 10 systems
  - PE: eight organ systems

- The observation discharge code 99217 has its own documentation requirements:
  - At the conclusion of observation, a summary, including an appropriate evaluation
  - Summary of the clinical course in the unit
  - MDM diagnosis reached
  - Discharge, or admit, discussion of continuing care, and follow-up plans

Additionally, observation stays require progress notes to demonstrate patient monitoring and response to treatment. Documentation best practices include:

- Documentation of comprehensive or detailed history and PE
- An order to "place in observation" or "provide observation care" with time and date
- Notation of medical necessity and risk stratification
- Treatment plan
- Progress notes for ongoing care
- Discharge note

Observation Cases

The two cases below demonstrate appropriate use of observation status. In each, a more prolonged evaluation requires care beyond that which can be provided in the ED is initiated, and yet expensive and unnecessary hospital admission is avoided.

Case Study: One-Day Stay

A 26-year-old woman presents to the ED at 8 am with shortness of breath and wheezing. She reports recent cold symptoms and a history of allergy-induced asthma but is not currently on inhaled steroids. Examination reveals diffuse wheezing throughout. She receives oral (PO) prednisone and several nebulizer treatments with minimal improvement. A formal dated and timed order is written, and the patient is placed in observation status for continued treatment. A chest x-ray is performed but reveals no focal infiltrates. After several additional rounds of nebulizer treatments, she gradually improves as reflected in the physician's progress notes. At 9:30 pm, the physician writes a discharge order and a short summary of the observation stay, noting that the final PE revealed clear lungs and outlining a plan for continued PO steroids with PCP follow-up.

This physician documented a comprehensive history and PE, a timed admit to observation order, several progress notes, and a brief discharge summary. The patient's clinical course would typically reflect moderate MDM, and the code 99235 is assigned.

Case Study: Two-Day Stay

On January 1st at 6 pm, a 56-year-old man presents to the ED with burning chest pain. He has a history of hypertension and is a heavy smoker. He is treated with sublingual nitroglycerin, and a full cardiac workup is initiated. The initial ECG demonstrates nonspecific ST-segment changes, and the patient's chest pain is relieved with a single dose of nitroglycerin. At 10 pm, he is placed in observation, and a formal order is documented in the record. His treatment plan includes two additional sets of cardiac enzyme tests and continued monitoring. Several progress notes are documented overnight showing that the patient is pain-free and serial ECGs reveal no acute changes. The next morning at 8 am, he undergoes a thallium stress test, which is normal. At 10 am, the physician documents a summary of the man's stay and plans for an outpatient gastrointestinal evaluation. A formal discharge order is also documented.

This physician has documented a comprehensive history and PE, a timed admit to observation order, several progress notes, and a discharge summary with plan. The patient's clinical course would typically reflect high MDM. The code 99220 is assigned for January 1st, and the code 99217 is assigned for the discharge on January 2nd.

Observation Billing Issues

Observation billing generally mandates that if the same physician provides the ED care and the observation care, then the ED services become a bundled and nonreportable component of the observation services. According to CPT:

> *Observation status that is initiated in the course of an encounter in another site of service (e.g., hospital emergency department, office, nursing facility) all evaluation and management services provided by the supervising physician in conjunction with initiating the observation status are considered part of the initial observation care when provided on the same date.*[7]

The term "same physician" has been interpreted by CMS to include all physicians of the same specialty reporting services under the same tax identification (ID) number. As a result, the observation codes are typically reported in place of the ED codes when the same providers are involved. Complex tax ID number configurations are beyond the scope of this chapter; however, providers interested in setting up independent observation groups are advised to seek advice from experienced health-care counsel.

Observation Reimbursement Issues

Observation services are typically valued at roughly 1.3 relative value units (RVUs) more than the comparable 9928x codes.[8] Note that the full reimbursement for a 2-day observation stay is determined by adding the initial day observation RVUs (99218 to 99220) to the discharge code 99217.

Financial Issues

Although the observation services are assigned higher RVU values than the ED codes, if the group must add new full-time equivalent (FTE) clinicians at their own expense due to initiating observation services, it can be challenging to ultimately turn a profit. If, however, the hospital is able to provide some support for the additional FTEs, the financial impact is mitigated. The observation financial feasibility calculation is as follows:

- Observation generates 1.3 RVUs more than the corresponding ED code
- 1.3 RVUs create an additional $50 in revenue
- Treat patient for 8 hours
- Five hours longer than usual yields an hourly rate of an additional $10/hour
- Several patients "observed at one time" might be generating $30/hour in additional revenue
- However, the additional FTE cost in salary and benefits is typically $130/hour

There are many different staffing and financial solutions related to observation services. Keep in mind the extra costs that may be associated with having to increase staffing to provide observation care. In conclusion, observation may be good for individual cases, if the group is already providing care and will require no staffing increase (i.e., an intoxicated college student). Observation may be seen as an extra hospital service, which can further build the perception of your group as a value-added partner.

Economics of a Fully Independent Unit

What are the economics of a fully independent observation unit? The first step in the process is to estimate the revenue generated by such a unit:

- 10-bed unit, turned 1.3 times daily
  - Blend of moderate and high MDM cases yields an average of 5.5 RVUs per case.
  - 71 RVUs at $34/RVU creates $2,400 in daily revenue or $100/hour.

Next, it is necessary to address the cost side of the equation:

- FTE cost: hourly salary benefits $130/hour plus $10/hour indirect management costs yields $140/hour.

If the unit is required to be covered by a board-certified emergency physician without any hospital support, it is very difficult to fully cover the costs. Some groups have developed solutions like providing physician coverage for new admits and discharges in the morning and evening with interim coverage by nurse practitioners (NPs) or physician assistants (PAs). Other groups have used family practice physicians, who may demand a lower salary.

MODERATE CONSCIOUS SEDATION

Emergency physicians provide important sedation services, both in support of their own procedures and as part of a teamed approach with consultants performing procedures in the ED. The coding rules surrounding moderate conscious sedation (MCS) are a bit complex. This section of text provides the tools necessary to understand them. The CPT defines sedation services along a continuum from anxiolysis to MCS to deep sedation and general anesthesia. There are no separate codes to report simple anxiolysis. Moderate conscious sedation implies the following criteria are met:

- Patient responds purposefully to verbal commands with light tactile stimulation.
- No interventions are required to maintain an adequate airway.
- Ventilation is adequate.
- Cardiovascular function is maintained.

The MCS codes are divided into two groups: MCS provided by the same physician who is performing the procedure, which requires the presence of an independent trained observer; and MCS provided by a physician in support of a second health-care provider performing

TABLE 93.5 ■ Moderate Sedation Time Requirement

Intraservice Time	Patient Age	Moderate Sedation Single Provider	Moderate Sedation Different Provider
		Code(s)	Code(s)
<10 min	Any age	Not reported separately	Not reported separately
10-22 min	<5 years	99151	99155
10-22 min	5 years or older	99152	99156
23-37 min	<5 years	99151 + 99153 X 1	99155 + 99157 X 1
23-37 min	5 years or older	99152 + 99153 X 1	99156 + 99157 X 1

the procedure. Each group of codes is then further stratified based on the age of the patient and the time involved in providing the MCS (**Table 93.5**).[3]

- MCS same physician: CPT codes 99151 to 99153
  - 99151—under 5 years old, first 15 minutes
  - 99152—5 years old and over, first 15 minutes
  - 99153—each additional 15 minutes
- MCS different physician: CPT codes 99155 to 99157
  - 99155—under 5 years of age, first 15 minutes
  - 99156—5 years old and over, first 15 minutes
  - 99157—each additional 15 minutes

In contrast to the more familiar 9928x ED codes, these codes are time based. As such, an understanding of the rules governing the activities counted toward intraservice time is required. Note that CPT has deviated from its typical requirement to meet the midpoint of a timed service and demonstrated that a minimum of 10 minutes is required to report moderate sedation services.[3] Intraservice time is defined as follows:

- Starts with the administration of the sedation agent
- Requires continuous physician face-to-face contact
- Ends at the conclusion of personal contact by the physician

Moderate Conscious Sedation Case Studies

The follow case studies demonstrate proper coding for the provided MCS services.

Single Physician Involved

A clinician who spends 12 minutes providing sedation with versed and fentanyl to a 38-year-old athlete with a dislocated shoulder would assign the following CPT codes:

- 23650—shoulder dislocation
- 99152—moderate sedation same provider

Two Physicians Involved

A clinician providing 28 minutes of sedation using IV ketamine to manage a 4-year-old undergoing a fracture reduction by orthopedics would assign the following CPT codes:

- 99155—MCS provided in support of another physician, age <5 years old, first 15 minutes
- 99157—MCS provided in support of another physician, each additional 15 minutes
- The orthopedic physician reports the fracture care code.

Moderate Conscious Sedation Billing Issues

Coverage and payment for MCS services vary greatly by payor. Medicare has designated the MCS codes as "status indicator A," meaning they are active codes that should be reimbursed. However, keep in mind that 99153 is valued at zero RVUs, so consideration should be given prior to billing this code to Medicare (**Table 93.6**).

TABLE 93.6 ■ Typical Suggested MCS Work RVUs	
CPT Code	Work RVUs
99151	0.50
99152	0.25
99153	0.0
99155	1.90
99156	1.65
99157	1.25

TEACHING PHYSICIANS

In 2002, Medicare made several significant changes to its longstanding rules governing teaching physicians (TPs). These changes no longer require the attending physician to completely redocument the evaluation performed by the resident. Instead, TPs are only required to record their involvement in the key aspects of the patient's care. Additional clarifications to the TP rules have also been made with regard to the definition of a "resident" and the level of the attending physician's involvement.

The TP guidelines typically apply to residents during the care of Medicare patients. Transmittal 1780 defines a resident as "an individual who participates in an approved graduate medical education (GME) program or a physician who is not in an approved GME program but who is authorized to practice only in a hospital setting."[9] The term includes residents and fellows in GME programs recognized as approved for purposes of direct GME payments made by the fiscal intermediary. Receiving a staff or faculty appointment or participating in a fellowship does not by itself alter the status of a resident. Additionally, this status remains unaffected regardless of whether a hospital includes the physician in its full-time equivalency count of residents. A medical student is not treated the same as a resident. Generally speaking, interns, residents, and fellows fall under the TP rules.

The TP must document his or her oversight or personal performance of the key/critical aspects of the patient's evaluation. The TP, within the realm of reasonable medical/clinical practice, is free to define the key/critical aspects of a patient's evaluation. This documentation might include the heart and lung examination of a patient with dyspnea or the abdominal examination of a patient with abdominal pain.

Case One

The TP sees and evaluates the patient without resident involvement. The TP's documentation must solely satisfy the requirements for the service billed.

Case Two

The TP and the resident see the patient jointly, either at the same time or in a staggered fashion. The TP's note should reference the resident's note. For payment, the composite of the TP's entry and the resident's entry together may be used to satisfy the documentation guidelines. Examples of *acceptable* TP documentation include:

- "I performed a history and PE of the patient and discussed his management with the resident. I reviewed the resident's note and agree with the documented findings and plan of care."
- "I was present with the resident during the history and examination. I discussed the case with the resident and agree with the findings and plan as documented."
- "I saw and evaluated the patient. I reviewed the resident's note and agree, except that the picture is more consistent with pericarditis than myocardial ischemia. Will begin nonsteroidal anti-inflammatory drugs."

Examples of *unacceptable* TP documentation include:

- "Agree with above" followed by legible countersignature or identity
- "Rounded, reviewed, agree" followed by legible countersignature or identity
- "Discussed with resident. Agree" followed by legible countersignature or identity
- "Seen and agree" followed by legible countersignature or identity
- "Patient seen and evaluated" followed by legible countersignature or identity

Best Practices

E/M services attestation: Develop a specific attestation for the E/M services and make sure to include some case-specific information demonstrating your involvement in the key/critical aspects of the patient's care. Have the key/critical aspects of the E/M of the patient been further defined? As defined by CMS, "critical or key portion means that part (or parts) of a service that the TP determines represent key or critical portions."[9] Under what circumstances may a TP bill for procedures? For minor surgical procedures (<5 minutes), the TP must be physically present during the entire service. For major procedures (>5 minutes), the TP must be physically present during the "key portions" of the service and be available to provide guidance during the entire procedure.

Procedural attestation: Develop a separate TP procedural attestation based on the length of time it takes to perform the procedure.

Teaching Physician and Critical Care Requirements

Must the TP be present in order to appropriately bill Medicare for timed services (**Box 93.6**)? In the absence of the TP, resident participation in timed services cannot be used for billing purposes. Likewise, teaching time does not count toward timed services.

Potential Update to the TP Rules

In an effort to reduce physician documentation burden, CMS in the 2019 Medicare Physician Fee Schedule Proposed Rule is proposing to eliminate duplicative documentation

---

BOX 93.6 ■ SUMMARY MENU OF TP ATTESTATIONS

- Separate attestation for supervision of E/M services 99281 to 99285
- Major and minor procedure attestations
- Personal TP direct provision of critical care attestation

requirements for TPs when the required information has already been documented by someone else. CMS specifically proposes the following:

> The medical records must document the extent of the teaching physician's participation in the review and direction of services furnished to each beneficiary, and that the extent of the teaching physician's participation may be demonstrated by the notes in the medical records made by a physician, resident, or nurse.[10]

If this documentation relief is enacted, TPs would be spared from redocumenting large components of the medical record, and the TP's involvement could be recorded by another physician, a resident, or nurse.

Medical Student Documentation

In another win for TPs, Medicare issued Transmittal 808 with an effective date of August 14, 2018, related to medical student documentation.[11] The transmittal clarifies that the TP does not have to redocument items in the medical record entered by medical students and, though the TP must perform the components of the medical service (such as physical exam and MDM), the TP is only required to provide his or her signature following the medical student's documentation.

Pub 100-08 Medicare Program Integrity

> If the teaching physician chooses to rely on the medical student documentation and declines to re-document the E/M service, contractors shall consider this requirement met if the teaching physician signs and dates the medical student's entry.[11]

What are the specific performance and documentation requirements for Medicare billing when a medical student has been involved in the care of a patient?

- Medical students may gather the ROS and past, family, and social history.
- Medical students may document the history, physical exam, and MDM.
- TPs must document their performance of the HPI, PE, and MDM.
- The TP must document his or her review and agreement with the student's documentation.
- Medical students may not perform procedures independently.
- Medical students may participate in procedures with a resident, provided the rules are satisfied with regard to attending-level supervision.
- Medical students may also directly assist the attending in the performance of procedures.

ADVANCED PRACTICE PROVIDERS: PAs/NPs

Many ED groups have incorporated advanced practice providers (APPs), such as PAs and NPs, into their practices. The CMS uses the designation nonphysician practitioner (NPP) to describe them. These NPPs frequently work in "fast-track" settings, seeing lower acuity patients, assisting with evaluations and workups in the main ED, and performing procedures. As the growth of NPP use has increased, it has become imperative to gain an understanding of the coding rules governing the reporting of NPP services.

On October 25, 2002, CMS released Transmittal 1776, which defined significant changes to the coding and billing processes associated with NPs and PAs.[12] Transmittal 1776 defined midlevel providers or NPPs to include NPs and PAs, and for this discussion, NPs and PAs are treated similarly for coding purposes.

When an ED patient receives E/M services by both an MD and an NPP, the E/M service may be billed under either the physician's or the NPP's national provider identifier (NPI) number if the MD documents a clinically meaningful face-to-face encounter. If the physician does not document a face-to-face encounter, the E/M service must be billed out under the PA's or NP's NPI number and will be reimbursed at 85% of the Medicare physician fee schedule.

Importantly, these provisions in Medicare Transmittal 1776 apply only to E/M services and do not apply to procedures. If the physician simply cosigns the record, the E/M service must be reported under the PA or NP's NPI for Medicare. At this point, private payor policies vary with regard to APPs. Some payors credential such providers and follow Medicare guidelines. Others do not, in which case the private payor will typically request that bills be submitted under the supervising physician. Groups are advised to check their private payor contracts for details regarding NPP credentialing.

Advanced Practice Provider Case Studies

The following four cases demonstrate proper coding for service provided by APPs.

Case One

A 32-year-old woman has a sprained ankle and is seen in the "fast-track" area of the ED by a PA who performs a level 3 E/M service. The patient's health insurance carrier does not credential PAs. The MD is available as needed for discussion of the case and cosigns the record based on hospital policy at the end of the shift having not seen the patient.

- Bill 99283 under the supervising physician

Case Two

A 69-year-old Medicare patient is seen in the "fast track" with a rash. The PA provides level 3 E/M services. The physician cosigns the record but has not seen the patient.

- Bill 99283 under the PA's NPI

Case Three

A PA sees a 67-year-old Medicare patient with a COPD exacerbation and documents a level 4 E/M service. The MD sees the patient and documents a face-to-face encounter, including a brief note regarding the lung examination and plan for nebulizer treatments.

- Bill 99284 under the MD's NPI number

Case Four

A 74-year-old Medicare patient presents for syncope. The MD personally performs and documents a 99285 service. The PA sutures a 2-cm scalp laceration from the resulting fall.

- Bill 99285 under the MD's NPI number
- Bill the scalp laceration repair (12001) under the PA's NPI number

Critical care services, as pointed out previously, are time-based services, and as such the shared visit construct does not apply. Scope of practice for NPPs is generally defined at the state level. The CMS has stated that NPPs are generally not limited in the types of services they may bill for as long as those services are medically necessary and fall under the scope of practice parameters for that particular state. In 2008, CMS issued Transmittal 1548 stating qualified NPPs may also report critical care services.[13] Keep in mind that because this is a time-based code, the "face-to-face encounter" aspects of Transmittal 1776 would not apply. If the NPP provides greater than 30 minutes of critical care services for a critically ill patient, the claim (for Medicare and similar payors) would be submitted under the NPPs NPI and reimbursed at 85%. In order for the MD to bill for critical care service, he or she must personally provide and document 30 minutes of care. Currently, some carriers are creating controversy by limiting reimbursement for certain PA services, such as fracture care and critical care. The American Academy of Physician Assistants website has an active advocacy registry and is an excellent resource for keeping tabs on this evolving area.

CARDIOPULMONARY RESUSCITATION

There is a lot of mystery surrounding the coding of CPR services. From a coding perspective, CPR consists of basic life support (BLS). The CPT states the goal of CPR is to restore the patient's breathing and circulation. CPR includes the following:

- Assessing the victim
- Opening the airway
- Providing ventilation (i.e., bag-valve-mask support)
- Restoring circulation (i.e., closed chest cardiac massage)

Importantly, the physician does not have to be the one manually performing the given services but rather would be directly supervising the provision of CPR. According to the American Medical Association (AMA), the publisher of the CPT manual, CPR may be reported whether "The physician does not have to physically perform the chest compressions or ventilation of the patient, but rather can direct the provision of CPR services."[14]

Another area of confusion relates to the minimum time requirement. The CPT does not specify a minimum time requirement for the provision of CPR. Of note, the reporting of CPR would not be appropriate for a simple dead on arrival proclamation. The procedure requires some amount of chest compressions and ventilatory support to be provided to the patient and documented in the chart.

The E/M level reported with CPR will be determined by the amount of history and PE, as well as MDM documented. As per the CMS table of risk, the assignment of a do-not-resuscitate (DNR) status or decision to de-escalate treatment is typically representative of high risk and will generally support higher level E/M services.[15] Because CPR is a separately billable service, a patient who is in "arrest" during the entire ED encounter would not have critical care (99291) also reported because once CPR time is subtracted out, there would not be enough time to satisfy the 30-minute minimum for critical care. Critical care and CPR would both be potentially reported if the patient survived and then went on to receive critical care services like pressors or vasoactive medications.

Case Study: CPR

An 82-year-old man arrives in cardiac arrest, having received two epinephrine and two atropine boluses en route; he is in an agonal rhythm with CPR in progress. Paramedics have been unable to intubate the man, and ventilation is being provided via a bag-valve-mask. The emergency physician directs the performance of BLS measures, orders an additional round of epinephrine and atropine, and intubates the patient. Despite these efforts, the patient's rhythm decays to asystole. After 17 minutes, the code is called. The physician documents a comprehensive history and PE with high-level MDM (**Box 93.7**).

- Codes assigned
    - 99285—E/M service
    - 92950—CPR
    - 31500—intubation

> **BOX 93.7 ■ CPR CODING PEARLS**
>
> - CPR may be reported for oversight of "codes" in the inpatient ward.
> - There are no minimum documentation requirements, though there should be a procedure note, and most institutions have a CPR flow sheet that must be signed by the supervising physician.
> - Intubation and most other significant procedures are separately billable with the CPR code 92950.
> - CPR is a high RVU service. In 2018, CPR 92950 was assigned 5.34 total RVUs.

ORTHOPEDIC PROCEDURES

Emergency physicians provide important and meaningful fracture care and are often the first to see, treat, and stabilize injuries involving fractures. The American College of Emergency Physicians supports the reporting of fracture care by emergency physicians when appropriately documented. The CPT and Medicare (CMS) recognize the provision of fracture care by emergency physicians without placing a specialty-specific limitation on reporting the codes for fracture care services.

Manipulations

The emergency physicians often provide reductions of fractures in their department. These reductions should be documented with a full surgical.

Case Study: Fracture Manipulation

A 12-year-old girl presents with a Colles fracture after falling off her bicycle. The clinician performs a detailed history and PE and documents a moderate-complexity MDM while screening for other injuries. He places a hematoma block, reduces the wrist fracture, and places the patient in a short arm splint. Instructions for orthopedic follow-up are given.

- Codes assigned
    - 99284—ED E/M service
    - 25605 with modifier -54—reduction of Colles' fracture
- Additional notes
    - Splint is bundled with the fracture care code.
    - There is no separate code for the hematoma block.

Many clinicians perform manipulations for displaced fractures (**Box 93.8**), such as:

- Finger fractures
- Toe fractures
- Metacarpal fractures
- Metatarsal fractures
- Distal tibial and fibular fractures
- Bimalleolar and trimalleolar ankle fractures
- Distal radius fractures

Nonmanipulated Fractures

Emergency physicians may manage fractures that will not require manipulation, such as injuries involving the fingers, toes, clavicle, or nose. To bill for the treatment of these fractures, the emergency physician must provide restorative and definitive care, that is, the same care as the specialist or follow-up physician would provide.

Case One

A 46-year-old man presents with a minimally displaced bimalleolar fracture after tripping and falling off a high curb. The physician performs a detailed history and PE, documents moderate MDM, and provides morphine for pain relief. The patient is placed in a short leg splint, which is directly overseen by the physician. Orthopedic follow-up is arranged for the next day, when casting will take place.

- Codes assigned
  - 99284—E/M service
  - 29515—short leg splint
- No fracture care code is assigned because the definitive care (casting, in this case) will be provided by the orthopedist.

Case Two

A 28-year-old man is hit in the face while playing basketball. He experienced a possible brief loss of consciousness, subsequent dizziness, and some nausea. CT confirms a nondisplaced nasal fracture and no intracranial injury. The emergency physician documents a detailed history and PE with moderate MDM. The physician orders pain medication, and an ice pack is provided. The physician also counsels the patient regarding the signs and symptoms that represent complications and reviews head injury instructions with the patient's brother.

- Codes assigned
  - 99284—E/M service
  - 21310—closed treatment of nasal fracture without manipulation

Splints

To stabilize injuries and provide patient comfort, emergency physicians often utilize splints, which reduce movement of the affected area or joint. Medicare requires the physician to directly apply the splint. Private payors may require documentation of direct supervision, such as a post-placement alignment and neurovascular check, or may default to the Medicare guidelines.

Splints commonly placed by emergency physicians include:

- 29105—long arm
- 29125—short arm
- 29130—finger
- 29515—short leg
- 29105—long leg

BOX 93.8 ■ FRACTURE CARE TIP

Remember to write a procedure note when performing these manipulations so that the coder can capture these high RVU procedures and bill appropriately. Note that most of the fracture care codes have a 90-day global, which includes multiple postreduction follow-up visits. To communicate to the payor that the ED physician provided only the operative portion of the care and will not be seeing the patient for the typical follow-up office visits, the -54 modifier is applied to the fracture care code. The application of the -54 modifier garners roughly 70% of the overall RVUs for the procedure for the ED physicians.

Additional Fracture Care Issues

Should the physician report the fracture care codes that carry the term "with anesthesia" if they sedate the patient to reduce pain from a fracture, or should the physician perform MCS? Although the CPT manual itself does not have a specific description of when to apply the "with anesthesia" codes, written correspondence from AMA personnel has stated that "with anesthesia" refers to procedures performed in the operating room (OR).[16] The additional significant RVUs applied to the codes carrying the term "with anesthesia" reflect the extra effort involved in the formal OR process, such as stand-by time for OR preparation, scrubbing, induction of anesthesia, and other surgical processes.

Is it acceptable to bill for x-ray readings if fracture care is also provided? Yes, as long as you have met the documentation requirements for the x-ray reading service, there is no prohibition against the same physician billing for both x-rays and fracture care. The CPT specifically lists the subcomponents that are considered bundled with surgical procedures, inlcuding local infiltration and metacarpal/digital blocks. Radiology services are not bundled.

Is there a difference, from a coding perspective, between open and closed fracture treatment? Yes. Open treatment of a fracture describes a process in which a surgical incision is made to reveal the fractured bones. Closed treatment is more commonly provided in the ED and does not involve making a surgical incision. Even if the patient has suffered an open fracture, the open fracture codes are only employed if the physician makes a formal incision as part of the treatment.

ULTRASOUND

Emergency physicians are increasingly incorporating ultrasound into day-to-day practices in an effort to increase the rapidity of diagnosing high-acuity conditions. As per the CPT, the documentation and coding requirements for ultrasound services include:

- *Medical necessity*: The medical record documentation must indicate why the test was medically necessary.
- *Interpretation*: A written report must be completed and maintained in the patient's medical record and describe the structures and organs studied, including an interpretation of the findings.
  - ☐ The report should identify the provider performing and interpreting the study.
- *Image retention*: Appropriate images of the relevant anatomy and pathology must be permanently stored and available for future review.

Current Procedural Terminology Coding Issues

All diagnostic ultrasound examinations require permanently recorded images.[8]
A final, written report should be issued for inclusion in the patient's medical record.[17]

Note that the ultrasound report does not have to be a separate sheet, but it ideally should have a distinct heading within the patient's record. Emergency physicians typically provide and document limited rather than complete ultrasound studies. As a result, the limited ultrasound codes are often used in the ED. The CPT states:

For those anatomic regions that have 'complete' and 'limited' ultrasound codes, note the elements that comprise a "complete" examination. The report should contain a description of these elements or the reason that an element could not be visualized (e.g., obscured by bowel gas, surgically absent).[8]

The following example of the components of a complete ultrasound of the abdomen was put forward by CPT:

A complete abdominal ultrasound (76700) would consist of real time scans of the liver, gall bladder, common bile duct, pancreas, spleen, kidneys, upper abdominal aorta, and inferior vena cava.[3]

Proficiency Pathways

There are two proficiency pathways commonly discussed relative to ED ultrasound: the residency-based pathway and the practice-based pathway. Importantly, CPT does not require an emergency physician to have credentials in ultrasound and by general tenet applies the litmus test of "any qualified provider" in reference to billing for medical services provided. Currently, CPT does not specifically require an emergency physician to be credentialed by a hospital or a specialty society for the provision of ultrasound services.

Residency-Based Pathway

The Accreditation Council on Graduate Medical Education mandates procedural competency for all emergency medicine residents in emergency ultrasound because it is considered a "skill integral to the practice of emergency medicine."[18] For those who did not receive residency training in ultrasound, a practice-based pathway exists to establish proficiency in the provision of ultrasound services. It typically includes:

- Didactics and hands-on training
- Ultrasound performance under supervision
- Credentialing
- Continuing medical education and continued proficiency

General Coding Parameters

Along with typically performing limited studies, the emergency physician usually provides the professional component of the ultrasound service and will append the -26 modifier to the ultrasound CPT code to designate that the service being reported is limited to the professional component. The hospital will then report the ultrasound code with a technical component modifier. Groups purchasing ultrasound equipment and wishing to bill for global ultrasound codes are advised to consult experienced health-care counsel.

Specific Ultrasound Applications

Special note is made of the FAST exam, which is a compilation of two (and sometimes three) distinct ultrasound studies. A FAST exam will typically involve the study of four intra-abdominal areas to ascertain the presence or absence of hemoperitoneum. This first component is reported with 76705. A second component investigates the heart and pericardiac structures for evidence of hemopericardium and is reported with 93308. The following is a list of typical emergency ultrasound applications:

- Trauma
- Cardiac

- Abdominal aortic aneurysm
- Intrauterine pregnancy
- Biliary
- Urinary tract
- Soft tissue and musculoskeletal
- Thoracic
- Ocular
- Procedural guidance

Table 93.7 represents a partial list of commonly performed ED diagnostic ultrasound services and their corresponding codes.

Case Study: FAST Examination

The patient is a 25-year-old male victim of a rollover motor vehicle collision. His blood pressure is 80/60 mm Hg, heart rate is 120 beats/minute, and his belly is firm. The physician performs and documents a FAST examination, evaluating both the abdomen for hemoperitoneum and the chest in a more limited fashion to ascertain the presence of cardiac tamponade. The FAST shows free fluid in the left upper quadrant. His blood pressure drops further despite the rapid administration of 2 L IV fluids. The patient is taken to the OR, where a ruptured spleen is discovered.

- Codes assigned
    - 76705—limited abdominal ultrasound
    - 93308—limited transthoracic echo

Note that the FAST examination can sometimes have a third component representing a further investigation of the mediastinal contents and lung, which is reported with code 76604.

TABLE 93.7 ■ Common ED Ultrasound Diagnostic Studies

Ultrasound Descriptor	CPT Code	CPT Definition
FAST: Evaluation for hemoperitoneum and hemopericardium, and possibly lung evaluation for pneumothorax	93308	Echocardiography, transthoracic, real-time follow-up or limited
	76705	Ultrasound, abdominal, limited (e.g., single organ, quadrant, follow-up)
	76604	Ultrasound, chest, real time with image documentation
Pregnancy transabdominal	76815	Ultrasound, pregnant uterus, limited
Pregnancy transvaginal	76817	Ultrasound, pregnant uterus, real time with image documentation transvaginal
AAA	76775	Ultrasound, retroperitoneal (e.g., renal, aorta, nodes); limited
Cardiac	93308	Echocardiography, transthoracic, follow-up or limited
Biliary	76705	Ultrasound, abdominal, limited (e.g., single organ, quadrant, follow-up)
Urinary tract	76775	Ultrasound, retroperitoneal limited
Post-void residual	51798	Measurement of post-void residual urine by ultrasound, nonimaging

TABLE 93.8 ■ ED Soft-Tissue Ultrasound Applications

Ultrasound Descriptor	CPT Code	CPT Definition
Neck	76536	Ultrasound, soft tissues of head and neck
Axilla	76882	Ultrasound, extremity
Chest wall	76604	Ultrasound, chest
Breast	76645	Ultrasound, breast
Back upper	76604	Ultrasound, chest
Back lower	76705	Ultrasound, abdominal, limited
Abdominal wall	76705	Ultrasound, abdominal, limited
Pelvic wall	76857	Ultrasound, pelvic (non-obstetric)
Extremity	76882	Ultrasound, extremity, non-vascular limited
Thoracic	76604	Ultrasound, chest

Ultrasound is also used to evaluate various areas of the body in an effort to delineate the presence or absence of a fluid collection or foreign body (**Table 93.8**). A nonexclusive list of ED soft tissue ultrasound applications is discussed next.

Case Study: Abscess Identification

An 18-year-old man presents with a firm indurated area over the right inner thigh. He has a history of methicillin-resistant *Staphylococcus aureus* skin infections and has had multiple abscesses drained in that area. Ultrasound is employed to evaluate for the presence of fluid. A collection consistent with an abscess is identified and drained using a typical incision-and-drainage procedure with a probe.

- Codes assigned
  - 76882—lower extremity ultrasound
  - 10061—incision and drainage complex

Ultrasound is also used in conjunction with many ED procedures to better define anatomy and provide real-time guidance for percutaneous procedures (**Table 93.9**). As with other procedures, both the ultrasound and treatment are reported, and separate entries within the medical record should individually substantiate both.

TABLE 93.9 ■ Ultrasound-Guided Procedures

Description	Ultrasound CPT Code	Procedure CPT Code
Peritonsilar abscess drainage	76942	42700
Foreign body (FB) removal	76942 if needle guidance used. Use soft tissue for localization of FB only	10120 or 10121
Lumbar puncture	76942	62270
Vascular access (requires real-time visualization)	76937	36555, 36556

Case Study: Central-Line Placement

A 29-year-old intravenous drug user presents with cellulitis of both lower extremities following skin popping. Multiple attempts at IV access are unsuccessful. The emergency physician utilizes ultrasound in real time to place a right internal jugular line.

Report procedure code 36556 and central line ultrasound code 76937. Importantly, the ultrasound guidance code 76937 requires real-time visualization of vascular needle entry, a dynamic technique rather than a static technique.

CONCLUSION

Successful leadership and management of an ED group in today's evolving and complex health-care environment depend on a working knowledge of both basic and advanced coding concepts.

REFERENCES

1. Brainyquote.com. Reimbursement quotes. 2020. Available at: https://i.brainyquote.com/quotes/dean_ornish_822512?src=t_reimbursement. Accessed October 30, 2020.
2. American Medical Association. CPT 2020: Professional Edition. 2019. Available at: https://www.amazon.com/Professional-2020-Current-Procedural-Terminology/dp/1622028988/ref=sr_1_1?dchild=1&keywords=CPT+Code&qid=1604092932&sr=8-1. Accessed October 30, 2020.
3. American Medical Association. *AMA CPT Professional. AMA Current Procedural Terminology*. Professional Edition. American Medical Association; 2018.
4. CMS.gov. 1995 Documentation Guidelines for Evaluation and Management Services. Available at: https://www.cms.gov/outreach-and-education/medicare-learning-network-mln/mlnedwebguide/downloads/95docguidelines.pdf. Accessed October 30, 2020/
5. Medicare Part B Extract Survey Data.
6. CMS Manual System. Pub 100-04. Transmittal 1760. 2009;290.1:25.
7. CGS Administrators. Observation Services: Fact Sheet. 2019. Available at: https://www.cgsmedicare.com/partb/mr/pdf/observation_serv_factsheet.pdf. Accessed October 31, 2020.
8. 2018 Medicare Physician Fee Schedule.
9. cms.gov. Medicare Carriers Manual Part 3: Claims Process—Transmittal 1780. 2002. Available at: https://www.cms.gov/Regulations-and-Guidance/Guidance/Transmittals/downloads/R1780B3.pdf. Accessed October 31, 2020.
10. cms.gov. Calendar Year (CY) 2019 Medicare Physician Fee Schedule (PFS) Proposed Rule. Available at: https://www.cms.gov/About-CMS/Story-Page/2019-Medicare-PFS-proposed-rule-slides.pdf. Accessed October 31, 2020.
11. cms.gov. CMS Manual System: Pub 100-08 Medicare Program Integrity—Transmittal 808. 2018. Available at: https://www.cms.gov/Regulations-and-Guidance/Guidance/Transmittals/2018Downloads/R808PI.pdf. Accessed October 31, 2020.
12. cms.gov. Medicare Carriers Manual Part 3: Claims Process—Transmittal 1776. 2002. Available at: https://www.cms.gov/Regulations-and-Guidance/Guidance/Transmittals/Downloads/R1776B3.pdf. Accessed October 31, 2020.
13. cms.gov. CMS Manual System: Pub 100-04 Medicare Claims Processing—Transmittal 1548. 2008. Available at: https://www.cms.gov/Regulations-and-Guidance/Guidance/Transmittals/downloads/R1548CP.pdf. Accessed October 31, 2020
14. acep.org. Cardiopulmonary Resuscitation (CPR) FAQ. Available at: https://www.acep.org/administration/reimbursement/reimbursement-faqs/cardiopulmonary-resuscitation-cpr-faq/#:~: Updated 2020. Accessed October 31, 2020.
15. CMS-Medical Learning Network. Evaluation and Management Services Guide. MLN Booklet, pg 20. 2020. Available at: https://www.cms.gov/outreach-and-education/medicare-learning-network-mln/mlnproducts/downloads/eval-mgmt-serv-guide-icn006764.pdf. Accessed October 31, 2020.
16. cms.gov. National Correct Coding Initiative's (NCCI) General Correspondence Language and Section Specific Examples. Available at: https://www.cms.gov/files/document/correspondence-language-manual-medicare-services-revision-date-january-1-2020.pdf. Revised January 1, 2020. Accessed October 31, 2020.
17. American Medical Association. CPT Changes, An Insider's View. 2007; 173.
18. ACEP.org. Policy Statement: Emergency Ultrasound Guidelines. 2008. Available at: https://emed.stanford.edu/content/dam/sm/emed/documents/specialized-programs/ultrasound/ultrasound_guidelines.pdf. Accessed November 3, 2020.

CHAPTER 94

FACILITY REVENUE CONSIDERATIONS

Caral Edelberg

Emergency department (ED) leadership is increasingly challenged to manage the delivery of both excellent clinical care and a solid financial performance. In many cases, particularly those in which the ED group contracts with the hospital, the individual overseeing the facility billing will be a nurse. However, where the physicians in a group are hospital employees, especially in academic settings, that individual can be the medical director or department chair. Many directors find this responsibility intimidating because few have a strong understanding of the processes that support optimal performance. The good news is that every leader can acquire this knowledge, and the information in this chapter will start the journey.

Revenue cycle management (RCM) is a hospital function. It typically falls under the purview of patient financial services (PFS) and the chief understanding of how to optimize the revenue in their EDs. In recent years, however, many outside vendors have joined with RCM to provide external coding and compliance services to assist in streamlining the RCM process. Nine process components of the revenue cycle—patient registration; emergency medical services (EMS), triage, and provider documentation; charging; coding; scrubber and release; bill drop; process monitoring; compliance auditing; and claim follow-up, payor audit management—provide an ideal conceptual framework for a discussion about the key processes that determine an ED's financial health (**Figure 94.1**). By understanding and actively engaging in these processes, ED leaders can monitor and drive change in these areas if improvements are needed.

The ED leaders will not be the revenue cycle process owner in most cases. But because they are accountable for financial outcomes in the ED, a working understanding of and the ability to speak the language will facilitate collaboration with others whose job it is to directly manage these processes. A working understanding will also allow the ED leader to communicate these important revenue concepts and expectations to the ED staff, whose support is essential for achieving success.

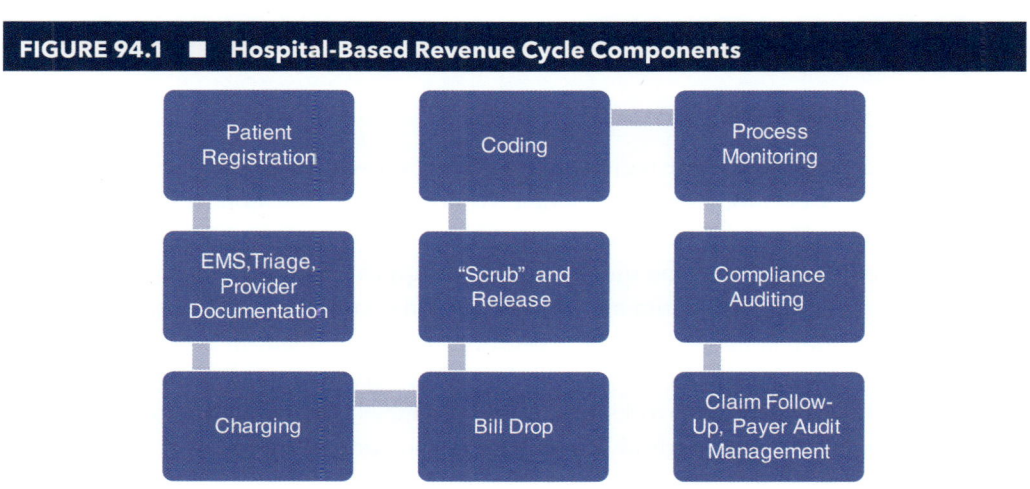

FIGURE 94.1 ■ Hospital-Based Revenue Cycle Components

REVENUE CYCLE AWARENESS

The Healthcare Financial Management Association and others define RCM as the coordination of "all administrative and clinical functions that contribute to the capture, management, and collection of patient service revenue."[1] The medical revenue cycle is a process of actions used to turn the medical claim into cash flow. The cycle includes receipt of claims, patient demographics, and insurance information. The claims are coded, and data entry of the information is accomplished. In other words, RCM is the process that manages claims processing, payment, and revenue generation. It unifies the business and clinical sides of health care by pairing administrative data, such as a patient's name and insurance provider and other personal information with the treatment a patient receives. These functions support generation of a clean claim, help optimize reimbursement, and are often the focus of compliance efforts.

While the ED leader's span of control and responsibilities places them in an ideal position to affect improvement in the revenue cycle, there are numerous hurdles to overcome. Resources are tight and some hospital chief executive and financial officers (CEOs and CFOs), and even some in executive leadership, believe that the work of the ED clinical and management staff and ED clinical processes should not be tainted by having to worry about functions traditionally left to the hospital finance group. ED leaders can overcome this notion as they gain knowledge, educate staff, and, through partnership with others, begin to affect improvements in ED revenue performance.

A note about what is meant here by the term "revenue": Revenue represents the expected dollar value or inflows from the delivery of ED services. These are often separate from the professional fee charged by the physician, though at times, especially when the physicians are employees of the hospital, these may be bundled. Services are provided and charged based on the fees listed in the ED charge master, which is simply a list of services and their charges. The aggregate charges for all ED services for a period represent revenue for that period. It is important to note that receiving payment is not a criterion for initial revenue recognition.[2] Actual reimbursement (payment) from payors and self-pay patients may be less because of contractual arrangements, write-offs for charity care or nonpayment, and payor denials or downcodes.

RCM PROCESSES IN THE ED

The ED-relevant processes in this cycle are sequential yet interdependent. Following are descriptions of each ED revenue cycle component and important issues to consider for effectively managing them.

Patient Registration

Complete and accurate patient registration information will help ensure that the ED is adequately reimbursed for services provided. Whether the registration staff reports to the ED manager or another department, or if registration is performed in a common registration area or at the bedside, the same quality standards apply. Emergency department clerks and patient representatives should have training based on written policies and procedures and clear expectations about the extent of information obtained, including supporting documentation like copies of of the patient's insurance card and government-issued ID. In some EDs, patient registration works closely with financial counselors who may interview selected patients after the medical screening exam or prior to discharge to investigate options for payment (e.g., veteran's benefits, Medicaid).

In addition to training, other factors that support excellence in patient registration and revenue optimization are:

- An automated registration system that is easy to use and requires input of the necessary data elements
- An audit of the registration staff's work on a regular basis to identify any deficiencies in patient demographics, payor information, and the accuracy of data entry. Error tracking and feedback to staff are key success factors.
- An established expectation for excellent customer service. The volume of patients and patient services are drivers of ED revenue. With their early interaction with the patient, registration staff members are in a key position to set the stage for a positive patient experience. Provision of excellent customer service is a critical element of patient satisfaction and will help to ensure a return visit if the need arises.

Emergency Medical Services, Triage, and Provider Documentation

Optimized documentation supports clinical care, medicolegal and risk management interests, data needs, quality reporting, and the revenue cycle processes that follow it. Good documentation is one of the most important components of the revenue cycle and the one over which the clinical staff has the most control.

All elements of documentation related to an ED patient encounter must be reviewed to assign the appropriate billing codes. The EMS report can establish medical necessity based on the patient's condition. Triage information provides details about the patient's condition upon arrival to the ED. Nursing notes provide both the admission status and the progress of the patient throughout the ED course with detailed information about managing the patient's problems following discharge. The emergency physician and advanced practice practitioners (APPs) provide the patient's history, examination notes, and the decisions made to provide diagnostic testing, medications, treatments, and disposition of the patient once the ED service is completed. All of these steps are required for optimal facility charging and coding. While nursing documentation is primarily used to determine facility resource utilization and the level of service provided, the EMS, triage, and physician/APP documentation are also required for facility procedure coding, orders, and *International Classification of Diseases, 10th Edition* (ICD-10) diagnostic coding.[3,4]

The use of electronic health records (EHRs) can be challenging for providers, and frequent feedback from the individuals who provide the coding service is essential. Providers need to be reminded when necessary portions of history, physical examination, and decision-making are not provided. Also, details about any diagnostic tests, surgical procedures, and any other noteworthy information that helps to accurately establish the type and amount of care provided are critical to establishing the necessity of medical treatment. Knowledge about the patient's condition throughout the ED stay is critical for the coding process and will be necessary for follow-up processes if claims are either downcoded or denied.

Documentation in the ED record captures resource utilization and establishes medical necessity for services provided. "Medical necessity" is an important factor in both documentation and coding. It simply means that a billed service must be reasonable, necessary, and appropriate for the diagnosis or treatment of a patient's illness or injury. Payment will be denied for a service that is not medically necessary. When documenting facility visit and procedural services, notation supporting resource utilization and medical necessity must be present—two factors that are considered by all payors in evaluating justification for payment.

In addition to training, other best practices that support excellence in clinical documentation and revenue optimization include:

- Provide nursing documentation education, especially as it relates to the ED's internal guidelines for determining the ED visit level. It is vital that both physician and nursing documentation be accurate and complete. Clinical documentation improvement (CDI) programs are frequently implemented to improve inpatient clinical documentation, but these programs are rarely extended to the ED. The ED leader can request that CDI consultants and the hospital's CDI nurses begin working with the emergency physicians and staff and evaluate the ED record content to optimize ED outpatient documentation. The Joint Commission, state regulations, and internal hospital policies also provide guidance on best practices for documentation. Nursing documentation can improve rapidly if inadequate documentation is tracked and reported to each nurse.
- Provide physician education on documentation requirements for professional visits, procedural services, diagnoses, quality measures, and hospital documentation requirements, such as documenting the reason for all services provided (e.g., image). For admissions, the physician should document the presence of patients' preexisting medical conditions—those that will be present on admission (POA). Medicare and some Medicaid programs and commercial payors will not pay for certain complications or conditions that occur during the admission (hospital-acquired conditions). The most relevant POA conditions for emergency physicians to document include presence of pressure ulcers, any injuries, diabetic imbalances, catheter-associated urinary tract infections, vascular access-related infections, and postoperative infections and vascular complications.
- "Hardwire" documentation prompts in paper or electronic documentation templates ensure data capture and modify documentation content as regulations/guidelines change. Clinical records in paper or electronic formats will require periodic revisions as services and other documentation requirements change. Build this task into the project plan for the ED's annual review and update of policies and procedures.
- Audit records and provide feedback on documentation quality and any deficiencies. Quantify dollars left on the table because of deficiencies. All providers, nurses, physicians, and APPS should receive timely notifications of encounters that are missing important documentation to allow them to ask questions and collaborate with other physicians to ensure improvement in all aspects of documentation.
- Establish a query program to educate staff and improve ED documentation quality.

Charging

When ED coding is performed by the hospital staff, charging for ED services is usually completed in the clinical area by clinical staff or charge analysts and includes identification of the correct Common Procedural Terminology (CPT) codes for the visit level and some procedures.[5] Coding is typically performed in the health information management (HIM) department by professional coders and includes the identification of additional CPT procedure codes, modifiers, *ICD-10* codes, and other reportable information such as treating physician and quality measures. Some HIM coders validate the "charges" submitted by the ED staff in addition to their "coding," and in some cases, HIM coders perform all of the charging and coding, eliminating the need for ED staff involvement.

When ED coding and charging are performed by outside vendors, most or all of the charging and coding processes are performed outside the HIM department and either entered into the billing system by hospital staff or interfaced between the coding vendor and the billing system. ED charges include visit levels, procedures, and supplies.

ED Visit Levels

The ED facility visit level or evaluation and management (E/M) service includes general visit services (nursing time, treatment room, medical record, billing, etc) and is usually reported with one of the five ED CPT codes, 99281-99285, or Critical Care, 99291. Medicare differentiates between two types of ED beds: type A and type B:

- Type A beds meet the Emergency Medical Treatment and Active Labor Act (EMTALA) definition of a dedicated ED and are open 24 hours a day, 7 days a week, per the CPT definition of an ED. The code set used to report visit levels in a type A ED is noted above.
- Type B beds also meet the EMTALA definition of a dedicated ED, but these beds are open and available less than 24 hours a day. Visit levels for Medicare patients cared for in this setting or area of the ED are reported using type B ED Healthcare Common Procedure Coding System or HCPCS codes G0380 through G0384 for levels 1 through 5.[6]

The remainder of this discussion on ED visit levels focuses on the type A ED beds. There are no specific nationally accepted guidelines or standards that direct hospitals on how to differentiate between the ED levels of service, 99281-99285. The Centers for Medicare and Medicaid Services (CMS) instructs hospitals to develop their own guidelines and has published 11 general guidelines that are used by EDs to calculate visit levels for all patients, irrespective of payor (Table 94.1).[7,8] However, many private payors have attempted to standardize ED facility criteria and use these criteria to audit coding for ED facility levels.

There are several different methodology options for a hospital to consider when developing their own internal guidelines. These guidelines may be developed internally or purchased, and they may be electronic or in the form of a paper description or checklist.

TABLE 94.1 ■ CMS General Guidelines for ED Facility Level Determination[4,5]	
1.	Follow the intent of the CPT codes reasonably, relating the intensity of hospital resources to the levels of effort represented by the codes
2.	Based on hospital facility resources, not on physician resources
3.	Facilitate accurate payments; be usable for compliance purposed and audits
4.	Meet the Health Insurance Portability and Accountability Act (HIPAA) requirements
5.	Only require documentation that is clinically necessary for patient care
6.	Not facilitate up coding or gaming
7.	Be written or recorded, well documented, and provide the basis for selection of a specific code
8.	Be applied consistently across patients in the ED or clinic to which they apply
9.	Not change with great frequency
10.	Be readily available for FI (or if applicable MAC) review
11.	Result in codes that could be verified by other hospital staff, as well as outside sources

Whatever method is selected, it must comply with the 11 general guidelines published by the CMS. The most common methodologies include:

- Point systems that assign values to different types of nursing work and resources
- Algorithms combining an acuity factor, such as the presenting problem and additional resource points
- The ACEP model, which is a clinically oriented table identifying nursing interventions and symptoms or presenting problems at each respective visit level[9]
- The American Hospital Association and American Health Information Management Association guidelines, which contain interventions specified for each level and the ability to increase one level higher if certain interventions or combinations of interventions are documented[10,11]

Whichever methodology is selected, clinical staff should be educated on its documentation requirements and the same methodology should be used for all patients and all payors. The method should be tested and validated to make sure it accurately reflects resource utilization in the ED. Audits of the methodology will be useful for monitoring accuracy of codes and charges over time. Most EDs track the resulting visit-level frequency distribution and perform focused audits when unexplained variances are identified.

The highest level of ED visit that can be reported is critical care. The CMS requires reporting of critical care "as defined by CPT code 99291."[5] To compliantly code facility critical care, the documentation must reflect the criticality of the patient's condition and interventions and that a minimum of 30 minutes of facility staff face-to-face time was spent with the patient. The CPT defines critical care as:

> ... the direct delivery, by a physician, of medical care for a critically ill or injured patient. A critical illness or injury is defined as one that acutely impairs one or more vital organ systems such that there is a high probability of imminent or life-threatening deterioration in the patient's condition.[12]

The critical care time must be calculated to ensure that a minimum of 30 minutes of care was provided. The time required to perform procedures that are separately billed must be subtracted from the total critical care time to determine the billable critical care time. Under the Outpatient Prospective Payment System (OPPS), the time that can be reported as critical care is the time spent by a physician and/or hospital staff engaged in active face-to-face critical care of a critically ill or critically injured patient.[13] If the physician and hospital staff or multiple hospital staff members are simultaneously engaged in this active face-to-face care, the time involved can only be counted once.[14]

Critical care is reimbursed at a higher rate by Medicare if trauma activation services are also provided. Other payors may reimburse the hospital for trauma activation as a separate payment. The trauma activation must be provided in a state or American College of Surgeons–designated trauma center and meet other requirements as set forth by the National Uniform Billing Committee (NUBC). The CMS will reimburse hospitals for HCPCS code G0390 (trauma response team activation associated with hospital critical care service) when a trauma team activation occurs and all NUBC conditions are met. These conditions include out-of-hospital notification of the patient's ED arrival from emergency medical services or interhospital transfer of caregivers and reporting under revenue code 068x, where x indicates the numerical level of the trauma center, 1 to 4. **Table 94.2** highlights the ED visit codes and their corresponding reimbursement.[15]

TABLE 94.2 ■ 2019 Medicare Facility Payments for ED Visit Codes[8]

CPT/HCPCS Code	Descriptor	APC	Relative Weight	Medicare Payment
99281	Level 1 ED visit	5021	0.8783	$69.87
99282	Level 2 ED visit	5022	1.6117	$128.20
99283	Level 3 ED visit	5023	2.8284	$224.99
99284	Level 4 ED visit	5024	4.5781	$364.17
99285	Level 5 ED visit	5025	6.6644	$530.13
99291	Critical care, first hour	5041	9.4855	$754.53
G0390	Critical care with trauma team activation	5045	11.7499	$934.66

Procedures

The second category of ED charges is procedures, which comprises:

- Surgical procedures usually performed by the physician or other clinician, such as wound repairs and fracture care, are coded based on physician documentation that is consistent with the CPT code descriptor for the procedure.
- Medical procedures that are performed by various caregivers, such as cardiopulmonary resuscitation or moderate conscious sedation, are usually coded based on a combination of physician and nursing documentation.
- Nursing procedures that are usually performed by the nursing staff (from the medicine section in the CPT manual) include intravenous infusions and injections, intramuscular and subcutaneous injections, Foley catheters, and others, and are coded based on nursing documentation and CPT and CMS directions.
- Diagnostic procedures that may be performed by ED staff or an ancillary service, such as electrocardiograms, are generally coded based on the physician documentation and orders.

Each type of procedure must be ordered by the physician, be medically necessary, and sufficiently documented. These procedures are "coded" using CPT codes. There are approximately 350 to 450 different procedures performed in EDs, and facility payment for them is separate from the ED visit charge. When a procedure is performed by the emergency physician, the facility may also submit a facility charge to cover the facility resources, including nursing staff time.

A complete discussion of procedure charging is beyond the scope of this chapter, but one set of procedures that bears separate mention is drug administration—specifically, injections and infusions. Medicare instructs hospitals to follow the CPT guidelines, but these guidelines are very complex and often confusing. The CPT defines a hierarchy of injection and infusion service types that are then coded based on the timing and sequencing of initial and secondary services (**Figure 94.2**).[16]

Infusions are time-based codes that require nursing documentation of start and stop time to determine the accurate CPT code. Some Medicare contractors allow the reporting

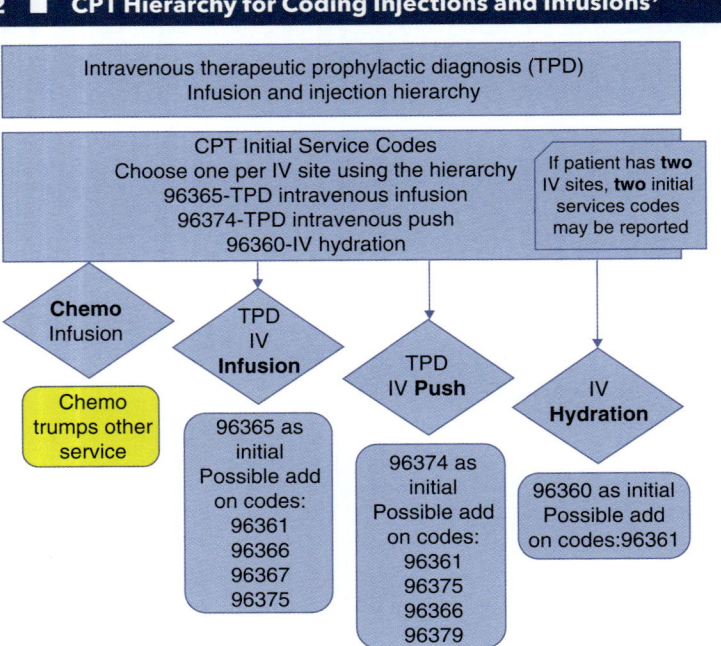

FIGURE 94.2 ■ CPT Hierarchy for Coding Injections and Infusions[9]

of an injection instead of an infusion when no stop time is documented, but others prohibit this practice and, absent a documented stop time, the infusion cannot be coded. The payment difference between an infusion and an injection is significant, so nursing documentation education in this area and ongoing feedback is critical to ensure accurate coding and optimal revenue capture. In addition, commercially available coding tools and education material can assist nurses and coders with this coding challenge. Medicare payments for the common ED drug administration codes and procedures[15] are noted in **Table 94.3**.

Supplies and Medications

The third category of ED charges, supplies, is captured in a variety of ways. Electronic capture using bar codes or an automated checkout system based on the chargemaster (see the next section, "The Chargemaster") are the preferred methods, but some EDs still use charge tickets or sticky labels placed on a charge sheet or card, and the charges are keyed into the billing system after the ED visit.

The cost of some supplies is accounted for in the procedure charge where the supply is used and not reported separately, but other supply items may be separately charged depending on payor direction; splints, crutches, and other orthopedic supplies are three such examples. In accounting for ED supplies, the cost of the supply item may be considered in the procedure for which the supply is a component part or charged separately, but the supply cost should not be included in a procedure charge and then also charged separately.

The accurate reporting of medication charges is another challenging aspect of supply charge capture. Not all medications are separately reimbursed; a consultation with the hospital or ED pharmacist and coder will be instructive. Reporting the medication dosage as the number of units is especially prone to error, and there are special rules associated with medications that Medicare classifies as "self-administered." Automated systems and skilled coders can assist with this medication charge process.

TABLE 94.3 ■ Common ED Procedures and Medicare Payments[3]		
CPT/HCPCS Code	**CPT Descriptor**	**2019 Medicare Payment**
96365	Therapeutic/prophylactic/diagnostic IV infusion, initial	$187.87
96366	Therapeutic/prophylactic/diagnostic IV infusion, add on	$37.89
96367	Therapeutic/prophylactic/diagnostic additional sequential IV infusion	$59.95
96368	Therapeutic/prophylactic/diagnostic concurrent IV infusion	$0.00—not paid by Medicare
96372	Therapeutic/prophylactic/diagnostic injection, SC/IM	$59.95
96374	Therapeutic/prophylactic/diagnostic injection, IV push	$187.87
96375	Therapeutic/prophylactic/diagnostic IV injection, new drug, add on	$37.89
96360	Hydration IV infusion, initial	$187.87
96361	Hydration IV infusion, add on	$37.89
10060	I&D abscess, simple	$175.38
10061	I&D abscess, complicated/multiple	$316.70
12001	Repair superficial wound(s)	$175.38
12002	Repair superficial wound(s)	$175.38
12011	Repair superficial wound(s)	$175.38
29125	Apply forearm splint	$106.97
29515	Application lower leg splint	$137.11
31500	Insert emergency airway	$204.93
51702	Insert temp bladder catheter	$106.97
62270	Lumbar puncture	$608.97
93005	Electrocardiogram, tracing	$56.60

The Chargemaster

All appropriate visit and procedural services are coded from a chargemaster or charge document master (CDM). The chargemaster is a master list of all billable and trackable services that are provided in the ED or other hospital departments. Items in the CDM are listed with a revenue code (indicating the department where the service was provided), a numerical charge code, a CPT code (or HCPCS code) and descriptor, and the fee for the item or service. Hospitals may add other CDM item categories depending on how the CDM is set up and maintained.

TABLE 94.4 ■ Hospital Revenue Codes Commonly Found on ED Bills

Revenue Code	Revenue Code Description
250	Pharmacy
260	IV therapy
270	Medical-surgical supplies
300	Laboratory, clinical diagnostic
320	Radiology diagnostic
350	CT scan
410	Respiratory services
450	Emergency room
451	ER EMTALA
68X	Trauma response: X = levels I-IV representing level of trauma center

Emergency department charges may be captured in a variety of ways. One option is to capture the charges during EHR documentation using business rules that pull documented data elements, map those elements to chargemaster items, and enter them into an electronic "charge ticket" with automatic extraction into the billing system. Another option is using a notation on a paper charge ticket, which is later keyed into the hospital billing system. **Table 94.4** lists common hospital revenue center codes.

In addition to training for individuals who perform the charging function, best practices that support accurate charge capture and revenue optimization include:

- Partner with HIM, compliance, and finance and share education and information about the charging function.
- Validate the ED visit-level calculation methodology to ensure it is an accurate measure of facility resource utilization. This process should be reviewed each year along with any CMS rule changes. If the ED's records are audited, have copies of the level assignment methodology available for auditors and request that they use it, rather than a different methodology.
- Reconcile the ED patient log with individual records to ensure that all patient records are accounted for and the charging is completed each day.
- Designate a time frame within which ED charges are entered into the billing system. The time interval is often referred to as the "bill drop cycle" and is measured with the date of service counting as day 0. Drop cycles range from 24 hours to about 5 days, but it is optimal to have ED charges completed within 24 to 48 hours of the visit so as not to slow the "coding process." Submitting late charges should be prevented if possible.

One charging scenario that seems to be especially problematic occurs when an attending physician or consultant comes to the ED to perform a procedure. The clinician may document a brief entry in the ED record and then dictate a procedure note. These procedures are difficult to charge without sufficient documentation, and the procedure transcript is rarely available to the ED charging staff. This charging should be assigned to coders, and a process designed to flag the chart and obtain the transcript in a timely manner should be implemented.

Additional best practices include:

- Maintain a complete and up-to-date chargemaster (CDM) for all services provided in the ED. The CDM should be reviewed at least annually for any necessary code and fee updates. All chargeable services/codes must be present—visit levels, procedures, and supplies unless some other supply-tracking process is used. Outdated codes should be deleted or inactivated. If coders or nurses identify documentation of a procedure in the clinical record that does not have a listing in the chargemaster, a request should be submitted to get the CPT code added as soon as possible.
- Maintain current ED CPT manual available online or in the ED's or institution's library. This resource will provide physicians, nurses, and others with an excellent reference for documentation requirements, information about what procedures are separately billable, and information about component services that might be included in the billable service.
- Determine who will perform the charging function—nurses, coders, or charge analysts—and provide them with ongoing education and monitoring. A charge manual with ED-specific guidelines for visit, procedure, and supply charging should be developed so all individuals performing the charging do it consistently. A query process should be established so that if the charge analyst has questions, he or she can go to the clinicians and resolve the issue. ED facility charging may be performed internally or outsourced.
- If an electronic charging system is used, create an interface into the billing system that will support an accurate, efficient billing process. A manual key entry process from a paper charge ticket is time consuming and subject to error.

Coding

In the context of a revenue cycle discussion, coding is the process of converting clinical information in the ED record into data that is recognizable by payors and their information systems. When coding an ED record, both the physician and nursing documentation (as described in the "Emergency Medical Services, Triage, and Provider Documentation" section) are used. In the coding process, coders use the documentation from an ED record and a coding system that has some level of automation and CPT and *ICD-10* code search capability. Coders often refer to the coding process as "abstracting" the record.

Some coding systems work with EHRs and employ a strategy called computer-assisted coding (CAC). Using CAC, inputs for coding some or all of the visit levels, procedures, and *ICD-10* diagnosis codes are automatically abstracted from documentation in the EHR. The appropriate codes are then identified using the system's business rules. A final validation of the codes assigned by the CAC through review of the documentation is necessary. Other coding systems allow a coder to review the ED record, either online or on paper, for evidence of resource utilization for the ED visit level, details about procedures performed, and diagnoses documented by the physician. The coder will then select the appropriate codes based on either online search capability or paper CPT and *ICD-10* code books.

Once the coder has completed or verified the CPT code selections in the abstract and billing systems, CPT code modifiers are added. Modifiers are two-digit alpha or alpha and numeric additions to the CPT visit and procedure codes that provide information for payors about the service and how the claim should be paid. These modifiers might identify an anatomical site on the body where a procedure was performed or explain to the payor that a separate visit and procedure were performed during the same encounter and both should be paid (a coder would append the -25 modifier to the visit level in this case). It is important to note that modifiers approved for use in physician coding may not apply to hospital ED facility billing, such as modifier -54 for surgical care only. In some cases, Medicare Administrative Contractors (MACs) require locally assigned modifiers for use in billing so it is important to know the differences.

The coder will finish coding the account by identifying the physician name that will appear on the claim, reporting quality measures if needed, and adding any other information that is required based on internal processes and policies. Outpatient quality measures are reported for patients who are discharged, transferred, or expire in the ED and are usually reported through registries. The ED leader most often will not provide direct supervision or be responsible for the coding process, but it is important that he or she understands the process and monitors coding outcomes because they impact ED revenue and compliance. From an ED perspective, best practices that support coding and revenue optimization include:

- Coders should use current coding references and payor information, and they need to understand what diagnoses are required to support medical necessity for the services that are charged and coded. There should be a process wherein the coder queries the ED nurse or physician if diagnostic or any other required information is missing, incorrect, or unclear.
- It is important that the charging and coding processes are coordinated so optimal billing can take place. It is the final step in the coding process that "drops" the bill. If the charging process has been delayed and the coding process is completed, the bill will drop without ED charges. This problem can be corrected after the fact, but back-end correction is time consuming and expensive. Missed charges will likely result in lower reimbursement, even if late charges are submitted. Coding should be completed only after all charges are entered into the billing system in a timely manner. It is important that sufficient staff are assigned to perform the charging and coding functions. Adequate resources will help prevent backlogs and misalignment of the charging and coding as described earlier.
- It is usually beneficial if a hospital's process includes a review and validation of the ED charging by the HIM coder, especially if the charging process is completed by busy ED nurses. Missed or inaccurate charges should be added or modified by HIM before the bill is sent.
- The ED leader should collaborate with HIM to ensure that timely compliant charging and coding processes and policies are in place.

Scrub and Release

At this point, code editor software, such as CMS's outpatient code editor (OCE), also known as the "scrubber," is run by the coder to validate that all information and codes are correct and complete. Errors and edits are resolved and the codes are finally extracted into the billing system where they are paired with ED charges for visits and any other charges from ancillary hospital departments. This phase of the RCM cycle has become increasingly valuable to avoid unnecessary follow-up for denied or suspended claims due to inaccurate billing. Numerous systems are available commercially to make the coding and editing process more efficient and help coders avoid coding errors, particularly with Medicare and Medicaid, which have very specific coding requirements that may change frequently for a local area.

Bill Drop

The hospital's billing or PFS department will ensure completion of the automated billing functions once charging and coding have been completed. The PFS's goals are to increase

FIGURE 94.3 ■ Sample UB-04 Form

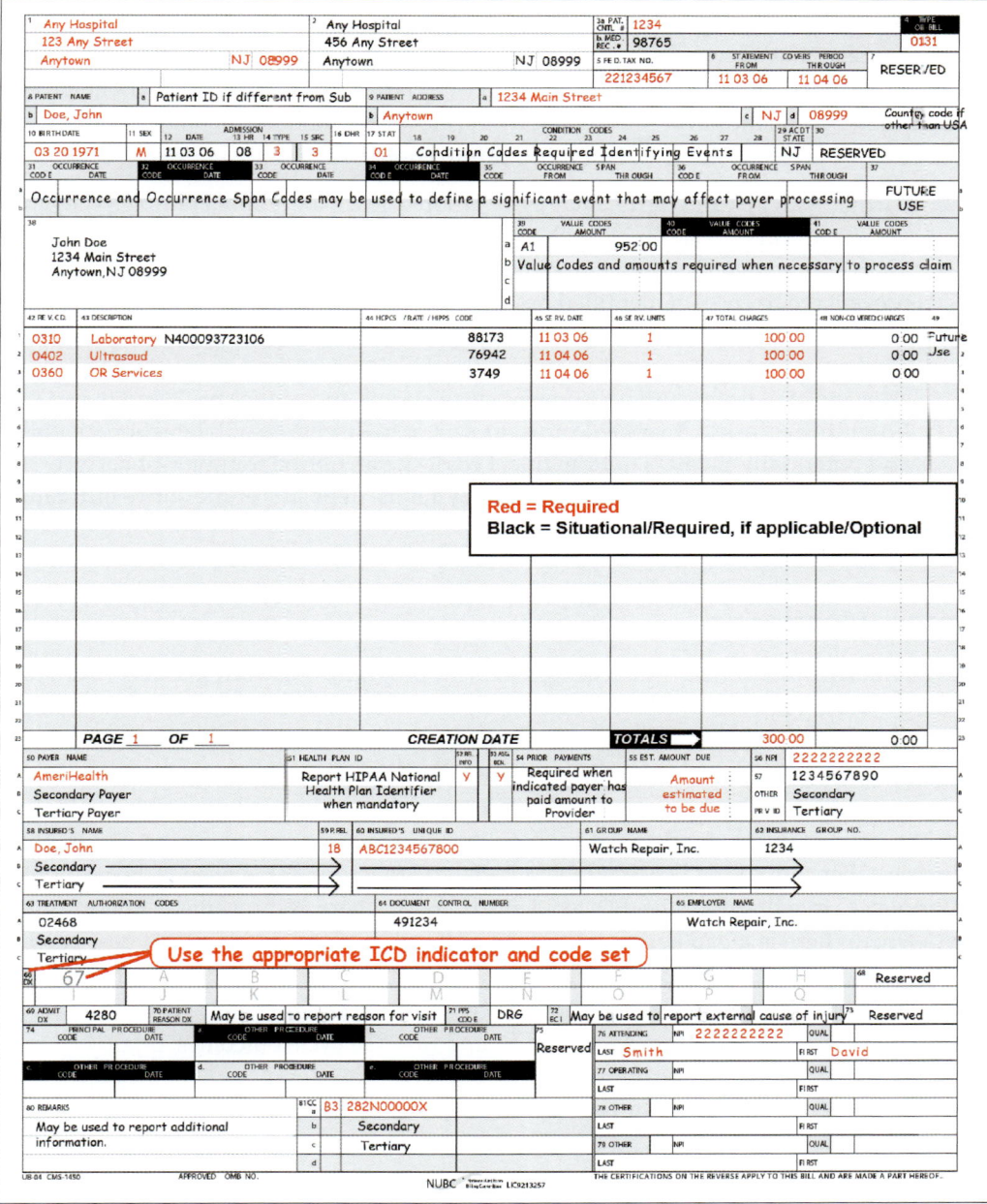

revenue and reduce denied claims through use of an efficient and accurate billing process. Once all charges and codes are in the billing system, an itemized bill for the ED encounter is created and a UB-04 claim is generated (**Figure 94.3**). A prebilling edit process is then run to validate information on the claim to ensure that it is accurate and ready for payor processing.[17]

It is important that the edits in the system are accurate and up to date. A portion of accounts that do not pass this edit process will end up in a sample claim form called "discharged not final billed" (DNFB) report.

Someone in PFS will work to categorize and identify responsibility for resolving the edits. Some of these edits will occur as the result of questionable demographic or payor information and documentation deficiencies or inconsistencies. Emergency clinicians may be called upon to review and help resolve these issues prior to submitting the claim. After all edit concerns have been fixed, a "clean claim" is submitted to the payor or clearinghouse (where the claim will be converted from a nonstandard format to a standard one or vice versa, depending on the payor's needs and the format of the submitted claim).

The contributors to billing and revenue optimization include:

- Partner with PFS and the revenue cycle group to learn more about billing issues and where clinical staff can support the process.
- Make sure someone is reconciling the DNFB list of patient accounts and take steps to prevent recurrences of identified problems.
- For high-volume EDs, consider a discharge desk where registration and discharge information can be reviewed and verified, and payments can be made. This additional step will help ensure clean claims and reduce back-end fixes. Providing access to financial counselors prior to discharge will benefit patients and potentially the ED's bottom line. Providing an option for point-of-service payment collection, which includes copayments, deposits, or the entire bill, can increase ED revenues.

Process Monitoring

Like monitoring in a clinical quality improvement program, monitoring aspects of the ED revenue cycle is required to ensure high-level performance, identify problems, and target improvement efforts. Monitoring efforts include auditing, reports analysis, benchmarking, and paying special attention to key ED performance indicators.

Benchmarking is the process of comparing internal processes and performance metrics with the industry's best (and sometimes looking at similar process benchmarks in other industries). Benchmarking is essentially an analytic practice that is used to help improve performance. It will allow the ED to identify areas where improvement opportunities exist—where there is a gap between the ED's performance and an identified best practice or benchmark. Once these opportunities are identified, performance can be improved by researching best practices and implementing those practices as appropriate in a particular setting. ED benchmarks will include clinical and revenue cycle outcomes, quality of care, time metrics, costs, and productivity.

While the ED leader will not be responsible for monitoring all aspects of the revenue cycle, there are areas that are appropriate for clinical leadership oversight. From an ED perspective, best practices for monitoring that can potentially enhance revenue include:

- Measure and monitor performance in all areas to ensure that registration, documentation, charging, coding, billing, and follow-up are optimal.
- Maintain knowledge of audit response time in order to avoid claim denials.
- Benchmark performance for key ED revenue cycle components and regularly compare current performance to benchmarks or performance targets.
- Examine any variances and try to determine the reasons; even infrequent variances indicate the need for process improvement.
- Review detailed reporting by provider (nurse and/or physician), coder, or biller to facilitate improvements. Dashboards offer a customizable automated display of performance measures or indicators and can provide the ED leadership with real-time and trended views of ED performance. Examples of ED indicators include the ED volume per day, the number of records charged and coded each day compared

with patient volume for the same day, visit-level frequency distributions, number of patients leaving without being seen, and the number of procedures per a given volume, such as per 100 visits.
- Conduct audits at regular intervals, and as needed, on a portion of ED records. These audits should include an evaluation of the quality of registration and documentation, including the physician's orders, charging, and coding. They also should provide feedback and education based on audit findings and track and trend results to show improvement. Start to finish audits should incorporate the "explanation of benefits" (EOB) document, so the outcome of charging, coding, and billing can be assessed together.
- Communicate the results of monitoring, share information, and educate physicians, nurses, and other ED staff on their performance versus best practices. It is especially useful to quantify lost revenue that resulted from less than optimal performance. Set goals for improvement and share results. The establishment of concrete performance goals will help gain buy-in from the ED staff.
- Consider adding a case manager to the ED staff. An ED registered nurse case manager with special training in CDI, disposition decision support (knowledge of medical necessity and admission criteria), discharge planning, charging, some coding, addressing patient concerns, and data analysis can assist and support the ED staff and management with not only monitoring each individual's performance but also in delivering optimal performance in the eight other ED revenue cycle processes.[18]

Compliance Auditing

The world of compliance has grown significantly as the coding and billing process has become more sophisticated and payors have developed electronic monitoring systems to identify anomalies in provider billing. The number of payor audits has increased—from targeted probes and educate process used by MACs to conduct prepayment probes and education processes to the Recovery Audit Contractors (RACs) who are tasked by the Medicare program to identifying improper payments. Initially, few, if any audits were conducted on ED facility levels of service by payors. More recently, however, private payors, Medicare, and Medicaid have developed a variety of systems to identify questionable E/M distribution or overcoding of the higher levels of service (99284, 99285, 99291) and request additional provider documentation to support the charges that are billed.

Internal audits are essential to ensuring correct documentation, coding, and billing. The RCM generally arranges for internal audits on a routine basis. However, it is beneficial for the ED to ensure that broad sample of claims are audited to identify specific areas requiring improvement in the ED. Generally, ED facility audits identify issues with coding of accurate E/M levels, infusions and injections, and, to a lesser degree, procedures.

Follow-Up

Issues requiring follow-up may be identified in any of the ED revenue cycle processes, but they are most often discovered after the billing process or during monitoring. During billing follow-up, an ED leader might be called upon to provide assistance with appealing payment denials and downcodes, payor audit defense, or follow-up on patient complaints regarding their bill. Other common areas of follow-up include:
- Analyzing and resolving problems identified during monitoring
- Improving processes where ongoing "fire-fighting" occurs

- Communicating information to ED staff and physicians
    - ☐ Motivating them to engage in process improvement and corrective actions
    - ☐ Informing them of improvement efforts and outcomes
    - ☐ Congratulating them on successes

Payor Denials

Payor denials in the ED may involve a single record at a time or multiple records. While this process can be time consuming, appeals are often successful so, depending on the extent of the denial, it is usually worth the time and effort to pursue the lost revenue. Appeals should include the provider name, patient name and ID number assigned to the claim by the payor, date of service, the original codes assigned, and the downcodes or issue presented by the payor. A discussion of the documented reason for the visit, presenting problem, risk factors, treatment provided, contributory factors, and discussion of the differential diagnoses should be provided. Some payors determine payment from the final diagnosis. If this is the case, provide supporting documentation to establish the elements of EMTALA and the "prudent layperson standard" that base treatment on presenting problem and show why the patient needed emergency treatment. The "prudent layperson standard" is required of all insurers and simply means that a prudent layperson would consider the presenting problem to be an emergency.

After the ED claim is received and adjudicated by the payor (meaning that the payor determines the "correct" payment amount based on the coded information on the claim, the patient's insurance benefits, and other contractual issues with the hospital or health system), the hospital will receive a response from the payor. The response will usually include a payment accompanied by a document called an EOB or remittance advice. Any variances between what was coded and billed and what the payor ultimately paid will be explained in this document. Payment may be made as submitted on the claim, less than submitted, or denied all together. If an ED visit level was paid at a lower level than the one submitted, it is called a "downcode." If a line item on the claim was not paid at all, it is called a "denial." Reasons for payor denials generally fall into three categories: registration errors, clinical issues, and billing errors.[19] ED nursing leadership is in a key position to address and affect improvements in registration and clinical denials.

When there is a difference between what was billed for an ED encounter and what was paid, the hospital can choose to accept what the payor provides in terms of reimbursement and write off the remainder or the hospital may appeal the difference in effort to recoup all or a portion of the payment that was denied.

In appealing an ED downcode or denial, clinical information will be required to build an argument that the claim was justified as submitted. Someone from the ED or HIM will audit or review the record to determine if the charges and coding were correct. If they were not, the record should not be appealed. If the coding was correct and PFS decides to appeal, they will request that the ED or HIM write an explanation as to why the service and claim for payment were correct and should be paid as submitted. This explanation will involve substantiating the medical necessity for the claim by documenting the patient's severity of illness and the intensity of service provided for the evaluation and treatment of the patient.

Payor Audits

It is important to note that all hospital EDs are being audited by payors. In this time of increased scrutiny of health-care spending and concerns about fraud and abuse, initiatives involving audits, payment denials, and takebacks are showing a strong return on investment for payors.

Audits usually involve a group of ED patient claims or records that the payor believes are incorrectly coded. Most often the concerns are related to visit levels coded at a level higher than the payor expected. The payor will often provide the hospital with patient names and account numbers in a letter and request that the hospital send records to the payor so they can perform an audit. In response, the HIM department will coordinate an audit of the same records to determine the accuracy of the coding. In a process similar to the management of denied claims, the hospital will want to build a response for each record that was coded correctly and prepare a rebuttal to the payor's audit concerns and downcodes.

The audit discussion may take place in writing, via e-mail, over the phone, or in person. Each record will be discussed. The ED medical director leader or ED nurse manager will work with HIM, the hospital compliance department, or the coding vendor to prepare the response. The ED must be able to defend the level of service (and perhaps procedure coding) from a clinical perspective and be able to demonstrate the visit-level methodology was accurately applied. The audit may get into a discussion of the methodology itself, if the payor believes it has led to the "incorrectly" coded visit levels.

The outcomes of audit discussions are highly variable. The payor may agree with the coding after an explanation and some or all of the claims will be paid as submitted, or the downcodes may stand. There is usually an appeals escalation process that the hospital can choose to pursue. As a part of the discussion, it will be important for HIM and the nurse manager to learn exactly what generated the payor concerns such as: Are there payor policies that the hospital was not aware of? Was a payor audit methodology used that was different from the hospital coding methodology? If the payor used the hospital's internal visit coding guidelines, did the payor apply them correctly?

Getting answers to these questions and applying them to coding practice as appropriate may help prevent future audits. It is important that the hospital adheres to the time frames specified by the payor in any rebuttal or appeal process. If a deadline is missed, there may be no other opportunity to reverse the payor's downcodes.

Patient Bill Complaints

Patient complaints about bills are not infrequent and usually occur because the patient believes that the fees on the bill are too high—either the visit level or a procedure. The ED or HIM should audit the record of the encounter to determine if the coding was correct. If not, it should be corrected and a new bill generated. If the coding was correct, how the level of service was determined should be explained to the patient. Often there is some negotiation, and the bill may be reduced. Patients may also be referred to PFS to discuss a payment plan or to charity care, if applicable.

If the coding is correct but other factors favor a reduction in the charges, they may be reduced per hospital policy. If the coding is found to be correct, do not change the CPT codes; a change would misrepresent the services provided. If the complaint involves some type of medical misadventure, a quality of care issue, or a public relations issue, the complaint should be forwarded to risk management and the appropriate ED individual who is responsible for managing patient complaints.

For managing follow-up on revenue cycle processes, the ED leader will usually have a supportive role. It is important, however, that leaders understand the issues and opportunities and provide support when requested by process owners. From an ED perspective, best practices for ED leadership that support follow-up and revenue optimization include:

- Identify drivers of issues creating a need for follow-up; solve problems, identify improvement opportunities, and then modify processes to reduce future concerns.
- When process and performance outcomes vary from benchmarks, investigate why, determine a solution, and make improvements where needed.
- If available, involve an ED case manager to research issues, drive improvement efforts, monitor progress, and communicate liberally.

- Gain a basic understanding of what terms are included in major payor contracts and government payment policies for ED services. For Medicare, this information will be found in the Medicare policy manuals, OPPS rules, and in individual contractor's local payment policies. For Medicaid, each state program has its own payment rules for visit levels and/or procedures; the leader should have a basic understanding of what this Medicaid reimbursement does and does not include.
- Work with PFS to assess reimbursement and manage downcodes and denials. Identify the drivers of these occurrences. Where improvement opportunities exist, modify processes to reduce future concerns.
- When working with payors to rebut an audit, either over the phone or face-to-face, prepare and document the "story" for each record, listen, and provide calm rational responses. These encounters are stressful, but they should not be taken personally. Many payor auditors are unfamiliar with ED coding, especially visit levels, and the audit discussion becomes an education session—this educational style interaction is not a bad thing, if it prevents a future discussion on the same issues.

COMPLIANCE, RULES, AND REGULATIONS

Compliance is a factor in each of the nine components of the revenue cycle discussed earlier. The compliance rules come from multiple directions and organizations, including Medicare, Medicaid, and their contractors and overseers: MACs; RACs; the Office of Inspector General (the OIG acts as a watchdog for CMS by promoting efficiency and compliance and by detecting fraud, waste, and abuse in CMS programs); OPPS guidelines; The Joint Commission; state and federal laws—especially those related to fraud and abuse; commercial payor rules and regulations; and even internal hospital policies.

The risks of noncompliance can be significant for hospitals and include, in escalating severity, take-backs of reimbursement, fines, placement on an OIG corporate integrity agreement oversight program, exclusion from the Medicare program, and jail time if the noncompliance is willful and in direct violation of federal laws. Noncompliance in any form will reflect poorly on the hospital and may result in decreased patient satisfaction and tarnished public relations.

The ED leader should be mindful of compliance when managing the department and, more specifically, when looking at processes and outcomes related to revenue and reimbursement. Nonclinical compliance issues will generally be related to documentation, charging, coding, and/or billing. Knowing the rules and having established policies and procedures in written form for staff to reference, as well as an internal compliance plan, will provide an excellent foundation for compliance. Department managers can help ensure compliance through effective systems and processes, education, audits, and monitoring. Clinical staff can help ensure compliance by providing thorough clinical documentation, by following hospital policies, and by monitoring all coding audits to ensure that problem solving is immediate and corrective action is taken.

Both HIM and PFS devote significant compliance efforts toward understanding and developing policies to support consistent application of Medicare, Medicaid, and other payor rules. It will be beneficial for the ED leader to understand basic information about these payor programs. Most payors audit a portion of an ED's claims and clinical records. Through awareness of program requirements and implementation of policies that support government payor rules, ED leaders can help prevent adverse outcomes that might result from this audit activity.

Medicare

The rules for coding and billing for commercial payors are not always readily available, but CMS has published the rules for charging and coding for Medicare beneficiaries. The

CMS's OPPS outlines these rules, which are updated annually. The OPPS is the payment system that CMS uses to pay hospitals for outpatient services provided for Medicare beneficiaries. Medicare payments are adjudicated regionally by a group of 15 MACS.[20] CMS allows its contractors some latitude in setting payment policies, so it is necessary for someone involved in ED coding and charging to be aware of these local policies. The OPPS rules for outpatient facility payments apply to services provided in EDs and hospital-based clinics, but not to physician services, which are paid based on a professional Medicare fee schedule.

The OPPS uses ambulatory payment classifications (APCs) to determine hospital payments. Ambulatory payment classifications are the outpatient counterpart to inpatient diagnostic-related groups (DRGs), and they are grouped under CPT/HCPCS codes that have a common dollar payment; each CPT code maps to an APC. Unlike DRGs, where one DRG is determined and paid for each inpatient admission, the ED or clinic can be reimbursed for multiple APCs for a single outpatient encounter.

Medicare uses the OCE in their claims-processing software. This editor will read the codes and modifiers on the ED claim and determine the correct payment for services rendered. The CMS correct coding initiative edits are part of the OCE. These edits look for line items that are not usually billed on the same claim, inconsistencies, and other errors that affect payment. Many hospitals have purchased this software and integrated it into their coding systems, which allows coders to validate outpatient coding and make any necessary changes before submitting the claim to Medicare.

The CMS states that they do not expect every hospital ED's visit-level frequency distribution to result in a normal bell curve. The CMS monitors these distributions to make sure hospitals are billing appropriately. As a result of ongoing CMS discussions regarding visit distributions, most hospitals also monitor their internal distributions for all payors and Medicare.

Medicaid

Medicaid is a shared federal and state health-care program that provides oversight and payment for medical services provided to poor and disabled individuals who are enrolled in the program. Medicaid payment rules vary by state. Hospitals closely track these rules and policies to help ensure compliance and reimbursement for services provided.

The intensity of Medicaid compliance oversight and auditing is increasing as health-care reform and other statutes allocate more funding to compliance efforts and detection of fraud and abuse in Medicaid programs.

Commercial Payors

Commercial payors' policies vary, but most follow CPT guidelines and reimburse EDs on a percentage of their charges. Hospital billing departments monitor all applicable payors' payment policies and rules when they are available. Many commercial payors should publish provider bulletins that contain important payment policy information, but most do not. In some recent publications, payors have announced reductions in hospital ED visit level payments as part of cost containment initiatives.

CLINICAL OBSERVATION

There are several services that might be offered in or near an ED that would affect reimbursement. Opening a fast-track area or an urgent care clinic are two, but providing observation is probably the most notably and frequently considered. The CMS defines observation care as an outpatient service with:

> ... a well-defined set of specific, clinically appropriate services, which include ongoing short-term treatment, assessment, and reassessment. These services are furnished while deciding whether the patients will require further treatment as hospital inpatients or if they will be discharged from the hospital.[19]

The CMS publishes very specific rules for observation documentation, coding, and reimbursement for Medicare patients. Many hospitals apply these CMS rules to records coded under other payor programs as well.

According to CMS, the patient is an inpatient starting when formal admission occurs. ED services, observation services, outpatient surgery, lab tests, x-rays, or any other hospital services are considered outpatient if the order to admit as an inpatient has not been written, even if they spend the night in the hospital. Observation services are hospital outpatient services until the physician decides to admit the patient. Observation services can be provided in the ED or another area of the hospital. The CMS acknowledges that the decision for inpatient hospital admission is a complex medical decision-based physician judgment related to the need for medically necessary hospital care. An inpatient admission is generally appropriate if two or more midnights of medically necessary hospital care are required.

For example: The patient comes to the ED with chest pain and remains in the hospital for two nights. The first night is spent in observation, and the doctor writes an order for inpatient admission on the second day. In this example, the patient would be considered an outpatient until formally admitted as an inpatient based on the physician's order.

If the physician writes an order for patient admission, and the hospital later determines it's changing the hospital status to outpatient, the doctor must agree, and the hospital must notify the patient in writing that the hospital status changed. The notification must occur while the patient is still a hospital patient before discharge.

To summarize, even a patient who stays overnight in a regular hospital bed may still be considered an outpatient. Any patient who receives outpatient observation services for more than 24 hours must receive a Medicare Outpatient Observation Notice, which alerts them that their status has been changed.

The observation service may be provided in a regular ED bed, in a special observation area of the ED, in a formal observation unit, or even in an inpatient bed on the floor. The process and rules for coding facility observation are the same irrespective of the location where the service is provided. The CPT has established three sets of observation codes[12]:

- Same-day services, 99234-99236
- An observation stay spanning more than one calendar date, 99218-99220, and an accompanying discharge code, 99217
- The second day of a 3-day observation stay, 99224-99226

For most facility observation coding, however, CPT codes are not used. Most hospitals report a charge with the observation revenue code (762) for commercial payors, or they report the same HCPCS code they use to report observation for Medicare patients, G0378 (hospital observation service, per hour).

Observation is paid under a Comprehensive Ambulatory Payment Classifications (C-APC). However, the individual observation services are identified on the claim form, and Medicare's claim editor converts the individual codes to the C-APC payment amount that has been set for a new APC 8011 for a payment of $2,379.80 with a relative weight of 29.9173 relative value units.

According to CMS Medicare for 2019[21]:

- Claim cannot contain a HCPCS code with status indicator T
- Claim must contain eight or more units of service for G0378 (observation services per hour)
- Claim must contain one of the following codes:
  - G0379 (direct referral of a patient for hospital observation care on the same date of service as G0378, 99281, 99282, 99283, 99284, 99285 [ED visits]); G0380, G0381, G0382, G0383, G0384 (type B ED visit Levels 1-5); 99291 Critical care; First 30 to 74 minutes, or G-0463 (hospital outpatient clinic visit for assessment and management of a patient provided on the same date of service or 1 day before the date of service for G0378). The payment for G0379 in 2019 is $530.13 with a relative weight of 6.6644.
- Claim does not contain a HCPCS code with status indicator J1 (Hospital Part B Services Paid Through a Comprehensive APC).

Facility observation is eligible for Medicare reimbursement if the previously mentioned conditions are met, at least 8 hours of observation are reported, and there is not a surgical CPT procedure code on the same claim. There are strict rules for calculating observation time, including a provision for subtracting the time for any separately billable procedure that requires active monitoring by the nurse. Like ED visits, most procedures provided during an observation stay are reported and paid separately.

CONCLUSION

Managing an ED and structuring processes and systems to achieve optimal financial performance will present some of the greatest challenges in an ED leader's career, but if managed successfully, the experience can be highly rewarding. Collaboration, education, and motivating key staff to engage in and support the process are the keys to pulling all of these RCM processes together to achieve financial success.

Under health-care reform, alternative payment models will be employed where payments will be bundled and hospitals will share financial risk with other providers. The details of how this will work and how the ED will fit into the picture remain to be seen. What is certain is that reform will present new challenges for ED nursing leadership and the need for positive outcomes in the revenue cycle processes discussed in this chapter will be no less important than they are now under a traditional revenue cycle model.

REFERENCES

1. LaPointe J. Exploring Key Components of the Healthcare Revenue Cycle, RevCycle Intelligence. 2017. Available at: https://revcycleintelligence.com/news/exploring-key-components-of-the-healthcare-revenue-cycle. Accessed October 8, 2020.
2. Income measurement. In: Walther L, ed. *Principles of Accounting*. Available at: https://www.principlesofaccounting.com. Accessed September 5, 2018.
3. The American Medical Association. *ICD-10-PCs 2021: The Complete Official Codebook*. Eden Prairie, Minn: Optum 360, LLC; 2020.
4. ICD10data.com. The Web's Free 2021 ICD-10-CM/PCS Medical Coding Reference. 2020. Available at: https://www.icd10data.com/. Accessed October 9, 2020.
5. The American Medical Association. *CPT 2021: Professional Edition*. Chicago, Ill: The AMAStore.com; 2020.
6. Medicare program—revisions to hospital Outpatient Prospective Payment System and calendar year 2007 payment rates; final rule. *Fed Regist*. 2006;71(226):68129-68139. 42 CFR Parts 410, 416, et al. Available at: htpps://www.cms.gov/quarterlyproviderupdates/downloads/CMS1506fc.pdf. Accessed June 27, 2013.
7. Medicare and Medicaid programs; interim and final rule. *Fed Regist*. 2007;72(227):66805. 42 CFR Parts 410, 411, 412, et al. Available at: https://www.cms.gov/quarterlyproviderupdates/downloads/CMS1392fc.pdf. Accessed June 27, 2013.
8. CMS. Medicare and Medicaid programs—interim and final rule. *Fed Regist*. 2007;72(27):66806-66807. 42 CFR Parts 410, 411, 412, et al. Available at: https://www.cms.gov/quarterlyproviderupdates/downloads/CMS1392fc.pdf. Accessed June 27, 2013.
9. American College of Emergency Physicians. ED Facility Level Coding Guidelines. American College of Emergency Physicians.

2020. Available at: https://www.cms.gov/Medicare/Coding/MedHCPCSGenInfo. Accessed October 9, 2020.

10. American Hospital Association. Coding Clinic. July 7, 2020. https://www.codingclinicadvisor.com/. Accessed October 9, 2020.

11. American Health Information Management Association. *ICD-10-CM Official Coding Guidelines*. 2018. https://www.cdc.gov/nchs/data/icd/10cmguidelines-FY2020_final.pdf. Accessed October 4, 2020.

12. Ganovsky M. Critical care billing, in reimbursement strategies. Presented at: ACEP's Emergency Department Directors Academy, February 6, 2020. https://www.acep.org/globalassets/sites/edda/media/nov19-presentations/th-23-reimbursement-issues---granovsky.pdf.

13. CMS.gov. Hospital Outpatient PPS. 2020. Available at: https://www.cms.gov/Medicare/Medicare-Fee-for-Service-Payment/HospitalOutpatientPPS/index?redirect=/HospitalOutpatientPPS. Accessed October 4, 2020.

14. Part B hospital (including inpatient hospital part B and OPPS). In: *Medicare Claims Processing Manual*. Section 160 Clinic and Emergency Visit; subsection 160.1 Critical Care Services (Rev. 2141, Issued 01-24-11, Effective: 01-01-11, Implementation: 01-03-11). Available at: https://www.cms.gov/Regulations-and-Guidance/Guidance/Manuals/Downloads/clm104c04.pdf. Accessed October 1, 2020.

15. Hospital outpatient prospective payment–notice of proposed rulemaking (NPRM). Reg. No. CMS-1695-P. Centers for Medicare & Medicaid Services. 2019. Available at: https://www.cms.gov/Medicare/Medicare-Fee-for-Service-Payment/HospitalOutpatientPPS/Hospital-Outpatient-Regulations-and-Notices-Items/CMS-1695-P.html. Accessed November 6, 2020.

16. Medicare program: hospital outpatient prospective payment and ambulatory surgical center payment systems and quality reporting programs. *Fed Regist*. 2017;82(217). 42 CFR Parts 414, 416, and 419. Available at: https://www.gpo.gov/fdsys/pkg/FR-2017-11-13/pdf/2017-23932.pdf. Accessed October 1, 2020.

17. Legg L. Pre-Bill Audits. Healthcare Resource Group. 2017. Available at: https://www.slideshare.net/HRGPROS/power-of-prebill-audits. Accessed October 1, 2020.

18. Edelberg and Associates. Available at: https://Edelberg.com. Accessed November 6, 2020.

19. CMS Transmittal 1745. *Medicare Beneficiary Policy Manual*. Ch 6, 20.6 Outpatient Observation Services Overview. 290.1. 2020. Available at: https://www.cms.gov/Regulations-and-Guidance/Guidance/Manuals/downloads/bp102c06.pdf. Accessed October 1, 2020.

20. A/B MAC jurisdictions as of October 2017. Centers for Medicare & Medicaid Services (CMS). Available at: https://www.cms.gov/Medicare/Medicare-Contracting/Medicare-Administrative-Contractors/Downloads/AB-MAC-Jurisdiction-Map-Oct-2017.pdf. Accessed November 5, 2017.

21. CMS.gov. Medicare Claims Processing Manual. 2020. Available at: https://www.cms.gov/Regulations-and-Guidance/Guidance/Manuals/downloads/clm104c23.pdf. Accessed October 1, 2020.

CHAPTER 95

BILLING AND COLLECTING

Jeffrey Bettinger, Elijah Berg

Billing and collecting for emergency services are crucial functions because they provide the revenue that supports emergency departments (EDs) and reimburses emergency physicians for the services they render to patients. Whether a practice is fully fee-for-service and self-supporting, is directly employed by the hospital, or requires a subsidy to meet its expenses, all of the legitimate revenue that is generated by the emergency physician should be collected. A sound, professional billing and collection process enhances contract security and provides support for appropriate ED coverage and competitive provider salaries.

BASIC STEPS

The billing process begins long before patient treatment with the establishment of contractual relationships between ED providers and insurance companies. The billing process continues with the ED visit, documentation of the visit on a medical record, and transfer of that record and insurance information from the hospital to the billing agent. Once the billing agent has received the record, it is coded for eventual payment of rendered services before being submitted to the appropriate payor for payment. Finally, the billing process ends when the practice receives appropriate payment.

Many processes are required between each of these steps to ensure that appropriate payment is received. But what are these steps, and how can providers and the billing agents that serve them guarantee that they are collecting appropriate revenue for services? This chapter addresses each of the billing steps in detail and will review benchmarks against which a practice can be measured, as well as common pitfalls that often negatively impact the emergency physician revenue stream. A glossary of terms is provided in **Appendix 95.1**.

ED Record Generation Types

There are a variety of commercially available and locally developed ED treatment records, as well as services and software applications that generate a complete patient record. They include paper and electronic templates, electronic health records (EHRs), scribe services, and voice recognition software. Benefits and drawbacks are associated with each type of record.

Paper Records

Paper records are generally quick to document and, if appropriately designed, incorporate checkboxes meant to enhance provider documentation, support code choice, and simplify billing processes. Relative to electronic and dictated records, paper records are not as easily interpreted by other providers (e.g., the admitting doctor). This difficulty is due to legibility issues and the relatively limited amount of history of the present illness and medical decision-making that is often documented on a paper record.

Commercial Records

Commercial records generally have a cost per encounter, while locally designed records require that an employee of the practice takes responsibility for keeping the record current with changes in:

- "Quality reporting" measures for the physicians
- "Core" measures for the hospitals
- Medicare Administrative Contractor interpretations regarding the required documentation elements

Dictated and Voice-Recognition Records

Dictated records are often expensive and are not always readily available at the time of dictation. While they offer the advantage of a legible printed record that provides other clinicians with good information about the clinical encounter, reimbursement can suffer due to the lack of consistency that a templated record provides and incomplete documentation on certain areas of the record.

Voice-recognition records can provide many of the benefits of dictated records at a lower cost, as well as structured templates that assist the clinician with a consistent documentation process.

Electronic Records

Electronic records provide an immediate typed record and usually cost less than a dictation service. Some EHRs can be completed relatively quickly (3 to 5 minutes) and include appropriate macros that assist the provider in fully documenting the clinical encounter to allow for appropriate reimbursement. Still others can be laborious and time consuming (up to 10 minutes) to document and do not include helpful reimbursement features. Because the choice of an EHR can have a significant impact on reimbursement and productivity, it is important for emergency physicians to provide as much input as possible in the selection of an EHR.

Gathering Demographic and Insurance Data

Unlike office-based practices, emergency physicians do not employ a secretary who verifies insurance information while registering the patient. In the ED, a hospital employee—typically an employee of the "registration" office—has a conversation with the patient, during which demographic information is gathered. These data include the patient's name, address, phone number, insurance (if any), and who is responsible for payment (e.g., for minors or work-related injuries). Upon completion of the registration process, the employee may or may not run an electronic insurance verification check in order to verify the accuracy of the data provided and to obtain copayment amounts.

The accurate gathering of insurance data is critical to the emergency physician practice, because the billing agent will be relying on these data for claims submission. It is not uncommon for a relatively low-wage registration clerk to fail to update a patient's insurance information at registration because the clerk wrongly assumes that there has not been a change in insurance since a patient's last visit. If, after receiving a statement, patients are frequently contacting the billing agent in order to provide up-to-date insurance information, then the hospital registration process may need to be improved.

Transmitting Information to the Billing Entity

Patient demographic information is usually printed on one of the pages of the ED record. While the actual record needs to be sent to the billing agent for both coding and billing, patient demographic data are usually transmitted electronically. Demographic data are usually exported by the hospital IT department in a file format that the billing agent can import directly into its billing software system in preparation for submitting claims and statements.

Health Plan Credentialing/Enrollment

Proper and timely credentialing or enrollment (i.e., Medicare) of ED providers is of the utmost importance. Once a contract between a payor and a group has been finalized, each individual provider within the group (physician/physician assistant/nurse practitioner) will be required to submit credentialing paperwork in order to be eligible to receive payment for the services rendered to the payor's beneficiaries. Medicare will allow providers to get paid for services going back 30 days prior to the credentialing application submission date (or the start date of the physician in the ED, whichever is later), but any services rendered prior to those dates will not be reimbursed. Some private payors will not allow any retroactive payments to be made, creating a significant financial penalty for physicians (groups) whose credentialing application is not complete and submitted prior to the rendering of care. It is important that the credentialing forms be completed prior to the provider's first shift, and there should be robust processes in place, as well as sufficient credentialing staff, to oversee the credentialing process.

Negotiating Payor/Provider Agreements

The choice to contract ("participate") with a payor should be considered very deliberately and acted upon only after review of all of the pertinent data. Rates that can be negotiated, the effect that nonparticipation will have on other parties (e.g., the hospital, medical staff, and patients), and federal and state laws that influence individual payors should all be reviewed and evaluated. Common considerations include

- Does the hospital Independent Physician Association or Physician Hospital Organization face a decrease in payment from the insurance company if the ED group does not participate?
- Does the insurance company honor reassignment of benefits for nonparticipating emergency physicians either based upon company policy or state law?
- How are the allowed payment rates amounts determined for nonparticipating providers?

Additionally, insurance companies offer different types of products (such as indemnity, health maintenance organization [HMO], and preferred provider organization [PPO] products) and each of these are governed by different rules. Each insurance product should be analyzed with all of these items in mind.

When opting to participate with a payor, it is crucial to negotiate for appropriate payment. Be armed with the cost of running a practice and compare the offered rates to other rates that have been negotiated with other payors. Sometimes contracts will identify in dollar amounts the different payments for each of the five ED evaluation and management (E/M) Current Procedural Terminology (CPT) levels (99281-99285), while other payors opt to group the five levels into three payment levels (e.g., 99281/2; 99283; 99284/5). Some payors use a strict payment/relative value unit (RVU) methodology, while others use one global case rate for all visits, and still others pay based upon a percent of what Medicare pays. There is no "correct" methodology. Ultimately, the group should compare the various reimbursement methods in order to find the method that yields the highest payment per visit. It is common to negotiate yearly escalators for a few years, after which time the group should revisit the negotiating table.

Diagnostic Coding

ED services that are provided to patients are submitted to the insurance company for payment using Current Procedural Terminology (CPT) codes and *International Classification of Diseases* diagnosis codes. Coding can be complicated, and many coding rules are updated on an annual basis. Certified professional coders who have received special training in emergency medicine coding will help to ensure optimal revenue and compliance with state and federal regulations. Code choice should be audited annually, and following audits physicians should receive feedback regarding documentation quality from coding and reimbursement perspectives.

Claim/Statement Generation

Claims go to insurance companies, and statements go to patients. Once a record is coded, the charges and diagnosis data populate the billing software system. The billing agent typically gets a demographic insurance data file electronically from the hospital registration system. This demographic data includes payment responsibility and insurance information and is reconciled against the patient account. Both statements and claims list the date of treatment, the services provided (e.g., CPT 99283 for the E/M level and CPT 12001 for the laceration repair), and line item charges that state the price the group is charging for each service. Statements should include a website and customer service number that patients can call with questions and to make payments. When patients fail to respond to a statement, follow-up statements are usually sent at 30 days and again at 60 days. Each subsequent statement should include increasingly strong language that indicates that payment or contact with the business office is expected.

Claim/Statement Submission

Claims are sent to insurance companies both electronically and on paper. All major insurance companies accept and expect claims to be submitted electronically. Electronic claims are submitted through an electronic data interchange (EDI). Some smaller insurance companies are not set up to accept electronic claims, and some companies require submission of a copy of the ED record with the claim (e.g., motor vehicle insurance and workers' compensation claims). Larger billing operations have EDI departments that submit claims directly to insurance companies. If the billing operation cannot electronically submit files directly to the insurance company, then a third-party "clearinghouse" is often hired to convert more standard electronic files into formats that will be accepted by individual insurance companies.

Posting Payments, Disallowances, and Write-Offs

Once payment is received on a claim or statement, the payment is posted (data entered) into the billing software system. Similarly, disallowance adjustments, denials of payment, and write-offs need to be posted in order to adjudicate each invoice. An invoice balance may occur, which requires appropriate action (see later in chapter). Posting may be performed in a manual or electronic fashion. With manual posting, personnel enter the information into the billing software system based on information supplied on the payor remittance advice or the patient statement. With electronic posting, data sent by the payor are entered into the billing software system by way of an electronic data interface. Quality control mechanisms should be in place to ensure accuracy throughout the posting process.

Balance Billing

If claims are submitted to a payor for which the group does not have a contractual agreement as to the payment rate, then in addition to deductibles and copays, there might be an additional balance that the patient will have to pay if the payor does not allow payment of the full charge. The process of sending statements (bills) to the patient or guarantor for this balance is known as "balance billing." In some states, balance billing is prohibited for certain insurance products. In situations where balance billing is prohibited, an attempt is often made to collect additional payments from the payor.

Accounts Receivable Management

For those accounts that remain unpaid, and for other accounts that have partial unpaid balances, the process of attempting to collect the remaining amounts owed is known as "accounts receivable (AR) management." Billing personnel use a variety of techniques in order to attempt to collect unpaid balances. These techniques consist of contacting payors, resubmitting claims, filing appeals, contacting patients for updated insurance information, filing grievances with state agencies, and possibly legal action. Billing personnel are dependent on tools within the billing software that allow identification and aggregation of accounts that require follow-up actions.

A substantial amount of AR is often the responsibility of the patient or guarantor. This AR is often known as "self-pay" or "patient responsible." This AR includes accounts that never had identified insurance and accounts that started out as third-party payor accounts but became self-pay after the payor determined that the patient was responsible for a copayment or deductible amount. Additionally, when payors deny payment for various reasons, the account often transfers to patient responsibility. Again, billing personnel use a variety of techniques in order to attempt to collect unpaid balances in these self-pay accounts. The most common technique is sending the patient or guarantor a series of statements asking for payment. Additional techniques include directly contacting patients by telephone, by publishing websites where the patient can make payments or leave updated insurance information, and by rechecking Medicaid or other databases to see if the patient has valid insurance.

Payment Denial by Payors

There are numerous reasons why payors refuse to remit payment for claims sent to them. Usually, the reason for denial is included on the remittance advice sent to the billing agent. Common reasons for payment denial include:

- No coverage in place on the date of service
- Incorrect patient identification information
- Duplicate invoicing
- Coordination of benefits with another third-party payor, often involving accident cases
- Another payor is the primary payor
- No authorization to be seen in the ED (uncommon with prudent layperson laws)
- ED visit deemed not an emergency (reasons may include the diagnosis submitted or a manual chart review)
- Patient exceeded policy limits for the number of allowed ED visits
- Certain procedures, such as electrocardiograms (ECGs), X-rays, and ultrasounds, may be deemed as "incidental" or "bundled" into the reimbursement of the E/M services, or the procedures may be deemed as "mutually exclusive" from the E/M services

Billing personnel should review each denied account to determine the appropriate follow-up action (see "Accounts Receivable Management" earlier in this chapter).

Modification of Claims by Payors

Many payors make changes to the CPT code set submitted on the claim. These modifications almost always result in payment reductions versus what is expected if each CPT code is paid individually. Follow-up actions by the billing agent are dependent upon whether a contractual relationship exists between the emergency physician and the payor and by state regulations. Common payment modifications include:

- *Bundling*: The payor includes payment for one submitted CPT code to be inclusive in payment for another submitted CPT code.
- *Denial*: The payor determines that one of the individual submitted CPT codes is not reimbursable.
- *Down coding*: The payor changes the level of E/M code to a lower code.
- *Modifier nonrecognition*: The payor determines that the submitted CPT code modifier is invalid for the services rendered.
- *Numerous visits on the same day*: The payor determines that only one ED visit or one observation visit is payable on the same day of service.

Billing personnel should review each denied account to determine the appropriate follow-up action.

Collection Agencies

Many emergency providers instruct their billing agent to transfer unpaid "self-pay" accounts after a defined period of time to a collection agency. At this stage, the account is generally categorized as having been written off as bad debt. The account is still owned by the emergency provider, but attempts at collection are now handled by a collection agency.

Most collection agencies use a combination of mailings and telephone calls in an attempt to collect payment. Often, the collection agent queries available databases in order to increase their ability to collect payment. The degree of aggressiveness of the collection agent varies by agent and by instructions from the emergency physician group.

Some emergency providers will sell their bad debt after the collection agent has unsuccessfully attempted to collect payments for a defined period of time. A third party will purchase the bad debt at a deeply discounted rate. The emergency provider no longer owns the account and may not have any input if patients feel aggrieved or dispute the account.

STANDARD BILLING REPORTS

Whether medical billing is performed by an in-house billing agent, or through an outsource vendor, almost all medical billing organizations create monthly summary reports. "Standard" billing reports typically contain limited variables and appear in a fixed format from month-to-month. A standard billing reports package may include:

- Aging report
- Collections analysis report
- Cash receipts and charges report
- Encounter-tracking report
- Time-to-collect report
- Coding acuity reports

| TABLE 95.1 ■ Sample Aging Report ||||||
| Client XYZ, Accounting Period January 20xx ||||||
	< 0-30 Days	30-60 Days	60-90 Days	90-120 Days	≥ 120 Days
Medicaid					
Self-pay					
Blue Cross					
X-HMO					
Y-Insurance					
Medicare					

Aging Report

Sometimes referred to as an "aged trial balance report," an aging report provides a one-line aging snapshot for individual payor AR at current, 30, 60, 90, and 120+ days. Accounts receivable represents gross amounts in patient accounts that are outstanding. See **Table 95.1** for an example of a typical aging report. The zero date is usually determined by the billing organization and may begin on the date that the service was provided, on the date of data entry, or on the date of actual claim submission. While some billing organizations choose to re-age an invoice to the zero date when financial class information changes, other billing organizations opt instead to keep the invoice in the original financial class regardless of the change of class.

Ideally, a billing organization will include aging data for each individual payor. The "current" period—0 to 30 days after claim generation—typically accounts for the largest component of AR on an aging report. However, because the current category can be artificially inflated by billing systems that re-age accounts to current after the primary insurance partially pays or denies payment, a truly accurate picture can only be had if invoices remain in their original age column, even if a change of financial class occurs.

For example, assume a payor denies payment due to lack of eligibility and the invoice is then reclassified as a self-pay account. If the system re-ages the account to current as a result of the change of financial class, the current AR will be falsely inflated providing an inaccurate snapshot of the current and total AR. Whenever possible, billing software reports should incorporate rules that do not allow a change of financial class to current following partial payment or denial.

Collections Analysis (Ratio) Report

A collection analysis report provides a snapshot of collected amounts and reflects any adjustments to the original charges by tracking payments and comparing them to the original charge. See **Table 95.2** for an example of a typical collections analysis report. This report typically includes columns for charges, receipts, disallowances, bad debt, and an AR balance. Not every billing agent is capable of tracking payments, disallowances, and write-offs back to the original charge. However, this process is the most accurate method of calculating collection rates.

All columns should also be expressed as a percentage of charges for each month in a 24-month period. The amounts in each row represent the receipts, disallowances, and bad

TABLE 95.2 ■ Sample Collections Analysis Report

Client XYZ

Month	Visits	Charge	Collections to Date	Average Collections Per Visit	Disallowances	Bad Debt	AR Balance

debt for invoices that are included in charges for the individual historic month. Occasionally, an organization will include a "collection agency receipt" column, although this is uncommon.

The most critical information in the collections analysis report can be found in the "collections per visit" column. This calculation avoids differences in collection percentages that can be artificially altered by different fee (charge) structures.

Cash Receipts and Charges Reports

Also known as the "transaction summary report" or the" collection and charges trending report," the cash receipts and charges report are actually two reports in one. The report should be evaluated as a 1-month review of payments and disallowances by financial class, as well as a multimonth account of summary charges and collections. **Tables 95.3** and **95.4** are examples of a typical cash receipts and charges report. Ideally, the cash receipts and charges report should follow strict calendar month accounting rules. While the single report should contain receipts and disallowances for all major financial classes, trending reports should track data for the previous three years and should contain encounter number information.

TABLE 95.3 ■ Sample Cash Receipts and Charges Report (Summary)

Month	Charges	Payments	Disallowances	Write-Offs	Volume
Jan 20xx					
Feb 20xx					
Mar 20xx					
Apr 20xx					
May 20xx					
Jun 20xx					

TABLE 95.4 ■ Cash Receipts and Charges Report (per Payor)					
Payer	Charges	Payments	Disallowances	Write-Offs	Volume
Medicare					
Medicaid					
Workers' compensation					
Tricare					

Encounter-Tracking Reports

One of the areas of potential revenue loss for emergency physician services is misplacement of information necessary to generate an accurate invoice. It is not uncommon to see ED records that were never received by the billing agent. Despite the fact that most records are transmitted to the billing agent electronically, important parts of the chart, such as templated records, transcriptions, nursing notes, and ECGs, often fail to reach the billing agent in a timely fashion, if at all. The results are absent, or diminished, revenue per encounter.

The ED log is the primary source document from which data are culled for the encounter-tracking report. See **Table 95.5** for an example of a typical encounter-tracking report. The federal and state laws and The Joint Commission requirements mandate that all ED patients be entered into the ED log. (All patients who present to the ED—including any admits—should be accounted for in the log.) Emergency department and billing agency personnel use this log as the initial control document against which all reconciliation is performed after date of service.

Personnel who are responsible for the encounter-tracking mechanism should never rely on notations such as left without being seen, against medical advice (AMA), and private medical doctor. Rather, patient records for these visits should be consulted to confirm that these visits are nonbillable encounters.

TABLE 95.5 ■ Sample Encounter-Tracking Report			
Date of Service	# Patients in Log	# Missing Records	# Incomplete Records
January 1			
January 2			
January 3			
January 4			
January 5			
January 6			
January 7			
January 8			
January 9			
January 10			

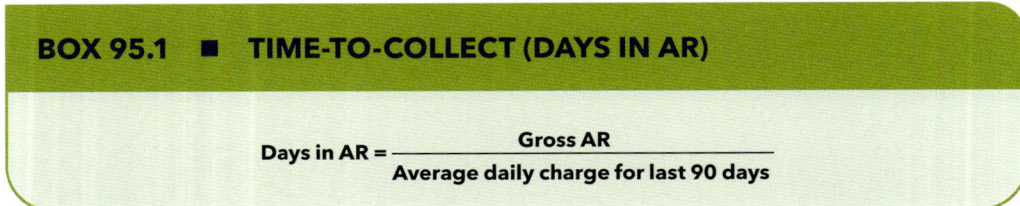

BOX 95.1 ■ TIME-TO-COLLECT (DAYS IN AR)

$$\text{Days in AR} = \frac{\text{Gross AR}}{\text{Average daily charge for last 90 days}}$$

Time-to-Collect Reports

The most common calculation used as a time-to-collect report is the days in AR calculation. Days in AR can be calculated by dividing gross, active AR, by the average daily charge for the previous 90-day period. While some analysts prefer net days in AR, net AR is a difficult calculation for emergency medicine (**Box 95.1**).

Coding Acuity Reports

Coding acuity can be evaluated by review and evaluation of a variety of reports. A coding reports package should include the following:

- *Procedure code analysis report.* Total and by provider.
- *E/M CPT codes distribution report.* Total and by provider (**Table 95.6**).
- *RVU reports*
- *CPT code distribution by payor*

Common Benchmarks

Coding and billing benchmarks should be established for key processes. While there are some national benchmarks against which a group can measure performance, it is important to determine benchmarks based upon local factors. For example, if a group treats an abundance of self-pay patients and is also nonparticipating with many insurance products for which patients are paid directly, then AR will take longer to collect compared to other practices. If the ED is relatively understaffed and uses an EHR that is quite laborious, then the percent of records completed at the end of a shift will be less than that of a well-staffed ED that uses an easy-to-use EHR.

Once a benchmark is established, it is important to measure and evaluate fluctuations in performance over time. One value of a benchmark is the ability to recognize a change in

TABLE 95.6 ■ Sample E/M CPT Code Distribution

Provider	Visits	99281		99282		99283		99284		99285		99291	
		Vol	%	Vol	%	Vol	%	Vol	%	Vol	%	Vol	%
Smith													
Jones													
Bass													
Robb													
Total													

> **BOX 95.2 ■ COMMON ED BILLING BENCHMARKS**
>
> - E/M distribution
> - Average charge
> - Unbilled charts
> - Days until bill submission
> - Accounts receivable aging
> - Outstanding accounts receivable
> - Days in accounts receivable

performance and identify the underlying cause for the change. Common coding and billing benchmarks and key performance indicators are listed in **Box 95.2** and discussed next.

Evaluation and Management Code Distribution

This local benchmark is based on the acuity of the patient population that presents to the ED for treatment. A tertiary referral center will have a higher acuity "right-shifted" distribution when compared with a community hospital. Medicare publishes state and national data that may provide some benchmarking data. However, it should be recognized that Medicare patients tend to be sicker than non-Medicare patients, so these data are not reliable for establishment of an "all-payor" benchmark. Once a benchmark is set, it is important to continually evaluate an all-payor and E/M distribution because patient acuity within the ED generally remains stable from month to month. Another general acuity indicator is the admission rate, where an increasing admission rate is consistent with a higher acuity distribution. A specific benchmark can be determined by having a statistically significant sample of records diligently audited by an experienced ED coder.

Average Charge

The fee schedule, E/M acuity distribution, and procedure coding determine the average charge. This metric is expected to remain stable from month to month, assuming no changes to the fee schedule.

Unbilled Charts

This very important metric can highlight "intradepartmental" operational opportunities. Less than 0.5% of patient records should go unbilled. There are a variety of operational pitfalls that can result in failure of coding or billing, such as a provider not completing a patient record or a record not transmitted to the billing agent. Unbilled records represent lost revenue. Paper processes are more prone to contribute to a missed benchmark than EHR-generated records. The key to measuring the rate of unbilled records is to reconcile the charts coded by the billing agent to the hospital's electronic ED log.

Days Until Bill Submission

"Days until bill submission" is the average number of days from the date of service until a bill is submitted. This is a good measure of the success of "front-end" processes that include chart completion, chart transmission to the billing agent, and the completion of coding and data entry. Increases in this number may highlight a backlog in any one of these processes. A reasonable benchmark for this process is between 9 and 14 days.

AR Aging

An aging report should be evaluated with several key performance benchmarks in mind. The gross AR data are of prime importance. Less than 20% to 25% of the gross, active AR should be older than 120 days. Individual payor data that reside in the >120-day category should also be evaluated and will be influenced by a variety of factors, including:

- Organization's dunning (statement and phone call cycle) philosophy
- Self-pay process
- Resetting of initial bill date when balance transferred to another payor
- Outstanding provider numbers
- Individual payor payment policies
- State timely payment laws
- Billing company AR management

Overall, an aging report should reveal a trend of steadily decreasing AR, with very little buildup of AR in the older aging categories. Importantly, the distribution of the aging categories should be stable from month to month. If there is an increase in the age of certain buckets, the underlying reason should be investigated.

Another important column is the amount of outstanding AR. As a rule, this report should reveal less than 2% outstanding AR at the 12-month period.

Ideally, the days in AR report will reveal the amount of charges that remain open. Total charges/average daily charge is the days in AR formula. Days in AR should typically fall between 40 and 60 days. Factors that may negatively impact the days in AR calculation include the following:

- Billing organization's dunning philosophy
- Efficiency of the billing operation
- Credentialing or enrollment delays or write-offs of Medicare AR
- Problem payors
- Physician nonparticipation and insurance not honoring reassignment of benefits
- Accuracy of initial patient insurance information
- Time at which AR is transferred to a collection agency

COMMON PITFALLS

When utilizing billing agents and collection services, advanced consideration of several processes can prevent common pitfalls.

Unbilled Visits

All visits should be reconciled to an ED log to ensure that a claim is submitted for each visit. Some of the common reasons that visits go unbilled include:

- Paper record is "broken down" before the clinician has had a chance to complete the record
- EHR is not completed
- Flaws in electronic transmission of charts to the billing agent
- Provider fails to fill out the record because he or she mistakenly thinks that a clinical encounter did not warrant completion of a record. This can occur in cases such as direct hospital admissions that are first seen in the ED, same-day visits, and patients who are seen by private physicians in the ED.

Provider Credentialing or Enrollment Problems

The most common credentialing problem occurs when providers fail to enroll in governmental plans in a timely manner, resulting in attendant write-offs for failure to obtain proper credentialing. Factors to consider include:

- Medicare will only allow the effective date of the provider number to be 30 days retroactive from the latter of the date that:
    - Application is received by Medicare
    - Provider begins providing services
- Many Medicaid plans do not allow for retroactive application of provider numbers.
- Certain Blue Shield health plans may only review a provider's enrollment on a predetermined schedule (e.g., once per month by a committee). These inherent delays may cause a period of nonpayment during which the claims may be considered to be out of network.

Fee Schedule Issues

Provider fees that are set below the usual and customary community fees for similar CPT codes will result in less than optimal reimbursement. A group's fee schedule should be reviewed annually at a minimum. Some contracts pay the group "the lesser of the contracted rate or provider charge." If charges are below the contracted payments (or usual and customary payment for nonparticipating providers), the group is losing revenue.

Managed Care Contracting Issues

Poor negotiation of expected payments in managed care contracts will negatively impact reimbursement rates. Successful negotiation of managed care contracts is critical to the financial success of an ED group. Contracts should be reviewed at least annually, and each product (PPO, HMO, etc.) should be evaluated individually. Groups should understand that insurance negotiation is similar to other types of negotiation, and strategic preparation should be undertaken prior to the negotiations. The insurance companies that represent the largest percentages of the payor mix should be especially well managed.

Coding Errors

Lack of attention to coding guideline clauses in managed care contracts can result in lower than average payment rates for bundled services. Payors often have policies that bundle in common ED procedures (such as ECGs) with the E/M payment. It is preferable for the payor not to have such policies. However, if these policies exist and cannot be removed from the contract, then bundled services payment rates should be negotiated.

Inaccurate Insurance Information

Sometimes, the demographic insurance data provided by the hospital to the billing agent include inaccurate demographic information. Submission of inaccurate data on claims that are submitted to payors will result in delays in collection of or nonpayment of receivables.

Acceptance of Noncontracted Payment Amounts

Even when insurance companies may have contracted to pay a certain amount for a particular service, they may actually pay less than the contracted amount. Processes for identifying payment discrepancies should be established. When payment discrepancies are noted, the go-forward payment rates should be corrected, and any back payments that are due should be obtained. Ideally, any underpayments will be identified at the time of payment posting. However, they can also be identified by an electronic or manual review and comparison of contracted payment rates to actual payments.

AR Management Issues

Lack of appropriate AR management by the billing organization will result in untimely payments and lost revenue. The billing staff should actively work unpaid claims. Claim status should be checked by way of payor websites or through direct contact with the insurance carriers. Rebilling of claims should be scheduled based upon payor payment cycles and should be followed closely.

CONCLUSION

Billing and collections is an integral part of the practice of emergency medicine. Revenue generated helps underwrite staffing of EDs with competent physicians and other emergency providers. The various processes involved with billing and collecting for emergency services are complex, with many areas of potential diminishment of eventual collected revenue. By understanding the complexity of the billing process, ED leaders can identify areas of weakness and institute corrective actions that allow for maximal collections of legitimate revenue for emergency services.

APPENDIX 95.1

Glossary of Terms

Term	Definition
Accounts receivable (AR)	Total outstanding charges awaiting payment. AR can be expressed as gross or net. Gross AR is the total, nondiscounted charges awaiting payment. Net AR is the total charges awaiting payment, discounted for expected adjustments.
Adjustments	Nonpayment credits that reduce the AR. Adjustments may include the following: disallowances, bad debt write-offs, small balance write-offs, courtesy adjustments, charge corrections, and timely filing limit write-offs.
Aged trail balance (ATB) report; also aging report	Billing report that lists remaining AR amounts from historic periods. ATB reports typically list remaining AR for the past four to six individual months, plus a summary value for all AR older than the oldest individual month (such as over 120 days).
Allowable	Expected payment per CPT code from any payor, including nongovernmental insurer or governmental payor such as Medicaid or Medicare.
Bad debt	Uncollectable charges, not including disallowances and other write-offs.
Balance billing	Process of sending a statement to the patient, or guarantor, to cover the portion of the account that was not paid by the insurer.
Bundling	Process where the insurer incorporates payment for one service into payment for a second billed service. This usually is seen by combining two or more CPT codes into one payment. Bundling edits appear on explanations of benefits (EOBs) as showing certain procedures as "incidental" or "mutually exclusive" and are common with EKGs, X-rays, ultrasound, and moderate sedation codes.

Charge ticket/fee ticket	A form that some ED physicians use to enable the physician to assign CPT codes for the patient visit and for any procedures performed during the visit.
Coding	Process of applying accurate CPT and *ICD-10* codes to the medical record.
Collection agency	Usually a separate company from the primary billing entity; collects payments on accounts that the billing agent has been unable to collect.
Conversion factor	Dollar value that when multiplied by the RVU, gives the allowable Medicare payment amount.
CPT (current procedural terminology)	Codes described in a manual published annually by the American Medical Association that codifies and describes all physician services for billing purposes.
Credit balance	Overpayments that have been received for an account.
Data entry	Input of data into the billing software system. Data entry is required for claim/statement generation, and also for updating any payment activity (payment posting).
Days in AR	Calculation derived by dividing the amount of active AR by the average daily charge (gross days in AR). Net days in AR is similar, but substitutes net AR and net charges.
Disallowance	Amount of AR that cannot be collected secondary to provider-contracted fee schedules with governmental or nongovernmental payors.
Down-coding	A process where the insurer pays for a lesser CPT code than the code submitted by the physician.
Dunning	Cycle of repetitious demands for payment.
Electronic claims submission	Transmission of billing claims to the insurer via electronic means.
Electronic funds transfer	Electronic transfer of funds from the insurer to the provider's bank account.
Electronic interface with hospital	A communication protocol that allows electronic transmission of patient demographic information from the hospital to the billing agent.
Electronic remittance	Direct electronic transmission of payment information from the payor's system to the billing agent's software system.
ED registration system	Software applications used by ED registration clerks to enter patient demographic data.
Encounter tracking	Use of control documents, and procedures, to verify that 100% of billable visits are accounted for.
CMS-1500 form	Standard claim form accepted by most insurers. There are both paper and electronic versions.
Hospital information system	Primary software application used by the hospital for patient demographic information and other accounting functions, including hospital billing and collections.
International Classification of Diseases, Ninth Edition (ICD-10)	Manual that codifies all diseases and injuries constructed and updated by the World Health Organization.
Lockbox	Banking arrangement where the deposits are sent directly to a post office box, opened by the bank, and deposited. Copies of payment information and correspondence are then sent to the billing agent.

Nonrecourse factoring	Sale, by the provider, of AR to a vendor who then owns the AR and attempts collection.
Percentage of AR greater than 120 days	Calculation derived by dividing the AR greater than 120 days old by the total AR, multiplied by 100.
Provider enrollment	Process of obtaining provider numbers for practitioners in order to receive payment from certain payors.
RBRVS (resource-based relative value system)	Payment system designed by the CMS that assigns relative weights for provider work, practice expense, and malpractice costs when calculating the total relative value unit (RVU) for each CPT code.
Recoupments	Process where the insurer reduces provider payment caused by overpayment on a previous account.
Secondary placement	Further attempt at collection by another vendor after the collection agency has finished working an account. The provider still owns the AR.
Statement	Invoice that is generally sent to the patient or guarantor.
Tax identification number (TIN)	A number that is assigned by the U.S. Internal Revenue Service and identifies provider groups. The TIN is listed on all billing claims.
Timely filing limits	Length of time that an insurer allows a claim to be submitted after the date of service.
Time-of-service (TOS) payment	Payment made at the time of the ED visit.
Ultimate collectability	Collection percentage expected to be achieved after all AR is adjudicated. Depending on the internal policy of write-offs of bad debt, ultimate collectability is usually expressed as a percentage 12 to 24 months after the date of service. This is often determined per payor class, and in total.

CREATING A CULTURE OF COMPLIANCE

CHAPTER 96

Edward R. Gaines III

It takes 20 years to build a reputation and five minutes to ruin it. If you think about that, you'll do things differently.

—Warren E. Buffet

Compliance is more than just coding and billing correctly. It entails addressing legal and regulatory standards while ensuring quality assurance (QA), risk management, and ethical responsibility. It's saying "the ends do not justify the means and that the 'means' matter."

Emergency medicine has unique and heightened exposure to federal and state penalties because of the volume of patients treated in the emergency department (ED) and the ever-growing proportion of patients who are insured by the government. Though government payor patients are the primary focus of the US Department of Justice (DOJ) and the US Department of Health and Human Services (DHHS) Office of the Inspector General (OIG), enforcement, penalties, and damages for commercial fraud can be significant as well. This is true in small community hospitals as well as in academic trauma centers, again because of the volume of transactions in the ED and the characteristics of "per-claim" penalties and damages under federal and state law.

Too often, emergency physicians talk about compliance *only* in terms of the prebilling and, specifically, the coding issues of compliance. While a focus on coding risk areas is absolutely essential, it is critical to pay particular attention to the post-billing compliance issues, which are particular importance to the federal government.

The federal False Claims Act (FCA), explained in detail later in this chapter, applies to any government payor, including Medicare, Medicaid, Tricare/CHAMPUS, and the Federal Employees Health Benefit Plan (FEHBP), also known as Federal Blue. The FCA penalties and overpayments are based on a *per-claim* methodology (e.g., Centers for Medicare & Medicaid Services [CMS] 1500 claim), where the ED volumes serve to provide "a multiplier effect" for claims that are, for example, found to be routinely up-coded. While these exposures certainly exist for an office-based or clinic practice, the volumes of government claims make the ED an attractive target for government investigators and qui tam relators (whistleblowers).

THE TRUE PURPOSE OF COMPLIANCE PROGRAMS

While participation in the government payor programs is voluntary, in a practical sense, it is mandatory for emergency medicine. Compliance programs should seek to protect both the ED group and the individual clinician. Medicare's provider transaction access number (PTAN) permits the physician's services to be billed and reimbursed by Medicare but, like a driver's license, it is revocable. Provider transaction access numbers are issued to ED groups; in turn, emergency physicians "reassign" their Medicare receivables to their employed or contracted groups. The group's PTAN is also revocable. Because both the individual clinician and ED group PTANs are listed on the CMS 1500 claim form, both the physician and the group are certifying to the truthfulness, accuracy, and completeness of that claim, though neither generally code the chart or send the bill for the services. The consequences of violating these certification statements on the claim form could be revocation of the PTAN, which would effectively eliminate the physician's or group's ability to practice emergency medicine.

Beyond protecting the individual and group practice, compliance programs with significant resources devoted to auditing and monitoring (coding and billing QA) should enhance the appropriateness of the group's revenue capture. Undercoding, which is coding that is lower than that supported by the medical record, is a significant issue for emergency medicine. Detecting and correcting both undercoding and overcoding are critical objectives of an effective compliance program. While the federal government may care less about undercoding and its associated decreased payments to the group, emergency clinicians and their partners certainly should care. Vigorous and continual QA programs with randomly selected claims and coding should serve to discover both over- and undercoding. Therefore, compliance is also about achieving the appropriate code capture and collecting all of the reimbursements that the group is entitled to—no more and no less.

The fact is that many of the good management practices that ED groups engage in can and should be part of an effective compliance program. What is required is the formalization of those practices into an effective corporate compliance program (CCP). The US DHHS (or HHS) OIG has repeatedly stated that only "effective" CCPs would receive "credit" by the agency (more on credit concept later). In fact, the truism in compliance is that it is better to have no policies and procedures (P&P) in place than to ignore those that already exist. In other words, there is more risk having a compliance program that is a "paper tiger" than having none at all—and having none at all is no longer an option for emergency physicians under the Patient Protection and Affordable Care Act of 2010 (PPACA, or ACA).

THE PATIENT PROTECTION AND AFFORDABLE CARE ACT OF 2010

The PPACA, Section 6401, requires that providers of Medicare and Medicaid services, as a condition of enrollment, "establish a compliance program that contains certain elements" as determined by the secretary of HHS. As of August 2018, HHS had not yet issued its final regulations on the CCP requirements for physicians and/or ED groups, and there is no indication that HHS will be issuing regulations in the near future. What if the emergency physician practices as "John Smith, MD, FACEP, LLC" (individual LLC) or bills under their social security number (SSN) instead of an employer identification number? It is expected that HHS will permit physicians to certify that their compliance requirements are being met through their ED group's CCP. Alternatively, if emergency physicians use their individual LLC or SSN, HHS may require them to have their own CCP that meets certain core elements.

Both emergency physicians and groups should avoid intentionally or unintentionally "certifying" their CCP if none exists. The Medicare provider/supplier enrollment form 855i (individual) explains in detail the significant criminal and civil sanctions, and penalties, including potential exclusion from the governmental reimbursement programs, that can occur as a result of false certification of information in the provider enrollment process. An ED group may fall into another potential trap by certifying that it meets the core CCP elements as a result of simply "bootstrapping" its ED coding and billing company's CCP, when the ED group has no independent program. The PPACA statutory compliance mandate creates an obligation on the entity or person who is enrolled in the Medicare/Medicaid program is providing the certification. To date, coding and billing companies cannot enroll in these governmental programs; thus, an "incorporation by reference" by the physicians will not suffice.

The Notice of Proposed Rule Making (NPRM), issued by HHS (2010), is based on the OIG's well-established compliance program guidance (CPG) for third-party billing companies (1998), individual physicians, and small group practices (2000). The HHS stated in the NPRM that it is considering whether certain additional elements, for example, "quality indicators," should be included as part of the provider's compliance program. At the time of publication of this chapter, it is the opinion of this author that most of the final requirements are known.

Now more than eight years after the passage of the PPACA, there exists an apparent statutory requirement but no implementing regulations from HHS and no indication that the same will be issued anytime soon. Emergency medicine groups should seek and obtain an experienced health-care counsel's advice on issues related to whether the ACA obligations pertain to them.

HEALTH-CARE FRAUD AND ABUSE LAWS

A review of the PPACA fraud and abuse provisions reveals an extraordinary breadth of stipulations, penalties, and consequences. For example, new provisions for Medicare and Medicaid administrative payment suspensions based on "credible allegations of fraud" were included in Section 6402 (h)(1), which requires that once "overpayments" are identified, the refund must be received by that payer within 60 days with a written explanation.

In the context of emergency medicine compliance, the federal FCA has greater importance than many of the other fraud and abuse laws. This is because of the disproportionately high numbers of Medicare and Medicaid patients treated in the ED. The FCA assesses penalties on one who "knowingly presents or causes to be presented" false or fraudulent claims to governmental payors. (These payors include Medicare and Medicaid but also include Tricare [CHAMPUS] and the FEHBP that has been administered by Blue Cross Blue Shield.

Under the FCA, the government is not required to prove specific intent to defraud. Instead, it must only prove by a preponderance of the evidence one or more of the following:

- The party knowingly allowed or encouraged falsity.
- The party had "deliberate ignorance" of the truth or falsity of the claim.
- The party had "reckless disregard" of the truth or falsity of the claim, including where one "knew or should have known" about the truth or falsity of the claim.
- "Abuse" is generally defined as practices that are inconsistent with sound medical or business practices, actions taken where there is no legal right to reimbursement or acts in which "specific intent to defraud" cannot be proven. Examples could include unknowingly billing a charge for service that should have been bundled into the primary service or rebilling claims without a legitimate basis for the rebill.

To illustrate, the CMS improper payment rate in FY 2017 fell below 10% (9.5%) for the first time and includes improper coding and insufficient or nonexistent documentation (**Figure 96.1**). For claims arising on or before August 1, 2016, and once the proof standards

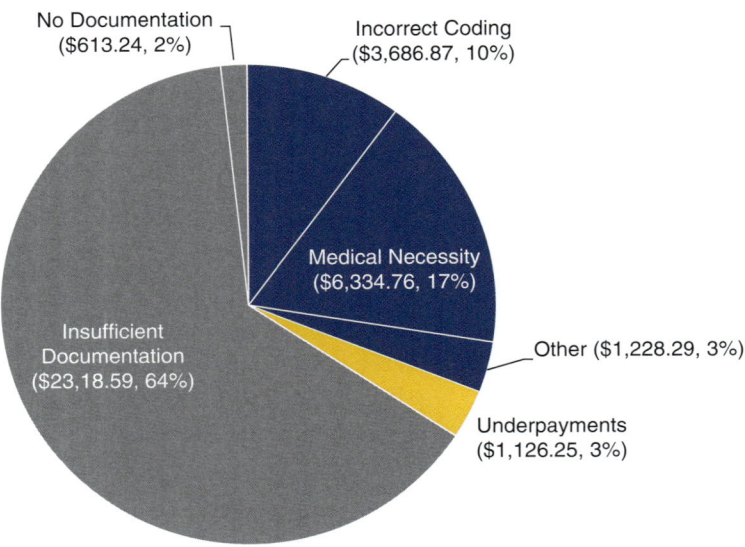

FIGURE 96.1 ■ Improper Payments

are met, the penalties are set at a minimum of $5,500 per claim and maximum $11,000 per claim. The maximum may be obtained if there was a specific intent to defraud:

- 100,000 annual visits to hospital ED system with a 30% governmental payor mix
- Assume a 1% FCA "knew or should have known" or "deliberate ignorance" of the truth or falsity of the claims of the 30,000 governmental payor claims
- Minimum penalty = 1% or 300 × $5,500 = $1.65 million
- Maximum penalty = 1% or 300 × $11,000 = $3.3 million
- Plus, treble damages of the difference; for instance, between CPT 99285 and 99284, per claim across the 300 claims. Examples:
  - If 300 Medicare claims were overcoded at CPT 99285 (2012) payment at $168, but should have been coded at CPT 99284 (2012) payment at $115, the overpayment per claim is $53.
  - That would be tripled for each claim to $159 ($53 × 3).
  - The "total overpayment" for that 300 patients would equal $47,000 (300 patients × $159.00 per patient).
  - This total overpayment under the FCA is only one part of the government claim. They could also demand the minimum penalty of $5,500 per CMS 1500. 300 × $5,500 = $1.65 million.
  - Total government liability = $1,697,000.

Congress required that the DOJ update the per-claim penalties in the FCA, and DOJ did so in February 2017. For claims arising on or after August 1, 2016, the range of FCA penalties would be as follows using the above examples:

- Minimum penalty = 1% or 300 claims × $10,781 per claim totaling $3.244 million
- Maximum penalty = 1% or 300 claims × $21,562 per claim totaling $6.468 million

As a result, ED coding and billing is a potentially attractive target for governmental investigators (as well as *qui tam* relators—see next section of this chapter). The myth that an ED group is a "small fish" to investigators should be dispelled.

The Qui Tam Relator

One of the key features of the FCA is that "whistleblowers" known as *qui tam* relators may file cases as the original source of the information. *Qui tam* is short for *qui tam pro domino quam pro seipso* (he who is as much for the King as for himself). Relators are typically current or ex-employees (including physicians and advanced practice providers [APPs]) of the entity that is the subject of the complaint. There is no requirement under the FCA that the relators must first access the internal compliance reporting methodologies—for example, internal "hotline" or compliance website—as a precondition to filing their case.

These cases are filed in federal district court in secret until the DOJ decides whether or not to join the case. During the time that the case is under seal, the entity against whom the complaint is pending has no independent knowledge of the complaint's existence. During review by the DOJ, the entity may or may not be asked to respond to the complaint. The case does not become a matter of public record until the seal is lifted by the DOJ; this opening may or may not be accompanied by an announcement that the DOJ is joining the relator's case.

US Department Of Justice

Providers and their coding and billing companies (B/Cs) should consider the DOJ as one of the principal assessors of their CCP. The DOJ is the entity that decides whether or not to take action in the whistleblower's case. If the entity (i.e., ED group) is contacted while the case is under seal, it may have the opportunity to present the CCP to the DOJ and explain how the compliance plan is truly effective despite the relator's complaints. Likewise, while the relator is not required to access internal compliance resources before filing their compliant, the entity may have legitimate arguments that it did not have sufficient opportunity to address the relator's issues internally before the complaint was filed.

If the DOJ becomes convinced that the entity's program was effective or becomes doubtful of the legal basis for the complaint, the DOJ may decline to take action, leaving the relator to proceed individually. The difference between litigating against an individual or the federal government cannot be overstated, as the latter has unlimited resources. If successful with the DOJ prosecuting their case, relators are entitled to 15% to 30% of the FCA recovery plus their attorney's fees. Prosecutorial discretion by the DOJ is significant—to decide whether or not to join a private relator's case or not—and that discretion is unlikely to be reviewable by a federal court. So, the goal would be to convince the DOJ to not join the case based in part on the strength of the compliance program.

The FCA multiplier has produced enormous penalties, including the following, according to the nonprofit organization Taxpayers Against Fraud. As of 2010, three hospitals were responsible for paying three of the FCA's top five largest settlements:

- #2 Tenet Healthcare: $900 million for outlier payments and upcoding in July 2006
- #3 HCA: $731 million for lab billing and upcoding in December 2000
- #5 HCA (2.5 years later): $631 million for kickback payments to physicians in June 2003

When the DOJ announced the largest whistleblower-related recovery in history, the bar was truly raised. *The Guardian* newspaper reported total expenses to Glaxo exceeded $4 billion, including fines, penalties, and legal and professional expenses. The relator, a former quality control manager of Glaxo, received $96 million in the fall of 2010.

Other Health-Care Fraud Statutes

The main health-care fraud statutes that should be considered in developing the CCP include the following:

- The Anti-Kickback Statute: 42 USC Section 1320a-7b(b) and Safe Harbor Regulations at 42 CFR Section 1001.952
- The Physician Self-Referral Law (known as the Stark Law after its author, Representative Fortney "Pete" Stark, D-CA) and Safe Harbor Regulations at 42 CFR Sections 411.350-389
- The Criminal Health Care Fraud Statute at 18 USC Section 1347 and 1349
- PPACA's new provisions (discussed more fully later in this chapter) regarding repayment of governmental payer refunds within 60 days
- States individual "FCA" provisions that may apply beyond state Medicaid programs—consultation with qualified and experienced health-care counsel is a must in these areas
- Additional information may be found at http://oig.hhs.gov/fraud/Physician Education/01laws.asp and http://oig.hhs.gov/fraud/emforcementactions.asp

Federal mail, wire fraud, and the Racketeering Influence and Corrupt Organizations Act statutes may also be cited in federal fraud and abuse cases.

Fraud and Abuse Liability

These sources of physician and group liability can come from the certification statements made by providers or the CMS 1500 claim form itself. The certification statements are the result of the provider/supplier attesting that all of the information in the enrollment and credentialing documents are accurate and subject to financial and legal penalties for false certification. Also, the federal government has used the CMS 1500 form to establish liability under the FCA **(Figure 96.2)**.

Block 31 of the CMS 1500 form includes the following: "I certify that the statements on the reverse apply to this bill and are made a part thereof." Note that the name of the physician is provided in that block, in addition to his or her "rendering provider" number (24.j.), National Provider Identifier, and the ED group's number in Block 33. Statements on the back of the CMS 1500 form include:

Notice: Any person who knowingly files a statement of claim containing any misrepresentation or any false, incomplete or misleading information may be guilty of a criminal act punishable under law and may be subject to civil penalties.

Notice: This is to certify that the foregoing information is true, accurate and complete.

Therefore, it is important to think of a "claim filed" as a "certification" of truth with significant FCA implications. The federal government has consistently enforced the standard that individual clinicians and their ED groups are responsible for the claims submitted on their behalf, regardless of who performs the coding, billing, and practice management for the physicians. The ultimate sanction against emergency physicians and their groups—in addition to the financial penalties and overpayments—is excluding them from Medicare and other programs.

One final point on the FCA relates to the implications for ED groups and their third-party B/Cs. Recall that the FCA applies to persons who "knowingly presents, or causes to be presented, a false or fraudulent claim for payment." The "or" is important because the OIG and DOJ have traditionally enforced the FCA provisions against both the ED groups

FIGURE 96.2 ■ Health Insurance Claim Form 1500

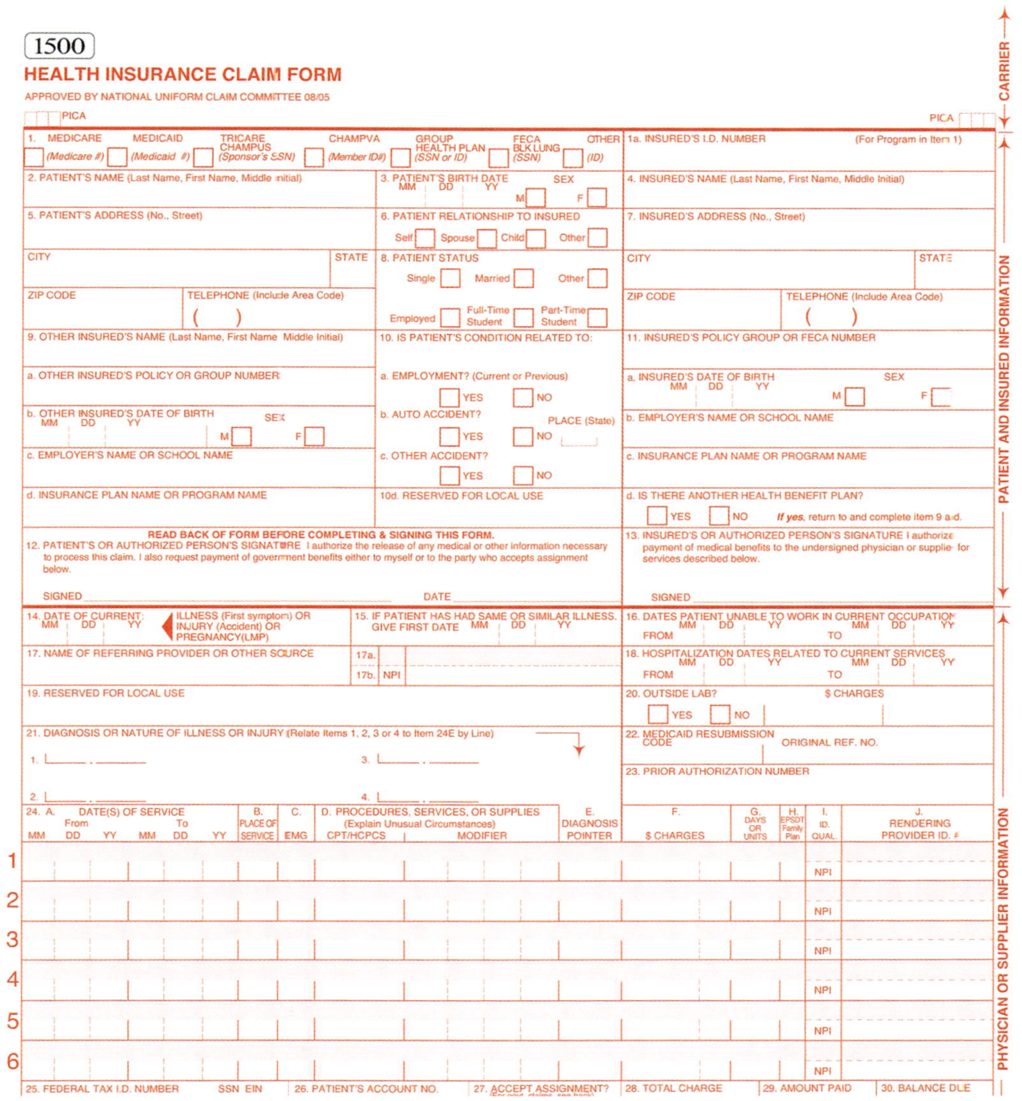
1500
HEALTH INSURANCE CLAIM FORM
APPROVED BY NATIONAL UNIFORM CLAIM COMMITTEE 08/05
PICA PICA
CARRIER
1. MEDICARE (Medicare #) MEDICAID (Medicaid #) TRICARE CHAMPUS (Sponsor's SSN) CHAMPVA (Member ID#) GROUP HEALTH PLAN (SSN or ID) FECA BLK LUNG (SSN) OTHER (ID)
1a. INSURED'S I.D. NUMBER (For Program in Item 1)
2. PATIENT'S NAME (Last Name, First Name, Middle Initial)
3. PATIENT'S BIRTH DATE MM DD YY SEX M F
4. INSURED'S NAME (Last Name, First Name, Middle Initial)
5. PATIENT'S ADDRESS (No., Street)
6. PATIENT RELATIONSHIP TO INSURED Self Spouse Child Other
7. INSURED'S ADDRESS (No., Street)
CITY STATE
8. PATIENT STATUS Single Married Other
CITY STATE
ZIP CODE TELEPHONE (Include Area Code) ( )
Employed Full-Time Student Part-Time Student
ZIP CODE TELEPHONE (Include Area Code) ( )
9. OTHER INSURED'S NAME (Last Name, First Name, Middle Initial)
10. IS PATIENT'S CONDITION RELATED TO:
11. INSURED'S POLICY GROUP OR FECA NUMBER
a. OTHER INSURED'S POLICY OR GROUP NUMBER
a. EMPLOYMENT? (Current or Previous) YES NO
a. INSURED'S DATE OF BIRTH MM DD YY SEX M F
b. OTHER INSURED'S DATE OF BIRTH MM DD YY SEX M F
b. AUTO ACCIDENT? YES NO PLACE (State)
b. EMPLOYER'S NAME OR SCHOOL NAME
c. EMPLOYER'S NAME OR SCHOOL NAME
c. OTHER ACCIDENT? YES NO
c. INSURANCE PLAN NAME OR PROGRAM NAME
d. INSURANCE PLAN NAME OR PROGRAM NAME
10d. RESERVED FOR LOCAL USE
d. IS THERE ANOTHER HEALTH BENEFIT PLAN? YES NO If yes, return to and complete item 9 a-d.
READ BACK OF FORM BEFORE COMPLETING & SIGNING THIS FORM.
12. PATIENT'S OR AUTHORIZED PERSON'S SIGNATURE I authorize the release of any medical or other information necessary to process this claim. I also request payment of government benefits either to myself or to the party who accepts assignment below.
SIGNED DATE
13. INSURED'S OR AUTHORIZED PERSON'S SIGNATURE I authorize payment of medical benefits to the undersigned physician or supplier for services described below.
SIGNED
PATIENT AND INSURED INFORMATION
14. DATE OF CURRENT: MM DD YY ILLNESS (First symptom) OR INJURY (Accident) OR PREGNANCY(LMP)
15. IF PATIENT HAS HAD SAME OR SIMILAR ILLNESS. GIVE FIRST DATE MM DD YY
16. DATES PATIENT UNABLE TO WORK IN CURRENT OCCUPATION FROM MM DD YY TO MM DD YY
17. NAME OF REFERRING PROVIDER OR OTHER SOURCE
17a. 17b. NPI
18. HOSPITALIZATION DATES RELATED TO CURRENT SERVICES FROM MM DD YY TO MM DD YY
19. RESERVED FOR LOCAL USE
20. OUTSIDE LAB? YES NO $ CHARGES
21. DIAGNOSIS OR NATURE OF ILLNESS OR INJURY (Relate Items 1, 2, 3 or 4 to Item 24E by Line)
1. 2. 3. 4.
22. MEDICAID RESUBMISSION CODE ORIGINAL REF. NO.
23. PRIOR AUTHORIZATION NUMBER
24. A. DATE(S) OF SERVICE From MM DD YY To MM DD YY
B. PLACE OF SERVICE
C. EMG
D. PROCEDURES, SERVICES, OR SUPPLIES (Explain Unusual Circumstances) CPT/HCPCS MODIFIER
E. DIAGNOSIS POINTER
F. $ CHARGES
G. DAYS OR UNITS
H. EPSDT Family Plan
I. ID. QUAL.
J. RENDERING PROVIDER ID. #
1 NPI
2 NPI
3 NPI
4 NPI
5 NPI
6 NPI
PHYSICIAN OR SUPPLIER INFORMATION
25. FEDERAL TAX I.D. NUMBER SSN EIN
26. PATIENT'S ACCOUNT NO.
27. ACCEPT ASSIGNMENT?
28. TOTAL CHARGE
29. AMOUNT PAID
30. BALANCE DUE

and their B/Cs (or revenue-cycle management companies). The B/Cs are brought in by virtue of the language "who knowingly present." The DOJ has simply argued that the groups have caused their B/C to knowingly present claims that violate the FCA. The government's position has been that both groups and the B/Cs were liable for FCA penalties. Because the Medicare reimbursement was made to the ED group under the group's provider number, the group was also liable for the Medicare overpayments.

In short, the federal government views the ED groups and B/Cs to be "joint and severally liable" for any FCA penalties. An ED group may have legal recourse against their billing company for contractual or common law indemnity and contribution for FCA penalties paid. In contrast, any overpayment liability penalties rest solely with the physician group, as it received the Medicare reimbursement directly. When as a result of an internal inquiry an ED group or B/C reasonably believes that the FCA standards have been breached, they may choose to participate in the OIG voluntary disclosure program (discussed later in the chapter).

Risk-mitigation strategies for ED groups in their relationships with B/Cs may include one or more of the following:

- ***Contractual indemnification for the coding and billing***: Given the FCA penalties multiplier and potential costs of an adverse decision, an ED group and its B/C may wish to obtain supplemental insurance to meet the indemnification obligations.
- ***Errors and omissions insurance***: It is necessary to determine the scope of coverage, limitations, exclusions, and self-insured retention, as well as potential exclusions for "fraud" and "intentional acts." What is the "best rating" of the insurer—AM Best ratings of A (excellent) or higher?
- ***ED group policies***: ED groups may wish to obtain their own policies to cover coding and billing errors or other compliance-related risks, for example, the Health Insurance Portability and Accountability Act (HIPAA) under a "cyber threats" policy or the Emergency Medical Treatment and Active Labor Act (EMTALA). Policies that cover defense costs in the event of a government investigation may be worth considering. Hospitals and professional advisors (e.g., certified public accountants or attorneys) may be excellent referral sources for insurance brokerage services in addition to professional and trade associations.

COMPLIANCE BILLING ISSUES

Chapter 93 provides explanations of the ED coding, reimbursement, and compliance issues related to evaluation and management (E/M) coding, coding of procedures, use of modifiers, and issues related to bundled and unbundled services. In addition, Medicare requirements for the nonphysician practitioner (NPP), APP, and physician at teaching hospital (PATH) are also discussed in detail.

Prebilling

The reader is referred to Chapter 24 to assist in creating a checklist of considerations when developing a CCP and the associated P&Ps. For example, the ED group should define an NPP policy to determine the level of supervising physician documentation necessary to bill at 100% of the physician's fee schedule. ACEP's 2004 "Fraud, Compliance and Emergency Medicine" report, while dated, provides an excellent outline of key issues to consider when creating a CCP.

Another resource for prebilling risk management is utilization of the CMS extract summary data file (available on the ACEP website under Practice Resources). This file permits an ED group to conduct a periodic or annual "outlier analysis" with comparisons against national data. This analysis allows some comparisons of the group's physicians to the state and national Medicare Part B data. The CMS summary data file uses a standard spreadsheet program that includes the coding and billing data for Medicare Part B patients only. (Note: The Medicare data is specialty-specific. As a result, physicians who were originally enrolled in Medicare in a specialty designation other than emergency medicine are not included.) **Table 96.1** reflects a hypothetical example of how this is achieved.

The comparison does not reveal whether there is a problem with the hypothetical "Dr. Brinkley's" coding and billing, but rather may be used to prompt further inquiry and analysis into her outlier critical care coding. Legitimate reasons might include practice in a trauma center or other high-acuity ED.

Emergency department groups must ensure that they do not employ or contract with practitioners who have been excluded from governmental reimbursement agencies. "Excluded" means debarred by the OIG, which may occur as a result of licensing board

TABLE 96.1 ■ National and State Acuity Statistics

Anywhere Medical Center, Florida

	CPT code	99281	99282	99283	99284	99285
State acuity	0.15%	1.68%	13.25%	21.50%	56.36%	7.06%
National acuity	0.29%	2.24%	17.15%	26.53%	47.50%	6.29%
Group acuity	0.86%	1.14%	27.02%	27.72%	37.93%	5.34%

Doctor	CPT Code Visits	99281	99282	99283	99284	99285	99291
Physician #1 DO	475	1.05%[a]	1.26%	29.47%[a]	25.05%	38.53%	4.63%
Physician #2 MD	54	3.70%[a]	5.56%[c]	79.63%[a]	9.26%	1.85%	0.00%
Physician #3 DO	477	1.67%[a]	1.25%	33.40%[a]	36.53%[a]	19.42%	7.72%
Physician #4 DO	369	0.54%[b]	0.54%	24.66%[b]	26.02%	44.17%	4.07%
Physician #5 DO	508	1.18%[a]	1.18%	27.17%[b]	27.36%	34.45%	8.66%[b]
Physician #6 MD	1,011	0.10%	0.79%	23.74%[b]	29.57%	39.86%	5.93%
Physician #7 MD	648	0.62%[b]	1.39%	29.17%[a]	28.40%	36.27%	4.17%
Physician #8 DO	607	0.66%[b]	1.32%	30.64%[a]	27.18%	36.74%	3.46%
Physician #9 MD	552	0.36%	0.36%	27.72%[a]	27.72%	36.78%	7.07%
Physician #10 MD	523	1.53b	1.53%	22.75%[b]	29.45%	42.07%	2.68%
Physician #11 DO	610	0.66%[b]	1.64%	24.43%[b]	25.74%	43.11%	4.43%
Physician #12 MD	429	1.17%[a]	3.03%	38.46%[a]	20.28%	32.87%	4.20%
Physician #13 MD	595	0.67%[b]	1.34%	23.53%[b]	34.45%[b]	39.33%	0.67%
Physician #14 MD	605	0.99%[a]	0.17%	18.51%	25.29%	43.64%	11.40%[a]
Physician #15 MD	290	1.03%[a]	0.34%	30.00%[a]	31.72%[b]	33.79%	3.10%
Physician #16 MD	69	0.00%	0.00%	21.74%	23.19%	46.38%	8.70%[b]
Physician #17 DO	698	1.29%[a]	0.86%	25.21%[b]	23.35%	43.12%	6.16%
Total	8,522	0.86%[a]	1.14%	27.02%[b]	27.72%	37.93%	5.34%

[a] Acuity greater than 2.
[b] Acuity between 1 and 2.

actions or a default on a health education assistance loan. Therefore, ED groups should establish a process to screen current and future employees and contractors against the OIG's list of excluded parties. Among the coding and billing risk areas noted in the OIG's 1998 CPGs for third-party billing companies, the following are most relevant to emergency medicine:

- Billing for services not actually documented
- Unbundling certain procedures that should be bundled under Medicare reimbursement policies and billing those procedures separately

- "Upcoding" or using a higher E/M code than is justified by the documentation (particularly with increasing E&M utilization)
- Failure to properly use modifiers

Postbilling

The postbilling issues for the risk analysis can be more thoroughly understood by reviewing several of the references included at the end of this chapter, including the OIG CPGs for third-party billing companies and for physician group practices. In addition, several regulations, the OIG CPGs, HIPAA, and the Health Information Technology for Economic and Clinical Health (HITECH) Act of 2009, have significantly increased the protections and associated penalties for protected health-care information (PHI) in both paper and electronic (ePHI) formats. Experienced health-care counsel and accountants are important resources to the ED group completing the "back-end" risk assessment and developing associated P&Ps. Significant postbilling risk considerations include:

- *HITECH Act's mandatory notification requirements*: Notification must be provided to other covered entities, patients, prominent media outlets, and to HHS (if more than 500 patients are involved) in the event of a "breach" of "unsecured PHI." (These terms are defined; see http://edocket.access.gpo.gov/2009/pdf/E9-20169.pdf.) Counsel should be consulted before P&Ps are developed and implemented.
- *PPACA's mandates*: Once "overpayments" are identified (after "reconciliation"), the overpayment must be paid to the governmental payer within 60 days with a written, pursuant to Section 6402. The "reasonable diligence" period to investigate and determine if a refund is in fact due is usually no more than six months. Once that period is complete and the refund is in fact due and owing, the amount must be repaid within 60 days of that determination date.
- *Fraud Enforcement and Recovery Act of 2009*: This act addresses ("reverse FCA") claims for a provider's failure to refund their governmental payers.
- *Waivers*: Waivers of coinsurance, "deductible," "prompt pay," "professional courtesy," and charitable care discount laws and regulations should be reviewed with counsel and P&P developed in each of these areas.
- *State "unclaimed property"/escheats laws and regulations*: Depending on the state, a returned refund check or low credit balance that is unclaimed whose owner cannot be located after a certain time known as the "dormancy period" belongs to the state and cannot be retained by the provider.

In addition to the RCM issues noted above, the ED group's risk analysis should consider other legal obligations, such as EMTALA wage and hour and antidiscrimination in hiring and terminations. Then the process of addressing each of the OIG's seven elements can and should be addressed with the goal of P&P development and implementation.

ELEMENTS OF AN EFFECTIVE CCP

The seven elements come from the US Sentencing Commission Guidelines (**Table 96.2**). See http://www.ussc.gov/Guidelines/2010_guidelines/index.cfm. The commission stated that organizations potentially subject to criminal sanctions would be given "credit" against model sentencing terms if the organization had an "effective" compliance program.

The OIG now encourages voluntary compliance. The HHS inspector general (IG) previously stated that, given the size and scope of health care, voluntary compliance was the only hope that the programs had to truly reduce fraud, waste, and abuse. In the CPG issued

TABLE 96.2 ■ OIG's Elements of Compliance

Element	Explanation: Organizations Must
Written policies and procedures	Implement written policies and procedures and standards of conduct (e.g., coding quality-assurance standards).
Compliance officer and committee	Ensure that each is scalable to the organization.
Effective training and education	Ensure training and education are conducted (online or live).
Effective lines of communication	Establish and include an anonymous reporting function (e.g., an employee hotline or other method of internal reporting).
Internal monitoring and auditing	Conduct internal monitoring and auditing (e.g., P&P for refunding miscoded claims and rebilling the appropriate E/M procedure).
Disciplinary enforcement	Develop standards through well-publicized disciplinary guidelines (e.g., P&P on the failure to report).
Mechanisms for responding to detected problems	Develop a response and prevention program (e.g., corrective action plans for coding and billing NPP services).

by the OIG (third-party billing companies [1998] and to individual physicians and small group practices [2000]), the agency established the seven elements of a CCP.

The PPACA requirements will substantially utilize the OIG's seven elements. Emergency medicine groups (and their counsel) should continually consult these requirements when developing and modifying their CCPs.

Element #1: Implementing Written Standards and P&Ps

These compliance standards and related P&Ps must include risk areas beyond coding and billing, including:

- *EMTALA.* The group should document its EMTALA training for clinicians, including the P&P review and coordination with the hospital.
- *HIPAA privacy and security.* The group should have a P&P regarding the storage/removal and transportation of ePHI on movable devices such as flash drives, portable hard drives, and laptops. For example, should laptops and other portable media be required to be encrypted to avoid possible disclosure under the HITECH Act? What about smart phones and tablets? Unlike laptops, many of these products have hard drives that cannot be encrypted. As such, under the HITECH regulations, these products are deemed "unsecured" and any ePHI that is lost or stolen from those devices may likely implicate HITECH Act reporting.
- *Equal employment opportunity (EEO) laws and regulations regarding age, race, and gender discrimination.* The group should ensure that its hiring and employee termination practices are compliant with EEO standards.
- *Wage and hour laws and regulations, the Employee Retirement Income Security Act requirements for health and welfare benefit plans, and workers' compensation laws.* The group should ensure proper classification of "exempt" and "nonexempt" employees for proper compliance with overtime pay rules.

As previously discussed, it is essential that the ED group demonstrates P&Ps to show effective coordination with the ED group's B/C in the areas of credit balances, refunds, and unclaimed property.

Element #2: Compliance Oversight

A 10-doctor emergency group may not be expected to have a full-time compliance officer and may instead designate one of the physicians or an administrative person in the group to serve in this role. However, an ED group of 50 or more physicians might be expected to have a full-time chief compliance officer (CCO). Another way to think of this requirement is as follows: A group receiving more than $10 million in Medicare/Medicaid reimbursements might be expected to have a full-time CCO. There are no bright line standards; however, ACEP and the Emergency Department Practice Management Association (EDPMA) both filed formal comments with the HHS NPRM, recommending scalability and flexibility of the compliance officer function, given the tremendous variety in sizes of groups and practice structure in the HHS final rules.

For larger organizations, particularly those organized under the state of Delaware law, the CCO should report to the board of directors or at least its audit committee. Compliance "best practice" ensures that the CCO periodically reports directly to the board or one of its committees. This periodic report typically includes risk areas like coding, QA sampling techniques, and associate and executive training and education results and mitigation techniques (e.g., specific coder education and retraining). An effective CCP along with periodic reporting by the CCO to the board may mitigate potential director and officer liability for noncompliance (under the *In Re: Caremark* 698 A. 2d 959 [Del. Ch. 1996] decision). In the Caremark case, the court found that the board had met its fiduciary duties and appropriately monitored company actions.

Element #3: Education and Training

Compliance education requires a process to ensure that organizational members are continually apprised of and are using the newest standards. Multiple formats should be considered, such as online webcasts, audio conferences, in-person conferences, periodic newsletters, learning management systems, and e-mail alerts that scale to the organization. Emergency physicians may attend or participate in educational sessions and presentations through their hospitals, ED groups, or their work with a state medical society or ACEP chapter. These programs should be documented in the ED group's "compliance binder" or in records supporting the compliance functions. For example, ACEP's Coding and Reimbursement Conference, certain *Scientific Assembly* courses, and EDPMA's annual Solutions Summit offer courses that could qualify as coding and compliance training. Certain hospital meetings and training courses may qualify as effective training in the areas of HIPAA and EMTALA. The training should be directly tailored to the general functions in which the employees are engaged. For example, prebilling or front-end employees may be grouped in the billing function.

Given the significant amount of material and the number of laws and regulations driven by PPACA, it may be advisable to divide the training into major topics. To illustrate, HIPAA's privacy regulations and the security standards mandated by the HITECH Act naturally can be combined into one online training course. It may be particularly effective to reiterate key areas through follow-up e-mail updates and newsletters, including specific examples of breaches of PHI that have been publicized.

Element #4: Developing Effective Lines of Communication

Traditionally, reporting for compliance meant the establishment of an "800" hotline (including an anonymous e-mail alert system) that employees could use to report compliance issues

> **BOX 96.1 ■ PRIVACY AND ETHICS QUICK TEST**
>
> - Does the action comply with the Company's policies and procedures?
> - Is the action legal?
> - How would the action look to your family and friends, our clients, and the general public if it was published on the front page of the newspaper?
> - Would the action make you feel bad if you did it?
> - If you know it's wrong, don't do it!
> - If you're not sure, ask until you get an answer.

anonymously. Anonymous reporting is viewed as critical for employees to avoid possible retaliation or retribution for raising questions, particularly when questioning their direct manager or senior management. These hotlines still exist but do not receive the majority of the compliance reporting traffic, with the exception of HR issues. Many companies provide wallet cards that include the reporting number and instructions (**Box 96.1**).

Retaliation: The Compliance "Cancer"

Again, the chief reason behind the anonymous reporting and hotlines of the 1990s was concern over retaliation and retribution. Retaliation by management against employees for reporting compliance issues can intimidate employees and prevent the reporting necessary to have an effective compliance program. Though managers may ask who raised the issues, it is critical that the CCO or the person serving in the compliance function maintains, to the greatest extent possible, the anonymity of the reporting individual. The CCO should clearly communicate that all questions, concerns, and issues should be raised, including human resources (HR) issues. These issues will then be triaged appropriately with the necessary inquiry or investigation.

Blanket guarantees of confidentiality to the reporting employee should be avoided. When a major compliance inquiry begins, it may be necessary to divulge the employee's name. For example, in the course of an internal inquiry or a self-disclosure and inquiry by the OIG, it is possible that the entity's counsel or OIG attorneys will request to speak directly to the person who raised the compliance issue. Therefore, it is recommended that the employee reporting the issue be told that confidentiality will be maintained to the greatest extent possible but will not be guaranteed throughout the process.

Failure to Report

In any ED group, and particularly those in multiple offices or states, the "failure to report" should be addressed in the organization's P&P. The failure to report should be considered a serious potential policy violation that results in corrective action or progressive discipline. To illustrate, in certain health-care organizations, operations managers certify that they have identified and forwarded all material compliance issues to the attention of the CCO or compliance function. Another strategy is to incorporate the fulfillment of compliance responsibilities into the manager's and employee's annual performance appraisals.

Element #5: Internal Monitoring and Auditing

Given the high proportion and number of governmental payor claims in the ED and "multiplier effect" of the FCA penalties, the ED coding QA P&Ps are crucial to an effective

CCP. The ability to capture the coding QA data is essential, even in a midsize ED group. The following issues and considerations should be defined in the group's internal QA and for those providing the coding and billing:

- *How will claims or records be selected for the QA process?* There must be a random selection process and an adequate sample size to ensure the coding accuracy rate within a defined margin of error.
- *How can random selection be achieved?* Use low-tech methods such as selecting a day of the week, the clients, and the coders to audit by using random number generator software (such as the OIG "RAT-STATs") to randomly select accounts or records to review. While there are many "random number generator" software packages available, the OIG's program is freely downloadable from the OIG website and use of the OIG software should support the legitimacy of the random selection.
- *What is the best way to target specific issues or concerns?* In addition to QAs that are part of the "official" QA scorecard of coding accuracy (because they are randomly generated), there are additional QAs known as "focused reviews" or "focused audits" that are not part of that official scorecard accuracy. These focused reviews are not randomly generated and usually are targeted to specific issues or concerns (e.g., critical care coding and billing, or the differences between "high moderate" [CPT 99284] and "low moderate" [CPT 99283] coding). Focused reviews are usually inward facing and used for specific coder and/or clinician feedback. While their purpose is similar to the official randomly selected QAs in improving accuracy, it is important not to mix their "nonrandom" nature with the truly randomly selected records and official QA accuracy standards.

Capturing the regular coding QA results in an appropriate database for internal and external reporting is essential. **Table 96.3** shows an issue-specific QA report used to conduct specific documentation reviews related to specific documentation and coding issues, such as electrocardiograms or laceration repairs (LAC). Errors are identified, claims refunded, and rebilled and corrective action and education taken with the coders.

In this example, one of the risk areas for ED coding (e.g., LAC coding) is selected for focused coder and client review. The LAC codes are entered into the billing application, and the universe of potential accounts is selected for a given month. Similar coder-focused reviews can be done in the risk areas of PATH and NPP coding and billing. Once the data are in a reportable database, internal management and client reports can be provided showing how specific issues such as PATH or NPP's were analyzed and additional education and training resulted from that focused review.

It is also important for the database to reflect that corrective action was initiated for each of the miscoded claims, particularly with governmental payors. If the regular coder QA reveals claims coded at 99284 that should have been coded at 99283, then it is important for the full refund to be made to the governmental payor. To avoid being denied as a duplicate claim, the claim must be rebilled to that payor, provided that the timely filing period has not expired. As discussed previously, the timeliness of the refund process is essential as well. Once the coding QA function determines that the case was wrongly coded and up to 6 months to determine the overpayment or credit balance after all insurances have remitted payment, the 60-day clock to repay the governmental payor begins to run. The refund form used for each Medicare MAC is usually available on the MAC website and must be used when issuing the refund to Medicare.

Element #6: Enforcement and Discipline

Enforcement of written compliance P&Ps is essential. In fact, OIG and DOJ officials have stated publicly that the organization's failure to follow their own internal P&P can be viewed by the government as evidence of "intent" to defraud the government. Recall that the penalties under the FCA rise from the minimum $10,957 per claim to as much as $21,916 per claim if the government believes that the provider's conduct was intentional. So, if an organization states that it will make appropriate inquiry or investigation of internal compliance issues, the organization should do so and document all stages of the inquiry, including reference to the internal P&P that may have been violated.

Enforcement and discipline may arise in several key areas of the ED group's P&P. For example, assume an employee fails to report material compliance issues, and the hospital or a third party audits the group. Management decisions, including failure to report and the disciplinary action, if any, will be closely scrutinized by the auditing organization. Because most health-care organizations have a policy prohibiting retribution, any manager who retaliates against an employee for bringing compliance issues forward should be addressed as a serious violation of P&P.

The difficulty occurs when attempting to determine whether the employee is being properly disciplined for HR issues or is being retaliated against. The CCO, HR, and management must assess these issues. Retaliation against the employee may, of course, turn that person from someone who makes an "internal complaint" into a relator (OIG whistleblower). Provisions of both the FCA and EEO laws prohibit retaliation against employees for raising legitimate compliance issues. Therefore, retaliation cannot only cause the ED group's entire CCP to be questioned, it can also expose the group to additional liability (in addition to the FCA liability, if any) under the FCA and EEO laws.

Element #7: Corrective Action Programs

When internal compliance issues arise, many in the organization may watch to see how the entity responds and if it follows the compliance P&P. Obtaining the appropriate reimbursements for ED groups is very complex and undergoes ongoing reviews, with frequent reimbursement of providers by commercial payors and health plans at incorrect contract rates. However, denials for one set of claims cannot be the basis for failure to address coding or billing issues identified for another set of claims. Instead, the response and prevention should come in the form of correction action plans.

Correction action plans or programs may be small, medium, or large, covering specific issues, coders, or a major subject matter like PATH that can stretch across many coders and clients. Once the issues are identified, a root-cause analysis should be conducted to determine the essential facts that gave rise to the problems. Depending on the nature of the issue, experienced health-care counsel may be critical in advising the ED group about disclosing the compliance issue to the government. So how should the disclosure be accomplished and to whom? The issue whether to disclose the compliance issue and the CAP to the government is critical to an effective CCP. Misconduct does not include inadvertent errors or mistakes. Such errors should be reported through the normal channels with the applicable carrier, intermediary, or other HCFA-designated payor (**Figure 96.3**).

Office of the Inspector General's Billing Company Guidance

If the issues are systemic and require detailed analysis of claims or coding over months or years, then the ED group should consider having their counsel write a letter to the MAC. The issue may or may not be referred to the OIG or DOJ for further review.

FIGURE 96.3 ■ Example of CMS Medicare Overpayment Form

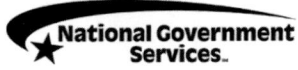

A CMS Medicare Administrative Contractor

MEDICARE

Jurisdiction 6 Medicare Part B MSP Overpayment Request Form

Claim(s)-Specific Data

Date of Service: _____ Overpayment Amount: _____

Beneficiary Health Insurance Claim Number (HICN): _____ Medicare Beneficiary Identifier (MBI): _____

Claim Control Number(s): _____

Immediate Offset Request: ☐ Allow National Government Services to set up an immediate recoupment for this overpayment request. By checking this box you acknowledge that an immediate recoupment payment arrangement constitutes a voluntary payment and that you may be waiving the right to potential payment of interest pursuant to Section 1893(f)(2) for the overpayment(s). **Note:** Although your overpayment will be offset upon completion of this request, please be aware that a demand letter will still be created for your records.

Reason for Overpayment

Medicare Secondary Payer (MSP)/Other Payer Involvement Select reason

07–MSP Group Health Plan Insurance: (working aged, disability, end-stage renal disease [ESRD])
08–MSP Auto No Fault Insurance
09–MSP Liability Insurance
10–MSP Worker's Comp. (Incudes Black Lung)
16–Other

Complete the following **primary** insurance information and **attach a copy of** the primary payer's Explanation of Benefits **(EOB)**.

Policy Information

Subscriber Name: _____
Relation to Patient: _____
Policy Number: _____
Group Number: _____
Injury Date (if applicable): _____
Related Diagnosis: _____

Insurer Information

Name: _____
Address: _____
City, State and ZIP Code: _____
Phone Number: _____

Contact Information

Provider Transaction Access Number (PTAN) and/or National Provider Identifier (NPI): _____

Provider Name: _____

Contact Name: _____ Phone Number: _____

Signature: _____
Provider, Administrator or CFO's signature (someone with authority is required to sign).

Mail this completed form and primary EOB to:

National Government Services
J6 Part B MAC MSP Overpayment Recovery Unit
P.O. Box 6475
Indianapolis, IN 46206-6475

Or Fax this completed form and primary EOB to: **315-442-4151**

Health-care counsel should also assist the ED group in deciding whether or not to disclose directly to the OIG pursuant to the OIG's self-disclosure protocol (SDP). If the root cause analysis shows evidence of more than negligence and shows recklessness or deliberate ignorance, then the SDP should be considered. The following "tips" are from the OIG's provider compliance training session as part of the Health Care Fraud Prevention and Enforcement Action Team initiatives. They are called "Tips for Success in the OIG Self-Disclosure Protocol":

- Follow all the requirements in the Federal Register and the 2008 "Open Letter" in your written submission. A common mistake is missing contractor [A/B MAC] information.
- Mail it to the address in the Federal Register: Assistant IG for Investigative Operations, HHS/OIG 330 Independence Ave. SW, Room 5409, Washington, DC 20201.
- Do not disclose prematurely. Your investigation and damages audit either needs to be completed or you commit to completing within three months after acceptance.
- Provide a complete description of the conduct and investigation:
  - What happened?
  - What is the time period?
  - Why did it happen?
  - Why is there potential legal liability for the conduct?
  - Who was involved?
  - How was the conduct discovered?
  - What corrective actions have been taken?
- Identify the fraud laws at stake. Just "federal laws, rules, and regulations" or "the Social Security Act," for example, is not sufficient.
- Stark-only conduct that does not also have a colorable anti-kickback claim is not eligible for OIG's protocol. The CMS has created its own disclosure protocol for Stark-only conduct—http://www.cms.gov/PhysicianSelfReferral.
- Expect that disclosure will result in a settlement agreement for an amount that is a multiplier of damages. Simple overpayments are not appropriate for the SDP.
- Full cooperation is essential.

If there is reason to believe that the FCA's standards of "reckless disregard" or "deliberate ignorance" are found in the inquiry, then the SDP is an appropriate avenue for disclosure. If, however, there was mere negligence or an innocent error in the claims, then the overpayment should be made to the A/B MAC.

CONCLUSION

As ACEP describes:

> *In simple terms, a compliance program is a quality-assurance strategy. An effective program establishes, implements, and enforces internal controls and monitors its conduct in order to prevent and correct inappropriate activity.*

Emergency department groups and their advisors can and should be able to establish truly effective compliance programs using the resources in this book, those referenced previously, and the government's own substantial resources. "Operationalizing" the CCP is the true work of compliance, and it is imperative to recognize that even the most vigorous CCP regularly determines issues and engages in corrective action. That there are compliance issues is not to say that the program is ineffective—rather, ineffective programs rarely uncover compliance issues or engage in corrective action. The E/M coding has subjective aspects that can be judged differently on subsequent review, and other coding and billing mistakes get made along the way. The ED revenue cycle is endlessly complex with potentially hundreds, if not thousands, of payors for a large multistate group. Compliance functions, including coding QA and other programs used in operations (e.g., refunds, patient services), may actually enhance appropriate revenue capture. In summary, compliance is not just about doing things right—it's about avoiding even the appearance of impropriety.

ADDITIONAL READING

- HHS Office of Inspector General Compliance. https://oig.hhs.gov/compliance/compliance-guidance/index.asp. Accessed October 23, 2020.
- OIG's compliance guidance to third party billing agencies. https://oig.hhs.gov/reports-and-publications/archives/enforcement/state_archive.asp. Accessed October 23, 2020.
- OIG's compliance guidance to individual physicians and small group practices. https://oig.hhs.gov/compliance/physician-education/01laws.asp. Accessed October 23, 2020.
- ACEP's Fraud, Compliance, and Emergency Medicine. https://www.acep.org/administration/reimbursement/compliance/reimbursement-compliance/. Accessed October 23, 2020.
- OIG advisory opinions. https://oig.hhs.gov/reports-and-publications/archives/advisory-opinions/index.asp. Accessed October 23, 2020.

CHAPTER 97

QUALITY AND REPORTING IN THE ERA OF PAYMENT REFORM

Zach Jarou, Adam Rodos, Pawan Goyal

Eighty-five percent of the reasons for failure are deficiencies in the systems and processes rather than the employee. The role of management is to change the process rather than badgering individuals to do better.

—W. Edwards Deming 1900–1993[1]

In its broadest sense, quality is the degree to which performance meets or exceeds expectations and variability is minimized. One of the earliest examples of quality assessment is the guilds of medieval craftsmen who developed strict rules for product quality. While the history of measurement is as old as civilization itself, the concept of "scientific management" was not introduced until the late 19th century when the division of labor within factories resulted in enormous increases in productivity, but at a cost to quality, which was often evaluated only after the final product was made.[2]

In the early 20th century, Walter Shewhart, a statistician for Bell Laboratories who today is recognized as the father of statistical quality control, observed that the quality of a finished product was dependent upon the processes used to create it. Quality was particularly important during World War II, when the government relied upon civilian manufacturers to produce safe military equipment.

Following World War II, many American companies abandoned statistical quality control, and Japan became home to the quality movement thanks to the teachings of W. Edwards Deming, a former mathematical physicist at the US Department of Agriculture. He was an expert statistician sent to Japan by the US War Department to study agricultural production problems in the war-damaged nation. By recognizing the importance of the relationships between workers and managers, Deming laid out a new "total quality management" approach that recognized implementing organization-wide processes that helped transform the Japanese manufacturing industry from one of the worst to one of the best in the world.

EARLY HISTORY OF HEALTH-CARE QUALITY

The roots of the health-care quality movement can be traced back to Florence Nightingale's work of the 1850s that linked mortality outcomes with hygiene standards. Harvard surgeon, Ernest Codman, was a pioneer in tracking outcomes of his surgical patients to determine the effectiveness of his treatments. Codman founded the American College of Surgeons (ACS) in 1913; four years later, the ACS launched its Hospitalization Standardization Program, which established the following minimum standards[3]:

- Creation of organized hospital medical staff
- Limiting medical staff membership to well-educated, licensed, competent, and ethical physicians
- Adoption of rules and regulations to ensure regular staff meetings and clinical reviews of various departments of the hospital
- Keeping of accurate and complete medical records for all patients, including chief complaint, past history, history of present illness, physical examinations, laboratory and radiology results, provisional diagnoses, treatments received, final diagnoses, condition on discharge, follow-up, or in the case of death, results of the autopsy
- Establishing supervised clinical laboratory and radiology departments

In 1919, only 89 out of 692 hospitals with more than 100 beds met the new ACS minimum standards, but by 1950, this number rose to 3,290, more than half of the hospitals in the United States. The increasing complexity of medical care provided in modern hospitals by nonsurgical specialists required extending the size and scope of the Hospital Standardization Program beyond what the ACS was able to support on its own. In 1951, the ACS joined forces with the American College of Physicians, the American Hospital Association, the American Medical Association, and the Canadian Medical Association to form The Joint Commission as a private, nonprofit organization.[4] Health care did not fall under federal supervision until 1965 when the Social Security Act of 1935 was amended to include Titles XVIII and XIX, which established the Medicare and Medicaid programs.[5,6]

Recent History of Quality

In response to the federal government "competing" with The Joint Commission to define new minimum standards, the majority of which had been already been achieved by most hospitals in the country, coupled with a belief that new levels of quality could be achieved, The Joint Commission redefined their mission to move beyond minimum standards and instead began to focus on defining the *optimal* achievable level of care.

The stage was set for quality measurement and quality improvement to become integral parts of health-care delivery. The Joint Commission and the federal government have continued to play a major role in the quality movement. But before addressing today's quality environment, it is important to understand what can and should be measured and how that information should be used.

QUALITY ASSESSMENT, ASSURANCE, AND IMPROVEMENT

As Thom Mayer explains, "Excellence is what we strive for, but consistency is what we demand."[7] The primary goal in health-care quality is to use scientific principles to identify and adopt best practices to improve consistency and improve outcomes.

To a layperson, quality health care might be considered "the care health professionals would want to receive if they got sick."[8] More formally, in 1990, the Institute of Medicine (IOM) defined "quality of care is the degree to which health services for individuals and populations increase the likelihood of desired health outcomes and are consistent with current professional knowledge."[9] (See **Box 97.1** for more information.)

> **BOX 97.1 ■ DIMENSIONS IN DEFINITIONS OF QUALITY[9]**
>
> 1. Scale of quality
> 2. Nature of entity being evaluated
> 3. Goal-oriented
> 4. Aspects of outcomes specified
> 5. Acceptability
> 6. Type of recipient identified
> 7. Role and responsibility of recipient asserted
> 8. Continuity, management, coordination
> 9. Professional standards
> 10. Technical competency of provider
> 11. Interpersonal skills of provider
> 12. Acceptability
> 13. Statements about use
> 14. Constrained by resources
> 15. Constrained by consumer and patient circumstances
> 16. Constrained by technology and state of scientific knowledge
> 17. Risk versus benefit tradeoffs
> 18. Documentation required

Quality assessment has solely to do with measurement. *Quality assurance* is a formal exercise of identifying problems, developing and implementing solutions, and performing follow-up to ensure that the corrective actions have been effective without introducing any unforeseen new problems. Finally, *quality improvement* is the continuous study and improvement of the processes of health-care delivery.

Quality-assurance programs do not guarantee or promise an error-free health system; however, they can serve four major purposes:

- To identify physicians whose care practices are so unacceptable that immediate actions are necessary to remove them from the workforce or no longer reimburse them for care delivered.
- To target physicians with below average performance who may benefit from interventions to bring their performance quality to an acceptable level.
- To improve the average quality of care provided by an entire community of physicians ("shifting the curve").
- To motivate and mentor others by recognizing physicians who achieve the highest levels of quality.[10]

See **Box 97.2** for desirable attributes of quality-assurance programs.

The Traditional Structure-Process-Outcome Model

In 1966, Avedis Donabedian, physician and founder of the formalized study of health-care quality and outcomes, published the earliest unified model for quality assurance in health care, highlighting a triad of structure, process, and outcomes.[11,12]

Structure is a measure of a health-care organization's resources and presumed capacity. How many clinicians are there? What training or certification do they have? What is the size and location of their care facilities? How is the organization governed? Does the organization have any special technical capabilities or accreditation? What are the staff-to-staff and staff-to-patient ratios? Are the employees engaged and passionate about the work they do?

Process is a measure of what is done for patients. Processes can be measured within a single episode of care or longitudinally as part of a health maintenance plan. Process measures are directly related to the actions taken by physicians and other members of the care team. Process measures seek to understand whether medicine is being practiced in

> **BOX 97.2 ■ DESIRABLE ATTRIBUTES OF A QUALITY-ASSURANCE PROGRAM**[10]
>
> - Addresses overuse, underuse, and poor technical and interpersonal quality
> - Intrudes minimally into the patient-provider relationship
> - Is acceptable to professionals and providers
> - Fosters improvement throughout the health-care organization and system
> - Deals with outlier practice and performance
> - Uses both positive and negative incentives for change and improvement in performance
> - Provides practitioners and providers with time line information to improve performance
> - Has face validity for the public and for professionals (i.e., is understandable and relevant to patient and clinical decision-making)
> - Is scientifically rigorous
> - Has a positive impact on patient outcomes can be demonstrated or inferred
> - Can address both individual and population-based outcomes
> - Documents improvement in quality and progress toward excellence
> - Is easily implemented and administered
> - Is affordable and is cost-effective
> - Includes patients and the public

accordance with "best practices," but they do not consider whether adherence or deviation from a defined process caused benefit or harm to the patient. Adherence to process measures can be facilitated in real time by clinical decision support tools.

Outcomes are a measure of the end result of the care provided. A pessimistic list of outcomes might include "the five Ds"—death, disease, disability, discomfort, and dissatisfaction. A more optimistic list of outcomes might include survival; states of physiologic, physical, and emotional health; and satisfaction. Many patient outcomes may be strongly influenced by nonmedical factors, including social determinants of health.

The relative value of measuring processes versus outcomes has been debated for decades. See **Table 97.1** for a comparison of the strengths and weaknesses of each type of measurement.

A Newer Model: Continuous Quality Improvement

A modern leader in the health-care quality movement was Harvard-trained pediatrician Donald Berwick. He proposed that health care should adopt the management principles that revolutionized manufacturing operations. His 1989 article in the *New England Journal of Medicine* urged us to move beyond "quality by inspection" (the theory of bad apples) to a system of "continuous improvement as an ideal in health care."[13]

Continuous quality improvement focuses on "shifting the curve," rather than "trimming the tails." The Japanese word *kaizen* captures the spirit of continuous improvement—"every defect is a treasure"—and that the discovery of imperfections should be welcomed as an opportunity to improve.

Inspired by leaders of the total quality-management movement, Berwick espoused that problems in health-care quality are not the result of unskilled, unmotivated, ill-willed, people; rather, they are byproducts of poorly designed systems. By shifting the blame away from individuals, an environment can be created for honest, open discussion about opportunities for improvement. Conversely, cultures based on fear can lead to job

TABLE 97.1 ■ Strengths of Process and Outcome Measurements[10]*

Dimension	Process	Outcome
Relevance to goal of health care	-	++
Appeal to practitioners and institutions	++	+
Appeal to patients and public	+	++
Can detect problems of overuse	++	-
Can detect problems of underuse	+	+
Can detect poor technical or interpersonal quality	++	-
Real-time review and timely intervention possible	++	-
Points directly to specific areas needing performance improvement	++	-
Reflects important trends over time	+	++
Usefulness during clinic visit	++	-
Usefulness during hospitalization	++	++
Usefulness for posthospital care (i.e., home health)	+	+
Minimizes intrusiveness for providers	-	++
Minimizes intrusiveness for patients	++	-
Reliable and valid assessment methods	+	+
Reliable and valid evaluation criteria	+	-
Relevant information recorded in billing or utilization data	+	--
Consensus on best practices	++ to --	NA
Consensus on best outcomes	NA	++
Can account for biological variability	-	+
Can account for patient preferences	--	+
Can account for patient behavior	--	-
Can assign accountability to multiple clinicians over time	-	--
Costs of measurement	+ to -	+ to --

* ++, strong; +, adequate; -, fair; --, poor; NA, not applicable.

dissatisfaction, the manipulation of information, and lack of new learning opportunities.[13] See **Box 97.3** for Berwick's four assumptions and eight key constructs, which serve as a health care-specific version of the principles outlined by manufacturing leaders, as summarized by the 1990 IOM Committee to Design a Strategy for Quality Review and Assurance in Medicare.[14]

> **BOX 97.3 ■ BERWICK'S MODEL**
>
> **Four core assumptions:**
>
> 1. People delivering health care work in organizations; organizational energy and lines of accountability are used for quality improvement and top leadership must be committed.
> 2. Workers wish to perform to the best of their capacity.
> 3. When performance is suboptimal, it is often the result of wasteful, needlessly complex, and undependable systems.
> 4. The interaction of individuals and the organizations and systems within which they practice can always improve.
>
> **Eight key constructs:**
>
> 1. All that is done is done for the benefit of the patient.
> 2. All that precedes the benefit to the patient must be involved in a relentless, systematic, and cooperative effort to improve care.
> 3. Activities are cyclic, involving continuous "planning, doing, checking, and acting."
> 4. The work of individuals and departments within health-care organizations as interconnected. People and departments serve as their own internal "suppliers" and "customers," and their interconnected activities are intended to benefit the external customer.
> 5. Constant improvement of every production process by everyone involved is the central focus. In this view, every health worker has two roles: first, doing their job and, second, improving the job.
> 6. Improvement occurs by integrating the voices of customers and of processes of care into the cyclical redesign of service and care.
> 7. Active, visible commitment of the highest leadership of the organization is necessary.
> 8. Practical techniques that facilitate learning and action

A MODERN HISTORY OF HEALTH-CARE QUALITY

In 1998, The IOM (today known as the National Academy of Medicine) launched a commission that published two landmark reports aimed at achieving a significant improvement in health-care quality through fundamental, sweeping redesign of the entire health system. One was *To Err Is Human: Building a Safer Health System*.[15] The other was *Crossing the Quality Chasm: A New Health System for the 21st Century*.[16]

To Err Is Human: Building a Safer Health System

Published in 2000, *To Err Is Human: Building a Safer Health System* was a monumental report that highlighted the significant toll of medical errors in terms of preventable deaths.[15] Two large studies—one in Colorado and Utah, the other in New York—estimated that adverse events occurred in 2.9% to 3.7% of hospitalizations and that 6.6% to 13.6% of those adverse events led to death. It was estimated that more than half of adverse events were directly related to preventable medical errors.

Not only do medical errors result in death, but they are also costly in terms of dollars spent fixing newly introduced problems or treating iatrogenic complications. Beyond dollars, the loss of trust by patients, the loss of morale by providers, and the loss of productivity by society must also be considered.

The report reiterated many of the concepts from Berwick's model of continuous quality improvement, stating that:

> ... errors can be prevented by designing systems that make it hard for people to do the wrong thing and easy for people to do the right thing" and that "as health care and the system that delivers it become more complex, the opportunities for errors abound. Correcting this will require a concerted effort by the professions, health-care organizations, purchasers, consumers, regulators and policy-makers. Traditional clinical boundaries and a culture of blame must be broken down.[15]

Finally, the report advocates for the adoption of voluntary error reporting systems, such as The Joint Commission's voluntary reporting of sentinel events like unexpected death or serious injury. Genuine investigation of errors is best achieved if protected from legal discovery. If physicians are fearful about discussing errors and ways to avoid them in the future, the system cannot be improved.

Crossing the Quality Chasm

In its 2001 report, *Crossing the Quality Chasm: A New Health System for the 21st Century*, the IOM boldly began with the statement that "current care systems cannot do the job; trying harder will not work."[16] They called for a "new health system" that addresses the current challenges of today's care environment, including 1) the increasing complexity of medical knowledge, drugs, devices, and other interventions, which are advancing more quickly than our ability to deliver them in a safe, efficient, effective manner; 2) the increasing complexity of patients who have an increased number of chronic conditions yet are living longer lives than ever before; 3) a disorganized, decentralized, complex care delivery system with poorly coordinated handoffs and abundant waste; and 4) slow adoption of potentially revolutionary health information technology.

The report calls upon all stakeholders to commit to six factors to improve quality (**Table 97.2**) and also provides principles for the redesign of health-care processes, including transitioning the work product of health care from "office encounters" to "continuous healing relationships"; customization based on patients preferences, needs, and values; shared decision-making; the free flow of information; evidence-based decision making; safety as

TABLE 97.2 ■ The Institute of Medicine's Aims for Quality Improvement[16]	
Factor	**Definition**
Safety	Patients should not be harmed by care intended to help them. Providers should not be harmed by those they are caring for.
Effectiveness	Care is evidence-based. Interventions should produce outcomes better than alternatives, including doing nothing.
Patient-centeredness	The patient's experience should be tailored to their individual needs and preferences.
Timeliness	Important to any service or experience. Patients should have access to information, screening, treatment, and follow-up in a timely manner.
Efficiency	Resources are deployed efficiently to optimize value of care delivered.
Equity	Goals of quality improvement apply not only to the individual but also to the health of the entire population.

TABLE 97.3 ■ Organizations Leading Health-Care Quality

Name	Abbreviation	Focus	Type of Organization
Agency for Healthcare Quality	AHRQ	Evidence-based tools and resources	Government–part of HHS
American Hospital Association	AHA	Promote quality health-care provision	Private not-for-profit
American National Standards Institute–Healthcare Informatics Standards Board	ANSI-HISB	Coordination of health-care informatics standards	Private not-for-profit
Centers for Medicare & Medicaid Services	CMS	Administrator/oversight body for Medicare, Medicaid, CHIP, HIPAA, and Quality standards	Government–part of HHS
International Organization for Standardization	ISO	Technical Committee (TC) 215–Health Informatics	United Nations Organization
National Committee for Quality Assurance	NCQA	The Healthcare Effectiveness Data and Information Set (HEDIS)	Private not-for-profit
National Library of Medicine	NLM	Translating biomedical research into practice and easy to read language as basis for electronic health record	Government–part of HHS–National Institutes of Health (NIH)
National Quality Forum	NQF	Health-care quality through measurement	Private not-for-profit
Office of The National Coordinator for Health Information Technology	ONC for HIT	Adoption of HIT and Health Information Exchange	Government–part of HHS
The Joint Commission	TJC	Accreditation and certification, national patient safety goals	Private not-for-profit

a system property; the need for health systems to be transparent to the public; anticipating rather than reacting to patient needs; continuous decrease in waste; and enhanced cooperation between clinicians to minimize redundancy, cost, and miscommunication. Purchasers and regulators were also encouraged to create infrastructure to make better use of health information technology and clinical decision support and to align payment policies to recognize, reward, and support quality improvement.

Quality in health care has become a global movement. Several US-based and global organizations have emerged as quality leaders in health care. (See **Table 97.3** for a list of organizations and their focus.)

BALANCING QUALITY WITH VALUE

Defining quality of necessity requires consideration of the value portion of the equation, meaning consideration of the cost of quality in a capacity-constrained medical environment.

A simple way of thinking of it is that is value in health care is a function of quality of health-care outcomes divided by the cost needed to produce those outcomes.

Until this point in the chapter, use of the term "quality" has referred to the quality of the clinical care provided. However, quality may mean different things to a patient, physician, payor, purchaser, or hospital administrator. In addition to "clinical quality," providers must also consider the "service quality" and "cost efficiency" of the care they provide.

The "Triple Aim"

Despite spending twice as much on health care as that of the next closest country, the US health-care system achieves comparatively suboptimal outcomes. A 2008 article titled "The Triple Aim: Care, Health, and Cost" suggests that decreasing the imbalance between resource allocation and outcomes requires a concentrated effort in three areas: 1) improving the individual experience of care, 2) improving the health of populations, and 3) reducing the per-capita costs of care for populations.[17]

The "Triple Aim" moves beyond the quality of care provided to an individual patient or by an individual hospital or department and sets its sights on improving the health of a population, while also reducing per-capita costs.

The Affordable Care Act

In 2010, under President Barack Obama, the Patient Protection and Affordable Care Act (the ACA) was signed into law, which codified the principles of the "Triple Aim." The ACA called for the Centers for Medicare & Medicaid Services (CMS) to issue rules for the implementation of accountable care organizations (ACOs) with the intention of creating coordinated high quality, high-value, patient-centered care. The ACA created new, incentivized quality programs, as well as strategies like the Transforming Clinical Practice Initiative to help achieve large-scale practice transformation.[18] See **Box 97.4** to learn more about practice transformation efforts specific to emergency medicine.

BOX 97.4 ■ ACEP'S EMERGENCY QUALITY NETWORK

ACEP's Emergency Quality Network (E-QUAL) engages emergency clinicians and leverages emergency clinician practices to improve clinical outcomes, to coordinate care, and to reduce costs in four learning collaboratives: improving sepsis care, reducing avoidable imaging, reducing chest pain hospitalizations, and reducing opioid-associated harm.

E-QUAL is inclusive of several well-established best practice sources, including ACEP's clinical policies, the Surviving Sepsis Campaign, Choosing Wisely, and other ACEP-sponsored and -supported products.

Due to the complexity and variety of quality-improvement requirements and new federal payment policies, front-line clinicians and emergency care leaders are not always up to date on the latest advances in ED quality-improvement practices. E-QUAL provides up-to-date education on the latest ED requirements in the diagnosis, treatment, clinical skills, and practice-transformation innovations related to sepsis care, reducing avoidable imaging, reducing chest pain hospitalization, and reducing opioid-associated harm.

Breakdown of 2018 E-QUAL EDs by zip code and hospital type: 1,017 departments are participating, across 48 states. Of these, 190 are rural, 77 are critical access hospitals (CAH), and 22 are safety net departments.

The "Quadruple Aim"

Recognition of the high rate of burnout among the US health-care workforce led to the proposal of the "Quadruple Aim" in 2014. Expanding upon the goal of the "Triple Aim" to improve the health of a population by improving their care experience while reducing per-capita costs, the initiative includes improved clinician work-life balance as a tenet around which we should build or modify our health-care systems.[19,20] Despite the work physicians and other clinicians do to help others, rates of attrition and burnout remain astonishingly high and continue to grow. In several specialties, including emergency medicine, burnout rates are estimated to be just under 50%.[21] Satisfied front-line workers who experience joy and meaning in what they do offer the greatest potential to improve the patient's experience of care while removing waste from the system. Chapter 125 provides a comprehensive discussion of burnout in emergency departments (EDs).

QUALITY IN THE ED

Emergency departments are places of controlled chaos. Patients arrive undifferentiated, and life-and-death decisions must be made with little time or information. The ED is a challenging high-stress, high-risk environment where the likelihood of making an error is significantly increased. The breadth and acuity of patients and disease processes being seen coupled with frequent task interruptions, all while attempting to coordinate a fragmented system, are some of the many unique challenges faced by emergency physicians. Quality-improvement efforts in the ED should focus on high-frequency, high-cost chief complaints and address the aspects of care in which the interests of multiple stakeholders align.

The challenges of providing quality care in the ED include making proper diagnoses, enlisting the support from hospital leadership, and operating within the gridlock created by overcrowding, boarding, difficult payor mixes, and the unfunded mandate created by the Emergency Medical Treatment and Active Labor Act. Considering what quality means in the ED, start by considering the structure, processes, and outcomes of emergency care.[22]

Structure of Emergency Care

The structure of emergency care has radically evolved over the past several decades. Today's EDs are small and large, urban and rural, academic and community, free-standing and hospital-affiliated. Some EDs specialize in the treatment of trauma, heart attacks, and strokes. A new initiative by the American College of Emergency Physicians (ACEP) on geriatric emergency department accreditation seeks to tailor care for the needs of our aging population, similar to what has been accomplished in the pediatric emergency space.

Hospitals located in critical-access areas must transfer a large number of their patients to other facilities, while other EDs have expanded to include fast-tracks, observation services in clinical decision units, ED-based critical care units, and psychiatric EDs. Commitment from hospital and health-system leadership is essential to address common patient-flow issues, including overcrowding, boarding, left-without-being-seen rates, and ambulance diversion time. Emergency medical services systems have also evolved to include integrated 911 dispatch, air medical transport, and injury-prevention efforts that can help coordinate regionalized care.

Most ED patients will be seen by physicians who have completed an Accreditation Council of Graduate Medical Education or American Osteopathic Association-accredited emergency medicine residency program and have obtained board certification by the American Board of Emergency Medicine or the American Osteopathic Board of Emergency Medicine. Patients in rural settings, however, may not have access to residency-trained, board-certified emergency physicians and may end up being seen by a physician trained in a different specialty or by a nurse practitioner (NP) or physician assistant (PA). In locations where there is no on-site emergency physician, one may be available for telehealth consultation.

In addition to the primary ED provider, many patients may require urgent or emergent care from on-call specialists, many of whom are in short supply. This is because there is little financial incentive for clinicians to provide care for under- or uninsured ED patients while being exposed to more liability than they would if caring only for patients they have prescreened during clinic hours.

The availability of point-of-care laboratory and ultrasound testing in the ED as well as hours and availability of 24-hour consultative ultrasound and magnetic resonance imaging also affect the type of care provided. Structural measures are a reflection of the system in which the physician is providing care, rather than a measure of any individual provider.

Processes and Outcomes of Emergency Care

In the ED, adherence to a large number of process measures is common, well-established practice. For example, "door-to-doc," "door-to-balloon," and "door-to-needle" times are widely recognized core measures. Some early process measures of ED quality—such as the collection of blood cultures in all patients diagnosed with pneumonia—were retired after further investigation demonstrated this intervention was not medically necessary, while other measures like sepsis bundles continue to be rigidly adhered to despite newer evidence questioning their value.[23]

Tracking the long-term outcomes of ED patients can be challenging given the episodic nature of the care provided. However, in light of the emphasis that has been placed on the dangers of ED crowding and boarding, throughput metrics have been added to CMS's list of core measures, including median length of stay time and boarding time. Patient surveys like Press Ganey or the Emergency Department Consumer Assessment of Healthcare Providers and Systems track outcomes related to patient satisfaction, a metric to which many emergency physicians have some portion of their salary tied. Other important outcomes in the ED include unplanned return visits after discharge, rates of missed diagnoses, and unexpected deaths.

HOSPITAL-BASED QUALITY PROGRAMS

With the exception of investor-owned freestanding facilities, EDs fall under the hospitals' quality-improvement programs and should be integrated into their overall efforts and structure.

Inpatients

Developed as a result of the Medicare Prescription Drug, Improvement, and Modernization Act of 2003, the Inpatient Quality Reporting (IQR) program was designed to improve the quality of inpatient care. By making quality-performance data publicly available on the

Medicare website, the program also equipped patients with the information necessary to make informed decisions when choosing a hospital.[24] With the passage of the ACA in 2010, the Hospital Value-Based Purchasing (HVBP) program built upon the infrastructure of the hospital IQR program to create the first federally implemented pay-for-performance program for acute inpatient care. Major components of the HVBP program include avoidance of health care-associated infections or hospital-acquired conditions, reducing rates of readmission, and improving the patient experience.[24]

BOX 97.5 ■ HOSPITAL-BASED QUALITY MEASURES (2018)*

Throughput:
- ED-1: Median time from ED arrival to ED departure for admitted patients
- ED-2: Admit decision time to ED departure time for admitted patients
- OP-18: Median time from ED arrival to ED departure for discharged ED patients
- OP-20: Door to diagnostic evaluation by a qualified medical professional
- OP-22: Left without being seen

Acute MI:
- OP-1: Median time to fibrinolysis
- OP-2: Fibrinolytic therapy received within 30 minutes of ED arrival
- OP-3: Median time to transfer to another facility for acute coronary intervention
- OP-4: Aspirin at arrival
- OP-5: Median time to ECG
- AMI-97: Primary PCI received within 90 minutes of hospital arrival

Stroke:
- OP-23: Heat CT or MRI scan results for acute ischemic stroke or hemorrhagic stroke who received head CT or MRI scan interpretation within 45 minutes of ED arrival

Sepsis:
- SEP-1: Severe sepsis and septic shock: Management bundle

Imaging:
- OP-8: MRI lumbar spine for low back pain
- OP-10: Abdomen CT–Use of contrast material
- OP-11: Thorax CT–Use of contrast material
- OP-14: Simultaneous Use of brain computer tomography (CT) and sinus computed tomography (CT)

Readmission reduction (30-day, all-cause):
- READM-30-AMI: Acute myocardial infarction (AMI) hospitalization
- READM-30-CABG: Coronary artery bypass graft (CABG) surgery
- READM-30-COPD: Chronic obstructive pulmonary disease (COPD) hospitalization
- READM-30-HF: Heart failure (HF) hospitalization
- READM-30-HWR: Hospital-wide all-cause unplanned readmission
- READM-30-PN: Pneumonia hospitalization
- READM-30-STK: Stroke hospitalization
- READM-30-THA/TKA: Elective primary total hip arthroplasty and/or total knee arthroplasty

Miscellaneous:
- OP-12: The ability for providers with HIT to receive laboratory data electronically directly into their ONC-certified EHR system as discrete searchable data
- OP-17: Tracking clinical results between visits
- OP-21: Median time to pain management for long bone fracture
- OP-27/HCP: Influenza vaccination coverage among medical personnel
- CAUTI: Catheter-associated urinary tract infection
- CLABSI: Central line-associated bloodstream infection

*Measures beginning with OP are part of the Hospital OQR Program, while the remainder are part of the IQR Program.

Outpatients

Building upon the success of the IQR program, CMS began to collect data on the quality of outpatient hospital-based care in 2009, as mandated by the Tax Relief and Health Care Act of 2006. Hospitals who do not report this data receive a 2% reduction in CMS reimbursement by applying a reporting factor of 0.98 to all Outpatient Prospective Payment System payments.[25] A list of emergency medicine-related inpatient and outpatient hospital quality measures can be found in **Box 97.5**.

QUALITY REPORTING FOR PROVIDERS

The first program to measure the quality of care by individual clinicians was the Physician Voluntary Reporting Program (PVRP).[26] Launched in 2006 with a core "starter set" of quality measures, the PVRP allowed CMS to understand the care provided to Medicare beneficiaries in a more granular way than the hospital-wide quality programs that were already in place.

In 2006, President Bush signed the Tax Relief and Health Care Act, which created the Physician Quality Reporting Initiative (PQRI).[27] Participation remained voluntary and the act introduced financial incentives for physicians, PAs, NPs, and other providers. Reporting clinicians were eligible to earn a bonus payment of 1.5% of their Medicare Part B income. At the time of implementation, 66 measures were included in the program. The initial PQRI was only authorized as a one-year pilot program, but it was renewed for two additional years by the passage of the Medicare, Medicaid, and SCHIP Extension Act of 2007. In 2008, the PQRI was made permanent, and incentive bonuses were increased to 2% through the passage of the Medicare Improvements for Patients and Providers Act.

The Health Information Technology for Economic and Clinical Health Act of 2009 created financial incentives for eligible professionals and hospitals to adopt, implement, or upgrade their electronic health record (EHR) systems.[28] Eligibility depended on those who could demonstrate "meaningful use," including the ability to capture and share information related to the quality of patient care. Providers who did not adopt certified EHRs by 2015 were subjected to negative payment adjustments.

With the passage of the ACA in 2010, PQRI became known as the Physician Quality Reporting System (PQRS). Unlike the previous voluntary programs, PQRS would apply negative payment adjustments to clinicians who did not participate. The ACA also leveraged the data reported by PQRS to apply a value-based modifier (VBM) to Medicare fee-schedule payments for all physicians by 2017 based on their performance on a composite of quality and cost-of-care measures.

The American Taxpayer Relief Act of 2012 enabled the creation of qualified clinical data registries (QCDRs) as a new way to report quality measures.[29]

THE MEDICARE ACCESS AND CHIP REAUTHORIZATION ACT OF 2015

The Medicare Access and CHIP Reauthorization Act of 2015 (MACRA) eliminated the sustainable growth rate (SGR) formula that had capped increases in payments for Medicare services to gross domestic product growth and created the Quality Payment Program (QPP). The QPP rewards the provision of high-quality, high-value care in lieu of volume-based

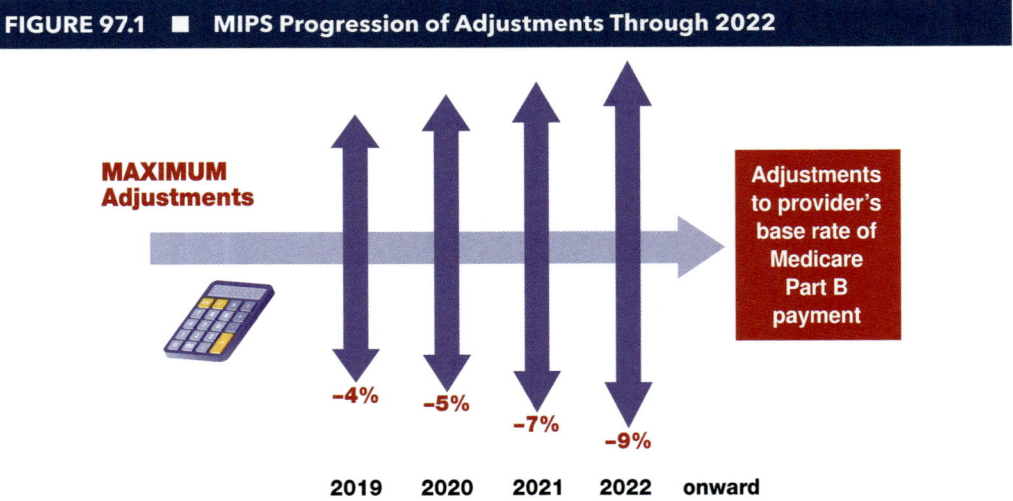

FIGURE 97.1 ■ MIPS Progression of Adjustments Through 2022

reimbursement. Providers participate in the QPP through either the Merit-Based Incentive Payment System (MIPS) or alternative payment models (APMs).[30] The QPP participation in 2018 applies to clinicians who both care for more than 200 Medicare patients annually and have greater than $90,000 in allowable Medicare Part B charges. By the year 2022, MIPS scores have the potential to positively or negatively adjust a physician's Medicare Part B payments by 9% (**Figure 97.1**).

Table 97.4 details the potential financial impact of these payment adjustments based on ED volume, but the positive-adjustment percentages could be less than the maximums listed due to the fixed dollar amount available for program administration. CMS has made APM participation attractive with a 5% positive payment adjustment without a corresponding risk corridor.

Merit-Based Incentive Payment System

Merit-Based Incentive Payment System participants receive a payment adjustment based on their performance in the four categories of quality, cost, improvement activities, and promoting interoperability (formerly advancing care information). These categories combine many of CMS's previous programs, including PQRS, Meaningful Use or the EHR incentive program, and the value-based modifier.[31] The relative weights of each category are determined by CMS and vary annually.[32]

TABLE 97.4 ■ Estimated MIPS Payment Adjustments by Visit Volume*

		Visit Volume (in Thousands)		
		40	60	120
Percent payment adjustment	4%	$62,720	$94,080	$188,160
	5%	$78,400	$117,600	$235,200
	7%	$109,760	$164,640	$329,280
	9%	$141,120	$211,680	$423,360

* Assuming 28% Medicare payer mix with average physician reimbursement per visit of $140.

TABLE 97.5 ■ MIPS Scoring and Payment Adjustments for 2019[27]	
Final Score	**Payment Adjustment**
>70	Positive adjustment*
	Eligible for exceptional performance bonus
3.1-69.9	Positive adjustment between 0% and 4%[a]
	Not eligible for exceptional performance bonus
3.0	Neutral adjustment
0.76-2.9	Negative adjustment between 0% and −4%[a]
0-0.75	Negative 4% adjustment

*Actual adjustment within the range determined by linear sliding scale, adjustments will increase to ±9% by the year 2020.

Providers can report to MIPS as 1) individuals, 2) groups of two or more clinicians who bill Medicare under the same tax identification number, or 3) virtual groups comprised of individuals or groups with fewer than 10 MIPS eligible clinicians who come together for the purpose of reporting to MIPS for a performance period. A performance period is defined by calendar year, and performance impacts Medicare payments for claims submitted beginning 24 months after the beginning of a reporting period. For example, performance year 2017 is defined as January 1, 2017, through December 31, 2018, and any payment adjustments based on data submitted during performance year 2017 would be applied to Medicare claims submitted beginning January 1, 2019. Payment adjustments are determined through the calculation of a final score, which incorporates performance scores from each of the four categories mentioned above.

Table 97.5 summarizes the payment adjustments based on the final score for performance year 2019. These tiers are determined annually by CMS.[33] Due to the budget neutrality requirement, any increase in allowed charges from positive payment adjustments must be offset by decreases in allowed charges from negative payment adjustments for each performance year. Positive payment adjustments, therefore, may be increased or decreased by a scaling factor that ensures neutrality and is calculated based on the distribution of scores for a given performance year. A final score greater than 70 makes one eligible for an exceptional performance bonus, for which a total of $500 million has been made available for performance year 2019.

Quality

Clinicians select six from among more than 300 approved quality measures on which to report, with at least one reported measure required to be an outcome or high priority measure. Measures are developed by CMS or medical specialty groups. The QPP measures denote CMS developed measures that may be pertinent to numerous specialties. An example of an emergency medicine relevant CMS measure is QPP 116: Avoidance of Antibiotic Treatment in Adults with Acute Bronchitis. A complete list of CMS-approved quality measures can be found at the CMS website.

In addition to the CMS-owned MIPS QPP measures, clinicians may also report clinical data via a CMS-approved QCDR. The CMS defines a QCDR as "an entity . . . that collects clinicians' clinical data for submission, such as regional collaboratives and specialty societies."[34] **Box 97.6** introduces ACEP's Clinical Emergency Data Registry (CEDR) as an example of one QCDR in the emergency medicine space. Each QCDR can develop up to 30

> **BOX 97.6 ■ ACEP'S CEDR: AN EMERGENCY MEDICINE QCDR**
>
> This is the first emergency medicine specialty-wide registry, designed by ACEP to measure acute care quality, outcomes, practice patterns, and trends in emergency care. CEDR is an evolving registry, which will support emergency physicians' efforts to improve quality and practice in all types of EDs even as practice and payment policies change over the coming years. The CEDR registry ensures that emergency physicians, rather than other parties, are identifying what practices work best for them.
>
> CEDR currently offers a choice for 44 measures to fulfill MIPS quality reporting requirements. National and comparative data generated by the CEDR registry will support evidence-based shared decision-making and guideline-informed physician practices. The advantages of participating in CEDR are:
>
> - Protection of revenue/ability to gain bonus
> - MACRA/MIPS compliance
> - Establish national benchmarks for EM-specific quality measures

measures for submission, or measures can be selected from several other areas, including Clinician and Group Consumer Assessment of Healthcare Providers and Systems surveys, National Quality Forum endorsed measures, and QPP measures. **Box 97.7** describes the making of one QCDR measure developed and reportable through CEDR. The list of CMS-approved QCDRs continues to grow with 141 approved for the 2018 reporting period.

If not reporting via QCDR, individuals may also submit quality data via the EHR or through submitted claims, while additional reporting methods for groups include administrative claims, the CMS Web Interface, or a CMS approved survey vendor. Regardless of submission method, measure performance is compared to specific benchmarks to determine how many points are awarded for that measure. Each measure is scored between

> **BOX 97.7 ■ ANATOMY OF A QUALITY MEASURE**
>
> **ACEP 24: Pregnancy test for female abdominal pain patients** (This QCDR measure is one of the 10 most frequently reported measures by ED groups.)
>
> **Inclusion criteria:**
> Females between 14 and 50 years of age who present to the ED with abdominal pain and have a serum or urinary pregnancy test ordered during the visit. This is reported as a percent with a higher percent indicating better performance.
>
> **Numerator:**
> ED patients for whom a pregnancy test (urine or serum) has been ordered.
>
> **Denominator:**
> All ED visits for female patients aged 14 through 50 years old who present with a chief complaint of abdominal pain.
>
> **Exclusion criteria:**
> Patients who have had a hysterectomy or who are currently pregnant.
>
> This measure highlights the opportunities and challenges of quality measure development and reporting. ACEP 24 has easily understood inclusion and exclusion criteria, and there is nothing controversial about evaluating for pregnancy in a female patient with abdominal pain.
>
> If a patient's history of a hysterectomy hasn't been recorded in a structured data field, the record won't be identified as containing an exclusion criteria and lack of ordering a pregnancy test in this patient will negatively impact performance. Or if the patient has a documented pregnancy test recorded prior to (but not during the ED encounter), measure performance will be negatively impacted. Finally, the measure is structured to identify pregnancy test order placement as a proxy for evaluation of pregnancy, though conceivably an order may be placed but no result obtained.
>
> This is not to say that the infrequent exceptions noted above invalidate the measure, but these examples highlight some of the difficulties in extracting performance data from the EHR.

3 and 10 points based on benchmarked performance with 3 points awarded for measures lacking benchmarks. Bonus points are available for submitting data directly from the EHR to a QCDR or the CMS Web Interface and for choosing to report on additional outcome or high-priority measures. As of 2018, bonus points will also be awarded based on the rate of improvement in a quality performance category.

Submitted measures must meet a data completion threshold, which varies based on measure type and submission mechanism but requires that a majority of the patients seen by the individual clinician or group are included in the submitted data set. Measures for which "performance is so high and unvarying that meaningful distinctions and improvement in performance can no longer be made" are labeled as topped-out measures for which a lower maximum measure performance score is available.[35] Topped out measures are subject to removal over a four-year cycle to ensure adequate time for the generation of additional reporting measures. The total quality performance category score is the sum of points earned for each of the required six quality measures and any bonus points earned compared to the maximum number of points possible. That percentage (between 0 and 100) multiplied by the weight of the quality category for the performance year determines the total quality performance category score. More information is available on the CMS website.

Improvement Activities

The improvement activity category assesses participation in clinical practice improvement activities that are categorized into the domains of care coordination, clinician and patient shared decision-making, use of patient safety practices, and expanding practice access.[36] Activities are selected from a CMS-approved list of over 100 options, many of which are pertinent to emergency medicine. Group size among other factors determine the number of required activities, and reporting can be done via several mechanisms, including QCDR (e.g., CEDR) and participation in a qualified registry (e.g., ACEP's Emergency Quality Network [E-QUAL]). More information is available at the CMS website.

Promoting Interoperability

In replacing meaningful use and the EHR incentive program, interoperability incentivizes patient engagement with the EHR and the sharing of health information among providers. Hospital-based clinicians, which include most emergency medicine clinicians, are currently exempt from promoting interoperability reporting, and the associated points are applied to the quality category. Approximately 15 total measures are available for reporting, and up to nine measures can be submitted for additional credit. Reporting for advancing care information occurs via attestation, QCDR or a qualified registry, or an EHR vendor. More information is available at the CMS website.

Cost

The cost performance category score is determined based on two measures: total per capita costs and Medicare spending per beneficiary. Both measures were reported previously as part of the VBM program. Since Medicare claims are used to calculate performance, no data submission is required. Costs included in these measures are subject to payment standardization, reflecting regional variation in allowed Medicare payment amounts for a given service. Cost category benchmarking is determined by claims data from that performance year, and CMS will assign points based on an individual's or group's performance compared to that benchmark.[37,38] The process for attributing beneficiary cost to a particular provider (attribution logic) and additional information about measure calculation is available at the CMS website.

Alternative Payment Models

The APM pathway for QPP participation, similar to MIPS, incentivizes the provision of high-value care but differs in that an APM is defined by a specific clinical condition, episode of care, or patient population. Clinicians who select the APM pathway earn an incentive bonus for receiving a threshold level of payments or seeing a threshold number of patients through the APM. If the threshold for APM participation is not met, most participating clinicians will be scored under MIPS. Comprehensive End-Stage Renal Disease Care, Comprehensive Care for Joint Replacement, and Bundled Payments for Care Improvement Initiatives are examples of currently approved APMs where payments are bundled for an episode of care, a procedure, or a group of patients with a specific disease process.[39] The opportunity for a 5% bonus on Medicare Part B payments without an associated risk corridor, contrary to MIPS where the potential exists for a payment reduction, incentivizes QPP participation via the APM pathway.

One can see many opportunities where APMs apply to care delivered in the ED. For starters, bundled reimbursements incentivize cost reduction, including the elimination of preventable ED visits. Using evidence-based clinical pathways supported institutionally by a multidisciplinary team can reduce hospital admission denials for patients presenting with complaints like chest pain by providing more accurate diagnoses such as pulmonary embolism. Cost savings achieved via treatment in concordance with evidence-based guidelines are then shared with the ED.

Other potential opportunities for participation in APMs include bundled payments for care related to an ED visit for a diagnosis like cellulitis or asthma. As piloted in Arkansas, an ED visit for asthma might trigger a bundled payment that includes all facility, professional, and diagnostic service charges for any asthma-related care over the next 30 days.[40] This incentivizes the use of guideline-directed medical therapy and follow-up with the goal of preventing a repeat ED visit or hospital admission. These examples illustrate several mechanisms under investigation by which ED clinicians might participate in APMs in the future.

ACEP proposed APM—Acute Unscheduled Care Model (AUCM): Enhancing Appropriate Admissions—was recommended by the Physician-Focused Payment Model Technical Advisory Committee to the Secretary of Health and Human Services in September 2018.[41] Though not yet approved by CMS, it represents a significant step toward emergency physician APM participation, something currently only available for those practicing in an area with an APM eligible ACO. The AUCM proposes shared savings based on three cost-reduction measures: decreasing hospital admissions and observation stays while ensuring safe discharge, coordination and management of postdischarge workups, and monitoring and reduction of post-ED discharge safety events.[35]

DEVELOPING AND VALIDATING MEANINGFUL MEASURES

In 2017, CMS launched the "Meaningful Measures" initiative to emphasize a set of principles to identify high-impact, high-priority areas to achieve CMS's four strategic goals:

- Improving the customer experience
- Ushering in an era of state flexibility and local leadership
- Supporting innovative approaches to improve quality, accessibility, and affordability

- Empowering patients and doctors to make decisions about their health care
- These four goals then are subjected to six cross-cutting criteria, including:
    - Eliminating disparities
    - Tracking measurable outcomes and impact
    - Safeguarding public health
    - Achieving cost savings
    - Improving access for rural communities

The final result of this framework includes 19 meaningful measure areas organized into six overarching categories of quality.[42]

CHALLENGES AND OPPORTUNITIES

This chapter began with a simple definition of quality: the degree to which performance meets or exceeds expectations, while minimizing variability. Health-care quality pioneers of the 19th and early 20th century established the firm precedent of establishing minimum standards around the provision of medical care. The 2000 publication of *To Err Is Human: Building a Safer Health System* brought a renewed focus on reducing medical errors and incentivizing the provision of high-quality care.[15] The passage of MACRA heralds a shift from volume to value-based payment with the establishment of MIPS and APMs that reward the delivery of high-value, cost-effective care to Medicare beneficiaries. While MACRA undoubtedly represents a significant step toward inextricably linking quality and health care, the complex nature of the product (health) and the production process (provision of health care) leaves many gaps and opportunities within the quality paradigm.

Access to Data

To be successful in quality measurement, it is essential to have access to the right data. There is usually a trade-off between the clinical relevance of data and the cost or ease with which it can be acquired. For example, billing and claims are usually cheap to obtain and readily available but may be less valid due to coding errors and the fact that information is lacking about the appropriateness (or medical necessity) for the care provided. Although manual chart abstraction can provide much more detail, this approach is expensive and time consuming.

Digital data sources like EHRs, picture archiving and communication systems, and laboratory information management systems have the potential to balance the granularity required for quality measurement through automated extraction processes. However, not all electronic health data are currently structured as coded variables. Finally, many hospitals may not wish to share their data with QCDRs due to security or strategy concerns. While the 21st Century Cure Act includes provisions to prohibit data blocking, many hospitals have limited IT resources, which can pose a significant barrier to obtaining timely access to data.

Harmonization, Evidence-Based Measures, and the Quadruple Aim

The lack of the harmonization among quality programs leads to confusion and threatens the clinician wellness that is a critical component of achieving the "Quadruple Aim." It is overwhelming to the average physician to have to track dozens of quality programs sponsored by dozens of organizations, when all the physician wants to do is the best thing for the patient. This is particularly disheartening when quality measures are at odds with the latest evidence-based medicine, causing physicians to feel a sense of loss of autonomy.

Attributing Individual Responsibility to Outcomes

The complex nature of health-care delivery underpins the challenge of incentivizing quality. Adherence to a seemingly straightforward short-term outcome measure, such as readmission to the hospital within 30 days of discharge after an episode of congestive heart failure, requires coordination among multiple caregivers who may not be part of the same hospital system. Additionally, patient education, access and adherence to medications, and scheduling and ensuring transportation to outpatient follow-up appointments can be challenging. Hospitals are incentivized to minimize readmissions from a financial reimbursement standpoint and also due to their requirement to publicly report unplanned readmissions on Medicare's "Hospital Compare"—a consumer-oriented website that shares how well hospitals provide recommended care to their patients.[43] Determining which of the many system components succeeded or failed in preventing a readmission remains difficult.

The EM Workforce

In today's medical system, care is provided by individuals with significant differences in their education and training requirements, including physicians, PAs, and NPs, who may or may not be required to be supervised by a physician. Although nonphysician clinicians may help reduce the dollars spent on staffing, using these providers may not save overall health-care dollars related to increased prescriptions, imaging, referrals, and other resource utilization. It will be important to track quality and resource utilization by clinician type and supervision models to identify opportunities for educational interventions and also to research and implement optimal staffing ratios for members of the health-care team.

Beyond MIPS: The Cost and Complexity of Measuring Quality

In March 2018, the Medicare Payment Advisory Commission (MedPAC) released a report which supported the elements of MACRA that repealed the SGR and encouraged the creation of APMs to deliver comprehensive, patient-centered care. However, the commission concluded that MIPS will not fulfill its goals, and it should be eliminated and replaced by a new voluntary value program for traditional (non-APM), fee-for-service Medicare.[44] MedPAC estimates that $2 billion will be spent during the first two years of MIPS for reporting costs alone. The committee also raises concerns that physicians can choose which measures to self-report and will understandably want to use measures for which they are already performing well, which may have little to do with providing high-value, patient-centered care and for which there will be little variability with which to differentiate performance.

In 2017, of the 403 MIPS measures, 113 met CMS's definition of being "topped-out," and the current plan to retire them will likely take several years. MedPAC also raises concerns that because the measures each physician can choose to report are highly variable, there is no way to easily enable patients to choose a high-value provider. In fact, many physicians submitting as part of a group may have their quality determined by clinicians from other specialties who reported the highest performance on their specialty-specific measures, which have nothing to do with care in the ED. Finally, CMS estimates that over half of clinicians will be exempt from MIPS reporting and payment adjustments.

CONCLUSION

Systems awareness and systems design are important for health professionals but are not enough. They are enabling mechanisms only. It is the ethical dimension of individuals that is essential to a system's success. Ultimately the secret of quality is love. You have to love your patient, you have to love your profession, you have to love your God. If you have love, you can then work backward to monitor and improve the system [45]

—Avedis Donabedian

Donabedian, considered by many to be the father of the modern health-care quality movement, illustrates the inherent limitations of improving the system without also focusing on the individuals who make up the system. Recognition of this same principle drove the expansion of the "Triple Aim" to the "Quadruple Aim." Enacting system improvements while fostering Donabedian's concept of love within the system offers perhaps the best chance for achieving a truly quality-driven health-care system in the United States.

REFERENCES

1. Deming WE. Total quality management. From a-z quotes. Available at: https://www.azquotes.com/author/3858-W_Edwards_Deming. Accessed October 31, 2020
2. Chandrupatla TR. Quality concepts. In: Chandrupatla TR, ed. *Quality and Reliability in Engineering.* Cambridge University Press; 2009:1–10.
3. Chun J, Bafford AC. History and background of quality measurement. *Clin Colon Rectal Surg.* 2014;27(1):5–9.
4. Roberts JS, Coale JG, Redman RR. A history of the joint commission on accreditation of hospitals. *JAMA.* 1987;258(7):936–940.
5. Marjoua Y, Bozic KJ. Brief history of quality movement in US healthcare. *Curr Rev Musculoskelet Med.* 2012;5(4):265–273.
6. Committee to Design a Strategy for Quality Review and Assurance in Medicare, Institute of Medicine. Hospital conditions of participation in Medicare. In: Lohr KN, ed. *Medicare: A Strategy for Quality Assurance.* Vol I. National Academies Press; 1990:119–137.
7. Urgent Matters, "The Risk-Free ED." Podcast interview of Thom Mayer by Jesse Pines. 2014. Available at: Available at: https://directory.libsyn.com/episode/index/id/3158537. Accessed October 31, 2020
8. Graff L, Stevens C, Spaite D, et al. Measuring and improving quality in emergency medicine. *Acad Emerg Med.* 2002;9(11):1091–1107.
9. Committee to Design a Strategy for Quality Review and Assurance in Medicare, Institute of Medicine. Health, health care, and quality of care. In: Lohr KN, ed. *Medicare: A Strategy for Quality Assurance.* Vol I. National Academies Press; 1990 19–44.
10. Committee to Design a Strategy for Quality Review and Assurance in Medicare, Institute of Medicine. Concepts of assessing, assuring, and improving quality. In: Lohr KN, ed. *Medicare: A Strategy for Quality Assurance.* Vol I. National Academies Press; 1990:45–68.
11. Donabedian A. Evaluating the quality of medical care. *Milbank Q.* 1966;83(4):691–729.
12. Agency for Healthcare Research and Quality. Types of quality measures. Available at: http://www.ahrq.gov/professionals/quality-patient-safety/talkingquality/create/types.html. Last Reviewed July, 2011. Accessed September 10, 2018.
13. Berwick DM. Sounding board: continuous improvement as an ideal in health care. *N Engl J Med.* 1989;320(1):53–56.
14. Berwick DM. Heal thyself or heal the system: can doctors help to improve medical care. Available at: https://www.ncbi.nlm.nih.gov/pmc/articles/PMC1054952/?page=3. Accessed November 20, 2020.
15. Committee on Quality of Health Care in America, Institute of Medicine. Kohn LT, Corrigan JM, Donaldson MS, eds. *To Err Is Human: Building a Safer Health System.* National Academies Press; 2000.
16. Committee on Quality of Health Care in America, Institute of Medicine. *Crossing the Quality Chasm: A New Health System for the 21st Century.* National Academies Press; 2001.
17. Berwick DM, Nolan TW, Whittington J. The Triple Aim: care, health, and cost. *Health Aff.* 2008;27(3):759–769.
18. Marjoua Y, Bozic KJ. Brief history of quality movement in US healthcare. *Curr Rev Musculoskelet Med.* 2012;5(4):265–273.
19. Bodenheimer T, Sinsky C. From triple to quadruple aim: care of the patient requires care of the provider. *Ann Fam Med.* 2014;12(6): 573–576.
20. Sikka R, Morath JM, Leape, L. The Quadruple aim: care, health, cost, and meaning in work. *BMJ Qual Saf.* 2015;24(10):608–610.
21. *Medscape National Physician Burnout & Depression Report 2018.* Medscape. 2018. Available at: https://www.medscape.com/slideshow/2018-lifestyle-burnout-depression-6009235. Accessed August 1, 2018.
22. Committee on the Future of Emergency Care in the United States Health System, Institute of Medicine. *Hospital-Based Emergency Care: At the Breaking Point.* National Academies Press; 2007.
23. Schuur JD, Hsia RY, Burstin H, et al. Quality measurement in the emergency department: past and future. *Health Aff.* 2013;32(12): 2129–2138.
24. Hospital inpatient quality reporting (IQR) program: overview. QualityNet at CMS.gov. Available at: https://www.qualitynet.org/dcs/ContentServer?c=Page&pagename=QnetPublic%2FPage%2FQnetTier2&cid=1138115987129. Accessed September 10, 2018.

25. Hospital outpatient quality reporting program. Centers for Medicare and Medicaid Services at CMS.gov. Available at: https://www.cms.gov/Medicare/Quality-Initiatives-Patient-Assessment-Instruments/HospitalQualityInits/HospitalOutpatientQualityReportingProgram.html. Updated July, 28, 2020. Accessed September 10, 2018.

26. CMS.gov. Physician Voluntary Reporting Program. 2005. Available at: https://www.cms.gov/newsroom/fact-sheets/physician-voluntary-reporting-program. Accessed October 28, 2020.

27. cms.gov. Program Overview: 2007 Physician Quality Reporting initiative (PQRI). Available at: https://www.cms.gov/Outreach-and-Education/Medicare-Learning-Network-MLN/MLNMattersArticles/downloads/mm5558.pdf. Updated June 15, 2013. Accessed October 28, 2020.

28. HHS.gov. HITECH Act Enforcement Interim Final Rule. 2009. Available at: https://www.hhs.gov/hipaa/for-professionals/special-topics/hitech-act-enforcement-interim-final-rule/index.html. Accessed October 28, 2020.

29. Congress.gov. H.R.8—American Taxpayer Relief Act of 2012. 2013. Available at: https://www.congress.gov/bill/112th-congress/house-bill/8/text. Accessed October 28, 2020.

30. Medicare Program; CY 2018 Updates to the Quality Payment Program; and Quality Payment Program: Extreme and Uncontrollable Circumstance Policy for the Transition Year. *Fed Reg.* 2017; 53568–54229.

31. Centers for Medicare and Medicaid Services. Quality payment program overview. Available at: https://qpp.cms.gov/about/qpp-overview. Accessed July 23, 2018.

32. Centers for Medicare and Medicaid Services. Computation of the 2018 Value Modifier. Available at: https://www.cms.gov/Medicare/Medicare-Fee-for-Service-Payment/PhysicianFeedbackProgram/Downloads/2018-VM-factsheet.pdf. Accessed November 20, 2020.

33. Centers for Medicare and Medicaid Services. CMS Hospital Value-Based Purchasing Program Results for Fiscal Year 2020. 2019. Available at: https://www.cms.gov/newsroom/fact-sheets/cms-hospital-value-based-purchasing-program-results-fiscal-year-2020. Accessed October 28, 2020.

34. Centers for Medicare and Medicaid Services. 2018 Merit-based Incentive Payment System (MIPS) Qualified Clinical Data Registry (QCDR) self-nomination fact sheet. Available at: https://www.hhs.gov/guidance/sites/default/files/hhs-guidance-documents/MIPS%20QCDR%20Self%20Nomination%20Fact%20Sheet%202017%2010%2016%20Remediated_7.pdf. Accessed August 6, 2018.

35. American College of Emergency Physicians. Acute Unscheduled Care Model (AUCM): enhancing appropriate admission. A Physician-Focused Payment Model (PFPM) for emergency medicine. Available at: https://aspe.hhs.gov/system/files/pdf/255906/ProposalACEP.pdf. Accessed September 6, 2018.

36. QPP.CMS.gov. Improvement Activities Requirements. 2020. Available at: https://qpp.cms.gov/mips/improvement-activities. Accessed October 28, 2020.

37. AbleHealth.com. A complete guide to MIPS scoring. 2020. Available at: https://ablehealth.com/2019/07/11/everything-you-need-to-know-about-mips-scoring/. Accessed October 28, 2020.

38. Centers for Medicare and Medicaid Services. 2020 Cost Measures Requirements. Available at: https://qpp.cms.gov/mips/cost. Accessed October 28, 2020.

39. Centers for Medicare and Medicaid Services. Innovation models. Available at: https://innovation.cms.gov/initiatives/index.html. Accessed July 23, 2018.

40. Pines JM, McStay FJ, George M, et al. Aligning payment reform and delivery innovation in emergency care. *Am J Manag Care*. 2016;22(8): 515–518.

41. A Federal advisory committee recommends ACEP-proposed alternative payment model. News release. American College of Emergency Physicians. 2018. Available at: http://newsroom.acep.org/news_releases?item=122951. Accessed September 10, 2018.

42. Moody-Williams J, Yong P, Long TG. Meaningful measures. Slide show. Centers for Medicare and Medicaid Services. 2017. Available at: https://www.cms.gov/Medicare/Quality-Initiatives-Patient-Assessment-Instruments/QualityMeasures/Downloads/Meaningful-Measures-webinar-slides-11-30-17.pdf. Accessed September 10, 2018.

43. Data.Medicare.gov. Hospital Compare Datasets. Available at: https://data.medicare.gov/data/hospital-compare. Updated October 28, 2020. Accessed October 28, 2020.

44. Report to the Congress: Medicare Payment Policy. MedPAC Medicare Payment Advisory Commission. 2018. Available at: http://www.medpac.gov/docs/default-source/reports/mar18_medpac_entirereport_sec.pdf?sfvrsn=0. Accessed September 10, 2018.

45. Best M, Neuhauser D. Avedis Donabedian: father of quality assurance and poet. *BMJ Qual Saf*. 2004;13(6):472–473.

ALTERNATIVE PAYMENT MODELS

Susan M. Nedza

CHAPTER 98

Will emergency physician payments eventually be based on patient outcomes rather than on the provision of services? The movement by public and private payers to adopt alternative payment models (APMs) that reward "value over volume" and progress beyond fee-for-service (FFS) models is accelerating. As the provider of symptom-driven acute unscheduled care services, emergency medicine does not easily fit into current programs focused on managing costs associated with populations of patients, inpatient procedures, and specific chronic diseases.

Yet emergency physicians have been indirectly impacted by programs that consider emergency department (ED) visits a failure of the system and are to be avoided. In addition, many emergency physicians are impacted directly by the pressure to avoid readmissions. Because these programs have not addressed the important value of clinical services, there has been a need to develop emergency medicine-specific APMs.[1] In response, the American College of Emergency Physicians (ACEP) developed the acute unscheduled care model (AUCM). In September 2018, the model was reviewed by the Physician-Focused Payment Model Technical Advisory Committee (PTAC), which recommended implementation to the secretary of the US Department of Health and Human Services (HHS).[2]

GENESIS OF ALTERNATIVE PAYMENT MODELS

How did APMs evolve? An examination of prior attempts to reform the payment and health-care delivery system will provide the answer. This is important because reform is a continuum that accelerated with the passage of the Patient Protection and Affordable Care Act of 2010 (PPACA).[3]

Medicare Demonstration Projects

In 1967, the Social Security Act of 1965 was modified. The Centers for Medicare and Medicaid Services (CMS) was granted "demonstration waiver authority," allowing it to research the potential impact and operational challenges of a proposed modification to the Medicare program.[4] These projects were real-world tests of new delivery methods, payment models for health-care providers, and benefit changes. Demonstration projects that led to significant changes to the Medicare program included the development of the Inpatient Prospective Payment System, the hospice benefit, and the skilled nursing facility and home health assistance prospective payment systems. Although these changes did not directly affect physician payment, they resulted in significant changes in the health-care delivery system and its funding. **Table 98.1** provides a list of demonstration projects that had an influence in the development of current APMs.

Unfortunately, the demonstration projects had several limitations. They often took years to plan, launch, and review, and they required congress to pass legislation that

TABLE 98.1 ■ CMS Demonstration Projects Informing Value Over Volume Initiatives		
Project	Focus	Result
Hospital gainsharing	Allowed hospitals and physicians to share in savings	Included protection for APMs from anti-kickback provisions like Stark
Premier hospital	Tested the impact of financial incentives for physician groups demonstrating high quality in acute myocardial infarction, CHF, pneumonia, coronary artery bypass graft, and total joint replacement	Provided rationale for hospital quality incentives and penalties
Physician group practice	Incentive payments to physicians based upon cost efficiency and performance generated from care coordination	Provided rationale for models in which the accountable entity is a group practice
Informatics for diabetes education and telemedicine	Impact of telemedicine to improve primary and preventive care in underserved inner city and rural areas	Introduced payment for telemedicine services

would allow CMS to implement changes to the Medicare program. They were prone to limited success, as stakeholders interested in maintaining the status quo could block implementation through the courts, modify the scope of changes, and protect constituents from disruption. As a result, changes to the Medicare program were often not timely, misaligned, and resulted in few savings. Congress remained in control of the program as the default was to modify Medicare through large spending or omnibus legislation, often on an annual basis.

Enabling Legislation

Medicare programs are implemented through enabling legislation, which grants designated officials the authority to take certain actions in order to carry out policies and laws. This legislation delegates rulemaking authority and stipulated responsibilities to those officials.

The Medicare Prescription Drug, Improvement, and Modernization Act of 2003

The Medicare Prescription Drug, Improvement, and Modernization Act included the first major pay-for-value program, the Hospital Quality Initiative (HQI).[5] The HQI required hospitals to submit data on 10 quality measures annually or face a 0.4% reduction in its annual payment update from CMS in FY 2005 to FY 2007.

The implementation of this act illustrated the unique place that EDs inhabit in the health-care system. The act included measures related to the care of patients with an acute myocardial infarction (AMI), heart failure, and pneumonia. As the physicians most likely to diagnosis these conditions, emergency physicians were moved to the frontline of compliance. Importantly, the measure required that pneumonia patients receive their first dose of antibiotics within four hours of arrival at the hospital. The time-based requirement quickly drove changes in the ED process of care and impacted ED throughput. Emergency physician practice was now linked to aggregate hospital revenue and not just revenue generated through the provision of ED services.

Tax Relief and Health Care Act of 2006

The earliest successful movement toward a focused quality-driven physician payment model occurred in the Tax Relief and Health Care Act of 2006.[6] This statute authorized the launch of the voluntary Physician Quality Reporting Initiative (PQRI). The PQRI did not fundamentally change the physician payment model, but it did pay a bonus for voluntarily reporting quality measures via claims. The initiative did not reward quality but "paid for reporting." It would later be modified and become the Physician Quality Reporting System and, ultimately, incorporated into the Quality Payment Program (QPP), defined in the Medicare Access and CHIP Reauthorization Act of 2015 (MACRA).[7]

Patient Protection and Affordable Care Act of 2010

The Patient Protection and Affordable Care Act signaled a significant change in Medicare payment policy, which contained many very important provisions including those authorizing the Hospital Readmission Reduction Program, the Accountable Care Organization (ACO) program, and the Medicare Shared Savings Program (MSSP). Two additional provisions included the creation of the Center for Medicare and Medicaid Innovation (CMMI) and granted authority to the secretary of Health and Human Services to implement programs without congressional approval.

The Center for Medicare and Medicaid Innovation

Congress created the CMMI to test innovative payment and health-care delivery models designed to reduce expenditures while preserving or enhancing the quality of care. Patient Protection and Affordable Care Act earmarked $10 billion in funding for CMMI for FY 2011 to FY 2019 and another $10 billion for each decade thereafter.

The CMMI is charged with analyzing models and disseminating the best practices of providers who meet the goals of these models. It also interfaces with stakeholders such as hospitals and specialty societies to develop additional models. The CMMI became the home for ongoing demonstration projects as well as those mandated by PPACA. They included the MSSP, ACO, and the Bundled Payments for Care Initiative (BPCI), among others.[8]

These programs have evolved into APMs and were recently adapted to meet the advanced alternative payment model (AAPM) requirements outlined in MACRA.[7] As of 2018, the center has launched 40 new payment models, involving more than 18 million patients and 200,000 health-care providers.[9] An example is the Geriatric Emergency Department Innovations: Transitional Care Nurses and Hospital Grant that tested the impact of targeted evaluation by geriatric ED staff to reduce the risk of inpatient admission.[10] This study informed the development of the ED-specific APM models, supported the inclusion of funding for care coordination, and justified the requirement for a safe discharge assessment tool.

Authority to Expand Programs

The PPACA granted the HHS secretary the ability to expand (including implementation on a nationwide basis) the duration and scope of a model through the rule-making process, if certain criteria were met. These criteria included a reduction in spending (without reducing the quality of care) and improving the quality of care. The CMS chief actuary would need to certify that the expansion would reduce program spending. It has been under this authority that the Comprehensive Care for Joint Replacement program was mandated at the national level based upon findings in earlier programs.[11]

Medicare Access and CHIP Reauthorization Act of 2015

In 2015, there was widespread agreement by stakeholders that the sustainable growth rate (SGR) method of rate setting for physician services was flawed and required replacement,

> **BOX 98.1 ■ ADVANCED APM CRITERIA**
>
> - Participants must use certified EHR technology.
> - Payment is based on quality measures comparable to those in MIPS.
> - APM entities must bear more than "nominal risk" for monetary losses.

which was accomplished with the passage of MACRA. The statute replaced the SGR process with the QPP, a value-based model for payment of services by Medicare Part B providers. The QPP provides physicians and groups two tracks for participation: the Merit-Based Incentive Payment System (MIPS) (see Chapter 97).

ADVANCED ALTERNATIVE PAYMENT MODELS

Advanced alternative payment models are a subset of APMs in which the participating organization (physician group practice or acute care hospital) bears greater revenue and risk opportunities. These financial incentives can include shared savings (upside risk) or losses (downside risk). It is the inclusion of downside risk that determines whether or not the organization is eligible for AAPM designation.

Requirements for AAPM Designation

There are three requirements for AAPM designation (**Box 98.1**). The nominal risk requirement is currently set at 8% of annual Medicare payments. The CMS will calculate target prices, and participants will be eligible for shared savings or shared losses. Physicians must meet sufficient participation requirements to be recognized as a Qualifying APM Participant (QP) eligible for an annual 5% Medicare Part B incentive (paid 2019–2024) and exemption for MIPS. This bonus is paid two years after the performance year. The definition of sufficient participation can be calculated in one of two ways, and the threshold scores continue to increase over time.[12] Understanding this methodology is critical because most emergency physicians would not reach QP designation by participation in current programs alone.

Beginning in 2019, participation in other payer AAPMs in addition to a CMS AAPM is included in the calculation for the QP status. **Box 98.2** lists CMS-recognized AAPMs for 2019. The inclusion of private payer APMs is designed to encourage Medicare Advantage plans to

> **BOX 98.2 ■ CMS-RECOGNIZED AAPMs FOR 2019**
>
> - Comprehensive Primary Care Plus (CPC+) Model
> - Medicare Accountable Care Organization (ACO) Track 1+ Model
> - Medicare Shared Savings Program (MSSP) Tracks 2 and 3
> - Next-Generation ACO Model
> - Oncology Care Model (OCM) 2-sided Risk
> - Comprehensive ESRD Care (CEC) 2-sided Risk
> - Bundled Payments for Care Improvement Advanced Model (BPCI Advanced)
> - Comprehensive Care for Joint Replacement (CJR) Track 1-CEHRT
> - Vermont Medicare ACO Initiative

adopt this payment methodology. If it is successful, ED groups may be asked to participate in these models during contract negotiations or by their hospitals.

Accountable Care Organizations

Accountable Care Organizations are groups of doctors, hospitals, and other health-care providers who voluntarily form partnerships to collaborate and share accountability for the quality and cost of care. The CMS uses claims data to attribute beneficiaries to specific providers who are affiliates of a Medicare ACO. The CMS payments to ACOs incorporate financial incentives for lowering spending and meeting specified quality goals for their beneficiary population. How broad is participation? As of 2018, CMS reported 10.5 million beneficiaries in an MSSP ACO and 1.4 million attributed to a next-generation ACO.[13] Although savings have been reported in these programs, the results have been skewed by the withdrawal of multiple participants and the lack of transition to accepting downside risk by some participants. A review of the structure and evolution of these programs that allows comparison across models is available through The Kaiser Family Foundation.

Bundled Payments for Care Initiative Advanced

The Bundled Payments for Care Initiative Advanced (BPCI Advanced) is the latest in a series of bundled payment programs and qualifies as an AAPM.[14] It is a voluntary model and covers 29 inpatient episodes (including procedures and medical conditions) and three outpatient episodes. The inpatient episodes are triggered upon either emergent or elective admission to the hospital, are diagnosis-related group driven, and are not initiated by ED providers. In BPCI, Medicare has established a total budget for all services provided to a beneficiary throughout a given episode of care. If the episode's spending on services is below budget, then the providers may share in Medicare savings; alternatively, if providers' costs exceed the budget, then the providers may incur losses.

Emergency Medicine Considerations

The lack of clarity in these models, the lack of direct impact on emergency medicine, and the focus on current day-to-day challenges have limited both awareness and planning for APMs, even by emergency medicine and population health leaders.[15] This is changing as hospital leadership is increasingly seeking to include emergency physicians as downstream providers in these programs. The drive for participation may be equated to seeking "in-network" participation with major payers. Unfortunately, hospitals do not always have the structure in place to integrate emergency physicians into these models, and the ED director is left to negotiate with these independent entities.

Successful participation by a hospital or a physician group requires collaboration with the ED group. This is driven by two factors. The first is the cost associated with readmissions during the 90-day episode window. A high readmission rate will result in missing the target price for the episode and the likelihood of owing CMS a reconciliation payment at the end of a performance year. The second is diagnostic accuracy. **Box 98.3** provides an example of a case where a rule-out myocardial infarction diagnosis leads to inappropriate assignment of a case to the BPCI Advanced for AMI. It is recommended that groups should actively audit their diagnostic accuracy and coding relevant to APMs.

It is becoming common for hospitals to include contractual obligations linked to achieving specific performance targets in ACOs, the Hospital-Acquired Condition program, and the Hospital Readmission Reduction program. Hospitals are also requiring participation in clinically integrated networks (CIN) because approximately one-third of the

> **BOX 98.3 ■ CASE STUDY**
>
> **Inappropriate Inclusion in a BPCI Advanced Bundle**
>
> A 74-year-old woman presents to the ED after being found lying on the floor of her home for 2 days. She is confused and dehydrated. A CT scan of the brain is negative, an ECG shows only sinus tachycardia, but she has an elevated sensitive cardiac troponin assay. The admission diagnoses include syncope, altered mental status, rule-out myocardial infarction, and dehydration. The hospitalist physician changes the order of these diagnoses in her note, and acute myocardial infarction (AMI) is now listed first.
>
> The patient receives IV fluids and her mentation improves. She undergoes extensive additional testing including a cardiac catheterization.
>
> She is discharged on day 6. Another hospitalist dictates the discharge summary and lists possible AMI as the final diagnosis.
>
> The hospital coding professional phones another physician who reviews the discharge summary and confirms the diagnosis. The case thus becomes eligible for inclusion in BPCI cases. The patient is discharged to a skilled nursing facility, deteriorates mentally, and is readmitted to the hospital. She is diagnosed with a subdural hematoma and undergoes surgery. She is discharged to a skilled nursing facility. The initial stay was coded as MS-DRG 282; her case is eligible for inclusion in the BPCI Advanced AMI case count.

quality measures used in this designation are ED-related. When viewed through a quality lens, participation provides access to data and an opportunity to improve outcomes and manage costs in the post-ED setting. Emergency physicians should actively seek partnership and accept leadership opportunities in ACOs and CINs because they represent a chance to educate colleagues about the challenges that are intrinsic to the practice of emergency medicine. This can also mitigate the risk that targets will be unachievable and result in financial penalties.

Integrating emergency physicians into these models is an imperative for both patients and for the success of the program. Department leaders should be proactive in seeking opportunities to partner with physician groups and hospitals in these endeavors.

PHYSICIAN-FOCUSED PAYMENT MODELS

MACRA creates incentives for physicians to participate in APMs through the development of physician-focused payment models (PFPMs). MACRA authorized the creation of the PTAC. The PTAC's mission is to make comments and recommendations to the HHS secretary on proposals for PFPMs submitted by individuals and stakeholder entities. In 2018, the secretary provided additional guidance to the PTAC regarding the types of models that would be of interest for testing or incorporating into current or future APMs.

Review Process

Individuals and stakeholders, such as specialty societies, submit proposed models to the PTAC. The models are then reviewed by the committee using 10 criteria (**Table 98.2**) that were defined in the MACRA final rule.[16] After a preliminary review by a subset of members of the committee, a discussion and vote is taken on each criterion, and a final recommendation is made. If the model is referred to the secretary of HHS, he or she must respond to the PTAC and provide a detailed rationale for not testing the model or a referral to CMMI for review and revision to enable implementation. Based upon this review, CMMI can undertake limited testing or develop a national model. All proceedings of the PTAC and the documents associated with its proposals are publicly available.

TABLE 98.2 ■ PTAC Evaluation Criteria	
Criterion	**Description**
Scope	Addresses an issue in payment policy a new way and includes entities for which opportunities to participate in APMs have been limited
Quality and cost	Improves health-care quality while decreasing cost
Payment methodology	Establishes payment methodology designed to meet goals
Value over volume	Provides incentives to deliver high-quality care
Flexibility	Provides the flexibility needed to deliver high-quality care
Ability to be evaluated	Provides evaluable goals for quality of care, cost, and other PFPM goals
Integration and care coordination	Encourages greater integration and care coordination across settings
Patient choice	Serves the unique needs and preferences of individual patients
Patient safety	Improves or maintains standards of patient safety
Health information technology	Encourages use of health information technology to improve care

Emergency Medicine Considerations

In 2017, Leavitt Partners identified that "no avenue for emergency physicians exists to participate in APM programs."[18] Emergency services for acute unscheduled care represent a segment of Medicare expenditures that has not yet received focused attention by CMS as the agency attempts to drive payment models that reward physicians for providing value over volume. ED leaders recognized the imperative to design emergency medicine-based APMs to fill this gap.[19] The reality that emergency physicians were unlikely to reach the QP thresholds in nonemergency medicine APMS increased the urgency for the development of such models. The PFPM statute provided the opportunity to respond to this challenge.

EMERGENCY MEDICINE-SPECIFIC APMs

In response to the lack of opportunity for emergency physicians to participate in non-ED-specific APMs, an ACEP task force developed two ED-centric PFPMs for submission to HHS. The task force included representatives from groups of all sizes, academicians, researchers, and health policy experts. **Box 98.4** lists the MACRA-aligned criteria the task force utilized in the design of the models.

Acute Unscheduled Care Model

The proposal, the *Acute Unscheduled Care Model (AUCM): Enhancing Appropriate Admissions*,[2] provides incentives to safely discharge Medicare beneficiaries from the ED by facilitating and rewarding postdischarge care coordination. It represents the next step beyond the Hospital Readmission Reduction program because it seeks to reward appropriate admissions to the hospital for Medicare beneficiaries who present to the ED for acute unscheduled care. The model ensures that emergency physicians who make the decision to provide safe, efficient

BOX 98.4 ■ MACRA-Aligned Criteria

- There is an opportunity for cost savings through improved efficiency while maintaining or improving the quality of care.
- Potential cost savings must be sufficient for the participating physicians and groups to assume a greater financial risk.
- The model could be implemented in all EDs regardless of geography, staffing model, or hospital type.
- The model is modular and allows for integration into other APM models.
- The model includes options regarding the assumption of financial risk.

outpatient care have the necessary tools to support this transformation and are rewarded for their decision-making. **Figure 98.1** provides the AUCM conceptual model.

An opportunity analysis of Medicare administrative data for an ambulatory Medicare population revealed variation in admission rates for high-volume, high-cost symptomatic conditions. In a review of 6.9 million Medicare FFS ED visits in 2014, 35.8% resulted in admission, 7.3% resulted in observation stays, and 54.7% resulted in discharges to home or the community. Significant variation seen in risk-adjusted admission rates across states, facilities, and clinical categories confirmed the opportunity.[20]

In patients discharged home to the community, there was a postdischarge event (i.e., death, repeat ED visits, inpatient admission, observation stay) rate of 8.8% at 7 days and 19.9% at 30 days. At the same time, as many as 45% of ED patients discharged home received no other Medicare services within 7 days of discharge; at 30 days, this rate remained as high as 17% for some categories of discharge diagnoses. This analysis identified significant variation in postdischarge care patterns as well.[20] The task force concluded that there was a significant opportunity to safely reduce hospital admission rates and to decrease costs associated with unscheduled post-ED return visits and admissions. The AUCM model is focused on rewarding clinicians for reducing costs in three ways:

- Reducing hospital inpatient admissions or observation stays
- Enhancing the ability of emergency physicians to coordinate, manage, and avoid unnecessary postdischarge services, when appropriate
- Avoiding post-ED visit patient safety events and their associated costs.

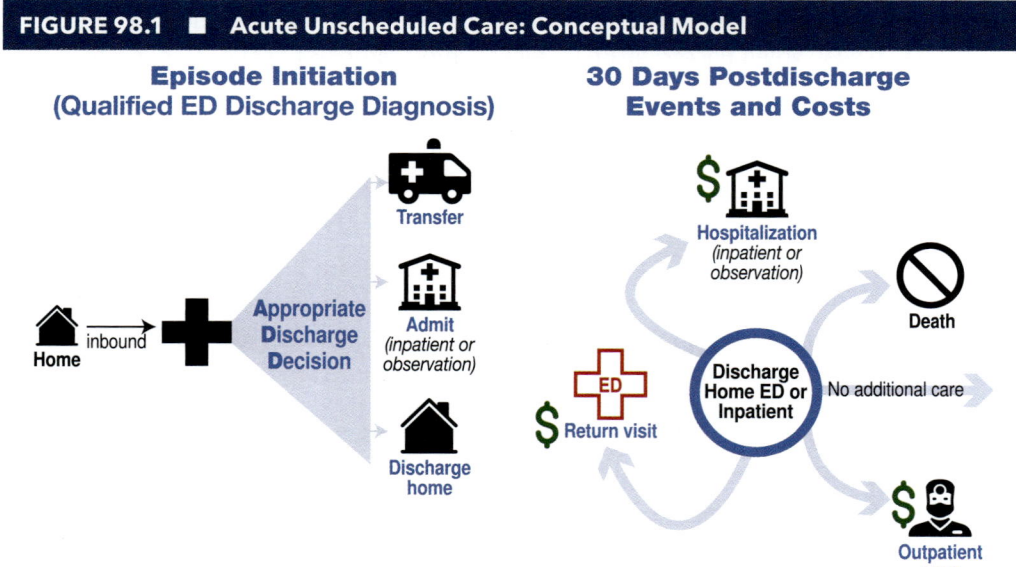

FIGURE 98.1 ■ Acute Unscheduled Care: Conceptual Model

The proposed monitoring of postdischarge events protects Medicare beneficiaries and ensures that attempts to decrease the cost of care do not result in decreased quality. This model honors patient preference to avoid hospitalization and observation stays (when appropriate) through the provision of transitional follow-up care in the home environment. The proposed payment methodology (**Figure 98.2**) is an episode-based, bundled payment model similar to BPCI Advanced. A qualified episode is triggered by the submission of a Medicare claim for an eligible visit by an emergency physician.

Medicare FFS claims for all items and services furnished during that clinical episode will continue to be processed under the relevant Medicare payment system rules. On an annual basis, Medicare FFS expenditures for the clinical episode will be subsequently reconciled against the final target price. Episode-level data is shared with participants to enable the development of quality improvement initiatives designed to focus on ED outcomes and cost of care.

How will safe discharge be made possible? The model also includes payment waivers for ED acute care transition services, telehealth services, and postdischarge home visits, which will provide emergency physicians with the necessary flexibility and tools to better coordinate care for their patients and which will be necessary to promote better outcomes. The model includes a set of outcome measures that can be calculated by CMS using claims data, registry data, and a set of patient safety measures. When combined, these measures set a minimum (floor) for qualifying for reconciliation payments as well as provide safeguards against inappropriate discharges that result in potential patient harm or additional cost.

Initially, the model focuses on episodes related to four high-volume ED undifferentiated presenting symptoms: abdominal pain, altered mental status, chest pain, and syncope. Starting in its third year, the model will expand to include additional diagnoses (excluding those that result in greater than a 90% admission rates per condition) as well as qualifying visits by dual-eligible beneficiaries. To maximize participation from both large and small physician groups, the model will include three options for risk sharing that enable emergency physicians to either take on downside risk immediately or ease into risk sharing over time.

The model guarantees savings for Medicare by building a discount into the target price for each episode and produces additional savings by reducing hospital

FIGURE 98.2 ■ Acute Unscheduled Care: Conceptual Model

Target Price
- Participant-specific episode benchmark is set using 3 years of historical data.
- Benchmark is risk-adjusted.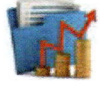
- Episode-specific target price is set by applying 1.5% to 3.0% discount benchmark.

Performance Period

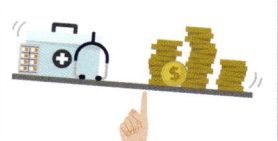

Services are reimbursed under traditional fee-for-service models for each episode.

Reconciliation Payment
- Actual spending during the performance period is compared to the target price for each episode.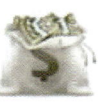
- Actual spending < target price → **positive** reconciliation payment
- Actual spending > target price → **negative** reconciliation payment
- Positive and negative reconciliation payments are capped at stop gain/stop loss.
- CMS makes positive or negative reconciliation payment to participant.

admissions and other postdischarge costs associated with each episode. A conservative 3% decrease in admission rates for these conditions could reduce annual Medicare spending by $314 million. Over time, a national 8% decrease in admission rates for just the four initial high-volume ED conditions could save Medicare over $840 million annually. Additional savings will be possible as new diagnoses and populations become eligible for inclusion.

TABLE 98.3 ■ Acute Unscheduled Care Model Specifications

Parameter	Specifications
Population	Medicare FFS beneficiaries. Dual eligible beneficiaries will be rolled into the model in year three
Qualifying ED visit/anchor events	An ED visit that results in: • Discharge home to the community • ED observation stay followed by discharge home to the community • Non-ED observation stay be followed by discharge (any location) • Inpatient admission followed by discharge (This includes stays where patients admitted to non-ED observation ultimately are discharged from inpatient status)
Qualifying episodes	All live ED discharges for which the first-listed ED diagnosis does not result in admission over 90% of the time nationally. • Model initial years (1-2): A select group of episodes for a basket of targeted symptoms or diagnoses (abdominal pain, chest pain, altered mental status, and syncope) • Model years three and after: All episodes of acute unscheduled care rolled into model
Postdischarge events of interest	In the 30 days following discharge home: • Return ED visits (treat and release) • Observation stays • Unscheduled inpatient admission • Death
Patient safety metrics	Repeat ED visit, inpatient or observation stay within 7 days for: • Injuries • Adverse drug reaction • Post-ED procedure complications
Cost metrics	Postdischarge costs for included services* within 30 days of the ED disposition decision
Waivers	Participants become eligible to provide telehealth services, receive care coordination payments, and supervise postdischarge visits
Exclusions	Deaths in ED, hospice and ESRD beneficiaries, Medicare beneficiaries with an inpatient admission in the 90 days prior to the qualifying ED visit or an ED visit in the 30 days prior to the index ED visit

*In alignment with BPCI-Advanced program.

Alternative Acute Care Model

The Alternative Acute Care Model (AACM) is designed to complement AUCM as it moves beyond the ambulatory population to focus on driving cost savings by avoiding ED visits by individuals residing in skilled nursing facilities. Cost savings would also be augmented by reducing the cost of transport between the ED and the facility. Emergency physicians would utilize telehealth to perform a rapid assessment of acute conditions and injuries.

This proposal expands upon the AUCM model by extending the emergency physician participation into the management of the long-term care population. Opportunities for savings in the care of this population depend on the use of telehealth to manage the ED–nursing facility interface, first to improve quality, and second, to allow for diagnosis, treatment, and follow-up care in a more cost-effective manner. **Table 98.3** provides details on the tenets of the model that are being tested. A preliminary analysis focused on identifying conditions for which a pre-ED evaluation would mitigate the transfer for evaluation and the cost included in ambulance transport.

It is anticipated that this model will be submitted to the PTAC or incorporated into discussions of the AUCM model with CMMI. The model's specifications will identify specific symptoms and injuries where care in place is possible, define specific eligible populations, quantify potential savings, and ensure alignment with other PFPM models currently undergoing evaluation through the PFPM process.

THE FUTURE

The CMS had set a goal of tying 50% of Medicare FFS payments to APMS by the end of 2018.[21] The current growth in national health-care expenditures will likely accelerate the movement to APMs regardless of which political party is in office. The QPP program will likely evolve as well. In June 2017, the Medicare Payment Advisory Commission cited concerns about the long-term viability of the MIPS program. Concerns included complexity of the program, the reporting burden placed upon providers (including hospitals), and the likelihood of limited savings to the Medicare program.[22] The 2020 executive branch made the explicit commitment to decrease this burden and recently signaled its intent to move away from process measures and increase the focus on cost measures.[23]

The AUCM that is currently being reviewed for testing or implementation fills an important gap in the CMS APM portfolio by providing a model to manage the cost and enhance the quality of acute unscheduled care. In September 2019, the HHS Secretary Alex Azar stated that "he believe[d] the core concepts of the AUCM should be incorporated into the APMs that . . . CMS is developing."[24] The AACM may drive new opportunities that will allow emergency physicians to reach into the out-of-hospital long-term care and home settings to provide evaluation and to recommend the treatment of acute and traumatic conditions without transport to the hospital ED. This model has the potential to disrupt the current model of emergency medical services in the process.

In the short term, ED groups should focus on how best to participate in hospital-based APMs. As inpatient spending still represents a significant share of Medicare expenditures, they should prepare for BPCI Advanced bundles to become mandatory. Success will depend on diagnostic accuracy at the initial visit and the avoidance of readmissions.

In the long term, the ED practice environment will increasingly be impacted by changes in payment methodology as programs span the continuum of care and payers coalesce and adopt models that focus on outcomes. This will require a culture change in the specialty as it will require the movement to accept accountability beyond the four walls of the ED. As APMs evolve, groups will no longer focus on achieving performance levels on ED-specific process measures but instead focus on impacting outcomes and driving cost-efficient post-ED visits. Compensation will be determined by the ability to coordinate care with post-ED providers to manage patients and impact the cost of care that follow ED visits.

This will require a culture change because it will require moving beyond the four walls of the ED and coordinating care and manage costs. The ED incentives will shift from valuing the intensity of services, increasing throughput, and admitting patients "just to be safe" or due to concerns about professional liability. The result for the health-care system will be integration of models focused on acute unscheduled care that reward emergency physicians for decision-making.

CONCLUSION

The time to develop an APM strategy is now. As speculative fiction writer William Gibson said in 2003, "The future is already here—it just not evenly distributed."[25] It is likely that APM adoption may occur at different rates due to variations in a local health-care market. For EDs in competitive markets, it is likely to occur quickly and across all payers as competitive forces drive the move from a volume-driven to value-driven health-care system.

REFERENCES

1. Medford-Davis LN. The imperative for emergency medicine to create its own alternative payment model. *Am J Emerg Med*. 2017;35(6):905–906.

2. Kivela P. Acute Unscheduled Care Model (AUCM): Enhancing Appropriate Admissions. 2018. Available at: https://aspe.hhs.gov/system/files/pdf/255906/ACEPResubmissionofAUCMtoPTAC.PDF. Accessed September 7, 2018.

3. US Government Publishing Office. Patient Protection and Affordable Care Act of 2010. 2010. Available at: https://www.govinfo.gov/content/pkg/BILLS-111hr3590enr/pdf/BILLS-111hr3590enr.pdf. Accessed September 7, 2018.

4. Cassidy A. The fundamentals of Medicare demonstrations. Background Paper No. 63. *National Health Policy Forum*. 2008. Available at https://www.nhpf.org/library/background-papers/BP63_MedicareDemos_07-22-08.pdf. Accessed August 8, 2018.

5. Medicare Prescription Drug, Improvement, and Modernization Act of 2003, HR 1, 108th Cong (2003). Available at: https://www.gpo.gov/fdsys/pkg/PLAW-108publ173/pdf/PLAW-108publ173.pdf. Accessed September 10, 2018.

6. Tax Relief and Healthcare Act of 2006. Government Publishing Office website. 2006. Available at https://www.govinfo.gov/content/pkg/PLAW-109publ432/html/PLAW-109publ432.htm. Accessed September 7, 2018.

7. Medicare Access and CHIP Reauthorization Act of 2015, HR 2, 114th Cong (2015). Available at: https://www.congress.gov/114/plaws/publ10/PLAW-114publ10.pdf. Accessed September 7, 2018.

8. Centers for Medicare & Medicare Services. About the CMS Innovation Center. Available at: https://innovation.cms.gov/about/index.html. Accessed September 7, 2018.

9. Centers for Medicare & Medicare Services. CMS Innovation Center: Report to Congress. 2016. Available at: https://innovation.cms.gov/Files/reports/rtc-2016.pdf. Accessed September 11, 2018.

10. Hwang U, Dresden SM, Rosenberg MS, et al. Geriatric emergency department innovations: transitional care nurses and hospital use. *J Am Geriatr Soc*. 2018;66(3):459–466.

11. Centers for Medicare & Medicate Services. Comprehensive care for joint replacement model. Available at: https://innovation.cms.gov/initiatives/cjr. Updated September 23, 2020. Accessed October 26, 2020.

12. Centers for Medicare & Medicare Services. Qualifying alternative payment model participants (QPs) methodology fact sheet. Available at: https://qpp-cm-prod-content.s3.amazonaws.com/uploads/560/2019%20QP%20Methodology%20Fact%20Sheet.pdf. Updated October 15, 2019. Accessed August 7, 2020.

13. Medpac.gov. Medicare Accountable Care Organization models: recent performance and long-term issues. 2018. Available at: http://www.medpac.gov/docs/default-source/reports/jun18_ch8_medpacreport_sec.pdf?sfvrsn=0. Accessed August 6, 2020.

14. Centers for Medicare & Medicare Services. BPCI Advanced. Available at: https://innovation.cms.gov/initiatives/bpci-advanced. Accessed September 11, 2018.

15. Wu A, Carter C, Pines JM. Emergency medicine stakeholder perspectives on value-based alternative payment models: a qualitative study. *Am J Emerg Med*. 2018. doi:10.106/j.ajem.2018.07.020

16. Centers for Medicare & Medicare Services. Medicare program; CY 2018 updates to the Quality Payment Program; and Quality Program: Extreme and Uncontrollable Circumstance Policy for the Transition Year. Document No. 2017-24067. 2017. Available at: https://www.federalregister.gov/documents/2017/11/16/2017-24067/medicare-program-cy-2018-updates-to-the-quality-payment-program-and-quality-payment-program-extreme. Accessed September 7, 2018.

17. US Department of Health & Human Services. Physician-Focused Payment Model Technical Advisory Committee (PTAC): Welcome. Available at: https://aspe.hhs.gov/ptac-physician-focused-payment-

model-technical-advisory-committee. Updated June 22, 2020. Accessed August 7, 2020.

18. Leavitt Partners. Medicare alternative payment models: not every provider has a path forward 2017. Available at: https://leavittpartners.com/press/leavitt-partners-releases-medicare-alternative-payment-models-not-every-provider-path-forward-white-paper/. Accessed September 7, 2018.

19. Harish NJ, Miller HD, Pines JM, Zane RD, Wiler JL. How alternative payment models in emergency medicine can benefit physicians, payers, and patients. *Am J Emerg Med*. 2017;35(6):906–909.

20. US Department of Health & Human Services. MEDPAR Limited Data Set (LDS)—Hospital National. Available at: https://www.cms.gov/Research-Statistics-Data-and-Systems/Files-for-Order/LimitedDataSets/MEDPARLDSHospitalNational. Updated August 3, 2020. Accessed on August 5, 2020.

21. Testimony of Patrick Conway. MD, to the US House Committee on Energy & Commerce Subcommittee on Health. 2016. Available at: https://docs.house.gov/meetings/IF/IF14/20160317/104683/HHRG-114-IF14-Wstate-ConwayP-20160317.pdf. Accessed October 26, 2020.

22. Medicare Payment Advisory Commission (MedPac). Report to the Congress: Medicare and the health care delivery system. 2017. Available at: www.medpac.gov/docs/default-source/reports/jun17_reporttocongress_sec.pdf. Accessed August 15, 2018.

23. Centers for Medicare & Medicare Services. 2021 Quality Payment Program Proposed Rule Overview Fact Sheet. Available at: https://www.sirweb.org/globalassets/aasociety-of-interventional-radiology-home-page/practice-resources/coding_pdfs/2021-qpp-proposed-rule-fact-sheet-1.pdf. Updated August 2020. Accessed August 7, 2020.

24. Davis J. Acute Unscheduled Care Model. American College of Emergency Physicians, Federal Advocacy Overview. 2020. Available at: https://www.acep.org/federal-advocacy/federal-advocacy-overview/APM/. Accessed August 7, 2020.

25. Anonymous. Broadband Blues. *The Economist (Business Section)*. 2001. Available at: https://www.economist.com/business/2001/06/21/broadband-blues. Accessed November 14, 2020.

CONTRACTS

SECTION 9

CHAPTER 99

NEGOTIATION SKILLS

Robert W. Strauss

Everything that we want or would like to own is currently owned by or under the control of someone else.

—Roger Dawson, author, trainer, speaker, professional negotiator

Negotiating entails the attempt to obtain a desired outcome. Few people enjoy the conflict inherent in negotiations. Many will avoid asking for more than is initially offered because of the potential for rejection and failure. However, most people are regular participants in the negotiating process, often unknowingly.[1,2] Any time one person interacts with another person to obtain an outcome that does not already exist, a negotiation is occurring. Negotiation is simply a form of conflict resolution. The conflict is simple: one wants an outcome that does not currently exist.

PRECONCEPTIONS ABOUT NEGOTIATION

The image of a stereotypical negotiation leaves many people feeling intimidated by the prospect of the conflict, since they believe they lack the skills or confidence necessary to be successful. In particular, women are more reticent than men to negotiate, with 2.5 times as many women as men describing great apprehension.[3,4] A study of graduating MBA students revealed "half of the men had negotiated their job offers as compared to only one eighth of the women."[5] This is more commonly due to how women who negotiate are treated rather than to their confidence. Examples that are routinely cited by men and women as creating anxiety include:

The aggressive salesman: A used car salesman or a merchant in a foreign bazaar haggles over the price of a desired object. After an emotional exchange, the parties settle on a price. If the agreement comes too easily, one party may feel as if they could have done better.

Asking for a raise: A hardworking employee enters the boss's office to ask for a raise. The employee feels underappreciated but is intimidated by the prospect of rejection. Embarrassed, the employee defensively apologizes and blurts out all the justifications for the raise. The boss simply says, "no!"

As a result of the anxiety felt during these interactions and the "social cost" of negotiating, many people perceive negotiating as distasteful or exceedingly complex. In reality, bargaining is learned at an early age. Children are masters because they inherently recognize that success is achieved by knowing what they want and demonstrating that they care about it (crying, temper tantrums, etc.).

APPROACHES TO NEGOTIATION

While all negotiators want to strike a deal that is personally beneficial, a completely one-sided negotiation can create significant long-term consequences and represents the "win-lose" style of negotiation: "I'm going to win and I really don't care what happens to you." This

> **BOX 99.1 ■ NEGOTIATION COMPONENTS**
>
> - Planning and preparation
> - Attitude
> - Information and aspirations
> - Time and deadline
> - Power

approach may be successful in the short term, but it runs counter to the development of the positive relationships necessary for ongoing collaboration. Adhering to a collaborative or "win-win" approach is more likely to create a solution satisfactory to both parties.[6] Thomas and Kilmann have devised a "Conflict Mode Instrument" that defines various forms of conflict resolution and negotiating styles.[7] Recognizing your own style and that of others can provide a significant advantage when determining your response to a situation.

Successful negotiation involves five components, which are listed in **Box 99.1**.[8,9]

Planning and Preparation

Thorough preparation is a key factor for successful negotiation. Among inexperienced negotiators, advance preparation is both the most important part of the process and the most neglected. Effective negotiators gather as much data as possible to formulate a plan. Advance research allows a person to formulate critical questions, consider potential answers to those questions, and compare the answers to personal goals.

Preparation may also allow a person to plan an approach that addresses the needs of the other side. Determining the other side's reasons for negotiating, political pressures, financial position, and likely strategy enhances the ability to formulate a solution that meets both sides' needs. For example, a person negotiating a contract to staff an emergency department (ED) should perform extensive research to gather detailed answers to multiple questions, a few of which are detailed in **Box 99.2**.

The issues and interests of each participant may be multifaceted. When considering hiring practitioners, there are the obvious considerations, such as money, title, and responsibilities. Other priorities depend on personal interests. For instance, a person with a young family

> **BOX 99.2 ■ NECESSARY ED DATA**
>
> **Planning for an ED practice requires gathering a substantial amount of current and projected information.**
>
> - Patient volume
> - Arrival times
> - Case mix: acuity
> - Payer mix
> - Fee schedule
> - Billing expense
> - Registration data
> - Documentation process
> - Flow metrics
> - Physician qualifications
> - Third-party contract details
> - Malpractice expenses
> - Business admin expenses
> - Physician qualifications
> - Provider costs
> - Leadership costs
> - Service support (lab, etc)

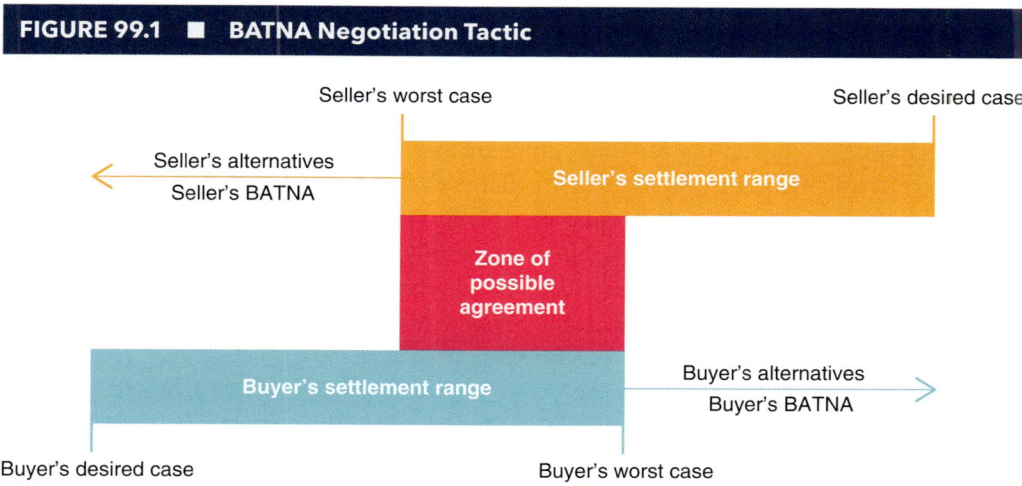

FIGURE 99.1 ■ BATNA Negotiation Tactic

might look for a consistent schedule, job security, and limited or no travel. Another person with an interest in building a career might want significant growth opportunities and have minimal interest in a long-term position.

Considerations in advance of a negotiation may include:[5]

- *Resources*: What can each side give to and get from the other?
- *Relative value*: What resources are of greater and lesser value to each party that can be traded? For example, trading time for money.
- *Risk preference*: What risk can each side tolerate or not tolerate? For example, consider an incentive plan or an "at-risk" plan, in which each side assumes some of the risk.
- *Time preference*: Does one side have urgent needs that can be negotiated, such as being willing to pay more or to pay a signing bonus for an early start?

BATNA

When developing a strategy, it is important to know not only your optimum realistic goal for a negotiated agreement but also your best alternative to a negotiated agreement (BATNA).[10,11] BATNA (**Figure 99.1**) explores and develops options if the desired agreement is not reached—a failed negotiation.

An example of BATNA could occur when a physician or nurse cannot come to acceptable terms when negotiating for a job in a desirable location.

- *BATNA 1*: Walk away.
- *BATNA 2*: Consider another slightly less desirable job at the same location while waiting for the ideal job to become available.
- *BATNA 3*: Take a slightly less desirable job under better terms at a nearby location.

Determining one's BATNA options in advance allows innovation when the predetermined bottom line (see aspirations and goals below) is not met, but one prefers to avoid walking away. Careful, thorough preparation is an effective way to mentally prepare for a negotiation. Understanding the needs and resources of both parties allows the adoption of a calm, assertive attitude that can help to communicate a sense of confidence and collaboration.

Attitude

It almost goes without saying that the attitude you bring to the negotiation is a key component in reaching a successful outcome.

Mental and Physical Preparation

People who exercise regularly recognize that being in good physical and emotional condition makes them more capable of dealing with day-to-day stresses.[12] This is particularly true when negotiating. Negotiating sessions can be intense and prolonged, so participants who are physically and mentally prepared have a distinct advantage.

Expectation and emotional attitude can play a significant role in the success of a negotiation. A negotiator with favorable expectations tends to project confidence and is more able to influence others. Alternatively, those who anticipate a negative outcome will likely communicate their low expectations nonverbally and work less hard to accomplish their aspirations.

Creating "Understanding by Identification"

It is difficult to negotiate when neither will trust.

—Samuel Johnson[13]

When trying to influence people and negotiate solutions, it is necessary to develop trust and convey respect. When both sides of a negotiation identify with each other, a foundation for understanding and a long-term relationship is established. For instance, leaders should avoid distinguishing themselves as different from those who provide services. Successful management teams do not "send down directives" or provide themselves with excessive personal amenities (e.g., special eating spaces, parking lots, luxuries, etc.) that separate themselves from those who deliver the product. Rather, they get close to those who deliver the service and inspire commitment to it. Management should be perceived as being a part of a team, with all participants being uniquely necessary for success.

The same principle applies during a negotiation. Early in the discussion/negotiation, it is important to be perceived as a peer of the other person. An identification of similarities unites the parties while emphasizing differences sets the two sides apart. Statements such as, "because I am a doctor/nurse," create a barrier to mutual respect and understanding. Instead, it is necessary to find areas of mutual interest to establish a bond of commonality.

Active Listening

Another key principle of successful negotiation is active listening.[14] It is difficult for most people to be mentally receptive to another's message until they themselves have been heard. A saying believed by this author is:

The one who does the most talking thinks the most was accomplished.

Although novice negotiators often want to speak right away and can be eager to set the tone and parameters, it may be more beneficial to allow the other side to speak first. Speaking last permits the other side to relax and establish their point of view. In turn, you'll have time to determine what the other side thinks is most important and incorporate those interests into your presentation. Many poor communicators wait for their turn to speak by preparing a rebuttal rather than listening. When thinking about one's own interests, it is impossible to listen actively.

Active listening is a technique in which the listener communicates what was heard by paraphrasing or restating what has been said. Done well, the original speaker's point of view is acknowledged and perhaps even validated. Active listening may involve the effective use of body language and eye contact to communicate concern and interest in what the other person is saying. Neurolinguist Suzette Hayden Elgin points out that particularly effective active listeners begin to move and breathe in sync with the speaker. Interested and intent listeners naturally tend to mirror the body positions of the speaker.[14]

Information and Aspirations

The Value of Information

Information creates powerful leverage in a negotiation.[15] Large corporations and governments may spend millions of dollars for research before entering major negotiations. Likewise, it is important that an individual takes the time necessary to perform the "homework" likely to lead to success. Those who accumulate relevant and specific information about the other side's needs and resources significantly increase the likelihood of a favorable outcome. A negotiation is somewhat like a game of poker—greater information about the other's position creates a substantial advantage. Facts may be separated into material facts and motivational facts. For instance, when considering a position as an ED director, helpful material and motivational facts that would improve the position of the candidate include those listed in **Box 99.3**.

Aspirations and Outcomes

Negotiating goals may be defined by two levels of aspiration: the optimum realistic goal (ORG) and the bottom line. The ORG is the set of parameters that would maximize the deal for the job seeker and could still be accommodated by the other side. The bottom line is the set of minimum criteria that must be provided for the job seeker to agree on a deal. In some instances, these two aspiration levels may be the same, meaning there is only one "non-negotiable" offer.

Siegel and Fouraker studied the relationship between expectation and outcome.[16] A group of Harvard students were divided into two groups. Members of group A were given a set of material facts and then told that their position would likely generate a profit of $2.10. Members of group B were given the exact same material facts but told that their position would likely yield a profit of $6.10. Individuals from groups A and B were then paired to negotiate against each other. Although it would have been reasonable to assume that each party would profit equally, the actual outcome was in line with the provided expectations, with members of group B negotiating a greater profit than members of group A. This result was one of the earlier experiments demonstrating that "negotiators who expect more achieve more."

In 1968, business pioneer Chester L. Karrass paired 120 skilled professional negotiators against each other in a classic negotiation.[17] Group A represented a man suing

---

BOX 99.3 ■ MATERIAL VS MOTIVATIONAL FACTS

Material facts
- Expectations
- Responsibilities
- Salary and benefits, including local market comparisons
- Start date
- Reasons why the previous director left

Motivational Interests
- Fears and concerns
- Interests
- Importance of timing (why now?)

> **BOX 99.4 ■ NEGOTIATOR ASPIRATIONS AND OUTCOMES**
>
> - Higher initial aspirations achieved higher awards, regardless of their power.
> - High initial aspirations did particularly well when paired with negotiators with low initial aspirations.
> - Unreasonably high initial positions did the best or deadlocked.

a pharmaceutical company because a drug he had taken caused hair loss and blindness. Group B represented the pharmaceutical company. The study compared initial demands (aspirations) with final outcomes. It also contrasted the negotiators' expectations of their opponents' demands with their actual demands. The conclusions are noted in **Box 99.4**.

Karrass's experiment demonstrated that expectation and aspiration have a direct bearing on outcome. In other words, the level of aspiration represents one's intended success. As an example, most people would like to earn more money than they currently make. Setting goals just slightly above the present salary allows potential success with minimal risk of disappointment. Setting a higher goal potentially achieves more, but with a greater risk of failure. As the experiment demonstrated, negotiators willing to strive for higher goals attained more.

Paradox of Lofty Goals[18]

Higher aspiration levels may allow one to simultaneously gain and lose more. That is, by asking for less, one is more likely to get most or all of the requested amount and simultaneously have minimal or no disappointment. A higher aspiration level (request) may lead to a greater gain while simultaneously creating the greater disappointment (loss/deficit) inherent in not getting all of what is desired (**Table 99.1**).

Assumptions

The Karrass experiment also demonstrated that one cannot make accurate assumptions about the other side's aspirations.[17] In other words, what is fair and reasonable to one person may not be fair and reasonable to another. A person's needs and expectations are unique. Initial assumptions about another's aspirations tend to be based on one's own personal constructs and beliefs. Therefore, all assumptions should be tested to determine the other side's actual aspirations. These assumptions may have to be modified as more data are gathered.

Feedback Changes Aspiration Levels

In a negotiation, perceptions about the outcome may fluctuate depending on the feedback and data that are obtained. Encouraging feedback such as "Yes," "Sure, that's fine," and a smile increases aspiration levels. Discouraging feedback such as "No! Are you kidding?" with a

TABLE 99.1 ■ The Paradox of Lofty Goals

Goal	Result (Gain)	Deficit (Loss)
4	4	0
8	6	2
12	8	4

scowl reduces aspiration levels. However, this type of negative feedback may be a purposeful ploy designed to lower expectations.

Time and Deadlines

Time is a powerful tool in a negotiation. It can be used effectively to modify outcomes. The impact of time can be broken down into three primary segments:

- Planning and preparation time
- Time during the negotiation
- Deadlines

Time

Understanding the strategic importance of time during a negotiation is a crucial element for success. Time can be used to build momentum, facilitate decision-making, and increase commitment.

An effective way to increase the other side's investment in making the deal is to achieve early mutual success. Sequencing easily agreed-upon issues early in the process leads to a greater commitment later when it may be necessary to work through more complex issues requiring concession. Early successes engender the atmosphere of collaboration necessary to tackle the tough issues. The more time both sides invest in the process, the more likely each will feel compelled to complete it.

The pace of the negotiation can enhance or limit success. Properly arranging the agenda and conducting the negotiation may facilitate momentum. If an urgent, time-sensitive negotiation begins to drag, momentum may be lost, and the deal may die. Even in less time-sensitive negotiations, long periods of inactivity between discussions may have a chilling effect on the eventual outcome. Alternatively, expanding the time between negotiations can be used to defuse an explosive situation. Given a little time, people can calm down and let anger dissipate.

Time pressures that appear to create time limits may be used to move the discussion forward. As an example, a person may state that the negotiation must conclude by a specific date. This stated deadline may be real or contrived to place pressure on the other side and accelerate the conclusion.

Deadlines

Early in the process, it may be advantageous to determine the other side's time limit. Deadlines are powerful tools; they create the incentive to settle because of the possibility of losing the opportunity or "deal" if the deadline is not met.[17] Sometimes individuals set arbitrary deadlines. It is important to clarify the reasons for a deadline and the consequences of going beyond it.

Difficult negotiations usually last to the deadline. Congress makes most decisions just before recess. Labor management negotiations often achieve resolution just before the strike, at "the 11th hour." This occurs for two reasons. First, large concessions are generally made at the last minute out of fear of imminent loss. Second, under the assumption that easy settlements do not achieve all possible concessions, the sides represented by the negotiators might be distrustful and disappointed with their leadership if the settlement was made without the appearance of a hard-fought effort.

The fear that a deadline may be used against one side leads some negotiators to avoid sharing their true deadlines. However, negotiators should be cautious when considering the use of a deadline or any negotiating ploy to "force a deal." Often, negotiations are part of a longer-term relationship. Using a ploy to force another into a one-sided deal creates the foundation for a poor partnership.

> **BOX 99.5 ■ FORMS OF NEGOTIATION POWER**
>
> - Power of weakness
> - Power of competition
> - Power of legitimacy
> - Power of expertise
> - Power of previous investment
> - Power of persistence
> - Power of limited authority

Harnessing Power

Inexperienced negotiators commonly feel the other side has more power. Novices may worry they are not as tough, smart, or experienced as their opponents. Because they are acutely aware of their own pressures and not those of the other side, inexperienced negotiators may believe the other side will "walk all over them." Much of the power wielded in a negotiation is "perceived" power. Positions are continually adjusting as the perceptions of relative power shift.

The degree to which one can alter those perceptions may determine the success or failure of the negotiation. Individuals will do less to promote the merits of their position if they believe their position is weak entering a negotiation. Conversely, those who believe they have a particularly strong position are more likely to pursue goals with conviction. The following are descriptions of some of the various forms of power and how they are used in negotiations (**Box 99.5**).

The Power of Weakness

It is not always disadvantageous to appear weak during a negotiation. In fact, it may be smart to act dumb and dumb to act smart. Consider Columbo, the bumbling detective, who, when walking away defeated, would turn around and ask, "Just one more thing . . ." A phrase such as, "Could you please go over that again?" will usually slow the other side down and reduce its momentum. This approach may result in the opponent revealing additional helpful information. Not quite getting it can be powerful. In some instances, it can even produce a concession.

A variation of the power of weakness is asking for help. This approach is most likely to work when the other side is seeking a win-win solution. Asking, "What would you do in my situation?" compliments the other side, gives it an opportunity to demonstrate its expertise, and encourages it to take the other point of view. This approach helps develop the lasting relationship most successful negotiators seek (**Figure 99.2**). As the other side reviews its position and tries to "help you understand," it may gain new insights that will enhance its own understanding.

The Power of Competition

Creating competition for a position, object, or service enhances its apparent value. A real estate broker uses the power of competition by suggesting there are other serious buyers looking at the house being considered. Interviewers create apparent competition when they tell interviewees how many candidates are looking at the position. Conversely, candidates may reveal the names of other prestigious companies that are wooing them.

Describing an opportunity as one of several options invokes the "power of competition" and may compel the other side to compete for the candidate who is now held in higher esteem. Alternatively, those who are or appear to be desperate lose bargaining power by

FIGURE 99.2 ■ **Negotiating Styles**

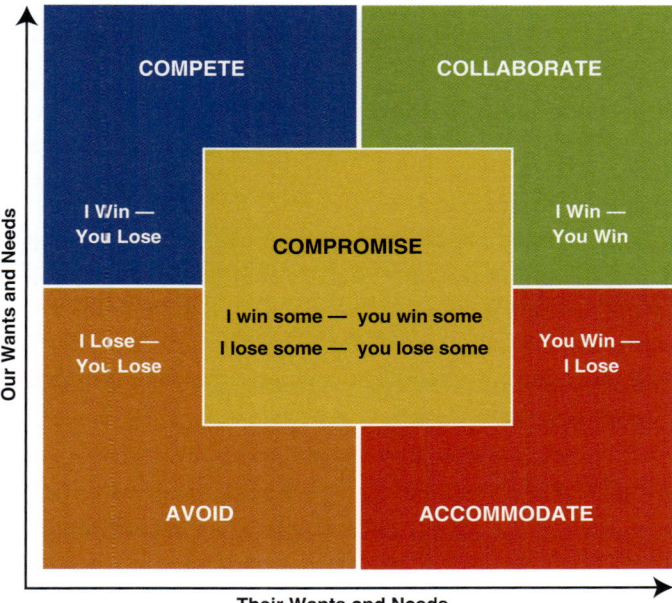

diminishing their value in the eyes of the other side. As an example, the following simple responses to the question, "Are you looking at other positions?" may create a very different perception.

Response A: "Not really, nothing seems very interesting. I'd really like to work here."

Response B: "Yes, I'm very excited about my opportunities. I've been offered several positions. As an example . . ."

The first response creates the impression that the job-seeker has limited opportunities and could be hired easily. Further, it demonstrates that this candidate is unexcited and disinterested. The second response creates the impression that this candidate has several offers and is in high demand. It is not clear whether the current position being discussed is of interest to them. In fact, the offer may have to be "sweetened" to get this candidate.

> . . . but this swift business
> I must uneasy make,
> lest too light winning
> make the prize light.
>
> —Prospero, *The Tempest*, Shakespeare, 1601[19]

As Shakespeare so wryly noted, another facet of the power of competition is that people generally are more satisfied with prizes that are earned and victories that are hard fought. A fish caught will taste better than a fish bought. A mountain climbed will have a better view than the same mountain driven. Consider the case of a provider who is considering other work opportunities.

Used for: Though the director becomes upset when a staff member looks at other opportunities, the practitioner contracts with another hospital for part-time work. Future negotiations with the director become easier and more successful because the practitioner is no longer at the mercy of the director.

Used against: When the provider mentions seeking other opportunities, the director nonchalantly states, "OK, let me know soon. I've got an interview with a superstar scheduled for next week."

Competition solutions include:[2]

- *Gain information*: Finding out how much competition exists allows one to more effectively respond to the situation. If the candidate learns their position, offer, or proposal is strong and is known to be the other side's first choice, negotiations are more likely to be successful.
- *Describe uniqueness*: Conversely, a candidate who is one of several must be prepared to describe how they are uniquely qualified to meet the employer's needs. The process of setting oneself apart from other competitors can create an advantage.
- *Develop options*: The candidate should be prepared to (honestly) describe other desirable opportunities. A candidate with many options is generally more respected than one with few or none.

The Power of Legitimacy

Outward manifestations of success create a perception of credibility and legitimacy.[2] In certain business settings, the people with whom one associates, the type of car driven, and the clothes worn convey a message of success and authenticity. Patients are more likely to hire a plastic surgeon who is well spoken, well dressed, and appears successful. Inherently, the surgeon communicates that their services are desirable to others with means. Alternatively, potential clients may be less likely to hire a plastic surgeon who drives a broken-down car and practices in an unattractive office in an undesirable part of the community.

Certifications by specialty boards, advanced training, publications, previous recognition, and a well-written curriculum vitae (CV) all validate an individual's achievements and successes. A polished CV confers legitimacy. A sloppy document, on the other hand, creates a negative impression and diminishes the conveyed information.

Used for: When presenting or negotiating, one should dress well, appear successful, bring documents that demonstrate achievements, and share written information that makes critical points.

Used against: An ED leader promotes a physical expansion of the department. In response, the hospital produces a bound report from a respected industry consultant that indicates the current space is more than adequate. As a result, the administrator concludes that the board will not support funding for additional space. Most people will assume that written document presented from a consultant is legitimate. Legitimacy solutions include:

- One must be careful not to accept all documents at face value, as the documents may have been specifically requested to legitimize a position.
- Finding or generating documents that are supportive of one's own position creates the appearance of legitimacy.

The Power of Expertise

A corollary to the power of legitimacy is the power of expertise.[2] The appearance of knowledge, experience, and expertise is an influential and powerful tool that can be used daily. Simply walking into a room wearing a white coat and a stethoscope creates the impression that the practitioner is an expert and knows what to do. Because of the appearance of expertise, patients allow staff members to perform invasive and painful procedures on them without questioning their competence.

Mastery of facts creates both expertise and confidence. Moore found that a confident approach enhances the perception of expertise in others, even when the track record of the expert is poor.[20] Therefore, one may appear to be an expert by having a command of information and a confident attitude.

Used for: A person walks into a negotiation to expand the ED with a full understanding of the facts, backed by supportive documents. The confidence in and knowledge of the information is persuasive.

Used against: The hospital calls in a consultant firm of architects with substantial credentials and a record of having undertaken multiple hospital renovations. The consultant recommends a less costly but impractical approach. Pleased with the new plan, the hospital prepares to move ahead. Further exploration of the consultant's background would have revealed broad experience in developing small specialty outpatient clinics but minimal experience in developing EDs.

Expertise solutions include:

- Recognize that most experts provide answers supporting the position of the person or organization that hires them.
- Avoid overconfidence in an expert. Most experts rely on previous work experience to guide future recommendations. Each set of circumstances is unique, and experts should consider the particular characteristics and nuances of a situation.
- Ensure that the experts demonstrate exactly how their recommendations address specific issues.
- Determine the experts' relevant experience, and find out if their solutions have led to the types of results that are warranted in the situation at hand.
- Use others' expertise to create an advantage. Actively collaborate with and guide the expert, demonstrating personal knowledge and expertise.
- Establish personal background and expertise early in or prior to the negotiation. When expertise is claimed during the debate phase, it is less likely to be accepted.

The Power of Previous Investment

The more time and effort put into a task, the harder it is to walk away. In economics, "sunk costs" are unrecoverable costs already incurred. Willingness to continue to work through a difficult negotiation, in large part, depends on the previous efforts expended.[21] Examples of the power of previous investment abound:

- In poker, it is called "chasing." Once a person has placed money into the pot, the decision of whether to continue to invest in this hand may be based more on the amount of money contributed than on a comparison of the odds of winning the next bet.
- As the United States lost more lives in Vietnam, it became harder to withdraw. The government became more committed to achieving a victory based on its past loss of lives than on a rational assessment contrasting the benefits of victory with the cost of future investment in lives and resources.
- Surrogate mothers may want to keep the baby they carried for 9 months.

Used for: The more time and effort spent agreeing on contractual issues, the more likely compromise will be achieved on the final issues. Early in a negotiation, it may be wise to postpone a difficult issue or an impasse. This can be deferred by saying, "This is obviously a difficult point for both of us. Let's work on some other issues and come back to it a little later."

In this instance, the frustration of an imminent breakdown in the negotiations can be replaced with the satisfaction of achieving early agreement on simple issues. Early agreement on less challenging matters will enhance the relationship and build the foundation necessary to work through the more contentious issue.

When it is time, the more challenging issue can be introduced by saying, "We have made so much progress and are virtually done with this agreement. Why don't we find a compromise on this final issue?"

At this point, both sides are more likely to make the extra effort to complete the deal. This phenomenon explains why incumbency in a contractual relationship is so powerful. A hospital may become so invested in a group or individual that it is difficult to change.

Used against: Either side can use this same approach. It may be difficult to walk away from a "bad deal" once a long-term relationship is established. The other side may extend the process timing so the investment of time and resources leads to significant compromises by you.

Previous investment solutions include:

- When the deal and relationship are both important, putting off more complex issues and instead addressing simpler issues first creates a foundation for success.
- When a a particular issue is more important than the relationship and walking away is acceptable, it may be disadvantageous to postpone the discussion.
- Incumbency may be used as an advantage by demonstrating the advantages of continuing the current relationship (e.g., market successes, ongoing projects, future potential).

The Power of Persistence

Persevering until success is achieved is one of the hallmarks of a good negotiator. Persistence requires creativity and discipline.[22] A proposal may need to be presented over and over in a variety of different ways before it is accepted. Repeated efforts to attain a specific goal send a powerful message of conviction.

It is important to be physically and emotionally fit to endure the rigors of persistence. A long and complex negotiating session can be exhausting. As the hours stretch on, there is a tendency to give in and say, "Okay, enough, I accept your . . .!"

Used for: The director of a busy ED proposes enhanced staffing, knowing that it will be expensive. The plan is met with stiff resistance from administration. Success may eventually occur after doggedly working with various leaders to demonstrate the long-term financial benefit to the organization. Persistence will pay off if the necessary changes are eventually approved.

Used against: The other side may tirelessly repeat the same solution, leading one to concede a little each time or even capitulate completely. Alternatively, a party that will not "take 'no' for an answer" may be perceived as stubborn and frustrate the opponent, possibly breaking up the negotiation.

Persistence solutions include:

- *Be well rested and in good physical shape*: Loss of concentration creates a significant disadvantage. Taking a break to refresh may be advantageous.
- *Take detailed notes*: It may be very helpful to refer to well-kept notes when a previously resolved issue is raised in an attempt to wear down a negotiator. Publishing notes and having the other side sign off on them is even better.
- *Learn to creatively restate objectives*: Because it may be necessary to persevere on an important issue, learn to restate the issue using different examples and

perspectives. This approach demonstrates that the issue is multifaceted, well thought out, and important to the presenter.
- *Be willing to persevere*: Persevere even in the face of persistent attack.

The Power of Limited Authority

Rather than displaying power and authority, some will refer a decision to a "higher authority." The technique is commonly used in the automobile sales industry. After haggling with a salesperson, a deal is struck. Hands are shaken and the buyer is relieved and psychologically committed to the deal. The salesperson says, "Everything is in order. I'll just get final approval from my manager." While the buyer has made a commitment, the salesperson has not. The salesperson returns saying, "I'm really sorry. My boss said that with the recent increases in overhead, we would lose money at that price. We could, however, do the deal for just $300 more." Once the decision to purchase the car is made, it is hard to walk away for just $300.

> *Used for*: The ability to defer to a "higher authority" may help avoid arriving at a hasty decision and allow time to consider its ramifications. The process can be used to bring parties to a well-considered and mutually beneficial conclusion. Deferred authority should not be used in a deceitful way or to force the other side into a deal that is unfair; to do so would ultimately erode the relationship.

> *Used against*: After negotiating and shaking hands on a deal to provide services, one side states, "I have to take this back to my Board. I am confident that it will be approved." A few days later she returns and claims, "The Board was tough, but I have good news. They agree to everything except the price. If you would just give a little—I think 8% would do it—we can close the deal right now." The other side has used the power of limited authority to attempt to create a more favorable deal.

Limited authority solutions include:

- *Establish authority early*: At the beginning of the negotiation, determine who has the authority to make the final decision for the other side. If the other person's authority is limited, clarify its scope.
- *Prevent the last-minute surprise*: If the other side describes limited authority at the last minute, it may be helpful to both play on pride and gain commitment by asking directed questions that encourage the other side to honor the deal as negotiated when speaking to their decision-makers.
- *Invoke one's own trusted advisor*: When surprised by the other side's limited authority, a powerful counter is to describe the need to obtain advice from your own trusted source. If the other side returns with a less favorable offer, balance may be achieved by describing the additional requirements suggested by your trusted advisor.

CRITICAL ASPECTS OF THE NEGOTIATION

Several aspects of the negotiation clearly influence success (**Box 99.6**).

The Starting Point

The "starting point" is the stated initial position in a negotiation.[24] There is often a direct relationship between the starting point and the final outcome.

> **BOX 99.6 ■ CRITICAL ASPECTS OF NEGOTIATION**
>
> - **The starting point**
>   - Starting high
>   - Starting low
> - **Concession behavior**
>   - The incremental nature of concessions
>   - Karrass on concession behavior
>   - The diminishing value of concessions
>   - The "too-easy" win
> - **Principled negotiations**
>   - Positional bargaining
>   - Principled bargaining
>   - Interests before positions
> - **Other techniques**
>   - The theory of "yes"
>   - Feel, felt, found

Starting High—Implying Self Confidence

Famed Yale psychologist Carl Hovland demonstrated that when trying to move or influence people, greater success is achieved if they are encouraged to go beyond the expected end point.[25] In other words, when trying to persuade a group to move from starting point A to end point X, targeting an additional end point beyond X, such as Z, was consistently more successful than targeting only end point X (**Figure 99.3**). Considering this in negotiation, it may make sense to begin a little higher than the anticipated goal. This is like the concept of encouraging others to adopt a shared vision. No matter how "right" a concept appears to be, you cannot assume that others will wholly embrace it.

In the Karrass negotiating experiment, the highest initial demands led to the highest settlements (**Box 99.7**).[17] Starting high may communicate to others a high self-esteem. In other words, starting high suggests confidence and self-assurance. Conversely, a "too-high" starting point suggests arrogance. Starting somewhat above the desired end point may help during the compromise phase of the negotiations. In many negotiations, opposing parties may think the other side is "starting high" and will work toward a compromise. If padding is anticipated, you may place yourself at a disadvantage if you start at your "bottom line." Then, resistance to concessions might be interpreted as unyielding rigidity.

Starting Low—Implying Flexibility

Starting low is the same concept from the opposite perspective.[2] In this situation, the purchaser of a service or product begins at a low point. This low offer may be meant to devalue the other person's position. Starting low carries some risk and should be done with sensitivity to avoid the insult inherent in asserting low value. If a low offer is made to counter a high starting offer, it may imply flexibility.

FIGURE 99.3 ■ Hovland's Order of Presentation

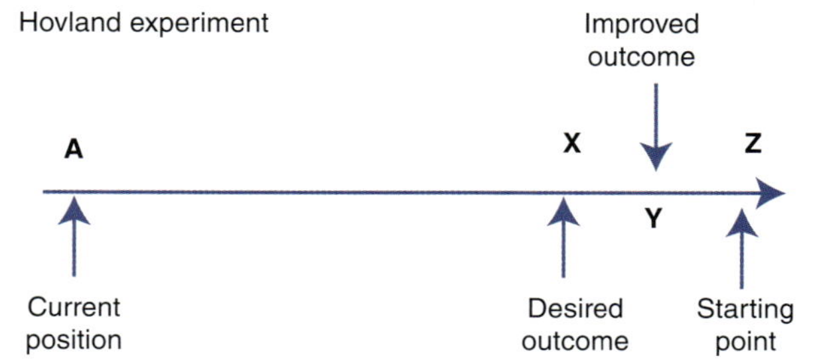

> **BOX 99.7 ■ ADVANTAGES OF STARTING HIGH**
>
> 1. Enhances others' perceptions of you
> 2. Allows room for negotiation
> 3. Improves the end result

As an example, assume a purchaser is interested in a piece of art that may be worth $7,500. The purchaser could make a low offer with implied flexibility, such as, "I'm not exactly sure what it is worth but given what I see, I think that $4,200 would be a fair price." This statement suggests flexibility to avoid alienating the seller. Concessions by the buyer will simultaneously allow the seller to "get something" more than the initial offer and allow the buyer to purchase the item for less than the starting point.

Concession Behavior

All negotiations involve compromise. Without compromise, there is no negotiation. Without flexibility, there is a risk of each side becoming trapped in an all-or-nothing position. Conversely, there may be a great cost if one's approach to making a deal is just to "give in" to the other side. To compromise or adjust goals in a negotiation is referred to as *concession behavior*. How one concedes dramatically influences the success or failure of the negotiation (**Table 99.2**).

- *Give to get*: When dealing with conflict or negotiating, the approach of "you have to give something to get something" engenders the belief that both sides should succeed. If one side achieves its goals, it is appropriate for that side to help the other meet its goals. This approach builds strong relationships.
- *My way or the highway*: This strategy is based on the belief that concessions are a sign of weakness and that long-term relationships have no importance at the negotiating table. The ancient Romans maintained peace by demonstrating a readiness to use overwhelming force (*Pax Romana*). They demanded complete concessions and gave none; they were willing to win at any cost.[26]
- *Get only*: The view of the former Soviet Union was a variation on this theme.[27] The classic Soviet style of negotiation was never to concede. By this theory, a concession was proof that the other side's position was weak, and more concessions were likely to follow.

The Incremental Nature of Concessions

The way negotiators make concessions communicates their end point. Those who concede easily and in large amounts are sending the message that they have great flexibility and

TABLE 99.2 ■ Alternate Views of Concession Behavior

View	Example	Belief
Give-to-get	Typical	Compromise and seek middle ground
My way or the highway	Pax Romano	Total concession by other party
Get only	Russian	Concessions demonstrate weakness

little commitment to their initial position. Novice negotiators may erroneously believe that a large concession will favorably impress the other side and lead them to a deal. Ironically, a large concession usually raises the aspirations of the other side, who may interpret easy, large concessions as a sign that more is available for the taking. As a result, they may ask for more concessions. Those who concede slowly and in a "stingy" manner reveal strong attachment to their position. This behavior sends the message that there is less room for flexibility and will lower the aspirations of the other side. Typically, negotiations are a back-and-forth process, with each side making concessions as they draw closer to a deal. The size and relationship of successive concessions influence the end point (**Figure 99.4**).

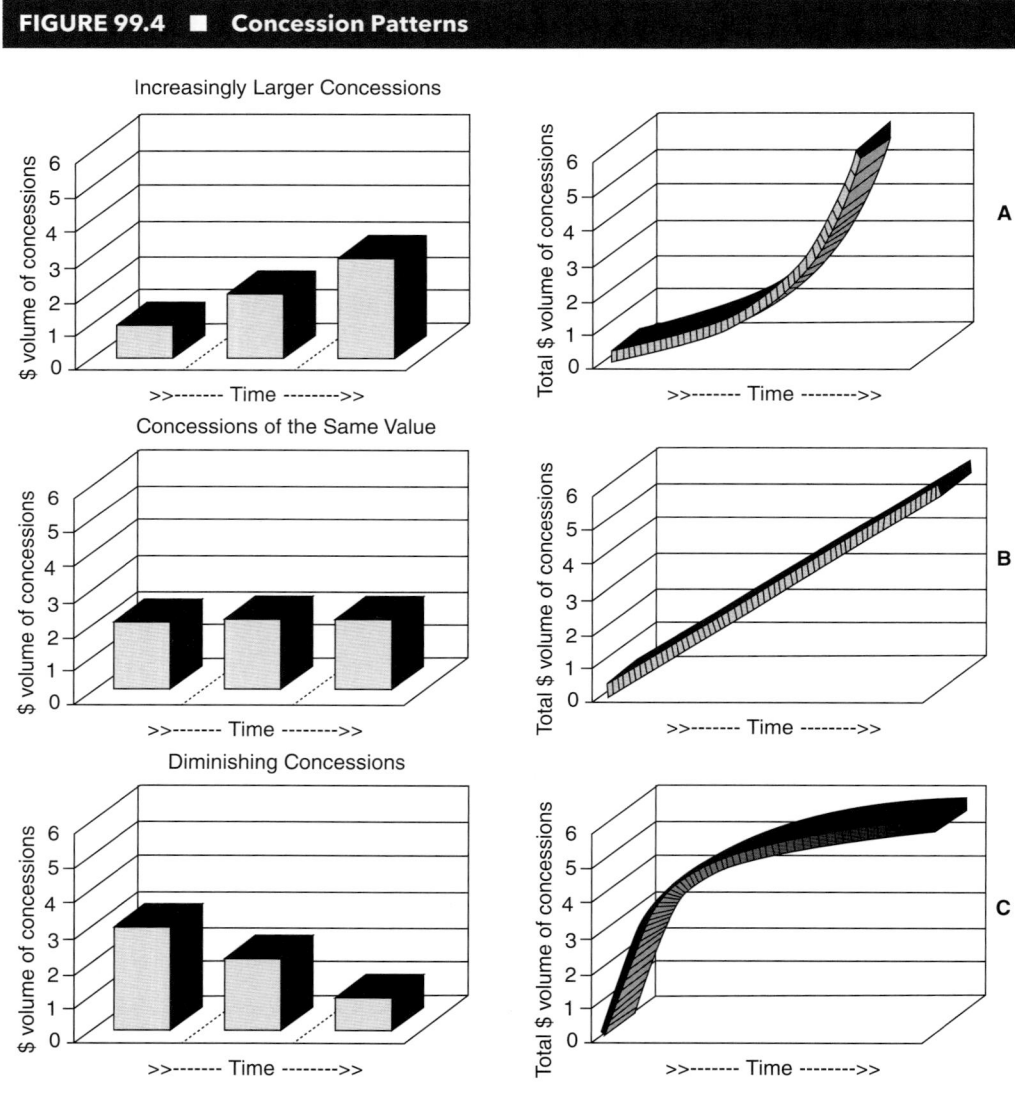

FIGURE 99.4 ■ Concession Patterns

(A) The negotiator gives increasingly larger concessions, perhaps to convince the other side to close the deal. However, this pattern may have the opposite effect. The unspoken message is that by holding out, the other side can get increasingly larger concessions. (B) Each of the concessions is similar in size. There is no message to suggest a limit to these concessions. The total value of the concessions is continuing to increase. (C) This pattern sends a different message. Each successive increment is smaller, suggesting to the other side that the end point is near. Thus, the total value of the concession is approaching a limit.

Karrass on Concession Behavior

In the Karrass experiment, early large concessions (sizable decline in demands) by the plaintiff's side led to the lowest settlements.[17] Early large concessions by the defendant pharmaceutical company (sizable increases in the offer) led to the highest settlements. Karrass found that:

- Losers tended to make the first and the largest concessions.
- Winners tended to make the smallest concessions. Those obstinately making small concessions occasionally deadlocked, but if they didn't deadlock, they won.

Winners also made smaller concessions as the deadline approached. Deadlines create increasing pressure for both sides. Most deals are made as the deadline nears, not before. The winners made smaller concessions at this point than the losers and therefore made better deals.

The Diminishing Value of Concessions

The value of services always decreases rapidly after those services have been performed. Once a concession or favor has been given, its future value decreases. The concept "they will really owe me a lot for this concession" has no place in negotiation.

This concept could also be referred to as the "Hungry Man Principle."[28] The wealthy man dying of hunger and thirst in the desert may say he'll give everything he has for water, food, and safety. Once these are provided and he is in the safety of his mansion, there is little likelihood he will live up to his promise and turn everything over to his rescuer. Because the value of the services (concessions) diminishes rapidly after they are provided, it is wise to ask for something in return immediately when asked for a concession. The following scenario illustrates this point:

Quite frankly I'm not sure we can concede on this point. I'll have to ask the group (higher authority). But if we gave you "X" instead, what can I tell them you will do for us?

In this way, the value of the concession is elevated. Conversely, things given away for nothing, even unimportant items or services, may set up a process of grinding away or "nibbling." Some negotiators will continue to ask for more until the other finally says, "Enough!"

If the other side recognizes that every time it requests something additional it has to give up something in return, it will be less likely to continue to ask. The value of a concession is increased by insisting on reciprocal concession, as illustrated by the following examples:

- The staff members agree to rotate on more weekend and night shifts, if leadership agrees to pay more for those hours and publish the schedule earlier.
- The physicians agree to lower a guaranteed stipend if the administrator will provide an acceptable incentive plan.
- The group accepts a restrictive covenant prohibiting them from approaching area hospitals if the hospital will accept a long-term contract.

The "Too-Easy" Win

It is possible to be less satisfied with a better deal and more satisfied with a worse deal (**Box 99.8**). This paradox can occur when a settlement is reached too easily. People often think, "If I got what I wanted so easily, I probably could have gotten even more."

For example, a house is placed on the market for $325,000. On the first day, a buyer says, "I'll take it for the full asking price." This is good because the seller got the full asking price. This is bad because the seller may believe the house was undervalued. Alternatively, if

> **BOX 99.8 ■ RESULTS OF THE "TOO-EASY WIN"**
>
> **Settlements made too easily may leave one party thinking:**
>
> - I could have done better.
> - There must be something wrong with this situation.
> - I do not trust them.

several offers were made between $250,000 and $295,000 over the course of 1 month, and then a buyer offers $315,000, the seller may feel very satisfied with an offer less than the original asking price.

When a negotiated purchase is made too easily, the purchaser may think, "I could have done better" and "I wonder if there's something wrong." For example, a person considers purchasing a used car advertised for $19,000. After inspection, the purchaser offers the low-ball price of $9,000 and it is accepted without hesitation. The purchaser may immediately think, "There must be something wrong with the car. I don't trust the seller. I could have gotten a better deal!" Alternatively, if the seller haggles for an hour and eventually sells the car for $12,000, the buyer is more likely to believe a good deal was struck. The "too-easy" win occurs when services or commodities that are typically negotiated are purchased without any struggle.

Principled Negotiations

In *Getting to Yes*, Fisher and Ury describe the concept of "principled negotiation"—the philosophy of focusing on interests rather than positions.[11] This approach advocates that parties avoid positional bargaining and instead focus on their own and the other party's interests.

Positional Bargaining

Positional bargaining focuses on narrowly defined outcomes. Solutions are more limited and less creative. In "hard" positional bargaining, more resistance to the position results in a greater commitment to the position. With further resistance, relationships may deteriorate. Hard positional bargainers typically see the other side as adversaries that must be overcome. The goal is winning; bonding and alliance are unimportant. The hard bargainer's demeanor may be distrustful, threatening, and insistent. The hard bargainer would like the other party to avoid conflict and simply acquiesce.

The "soft" bargainer would like to maintain the relationship and cares less about the outcome. The soft bargainer's demeanor may be trusting, yielding, self-deprecating, and solicitous. This accommodating approach steers clear of the confrontation and disagreement and instead focuses on maintaining the relationship. Accommodation accomplishes one goal—an agreement without confrontation—but often at great cost.

Principled Bargaining

Negotiations based on interests rather than positions generally produce wiser and more nuanced outcomes. This type of bargaining focuses the discussion on problem-solving based on objective standards. Adhered to, interest-based bargaining avoids getting bogged down in personalities, positions, and narrowly defined solutions and instead seeks options to meet the needs of both sides. The interests of both parties become the focus, and the goal is a judicious outcome achieved in a cordial environment. Consider the following example:

A physician, eager to join a group, is negotiating for an open position. The physician expresses determination to get a certain amount of money and is inflexible. The group would like to hire the physician but cannot afford the requested amount in the present reimbursement environment.

Positional bargaining will lead to frustrating concessions by one or both sides, or to deadlock. Alternatively, an open-minded focus on the interests of the parties might reveal their underlying issues. For the physician who might need a certain amount of money, the group might offer partnership, help secure a loan, or find additional sources of income such as an administrative stipend from the hospital. For the group, the physician might work additional shifts, work higher-paying night/weekend shifts, forego unneeded benefits, or provide administrative support that will save the group money.

Interests *Before* Positions

Occasionally, there is only one solution to a problem, forcing one side to adopt a hard position. When a position is essential, it is often helpful to describe the underlying issue before stating the position. By putting interests before the conclusion, the other side has an opportunity to listen and understand the reasoning.[11] The following examples demonstrate the difference between the two approaches.

- *Position before interest*: Leader A says to Leader B, "We're going to have to find a way to pay our practitioners more money because we are unable to recruit." Leader B may focus on and reject the stated position (the request for more money), overlooking the interest, which is recruiting quality practitioners in a competitive market.
- *Interest before position*: Leader A to Leader B, "Alice just turned in her resignation. She got a great opportunity at a nearby hospital and she will be leaving in 2 months. It's unfortunate because she's an excellent practitioner who is respected by the medical and nursing staff. Some of the medical staff and out-of-hospital care personnel specifically send their patients here because of her abilities. I'm sure you remember that the utilization program she developed has been the critical factor in our success with the managed care contracts. We've tried to recruit a replacement, but it's difficult to attract quality practitioners like Alice. In fact, other members of the group are considering following her lead. To keep our current staff intact, we must be able to attract a replacement for Alice. To do this, we're going to have to find a way to pay our staff more so we can be competitive with nearby facilities."

Identifying the issue/interest first and providing the other side an opportunity to understand the common interests forms the foundation for collaborative problem-solving. When the other side finally hears the position, "paying more," they are more likely to participate in the solution.

Other Techniques

The Theory of "Yes"

The theory of "yes" simply entails acknowledging the other's point of view, not necessarily agreeing with it. This is a critical distinction. Repeating the other's perspective, goals, and aspirations affirms an understanding of the other's point of view without giving in to it. Examples include:

- "Yes, I can see that that is important to you. Let's discuss it further."
- "Sure, I can understand based on your situation why you would ask for that. Let's review the ramifications."
- "I get it; so you're saying . . . Is that correct? I'd like you to elaborate on this portion of it."

Saying yes and incorporating the other side's idea into a response acknowledges its point of view and validates and demonstrates appreciation of its concern. Starting with a form of "yes" opens the door to consideration of options and encourages forward movement. Alternatively, when negotiators respond to a proposal by shaking their head or saying "no," they are implying that the proposal has no merit. "No" is often interpreted as a lack of concern or understanding that shuts down the discussion and forces the other side to become more positional.

While it is not necessary to accept a proposal, it is helpful to accept the other's perspective and the validate the underlying issue. When their perspective is acknowledged, the other side becomes more receptive.

Feel, Felt, Found

The "feel-felt-found" technique is another way to acknowledge the other's view, even when personal experience would suggest the other is wrong.[2] Affirming by using the feel-felt-found technique incorporates the other's concerns as if they are one's own, decreases positional approaches, and moves the discussion forward. In the following example, the concept of direct patient billing is rejected.

Statement: "I'm very concerned that billing the patients directly as your fee-for-service proposal suggests would create a stir in this community. Patients would think we're too expensive."

F-F-F Response: "I understand how you feel. When we started separate billing at XYZ Hospital, our patients initially felt the same way. We directly bill the third parties whenever possible. Because of the increased reimbursement, we've brought in top-notch doctors, the quality of service has improved dramatically, and patient satisfaction is in the 97th percentile. As a result, we have found that the concern has not been realized."

OVERCOMING OBSTACLES

Negotiating does not come easily to many and is difficult for everyone at times. In the nursing profession, unionization has been an increasingly common means of deferring the burdens of negotiation to parties who are more comfortable and skilled in the activity.

Difficulties in negotiation can appear in many forms. Some negotiators adopt an "all or none" attitude. Some become emotional and blaming. Still others resort to ploys to accomplish their end. To effectively negotiate, one must recognize when the negotiations are sidetracked and initiate methods to realign the interests of the parties (**Table 99.3**).

TABLE 99.3 ■ Effective Responses to an Unreasonable Request for Clinician Coverage

Restating their position	"So, you would like to have double physician coverage 24 hours a day for our 12,000-visit ED."
Acknowledging and validating their position	"Yes, and I know that your proposal is driven by a desire to eliminate waiting times and provide excellent customer service to our patients."
Emphasizing your expertise	"It is our experience that the number of providers is not the constraining factor for waiting times and patient experience."
Opening up the discussion	"Let's consider some of the other ramifications of the proposed provider staffing as well as additional solutions."

Breaking Deadlocks

Deadlocks cause great stress, test resolve, and reduce aspirations, all while jeopardizing the potential for a successful outcome. Sometimes during a negotiation, there seems no way back to meaningful dialogue. Good negotiators figure out a way to walk back "in the door" without losing face and help the other side to do the same thing. Deadlock breakers work because they refocus the parties on meaningful discussion.[2,30] The following approaches are potentially successful methods of breaking deadlocks:

- *The set aside*: The "set aside" is the postponement of difficult issues until a later time when mutual trust has developed and earlier successes have been achieved. When a difficult issue that is likely to become an impasse arises early in the negotiation, it can be set aside by saying, "I understand how you feel about this issue. I would like to think about it. Let's set it aside and talk about some of the other issues first." Later, when both sides have invested more time and consideration, it is likely both parties will be more willing to compromise to achieve agreement. Reordering the agenda allows the group to regain forward momentum by dealing with different, less contentious issues.
- *Take a break*: Taking a break allows either or both parties to momentarily let go of the intense focus that may be required during a negotiation. Its intent is to allow everyone to "cool down."
- *Caucus*: Caucus is like taking a break but has the specific purpose of allowing members of a team to privately confer. Away from the bargaining table, a person is free to reexamine each side's interests. It is an excellent way to decompress a situation.
- *Ask for help*: This approach entails simply stating the problem that's causing the impasse and then asking for help getting beyond it. A form of the question, "What would you do in my position?" may be very effective. Asking for advice flatters the other party while encouraging it to see your side of the issue. Ideally, the other party will look at methods to solve the problem.
- *Modify the team*: Adding a new participant may create an opportunity to bring greater objectivity to the negotiations. A new "objective" participant will be less encumbered by preconceptions and emotional attachment to the previous positions. However, this approach does add risk if the third party is not familiar with or sympathetic to your point of view.

Deadlock breakers are effective because they allow both parties to begin to move forward together. Once both parties begin to negotiate after a significant deadlock, there is great relief and significant potential for bilateral concessions.

Negotiating Ploys

The term *ploy* has negative connotations, as ploys are frequently used to gain advantage or "win" at the expense of the other party. A "win-lose" may result in short-term gains but undermine the long-term relationship. In most instances, it is best to avoid using negotiating ploys and techniques. Unless one is very adept, others will recognize them and be put off by their use. Experienced negotiators may turn a ploy against its user. It is necessary to be aware of these techniques in order to recognize them when they are being used and avoid falling prey to them.

Bait and Switch

The bait-and-switch technique is common in everyday life. The underlying concept is to lure the prey (potential buyer) with the bait (an attractive offer or a deal that is too good to be true). Once the prey has been enticed to buy and is psychologically committed to the offer, the switch is made. A less attractive or somehow diminished model is substituted, and the buyer makes a less advantageous deal.

> *Everyday example*: An advanced digital camera is advertised for a very low price. The buyer has wanted this particular model, and this is the best deal yet. Excitedly, the buyer arrives eager to purchase the camera, only to find that the store has "run out of the sale model." The buyer is told that for a few dollars more a deluxe brand is available. The technique is often successful. The buyer is there, committed to a product, and ready to buy.

> *Contract example*: A physician reaches an oral agreement and commits to joining a group with the understanding that she will achieve partnership within 2 years. The conditions of partnership are never explicitly discussed. She gives notice to her current employer and prepares to move to the new location to join the new group. The written contract arrives and does not mention partnership.

Bait-and-switch solutions include:

- *Take assiduous notes*: Diligently record information when discussing the various aspects of the deal. Sending a copy of the notes to the other side for review will codify the verbal understanding. It is possible that the notes may be the only record of the discussion.
- *Get it in writing*: The best method of preventing a bait and switch is to document the agreement in writing, with explicit details covering all aspects of the understanding.
- *Create penalty and termination clauses*: A bait and switch may be prevented by incorporating a penalty clause or addressed by invoking a termination of the agreement based on noncompliance or nondelivery.

Good Guy–Bad Guy

The tough and irate "bad guy" is aggressive and demanding, perhaps even threatening. The pleasant, soft-spoken "good guy" intervenes and offers to protect you, the "innocent" negotiator, from the bad guy. Even if the good guy is not making a great offer, it is much easier to deal with the nice guy rather than to have to deal with the jerk again. This is a classic setup to gain key concessions.

> *Everyday example*: The surly cop begins to rough up the suspect. The gentle, brotherly good cop rescues the suspect, temporarily stopping the bad cop. The good cop does not know how long he can hold off the bad cop and suggests that the suspect cooperate before the other guy loses control completely.

> *Everyday example*: In the family setting, a stay-at-home parent says, "If you continue to behave like that, I'm going to have to tell your father (mother) when he (she) gets home." The parent is playing the good guy, implying "do it my way and it will be easy for you." The other parent is cast as the bad guy to modify the child's behavior.

> *Contract example*: Two physicians representing a group are negotiating a contract with a hospital administrator who is desperate to get ED coverage. One member of the physician team gets angry over the compensation package and storms out of the room. As the other physician picks up his papers to leave, he says, "Gee, I am really sorry this happened. We were so close to a deal. This is a sensitive issue for him. If there was something you could give, maybe I could get him back."

Good guy–bad guy solutions include:

- *Recognize it*: The good guy and bad guy are on the same team. They are partners with the same goal—to get the best deal. Avoid being drawn in by it.

- *Avoid responding by trying to appease*: Placating is responding to a bully. The other side will win and will continue to use this technique until it does not work anymore.
- *Refer to the interest, not the position*: If the bad guy tries to maneuver the negotiation into positional bargaining, that is, "my way or we are done," refocus the discussion on the underlying interest.
- *Identify the ploy and create embarrassment*: "Hey, you guys aren't going to use the old good guy-bad guy technique on me, are you?" Once caught, they will probably smile, deny it, and get back to the discussion in a more fruitful manner.

Splitting Behavior–The End Run

The underlying principle of splitting behavior is playing team members against each other and reducing their aspirations. This technique can create conflict within a group and lead to concessions by individual members of the group. The end run is similar in that it attempts to split the other side by going around the negotiator(s) and appealing to another decision-maker. There are legitimate reasons for the end run, including trying to break a deadlock, bringing a more collaborative person into the discussion, and involving the decision-maker. There are also deceptive and improper reasons for using the end run and splitting behavior, including creating conflict to gain an advantage. To successfully counter this technique, it is necessary to first recognize it.

Everyday examples: A couple purchasing a car exposes areas of disagreement. The salesman recognizes this conflict and plays one against the other to enhance his profits. Another common example is a child asking the second parent's permission to do something to which the first parent has said no.

Contract example: A physician is empowered by the group to negotiate for it. The other side goes directly to the group and states it is impossible to deal with that physician and the group is at risk of losing the opportunity. If the ploy is unrecognized, the physician and the group are put at a significant disadvantage. In a unionized nursing environment, laws protect the represented parties from tactics of addressing the nursing body directly by circumventing the negotiating entity.

Splitting behavior solutions include:

- *Determine your negotiating approach prior to the negotiation*: Revealing internal disagreements in front of the other side will demonstrate significant weaknesses in position and resolve. Define areas of concession privately in advance of negotiation meetings.
- *Do not get sucked in*: Those not part of the primary negotiating team should not make decisions apart from the selected negotiator(s) and should reaffirm the group's decision-making process.
- *Modify the group*: Agree to send an additional person, not a replacement. By offering to expand the group, the alleged concern is addressed without undercutting the team.

Silence

Difficult moments in a negotiation can often be successfully managed with silence. As tension mounts and deadlines approach, most people will have a strong desire to act. It may be beneficial to resist the temptation to speak and allow the other side to fill the void. The person who speaks less listens more. Further, the discomfort caused by one person's silence may cause the other side to reconsider a hard position and begin to concede.

Contract example: A physician negotiates on behalf of the group. After presenting multiple ways in which the group can provide quality care in a financially responsible way, the other person is silent and appears disapproving. The physician, having assumed responsibility for the group, becomes increasingly fearful that he has angered the other party and that the group will suffer significantly as a result. The ploy of silence causes the physician to make early concessions.

Silence solutions include:

- ***Wait comfortably***: Take a couple of slow deep breaths, relax, and wait for the other person to speak again.
- ***Distract with humor***: If the other side is intent on winning the battle of silence, allow the victory by speaking first in a way that will not include concessions. Talk about an unrelated incident in the ED or a recent event. The key is to make it light and engaging so that the other person will feel good about reentering the discussion.
- ***Give time to think***: If the other negotiator is unwilling to make a comment or a counterproposal, simply acknowledge that they may need time to consider the proposal and even discuss it with others. Offer to set a time for a follow-up meeting with the goal of settling this item.

The Ultimatum

The risk of nonagreement is present in every negotiation. The risk becomes reality if the sides cannot find a mutually acceptable solution. Some negotiators will threaten nonagreement as a ploy to accomplish their objectives.

The key to effective threats is believability. They are meant to lower the opposition's aspirations. The normal response is to become defensive and anxious. Ultimatums should be avoided because they always build resentment. Threats are the classic game of chicken: *Who will blink first?* While not recommended, ultimatums should only be used when nonagreement (walk-away as a BATNA) is a real option. Even then, it should be done in a way that allows the other side to acquiesce without loss of face.

Brinkmanship is an extreme example of threats and ultimatums. This tactic is considered the ultimate game of chicken in which one or both sides threaten extreme measures unless its demands are met. The threats can be in the form of verbal attacks or veiled in the righteous air of trying to save the deal. The Cuban Missile Crisis, which threatened nuclear war, was a successful example. The Peloponnesian War was an unsuccessful example, leading to the eventual fall of Athens. More recently, US President Donald Trump threatened North Korea by saying:[31]

[Further threats] will be met with fire and fury like the world has never seen.

Ultimatum/threat solutions include:

- ***Take a deep breath and maintain control***: The normal response is to get upset and feel the need to either acquiesce or get up and walk out. Instead of being thrown off balance, take a deep breath, acknowledge that the issue is important to both sides, and ask the other side to elaborate its interest.
- ***Use the power of silence***: Let the room fill with silence. Angry, threatening individuals depend on a defensive reaction from the other side. Silence may lead to discomfort.
- ***Focus on the interest, not the position***: The threat is a position. Identify the mutual interests and work toward resolution.

The Nibble

The definition of the "nibble" is to chew off a little more after the deal is completed.[32] This technique is successful because once agreement is achieved, both sides become psychologically committed to the deal, lose their walk-away power, and let their guard down. Once a deal is done, there is a tendency to give even more to "sweeten the relationship." Therefore, if someone asks for a little more after a deal has been struck, he or she usually receives it. Recognizing this phenomenon, the other side can add more and more, slowly changing the deal. The nibble may be preceded by words such as, "Of course you are including . . .," or "And by the way . . .," or "Oh yes, there is just one more minor detail . . ."

> *Everyday example*: The seller concludes a deal to sell his house and shake hands. The buyer says, "Of course, you are leaving the refrigerator." The seller agrees and then the buyer adds, "Just one more minor detail—we assume you will replace the old fence." This nibbling process could continue until the seller stops it. Each time one acquiesces to an additional request, the behavior is reinforced.

> *Contract example*: The ED group has recruited a new practitioner. After coming to agreement, the new staff member says, "Oh, by the way, to whom should I give the bill for my moving expenses?" Or, "Of course you will be paying for my license and dues, won't you?" This ploy works because the group has made a psychological commitment. To say no might undo the deal.

Nibble solutions include:

- *Recognize the ploy*: The most important step in protecting against the nibble is to recognize it. Congratulate the other side on the deal it has already negotiated and point out the nibble. "You negotiated a fantastic deal. You're not going to nickel and dime me now, are you?"
- *Just say no*: Some people will continue to nibble until you say enough. "We've made a deal. If you would like to discuss additional items, I would be willing to reopen the negotiations."
- *"Tit-for-tat"*: Ask for a reciprocal concession. If they ask for more, so should you, "Sure I'd be willing to . . ., if you'll . . ."

The Flinch

The "flinch" is a physical reaction demonstrating strong rejection of a proposal. It is powerful ploy designed to create embarrassment and concession. The flinch may be manifested verbally and/or nonverbally and may include a wince, moan, exaggerated gesticulation, or exclamation. The more dramatic the flinch, the more effective it becomes. Upon hearing the offer, the flinching party may respond immediately with a look of astonishment and disbelief while simultaneously uttering, "You want *what*?"

The flinch is a particularly effective ploy when used on someone who would never purposely use the flinch, and it may be a prelude to a very poor offer.

> *Everyday example*: In an antique shop, a buyer decides to bid on a desired object and offers a reasonable price, at which point the dealer drops his jaw, throws his hands in the air, and claims, "That's ridiculous!"

> *Contract example*: A physician group is presenting a proposal to staff an ED. Upon stating the support requirements, the other party suddenly stands up, with arms thrown in the air and a stunned expression, and yells, "You've got to be kidding! There is no way we can do this deal." The representative of the group immediately develops a sinking feeling in his stomach as aspirations plummet. The immediate reaction is to try to figure out how to change the deal to make it more appealing.

The flinch solutions include:

- *Recognize the ploy*: Avoid appeasing the "apparently" upset person.
- *Calmly reassert the value proposal*: Be prepared to restate calmly and clearly the value of the product or service. "Perhaps I didn't fully clarify the financial reward you and your institution will achieve by contracting with us."
- *Ask for a reciprocal concession*: If giving something to the flinching person, ask for something of equal value.

Puppy Dog Technique

The "puppy dog" technique is a trial offer of a desired object. "Why don't you take the puppy home over the weekend and show it to the kids? If they don't like it, you can bring it back next week." Once the puppy dog is home, the kids will naturally fall in love with it and the deal is closed. This ploy is the same as the 30-day trial period; it is rare for the purchaser to return something within the trial period.

Everyday example: The trial offer is frequently used in television infomercials. A company promotes guaranteed exercise equipment and promises a full refund of the money minus (expensive) shipping costs if the purchaser is dissatisfied. Once purchased, the equipment may be used a great deal initially. Even if not used, most people will rationalize that they will start using it soon.

Contract example: As a recruitment tactic, a nurse is invited to perform a shadow shift on a low-volume day with a highly talented, particularly likable and entertaining charge nurse. Afterward, they and others have a wonderful dinner. The person being recruited leaves with a particularly, perhaps unrealistically, favorable opinion.

Puppy dog technique solutions include:

- *Develop criteria for acceptance*: Determine what will make the deal acceptable and unacceptable before accepting any trial. It is easy to rationalize what may ultimately be a bad situation once in the middle of it. Those who are more deliberate are less likely to fall prey to this technique.
- *Predetermine walk-away criteria*: Before the trial period begins, determine exactly how to evaluate it and in what situation you'll say "no."

Funny Money

"Funny money" is a term used to describe changing the cost basis to an insignificant quantity or increment. By concealing the value, the funny money ploy attempts to create the perception that a desired object is less expensive than it is.

Everyday example: To hide the true cost of a product, an advertiser may convert the payment to a daily cost. "For only $1.78 a day, you can enjoy . . ." The annualized payment of $650 may be more than the purchaser can afford.

Everyday example: When purchasing a house, the realtor might say, "It will only cost you five dollars more a day. Are you going to let five dollars keep you from living here?" It is considerably more than five dollars. On a 30-year mortgage, five dollars a day will cost the buyer $54,750 in increased principal plus approximately $51,058 in interest (at 5%), or a total cost of $105,808 to the buyer.

Contract example: The hospital foundation comes to the physician group and says, "You have been very successful here. We would like your group to donate only one dollar an hour for the period of time that you've held the contract." While a dollar an hour seems small, if a "single coverage" group has been present for 10 years, the cost would be $87,600.

Funny money solutions include:

- ***Determine the true cost***: Before saying yes, calculate the true total cost by translating it into real money—not pennies per hour, but dollars per year.
- ***Correct the time frame***: Use the total time frame for which payment will be made.

CONCLUSION

This chapter has provided basic negotiation theory and a few practical applications. The skill to negotiate is the result of observation, practice, and study. The success of negotiation should not be measured by short-term gain at the expense of the other side. Rather, it should be measured by the development of a long-term and mutually beneficial relationship that is built on trust and the desire to achieve common goals. In a successful negotiation, both parties feel they have achieved their goals and want to do business with each other in the future.

Special thanks and note of appreciation to John (Jack) G. Keene, MD, FACEP, for cowriting a previous version of this chapter.

REFERENCES

1. Haden-Elgin S. *The Gentle Art of Verbal Self Defense* (Revised and Updated). New York, NY: Fall River Press Edition; 2009.
2. Dawson R. *The Secrets of Power Negotiating: Inside Secrets from a Master Negotiator*. Pompton Plains, NJ: Career Press; 2011.
3. Babcock L, Laschever S. *Women Don't Ask: The High Cost of Avoiding Negotiation – And Positive Strategies for Change*. New York, NY: Bantam Books; 2007.
4. Babcock L, Dunbrooke S. *Women Don't Ask: Negotiation and the Gender Divide (Audible Audiobook)*. Newark, NJ: Audible Studios; 2012.
5. Bowles HR. *Why Women Don't Negotiate Their Job Offers*. Brighton, Mass: Harvard Business; Review June 19, 2014. https://hbr.org/2014/06/why-women-dont-negotiate-their-job-offers. Accessed July 5, 2018.
6. Nierenberg GI. *The Art of Negotiating*. New York, NY: Cornerstone Library Publications; 1968.
7. Thomas-Kilmann Conflict Mode Instrument – CPP, Inc. Available at: https://www.cpp.com/en-US/Products-and-Services/TKI. Accessed July 10, 2018.
8. Strauss RW. Negotiation skills. *Am Coll Emerg Phys*. Emergency Department Directors Academy. 2004-2019.
9. Wertheim E. Negotiation and resolving conflicts: an overview. College of Business Administration, Northeastern University. Available at: https://www.europarc.org/communication-skills/pdf/Negotiation%20Skills.pdf. Accessed July 22, 2018.
10. Mnookin TH, Peppet SR, Tulumell AS. *Beyond Winning: Negotiating to Create Value in Deals and Disputes*. Cambridge, Mass: Belknap Press of Harvard University Press; 2004.
11. Fisher R, Ury W. *Getting to Yes*. New York, NY: Penguin Books; 2006.
12. Exercise, yoga, and meditation for stress management. In: Dasgupta A. *The Science of Stress Management: A Guide to Best Practices for Better Well-Being*. London, United Kingdom: Rowman and Littlefield; 2018.
13. Johnson S. *Rasselas, Prince of Abyssinia*. London, United Kingdom: Cassell and Company; 1889. Chapter 37. Available at: http://www.gutenberg.org/files/652/652-h/652-h.htm. Accessed June 30, 2018.
14. Active Listening: a negotiators best tool. 2010. Available at: https://www.karrass.com/blog/active-listening-a-negotiators-best-tool/. Accessed June 23, 2018.
15. When negotiating—information is power. 2010. Available at: https://www.karrass.com/en/blog/when-negotiating-information-is-power/. Accessed June 25, 2018.
16. Siegel S, Fouraker LE. *Bargaining and Group Decision Making*. New York, NY: McGraw-Hill; 1960.
17. Karrass C. *The Negotiating Game*. New York, NY: Harper Collins; 1994.
18. Strauss RW, Keene JG. Negotiation skills. In: Salluzzo R, Strauss RW, Mayer T, et al, eds. *Emergency Department Management: Principles and Applications*. Philadelphia, Pa: Mosby; 1997.
19. Shakespeare W. *The Tempest (Folger Shakespeare Library)*. New York, NY: Simon and Schuster; 2015.
20. Radzevick JR, Moore DA. Competing to be certain (but wrong): social pressure and overprecision in judgment. Carnegie Mellon University. 2009. Available at: http://www.gsb.stanford.edu/facseminars/events/marketing/documents/ob_01_09_moore.pdf. Accessed May 11, 2011.
21. Kuntsler JH. The psychology of previous investment, raise the hammer. 2005. Available at: http://www.raisethehammer.org/article/181. Accessed June 3, 2018.
22. St. John B, Haines AP. *Micro-Resilience: Minor Shifts for Major Boosts in Focus, Drive, and Energy*. New York, NY: Center Street; 2017.
23. Karrass C. *Business as in Life-You Don't Get What You Deserve, You Get What You Negotiate*. Beverly Hills, Calif: Stanford Street Press; 2013.
24. Shell GR. Step 3: Opening and making concessions. In: *Bargaining for Advantage: Negotiating Strategies for Reasonable People*. New York, NY: Penguin Books; 2006.
25. Hovland CI. *The Order of Presentation in Persuasion*. New Haven, Conn: Yale University Press; 1957.
26. Cohen H. *You Can Negotiate Anything*. New York, NY: Bantam Book; 1982.
27. Rowny E. Negotiating with the Soviet Union: the diplomatic discussion? Available at: https://www.bu.edu/iscip/pubseries/PubSeries1rowny.pdf. Accessed, July 16, 2018.

28. Strauss RW. Negotiation skills. In: Strauss RW, Mayer TA, eds. *Strauss & Mayer's Emergency Department Management*. Philadelphia, Pa: McGraw-Hill; 2013.

29. Strauss RW. Conflict management. *Am Coll Emerg Phys*. Emergency Department Directors Academy. 2004-2019.

30. Malhotra D. *Negotiating the Impossible*. Oakland, Calif: Berrett-Koehler Publishers; 2016.

31. Foreman A. A brief history of brinkmanship. *Wall Street Journal*. August 23, 2017. Available at: https://www.wsj.com/articles/a-brief-history-of-brinkmanship-1503507520. Accessed July 22, 2018.

32. Karrass C. *Give and Take: The Complete Guide to Negotiating Strategies and Tactics*. New York, NY: Harper Collins; 1993.

CHAPTER 100

CONTRACTS WITH PHYSICIANS

Robert W. Strauss, Leslie S. Zun

Successful contracts do not achieve vague or indeterminate goals. They require both sides to define optimum realistic goals, seek an opportunity to meet those goals, and then negotiate an agreement that holds the parties accountable for accomplishing those goals.

Individual practitioners, physicians, and advanced practice providers (APPs) generally enter into contractual relationships with hospitals, multispecialty medical groups, and emergency physician groups.[1] There are many components to negotiating a successful contract. This chapter addresses the pertinent contractual issues between providers and hospital or groups, as listed in **Box 100.1**.

Note that sample language is used several times in this chapter. Its purpose is to familiarize the reader with the types of language that may be used to convey contractual intent. The sample language is not meant to be definitive, complete, or used in a contract by the reader. Before accepting any contract language, the reader should consult advisers with expertise in contract law in the state in which the contract is to be executed.

POSITION EVALUATION

Prior to entering a negotiation, practitioners should gain a thorough and realistic understanding of the position they are considering and compare that with their predetermined goals. (**Appendix 100.1** contains 21 questions that may be utilized by an employment seeker to consider the position being contemplated.) There are many opportunities to gain information well in advance of the contractual discussion.

BOX 100.1 ■ CONTRACTUAL ISSUES

- Evaluation of the position
- Contract necessity
- The negotiation process
- Role of legal counsel
- Letter of intent
- Key contract clauses
- Pearls and pitfalls

Emergency Department Observation

The considering practitioner can spend time in the emergency department (ED) reviewing the different shift operations to observe processes such as:

- Organization of care
- Use of the electronic health record
- Flow efficiency of information, clinicians, patients
- General approach to patients
- Interaction among staff
- Process of admission and discharge
- Relations with non-ED medical staff
- Support services (imaging and lab) operations
- Teaching activities
- Safety

Communication With Key Stakeholders

After obtaining advance permission, invaluable information can be discerned by speaking with the staff members, group members, and administrators who interact with the ED. Asking key questions will help to ascertain the level of respect and understanding for the ED and the plans for future growth and resources. See **Appendix 100.1** for questions regarding relationships with key stakeholders.

If possible, it may be quite valuable to speak with practitioners who have left the group to determine the reason for their departure.

Professional Growth Opportunities

Many graduating residents approach a new job with an attitude of "I just want to settle in, hone my skills, make a decent salary, and prepare for the board examination." This thinking is often short-lived; over time, many practitioners develop an increasing desire to do more. Growth opportunities may come in several forms such as increased responsibility, a leadership position, greater involvement in organized medicine, and partnership within the group. A thoughtful approach to a new job requires applicants to consider their intermediate and long-term goals in advance. Once an individual's professional growth goals are defined, "key question #7" becomes germane:

> *Will the people with whom I will be working understand where I want to go, and will working with them help me to get there?*

CONTRACT NECESSITY

There are several reasons to form a contractual relationship between physicians and the staffing group or hospital, yet there are some practitioners who work without a contract, citing the arguable advantage of enhanced flexibility. For instance, without a contract, a practitioner might sever the relationship with brief or no notice. Of course, the converse is true as well; a practitioner without a contract might not have the security that comes with well-defined terminations processes.

In most circumstances, a written and executed contract is recommended. The contract protects interests, clarifies responsibilities, details compensation, identifies restrictions, and defines termination processes. Further, the contract generally contains provisions to resolve disputes arising between the parties in case of disagreement or perceived breach (failure of performance). The written contract supersedes and generally replaces all discussions and preceding agreements. Another reason to clarify the intent of parties with a written contract is to satisfy inquiries by regulatory authorities or aggrieved parties that may request a copy of the contract in order to verify or establish the basis of the relationship between the parties.

Although the contract is intended to outline the "four walls" of the relationship, it will not address all eventualities that may arise during the life of the contract. A successful relationship based on mutual respect, understanding, and trust will provide a critical foundation when an issue not contained in the contract arises.

CONTRACT NEGOTIATION PROCESS

The negotiation process is a critical aspect of contracts.[3] The approach that each party takes in the negotiation will influence the success of the process. Some may contend that *everything* is negotiable. However, entering a negotiation with everything "on the table" creates an adversarial approach to all contract issues. It may be desirable to define the critical interests ("make or break" issues) and focus primarily on those. Effective planning will help define which compromises a practitioner can make while still maintaining the integrity of an acceptable deal.

Concluding the Negotiation

The decision makers should perform the negotiations. For the group or hospital, the decision maker may be the medical director, president, COO, legal counsel, and so on. It is problematic for a practitioner to negotiate with a person who will defer decision-making to a higher authority.

Positive Process

The negotiation process should use productive strategies and avoid adversarial approaches. Use techniques that deal with interests, not personalities or power positions.[4] Both parties should search for mutually beneficial solutions or options and agree on objective criteria and predetermined time frames. The parties should avoid tactics and ploys that, if discovered, will create resentment, including "take it or leave it," win-lose, bidding one deal against another, and secret deals.

The negotiation process may take weeks to months to complete (**Table 100.1**). Shorter processes occur when there is little to negotiate, that is, there is a single "set" contract with

TABLE 100.1 ■ Contract Relations Time Frame		
Activity	**Time**	**Total Time**
Initial interview	0	0
Second meeting	4 weeks	4 weeks
Letter of intent	1 weeks	5 weeks
Review issues	2 weeks	7 weeks
Legal counsel drafts document	2 weeks	9 weeks
Review document	2 weeks	11 weeks
Revise document	2 weeks	13 weeks
Sign document	1 weeks	14 weeks

little or no variation. Conversely, complex contracts with multiple components and variations generally take longer. However, contracting processes that require several months may never be concluded, as it is likely that if the parties do not agree to terms after this length of time, they will not agree at all.

The negotiation will get off to a better start if both parties are thoroughly prepared, which entails substantial planning. The parties should proceed in a systematic manner by determining goals in advance.

CONTRACT PREPARATION

Contract preparation requires expertise and multiple steps. It is important to take appropriate care up front to make goals and negotiations clear and attainable.

Legal Counsel

Legal counsel plays a critical and necessary role in contract preparation. Attorneys are expert in the interpretation, writing, and enforcement of contracts. Legal counsel generally performs the essential function of contract review and modification. The primary role of counsel is to ensure that the intent of both parties is reflected in the contractual language of the document. Practitioners should direct the attorney through clear communication of their interests and their relative importance. Without that clarity, a poorly directed attorney may aggressively seek to achieve the practitioner's interests at all costs, including the potential loss of the opportunity.

Some practitioners will use legal counsel to provide a broader range of services, including assisting in contract negotiations, creating a contract *de novo,* and even establishing a corporate entity for the practice. This expanded role can be costly.

Drafting the Contract

The parties must consider whose counsel will prepare the contract. Generally, the hospital or group may have a "boilerplate" contract that is provided for consideration. However, either party may elect to prepare the contract. Contract preparation usually involves substantial legal cost and time but provides the advantage of ensuring that the authoring party's perspective on the terms and conditions is written into the language of the contract. It is essential that the chosen counsel is experienced in the drafting of contracts related to the health-care profession in general and emergency medicine practitioners, in particular.

Obtaining Legal Counsel

Appropriate legal counsel should be secured to perform the aforementioned duties. It is important to find an expert in health-care contract law rather than a cheaper expert in real estate law. An attorney may be found by asking your associates or mentors or contacting the local bar association for a referral. Alternatively, the American College of Emergency Physicians or its state chapter may be a referral source for legal services.

Legal costs can vary depending on geographic location, size of the firm, and scope of work to be performed. The preparation and review process can take a few hours or hundreds of hours. It is both reasonable and wise to ask an attorney to estimate the cost of contract review and what will be provided for the fee. Money well spent early in the process may prevent contractual and monetary losses later.

Letters of Intent

During the contract-negotiation process, the involved parties may draft a letter of intent (LOI). Letters of intent describe the general terms of the agreement the parties intend to (but are not guaranteeing they will) execute. Such documents simply imply that both parties are sincere about moving the process forward and signing a formal contract. Letters of intent are usually short documents that delineate the basic underpinnings of the desired relationship and generally describe compensation, benefits, start dates, duties, and responsibilities. In addition, the LOI usually defines the time frame for contract completion.

Some institutions require a lengthy process and multiple reviews prior to a contract offer. Letters of intent also require careful review as they set the tone for the contract. If a formal contract is not completed by the time services begin, the LOI may serve as an enforceable document. Thus, it should contain sufficient detail so that the terms of the relationship can be understood. Most often, the formal contract will contain language that supersedes prior discussions and documents, including LOIs.

KEY CONTRACT CLAUSES

A list of key provisions typically found in contracts between physicians and hospitals/groups is provided in **Box 100.2**.[5-7] While a contract can never address every potential eventuality, it is meant to define the expectations and responsibilities of all parties. Therefore, the explicit details should be fully understood by all signatories.

Requirements

The requirements section of a contract describes the credentials the provider must possess in order to work for the group or hospital and may include a medical license, drug enforcement administration membership, board certification, special training, academic appointment or medical staff membership, and privileges.

Some groups or hospitals may require a physician to have and maintain specific board certification or acquire it by a specific date. Successful completion and maintenance of additional educational requirements may be necessary for institutions seeking specific categorizations (i.e., comprehensive, advanced, basic, limited), designations (i.e., stroke, trauma), or certifications (i.e., procedural sedation).[8-11]

BOX 100.2 ■ KEY CONTRACT CLAUSES

- Requirements
- Status/relationship of the parties
- Professional liability insurance
- Compensation and benefits
- Payment clause
- Physician duties and responsibilities
- Hospital duties and responsibilities
- Group duties and responsibilities
- Bylaws, policies, and procedures
- Indemnification and hold harmless
- Term
- Termination
- Breach
- Dispute resolution
- Restrictive covenants
- Miscellaneous issues

The American Board of Emergency Medicine (ABEM) addresses requirements for additional certifications in a policy statement:

> [F]or ABEM-certified physicians who are participating in MOC, ABEM strongly opposes the use of certificates of completion of courses such as APLS, ACLS, ATLS or other similar courses, or the completion of a specific number of CME hours in a specified content area of Emergency Medicine, as requirements for privileges, employment, or qualification by hospitals, city or state agencies, or any other credentialing organization to provide care for designated disease entities encompassed by the practice of Emergency Medicine.[12]
>
> ABEM Maintenance of Certification (MOC) requires adherence to state CME requirements as well as participation in Lifelong Learning and Self-Assessment Activities.

To be eligible for certain positions within an institution or department, the clinician may be required to have special training, such as a fellowship in research, emergency medical services (EMS), or administration. The providers generally must obtain and maintain medical staff membership and/or an academic appointment in order to comply with the contract.

Sample Language

"_____" (The physician/APP) represents and warrants that, to carry out duties and responsibilities hereunder, he/she shall:

A. Hold a currently valid and unlimited license to practice medicine in the State of . . .
B. Apply for, be awarded, and maintain in good standing membership on the staff with clinical privileges in emergency medicine or have received and maintained temporary privileges, all in accordance with hospital policies.
C. Be board certified or board prepared in emergency medicine or have completed . . .

Relationship of the Parties

The relationship of the parties may be that of independent contractor or employer/employee. Each arrangement has significant ramifications for both sides regarding compensation, benefits, responsibilities, internal revenue service (IRS) rules, and so on. These differences must be clearly understood when entering a contractual relationship.

Sample Language

Independent contractor: The independent contractor and its provider(s) shall perform all obligations imposed by this agreement. Nothing in this agreement shall be construed to create the relationship of employer and employee between hospital/group and the independent contractor. The independent contractor shall not be entitled to receive employee benefits. The hospital/group shall not have or exercise any control or direction over the manner, means, and methods by which the independent contractor shall perform work pursuant to this agreement. The independent contractor shall have the exclusive right and obligation to direct the manner, means, and methods used to provide service pursuant to this agreement. Independent contractors at all times:

A. Shall not have authority to bind the hospital/group in any manner
B. Shall not hold themselves out as officers, agents, or employee of hospital/group

There may be an additional relationship or status beyond that of employee or independent contractor, such as partner, stockholder, or profit sharer. This enhanced status may take the form of an optional buy-in period and amount after meeting

TABLE 100.2 ■ Typical Components of PLI Contract Language Clause	
Component	**Description**
Type of insurance	"Claims-made" or "occurrence"
Coverage limits	Amount per case, amount per year (typical $1M-$3M)
Coverage exclusions	Fraud, criminal acts, abusive behavior, etc.
Duties of parties	Notification of claim or summons and complaint
Consent authority	Party with right to determine settlement of a case
Premium payment responsibility	Payment by group, hospital, or individual
Tail payment responsibility	Payment by group, hospital, or individual

distinct criteria. It is imperative that if any additional relationship exists, the terms and conditions are unambiguous at the outset and clarified in the language of the contract. Some partnership agreements are expressed in vague terms, such as "After satisfactorily completing 2 years of employment, the physician may be offered shares in the partnership." The terms are so ambiguous that both sides may in good faith have differing interpretations of "satisfactorily," "may," and "shares," creating eventual disappointment, dissatisfaction, and hostility.

Professional Liability Insurance

Malpractice insurance is available in two forms: occurrence and claims-made. The contract may reflect the professional liability insurance (PLI) components as described in **Table 100.2**.

Sample Language

The physician shall maintain and keep in full force and effect throughout the term of this agreement PLI coverage in the minimum amounts of 1 million/3 million dollars ($1,000,000 per event/$3,000,000 aggregate) or other amount as may be specified by staff regulations or hospital requirements. The physician shall provide documentation of such insurance to the hospital/group.

Compensation and Benefits

Generally, the professional fees charged for care rendered by the practitioners are assigned to the group or hospital. This assignment allows the group or hospital to bill, collect, and pay all providers in a consistent manner.

Compensation and benefits depend on the relationship of the parties, that is, employee or independent contractor. Employees receive a salary and benefit package. An independent contractor receives hourly compensation inclusive of the cost of benefits. Theoretically, the independent contractor receives a higher hourly rate to compensate for the cost of benefits that are provided separately to the employee.

It is important to calculate the cash value of the benefits and other components when comparing an employee to an independent contractor relationship. Benefits specific to employee relationships may include insurances (liability, life, health, dental, vision, unemployment, and disability), paid time off (vacation, personal days), continuing medical education, license, dues and fees (professional membership, journals, hospital dues), and vesting in a pension plan or other retirement plans. Many employee contracts define required minimum hours of work.

The contract usually specifies the amount and timing of compensation increases, which may take the form of salary raise, bonus/incentive, or hourly rate increase. Ideally, increases are based on objective performance evaluations. The increase may also be tied to the financial performance of the group or department.

Profit sharing and incentives can be powerful motivating tools. Both employee and independent contractor relationships may be structured to incorporate bonuses, incentives, and profit sharing. The amount and timing of the disbursement should be clearly defined in the contract and based on objective and measurable criteria, such as productivity, quality, service, and administrative contributions to the ED. These incentives may be tied to an annual or biannual evaluation.

Payment Clause

The payment clause describes the timing and method by which the practitioner will be paid and should be unambiguous.

Sample Language

Compensation shall be payable to the practitioner monthly, in arrears, on or before the 14th day of the month following the month in which service is rendered by the practitioner.

Practitioner Duties and Responsibilities

Practitioner duties and responsibilities will vary according to the institution, its requirements, and the associated job description and may include:

- Clinical duties related to the ED, such as minimum or maximum number of hours per month, requirement to complete bridging orders to admit patients, on-call schedule for backup, timing of medical record completion, examination of employees, teaching of residents, students, or nurses, and so on
- Professional obligations, such as initially attaining and then continuously maintaining board certification, malpractice insurance, medical staff membership, Medicaid and Medicare participation
- Administrative duties related to the ED, such as committee participation, EMS involvement, performance improvement, management of complaints, commitment to research, and so on

Each of these responsibilities, which should be clearly delineated in a contract, may be tied to administrative stipends, bonuses, or an incentive system; alternatively, they may stand alone as a requirement for employment. In today's changing health-care environment, the duties and responsibilities may require regular review and updating.

Sample Language

When scheduled for service, the physician will provide emergency medical treatment to patients in the department, including:

A. Evaluating the medical needs of all patients presenting to the department for medical care
B. Generating and maintaining medical records in form and content consistent with policies and procedures of the hospital, established from time to time, for all patients treated in the department

C. Adhering to core measures
D. Responding to in-house emergencies, defined as respiratory or cardiac arrest, provided that (at the physician's sole discretion) the acuity of the patients in the ED allows the physician to attend to the in-house emergency without compromising the care of the patients currently in the ED (This clause is most commonly seen in hospitals with low-volume EDs and no availability of other 24 × 7 inpatient staff, such as hospitalists or residents.)

Hospital Duties and Responsibilities

The hospital has responsibilities to the ED providers for the provision of certain personnel, equipment, and services. The contract may specifically describe the type and number of personnel, including clerical, nursing staff, essential support services (lab, imaging), and administrative staff. Equipment, supplies, maintenance, fixtures, and utilities are generally the responsibility of the hospital. The contract may designate meeting and office space. The hospital also has the responsibility for insurance of the premises.

Sample Language

The hospital shall provide and maintain for the provider(s) suitable office space, equipment, supplies, and utilities as shall be necessary for the proper functioning of the ED.

The hospital shall, at its own expense, furnish usual and customary mail service, laundry service, gas, water, and electricity for light, power, and telephone, as may be required for the proper operation and conduct of the ED.

The hospital shall provide, at its own expense, staff (including technicians, clerks, registrars, nursing personnel, and other employees) as required for the efficient and proper operation of the department. All salaries, benefits, and other obligations attributable to such employees shall be paid by the hospital in accordance with its usual personnel policies.

Group Duties and Responsibilities

The group has certain responsibilities when contracting with individual physicians, including operating group scheduling, certain performance improvement processes, hospital contract fulfillment, and financial management of the group.

Bylaws, Policies, and Procedures

The contracting physician should be provided with all pertinent bylaws, policies, and procedures of the group and hospital before the contract is signed. Ideally, these documents should be incorporated by reference into the contract. There may be hospital, group, medical staff, and department policies and procedures. The providers will be held to these standards and should review and understand them.

Sample Language

Provider hereby agrees to follow established procedures to ensure the consistency, quality, and appropriateness of all emergency services. Further, provider agrees to abide by all standards as set forth by hospital policies and procedures, medical staff bylaws, The Joint Commission, the Centers for Medicare and Medicaid Services, Emergency Medical Treatment and Active Labor Act (EMTALA) guidelines, and so on.

Indemnification

Indemnification clauses create a contractual obligation to reimburse one party for financial losses caused by the acts of another party. An indemnification clause might obligate a physician to reimburse the hospital for its costs associated with defending a malpractice case that was eventually determined to be the fault of the physician only. Another example might include paying the hospital's EMTALA fine, if the physician was found to be primarily at fault. One must be careful when reviewing and signing an indemnification clause, as it is uncommon for a professional liability insurer to pay for associated losses.

The American College of Emergency Physicians strongly opposes indemnification clauses in medical contracts and specifically discourages physicians from seeking employment with institutions/groups that shift liability to the physician[13]:

> *Physicians should seek alternate employment when indemnification or any other contractual shift of liability is contained in a potential employment agreement. Medical industry standards are heavily against having indemnification clauses in physician contracts; contractual indemnification may void medical malpractice insurance coverage, and indemnification clauses provide an unacceptable potential for physicians to incur significant personal financial losses.*

When present in a contract, an indemnification clause should be mutual.

Sample Language

Physician (hospital) agrees to indemnify and hold the hospital (physician/group), its directors, agents, and employees harmless against any and all loss, damage, liability, and expense, including court costs directly resulting from or arising out of the dishonest, fraudulent, negligent, or criminal acts of the physician. This includes but is not limited to any act or error of omission, misconduct, EMTALA violations, malpractice judgments, hostile workplace infractions . . .

Term

Contracts may be for 1 year or several years and may contain an "evergreen clause," which allows automatic continual renewal unless one party gives notice or requests renegotiation within a predetermined time frame. Typically, the time frame for notification of renegotiation or termination occurs between 60 and 180 days prior to the end of the current contract. An evergreen clause may be advantageous for any party that does not want to undertake a regular and sometimes extended contract renegotiation. If terms require reconsideration, the discussions generally occur during this window.

Sample Language

Group (Hospital) hereby contracts with _____ (Provider). Unless terminated in accordance with Section (Termination Section), this agreement shall remain in full force and effect for a term of 3 years commencing on (date). Unless either party gives written notice of intent to not renew this agreement to the other party at least ninety (90) days prior to the termination date of this agreement, this agreement shall automatically be renewed for (number) year(s) on the terms and conditions set forth herein.

Termination

Many contracts contain a "no cause" termination clause that entitles the hospital or group to terminate the practitioner without cause within a certain time frame, usually

90 days. This clause is commonly reciprocal, allowing the practitioner to terminate the relationship with a 90-day notice. Since the inclusion of a "no-cause" termination clause may allow a party to arbitrarily terminate the relationship, the practitioner should assess how frequently and in what circumstances this clause has been invoked in the past.

All contracts should contain language that the contract can be terminated "for (reasonable) cause." For the hospital or group, the cause may be impairment, loss of license, professional misconduct, disability, and so on. For the practitioner, the cause may be breach of contract, nonpayment of monies, or change in the working conditions, and so on.

Sample Language

Either party may terminate this agreement, for any reason or for no reason whatsoever, upon 90 days written notice. Notwithstanding the foregoing, this agreement shall terminate as follows:

- **A.** If practitioner becomes disqualified to practice the specialty of emergency medicine in (state), hospital/group may terminate this agreement immediately upon notice to practitioner.
- **B.** If practitioner loses staff/clinical privileges at hospital, hospital/group may terminate this agreement immediately upon notice to practitioner.
- **C.** If practitioner fails to comply in any material respect with the terms of this agreement and such failure continues for 30 days after written notice thereof to practitioner, hospital/group may terminate this agreement immediately upon notice to practitioner.
- **D.** If hospital/group fails to comply in any material respect with the terms of this agreement and such failure continues for 30 days after written notice thereof to hospital/group, practitioner may terminate this agreement immediately upon notice to hospital/group.

Failure of Performance

In the termination sample language (C and D above), there is reference to failure of performance (breach) and an opportunity to address and correct the problem (cure). Breach in this example is material, or serious and significant. If departmental policy required physicians to dress neatly and conservatively with a white coat and a tie and a physician wore a "loud" tie, this would not be a material breach. On the other hand, a physician who refused to complete medical records within the time frame defined in policy or bylaws may be in material breach of the contract.

Note in the sample language that a 30-day "cure" period, or opportunity to resolve the material breach without immediate termination, is available. In certain circumstances, if the issue leading to notice of termination is addressed, this clause allows a continuation of what may be an otherwise mutually beneficial contractual relationship.

Dispute Resolution

A mechanism for dispute resolution should be established in the contract. Without a specific dispute resolution process, unresolved issues may involve the court system with its attendant consumption of time and resources. Resolution options include mediation, arbitration, grievance procedures, and specific dispute resolution policies. The mechanism should be contractually specified and include the process, cost, timing, and method of resolution.

Restrictive Covenants

Restrictive covenants are common in emergency physician contracts. The enforceability of these covenants varies greatly between, and even within, states. Certain jurisdictions allow only limited restrictive covenants. There are five basic types of restrictive covenants: tortious interference, outside practice, hiring restriction, noncompete, and confidentiality (**Table 100.3**).

Tortious Interference

Tortious interference is a legally actionable, intentional interference with a contractual relationship. For example, physicians under contract with a group may not interfere with that group's contract with the hospital to obtain the contract for themselves. Further, the physician who commits the tort (*tortfeasor*) may not disrupt the ability of the group to perform its contractual obligations. This restrictive covenant is common in business relationships and, while it may to some degree reduce marketplace competition, it has the effect of stabilizing a work situation. If tortious interference is proven, punitive damages may be awarded. The most typical examples are:

- A. *Interference with a contract*: An individual wrongfully comes between two parties in an existing contract
- B. *Interference with business*: An individual makes false claims against a party to disrupt the relationship

Outside Practice

Many contracts restrict a practitioner from working in a competing practice or hospital while under contract with the current hospital/group. The argument for this type of restriction is that a practitioner should not be permitted to participate in a practice directly competitive with the primary ED. An example might include working at a nearby competing urgent care center or practicing in both competing hospitals of a two-hospital town. The argument against an outside practice restriction is that patients do not seek out an individual emergency care provider and therefore this restriction is immaterial.

> *Sample language:* During the term of this agreement, Physician shall not practice emergency medicine within a "__" mile radius of hospital without written consent of hospital.

In an academic setting, this clause may attempt to prevent a member of the faculty from conflicts of commitment.[14] The restricted activities may include activities such as consulting, providing expert testimony, and moonlighting.

TABLE 100.3 ■ Types of Restrictive Covenants	
Restriction	**Intends to Prevent**
Tortious interference	Intentional interference with contractual relationship
Outside practice	Practice that competes with primary facility or obligations
Hiring restriction	One party from hiring a valuable employee of other party
Noncompete	Physician from providing certain services after contract termination
Confidentiality	Prevents practitioner from sharing proprietary information including intellectual property

Sample language: *The physician may not engage in teaching, consulting, or practice of his or her specialty outside the hospital.*

The Association of American Medical Colleges defines conflict of commitment as:

The term conflict of commitment relates to an individual faculty member's distribution of effort between obligations to one's academic appointment (normally "full-time" in teaching, research, and/or patient care) and one's commitment to "outside" activities. . . . A conflict of commitment arises when these [outside] or professionally removed activities (e.g., outside teaching or business) come to interfere with the paramount obligations to students, colleagues, and the primary missions of the academic institution by which one is appointed and salaried.[12]

Hiring Restrictions

Hiring restrictions prevent the hospital from hiring providers or employees of a current group during or after termination of the contract. From the point of view of the group and its members, including a hiring restriction may prevent a hospital from terminating the contract with the group and "cherry-picking" (keeping select) providers. The following example demonstrates the value of a hiring restriction for members of a group.

A hospital with the only ED in the region terminates the agreement. Several emergency physicians and their families have been recruited by the group to the location. Several practitioners who have committed to the area are approached by the hospital and offered a contract with less generous terms. The practitioners may now have to move to seek employment. The hospital might have been more circumspect about terminating the group if they could not selectively hire the clinicians after termination of the agreement between the hospital and the group.

Noncompete Clauses

Many contracts restrict terminated physicians from working at a hospital (or within a set distance from the hospital) for a set time period. In emergency medicine, as elsewhere, noncompete language is hotly debated. Noncompete clauses are unenforceable in certain states. When written in states that enforce noncompete clauses, the clause must:

- Impose reasonable restrictions that protect the legitimate interests of the employer
- Provide sufficient consideration to the employee

The arguments for noncompete language relate to the legitimate business interests of a hiring entity. The following examples demonstrate ways in which an appropriately crafted noncompete clause could restrict an entity from unscrupulous behavior.

- A competing hospital or group wishes to hire a well-known community practitioner who has made substantial inroads with EMS providers. A noncompete clause could prevent the practitioner from leaving his or her current position, which would confer a competitive advantage to the new institution or group.
- A hospital or group spends substantial human and capital resources to recruit, hire, and build programs and facilities for a group of practitioners. A noncompete clause could prevent a competing hospital or group from hiring practitioners away from a nearby institution.
- A noncompete clause could prevent a hospital currently contracted with a group from terminating the contract and then "cherry-picking" individual practitioners. (This is similar to the hiring restriction clause.)

The arguments against noncompete language include that the language can be:

- Unduly restrictive and may limit a practitioner's ability to earn a living
- Against "public policy" by limiting the region's access to (emergency) practitioners

The language in the contract may state that the physician agrees not to provide services to other hospitals within a specific radius for a specific time period.

Sample language: *Physician covenants and agrees that he/she will not, for a period of 1 year after termination of this agreement (whether by expiration of the term or by earlier termination in accordance with the termination section of this agreement), directly or indirectly engage in, solicit, or perform any work for the hospital (or any affiliate thereof) or engage in the practice of medicine within 5 miles of hospital. This restrictive covenant survives the termination of this agreement.*

Confidentiality

Contracts may have a clause that restricts the physician from sharing confidential information such as trade secrets or intellectual property with another hospital or competing group. It may be difficult to determine what is proprietary information, what is in the public domain, and which institutions or groups are competitors. To avoid confusion or later disagreement, the contract should explicitly state what is considered confidential, proprietary, intellectual property, and a competitor.

Sample language: *During the term of employment with the company and after termination of practitioner's employment with the company, practitioner shall not (i) use any confidential information of or concerning the company or the related companies except for the company's benefit or (ii) disclose or divulge to any third party any confidential information relating to the company or the related companies, except as otherwise required by law. "Confidential information" shall mean. . . .*

Definitions

Many other boilerplate clauses may be seen in contractual relationships between practitioners and hospitals/groups. The following definitions include typical examples of some of these other clauses.

Agreement: The term "agreement" shall mean this emergency service agreement and any amendment(s) hereto as may be from time to time adopted as hereinafter provided.

Department: The term "department" shall mean the ED of the hospital, including, without limitation, the emergency treatment area and the administrative offices for the department.

Modification: Describes the method by which the agreement may be modified or amended and generally requires the mutual written agreement of both parties.

Maintenance of records: By federal mandate, certain books, documents, and records must be maintained and accessible for review for a minimum period of time, often 4 to 7 years. This type of clause in a contract stipulates each party's responsibility to comply with these mandates.

Obligations to comply with laws: This "catch-all" clause obligates the parties to comply with "all" applicable federal, state, and local statutes.

Notice: Designates to whom and the method by which formal notices and demands permitted in the contract may be delivered.

Assignment: Defines the degree to which the parties may transfer the responsibilities described in the contract to another nondesignated party.

Entire agreement: Defines the executed agreement to be the understanding of the parties and usually includes a statement that the present agreement supersedes previous representations and agreements.

Severability: A legal concept used in a contract to allow the remainder of the agreement to remain enforceable if any provision within it is declared invalid, illegal, or unenforceable.

Addenda: Any and all additions, appendices, or addenda should be referenced in the body of the contract, understood, and present at the time of signature.

PEARLS AND PITFALLS

A few key concerns that should be considered in the development of a contract are discussed next.

Fraud Alert of May 1992

The May 1992 Fraud Alert of the Healthcare Financing Authority attempts to restrict hospitals from directly or indirectly paying physicians for hospital admissions.[15] The application of the fraud alert to emergency medicine addresses the issue of payment. Any relationship between the hospital or group and the physician that can be interpreted as an incentive to admit patients is subject to this Medicare fraud and abuse statute. Additionally, a hospital that performs billing and collecting services in the name of the physician and keeps a portion of that money greatly in excess of the normal reasonable cost of billing may also be subject to scrutiny under the fraud and abuse statute.

References

Before the agreements are signed, both sides should obtain references. It is advisable for both parties to request a letter in writing and personally communicate with the references. A personal phone call permits commentary that a person may not be willing to put in a letter of reference. The National Practitioner Data Bank and State Medical Society should also be queried. The practitioner should provide professional training and residency recommendations, and the hospital or group should provide a list of physicians who currently work or have previously worked at the institution.

Right Questions

It is appropriate that some difficult questions are asked about the background of the physician or hospital early in the negotiation process. Practitioners should be asked about their malpractice history, lapses in training or employment, and "skeletons in their closets" (**Box 100.3**). Practitioners may wish to ask hospitals and groups about unhappy physicians or clients, pending or settled lawsuits, financial stability of medical malpractice carrier or self-insured trust, and reasons that physicians have left.

BOX 100.3 ■ EXAMPLES OF RIGHT QUESTIONS

- **License:** Suspended, revoked, or limited
- **Medical privileges:** Suspended, denied, revoked, or reduced
- **Specific clinical privileges:** Granted with limitations or denied
- **Medical liability:** Claims or cases pending

CONCLUSION

Many providers are intimidated by contracts and do not take the time to understand them. The contract process should be positive and collaborative, allowing all parties to establish their goals in advance, understand the contract terms and conditions, review the contract, and work closely with counsel to ensure the contract language matches intent. An effective contracting process can form the foundation of a satisfactory relationship that lasts for many years.

APPENDIX 100.1: STRAUSS'S 21 ESSENTIAL QUESTIONS TO ADDRESS WHEN CONSIDERING A JOB

Your Contract

1. **Employee or independent contractor?**
   a. If an employee:
      i. Will you be group employed?
      ii. Will you be hospital employed?
   b. If an independent contractor (IC):
      i. Will the IC status stand the IRS tests (either meet the 20-rule test or Section 530 relief)?
      ii. When considering your compensation package, is it "apples to apples?" Does the additional hourly rate as an IC permit you to purchase the benefits you would have gotten had you been an employee?

2. **If offered employee status, what are the benefits and their value?**
   a. Can vacation and other PTO accrue and be used after the year in which it was earned? Upon termination, does accrued PTO have a cash value?
   b. CME dues?
   c. Insurance (health, life, disability, etc.)?

3. **Is there a pension or other retirement plan?**
   a. What is the contribution by employer/employee, including matching programs?
   b. What is the eligibility period and vestment schedule?
   c. Is there an opportunity to control the investment of the funds?

4. **Malpractice**
   a. What type is available?
      i. Occurrence?
      ii. Claims made: How is "tail coverage" managed?
   b. What are the required limits?
   c. What is the malpractice record of the group?
   d. What processes does the group/hospital employ to support sued practitioners (i.e., litigation support program)?

5. **Term: Length of contract?**
   a. Yours—Is it an "evergreen" contract (automatic renewal)?
   b. Group's contract with the hospital

i. What is the actual term?
ii. Is the contract likely to be renewed at term?

6. **Termination of the contract between you and the group**

    a. "Not-for-cause" termination

       i. Is it equal (i.e., you get and must give 90 days)?
       ii. How frequently has the group used this termination procedure?
       iii. In what specific situations has a "not-for-cause" clause been executed by the group?

    b. "For-cause" termination

       i. What are the causes and are they reasonable?
       ii. Is there a "cure" period?

YOUR GROWTH POTENTIAL

7. **Personal growth opportunities**

    a. What do you want?

       i. Departmental leadership roles (director, CQI, education)
       ii. Community leadership roles (EMS)
       iii. Academic positions (research, teaching)
       iv. Specialty involvement (ACEP, ABEM, SAEM, AAEM)

    b. Do the people with whom I will be working understand where I want to go and will working with them help me to get there?

HOSPITAL ISSUES

8. **Relationships and issues with administration**

    a. Are emergency providers integrated into the hospital committee structure?
    b. When being recruited, are you interviewed by senior hospital management?
    c. How does the administrator envision the ED in the hospital's strategic plan?

9. **Hospital financial status**

    a. Review online search programs (e.g., ahd.com)
    b. Do you know the hospital's performance metrics (average daily census, length of stay, HCAHPS scores, CMS performance)

10. **Local/regional competition to hospital/ED—hospital market share and trends?**

11. **Facility operations**

    a. Does the ED structure (layout) contribute to efficient patient care?

       i. Recent or planned renovations?

    b. What information technologies and operational processes/programs support efficient practice?

       i. Information and data tracking systems?
       ii. Bedside registration/rapid triage?

iii. Does the EMR enhance documentation and discharge processes (MD and RN)?
iv. Are there scribes?
v. Are there routine demand/capacity analyses?
vi. How does the facility measure/analyze ED saturation (NEDOCS, ED Safe-T, other)?
vii. Do the operations of essential services (lab, imaging, transport, etc.) facilitate efficient patient flow?

12. **Nursing**
    a. Nursing leader
        i. What is the tenure of the previous and current ED nursing leader?
        ii. Does nursing leadership collaborate with the medical director?
        iii. When interviewing, do you have the opportunity to meet with the nurse leadership?
    d. Nursing staff
        i. Stability of staff—What is the turnover rate?
        ii. How are staffing ratios determined and maintained (e.g., state law or facility decision)?
        iii. Do nurses enjoy working in this ED with these providers?
        iv. Do the nurses understand and believe in customer service?
        v. Is the nursing staff unionized?
        vi. What are the employee engagement scores?

13. **Your hospital responsibilities**
    a. Do the emergency physicians write "admission/bridging orders?"
    b. Are you encouraged to be a member of a hospital committee?
    c. Out-of-ED care
        i. Must you respond to "floor codes" or unattended deliveries and, if so, in what situations?
        ii. Must you respond to floor nonemergencies?

14. **Medical staff relationships**
    a. Is there executive committee participation by the ED leader?
    b. If there are hospitalists
        i. What is the transfer of care process?
        ii. How are admission disputes managed?
    c. What surgical/medical subspecialty coverage exists?
        i. Ease of consult access?
        ii. Ease of admissions?
    d. What diagnostic and interventional imaging services exist and what are the hours of availability?
    e. EMTALA
        i. Do the hospital's physicians understand their EMTALA obligations?
        ii. What recourse is available to address EMTALA issues (e.g., CMO, administrator on-call)?

GROUP ISSUES

15. **Group/individual incentives—Do incentives exist?**

    a. Type
        i. Productivity incentive plan?
        ii. Group or individual bonus plan?
        iii. Partnership/equity plan?
        iv. Compensation tied to patient experience scores?
        v. Length of stay targets?

    b. Participation methodology
        i. Is there a defined and objective methodology for participation?
        ii. How is it determined?
        iii. Who participates?
        iv. What is the group's history of distributions to date?

16. **Group change management—democracy of decision-making**

    a. What are the group's long-term goals?
    b. How are members of the group integrated into departmental decision-making?
    c. What specific issues/changes have incorporated the group members in decisions/implementation?
    d. How much input and control do individual practitioners have in this environment?

17. **Director participation—Does the director . . .**

    a. Work clinical shifts?
    b. Have specific defined administrative expectations?
    c. Vote on the executive committee?
    d. Direct the ED ("home rule" vs hospital committee)?

18. **Group member participation—What are the . . .**

    a. Shift responsibilities?
    b. Administrative expectations?
    c. Hospital committee responsibilities?
    d. Medical staff membership requirements?
    e. Community/EMS requirements?
    f. Society memberships and contributions?

19. **Scheduling**

    a. Who does it and is it fair?
    b. How are vacation, holidays, and sick days allotted and covered?

20. **Performance improvement/error reduction**

    a. What is the plan and how comprehensive is it?
    b. Does the ED have standards and guidelines?
    c. How often is feedback given? Is it objective, honest, supportive, and fair?
    d. Is there an interdisciplinary team approach?
    e. How are complaints managed?
    f. When deficiencies are identified, how are they managed?

21. **Patient experience of care/customer satisfaction**
    a. Do the members of administration and the ED staff have consistent goals?
    b. What methods are used to measure/monitor satisfaction?
        i. ED PECS
        ii. Proprietary service
    c. Is group feedback or individual feedback preferred?
    d. What are the patient experience ratings and trends over the last two years?
    e. Are incentives/disincentives used to improve performance?
    f. Is there a 360-degree evaluation process?

REFERENCES

1. Branagan A, *Making Sense of Business: A No-Nonsense Guide to Business Skills for Managers and Entrepreneurs*. Philadelphia, Pa: Kogan Page; 2009.
2. Getty JP. (December 15, 1892-June 6, 1976). Available at: https://www.quotes.net/quote/51459. Accessed August 8, 2018.
3. Strauss RW. Negotiation skills. In: Strauss RW, Mayer TA, eds. *Strauss & Mayer's Emergency Department Management*. Philadelphia, Pa: McGraw-Hill; 2013.
4. Fisher R, Ury W. *Getting to Yes*. New York, NY: Penguin Books; 2006.
5. Wood JP, Shufeldt JJ, Rapp MT. *Contract Issues for Emergency Physicians*. Irving, Tex: Emergency Medicine Residents Association; 2007.
6. Clouson JP. Key contract clauses. In: Strauss RW, ed. *Contracts: A Practical Guide for the Emergency Physician*. Irving, Tex: American College of Emergency Physicians; 1990.
7. Strauss RW, Zun L. Contracts with physicians. In: Strauss RW, Mayer TA, eds. *Strauss & Mayer's Emergency Department Management*. Philadelphia, Pa: McGraw-Hill; 2013.
8. Kocher KE, Sklar DP, Mehrotra A, et al. Categorization, designation, and regionalization of emergency care: definitions, a conceptual framework, and future challenges. *Acad Emerg Med*. 2010;17(12):1306-1311.
9. The Joint Commission, Certification for Primary Stroke Centers. 2020. Available at: https://www.jointcommission.org/certification/primary_stroke_centers.aspx. Accessed January 6, 2020.
10. American Trauma Society. Trauma Center Designations and Levels. 2000. Available at: https://www.amtrauma.org/page/traumalevels. Accessed January 6, 2020.
11. American College of Emergency Physicians Policy Statement. Procedural sedation in the emergency department. *Ann Emerg Med*. 2017;70(6):945-946.
12. American Board of Emergency Medicine Policy Statement. Policy on third party standards. 2012. Available at: https://www.abem.org/public/docs/default-source/policies-faqs/policy-on-third-party-standards.pdf?sfvrsn=4. Accessed July 18, 2018.
13. American College of Emergency Physicians. Indemnification clauses in emergency medicine contracts: an information paper. 2016. Available at: https://www.acep.org/globalassets/uploads/uploaded-files/acep/clinical-and-practice-management/resources/medical-legal/indemn-clause-ip_final_apr_2016.pdf. Accessed June 3, 2018.
14. AAMC. Guidelines for dealing with faculty conflicts of commitment and conflicts of interest in research. *Acad Med*. 1990;65(7):487-496.
15. Fraud Alert of 1992 may be found online at: https://oig.hhs.gov/fraud/docs/alertsandbulletins/ 121994.html. 1992. Accessed June 21, 2013.

CHAPTER 101

CONTRACTING WITH HOSPITALS

Robert W. Strauss, Thom A. Mayer, David W. Singley

Emergency department (ED) staffing and management services are almost always provided through an exclusive contract between the hospital and physician group or practice management organization. Some hospitals, particularly academic medical centers, choose to employ or directly contract with individual emergency physicians. This chapter will focus on the more common form of ED contracting through an agreement between the hospital and a physician group for staffing and management of the ED's clinical and professional services.

When entering a legal contract with a hospital, it is advisable for physician groups to obtain legal counsel, preferably with experience in medical law. An old adage, "The man who represents himself has a fool for a lawyer," applies. There are numerous legal, compliance, performance, and regulatory issues involved in relationships between hospitals and physicians. Effective legal counsel will help the parties ensure that the agreement is clear, enforceable, and in compliance with the complex laws and regulations governing the health-care industry and the state in which the services are rendered.[1] While counsel should always be used to ensure that the intent of the parties is legally specified, counsel does not obviate the requirement that the physician group has all of the following:

- Requisite working knowledge of contracts
- Insight into key contract terms
- Involvement in the contracting process
- A good understanding of all the business ramifications of the contract terms

THE CONTRACT

An emergency services contract is a written document agreed to by at least two parties that describes the requirements, duties, and responsibilities of each.[2] A service contract has a start date, an end date, and a "consideration" (value exchanged). Hospitals use an emergency services agreement (ESA) when they wish to outsource their emergency physician services to an outside party in order to, at minimum, provide care and treatment for patients presenting to the ED. The ESA is designed to create clear and detailed expectations between the parties and describes the specific services that are to be provided, including "how much," "how long," "where," and for "what consideration." Consideration in law requires an agreement regarding the mutual exchange of something of value, such as payment, services, and so on.[3]

A contract documents and governs what happens to the relationship when certain events occur. For instance, if the contracting parties choose to terminate the agreement at any point in the future, the contract should define the obligations of both parties during and after the dissolution. Well-written contracts provide pathways for resolving most disagreements, usually within specific time frames. Contract-related lawsuits between the parties are more often related to poorly described expectations than to blatant disregard for clearly understood responsibilities. Time spent defining and documenting expectations is well worth the effort and prevents confusion, misunderstanding, and blame later.

Relationships

> *Negotiating a contract can be the first major test of a relationship or a major challenge in an established relationship. How the parties approach the task and resolve the areas of conflict leaves an indelible stamp on the relationship. In many ways it sets the tone for almost all future interactions . . . If the parties are able to engage each other in collaborative problem solving, everyone will expect that type of interaction when future issues arise.*[4]

In service businesses, relationships are critical to success. While this chapter focuses primarily on the contractual clauses and definitions of an agreement, it is actually the relationship between the parties that will, in the end, most often determine the longevity of the contract. With a long-standing collaborative partnership, difficult periods can be successfully navigated. Without a good relationship, a contract always remains fragile at best.

However, a good relationship does not take the place of a good contract. There are situations in which the relationship has worn to the point of near separation, and it can only be salvaged by the meticulously drafted contract, which requires the parties to live up to their promised performance. While the specific terms of the contract may seem obvious, the details are important to ensure there is a common understanding of what is expected.

The Contracting Process

To begin the process, the basic and "easy" contract provisions can be sketched out. The hospital often takes the lead by having its legal counsel provide a draft template contract to the physician group. Hospital administrators have many contracts to manage and prefer consistency in their approach, structure, language, and process of contracts. The key issue for a physician group is not who controls the drafting of the contract, but rather the ultimate terms of agreement. From a negotiating standpoint, it is common for hospitals to assert, "Our contracts are all the same for hospital-based groups, so they cannot be amended." This is almost never an accurate statement, with the possible exception of certain language regarding contracting with insurance payers.

Though an overall "meeting of the minds" may be understood at a "handshake" level, the real negotiations take place when the language of the contract is hammered out. The contract is designed to keep both parties on the agreed-upon path. The contract must also spell out what happens when either party deviates from the contractual terms. Though parties enter into a contract in good faith and generally with high hopes, it is rare that these relationships last in their original form. As a result, the process of managing disagreements and changes must be addressed in the contract, usually in the form of an amendment.

During the "honeymoon" period when the relationship is strong, it may be difficult to work through these adverse scenarios. This process of conjuring up all the bad things that could possibly happen and addressing how they are to be handled is one of the first real tests of the partnership. It is easier to calmly address concerns and potential changes in advance.

Finalizing a contract requires leaders to focus on the important terms that define the "good" and "bad" times. A contract generally involves some compromise from both parties, each of whom may have to settle for terms they do not particularly like. Before undertaking the contract negotiation, the physician group and hospital should each understand their own realistic goals and bottom lines (must-have deal breakers).[5]

Understanding acceptable outcomes prior to negotiations allows each party to effectively work through difficult issues and compromise without losing focus on what is important and necessary.

CONTRACT CLAUSES

There are a number of key contracting terms that physician groups must address when developing an agreement with the hospital.

Term

The term or length of the contract is the time during which each party's contractual obligations are in effect. Generally, at the conclusion of the term, the parties are no longer obligated to each other, unless the contract is renewed under the same or newly negotiated conditions, or the contract stipulates postcontractual obligations (survival clauses), such as:

- Payment of monies due as defined within the contract
- Confidentiality related to proprietary information or intellectual property
- Noncompetition or nonsolicitation clauses[6]

If the contract expires, the entire business and livelihood of the group may simply end, at least at that location, unless other business opportunities are developed. As such, many groups attempt to obtain the longest term available (e.g., 3-5 years). However, many hospitals prefer or are bound to a one- or two-year contract. When a longer term is not possible, an "evergreen" clause can ensure that the contract will automatically renew if not specifically terminated according to the terms of the agreement. For instance, an initial two-year contract with automatic two-year renewals, upon mutual approval, can be used to extend a short-term contract.

Termination

There are many reasons why both parties may want to end a contractual relationship, including:

- Promised services are not delivered.
- Delivered services do not meet acceptable standards.
- There is an unacceptable deterioration in the relationship.
- An alternative organization (hospital, group) is preferable.

For instance, if the group is unable to fully recruit, staff, and retain acceptable practitioners to meet its coverage obligations, the hospital may become dissatisfied with a real or perceived unmet promise. Alternatively, the hospital may not be able to maintain adequate specialty coverage or provide enough nursing and essential support staff to safely and efficiently manage the ED census. Termination in advance of the contracted term can occur "for cause" or "without cause."

For-Cause Termination

A "for-cause" termination is one in which a party asserts that the other party has not delivered on a significant contractual obligation or has committed a "breach" of the contract. The specific reasons that either party may invoke a for-cause termination are often considered in advance and usually defined in the contract. One party must only provide written notice of the intent to terminate the contract and identify the reasons or contractual breach. There are multiple causes for termination, including financial insolvency, breach of obligations, duties or policies, conduct injurious to the other party, disclosure of confidential information, material violation of the law, failure to maintain the ability to contract with Medicare and Medicaid service or other insurance payers, and so on. When defining the process of a for-cause termination, the contract should contain:

- Specific examples of "cause"
- The method of how the breaching party is to be given notice
- Whether breaching party has an opportunity to "cure" or fix the alleged breach over what period of time and in what circumstances
- The time period until services are discontinued (e.g., immediate, 30 days after receipt of notice, etc.).

Cure Provision

In certain circumstances, it is preferable to have a "cure" provision in the contract. A cure is defined as a limited right over a specific period of time (30 days, for example) during which the breaching party has the opportunity to resolve a correctable breach. While many of the specific reasons for termination are written into the contract, not every problem can be anticipated.

Example: A contract states that all providers must continuously maintain malpractice insurance. However, a physician loses his malpractice insurance simply because a check was not cleared in time. If the practitioner does not work until this breach is rectified (perhaps 24 hours later), a devastating and unnecessary termination may be avoided. Both parties should permit the opportunity to review claims of a possible breach.

Termination Without Cause

Most contracts also contain provisions for termination "wthout cause" (sometimes called "not-for-cause" termination). Termination without cause allows either party to end the contractual relationship without providing a reason. Prior to the cessation of obligations, the terminating party must give a contractually defined notice period (the time period between when the other party is notified and the effective date of termination). During this notice period, all the parties must continue their contractual obligations. Hospitals and physician groups may want this type of termination clause in their contracts to ensure flexibility. This clause limits the value of the term section of the contract because termination without cause, once exercised, immediately redefines the terms.

Example: A physician group and a hospital enter into a five-year emergency services contract, but the contract also contains a 180-day termination-without-cause provision. During the term, that provision is exercised, transforming the agreement immediately into a 180-day contract, irrespective of the remaining term. In this case, either party may cancel the contract without reason in 180 days.

From one point of view, both parties may wish to avoid a without-cause provision to "lock in" the relationship. However, hospitals may desire such a clause to ensure that they have maximum future flexibility to determine the group that will staff and manage its ED. Physician groups may desire a without-cause provision, particularly when there are uncertain business issues.

Example: A physician group's estimate of the costs of and collections from services proves inaccurate and the business becomes unviable. Rather than lose money for the term of the contract, the physician group may exercise termination without cause.

This without-cause language allows both parties to address future unknowns and avoid potentially contentious initial negotiations.

Example: A hospital is instructed by its board that an initial subsidy to the physician group must end in 30 months. Uncertain about its long-term prospects, the group unsuccessfully advocates for a subsidy throughout the term of the contract. At the end of 24 months, the group still needs financial support to survive. As a result, it exercises its 180-day notice of termination without cause, which allows the group to avoid a financially nonsustainable relationship. As an alternative, if the group becomes a critical hospital partner, the without-cause language could lead to renegotiation.

The initial inclusion of this language allows the group to take the risk of entering into this relationship. As a general rule of thumb, termination without cause is less desirable to the party with the more favorable contract. That party desires the longest term possible. Without-cause provisions are generally between 90 and 180 days from the written notice provided by either party. (Given the length of time required for hospital credentialing or starting a new group, less than a 180-day notice may be impractical.)

Performance Standards

The parties should clearly delineate the anticipated services to be performed by each party under a contract.[7] Most ESAs will go to great lengths to detail specific requirements. For instance, the hospital may contractually define the required physician qualifications, physician credentialing and privileging process, physician staffing coverage and backup, administrative responsibilities, quality and performance obligations, CME or certification requirements, and so on.

Increasingly, hospitals stipulate specific contractual performance standards that detail what the physician group is expected to achieve. For instance, the hospital may contractually list operational metrics that must be met, such as "door-to-doctor" times and patient experience scores. Specific performance metrics might include:

- 100% achievement of core measures
- Full participation in the Merit-Based Incentive Payment System
- Efficient use of medical imaging
- <1% of patients who leave prior to receiving a medical screening examination
- <150 minutes average length of stay (LOS) for discharged patients
- Compliance with practice care guidelines
- >80th percentile patient experience of care survey (ED PECS) scores

While these types of performance standards appear straightforward, they may be quite difficult to achieve without collaboration and teamwork. Prior to agreeing to be accountable for a specific outcome, the responsible party must have significant control over the process and the cooperation of other divisions, services, and staff. For instance, achieving a "door-to-doctor" time of less than 30 minutes may not be possible if patients are not triaged and placed into a bed within a 20-minute time period. Further, the admission LOS could be prolonged by inpatients boarding in the ED, creating a bottleneck that delays the entrance of waiting room patients. Regardless of the cause of ED boarding, the physician group may have little or no ability to hit the "required" contractual target. A more accurate and controllable metric is the "bed-to-doctor" time, which helps emphasize a combination of physician staffing and flow.

Example: The hospital insists on contract language requiring the physician group to ensure that discharged patients have an overall LOS averaging 120 minutes or less. Since *the hospital is responsible for providing all of the staff and equipment, the control of many necessary resources (e.g., nursing, laboratory, imaging) are in its hands. If these resources are inadequate, the physician group could assume responsibility for performance it cannot control. If the performance standard is contractually promised, the group may find itself in breach of the contract and ultimately have its contract terminated for cause. Therefore, the physician group should anticipate and hold the hospital responsible for the resources and related processes that it controls.*

Contractual performance standards should reflect each party's level of control over the measure. It is appropriate to identify who is responsible for which component and outline measurable and monitored performance expectations for each responsible party.

Example: *The hospital and physician group agree to an ED PECS score in the 75th percentile. Should scores not reach the delineated target, both parties agree to collaborate in hiring a mutually acceptable patient experience consultant. Both the hospital and group agree to adopt the consultant's recommendation and actively participate in any suggested improvement activities.*

Example: *The hospital and physician group agree to achieve a discharge LOS of 150 minutes. Should the LOS cycle time between decision to admit and left the ED exceed 10% of the target, the physician group is not obligated to achieve the discharge LOS target until this measure is addressed.*

Group Responsibilities

Hospitals will contractually require the physician group to address several critical clinical and administrative needs. It is common for hospitals to define the number and types of physicians and other providers that the group must contractually provide. The contract might only outline vague requirements, that is, the "group must provide enough emergency providers to adequately staff the hospital ED." Alternatively, the contract could specify the number of shifts, the types of providers covering those shifts, and even aspects of the provider schedule. A more objective method to determine coverage is to link it to a demand–capacity analysis (see Chapter 33). Similarly, the hospital should be held responsible for nurse, technician, clerical, and support staff based on the same analysis. If specific staffing requirements are a component of the contractual responsibilities, those obligations should be tied to market variation, such as volume growth or contraction.

The contract might also stipulate the specific qualifications of the providers (e.g., board certification in emergency medicine) and ongoing training or demonstration of competency (e.g., in stroke care or procedural sedation). Other contractual responsibilities required by the hospital might include:

- Provision of a medical director, advanced practice providers (APPs), and scribes
- Attendance at medical staff and hospital meetings
- Emergency physician completion of admission or transition orders
- Responsibility for in-house codes or unattended obstetrical deliveries
- Education in-services to the ED staff
- Participation in quality programs
- Emergency medical services outreach and leadership involvement

All of these obligations should be clearly laid out in the contract with an understanding of the resources required to execute the obligations.

Overly rigid legal wording can inadvertently cause a "technical breach" when the parties' actual intent was different. As a result, it may be wise to use language such as, "... will use reasonable efforts to...."

> **Example:** *A contract may stipulate that the "group will comply with all Joint Commission, EMTALA, medical staff, and state regulatory standards." However, a physician might be unaware of, or not have the resources to accomplish, a new minor hospital standard. This "minor infraction" should not be cause for a breach by the group, particularly if the group makes "reasonable efforts" to address all protocols and standards.*

Hospital Responsibilities

In order for the group to effectively fulfill its role, the hospital must provide certain resources and perform its agreed-upon contractual duties. As such, the contract should define the hospital's performance requirements. Among the most common obligations include the adequate provision of the following:

- Staffing (nurses, essential support services/technicians, lab and radiology turnaround targets, unit secretaries)
- Supplies and medical equipment
- Registration services that are accurate and timely
- Office space for medical director that includes telephone and Internet
- Physician's on-call room/office
- Medical staff on-call list
- Tools for communication
- Computers for documentation and an integrated electronic health record

It is also prudent to contractually define the hospital's performance responsibilities using measurable criteria. Further, there are several performance criteria that can only be met through collaborative efforts of both the hospital and group.

> **Example:** *In the example cited previously, the hospital and group contractually agree to a door-to-doctor time of 30 minutes or less. To accomplish this goal, both parties must be accountable for the processes that they control. As such, the hospital may contractually be held to an average arrival-to-bed time of less than 15 minutes, and the group may contractually be held to an average bed-to-provider time of less than 15 minutes.*

Financial Obligations

The emergency services contract between a hospital and physician group contains a section that details the financial commitments of each of the parties. All financial relationships affecting ED patient billing should be disclosed during contract discussions. For instance, the hospital should describe its intention to provide the following:

- Free ED care to all employees and their families
- Free ED care to community physicians and their families
- Write-offs to any complaining patient or family member
- Reduced charges to special groups
- Pursuit of preferred provider agreements with significant commercial insurers

While the hospital may decide to adopt policies to address the listed business practices, the group must take particular care that the imposed practices do not run afoul of current health-care laws related to compliance and Stark regulations. A legal review of the contract is critical to ensure compliance. Any time there is an exchange of money (including "in-kind" payments) between a hospital and a physician or physician group, legal counsel should ensure that the exchange is allowable and reasonable. For instance, it would not be reasonable or allowable for a hospital to:

- Pay a group for more hospital admissions
- Provide the group with a start-up loan with no intention of obtaining repayment
- Discourage a group from providing a medical screening examination to patients with no means of payment
- Split fees or obtain a "kickback"

If the ESA does not require financial support from the hospital, then the financial section may be brief, perhaps only requiring an approved fee schedule and description of the relationship when contracting with managed care entities.

Alternatively, the hospital might provide funding, such as a medical director stipend or a monthly stipend, to support a practice that is unable to support itself based on patient billing alone. In that case, the amount, timing, and payment terms must be clearly described. The financial obligations of both parties should be clearly defined, as they can often lead to misunderstandings and complications. There is a saying, "You name the price, and I'll name the terms." This means that different levels of financial support may lead to different practice models. For instance, certain subsidies may be necessary to support a contract that requires the following:

- Group to use only board-certified emergency physicians
- Medical director to spend 75% of his or her time administratively
- Group to participate in all managed care contracts with which the hospital contracts
- Group to give free care to multiple categories of patients

Obligations, performance standards, penalties (for not achieving standards), and changing payer mix, volume, and acuity levels may all erode finances, which in turn may compromise the relationship. The financial terms and obligations of the contract should address the expected market conditions, account for likely variations, and provide an opportunity to revisit the contract in the event of unexpected market changes.

Exclusivity

The hospital generally grants the physician group an exclusive contract, permitting and requiring it to provide services to all of the patients presenting to the ED. From a business standpoint, exclusivity provides the group with a "monopoly" on all emergency services provided at the hospital. If exclusivity did not exist in the contract, the group might have to compete with other sets of physicians on the medical staff, significantly decreasing the value of the "business." The typical exception to this exclusivity clause allows the private medical staff to see their own patients in the ED. (It should be noted that patients waiting to see their private physicians in the ED are the responsibility of the emergency physician group.) However, with the increasing use of hospitalists, fewer private clinicians see their own patients in the ED.

Restrictions

There are other forms of exclusivity, that is, there are restrictive covenants that the hospital may require of the group, including the following:

- ***Outside practice restriction:*** This restriction prevents the group and its providers from working at other facilities that may directly compete with the hospital. For instance, an emergency physician group would be precluded from opening or providing clinical services for an unaffiliated private urgent care center in a particularly affluent community 1 mile from the hospital. The outside practice restriction should not unreasonably limit a physician's practice.

- *Nonsolicitation*: The group may not hire staff away from the hospital. An emergency physician group might otherwise attract some of the best clinical and administrative staff away from the hospital. A nonsolicitation agreement could also prevent the hospital from selectively hiring the group's providers.
- *Noncompete*: This provision could prevent members of the group from practicing in a competing facility upon termination of the hospital relationship. This is an example of the hospital attempting to protect its interests against competitive organizations. Noncompete restrictions are not valid in every state. In states where noncompete clauses are permissible, the time period and geographic boundary must be "reasonable."
- *Noninterference*: Noninterference clauses are related yet distinct from noncompete clauses in that they restrict the group's providers and the hospital from interfering with the contractual relationship.
- *Restrictive covenants*: These covenants, which are usually between the physician group and the providers (emergency physicians and APPs), restrict the ability of the clinician to provide service to the hospital in the event the contract is terminated. However, some hospitals insist on a clause indicating that the group will neither have nor enforce restrictive covenants.

Termination of Medical Staff Privileges

The two forms of termination of medical staff privileges addressed here are the "clean sweep" provision and the hospital request for individual provider termination.

The "Clean Sweep" Clause

In exchange for the exclusive right to practice emergency medicine at the hospital, the hospital will generally request the resignation of the entire group and its practitioners—the "clean sweep"—if and when the contract is terminated. From the hospital's point of view, it is necessary to provide a new "replacement" group with the same exclusivity enjoyed by the previous one. If emergency physicians were not required to resign their privileges, theoretically, there could be two or more groups simultaneously competing for the same patients. Hence, the concept of exclusivity as described previously.

Note that a "clean sweep" combined with a "noncompete" restriction could prevent a terminated physician from practicing in or near the community. However, the hospital may want certain physicians from the group to continue to practice in the ED as members of the new entity. To accomplish this, a contractual variation might require physicians to resign their privileges "at the discretion of the hospital or its representative." This exception would allow an emergency physician to continue to practice at the hospital, if the hospital chose to allow it.

Seen in a positive light, some clinicians could maintain their practice in the community. Seen more negatively, this variation could allow a hospital to terminate a group and then "cherry pick" certain providers to the detriment of the group and its nonretained members. To prevent this, the group may include its own restrictive covenant clause in its contract with its individual practitioners, the hospital, or both. (See Chapter 100 for a more in-depth discussion on this topic.)

Request for Individual Provider Termination

Whether an employee of the hospital, an employee of an emergency group, or an independent contractor (IC), the ED clinician is generally assumed to be an "agent" of the hospital. As a result, the hospital is often perceived to be responsible for the physician's negligence when working in the hospital's ED. Many hospitals press for a contract provision that allows the removal of a specific physician. The hospital typically exercises this right when a physician's performance is deemed to be detrimental to the facility or its patients. Under this provision, the group must comply, unless it is able to convince the hospital to modify its position by implementing an internal review process and, when necessary, monitoring corrective action. The language of the modification clauses could be specific and include:

- Performance metrics that define the hospital's potential concerns
- Communications to alert the group of a concern
- Agreed-upon internal review processes
- Cure opportunities for the clinician, such as a corrective action, to address the concern

When the hospital insists on language about terminating individual providers, the group should add parallel language to the clinician's contract that requires resignation without the benefit of the medical staff's "due process." In this situation, the physician's hospital privileges are then terminated upon separation from the group. Hospitals may perceive this clause as necessary to secure their ability to terminate emergency clinicians with significant clinical or behavioral problems and avoid the group's potential opposition to such a request.

Most physician groups perceive this type of termination provision as heavy handed and unnecessary; some might insist on the modifying clauses (above) to ensure the hospital does not make overly hasty, reactive, or "knee-jerk" decisions. The language should foster a collaborative approach to address resolvable issues.

> **Example:** *If the hospital has a significant concern about an individual physician's performance, it will notify the group. The group is obligated to investigate and, when confirmed, will develop a mutually acceptable plan to address the concern.*

Other Contract Clauses

Independent Contractor Status

It is necessary to define the relationship of the parties for several reasons that address who is responsible for the clinician's performance related to malpractice and the US Internal Revenue Service (IRS). Hospitals engage nonemployed physician groups as ICs. This relationship somewhat limits the liability of both parties for the actions of the other (see Chapter 102). If the clinician is to be treated as an IC, the contract between the hospital and group, as well as the agreement between the group and its clinicians, should consistently cite and treat providers as ICs. The more control the hospital exercises over the group, its physicians, and their activities, the more likely the group and its clinicians may be seen as employees. This IRS reclassification could have profound effects on the hospital, group, providers, and taxes and pension plans, which if disqualified would be subjected to taxes and penalties.

Indemnification

Physician groups are frequently asked to "indemnify" and "hold harmless" the hospital against acts of the physicians and the group itself. This means that the hospital is asking the group to assume responsibility for physicians' actions. Unfortunately, though the physician or group may injudiciously agree to indemnify the hospital, virtually no malpractice insurance will provide that coverage. This noncoverage could leave the physician (group) bare and personally responsible for these costs. If the hospital asks a group for this coverage, it may be wise to ask for the hospital's help finding an insurance company that will provide it. When indemnification contract language is used, the group should confirm that the contract includes parallel or bilateral language ensuring indemnification by both the group and the hospital (same language that each party indemnifies the other for its acts).

Insurance

A clause in the contract defines the professional liability insurance responsibilities of the group. The provisions typically describe the limits, type (occurrence, claims made), and other stipulations ("tail" requirements). The hospital is also required to carry insurance. Other insurance requirements may also be listed in this section of the contract, including general liability, worker's compensation, and so on.

Arbitration

Service contracts generally contain a clause that defines the method of resolving contract disputes. An arbitration clause is often the chosen solution. Arbitration is a legal process to avoid litigation when trying to resolve legal disputes (a contract disagreement). There are many potential benefits of arbitration, including:

- Streamlined process
- Arbitrator more knowledgeable than most juries
- Frequently, but not always, less expensive
- Private proceedings

The key, of course, is to avoid a lawsuit or the need for arbitration altogether. However, arbitration can be an effective deterrent, encouraging both parties to work out their differences and avoid the fight.

CONCLUSION

The emergency services contract between the physician group and the hospital defines the business relationship of the parties. The contract itself establishes and governs the formal legal relationship and clarifies the expectations and responsibilities of each party. Developing a "good" contract that is clearly understood by both parties takes a great deal of time and relationship building before the term begins. The emergency physician group entering into a contract for services with a hospital should retain competent counsel familiar with health-care law to ensure the following:

- The intent of the parties is met in the contract language.
- The physician group recognizes the legal ramifications of its contractual commitments.
- The hospital's obligations are clearly defined.
- Critical contract elements are meticulously addressed.
- Termination provisions are evenhanded.

An in-depth, working understanding of contracts, their purpose, and implementation prepare a group to negotiate a solid contract, perform successfully, and establish a long and successful relationship with its hospital business partner.

REFERENCES

1. Shubov E. *Physician Employment Contracts: The Missing Module.* Advocate Press; 2019

2. Wood JP, Shufeldt JJ, Rapp MT. *Contract Issues for Emergency Physicians.* Emergency Medicine Resident's Association; 2007.

3. Wikipedia. Consideration under American law. 2019. Available at: https://en.wikipedia.org/wiki/Consideration_under_American_law. Accessed February 1, 2020.

4. Keene JG, Dresnick SJ. Contracting with hospitals: monetary and legal issues. In: Salluzzo RF, Mayer TA, Strauss RW, Kidd P, eds. *Emergency Department Management: Principles and Applications.* Mosby (Elsevier); 1997:290.

5. Fisher R, Ury WL, Patton B. *Getting to Yes.* Penguin Books; 1991.

6. Law Insider. Post contractual obligations confidentiality communication: sample clauses. 2020. Available at: https://www.lawinsider.com/documents/eRrKWBw7YY5#post-contractual-obligations-confidentiality-communication. Accessed January 31, 2020.

7. Welch SJ. *Quality Matters: Solutions for a Safe and Efficient Emergency Department.* The Joint Commission Resources; 2009.

8. Khare R, Powell ES, Reinhardt G, et al. Adding more beds to the emergency department or reducing admitted patient boarding times: which has a more significant influence on emergency department congestion? *Ann Emerg Med.* 2009;53(5):575–585.

CHAPTER 102

EMPLOYEE VS INDEPENDENT CONTRACTOR

Robert W. Strauss

> ... the goal is to grant as much information and independent decision-making ability to employees or contractors as possible.
>
> —Timothy Ferriss, *The 4-Hour Workweek*

Before the development of a contract between a physician and a contract group (or hospital), it must first be determined whether the physician will be treated as an employee or independent contractor (IC). This distinction is critical to the contractual relationship.

The sample language used in this chapter is meant to familiarize readers with the type of verbiage that may be used to convey contractual intent. The sample language is not meant to be definitive, complete, or used in an official capacity. Before accepting any contract, emergency clinicians are encouraged to consult advisers with expertise in contract law in the state in which the document is to be executed.

EMERGENCY PHYSICIAN COMPENSATION

Regardless of the physician's classification, the total amount of money available for compensation and benefits is generally the same after deducting for professional liability insurance and group overhead (**Table 102.1**). Additionally, clinical and professional responsibilities are generally the same regardless of the classification.[1]

Emergency physician compensation is commonly based on an hourly rate or productivity payment. The traditional US employee setting is a 40-hour workweek over 52 weeks. An emergency physician may choose to work more or fewer hours, and as such, payment calculations based on a traditional workweek are not applicable. Treating emergency physicians the same, though they may have varying hours, creates further complexity when calculating the value of benefits and business expenses, such as those for continuing medical education (CME), travel, and transportation.

The differences between employees and ICs are most evident when addressing taxes and benefits (**Table 102.2**). Independent contractors are permitted greater individual flexibility with business deductions than employees. Additionally, ICs may develop individualized benefits that include retirement plans and various types of insurance. An employee will generally be confined to the precise benefit package to which other members of the group are entitled. Therefore, the restrictions of a group plan may or may not be advantageous to an individual employee. On the positive side, an employee can often take advantage of

TABLE 102.1 ■ Comparing Employee and IC Salary and Benefits

	Employee	IC*
Paid hours worked	1,692	1,692
Paid hours NOT worked		
• Vacation (4 weeks)	144	0
• CME (1 week)	36	0
• Hourly rate	$150	$182
• Salary	$280,800	$307,944
• Malpractice	$20,000	$20,000
Benefits		
• Health	$8,000	0
• Disability	$1,500	0
• Life	$500	0
Miscellaneous		
• Dues	$1,000	0
• CME	$2,000	0
• Pension (3% salary)	$14,200	0
Total value	**$328,000**	**$328,000**

*Figures are rounded.

premium reductions offered with group benefit plans, and the discounted group rates available to an employee may not be available to an IC.

The disparity of hours and diverse financial needs cause some emergency physician groups to treat their providers as ICs. However, converting from employee to IC status may present some problems if physicians are currently considered employees of that practice. Physician groups are advised to seek the expertise of a tax planner before making any decisions regarding this complex issue.

TABLE 102.2 ■ Tax and Benefit Treatment of Employees and ICs

	Employer/Employee	IC
Income tax	Employer withholds each payroll period	IC calculates and pays quarterly
Employment tax	Employer contributes 50% and withholds 50%	IC pays 100% (50% is tax deductible)
Benefit plan	Employer defines; group plans may be more robust and less expensive; employees have minimal decision-making power	IC defines; ICs can avoid unnecessary expense (i.e., spouse has adequate health insurance)
Retirement plan		None
Business deductions	Limited; may deduct certain expenses in excess of 2% of adjusted gross revenue	Broader opportunities for business deductions

Physician Classification

Because physicians within a group may have different needs, it can be difficult to find a single set of plans that works for everyone (**Box 102.1**).[2] For example, an unmarried physician with few expenses may prefer to maximize their contributions to a retirement or pension plan, whereas a physician who is married with a large mortgage and family may wish to devote their entire paycheck to living expenses. Such a physician may be unable or unwilling to put money into a retirement plan. Similarly, a physician might have a spouse who already has full health insurance coverage through their employer. This physician might wish to forego any deductions that would be contributed to health insurance.

Advantages of Employee Status

It is human nature that people are most comfortable with the status quo; it is easier to accept that which is familiar. Since medical residents are considered employees, most prefer to remain that way even after they graduate from their training program. Multiple aspects of the employee classification—that is, dealing with benefits, tax payments, write-offs, retirement plans, and so on—are addressed simply by virtue of the employee relationship and involve no complex decision-making. This simplicity is very attractive to many practitioners.

The benefits of an employee relationship can be substantial. Employees may receive multiple "free" benefits, including paid vacation and sick time. Insurance fees may be paid by the employer and at a lower cost because of participation in a group plan. Taxes are automatically withheld and paid by the employer. There is little or no financial risk, as most of these payments are known in advance. Employment-based group retirement or pension plans, if any, are managed by the employer. Also, an employee relationship can be structured to include bonuses and incentive payments.

Further, the transition from employee (as a resident) to IC status (postresidency) is fraught with unknowns, complex decisions, deadlines, and benefit determinations. Finally, there may be significant penalties should the Internal Revenue Service (IRS) subsequently reclassify the IC as an employee.

BOX 102.1 ■ IRS WORKER CLASSIFICATION[2]

People such as doctors, dentists, veterinarians, lawyers, accountants, contractors, subcontractors, public stenographers, and auctioneers who are in an independent trade, business, or profession in which they offer their services to the general public are generally ICs. However, whether these people are ICs or employees depends on the facts in each case. The general rule is that an individual is an IC if the payer has the right to control or direct only the result of the work and not what will be done and how it will be done. The earnings of a person who is working as an IC are subject to self-employment tax.

You are not an IC if you perform services that can be controlled by an employer (what will be done and how it will be done). This applies even if you are given freedom of action. What matters is that the employer has the legal right to control the details of how the services are performed.

Advantages of IC Status

Conceptually, ICs are their own boss. In other words, the hiring entity (the contract group) hires providers' services, rather than the providers themselves. Independent contractors are generally paid a higher hourly rate than employees, since the employer is no longer responsible for overhead costs associated with withholding taxes or paying benefits. From these additional payments, the IC must independently pay taxes (state, local, federal, Social Security and Medicare, etc.), benefits (health and other insurances), and business expenses, and make contributions to retirement plans. Most ICs separately hire accountants to advise them on the more complex management of payments required by nonemployees.

While there is simplicity and limited risk associated with employee status, there are unique benefits to IC classification. Simply stated, the advantages are flexibility, self-determination, and enhanced contributions to retirement savings.

Business Expenses

Independent contractors have greater opportunities to deduct business expenses, such as car expenses (when used to commute for work, other than back and forth from home to the office), equipment purchases, education, and associated travel and lodging. To be clear, to qualify as a business expense, the purchase must be legitimate; providers must avoid masquerading personal expenses as business expenses. Discussing a medical situation over lunch with a friend would not be deductible as a business-related meal. The IRS specifies:

> *To be deductible, a business expense must be both ordinary and necessary. An ordinary expense is one that is common and accepted in your trade or business. A necessary expense is one that is helpful and appropriate for your trade or business. An expense does not have to be indispensable to be considered necessary. It is important to separate business expenses from the following expenses: the expenses used to figure the cost of goods sold, capital expenses, and personal expenses.*[3]

Regarding personal vs business expenses, the IRS goes on to say:

> *Generally, you cannot deduct personal, living, or family expenses. However, if you have an expense for something that is used partly for business and partly for personal purposes, divide the total cost between the business and personal parts. You can deduct the business part.*[3]

Taxes

Employment taxes, or Federal Insurance Contributions Act (FICA) taxes (i.e., Social Security and Medicare), on adjusted gross income are the same for both employees and ICs. In an employment model, the employer pays half of the taxes, and the employee pays the other half as a payroll deduction. Under Section 2042 of the Small Business Jobs Act, ICs are permitted to deduct half of their self-employment taxes:

> *. . . you can deduct the employer-equivalent portion of your Self-Employment tax in figuring your adjusted gross income. Wage earners [employees] cannot deduct Social Security and Medicare taxes.*[4]

Deferred Income

Deferring pretax money is considered one of the major advantages to IC classification. As an example, using the year 2018:

- Employees could contribute a maximum of $18,500 ($24,500, if older than 50 years). The employer could contribute as much as $33,000 for a potential total contribution of $50,000 ($55,500, if older than 50 years). However, it is uncommon for employers to maximize contributions to the employee's benefit plan, and most that do only "match" a small percentage of the employee's salary.
- Independent contractors can defer $55,000 into a pretax retirement plan through a combination of four plans (401k, SEP IRA, defined benefit plan, or simple IRA). By using a defined benefit plan, ICs can contribute substantially more than $55,000, depending on their age.

The importance of a disciplined approach to investing pretax money is demonstrated by the following example. It assumes an average 7% rate of return over time, creating a significant potential advantage to the IC. **Table 102.3** assumes the following:

- The IC annually contributes $50,000 pretax to a retirement plan.
- The employee contributes $18,000 pretax to a 401k plan plus an additional $32,000 of their gross income ($18,000 after federal and state taxes). The employee invests an annual total of $36,000.
- The difference is $14,000 annually.
- The annual investment rate of return is 7% (10%).

Over 30 years of steady pretax investments of $50,000 (IC) or $36,000 (employee) with an annual rate of return between 7% and 10%, the IC will accumulate between $1.3 and $2.3 million more than the employee.[5]

Additional factors, not included in this example: Some employers will contribute to their employees' plans, increasing the pretax investment and decreasing the differential. In contrast, ICs may utilize a defined benefit plan to defer substantially more than $50,000 annually, increasing the differential.

TABLE 102.3 ■ Employee vs IC Retirement Planning

	Employee	IC	Differential
Gross income	$300,000	$300,000	
Net income	$250,000	$250,000	
Pretax contribution	$18,000	$50,000	
After-tax contribution	$18,000	0	
Total contribution	$36,000	$50,000	
Annual interest earnings	7%	7%	
Total after 30 years	$3.4 million	$4.7 million	$1.3 million
Annual interest earnings	10%	10%	
Total after 30 years	$5.9 million	$8.2 million	$2.3 million

Accounting Fees

The complexities and deductions associated with the IC model generally require the involvement of an accountant. Among the many calculations required are quarterly estimates and tax payments, determination of business expenses (if any), benefit deductions, and management of deferred income. These additional steps require regular attention and must be managed accurately to avoid IRS reclassification and penalties.

INTERNAL REVENUE SERVICE

The IRS intermittently turns its attention to the issue of employee vs IC, particularly within the medical field. It scrutinizes the IC designation and occasionally challenges its use by various contract management groups.[6] The IRS's interest in the designation relates to two issues: collecting taxes sooner and ensuring proper classification and payments.

Employment taxes are paid biweekly; the IC's taxes are paid quarterly. Further, the large pretax deductions of the IC only generate taxable income when withdrawn at retirement, which may be decades later. Additionally, the IRS believes that ICs generate less tax revenue. This is generally true because the employee's tax is paid on all of an employee's income, whereas tax is paid only on an IC's income after deductions (sometimes large) have been taken. These deductions include business expenses (car lease payments, CME, etc.) and health benefits.

There is substantial evidence of improper tax classification leading to the nonpayment of taxes by some who do not comply with IRS requirements. Employees have taxes paid on their behalf throughout the year based on actual income earned, whereas ICs make quarterly payments based on reasonable estimates of income. Therefore, ICs retain greater use of their money throughout the year and leave the government with delayed and possibly less revenue and interest earned. The IRS estimates that more than $50 billion in tax revenue is lost annually due to the "misclassification of ICs and related underpayment of taxes" and related underpayment and nonpayment of payroll taxes.[7,8]

Currently, the US Department of Labor believes that as many as 30% of ICs are "misclassified" and should be employees.[9] Further, ICs are widely believed to understate their earnings and overstate their deductions. Although physicians make up only a small portion of the total number of ICs, physicians are high-income earners with high visibility; therefore, they are intermittently subject to greater scrutiny.

COMMON LAW TESTS

Common law tests are used as guides by the IRS to determine the classification of a worker, employee, or IC. There are 20 tests (facts) that reveal the degree of a worker's control and independence. The less independence the worker has, the more likely the worker is to be classified as an employee.

Generally, an IC is a person who is compensated by individuals or businesses for work performed. The IC maintains control over the practices, processes, and procedures by which the work is completed. Conversely, an employee's method of work and practices are controlled by the employer. The 20 tests fall into three categories: behavioral, financial, and relationship (**Table 102.4**).[6]

Emergency physicians who are either considering or already have a current IC designation are encouraged to recognize and understand the criteria by which the IRS determines the proper classification. Although the election of IC status may not present any

TABLE 102.4 ■ Common-Law Facts to Determine Employee vs IC Status

Determining Facts	Determining Questions	Suggests Employee If:
Behavioral	Does the company control or have the right to control the details of the individual's work (i.e., what the worker does, how the worker does the job)?	The hiring entity control individual's: • Time and location of work • Tools and equipment • Supplies and services • Specific work product • Order and sequence of work • Hiring of assistants
Financial	Are the business aspects the worker's job controlled by the payer? (These include things like how the worker is paid, whether expenses are reimbursed, who provides tools/supplies, etc.)	The hiring entity: • Reimburses all business expenses • Owns and controls the facility and the individual's work location • Prohibits work elsewhere in the market • Pays by the hour • Limits profit/bonus opportunity
Type of relationship	Are there written contracts or employee-type benefits (e.g., pension plan, insurance, vacation pay)? Will the relationship continue, and is the work performed a key aspect of the business?	The hiring entity: • Provides benefits • Expects an ongoing relationship • Directs and controls performance

initial problems, a subsequent IRS audit could challenge the designation. An IRS audit with an adverse outcome could result in significant penalties and interest.

An employer has the duty to withhold taxes from an employee. If an employer is found to have improperly classified an employee as an IC, the employer may be found liable for those taxes and associated penalties, even if the previously designated IC had properly paid the taxes. Further, a "qualified" retirement, pension, or profit-sharing plan may be disqualified, leading to federal tax payments and significant associated penalties.

The specific common law test used by the IRS to determine the appropriate designation of the worker is listed in **Table 102.5**.[10] These issues should be addressed when developing contract language. For instance, the IC contract should avoid the obvious and all-too-common mistake of labeling the contract an "*employment*" agreement." A casual review of the common law tests would suggest that emergency physicians rarely comply with all of the standards. Fortunately, the IRS does not expect 100% compliance; rather, it looks for what it deems "substantial" compliance. There is no formula or clearly defined precedent that is used when applying these standards. Only an IRS audit, which considers all of these factors, can determine the outcome.

The 20 common law tests used by the IRS cover a broad spectrum of working relationships, industries, and occupations. As a result, some of them are not applicable to the practice of emergency medicine. Criteria carry different weights, and the importance applied to each individual test is somewhat arbitrary. Although there are numerous IRS rulings regarding designation, the courts have determined that IRS rulings do *not* set precedent. This is somewhat unusual; rulings in legal cases typically do create precedent. Therefore, an IRS investigator is not obligated to rely on determinations made in similar cases. Each common law test should be considered in light of its application to a specific emergency physician.

TABLE 102.5 ■ IRS 20-Factor Test[10]	
1. Instructions	Is the worker required to comply with an employer's instructions about when, where, and how to work?
2. Training	Is training required? Does the worker receive training from or at the direction of the employer, including attending meetings and working with experienced employees?
3. Integration	Are the worker's services integrated with activities of the company? Does the success of the employer's business significantly depend upon the performance of services that the worker provides?
4. Services rendered personally	Is the worker required to perform the work personally?
5. Authority to hire, supervise, and pay assistants	Does the worker have the ability to hire, supervise, and pay assistants for the employer?
6. Continuing relationship	Does the worker have a continuing relationship with the employer?
7. Set hours of work	Is the worker required to follow set hours of work?
8. Full-time work required	Does the worker work full time for the employer?
9. Place of work	Does the worker perform work on the employer's premises and use the company's office equipment?
10. Sequence of work	Does the worker perform work in a sequence set by the employer? Does the worker follow a set schedule?
11. Reporting obligations	Does the worker submit regular written or oral reports to the employer?
12. Method of payment	How does the worker receive payments? Are there payments of regular amounts at set intervals?
13. Payment of business and travel expenses	Does the worker receive payment for business and travel expenses?
14. Furnishing of tools and materials	Does the worker rely on the employer for tools and materials?
15. Investment	Has the worker made an investment in the facilities or equipment used to perform services?
16. Risk of loss	Is the payment made to the worker on a fixed basis regardless of profitability or loss?
17. Working for more than one company at a time	Does the worker only work for one employer at a time?
18. Availability of services to the general public	Are the services offered to the employer unavailable to the general public?
19. Right to discharge	Can the worker be fired by the employer?
20. Right to quit	Can the worker quit work at any time without liability?

Relationship of the Parties

In an IC relationship, the hospital or the group should not have significant control over the physician's practice. The greater the control, the more likely the relationship is to be that of an employer–employee and the greater the risk of subsequent reclassification. To clarify the intention of the relationship, IC contracts often contain language describing that intention.[11]

> *Example:* None of the provisions of this agreement are intended to create, nor shall they be construed to create, any relationship between the hospital (group) and the physician other than that of independent entities contracting with each other solely for the purpose of affecting the provisions of this agreement. Neither of the parties hereto nor any of their representatives will be construed to be the agent, employer, or representative of the other.

> *Example:* Each party to this agreement retains its own identity and full autonomy in carrying out its responsibilities in the management of its affairs. Neither party will act as the agent or employee of the other party, except as specified in this agreement. Neither the hospital (group) nor the physician will be liable to any other party for any act, or failure to act, of the other party to this agreement.

Compliance with Company Policies

> *An Employee receives instructions about when, where and how the work is to be performed. An Independent Contractor does the job his or her own way with few, if any, instructions as to the details or methods of the work.*[12]

Does the party receiving the benefit of the service have the right to control the details, manner, and method of the work? Does the hospital or group provide instructions about how the work is to be accomplished? Control of practice, activity, and specific work instructions are more consistent with an employer–employee relationship. The IRS recognizes that an insistence on adherence to recognized standards, such as licensure requirements, federal mandates, regulatory and Centers for Medicare and Medicaid Services guidelines, and so on, is not the same as an employer controlling the activities of an employee. However, an organization's mandates on meeting attendance, strict adherence to educational policies, and participation in quality-review processes meant to change practice are more consistent with employee status. Contracts for ICs should clearly state the following:

> *Example:* The physician will be solely responsible for the method and manner in which care is rendered, and that care shall be consistent with the standard of medical practice.

Training

> *Employees are often trained by a more experienced employee or are required to attend meetings or take training courses. An Independent Contractor uses his or her own methods and thus need not receive training from the purchaser of those services.*[12]

Mandatory "local" institutional training beyond orientation generally indicates an employee relationship. An employee is more likely to receive training in the particular manner requested by an employer. The training concept is distinct from required prequalifications, such as "must be residency trained in emergency medicine . . ." An orientation to the workplace and its specifics does not qualify as training. An IC should already possess the skills necessary to render appropriate care. Therefore, the IC contract should include a statement like the following:

> *Example:* The physician possesses the skills and training necessary to perform the services described herein.

Integration

Services of an Employee are usually merged into the firm's overall operation; the firm's success depends on those Employee services. An Independent Contractor's services are usually separate from the client's business and are not integrated or merged into it.[12]

Integration of a particular worker's services into a business operation suggests that the worker is an integral part of the business and is therefore an employee. In other words, when the success of a business or a business project is dependent upon the performance of a particular individual, that individual is usually deemed an employee. In emergency medicine, the job can usually be performed by one of many (interchangeable) providers. When drafting an IC contract, language stating that the "group provides physician staffing" for the emergency department (ED) should be avoided. Instead, to maintain the IC relationship, the contract between a group and a hospital should state that it "provides physician recruiting and scheduling services."

Services Rendered Personally

An Employee's services must be rendered personally; Employees do not hire their own substitutes or delegate work to them. A true Independent Contractor is able to assign another to do the job in his or her place and need not perform services personally.[12]

A contract requiring the contracted individual to provide all of the work alone suggests that the worker is an employee. The ability to subcontract the service is more consistent with an IC. However, the nature of emergency medicine prevents subcontracting. Contractually, agreements between ICs and groups or hospitals should *avoid* the use of the phrase "personal services agreement." Since most ICs do provide services on an individual basis, it is fortunate that the IRS seldom attaches great significance to this section of the 20 tests.

Hiring, Supervising, Paying Assistants

An Employee may act as a foreman for the employer but, if so, helpers are paid with the employer's funds. Independent Contractors select, hire, pay, and supervise any helpers used and are responsible for the results of the helpers' labor.[12]

This requirement is similar to the "services rendered personally" test discussed previously. An IC could subcontract with an assistant, whereas an employer would be more likely to *provide* an assistant. In other words, if the entity contracting with the physician also hires, supervises, or pays a physician's assistant or a scribe to support the physician, that factor suggests control over the physician's work environment.

Alternatively, a worker's practice of hiring assistants and paying them out of personal funds usually indicates that the worker is an IC. While it is uncommon for emergency physicians to hire and pay their own advanced practice providers (APPs), most do directly supervise these clinicians. Similarly, some groups require physicians to pay for their scribes. Those practitioners seeking IC status may wish to include language allowing the use of qualified assistants.

Example: The physician shall have the right to hire any assistants necessary to carry out the duties of this contract, as long as the cost is borne by the physician and the presence of such an assistant is in compliance with the rules and regulations of the hospital (group).

Continuing Relationship

An Employee often continues to work for the same employer month after month or year after year. An Independent Contractor is usually hired to do one job of limited or indefinite duration and has no expectation of continuing work.[12]

A long-term or continuing relationship without variation is consistent with an employer–employee relationship. This would be true of a physician who works a consistent schedule month after month in the same hospital ED without variation. Independent contractors may work for a hiring entity at irregular intervals. Arguably, a practitioner who works a varying schedule based on the changing desires of the IC or the needs of the hiring entity could be considered an IC. An IC relationship is more likely when a physician works at more than one institution or hospital.

Set Hours of Work

An Employee may work "on call" or during hours and days as set by the employer. A true Independent Contractor is the master of his or her own time and works the days and hours he or she chooses.[12]

It is necessary to schedule hours to ensure consistent and constant (24/7) coverage of the ED. Employees tend to have set hours of work with minimal deviation. Further, when the hiring entity exercises control by determining work hours without input from the practitioner, the scheduling process appears to create an employer–employee relationship. Conversely, ICs have no set hours and generally determine their own availability. Contracts containing both minimum and maximum hours of work create an "in-between" state. Contracts for ICs should contain language stipulating that the ultimate right to control hours rests with the physician, not the scheduler. However, to account for the necessities of the scheduling process, the contract between the IC and the entity may specify:

> **Example:** *For the convenience and necessity of providing coordinated service, the physician will submit, in advance, a list of (un)available workdays.*

Full-Time Requirements

An Employee ordinarily devotes full-time service to the employer, or the employer may have a priority on the Employee's time. A true Independent Contractor cannot be required to devote full-time service to one firm exclusively.[12]

While many practitioners provide the majority of their work within a single institution, the requirement to perform all gainful work at a single facility, or a stipulation placing substantial limitations on work performed elsewhere, suggests the control that an employer has over an employee. A full-time worker is generally considered to be an employee rather than an IC. While the contract with an IC may describe the minimum or maximum number of hours that the physician will work, the use of the term "full-time," as well as language that restricts the practitioner's opportunities to work elsewhere, should be avoided. Allowing a practitioner to work at other (noncompetitive) institutions independent of the current contractual relationship is consistent with an IC relationship.

Employer's Premises

Employment is indicated if the employer has the right to mandate where services are performed. Independent Contractors ordinarily work where they choose. The workplace may be away from the client's premises.[12]

Performing work on the premises of the hiring entity, particularly when it could be done elsewhere, usually indicates employee status. The importance of this factor somewhat depends on the nature of the work itself. If the hiring entity can compel the practitioner to work at specific locations at specific times, that practitioner is more likely to be considered an employee. Emergency physicians contracting with a group (or groups) for work at more than one facility are less likely to be considered employees. To establish an IC relationship, the contract could state:

Example: (Group) is contracting to recruit and schedule physicians at (hospital) and (physician) is desirous to provide services at (hospital).

Order or Sequence Set

An Employee performs services in the order or sequence set by the employer. This shows control by the employer. A true Independent Contractor is concerned only with the finished product and sets his or her own order or sequence of work.[12]

A worker is usually considered to be an employee when the group is allowed to determine the sequence in which their duties are performed. Because emergency physicians determine the order in which patients are seen and the order of care for each patient, the IRS does not use this test as a criterion to define the emergency physician as an employee. The same contract language suggested in the "instructions" test factor (above) is applicable here.

Example: The physician will be responsible for the method and manner in which care is rendered, and that care shall be consistent with the standard of medical practice.

Oral or Written Reports

An Employee may be required to submit regular oral or written reports about the work in progress. An Independent Contractor is usually not required to submit regular oral or written reports about the work in progress.[12]

If the group or hospital requires the worker to provide regular detailed status reports (distinct from medical record documentation), the worker can be considered an employee. Independent contractors are generally not required to prepare and submit reports. Many groups do require administrative reports from their medical directors, however. Medical director responsibilities should be delineated in a separate document and not listed in the primary contract if the physician wishes to avoid classification as an employee. The classification may be more complicated for medical directors, who generally have certain contractual duties beyond the provision of clinical care. Medical directors who wish to be classified as ICs could potentially have two coexisting contracts: an employee contract defining their administrative duties and compensation and a separate IC contract addressing purely clinical responsibilities. In any case, the successful navigation of these complexities requires the input of legal counsel.

Payment by Hour, Week, or Month

An Employee is typically paid by the employer in regular amounts at stated intervals, such as by the hour or week. An Independent Contractor is normally paid by the job, either a negotiated flat rate or upon submission of a bid.[12]

Workers paid by the hour, week, or month are usually employees. Workers paid by procedure or the percentage of collections and those with the potential for both profit and loss usually are ICs. Since many emergency physicians are paid based (at least in part) on an hourly rate, this form of compensation could be contractually defined as a "minimum guarantee." If the physician receives compensation beyond the guaranteed amount—relative value unit (RVU)-based compensation—IC status is suggested.

Business Expenses

An Employee's business and travel expenses are either paid directly or reimbursed by the employer. Independent Contractors normally pay all of their own business and travel expenses without reimbursement.[12]

The IRS has, in the past, paid particular attention to this common law test. Payment of travel and CME expenses and malpractice premiums by the worker suggests that the worker is an IC. Alternatively, the routine payment of travel and business expenses by the hiring firm suggests an employer–employee relationship. Contracts for ICs may state that the "physician is responsible for any business and travel expenses he or she incurs."

As a business expense, the IC physician may wish to contractually reimbursement the group on a monthly or quarterly basis for the cost of malpractice insurance. Groups will occasionally compensate the IC in an amount consistent with the cost of malpractice insurance and then deduct that amount from their payments.

Example: To provide convenience and ensure premium payments, the group/hospital may at physician's request deduct a certain amount for malpractice insurance on a monthly basis.

Tools and Materials

Employees are furnished all necessary tools, materials, and equipment by their employer. An Independent Contractor ordinarily provides all of the tools and equipment necessary to complete the job.[12]

The provision of one's own training, tools, and equipment usually is an indication of IC status. The contract should clearly state:

Example: Other than the equipment that will be provided by the hospital, the physician will be responsible for training and providing personal equipment.

Significant Investment

An Employee generally has little or no investment in the business. Instead, an Employee is economically dependent on the employer. True Independent Contractors usually have a substantial financial investment in their independent business.[12]

A significant investment in one's own business or facility, separate from the hiring entity, suggests IC status. Emergency physicians seldom invest in the particular facility in which they practice. However, the contract may reference the "significant investment" the physician has made by securing training, expertise, equipment, insurance, and so on. If an office is provided to the physician, avoid listing the office as a contractual obligation by the company (group), because the physician is not "investing" in the acquisition or the ongoing maintenance of such an office.

Profit/Loss Potential

An Employee does not ordinarily realize a profit or loss in the business. Rather, Employees are paid for services rendered. An Independent Contractor can either realize a profit or suffer a loss depending on the management of expenses and revenues.[12]

The potential to realize a profit or loss is an important and sometimes pivotal factor in distinguishing between an employee and an IC. Employees generally cannot realize a profit or loss as a result of their work and are compensated at a fixed rate regardless of the money earned or services rendered. The IRS tends to agree with a physician's IC designation if the work may lead to a profit, loss, or variable payment, such as that realized in an RVU-based performance incentive program. When possible, the IC's contract should describe compensation beyond a pure hourly rate by including variable compensation scenarios, such as a percentage of the receipts, base plus bonus, RVUs generated, and so on.

Working for More Than One Hiring Entity

An Employee ordinarily works for one employer at a time and may be prohibited from joining a competitor. An Independent Contractor often works for more than one client or firm at the same time and is not subject to a non-competition rule.[12]

Physicians who work for more than one group or hospital are typically ICs. Those who work for a single group or hospital run a greater risk of being classified as employees, particularly if there is no variation in their work location, hours, schedule, and so on. Groups and hospitals that require the physician to work only for them are more likely to be classified as employers. Correspondingly, if the physician is required to work only for a single entity, it is unlikely that the IRS will classify that practitioner as an IC. The less dependent a physician is on a single hospital or group, the more likely that physician is to be an IC. Those wishing to be classified as ICs may request that their contracts with the group or hospital state:

Example: *Physician is free to perform services at other places when not scheduled to work at the designated hospital.*

Groups with multiple practice sites may establish each as a separate legal entity and sign separate contracts and paychecks for each. The IC contract may contain specific wording that allows the physician to make independent decisions regarding their places of work.

Services Available to the Public

An Employee does not make his or her services available to the public except through the employer's company. An Independent Contractor may advertise, carry business cards, hang out a shingle, or hold a separate business license.[12]

Employees tend to work for a single specific hiring entity, while ICs have the opportunity to be hired by multiple entities.

Right to Discharge

An Employee can be discharged at any time without liability on the employer's part. If the work meets the contract terms, an Independent Contractor cannot be fired without liability for breach of contract.[12]

The group or hospital's right to fire a physician "at will" for reasons other than nonperformance implies an employer–employee relationship. Alternatively, ICs generally cannot be fired if they continue to meet their contractual requirements. An IC contract can address this issue by including a provision such as:

Example: *Hospital or group has the right to request that the physician not be scheduled.*

Right to Terminate

An Employee may quit work at any time without liability on the Employee's part. An Independent Contractor is legally responsible for job completion and, on quitting, becomes liable for breach of contract.[12]

An employee can usually terminate a contract with their employer "at will" without liability after providing a contractually predefined written notice. Independent contractors are responsible for fulfilling their obligations and may be subject to legal action if they do not. This criterion is not significant as applied to emergency physicians.

INTERNAL REVENUE SERVICE CHALLENGES

Section 530 Relief

In the event that an IRS audit determines a physician to be an employee rather than an IC, the decision can be appealed by seeking relief under Section 530 of the IRS code. Section 530 relief, if granted, permits IC designation to stand even though there may not be substantial compliance with the common law tests. To gain relief, the taxpayer must have had a reasonable basis for not treating individuals as employees. A reasonable basis is said to exist if there is a letter ruling, or if workers are recognized as ICs by either a previous audit or a long-standing practice within a particular industry.

To obtain Section 530 relief, the taxpayer must also have treated all individuals in similar positions in the same manner—and must have done so since 1978 or the inception of the practice. Additionally, all tax returns since that time must have been filed as if the individual workers were, in fact, ICs.

There have been several emergency physician-related cases in which Section 530 relief has been granted. Assuming that the other conditions to obtain this relief are met (**Box 102.2**), the major argument has been that a significant segment of the industry treats emergency physicians as ICs. Although this argument has been upheld in numerous cases, there have also been cases in which Section 530 relief has been denied.

Contractual Issues

When the IRS challenges an emergency physician's IC designation, it will closely examine the physician's contract. To this end, physicians who claim IC status should address these major areas of concern within their contracts. Of particular importance are the nature

---

BOX 102.2 ■ CONDITIONS NECESSARY FOR SECTION 530 RELIEF

Taxpayer must have had a "reasonable basis" for not treating individuals as employees.

- Judicial precedent, published ruling, or letter
- Past audit
- Other individuals in similar positions also not employees
- Long-standing, recognized practice of a significant segment of the particular industry
- Treatment the same since 1978 (or since inception of the practice)
- All tax returns filed as if individual not an employee

of the relationship and the method of tax payment. The contract should clearly state that the physician is an IC and will be treated as such under the IRS code. Any use of the word "employee," "employer," or "employment" should be avoided. The contract should additionally state that the physician is personally responsible for any and all taxes, including state and federal unemployment tax.

CONCLUSION

The decision to designate an emergency physician as an IC rather than as an employee is frequently a complex one, and any group or individual that chooses the IC status must be aware of the potential for an adverse ruling by the IRS.[4] Audits are more likely to be favorable if the common law tests are substantially addressed within the group/hospital contract. If requested, the IRS will issue a ruling on the group's classification before an audit; this strategy is not generally recommended.

Emergency physicians should realize that the goal of the IRS is to increase tax revenue and that, as well-paid professionals, physicians will continue to be closely scrutinized "targets" of the organization. The decision to become an employee or an IC requires both a thorough working knowledge of the regulatory issues and advice from the appropriate legal, financial, and tax advisors.

With gratitude to Stephen J. Dresnick, co-author of a previous version of this chapter, and to Scott M. Slovin, Esq, tax attorney and partner at Wood & Lamping, LLP, for his thoughtful and discerning review.

REFERENCES

1. Dresnick SJ, Crook PL. Employee versus independent contractor status. In: Strauss RW Jr, ed. *Contracts: A Practical Guide for the Emergency Physician*. American College of Emergency Physicians; 1990.

2. US Internal Revenue Service (IRS). Independent contractor defined. Available at: https://www.irs.gov/businesses/small-businesses-self-employed/independent-contractor-defined. Updated January 23, 2020. Accessed August 6, 2020.

3. US Internal Revenue Service (IRS). Definition of business expense. Available at: https://www.irs.gov/businesses/small-businesses-self-employed/deducting-business-expenses. Updated March 16, 2020. Accessed August 6, 2020.

4. US Internal Revenue Service (IRS). Self-employment tax (Social Security and Medicare taxes). Available at: https://www.irs.gov/businesses/small-businesses-self-employed/self-employment-tax-social-security-and-medicare-taxes. Updated February 12, 2020. Accessed June 30, 2020.

5. Tools and calculators: retirement planning. Edward Jones: Making Sense of Investing (website). Available at: https://www.edwardjones.com/preparing-for-your-future/calculators-checklists/calculators/retirement-savings-calculator.html. Accessed January 8, 2019.

6. US Internal Revenue Service (IRS). Independent contractor (self-employed) or employee? Available at: https://www.irs.gov/businesses/small-businesses-self-employed/independent-contractor-self-employed-or-employee. Updated July 31, 2020. Accessed August 6, 2020.

7. American Rights at Work. Billions in revenue lost due to misclassification and payroll fraud. 2010. Available at: http://americanrightsatwork.org/20100809-908-116-116_iz3k7tgw3o0jvrspii2ipv-2/. Accessed September 12, 2018.

8. IRS expected to crack down on worker misclassification in construction industry. Jobs with Justice. 2010. Available at: https://laporte.com/knowledgecenter/tax-services/irs-expected-to-crack-down-on-worker-misclassification-in-construction-industry. Accessed September 13, 2018.

9. US Government Accountability Office. Employee misclassification: improved coordination, outreach, and targeting could better ensure detection and prevention. Report No. GAO-09-717. 2009. Available at: http://www.gao.gov/products/GAO-09-717. Accessed December 13, 2018.

10. Regent University. Independent contractors: IRS 20-factor test. 2020. Available at: https://www.regent.edu/admin/busoff/pdf/20-questions1099test.pdf. Accessed August 4, 2020.

11. Clousson JP. Key contract clauses. In: Strauss RW Jr, ed. *Contracts: A Practical Guide for the Emergency Physician*. American College of Emergency Physicians; 1990.

12. Texas Workforce Commission (TWC). Appendix E: TWC independent contractor test. Texas.gov. Available at: https://twc.texas.gov/news/efte/appx_e_twc_ic_test.html. Accessed October 13, 2018.

CHAPTER 103

EQUITY, PARITY, AND GROUP STRUCTURE

Thom A. Mayer, Robert W. Strauss, Jay Kaplan With Mark Reiter, Joel Stettner

Emergency medicine is by necessity a group practice. The requirement of a team of multiple physicians to staff an emergency department (ED) has resulted in numerous models of emergency medicine group practice. These models most commonly include physicians employed by or contracted with the hospital or medical group practices; democratic physician groups (ranging from single hospitals to multiple sites); sole proprietorships; regional or local groups; and large, multihospital national groups.

The type of ED group at a specific hospital varies widely, often because of factors like the history of the ED at that institution; preferences of the CEO, board, and medical staff; and the availability of emergency physician resources within a given geographic area. The taxonomy of emergency medicine groups has been inconsistently defined and inadequately articulated.[1] Nonetheless, it is common for emergency physicians to have deeply held views on the best structure, ranging from small "democratic groups" to physician groups providing services in multiple states and multiple specialties (**Box 103.1**).[2,3]

QUALITY IN EMERGENCY MEDICINE

Woven into this group structure concept is the notion of emergency medicine as not only an art and a science but also a business.[4] The primary goal of the ED should always be quality patient care. However, quality patient care itself has multiple definitions and is an ever-changing, "moving target." In traditional thinking, "making the right diagnosis, and providing the right treatment" was considered "quality." However, current and emerging concepts in the health-care environment affirm that the definition of quality also involves

BOX 103.1 ■ PRIMARY GROUP STRUCTURES

ED structures:
- Hospital employees (or independent contractors)
- Physician group practice employees
- Democratic groups
- Partnerships
- Corporate models—single hospitals
- Corporate models—multihospital groups
- Sole proprietorships

ED diversification:
- Hospital medicine
- Pediatric hospitalists
- Surgical hospitalists
- Obstetrical hospitalists
- Anesthesiology
- Radiology
- Pathology

a careful understanding of, and effective and satisfactory response to, the multiple and diverse customers involved in the delivery of health care.[5,6]

These customers include families, payers, EMS providers, medical staff members, administration, and the hospital board, as well as internal stakeholders, including emergency physicians, emergency nurses, technicians, and other essential personnel. In addition to clinical and service quality, elements of patient safety, flow, and the ability to form and grow close partnerships with the hospital, its nurses, and the medical staff also help to define quality care.[7]

When physicians are tasked with maximizing potential revenues while providing care in an increasingly resource-constrained environment, "quality patient care" begins to look more like a confusing, confounding witches' brew than a clearly defined entity. Regardless of the group structure, however, all these elements of quality must be considered and addressed as fundamental responsibilities.

The Changing Health-Care Environment

Dramatic and rapid changes changes in the health-care environment have resulted in fundamental structural alterations in the way medical care is planned, organized, financed, and delivered in the United States. These changes have been driven partially by legislative changes, with a major drive coming from the marketplace participants themselves.

Value-based programs have replaced volume-based and fee-for-service reimbursement as the US health-care system seeks to deliver the highest possible quality at the lowest possible cost. Indeed, "becoming the high-quality, low-cost health care provider" has become the mantra of health-care boards and their leadership teams. Emergency physician groups must be aware of this and be responsive to the demands placed on the system and on themselves by the system's stewards.[8,9]

As emergency medicine has continued to develop, both as a clinical specialty and as an important component of the overall health-care environment, it has become increasingly clear that the application of sound business principles to the clinical practice of emergency medicine is not just an attractive option but rather an *absolute requirement* for a successful practice. As the attention to and understanding of emergency medicine have grown, the multitude of stakeholders has, at a seemingly exponential rate, placed increasing demands on emergency providers and their groups.

For the ED, this new set of expectations has created an even more important need for a sound understanding of business principles. These expectations include quality, physician stability in a changing market, cost-effectiveness, contracting experience, responsiveness to changing health-care requirements, and the ability to function effectively in a team model as opposed to an independent environment. Consistency of practice and standardization of care are no longer options but necessities.

Consequently, it is critical that the group structure holds physicians accountable for the measurable delivery of quality care that can be accomplished reliably, predictably, and demonstrably. Now more than ever, provider accountability is a core feature of successful physician groups, particularly in the ED.

DEFINITIONS

Before we continue discussing these issues in emergency medicine, here is a review of relevant definitions.

Group structure: Group structure refers to the organization and the relationships between emergency physicians and the institutions they serve. The structure must address the functional elements of the group, including the diverse professional, personal, financial, and fiduciary components. Specific definitions for types of group structure are included in the following sections, including hospital employees or individual independent contractors, democratic groups, partnerships, corporate models for both single hospitals and multihospital groups (MHGs), and sole proprietorships.

Equity: Equity is derived from the Middle English term meaning "fair or reasonable." The current definition is 1) the quality, state, or ideal of being just and 2) the money value of a property beyond any liability associated with it.[10] The etymology of this word is instructive, as the term "equity" is often associated with "ownership" in the current context of emergency medicine practice. To say that one wants equity usually means that one wants a piece of the action. Too often, it is assumed that this only means a share of the profits, but the definition clarifies that any monetary value associated with ownership must take into account the liability contingent as well, including both profits and losses.

The derivation of the term "equity" suggests fairness, justness, and equality, which raises important issues with regard to emergency medicine's group structure. Emergency physicians within a group manage the same patients in the same environment and by nature want to be in an environment that is fair, reasonable, and just. Emergency physicians desire a situation in which their voices can be heard, particularly amid the current changes in health care. As emergency physician groups begin to address the issue of equity, it is often important to weigh the time, energy, effort, and dollars that were spent in building the practice. The goal of providing equity for the more junior partners requires careful consideration about how to value the "sweat equity" expended by the founding physicians in obtaining and developing the contract.

However, the concept of equity in a group practice must always ensure that what is best for the patient is central to the group's and individual practitioner's mission. The goals of the group should never supersede the fundamental purpose of providing quality care and caring to those who entrust their well-being to the practitioners.

Vesting: Vesting is Latin in origin, from the word meaning "to clothe or place in vestments." In current use, vesting usually refers to a time, performance, commitment, or financial schedule by which new members are assimilated into the equity structure of an existing group. Such vesting schedules not only apply to emergency physicians but also to other physicians and to other professionals, such as accountants, lawyers, architects, and others. The origin of the term is again instructive: Vesting new members into a group involves "clothing" them in higher positions within the group, as well as taking on associated responsibilities.

Parity: Parity is also Latin in origin and has a simple meaning—"equality." In essence, the term parity among practitioners simply means that individuals of a group are treated in an equal fashion. Although the terms equity and parity are often used synonymously, they are not the same. In fact, the concept of a vesting schedule or advancement to senior physician status limits true parity, at least at the outset of the relationship. If a physician must be vested into partnership over a period of years or at a financial cost, equality isn't truly equal – it is only subject to a consistent treatment.

Application and interpretation of the term "parity" are subject to substantial variation. For example, the concept of parity may be applied in a way that treats and pays each partner in exactly the same fashion and at exactly the same level, regardless of contribution or effort. However, many groups have redefined parity to include productivity-based incentive plans that recognize variable contributions made by different physicians at the same level of the group structure. Although this is a concept that cuts across the principle of strict equality (parity), many believe that this variation addresses the issues of fairness in a more reasonable fashion and holds physicians accountable for the volume and quality of their work.

Stock: The commonly accepted definition of this term (in this context) relates to the shares of a given corporation offered for purchase or transfer to attain equity status with the group. Yet, the unavoidable analogy of the tree trunk as the foundation on which the tree exists has important connotations as it relates to current understanding of ED groups.

ESSENTIAL GOALS OF EMERGENCY MEDICINE GROUPS

The goals of emergency physician groups vary, but the following goals are appropriate for an emergency physician group, regardless of its specific structure:

- Provide quality patient care for every patient, every time.
- Provide quality service to diverse groups, including the patient's family, the medical staff, administration, and EMS.
- Provide personal and professional growth opportunities for individuals in the group.
- Provide a practice opportunity that is intellectually stimulating and emotionally fulfilling, engendering a long career in emergency medicine.
- Provide the ability for the group to be responsive to rapid health-care changes.
- Provide a practice that is economically viable and fiscally sustainable.
- Provide a fair and equitable practice opportunity.
- Provide an environment in which the opinion of the emergency physician can be voiced in a meaningful fashion.

The importance of each of these goals will vary among individual emergency physicians and across different emergency physician groups. Critical questions should be asked when assessing a group's intentions and achievement of goals.

Quality Service

Quality patient care is a distinction that should form an essential benchmark for any ED group.

- Does the group hire only qualified, experienced emergency physicians, or is it more interested in simply filling shifts with warm bodies?
- Does the group actively define, distribute, and ensure individual accountability for its patient care objectives and protocols? As an example, is there a protocol that requires practitioners to "hand off" patients at the changes of shift in a manner that meets the highest standard of safety, care, and communication?

The concept of quality of service also extends to other internal and external customers of the ED environment.

- Does the group value the building of outstanding staff relationships as much as it does a physician's clinical competence and technical skill?
- Does the group address the needs of these diverse interests?
- Does the definition of quality for the group include a high degree of professionalism with family members, nurses, medical staff, and EMS?

Growth Opportunities

Providing personal and professional growth opportunities for the emergency physicians in the group is an area of increasing importance.

- Does the group have a recognized structure for ensuring that the individual can develop their personal and professional career goals and objectives? Or, is the physician going to be considered an "FTE" (full-time equivalent) whose very function is to comply with the dictates of senior management?
- Are there defined administrative paths that physicians can pursue as their knowledge and experience expand?
- Does the group have a philosophy of growth that might allow the individual an opportunity to assume a position as a medical director or chair?
- Is the personal growth of the individuals comprising the group an issue of central importance to the group's leadership?

Practice Environment

An intellectually stimulating and emotionally fulfilling practice environment is important to most emergency physicians. For those just out of residency, practicing in an environment where multiple ill or injured patients are seen can be particularly helpful when preparing for and passing the board examination in emergency medicine.

- To what extent does the group and the structure provide the emergency physician the opportunity to update the skills, abilities, and expertise found in recent developments in emergency medicine?
- Is there support for and encouragement of continuing medical education (CME)?
- Does the group provide these opportunities itself, online, or at group-sponsored meetings?

Responsiveness to Change

It is also important that the group responds to the rapid changes occurring in the health-care environment. For example, the group's structure must allow it to quickly and efficiently adapt to health-care reform (e.g., accountable care organizations [ACOs], new billing and coding structure, etc.), including negotiating favorable contracts that allow the hospital to obtain its objectives. Similarly, the group must have the capacity to determine which, if any, practice diversification opportunities (e.g., urgent care, freestanding ED services, chest pain centers, geriatric and pediatric EDs, etc.) it should pursue.

- What internal or external expertise does the group have to address the changing health-care environment?
- How has the group fared during recent regulatory, financial, and other system changes?

Economic Viability

One of the most often ignored aspects of ED group structure is the necessity of providing a practice that is economically sustainable. For example, an ED without experienced leadership that does not apply sound business principles to its practice may be doomed to fail despite its other attractive attributes. Regardless of the specific structure, each emergency physician group must ensure that the business knowledge and expertise required for successful practice are maintained throughout the life of the group. In many cases, this expertise will reside with individual group members. In others, it must be sought through consultants, advisors, or affiliation agreements.

Fair and Equitable Practice

The last two goals for the emergency physician group—fairness and ensuring that the voice of each group member is heard—have become the source of substantial controversy. Among the most important questions that emergency physicians ask are:

- Does my opinion matter?
- Will our voices be listened to when considering scheduling, departmental operational decisions, group structure changes, long-term development, and financial issues?

Although seemingly straightforward, these issues of fairness can be difficult and confusing since what constitutes fairness for one person may seem grossly unfair to another. For example, a recent residency graduate may operate under the theory "same patients, same acuity, same shifts." As such, the new physician should have the same voice in the departmental structure and financial disbursements as the senior partners in the group. Conversely, senior partners may believe in the theory "we struggled, assumed risk, and built this practice that allows you to be successful." They might contend that the 10 years they spent building the practice and strengthening its integration into the hospital and the community implies a more long-term vesting schedule for financial disbursements. Those same partners may feel comfortable ensuring the "new" group member has an equal voice in departmental operations while insisting on a more graded integration of that new member into the business and financial structure of the group.

GROUP STRUCTURE ALTERNATIVES

Of necessity, any classification of emergency physician groups is somewhat arbitrary. The intention of the following classification is to list not only structural but also functional categories that allow the creation of taxonomy of emergency physician groups. What such groups are called is far less important than how they operate on a daily basis. As emergency physicians approach practice opportunities, it is incumbent on them to determine which structure best meets their professional, personal, philosophical, and financial needs. In many cases, groups may have features of more than one of the structures described below.

Ideally, the taxonomy should allow emergency physicians to classify existing groups, as well as look creatively at the formation of new ED groups when those opportunities present themselves. The primary goal of the following classification system is to create a framework for comparison and to describe potential advantages and disadvantages. In many cases, there are overlapping structural elements; absolute distinctions cannot be made. Without exception, functionality, not strict taxonomy, determines the success or failure of the emergency physician group. Each of the following group structures will be characterized by general description, advantages, disadvantages, and overall assessment.

Hospital Employees

Emergency physicians may be contracted directly with the hospital in either an employment relationship or as independent contractors. This discussion focuses primarily on hospital-employee structures as it is far more common. In employee relationships, the hospital usually provides a detailed employment contract with clearly defined terms and benefits. As the employer, the hospital withholds taxes, specifies hours of service, and establishes the parameters of practice for the physician.

All of the emergency physicians required to staff the department are directly contracted by the hospital. The hospital typically handles recruitment, credentialing, and recontracting. To ensure that departmental administrative duties and tasks are performed, the hospital will select and contract with one or several emergency physicians to assume various leadership positions, such as quality oversight, EMS director, and (associate) medical director/chair.

While the employment relationship with the hospital may be straightforward, the relationships among the physicians may be less clear. Still greater confusion will occur if the contractual relationships, requirements and obligations, and financial structures vary widely from physician to physician.

Certain health-care organizations have increasingly chosen to employ primary care and specialty physicians, including emergency physicians. This approach to physician employment is a strategy to ensure coverage, control resource utilization, and capture profit margins.[11] The advent of single-service providers such as ACOs and value-based contracting programs can decrease competition and costs.

Advantages

There are some advantages to these relationships (**Table 103.1**). First, if the physician affiliation with the hospital is the same for all, there will be less competition among the physicians. Second, hiring the physicians allows the hospital to utilize a single taxable entity for all its employed physicians. This can be of theoretical and practical significance to the hospital, the physician, and the IRS. Third, there is no "middleman" involved in the transaction or relationship, so there is a direct passage of salary to the physician. However, this may or may not maximize the emergency physician revenue because the determination of salaries may not be directly related to revenue, and the collection of revenue by the hospital depends solely on the hospital's ability to bill and collect for emergency physician services.

Some emergency physicians prefer this direct hospital relationship because it eliminates "dependence" on other physicians, contract groups, or a contract that must be renewed intermittently. Some emergency physicians who prefer this relationship might assert they have greater power and control over their personal practice as they do not have to conform to

TABLE 103.1 ■ Emergency Physicians as Hospital Employees or ICs

Advantages	Disadvantages
Less competition between physicians	Labor intensive for the hospital
Single taxable entity per physician	Frequency of negotiations
Perceived independence	Lack of ED physician recruitment infrastructure
Rapid decisions on contract changes, coverage, etc.	Multiple, sometimes dissimilar contracts
	Little group cohesiveness
	Lack of authority for medical director
	"Group" may lack leverage in negotiating with the hospital
	Poor billing for professional services on the part of the hospital

a group's rules, scheduling requirements, and programs. The physicians are only responsible for their own day-to-day practice.

An additional potential advantage is that the physician can make quick, independent decisions when contracting with the hospital. For example, when any change of the relationship is considered, such as the compensation rate, benefits, work hours, and conditions, employed physicians need only consult themselves, their business advisors, and their families to determine their negotiating stance.

Disadvantages

There are several potential disadvantages of a direct employee or independent contractor relationship with the hospital. Recent surveys conducted by hospital administration publications demonstrate a continuing trend toward outsourcing contracting with specific defined entities to provide hospital-based physician services.[12]

First, hospitals have increasingly found that physician–employment relationships may be difficult and quite different from their more typical labor relationships with nurses, technicians, housekeepers, and so on. The physician relationships may involve multiple and frequent negotiations with individual physicians, rather than a single negotiation with a person representing a group of physicians.

Second, it may be increasingly difficult for hospitals to successfully recruit and retain sufficient numbers of emergency physicians, particularly when the number of board-certified emergency physicians is increasing slowly and those available are choosing to limit the number of hours worked.[13]

Third, in attempting to meet the needs of a diverse group of physicians from different specialties, the hospital often finds itself with multiple, varying employee/independent contractor relationships and payment/incentive structures. These variances may be difficult to justify from the standpoint of corporate compliance and the IRS.

Fourth, a group of individually employed physicians may have little or no group cohesiveness. Instead, the emergency physicians may operate independently because they feel little allegiance to an administrator to whom they report, as opposed to an ED director or group. This can result in a less collegial interaction among the emergency physicians, due in part to this lack of group camaraderie.

Fifth, emergency physicians who are individually contracted with the hospital have little or no leverage or power in contract negotiations with the hospital. As a result, they may be less effective when advocating for additional resources, increasing hours of physician coverage, and responding to market pressures.

Whether intentionally or not, hospital administrations are in a strong negotiating position when dealing with employed physicians, potentially permitting a "divide-and-conquer" strategy. Under such circumstances, it may be easy for the hospital administration to terminate and replace an emergency physician on very short notice. This is true both of the individual physicians and of the overall "group" of individuals.

When considering practice diversification or additional contractual relationships, hospital-employed physicians have limited capital and access to resources to diversify and expand their practices. Thus, this group of emergency physicians will find significant limitations and restrictions should they wish to grow, either internally (fast-track services, chest pain EDs, trauma center verification, and others) or externally (off-site freestanding clinics, additional ED contracts, and so on).

One of the most important potential disadvantages of hospital-employed physicians is that hospitals' billing processes and personnel can be notoriously untrained and ineffective at billing and collecting for emergency physician professional services. This is particularly true if the hospital assesses billing revenue when considering clinician salary and benefits.

Further, the collection procedure from the hospital is often inadequate to build a substantial revenue base for the emergency physician group practice. Given the increasingly difficult economic environment in which hospitals exist, the added financial pressure from poor billing procedures increasingly causes hospitals to view the employed ED physician group as a "loss leader" instead of a revenue center for the hospital. This perspective generally leads to limited support and capital expenditures.

A functional variation of the emergency physician as an employee of the hospital is often seen in academic medical centers. In most cases, emergency medicine faculty are employed by the institution or by a faculty practice plan and have a reporting relationship through a designated chair of the department. Many such departments have a combined structure that involves simultaneously being hospital employees with reporting structures through a semi-independent department and financial payments through faculty practice plans.

Overall Assessment

In assessing the hospital-as-employer structure, there is no ownership of the practice revenues or accounts receivable by the group or individuals. Instead, ownership and control, to the extent they exist, reside with the hospital or the administrator. There is usually a director or chair identified as having responsibility for overall operations, but the contractual structures may vary within a single institution, and it may be difficult to tell where control lies. At one extreme are academic medical centers in which the chair of the department has a discrete aspect of control. At the other extreme are medical directors or chairs whose contracts do not give them substantial control/authority over the individuals for whom they are responsible.

Similarly, the responsibility for the provision of services varies widely under this model. The physicians may perceive that their responsibility is solely to themselves and their patients. In this setting, there is little to no control over operational issues such as other hospital personnel, hours of coverage, quality, metrics, or advocacy for improvements.

Profit distribution is generally not a consideration because (a) the contractual structure often results in a cash shortfall for the hospital and (b) should profits exist, they would probably go into the institutional coffers. When a faculty practice plan is in place, "profits" or moneys collected above a baseline may be distributed based on a variety of incentives.

Liability is limited to the individual physician's professional liability, which is usually covered under the hospital's master malpractice insurance policy. It is critical for the physician to ensure that reporting endorsement or "tail" coverage is contractually provided by the hospital should the physician leave the practice. The issue of *investment* of time, energy, and effort may or may not be appreciated by the hospital (employer).

In summary, there are advantages to physicians working as employees of the hospital, particularly in academic medicine, and there are institutions in which this model has operated successfully. However, as reimbursement becomes an increasing issue, hospitals will try to achieve the delicate balance between owning the emergency physician practice and creating incentives to ensure a fully engaged group. It will be more difficult for hospitals that do not have the expertise necessary to maximize billing and collections for the ED physician component. Moreover, as hospitals become increasingly aware of the importance of management/leadership training and mentoring, customer service, flow, and evidence-based guideline development and implementation, they will have to find a way to incorporate these resources.

Physician Group Practice Employees

As the growth of the group practice alternative increases, many emergency physicians may be offered opportunities to practice with large group practices. Most of these groups regard their physicians as employees, but some regional practices provide independent contractor jobs.

Physician group practices may have their own hospitals or they may practice in for-profit or not-for-profit hospitals, but it is rare for group practices to employ emergency physicians unless they own and operate the hospital or ED. These groups typically have defined leadership structures, including medical and administrative personnel who manage the business aspects of the practice.

Advantages

Group practice models have many of the same advantages as the hospital employees model, including excellent benefit and retirement packages, clear definitions of hours worked, favorable schedules, and good relationships with other employees, including the nursing and essential services staffs (in models where the hospital is owned by the physician group practice). When the group practice includes the entire medical staff, responsiveness of on-call physicians may be dramatically improved. The responsibilities of physicians in administrative roles are usually clear and recognized in the medical staff structure. Depending on the geographic area, the type and nature of the patients may be quite different from those in nearby community hospitals, and, in many cases, nearly all of the patients are insured.

Disadvantages

Like hospital employees, emergency physicians in this model do not own equity in the form of ownership of the accounts receivable, so there is no accrued financial return upon leaving the group. For patients who require admission but are not part of the group practice plan, arrangements may need to be made for transfer.

Overall Assessment

Many emergency physicians have found group practice employment a favorable model in which to practice. However, this depends on local circumstances and individual physician preferences.

Democratic Emergency Physician Groups

The essential feature of democratic physician groups ("pure" democratic groups and groups with defined equity) is that all members (sometimes after a certain trial, "earn-in," or probation period) share in the decision-making efforts of the group and, in most cases, its ownership. This usually applies not only to decisions on the type, number, and specific emergency physicians to be hired but also to financial decisions, group expansions, contractual relationships with the hospital, and policies and procedures.

Most democratic groups are partnerships, but not all partnerships are democratic groups because a small number of partners may be owners of the contractual relationship. Many democratic groups rotate or elect the chair or medical director on an ongoing basis, while others allow physician leaders to remain in their roles for extended time periods. However, this turnover of the leadership position feature is not essential to be considered a democratic group.

The most common description of partnership democratic groups is summarized by the concept of "equal voice, equal pay, and equal responsibility." However, as with all partnerships, equal responsibility comes with equal exposure to potential liabilities, such as changes in reimbursement, decreased volume, altered market share, and the rising tide of expectations and demands that hospitals place on emergency physician groups. Most democratic groups contract as a discrete entity with the hospital to provide emergency physician staffing and management services. Finally, a common feature of democratic groups is the availability of contractual and financial information—"open books" (including medical director fee compensation)—among all partners.

Advantages

The advantages of small democratic groups (**Table 103.2**) certainly begin with the capacity for shared decision-making and investment and motivation on the part of the emergency physicians to make the practice successful. Because each individual within the group has the capacity to guide the group's direction, there is strong incentive for the individual to perform at the highest possible level to ensure the success of all members. As owners, members of a democratic group may be the most motivated to meet the long-term needs of the hospital and are likely to live and work within the community for much of their careers.

Similarly, ownership of the group is commonly shared in a democratic or quasi-democratic fashion. In larger democratic groups, individual input at the local level remains while decisions by a chosen group of representative peers guides the group on a more global/organizational level. Physicians who "own part of the rock" perceive themselves as "owners" rather than "renters." Unvested physicians may feel their only responsibility is to work their hours, while owners are more likely to see themselves as an integral part of the social fabric of the ED and the hospital medical staff in general.

Theoretically, members of a democratic group may achieve higher compensation for the individual physicians by eliminating costs associated with an operational or business "middleman." This presupposes that the business acumen, financial expertise, and resources are available within the group (or through contracting with a management services provider) to optimize potential revenues. The costs of these services may or may not lead to enhanced net revenue. When such expertise is available (either internally or externally), higher compensation may result with all other costs being equal (i.e., cost of recruiting, educational resources, business resources, and so on).

Recruitment may be easier for democratic groups because some data suggest that board-certified or residency-trained emergency physicians prefer a group practice option when it is available within their desired geographic area. In addition, retention of the group members may be easier if they view themselves as owners.

Self-direction is another potential advantage of democratic groups. These groups have the capability of answering their own key questions, creating a greater sense of

TABLE 103.2 ■ Democratic Groups

Advantages	Disadvantages
Shared decision-making	Potential of labor intensity of decision-making
Common investment and motivation	Breaking logjams when consensus cannot be reached
Profit from cutting out the "middleman"	Rotating medical directors
Defined team approach	Potential to underfund administrative time
Recruitment advantages	Potential for "analysis paralysis"—is a 9-1 vote a tie?
High retention rates	More limited capital and access to resources
"Open books" information policy	Single-signature contracting
	Physician accountability in dealing with outliers
	"Supermajority" clauses

empowerment. The group can decide how administrative responsibilities will be handled and funded. Questions that a democratic group must address include:

- Will there be a single medical director or chair with all of the administrative duties, or will there be a medical director with additional administrative duties split up among the members?
- Does the office of the chair or medical director rotate, or does it reside with a single individual over a prolonged period of time?
- How will the group fund the considerable administrative time needed to successfully manage the contract in a complex and demanding health-care environment?
- How are decisions made regarding the physician administrators' hours to be worked or shifts to be covered?

Disadvantages

The disadvantages of democratic groups begin with the labor intensity of such structures. Although this is especially true for small democratic groups, this challenge may be mitigated in larger practices that can create an effective internal management services division.

With complete democracy, decision-making and rapid response to change can be impeded by the lack of a single leader capable of committing to that decision or change. Some hospital administrators would rather have a single person who can make decisions, a "go-to person," rather than the potentially slower process of having all members of the group participate in each decision. Overly inclusive decision-making can result in "analysis paralysis." Hospitals moving toward value-based models increasingly insist on a rapid response and "single-signature capability" to quickly contract with insurance companies. Prolonged debate by a group to gain detailed consensus could impair the hospital's ability to move quickly into managed care relationships.

Ineffective groups do not decide how administrative responsibilities will be handled and funded (see questions above). Effective groups will often elect a core group of physicians empowered to lead the group and make decisions on behalf of the group. It is particularly important for the group to define:

- Stable leadership structure with decision-making authority
- Adequate protected and paid time for its leaders and to fund the considerable administrative time needed to successfully manage the contract

Structuring the relationship of the group to encourage a long-term commitment is an important part of all ED practices. To attain the greatest potential benefit of a democratic group requires a long-term commitment from each of the members. The required commitment provides substantial incentive for group members to remain at the facility for the long term. However, it might also limit the ability of physicians to leave the group and move to other practice opportunities.[14]

The capital access required for expansion may be limited in small democratic groups. As a result, many small groups have formed alliances to bring in or outsource critical resources. This gives these groups broader exposure to business expertise, access to capital, and sharing of resources like recruiting, quality improvement, and physician billing services. In addition, emergency group coding/billing vendors and ED management companies have become increasingly sophisticated, allowing the small groups contracting with a vendor access to a similar level of resources available to the largest groups.

A particularly significant issue for democratic groups is ensuring a mechanism of physician accountability. When all physicians are "equal," the medical director or the group as a whole must have the authority to deal with those who do not meet the group's or hospital's expectations. Partnership should not guarantee job security. Physicians who

> **BOX 103.2 ■ CASE STUDY: PHYSICIAN ACCOUNTABILITY**
>
> - The ED group is democratic and "open books." As a member, you believe that this is the ideal practice model for emergency medicine.
> - However, the CEO insists on a contractual performance clause tied to customer satisfaction scores.
> - Despite an aggressive customer service focus, two of the eight partners have low scores, and they are getting worse.
> - The group requires a "supermajority" of 75% of the partners to eliminate a partner.
>
> - Issues:
>   - Are the outlier partners putting the contract at risk?
>   - Does the medical director have the authority to counsel and mentor the physicians, or is it strictly a "one-person, one-vote" group?
>   - What happens if the outlier physicians refuse to change?
> - If a small group of physicians has consistently poor metrics, will they be allowed to pull down the entire group or will they be forced to increase their results?

are too slow, are not committed to patient satisfaction, or do not practice quality medicine have to be held accountable. As the case study in **Box 103.2** indicates, this is an increasingly important topic. Some groups require a "supermajority" of two-thirds or three-fourths of all voting members to deal with outlier physicians who consistently underperform. Since one outlier physician can put a group's contractual relationship at risk, mechanisms must exist to address these problems.

Overall Assessment

Regarding ownership, democratic groups create a sense of parity. Thus, fully vested partners usually have an equal share and an equal voice in department operations. In most cases, such groups have defined structures for junior physicians to progress to senior physician status, including various types of cash buy-ins, "sweat equity," deferral of bonus payments, and initially increased hours of clinical coverage.

Similarly, the concepts of control and responsibility are equally distributed within a democratic partnership. Shared decision-making, with its strengths and weaknesses, is an essential part of a democratic group. In most cases, the responsibility for ensuring that the group's contractual and philosophic obligations are met is also shared. A central issue for members of a democratic group is the openness of the financial books, including the ability to know the revenues, expenses, and profit distribution. Although the distribution of profits may differ among members, an important feature of these groups is open review, discussion, and debate. Similarly, the liability and investment are usually equally shared among members of democratic groups.

Partnerships

A partnership is an association of two or more persons as co-owners of a business for profit. A partnership may be similar to a democratic group but with fewer and potentially unequal partners. Partnerships may involve a single hospital or an MHG. Partners share the profits and losses of their business and participate in management according to a predetermined agreement or formula, perhaps based on prorated ownership of shares. The partnership agreement reflects the relationship, establishes the culture of the organization, sets a tone of collegiality and respect, sets forth guidelines for running the business, and delineates ways in which the partnership can be dissolved or modified to meet the changing needs of the partners. A partnership agreement also:

- Delineates the purpose, definitions, and terms of the organization
- Lays out specific capital contributions and accounts
- Addresses the governance of the organization, including reporting lines of authority and limitations, compensation, distributions, and liabilities
- Defines noncompete clauses and terms for dissolution of a partner's participation
- Refrains from defining day-to-day operational management
- Defines the compensation structure

The partnership agreement often requires changes over time, particularly when additional partners or hospitals are added.

Partnerships pay no income tax directly, and profits and losses are passed onto the individual partners. Partners are generally liable for the acts of their partners, although individual partners can also incorporate to limit their liability. In some states, only licensed professionals can participate as partners in a professional practice. In others, both professionals and nonprofessionals can legitimately act as partners.

Advantages

The advantages of a partnership structure (**Table 103.3**) include a lack of the legal encumbrances found in more formal corporate structures, the lack of a separate tax structure, and the avoidance of double taxation on profits generated by the business. In addition, when properly conceived and implemented, the partnership can establish a culture based on collegiality, respect, and adaptation, formalized through written guidelines for resolving differences among physicians. A partnership offers both an important long-term perspective and an opportunity for individual growth. When a partnership reaches a certain size (the precise level is open to debate), it may also provide financial leverage, including benefits, contracting flexibility, development of related business entities for professional liability insurance, billing, and the ability to absorb partners elsewhere in the group should an individual hospital contract be lost.

Disadvantages

The disadvantages of partnerships may be similar to those of a democratic group. The lack of internal human or capital resources as well as leadership skills may limit the partnership's ability to respond to changing environmental conditions. Further, if a clearly defined decision-making structure and partnership agreement is not in place before signing the initial hospital contract, the partnership may be limited in its ability to effectively address a specific need.

TABLE 103.3 ■ Partnerships

Advantages	Disadvantages
Simple legal structure	Potential lack of a clearly defined decision-making structure
Lack of separate tax structure	Verbal versus written agreements
Firm culture of group	Lack of clear pathways to adding additional partners
Ability to customize benefit plans	Management of accounts receivable when partners leave
Development of related businesses	Physician accountability issues

As an example, occasionally emergency physicians have a verbal agreement to create a partnership but have not completed the complex negotiations necessary to form a legal partnership that delineates the precise details of the partnership. The ideal solution for this potential problem requires a partnership agreement to be set up in advance that clarifies such issues as how new partners will be brought into the group, whether based on longevity, hours worked, financial contribution, attainment of board certification, and so on. Like democratic groups, partnerships need a clear and functional mechanism to define how physician accountability will be handled and by whom.

Overall Assessment

The partnership is owned by the partners as defined in the agreement itself. Similarly, control resides with the management structure as defined by partners in their preexisting agreement. In most circumstances, the partnership has a specific administrative structure delineated at the individual hospital level. When partnerships cover multiple hospitals, a central governing board of directors or management team usually exists. This entity usually has the responsibility for ensuring the contractual obligations of the partnership are met in a timely and appropriate fashion. Profits may be disbursed in several different ways according to the relationship delineated in the partnership agreement.

Single Hospitals

A corporation is a legal entity that is separate and independent from its stockholders. Emergency medicine corporations are usually structured as professional or personal services corporations like those in law, engineering, architecture, accounting, actuarial sciences, and consulting. Corporations are usually characterized by the principle of limited liability, meaning that individual shareholders are not liable for the acts of other shareholders or for the debts or liabilities of the corporation. However, individual shareholders are liable for their own negligence or wrongdoing. Corporations are subject to the laws of the state in which they legally reside and are subject to stipulated accounting requirements. Generally, corporations are structured like partnerships, with the specific formative details determined by the individual physicians who form the original partnership or corporation. Corporate profits are usually distributed prior to the end of the year to avoid additional ("double") taxation to the shareholders.

Most corporations allow emergency physicians to purchase stock and do not specifically limit the number of shareholders. Most require a specific stock repurchase agreement (when the stock is "privately held") to allow buyback of stock if a shareholder leaves the group. The precise language regarding these stock repurchase agreements is generally determined in advance to clarify the stock valuation procedure to be followed in the event the corporation is liquidated or shareholders leave the corporation to pursue other career opportunities or to retire.

Advantages

Corporate models with specified buy-in arrangements offer advantages like those of a partnership arrangement. Physicians usually have strong incentives to pursue stock purchase agreements and ensure the corporation is successful. Profits are usually distributed according to a predetermined formula. Liability is limited for stockholders, and the corporate structure avoids risks of double taxation.

Disadvantages

Disadvantages include the need for certain legal and accounting fees to meet state and local regulations, potential corporate licensing fees in certain states and jurisdictions, and the need for the shareholders to abide by corporate bylaws (or revise them to meet their needs).

Overall Assessment

While generally less common than partnerships, it can be a very successful structure for those inclined to pursue this option.

Multihospital Groups

Although partnerships and corporations may each operate at multiple sites, "MHG" is used here to describe larger corporate entities, often operating in several states. Individual emergency physicians may work for MHGs as employees or independent contractors. While physicians may have significant ability to influence the local practice, they will have limited ability to control the larger entity unless they achieve status as a medical director or regional medical director. Multihospital groups vary widely in their size and sophistication.

A significant goal of MHGs is to take advantage of their size to provide "economies of scale" and "consistency of resources." Rather than outsourcing services, they typically create and provide a broad range of internal programs (**Box 103.3**). These resources may strengthen the practice of emergency medicine and provide substantial benefit for both the patient and the emergency physician, assuming they are actually delivered and not just advertised.[15]

Many MHGs have expanded their service lines to include hospital medicine, anesthesiology, radiology, surgical and pediatric hospitalists, pathology, and even post-acute care. As these product lines develop (provided they align with strategic incentives with the hospital and produce measurable results), the group will be able to embed more deeply within the institution as well as reduce the need for subsidies for these services—a very powerful strategy in these capital-constrained times. To achieve similar advantages, some smaller groups of various structures and even some larger partnerships have affiliated to pursue this strategy. However, it is simply easier to create practice integration with the shared infrastructure, billing, recruiting, and performance improvement capabilities of a large organization that has capital to invest.

Advantages

Among the major advantages of large MHGs (**Table 103.4**) is the ability to deliver highly sophisticated and value-added services to each institution, including small ones. Although some smaller groups have been successful in accessing additional resources, it may be difficult to create these services anew in a cost-effective manner and to maintain them may require substantial, dedicated, and ongoing resources and efforts.

BOX 103.3 ■ INTERNAL PROGRAMS BY MHGS

- Professional leadership training
- Customer service training and support
- Recruiting and credentialing programs
- Risk reduction and management
- Patient safety and error reduction programs
- Clinical decision support systems
- Quality improvement programs
- Benefit packages
- CME opportunities
- Informatics programs, emergency medical record support, scribe systems
- Practice diversification potential
- Billing, coding, reimbursement strategies
- Wellness programs
- Nursing support programs
- Integrated service programs (e.g., hospital medicine, anesthesia, radiology, etc.)

TABLE 103.4 ■ MHGs	
Advantages	**Disadvantages**
Potential to deliver a wide range of value-added services	Profit margins must be fair and competitive
Economies of scale	Lack of formal equity ownership
Billing expertise may create better returns	Potential corporate practice of medicine issues
Single contractual entity	Potential recruitment and retention issues
Ability to mentor medical directors	
Multiple product lines	

Large MHGs have experience with multiple payers and often have the ability to effectively negotiate. Economies of scale create relatively robust support systems at a lower than usual cost, leaving the net revenues available for distribution to providers. As a result, physician compensation can be at or above market rates. Further, nuanced productivity-based payment systems are frequently available for the practitioners.

Multihospital groups have large internal support structures that provide practitioner and medical director recruitment, training, and ongoing mentoring. They often develop large collaboratives among their medical directors to share issues and problems and come up with solutions that can be shared. The MHG offers the potential advantage of broader support for scheduling and coverage constraints to the hospital when a rapid change in coverage or practitioner replacement, including the director, is required.

For the individual physician, multiple practice sites allow a practitioner to continue to work for the same group when the physician chooses to change the practice location. In this way, the physician can stay with a familiar organization and maintain whatever seniority and goodwill has been earned. Another critical advantage provided by most large MHGs is the opportunity for internal career advancement as leadership opportunities become available. Examples include positions as directors, associate directors, regional medical directors, and risk management coordinators.

Disadvantages

The most common criticism of MHGs is they may be driven by profitability for the shareholders. These groups operate with an intended profit margin. The requirement for profitability may take away from monies that might otherwise be used for physician salaries. Alternatively, and ideally, additional profit margins are generated by significant economies of scale, particularly in the areas of billing and collections, professional liability insurance, expenses related to recruiting and providing physicians, and so on.

For a physician who desires practice equity or ownership, MHGs offer very limited options. Those physicians may be less likely to commit to a long-term relationship with a hospital. Occasionally, senior members of the group may be offered equity positions. Some MHGs have acquired smaller emergency physician groups, providing principles/members of the smaller group with equity in the larger group through stock buyouts.

Overall Assessment

The issues of ownership and investment in an MHG structure are under the control of the group itself. The individual practitioner is not subject to the group's liability, that is, financial losses pertaining to the contractual relationship. However, "local" control, responsibility, and profits (when incentive-based productivity programs exist) may be under the control of the members of the group. Multihospital groups create "economies of scale" and often develop and provide attractive positions for career advancement.

Sole Proprietorship

A sole proprietorship in emergency medicine usually consists of an individual physician (occasionally more than one individual—a "limited proprietorship") who forms a corporation and holds a personal services contract with the hospital or health-care system. The sole proprietorship simply means that 100% of the ownership of the entity/corporation resides with a single individual who is responsible for staffing and managing the ED with qualified emergency physicians. The contract may also specify additional services, including performance improvement processes, risk management, nursing in-services, occupational health, direction of EMS, and so on. Under this model, the sole proprietor assumes the risk and management responsibility for ensuring the contractual obligations are met. There may be substantial financial risk at the outset of the contract, particularly if the terms are fee-for-service, where start-up costs can be considerable.

Although sole proprietorships are responsible for the overall contractual relationship, staffing, and management of the ED, the specific structure and leadership can vary. Physicians within the group can be hired as employees or independent contractors. Sole proprietors may operate in an autocratic fashion or as benevolent leaders. In the former, all ownership, control, responsibility, profit disbursement, decision-making, and liability reside with a single individual. In the latter, sole proprietors may share control, decision-making, responsibility, and profit disbursement but not liability.

Advantages

The primary advantage of sole proprietorships (**Table 103.5**) is the ease of decision-making and the availability of a single, clearly identified individual with whom the hospital administration can work to reach decisions.

Similarly, in third-party reimbursement negotiations, this single-signature approach can help ensure the physician group will readily participate in prescribed agreements. Sole proprietorships have clear lines of authority for business decisions and for operational decisions regarding the ED. Assuming a well-structured and financially successful contractual relationship with the institution, the sole proprietor will try to maintain a long-term commitment

TABLE 103.5 ■ Sole Proprietorships

Advantages	Disadvantages
Single, clearly defined voice for the hospital	Potentially unfair physician compensation
Single-signature contracting with payers	Vulnerable structure that could collapse if the sole proprietor dies or becomes incapable of providing service
Clear lines of authority	Requires clear, fair, adaptable contracts with both the hospital and its clinicians
Dealing with physician accountability	Performance may suffer if physicians are not empowered to share in decision-making
Can address parity of physicians and fairness	Liability clearly resides with the sole proprietor

to provide services. In the best of circumstances, sole proprietorships will adapt and change their structure to meet the needs of the individuals within the group, the hospital client, and the community, provided that the sole proprietor recognizes the need and has the capacity to adapt. Finally, sole proprietorships can be operated in such a way that they incorporate the best features of groups with shared decision-making.

Disadvantages

One of the disadvantages of a sole proprietorship is that both the hospital administration and the physicians "have all their eggs in one basket." If the sole proprietor dies or becomes disabled, incapacitated, or incapable of providing service in any way, the structure of the contract would require reconsideration.

Under certain circumstances, sole proprietorships can be unfair to the practitioners in a number of ways, not the least of which are financial and undue exercise of power by the individual holding the contract. If substantial patient care revenues are directed to the sole proprietor, physicians working clinically could receive inappropriately low compensation that is well below the market value. As such, the structure of relationships with the sole proprietor is in the most critical aspect of the contract. The relationship defined by the contracts with both the hospital and the clinicians should be clear, fair, equitably applied, and capable of adaptation based on the changing needs of the parties. Sole proprietors who are unable to react to these changes place themselves and their groups at a disadvantage.

If the group's physicians are not empowered to substantially share in the decisions and financial success of the group, their performance may suffer due to dissatisfaction, lack of incentive, and poor retention. If members of the group do not perceive themselves to be vested in the ED and hospital, they may be less likely to be committed to a long-term relationship with the hospital and community.

Overall Assessment

In a sole proprietorship, both the ownership and liability clearly reside with the sole proprietor. However, control may vary widely, from a situation in which the sole proprietor exercises complete dictatorial control to one in which he or she develops a structure and mechanism to ensure that individual physicians have a voice in management decisions, application of business principles, recruiting, and so forth. Similarly, the responsibility for meeting contractual obligations could either be handled by a single individual or shared among physicians in the group. Finally, profit disbursement can be highly variable, from "none" to formulas tying compensation to a productivity/fee-for-service or modified fee-for-service approach based on billing and collection information.

CONCLUSION

The elements of group structure and function are essential to an understanding of practice opportunities in emergency medicine. Although no specific taxonomy has previously existed for emergency medicine group structure, there have been attempts to help identify the ways in which emergency medicine practices respond to the needs of their constituents. This chapter provides a classification system that broadly represents the ways in which emergency medicine is practiced. Understandably, some groups do not easily fit within a single category and may span several.

In choosing a setting in which to practice emergency medicine, analyzing the group structure according to the precepts described here may be of some assistance. However, for most practitioners, the most important factor leading to the choice of a practice opportunity is *location*. When location is the primary factor, choices will be limited to the types of practice available within that geographic setting.

Over 25 years ago, Mayer and Cohen offered four essential questions to help address whether or not an emergency physician should affiliate with a group[16]:

- Is the group's primary commitment to quality medical care for every patient?
- Are the principals of the group practicing emergency physicians?
- Does the group foster growth and development for individual emergency physicians, as well as the practice of emergency medicine as a whole?
- Is the distribution of resources and compensation fair?

These questions are as pertinent today as they were 25 years ago, and they constitute a reasonable checklist by which an emergency physician can assess practice opportunities. The taxonomy offered here is intended to be functional in nature. It is ultimately the responsibility of individual emergency physicians to determine how to choose a practice that meets their own needs, those of the profession, and those of their family.

REFERENCES

1. Larsen LC, Allegra JR, Franaszek J. Equity buy-in structures of emergency medical group practice. *Am J Emerg Med*. 1993;11(1):28-32.
2. Sims J. The Good, the bad and the ugly. 2011. Available at: www.acep.org/Content.aspx?id=79270. Accessed July 1, 2013.
3. AAEM, Vision Statement, https://www.aaem.org/about-us/our-values/vision-statement Published 2020, American Academy of Emergency Medicine, Accessed, June 9, 2020.
4. Mayer T, Jensen K. *Hardwiring Flow*. Gulf Breeze, Fla: Fire Starter Press; 2010.
5. Roski J, McClellan M. Measuring healthcare performance. Now, not tomorrow: essential steps to supportive healthcare reform. *Health Aff*. 2011;30:682-689.
6. Kahn CN. Payment reform will not transform healthcare delivery. *Health Aff*. 2009;28:216w-218w.
7. Mayer T, Cates R. *Leadership for Great Customer Service: Satisfied Patients, Satisfied Employees*. Chicago, Ill: Health Administration Press; 2004.
8. Pauly M. The trade-off among quality, quantity and cost: how to make it—if we must. *Health Aff*. 2011;30:574-580.
9. NEJM Catalyst. What is value-based healthcare? Available at: https://catalyst.nejm.org/doi/full/10.1056/CAT.17.0558. Accessed June 9, 2020.
10. James BC, Savitz LA. How intermountain trimmed healthcare costs through robust quality improvement efforts. *Health Aff*. 2011;30(6):1185-1191.
11. *Webster's III New Riverside University Dictionary*. Boston, Mass: Riverside Publishing; 1994.
12. Staiger DO, Auerbach DI, Beurhaus PI. Trends in the work hours of physicians in the United States. *JAMA*. 2010;303(8):747-753.
13. Iglehart JK. Doctor-workers of the world unite! *Health Aff*. 2011;30:556-558.
14. Modern Healthcare 32nd Annual Outsourcing Survey. Available at: www.modernhealthcare.com/article/20100920/DATA/100919950. Accessed September 20, 2010.
15. Mayer TA, Cohen RL. Entrepreneurism and benchmarks of emergency medical practice. *Ann Emerg Med*. 1984;13(12):1161-1163.

LEGAL AND REGULATORY ISSUES

SECTION 10

CHAPTER 104

EMTALA FOR EMERGENCY DEPARTMENT LEADERS

Robert A. Bitterman

EMTALA, the Emergency Medical Treatment and Active Labor Act, governs virtually every aspect of hospital-based emergency services.[1,2] Consequently, medical and nursing leaders of the emergency department (ED) are charged with achieving overall compliance with EMTALA as it relates to this primary access point. Additionally, hospital leaders frequently look to the ED leaders as the most knowledgeable resources on EMTALA and expect them to assist the hospital, its legal counsel, compliance officer, risk manager, and medical staff leadership to ensure that the hospital complies with the law.

Department leaders should ensure all EMTALA issues related to the ED and the organization are adequately addressed in both policy and practice. A compendium of the key issues—an EMTALA compliance checklist—is included in **Box 104.1**. A best practice

---

BOX 104.1 ■ EMTALA COMPLIANCE CHECKLIST

1. Adopt (and enforce) organization-wide and ED-specific EMTALA policies.
2. Educate all appropriate staff and care providers.
3. Define the organization's medical screening exam (MSE) process, including identifying "DEDs" and designated "QMP" to perform the MSE.
4. Establish the organization's patient stabilization procedures and documentation.
5. Ensure access to the MSE, stabilizing care, on-call specialists, and/or transfer to a higher level of care is unencumbered.
6. Review ED/outpatient registration and payment collection procedures and address any delays on account of or to inquire about the patient's insurance status or other demographics.
7. Maintain processes and procedures regarding patient refusal of the MSE, stabilizing treatment, or transfer.
8. Evaluate the current ED physician on-call system to validate its effectiveness and compliance with written duties and responsibilities; establish a process for routine monitoring and reporting of compliance failures.
9. Ensure a uniform system, with standardized documentation, for transferring patients out of the facility.
10. Establish clear and specific written guidelines for accepting or rejecting patient transfers from other facilities.
11. Ensure appropriate documentation requirements are being met for all ED patient records, a clear and concise central log for patients presenting to the facility, transfers out of the facility, and on-call lists for specialists.
12. Verify that all required signage related to EMTALA is clearly visible in areas used for MSEs, including but not limited to the ED, L&D, and behavioral health intake centers.
13. Monitor and evaluate the organization's quality assurance review processes related to EMTALA compliance.
14. Maintain agile and actionable policies and procedures to report suspected EMTALA violations to CMS.
15. Review the potential application of EMTALA to the organization's outlying emergency care access points (e.g., UCCs, free-standing emergency departments).

16. Research and consider the relationship between federal and state EMTALA laws, as well as medical malpractice liability insurance coverage.
17. Review disaster management plans and public health emergency responses for EMTALA issues.
18. Draft and utilize legally approved EMTALA forms to achieve/document compliance.

BOX 104.2 ■ TYPICAL MEMBERS OF A HOSPITAL EMTALA COMPLIANCE COMMITTEE

- Legal counsel
- Compliance officer
- Risk manager
- Physician vice president of medical affairs or chief medical officer
- Medical, nursing, and/or administrative director of the ED
- Medical, nursing, and/or administrative director of labor and delivery
- Transfer center coordinator (if the hospital operates a transfer center; if not, then a leader who is intimately involved with transfers to and from other hospitals)
- Medical staff member: a physician who actively participates in the hospital's ED on-call coverage
- Patient-access leadership

to achieve compliance is to form a hospital EMTALA compliance committee **(Box 104.2)** to ensure that each item on the list is appropriately addressed.

ADOPTING AND ENFORCING EMTALA POLICIES

The Centers for Medicare and Medicaid Services (CMS) requires written policies and procedures governing organizational EMTALA compliance. An ED-only EMTALA policy or a solely hospital or ED transfer policy is not adequate.[3,4] Therefore, ED leaders must work with hospital administration, legal counsel, and risk managers to ensure that organizational EMTALA and ED policies conform and are current and operational. Department leaders should also be prepared to serve as subject matter experts in training and maintaining compliance with these policies. Specifically:

- ED-specific policies should include triage and medical screening processes, labor-and-delivery (L&D) encounters, interactions with emergency medical services (EMS), patient transfers, accepting transfers from other facilities, on-call practices, and admission processes. These ED policies should also include systems to handle volume surges and crowding situations.
- All EMTALA-related policies must be critically reviewed by knowledgeable individuals who are capable of recognizing potential medical and legal pitfalls. "Failure to follow your own rules"—that is, ill-conceived written policies and a failure to abide by them—is a primary source of litigation under EMTALA. Plaintiffs' counsel routinely aim to prove that the organization caused harm by deviating from its own established triage or medical screening policies ("disparate treatment" claims under EMTALA or state laws).

- Failure to enforce EMTALA policies or censure noncompliant behavior is itself a violation of the law.

Educating Appropriate Staff

It is essential to educate all caregivers on potential EMTALA issues. Most individuals who work in health care, even those within the ED, have little knowledge of the breadth of the law and its impact on medical practice. The CMS requires that organizations provide EMTALA education to all employees, particularly on issues related to emergency care capabilities, specialty services, and patient transfer, including:

- Education of all facility personnel, including medical staff, administration, nurses, clerical staff, volunteers, and security, in basic EMTALA awareness
- Special EMTALA training for ED L&D caregivers
- Mandatory EMTALA training for all new members of the medical staff as a condition of privileges; continuous training for all members of the staff
- In-depth training for all providers who accept transfers into and out of the hospital, including:
    - Administrators responsible for ED operations or transfer systems, such as physician referral lines or transfer centers, and those taking administrative call for the facility
    - Medical staff leadership and bylaws committees
    - Legal counsel, compliance, and risk personnel

MEDICAL SCREENING EXAMINATIONS

The CMS requires that a medical screening examination (MSE) and stabilizing treatment must be provided to any individual who presents to a dedicated emergency department (DED) seeking care. The law does not state for an "emergency condition," as it is the purpose of the MSE to determine whether each individual case is indeed an emergency (as defined by the statute).[2] Organizations are responsible for addressing the primary medical screening requirements, including where the MSE is conducted, who can conduct the exam, and how standard screening is defined. Uniformity is a requirement. All patients should get the same MSE (process) based on their chief complaint and medical condition, regardless of their status or ability to pay.

Identify DEDs

It is important to determine which areas of the hospital are considered CMS DEDs (and therefore must comply with EMTALA). Specifically, organizations must examine whether their ED, L&D, psychiatric screening or intake center, walk-in clinics, or urgent care centers (UCCs) meet the legal definition of a DED and must comply with the law.[5]

Designate Qualified Medical Personnel

The governing body of the institution must formally designate in writing who is qualified to perform screening examinations in each of the facility's DEDs.[5] Appropriate qualified medical personnel (QMP) may include physicians or advanced practice providers (APPs). In L&D, specially trained nurses may be the designated QMP to rule out active labor in patients with labor-related complaints. When a nurse is the QMP on an L&D unit, there must be 24-hour backup from an on-call obstetrician (who must be called for each case and is the final medical decision-maker in all instances). Labor and delivery nurses should not be placed in the position of ruling out other potential emergent medical conditions that are not labor related. These should be escalated to an advanced provider on site.

Define the Hospital's Standard Screening Process

The facility must clearly define and adhere to a standard MSE process for patients presenting to the DED. The scope of the MSE must be "reasonably calculated" to exclude the presence of an emergency medical condition (EMC); this includes utilizing necessary tests, ancillary services, and on-call specialists when necessary.[5] Emergency department leaders must ensure that policies, procedures, and protocols are drafted carefully to address multiple at-risk presentations, including fever, repeat and abnormal vital signs, chest pain workup protocols, and so on.

Address the Treatment of "Nonemergencies"

The screening of patients with complaints that appear to be "nonemergencies" is also governed by EMTALA and should be no different than for those with obvious emergencies.[5] While the *scope* of the diagnostic studies for the MSE may vary depending on the nature of the patient's complaints, the *process* of screening patients should not vary. Potential problem scenarios, such as those that should be specifically addressed in policy and for which education should be provided, frequently include forensic evidence collection (e.g., police blood alcohols, evidence collection for alleged rape) and referrals for procedures from outside providers. In these instances, if the patient declines the MSE, hospital policy should require the patient to sign a waiver form (**Figure 104.1**) to document that the individual was not denied but rather declined their "federal right to a MSE."

PATIENT REGISTRATION AND TRIAGE

The collection of insurance information and other nonessential demographics should never delay an MSE. In fact, only information that is reasonably necessary to provide care should be collected prior to the exam. Triage is the primary touch point for persons seeking care at the DED. Triage staff and patient-access personnel must be extensively trained and well versed on all matters related to EMTALA. Triage by the registered nurse does not constitute an MSE unless specifically outlined (for specific circumstances) in the institution's QMP policy and procedures. Additionally, organizations should implement clear and comprehensive patient registration and triage policies that address the potential EMTALA issues that may arise (**Box 104.1**). All providers and staff at any patient-access point must be intimately familiar with these policies.

Private or "VIP" Patients

In some hospitals, members of the medical staff may meet their private patients in the ED. These patients are examined and treated by this medical staff member instead of an ED provider on duty. This practice is entirely appropriate to maintain physician–patient relationships and is allowable under EMTALA. However, the hospital should have prearranged procedures for handling private patients that ensure no delay of the patient's MSE. Delays in treatment can result in patient morbidity or mortality as well as organizational liability under EMTALA for failure to provide an "appropriate" MSE.

All private patients should be triaged according to the organization's established protocols. An emergency provider should see the patient in the order consistent with the usual practice of the ED, generally in the order of acuity and time of arrival.

FIGURE 104.1 ■ **Sample Refusal of Screening Exam and Treatment Form**

PATIENT DENIAL OF REQUEST FOR A MEDICAL SCREENING EXAMINATION/PHYSICIAN ORDER CONFIRMATION

Under federal law, the hospital's emergency department must provide a medical screening exam to determine if an emergency medical condition exists for any individual who requests examination or treatment. At General Hospital, this exam is performed by a physician. If you want to receive a medical screening examination, please tell your nurse. If you do not wish to have a medical screening examination, please check the appropriate statement below and fill out the information requested.

I am presenting to the emergency department for:

☐ Laboratory test(s) ordered by my physician, or

☐ Radiological procedure (x-ray, CT, MRI, or nuclear medicine) ordered by my physician

☐ Scheduled out-patient visit for _____, to see Dr _____.

☐ Other _____

I do not request a medical screening examination to determine whether I have an emergency medical condition, nor do I request treatment for a medical condition at this time. I understand that the hospital is willing to provide me with such an examination and treatment should I ask for it. Furthermore, I am not asking the hospital, its personnel, or the emergency department physician to analyze the laboratory test or radiological procedure results.

Print name: _____

Date of birth: _____ SS# _____

Signature: _____

Parent or guardian in case of minor: _____

Address: _____

City, state, zip: _____

Date: _____ Time: _____

Witness: _____

<u>Confirmation of order: (to be completed by clinical staff)</u>

Ordering MD: _____

Test ordereed: _____

Select one: _____ Verbal order called to department
_____ Written order sent with patient

Confirmed by: _____

- If the private provider comes to the ED and sees the patient before an emergency provider, then the examination by the private provider will generally constitute the required MSE.
- If the patient's primary provider has not arrived by the time the emergency provider would normally examine the patient, the emergency provider should perform an MSE. Upon examination by the emergency provider:
  ☐ If no EMC is evident, the patient can wait for their primary care provider to arrive.

☐ If an EMC does exist, the emergency provider should undertake appropriate stabilizing treatment until the patient's provider arrives, at which point an appropriate transition of care can occur.
- If at any point the patient's condition deteriorates, an emergency provider should be consulted to screen and assist with stabilizing treatment.

Minors

The organization must conduct an MSE on any unaccompanied minor who requests treatment or on whose behalf a request is made (even if it comes from a layperson, another minor, law enforcement, or the EMS staff), irrespective of whether consent has been obtained from the parent or legal guardian.[5,6] Consent is a creation of state law, and it is preempted by federal law (EMTALA) under the supremacy clause of the US Constitution. The MSE should never be delayed to obtain consent or demographic information.

If the MSE reveals no EMC, caregivers can—and generally should—wait to obtain proper consent from the minor's parents or legal guardian before proceeding with further treatment. If an EMC does exist, stabilizing treatment should be provided as needed while prudent attempts are made to gain consent.

Labor and Delivery

If L&D is used to perform screening examinations to rule out active labor, the process must be uniform for all patients, and the interplay between L&D and the ED must be clearly defined in advance. Both departments must conform to the same EMTALA requirements. Documentation is critical since there is a great deal of confusion regarding "labor," "active labor," "false labor," and what exactly is required to screen pregnant women.

EMERGENCY MEDICAL SERVICES

Hospitals in the jurisdictions of the First and Ninth Circuit Court of Appeals must address EMTALA issues, which may stem from EMS direction by their ED telemetry stations. The states and US territories controlled by the ninth circuit are Arizona, California, Hawaii, Idaho, Montana, Nevada, Oregon, Washington, Guam, and the Northern Mariana Islands. The states and territories controlled by the First Circuit include Maine, Massachusetts, New Hampshire, Rhode Island, and Puerto Rico.[7]

Hospital-Based Telemetry Control

Appellate courts hold that any telemetry radio contact to the hospital's ED constitutes "coming to the ED" and a "request for examination and treatment of a medical condition." EMTALA is "triggered"; therefore, the hospital is required to provide the patient an MSE and stabilizing treatment (unless the hospital is already on diversion). If instead the hospital directs EMS personnel to take the patient to another facility for *any reason* (not including community trauma protocols, etc., but including reasons like managed care status, indigent status, doctor preferences, etc.), the decision can be subject to a retrospective analysis to determine if the hospital violated EMTALA.

Thus, the hospital could face potential civil litigation under federal law and fines or termination from Medicare because of its physician's judgment. This is an enormous expansion of hospital liability that applies regardless of state-enacted statutory liability protections; federal law supersedes state law because of the supremacy clause of the

Constitution.⁷ In US jurisdictions other than the First and Ninth Circuit Court of Appeals, diversion of EMS *before* arrival on hospital property is not an issue governed by EMTALA.

EMS on Hospital Property

EMTALA controls the hospital's initial contact with EMS providers once they come to the ED (actually, once they are anywhere on hospital property).[5,6]

Medical Screening Examination

The hospital may not divert the ambulance off hospital property, regardless of whether or not the hospital is capable of handling the patient's emergency condition. First, the emergency physician (or other QMP) must perform an MSE before any patient can be transferred away from the hospital. (However, the location of the MSE is not defined, and it is not a violation of the law if the emergency physician performs the MSE in the back of the ambulance and then immediately transfers the patient to a more appropriate facility, provided the transfer is done according to the "appropriate transfer" rules discussed later in this chapter.) Triage itself does not count as an MSE under federal law, and triage nurses are not allowed to divert the ambulance away for *any* reason.

Early Triage of EMS Patients

Even when the hospital is overwhelmed, all EMS patients must be triaged shortly after arrival to the ED. Previously, some overcrowded EDs ignored ambulance patients and left EMS personnel to care for them until the hospital accepted the patient, a practice CMS calls "EMS parking." These hospitals and EDs erroneously believed that, unless they accepted responsibility for the patient, they had no EMTALA duty to provide care. The CMS issued a memorandum reminding hospitals that their EMTALA obligation begins the moment the patient "comes to the ED," not when the hospital "accepts" the patient.[8]

In a clarifying memo, CMS later acknowledged that certain circumstances (e.g., an influx of multiple trauma victims) could make it reasonable for the hospital to ask the EMS provider to continue to care for the patient until the ED staff becomes available. However, it is still mandated that "even if a hospital cannot immediately provide an MSE, it must still triage the individual's condition immediately upon arrival to ensure that an emergent intervention is not required and that the EMS provider staff can appropriately monitor the individual's condition."[9]

Emergency department leadership should review the two CMS memos defining the interactions with EMS, and educate the entire staff on these issues. The practice of "parking" EMS patients may also violate Medicare regulations, which require hospitals to "meet the emergency needs of patients in accordance with acceptable standards of practice."[10]

STABILIZATION REQUIREMENTS

If it has the capability to do so, the hospital must stabilize the patient's EMC prior to transfer or discharge from the ED. This stabilization includes utilizing the services of the physicians on call if their expertise is needed.[2,5,6]

- CMS regulations state that admission to the hospital ends the application of the law, but there are caveats to the "admission defense" for hospitals.[5]
    - The admission must be in "good faith" and not a ruse to circumvent the hospital's obligations under EMTALA.
    - The patient must be formally admitted. This essentially means that the patient is admitted with the *intent* to:

- Occupy an inpatient bed
- Receive inpatient hospital services
- Stay overnight in the hospital—even if it does not happen (e.g., if an admitted patient boarded in the ED is eventually transferred or improves and can be discharged before an inpatient bed actually becomes available)
  - ☐ An actual written admission order will be required to claim EMTALA ends.
  - ☐ Admission to observation status does not count as admission for purposes of ending the application of EMTALA. This includes patients "admitted" to an ED observation center or chest pain center.
  - ☐ If an individual develops an EMC while an inpatient, EMTALA does not apply to that hospital or its medical staff.
  - ☐ CMS regulations also state the other hospitals do not have to accept transfers of inpatients under EMTALA, even if the transferring hospital cannot stabilize the patient and the potentially accepting hospital can. Hospitals asked to accept inpatients in transfer have no legal obligations under EMTALA, according to CMS, and therefore can choose to accept insured patients and reject uninsured patients with no federal consequences.[5,6]
- CMS's inpatient regulations do not apply to civil litigation in Michigan, Ohio, Tennessee, and Kentucky.[11]
  - ☐ The Sixth Circuit Court of Appeals rejected CMS's inpatient regulations in the case of *Moses v. Providence Hospitals*.[11] The Sixth Circuit holds that the EMTALA stabilization requirement applies to the discharge or transfer of inpatients, exactly as it applies to the discharge or transfer of ED patients. Thus, in these four states, patients sent home or transferred even after prolonged stays must be stable under EMTALA, and the hospital is subject to civil liability and regulatory sanctions exactly as in the case of ED patients—markedly expanding potential liability and regulatory penalties against the hospital and discharging physicians.
  - ☐ Additionally, since EMTALA still applies to inpatients in these four states, more capable hospitals still have an EMTALA obligation to accept inpatients in transfer when the admitting hospital is unable to manage the inpatient's emergency condition.[11]

No Delay for Insurance Information/Authorization

A core principle of EMTALA is nondiscrimination. Therefore, hospitals cannot discriminatorily provide emergency services based on an individual's insurance status or ability to pay. In other words, hospitals cannot deny or delay access to the MSE, stabilizing care, on-call physicians, or accepting patients in transfer for economic reasons.

- **MSE:** The screening examination must not be delayed because of an effort to obtain authorization for coverage or payment from a third-party payer.[2,5]
  - ☐ Do not delay the MSE by asking questions about insurance, seeking authorization for payment from a third-party payer, requesting copayments or signatures on Medicare's advanced beneficiary notification (ABN) forms.
  - ☐ Do not attempt to influence the patient by bringing payment or coverage issues to the patient's attention prior to screening.
  - ☐ First triage patients. Then examine and treat them in the order determined by their medical acuity. Blind the clinical staff to the patient's payer status until disposition, that is, triage decisions should be made without knowledge of the patient's payer status.
  - ☐ Ensure that triage and patient-access staff know how to handle patients who ask about insurance or financial questions regarding their ED visit, such as whether

their insurance will cover the visit or how much it will cost to receive care in the ED. These staff members should be trained to neither discourage nor coerce the patient in any way. Staff should encourage patients to stay and defer economic discussions until after an MSE and any necessary stabilizing treatment is performed.
- **Stabilization:** Once it is determined the patient has an emergency condition, further treatment must not be delayed while obtaining authorization from payers for further care, admission, or transfer of the patient. This includes the involvement of on-call physicians and other hospitals accepting patients in transfer.

After the MSE and initiation of stabilizing treatment, economic considerations can be taken into account while determining the patient's future care.

REGISTRATION AND PAYMENTS

Hospitals may conduct reasonable registration procedures in the ED, including collecting insurance data (but not cash or other forms of payment) at the time of registration, as long as the process does not delay triage or the MSE.[5,6] During the registration process, the patient can sign the hospital's usual "informed consent to be examined" form and routine paperwork that holds the patient financially accountable for any charges not covered by their insurance carrier.

The key to an effective and permissible process is to create parallel tracks for medical and financial issues and ensure that the financial track never interferes with clinical care in any way. Bedside registration is probably necessary under the existing regulatory scheme to avoid "no-delay" violations, as CMS considers any delay in access to the MSE for the purpose of completing registration to be against the law. Waiting for treatment because of volume and capacity constraints is not a violation; however, delaying an exam to conduct registration practices other than those necessary to initiate a patient encounter is likely a violation.

CMS warns hospitals not to coerce patients into leaving before they receive their federally guaranteed right to an MSE, stating "reasonable registration processes may not unduly discourage individuals from remaining for further evaluation."[6] Collection of copays, down payments, ABNs, or signatures on managed care forms may constitute such "economic coercion" if not done very carefully. Hospitals must also ensure that staff behavior does not create a "hostile environment" or "constructive denial" of the MSE.

PATIENTS WHO REFUSE CARE

Patients who leave before an examination, treatment completion, or against medical advice present high-risk medicolegal encounters for EDs. These situations also place the hospital in a difficult position with respect to EMTALA; hospitals must be able to demonstrate that they did not deny any individual their federally mandated right to an MSE and stabilizing treatment. Patients with capacity have the right to make decisions about their own health care. It is incumbent upon the members of the medical team and, in particular, the clinician in charge to ensure and demonstrate that those rights are addressed.

Written Informed Consent

The hospital must take all reasonable steps to obtain the patient's informed written consent for refusing the examination, treatment, or transfer. (This requirement legally applies only to the stabilization or transfer of patients the hospital determines to have an EMC. It does not apply to patients refusing the MSE).[1,2,5,6]

Avoidance of "Constructive Denial" of the MSE

All staff must be prepared to deal with patients considering or intent on leaving the ED without receiving or completing an examination or treatment. Staff must never be seen as "encouraging patients to leave" or "unduly discouraging them from staying."[6]

Refusal Form

The hospital must explain its legal obligations under the law and the risks and benefits of refusing the examination. It must also determine if the patient has the capacity to refuse and then obtain the patient's signature (see Chapter 105). The emergency physician or the patient's private physician should always be involved in this process.[1,6] If the patient declines to sign the refusal form, then a hospital representative should sign a statement indicating that the patient was offered but refused the examination and refused to sign the form.[6]

Patients Who Leave Before Treatment is Complete

Patients who leave before treatment is complete include those who have arrived in the ED (therefore are included in the central EMTALA log) and subsequently:

- Leave prior to triage
- Leave before being seen by a provider
- Elope without notice
- Leave against medical advice

Hospitals must create systems that clearly demonstrate that patients who left the ED before their treatment was completed did so voluntarily or without notice and that those patients were offered the opportunity to have an MSE and stabilizing treatment without delay.

HOSPITAL ON-CALL PHYSICIAN REQUIREMENTS

EMTALA governs the hospital's physician on-call backup system for the ED.[3-5] The hospital and medical staff must provide guidelines by which physicians must take call, including how often. The guidelines must provide an easily accessible schedule that clearly outlines on-call coverage for the ED. The ED must know *prospectively* whether a particular specialty has coverage available for each 24-hour period. This information is critically important to notify local EMS providers of the services available for transferring patients to other facilities and for accepting or rejecting patients from other hospitals.

Additionally, the hospital must explicitly define the duties and responsibilities of the physicians when they do take call so that all stakeholders know in advance exactly what it means to be "on call" for the hospital. Under EMTALA, the on-call system is the responsibility of the hospital board, although an astute board will look to the medical staff for governance and oversight. This duty also means the hospital is directly liable under the law if harm comes to patients due to any failure of the on-call system. Emergency department leaders should work collaboratively with the hospital to maintain a call system that meets the needs of their patients and providers. Department and hospital leaders must partner effectively to address opportunities or barriers that arise as a result of a need for on-call services.

Barriers and Challenges

Examples of potential issues or barriers that may arise relative to the on-call system include the following:

Medical Staff Commitment

The medical staff bylaws, or rules and regulations, must include a commitment in writing to:

- Provide on-call services to the ED.
- Align hospital privileges and on-call duties.
- Provide mandatory EMTALA training for all new members of the medical staff as a condition of privileges, with continuous training for all existing staff.[12]

Administration of the Physician On-Call List

The system must:

- Determine which providers must take call and how often. Generally, all medical specialists represented on the clinical staff should provide some on-call coverage.
- Address the issue of whether "senior" physicians must take call.
- Differentiate call duties for one's private practice versus call for the ED.

Maintenance of an Accessible On-Call List

Maintaining an accessible on-call list of ED providers includes the following requirements:[3,4]

- The list must be posted in the ED.
- It must include the name of the individual physician on call each day for each specialty. The hospital may not list only the name of the physician's practice group and/or the practice phone number.[5,6]
- The hospital must define the method by which physicians can make changes in the call coverage and how the ED will be updated.
- The hospital must maintain a copy of the daily on-call physician list for 5 years.[3,4]

Simultaneous On-Call Duties

Providers with simultaneous on-call duties (e.g., elective surgery or simultaneous on-call duties for more than one hospital) must ensure that:

- Elective surgery schedules do not materially affect the provider's ability to meet their on-call duties.
- Hospitals are aware when they are on call simultaneously for another hospital, and written policies and procedures are in place to ensure that patients presenting to the DED with an EMC are provided the care required under EMTALA.[5,6]

Response Times

Under federal law, the hospital must require the on-call physician to respond "within a reasonable period of time" for EMTALA cases, though it encourages hospitals to adopt specific periods "in minutes."[5,6] Some states, such as Missouri and New Jersey, require on-call physicians to respond within 30 minutes in certain circumstances.[13] It is critical that ED leaders understand their state laws.

- ***EMTALA governs the request to appear to help stabilize patients with EMCs.*** Thus, the EMTALA emergency response time written in the medical staff bylaws (such as "30–45 minutes") applies to these cases when the emergency physician requests the presence of the on-call physician ASAP. It is necessary to differentiate phone response times from physical response times. Every on-call physician should be able to return a page from the ED within 15 minutes. The conversation between the emergency physician and the on-call physician should then end with a mutual understanding about whether the on-call physician needs to physically come into the ED to attend to a patient and, if so, a reasonable expected time of arrival.[1]

- ***Procedure to follow when the on-call physician is unable or unwilling to respond:*** The hospital must have written procedures that can be followed when a particular specialty is not available or the on-call physician cannot respond because of circumstances beyond their control.[6] The written policy should also define the actions the ED should take if the on-call physician refuses to come into the ED when requested. If it is necessary to transfer a patient because the on-call physician refused or failed to come to the ED, the hospital is required to include the name and address of that provider on the transfer documents (**Figure 104.2**).[2,5,6] Failure to send the name and address of the on-call physician under these circumstances is itself a violation of the law, and the sending hospital can be fined or terminated from Medicare for failure to comply.[2,5,6]

- ***Notification of unavailability:*** The on-call physicians must be required to notify the hospital or the ED promptly if they are unable to respond.

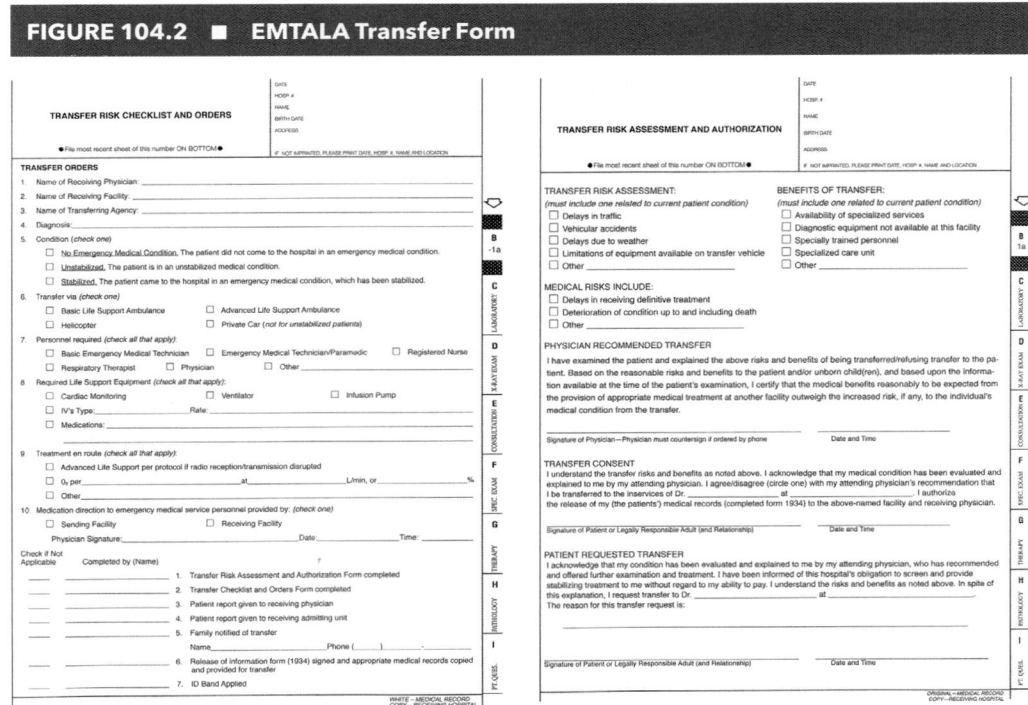

FIGURE 104.2 ■ **EMTALA Transfer Form**

Meaning of "On-Call"

The hospital must define, in writing, exactly what it means to be "on call."

- Is the on-call physician available only to consult, or is the clinician expected to come to the ED when necessary to examine and stabilize patients with emergency conditions? Under EMTALA, the hospital must contractually or through the medical staff bylaws require on-call physicians, when requested, to physically present to the ED to help medically screen or stabilize emergency patients.[3,5,6]
- Are on-call physicians required to respond to in-house emergencies when requested by the patient's admitting physician, or are they only required to respond to emergencies in the hospital's ED? Everyone at the hospital needs to know in advance so that the staff is not trying to figure out who is responsible for patient management while the patient is deteriorating or dying.
- The hospital must define the on-call physician's role in accepting or rejecting EMTALA-related transfers on behalf of the hospital (and specifically differentiate this from physicians accepting patients in the capacity of their own private practice).
- On-call physicians must carry out their EMTALA duties regardless of the patient's insurance status.

Advanced Practice Providers On-Call

Institutions must define the role of nurse practitioners and physician assistants—APPs—in a manner that is consistent with EMTALA standards. Some physicians (e.g., pediatricians, orthopedic surgeons, internists, cardiologists) routinely use APPs in their practices and interactions with the ED. EMTALA and CMS's regulations distinctly require the hospital to provide on-call *physicians*, so it is clear that the hospital may not allow a midlevel provider to take ED call instead of a physician.[2,5,6] Critical-access hospitals, while subject to EMTALA's requirements, may allow APPs to take ED call in certain circumstances.[14]

Thus, it is perfectly appropriate to list the name of the on-call physician on the call panel and the name of the physician's APP. For routine admissions or follow-up care, the emergency physician can contact the APP to arrange the necessary services. However, for true emergencies or other instances during which the emergency physician wants a phone consultation with the on-call specialist or needs the specialist to come to the ED, the emergency physician must be able to contact the specialist directly at any time.

The choice of which on-call provider to summon to the ED must *always* rest with the physician examining the patient. The CMS agrees, holding that the decision of whether the on-call physician must come to the ED rests with the emergency physician who has personally examined the patient.[6]

Sending ED Patients to an On-Call Physician's Office

Occasionally, providers may wish to send an ED patient directly to an on-call physician's office for acute intervention. This is considered a transfer under EMTALA. The CMS looks askance at transferring patients to a physician's office for acute procedures that could have been handled in the hospital.

Ophthalmologists may be an exception because, although the ED may have rudimentary eye tools, ophthalmologists typically have much better equipment in their offices for examining patients with eye complaints. In essence, movement to the office in these cases becomes a medically indicated transfer to a higher level of services than the hospital can provide. CMS accepts such movement, as long as the ED arranges a formal transfer in compliance with EMTALA.

Sending orthopedic cases (e.g., displaced fractures that need reduction) to an orthopedic surgeon's office is standard practice in many hospitals. However, it is frowned upon by CMS and subject to investigation if the process is abused. An argument can be made that since EMTALA only applies if the EMC is unstable at the time of transfer, it is reasonable for the emergency physician to transfer a stable patient with a fracture to the orthopedic surgeon's office for further treatment. The decision rests solely on the examining emergency physician. If the fracture cannot be adequately splinted, the patient has accompanying injuries or is too uncomfortable to be moved, or the emergency physician believes the injury prohibits the patient from traveling, then the orthopedic surgeon should be required to care for the patient in the ED.

On-Call Physician Follow-Up

Hospitals must define the on-call physician's role in providing follow-up care for ED patients. Obtaining follow-up care for discharged ED patients, particularly indigent persons and Medicaid recipients, is a significant problem for nearly every hospital. However, EMTALA does not reach the on-call physician's office in this scenario. If the patient does not have an EMC or is stable at the time of discharge, EMTALA does not apply from that point forward, and the on-call physician has no legal duty to see the patient in the office.

Commitment to Community

The real issue in ED follow-up is the level of commitment the hospital and medical staff want to make to their community. If the administration, board, and medical staff are comfortable with their decision, and if they have acted in the best interests of the patients they serve, they should have no trouble defending their actions to CMS or anyone else. Typically, the hospital expects the on-call physician to follow up with the ED patient to address the issues for which the patient presented or at least see the patient once when deemed necessary by the ED.[1]

No matter what the hospital and physicians decide regarding ED follow-up duties, those responsibilities must be explicitly defined in the medical staff bylaws or hospital rules and regulations so that everyone understands, *in advance*, what it means to be on call.[6] Discharge instruction sheets should also include a fail-safe clause advising patients to return to the ED if their condition deteriorates before seeing the referral specialist or if the follow-up arrangements disintegrate for any reason. Such a statement could help the hospital avoid liability when the on-call specialist fails to implement the prescribed follow-up plan.

On-Call System and Physician Response

Every hospital knows its uncooperative physicians. The hospital should act to correct those behaviors before they cost a patient's life or spark adverse publicity for the hospital, a government investigation, or a protracted court battle.

Emergency department leaders—in collaboration with the medical staff leaders—should monitor the on-call physician response times as part of their ongoing quality-improvement program. The ED should objectively document the time the physician was called and the time the physician responded. There should be no editorializing in the medical record—the times speak for themselves.

Transferring Patients Out of the Institution

To create an effective system, ED and hospital leaders must consider the following requirements:

- *Formalize*: The hospital must have a formal, designated system.
- *Transfer packets*: The institution should create a packet that includes transfer instructions, a transfer checklist or algorithm, and transfer forms.
- *Uniformity*: Use the EMTALA transfer forms for all transfers—whether the patient is stable or unstable—and for transfers out from inpatient units as well as the ED. Uniformity ensures that forms are always completed for patients who are retrospectively determined to have been unstable, and the examining physician's judgment at the time of the transfer is documented.
- *EMTALA transfer forms*: Use EMTALA transfer forms even when transferring patients from satellite facilities, such as an UCC or freestanding ED, back to the main hospital. Legally, these repatriations are called "movement" back to the main hospital; they do not meet the definition of a "transfer" under EMTALA. Uniformity avoids error and ensures compliance with state laws and acceptable standards of care.
- *Economic transfers*: These include managed care transfers and lateral psychiatric transfers to state or private institutions. The question of stability will be reviewed retrospectively. If the transfer is perceived by the reviewing agency as an economically motivated transfer, the hospital and transferring clinicians may be subjected to EMTALA liability plus fines and malpractice claims. Economically motivated transfers are not illegal per se, but they will be highly scrutinized by enforcement agencies.
- *Appropriate transfers*: Clinicians must always comply with the statutorily required transfer elements, which CMS refers to as "appropriate" transfers under the law (**Box 104.3**).[2,5,6]
- *Informed consent*: Obtain the patient's informed consent to the transfer.
- *Rechecks*: By protocol, the ED should always reevaluate the patient and recheck and record the patient's vital signs just before the transfer occurs. Any unexpected change or instability must be communicated to the transferring physician. Failure to do so is a common error and a frequently cited violation by CMS.[1]
- *Keeping records*: Maintain the records of all transfers for 5 years.[3,4]

Accepting Transfer Patients From Other Facilities

EMTALA requires hospitals to accept transfers when they have the capability and capacity to treat the patient's emergency condition when the transferring hospital does not. The duty

---

BOX 104.3 ■ "APPROPRIATE" TRANSFERS

- Stabilize the patient whenever possible.
- Complete a physician certificate of transfer, including the risks and benefits of transfer.
- Arrange for another hospital (and physician) to accept the patient in transfer.
- Send appropriate data to the accepting facility (medical records, test results, transfer forms).
- Arrange the transfer through qualified personnel and transportation equipment.

> **BOX 104.4 ■ RECOMMENDATIONS FOR THE FACILITY ACCEPTING A TRANSFERRED PATIENT**
>
> - Have a formal system for accepting or rejecting transfer requests, and document the reasons for any refusal to accept a patient in transfer.
> - Accept all appropriate requests for transfer, regardless of whether the patient is an ED patient or an inpatient of the hospital.
> - Maintain records of all transfers for 5 years.
> - Report all EMTALA transfer violations (receipt of inappropriate transfers of unstable patients) to CMS.

to accept rests with the hospital, not physicians, even though the hospital typically must work through its medical staff to appropriately accept or reject requested transfers.

Hospitals absolutely must directly and vigorously address "inappropriate" refusals of requested transfer by the receiving institution. It is a frequent violation cited by CMS and a liability claim in civil court. As a result, accepting institutions must consider the following:

- *Designate responsibility*: The receiving hospital should designate who can accept or reject patients on behalf of the institution. (Differentiate this from physicians accepting patients in the capacity of their own private practice.)
- *Emergency physicians*: It is recommended that hospitals use their ED physicians, rather than specialty on-call physicians, to accept patients transferred from other facilities. If involvement of the on-call physicians is necessary, then add a hospital representative to the acceptance process, such as a nursing supervisor or transfer nurse. *Never* use the on-call physicians alone; all it takes is one uninformed or uncooperative on-call provider to violate EMTALA.
- *Defining capabilities*: Define the resources and capacity of the institution and the times when those resources may or may not be available. When necessary resources are not available, the hospital must inform the individuals charged with accepting or rejecting transfers.
- *EMS bypass*: Include a system for rerouting or closing the ED to EMS. (This is similar to defining the capacity of the institution. There are some exceptions, such as when the hospital is a formally designated trauma center.[5,6])
- *Documentation*: Use a transfer acceptance/rejection form to document all transfer requests from other facilities (especially document refusals and reasons for refusal).
- *Education*: Educate nearby facilities on the proper procedure for transferring patients to the receiving facility, including informing them of who is authorized to accept patients on behalf of your institution.
- *Inpatient transfers*: Address the issue of accepting inpatient transfers from other hospitals (**Box 104.4**). Which inpatient transfers, if any, must a hospital accept? Who should accept or reject inpatient transfers? Determine the admitting medical staff members who will care for the admitted patient (not the emergency physicians). The *Moses* case is instructive if your hospital is in Michigan, Ohio, Tennessee, or Kentucky.[11]

DOCUMENTATION REQUIREMENTS

EMTALA has documentation mandates. These include a centralized log, a record of all transfers, and on-calls lists.

Centralized Log

- The hospital must maintain a central log of each person who presents to the hospital DED seeking medical care, whether or not the patient is actually seen.[3,4,6]
- The elements of the log should contain, at a minimum, the date, time of presentation, name, age, sex, presenting complaint, diagnosis, disposition, and time of discharge.
- If L&D is used to evaluate patients with potential contractions, then L&D must also maintain the exact same log as the DED. If off-campus facilities must comply with EMTALA, they also must keep the log.
- CMS does not state how long the log must be kept, but the recommended minimum is 5 years.

Transfers

- A record of all transfers into or out of the hospital must be maintained. The hospital must be able to retrieve a listing of these transfers at CMS's request.[3,4,6]
- A record of all transfers out of the hospital from inpatient settings must also be included, not just transfers out of the ED.
- CMS requires that transfer records be kept for a minimum of 5 years.[4,6]

On-Call Lists

- On-call lists must be maintained for 5 years.[3,4,6]
- Must contain a specifically named individual physician, not a group name.

OTHER CRITICAL ISSUES

Other critical issues must be addressed to comply with the EMTALA standards. Several of the more common ED issues are listed below.

Required Sign-in Areas

- The hospital must post signs in any area meeting the definition of a "DED." These areas typically include the ED entry areas, ED registration areas, or other areas by which patients may seek access to emergency care at the hospital, such as L&D, psychiatric intake centers, or off-campus freestanding EDs.[3,4,6]
- The content and size of the signs are specified by CMS. A sample sign is available in the ACEP EMTALA book.[1]
- The signs should be in all languages consistent with the hospital's service population.

Hospital Quality-Assurance Reviews

- As part of its standard quality-assurance plan, the hospital should review its screening processes and a number of transfers out of the institution for compliance with EMTALA.
- Quality assurance of EMTALA compliance is an institutional responsibility, not solely that of the ED. It should encompass the entire organization and be reported to the hospital's quality-assurance committee.
- State agency or CMS investigators always review the hospital's quality-assurance practices related to EMTALA.[1]

Reporting Suspected EMTALA Violations

- A hospital must report to CMS or the state survey agency any time "it has reason to believe it may have received an individual who has been transferred in an unstable EMC from another hospital in violation of the requirements of [EMTALA] section 489.24(d)."[3,4,6]
- The responsibility to report violations rests with the *hospital*. Physicians who receive a transferred patient in violation of EMTALA should report the incident to the hospital's designee (legal department, risk management, or corporate compliance).
- The hospital and legal counsel must investigate the case, obtain appropriate physician input, and decide whether to report the offending institution and physicians to CMS. It is entirely appropriate to contact the transferring institution to gather information and request its input on the events in question.
- CMS's interpretive guidelines now require the hospital to report the incident within 72 hours of when it has "reason to believe" it received an inappropriate transfer of an unstable patient.[3,4,6] Until a reasonable investigation of the incident has been conducted, the hospital may argue that it did not have a "reason to believe" it received such a transfer, so it may not have to report the case within 72 hours of actually receiving the patient in transfer.
- As a general rule, it is strongly recommended that hospitals do not "self-report." They should "self-correct" instead.

Potential Application to Outlying Facilities

- CMS's current regulations rescinded previous regulations related to the application of EMTALA to off-campus facilities. However, facilities that meet the regulatory definition of a DED still must comply. Included in the CMS definition of a DED are freestanding EDs and psychiatric-intake centers. It may or may not also include provider-based UCCs that accept walk-in, unscheduled patients for evaluation and treatment. CMS intended the new regulations to include UCCs, but the actual language of the regulations coupled with the definition of an EMC in the statute probably excludes them from EMTALA mandates. Read CMS's interpretive guidelines on when an UCC is considered a DED.[6]
- Hospitals must still implement written policies, protocols, and procedures at the off-campus department for addressing patients who present with or are determined to have EMCs.[5,6] These facilities are no longer required to transfer patients back to the main campus facility or enter into transfer agreements with other nearby hospitals that may be able to treat the patient's EMC.
- Hospital-owned and operated ambulances, including air ambulances and helicopter services, will generally be considered in compliance with the law if they operate within state or local protocols.[6]

State EMTALA Laws and Liability Insurance

Organizations and ED leaders must:

- Determine if their state has an "EMTALA equivalent" law, how it differs from the federal law, and how it may affect their compliance plan or liability. For example, California and Florida both have stricter versions of EMTALA.
- Determine if their personal or institutional medical malpractice liability insurance covers EMTALA lawsuits or will cover defense costs associated with an EMTALA investigation, Quality Improvement Organization hearing, or prosecution for civil or monetary penalties or termination from Medicare.
- Examine the indemnity provisions in state law, common law, and contracts with physicians/hospitals.

Disasters and Public Health Emergencies

- The Pandemic and All-Hazards Preparedness Act changed the EMTALA regulations in Section 1135 of the Social Security Act.[15]
- The implementing regulations specify that EMTALA sanctions do not apply to either inappropriate transfers of unstabilized individuals or the redirection of persons to another location before an MSE in times of certain disasters or public health emergencies as defined by the Act.[16]
- Waiver is limited to the 72-hour period beginning with the implementation of a hospital disaster protocol, unless the emergency involves a pandemic infectious disease, in which case the duration of the waiver will be determined by Section 1135(e) of the Act.[6,17]

Hospitals need to familiarize themselves with governing regulations and EMTALA in order to understand under what circumstances they can forgo compliance.[6,15-18]

CONCLUSION

Emergency department leaders must understand the broad scope of EMTALA and implement appropriate policies and procedures to ensure compliance with the law. Start with the EMTALA compliance checklist provide herein (**Box 104.1**) and then work with the hospital, its legal counsel, compliance officer, risk manager, and medical staff leadership to ensure that each issue is adequately addressed through policy, education, and in practice.

REFERENCES

1. Bitterman RA. *Supplement to Providing Emergency Care Under Federal Law: EMTALA.* American College of Emergency Physicians; 2004.
2. Emergency Medical Treatment and Active Labor Act, 42 USC § 1395dd (1986).
3. EMTALA "related" requirements. 42 USC § 1395cc(a)(1).
4. EMTALA regulations for "related" requirements. 42 CFR § 489.20.
5. EMTALA regulations. 42 CFR § 489.24.
6. *CMS State Operations Manual: Appendix V—EMTALA interpretive guidelines—responsibilities of Medicare participating hospitals in emergency cases.* Centers for Medicare & Medicaid Services; Rev. 191. 2019. Available at https://www.cms.gov/media/423786. Accessed March 3, 2020.
7. See the cases of *Arrington v Wong*, 237 F.3d 1066 (9th Cir. 2001) and *Morales v Sociedad Espanola De Auxilio Mutuo Y Beneficencia, et al.* 524 F.3d 54 (1st Cir. 2008).
8. EMTALA—"Parking" of Emergency Medical Service patients in hospitals. Ref S&C-06-21. Center for Medicaid and State Operations/Survey and Certification Group. 2006. Available at http://www.cms.hhs.gov/SurveyCertificationGenInfo/downloads/SCLetter06-21.pdf. Accessed March 3, 2019.
9. EMTALA issues related to emergency transport services. [Emphasis added.] Ref S&C-07-20. Center for Medicaid and State Operations/Survey and Certification Group. 2007. Available at http://www.cms.hhs.gov/SurveyCertificationGenInfo/downloads/SCLetter07-20.pdf. Accessed March 3, 2019.
10. EMTALA regulations. 42 CFR § 482.55.
11. *Moses v Providence Hosp. and Medical Ctrs., Inc.*, 561 F.3d 573 (6th Cir. 2009). See also Bitterman RA, Fish MB. Sixth circuit: admission to the hospital does not end EMTALA liability. *Emerg Depart Legal Letter.* 2009;(7):73–76.
12. 70 Federal Register 4870 (January 31, 2005).
13. MO. 19 CSR 30-20.021; and NJ Stat. 8.43G-12.5b.
14. See 42 CFR 485.618(d)(1), Personnel Standards; and CMS S&C-07-27, July 13, 2007. Emergency Medical Screening in Critical Access Hospitals. Available at: https://www.cms.gov/Medicare/Provider-Enrollment-and-Certification/SurveyCertEmergPrep/Downloads/1135-Waivers-At-A-Glance.pdf. Accessed March 3, 2019.
15. Pandemic and All-Hazards Preparedness Act, Pub. L. 109-417. Section 302(b).
16. Waiver of EMTALA sanctions in hospitals located in areas covered by a public health emergency declaration. Ref S&C-08-05. Center for Medicaid and State Operations/Survey and Certification Group. 2007. Available at http://www.cms.gov/SurveyCertificationGenInfo/downloads/SCLetter08-05.pdf. Accessed March 3, 2019. Revised December 14, 2007.
17. EMTALA requirements and options for hospitals in a disaster. Ref S&C-09-52. Center for Medicaid and State Operations/Survey and Certification Group. 2009. Available at http://www.cms.gov/SurveyCertificationGenInfo/downloads/SCLetter09_52.pdf. Accessed March 3, 2019.
18. EMTALA regulation changes and H1N1 pandemic flu and EMTALA waivers. Ref S&C-10-05. Center for Medicaid and State Operations/Survey and Certification Group. 2009. Available at: https://www.cms.gov/Medicare/Provider-Enrollment-and-Certification/SurveyCertificationGenInfo/Downloads/SCLetter10_05.pdf. Accessed March 3, 2019.

CHAPTER 105

CONSENT TO AND REFUSAL OF MEDICAL TREATMENT

Matthew M. Rice, James E. George, Robert W. Strauss

> *Though the doctors treated him, let his blood, and gave him medications to drink, he nevertheless recovered.*
>
> – Leo Tolstoy, *War and Peace*

Generally, clinicians have a duty to treat someone with whom a professional relationship exists. Hospitals have a duty to render reasonable emergency care to presenting patients. As codified under the Emergency Medical Treatment and Active Labor Act (EMTALA), hospitals cannot refuse to perform medical screening examinations and stabilization of patients. Thus, clinicians staffing hospital emergency departments (EDs) have a duty to provide care to all presenting patients.

However, some patients do not consent to the treatment offered. When patients refuse care, ED management becomes more complicated, and staff may become confused by the presence of patients who could benefit from treatment but refuse it. Though seemingly simple, even experienced ED personnel find various consent issues complex, especially when they deviate from the routine patient visit. Thus, staff and patients are best served when ED leadership is knowledgeable about and can provide support to address various consent-related scenarios in emergency care.[1,2]

GENERAL CONCEPT OF CONSENT

Health-care professionals must thoroughly understand the process and confounding factors related to obtaining the patient's (guardian's, responsible party's) permission for medical treatment (**Box 105.1**). This is referred to as *consent*. It can be viewed as a balance between ensuring medical care to all and the American legal right to exercise individual freedom. In the United States, the health-care system, patients, and physicians are afforded basic rights and responsibilities through the "contractual" relationship they establish when seeking and providing care. Consent initiates both the patient's and medical professional's responsibility, in which the patient grants permission for the medical professional to render responsible care. By virtue of that consent, ED providers have a fiduciary, ethical, and clinical relationship with patients—bound by good faith and trust—to provide advice and services.

> **BOX 105.1 ■ CONSENT SCENARIO**
>
> During a department staff meeting, an administrative clerk asks the new ED director why doctors often ask for "consent forms" when performing procedures on ED patients. After all, the patients sign "consent to treatment" forms at registration. Shouldn't that form be all that is necessary during the visit?

Patients may decide to provide or withhold consent based on what, in their opinion, is medically "right" for their health. If consent is provided, patients accept responsibility for participating in their health maintenance by complying with their health providers' healthcare recommendations and being responsible for associated costs of care. Thus, patients "consent" to participate in their health care and to be responsible for services provided. This helps protect providers and staff from later being accused of inappropriately administering treatments or touching the patient without consent (called "battery"). Providing consent to care helps establish a contractual relationship between physicians and patients.[3,4]

Express and Implied Consent

There are two major types of consent—express and implied. Express consent is typified in the vast majority of ED visits when patients give health professionals explicit permission to provide care. This normally occurs when a patient, arriving in an ED "asking for help," expresses their desire to receive care prior to providing written consent. This consent is memorialized in the "front-end" ED documents, which are routinely signed by patients during the registration process in the form of a general consent for treatment.

Implied consent is also routinely given in the ED, even though the words are not spoken. Implied consent refers to actions taken by a patient that suggest they want help. Certain actions by patients are considered so routine and generally understood that specific express consent is not necessary because the patient's actions imply their consent to proceed. By simply presenting to an ED, a patient is providing an implied request for medical assistance. Other classic examples of implied consent include the patient rolling up their shirtsleeves prior to an injection, opening their mouth for a dental evaluation, undressing and positioning themselves for an examination, or extending an arm for blood collection. Thus, during a routine patient encounter, it becomes unnecessary to continuously ask for permission to perform all routine ED tasks.[5,6]

Emergency Doctrine

The law recognizes and society understands that special circumstances exist when patients are not able to express themselves during an emergency. Under such cases, an exception to usual consent—the "emergency doctrine"—applies. According to the emergency doctrine, when a medical emergency arises there is a societal expectation that most individuals would want to be treated. Medical professionals can then assume there is an "implied consent" to evaluate and treat a patient who is not capable of providing express consent. Legally, an emergency medical condition exists when there is an immediate threat to life, limb, or health and the hazard to the patient will increase without immediate intervention. When the patient is capable of understanding treatment options and has the ability to participate in decision-making, then express consent should be obtained for further care.[7,8]

Consent Beyond Routine Care

Obtaining initial patient consent does not automatically create consent for more complex treatment. If more than a routine patient evaluation, assessment, and intervention are required, an additional "informed consent" should be obtained when possible. Informed consent is a process that is more complex than signing a general consent-to-care form. Clinicians should inform patients, who have the capacity to make decisions, of the recommendations for evaluation and treatment with a description of the known risks and

> **BOX 105.2 ■ CONSENT FORM: SUGGESTED CONTENT**
>
> - Procedure recommended by the physician in technical and lay terms
> - Benefits and risks, including likely complications associated with the recommended procedure with statistical risk
> - Alternatives to the recommended procedure, including doing nothing
> - Risks and benefits of the alternatives

benefits. Alternative choices to those recommended treatments should also be presented to the patients, with known risks and benefits, including no further treatment **(Box 105.2)**.

Providers and institutions may have different opinions about what specific care and procedures require informed consent. However, all agree that the process improves communication and affords some protections to patients, providers, and health-care institutions and their employees. The informed consent process is usually recommended for invasive procedures that are less routine, more complex, and are associated with greater risk **(Box 105.3)**. More invasive procedures generally carry a higher risk for potential complications. The greater the stability of a patient's medical condition, the more important it is to have a patient agree to the procedure prior to providing care. This consent helps to demonstrate that the patient agreed to the treatment and understands its associated benefits and risks.

Hospitals have standardized "informed consent" forms that are signed and witnessed. Various forms are more complete than others, and some actually incorporate lists of potential complications from certain procedures and the statistical likelihood of those complications occurring. All forms should include both the technical and layperson terms that describe the recommended intervention and the associated risks and benefits, especially the most common and highest risk complications. The process of obtaining consent and the documentation of the process are necessary and important administrative, clinical, educational, and medical–legal activities.

As important as these processes are, emergency care providers must clearly remember that any patient presenting to an ED, implicitly or expressly seeking assistance for a medical condition, has provided initial permission to begin the medical care process. Therefore, care should *not* be delayed for the sake of administrative procedures when immediate stabilization of a patient's medical condition is necessary. Society expects emergency patients to receive timely life-supporting services as evidenced by federal statute (EMTALA), ethical principles, common law, and professional standards. Nonetheless, the interactions and processes used when providing care in emergent situations must be documented appropriately to memorialize what transpired. In addition to a signed form, informed consent should be thought of as a well-documented process that mirrors the

> **BOX 105.3 ■ PROCEDURES REQUIRING INFORMED CONSENT**
>
> - Sedation—moderate and deep
> - Thrombolytic administration
> - Thoracostomy
> - Central venous line placement
> - Spinal tap
> - Thoracentesis; paracentesis
> - Arthrocentesis

> **BOX 105.4 ■ SURROGATE DECISION-MAKERS**
>
> - Spouse (not divorced or legally separated)
> - Majority of adult children (not just one of several children)
> - Parents of an adult
> - Domestic partner
> - Sibling
> - Close friend
> - Attending physician
> - Priority of authority depends on state law.

patient's management. This process focuses on giving the patient as much information as is reasonable to make informed decisions.[9,10]

Predetermined Decisions

Some patients present with documents that clarify their predetermined medical decisions. These documents contain information about what patients "would have considered appropriate," if they are currently incapable of expressing their desires and consenting to treatment. In such circumstances, decisions might be conveyed through a *living will*, a document authorized by patients while they are capable of making decisions. These living wills indicate what the patients would desire (consent to) if their medical condition prevents them from expressing their desires at a later time. However, these documents may be "revoked" or invalidated at any time by a competent patient or surrogate.

Surrogate Decisions

A court or a patient may appoint a surrogate or guardian to specifically provide information and make medical decisions, including consent to medical care. Once appointed, the guardian is authorized to make various legal decisions in the best interest of a patient. Similarly, a patient may have authorized another individual through a *power of attorney* to provide consent for medical care decisions. When there are no specifically authorized decision-makers for impaired patients, other surrogates may offer assistance in decision-making based on their relationship to the patient. Such surrogates, in a close legal or familial relationship to the patient, may legitimately assist as decision-makers. Various states recognize certain individuals as having priority as the primary surrogate in such cases **(Box 105.4)**.[11,12]

REFUSAL TO CONSENT AND LEAVING AGAINST MEDICAL ADVICE

In most circumstances, patients have the right to refuse care. As an exception to this, physicians and nursing caregivers at times may use their judgment to overrule the patient's refusal when it is in the best interest of the patient. However, refusal to consent to medical care is often frustrating for emergency care providers and staff. Each time a patient refuses care, normal operations and procedures are disrupted and, because emergency caregivers are dedicated to doing what is best for patients, there is a toll on ED staff's time and emotions. Refusals of care also place patients and institutions at risk of harm and litigation. Department and hospital leaders are challenged to manage concerns raised by these occurrences. Therefore, ED staff understanding of the associated legal principles makes them more capable of effectively managing these difficult events.

> **TABLE 105.1 ■ Two Cases of Refusal to Consent for Care/AMA**
>
> In the monthly ED quality improvement meeting, two cases are referred from the hospital risk manager for review. Both concern the refusal of patients to accept care.
>
> **Case #1** involved a member of the hospital board of directors, a local business owner, who was being treated for chest pain. Initial vital signs and an EKG were normal. However, the patient would not allow further evaluation or hospital admission despite the emergency physician's concern that he was experiencing acute coronary syndrome. The patient was feeling better and, though aware of staff concerns, insisted on leaving to attend an important business meeting. He later returned, unstable, with acute MI. Subsequently, many individuals in the hospital and community began asking questions.
>
> **Case #2** involved a 21-year-old trauma patient who had been in a high-speed car crash. He presented intoxicated, disoriented, and combative. He did not remember "everything that happened" in the ED because of his serious condition. Nonetheless, he complains that he was forced to receive care that he did not want. He now has officially complained to the hospital and refuses to pay his hospital medical bills. Further, he is threatening to "sue" if his ED bill is not eliminated.

Competency and Capacity

To begin, it is necessary to understand the differences between the legal and medical concepts of competency and capacity. Put simply, the legal system determines competency; the medical system determines capacity.

The principles of law supported through court decisions have generally held that adults are masters of their own body, and they have the right to determine their own destiny in health-related matters. In most circumstances, adult patients may ethically and legally refuse treatment totally or in part. But the patient's right to agree to or refuse care depends on the ability of the patient to make decisions appropriately. The legal process refers to this ability as competency. Thus, competent adults presenting for care may terminate, or modify their requests for and compliance with, care at any time. Incompetency, as determined by the legal system, limits the patients' rights and permits others to make substituted judgments on their behalf. The "others" may include the medical professionals who are providing emergency care.

Assessing competency is the key to assisting the legal system in determining whether a patient's rights were adhered to or abused (**Table 105.1**). Interestingly, competency may be decided retrospectively when defined by courts and judges based on various forms of presented evidence. Much of that evidence comes from medical and nursing professionals who assess capacity.

Physicians and nurses are skilled in assessing cognitive "capacity"—the ability to:

- Understand information
- Form intentions on the basis of relevant facts
- Reach a rational decision based on the facts

In emergency settings, a patient's cognitive capacity can and must be rapidly assessed. This capacity may be accomplished using various tools, such as the Mini-Mental Status Exam **(Box 105.5)**. This particular tool is very helpful in assessing any patient who cannot express their consent for care or who is refusing care.[13,14]

> **BOX 105.5 ■ MINI-MENTAL STATUS EXAM**
>
> - Orientation (time, person, place)
> - Registration of information (repeating the names of three items)
> - Naming (What is this?)
> - Reading (Please read what this says.)

> **BOX 105.6 ■ COMPONENTS OF REFUSAL DOCUMENTATION**
>
> - Nature of the circumstances, especially the clinical data
> - Recommended care, including the expected benefits and risks
> - Alternatives offered, including expected benefits and risks
> - Care accepted and refused
>   - Patient's reasoning for his or her decision to refuse care
>   - Any input from family or friends
>   - Description of staff's attempts to inform the patient of risks and benefits of the patient's care choices
> - Assessment of the patient's capacity to make decisions
> - Specific care offered and accepted by the patient (e.g., antibiotics at discharge, follow-up arrangements, staff requests for the patient to return if …)

Emergency department staff must make rapid decisions about a patient's cognitive ability, often with very little data or input from family or friends. The patient with an altered mental status because of alcohol, drugs, a head injury, or a medical or psychiatric illness may be incapable of making appropriate decisions that he or she might reasonably make when not impaired. Thus, the patient with diminished cognition and therefore diminished capacity cannot rationally make decisions. When such patients refuse treatment or make unreasonable decisions about care, they should be considered incapacitated if those decisions are not in their best medical interest or are at odds with choices that a reasonable person would likely make.

If the patient is cognitively incapacitated, the care team's judgment and actions should be focused on providing the care that would be given to the "average reasonable person in a similar circumstance." As time is available during or after stabilizing a patient's emergency condition, the medical care providers and nurses should engage in a well-documented more detailed ongoing assessment of the patient's capacity.

Respect for a patient's rights is critical. A health-care provider's desire to help a patient should not overshadow the rights of a patient who has a normal cognitive capacity to make reasonable informed decisions, even if the patient's decisions are counter to usual and best medical practices. In such cases, the patient's "informed refusal" should be carefully documented. The documentation should include the components listed in **Box 105.6** and clearly define the patient's capacity to refuse the care offered **(Box 105.7)**.[15]

> **BOX 105.7 ■ ELEMENTS TO CONSIDER WHEN ANALYZING A PATIENT'S CAPACITY TO REFUSE CONSENT**
>
> - Does the patient know he or she has a choice?
> - Does the patient understand the particular treatment being offered, associated risks, and relevant information about the care?
> - Does the patient appreciate the medical situation and its consequences?
> - Is the patient able to make a coherent and reasonable decision?
> - Can the patient communicate his or her decision, verbally or nonverbally?

> **BOX 105.8 ■ AMA FORM COMPONENTS**
>
> - Clinical scenario is explained
> - Patient's capacity to understand
> - Admission or treatment that is medically advised
> - Admission or treatment is refused
> - Potential consequences of refusal are explained
> - Patient takes responsibility for adverse outcomes

A standardized, signed, and witnessed against medical advice (AMA) form is useful in any refusal of care event (**Box 105.8**). However, a form is not a substitute for a well-documented clinical note of the events and circumstances. Too often, impassioned providers and staff have AMA forms signed and then neglect to carefully document their full efforts and processes to render care. As a result, the record may fail to demonstrate how much ED staff cared about a *"recalcitrant patient."* Emergency clinicians, who are well educated in the refusal of consent processes, find the refusals less stressful and are able to appropriately address the processes, people, and documentation. Importantly, the ED staff is better able to provide the best care, given the patient's choice.[16,17]

Case One Review

The businessman (hospital board member) with chest pain was assessed. He possessed normal mental capacity. He was informed of the risks of refusing recommended care (admission and continuing management), as well as the risks and benefits of alternative choices, including leaving AMA, and was allowed to leave the ED. Prior to leaving, the staff members continued to demonstrate their best interpersonal skills to ensure the patient was aware of all his medical options. The family and the patient's primary care practitioner were enlisted to assist the patient in understanding the issues and participated in developing reasonable outpatient options for care to further assist the patient's decision-making.

It is important that patients refusing recommended treatment are not abandoned but rather given continued care (prescriptions, etc.), encouraged to return to the ED at any time, and provided with a timely, specific follow-up appointment arranged with an appropriate physician. Such patients should also be warned not to place others at any risk from the current health situation, that is, driving while having a possible heart attack. These efforts demonstrate the caring of the staff.

Case Two Review

Given that reasoning and logic were futile in the incapacitated patient, the health-care providers were obligated to provide the best care through an implied consent to save "life and limb." Simply having the impaired patient sign an AMA form and allowing him to refuse care places the patient and the ED staff at risk.

The list of scenarios of patients presenting to an ED with diminished mental capacity is extensive. When patients with diminished capacity refuse reasonable recommended emergency care, medical care should be provided in a safe and logical manner with the goal of preserving life and limiting disability. In general, the intoxicated, traumatized, or otherwise incapacitated patient with life-threatening injuries should be provided with life-supporting care until the patient is stable. These efforts should continue until the patient has the clear capacity to understand and either accept or refuse further care, until an appointed surrogate (legal representative) for the patient intervenes for the patient or until further care would be futile under the circumstances.

Incapacity to consent to care at the time it is rendered does not relieve patients of their subsequent responsibilities. When reasonable care is provided, a patient is responsible for any associated financial obligations. More importantly, irrespective of the financial issues, the skilled ED team has minimal risk from litigation when lives were saved, even if the care is retrospectively criticized by those who most benefited.[18]

Special Circumstances

"Special circumstances" add nuance and complexity to the issue of refusal of consent. Some of these circumstances include:

- Personal and religious beliefs that conflict with established medical care
- Intoxication
- Incarceration (patients transported by the police against their will)

Personal/Religious Beliefs

A classic religious conflict is exemplified by Jehovah's Witnesses who may refuse blood transfusions because of their beliefs. Case law addressing these circumstances varies. Some decisions support the right of the individual patient's refusal to be treated with a life-saving transfusion, if that patient is determined to have capacity, even if death is an end result. Other legal decisions (fewer in number) support blood transfusions in life-and-death emergencies against the will of the patient, who is determined to have capacity. The circumstances are even more complicated when others' lives are involved. Examples include pregnant patients (placing the life of the unborn child at risk) and children receiving transfusions.

When there is doubt, the general rule is to perform life-saving measures, such as transfusions, rather than simply watching. If subsequently subjected to legal scrutiny, it is better to defend saving a life than to defend doing nothing and allowing a person to die. When time permits, it may be helpful to seek second opinions from other medical professionals and hospital administrative/legal personnel. Substituted judgment (someone other than the patient making consent decisions) from spouses, family, or close colleagues, or from courts or court-appointed guardians, is also helpful in such difficult situations. When the patient is a minor, ED treatment issues surrounding consent and refusal are complicated. It is appropriate to provide life-saving care to the minor while the complexities of the legal processes are sorted out administratively.[19,20]

The Intoxicated Patient

Patients who are intoxicated present special problems. There is no absolute standard that defines when an intoxicated patient can be objectively determined to possess the cognitive capacity to make decisions they would otherwise make if sober. Some intoxicated patients function normally with high serum alcohol levels, even when state laws define them as being unable to safely operate a motor vehicle. Nonetheless, there is no specific level of alcohol or other drugs and medications that is routinely used to determine the capacity or inability of an individual to function and make decisions.[21]

In some states, it is illegal to drive with any drug impairment, irrespective of the type of drug. Yet some patients seem to function reasonably well and make reasonable decisions with various levels of alcohol and drugs. It is therefore imperative that emergency physicians carefully and objectively assess the cognitive state and capacity of a patient who refuses to give consent when there is a suspicion of alcohol or drug impairment. Again, if subjected to legal scrutiny, it is better to defend restraining or saving a patient against the patient's will than to defend allowing an "intoxicated" patient to die or harm him- or herself.

Experienced ED providers and nurses will consider mildly to moderately intoxicated patients "incapacitated," when in the face of grave and immediate danger those patients refuse care. Until it is clear that the patient has capacity to make reasonable decisions, restraints may be required to appropriately assess and stabilize the patient. The greater and more immediate the risk to the welfare of the intoxicated patient refusing care and treatment, the more likely that such standard and appropriate emergency care will be successfully defended from subsequent legal scrutiny. If after assessment, emergency stabilization is not required, it may be reasonable to allow the patient to reach a stable cognitive level to enhance his or her ability to make better informed decisions about further care.

An intoxicated patient, restrained for appropriate evaluation and stabilization, may later claim assault and battery or false imprisonment. However, the risk of such litigation being successful is minimal. Rather than being indiscriminate, decisions to intervene and provide care to impaired patients should be reasonable, evidence based, and well-documented when care is provided without a patient's express consent.[22,23]

The Incarcerated Patient

Patients who are brought to EDs by police for assessment or treatment should be treated as any other patient with similar medical problems and in a similar state of cognitive capacity (unless specific laws compel the medical professional to act differently). A patient who refuses care for injuries received during or prior to "arrest" should be treated in the same fashion as a similar patient not under arrest. If the patient is brought to the hospital for administrative medical reasons (that is, he or she is a body packer or a drug or alcohol level needs to be obtained), the patient should be treated as any patient relative to their rights and responsibilities. However, when a patient is under arrest, the police, who represent the "state," may have the right and obligation to have an arrested patient assessed for medical problems.

In most circumstances, the state cannot force patients to make a decision about their health rights, if it is not an emergency situation or without a court order. Thus, while ED professionals should be cooperative with police, they should follow the same standards that they use with patients who have similar medical problems. If a court order compels the care team to perform certain procedures to obtain or preserve evidence, the order permits the clinicians to proceed with providing care according to best medical judgment. In these circumstances, the physician continues to be responsible both for determining the correct medical care and for the outcome of that care.[24,25]

MINORS AND CONSENT

Legal issues surrounding minors may be difficult, emotional, and confusing for medical professionals (**Table 105.2**). Part of the confusion stems from the state-by-state variation in

TABLE 105.2 ■ Case of Minor and Consent
While working in the ED, a resident approaches the attending physician and describes the following presentation.
Case #3 involves a 2-year-old boy diagnosed with first-time diabetic ketoacidosis, which requires admission to the hospital. The mother is a 16-year-old single parent, living alone with no family to support her. She wants to leave against advice with her baby because she has to go to work to support her child, but she promises to bring him back if he gets worse.

consent laws for minors. Understanding several basic legal principles can lessen some of the confusion. The legal system often treats adults and minors differently, especially related to medical decisions. Adults have a right to make their own health-care decisions, whereas minors may not, except under certain circumstances. A minor is legally defined as a person younger than the age of legal competence. Generally, that is 18 years of age, with notable exceptions. For a patient younger than 18 years old who seeks emergency care, there are special considerations concerning consent to treat.

Emancipated and Mature Minors

As a general rule, consent from a parent or legal guardian should be obtained when providing nonemergent care to a patient younger than 18 years old. All states have exceptions to this rule, and ED clinicians must be aware of the laws of the state in which they practice. Emancipated ("mature minors") may be treated more like adults. Emancipated minors are those individuals who are usually between 15 and 18 and are considered self-reliant and living independently. The more independent they are, the more likely they will be considered emancipated and able to provide consent for their own medical care. Thus, a 16-year-old who is economically supporting him- or herself, and living independently, would generally be considered to be an emancipated minor.

Other examples of the "mature minor doctrine" may include a minor who is married, in the military, or a parent, even if unmarried. Proof of independence or of emancipation is not required when health-care professionals must decide if a minor can consent to his or her own care. Rather, the health-care professional may depend on any reasonable information provided by the minor when asserting emancipation.

Mature minors are allowed to consent to or refuse treatment if sufficiently mature to understand and appreciate the risks and benefits of the proposed medical care. The determination of maturity includes age, experience, education, judgment, and conduct. Many states statutorily permit minors as young at 13 years old to consent to treatment without parenteral consent. Common areas in which state laws allow mature minors to independently consent to medical treatment include care related to pregnancy, contraception, mental health, venereal diseases, and drug-related problems.[20,26]

It is generally appropriate to ask the minor patient if a parent or guardian may be contacted to discuss the minor's care. If the minor patient refuses this request, the law requires that minors should be treated when they present with a medical problem that does not *require* parental consent for treatment. When the issue of consent by the minor is unclear, medical care should be started and the process and degree of informing parents can be decided in discussion with the patient.[21,27]

Parental Rights

Generally, and unless prohibited by law, adults responsible for minor patients should be contacted in a timely manner by health-care professionals to inform them of issues and to seek consent for the minor's care. But in true emergencies, treatment of any minor should be undertaken even without parental consent, if treatment delay could result in a poor outcome. Delayed or untimely life-saving care would create greater moral and legal jeopardy than providing proper treatment without consent.

State's Rights

Though parents may refuse care for themselves, it does not necessarily follow that they can refuse care for their children. In fact, pediatric emergency care may be ethically

> **BOX 105.9 ■ CONSIDERATIONS WHEN TREATING MINORS AGAINST PARENTAL CONSENT**
>
> - Will the child be harmed by withholding treatment?
> - Is the treatment appropriate in the substituted judgment of the doctor?
> - Would the child have agreed to the treatment if he or she possessed the same knowledge as the physician?
> - Do the potential benefits of the treatment outweigh the risks?

and statutorily required even when parents refuse to consent. The "state" also has rights and responsibilities to protect minors. When parents' decisions are in conflict with societal expectations about proper health care for their children, clinicians must consider the welfare of the child and, if necessary, use the state's authority to ensure the child's welfare. The health-care team can intervene to protect the minor through various means, including court orders or police actions. Such decisions must always balance the interests of the parents against the interests of the child **(Box 105.9)**. A common rule to follow is:

> *The more likely it is that withholding immediate care will lead to a bad medical outcome, the more important it is to provide that care, even if against parental consent.*

Or alternatively:

> *The less likely it is that death or disability will occur if care is delayed — and the greater the risk and potential for complications associated with providing that care — the more important it is to obtain parental or surrogate consent (including a court order) for a minor's care.*[28,29]

Case Three Review

> *A child has been newly diagnosed with diabetes. The standard of care requires her admission to the hospital. However, the mother refuses such admission, and the clinical staff finds it necessary to contact child protective services to ensure the child's wellbeing.*

In such cases, the child is often taken into protective custody, allowing legally appointed guardians to make more appropriate medical decisions in the patient's best medical interests.

CONCLUSION

Consent is a concept that brings together the medical and legal issues at the core of individual rights and responsibilities for health care. The concepts surrounding consent are key to preventing and resolving ED problems associated with an individual's authorization and refusal of health care. Although there is variability among states regarding some consent issues, most principles are very similar. A working knowledge of the general principles, and the specific regulations of the state in which the provider practices, will assist patients in receiving—and ED staff in providing—the best and safest medical care. It will also provide practitioners and nurses with the comfort of understanding the associated legal issues. Familiarity with these principles and laws will best support medical decisions when difficult situations involving refusal of care arise. The right decisions related to consent in emergency medical care will result from focusing on quality medicine while keeping in mind patient rights.

REFERENCES

1. *Thompson v Sun City Community Hospital*, 688 P2d 605 (Ariz 0 1984).
2. *Findby v Board of Supervisors*, 230 P2d 526 (Ariz 1951).
3. Emergency Medical Treatment and Active Labor Act, 42 USC § 1395dd (1986).
4. EMTALA Final Regulations. 68 Federal Register 53221-53264; 2003. Available at: http://www.access.gpo.gov/su_docs/fedreg/a030909c.html. Accessed June 29, 2013.
5. Bitterman R. Medicolegal and risk management. In: Marx JA, Hockberger RS, Walls RM, eds. *Rosen's Emergency Medicine: Concepts and Clinical Practice*. Vol. 2. Mosby Elsevier; 2006:3165.
6. *Schloendorff v Society of New York Hospital*, 211 NY, 105 NE 92, 93 (1914).
7. Wikipedia "Consent". Available at: https://en.wikipedia.org/wiki/Consent. Updated October 18, 2020. Accessed October 27, 2020.
8. Rice M. Legal issues in emergency medicine. In: Rosen P, Barkin R, eds. *Emergency Medicine, Concepts, and Clinical Practice*. Mosby Year Book; 1998:238-239.
9. Siegel DM. Consent and refusal of treatment. *Medical Legal Issues Emer Med Clin North Am*. 1993;11(4):833-840.
10. *Dunham v Wright*, 432 F2d 940 (1970).
11. *Canterberry v Spence*, 464 F2d 772 (DC Cir), cert denied 409 US 1064 (1972).
12. *Sullivan v Montgomery*, 279 NYS 575 (1935).
13. White C, Rosoff AJ, leBlang TR. Informed consent to medical and surgical treatment. In: American College of Legal Medicine Textbook Committee, ed. *Legal Medicine*. 7th ed. Mosby; 2007:337-343.
14. Informed consent in medical malpractice. 55 Calif. L Rev 1396 (1967).
15. Plante ML. Some legal problems in medical treatment and research, an analysis of "informed consent". *Ford Law Rev*. 1968;36 (40).
16. Moskopo JC. Informed consent in the emergency department. *Emerg Med Clin North Am*. 1999;17(2):327-340.
17. Siner DA. Advance directives: emergency medical, legal, and ethical implications. *Ann Emerg Med*. 1989;18(12):1364-1369.
18. Peters DA. Advanced medical directives: the case for the durable power of attorney for health care. *J Leg Med*. 1987;8(3):437-464.
19. Grisso T, Appelbaum PS. *Assessing Competence to Consent to Treatment: A Guide for Physicians and Other Health Professionals*. Oxford University Press; 1998.
20. Simon JR. Refusal of care: the physician–patient relationship and decisionmaking capacity. *Ann Emerg Med*. 2007;50(4):456-461.
21. Drane JF. Competency to give an informed consent: a model for making clinical assessments. *JAMA*. 1984;252(7):925-927.
22. Appelbaum PS. Assessment of patient's competence to consent to treatment. *N Engl J Med*. 2007;357(18):1834-1840.
23. Mayer D. Refusal of care and discharging "difficult" patients from the emergency department. *Ann Emerg Med*. 1990;19(12):1436-1446.
24. *Cruzan v Director, Missouri Department of Health*, 497 US 261 279 (1990).
25. *Wons v Public Health Trust*, 500 So2d 679, 686 (Fla Dist Ct App 1987).
26. *Truman v Thomas*, 611 P2d 902 (Cal. 1980).
27. Wear S. *Informed Consent: Patient Autonomy and Clinician Beneficence Within Health Care*. 2nd ed. Georgetown University Press; 1998.
28. Knight S, Olson LM, Cook LJ, et al. Against all advice: an analysis of out-of-hospital refusals of care. *Ann Emerg Med*. 2003;42(5):689-696.
29. Roth LH, Meisel A, Lidz CW. Tests of competency to consent to treatment. *Am J Psychiatry*. 1977;134(3):279-284.

CHAPTER 106

EMERGENCY DEPARTMENT DOCUMENTATION

Diana Nordlund, Charles Grassie, Joanne E. Navarroli, Kay Bleecher, Robert W. Strauss

One of the most important aspects of patient care in the emergency department (ED) is high-quality documentation of the patient encounter. Thorough, accurate medical records (MRs) are critical to a hospital's ability to comply with the Centers for Medicare and Medicaid Services (CMS) and Joint Commission (JC) standards. Effective documentation improves continuity of care, reduces errors and delays, enhances the accuracy of billing and coding, permits precise metrics, aids in the defense of negligence claims, and helps resolve complaints from patients, family, and other providers.[1-5]

Organizations have established specific requirements for meeting regulatory agency compliance standards, federal and state laws, accreditation regulations, and professional practice standards for the documentation of particular implications.[1] It is imperative that dyad ED leadership teams (comprising the lead physician and nurse) ensure that all members of the patient-care team are held accountable for appropriate documentation.

The MR is primarily used as a communication tool that tells a clear, complete story about every patient encounter.[5,6] The MR is also considered an official medicolegal document. Each entry communicates how the patient's condition is changing, and medicolegal inferences are derived from what is or what is not documented.[6] High-quality documentation demonstrates quality of care and regulatory compliance as well as billing, research, quality improvement, and risk utilization.[4-6]

The vast majority of ED documentation in the United States is in the form of an electronic health record (EHR). According to the Office of the National Coordinator for Health Information Technology, the term *EHR* should be used because these records go beyond data collection "to share information with other health care providers . . . so they contain information from all the clinicians involved in the patient's care."[7]

ELECTRONIC HEALTH RECORDS

Electronic health records, also called electronic medical records, encompass the contemporaneous digitalization of privileged patient information. As EHRs have evolved over the past 10 years, so too have CMS requirements for reporting information. Initially, EHR use was simply "encouraged;" presently, the new rules state that "all Medicare-eligible hospitals, dual-eligible hospitals, and critical-access hospitals are required to use 2015 edition certified electronic health record technology."[8] In part, the change is intended to increase "interoperability and improve patient access to health information."[8] New requirements include but are not limited to the following:

- Documentation of the entire patient encounter (e.g., consents, diagnostic data, and discharge instructions) as well as additional communications (e.g., follow-up calls)
- Computerized provider order entry
- Documentation of differential diagnoses, with appropriate laboratory and imaging reports and data
- e-Prescribing
- Utilization functions like the management of ED patient flow, interprovider access to records, and intrinsic quality-control mechanisms

Advantages

Electronic health records are touted as the solution to "reduce errors, bring down costs, ensure privacy, and save lives."[9] The proposed benefits of EHRs include[10]:

- Immediate and universal availability
- One centralized record that allows seamless coordination of care
- Improved patient and provider convenience (such as e-Prescribing)
- Improved safety secondary to intrinsic cross-checks and decision support
- Improved efficacy, privacy, and security
- Improved health-care delivery at a reduced cost

Disadvantages

The implementation of EHRs has been neither easy nor inexpensive. The American Recovery and Reinvestment Act (ARRA) required all Medicare/Medicaid hospitals to have an EHR in place by 2014.[11] The ARRA provided billions of dollars to implement the Health Information Technology for Economic and Clinical Health (HITECH) Act to ensure the adoption of this new technology.[11,12] Initially, HITECH created disadvantages by requiring:

- Adherence to defined record structure, inputting required "core" information
- Interprovider information exchange
- Implementation of computerized provider order entry
- Performance of routine security checks
- Presumably, an adequate number of computerized mobile workstations[12]

As HITECH evolves, additional disadvantages are being cited, including:

- An inability to improve the quality, safety, and efficiency of patient care
- Interoperability, interface, software, and workflow challenges
- Utilization of an expensive provider (physician) to perform duties that can be performed in a more cost-efficient manner
- Changes in administrative priorities[13]

Although challenges persist, so do the increasing usage mandates. Preparation for implementation can take months to years, and the go-live process can create dramatic delays in ED care delivery—even with intensive preparation. The transition may require double staffing for a matter of weeks due to decreased productivity, and previous productivity levels may never again be achieved. Some suggest that EHRs require the physician or nurse to spend even less time at the patient's bedside.

Finally, clinicians often find that the complicated data-input systems, frequent hard stops, difficult record access, inability to review contemporaneous charting by other providers (such as residents and nursing staff), and a duplicative and ineffective final MR to be cumbersome and frustrating—at least in the initial stages of implementation. From a medicolegal perspective, a poorly designed or improperly implemented electronic template can provide an incomplete or inaccurate record of the clinician's impressions of the patient encounter, just as a paper template can.

Scribes

Scribes, paid assistants who work directly with emergency physicians and occasionally advanced practice providers (APPs) to facilitate accurate and efficient documentation, can enhance the efficacy of EHRs. A preliminary review of scribe use suggests that the increase in physician productivity more than recoups the cost of implementation.[14] Scribes may also enhance clinician satisfaction.[14,15] In addition, scribes may handle adjunct tasks, such as retrieving past records, lab results, and other duties as assigned (see Chapter 25).

REGULATORY STANDARDS

Today's EHR utilization is governed largely by the CMS and JC. Therefore, everyone who interacts with the EHR must comply with their standards.

Documentation

CMS standards mandate that EHR users must comply with Comprehensive Error Rate Testing (Part A and Part B) and a durable medical equipment Medicare administrative contractor, both of which clarify that the purpose of medical documentation is to facilitate[16]:

- The ability of the physician to plan the patient's immediate treatment and monitor the patient's health care over time
- Interprovider communication and continuity of care
- Accurate and timely claims review and payment
- Appropriate utilization review and quality-of-care evaluations
- Collection of data that may be useful in research and education

CMS goes on to describe the general elements to be contained in all MRs, including:

- Details of each patient encounter by licensed independent providers, including:
  - ☐ The reason for the encounter and legible history, physical examination findings, and prior diagnostic test results
  - ☐ Documentation of medical necessity for diagnostic studies and durable medical equipment; if not documented, the rationale for ordering tests and other ancillary services should be easily inferred
  - ☐ A plan for care, including laboratory tests, imaging studies, and medications
  - ☐ Additional resources needed to assist the patient with recovery, such as physical, occupational, and speech therapy; dietary needs; and other specialty services
  - ☐ Access to information about the patient's acuity and needs
  - ☐ Assessment, clinical impression, or diagnosis
  - ☐ The patient's progress, changes in treatment, and any diagnostic revisions
  - ☐ Clinician access to past and present diagnoses

- Identification of risk factors
- Appropriate use of the CPT and ICD codes

■ Documentation of each patient encounter by nurses should include:[6,17]
- Initial and ongoing assessments
- All patient education, including patient's understanding
- Response to all medications, treatments, and interventions, including progress or a decline in the patient's condition
- Any relevant statements made by the patient
- Use of appropriate abbreviations and terminology

Department leaders must maintain an ongoing awareness of the ever-changing guidelines and regulations of the CMS and JC. These organizations dictate standard ED practice via multiple methods, including nonpayment, financial penalties, and incentives. Suffice it to say that compliance with documentation standards is a prerequisite for a successful ED. Practitioner education and feedback mechanisms are imperative.

Control of the MR

The increasing complexity of the type and amount of data stored in the MR and the manner of production and storage of these records have led to an increasingly regulated and frequently litigated environment. Existing regulations attempt to balance confidentiality, access, cost, and accountability. Department leaders must be aware of the common issues of ownership, control, retention, and release of the MR and other forms of health information.

Ownership

The health-care entity (the hospital, clinic, or private practitioner) owns the MR in its physical form. Nonetheless, the patient has rights to the information contained within the record. Other parties may be granted nonproprietary access for medical, administrative, or legal reasons. The record-owning facility is responsible for the maintenance, integrity, compliance, confidentiality, and retention of the record. Most institutions will carefully monitor MR access to ensure that any record requests are based on legitimate medical need. Those who unnecessarily access records risk dismissal (see Chapter 107).

Amendment

Beyond normal, authorized chart entries, there are strict limitations on a party's permission to alter the MR. Standard procedure requires providers to amend chart mistakes by making single line through the incorrect entry, noting the date, time, and authentication of the change. This policy works well for minor errors discovered contemporaneously, but it is less acceptable for substantive errors or additions made after the fact, especially in the event of an adverse patient outcome. Many health-care institutions have policies about what, if any, chart amendments are permitted. Any change to a chart that may be involved in malpractice litigation is extremely risky. Furthermore, once a record leaves the immediate realm of care delivery, alterations and amendments can be discovered.

Whether electronic or tangible, copies of the original record are usually accessible as part of processing and storage. Further, individual keystroke changes by the "logged in" party can be accessed through forensic investigations. Aside from possibly leading to criminal charges, any alterations in the defendant's favor will seriously impair the credibility of the clinician and may lead to an unfavorable result.

Federal law protects patients' rights to access their MR for any reason and outlines a procedure for handling such requests.[18] A responding health-care entity has 60 days to determine whether or not the record is accurate/complete and act accordingly, whether by amending the chart (and taking reasonable action to notify parties who had previously received or relied on the relevant health information) or formally denying the request.[18] Recordkeeping and release requirements still apply.

Retention

State laws generally govern how long MRs must be retained, with various requirements based on the age of the patient and provider status. Regardless of the individual state statute, federal regulations like those mandated by the Health Insurance Portability and Accountability Act of 1996 (HIPAA) must be considered. HIPAA rules "require a covered entity, such as a physician or entity that bills Medicare, to retain required documentation for six years from the date of its creation or the date when it was last modified, whichever is later."[19-22] However, if a particular state law requires a longer retention of the record, the entities retaining the records within that state must follow the statute.[19]

With HIPAA requirements for the retention of protected health information (PHI) continually being updated, facility compliance officers should regularly verify the "current" requirements. CMS requires patient records to be kept for a minimum of 5 years for billing and 10 years for Medicare-managed programs.[20] Additionally, HITECH does address health-information retention and management, most specifically related to data protection, mandated disclosure of inadvertent release, and applicable penalties.

Furthermore, the American Medical Association (AMA) issued an ethics opinion on MR retention. Although emergency physicians generally do not take responsibility for chart storage and access (a task that instead falls to the hospital), the AMA policy still bears consideration.[23] The following guidelines can assist physicians in meeting their ethical and legal obligations.[24]

- When deciding whether to keep certain parts of the record, it may be helpful to consider whether a physician would want the information if seeing the patient for the first time.
- Even if a particular record is no longer needed for medical reasons, the physician should consult state laws regarding the minimum length of time a record must be kept.
- In all cases, MRs should be kept for at least as long as the statute of limitations for medical malpractice claims.
- The time of record retention should be measured from the last professional contact with the patient.
- If the patient is a minor, the statute of limitations for medical malpractice claims may not apply until the patient reaches the age of majority.
- If the patient expires, the onset of the statute of limitations may be delayed until an executor of the estate is appointed. While state laws vary, the statute of limitations does not usually begin until a "reasonable person should have discovered the negligence."
- Immunization records must be maintained and accessible.
- The records of any patient covered by Medicare or Medicaid must be kept for at least six years.
- In order to preserve confidentiality when discarding old records, all documents should be destroyed.
- Before discarding old records, patients should be given an opportunity to claim the records or have them sent to another physician.

The ED policy on MR access and retention must be consistent with hospital protocols, state law, federal law, and applicable regulatory body requirements. An understanding of and compliance with locally applicable regulations is required.

CONFIDENTIALITY AND DISCLOSURE

The laws regulating the protection and release of PHI are extensive and complex. HIPAA governs the access, release, use, and management of medical information.[25] For more detailed information on HIPAA and its application, see Chapter 96.

Medical providers are commonly confronted with situations in which they must choose whether or not to release a patient's health information. Emergency clinicians may field inquiries from law enforcement, local health-delivery organizations (such as EMS), and families. Privileged health information must not be released to law enforcement or other parties without a compelling reason or statutory requirement. It is prudent to have policies in place to avoid unwarranted disclosures.

In most states, there is an affirmative duty to disclose information to a third party without permission in certain circumstances. For instance, a patient statement such as, "I feel like going out and killing someone," it is likely privileged information. However, if the patient states, "I'm going out and killing my brother Paul," the clinician probably has an affirmative third-party duty to warn Paul. The difference is an explicit, identifiable victim.[26] When in doubt, a quick call to your hospital administrator or counsel is warranted.

Electronic Transmission

The advent of the EHR and standard, readily accessible digital communications technology poses a number of new challenges to confidentiality and disclosure. Many years ago, proper precautions may have amounted to keeping discussions of privileged information out of elevators, cafeterias, and other semipublic areas. Now it is necessary to consider email, cell phone cameras, social networking sites, blogs, and other media. Failure to enact proper protocols can result in disastrous consequences, including patient rights violations, employee termination, federal fines, and civil liability.

A properly authorized photo (or other information, such as an x-ray or ECG) should be communicated using an approved email server. As the adage goes, "A picture is worth a thousand words." That picture and its transmission must be authorized, confidential, and sent from one HITECH-compliant email server to another.

It must be noted that the standard web-based email services make no claim of confidentiality. Email can easily be misrouted—either intentionally or inadvertently—intercepted, copied, and disseminated. HITECH makes it clear: Any email communication containing any privileged patient data or other sensitive information *must* be transmitted on a secure server with encryption.[12,24] A confidentiality disclaimer addendum on a nonencrypted email is *not* sufficient protection. Any information shared must be clearly identified on a signed, witnessed transfer-of-information document. When sharing information about minors, the permission-to-share form must be signed by a parent or legal guardian.[12,24]

Social Media

Facebook, Twitter, and LinkedIn are the tip of the iceberg when it comes to the enormous number of web-based social media networks. Add to that the panoply of personal and professional blogs, and the ease of instant, widespread information dissemination is obvious. The repercussions of this immediate access are apparent when one reads news stories about hospitals firing staff for posting online comments related to the workplace.[27]

For example, naive clinicians occasionally share data on patients using semitransparent language: "Hypothetically, if I were taking care of a problem like this (picture included) what would you recommend?" While many of these sites are actively monitored by other clinicians, they may also be scrutinized by attorneys who understand HIPAA. Consequently, many hospitals block access to social networking sites in the workplace and issue no-tolerance policies forbidding all work-related postings. Although it may seem obvious, it bears repeating that even seemingly innocent comments can have serious consequences. Professional reputations may hang in the balance.

Images and Photography

Readily accessible handheld digital devices, whether in the hands of clinicians, patients, or families, also pose confidentiality issues. Eager nurses, attending physicians, and residents may wish to photograph a particular injury or condition for teaching purposes. Alternatively, patients and families may wish to document "before and after" photos or record an image to share with absent loved ones. Either way, confidentiality ramifications must be considered.

For the awake, competent, adult patient, it is easy to request permission to obtain a photograph for teaching purposes. However, if the patient is a minor, incompetent, unconscious, or otherwise cannot give consent, consent is *not* implied. Even if absolute care is taken to ensure that no identifying information is contained in the image, the possibility of policy or ethical violations remains. For example, in 2010, a Los Angeles hospital fired several employees after photographs were taken of a dying patient and posted on Facebook.[28]

While there is little question about obviously inappropriate photography (e.g., no educational value or an intentional violation of patient dignity), there remains a gray area. At times, a legitimate image may comply with HIPAA privacy regulations but still conflict with institutional or ethical policies. In general, photographs should only be taken with express patient permission. A parent or legal guardian may provide valid consent for a legally incompetent patient. If valid consent cannot be obtained, the best policy is to forbid photography in any form by staff. Furthermore, many hospitals have issued blanket policies regarding camera usage of any kind (whether by staff or patients) in clinical care areas.

METADATA

Department leaders must also be aware of the global digitalization of metadata, the hidden blueprint of a document that reflects information about authors, tracked changes, undo/redo history, hidden text, and the dates and times of any modifications.[29,30] In the health-care context, legally discoverable metadata also includes:[29,30]

- If, when, for how long, and under what username a radiographic image, laboratory test, or other electronic data was accessed
- Duration and location of telephone calls made from hospital extensions
- Websites visited via hospital servers

With the advent of universal EHRs, it is even more evident that nearly every aspect of medical charting, including the chronology of the patient encounter itself, is legally discoverable. A data trail is created each time the patient chart is opened, viewed, or edited.[29,30] It behooves ED leaders to educate practitioners about this digital blueprint and its ramifications for patient privacy and litigation purposes.

COMMON CHARTING MISTAKES

There are certain aspects of care that have specific documentation requirements to which all members of the ED team must adhere. These areas include high-risk situations; medication reconciliation; pain assessment, management, and reassessment; patient safety, including the use of restraints; infection and fall prevention; and reporting/recording critical results.[1-6]

A legible, accurate, and complete MR is one of the best possible protections in the event of medical malpractice litigation. Alternatively, a poorly documented chart can lead to a clinician's downfall. For this reason, an awareness of the common pitfalls of charting is highly relevant to successful ED management.

Common charting mistakes that can have medicolegal implications include but are not limited to the use of unapproved abbreviations and the omission of pertinent health and medication information. These mistakes include any changes in a patient's condition that arise from treatment. All members of the medical team should avoid using vague language, including words like "appears," "obviously," "nervous," "well," and so on.

Wrong Chart

Emergency physicians and nurses must manage multiple patients (and their charts) simultaneously. Dangerous errors occur when information is inadvertently recorded on the wrong chart. In the event that documentation has occurred in the wrong chart, the clinician should follow the facility's procedure to "unchart" and then immediately document the information in the correct patient record. With most EHR systems, documentation is accomplished with a series of checkboxes, drop-down tabs, and free-text fields. When "uncharting," it is necessary to know where a checkbox is associated with free text in a separate section.

It will be difficult to explain to the plaintiff's attorney why the physician or nurse authenticating the MR did not actually participate in the patient's treatment. Extraordinary care must be taken to ensure that the correct chart is being accessed every time.

Inadequate Provider Review

Far too many practitioners authenticate a record before verifying its contents. This also applies to the supervision of residents and APPs. Ultimately, a clinician's signature confirms that they have read, understood, and concurred with the record. Not only is examination of the record an important aspect of resident education and APP supervision, it is also unlikely that a response like "I never read it" will lead to a successful malpractice defense.

The MR passes through many hands before the conclusion of the medical encounter. Notations made by nurses, ED technicians, and residents *must* be reviewed, and any discrepancies should be addressed by the attending physician. First, notations by subordinate staff can be a valuable source of information. Second, malpractice defenses have floundered on interprovider inconsistencies. Ultimately, the attending physician is responsible for the entire substance of the record. Ignorance is not an excuse.

Overinclusive Electronic Templates

While the theory behind the prefilled EMR template is one of efficiency and completeness, care must be taken to avoid inadvertently documenting findings that were not objectively obtained. Importantly, this misinformation may have implications for the patient when subsequent caregivers rely on it. In addition, inappropriately exhaustive documentation not only subjects the physician and nurse to allegations of fraud, it also discredits the rest of the MR. In the courtroom, a discredited MR equates to a failed defense.

Loaded Adjectives

For difficult patients, direct quotes and careful descriptions of actions are preferred over subjective labels like "abusive," "hysterical," or "rude to staff." Whenever possible, providers must avoid categorical and critical adjectives and instead document objective medical observations. For example, "slurred speech," "ataxic gait," and "aroma of ethanol" are recommended over "obviously drunk" or "appears intoxicated."

Poor Documentation

Most physicians, nurses, and attorneys are familiar with the adage, "If you didn't document it, you didn't do it." This cliché is often exploited by plaintiffs' attorneys. It is imperative for ED providers to understand factors associated with practice-specific documentation. Emergency physicians and other licensed independent providers typically record their initial findings but may not completely document patient reevaluations, family discussions, informed consent, and communications with other participating providers.

Although nurses may reliably document initial and ongoing patient assessments, they may fail to completely record factors like allergies and medications; interventions and observations, such as community-acquired pressure wounds from another facility; and a change in the patient's condition and what was done to address it.[31] When a patient's condition changes, nurses must also document adherence to the facility chain-of-command policy if initial or subsequent requests for intervention go unanswered.[32]

Missing documentation has implications for patient care, billing, and medicolegal support. Informed consent, refusal of care/against medical advice, and provider sign outs are frequent topics of risk-management seminars. While a successful litigation defense can result by establishing a clinician's "usual practice" and eyewitness testimony, documentation regarding key aspects of care that frequently lead to risk-management complaints is a sensible addition to any physician's usual practice. Missing documentation in a nurse's practice may create the appearance of inappropriate treatment or even a cavalier attitude toward standards of care. These perceptions may form the basis of a lawsuit.[17,32] When documenting communication between providers and nurses, it is important to carefully record specifics, such as the actual vital signs that were reported.[32] Medical records that do not document any clinical interaction, intervention, or monitoring after the initial patient encounter are inadequate in all but the briefest and least acute of ED visits.

Poor Rationale

If a patient's cooperation or mentation prevents an effective review of systems, the practitioner must document why the evaluation could not be obtained. If a CT scan for pulmonary embolus was considered but not performed, the rationale for that decision must be recorded. While ED providers are not expected to be right 100% of the time, they are expected to exercise a reasonable degree of judgment, care, and clinical acumen when diagnosing and treating patients. Documentation of all pertinent medical decisions and an explanation of any limitations and omissions are imperative.

Ignoring Abnormal Vital Signs

Occasionally, when preparing the discharge of a patient with initially normal vital signs, the treating nurse notes that the repeat vitals reflect tachycardia, tachypnea, or a low-grade temperature. In such cases, an explanation of abnormal vital signs is necessary. Particularly if the patient is low-risk and discharge is appropriate, documentation is essential to demonstrate the clinician's awareness and consideration. Additionally, two common documentation errors should be addressed:

- Pediatric patients require a full set of vital signs, including blood pressure and weight. According to JC standards, a child's weight must be documented in kilograms, not pounds.[33]

- The frequent "normal" adult respiratory rate documented by many triage personnel as 20 breaths per minute is *not* normal. A resting respiratory rate of 20 breaths per minute in the average adult is tachypneic.

Provider Bias

Occasionally, the MR becomes a battleground for frustrated caregivers struggling with a colleague, consultant, or admission problem. A plaintiff might not need expert testimony if their attorney can demonstrate two "experts" arguing and blaming each other in the MR. Such challenges and disagreements are well known, but details about the potentially inappropriate behavior of a team member have no place in the MR. Despite frustrations, it is advised to follow the facility policy for reporting an individual instead of recording critical or belittling remarks.

Similarly, labeling patients (e.g., "frequent flyer," "whiner," "jerk," or any other derogatory term) is a form of bias that must never be used in the record. Instead, documentation should be objective in nature and used only to describe behaviors, language (use direct quotes as necessary), and even odors. When it is appropriate to record the timing, duration, and substance of an action or discussion that has implications for patient care, such documentation must be pertinent and objective. If the interaction with a patient or another provider was inappropriate, there are other avenues toward resolution within the healthcare system that do not involve the MR.

Chart Amendments

While this rule of documentation may seem obvious to most caregivers, some may decide to "buff" a chart after a patient suffers an adverse outcome or files a suit. Not only does this subject the practitioner to potential *criminal* liability, it is foolhardy in the event of litigation. Even the most well-intentioned, scrupulously documented efforts to correct or amend such a chart can be made to look self-serving and duplicitous in the courtroom. Such *ex post facto* changes must not be done. After the alteration, the hospital IT department may be called up to retrieve any part of the chart with time and date stamps. Intentional modifications to the MR after the fact, even for the purpose of clarity, can destroy a provider's credibility when defending their actions.[28,29] Some malpractice insurance companies may even consider this action cause for cancellation of the malpractice insurance contract.

Unacceptable Abbreviations

With the advent of EHR checkboxes, drop-down lists, macros, and preinserted phrases, the use of abbreviations has diminished. However, free-text insertions (typed or dictated) are still common components of the MR. To eliminate confusion and ensure common comprehensions, JC standard states:

> *The hospital uses standardized diagnosis and procedure codes and ensures the standardized use of approved symbols and abbreviations across the hospital.*[34]

This requires facilities to establish lists and policies regarding abbreviations. In addition, this standard states that:

> *Abbreviations are not used on informed consent and patient rights documents, discharge instructions, discharge summaries, and other documents patients and families receive from the hospital about the patient's care.*[34]

The Institute for Safe Medication Practices publishes a list of error-prone abbreviations, symbols, and dose designations that have been deemed dangerous or frequently misinterpreted.[35] Therefore, providers who are documenting in the chart, particularly those ordering medications, need to be aware of the facility's approved/do-not-use lists. Nurses also need to clarify any orders that create uncertainty.

Medicolegal Pitfalls

In the ED, high-quality, accurate documentation provides the best defense against the possibility of legal action. All providers are at potential risk for malpractice, and many might not even learn about a legal action or a pending case for two or more years after an adverse event occurs.[6] Due to this risk, it is imperative that all providers ensure proper and accurate documentation, including physician- and nursing-sensitive indicators. Because the ED record is a legal representation of a patient visit, the important aspects of documentation and communication must be addressed.

CONCLUSION

The documentation dilemma continues to plague the medical profession. When asked what they like least about their jobs, emergency providers often respond, "Paperwork!" with emphasis and without hesitation. However, "paperwork" is an indispensable part of healthcare delivery. Thorough documentation reduces the risk of litigation and demonstrates high-quality care. Increased attention to documentation during training further indicates the importance of quality documentation.[36] While nursing education has emphasized documentation principles since the era of Florence Nightingale, these standards have evolved to become an integral and legal part of the patient record.[37]

When approached carefully, documentation provides an opportunity for enhanced interprovider communication, streamlined continuity of care, more effective billing practices, improved risk management, and better outcomes. It further decreases vulnerability to misinterpretation and risk.

REFERENCES

1. Nielsen G, Peschel L, Burgess A. Essential documentation elements: quality tool for the emergency department nurse. *Adv Emerg Nurs J*. 2014;36(2):199–205.

2. Emergency Nurses Association. *Emergency Nursing: Scope and Standards of Practice*. 2nd ed. Emergency Nurses Association; 2017.

3. American College of Emergency Physicians. Patient medical records in the emergency department. ACEP. 2018. Available at: https://www.acep.org/patient-care/policy-statements/patient-medical-records-in-the-emergency-department. Accessed January 5, 2019.

4. Lorenzetti DL, Quan H, Lucyk K, et al. Strategies for improving physician documentation in the emergency department: a systematic review. *BMC Emerg Med*. 2018;18(1):36.

5. Guth T, Morrissey T. Medical documentation and ED charting. CDEM Curriculum. Available at: https://www.saem.org/cdem/education/online-education/m3-curriculum/documentation/documentation-of-em-encounters. Updated 2015. Accessed January 10, 2019.6.

6. Di Leonardi BC, Miller-Hoover SR. Professional nursing documentation. RN.com. 2015. Available at: https://lms.rn.com/getpdf.php/2163.pdf. Accessed January 10, 2019.

7. Garrett P, Seidman J. EMR vs EHR—what is the difference? HealthITBuzz. 2011. Available at: https://www.healthit.gov/buzz-blog/electronic-health-and-medical-records/emr-vs-ehr-difference. Accessed January 11, 2019.

8. Centers for Medicare and Medicaid Services. Promoting interoperability (PI). CMS.gov. 2019. Available at: https://www.cms.gov/Regulations-and-Guidance/Legislation/EHRIncentivePrograms. Accessed August 15, 2020. Updated July 13, 2020.

9. Remarks of President Barack Obama: Address to Joint Session of Congress. 2009. Available at: https://obamawhitehouse.archives.gov/the-press-office/remarks-president-barack-obama-address-joint-session-congress. Accessed September 18, 2020.

10. Centers for Medicare and Medicaid Services. Electronic health records provider. CMS Fact Sheet. 2015. Available at: https://www.cms.gov/Medicare-Medicaid-Coordination/Fraud-Prevention/Medicaid-Integrity-Education/Downloads/docmatters-ehr-providerfactsheet.pdf. Accessed January 17, 2019.

11. University of South Florida. Federal mandates for healthcare: digital record-keeping requirements for public and private healthcare providers. USFHealth/Online. Available at: https://www.

usfhealthonline.com/resources/healthcare/electronic-medical-records-mandate/. Accessed January 11, 2019.

12. Rouse M. HITECH (Health Information Technology for Economic and Clinical Health) Act of 2009. HealthIT. Available at: https://searchhealthit.techtarget.com/definition/HITECH-Act. Updated January 2018. Accessed January 10, 2019.

13. Graber ML, Bailey R, Johnston D. Goals and priorities for health care organizations to improve safety using health IT. The Office of the National Coordinator for Health Information Technology (ONC). 2016. Available at: https://www.healthit.gov/sites/default/files/task_9_report.pdf. Accessed January 11, 2019.

14. Danna J. Scribes hold the key to ED efficiency. *Emerg Physicians Monthly*. 2016. Available at: http://epmonthly.com/article/scribes-hold-the-key-to-ed-efficiency/. Accessed August 15, 2020.

15. American College of Emergency Physicians. The use of scribes in the emergency department. *ACEP Now*. 2012. Available at: https://www.acepnow.com/article/use-scribes-emergency-department/?singlepage=1. Accessed January 10, 2019.

16. Centers for Medicare and Medicaid Services. Complying with medical record documentation requirements. Medicare Learning Network; ICN 909160. 2017. Available at: https://www.cms.gov/Outreach-and-Education/Medicare-Learning-Network-MLN/MLNProducts/Downloads/CERTMedRecDoc-FactSheet-ICN909160.pdf. Accessed January 11, 2019.

17. American Nurses Association. ANA's principles for nursing documentation: guidance for registered nurses. 2010. Available at: https://www.nursingworld.org/~4af4f2/globalassets/docs/ana/ethics/principles-of-nursing-documentation.pdf. Accessed January 11, 2019.

18. Cornell Law School. 45 CFR § 164.526 Amendment of protected health information. Legal Information Institute [LII]. Available at: https://www.law.cornell.edu/cfr/text/45/164.526. Accessed January 17, 2019.

19. The Office of the National Coordinator for Health Information Technology. State medical record laws: minimum medical record retention periods for records held by medical doctors and hospitals. Available at: https://www.healthit.gov/sites/default/files/appa7-1.pdf. Accessed September 18, 2020.

20. Centers for Medicare and Medicaid Services. Medical record retention and media formats for medical records. *MLN Matters*. No. SE1022. 2012. Available at: https://www.cms.gov/outreach-and-education/medicare-learning-network-mln/mlnmattersarticles/downloads/se1022.pdf. Accessed January 17, 2019.

21. Centers for Medicare and Medicaid Services. CMS records schedule. CMS.gov. Available at: https://www.cms.gov/Regulations-and-Guidance/Guidance/CMSRecordsSchedule. Updated October 3, 2017. Accessed January 11, 2019.

22. Cornell Law School. 45 CFR § 164.306 Security standards: general rules. Legal Information Institute [LII]. Available at: https://www.law.cornell.edu/cfr/text/45/164.306. Accessed January 11, 2019.

23. American Medical Association. Management of medical records: code of medical ethics opinion 3.3.1. AMA Ethics. 2016. Available at: https://www.ama-assn.org/delivering-care/ethics/management-medical-records. Accessed January 11, 2019.

24. US Department of Health and Human Services. HITECH Act enforcement interim final rule. HHS.gov. 2017. Available at: https://www.hhs.gov/hipaa/for-professionals/special-topics/hitech-act-enforcement-interim-final-rule/index.html. Accessed January 11, 2019.

25. Centers for Medicare and Medicaid Services. HIPAA basics for providers: privacy, security, and breach notification rules. Medicare Learning Network; ICN 909001. 2018. Available at: https://www.cms.gov/Outreach-and-Education/Medicare-Learning-Network-MLN/MLNProducts/Downloads/HIPAAPrivacyandSecurity.pdf. Accessed January 10, 2019.

26. *Tarasoff v Regents of the University of California,* 17 Cal. 3d 425, 131 Cal. Rptr.14, 551 P.2d 334 (1976).

27. Fierce Healthcare. Hospital worker fired over Facebook comments about a patient. Fox 2 News. 2010. Available at: https://www.fiercehealthcare.com/healthcare/hospital-worker-fired-over-facebook-comments-about-patient#:~:text=An%20employee%20at%20Oakwood%20Hospital,parent%20company%20Oakwood%20Healthcare%2C%20Inc.&text=The%20hospital%20fired%20her%20instead. Accessed August 15, 2020.

28. Fierce Healthcare, Photos of dying patient posted to Facebook get four hospital workers fired. 2010. Available at: https://www.fiercehealthcare.com/healthcare/photos-dying-patient-posted-to-facebook-get-four-hospital-workers-fired. Accessed August 15, 2020.

29. Mitchell M. "Audit Trail" metadata discoverable in med mal suit. Law.com/The Legal Intelligence. 2017. Available at: https://www.law.com/thelegalintelligencer/almID/1202783488269/?slreturn=20190021163519. Accessed January 17, 2019.

30. Meyer JF, Tome JP, Neubecker L. Patient medical records: metadata as evidence in litigation. Enigma Forensics, Volume 101 #8. 2013. Available at: https://enigmaforensics.com/blog/patient-medical-records-metadata-litigation/. Accessed August 15, 2020.

31. Nurses Service Organization. 7 common pitfalls to avoid in charting patient information. 2018. Available at: https://www.nso.com/Learning/Artifacts/Articles/7-Common-Pitfalls-to-Avoid-in-Charting-Patient-Information. Accessed August 15, 2020.

32. Myers V. Defending yourself through documentation. *Am Nurse*. 2014. Available at: https://www.myamericannurse.com/defending-yourself-through-documentation/. Accessed January 17, 2019.

33. The Joint Commission. Preventing pediatric medication errors. *TJC Sentinel Event Alert*. 2008;(39). Available at: https://www.jointcommission.org/assets/1/18/SEA_39.PDF. Accessed January 17, 2019.

34. Joint Commission International. Use of codes, symbols, and abbreviations. 2018. Available at: https://www.jointcommissioninternational.org/use-of-codes-symbols-and-abbreviations/. Accessed January 17, 2019.

35. Institute for Safe Medication Practices. List of error-prone abbreviations. ISMP. 2017. Available at: https://www.ismp.org/recommendations/error-prone-abbreviations-list. Accessed January 10, 2019.

36. Centers for Medicare and Medicaid Services. Guidelines for teaching physicians, interns, and residents. Medicare Learning Network; ICN 006347. 2018. Available at: https://www.cms.gov/Outreach-and-Education/Medicare-Learning-Network-MLN/MLNProducts/Downloads/Teaching-Physicians-Fact-Sheet-ICN006437.pdf. Accessed January 11, 2019.

37. Chelagat D, Sum T, MPhil M, Chebor A, Kiptoo R, Bundotich-Mosol P. Documentation: historical perspectives, purposes, benefits, and challenges as faced by nurses. *Int J Hum Soc Sci*. 2013;3(16):236-240.

REPORTING REQUIREMENTS CONFIDENTIALITY, DATA BREACHES, AND HIPAA

CHAPTER 107

Howard A. Peth Jr, Denise Bayer

I will respect the privacy of my patients, for their problems are not disclosed to me that the world may know.

—Hippocrates (modern version)[1]

Medical professionals have an obligation to protect the privacy of their patients. It is this duty that forms the foundation of the patient relationship, and a failure to respect it will lead to patient harm. To effectively treat patients and provide them with the best possible care, health-care professionals must use data beyond objective assessments and test results. They must also rely on subjective information, which includes details about the patient's lifestyle, habits, and recreational activities. For patients to share that information, they must have confidence that health-care professionals will keep the private details of their lives private. The American College of Emergency Physicians and the Emergency Nurses Association have published policy statements that demonstrate their ongoing commitment to patient privacy in the fields of emergency health care.[2,3]

Although it has been updated over the years to reflect the current society, both the classic and modern versions of the Hippocratic Oath articulate the importance of patient confidentiality. The classic version states:

What I may see or hear in the course of the treatment or even outside of the treatment in regard to the life of men, which on no account one must spread abroad, I will keep to myself, holding such things shameful to be spoken about.[1]

Just as physicians have taken on oath to uphold the privacy of their patients, so have nurses. A modified version of the Hippocratic Oath, the Nightingale Pledge is a statement of the ethics of the nursing profession. Nurses recite the pledge at the completion of their studies and commit to "hold in confidence all personal matters committed to my keeping and all family affairs coming to my knowledge in the practice of my calling."[4]

HEALTH INSURANCE PORTABILITY AND ACCOUNTABILITY ACT

In response to fears that confidential patient health information was vulnerable to compromise, the US Congress passed the Healthcare Insurance Portability and Accountability Act (HIPAA).[5] The HIPAA is a complex federal law that has continued to evolve and expand its scope over the past two decades. The original act, passed in 1996,

TABLE 107.1 ■ Major HIPAA Milestones	
1996	Original Healthcare Insurance Portability and Accountability Act was signed into law.
2003	HIPAA Privacy Rule becomes effective.
2005	HIPAA Security Rule becomes effective.
2009	HIPAA Breach Notification Rule becomes effective.
2013	HIPAA Final Omnibus Rule becomes effective.

was primarily intended to improve the portability and accountability of health insurance coverage for employees between jobs. In addition, it was intended to reduce waste, fraud, and abuse in health insurance and health-care delivery. For a brief time line of the major milestones related to HIPAA, see **Table 107.1**.[6]

Today, after several updates, HIPAA has become synonymous with patient privacy in and governs the management and release of confidential information, referred to as protected health information (PHI).[7] It is important for health-care professionals to understand its definition (see **Box 107.1**).[8,9]

Failure to comply with HIPAA may result in significant civil monetary penalties to both individual health-care professionals and institutions. The American Recovery and Reinvestment Act of 2009, subsection Health Information Technology for Economic and Clinical Health (HITECH) Act of 2009, provides for significant civil monetary penalties—up to $1.5 million—for the most egregious conduct.[10] In addition, all 50 states recognize a right to privacy of one's personal information under either common or statutory law.

The Privacy Rule

Historically, patient medical records consisted of handwritten notes tucked safely away in physicians' offices. The emergence of the electronic health record, by virtue of its broad accessibility and potential for unfettered distribution, engenders many privacy concerns. Today, confidential patient information is vulnerable to exposure in ways never before contemplated by our forbearers in health care. A single touch of the "send" button on a computer can transmit a patient's PHI to an unlimited number of recipients within seconds.

The HIPAA Privacy Rule establishes national standards to protect individual's medical records and other personal health information (**Box 107.2**).[11] It also establishes when PHI may be used and disclosed. The HIPAA mandates that PHI may not be accessed by or disclosed

---

BOX 107.1 ■ PROTECTED HEALTH INFORMATION

- **Disclosure:** the release, transfer, provision of, access to, or divulging in any other manner of information outside the entity holding the information
- **Health information:** any information, whether oral or recorded in any form or medium, that is both:
  - Created or received by a health-care provider, health plan, public health authority, employer, life insurer, school or university, or health-care clearinghouse, *and*
  - Relates to the past, present, or future physical or mental health or condition of an individual; the provision of health care to an individual; or the past, present, or future payment for the provision of health care to an individual.

> **BOX 107.2 ■ PRIVACY RULE NATIONAL STANDARDS SUMMARY**
>
> - It gives patients more control over their health information.
> - It sets boundaries on the use and release (disclosure) of health records.
> - It establishes appropriate safeguards that health-care providers and others must achieve to protect the privacy of health information.
> - It holds violators accountable with civil and criminal penalties that can be imposed if they violate patients' privacy rights.
> - It strikes a balance when public responsibility supports disclosure of some forms of data (e.g., to protect public health).

to anyone without the patient's written consent, unless there is an explicit exception (**Box 107.3**).[9]

Privacy Compliance vs Reporting Obligations

While the HIPAA Privacy Rule does generally require patient consent for the disclosure of their PHI, it does allow for certain circumstances that do not require consent. As stated previously, the rule was designed to strike a balance when public responsibility supports disclosure of certain data (e.g., to protect public health). Subject to the requirements of 45 CFR §164.512(c), (e), and (f), HIPAA expressly authorizes the disclosure of PHI that is required by law.[12]

As federal law, HIPAA preempts state law when the state's privacy standard is less stringent than the privacy standard established under HIPAA.[9] However, when the state establishes a more stringent standard, that more rigorous standard will be upheld.[13] Under HIPAA, states retain their traditional authority to enact legislation that promotes public health and safety. Competing policy considerations have resulted in the enactment of a diverse body of law, and there is no uniform national reporting statute.

Subject to the requirements of 45 CFR §164.512(c), (e), and (f), HIPAA expressly authorizes disclosures of PHI that are required by law.[11,12] While there is nothing complex about any of the state reporting laws, there is enough variation among the states that an innocent misstep can lead to potentially adverse consequences.

Law Enforcement

When HIPAA first took effect in 2003, there was a great deal of confusion about what patient information ED staff were permitted to provide to law enforcement personnel.

> **BOX 107.3 ■ DISCLOSURE NOT REQUIRING PATIENT CONSENT**
>
> - Disclosures required by law
> - Disclosures for public health activities
> - Disclosures about victims of abuse, neglect, or domestic violence
> - Disclosures about decedents
> - Disclosures for cadaveric organ, eye, or tissue donation purposes
> - Health oversight activities
> - Judicial and administrative proceedings
> - Law enforcement
> - Research
> - Serious threat to health or safety
> - Essential government functions
> - Workers' compensation

> **BOX 107.4 ■ PHI FOR LAW ENFORCEMENT**
>
> **Information that may be disclosed in response to official law enforcement requests includes:**
>
> - Name and address
> - Date and place of birth
> - Social security number
> - ABO blood type and Rh factor
> - Type of injury
>
> - Date and time of treatment
> - Date and time of death, if applicable
> - Description of distinguishing physical characteristics, including height, weight, gender, race, hair and eye color, presence or absence of facial hair (beard or moustache), scars, and tattoos

HIPAA permits disclosures as required by law, including the reporting of certain types of wounds and other physical injuries. In addition, staff may disclose PHI in response to a law enforcement official's request for information, such as identifying or locating a suspect, fugitive, material witness, or missing person, provided that only the information listed in **Box 107.4** is given.[8,12]

When law enforcement officials produce a legal document (court order, subpoena, grand jury summons, or administrative agency order) demanding access to PHI, ED staff should direct the official to the hospital attorney, risk manager, or their supervisor. The attorney/administration will ensure that the hospital's response to the court order or subpoena complies with HIPAA requirements and that the patient's rights are afforded the full protection of the law. A court order or subpoena does not entitle law enforcement personnel to anything more than the specific object of the order. Hospital staff should not engage in any verbal discussion of the patient's case.

Reportable events are grouped into two categories pertinent to the care of emergency patients. They include reports in which a patient presents as a suspected or known victim of abuse, neglect, or violence and poses a risk to public health and safety. State reporting statutes often require inclusion of specified items of information that, if available, must be documented in the report. In such circumstances, emergency care providers are ethically constrained to disclose *only* the private information specifically required by the statute, with nonrequested information kept in confidence insofar as possible.[11] Specific reporting processes are mandated when the patient is the victim. Examples include child abuse, human trafficking, domestic violence, sexual assault, and so on.

Child Abuse and Neglect

Mandatory reporting laws in all 50 states require emergency physicians, nurses, and social workers to report all cases of actual or suspected child abuse or neglect to appropriate agencies immediately upon discovery. Most states have a 24-hour child abuse hotline that ED personnel can use to report cases directly to the designated agency. Though all 50 states have mandatory reporting requirements, state laws may vary. It is imperative that all ED healthcare professionals understand their obligation for reporting of child abuse and neglect.

In nearly every state and US territory, failure to report suspected abuse or neglect as required by law is punishable by fine or imprisonment.[14] This failure to report may also result in adverse action by state boards of medicine and/or nursing. Sadly, the worst consequence of a failure to intervene on behalf of an abused child can be the child's death. All states provide immunity to physicians and nurses whose reports are based on a good-faith belief.

Sexual abuse of children may present to the ED only after several months or years of repetitive incidents. Those cases that are eventually identified are likely to represent only the tip of the iceberg. Emergency clinicians may serve as the only point of access for many victims of child sexual abuse and are their only hope of rescue. If practitioners are to succeed in identifying the victims in need of intervention, it is imperative that they develop a high level of attentiveness to the possibility of sexual abuse in pediatric patients.[15]

The Child Abuse Prevention and Treatment Act defines sexual abuse of children to include rape, molestation, engaging in sexually explicit conduct or simulation of such conduct, producing visual depiction of sexual conduct, inducement of prostitution or other form of sexual exploitation of children, child pornography, or incest with children.[16] In addition to notification and activation of a state's designated child protective agency, the sexual abuse of a child necessitates both an evidentiary forensic examination and the involvement of law enforcement authorities.

Many states have adopted programs that use specially trained sexual assault nurse examiners. The sexual assault response team (SART) is another successful program devoted caring for victims and collecting evidence that will aid in the prosecution of the perpetrator. The success of these initiatives is dependent on the support of the hospital administration, close collaboration with local law enforcement, and strong professional and emotional support from the ED medical staff.

HIPAA allows for the disclosure of PHI to report known or suspected child abuse, neglect, exploitation, and sexual abuse, if the report is made to a public health authority or other appropriate government authority that is authorized by law to receive such reports. This disclosure does not require the consent of the patient, parent, or guardian. In some situations, health-care providers may restrict parents' or guardians' access to a child's medical information if releasing PHI to the child's guardians may pose a danger to the child or to another person. Likewise, health-care providers may refuse to disclose a child's PHI to a parent or guardian if the providers reasonably suspect that the parent or guardian is abusing the child.[12]

Case One

At a high-volume urban ED, Jean White, registered nurse, informs Dr. Brenda Smith that her next patient is Mary, a 4-year-old girl with a urinary tract infection (UTI). Dr. Smith enters the examining room to evaluate Mary, who is accompanied by her mother. The mother informs Dr. Smith that Mary has been having "a lot of trouble with UTIs" and that she was seen in the ED 4 months ago and diagnosed with a UTI. However, a review of the prior ED record shows that Mary's previous urine sample indicated no evidence of a UTI. Upon Dr. Smith's genital examination, Mary, who has been calm and cooperative, suddenly starts kicking and screaming.

While awaiting the results of Mary's urinalysis testing, Dr. Smith proceeds to see her next patient who happens to be Mary's 28-year-old father, John. He tells Dr. Smith that he has had a painful urethral discharge for a week and, upon the physician's questioning, admits that he has been having an affair with another woman. Dr. Smith obtains urethral swab specimens from John, and when exiting the examination room, Dr. Smith hears the patient call out, "Can my daughter get this infection from me?" In the meantime, Mary's urinalysis reveals an absence of bacteria indicative of a UTI. What is Dr. Smith's next step?

Case Resolution

Dr. Smith has enough information under an objective "reasonable person standard" to report Mary's case to her state's child abuse hotline. She is not accusing Mary's father, John, of sexual abuse, but it would be appropriate for child protective services and the SART nurse to initiate an investigation.

Adult Exploitation

Human trafficking is increasingly recognized as a form of exploitation.[17] It is a significant national and global human rights violation. Victims of trafficking may be lured with promises of a better life. They are instead enslaved. Many states are implementing laws requiring signage in EDs describing the possible presentations of trafficking to encourage reporting. This problem is too large and complex to be addressed briefly by this chapter. For those with an interest in pursuing more information on this topic, multiple organizations may be accessed from an online search.

Intimate Partner Violence

Intimate partner violence (IPV) is abuse or aggression that occurs in a close relationship. The term "intimate partner" includes current and former spouses and dating partners. Intimate partner violence can vary in frequency and severity and occurs on a continuum, ranging from one episode that might or might not have a lasting impact to chronic and severe episodes over a period of years.[18] Intimate partner violence includes four types of behavior: physical violence, sexual violence, stalking, and psychological aggression.[19]

An estimated 10% of women and 4% of men in the United States report experiencing physical violence, rape, or stalking from an intimate partner in their lifetime.[19] Unfortunately, despite the fact that IPV victims routinely use the ED for health care, they are often unlikely to be identified or receive intervention for IPV in the ED. All clinicians should be trained and aware of signs of IPV, which are summarized in **Box 107.5**.[20]

Under HIPAA, reporting of IPV is permitted subject to the constraints of state law.[12] However, the states are not united on the issue of mandatory versus patient-authorized reporting of IPV. In states with mandatory IPV reporting statutes, it is often controversial if patient consent is needed for emergency physicians and nurses to report all incidents of IPV. In such jurisdictions, the victim should be informed of the physician's statutory obligations, and no disclosure of PHI greater than is absolutely necessary to comply with the statute is permitted. The physician's discussion with the patient be documented in the medical record. In addition, it is recommended to confer with the hospital risk manager/privacy office/attorney for further guidance.

Case Two

Mrs. Johnson, a 42-year-old woman, arrives to the ED via ambulance after an "argument" with her husband. He reportedly struck her in the face because "dinner was not ready on

---

BOX 107.5 ■ SIGNS OF INTIMATE PARTNER ABUSE

- Monitors what intimate partner (IP) is doing all the time
- Criticizes IP for little things
- Constantly accuses IP of being unfaithful
- Gets angry when drinking or using drugs
- Controls how IP spends IP's money
- Controls IP's use of needed medicines
- Humiliates IP in front of others
- Destroys IP's property or things IP cares about
- Threatens to hurt IP, the children, or pets, or does hurt IP (by hitting, beating, pushing, shoving, punching, slapping, kicking, or biting)
- Uses or threatens to use a weapon against IP
- Forces IP to have sex against IP's will
- Blames IP for his or her violent outbursts

time." Finally, he threw her against the kitchen wall and then ran out of the house. She states that her husband has struck her before, "but it was never this bad." Her three young children witnessed the episode. Further questioning reveals that Mrs. Johnson moved to the area several years ago with her husband because of a job transfer. She has no local extended family. In addition, her husband's possessiveness has made it very difficult for her to make new friends. She has been very depressed by her circumstances. She has limited access to health care and no family physician. Her ED evaluation reveals facial swelling with bilateral periorbital hematomas. Imaging studies are negative for any fractures. What are the emergency physician's reporting requirements?

Case Resolution

Depending on the state in which Mrs. Johnson's IPV incident occurred, her ED provider may need her consent to report the assault to law enforcement. Her provider must inform the patient that they are willing to notify law enforcement with her consent. Alternatively, if she is in a mandatory reporting state like California, the ED provider should gently inform her that the state requires disclosure. The ED may be Mrs. Johnson's only resource, and her future safety may depend on the interventions offered to her during this visit. The evaluation should include an assessment of her immediate safety needs, social service consultation, a crisis intervention counselor, immediate arrangements for placement in a women's and children's shelter, medical and mental health follow-up, and law enforcement assistance.

Sexual Assault

In contrast to sexual crimes against children, for which mandatory reporting is always required, mandatory reporting does not apply when the victim of sexual assault is an adult. In the adult, a forensic examination requires consent. Sexual assault may take many forms along a continuum from offensive touching of another's body to sexual intercourse. Although victims of sexual assault frequently do sustain significant injuries at the hands of their perpetrators, injuries are not required elements of the crime.

The vast majority of sexual assaults are never reported. When these crimes *are* reported and prosecuted, many victims find the legal proceedings to be humiliating. The identification and apprehension of a sexual predator may wholly depend upon DNA analysis of the assailant's body fluids. After the collection of forensic evidence, the victim still may defer the decision to press charges. Stabilization of victims of sexual assault includes a safety assessment before an ED disposition is made. In addition, social services and rape crisis services should be made available to the patient.

Statutory rape laws are rooted in the belief that sexual activity between individuals below a certain age is coercive. However, there is no uniform age below which statutory rape is said to occur. In fact, only 12 states have clearly defined age limits for the age of consent. Among those states, there is no consensus on what that age is—it ranges from 16 to 13 years of age.[21,22]

In the case of sexual assaults, the disclosure of PHI should only be done with patient consent, unless the health-care provider is required by law to report the event regardless of patient consent. Most states do not require or mandate reporting of adult sexual assaults; instead, reporting is based on patient consent.

Elder or Dependent Adult Abuse and Neglect

In most states, emergency physicians and nurses are mandatory reporters who must file an immediate report if, within the scope of their employment, they are made aware of neglect

TABLE 107.2 ■ Definitions of Elder Abuse

Term	Definition
Physical abuse	Use of physical force that may result in bodily injury, physical pain, or impairment
Sexual abuse	Nonconsensual sexual contact of any kind with an elderly person
Psychological abuse	Infliction of anguish, emotional pain, or distress
Neglect	Refusal or failure to fulfill any part of a person's obligations or duties to an elder
Abandonment	Desertion of an elderly person by an individual who has assumed responsibility for providing care or by a person with physical custody of an elder
Financial or material exploitation	Illegal or improper use of an elder's funds, property, or assets
Self-neglect	Behaviors of an elderly person that threaten his or her own health or safety

or abuse. While there is variation in state laws on who is defined as a mandatory reporter, the Center for Disease Control and Prevention (CDC) has defined elder abuse as "an intentional act, or failure to act, by a caregiver or another person in a relationship involving an expectation of trust that causes or creates a risk of harm to an older adult."[23] The CDC further defines several types of elder abuse (**Table 107.2**).[23] State laws vary on who are mandatory reporters and where reports are to be filed. Typically, these reports are made to state social services agencies or local law enforcement authorities. Most states allow telephone reports via toll-free 24-hour abuse hotlines.[24]

Finally, in most states, adults with physical or mental limitations (including physical or developmental disabilities that render them unable to carry out normal activities or protect their rights) who are between the ages of 18 to 64 are considered vulnerable or dependent adults. As a result, these dependent adults, if abused, may fall within the purview of elder abuse reporting laws. All states have criminal penalties for mandatory reporters who knowingly and willfully fail to fulfill their obligations.

HIPAA allows for the disclosure of PHI to report known or suspected elder abuse, neglect, exploitation, and sexual abuse, if the report is made to a public health authority or other appropriate government authority that is authorized by law to receive such reports. This disclosure does not require the consent of the patient or guardian.[15]

Violence

Emergency physicians and nurses must comply with mandatory state reporting statutes pertaining to violent crimes. HIPAA allows doctors and nurses to use or disclose PHI to report violent crimes, such as gunshot wounds and stabbings, to local law enforcement pursuant to applicable state statutes. The reporting may only occur to the extent that the disclosure is required by law, and the disclosure is limited to the relevant requirements of the law.[8,12] Physicians may encourage victims of violence (that does not trigger a mandatory physician report) to file charges directly with the local authorities. The ED record, including x-rays and photographs, help document the victim's injuries.

REPORTS RELATED TO PUBLIC HEALTH AND SAFETY

Communicable Diseases

Reporting of communicable diseases to public health authorities is vital for containing infectious diseases before they spread into the wider community. Specifically, public safety reports related to communicable diseases:

- Help to identify contacts of an index patient who may need treatment.
- Alert epidemiologists to the presence of vectors in the environment that are involved in the propagation of infectious diseases.
- Help epidemiologists assess the effectiveness of vaccination programs and other preventive measures.

Vigilant surveillance is also vital to protecting the community in the event of bioterrorism. HIPAA allows the disclosure of PHI to:

- Public health departments for surveillance of communicable diseases and other information important to the public health and safety[12]
- Persons who may have been exposed to a communicable disease or may be at risk of spreading a disease or condition[12]
- Food and Drug Administration for postmarketing surveillance, reports of adverse drug events, and problems with medical devices[12]
- Authorized federal officials for the conduct of lawful intelligence, counterintelligence, and other national security activities[12]

Most infectious diseases today are diagnosed or confirmed by pathologists and laboratory personnel who submit mandatory communicable disease reports. However, when an emergency physician has occasion to suspect a high-risk diagnosis, such as meningococcemia, anthrax, or other disease specified by state statute, a report to the state health department must be made immediately.

Department of Motor Vehicles

There is no national consensus, legally or scientifically, that guides practitioners when addressing the potential hazards posed by drivers potentially impaired by medical conditions. To effectively balance the ethical obligations to their patients against the diverse demands of the states, emergency physicians should be familiar with their own state's reporting requirements and protections. The American Medical Association's (AMA) Ethical Opinion 8.2, "Impaired Drivers and Their Physicians," provides invaluable guidance for emergency physicians when balancing the interests of their patients and public safety:[25]

To serve the interests of their patients and the public within their areas of expertise, physicians should:

    (a) Assess at-risk patients individually for medical conditions that might adversely affect driving ability using best professional judgment and keeping in mind that not all physical or mental impairments create an obligation to intervene.

    (b) Tactfully but candidly discussing risks with the patient and, when appropriate, the family when a medical condition may adversely affect the patient's ability to drive safely. Help the patient (and family) formulate a plan to reduce risks, including options for treatment or therapy if available, changes in driving behavior, or other adjustments.

    (c) Recognize that safety standards for those who operate commercial transportation are subject to governmental medical standards and may differ from standard for private licenses.

(d) Be aware of applicable state requirements for reporting to the licensing authority those patients whose impairments may compromise their ability to operate a motor vehicle safely.
(e) Prior to reporting, explain to the patient (and family as appropriate) that the physician may have an obligation to report a medically at-risk driver:
 1. When the physician identifies a medical condition clearly related to the ability to drive
 2. When continuing to drive poses a clear risk to public safety or the patient's own well-being and the patient ignores the physician's advice to discontinue driving
 3. When required by law
    (a) Inform the patient that the determination of inability to drive safely will be made by other authorities, not the physician
    (b) Disclose only the minimum necessary information when reporting a medically at-risk driver, in keeping with ethics guidance on respect for patient privacy and confidentiality"[25]

In states where there is no department of motor vehicles (DMV) reporting statute and physicians are not authorized to report medically impaired patients' PHI, the AMA ethical opinion described above provides a prudent algorithm for the physician. The physician considering disclosure must nonetheless be aware that federal law under HIPAA prohibits the disclosure of PHI to the DMV without the patient's consent.

Emergency department providers may face the additional risk of liability to nonpatient third parties. A provider may be held liable if a discharged patient with a seizure disorder (or other disorder involving altered mental status) has a subsequent event resulting in the injury or death of a third party.[26] Liability is mitigated by providing a warning to the patient to stop driving accompanied by careful documentation in the ED record.[26]

Case Three

Mr. Green is a 22-year-old man who presents to the ED via ambulance. He was a restrained driver involved in a single-vehicle collision with a tree. When medics responded to the scene, he was awake but confused. His blood sugar in the field was 120 mg. On arrival, he is alert but has no memory of the event. He informs his ED nurse that he was just driving home after working a night shift. He also states that he has a 2-year history of epilepsy and that he has not had a seizure for the past 18 months. His doctor has prescribed carbamazepine for his seizures, which he states he takes every day as directed. For the past 3 weeks, his job has required him to work nights, and he has not been sleeping very well. Other than a few bruises, he has no significant injuries. What is the ED provider's best strategy in addressing Mr. Green's driving impairment?

Case Resolution

The reporting requirements will depend on whether Mr. Green lives in one of the six mandatory reporting states for lapses of consciousness while driving. If he lives in a mandatory reporting state, the ED providers must report Mr. Green's episode to the DMV or other appropriate state agency. Otherwise, if he lives in a permissive reporting state, a report to the DMV is not indicated at this time. Until this incident, Mr. Green had achieved good control of his seizure disorder. Close follow-up with his treating provider and addressing his recent change in sleep habit will likely accomplish good seizure control for Mr. Green. In the meantime, an admonition to refrain from driving—documented in the record and in combination with Mr. Green's agreement not to drive—is very important.

DEATH IN THE ED

State laws vary in their treatment of a person's right to privacy following their death. However, patient privacy rights do not end upon death under HIPAA, which preempts any state law to the contrary. Legal provisions allow the disclosure of a deceased patient's PHI for the purpose of identifying a deceased person, determining the cause of death, or responding to other duties as authorized by law.[8,12]

Emergency department staff may disclose PHI to funeral directors as necessary to carry out their duties with respect to the decedent.[12] Finally, ED staff may use or disclose PHI to organ procurement organizations or other entities engaged in the procurement, banking, or transplantation of cadaveric organs, eyes, or tissue.[12] Any other disclosures of a person's PHI require the authorization of the patient's legal representative. The HIPAA Privacy Rule protects the individually identifiable health information about a decedent for 50 years following the date of death of the individual.[8]

CONCLUSION

The primary objective of the HIPAA Privacy Rule is to establish minimum federal standards for safeguarding the privacy of individually identifiable health information. However, there is no uniform national reporting statute, and reporting requirements vary unpredictably across state lines, which can create a significant challenge when trying to understand and comply with HIPAA regulations. In addition, there are significant financial and civil penalties to both organizations and individuals for failure to comply with HIPAA, making it important that we all know and understand our roles.

In this era of high interstate mobility among physicians and nurses, medical directors and nurse managers should be alerted to the possibility that newly recruited clinicians will likely have some confusion about the reporting requirements of their new state. All hospitals are required to provide education to their staff regarding HIPAA regulations. It is suggested that this training be done often and in small doses. While there are many resources available to help staff understand HIPAA rules and regulations, common hospital resources, including policy and procedure manuals, legal counsel, risk management, and privacy officers, should not be overlooked.

REFERENCES

1. Wikipedia. Hippocratic Oath. Available at: https://en.wikipedia.org/wiki/Hippocratic_Oath. Updated October 21, 2020. Accessed October 24, 2020.
2. Confidentiality of patient information. Policy statement. American College of Emergency Physicians. 2017. Available at: https://www.acep.org/patient-care/policy-statements/confidentiality-of-patient-information/#sm.0000tfwbklrn3dqaquf2pq16ut24s. Accessed January 21, 2019.
3. Gurney D, Gillespie GL, McMahon MP, et al. Nursing code of ethics: provisions and interpretative statements for emergency nurses. *J Emerg Nurs*. 2017;43(6):497–503.
4. The Nightingale Pledge. Available at: https://www.countryjoe.com/nightingale/pledge.htm. Accessed January 21, 2019.
5. Moskop JC, Marco CA, Larkin GL, et al. From Hippocrates to HIPAA: privacy and confidentiality in emergency medicine—part II: challenges in the emergency department. *Ann Emerg Med*. 2005;45(1):60–67.
6. HIPAA for professionals. US Department of Health and Human Services. Available at: https://www.hhs.gov/hipaa/for-professionals/index.html. Last Reviewed June 16, 2017. Accessed January 21, 2019.
7. HIPAA Journal. What is Protected Health Information. 2018. Available at: https://www.hipaajournal.com/what-is-protected-health-information/#:~:text=Protected%20health%20information%20includes%20all,healthcare%20services%20or%20healthcare%20coverage. Accessed October 24, 2020.
8. 45 CFR §§160.103; Definitions. 2013. Available at: https://www.law.cornell.edu/cfr/text/45/164.103. Accessed October 26, 2020.
9. 45 CFR §§164.502—Uses and disclosures of protected health information: General rules. 2013. Available at: https://www.law.cornell.edu/cfr/text/45/164.502. Accessed October 24, 2020.

10. HIPAA Journal. HHS Changes HITECH Act Penalties for HIPAA Violations. 2019. Available at: https://www.hipaajournal.com/updated-hipaa-penalties-hitech-act/. Accessed October 24, 2020.

11. What does the HIPAA Privacy Rule do? US Department of Health and Human Services. Last Reviewed July 26, 2013. Available at: https://www.hhs.gov/hipaa/for-individuals/faq/187/what-does-the-hipaa-privacy-rule-do/index.html. Accessed January 21, 2019.

12. 45 CFR §§164.512.

13. US Constitution, Article VI, "Supremacy Clause."

14. Penalties for failure to report and false reporting of child abuse and neglect. Child Welfare Information Gateway. 2019. Available at: https://www.childwelfare.gov/topics/systemwide/laws-policies/statutes/report/. Accessed January 21, 2019.

15. Pelletier HL, Knox, M. Incorporating child maltreatment training into medical school curricula. *J Child Adolesc Trauma*. 2017;10(3):267–274.

16. 42 USC §5106g(4).

17. Emergency Nurses Administration. Human trafficking awareness in the emergency care setting. Joint Position Statement. Emergency Nurses Association. 2018. Available at: https://www.ena.org/docs/default-source/resource-library/practice-resources/position-statements/humantraffickingpatientawareness.pdf. Accessed October 24, 2020.

18. Preventing Intimate Partner Violence. Centers for Disease Control and Prevention. 2020. Available at: https://www.cdc.gov/violenceprevention/intimatepartnerviolence/fastfact.html. Accessed October 24, 2020.

19. Breiding MJ, Basile KC, Smith SG, et al. *Intimate Partner Violence Surveillance: Uniform Definitions and Recommended Data Elements*. Version 2.0. National Center for Injury Prevention and Control, Centers for Disease Control and Prevention; 2015.

20. The United States Department of Justice. Office of Violence Against Women (OVW). 2020. Available at: https://www.justice.gov/ovw. Accessed October 24, 2020.

21. Baldwin L. Statutory Rape Laws and Charges. Nolo. 2020. Available at: https://www.criminaldefenselawyer.com/resources/criminal-defense/sex-crimes/statutory-rape-charges-punishment-defense. Accessed October 24, 2020.

22. Glosser A, Gardiner K, Fishman M, et al. *Statutory Rape: A Guide to State Laws and Reporting Requirements*. The Office of the Assistant Secretary for Planning and Evaluation, US Department of Health and Human Services. 2004. Available at: https://aspe.hhs.gov/system/files/pdf/75531/report.pdf. Accessed January 28, 2019.

23. CDC. Preventing elder abuse. Available at: https://www.cdc.gov/violenceprevention/elderabuse/definitions.html. Updated May 12, 2020. Accessed October 24, 2020.

24. 2013 Nationwide survey of mandatory reporting requirements for elderly and/or vulnerable persons. National Adult Protective Services Association. 2015. Available at: http://www.napsa-now.org/wp-content/uploads/2014/11/Mandatory-Reporting-Chart-Updated-FINAL.pdf. Accessed October 24, 2020.

25. Impaired drivers and their physicians: code of medical ethics opinion 8.2. American Medical Association. Available at: https://www.ama-assn.org/delivering-care/ethics/impaired-drivers-their-physicians. Accessed January 24, 2019.

26. AMA. Impaired Drivers and Their Physicians—Code of Medical Ethics Opinion 8.2. American Medical Association. Available at: https://www.ama-assn.org/delivering-care/ethics/impaired-drivers-their-physicians. Updated 2020. Accessed October 24, 2020.

DISPOSITION, DISCHARGE, AND FOLLOW-UP

William Sullivan, Paul Allegretti, Joanne E. Navarroli

Upon concluding a patient's emergency department (ED) visit, the medical provider must decide whether the patient should be admitted, transferred, or discharged. This decision is often multifactorial, considering not only a patient's condition and predicted stability, but also incorporating social factors and the many regulations applicable to ED care.

EMERGENCY MEDICAL TREATMENT AND ACTIVE LABOR ACT

The Emergency Medical Treatment and Active Labor Act (EMTALA) applies specifically to evaluation and medical treatment of ED patients (see Chapter 104).[1] Prior to the enactment of EMTALA, uninsured individuals routinely received disparate care at private hospitals or were transferred to public hospitals in unstable condition. For example, **Table 108.1** shows a study of 467 individuals transferred to one public hospital prior to EMTALA's enactment.[2] EMTALA was crafted not only to ensure that hospitals provide an initial screening exam to individuals seeking medical care but also to to ensure that they put forth their best efforts to stabilize an individual prior to making a disposition.

EMTALA requires that an individual be screened for an "emergency medical condition," defined as:

> *A medical condition manifesting itself by acute symptoms of sufficient severity (including severe pain) such that the absence of immediate medical attention could reasonably be expected to result in placing the health of the individual (or, with respect to a pregnant woman, the health of the woman or her unborn child) in serious jeopardy, serious impairment to bodily functions, or serious dysfunction of any bodily organ or part; or with respect to a pregnant woman who is having contractions that there is inadequate time to effect a safe transfer to another hospital before delivery, or that transfer may pose a threat to the health or safety of the woman or the unborn child.*[3]

TABLE 108.1 ■ Patient Transfer Demographics Prior to Enactment of EMTALA	
Reason for/Condition on Transfer	**%**
Uninsured	87
Unstable condition	24
Died on admission	9.4
Died on admission (nontransferred patients)	3.8

Proper Disposition

The proper disposition of an individual depends upon whether that individual is deemed to have an emergency medical condition. Once an emergency medical condition is identified, the hospital must attempt to stabilize the patient. When the patient is stabilized, EMTALA no longer applies. EMTALA defines "stabilization" as treatment that ensures:

> ... *within reasonable medical probability, that no material deterioration of the condition is likely to result from or occur during the transfer of the individual from a facility" or, with regard to a pregnant patient having contractions, as delivery of the child, including the placenta.*[4]

A hospital must use all of its resources to provide stabilizing treatment. If the hospital lacks the capability to manage a particular emergency medical condition, it must arrange for an appropriate transfer of the individual to another facility that can provide a higher level of care.

"Individual" or "Patient"

EMTALA repeatedly uses the term "individual" rather than "patient." The reason for this distinction is important, as the law is specifically intended to apply to outpatients seeking care in the ED. A "patient" is defined as an individual who has been admitted to the hospital or has begun to receive outpatient services as part of a hospital encounter. With few exceptions, EMTALA does not apply to admitted (inpatient) patients. Another important point is that patients who are kept in a hospital under "observation" status are *not* considered "admitted" for purposes of EMTALA. The Centers for Medicare & Medicaid Services (CMS) interpretive guidelines clearly state that "placement in an observation status of an individual . . . does not terminate the EMTALA obligations of that hospital or a recipient."[5] Subsequent court opinions have bolstered this determination. For example, in *Dicioccio v Chung*, the court held that "CMS regulations and guidance make clear that admission for observation does not end a hospital's EMTALA obligations."[6]

This legal framework established by EMTALA helps to shape the disposition process of patients who have been evaluated in the ED.

THE DISPOSITION PROCESS

Many factors must be considered when determining whether a patient should be discharged, admitted, or transferred. While there is no standard algorithm for making such decisions, some of the many medical, social, and personal issues discussed here may play a role in the disposition process.

Unstable Patients

Patients who remain unstable despite treatment in the ED should be admitted to the hospital or transferred to a facility capable of managing the patient. This rule is not only medically appropriate, it is also a legal requirement. Acute strokes, myocardial infarctions, and respiratory failure are all examples of unstable emergency medical conditions that warrant hospital admission.

In some instances, a hospital may be unable to stabilize a patient's emergency medical condition. Consider a patient suffering an acute myocardial infarction who has failed thrombolytic therapy and requires urgent cardiac catheterization. If no primary coronary intervention is available at the facility where the patient presented, transfer to a facility capable of performing the procedure may be warranted.

Federal EMTALA laws also impose requirements regarding the transfer of patients between facilities. If a patient with an emergency medical condition is to be transferred to another facility, the patient must request the transfer in writing, or a physician must certify that the risks of transfer are outweighed by the benefits.[7] The transfer must also be "appropriate" under EMTALA laws, meaning that all of the following is done:

- The transferring facility has taken steps to minimize the risk of transfer to the patient.
- The receiving facility is capable of accepting the transfer and has agreed to accept the transfer.
- The transferring facility sends copies of all pertinent medical records to the receiving facility.
- The transfer is made using qualified medical personnel and transportation equipment.[8]

Most hospitals have formal transfer paperwork that highlights each of these requirements and must be signed by both the physician and the patient.

Stable Patients

Just because a patient has been stabilized does not mean that they can be safely discharged. Recall that the definition of "stability" under EMTALA is that "no material deterioration" is likely to occur after a patient has been discharged. However, because even stable patients can decompensate, there are several additional factors to consider when determining if discharge is appropriate.

Presenting Complaint

In some instances, the presenting complaint alone may guide a patient's disposition. Self-limited issues, such as paronychia or joint sprains, seldom require admission, whereas patients with complaints involving potentially serious illnesses, such as chest pain or dyspnea, are more likely to be admitted, even if clinically stable. Some practitioners may consider certain complaints as "admissible" solely because of the potential for adverse outcomes.

> *Example:* Febrile patients less than 28 days old have a substantial likelihood of serious bacterial illness and few reliable indicators upon which to base discharge decisions. Most clinicians would consider a documented neonatal fever as an admissible diagnosis, even though the patient might appear stable. Conversely, older children with fevers are routinely discharged. A patient with an open fracture may be clinically stable but will most likely require admission for intravenous antibiotics and operative wound cleansing to minimize the chances of infection.

Likelihood of Deterioration

Although a presenting complaint may justify admission, a patient's diagnosis, response to treatment, and potential to deteriorate are other considerations that may warrant inpatient treatment. Several examples may help to illustrate the point:

- A patient with exercise-induced asthma who ran out of a rescue inhaler might be discharged after a single albuterol treatment. Another asthma patient with multiple intubations, who has not responded to home therapy, and who demonstrates low

oxygen saturations and retractions, may require admission to the intensive unit—even if the patient's respiratory status stabilizes while in the ED.
- A suicidal patient with a plan and who has a history of prior failed suicide attempts is at an increased risk of further suicide attempts. Such a patient likely warrants admission for psychiatric evaluation and treatment, even if the patient denies suicidal ideation.
- Patients with known cardiac disease who experience an increase in anginal symptoms are at a higher risk for the compensation and may require admission even if they are asymptomatic and have a negative workup in the ED.
- A patient with persistently low blood pressure or elevated heart rate, even in the absence of a firm diagnosis, may require admission because the underlining etiology for those abnormalities may make deterioration more likely without close monitoring.

As these examples illustrate, patients who are clinically stabilized in the ED may still require admission based on factors that create an increased risk of decompensation upon discharge. If, in the physician's professional opinion, a patient is deemed at higher risk for the compensation, documenting that determination and the reasons for it will help to justify the physician's disposition decision.

Social Issues

Social issues like age, insurance, income, habitat/living arrangements, comprehension, and other medical/mental health problems can influence the disposition process. Patients with low health literacy or comprehension difficulties may require admission for more serious diagnoses:

- Newly diagnosed with diabetes, a patient has an elevated blood glucose level and may require hospitalization, where they can be monitored and educated on disease management and the importance of following a diabetic diet.
- Social support can be an important factor in the recovery of depressed patients. A patient who lives alone, suffers fractures to multiple extremities, and is unable to perform activities of daily living may be unsafe to discharge home despite being clinically stable. Instead, hospitalization may be necessary for rehabilitation or to arrange for placement in a rehabilitation facility.
- A child who has sustained physical abuse may need to be placed into protective custody until alternate living arrangements can be made.
- A patient may need assistance with obtaining medications, traveling to follow-up appointments, and finding a home caregiver who is able to assist with aftercare.

Although none of these social or medical situations alone might require a hospital admission, when combined with other factors, a patient's social situation may provide additional evidence to support their ultimate disposition.

Medical Provider's Risk Tolerance

No two providers practice medicine in precisely the same manner. It is not uncommon during a shift change for one physician to discharge a patient who was deemed necessary for admission by another physician. A provider's perception of medicolegal risk is difficult to quantify, yet it can often affect disposition decisions. Providers with higher risk tolerance may be more inclined to discharge patients, while those with lower risk tolerance may be less willing to discharge those who have even a small possibility of deterioration.

Because every case is unique, there can be few absolute guidelines on which patients should and should not be admitted to a hospital. However, over time, the percentage of patients that a given provider chooses to admit or discharge may establish that the provider is an outlier when compared to other practitioners in the group. Under such circumstances, providing objective data about disposition patterns within a group, constructively addressing litigation concerns, and educating the clinician on the outcomes of questionable disposition decisions may help improve the decision-making processes.

ADMISSION

Transferring the care of an ED patient to the admitting inpatient team is an important clinical and service process that requires careful consideration.

General Considerations

The emergency physician is often considered the "gatekeeper" for patients who may need admission to the hospital. According to estimates from the Agency for Healthcare Research and Quality, in 2016, 13% of the 144 million ED visits resulted in admission. The aggregate charges for hospital admissions were $1.67 trillion with average charges of $46,977 per admission.[9] To reduce the expense associated with these cases, federal regulations delineate specific criteria that must be met to justify a hospital admission for purposes of payment under Medicare Part A.[10]

A licensed practitioner who has admitting privileges at the hospital must sign an order of admission at or before the time of the inpatient admission. This order may not be delegated to other individuals who are not authorized to admit patients at the hospital.[11] In other words, unless advanced practice providers have admitting privileges, under these regulations, they are not permitted to sign admission orders.

The admitting physician must also expect that a patient will require hospital care "crossing two midnights" based upon "such complex medical factors as the patient's history and comorbidities, severity of signs and symptoms, current medical needs, and risk of an adverse event."[12] The patient's medical record "must contain information to justify admission and continued hospitalization, support the diagnosis, and describe the patient's progress and response to medications and services."[13]

Full Admission vs Observation Status

Determining whether a patient requires full admission or should remain in the hospital under observation is often a decision that is made collaboratively with the admitting physician. Patients who require hospitalization for at least two midnights under CMS regulations generally justify full admission to the hospital. Importantly, the time counted toward Medicare's two-midnight minimum begins when the patient *first receives care* in the ED. For example, if a patient arrives in the waiting room at 11 p.m. but is not evaluated until 1:00 a.m., the intervening midnight is *not* counted toward the two-midnight minimum. However, if a patient is evaluated upon arrival and orders are initiated, the intervening midnight counts as one of the two midnights necessary for a full admission. These requirements generally do not apply to patients who are not on Medicare.

Documentation

It is important to document the reasons why any patient requires admission, including their history and comorbidities, the severity of the presenting signs and symptoms, their current medical needs, and the potential for an adverse event.

Example: A stable patient with pneumonia may be eligible for outpatient management. But a patient with pneumonia who has preexisting COPD requiring supplemental oxygen, an elevated CURB-65 score, respiratory acidosis, and clinical dehydration, not only justifies full admission but may require treatment in the ICU.

A short note documenting complicating circumstances and necessary treatment will not only assist the admitting physician in formulating a plan of care, it will also help justify the patient's admission status. Under Medicare rules, admission is not appropriate for care that can be provided outside of the hospital, and factors that are considered "matters of convenience" are not considered when determining if a patient meets inpatient criteria.

Observation Status

Observation status is appropriate if the patient is being kept in the hospital to exclude diagnoses or the plan of care includes "observing" a patient. Under Medicare rules, a patient who is not expected to require hospital care for at least two midnights should generally be kept under observation status. During this time, the patient can be assessed to formulate a treatment plan and determine whether additional hospitalization is necessary.

Example: When managing a patient with chest pain and a normal ED workup, hospitalization under observation status is generally appropriate to perform serial cardiac enzyme testing and cardiac monitoring. If, at the end of the observation period, the patient is asymptomatic and has normal cardiac enzymes, discharge may be appropriate. However, if the cardiac enzymes are trending upward or an arrhythmia develops, inpatient admission may be required for further evaluation and treatment.

Observation services are generally not appropriate solely for matters of convenience, such as transportation issues or routine outpatient surgery preparation. As with those being admitted to the hospital, the justification for keeping a patient under observation status should be clearly documented.

Financial Implications

Hospitals receive substantially less reimbursement for patients placed in observation status. Furthermore, patients placed in observation may be responsible for significant copays. These pressures may create an incentive to classify observation patients as inpatients. However, hospital admission records are routinely audited, and insurance companies routinely deny payment for inappropriate hospital admissions. Federal authorities will not hesitate to file legal actions against hospitals or groups that engage in "upcoding."

Example: In one case, a large ED management group paid $60 million to settle allegations of upcoding hospitalist services.[14] In another case, a hospital chain paid $260 million to settle claims that it threatened emergency physicians with termination if they did not meet arbitrary admission quotas of 50% for all patients over age 65 and 15% to 20% of patients overall.[15]

So contentious is the financial battle over payment for inpatient versus observation services that in 2016, the Notice of Observation Treatment and Implication for Care Eligibility (NOTICE) Act passed.[16] This Act requires hospitals to provide a Medicare Outpatient Observation Notice ("MOON") informing Medicare patients that they may be responsible for significant copays if they remain in the hospital under observation status.[17]

There is no simple answer for how to classify a patient's admission status. Whether an individual requires an overnight stay or an extended hospitalization, clearly documenting the patient's history, comorbidities, complicating factors, treatment, and risk for adverse events will improve medical decision-making, assist the admitting physician in formulating a treatment plan, and allow the hospital to receive maximum compensation for the services that it provides.

Patient Boarding

In certain circumstances, patients admitted to the hospital are not immediately transferred to the admitting unit (e.g., the medical floor). During volume surges, admitted patients may sometimes be kept in the ED pending inpatient bed availability. This process, known as "patient boarding," has many deleterious effects on patient care. ED boarding:

- Significantly increases throughput for all ED patients[18]
- Is associated with an increased overall length of hospital stay
- Nearly doubles the chance of dying in the hospital for those who board longer than 12 hours[19]
- Contributes to ED workplace stress, professional dissatisfaction, and physician burnout[20]

Professional organizations, including the American College of Emergency Physicians, the American Academy of Emergency Medicine, and the Emergency Nurses Association, have policies against patient boarding, but this problem nevertheless continues to occur on a regular basis.[21-23] In a National Public Radio article in November 2019, two ED physicians note that ED boarding remains a medical crisis, flatly stating, "Emergency rooms shouldn't be parking lots for patients."[24]

Responsibility for Boarded Patients

Because the causes of patient boarding are multifactorial and can involve several departments, it is unlikely that any specific ED policy will alleviate this insidious problem. From an administrative standpoint, creating policies directed toward the management of boarded patients will help streamline care until these patients can be transferred to a medical floor.

To avoid confusion over the patients' medical care team, hospital boarding policies should clearly state that boarded patients are the responsibility of the admitting physician.[25] Emergency physicians should not provide routine care for admitted patients boarded in the ED. Doing so can be a significant liability risk.

Emergency physicians do not receive hospital credentialing for routine inpatient medical care. A hospital that allows (or requires) emergency physicians to practice medical care outside of their training and credentialing may be accused of violating its bylaws. Medical malpractice insurance policies rarely protect emergency physicians for inpatient care; this caveat gives malpractice insurance companies a reason to deny coverage for an adverse event associated with a boarded inpatient.

Boarding Policies

Hospital policies should also establish clear contingency plans to address patient boarding in the ED by:[26,27]

- Developing alternate staffing plans, including additional physicians, nursing, and support staff, to provide proper care to patients boarded in the ED
- Creating a "bed coordinator" who actively monitors admission bottlenecks and expedites inpatient discharges

- Instituting a policy of early discharges for admitted patients to create beds for ED patients, who are more often admitted in the afternoon and evening
- Addressing potential outpatient needs (home oxygen, prescriptions, durable medical equipment, transportation, home health care) early in the admission process
- Modifying surgical schedules to distribute procedures evenly throughout the week
- Distributing boarded patients to inpatient hallway beds when boarding has a significant detrimental impact on ED operations
- Moving patients from a hospital bed to a "discharge lounge" while they are awaiting discharge
- Decreasing turnaround time for bed and room cleaning after a patient has been discharged
- Transferring boarded patients to other facilities when no inpatient beds are available

TRANSFER

In some cases, a patient may have an emergency medical condition that is unable to be stabilized at the presenting facility.

Example: A patient with an acute aortic dissection presents at a facility without a cardiothoracic or vascular surgeon. Even though the hospital has an operating room, it lacks the capacity to provide stabilizing treatment. In other cases, a patient may require specialty care that is unavailable at the presenting facility. A patient with a retinal detachment may require transfer if there is no ophthalmologist on staff.

Even patients requiring seemingly straightforward management may require transfer under certain circumstances.

Example: Any patient requiring admission would need to be transferred from a freestanding ED. A patient requiring intubation and mechanical ventilation may require transfer from a critical-access hospital without the availability of an intensivist or another physician skilled in ventilator management.

EMTALA has several requirements regarding the transfer of patients between facilities. If a patient with an emergency medical condition is to be transferred to another facility, the patient must either request the transfer in writing, or a physician must certify that the risks of transfer are outweighed by the benefits expected from the provision of appropriate treatment at another facility.[28] The transfer must also be "appropriate" under EMTALA laws, meaning:

The transferring facility has taken steps to minimize the risk of transfer to the patient, that the receiving facility is capable of accepting the transfer and has agreed to accept the transfer, that the transferring facility sends copies of all pertinent medical records to the receiving facility, and that the transfer is made using qualified medical personnel and transportation equipment.[29]

To comply with EMTALA, most hospitals have formal transfer paperwork that specifically lists each of these requirements and must be signed by both the physician and patient.

Receiving Hospital Responsibilities

The hospital receiving the transferred patient also has EMTALA-imposed duties. Hospitals with specialized capabilities or facilities may not refuse to accept an appropriate transfer of an individual requiring such capabilities, assuming the receiving hospital has the capacity to treat the individual.[30] A receiving hospital may refuse requests for "lateral transfers" in which the same stabilizing services are available at both the sending and receiving hospitals.

EMTALA lists examples of "specialized capabilities" that may require hospitals to accept patient transfers, such as burn units; trauma units; neonatal ICUs; or, with respect to rural areas, regional referral centers.[30] Much to the chagrin of tertiary care centers, if a hospital has the capacity to provide necessary services that are not available at a sending hospital, the receiving hospital must accept the transfer.

Example: If a sending hospital has obstetrical services but the obstetrician is not on call, a receiving hospital with obstetrical services cannot refuse the transfer. If the sending hospital has obstetrical services but no high-risk obstetrical services, and the patient is deemed "high risk," then a receiving hospital that provides high-risk obstetrical services may not refuse transfer.

CMS Citations

CMS regularly cites hospitals for what it considers to be inappropriate transfers and lists a summary of its cases on the Internet.[31] Recent allegations of improper transfers resulting in settlements with the Office of the Inspector General include:

- $90,000 settlement when a patient complaining of dizziness, black stool, yellow skin, and stiff muscles was transferred with low blood pressure and no blood transfusion, then died shortly after arriving at the receiving hospital. *[Note: In some cases, transfer of an unstable patient may be necessary; here, however, the hospital apparently did not utilize all of its resources to stabilize the patient (i.e., providing a blood transfusion) prior to transfer.]*
- $180,000 settlement based in part on a hospital's refusal to accept a patient requiring ICU care when the transferring hospital did not have an ICU. The on-call physician allegedly stated that "the referring facility could manage the patient." *[Note: A receiving facility must accept an appropriate transfer when it has specialized capabilities not available at the sending facility.]*
- $52,414 settlement when a hospital with psychiatric facilities refused to accept a suicidal patient in transfer because the patient had out-of-network insurance. *[Note: A receiving facility's duty to accept an appropriate transfer may not be influenced by payment issues.]*
- $90,000 settlement when an emergency physician transferred an intubated patient to another facility for a transvenous pacemaker insertion, rather than asking the hospital's on-call cardiologist to come to the ED to do so. *[Note: Sending hospitals must utilize all available resources to attempt to stabilize the patient prior to transfer. If a hospital can perform a procedure, it must do so.]*
- $42,500 settlement when a hospital refused to accept the transfer of a patient who lived in another county. *[Note: EMTALA duties apply to transfer from any hospital within the United States, not just to hospitals within a given catchment area.]*

DISCHARGE

Approximately 80% of ED patients are discharged.[32] Once the decision has been made to discharge a patient, the discharge process should summarize the treatment received in the ED and provide recommendations for follow-up care. During this process, providers can emphasize important points in the written discharge instructions and can assess a patient's understanding and ability to follow through on any recommendations.

> **BOX 108.1 ■ PATIENT DISCHARGE INFORMATION**
>
> - Presumptive diagnosis and/or a presumptive explanation of symptoms
> - Expected course of the (presumptive) disease process
> - Signs or symptoms that should prompt a return visit
> - Provider's recommendations for treatment and follow-up care
> - Short description of the ED tests including results (in selected cases)
> - Lifestyle modifications

Discharge Instructions

The content for discharge instructions can vary widely, but it should ideally include the information listed in **Box 108.1.**

Presumptive Diagnosis

Although hospitals, insurers, and patients may pressure the clinician to provide a firm diagnosis, doing so may be difficult and detrimental to the patient's continuing evaluation and care. An ED evaluation can either confirm a diagnosis or alert the patient that an etiology for their symptoms is uncertain. Discharge instructions should reflect the clinician's thought process. For example:

- After an evaluation in the ED for a cough, discharge instructions—attributing the cough to a viral upper-respiratory infection (as opposed to pneumonia) and noting that a chest x-ray was normal—may preclude further workup for the evaluation of infectious etiologies.
- Diagnosing a patient with undifferentiated abdominal pain and nausea as having "gastroenteritis" may provide a proper billing code, but it can also provide the patient with premature closure for those symptoms. If the patient with undifferentiated abdominal pain is instead suffering from early appendicitis, follow-up care may be delayed based on the assumption that the "gastroenteritis" will eventually improve.

Explaining to the patient that a diagnosis is provisional and may require further evaluation will augment their understanding of the issue. Drawings, analogies, or demonstrations may help emphasize that the cause of the patient's symptoms is still uncertain.

Expected Disease Process

Discharge instructions should explain what patients can expect from their disease process and how prescribed medications are expected to work. While some physicians may become frustrated with those who return after several hours because their symptoms have not improved, in many cases, those return visits can be related to a breakdown in the prior discharge process.

> *Example:* Discharge instructions after a motor vehicle accident may explain that an increase in myalgias should be expected over the following 24 to 48 hours. Wound care instructions should ideally tell a patient not only when to have sutures removed but also what types of symptoms should prompt a return visit. Explaining that antibiotics may not begin to work for 24 to 48 hours reinforces the fact that symptoms may also not improve

immediately. Warnings that a wound should not get wet for the first 2 days, that a fracture will take 6 to 8 weeks to heal, or that an individual with uncontrolled seizures should not drive a car allow patients to plan their daily activities accordingly. Similarly, a statement that generalized abdominal pain may resolve spontaneously or may get worse, coupled with recommendations for each contingency, will impress upon the patient that timely follow-up is important when symptoms do not resolve.

High-Risk Signs and Symptoms

Highlighting symptoms that may represent worsening of a condition will improve patient understanding. However, it is logistically impossible to list every symptom that could possibly result in deterioration. Failure to list the actual symptom that was the cause of the patient's worsening condition could later be used as an allegation of negligence against the physician and hospital. For this reason, in addition to specific symptoms warranting return visits, discharge instructions should contain some type of "catch all" language that encourages return visits based upon a "reasonable person" standard.

Provider Recommendations

Recommendations for treatment and follow-up care are critical aspects of discharge instructions. Provider recommendations explain what must be done for the patient to get better and what steps to take if symptoms do not improve. Recommendations may also explain why certain treatments were not offered.

> **Example:** *An explanation that antibiotics were not prescribed because they do not work in patients with viral upper-respiratory infections and may even cause future bacterial resistance could alter a patient's incorrect assumptions that doctor visits and antibiotic prescriptions are necessary every time a cough develops.*

Most discharged patients require some type of follow-up care after leaving the ED. By providing a location and contact information for the appointment, follow-up compliance will improve and simultaneously demonstrate the provider's concern about the patient's continuing well-being. Although contacting the follow-up physician to make an appointment for the patient may further enhance compliance, it may not always be feasible in a busy ED.

In most cases, an appointment for follow-up care should be no more than 1 week in the future unless directed otherwise by the follow-up physician. When symptoms have a significant potential to result in a serious problem, such as undifferentiated abdominal pain, follow-up examinations either at the primary care physician's office or in the ED in 12 to 24 hours are not unreasonable.

If a patient does not follow a provider's discharge instructions and suffers a bad outcome as a result, their noncompliance could be used as an "affirmative defense" to any claims of medical malpractice (see Chapter 113 for more details).

> **Example:** *If a patient with a complex hand laceration is discharged with a prescription for antibiotics and told to follow up with a hand surgeon in 48 hours but fails to fill the prescription and does not follow up, future malpractice claims could potentially be reduced or completely barred.*

If a patient is visiting from out of town or does not have a local physician, it may be difficult to coordinate follow-up care from the ED. Adding a notation about testing results to the discharge instructions may help future providers determine the most appropriate course of action.

> **Example:** *A discharge notation like "Lab testing (e.g., CBC, Chem 12, lipase, cardiac enzymes) were all normal, and a CT scan of the abdomen and pelvis showed no abnormalities other than*

a simple liver cyst" will help the follow-up physician determine what additional testing (if any) must be performed. The notation also describes what testing was performed in case the follow-up physician needs copies of test results.

Including selected test results may help alleviate a patient's health concerns. A patient evaluated for a cough whose family member recently died from lung cancer will likely be relieved to see a specific notation on the discharge instructions that a chest x-ray showed no obvious signs of lung cancer.

Discharge instructions may also include suggestions for lifestyle modifications, such as smoking cessation and diet modifications, and may even remind patients about safety issues, such as use of a seat belt or bicycle helmet. To be effective, these discussions should demonstrate concern for a patient's welfare, rather than blame for their situation.

Pain Management

More than 2 million ED visits each year result from the misuse and abuse of prescription analgesics.[33,34] Drug-related deaths have quintupled since 1980 and have now surpassed trauma as the leading cause of death due to injury.[34] The percentage of all deaths attributable to opioids increased 292% (from 0.4% to 1.5%) between 2001 and 2016; in 2106, 20% of deaths in patients 24 to 35 years old involved opioids.[35] As a result, the US Department of Health and Human Services is taking aggressive action to reduce opioid overuse by encouraging prescribers to utilize Prescription Drug Monitoring Programs (PDMPs) and prescribing guidelines.[36] Currently, all states except Missouri have some type of PDMP, and of those states, 41 also have laws requiring providers to check the PDMP under varying circumstances.[37]

Discharge instructions for acute pain should include safe, effective, first-line analgesics like acetaminophen, NSAIDs, antidepressants, anticonvulsants, and topical pain patches in addition to nonpharmacological pain management interventions, such as yoga, heat/cold therapy, and relaxation treatment.[38] CDC guidelines recommend that patients with chronic pain receive prescriptions for no more than 50 morphine milligram equivalents (MME) per day, noting that dosages above this amount double the risk of overdose death. Concurrent use of opioids and benzodiazepines in chronic pain patients is also discouraged.[39] Unfortunately, many hospitals and pharmacies apply chronic pain prescription guidelines to patients with any pain whatsoever, prompting worried calls from pharmacists when a prescription for acetaminophen/codeine tablets exceeds the 50 MME threshold.

If opiates are prescribed for acute pain, they should be prescribed in limited quantities from the ED and may include warnings about overdose. In 2018, US Surgeon General Jerome Adams recommended coprescription of naloxone with opioids to any patient deemed "at risk of opioid overdose."[40] Several states have since passed laws regarding coprescribing naloxone with opiates even though naloxone is available over the counter.

Practitioners are urged to exercise care in the amount of narcotics they prescribe and consider one of the many nonopioid treatments for patients being discharged from the ED. Recommending naloxone for patients prescribed higher doses of opiates may also prevent an inadvertent overdose.

Templated Discharge Instructions

Many commercial programs and electronic medical records create detailed discharge instructions when a diagnosis is entered. Although the information provided by these programs may be useful, discharging clinicians should review the data to determine whether it is up to date and appropriate for the patient's condition.

Example: In some programs, antibiotics are specifically recommended for bronchitis. Such recommendations may prompt patient complaints or return visits because the patients did not receive the antibiotics that the discharge instructions described.

A patient's comprehension of discharge instructions largely determines their compliance with discharge planning. In fact, one study showed that comprehension was the *only* determinant of patient compliance with discharge instructions, exclusive of age, language, education, years in an English-speaking country, reading ability, format of discharge instructions, follow-up modality, and association with a family physician.[41] Comprehension, in turn, was associated with reading ability and English as the patient's primary language.[41] Unfortunately, a majority of patients read at the 7th grade level or below.[41,42] Even when discharge instructions are created to meet an average person's reading level, only 72% of patients are able to read their instructions, and nearly half are incapable of fully understanding preprinted discharge instructions.[43,44]

Patient comprehension of verbal discharge instructions is also less than adequate. When interviewed after being discharged from an ED, between 40% and 78% of patients had deficient comprehension of at least one aspect of their discharge instructions, and many illustrated deficient comprehension in multiple areas.[45]

Compounding matters, patients are seldom aware that they do not comprehend ED discharge instructions. Less than 30% of patients with comprehension deficiencies perceive their own inability to understand.[45,46] The most common source of misunderstandings in ED discharge instructions is the physician's recommendations for post-ED care, which totals one-third of all comprehension deficiencies.[47] Not only does confusion about follow-up care tend to decrease compliance, it is also the largest source of legal liability related to the discharge process.

Improving Comprehension and Compliance

Patient comprehension and compliance may improve when written instructions are supplemented with verbal discharge instructions.[48] However, even the content of verbal discharge instructions is often inadequate. One study revealed that in only 22% of encounters did the physician confirm the patient's understanding of the discharge instructions, and in most of those cases, the confirmation was judged to be of "minimal" quality.[49]

A patient's comprehension of discharge instructions can be assessed by asking if the patient has any questions about the visit or the treatment plans and by using a "teach-back" approach, in which the patient explains the discharge instructions back to the ED staff. Both processes can help clarify any miscommunication that occurred during the clinical encounter.[50]

Legal Cases Involving Discharge Instructions

Inadequate or poorly understood discharge instructions and conflicts between written and verbal recommendations are the largest sources of liability in the ED discharge process. Several cases are illustrative of the potential sources of such liability.

In *Marsolino v Patel*, discharge instructions to "[f]ollow-up in 4 to 6 weeks," were alleged to be too vague. However, the case was dismissed because the plaintiffs could not establish a causal link between the plaintiff's injuries and the discharge instructions. In this case, had the patient been able to show that an injury could have progressed with earlier follow-up evaluation or other recommendations, the case would likely have progressed to trial.

In *Bevan v Valencia*, a patient with a heroin overdose received preprinted discharge instructions describing signs and symptoms of heroin overdose and written instructions stating that the patient should return to the hospital if her symptoms worsened or did not improve. She later died of opioid toxicity. A subsequent lawsuit alleged that the instructions were inadequate. The court ruled that the instructions were neither unreasonable nor inadequate and "if heeded" could have prevented the patient's death. This case emphasizes the importance of the "catch all" discharge instructions: Return if symptoms worsen, new symptoms develop, or any problems occur. Had those instructions not been present, the court ruling may have been different.

Guadagno v Lifemark Hospitals of Florida involved a patient who suffered a greater trochanter fracture in a minibike accident.[53] The patient was discharged on crutches and instructed to follow up with the orthopedist 3 days later. He remained on bed rest for 3 days and then died from a pulmonary embolism in the orthopedic surgeon's parking lot. The family sued, alleging that the discharge instructions included no advice on how to prevent deep vein thrombosis (DVT). The appellate court ruled in the physician's favor, noting that there was no evidence showing how the allegedly inadequate discharge instructions caused the patient to develop DVT and pulmonary embolism.

Written vs Verbal Discharge Instructions

In *Clelland v Haas*, written discharge instructions were alleged to be inadequate because they did not recommend that the patient return if her symptoms worsened.[54] While the emergency physician testified that he verbally told the patient to "return to the ED or call her doctor if her symptoms returned or worsened," those instructions were not included in the chart, and the patient denied ever receiving them. A jury ruled in the doctor's favor, but when reviewing the case, the appellate court noted that the jury's determination amounted to a "credibility call." In other words, had a jury not believed that the physician told the patient to return if worse, the physician would likely have been found liable for malpractice.

In *McPherson v Abraham*, a patient fell and injured his wrist while playing basketball. x-rays of his wrist in the ED were reported as "negative."[55] Discharge instructions advised the patient to follow-up in the hospital's orthopedic clinic in 5 days, but the patient stated that he was told to return "only if he had further problems." Six months later, he was found to have a nonunited scaphoid bone fracture. The case was dismissed due to a tolling of the statute of limitations. Had the case not been dismissed, the discrepancy between the written and verbal instructions would likely have allowed the case to progress to trial.

In *Doll v Kester*, a morbidly obese patient sought care for chest pain.[56] The patient's pain was reproducible, and a workup including labs, electrocardiography, and a chest x-ray. He was diagnosed with musculoskeletal pain and instructed to follow up with his primary physician in 2 to 3 days. The discharge instructions also stated that the emergency physician would call if there were any discrepancies in the x-ray reading. The x-ray was interpreted by the radiologist as showing cardiomegaly, but the patient was not called. He died several weeks later from a presumed heart attack. The family sued because the doctor did not follow the statements in the discharge instructions. A jury decided in favor of the physician, and a post-verdict appeal affirmed the jury verdict, stating that the physician's failure to follow through on the discharge instructions had no effect on the outcome. In this case, cardiomegaly on a chest x-ray likely had no clinical significance and would not have changed the patient's management. However, had there been a more serious discrepancy like a pneumothorax or free air under the diaphragm, the physician's failure to follow the discharge instructions may have been used to demonstrate negligence.

Other Cases

In *Desimini v Bristol Hospital*, the Connecticut appellate court held that doctors do not have a duty to provide discharge instructions to a patient's family members because doing so could potentially violate Health Insurance Portability and Accountability Act laws and could put the doctor in the position of having to decide which of several relatives to advise.[57]

The authors have also reviewed cases not included in the appellate databases in which physicians were accused of negligence for failing to provide patients with a time frame in which to seek further care. Specifically, one case involved a patient who suffered a laceration to his hand, which was sutured in the ED. Discharge papers instructed him to "return if redness, swelling, or other signs of infection develop" but did not specify that he should return "immediately" if those symptoms occurred. The case was settled by the emergency physician's insurer.

DISCHARGES AGAINST MEDICAL ADVICE

While most patients are discharged from the ED on the order of a medical provider, approximately 2% of patients in the United States choose to leave a hospital against medical advice (AMA).[58] In most circumstances, a patient has the right to refuse further medical care, even if that refusal may result in the patient's death. Those who leave AMA are up to seven times as likely to be readmitted in the following 30 days and also have higher 30-day mortality rates.[59] Medical providers may incur liability both for treating patients against their will and allowing them to leave without treatment, making it in the best interest of all parties to avoid such situations (see Chapter 105).

Why Patients Leave AMA

Understanding the reasoning behind a patient's decision to leave AMA can be an important factor in helping convince them that proceeding with proposed care is the most reasonable course of action. Certain demographics make patients more likely to leave AMA. Those who are discharged AMA tend to be male, uninsured, suffer from alcohol or drug abuse (totaling 11.7% of all AMA discharges), and have previous instances of AMA discharges (odds ratio: 170).[60-62]

Patients who leave AMA commonly cite one of several reasons for leaving, including personal or family issues, financial concerns, feeling well enough to leave, dissatisfaction with the physician or treatment received, becoming "fed up," and dislike of hospitals in general.[63] One study showed that the date of issuance of welfare checks was a significant predictor of AMA discharges.[64] Eighty-two percent of patients leave AMA because they do not agree with a physician's treatment plan, and 96% of patients who return to the hospital after leaving AMA have the same chief complaint.[65,66] A smaller study of interviews with patients, nurses, and physicians showed seven themes involving AMA discharges (**Box 108.2**).[67]

BOX 108.2 ■ MAJOR REASONS PATIENT LEAVE AMA

- Drug addiction
- Pain management
- Preexisting obligations outside of hospitals
- Wait time
- Doctor's bedside manner
- Teaching hospital setting
- Poor physician-patient communication

Convincing a Patient to Remain in the Hospital

The best way to avoid complications from AMA discharges is to convince the patient to stay in the hospital or follow the recommended treatment plan. Addressing the issues that create a desire to leave AMA may resolve the problem. Document any attempts to mitigate the patient's circumstances. In some cases, time may be an ally. Bargain with adamant patients to wait an extra hour before leaving, after which time you will agree to let them leave. While they're waiting, offer them a meal. The time waiting may allow the patient to vent emotions, understand the seriousness of the problem, and reconsider their decision to leave.

Family issues and preexisting obligations outside the hospital have been shown to increase a patient's desire to leave AMA. Perhaps there is no one at home to care for a family member or pet. Helping the patient to arrange for that care may encourage them to remain in the hospital for treatment. Perhaps the patient believes that he or she will suffer adverse employment consequences for missing work. A call (with permission) to the patient's employer or a note on hospital letterhead explaining the issue may resolve that issue. Financial concerns also increase the chances of AMA discharges. Reiterate to the patient that finances are not taken into consideration when recommending emergency medical care. A hospital financial counselor may be able to help the patient apply for government insurance, provide a discount for the services provided, or establish a payment plan that meets the patient's budget.

If the patient's symptoms have resolved, explain why allowing the proposed treatment is in their best interests. Consider printing out medical articles that substantiate the proposed treatment, if possible.

Should a Patient Be Allowed to Leave AMA?

A patient's *desire* to leave AMA does not necessarily mean that they should be *permitted* to go. From an ethical standpoint, an AMA discharge is a choice between paternalism and patient autonomy. In some cases, a decision to hospitalize a questionably suicidal patient against their will becomes a dilemma of choosing between potentially being accused of battery and false imprisonment or being accused of malpractice and wrongful death if the patient leaves and commits suicide. Other considerations should be made before a patient is permitted to leave AMA.

Patient Capacity

Patients who refuse treatment must have the capacity to decide. In this regard, capacity should be considered on a continuum: The more important the decision, the more stringent the criteria for capacity should be. Assessment and documentation of capacity may be considerably different for a patient who refuses wound care as compared to a patient who refuses treatment for an ST-elevation myocardial infarction revealed on an ECG.

Clinicians should also note the difference between "capacity," which is the ability to make a decision, and "competency," which is a retrospective determination made by a court. Patients are presumed *competent* to make a decision until there is convincing evidence to the contrary. If a patient is making a decision against their own interests, it is important to document factual information showing why they do not have the *capacity* to make a decision.

Legal Capacity

Legal capacity generally requires an individual to be at least 18 years old or an "emancipated minor," such as being married, pregnant, or a parent. Some states also give children the legal capacity to consent to treatment for specific health issues as a matter of public policy. Other examples of emancipated minors in some jurisdictions include those living separately from their parents, those who are self-sustaining economically, and minors in active military service.

> ***Example:*** *If a child is a victim of a serious traumatic injury, physical or sexual abuse, or may be intoxicated, it would be against public policy to withhold medical care solely because the patient had not reached the age of majority. In each of these cases, minors may have legal capacity. Since definitions of legal capacity vary between states, each practitioner should be familiar with their own state's laws. Even if a patient does have legal capacity, the patient still must demonstrate clinical capacity.*

Determining Decision-Making Capacity

Clinical or "decision-making" capacity generally requires that a patient be able to understand the diagnosis, the proposed medical care, and the implications of proceeding with or refusing such care. Patients should have both legal and clinical capacity before being allowed to leave AMA.

Many factors can affect a patient's decision-making capacity, including dementia, psychiatric issues, metabolic problems, head injuries, drug use, and alcohol use. The Folstein Mini-Mental State Examination (MMSE) has been shown to be an effective screening tool for determining clinical decision-making capacity. A score of less than 21 (out of 30) on the MMSE appears to be 100% specific and 69% sensitive in identifying patients who lack decision-making capacity, while a score of less than 24 may be 83% sensitive and 90% specific in identifying patients without decision-making capacity.[68]

Decision-making capacity may be transient. Patients may have no decision-making capacity during acute psychosis but may quickly regain capacity after taking their medications. Alcohol intoxication may impair decision-making, but capacity will return as the alcohol is metabolized. Elderly patients with "sundowning" may lack capacity at night but have full decision-making capacity during the day. If a patient choosing to leave AMA appears to have decision-making capacity, note this clinical assessment on the chart along with the reasons for their departure. If a patient lacks decision-making capacity, document specific reasons why you believe this to be the case. For example, if an intoxicated patient wishes to leave AMA, consider a chart entry such as:

> *Patient continues to appear intoxicated with slurred speech and unsteady gait. Walked into door when brought to bathroom. Speech often unintelligible. Staggering gait. States "I don't care" when asked about implications of decision. Currently lacks capacity and will not be allowed to leave pending improved cognition.*

If a provider believes that a patient does not have decision-making capacity and the patient chooses a course of action that may be potentially harmful, it is usually best to proceed with treatment. In the context of AMA discharges, that treatment may involve preventing the patient from leaving and even restraint and sedation if necessary. Under these circumstances, it may be helpful to consult with hospital administration, hospital legal counsel, members of the hospital ethics committee, or a psychiatrist.

Discharging a Patient AMA

If a patient has decision-making capacity, is not at significant risk of self-harm or harm to others, and still wishes to leave AMA, the provider should provide explicit information about the consequences of this decision, including the tentative diagnosis, benefits of the proposed treatment, major risks associated with refusing the proposed treatment, and reasonable alternatives to the proposed treatment.[69]

Discussions should be relatively specific to a patient's complaints and symptoms. Generic admonitions like "You could get worse or die!" may be insufficient. Although risks of death and permanent disability may be included in a list of potential consequences, the risks of refusing care must be relatively specific to the patient's condition.

> *Example:* In a patient with chest pain, risks may include "a heart attack, a blood clot in the lungs, a rupture of the main blood vessel in the chest, worsening breathing, abnormal heart rhythms, loss of consciousness, other similarly serious medical problems, permanent disability, or even death." In Lyons v Walker Regional Medical Center, *a patient was transferred to the ED from jail with abdominal pain and hematemesis.*[70] *He refused a nasogastric tube and indicated a desire to leave the hospital before his labs had returned. As the patient signed the AMA forms, the nurse cautioned, "After signing out AMA, you understand that you could die or something else could happen to you." The patient's labs returned shortly after his departure, demonstrating diabetic ketoacidosis. He later died in jail. The Alabama Supreme Court held that the "blanket statement" made by the nurse was insufficient to put the patient on notice of the seriousness of his condition; therefore, the AMA obtained in the ED was invalid.*

To illustrate further, note how disclosure of pertinent information may affect compliance with a yard sign stating "Stay off the grass" as compared to one stating "Stay off the grass because there are land mines buried nearby." Exaggerating risks involved with AMA discharge or making untrue statements to abort the AMA process should be discouraged.

> *Example: Asserting that an insurer will refuse payment if a patient leaves AMA would be inappropriate. Several studies of hundreds of AMA discharges have shown that not a single patient was refused coverage because they left AMA.*[71,72]

A "teach back" method like that used in normal patient discharges can help the medical providers ensure that patients understand the implications of their decisions. Note any responses the patient gives you in the chart–in quotes if appropriate. Consider the following:

> *Example: Verbalizes understanding of tests showing possible cardiac injury, pulmonary embolism or aortic dissection, and the risks and alternatives of leaving AMA. Stated "I want to spend the holidays with my family" and "If I'm going to die, I'd rather die at home."*

Should this patient suffer an adverse outcome and these statements become a part of legal proceedings, they would provide quite persuasive evidence that the patient understood his condition and accepted the risks involved.

Discharging Children AMA

Parents (or custodians) may wish to refuse care on behalf of their child or remove the child from the ED. This situation presents a more challenging dilemma. On one hand, parents may legally control medical decisions for their children. On the other hand, under the doctrine of *"parens patriae"* ("country as parent"), state courts and state agencies may override a parent's decisions when a child's health is in jeopardy. The terminology frequently used in court decisions invoking *parens patriae* specifies that actions must be in "the child's best interests."

The concept of *parens patriae* has remained constant through the decades. In *Prince v Commonwealth of Massachusetts,* the US Supreme Court stated: "Parents [are] free to become martyrs themselves. [They are not free] to make martyrs of their children."[73] A 2020 New

Jersey Superior Court decision concisely explained the concept of *parens patriae* (citations omitted):[74]

> *It is axiomatic that parents have a constitutionally protected right to the care, custody, and control of their children. But that right is not absolute. It is a right tempered by the State's parens patriae responsibility to protect children whose vulnerable lives or psychological well-being may have been harmed or may be seriously endangered by a neglectful or abusive parent.*
>
> *If a child's health is at risk from a parent's refusal of recommended medical care, it is reasonable to take protective custody of the child in order to protect the child's health. Involving State child protective agencies and hospital administration early in such process would be advisable to minimize potential legal liability.*

Documenting the AMA Process

Unfortunately, physicians frequently neglect to adequately document the AMA discharge process. Eighteen percent of the charts of patients leaving AMA in a rural community setting included no AMA discharge documentation.[75] Documentation of a patient's clinical decision-making capacity ranges from 23% to 67%.[76] Documentation of patient's comprehension of their diagnosis, proposed treatment, alternative therapy, and clinical consequences of refusal occurs in approximately 36%, 44%, 2%, and 57% of cases, respectively.[76]

A similar study at a large county hospital showed that of 319 AMA discharges, only 29.6% of charts reflected an assessment of patient decision-making capacity.[77] Another study at an urban academic medical center showed documentation of a risk/benefit discussion in 69% of cases, documentation of informed consent in 63% of cases, and attending physician notification of the AMA discharge in 72% of cases.[78]

Sample AMA Chart Documentation

Below is sample wording used by the authors for patients being discharged AMA.

_____ (Patient) desires to leave the ED AMA prior to completion of recommended medical testing, treatment, and potential stabilization of patient's medical condition.

- I have recommended [LIST RECOMMENDATIONS HERE: e.g., further testing, hospital admission, specialty evaluation, transfer to higher level of care].
- Risks of leaving AMA discussed with the patient, including but not limited to the possibility of [INSERT ANY SPECIFIC RISKS HERE], worsening symptoms, increasing discomfort, permanent disability, and even death. Patient has a normal mental status and good decision-making capacity, understands these risks, can explain these risks, and agrees to hold harmless the hospital, physician, and staff for any adverse outcome that may arise from the patient's decision.
- The patient was given an opportunity to ask questions about the decision to leave AMA, and all questions were answered to the patient's satisfaction.
- The reason the patient still wishes to leave AMA is because [LIST REASON HERE. USE PATIENT'S OWN WORDS WHEN POSSIBLE].
- The patient was therefore allowed to leave AMA and was encouraged to seek further medical care as soon as possible, including returning to the ED at any time to complete evaluation and treatment.

Completing AMA Paperwork

After the patient has been informed of the consequences of their decision, the physician should attempt to have them sign a written refusal of care/AMA form. Recall that EMTALA requires that patients receive a screening exam and any necessary stabilizing treatment. One of the ways in which EMTALA duties are satisfied is if a patient refuses to consent to treatment.

However, EMTALA requires that the patient be informed of the risks and benefits of the treatment prior to the refusal and that the provider/hospital "take all reasonable steps to secure the individual's written informed consent to refuse such examination and treatment."[79] The presence of a signed AMA document creates a "rebuttable presumption" that the patient was presented with and understood the information contained on the form. Should the appropriateness of an AMA discharge later be challenged, the patient or family member would then need to present evidence to overcome the presumption that refusal of care was an informed refusal.

One study showed that in 42% of AMA discharges, no AMA form was signed by the patient.[80] If a patient refuses to sign an AMA form, the physician should note the interaction in the medical records. A copy of the completed but unsigned AMA paperwork will demonstrate that a good faith attempt was made to have the patient sign the form and will show what risks were conveyed.

Follow-Up Care of the AMA Patient

A study of provider attitudes at a large county hospital showed that 6% of attending physicians, 16% of residents, and 36% of nurses believed that patients who leave AMA should not receive prescriptions or follow-up care.[81] These sentiments are inappropriate.

Patients who leave AMA should be provided with the same treatment that would be provided to those who are formally discharged under similar circumstances. Patients with chronic back pain who leave AMA because they are not given narcotics need not necessarily receive a prescription for narcotic medications, especially if the physician believes that such a prescription may jeopardize the patient's health. However, a patient who lacks an essential medication, such as an asthma inhaler, should generally be provided with an appropriate prescription. If a patient is only willing to accept alternative but less-than-optimal treatments, note any care that was provided and why the more appropriate therapies were not given.

While physicians should make reasonable efforts to provide alternative treatments, they should not allow themselves to be coerced into providing inappropriate care solely because a patient threatens to leave AMA. A patient's assertion that if they do not get azithromycin for their cough, they will leave should not result in a prescription for a different antibiotic; instead, it should prompt a discussion of why antibiotics are an inappropriate therapy for coughs.

An outright refusal to provide appropriate treatment to patients who leave AMA is medically unjustified and would likely be viewed as vindictive and unprofessional by a court, jury, or licensing board. Recall that AMA decisions are often based on factors other than a patient's disagreement with the physician's medical judgment.

> **Example:** *While discussing the case of* Drummond v Buckley, *the Mississippi Supreme Court stated that "[s]urely, it cannot be suggested that supposed medical professionals would withhold proper service because a patient . . . exercised his prerogative not to follow medical advice."*[82]

Legal Cases Involving AMA Discharges

Several legal case summaries illustrate medical malpractice issues that providers face related to AMA discharges. The first, *Sawyer v Comerci*, involved a patient with right-sided abdominal pain, an elevated white blood cell count, and blood in his stool.[83] The emergency physician recommended admission, but the patient had a business appointment the following day and refused. The physician's notes stated that the patient and his wife "were hard to talk with" and "do not seem to understand the possibility of the seriousness of his condition." The patient's primary care physician agreed to see him either the next morning or after he was discharged. No AMA form was signed. The patient never followed up and died 5 days later. A lawsuit was decided in the physician's favor but was appealed. The Virginia Supreme Court criticized the lack of the emergency physician's documentation, stating that there were no entries indicating that the patient should have been admitted and no evidence that he "understood the severity of his condition and the consequences that might ensue if he were not admitted to the hospital." Because the patient was not provided with sufficient information before being discharged, he could not be held responsible for his decision to leave AMA.

In *Zablotny v State Board of Nursing*, a nursing supervisor allowed an admitted patient to leave the hospital AMA.[84] Two hours earlier, the patient was reportedly confused and needed restraints, although an evaluation by the nursing supervisor showed that the patient was "quiet, lucid, rational, and mentally competent." After signing AMA papers, the patient was discharged into a "blizzard" wearing nothing but a button-down shirt, pants, and moccasins. He was found buried under a foot of snow the following day, having died from hypothermia and opiate toxicity. The state nursing board suspended the nurse's license for 2 years. On appeal, the reviewing court held that the nurse had "engaged in unprofessional conduct by failing to provide the patient with accurate and complete information about the risks he faced upon leaving the hospital AMA." The license suspension was upheld.

In *Ingutti v Rochester General Hospital*, which seems to be an outlier opinion, a patient admitted with pancreatitis and alcohol intoxication, who "was confused with direction" and signed the wrong date and time on his AMA form, was nevertheless allowed to leave a hospital AMA.[85] He was found 2 hours later walking in the snow with frostbitten fingers that required amputation. He later sued for damages, but the appellate court dismissed the case, ruling that the hospital had "no duty to prevent plaintiff from leaving the hospital AMA [or] to ensure plaintiff's safe return home . . . ." There was a compelling dissent to this case questioning the reasoning for the majority's opinion.

CONCLUSION

Deciding on a patient's disposition is sometimes easy, sometimes impossible, but never without risk. Thorough documentation of the provider's thought processes will improve medical decision-making and provide a firm basis for follow-up care. Adhering to legal and regulatory guidelines and making sound decisions based upon a patient's clinical status, symptoms, physical findings, and potential complicating factors will provide the best outcomes for the patient's ED visit.

REFERENCES

1. 42 U.S. Code § 1395dd et seq.
2. Schiff R, Ansell DA, Schlosser JE, et al. Transfers to a public hospital. *N Engl J Med*. 1986;314(9):552–557.
3. 42 U.S. Code § 1395dd(e)(1).
4. 42 U.S. Code § 1395dd(e)(3).
5. Inpatient Prospective Payment System (IPPS) 2009 final rule revisions to Emergency Medical Treatment and Labor Act (EMTALA) regulations. Ref S&C-09-26. Center for Medicaid and State Operations/Survey and Certification Group. 2009. Available at: https://www.cms.gov/Medicare/Provider-Enrollment-and-Certification/SurveyCertificationGenInfo/Downloads/SCLetter09-26.pdf. Accessed August 15, 2020.
6. 232 F.Supp.3d 681 (E.D. Pa., 2017).
7. 42 CFR 1395dd(c)(1).
8. 42 CFR 1395dd(c)(2).
9. National statistics on emergency departments and hospitalizations, 2016. Agency for Healthcare Research and Quality (AHRQ). Available at: http://hcupnet.ahrq.gov/. Accessed April 16, 2020.

10. 42 CFR § 412.3.
11. 42 CFR § 412.3(b).
12. 42 CFR § 412.3(c).
13. 42 CFR § 482.24 (c)
14. US Department of Justice, Office of Public Affairs. Healthcare service provider to pay $60 million to settle Medicare and Medicaid False Claims Act allegations. Press Release No 17-151. *Justice News*. February 6, 2017. Available at: https://www.justice.gov/opa/pr/healthcare-service-provider-pay-60-million-settle-medicare-and-medicaid-false-claims-act. Updated April 27, 2017. Accessed May 3, 2020.
15. US Department of Justice, Office of Public Affairs. Hospital chain will pay over $260 million to resolve false billing and kickback allegations; one subsidiary agrees to plead guilty. Press Release No. 18-1252. *Justice News*. September 25, 2018. Available at: https://www.justice.gov/opa/pr/hospital-chain-will-pay-over-260-million-resolve-false-billing-and-kickback-allegations-one. Updated February 13, 2019. Accessed May 3, 2020.
16. NOTICE Act, HR 876, 114th Cong (2015–2016). Available at: https://www.congress.gov/bill/114th-congress/house-bill/876. Accessed May 3, 2020.
17. Medicare outpatient observation notice (MOON) instructions. CR9935. Centers for Medicare and Medicaid Services. 2017. Available at: https://www.cms.gov/Medicare/Medicare-General-Information/BNI/Downloads/CR9935-MOON-Instructions.pdf. Accessed May 3, 2020.
18. Krall SP, Guardiola J, Richman PB. Increased door to admission time is associated with prolonged throughput for ED patients discharged home. *Am J Emerg Med*. 2016;34(9):1783–1787.
19. Singer AJ, Thode HC, Viccellio P, et al. The association between length of emergency department boarding and mortality. *Acad Emerg Med*. 2011;18(12):1324–1329.
20. American Academy of Emergency Medicine (AAEM). Position statement on ED boarding. 2007. Available at: https://www.aaem.org/resources/statements/position/position-statement-on-ed-boarding. Accessed April 18, 2020.
21. American College of Emergency Physicians (ACEP). Boarding of admitted and intensive care patients in the emergency department. 2000. Available at: https://www.acep.org/patient-care/policy-statements/boarding-of-admitted-and-intensive-care-patients-in-the-emergency-department/. Revised June 2017. Accessed April 18, 2020.
22. American Academy of Emergency Medicine (AAEM). Position statement on ED boarding. 2007. Available at: https://www.aaem.org/resources/statements/position/position-statement-on-ed-boarding. Accessed April 18, 2020.
23. Emergency Nurses Association (ENA). Position statement: crowding, boarding, and patient throughput. 2017. Available at: https://www.ena.org/docs/default-source/resource-library/practice-resources/position-statements/crowdingboardingandpatientthroughput.pdf. Accessed April 18, 2020.
24. Dalton C, Tonellato D. Opinion: emergency rooms shouldn't be parking lots for patients. National Public Radio (NPR) Shots. 2019. Available at: https://www.npr.org/sections/health-shots/2019/11/30/783278033/opinion-emergency-rooms-shouldnt-be-parking-lots-for-patients. Accessed April 25, 2020.
25. American College of Emergency Physicians (ACEP). Responsibility for admitted patients. 2018. Available at: https://www.acep.org/patient-care/policy-statements/responsibility-for-admitted-patients/. Revised April, 2020. Accessed April 25, 2020.
26. American College of Emergency Physicians (ACEP). Boarding of admitted and intensive care patients in the emergency department. 2000. Available at: https://www.acep.org/patient-care/policy-statements/boarding-of-admitted-and-intensive-care-patients-in-the-emergency-department/. Revised June 2017. Accessed April 18, 2020.
27. Rabin E, Kocher K, McClelland, et al. Solutions to emergency department "boarding" and crowding are underused and may need to be legislated. *Health Aff*. 2012 31(8):1757–1766.
28. 42 CFR 1395dd(c)(1).
29. 42 CFR 1395dd(c)(2)
30. 42 CFR 489.24 (f).
31. US Department of Health and Human Services, Office of Inspector General. Civil monetary penalties and affirmative exclusions. Available at: https://oig.hhs.gov/fraud/enforcement/cmp/cmp-ae.asp. Accessed May 3, 2020.
32. National Statistics on Emergency Departments and Hospitalizations. 2016. Agency for Healthcare Research and Quality (AHRQ). Available at: http://hcupnet.ahrq.gov/. Accessed April 16, 2020.
33. Surmaitis RM, Amaducci A, Henry K, et al. Perception and practice among emergency medicine health care providers regarding discharging patients after opioid administration. *Clin Ther*. 2018;40(2):214–223.
34. Kronick R. AHRQ data reveal wider impact of opioid overuse. *AHRQ Views*. October 9, 2014. Available at: http://www.ahrq.gov/news/blog/ahrqviews/100914.html. Accessed April 24, 2020.
35. Gomes T, Tadrous M, Mamdani MM, et al. The burden of opioid-related mortality in the United States, *JAMA Netw Open*. 2018;1(2):e180217.
36. US Department of Health and Human Services. Addressing prescription drug abuse in the United States: current activities and future opportunities. 2013. Available at: https://www.cdc.gov/drugoverdose/pdf/hhs_prescription_drug_abuse_report_09.2013.pdf. Accessed April 24, 2020.
37. Pew Charitable Trusts. When are prescribers required to use prescription drug monitoring programs? 2018. Available at: https://www.pewtrusts.org/en/research-and-analysis/data-visualizations/2018/when-are-prescribers-required-to-use-prescription-drug-monitoring-programs. Accessed April 24, 2020.
38. Tick H, Nielsen A, Pelletier KR, et al. Evidence-based nonpharmacologic strategies for comprehensive pain care: the Consortium Pain Task Force white paper. *Explore (NY)*. 2018;14(3):177–211.
39. Dowell D, Haegerich TM, Chou R. CDC guideline for prescribing opioids for chronic pain–United States, 2016. *MMWR Recomm Rep*. 2016;65(1):1–49.
40. US Department of Health and Human Services. U.S. Surgeon General's advisory on naloxone and opioid overdose. HHS.gov/Office of the Surgeon General. 2018. Available at: https://www.hhs.gov/surgeongeneral/priorities/opioids-and-addiction/naloxone-advisory/index.html. Accessed April 24, 2020.
41. Clarke C, Friedman SM, Shi K, et al. Emergency department discharge instructions comprehension and compliance study. *CJEM*. 2005;7(1):5–11.
42. Spandorfer JM, Karras DJ, Hughes LA, et al. Comprehension of discharge instructions by patients in an urban emergency department. *Ann Emerg Med*. 1995;25(1):71–74.
43. Logan PD, Schwab RA, Salomone JA, et al. Patient understanding of emergency department discharge instructions. *South Med J*. 1996;89(8):770–774.
44. Williams DM, Counselman FL, Caggiano CD. Emergency department discharge instructions and patient literacy: a problem of disparity. *Am J Emerg Med*. 1996;14(1):19–22.
45. Engel KG, Heisler M, Smith DM, et al. Patient comprehension of emergency department care and instructions: are patients aware of when they do not understand? *Ann Emerg Med*. 2009;53(4):454–461.e15.
46. Logan PD, Schwab RA, Salomone JA, et al. Patient understanding of emergency department discharge instructions. *South Med J*. 1996;89(8):770–774.

47. Engel KG, Heisler M, Smith DM, et al. Patient comprehension of emergency department care and instructions: are patients aware of when they do not understand? *Ann Emerg Med.* 2009;53(4): 454–461.e15.
48. Spandorfer JM, Karras DJ, Hughes LA, et al. Comprehension of discharge instructions by patients in an urban emergency department. *Ann Emerg Med.* 1995;25(1):71–74.
49. Vashi A, Rhodes KV. "Sign right here and you're good to go": a content analysis of audiotaped emergency department discharge instructions. *Ann Emerg Med.* 2011;57(4):315–322.e1.
50. Choudhry AJ, Baghdadi YMK, Wagie AE, et al. Readability of discharge summaries: with what level of information are we dismissing our patients? *Am J Surg.* 2016;211(3):631–636.
51. *Marsolino v Patel*, E041922 (Cal. App. 5/11/2009).
52. *Bevan v Valencia*, 15–73 KG/SCY (D. N.M. 2017).
53. *Guadagno v Lifemark Hospitals of Florida*, 972 So.2d 214 (Fla. App., 2007).
54. *Clelland v Haas*, 774 So.2d 1243 (La. App., 2000).
55. *McPherson v Abraham*, 13 AD3d 422, (N.Y. App. Div., 2004).
56. *Doll v Kester*, 19A-CT-663 (Ind. App. 2020).
57. *Desimini v Bristol Hospital*, 927 A.2d 1004 (CT 2007).
58. Kraut A, Fransoo R, Olafson K, et al. A population-based analysis of leaving the hospital against medical advice: incidence and associated variables. *BMC Health Serv Res.* 2013;13:415.
59. Glasgow JM, Vaughn-Sarrazin M, Kaboli PJ. Leaving against medical advice (AMA): risk of 30-day mortality and hospital readmission. *J Gen Intern Med.* 2010;25(9):926–929.
60. Jasperse N, Grigorian A, Delaplain P, et al. Predictors of discharge against medical advice in adult trauma patients. *Surgeon.* 2020;18(1): 12–18.
61. Kraut A, Fransoo R, Olafson K, et al. A population-based analysis of leaving the hospital against medical advice: incidence and associated variables. *BMC Health Serv Res.* 2013;13:415.
62. Ibrahim SA, Kwoh CK, Krishnan E. Factors associated with patients who leave acute-care hospitals against medical advice. *Am J Public Health.* 2007;97(12): 2204–2208.
63. Ding R, McCarthy ML, Li G, et al. Patients who leave without being seen: their characteristics and history of emergency department use. *Ann Emerg Med.* 2006;48(6):686–693.
64. Anis AH, Sun H, Guh DP, et al. Leaving hospital against medical advice among HIV-positive patients. *CMAJ.* 2002;167(6):633–637.
65. Dubow D. Emergency department discharges against medical advice. *J Emerg Med.* 1993;11(3):333.
66. Reinke DA, Walker M, Boslaugh S, et al. Predictors of pediatric emergency patients discharged against medical advice. *Clin Pediatr.* 2009;48(3):263–270.
67. Onukwugha E, Saunders E, Mullins CD, et al. Reasons for discharges against medical advice: a qualitative study. *Qual Saf Health Care.* 2010;19(5):420–424.
68. Kahn DR, Bourgeois JA, Klein SC, et al. A prospective observational study of decisional capacity determinations in an academic medical center. *Int J Psychiatry Med.* 2009;39(4):405–415.
69. The Sullivan Group, Do's and Don'ts of AMA: Patients Who Leave Against Medical Advice. Published 2020, https://blog.thesullivangroup.com/ama-patients-who-leave-against-medical-advice, Accessed October 1, 2020
70. *Lyons v Walker Regional Medical Center*, 791 So. 2d 937 (2000).
71. Widger HN, Propp DA, Leslie K, et al. Insurance companies refusing payment for patients who leave the emergency department against medical advice is a myth. *Ann Emerg Med.* 2010;55(4):393.
72. Schaefer GR, Matus H, Schumann JH, et al. Financial responsibility of hospitalized patients who left against medical advice: medical urban legend? *J Gen Intern Med.* 2012;27(7):825–830.
73. *Prince v Commonwealth of Massachusetts*, 321 U.S. 158 (1944).
74. *N.J. Div. of Child Prot. & Permanency v S.R. (In re Guardianship of Me.R.)*, A-1741-18T3, N.J. Super. App. Div. (2020).
75. Moyse HS, Osmun WE. Discharges against medical advice: a community hospital's experience. *Can J Rural Med.* 2004;9(3):148–153.
76. Dubow D, Propp D, Narasimhan K. Emergency department discharges against medical advice. *J Emerg Med.* 1993;11(3):333.
77. Stearns CR, Bakamjian A, Sattar S, et al. Discharges against medical advice at a county hospital: provider perceptions and practice. *J Hosp Med.* 2017;12(1):11–17.
78. Tummalapalli SL, Chang BA, Goodlev ER. Physician practices in against medical advice discharges. *J Healthc Qual.* 2019.
79. 42 U.S. Code § 1395dd(b)(2).
80. Henson VL, Vickery DS. Patient self-discharge from the emergency department: who is at risk? *Emerg Med J.* 2005;22(7):499–501.
81. Stearns CR, Bakamjian A, Sattar S, et al. Discharges against medical advice at a county hospital: provider perceptions and practice. *J Hosp Med.* 2017;12(1):11–17.
82. *Drummond v Buckley*, 627 So. 2d 264 (1993).
83. *Sawyer v Comerci*, 2002 VA 411 (2002).
84. *Zablotny v State Bd. of Nursing*, 156 A.3d 126 (Me. 2017).
85. *Ingutti v Rochester Gen. Hosp.*, 114 A.D.3d 1302 (N.Y. App. Div. 2014).

MALPRACTICE

SECTION 11

RISK MANAGEMENT: CHALLENGES AND OPPORTUNITIES

Graham Billingham, Michelle Hoppes, Sue Dill Calloway

Health-care risk management arose from the insurance crisis of the 1970s. During that period, liability premiums skyrocketed, due in part to the dissolution of the doctrine of charitable immunity, which historically protected a hospital's assets from lawsuits.[1] Thus, risk management has historically been about protecting the hospital and preventing financial loss. It has evolved to include a primary focus on protecting the patient and preventing harm. This protection is called "value protection" and remains a challenge today. The current focus is not only about value protection but also about value creation: the ability to demonstrate the return on risk improvement or the upside of risk management.

Like the malpractice crisis of the 1970s, the patient safety movement today is creating change in risk management. One of the greatest catalysts was the Institute of Medicine's 1999 report, *To Err Is Human: Building a Safer Health System*. This report provided insight into the growing problem of medical errors, which then led to the rise in mounting regulations and government scrutiny.[2] Today, providers must meet an unprecedented and increasingly prescriptive standard of care. The evidence used to determine if a provider acted in a reasonably prudent manner may include standards created by regulatory and accrediting agencies. Even more important and challenging is the need to transform the hierarchical health-care environment into a culture of patient safety.

The effective implementation of risk management requires leadership to establish a culture of patient safety and risk reduction. They must recognize that the majority of risk issues are a result of system failures that must be managed within a "just-culture" framework. This framework is based on a shared accountability, in which there is a balanced approach between the focus on system issues and human error. In this culture, everyone must understand that risk is, for the most part, both predictable and preventable. This belief system enhances the adoption of prevention tools to decrease variation and to standardize operational process.

Risk management is interdisciplinary and affects all aspects of the organization. Problems in the emergency department (ED) can stem from operational, clinical, or communication issues, which all contribute to system errors. Through the implementation of a proactive approach to risk management and patient safety, adverse outcomes can and have been prevented.

CASE STUDY

A proactive risk-management program requires the development and execution of strategies to address the high-risk areas. In order to demonstrate the risk-management process, the following case study will be used throughout this chapter:

Case study: A 38-year-old woman presents at triage with a chief complaint of stabbing chest pain and nausea. She has a history of dyspepsia and reports eating at a local food stand earlier today. An ECG reveals a normal sinus rhythm, and an initial set of enzyme tests are negative. She is given a GI cocktail and reports some relief. She is discharged home with instructions to follow up with her primary physician in 3 days.

The patient returns the next day in cardiac arrest from an acute myocardial infarction (MI) and cannot be resuscitated. Subsequent details reveal a history of smoking and a family history of early heart disease.

RISK-MANAGEMENT PROCESS

Identification of Risk

It is leadership's responsibility to ensure that appropriate methods are in place to identify potential threats in a timely and effective manner. Identification of risk can come from a variety of sources, including:

- Complaint or notification by physician, nurse, or patient/family member
- Complaint by a consulting service
- Bad outcome (death, serious morbidity)
- Wrong site or wrong medication
- Sentinel events, which are events that result in serious injury or death

Identification should answer the following question: How does a health-care system know that there was a problem? In other words, what is the reporting system, and to whom is the problem reported? Multiple systems of identification, including anonymous methods, are critical to the success of any risk program. Examples include a complaint line, an anonymous call-in line, and incident reports.

Case study (continued): The problem was identified as a serious safety event through the occurrence-reporting process, which indicated that a young woman with chest pain was treated and discharged, returned within 24 hours in cardiac arrest, and expired. This patient record was flagged for immediate review at the ED quality improvement (QI) meeting. The risk-identification process in this case worked well.

Analysis of Risk

Risk analysis lies in establishing who is impacted and how. Only after studying the effects of the identified risk and the impact on the providers and the organization can solutions be created and implemented. The analysis can also be used to create a risk hierarchy. This prioritization can focus efforts on the highest-risk issues to achieve maximum impact. A frequent barrier to executing a risk program occurs when leadership does not agree on the exact etiology of the problem. A three-step approach is helpful for achieving the best results (**Box 109.1**).

BOX 109.1 ■ DETERMINING THE ETIOLOGY OF THE RISK

- What is the problem that we are trying to solve or understand?
- What tools are we using to analyze the issue that will help lead to the best possible solutions and alternatives?
- What is leadership's understanding and ultimate recommendation for prevention?

Case study (continued): *Case analysis indicated a failure to consider the diagnosis of acute MI, with the contributing factors of failure to 1) obtain a complete history of risk factors, 2) perform serial enzymes and ECGs in a patient who presented with chest pain of a duration less than 2 hours, 3) perform or arrange for a postdischarge stress test in a patient at risk for acute MI, and 4) observe to allow the pain etiology to be defined. Case analysis indicated lack of compliance with many of the key diagnostic tools for a patient presenting with chest pain. Further analysis revealed a pattern of missed MIs in young women within the health system. One of the interesting findings was that, far from being atypical, many of these patients presented with chest pain and had cardiac risk factors.*

Treatment of Risk

Risk treatment involves the deployment of successful countermeasures that directly result in a reduction of risk. The program should be flexible and tested at short, frequent intervals. Although this flexibility allows several solutions to be considered initially, it also enables the most effective solutions to emerge.

Case study (continued): *Treatment of this risk pattern included implementing a process to emphasize the early identification of female patients at risk for cardiac disease. The process included the implementation of a uniform approach to these patients by using a chest pain bundle, including serial ECGs, serial cardiac enzymes, and stress testing.*

Prevention of Risk

The evaluation of risk reduction is the process by which these strategies are measured for their effectiveness. It is critical for the evaluation process to be consistent in its approach and design. Successful strategies can then be modified as necessary and used to create programs that prevent adverse outcomes.

Case study (continued): *Evaluation of the risk treatment in this case included a multistep process to discern the effectiveness of the new countermeasures. Specifically, the program included a triad of web-based education followed by clinical audits and a benchmarking analysis. The program reviewed the expected behavioral changes to ensure compliance with the key metrics for diagnostic evaluation.*

Risk prevention is the key to protecting and avoiding adverse events while ensuring a focus on patient safety. Department leaders must be prepared to emphasize both the proactive and reactive risk-management issues. Prevention is the proactive component of risk management (**Box 109.2**).

BOX 109.2 ■ RISK-PREVENTION TECHNIQUES

- Developing and adopting clinical protocols in high-risk areas
- Implementing algorithms that outline the clinical and operational aspects of care in the high-risk conditions
- Creating pathways and order sets to ensure the delivery of care within established standards
- Hardwiring best practices in relation to operational excellence
- Measuring what is expected through audits and indicators
- Regularly evaluating established metrics

> **BOX 109.3 ■ ADDRESSING A CRITICAL EVENT**
>
> 1. Ensure that the immediate needs of the patient and event specifics are being handled.
> 2. Ensure the clinical providers are aware/involved.
> 3. Notify applicable leaders.
> 4. Minimize damage to equipment and the environment.
> 5. Do not disconnect or change any lines, equipment, cables, and so on, involved in patient care unless required to avoid further damage/injury.
> 6. Sequester all equipment attached or contiguous to the injured patient, as well as all documents, disposable products, packaging, and medications/vials that may have been involved.
> 7. Ensure patient/family support, and determine the disclosure process.
> 8. Direct or conduct immediate debriefing of the event with those involved.
> 9. Determine if notifying public relations is applicable or if any regulatory reporting is require (FDA, medical examiner, CMS, police, etc.)
> 10. Involve claims manager/insurance company as applicable.
> 11. Determine the members of the investigative team, and immediately mitigate the potential for further harm or recurrence.

Case study (continued): Prevention in this case included a change in approach to the triage and treatment of young females with chest pain. It also resulted in discontinuing the ED's use of GI cocktails to differentiate ischemic heart disease.

CRITICAL EVENT MANAGEMENT

Handling serious safety, critical, and sentinel events are core competencies of successful risk-management programs. These terms are often used interchangeably; however, certain differences should be noted. A serious or critical event is usually described as a deviation in practice that causes serious harm to the patient. A sentinel event is usually described as an unexpected occurrence involving death or serious physical or psychological injury, or the danger thereof. The steps to take when a critical event occurs are listed in **Box 109.3**. There are many tools that can be used to reduce risk when managing a critical event.

Barrier Analysis

Barrier analysis focuses on the administrative or physical controls designed to prevent or inhibit an undesirable event from reaching a patient. There are generally three modes of barrier failure: the barrier fails to protect, the barrier was not in place, or the barrier was circumvented. Another purpose for this type of analysis is to establish the barriers that should have been in place already as well as those can can be installed to increase safety in the future. This process allows the team to review the current and missing barriers and determine probable causal factors. Examples include:

- Administrative barriers
    - ☐ Practice guidelines
    - ☐ Policies and procedures

- Training methods
- Peer review and monitoring
- Physical barriers
  - Safety devices
  - Human factors design
  - Locked doors
  - Redundancy
  - Alarms and reminders

When considering barrier analysis, it may be necessary to specifically look at 1) what physical, human, or system controls were in place to prevent the event; 2) which barrier failed; 3) which barrier succeeded, and 4) what other controls might have prevented the problem.

Change Analysis

Change analysis analyzes the difference between what actually happened, what should have happened, and any best practice or ideal situation that can be implemented to mitigate future crises. The process includes:

- Determining the actual and ideal situation
- Reviewing similar processes that were event-free
- Comparing the process when event-free and when not
- Identifying the differences
- Integrating the differences into contributing causal factors

Event and Causal Factor Charting

Event and causal factor (ECF) charting is used to illuminate the causes that led to the event. ECF, which is useful for evaluating complex situations, can reveal the events from start to finish, including broken barriers, inappropriate actions, and causal factors. The technique was originally developed by the National Transportation Safety Board to use in accident investigation. It provides a structure for integrating findings and contributing factors into a pictorial flowchart. The most important part of using the ECF chart is defining the sequence of events and their relationship to the causal factors. This chart can be started as soon as the investigator starts the interviews and review process.

Failure Mode and Effects Analysis

Failure mode and effects analysis is a hazard-identification technique in which all known failure modes or features of a system are considered, and undesired outcomes are noted.

The Five "Whys"

The "five whys" constitute a questioning process designed to investigate the details of a problem or solution and peel away the layers of symptoms. The technique was originally developed by Sakichi Toyoda, the founder of Toyota Industries, who stated, ". . . by repeating 'why' five times, the nature of the problem as well as its solution becomes clear." This process brings clarity to a problem statement, gets to the root cause, and produces a potential solution. First, determine the starting point (an assumed root cause), and write it at the top of a document. Then, ask why the root cause occurred. Finally, repeat the question until no new answers result. This method often requires five rounds.

Fishbone Diagram

The fishbone analysis is used to identify the causes, factors, or sources of variation that led to the event. It is often used in concert with brainstorming and the five whys. This process groups causes into categories with a corresponding arrow indicating how they cascade toward the event. Fishbone diagrams are simple to create and can be drawn on a whiteboard or easel paper during a brainstorming session. The "spine" of the fish represents the sequence of events leading to the undesirable outcome (**Figure 109.1**). The fish "bones" represent selected categories that are considered contributors to the sequence. The category sets often include:

- The "four Ms"—**m**ethods, **m**achines, **m**aterials, and **m**anpower
- The "four Ps"—**p**lace, **p**rocedure, **p**eople, and **p**olicies
- The "four Ss"—**s**urroundings, **s**uppliers, **s**ystems, and **s**kills

As a brainstorming process, this tool is less likely to be based on evidence than on assumptions.

Fault Tree Analysis or Logic Tree

A fault tree analysis is a method of examining the logical combinations of various system states that lead to a particular outcome. Fault tree diagrams (**Figure 109.2**) can show how human errors contribute to system failures by providing a graphic representation of error sequences that can be understood by engineers and safety personnel. The question, "How could an event occur?" is asked and answered first. The question, "Why?" follows to identify the failure modes. The logic tree is cause-and-effect based, requiring evidence to back up the assertions. This approach requires an in-depth understanding of the flaws in the system that contributed to poor decisions.

The failure of the process to achieve its designed objective has to do with the links between its steps. Many believe that the logic tree's strict adherence to representing these tightly coupled relationships makes it a more accurate tool than others.

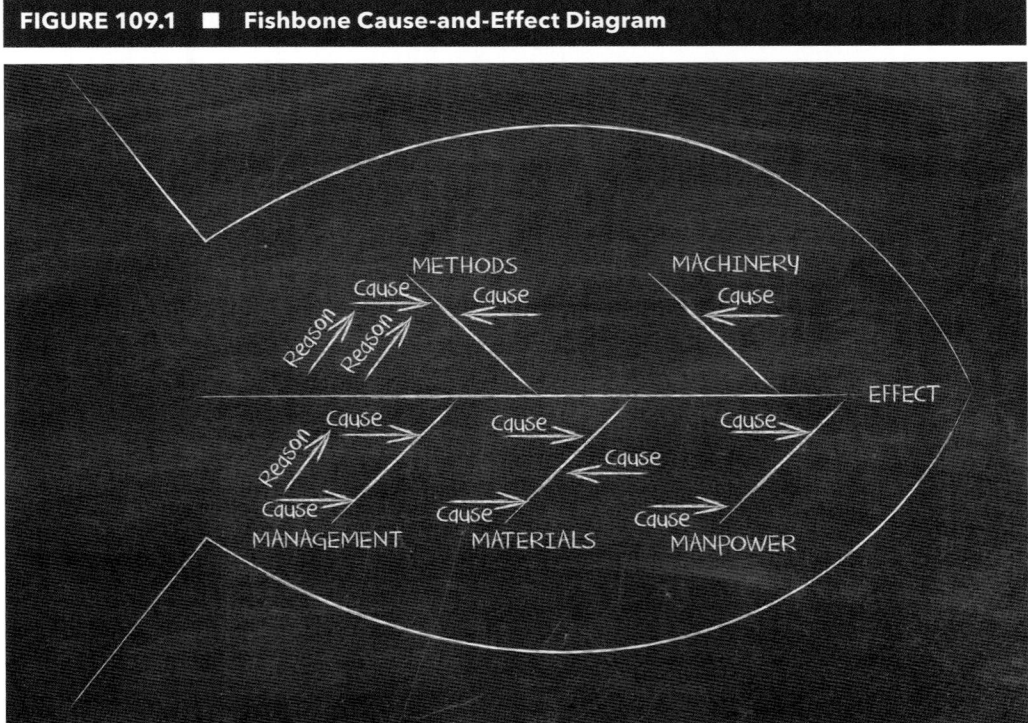

FIGURE 109.1 ■ Fishbone Cause-and-Effect Diagram

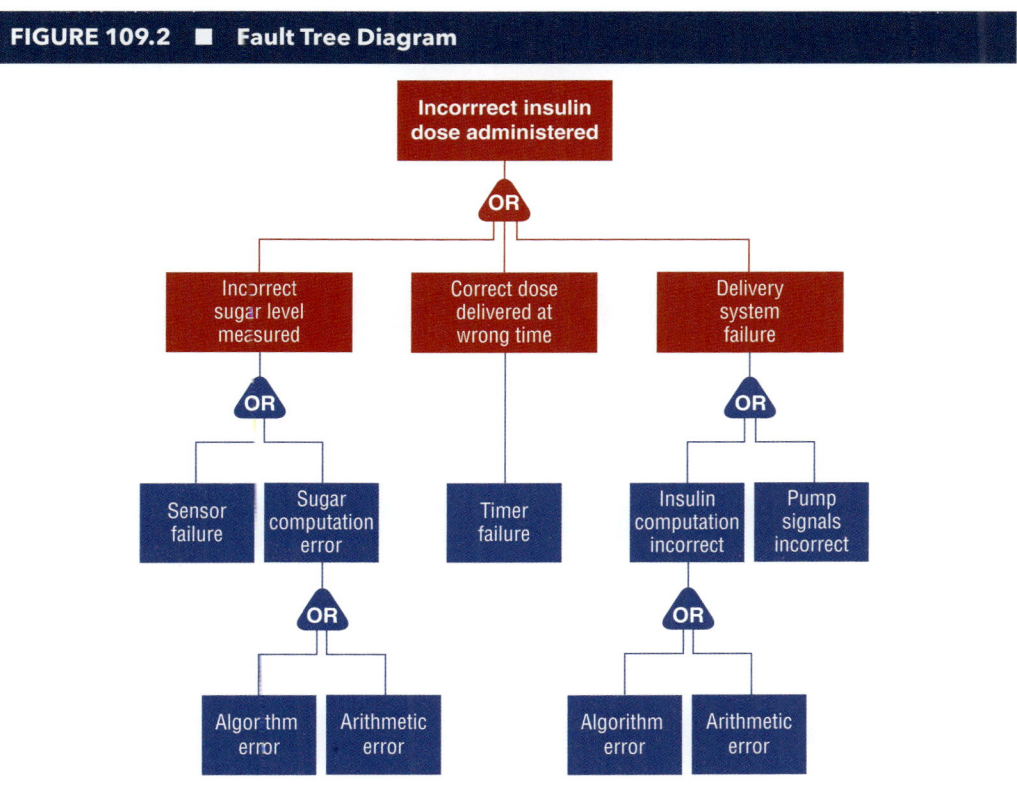

FIGURE 109.2 ■ Fault Tree Diagram

THE RISK-MANAGEMENT LEADER

To implement a risk-management process, the ED group must formally appoint an individual who can fill the leadership role by collaborating with the hospital risk manager. Even though there is significant overlap, it is important to distinguish between the functions of risk management and those of QI. A frequent and distinguishing difference in function describes risk management as critical event investigation and prevention and QI as compliance with and measurement of regulatory standards. The difference in function is often defined within the culture of the organization. It is not unusual for one individual to implement the functions of risk management and QI.

Traditionally, risk managers have identified both internal and external threats and have developed control measures and monitoring systems to mitigate them. The risk manager also plays the role of champion, communicator, and referee among different factions within the organization. A successful strategy usually requires a multidisciplinary approach with representation by claims, QI, patient safety, operations, finance, and leadership. It is the role of the ED leader to ensure the integration of these disciplines.

Typical tasks include prevention, management, and detection, specifically, preventing and managing risks as they occur and detecting threats before they reach the patient. Buy-in from the senior management team is essential to the success of any plan. Under current healthcare reform, the role of the ED risk-management leader will likely expand on and support the organization's strategic planning process.

MALPRACTICE CLAIMS

To fully support risk reduction, it is important to understand both existing and emerging threats. In the last several years, there has been a marked shift in ED malpractice claims from clinical

BOX 109.4 ■ OPERATIONAL RISKS LEADING TO MALPRACTICE

- Failure to orient and supervise
- Unaddressed prolonged waiting times and poor patient satisfaction
- Communication barriers
- Failure to decrease practice variation through guidelines and monitoring
- Delays in care and treatment
- Prolonged lab and X-ray turnaround
- Inadequate handoffs
- Lack of equipment or resources
- Inadequate documentation of the medical decision-making
- Poor teamwork
- On-call provider shortages
- Failure to address abnormal vital signs, physical or laboratory findings
- Overreliance on technology
- Repeat visits without thorough review
- Inadequate imaging/ED interface
- Inconsistent approach to assessment and reassessment
- Inadequate discharge planning
- ED boarding of admitted patients
- Admission to the wrong level of service or location

to operational risk because a significant portion of ED provider experience stems from the operational environment. It is important to note, however, that many of the problems that arise from systems issues can be mitigated. Examples of operational risks (beginning at triage and ending at discharge) that frequently lead to claims of medical malpractice are listed in **Box 109.4**.

Clinical high-risk areas in the ED have remained quite consistent over the years. The top areas of loss from a clinical perspective include missed or delayed diagnoses (**Table 109.1**). Patients with the conditions listed can present in an early stage or with unusual symptoms that make the diagnosis difficult to recognize. Obscure presentations are particularly true for meningitis and appendicitis; however, the cases that are most costly to settle are those that present in a typical manner but are mismanaged or misdiagnosed.

The Physician Insurers Association of America, now the Medical Professional Liability Association, has conducted a large-scale study (4,341 closed ED claims from 1985 to 2008) that defines the frequency and severity of the most common malpractice cases. The study indicates that the ED ranks 16th among 28 physician specialties in paid claims and 15th in

TABLE 109.1 ■ High-Risk Presentations

Presenting Complaint	Possible Diagnoses
Chest pain	MI, pulmonary embolism, or aortic dissection
Headache	Cerebrovascular accident, meningitis, or subarachnoid hemorrhage
Abdominal pain	Intestinal obstruction, appendicitis, aortic aneurysm, ectopic pregnancy, or testicular torsion
Pediatric fever	Sepsis and meningitis
Wounds	Retained foreign body, lacerated tendon or nerve, or missed fracture

the number of claims reported.[3] Other insurers report head injuries, strokes, spinal injuries, obstetrical conditions, respiratory distress, and infections as complaints with significant incidence and high-dollar payments.[4] Unfortunately, suicides are among an emerging group of claims risks and new challenges.

MITIGATING HIGH-RISK SITUATIONS

There are numerous high-risk areas in the ED from a clinical and operational perspective. Following are examples of operational issues and risk-reduction recommendations.

Supervision

The adequate supervision of providers with different levels of training is paramount to reducing risk. Supervision is an ongoing process that requires an initial orientation, direct oversight, chart review, and feedback. Medical and nursing students are unlicensed practitioners and require the most direct supervision. Attending physicians must be involved in all aspects of the care these trainees provide.

Department leaders must be familiar with the individual state laws defining the practice of physician assistants (PAs) and nurse practitioners (NPs); these responsibilities and liability vary by state. For example, the NP has an independent license, whereas the PA is a dependent extender under the physician's license in some states. In other states, PAs are recognized as licensed practitioners (see Chapter 24).

Residents rotating through the ED and those accepting patients from the ED are, by definition, phsyicians in training and have a broader scope of practice than PAs and NPs. However, it is important to remember that their backgrounds and training will differ from specialty to specialty. Further, there is individual variation among the skill levels of the residents themselves. Risk can be decreased by having all of the following:

- A consistent approach
- Guidelines that delineate scope of services
- Appropriate oversight with review of diagnosis and treatment
- Requirements for presenting cases to the attending
- Documentation guidelines

Common resident risk areas involve practicing beyond their scope of expertise, an over-reliance on technology, handoffs between providers, fatigue, and inadequate documentation. To reduce this risk, ED leaders may implement the processes listed in **Box 109.5**.

BOX 109.5 ■ PROCESSES DESIGNED TO REDUCE RISK

- Attending oversight for all high-risk conditions
- Comprehensive new provider orientation
- Review of 30 charts for adequate documentation
- Implementation of an auditing process to ensure compliance with the standards of care

> **BOX 109.6 ■ MITIGATING RISK DURING DISCHARGE**
>
> - Provide discharge instructions written in the patient's language and reviewed with both the patient and the family.
> - Include specific appointment information.
> - Explain specific recommendations, and clarify what to watch for and when to return.
> - Establish a "call-back" program, which should be used for high-risk conditions and allow for adequate follow-up, documentation of patient compliance, and a chance to address any patient complaints.
> - Ensure that all discharge paperwork instructs patients to return to the ED immediately in the event of worsening symptoms.

Discharge Instructions

The conversation had with the patient during discharge is sometimes referred to as the "last chance to get it right." A significant percentage of ED claims include allegations that the discharge instructions were not inadequate. To mitigate risk through effective discharge instructions, ED leaders can implement the processes listed in **Box 109.6**.

Risk Assessment

One of the first steps to protect against and reduce ED risk is to perform a risk assessment that can help identify problem areas, prioritize action plans, and develop countermeasures to offset risk. The risk assessment can also be used to monitor and track improvements in performance and benchmarks. Many of the systems issues will require an interdisciplinary approach among nurses, administrators, and providers. Risk-management leaders in the ED should start by completing an analysis to help illuminate the department's risk profile (**Table 109.2**).

Risk-Management Planning

Upon completing a risk assessment, a plan should be developed to address the findings. Each plan should include, at minimum, the elements listed in **Box 109.7**. With an increasing emphasis on cost containment, reimbursement, and waste elimination, it is imperative that ED leaders demonstrate the return on investment (ROI) of an effective risk-management program to the C-suite. Evaluating claims-related losses and reducing risk expenses can create direct financial returns. Equally important but harder to demonstrate are the soft costs associated with risk management. These include:

- Increased customer satisfaction
- Decreased medical errors
- Decreased complaints
- Improved provider satisfaction
- Effective methods to demonstrate the ROI, including:
    - ☐ Clinical audits to objectively measure process and outcomes
    - ☐ Operational indicators to objectively measure and benchmark system issues
    - ☐ Comparing the frequency and severity of claims to improvements in the ED risk profile

TABLE 109.2 ■ Components of an Effective Risk-Assessment Process

Major Program Components	Elements

Operations and leadership structure	• Patient flow (e.g., average length of stay <3 hours)
	• Efficiency metrics (e.g., door-to-triage <5 minutes)
	• Patient satisfaction (e.g., scores >85%)
	• Diagnostic turn around (e.g., troponin <30 minutes)
	• Communication and teamwork:
	  ○ Use "situation, background, assessment, response."
	  ○ Create handoff checklists.
	  ○ Implement simulation training.
	  ○ Ensure preliminary radiology reports are in the permanent record.

Documentation	• Fully address the patients' chief complaints. • Review allergies, medications, and old records. • Address and decode abnormal vital signs, lab, and X-ray findings. • Adequately examine the affected area. • Discuss the case with consultants, as necessary. • Repeat abnormal vital signs before discharge. • Include medical decision-making thought process. • Provide adequate discharge instructions.
Provider hiring and orientation	• Include complete application and reference check. • Determine history of malpractice claims, patient complaints, drug/alcohol abuse, and a criminal background check. • Provide formal orientation to the practice and its setting. • Implement double coverage shifts for a period of time. • Perform mandatory chart review. • Assign a mentor. • Ensure participation in quality improvement.
Provider evaluation	• Perform competency assessment and care evaluation. • Perform mandatory chart audits. • Ensure participation in peer review and high-risk CME. • Determine procedural competency. • Address unacceptable behavior immediately. • Use scorecards to benchmark and provide feedback.
Complaint management	• Timeliness: Respond to and meet in person within 24 hours. • Integrate and coordinate with hospital quality/complaint process. • Consider a written response offering a careful explanation and apology when appropriate (see Chapter 76).

Critical event investigation	• Address:
	  ○ Immediacy of reporting
	  ○ Investigation and management (checklist)

(Countinued)

	○ Disclosure ○ Resolution ○ Data tracking and analysis ○ Education and training
Clinical high-risk areas	• Chest pain: Consider serial enzymes prior to patient discharge and, when appropriate, serial ECGs and stress testing. • Stroke: Implement a door-to-CT time of 25 minutes, as recommended by the American Heart Association. • Pediatric fever: Ensure appropriate door-to-antibiotic time. • Abdominal pain: Ensure timely follow-up 8 to 24 for discharges with ongoing pain; institute a liberal CT policy, especially in the elderly.

TABLE 109.2 ■ (Continued)

CASE STUDY (CONTINUED)

Several important lessons arise from this case study.

Focused Review

The Emergency Physician Insurance Company gathered information and analyzed claims to determine potential contributing factors and areas of focus. The review particularly concentrated on chest pain, the diagnosis associated with highest payout in national claims involving the ED. Potential contributing factors included:

- The majority of missed MIs were in women between the ages of 35 and 55.
- High-risk cases involved discharged patients who presented with chest pain. Areas of focus included:
  - ☐ Enzyme and ECG frequency before discharge
  - ☐ Documentation of risk factors
  - ☐ Physician medical decision-making and rationale for discharge
  - ☐ Outpatient stress testing

BOX 109.7 ■ RISK-MANAGEMENT PLANNING

- Invest adequate time and resources to implement the risk-management plan.
- Identify and empower physician and nurse leadership to execute the plan.
- Ensure that the plan is multidisciplinary and is integrated in the hospital's plan.
- Involve all operational areas that impact the care of the ED patient.
- Establish guidelines for the treatment of high-risk chief complaints.
- Establish a culture of transparency, trust, and patient safety.
- Provide ongoing risk education.
- Establish a chart audit and feedback process that involves all providers.
- Establish a formal disclosure process to address chief complaints.
- Establish a "call-back" system to identify problems and ensure compliance.
- Build a customer service program that emphasizes communication.

Medical Record Audit

Based on the audit findings, the risk-management team conducted a review of relevant literature, standards of practice, and medical-legal issues. The review resulted in the creation of a clinical risk-management medical record audit tool. The tool was piloted and then used to review more than 2,000 medical records of patients over the age of 35 who were discharged from the ED with a primary complaint of nontraumatic chest pain. The record audits were completed among different ED groups and in multiple states. The primary audit included documenting and assessing related risk factors, diagnostic tests, medical decision-making, and discharge protocols.

Identified Opportunities

The audit identified opportunities for improvement in several specific areas. Based on the results, a number of interventions were implemented, such as:

- Review of individual group results with physician leaders
- Benchmarking among participating groups
- Reduction in practice variation through the use of clinical protocols
- Education on MI care and atypical chest pain in women
- Change in operational and/or system issues
- Establishing achievable benchmark targets

The Results

Over a three-year period, the same groups performed two more audits; their outcomes demonstrated a 20-point increase (40% improvement). The next step in the process will be to compare the specific indicators against claims frequency and severity. This further study will determine if there is an ROI or value creation.

CONCLUSION

Risk management is about value protection and value creation. By completing comprehensive risk assessments in the ED, understanding the overall risk profile, and diminishing threats, department leaders can do both. Protecting value includes ensuring patient safety and preventing financial loss. Creating value includes demonstrating the ROI in measurable terms, such as direct financial impact, increased patient and provider satisfaction, and improved operational and clinical outcomes. By careful planning, prioritization, and execution, an effective program will mitigate threats before they happen and enhance patient safety in the ED.

REFERENCES

1. Orlikoff JE, Fifer WR, Greeley H. *Malpractice Prevention and Loss Control for Hospitals*. Chicago, Ill: American Hospital Association; 1981.
2. Kohn LT, Corrigan JM, Donaldson MS, eds. *To Err Is Human: Building a Safer Health System*. Washington, DC: National Academy Press; 2000.
3. Brown TW, McCarty MC, Kelen GD, et al. An epidemiologic study of closed emergency department malpractice claims in a national database of physician malpractice insurers. *Acad Emerg Med*. 2010;17(5):553–560.
4. Kachalia A, Gandhi TK, Puopolo AL, et al. Missed and delayed diagnoses in the emergency department: a study of closed malpractice claims from 4 liability insurers. *Ann Emerg Med*. 2007;49(2):196–205.

RISK MANAGEMENT IN PRACTICE

Gregory L. Henry, Diana B. Nordlund

The term "risk management" has become a buzzword in many corporate communities. Practitioners of the healing arts should not forget that the only true risk is to the life and well-being of the patient. Health-care risk management is better approached as risk reduction that controls practice variables and maximizes the patient's chances of a satisfactory outcome. To view risk management as any more or any less is to disregard the traditional duties placed on physicians since the time of Galen. Accordingly, acting in the best interest of the patient is generally in both the short- and long-term best interests of the health-care professionals and the institutions they represent.

Traditionally, risk managers have used incident reports, patient complaints, and reported adverse outcomes as the impetus to begin to "manage risk." Thus, in its more traditional form, risk management is reactive and not proactive. It has been the administrative branch of the hospital where "bad outcomes" or "bad practice" were mitigated, if not repaired, on an after-the-fact basis. The risk was viewed as the threat to the institution and provider and not to the health of the patient. In the past, it was the rare institution that combined its risk management and quality improvement functions in such a way that led to true change.

The newer trends in risk management take a different view. Intelligent risk managers know that their job is proactive, not reactive, and requires close collaboration with the clinical leadership.

ORGANIZING SYSTEMS TO MITIGATE RISK

Before risk can be approached in a meaningful way, several concepts must be internalized. The first plank in the platform of risk management is that good things happen only when planned and bad things can happen all by themselves. Institutions have spent too much time providing the latest bit of equipment and not enough time analyzing the physical journey of the patient through the maze of the health-care institution. Studying the sojourn through the medical system from the patient's perspective is key to understanding risk.

The second major principle of risk management is that most of the problems are systems-based, rather than due to incompetent or malevolent actions of health-care providers themselves.[1] Few providers want anything for the patient but a rapid return to health. Still, precious little time is spent coordinating the activities of the various departments through which a patient must pass. Miscommunications between the emergency department (ED) and radiology, poor follow-up by on-call physicians, and failure to properly relay information between the nurses and physicians—these are the types of system failures that frequently characterize risk-management disasters.

The reasons for these system failures are multiple. Due to super-specialization, seemingly every technical aspect of the patient's care is performed by a different individual. These clinicians often perform their tasks well but without considering the overall needs of the patient. The headlong race for technologic superiority and efficiency frequently leaves the person who matters the most—the patient—in a bewildering maze. If each individual feels that it is someone else's job to oversee, coordinate, and integrate the separate components of the patient's care, medicine is doomed to remain fractured and risk-prone.

Pearl: *Good things happen only if they are planned. Bad things happen all by themselves.*

Recognizing the importance of start-to-finish planning of the health-care encounter allows the system to recognize and analyze both successes and failures. Rather than a reactive, blame-based structure, a proactive system that analyzes and replicates good outcomes holds more promise. Thus, the final plank of the risk-management platform is as an early detection system for the system's policies, procedures, and outcomes. Risk management should play a key role in creating the seamless thread of integrated medical care. It should be considered risk management's duty to bring such systems-based problems to the attention of the institution's leaders. The intelligent and humane provision of health care as viewed by patients is the only reason for our existence. The way we can know that we are indeed providing such care is through the feedback loop provided by risk management.

Application of Resources

A valid test of an institution's commitment to improving its system is the resource base allocated to the project. It takes both time and effort to monitor, study, and continuously improve medical systems. Additionally, it takes the human touch—a willingness to not merely study averages and percentages, but also to look at each and every human being who enters the system as the final assessment. It is the outcome, no matter how great or small the problem, that reflects the level of performance.

The concept of zero defects, which has become the watchword in all manufacturing industries, must now become the credo of health-care institutions. We must move to the point where unhappiness on the part of the patient with regard to our service should be considered unacceptable. Understanding the variability in all human systems, each health-care provider must be trained to handle online complaints about the system. Often, the most satisfied patients are those who have had some type of minor problem in the system that, once brought to the attention of the health-care personnel, has been properly and satisfactorily resolved.

Elements of Effective Risk Management

No single method avoids all risk in all EDs. However, the principal elements of risk reduction can be summarized as follows:

- Patients come to health-care institutions anxious, afraid, and with a somewhat diminished capacity to understand what is happening. It should be expected that medical providers will go the extra mile by providing explanations that reassure their patients.
- Every health-care provider is a risk reducer who does what is necessary to see that the patient's needs are met.
- When it is apparent that a patient's needs have not been met, each member of the medical team is responsible to reduce risk in real time, both at the bedside and within the system hierarchy.
- Open communication with the patient, no matter what the outcome or circumstances, is the best way to show concern. Whenever conflict is identified, rapid action on the part of both the provider and institution to correct the situation is in the best interests of everyone involved.

- To definitively manage risk, one needs a structured, organized system that not only responds to a particular patient's problem but also analyzes the root cause and can effectuate change based on its analysis.

Pearl: Everyone on the team is a risk reducer.

HIGH-RISK BEHAVIORS AND ISSUES

Although any interaction between a patient and the health-care system may result in litigation, it is clear that certain situations lend themselves to system failures. In some malpractice cases, there is no easily definable pattern. There is an outcome that could not be predicted or proactively mitigated. Disease is infinitely variable, and it is inevitable that some cases will have poor outcomes even in the best of hands. However, in approximately 95% of cases, there is a clear failure in either medical decision-making or system logic. Such failures (**Box 110.1**) can be and should be avoided by proper communication and advance action.

Change of Shift

The transition of care between providers at shift change is fraught with risk for both providers and patients. A casual passing of the baton from one physician, advanced practice provider, or group of nurses to the next can allow the critical details to "fall between the cracks." The oncoming clinician often anchors (assumes as a correct foundation for further management) on the off-going physician's impression and diagnosis. Also, the perhaps weary off-going clinician may not be immune to the perils of end-of-shift cognitive decline. Thus, risk increases.

Pearl: Change of shift is the dangerous time in the department.

Change of shift should not result in a lower standard of care. If, for any reason, the clinician cannot properly complete the workup of a patient and care must be transferred to another physician, a proper and orderly transfer of responsibility must take place. It is important that the transition notes describing the patient's condition include the fact that care has been transferred to another specific clinician at a specific time. Similarly, the oncoming clinician should acknowledge the condition of the patient and the program that will be followed. The clinician assuming care also assumes responsibility for the appropriate disposition.

In addition, nurses who are going off shift or leaving for break should ensure that the patient's care has been properly transferred to another nurse who will ensure that the appropriate course will be followed. The transfer of responsibility at the change of shift should be a formal and orderly process involving the patient as well as the health-care

BOX 110.1 ■ HIGH-RISK SITUATIONS

- Change of shift
- Return visits and transfers
- Private patients in the ED
- On-call physicians
- Against medical advice
- Left prior to medical screening examination
- In-house emergencies
- House staff in the ED
- Telephone orders from primary care providers
- Telephone advice

personnel. The patient and family should never have any doubt as to who is in charge of the patient's care and disposition.

Pearl: The patients must continuously know who is responsible for their care.

Return Visits and Transfers

Patients who return to the ED with repeat visits are often viewed as a medical annoyance. In truth, however, these cases are precious opportunities to reduce risk. Studies that have analyzed return visits have found that most patients were poorly instructed, the disease process had taken an unexpected turn, or the initial diagnosis was wrong.[2,3] This is potentiated by the fact that follow-up is almost universally an important part of the ED visit. Yet obtaining timely follow-up care can be extremely difficult (if not impossible) for many patients. The inability to access the primary and clinic-based specialty health-care system is a legitimate reason to return to the ED.

Patients transferred from other institutions have a similar risk of diagnosis anchoring that can represent a true impediment to good outcomes. Clinicians often rely too heavily on the initial workup and diagnosis, resulting in substantive delays and errors.

Pearl: Return visit and transferred patients have the most dangerous condition of all: a diagnosis.

Experienced emergency personnel realize that these patients must be viewed as entirely new. It is proper for a provider to refer to previous histories and physical examinations and to be aware of prior diagnoses, yet it is also critical that an independent history and physical forms the basis of the current clinical impression and plan. It may also be important for radiologists to review studies despite a prior (and possibly incorrect) interpretation from a prior encounter.

A rule that more and more emergency physicians are beginning to follow is that when a patient appears for the third time, admission should be strongly considered. It is troublesome when a patient comes repeatedly to an ED; these patients may have ongoing medical problems that are unclear. Repeat visits indicate:

- The correct diagnosis has not been recognized—and the appropriate treatment has not been initiated.
- The patient does not understand the nature of the illness and the course of the disease.
- Discharge and follow-up instructions were ineffective.

"Private" Patients in the ED

An important concept in both philosophy and law is that doctors do not "own" patients. Rather, the opposite is true: patients own doctors. Doctors, and indeed the entire clinical team, are the retained agents and servants of their patients, who can change health-care institutions and physicians whenever they so choose.

Emergency physicians have an absolute obligation to understand the status of their patients. Nurses have a similar duty to evaluate patients expeditiously, including those who are waiting to be seen. The Emergency Medical Treatment and Active Labor Act (EMTALA) clearly states that each patient who presents must be evaluated to determine if an emergency medical condition exists. There is no exception in the law for a patient whose "own doctor" is en route to provide care.

The hospital must clearly convey to the medical staff at all levels that every ED patient will be evaluated and, if necessary, treated before the arrival of private physicians. The private attending physician has no right to jeopardize the care provided because of ego issues. After the appropriate triage, medical screening examination, and necessary stabilizing treatment has been provided, care may be formally transferred to a private physician when he or she arrives.

> **Pearl:** No one is a private patient in the ED until their private physician is present and has taken charge.

If the hospital, for the sake of convenience or political purposes, wishes to provide an area where private attending physicians may meet their patients for nonemergent conditions, that area should be away from any part of the hospital governed by EMTALA.

On-Call Physicians

The Joint Commission has classified EDs into four levels of care: Levels I and II are required to have on-call lists for the broadest range of physician specialists. The hospital and by extension the medical staff have a direct obligation to care for patients who have come to the ED. On-call physicians play an essential role in the functioning of this system. When such physicians do not respond to calls to the ED or refuse to carry out follow-up care for ED patients, EMTALA violations may exist (see Chapter 104).

EMTALA (colloquially deemed the "anti-dumping law") was drafted in response to economically motivated shunting of patients. It is an attempt to channel hospital and medical staff resources to provide the greatest protection for the patients within the system confines. If such systems cannot be organized in a cooperative venture between the hospital and the governmental administration, there is no question that further federal action will move to secure such benefits for the denizens of the United States. Several key points of the on-call panel are described in **Box 110.2**.

Since the statute's inception, the reach of EMTALA has continued to expand. The Centers for Medicare and Medicaid Services has issued official guidance that the EMTALA mandate extends to hospital-affiliated urgent care providers, regardless of proximity to that hospital's dedicated ED.[4,5] Additionally, EMTALA penalties have been settled on behalf of psychiatric patients boarded in the ED and transferred to a state-run institution rather than being admitted in the hospital's own inpatient psychiatric unit.[6,7] Thus, a working knowledge of EMTALA and its application within the health-care system is an integral part of risk reduction.

BOX 110.2 ■ ON-CALL PANELS: CRITICAL POINTS

- The on-call list is the responsibility of the hospital, not the ED. It is incumbent on hospital administrations to secure the services of physicians and to ensure proper entry of patients into the health-care system.
- Care delayed is care denied. When on-call physicians are not available within a reasonable period of time and patients suffer harm secondary to such lack of care, the on-call provider, institution, and the system are culpable.
- The practice of consultant physicians screening potential patients by inquiring about their financial status or ability to pay is legally prohibited under EMTALA.
- Continuity of care and outpatient follow-up for emergency patients are paramount. In addition to seeing patients in the ED upon request, members of the on-call panel must accept patients for outpatient management of care for the acute illness for which they are referred.

Against Medical Advice

Patients who decline to follow carefully considered medical advice are at risk. These patients have essentially indicated that they either do not trust or do not prioritize the professional judgment of the emergency personnel providing it. Against medical advice (AMA) situations illustrate two divergent legal concepts: patient autonomy and the physician's duty to protect (see Chapter 105).

The patient's right to self-determination is well established. An adult of sound mind has the right to refuse any medical care. Conflicts may arise with communication and informed decision-making if the patient does not understand what is presented by the clinician and therefore does not make an informed decision. Thus, it is essential that providers understand the major pitfalls (**Box 110.3**).

The first duty of the emergency provider is to properly document the mental capacity of the patient who refuses care. A patient who is encephalopathic lacks capacity; therefore, the substitute judgment of the health-care professional may be appropriate. If, however, the patient is awake and alert, can carry on a reasonable conversation, and has the mental ability to act in his or her own self-interest, the criteria for competency are usually met.

Second, in informed refusal cases, it is often claimed that hospital personnel did not inform the patient in a manner that could be understood. It is important to inform and document that the patient was told in no uncertain terms of the recommendation of the health-care professionals and the fact that such discussion was held in terms that the patient could easily understand. Euphemisms should not be used. If the medical staff is afraid of sudden death, the term "death" should be used. If the clinician is afraid that injury to a limb might result in amputation, use of terms that clearly indicate that the limb may need to be removed should be used and recorded on the chart.

Third, patients must be properly informed if there are alternative modes of treatment that would solve the problem, and they should be given opportunities to use these therapies if they are available. When no alternatives exist, this fact should also be documented.

Fourth, family involvement is crucial. If a patient dies and a malpractice lawsuit results, that suit will be initiated by the patient's family. Whenever possible and allowed by the patient, family or friends who are with the patient must be made aware of the provider's recommendations and the patient's refusal. The hard-driving executive who may wish to deny his own chest pain is usually brought into more realistic thinking when he must deny care in front of his wife and children. Should the patient expressly forbid the medical staff from speaking to family or friends, this must also be carefully documented. It is perfectly reasonable to inform the family that you have been denied the option to speak to them by the patient. This allows the family to understand that the patient, not the physician, is refusing to discuss the problems.

Last, and least important, is the patient's signature. The signature line on the chart is no replacement for a properly documented record. Many times, patients who leave AMA do so in a hostile atmosphere and refuse to sign. The fact that the patient refused to sign

---

BOX 110.3 ■ KEY POINTS IN AMA

- Age
- Capacity
- Giving the patient a diagnosis
- Alternatives
- Involvement of family

the document should also be noted. The myth has long been advanced that as long as a signature is present, the patient has waived his or her rights and has relieved the health-care personnel of legal responsibility. This interpretation is not correct. Documentation of AMA requires the previously listed four parts of the process. A signature is not a substitute for a legal process, and proper documentation is crucial if these situations are to be adjudicated in favor of the health-care team (see Chapter 105).

The attitude with which a physician approaches a patient in an "AMA" situation is critical to success. A "take it or leave it" attitude combined with ultimatums frequently results in noncompliance on the part of the patient. Such situations should not be confrontational. AMA cases should be rare. If a physician has an AMA each shift, something is wrong.

Left Prior to Medical Screening Examination

The patient who leaves without being seen or prior to medical screening examination (LPMSE) constitutes a much different medicolegal problem than the patient who leaves AMA. Patients who leave AMA often represent a doctor–patient communication problem. In the LPMSE situation, the doctor was not even given the opportunity to form a doctor–patient bond. Large numbers of patients who LPMSE are due to system problems and usually represent prolonged waiting times. Patient dissatisfaction, a cause of malpractice lawsuits, is known to increase with excessive waits.[8-11]

Hostility is the basis of miscommunication and lawsuits. Substantial or rising LPMSEs should prompt a system's review to determine exactly why the patient flow is less than adequate. Long waits for lab tests and x-rays, difficulty in freeing beds because of inadequate or poor admission procedures, or delays in obtaining needed consultations should all be reviewed to determine why patient flow is inadequate to meet demands. In these situations, documentation is still critical. Obviously, a provider who did not have the opportunity to evaluate a patient cannot create meaningful notes, so this task will fall to the ED staff person who, in the context of his or her clinical role, did see the patient during the truncated ED stay.

> ***Pearl:*** *The last health-care professional to see the patient writes the notes.*

It is a common misconception that if a patient leaves at any point prior to the conclusion of treatment, and particularly before a screening examination is completed, then the provider is no longer responsible for managing the medical information received after the patient's departure. In fact, an important part of risk reduction is ensuring that the ED has a system in place to manage information for patients who do not complete their visits. This includes those patients who are not seen by a physician but have had per-protocol lab testing or other diagnostics initiated. Setting aside the EMTALA implications of care deemed denied to patients due to unreasonable wait times, the health-care system has an obligation to follow up on even per-protocol orders placed without the benefit of physician input. Further, the physician under whose name the orders are placed will certainly be a potential defendant in any legal matters arising from the associated encounter.

In-House Emergencies

The emergency physician is occasionally involved with patients who are doing poorly on the medical and surgical floors. These in-house emergencies vary from cardiopulmonary arrest situations to assessing patients who have fallen out of bed to pronouncing patients dead. All such situations, however, have the potential for liability. When emergency physicians are called out of the ED, they are no longer able to provide immediate care to those who come through the ED doors. This absence may spell disaster. Therefore, leaving the ED should be an infrequent event and one that is prompted by true medical necessity. It is wise for the emergency physician to never contractually guarantee to answer in-house emergencies. The physician is by such action guaranteeing to be in two places at once.

Pearl: Never agree to be in two places at the same time.

It is advisable for the emergency physician to agree to respond to in-house emergencies, as would any other physician in the hospital. Part of the test of a Good Samaritan action is that it is performed outside the usual practice setting of the physician and that the physician has no established duty to provide such services. A contractual link might invalidate a physician's eventual Good Samaritan defense. It is also wise for the emergency physician not to be paid per patient for responding in such events. Direct payment for medical services on a prearranged basis will also invalidate a Good Samaritan defense. Some states may not recognize the Good Samaritan defense if the patient is already in a hospital. In those states, the emergency physicians may bill for the services provided without concern for changing their Good Samaritan status.

It is not the role of emergency physicians to solve all problems of the hospital merely because they are available 24 hours per day. Should a patient become ill on the floor, hospital rules and regulations should clearly delineate the responsibilities of the primary attending physician. If indeed the primary physician cannot attend to the patient for some reason, such patients can be brought to the ED, where the emergency physician has proper facilities and equipment and is not forced to leave the site of primary obligation.

House Staff in the ED

House staff working in the ED are often trained under two erroneous concepts:

- Young doctors learn from their mistakes.
- If young doctors are not ready now to see patients on their own, how can they be "graduated" from the program?

The premise of learning by mistakes is unsound educationally and morally. No one wants pilots to learn by their mistakes as they land their 747 without supervision. Educational theory would dictate that the only thing learned from mistakes is how to make mistakes. The great advantage of emergency medicine is that each patient can be supervised in an online, real-time manner by an attending physician who can help the resident work through the decision process and intervene when the situation requires. No hospital gives a "training discount" reduction to patients because they have been seen by a resident in an unsupervised manner. The resident is a physician in training. Overall responsibility for every patient in the ED is borne by the attending physician. It is a cowardly—and legally unsound—act for an attending physician to blame the outcome of a case on the resident. Residents should be concurrently monitored and actively supervised by an attending physician while in the department.

Pearl: Residents are just doctors in training.

A resident rotating through the ED from a specialty other than emergency medicine should be supervised in the same manner as an emergency medicine resident but considered to be less familiar with ED policies and procedures. Retrospective review of charts, although useful as a teaching tool, is no substitute for hands-on evaluation of patients. Billing for residents' services that are not directly supervised by the physician doing the billing should be considered an extremely high-risk activity. The attestation statements signed by physicians who sign up with various insurance companies generally state that they will charge for only those services that they personally render or directly supervise. The federal government and many states actively pursue physicians under a doctrine of fraud when they have rendered bills for services in which they have not been *directly* involved.

Residents frequently feel that because their malpractice coverage is paid for by the institution and they are covered under a doctrine of respondent superior, they are immune from the ravages of lawsuits. This misapprehension should be corrected; residents certainly may be (and are often) sued and are not exempt from being reported to the National Practitioner Data Bank.

A challenging and often volatile situation involves off-service residents who are called down from the floor to evaluate patients in the ED. These physicians are still residents and are responsible to the physician in charge. It is often said by attending physicians on medicine and surgery services that their residents can function without reference to the emergency physicians and that they are essentially functioning "as their agents." Such physicians are rarely willing, however, to sign statements that they will assume all responsibility, pay all costs, and have all reported losses against their name in the National Practitioner Data Bank.

The emergency physician bears the liability of all patients in the department until they have been properly transferred to another attending physician. The resident, no matter how advanced or from what service, cannot relieve physicians of their responsibility to act in the best interests of the patient. Disputes regarding how a patient should be dispositioned should be resolved by the emergency physician and the physician in charge of that resident. All dispute resolutions should be between parties of equal power who will bear equal responsibility. If an emergency physician believes a patient should not be discharged, that patient does not leave the ED regardless of the off-service resident's decision.

Telephone Orders From Private Physicians

Outside physicians frequently do not appreciate the extent of liability that the hospital and emergency physicians may incur when a patient is treated without being examined by the emergency physician. Physicians may see patients in their office and wish for them to have a medication or treatment that is not conveniently available in their outpatient setting. As a result, such patients may be sent to EDs with telephone orders given to emergency personnel. This practice should be discouraged and eliminated whenever possible. There is no section of the hospital as tightly regulated by federal law as the ED. There is no exemption in the EMTALA statutes for patients being sent from outside physicians' offices. Although this practice still occurs, it is anachronistic and dangerous. Federal law requires that every patient who enters the ED requesting examination or treatment for a medical condition receives a medical screening examination. Nowhere does it indicate that patients may be treated without such an evaluation.

Pearl: *The telephone is your enemy.*

Should the hospital wish to run an outpatient clinic for the convenience of its own physicians, such a clinic should be set up separately from the ED and strict criteria should be laid out as to what can and cannot be done without concomitant physician evaluation.

Similar situations exist with regard to requests by medical staff, particularly screeners and gatekeepers from health maintenance organizations (HMOs), for the emergency physician to "just take a quick look" at a patient. Medicolegally, there is no such thing. When the emergency physician has agreed to see anyone to determine whether an emergency exists, a doctor–patient relationship is established. Such a visit must be memorialized with a chart. There is no exemption in EMTALA declaring that if a patient is being "looked at" for an HMO or a preferred provider organization, the usual duties incumbent on the emergency physician are waived.

Telephone Advice

Many health-care personnel are not aware that a doctor–patient relationship can be established with the telephone. A patient need not physically enter the ED for such a relationship to exist. As soon as the patient requests medical advice and the health-care professional is willing to give that advice, a doctor–patient relationship is established. The rule for the ED should be: We do not give telephone advice. Numerous studies have documented the poor quality of telephone advice, and common sense would dictate that with a patient not present, the most important clues to correct diagnosis and treatment are gone. It is both acceptable and advised that inquiring patients be politely and compassionately told that the ED is open 24 hours per day and will unhesitatingly evaluate them for an illness. No patient asks a casual question. People seek advice from EDs hoping to do something with that information.

> *Pearl:* ED telephone advice: do not give it.

In no circumstance should advice be given that does not directly state that the patient must be seen and evaluated before any type of medical diagnosis or specific treatment can be given. Telephone advice reiterates the adage that you get exactly what you pay for. Note that many health-care systems do operate a protocol-driven telephone-based nurse hotlines; this is different than ED nurses doing it "off the cuff" as discussed above.

PRACTICAL TIPS FOR MANAGING RISK

A practical approach based to risk reduction can dramatically reduce risk to the patient and clinicians. The clinician should be attentive to aspects of care that influence the interaction between the patient (and family) and the staff.

Perception Is the Only Reality

The patient's perception of the care received is influenced by each aspect of the process. The health-care institution that wishes to reduce risk should begin by sampling the product. Physical access into the system—parking, moving sick patients into the ED—should all be user-friendly. It should be considered the height of embarrassment for a family member to be struggling to get a sick patient out of a vehicle and hospital personnel unavailable to lend a hand. Such an introduction sets the tone for a relationship that is adversarial as opposed to therapeutic. Hospital EDs often convey an atmosphere of institutional mediocrity.

It is well-documented that patients are strongly influenced by how the health-care professionals appear. Clean uniforms with proper name tags and other markers of identification are essential. The usual rules of human interaction and polite social discourse often seem to be suspended in EDs. Physicians no longer shake hands with their patients and identify themselves. Some physicians ignore present family members instead of recognizing their presence and understanding their role in the process. It is the wise physician who makes friends with both the patient and the family.

The patient's first impression of the health-care provider is formed much like the impression of the institution itself. Patients of all socioeconomic ranks have an amazingly similar view of how physicians and nurses should be dressed. This so-called doctor camouflage is an important element in setting the tone for the doctor–patient interaction. Patients are willing to expose the most intimate details of their lives not because of who we are personally but because we represent a profession with a code of ethics and an oath of devotion to the patient's problems. It is mandatory that the patient believes in the provider. Any hint that information obtained would be used for purposes other than the advancement of the patient would certainly shut down communications.

Pearl: Attitude is felt, not stated.

Frustration Leads to Complaints

The two most prevalent complaints of patients who have been to an ED are that they waited too long and that the doctor "never told them anything." Both of these factors lead to frustration, which creates an atmosphere in which hostility can exist. It is appropriate for a physician and other members of the health-care team to apologize to a patient for any delay in being seen. Most clinicians would like to see every patient immediately. By recognizing that no one wants to wait and that the patient's time is just as valuable as the physician's, hostility can be reduced. Physician empathy forms patient perceptions more than any specific corrective action.

With regard to the second major complaint—"the doctor never told me anything"—the corrective actions are obvious. The moment of discharge for a patient is indeed the moment of truth. It is incumbent on the emergency physician and other health-care personnel to make certain that the patient understands the discharge instructions and the diagnosis. Practical matters, such as where the patient is to go, what the patient is to eat, where the patient can obtain medication, and whether the patient needs a note for work, are the real-life nuts and bolts issues with which the patient must deal when being discharged from the ED. Directly asking patients and their families how these everyday matters will be taken care of not only shows human concern but also allows the physician to proactively analyze the effectiveness of the prescribed therapy in the post-encounter therapeutic environment.

Discharge Is the Last Opportunity to Ensure Appropriate Care

Last, it is important for the physician to ask the patient if there are any other specific issues requiring assistance. All patients enter an ED with a specific program in mind. They have specific ideas of what will or will not be accomplished and set notions of desired outcomes. It is impossible to serve the wants and needs of patients without specifically asking what they would like. There is no better risk-management strategy than at the time of discharge to make sure that the patient and the family are comfortable with the diagnosis and the health-care program advocated and that they have the ability to carry out such a program in their daily lives.

Approximately 50% of lawsuits in emergency medicine are related in some way to either the discharge program or the inability to enter the patient into a coordinated health-care system. Virtually all cases of meningitis, missed fractures, abdominal pain, and wounds have to do with how patients are instructed and how they view their own role in the follow-up care.

Pearl: Discharge is the moment of truth.

Attitude Is Pervasive

The best weapon that any physician has in the risk-management war is attitude. The physicians who are secure and happy in their work tend to convey that attitude to the patients and the staff. Attitude, like anything of importance, begins at the top. Nurses and ancillary health-care personnel, as well as clerical personnel, often pick up their tone in the behavior from the physician on duty. Physicians who go out of their way to be kind to staff and patients often find such attitudes infectious. This attitude should be expressed not only to patients but to all members of the health-care team. Merely going through technical hoops and making certain that the process has taken place is no substitute for patient satisfaction, and the physician who can judge satisfaction separate from process will be well equipped to manage risk.

CONCLUSION

Risk is created—or avoided—one patient at a time. It is an intensely personal decision on the part of each patient and the patient's family to bring legal action against a health-care professional and a health-care organization. The simple fact that "they like you" can mean the difference between a lawsuit and a patient who is still your friend despite the outcome. Emergency medicine is, by its very nature, in the bad outcome business. Emergency departments are the place where families receive the news of their child's death, a family member's permanent paralysis, or other incurable lifetime disabilities. No patient is truly prepared for the news that emergency physicians bring.

The current maxim is that someone must be responsible. Should any evil befall a person or a family, someone must be to blame, and someone must pay. These factors, along with the general technologic isolation of modern medicine, have made it an ideal target for all failings. The corridors of the great health-care institutions—like our schools, our prisons, and our gigantic workplaces—have become sterile and devoid of perceptible caring. The degree to which clinicians can individualize and personalize health care will determine its ability to prophylactically manage risk. Demonstrating that ED providers are true advocates for the patient's well-being will go further than anything else to prevent the hostility and disappointment that frequently are dissipated through legal channels.

REFERENCES

1. Leape L. Why Do Errors Happen? How Can We Prevent Them? Harvard School of Public Health. Available at: http://www.ihi.org/education/IHIOpenSchool/resources/Pages/Activities/WhyDoErrorsHappen.aspx. Updated 2018. Accessed August 7, 2020.
2. Sheikh H, Brezar A, Dzwonek A, Yau L, Calder LA. Patient understanding of discharge instructions in the emergency department: do different patients need different approaches? *Int J Emerg Med.* 2018;11(1):5.
3. Boonyasai RT, Doggett D, Bayram JD, Connor C. Improving the Emergency Department Discharge Process: Environmental Scan Report. Agency for Healthcare Research and Quality. AHRQ Pub. No. 14(15)-0067-EF. 2014.
4. *Friedrich v S. County Hospital Healthcare,* C.A. No. 14-353 S (D.R.I. Nov. 1, 2016.
5. Emergency Department Legal Letter. 2018;29(5):49–52.
6. Bitterman RA. Feds declare emergency physicians incapable of performing the MSE on psychiatric patients. *ACEP Now.* 2017;36(10):20–21.
7. Bitterman RA. When is a psychiatric patient stable under federal law, EMTALA? *Bloomberg Law.* 2018. Available at: https://news.bloomberglaw.com/health-law-and-business/when-is-a-psychiatric-patient-stable-under-federal-law-emtala. Accessed March 8, 2020.
8. Sonis JD, Aaronson EL, Lee RY, et al. Emergency department patient experience: a systematic review of the literature. *J Patient Exp.* 2018;5(2):101–106.
9. Pitrou I, Lecourt A-C, Bailly L, et al. Waiting time and assessment of patient satisfaction in a large reference emergency department: a prospective cohort study, France. *Eur J Emerg Med.* 2009;16(4):177–182.
10. Bleustein C, Rothschild DB, Valen A, et al. Wait times, patient satisfaction scores, and the perception of care. *Am J Manag Care.* 2014;20(5):393–400.
11. Sayah A, Rogers L, Devarajan K, et al. Minimizing ED waiting times and improving patient flow and experience of care. *Emerg Med Int.* 2014;2014:981472.

CHAPTER 111

MEDICAL MALPRACTICE INSURANCE

William Montei, Ed Boudreau

Although the underlying principles of medical professional liability insurance remain constant, some adjustments have been made in response to changes in the emergency practice environment. Emergency care providers should be familiar with the most up-to-date types of insurance, deductibles, tail coverage, prior acts coverage, and the acronyms and abbreviations widely used in the insurance industry.

What happens when physicians receive a certified letter notifying them of a lawsuit naming them as defendant? How will they react? What will it do to them personally and professionally? How will their performance change? Emergency department (ED) leaders need a plan to address these issues before they happen.

GOOD NEWS vs BAD NEWS

The good news is that, when an untoward event occurs in the ED, it is usually known almost immediately. It is the nature of the practice. A physician attends to the patient for a very short period of time—a "relationship" that lasts from a few minutes to a few hours at most. As such, decision-making in the ED is compressed into a very small time frame.

The bad news is that untoward events can be very costly. Although the frequency of malpractice claims is not much higher in emergency medicine than in other specialties, the severity and cost of the claim can be substantially higher. The Physicians Insurers Association of America database for the years 1985 to 2007 shows the average medical liability indemnity payment for emergency medicine was just over $185,226 with a per-physician premium among the top 10 most expensive medical specialties.[1] According to a more recent study using closed claims data from the American Society for Health Care Risk Management and AON, the average indemnity payment climbed to $303,000 in the years 2013 to 2018.[2]

Because the period of potential exposure to a medical malpractice claim is so condensed, the time it takes for the patient to learn of any consequential damage is relatively short. As a result, the time to bring an action against the attending emergency physician can be considerably less than for those in other medical specialties. Information gathered earlier and with more certainty is easier for an insurance company to manage and price.

The Increasing Importance of Operational Efficiency

On the other hand, the risks for ED providers are becoming less about the medicine itself and more about the practice environment:

- Are admissions to the hospital handled quickly?
- Is the transfer of care from the ED to the hospital staff managed well?
- Do intradepartmental handoffs communicate all relevant information?

- Do the electronic medical record tracking system, computer physician order entry system, and picture archiving and communications system aid or hinder patient management?
- Is there access to specialists at all times and within reasonable time frames?
- Is the ratio of advanced practice providers to the number of emergency physicians reasonable?
- Are the responsibilities of all patient caregivers clear, and are staff supervised well?

These questions have little to do with medical decision-making. Rather, they are systemic risks that have more to do with ED operations and the relationship the physicians, nurses, and other staff have with the hospital than with their relationships with the patient. These potential pitfalls are a poignant microcosm of the health-care system in general, where poor funding, diminishing resources, and competing interests coalesce at the very moment of acute need by the patient.

These risks are real, significant, and evolving rapidly. Risks that do not have a long traceable history, especially those that are proliferating, are very difficult to measure and price. Poorly controlled forces within our health-care system are adding risks that will undoubtedly lead to significant increases in malpractice insurance premiums for emergency physicians.

Selecting the Right Insurance Carrier

Making the best decision on the purchase of malpractice insurance is not simple, and the willingness and ability of insurance companies to bear the risk of the ED is diminishing. Some physician groups take little time to understand the importance of the malpractice insurance; for many, cheaper is always better. Yet there are significant differences among carriers that should be known. These differences include coverage, claims handling, risk mitigation, and risk management. The ED leader must understand the endemic and growing risks within the medical profession and recognize the fickleness of the insurance market. It is not always a matter of cost; in some instances, it may come down to group survival.

THE INSURING CONTRACT (MALPRACTICE POLICY)

There are two dominant types of medical professional liability insurance: occurrence policies and claims-made policies. Both are defined by the "trigger" of when a claim is made (reported) and therefore whether it is covered or not.

Occurrence Policies

Occurrence policies provide coverage to a policyholder as long as the alleged malpractice event "occurred" during the active policy period, which is the time that the policy was in effect (premiums were being paid). As a result, if an event occurs during the active policy period but is reported after the active policy period—that is, when premiums are no longer being paid to the insurance company—an occurrence policy obligates the insurance company to provide "prior acts" coverage.

Claims-Made Policies

A claims-made policy provides coverage from the start date, referred to as the "retroactive date," through the continual renewals of the policy (as long as premiums are paid). However, the original insurance company will not cover a "prior acts" claim if the claim is made after the insured provider is no longer paying premiums (or switches to a new company). The notable exceptions to this coverage responsibility are:

- The subsequent insurance company adopts the original "retroactive date."
- A "tail," also known as "extended reporting period coverage," is purchased. In other words, if not covered by a subsequent insurer, the "claims-made" policyholder must purchase a "tail" to obtain insurance for events that occurred during the active policy period but are reported after the active policy period. Tail coverage effectively converts a claims-made policy to an occurrence policy. (See **Appendix 111.1** at the end of this chapter.)

A critical nuance of claims-made policies is that insurance companies do not all define a "claim" the same way. Some consider incident reports (the report of an incident that might lead to a claim) as a reported claim, some limit reported claims to a formal demand for damages by a plaintiff, and there are variations in between.

Avoiding Coverage Gaps

To avoid a gap in coverage, it is important to clarify how the current and potential new insurance companies interpret and address "claims" and "incidents." A physician leaving a claims-made carrier should strongly consider purchasing tail coverage. Optionally, the new carrier might agree to cover any claims that have not previously been reported (during the time the physician was covered by the previous carrier). It is critical to define what will and will not be covered because the new carrier may only cover those situations for which there is an incident report and deny coverage for any other claim. The physician could find him- or herself without coverage—or "in the gap."

In this instance, gaps in coverage occur when a claim is denied by both the previous and the current insurer because of the different language used by each to define a valid reported claim. When this "gap" occurs, the "character" of the new company will determine how difficult it will be to resolve the situation.

What Is Covered?

Most practitioners maintain a medical liability policy, and most demands for damages related to a medical event are covered; however, the definitions of "demand for damages" and "medical events" may differ significantly among insurance companies, and some incidents may not be covered. It is critical for the insured physician or group to become familiar with what is covered in the policy. The differences are real, and unfortunately, can be "economically tangible." These nuances can lead to another type of gap in coverage, that is, holes in the coverage language that the insurance company can use as an argument to deny coverage.

Generally, gaps in coverage are rare. Most insurance companies wish to maintain a positive reputation in the industry and try to eliminate coverage gaps. But when liability shifts from an individual's medical risk to system risk (that of multiple individuals or organizations), the stakes increase and language becomes critical. Courts, judges, and juries tend to give leeway to the plaintiff and keep the insurance company involved, but that should not be relied upon. The insured practitioner should ensure that the policy form is consistent with the industry standard. The character of an insurance company matters; however, a practitioner can only rely on the reputation of the company to a certain extent, so it may be a good idea to get an expert opinion.

Coverage exclusions are generally detailed in the policy. Typical exclusions are illegal and "immoral" activities, such as misrepresentations, alterations of records, sexual improprieties, criminal activities, and so on.

DEDUCTIBLES AND SELF-INSURED RETENTIONS: SAVINGS OR NO SAVINGS?

The desire to lower the cost of malpractice insurance has led groups to explore cost-saving measures such as deductibles and self-insured retentions (SIRs). While SIRs and deductibles are similar, there are important distinguishing features.

Deductibles

A deductible is a transaction directly between the insured and the insurance company. It creates an obligation for the insured (group) to pay a portion of a claim and sometimes a portion of the litigation expenses. Since the deductible is a transaction between the insured and the insurance company, the company is still obligated to pay the claim and all expenses up to the limits of coverage. Subsequently, the insurance company will seek recovery of the deductible from the insured.

For participation in the payment of the claim and its costs—the deductible—the insured receives a discount on the premium, a form of "savings." Yet most deductibles are within what is called the "working layer." The vast majority of claims result in payments that are significantly less than the limits of the policy coverage; in fact, for emergency medicine, most payments are less than $500,000. Unless a group has very few claims, it is easy to appreciate that paying the first portion of several claims could quickly overcome any savings in premiums. That savings would be even more quickly consumed if the deductible included litigation expenses. If a group or individual considers a deductible, it is important to reflect on the following points:

- Ensure that the deductible has an aggregate defining the most that a group is responsible for contributing during a policy year.[a] Compare the aggregate to the savings and judge the "risk tolerance" accordingly.
- Exercise care when considering inclusion of litigation expenses in the deductible. The litigation expenses are significant at times, and the philosophy of the insurance company regarding how hard it fights claims will have a bearing on what the insured must contribute.
- Remember that the insurance company controls the claim. An individual or group may be able to influence the insurance company (especially if the coverage includes a "consent to settle"), but it is still the insurance company's obligation to pay the claim.[b]

In short, be cautious about deductibles. Unless it is an exceptional group with few losses and an ideal environment, it is the opinion of the authors that the potential gain is significantly outweighed by the potential losses. Deductibles that work well are always between insurance companies and insureds who have a good sense of partnership. Character matters on both sides of the equation when deductibles are involved.

---

[a] Deductibles are paid per claim. If there are three claims, the insured pays the deductible on those three claims. An aggregate caps the total amount of deductibles paid, regardless of the number of underlying paid claims.

[b] A "consent to settle" clause in the insuring contract essentially states that a claim cannot be settled (paid) unless the insured agrees, or "consents." Physicians have little control over the litigation process, and even less in influencing settlement negotiation. A "consent to settle" clause in the insurance policy assures the physician that a claim cannot be paid unless he or she agrees.

Self-Insured Retentions

An SIR is a portion of a claim that is the sole responsibility of the insured. Whereas a deductible is part of the policy limit and paid by the insurance company, an SIR is paid by the insured directly to the claimant (plaintiff) and is separate from the policy limit.[c] An SIR demands substantial cooperation between the insured and the insurer, because the two entities are responsible for the claim payments.

Though it can vary, in general the insured is responsible for defending the claim. Finally, because the expense of an SIR is typically significantly higher than a deductible, the insurer's requirements for collateral or some other proof of financial responsibility are much more stringent. Since the insured's potential obligations from SIRs will accumulate over a period of years, a $250,000 SIR could result in a requirement for $1 million of collateral. Self-insured retentions are rare—most groups that use them are reasonably able to simply self-insure. Typically, SIRs are pursued by those groups large and sophisticated enough to have staff that can oversee a portfolio of claims. Self-insured retentions are not for the faint-hearted: they need a high level of internal expertise and a trustworthy partner for the loss exposures that occur above the SIR limit.

COVERAGE AND CLAIMS: THINGS TO LOOK FOR, THINGS TO THINK ABOUT

Several aspects of malpractice insurance should be carefully scrutinized by the insured. Lack of attention can lead to unanticipated costs.

Coverage Limits

The typical insurance policy has limits of $1 million/$3 million per physician.[d] There are jurisdictions where it may be wise to carry higher limits, such as $2 million/$6 million, and others where a smaller limit is preferable. Often, the coverage limit is dictated by a patients' compensation fund or a statutory mandate required to practice medicine in a state. When there is choice of coverage limits, the decision of how much insurance to purchase is fundamentally based on the risk tolerance of the insured.

The insurance company is only obligated to pay a claim up to the limits of the policy. If damages exceed these limits, the insured is responsible for the difference. It is rare for a plaintiff to pursue a physician for excess damages. Typically, the plaintiff attorney will target the limits of every defendant named in the suit: the hospital, physicians, and ancillary providers. The biggest awards for a case usually involve a hospital—the so-called "deep pocket." It simply is not in the attorney's best interest to pursue one of the defendants once the limits have been offered. It is the legitimate threat of pursuing an award in excess of the limits that brings the physician and their insurance company to the negotiating table.

The logic behind lower limits is to pay lower premiums and reduce the target for the plaintiff attorney. The argument goes, "If there is not much available by way of limits, there will be less incentive for the plaintiff to aggressively pursue amounts above those limits."

---

[c] Thus, if you purchase $1 million/$3 million coverage with a $500,000 SIR, the insured is responsible for the $500,000 SIR. The insurer is only responsible for the amount above the SIR.

The total settlement sought will simply be aggregated with the other providers' limits. The strategy worked in Florida, where the traditional $1 million/$3 million limits were universally accepted, until one company offered only $200,000 limits at a substantial savings of premiums. The hospitals soon bore the brunt of the liability, and now the typical physician coverage in Florida is $200,000/$600,000.

This strategy carries inherent risk because there are times when a jury renders a judgment that exceeds the policy's limits. Companies that are aggressive about defending physicians, especially when there is a compelling argument that there was no negligence, will have provisions in their "reinsurance" for such verdicts. When looking at a professional liability carrier, it is reasonable to ask if they carry that kind of reinsurance coverage.[d]

In the event of an excess verdict, in which the plaintiff threatens to pursue the policyholder, the policyholder can bring a "bad faith" action against the insurance company for not properly handling the claim. While rare, these actions are more likely to occur when the insurance company had an opportunity to settle the claim within policy limits.

Consent to Settle

The "consent to settle" clause, included in some professional liability policies, requires the insurer to seek the insured provider's "consent" prior to settling a claim. It may be important to consider inclusion of this clause for the physician who may strongly believe that the claim against him or her should be fully litigated. However, it is equally important to understand that if the provider refuses to settle (nonconsent), costs of settlement and defense costs beyond the settlement recommended by the insurer may become the responsibility of the insured provider.

Physicians and physician groups must work diligently to minimize their liabilities. Insurance companies underwrite very carefully, and claims, especially multiple paid claims, will impact both the group's premium and their insurability. Groups with poor claims history can be forced into residual insurance markets, called "high-risk" insurers, in which the cost of coverage may be prohibitively expensive.

Incident Reporting

It is wise to report any medical incident that has the likelihood of being brought forward by the patient as a claim. Insurance companies will not penalize groups for incident reports; at the very least, most insurers will create a file in case the incident does develop into a claim. Beyond that, many insurance companies recognize incidence reports as an opportunity for risk management review and education, which in turn help physicians reduce their exposure to lawsuits. Lowering an individual's risk profile is an absolute necessity, since every paid claim is reported to the National Practitioner Data Bank (NPDB), medical examining boards, hospital administrations, and other oversight bodies.[e]

---

[d] Reinsurance, which is essentially insurance for insurance companies, can be very complex. It is difficult to judge the quality of the reinsurance program. At best one can only judge the quality of the reinsurers themselves. If asking about the coverage for excess verdicts, it is called ECO/XPL coverage (extra contractual obligations/excess policy limits) in insurance parlance.

[e] The NPDB is a federally formed repository of medical malpractice paid claim information. It is available to hospitals and others who use the information to evaluate physicians. With regulatory oversight and the resulting penalties at an all-time high, the data is no longer overlooked by hospitals when granting hospital privileges.

USING BROKERS (AGENTS) vs GOING DIRECT

There are insurance companies that exclusively use brokers (agents), others that work directly with insured providers and their groups, and still others that contract with providers using both methodologies. There is no absolute answer to the question of which path to follow—it depends.

Eliminating a broker or agent from the transaction does not eliminate the entire cost of the brokerage fee from the premium. Brokers do perform certain valuable functions and, in the absence of the broker, the company must perform these functions at a cost. There is never a one-to-one recoupment of the brokerage fee.

The primary question of whether to use a broker or purchase directly from the company has more to do with the quality of service provided by the broker. It is important to ensure that the broker:

- Understands the professional liability market
    - Knows the pricing structure
    - Is aware of the pricing trends around the country
    - Has specific knowledge of the emergency medicine specialty
- Knows the particular risks of the ED specialty and is familiar with the risk programs of the carriers being represented and how they may apply to the group
- Knows the various policies and coverages, is capable of walking the insured through those nuances, and can demonstrate that there are no gaps in coverage
- Offers a full line of insurance products and services, applicable knowledge and expertise, and will meet face-to-face with the provider or group to fully describe the coverage
- Knows the insured/group, spends time listening and understanding the group's risk appetite, and works diligently to match the right insurance company and policies with the group

Single-line (malpractice only) brokers are of little value unless they also can competently bring the services listed above. All too often, malpractice-only brokers can sell only on price. They have limited knowledge of the market, based purely on what they can display in a spreadsheet rather than the wisdom of experience and advocacy. When selecting a broker, consider all of the following:

- Boutique brokerage firms are often more personal and helpful compared to larger firms. Larger firms may have access to more options but may pay less attention to smaller clients—and it is essential that the broker can (and does) pay attention to the insured client.
- The broker must offer specific knowledge of the professional liability market as well as a broader insurance expertise. He or she should provide multiple options with multiple companies.
- When working with a single-line broker, make sure the broker is listening and matching the client's needs with available options, rather than just presenting a single option. The cheapest policy is rarely the best fit.
- Make sure that the broker's firm has the wherewithal to serve the group's business as it evolves and grows. If the group will ultimately need more sophisticated insuring instruments or will eventually self-insure, it is important to select a broker who can provide the expertise needed through each stage.

Many professional liability insurance companies do not use brokers but market directly to the group. There are many well-run companies that have the right philosophy, first-class service, longstanding histories, and an excellent rapport with their insured clients. When working with one of these companies, it is important to:

- Be comfortable with the policy form. If advice is needed, most qualified brokers will work with the insured on a fee-for-service basis. Alternatively, the insured can find a coverage attorney.
- Know the company. There are a lot of factors that make an insurance company a good fit. *The size of the company does not necessarily matter.* Good management, strong advisors (such as actuaries, auditors, reinsurance brokers, and investment advisors), the right ownership, and consistently positive financial results are far better indicators of a successful relationship than the size of the company.

INSURANCE COMPANIES ARE DIFFERENT

Price should not be the dominant factor involved in a purchase decision for medical malpractice insurance. The character of an insurance company is a critically important factor. How hard will it fight a nonmeritous claim? How will it price risk over the long run? What will be the company's continued willingness to provide insurance loss? The company's philosophy and character are major distinguishing factors as they defend the reputation and livelihood of its insured providers.

Thus, in evaluating an insurance company, that company's focus must be balanced: they must be advocates for their insured as much as they are advocates for their owners. There are three factors that reveal how that balance is met: ownership and management, risk management, and claims litigation.

Ownership and Management

The manner in which a company is organized may affect its alignment with the interests of the insured.

Publicly Traded Companies

Particularly in a difficult and volatile market, the expectation of consistent profits may lead to decisions that run counter to the best interests of insured physicians.[f] Difficult markets tend to create more conservative pricing positions, and large risk-averse companies may underwrite fewer policies. Insurers that have more than one line of business may direct their attention away from medical malpractice to more profitable lines of business, leaving insured physicians with few options.

However, some publicly traded companies that are exclusively devoted to medical malpractice have created leadership and boards with substantial physician influence. These organizations may do more than others to support physicians, even in difficult markets.

Mutual Insurance Companies

Mutual insurance companies are technically owned by their policyholders, and physicians typically control their governance structure. Mutual insurance companies dominate the market; however, there are differences among them that should be understood. Larger companies that offer several types of insurance in multiple states may be less engaged with individual

---

[f] This will be true for subsidiary insurance companies of publicly traded holding companies as well, though they may, based on the nature of the holding company, have a greater appetite for risk over the long term. One must always remember, though, that they have the same profit objectives.

policyholders. Unless very well organized, the larger companies have the same potential as any large corporation to distance themselves from the clients they serve: the insured.

Risk Retention Groups

Risk retention groups (RRGs) are essentially confederacies of like-minded, same-specialty physicians who underwrite some or all of their own malpractice insurance. Their focus and energy are specialty-specific. Because RRGs are focused on the specialty, the board, philosophies, budget, pricing, and profit are directed to the benefit of the insured. Risk retention groups rely on capital contributions from their owners and do not typically have the reserves of larger insurance companies.

Success requires experienced management and strong financial partners (reinsurers, investment advisors, auditors, and so on). Risk retention groups are the strongest advocates for their insured owners, simply because the owners are the clients, and therefore, the owners become more involved than in most other insurance companies. Advantages include:

- Ability to file in one state but provide insurance in multiple states
- Control over litigation by members of the RRG
- Capacity to create consistent rates
- Fewer fees
- Like-minded leadership

When developing or joining an RRG, the insured group must fully understand the management team and its control. Risk retention groups have an attorney-in-fact (AIF) who is responsible for the company's management. The AIF may have an effective working relationship with the insured physicians, or alternatively, may be controlled by a separate organization with inherent conflicts of interest (maintaining profits of the separate organization). The relationship between the AIF and the RRG should be sound, clear, and reasonable. Prior to joining an RRG, it is important to ask about the relationship, look at the history, and consider possible conflicts of interest.

Risk Management

The approach to risk management (loss prevention) is the second critical factor in the evaluation of an insurance company. There are several types of risk management that may be offered, such as mandated and volunteer educational webinars and conferences, practice evaluations, and so on. Some companies will give a discount for taking courses focused on risk reduction.

Emergency medicine has become very complex and is associated with a growing risk that raises the potential for lawsuits, perhaps more than in other specialties. Clearly, an insurance company that has a firm grasp of the evolving risks in the ED will be in a much better position to manage a claim than one that does not. Insurance companies that have programs specific to emergency medicine and offer advice on provider, group, and system (institutional) risk are the most helpful to emergency physicians.

Claims Litigation

The final factor to be considered when evaluating an insurance company is its approach to claims. How much participation and control does the company grant the physician when considering a settlement or making expert witness or trial decisions? Some companies aggressively litigate most claims, while others aggressively seek resolution outside of litigation (settling every claim prior to trial whenever possible).

Savvy claims specialists will know when a claim has little chance for success prior to expensive discovery. It is inadvisable to pursue a claim to trial when it is quickly recognized as a weak case with a very high likelihood of a large loss. Generally, it is prudent to pursue claims that have significant potential for success and settle the ones that do not.[g]

CONCLUSION

Emergency medicine is unique among specialties. The inherent practice risks are evolving in ways that are distinct from those seen in other specialties. When purchasing malpractice insurance, the single most important goal should be to find an effective, involved partner who will help to both mitigate risk and manage the inevitable incidents and claims.

Where does price fall in the equation? It should be somewhere in the middle. List all the factors that are important and then determine an acceptable range of premium expense compared to the current or expected premium. Ensuring that a group has the best affordable malpractice insurance is a critical factor in a group's long-term success. It is necessary to do the proper homework, including discussing options with a broker or advisor, researching the company being considered, and of course, conferring with peers.

Most importantly, consider the purchase of malpractice insurance as an investment that can help preserve the group's reputation as well as reduce the potential for losses. The right malpractice insurance relationship can even protect and enhance the relationships with the group's hospital, but the bottom line is that it can help the group practice better medicine, which in the final analysis is the best protection of all.

APPENDIX 111.1: THE CLAIMS-MADE POLICY

The claims-made policy has been present in the medical malpractice industry since the early 1970s, when the cost of claims (severity) skyrocketed and insurance companies refused to write occurrence policies for physicians. The St. Paul Insurance Company is recognized as the major force behind the transition from occurrence coverage to claims-made coverage (**Box 111.1**). Most companies followed this lead, including the physician-owned companies that were formed during that period. Though claims-made policies are viewed as more favorable to the insurance company than to the physician, these policies have a number of features and characteristics that may actually cost less for the practitioner over the duration of the policy.

Many physicians misunderstand claims-made policies. It is important that the decision-making provider take the time to understand the mechanics of policies so that when terms like "nose coverage," "tail," and "step-rating" are bandied about, he or she is conversant. Further, when the policy moves into the second year, the increase in premium will not invoke surprise or anger.

The premium increase in a claims-made policy is one of its distinctions when compared to an occurrence policy. The pattern of year-by-year claims reporting is fairly stable

---

[g] To clarify this statement: this philosophy is directed to emergency medicine and relates specifically to medical incidents that do not have issues related to systemic risk and where there are gray areas of responsibility. Discovery is always necessary in those instances.

BOX 111.1 ■ OCCURRENCE vs CLAIMS-MADE COVERAGE

Occurrence policies cover claims based on when they occur. For a policy written from January 1, 2011 to January 1, 2012, a claim occurring in June 2011 but reported in 2014 would be covered. Occurrence policies, therefore, require the company to project the potential future liabilities and associated costs years before the actual costs are known.

Claims-made policies cover claims that are reported during the policy period only. Using the example above, a claim occurring in June 2011 and reported in 2014 would not be covered unless the insured provider still had that specific policy in force or the provider has purchased "tail coverage."

(**Figure 111.1**). The premiums are based on estimates of expected claims. Theoretically, over a five-year period, the "steps" of the claims-made premiums should equal an occurrence policy.

Figure 111.2 shows how years are actually charged. In the first year, very few claims will occur, and will be only for care during that year (in red). In the second year, more patients from the first year (34%) are likely to make a claim (in blue). Additionally, the second year adds another 26% of likely claims from new patients. This continues until the fifth year, when policy is mature. At this point, the premium has its "full complement of steps" from the current and previous years.

Tail Policies

"Tail policies" are extended reporting endorsements, which means that they essentially convert the policy into an occurrence policy. These policies are purchased when a group or physician wants to terminate their coverage but insure their future obligations. At the end of a policy year, there are still claims that may be made that have not been insured. This requires "tail" coverage. For example, at the end of the sixth year, insurance for the first and second year will have been fully purchased; however, for claims not yet submitted from the third year to the sixth year, insurance has to be purchased.

Figure 111.2 shows the general method of calculation of the tail policy premium to address the uninsured remainder, in this case 131 (74 + 40 + 19 + 8). Simply stated, this covers the unpaid increments for the years during which care was rendered, but premiums were not fully paid in advance. (Note: these numbers are theoretical and other factors influence the actual premiums charged, such as real actuarial trends, company operating expenses, and the insurer's "risk margin.")

FIGURE 111.1 ■ Year-by-Year Reporting Pattern of a Claim

Accident year	Report year 1 — 26%	Report year 2 — 34%	Report year 3 — 21%	Report year 4 — 11%	Report year 5 — 8%
1					
2					
3					
4					
5					
6					

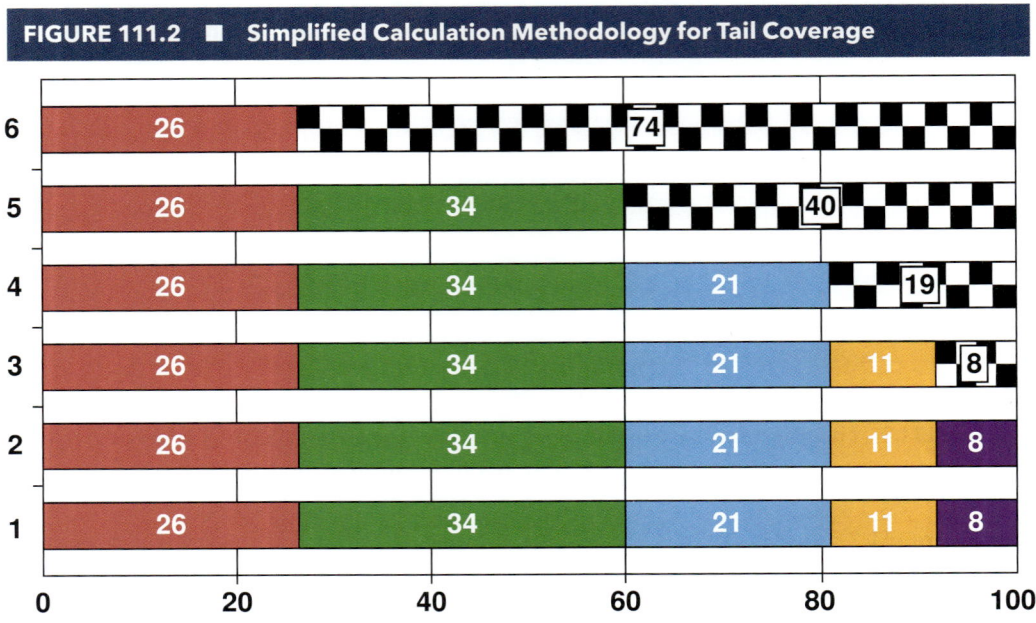

FIGURE 111.2 ■ Simplified Calculation Methodology for Tail Coverage

The risk margin is the amount that the insurer must keep in reserve to address the uncertainty of future claims. With time, the uncertainly decreases and the required reserve should also decrease, all else being equal. The case can be made that as a result, the actual premiums paid for a mature claims-made policy might be less than an occurrence policy. However, **Figure 111.2** shows that there is still considerable liability uncertainty and most insurance companies are conservative.

"Free Tail"

Most companies that offer claims-made policies will offer "death, disability, and retirement" coverage. If a physician dies, is disabled, or retires, the insurance company will issue an extended reporting endorsement without additional charge (the latter two under certain conditions). This feature is of great benefit to individual physicians, saving up to two times the mature premium or more. Of course, it is not really "free." The tail is paid by the premiums of the company's other insureds. Because it is spread across many insureds and is based on estimates of future events, the underlying cost is fairly nominal (2% to 6% of the premium), and most physicians would not be aware of this component within their premium.

APPENDIX 111.2: EMERGENCY MEDICINE BUSINESS TRENDS AND IMPACT ON INSURANCE

Large contract management groups continue to grow by merging with or acquiring emergency medicine practices of various size. Groups join for many reasons, including retirement of their founders, pressure from hospitals to improve performance, challenges in recruitment of new providers, increasingly complex billing and reimbursement processes, and increases in the cost of providing benefits to employees. In other cases, emergency physicians were forced by their hospitals to become hospital employees. The result of these market forces has led to substantially fewer independent emergency medicine practices.

Overall, the number of independent medical practices has declined dramatically, and as a result, physicians no longer require insurance from a multi- or single-line company.

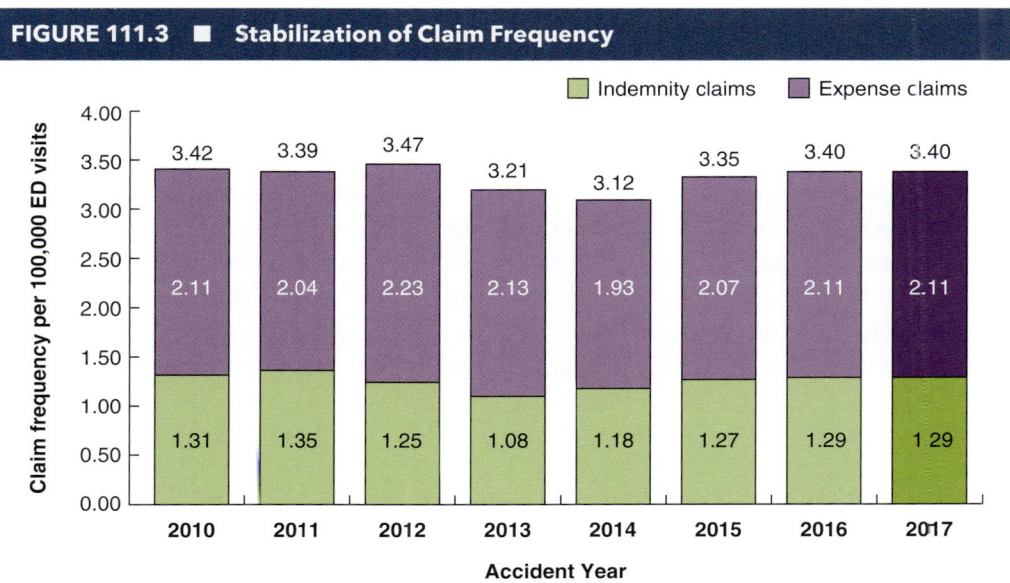

FIGURE 111.3 ■ Stabilization of Claim Frequency

Insurance companies and brokers have faced substantial pressure to maintain their own revenue in an increasingly smaller market. The impact on the overall insurance industry has been felt most acutely when the hospital or health system had their own self-insurance product. Simultaneously, the impact of tort reform has stabilized claim frequency (**Figure 111.3**), while the severity of claims has increased (**Figure 111.4**).

Because malpractice premium dollars are being taken out of circulation and trends for expense are reasonably controlled, the market has shifted dramatically.

Climate Change and Malpractice Insurance

To understand the concept of climate change and malpractice insurance requires an understanding of how insurance companies are structured. A malpractice liability insurance company may be a stand-alone company or may be a division of a much larger insurance entity. Larger companies with extensive financial resources and reserves can operate entirely with their own funds. Smaller companies may have to purchase "reinsurance" to spread the risk. Most reinsurance companies manage a portfolio of risk spread between

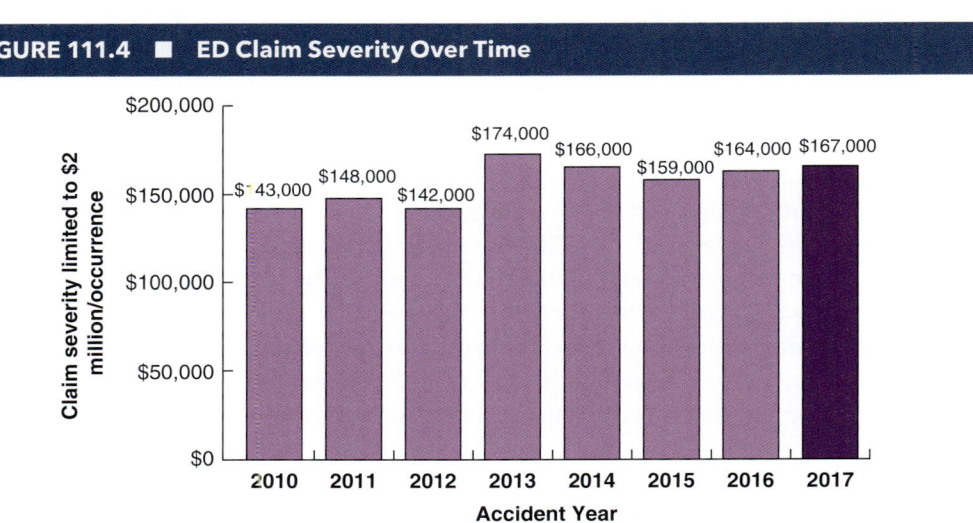

FIGURE 111.4 ■ ED Claim Severity Over Time

liability insurance and property/casualty insurance, and some of these companies have more money than a small country and are constantly assessing the world of risk and how to focus their investment in risk contracts.

Companies with broad insurance portfolios may have incurred extraordinary property loss in recent years due to worldwide hurricanes, earthquakes, and floods. Compared to those risks, professional liability insurance may be a relatively stable, predictable place to invest. Further, the market for liability insurance has decreased in size, creating a "soft market." While insurance companies hope for an ending of the soft market (increasing profits), many predict that the current market conditions are the new normal. For independent groups purchasing liability insurance, this means that the cost of purchasing malpractice insurance is relatively low. If purchased on price alone, a small effort can create great savings. When purchasing malpractice insurance, there are several critical questions that must be asked and answered.

Questions That Should Be Answered Before Selecting a Carrier

- *Is this a purchase with a long-term view of the business relationship?* If this purchase is viewed as a commodity and price is the major concern, the purchaser must be willing to live with the fluctuations in the market. Then, it may make sense to engage a broker to find the best price from a "credible" company. "Credible" is measured by a rating assigned by a rating agency, such as AM Best or Demotech. Insurance brokers are at risk for a bad recommendation and will tend to eliminate unrated companies and any form of self-insurance. The long-term relationship will be between the insured and the broker (and less so with the insurance company). This relationship works particularly well for groups with little energy for researching and directly contracting with insurance companies themselves. A cost-focused group may also use a broker when the group has good internal risk management processes, a good liability track record, and the belief that the malpractice risk is low.

- *Does the hospital require the group to obtain insurance from a carrier with a specific rating from a specific rating agency?* Some hospitals have very specific requirements for liability insurance, perhaps appearing in the medical staff bylaws or in the contract with the emergency medicine group. For example, a hospital may mandate that malpractice insurance is obtained from a company with an A rating or greater from the AM Best Company. It is essential that the group (and its broker) recognize any requirements prior to researching insurance companies and costs.

- *Should insurance be purchased from a publicly traded company, a mutual company, or an RRG?* This is less important when faced with current soft market conditions. Previously, emergency physicians were faced with multiple liability insurance companies refusing to write policies for them. In hard market conditions, when insurance carriers have a monopoly in a state, they have been known to dramatically increase their rates; in Ohio, for example, there was only one carrier who would write insurance for emergency physicians. That company increased its premiums between 50% and 75% every year for five years. Should difficult market conditions return, it might become quite important to determine which type of company is focused on the group's best interests.

- *Is the group large enough to self-insure?* This determination exceeds the scope of this chapter. As a rule of thumb, unless the group's annual premium is in excess of $1 million, the cost of setting up a self-insurance vehicle is likely to be prohibitive. If considering self-insurance, the group should get advice from an insurance professional and legal counsel. The types of insurance vehicles available for protection are only limited by one's imagination but should be done with eyes wide open and a full understanding of the implications.

- *What other things can the insurance company provide?*
  - □ *Risk management education*: Does the insurance company provide risk management education programs? What programs exist, and are any specifically dedicated to emergency medicine? Does the company provide CME with its mandatory education requirements? As risk management education becomes more important for licensure, will the company customize their education to help the group accomplish those objectives? As an example, many states have specific CME requirements in order for licensure which address opiate education and prescription. Some insurance companies, recognizing the potential risks involved, have developed CME specific to help policyholders meet those requirements. Does the company provide real-time consultation for policyholders with a perceived risk-prone circumstance for which they need advice? Will the company provide education on site?
  - □ *Dividends*: Does the company provide a dividend? How often have dividends been issued to policyholders (applies primarily to mutual companies or RRGs)? Are the dividends issued in cash or are they deducted from subsequent premiums?

What to Do When That Letter Arrives

Claims and potential claims come in a number of forms. Determine what the insurance company considers a claim. A letter from a patient requesting payment for funeral services because of failure to tell them about the nodule on the chest x-ray should be responded to with equivalent attention as a filed lawsuit.

The emergency group's management should have an established relationship with the claim's management staff of the insurance company (**Figure 111.5**). Some groups and insurance companies have a checklist for everyone in the practice to use when they receive notification of a claim (**Figure 111.6**). Remember that claim notifications may be sent to the hospital and routed through interdepartmental mail, the provider's home, or the practice office.

Your carrier very likely has a "first report of injury" form that must be completed when the provider or administrator of the department becomes aware of an adverse event that has potential to develop as a claim/suit. The typical response to notification of a new claim is tremendous curiosity and angst about what happened. Clinicians should resist the temptation to access the patient record until they coordinate with the claims manager. Metadata from an electronic record, including the time, date, and identity of anyone who has accessed the record, are routinely available to the plaintiff's attorneys. Further, the hospital

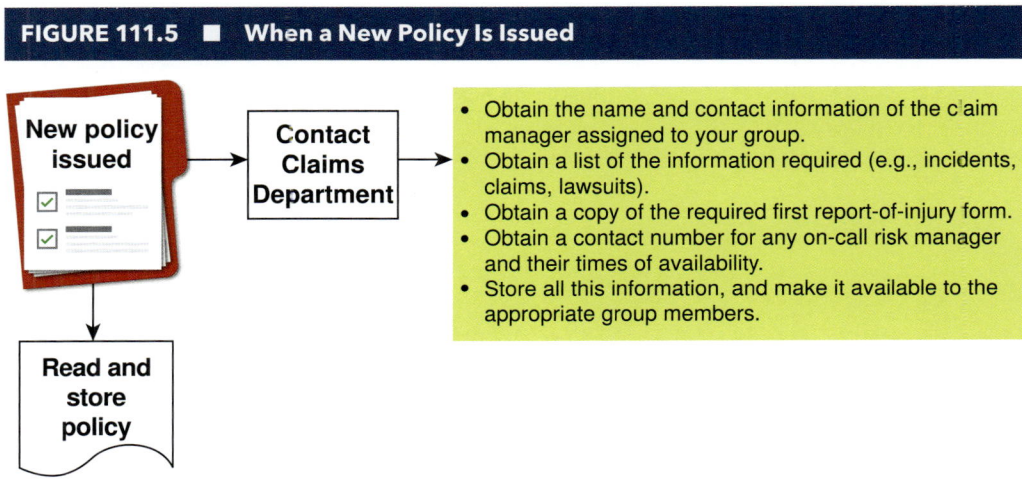

FIGURE 111.5 ■ When a New Policy Is Issued

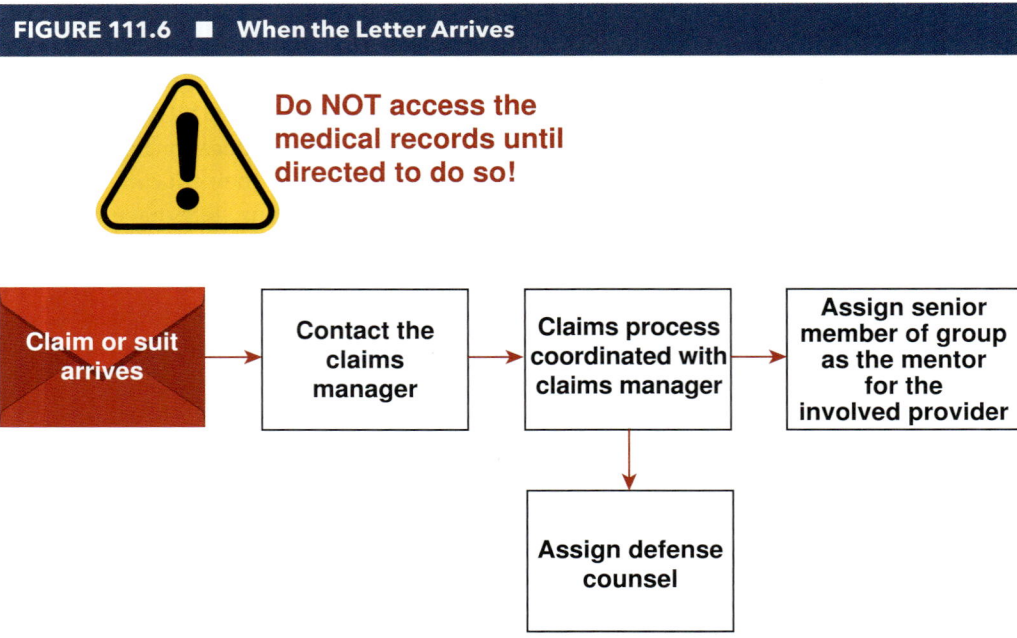

FIGURE 111.6 ■ When the Letter Arrives

risk management division should be notified. The clinician may wish to coordinate that notification with the insurance company's claims manager.

The provider should have someone to turn to for support. A senior member of the emergency group may be assigned as a mentor to the provider, a process that must be coordinated with the claims manager and the defense counsel.

Many defense attorneys and claims managers will provide substantial support. They will, however, have their limits. A member of the group will provide a degree of comfort that a noncolleague cannot. Since it would be very common to have the ED group corporation as a codefendant in the suit, having another member of the group attend depositions and provide support could make this experience less overwhelming.

Choosing an insurance carrier and contract is only the start of preparation. The remainder of preparation requires an established relationship with the claims manager of the company and knowing what is required when an event occurs.

REFERENCES

1. Brown TW, McCarthy ML, Kelen GD, et al. An epidemiologic study of closed emergency department malpractice claims in a national database of physician malpractice insurers. *Acad Emer Med.* 2010;17(5):553–560.
2. Aon, "Thought Leadership: 2019 AON/ASHRM Hospital and Professional Liability Benchmark Analysis." 2020. Available at: https://www.aon.com/risk-services/thought-leadership/2019-report-hospital-professional-liability-overview.jsp#:~:text=Now%20in%20its%2020th%20edition,compared%20to%20an%20industry%20benchmark. Accessed September 7, 2020

CHAPTER 112

MALPRACTICE: THE PERSONAL TOLL

Louise B. Andrew

Jane A. is a 35-year-old emergency physician who has practiced in the emergency department (ED) since completing her residency seven years ago. She loves medicine, especially the opportunity to help complete strangers in their time of greatest need, and prides herself on her attention to detail, conscientiousness, and meticulous documentation. She is generally regarded as one of the best physicians in the practice, both for her clinical acumen and empathic approach to patient care.

Jane is stunned when in the middle of a busy shift a process server accosts her with a medical malpractice claim in which she is named as defendant. Her concentration is broken, and she takes a break to review the claim. She does not remember the patient, whom she saw for a few minutes at the end of a shift before transferring care to an oncoming clinician. When Jane later obtains the medical records, she discovers that the physician who assumed care of the patient did not sign the chart. Neither that physician nor any of the other providers who were consulted during the disposition of the patient were named in the lawsuit.

Over the next four years, Jane defends herself admirably but is ultimately deemed negligent. Unfortunately, she did not handle her testimony well, and her lawyer could not prove to the jury that substantial decisions were made by other physicians involved in the case. Her health suffers, and she seriously contemplates the difficult decision to leave medicine.

Until recently, estimates regarding the frequency of malpractice claims against emergency physicians were sheer guesswork. Physicians have been reluctant to share their personal experiences with malpractice litigation due to fear of repercussions, including the loss of their professional reputation. Although liability insurers have had access to accurate figures, even statistics they were willing to share were flawed because of the failure to aggregate data and the difficulty in parsing out claims that actually resulted from emergency care.

CLAIM FREQUENCY

A comprehensive cross-specialty survey of 5,282 physicians by the American Medical Association revealed that 42% had been sued for malpractice at some time in their careers, with an average of 95 claims for every 100 physicians surveyed.[1] Variations in claims frequency among specialties were dramatic. Emergency physicians ranked fifth in claims frequency, with 109 claims per 100 physicians. Nearly 50% of respondents reported experiencing at least one claim, and 30.9% had been sued several times. In the year covered by the study (2007-2008), 8.7% of the emergency physicians surveyed had been sued, and more than 75% of emergency physicians older than 55 had experienced claims.

Aggregate outcomes data for emergency medicine malpractice claims from 1985 to 2007 were reported in a separate study done at Johns Hopkins using the Physician Insurers Association of America, whose members insure 60% of physicians nationwide.[2] The data revealed that 64% of claims closed without payment, 29% closed by way of settlement, and

7% tried to verdict, with 85% adjudicated in favor of the physician. Figures for emergency medicine were similar to those from other specialties. (In other words, the average indemnity payment for settled claims, adjusted for inflation, was $175,545; the average payment for adjudicated claims was $393,350.) Although this study found that overall claims as well as paid claims were trending down over the period studied, the average indemnity payment as well as expenses per claim had steadily increased. This study included cases generated from EDs and involved adult patients, but it could not isolate the lawsuits actually brought against emergency physicians.

Emergency Physician Claims

An unpublished all-member survey undertaken by the American College of Emergency Physicians (ACEP) in 2010 showed that most of the organization's members had been named in a malpractice claim at least once. Almost 10% of respondents had been named five or more times. The survey also suggested that more than 85% of these cases resulted in a defense verdict. Of all respondents, 60% had experienced litigation stress, although few had received any education in coping with it.

The specter of medical malpractice claims affects all US physicians and is a significant source of distress and anxiety for practitioners in specialties like emergency medicine, in which the frequency of claims is relatively high and the ability to mitigate adverse outcomes is relatively low. An idealistic physician with a limited understanding of litigation stress and poor access to available resources may be devastated by a malpractice claim.

The number of practitioners who choose to leave the ED or medicine altogether, who suffer posttraumatic stress, or who even choose death by suicide as a result of malpractice litigation will remain unknown unless and until more comprehensive data can be collected. It is almost a certainty, however, that productivity and job satisfaction are dramatically reduced in those who experience litigation—as well as in those who merely contemplate the probability.

THE CONSEQUENCES OF LITIGATION

Medical malpractice stress is a variant of litigation stress, which is experienced by many individuals who are involved in legal proceedings. However, physicians may suffer inordinately. Litigation stress is characterized by some degree of shock, dismay, or anger, especially early in the case; a sense of abandonment and aloneness; and often a sense of lost control. Psychiatric symptoms include hyperactivity or immobility, hypervigilance, restlessness, insomnia, exacerbations of feelings of paranoia and persecution, depression, and despondency.[3] Some degree of litigation stress is even experienced by plaintiffs.

Physician Predisposition to Malpractice Stress

American psychiatrist George Vaillant and others who have studied the psychology of physicians note that medical practitioners, more than other professionals, are significantly more likely than matched controls to have poor marriages, engage in drug or alcohol use, and undergo psychotherapy.[3] The choice of medicine, Vaillant concludes, may have been preordained in those who from an early age served as caretakers of an ill or incompetent parent. He postulates that those who had been deprived of a normal childhood may vicariously identify with their patients, giving them the nurturance they had once craved for themselves.

Furthermore, young and aspiring physicians are typically conscientious, compulsive (sometimes obsessively so), perfectionistic, eager to assume excessive responsibility, and inclined to deny their own needs. These personality characteristics are actively reinforced in the process of medical education. In the setting of litigation, however, these traits dramatically increase the vulnerability of physicians to stress. As a result, the typical litigation stress syndrome common to any defendant becomes compounded in physicians by feelings of guilt, shame, illness, apathy, and withdrawal.

More than other professionals, the self-esteem of physicians is tied to their occupation and successful clinical encounters.[3] Many physicians believe that their worth as a person depends on professional excellence and selfless dedication. This ideal of perfection and devotion to others may imbue physicians with a sense that they are invulnerable (protected from malpractice) based on all of the "good" that they accomplish. When this myth of invulnerability is shattered by a malpractice case, it can be a great insult to their self-image.[4]

Every step in the litigation process is perceived by the defendant physician as an attempt to prove intentional wrongdoing (by another professional with motivations far less noble). From the service of process, which may occur in full view of colleagues and patients in the midst of a busy workday, to the wording of the claim (rife with terms like "willful," "wanton," and "reckless") to discovery, deposition, settlement, and trial tactics, every step is intended to—and does—rub salt into the open wound.

Practice and Behavioral Changes

Charles and Frisch found that more than 95% of physicians undergoing litigation will experience some physical or emotional reaction.[6] Sued physicians may experience the onset or exacerbation of preexisting illnesses, especially gastrointestinal, cardiac, and emotional disorders. Even more than physical effects, sued physicians are likely to experience changed practice styles, altered professional and personal relationships, and changed life plans. Physicians may contract their practices in a variety of ways following a malpractice suit. They often become reluctant to care for plaintiffs or families of plaintiffs, manage high-risk patients, and expand into new and unfamiliar practice areas or use new techniques that may initially be associated with errors. Emergency physicians are less able to limit their practices following a malpractice case than other clinicians; as a result, they may cope less effectively.

Sued physicians often emotionally distance themselves from patients and develop more defensive practices, such as ordering more tests, consultations, and invasive procedures (either for reassurance or to detect complications earlier). They become more obsessive about their documentation, admit inpatients more liberally, and generally second-guess their decisions in an attempt to avoid further litigation. Ironically, these changed practice styles increase the distance between patient and physician and therefore increase the likelihood of subsequent claims. In fact, secondary claims are especially likely to occur in the period immediately following the notice of a first malpractice case.[5]

Personal and professional habits and relationships are also typically altered. Sued physicians pursue less recreation and indulge in more rumination about the case and how it might have been avoided. They often isolate themselves from potential sources of support, such as professional colleagues and family. They will participate less in important decisions being made in the practice.

Medicine is a hierarchical system in which decisions about training, credentialing, hiring, licensure, and liability coverage are often made subjectively and without clearly defined criteria. Sometimes even before the case has resolved, physicians who have been sued may find themselves scrutinized in minute detail by authorities, who may determine that the physician should be fired or have their license restricted. Sued physicians are also more likely to consider changing their practice setting or specialty.[1]

MITIGATING MALPRACTICE STRESS

Support for a physician undergoing litigation may not be readily available. Colleagues and associates may fail to offer empathy or understanding, especially if they have not personally experienced a claim. Other physicians, hospital administrators, and even practice partners may assume an adversarial stance, particularly if they fear that they may be implicated in the case. Furthermore, clinicians who have never been sued may harbor the mistaken belief that bad outcomes and malpractice suits only happen to physicians who make mistakes.[6]

Resources

Excellent resources are available for physicians undergoing the stress of malpractice. They include:

- Charles and Frisch's *Physician's Guide: Adverse Events, Stress and Litigation* provides tools for dealing with the emotional aspects of both adverse events and litigation.[5]
- Ilene Brenner's *How to Survive a Medical Malpractice Lawsuit* focuses on tactical approaches for defendant physicians.[6]
- Some liability carriers (e.g., The Doctors Company) make helpful information on litigation available to their insured.[7] Others (e.g., NorCal) make resources available to any physician.[8]
- The Sara Charles MD Physician Litigation Stress Resource Center offers valuable insights on its website (https://www.physicianlitigationstress.org).
- MD Mentor: This website (http://www.mdmentor.com) provides a variety of resources, including personalized litigation stress support for health professionals.
- ACEP (https://www.acep.org) offers information relevant to litigation stress, including a paper called "So, You Have Been Sued," a primer on malpractice litigation, and a peer support network.

Sharing Privileged Information

As an example, Charles, a practicing psychiatrist, strongly advocates for the critical importance of personal sharing by physicians after any adverse event, including litigation.[5] Conversely, risk managers and lawyers firmly discourage such sharing, citing the possibility that the disclosure of information may result in an advantage to the plaintiff or even significant prejudice to the case if any admission of fault becomes discoverable.

However, what is most beneficial to a physician undergoing litigation is not the sharing of facts, but rather the sharing of feelings engendered by a claim; such limited disclosure is not likely to entail legal risk. Nonetheless, discussions with a defendant's attorney, spouse, personal physician, counselor, or clergy are legally privileged and confidential and may allow for critical unburdening (including factual) without the risk of discovery by the plaintiff. Even in this setting, however, patient confidentiality must be maintained.

Additional Counsel and Healthy Pursuits

Some physicians seek personal advice and may consider hiring a coach or personal co-counsel when:

- The settlement amount under consideration may exceed policy limits.
- Negotiations by a third party with the insurer seem prudent to ensure that the assigned attorney is representing the physician's best interests.
- Defendant physicians seek to better understand the malpractice process or desire additional coaching to prepare for deposition and trial testimony.

Some liability carriers and medical societies or physician health plans make counseling available to defendant physicians. ACEP sponsors a counseling program that can help physicians facing litigation sort out available options.

A typical medical malpractice claim can last for years and psychologically retraumatize the defendant with each new litigation-related activity, such as additional claims, naming experts, depositions, settlement negotiations, and the trial itself. Sued physicians should be advised to make substantial efforts to pursue a healthy lifestyle, including attention to nutrition, exercise, and the pursuit of pleasurable activities, especially those involving family and friends. Active involvement in the case through partnering with the legal team, researching medical literature, and preparing for testimony must be balanced by healthy activities to prevent the case from becoming all-consuming.

Medical Director Support and Responsibilities

For emergency physicians, scheduling becomes particularly tricky because no one can be at their best in a deposition or courtroom after a series of night shifts. Department directors must be prepared to accommodate a defendant physician whenever possible and even exert pressure on others to make allowances. A director can help defendant physicians enormously by reassuring them that the mere existence of a malpractice claim does not necessarily reflect any shortcoming or error; rather, legal action is typically the result of a variety of factors, many of which are beyond the physician's control. Further, the director can assure the physician that many of their colleagues have successfully transcended malpractice claims. If the director has personally experienced malpractice litigation, this can be a very validating fact to share.

On the other hand, if a defendant physician acts in a maladaptive manner—that is, withdrawing, antagonizing staff or patients, obsessively second-guessing clinical decisions, interfering with good patient care, or exhibiting symptoms of physical or emotional illness or impairment—the director must intervene in a supportive yet firm manner to avoid harm. Such intervention can be career affirming and, in some cases, even lifesaving.

Pitfalls to avoid include ignoring the struggling practitioner or declining to discuss the issues due to concerns about embarrassing or singling out the physician. Not to address one of the most significantly painful events in a physician's life risks making them feel even more ostracized and alone in defending against a claim. Specific responsibilities of a medical director include ensuring that all practitioners:

- Are educated in risk and litigation stress management
- Familiarize themselves with their liability coverage and the terms of their liability contract
- Understand the resources available to help physicians deal with the adverse effects of litigation
- Have access to professional assistance when dealing with the predictable effects of litigation
- Acknowledge that malpractice litigation is not a personal indictment but rather a completely predictable hazard of current practice

CONCLUSION

Emergency physicians can anticipate being involved in malpractice litigation during a typical practice career. Physicians are on the whole uniquely susceptible to the adverse effects of litigation stress because of several psychological vulnerabilities, including a tendency toward perfectionism and an exaggerated sense of responsibility, which may be exacerbated by fragile self-esteem and poor self-care practices. Most of a typical physician's responses to litigation are maladaptive and may include physical or emotional illness.

There are a number of resources available to physicians experiencing litigation stress, including education, sharing of feelings in a legally protected environment, medical intervention, coaching, and personal counseling. Department leaders should be aware of these lifelines and share them with the physicians in their practices. Further, ED directors should vigilantly watch for signs of impairment or stress that adversely affect any clinician facing a malpractice claim.

REFERENCES

1. Editorial, Medical liability: Lawsuit chances take a toll. *AMNews*. September 6, 2010. Available at: https://amednews.com/article/20100906/opinion/309069955/4/ Kane CK. Medical Liability Claim Frequency: A 2007-2008 Snapshot of Physicians. AMA Center for Economics and Health Policy Research. 2010. Accessed September 9, 2020.

2. Brown TW, McCarthy ML, Kelen GD, Levy F. An epidemiologic study of closed emergency department malpractice claims in a national database of physician malpractice insurers. *Acad Emerg Med*. 2010;17(5):553–560.

3. Vaillant GE, Sobowale NC, McArthur C. Some psychological vulnerabilities of physicians. *N Engl J Med*. 1972;287(8):372–375.

4. Rafuse J. Physicians' fear of legal action becoming pervasive, lawyer tells Ottawa conference. *CMAJ*. 1995:152(4):573–575. Available at: https://www.ncbi.nlm.nih.gov/pmc/articles/PMC1337727/. Accessed September 9, 2020.

5. Charles SC, Frisch PR. *Physician's Guide: Adverse Events, Stress and Litigation*. Oxford: Oxford University Press; 2005.

6. Brenner IR. *How to Survive a Medical Malpractice Lawsuit: The Physician's Roadmap for Success*. London: BMJ Books; 2010.

7. Thee Doctors Company: Education and CME. 2020. Available at: https://www.thedoctors.com/patient-safety/education-and-cme/. Accessed September 19, 2020.

8. Andrew LB, Dearmin S. Adverse medical events, second victims and litigation stress. Professional Wellness Resource Center webinar. Norcal Group. Available at: https://www.norcal-group.com/wellness. Accessed January 12, 2020.

MEDICAL MALPRACTICE

William Sullivan

CHAPTER 113

The topic of medical malpractice evokes strong emotions from most physicians. There are often feelings of anger over being sued for what was perceived to be reasonable medical care. Fear may surface as physicians enter a process with which they are likely unfamiliar. Depression is also common due to the extended litigation process, the likelihood of a medical malpractice insurance premium increase, the perception of personal failure, and the social isolation that often accompanies medical malpractice lawsuits.

WHAT ARE THE CHANCES OF BEING SUED FOR MEDICAL MALPRACTICE?

Statistics vary on the extent and outcome of medical malpractice litigation in the United States. The National Practitioner Data Bank's Data Analysis Tool[1] shows that from 1991 to 2003, the total number of paid malpractice claims against physicians remained fairly stable, ranging between 14,110 and 16,117 paid claims per year. During that same time frame, the total amount paid in claims for US physicians nearly doubled from $2.3 billion to $4.35 billion.[2] When adjusted for inflation using 2018 dollars, the trend was less steep, increasing from $4.21 billion to $5.92 billion.[2] Since 2003, the number of reported claims against physicians has shown a steady downward trend. Between 2004 and 2018 (the most recent year of reporting), the number of medical malpractice payments made on behalf of physicians decreased from 14,517 payments in 2004 to 7,627 payments in 2018.[1] Similarly, the total amount of payments made on behalf of physician defendants steadily decreased from $4.42 billion in 2004 to $3.11 billion in 2018 (or from $5.83 billion to $3.11 billion in inflation-adjusted 2018 dollars).[2]

Data published by the Physician Insurers Association of America show that from 2006 to 2015, 18% of all claims originated from emergency department (ED) care, only 23.6% of claims for emergency medical care resulted in payment to a plaintiff, and that paid claims averaged approximately $336,000 per incident.[3] The largest indemnity payment for emergency medical care in this study was $2.0 million.[3] Among the 7% of total claims that proceeded to trial, 87.5% of cases were decided in favor of the physician.[4] While the odds of prevailing at trial are firmly in a physician's favor, the risk of an adverse judgment is significant. The average verdict in cases where a plaintiff wins at trial is $1.12 million, while the average settlement prior to trial is $341,000.[4] Considering that there are more than 135 million ED visits each year in the United States, the statistical odds of an emergency physician being involved in a malpractice lawsuit seem to be quite low.[5] However, each year roughly 7.6% of emergency physicians face a medical malpractice claim and each year approximately 1.5% of emergency physicians make some form of payment to a malpractice plaintiff.[6]

Even when physicians prevail in a medical malpractice lawsuit, the costs of defending medical malpractice claims are substantial. The average cost associated with defending a claim in 2015 was $78,906 for a settled claim, $191,341 when the defendant won at trial, and $262,141 when the plaintiff won at trial. Even when a malpractice claim was ultimately dropped, it cost an average of $30,475 to defend a physician's care.[4]

Subspecialties in Law

Just as with medicine, the field of law has multiple areas of concentration. Criminal law, tort law, family law, admiralty law, contract law, estates and trusts, tax law, patent law, and sports law are just a small sample of the multiple areas of legal concentration, each with its own pleading requirements and nuances. Contrasting two fields of law—criminal law and tort law—may help to illustrate the many potential differences in the requirements and liabilities involved.

Criminal Law

In criminal actions, the state brings charges against an individual for allegedly violating a law. The goal of a criminal action is to deter defendants from pursuing similar conduct in the future and to punish defendants for the crimes that they have committed. Punishment for criminal law may involve fines or even incarceration. Guilt of a criminal action must be proven beyond a reasonable doubt.

Tort Law

In contrast to criminal law, tort law pits one party against another party. The goal of a tort action is to reasonably compensate a plaintiff for damages caused by a defendant's negligence. In most cases, damages are monetary, although in some cases damages may involve a transfer of property or even punitive damages. Liability for a tort action generally must be proven "more likely than not" or by a "tipping of the scales."

Medical Negligence

Like medicine, areas in concentration in law can be subspecialized. Medical malpractice is a subspecialty of tort law based on a negligence theory. To win an allegation of negligence, a plaintiff must prove four elements: the defendant owed a duty to the plaintiff, the defendant breached a duty to the plaintiff, the plaintiff suffered damages, and the defendant's breach of duty caused the plaintiff's damages.

Although some medical malpractice cases are governed by federal rules, the vast majority of medical malpractice actions occur in state courts and are therefore governed by state law. The law applying to a medical malpractice action is important because each state has its own legal requirements regarding issues such as statutes of limitation, burden of proof on the plaintiff, expert witness qualifications, and malpractice awards.

NEGLIGENCE

Four conditions must be met before a person can be found legally negligent (**Box 113.1**):

- Duty
- Breach of duty
- Causation
- Damages

Case One: "I gave medical advice to someone who phoned the emergency department. Later, I heard that the patient was admitted at another hospital and died. Now our director received a subpoena wanting to know which doctor was working the night that the patient called. I can't be sued for giving someone informal medical advice over the telephone, can I?"

> **BOX 113.1 ■ REQUIRED COMPONENTS OF NEGLIGENCE**
>
> - **Duty of care:** Duty arises when there is a legal relationship between the parties creating an obligation to exercise the same reasonable care that another person in the same situation would exercise.
> - **Breach of duty:** One party by omission (doing nothing) or commission (doing something) does not perform the required standard of care consistent with the "duty."
> - **Causation (proximate cause):** The breach of duty directly caused or led to the plaintiff's loss or injury.
> - **Damages:** The harm, injury, or loss caused by the breach of duty.

Duty

Generally, the inquiry into whether medical malpractice occurred begins with a determination as to whether a physician had a duty to treat the patient. In most cases, a physician–patient relationship must be established before a physician can be held responsible for a patient's care.

A physician–patient relationship may be created in many ways. First, under Emergency Medical Treatment and Labor Act (EMTALA), a hospital is required to provide a medical screening examination to any patient who comes to the ED and requests medical evaluation.[7] While EMTALA does not impose upon physicians the duty to provide a medical screening examination as a prerequisite to providing services, hospitals often require that emergency physicians contractually agree to evaluate all patients seeking care in the ED. Once a physician evaluates a patient in the ED, a physician–patient relationship is created and a duty to the patient is established.

A physician–patient relationship may also be established by providing telephone advice to patients. For example, in *Cogswell v Chapman*, the New York Appellate Court held that "a doctor–patient relationship can be established by a telephone call . . . when such a call 'affirmatively advis[es] a prospective patient as to a course of treatment' and it is foreseeable that the patient would rely on the advice."[8] Providing medical advice over the telephone may also create multiple opportunities for errors. Those calling the ED for medical advice often do not identify themselves. No medical or medication history is readily available. Callers are unable to be examined. Providers rarely, if ever, document the recommendations over the telephone in a patient's chart. Should a patient suffer an adverse outcome based upon medical advice given over the telephone, it would be difficult to defend a malpractice claim based on undocumented advice given to an anonymous caller. For these reasons, hospitals often instruct callers seeking medical advice to contact their primary care physician or, if callers believe they are having an emergency, to come to the ED for evaluation.

Consider a patient who phones the ED seeking advice about what to do for "dark urine" after playing football outside with his child all day. Advice that the patient is probably dehydrated and should drink more fluids may seem reasonable, until the patient is admitted several days later for renal failure due to rhabdomyolysis.

A physician–patient relationship may be established by providing informal medical advice to nonpatients, depending upon what advice was given and what reliance the patient would have placed on the advice.[9,10] Physician–patient relationships may also be created when specialists make medical recommendations regarding patient care to emergency physicians over the telephone (such as when on-call for the hospital ED) or by contractual agreements between physicians and hospitals or insurance plans.[11-14]

Physicians generally do not have a duty to nonpatients. Exceptions may occur in some states where legal precedent requires a physician to warn nonpatients of a specific danger. For example, in *Tarasoff v Regents of University of California*, the California Supreme Court held that "once a [medical professional determines or] reasonably should have determined that a patient poses a serious danger of violence to others, he bears a duty to exercise reasonable care to protect the foreseeable victim of that danger."[15] Conversely, in *Tedrick v Community Resource Center Inc.*, the Illinois Supreme Court affirmed prior holdings that "the duty of care owed by a health-care professional runs only to the patient and not to third parties."[16] Ascertaining whether a specific duty to third parties exists in a given state will help practitioners determine the potential scope of duties to patients and third parties.

Breach of Duty

To prove medical malpractice once a duty to a patient has been established, a plaintiff must prove that the physician breached that duty. In legal terminology, the patient must prove that the physician failed to act in accordance with the standard of care. While the specific definition of the standard of care varies among states, those definitions all focus upon a "reasonable person" standard.

Standard of Care

In general, "standard of care" is defined as exercising the skill, care, and knowledge that a reasonably well-qualified practitioner *in the same specialty* would apply under the same or similar circumstances. Note that the standard of care does not require perfect or even high-quality care. Failing to meet the standard of care is equivalent to negligence, which is a failure to act *reasonably*.

Tort reform in some states has raised the standard of proof that a plaintiff must meet before a breach of duty can be proven. For example, Georgia law requires patients who file a medical malpractice claim arising out of care in the ED to prove by "clear and convincing evidence" that a medical provider's actions "showed gross negligence."[17] In other words, instead of proving only that a provider did not act "reasonably," a medical malpractice plaintiff in Georgia must prove that the provider failed to "exercise even a slight degree of care," which is the current legal definition of gross negligence in Georgia.[18] Georgia's heightened pleading requirements have withstood legal challenges all the way to the Georgia Supreme Court.[18]

Also note that the standard of care is very situation-specific. For example, most emergency physicians would likely assert that the standard of care requires aspirin be given to all patients suffering from an acute ST-segment elevation myocardial infarction. However, whether the standard of care was actually met in such a situation may depend upon multiple other factors, such as a patient's allergy to aspirin, the symptoms the patient has with the allergy, or whether the patient took aspirin before calling the ambulance.

Expert Witnesses Define Standard

In a medical malpractice trial, the standard of care is most commonly defined by an expert witness. Expert witnesses help a jury understand topics, facts, and terminology beyond the comprehension of an average layperson. Using the example of a heart attack, an expert witness may describe how myocardial infarctions occur, the risk factors for heart attacks, the symptoms of a heart attack, how a heart attack should be diagnosed or ruled out, how heart attacks should be treated, whether certain actions were likely to make the heart attack worse, and the prognosis or long-term consequences from treated or untreated heart attacks.

> **BOX 113.2 ■ EXPERT WITNESS GUIDELINES FOR THE SPECIALTY OF EMERGENCY MEDICINE**
>
> - Be currently licensed in the United States
> - Be board certified in emergency medicine
> - Be actively engaged in clinical practice of emergency medicine for 3 years immediately preceding the date of the event giving rise to the case
> - Possess current experience and ongoing knowledge in the area in which he or she is asked to testify
> - Avoid providing medical testimony that is false, misleading, or without medical foundation
> - Provide a thorough review of pertinent medical records and contemporaneous literature concerning the case being examined
> - Be willing to submit the transcripts of depositions and testimony to peer review

Within the scope of an expert's testimony is whether or not a medical practitioner breached a duty to a patient. The expert can be used to establish a physician's duty to a patient and can also be used to show how a physician breached that duty. For example, an expert may say that it is the duty of a physician to give aspirin to a patient who suffers an acute myocardial infarction and that the failure to do so breaches the standard of care.

Acting as an expert witness is not a task that should be taken lightly. The American College of Emergency Physicians (ACEP) has set forth guidelines for providing expert witness testimony.[19] **Box 113.2** describes a partial list of the ACEP guidelines and requirements of an expert witness.

In addition, it is important to note that physicians who provide inappropriate expert testimony may be subject to discipline by both ACEP and state medical boards.

Physician Admissions of Negligence

Expert testimony is not the only means by which a breach of duty can be established in a medical malpractice lawsuit. Another way in which plaintiff attorneys can prove that a physician breached the standard of care is by a defendant physician's own admissions. For example, in *Thomas v Corso* during sworn testimony, a physician admitted that if he had administered treatment sooner, he "might have" been able to save a patient's life and that the lack of treatment increased the danger of the patient dying.[20] The Maryland Appellate Court held that those admissions, coupled with additional testimony, "are sufficient to justify a jury finding of a substantial possibility of survival which was destroyed by [the doctor's failure] to examine, diagnose, and treat [the patient]."[20]

In *Colbert v Georgetown University*, a surgeon admitted to a patient that he "should have performed a mastectomy 2 months earlier" and that he had performed the "wrong operation" on a patient with multicentric breast cancer.[21] The DC Appellate Court held that the physician's "admission of negligence demonstrates that the standard of care was breached."[21] Similarly, in *Robertson v LaCroix*, the Oklahoma Court of Appeals held a "defendant's statement that he 'just made a mistake and got over too far' [during surgery for a hysterectomy] is more than a mere statement of mistaken judgment; it constituted an admission of negligence during the performance of the surgery."[22]

Breach of duty can be proven in more subtle manners as well. For example, suppose that during a deposition, the defendant physician is asked to describe the responsibilities of an emergency physician. The emergency physician testifies that an emergency physician's job is to "evaluate the patient, rule out and/or stabilize any life-threatening processes, and then arrange for follow-up care." If the patient involved in the lawsuit died in the ED, then the physician may have admitted a breach of duty because he did not "rule out" or "stabilize" the patient's life-threatening process. Adequate preparation for a defendant physician's deposition with a competent defense attorney or even a witness preparation consultant cannot be emphasized enough.

Violation of a Statute

Violation of a statute is another way that a plaintiff may prove breach of duty. If a physician makes a false representation on an EMTALA transfer form or performs an inappropriate cursory medical screening exam in violation of EMTALA, then the violation of the statutory provisions alone may be sufficient to prove a breach of the standard of care.[23] Similarly, reviewing a patient's medical information without a permissible reason may be sufficient to prove a breach of the Health Insurance Portability and Accountability (HIPAA) statutes.[24] In some jurisdictions, hospital licensing regulations, accreditation standards, and hospital bylaws can be used as evidence of the standard of care against a defendant hospital.[25]

Medical literature and product inserts may be sufficient to establish a rebuttable presumption of the standard of care in a few states, but generally these documents require expert testimony establishing that physicians relied upon the information.[26-28]

Res Ipsa Loquitur

The theory of *res ipsa loquitur* is also a means by which a plaintiff can show that a breach of duty occurred. The term *res ipsa loquitur* literally translates to "the thing speaks for itself." In order to allege negligence using *res ipsa loquitur*, a plaintiff must suffer injuries while under exclusive control of the defendant, those injuries must typically not occur in the absence of negligence, and the plaintiff must not have contributed to those injuries.[29] The classic example of a *res ipsa loquitur* case is a surgical sponge left inside a patient after surgery. In the ED, examples might include a patient's tooth being broken during intubation or a patient death during conscious sedation. *Res ipsa loquitur* may be inapplicable or limited in its applicability in some states. For example, Texas courts generally do not allow a res ipsa loquitur in medical malpractice cases unless the alleged injuries are so obvious that no expert testimony is required.[30] Similarly, Louisiana courts determine whether the *res ipsa loquitur* defense may be used in medical malpractice actions.[31]

Causation

> ***Case Two:*** *"A patient fell onto an outstretched hand and had pain along the distal radius. There was no wrist fracture on the x-ray, but I put the patient in a thumb spica splint and referred the patient to the orthopedist the following day. Now I learned that I completely missed an obvious scaphoid fracture on the x-ray, and the patient needed surgery to fix it. Am I liable?"*

Even though a physician may have breached a duty to a patient and the patient may have suffered damages, in order to be held liable for medical malpractice, a physician's breach of duty must have *caused* the patient's damages. There are two aspects of causation that must be proven: actual cause and proximate cause.

Actual Causation

The concept of actual causation is sometimes called the "but for" test, meaning that "but for" the alleged act of negligence, the patient's injury would not have occurred. Using the case study above, if a physician misses a fracture on an x-ray in a patient who later requires surgical repair for the injury, liability for malpractice may not follow if the patient would have needed surgical repair anyway. Using the example above, the fact that the doctor misread the x-ray probably had no bearing on whether the patient required surgery. Many scaphoid fractures require surgical management. Scaphoid fractures are treated by thumb spica splinting and prompt orthopedic referral, which is precisely what the physician in this case did. Therefore, the physician's actions did not "cause" the patient to need surgery, and a malpractice claim for this injury would likely fail.

Proximate Causation

The concept of proximate causation means that there must be a direct temporal relationship between the allegedly negligent act and the patient's injury. If the patient in Case Two was properly splinted, then fell again and reinjured the wrist, had surgery, developed a wound infection after surgery, then developed osteonecrosis, it would be difficult to prove that the misread x-ray was a proximate cause of the patient's osteonecrosis. There were simply too many other intervening factors between the negligent act and the patient's injury. If the plaintiff cannot prove both actual causation and proximate causation, the malpractice case will fail.

Damages

The presence of damages resulting from a physician's medical treatment is probably the largest factor in determining whether or not a medical malpractice case will be filed against a physician. From a legal standpoint, damages are one of the elements of medical negligence that must be proven in order to be successful in a medical malpractice lawsuit. For example, in the phone call scenario (see Case One), if the patient died, the patient's estate and family may sue the physician for all damages related to the patient's death.

However, if the patient thought that the emergency physician did not understand the situation (misdiagnosed his condition?) and immediately went to a hospital down the street where he was appropriately diagnosed with a myocardial infarction, was taken to the angiography suite, and was successfully stented with no residual effects on his cardiac output, the patient arguably has few if any damages over which to sue the first physician.

Types of Damages

Damages can be divided into "economic," "noneconomic," and "punitive" damages. Economic damages are compensation for financial losses the patient sustains and may include past medical bills, lost earnings, and costs of future medical care. Noneconomic damages are compensation for the "pain and suffering" that a plaintiff endures. For example, a patient who is paralyzed due to a physician's negligence may be awarded compensation for being confined to a wheelchair the rest of his or her life. Punitive damages are sometimes awarded to plaintiffs as punishment when a defendant's actions are particularly egregious. The distinction between types of damages is important because different states may have laws affecting how certain types of damages are awarded. Some states do not allow punitive damages in medical malpractice cases. Some states limit noneconomic damages at a specific dollar amount. Some states have no limit on any of damages that can be awarded.

Costs of Pursuing a Malpractice Claim

From a practical standpoint, damages are important in determining whether or not an attorney will file a malpractice case on a patient's behalf. Medical malpractice cases are very time-consuming and costly to pursue. According to the National Practitioner Data Bank, from the time an alleged incident of malpractice occurred, an average medical malpractice lawsuit takes 4.75 years to resolve.[32] In order to pursue a medical malpractice case, a plaintiff's attorney must obtain and review hundreds and sometimes thousands of pages of medical records, retain and pay experts to interpret those records, perform multiple depositions and pay to have those depositions recorded and transcribed, and often retain multiple expert witnesses to testify about a defendant physician's negligence. These costs can easily total $50,000 or more.

Medical malpractice cases are almost always managed on a contingency basis, meaning that potential plaintiffs do not pay the attorney an hourly fee but rather agree to give the attorney a certain percentage of any judgment obtained. Therefore, in order to proceed with a case, plaintiff's attorneys must personally pay for all costs of litigation as those costs are incurred. In a case with minimal damages, it would be fiscally unsound for an attorney to spend tens of thousands of dollars to pursue a potential judgment of only a few thousand dollars. Even in a case with $100,000 in potential damages, a plaintiff's attorney may not be willing to risk 4 years of litigation and $50,000 or more in litigation expenses for the chance to win 33% of any remaining judgment after the litigation expenses have been reimbursed.

INTENTIONAL TORTS

Intentional torts differ from negligent acts based upon intent of the actor. With negligence, there is no desire for consequences to occur, whereas intentional acts are performed with a desire for certain consequences to occur, or a belief that the consequences are substantially likely to result. While there are many intentional torts, only a few are typically seen in medical malpractice litigation (**Box 113.3**).

The term "assault" is generally defined as intending to and actually causing the perception of a harmful or offensive touching without consent. In a medical scenario, assault may occur if a provider threatens to punish a patient by performing some harmful act or threatens any action with sexual overtones.

"Battery" occurs when a person intends to cause and actually does cause harmful or offensive physical contact without consent. One of the most often cited court opinions regarding medical battery was created in 1914 when the New York Court of Appeals held that "Every human being of adult years and sound mind has a right to determine what shall be done with his own body; and a surgeon who performs an operation without his patient's consent commits an assault, for which he is liable in damages."[33]

In the medical field, battery most often arises because informed consent was not obtained or because physical contact was beyond the scope of consent. For example, battery cases have been brought against medical providers when an episiotomy was performed without permission, when a surgeon other than the one authorized by a patient performed a surgery, when a "do-not-resuscitate" patient was put on life support after suffering a cardiac arrest, and when an enema and anal probe were used at the direction of police on a patient suspected of harboring narcotics in his abdomen.[34-37]

"False imprisonment" occurs when a person is confined within boundaries fixed by another person without consent, without authorization, and without reasonable means of escape. Claims of false imprisonment usually arise from improper psychiatric commitments. In *Sassali v DeFauw*, a court held that failure to comply with procedures for

> **BOX 113.3 ■ INTENTIONAL TORTS IN MEDICINE**
>
> Intentional torts are intentional acts that cause harm, even though the harm itself may not have been intentional. Examples in medicine include assault, battery, and false imprisonment.

filing emergency detentions under the Illinois mental health code could amount to false imprisonment.[38] In *Riffe v Armstrong*, a psychiatrist's untrue assertions that he personally examined a patient before filing commitment papers were sufficient to substantiate a claim for false imprisonment (in addition to several other legal claims).[38]

Intentional tort claims against a physician may have several legal advantages for potential plaintiffs and additional implications for medical malpractice defendants. When alleging that an intentional tort occurred, no expert witness is needed to establish the standard of care. A jury is deemed capable of deciding whether a defendant violated statutory language. Commission of an intentional tort may subject a defendant to criminal liability in addition to civil liability. In other words, a conviction for assault or battery could subject the defendant to incarceration. Claims such as sexual assault or physical battery also may proceed solely upon a patient's accusations, and such claims are often inflammatory to jurors. Finally, malpractice insurance may not cover a physician for what are deemed to be criminal or intentional acts.

SUBPOENAS: COMING UNDER A COURT'S JURISDICTION

Case Three: "Great! A sheriff just served me with a subpoena, and I have no idea what the case is about. What should I do?"

In most cases, courts do not have the ability to just demand that a nonlitigant just show up in court. A subpoena is an order that creates a duty to appear in court and testify or to produce documents with evidence relevant to a case. The word *subpoena* comes from the Latin phrase *sub poena* meaning "under penalty." If you receive notice of a subpoena and do not comply, the court may have the ability to sanction you.

Subpoenas can be issued for a variety of reasons. A subpoena for documents (called a *subpoena duces tecum,* which is Latin for "bring with you under penalty of punishment") is issued so that a party to litigation can obtain documents or other tangible evidence that relates to the issues being litigated. For example, an insurance company may subpoena records regarding a patient's medical history. Defendants to a lawsuit may subpoena medical records and insurance information for someone who is suing them for injuries. Malpractice plaintiffs may subpoena records of physicians who provided care after an alleged malpractice event.

A subpoena for documents will request that you send documents to the entity whose address is listed on the subpoena and will make it clear that the subpoena does not require your personal appearance in court. There will be a deadline to comply with the subpoena for documents, but provided that you mail any documents in your possession to the requesting party, you have fulfilled your duties under the subpoena. There is no requirement that you search for documents not in your possession. If you do not have the documents that are requested, sending the requesting party a notice to that effect will usually be sufficient to fulfill the subpoena request.

Health Insurance Portability and Accountability may affect a physician's response to a subpoena for medical records. Disclosure of patient information for legal proceedings is considered a "permitted disclosure" under HIPAA for which a patient's authorization is *not* required.[40] However, when releasing protected health information pursuant to a subpoena without a signed release, there are multiple other requirements that must be met in order to comply with HIPAA, including receiving satisfactory assurances that the patient has been given notice of the subpoena or that the party serving the subpoena has attempted to obtain a protective order for the information being disclosed.[41] Since a subpoena for records is not a mandatory disclosure under HIPAA, it is probably best to obtain a signed patient release and/or a court order before releasing a patient's medical records in response to a subpoena. From an emergency medicine standpoint, emergency physicians generally do not keep copies of patients' medical records. Those records are stored in the hospital's medical record system. Therefore, to respond to the subpoena, it may be sufficient to write a short letter to the requesting party stating that the records in question are not within your possession or control.

Keep in mind that a subpoena for medical records may be the first step in the process of a patient obtaining information to file a lawsuit. Avoid any temptation to ever alter medical records, either before or after receiving a subpoena, and never send original files to the requesting party. Be aware that electronic medical record systems include auditing software that automatically track changes made to medical records.

> **Case Four:** *"The subpoena is demanding that I show up at some law office to a deposition. Do I have to go?"*

In addition to requesting documents, subpoenas may be issued to compel a witness to testify either in a deposition or in court. Chances are that if you were involved in a patient's care, you are going to be named as a defendant in a malpractice lawsuit. If you are a party to a lawsuit and an attorney wants you to testify, you probably will not receive a subpoena. You are already subject to the court's oversight by virtue of your involvement in the lawsuit. When it is time for you to be deposed, you or your attorney will receive a "notice of deposition" that lists the place, date, and time at which you will have to appear. Just as with subpoenas, you are subject to sanctions if you receive a notice of deposition and do not show up. There is usually a significant amount of flexibility in the timing of the depositions, so if you receive one for a time that creates a conflict for you, let your attorney know as soon as possible.

Subpoenas are issued to nonparty witnesses in both criminal and civil cases. For example, if the caption of the case lists "People of the State of _____" as the plaintiff, then it is a good bet that this will be a criminal case. The defendant in the case caption may not be a patient you treated but may instead be the person who *injured* the patient you treated. In criminal cases, an attorney (almost always a prosecutor) will subpoena a physician to provide medical testimony involving a potential crime. That testimony may be describing a patient's injuries or telling a jury about statements the patient made during treatment. In a civil personal injury case, a treating physician may be called to testify about the injuries a patient suffered in a traffic accident or a slip and fall. There are some instances in which a physician may receive a subpoena to testify in a medical malpractice case without being named as a defendant. For example, if a patient received care prior to arriving in the ED in cardiac arrest, the emergency physician treating the patient may receive a subpoena to testify about any statements the family made, any care the patient received in the ED, and the results of any testing that was performed.

If you have treated a patient and there is a possibility that you could be named in a lawsuit, be careful about any testimony you provide. Admissions made during a deposition could form the basis for an attorney to add you to the list of defendants in a malpractice lawsuit. If you receive a subpoena regarding a patient you treated who suffered a bad outcome, it would be wise to notify your malpractice insurer. By doing so, you protect yourself in the event that a claim is brought against you. In addition, the insurer will provide you with an attorney that will protect your interests should you be required to testify.

Fact Witnesses vs Opinion Witnesses

If you receive a subpoena, it is important to note whether you are being called to testify as a fact witness or an opinion witness. "Fact witnesses" are called to testify about facts relating to a case, as in what the witness observed or heard. Fact witnesses might testify about traffic conditions just before an accident or about the statements someone made after an accident occurred. Factual testimony about a patient might include the fact that the patient was sweating, shaking, complaining of the worst headache of his life, or had a blood pressure of 180/110. Anyone with knowledge of relevant facts can be called to testify as a fact witness.

"Expert witnesses" are called to give testimony regarding opinions that are formed after reviewing a given set of facts. Experts must be qualified by their knowledge, experience, expertise, and/or training regarding the subject matter. For example, an engineer may have expertise in stress tolerance of metals but would probably not be qualified to testify about whether a surgery went awry. Medical opinion testimony might include opinions that a blood pressure of 180/110 constitutes hypertension or that a subarachnoid hemorrhage may be in the differential diagnosis of a patient who complains of the worst headache in his or her life. In general, only expert witnesses may give opinion testimony. As will be seen in the next section, the classification of a deponent as a fact or expert witness may have significant implications.

Responding to a Subpoena

Each state has specific rules regarding how to respond to a subpoena. While these rules may vary to some degree, if you are served with a subpoena, in most cases, you must appear at the stated date and time. A subpoena will always list the name, address, and phone number of the entity requesting the witnesses' testimony. There is often some leeway in scheduling a deposition, especially if the witness is on vacation or otherwise unavailable during the scheduled date. Court testimony is less flexible, but in some cases, a testifying physician may be allowed to be "on call" when the physician agrees to be available and show up to court when called rather than being forced to sit at trial.

You may be able to find some online information about the case in which you are being called to testify. The federal Public Access to Court Electronic Records site has information and filings on federal cases (www.pacer.gov). Information about cases filed in state courts may be available through the court clerk's website in the county in which the case was filed.

Parties serving a subpoena must include compensation to the witness for attending the deposition. In cases filed in state courts, the amount of compensation varies from state to state. Subpoenas in federal court are governed by Federal Rule of Civil Procedure 45. The rule—Rule 45(b)(1)—requires that a party issuing a subpoena requiring personal appearance "tender[] the fees for one day's attendance and the mileage allowed by law," except when the subpoena is issued by the United States or any of its officers or agencies. US Code Section 28 USC §1821 delineates mileage and witness fees for federal cases. The federal witness fee for 1 day of testimony is currently $40. Federal witness fees may also include tolls, parking fees, and a "subsistence fee" as described in the statute.

The compensation for providing deposition testimony may change considerably if a witness is providing *opinion* testimony. State law generally provides that physicians deposed in their professional capacity are entitled to a "reasonable and customary fee" for time spent at the deposition. The definition of "reasonable and customary" depends on the specialty and stature of the physician being deposed but can range from hundreds to *thousands* of dollars per hour. Physicians with more knowledge and specialization are entitled to higher fees to compensate them for their expertise and for the time away from their practice. This is where the difference between a fact witness and an opinion witness becomes important. Some attorneys may attempt to circumvent paying a reasonable fee to a physician acting as an opinion witness by stating that the physician is being called as a "fact witness" only. Do not be misled. If you are a witness to a motor vehicle accident, you are a fact witness.

If you are being asked questions relating to medical diagnosis or treatment, you are being questioned in your professional capacity and are entitled to reasonable compensation. Make sure that you agree on the compensation you will receive in writing before you provide testimony. If an attorney persists in demanding your appearance but refusing to provide you with a reasonable fee, you are still required to attend the deposition, but you are not required to provide opinion testimony.

Questions relating to medical treatment or requiring medical knowledge can be met with a response to the effect of "Prior to the deposition you made it clear I would be a fact witness [or you paid me the fees to act as a fact witness]. I was not retained as an expert witness, nor did I receive a reasonable fee for my time, so I haven't had the opportunity to review all of the information and I don't feel comfortable rendering an opinion on that matter."

In summary, if you receive a subpoena, you are required to respond to it. If there is a question about whether you are allowed to disclose confidential patient information or whether you could be named in the lawsuit, it is probably a good idea to contact your malpractice insurer or an attorney first.

MALPRACTICE LITIGATION

Case Five: "*A sheriff is at the front door of my home holding an envelope full of legal papers and asking to speak with me. What should I do?*"

If a patient has suffered an injury and that injury may be a result of medical negligence, an attorney may decide to file a lawsuit on the patient's behalf. The typical course of medical malpractice litigation is discussed in the next sections of text, and it is listed in **Box 113.4**.

The Complaint

A complaint is the legal document that sets forth claims alleged by the patient, paragraph by paragraph. The complaint should state facts, which if proven, are sufficient to show that 1) the physician had a duty to the patient, 2) the physician breached the duty to the patient, 3) the patient suffered damages, and 4) the breach of duty caused the patient to suffer damages. If the patient is unable to prove each of the elements of a medical malpractice claim, then the claim will fail.

The complaint must be filed within the statute of limitations or it is subject to dismissal. Once the complaint is filed, then it must be served upon any defendants. With physicians, in most cases, a process server or a sheriff must personally hand the complaint to the physician. This is called "personal service." Without personal service, a malpractice complaint is subject to dismissal. Some physicians may attempt to avoid being served with a lawsuit in the hope that they can avoid a lawsuit. Rarely do such tactics work. The best course of action is to accept service from the process server, such as the sheriff in Case Five, and move forward with the litigation.

BOX 113.4 ■ PRETRIAL MALPRACTICE LITIGATION

- The complaint
- The summons
- The answer
- Discovery
- Depositions
- Motions practice

Being served with a malpractice complaint is a traumatic experience. The allegations contained in the complaint generally follow a legal format in which the allegations may appear exaggerated and are not necessarily true. A complaint only contains the accusations that must be proven for the plaintiff to win the case. If served with a malpractice complaint, it is wise to notify the medical malpractice insurer and/or an attorney about the complaint as soon as possible. In addition, because coverage in some medical malpractice insurance policies is bound when a claim or potential claim is *reported*, it may also be prudent to notify one's malpractice insurer about threats or bad outcomes that are substantially likely to result in a claim. Sometimes a resolution to such a situation can be achieved without resorting to litigation, which benefits all parties.

The Summons

When a complaint is served on a defendant, it will contain a summons. The summons will state something to the effect that "your failure to appear in response to this summons will subject you to punishment for contempt of this court." In other words, if a doctor receives a summons and the doctor (or a representative) fails to attend the scheduled court hearing, the court has the ability to enter sanctions or a judgment against the physician. Again, if served with a summons, a physician should promptly notify his or her insurance carrier or attorney.

The Answer

Once served with a complaint, defendants have a limited amount of time to respond to the allegations contained in the complaint. In many cases, a response must be made within 30 days. If the deadline is not met, the defendant risks having all allegations in the complaint presumed true and a default judgment entered against him or her in the case.

An answer responds to each allegation in the complaint by admitting the allegation, denying the allegation, or making a statement that the defendant lacks the necessary knowledge to determine whether the allegation is true or false. For example, an allegation in the complaint may state that the defendant physician is licensed to practice medicine in a given jurisdiction or that the physician provided medical treatment to the plaintiff on a given date. Answers to a complaint must be truthful, and a defendant who answers a complaint untruthfully may be subject to court sanctions. Allegations that are admitted no longer need to be proven during the remainder of the litigation. Allegations that are denied must generally be proven by a preponderance of the evidence.

Affirmative Defenses

Case Six: "*I just received notice of a malpractice case, but I saw that patient three years ago! Doesn't the statute of limitations prevent me from being sued?*"

The statute of limitations is one of multiple "affirmative defenses" that may be pled in response to a lawsuit. Essentially, an affirmative defense states that "even if everything that the plaintiff alleges is true, there is a justifiable reason for my actions and therefore I still win the lawsuit." An affirmative defense may give a court reason to dismiss a lawsuit or to reduce a judgment, but an affirmative defense cannot prevent a lawsuit from being filed. A simple example of an affirmative defense in a criminal case is "self-defense." While a criminal defendant may be charged with homicide for shooting and killing another person, if that defendant can show that he acted in self-defense, the allegations of criminal conduct may be negated.

There are multiple affirmative defenses to civil lawsuits. In federal courts, the list of affirmative defenses to civil claims is found in the Federal Rule of Civil Procedures.[42] There are 18 listed affirmative defenses, but the Federal Rules also allow a party to "affirmatively state any avoidance or affirmative defense" to any papers filed with the court, so the list of 18 affirmative defenses is not exclusive. Once a lawsuit is filed, the defendant must answer the allegations and then may raise any additional applicable affirmative defenses. From a procedural standpoint, it is important to note that affirmative defenses must be raised very early in the course of the lawsuit, generally along with the answer to the complaint. Failure to file affirmative defenses early in the litigation may give the courts reason to waive (not consider) the defense when deciding the outcome of the case.

While a comprehensive review of the affirmative defenses to civil lawsuits is outside of the scope of this text, a discussion of the statute of limitations and comparative negligence—two common affirmative defenses used in malpractice lawsuits—may illustrate how affirmative defenses can be used by a malpractice defendant.

Statute of Limitations

Each state has created a list of time frames within which lawsuits must be filed. The idea behind such statutes is that plaintiffs should seek compensation on a timely basis to preserve evidence and to ensure the availability of witnesses. Similarly, such statutes anticipate that at some point defendants should be able to wipe the slate clean without fear of being embroiled in a lawsuit long after an alleged harm has been suffered.

The time frame within which a medical malpractice lawsuit must be filed can range from as little as 1 year to 5 years or more. In addition, multiple other factors may "toll" the statute of limitations. For example, the statute of limitations generally does not start until a patient knows—or should have known—about the potential injury they suffered. In many cases, the knowledge of an alleged injury corresponds to when a patient seeks care in an ED. However, this is not always the case. Consider a patient who seeks care for coughing or shortness of breath, who receives a chest x-ray, and who is discharged home with a prescription for antibiotics after being told his chest x-ray is normal. In reality, the chest x-ray shows a suspicious lung nodule. One year later, the patient is diagnosed with metastatic cancer due to the lung nodule. Under such circumstances, the statute of limitations would likely begin when the patient found out about the cancer, not one year earlier when the initial x-ray was performed.

Another factor that may toll the statute of limitations is a patient's age. In many states, the statute of limitations does not start until a patient reaches the age of majority, usually 18 years old. This may mean that in some states, a patient could wait more than 18 years to file a lawsuit without the suit being barred by the statute of limitations. Fraudulent concealment of wrongdoing will also stop the statute of limitations from running. For example, hiding the fact that a medication overdose was accidentally given will likely stop the clock on the statute of limitations if the patient was not aware of the error (in addition to raising licensure and criminal law issues).

From an emergency medicine management standpoint, it is important to note that a provider is not immune from liability simply because the statute of limitations seems to have lapsed. There are multiple scenarios under which the statute of limitations may be tolled and other reasons that a court may extend the statute of limitations. For this reason, it is important to maintain appropriate malpractice insurance even if the statute of limitations seems to have run. Claims-made medical malpractice insurance policies should include "extended reporting coverage" or "tail insurance" to protect against potential malpractice claims that could occur years after an alleged event occurred.

> ***Case Seven:*** *"The patient didn't fill the prescription I gave him for anticoagulants. How can he sue me because he later developed a pulmonary embolism?"*

Contributory Negligence/Comparative Fault

This affirmative defense means that a plaintiff who contributes to his or her own injuries may be prevented from collecting damages from defendants in a lawsuit. For example, suppose a patient is diagnosed with pneumonia in the ED and given a prescription for outpatient antibiotics. Three days later, the patient returns to the hospital in septic shock and dies from the previously diagnosed pneumonia. A medical malpractice lawsuit may allege that the physician was negligent in discharging the patient. Affirmative defenses to that lawsuit might allege that the patient was comparatively negligent because he never filled the prescription for outpatient antibiotics and did not follow the discharge instructions to return immediately if his symptoms worsened.

Similarly, allegations that a physician did not obtain a proper medical history could be met with affirmative defense that the patient was negligent in providing an adequate history. Allegations that a patient suffered damages because a physician prescribed outpatient medications to which the patient was allergic could be met with an affirmative defense that the patient was negligent in taking the medications after seeing the name of the medication on the prescription. As with the statute of limitations, a patient's comparative negligence does not prevent the patient from filing a lawsuit, but it may negate the allegations in the lawsuit or diminish any malpractice award.

The effect of this affirmative defense varies between states. Contributory negligence applies in a minority of states and prevents plaintiffs from recovering *any* damages if they are in any way responsible for their injuries. Comparative negligence applies in a vast majority of states and may allow a plaintiff to recover some damages depending upon the degree to which the plaintiff's actions contributed to his or her injuries. In states that use the doctrine of comparative negligence, a patient may be barred from recovering any damages if he or she is more than 50% responsible for the damages suffered. In states that allow pure comparative negligence, courts will simply diminish the amount of damages by the percentage of a plaintiff's negligence as determined by a jury. For example, if a jury determines that a heart attack victim is 60% liable for his own injuries for failing to follow up with a cardiologist and failing to have an outpatient stress test as recommended, depending on how the specific state law applies the doctrine of comparative fault, the patient could receive no award of damages at all or could receive 40% of the damages awarded by a jury.

In emergency medical practice, the doctrine of contributory negligence and comparative fault should emphasize why it is important to provide patients with adequate follow-up instructions. Not only do good follow-up instructions significantly improve a patient's medical care, but a patient who fails to abide by follow-up recommendations may be prevented from collecting a subsequent judgment in a medical malpractice case.

Discovery

Once a complaint and answer have been filed, the "discovery" phase of a lawsuit begins. Discovery allows both parties to discover all of the facts about the case so that each party can formulate its version. Failure to comply with discovery requests may result in sanctions from the court. For example, in *Borrero v Lake Erie Women's Center*, a women's health clinic, hospital, physician, and midwife were ordered to pay $72,861.53 in sanctions when they failed to produce clinic protocols in their possession that were requested by a plaintiff during discovery.[43] Discovery violations may also create a jury impression that defendants are attempting to hide their guilt by not disclosing pertinent documents. In many jurisdictions, jury instructions include a statement that missing evidence may be presumed to contain information detrimental to the case of the party who did not produce it.

Discovery can either be written or verbal. Written discovery comes in the form of interrogatories and requests for production. Verbal discovery is called a "deposition."

"Interrogatories" are a set of written questions presented to the opposing party regarding pertinent facts in the lawsuit. Answers to interrogatories are considered sworn testimony and must be made under oath affirming that they are true. The answers given to interrogatories may be taken as fact by courts and juries. Questions typically used in interrogatories include requests such as "state the exact dates and places on and at which you provided medical care to the plaintiff" or "identify and list specific provisions of all medical literature which will be used in defending any of the allegations set forth in the complaint." If an answer to an interrogatory cannot be determined, there is an ongoing duty to supplement the answers if additional facts become known.

"Requests for production" of documents impose a duty on the parties to disclose all such documents within its possession or control. For example, a plaintiff may want to review medical records, office schedules, billing records, or other medical records related to the patient's injuries. Defendants may want to review medical records from other health-care providers, insurance claims, unemployment/disability claims, employment records, and any bills related to treatment for the alleged injuries. Failure to provide an opposing party with requested documents, even if those documents are damaging to one's case, may give rise to sanctions from the court. Destroying or modifying documents (most commonly medical records) without signing and dating the changes may lead to charges of "spoliation of evidence," will likely force settlement of the lawsuit, may void medical malpractice insurance coverage, and can be cause for additional sanctions, including actions against a physician's medical license.

Depositions

Depositions are typically a set of oral questions from an opposing attorney that are answered under oath. Depositions are an important way of uncovering information in that the opposing attorney has the ability to ask follow-up questions based on answers given by the person being deposed (the "deponent"). Those answers can be used to prove the case against the deponent or to discredit the deponent in court.

Attorneys use depositions for several reasons (**Box 113.5**). First, attorneys use depositions to gather further facts that they can use to bolster their case. Physicians may be asked about proper workups for given conditions or about their differential diagnosis for a patient with certain symptoms. Physicians may also be asked about who else was involved in the case and what those other parties did or did not do. Second, attorneys use depositions to lock the deponent into a specific fact pattern. For example, if a physician during testimony states

---

BOX 113.5 ■ GOALS OF DEPOSITIONS

1. Gather additional facts about a case.
2. Lock the defendant into a single version of facts about a case—if discrepancy occurs later in case, the opposing attorney can use deposition testimony to impeach the witness.
3. Attempt to obtain admissions by the defendant that can later be used at trial.
4. Determine how a witness will likely appear to a jury.

that a patient provided a particular history but, then during trial, describes a different history provided by the patient, the attorney will use the discrepancy in testimony to allege that the physician is not trustworthy, has a poor memory, and that his testimony cannot be believed—a process called "impeachment."

Finally, attorneys use depositions to determine how well a deponent will come across as a witness in court. A deposition is a dress rehearsal for court. Juries tend not to like a witness who comes across as being angry, arrogant, conceited, defiant, or evasive. Attorneys are more likely to continue litigation against deponents who possess those qualities because those qualities tend to create a negative impression on juries and make a negative verdict more likely. Conversely, a deponent who comes across as being sincere, calm, humble, honest, and caring about the patient is more likely to make a positive impact on a jury. Performing well at a deposition may make a physician less of a target in a medical malpractice case and may even cause the case to be dropped.

Motion Practice

"Motions" are court documents that provide the court with a party's request to take some action and a substantiation of those requests through facts, argument, and higher court opinions. Parties can enter a motion for the court to take almost any action, but two of the more common motions during litigation are motions to dismiss and motions for summary judgment.

A "motion to dismiss" is an argument that the allegations in the complaint are insufficient to proceed with the case. For example, if a plaintiff's complaint states that a patient was injured by a physician's negligence, but does not show how the physician had a duty to treat the patient, then the complaint would likely be dismissed through a motion to dismiss. Such a situation might occur in a "shotgun" lawsuit in which all physicians named in the chart are sued, but relatively few of them ever treated the patient. In a motion to dismiss, any facts alleged by the nonmoving party are assumed to be true, making the burden of proof heavily against the party submitting the motion.

Once a defendant files a motion to dismiss, the plaintiff is given time to file a written response to the allegations in the defendant's motion, and the defendant is then given time to reply to the plaintiff's response. After the written briefs have been submitted, a hearing is held where the judge hears any additional oral arguments the parties wish to make and then makes a ruling. If the motion is granted, the plaintiff's case is dismissed. If the motion is denied, the case then progresses to further discovery.

A "motion for summary judgment" is usually filed after all of the evidence has been presented from both parties in discovery. The motion for summary judgment alleges that one party is unable to prove all aspects of its case and that judgment should be rendered in favor of the moving party "as a matter of law." Summary judgment motions dispose of cases that do not involve "issues of fact." Defendants may argue that the evidence presented is insufficient for a plaintiff to prove all elements of his case. Plaintiffs may argue that a defendant has no defense to the plaintiff's claims. If a material issue of fact exists, the summary judgment motion must be denied, because a jury or trial judge is the only entity that can decide an issue of fact after all evidence has been set forth in the case.

As with motions to dismiss, in a summary judgment motion, a substantial burden of proof is placed upon the party submitting the motion. When the motion, response, and reply briefs have been submitted, a hearing is held. There the judge hears oral arguments and then makes a ruling in the case. If the summary judgment motion is granted, the case is dismissed. If the motion is denied, then the case progresses to trial.

GOING TO TRIAL

A trial is an opportunity for both parties to present their versions of the case to the "fact finder"—either a jury or a trial judge. Between 7% and 15% of medical malpractice claims result in a trial.[44,45] As litigation progresses, most cases are either abandoned (60%) or settled (27%).[44,45] If a medical malpractice case progresses to trial, the odds of winning are strongly in the physician's favor. Of the ED malpractice claims taken to trial, 85% result in defense verdicts.[44]

In order to win at trial, the plaintiff must prove the same four elements of negligence: duty, breach, causation, and damages. The defendant then tries to counter the plaintiff's allegations in an attempt to show that at least one of those elements was not proven or that some other defense exists. The fact finder decides which version of the factual dispute is more likely. The components of a trial are listed in **Box 113.6.**

Voir Dire

If either party demands a trial by jury, the jury must be selected before the trial begins. The process of jury selection is called *voir dire*, meaning "to say what is true." During *voir dire*, potential jurors are questioned about possible biases that may affect their ability to render an impartial verdict. For example, a juror whose family member recently died from alleged medical malpractice may have a bias against medical providers that would prevent the juror from being impartial during trial. Similarly, a juror whose life was saved at a hospital named as a defendant in a lawsuit may be biased in favor of the same hospital during trial.

Jurors who are likely to have a bias in the case may be excused from serving on the jury by the judge "for cause." In addition, plaintiff and defendant are each allowed several peremptory challenges wherein a juror can be excused from serving on the jury for almost any reason. Once a jury has been seated, the trial begins with opening statements.

Opening Statements

A trial begins with an opening statement. An opening statement is the attorney's summary of what he or she believes that the facts of a case will show. It is used to give the jury a flavor of what the case is about. Consider opening statements as the *Cliff's Notes* of the case. Arguments about the facts cannot be introduced during opening statements. Once each side has had an opportunity to present a synopsis of its version of the case, testimony begins.

Fact Testimony

The testimony in a case allows each side to explain its version of the events that occurred. During "direct examination," the lawyer helps guide the witnesses through the version of the story to be told. After the witness has finished telling his or her story, "cross examination"

BOX 113.6 ■ COMPONENTS OF TRIAL

- Opening statements
- Fact testimony
- Opinion testimony
- Closing arguments
- Verdict

allows the opposing attorney to discredit the witness's testimony by bringing out facts that conflict with the story presented or by demonstrating a witness's lack of knowledge about certain facts.

Most witnesses testify about facts relevant to a case. For example, a patient's spouse might testify about the pain a patient was experiencing or about what a physician told them in the hospital. An office secretary might be called as a witness to testify that the patient failed to show up for many follow-up appointments just prior to his or her adverse medical outcome. A jury need not believe a fact witness's testimony and may completely ignore the testimony as being untrustworthy.

Opinion Testimony

Interspersed with fact testimony will be opinion testimony from expert witnesses. As with fact witness testimony, opinion witness testimony may be entirely ignored as having little credibility or may be given great deference by the fact finder. An expert witness testifies about subjects that are deemed to be outside the understanding of the fact finder and may provide opinions as to whether a defendant's actions or inactions contributed to the plaintiff's alleged injuries. Expert opinions must generally be disclosed prior to trial and should have some scientific basis. An expert would likely be prevented from testifying about an opinion that did not have a scientific basis, such as an assertion that the standard of care requires that all ED patients receive care within 5 minutes of their arrival.

The threshold of admissibility that must be met by an expert's opinions varies by state and federal law. Two of the most used standards for determining admissibility of expert witness testimony are the Frye standard and the Daubert standard.

The Frye Standard

The *Frye* standard is based upon the 1923 case *Frye v United States*.[46] In Frye, a defendant attempted to use the results of a "blood pressure deception test" to show that he had not committed murder. The defendant's expert argued that systolic blood pressure always rises in a predictable pattern when one is attempting to deceive an examiner due to fear of being caught in a lie. The expert had performed this test on the defendant prior to the trial and the defendant wanted to use the results of this test as evidence of his innocence. The trial court denied the defendant's request and the appellate court affirmed, stating that:

> *While courts will go a long way in admitting expert testimony deduced from a well-recognized scientific principle or discovery, the thing from which the deduction is made must be sufficiently established to have gained general acceptance in the particular field in which it belongs.*

This "general acceptance" rule was fairly well accepted for the next 70 years until the Daubert standard was created. While the two standards are not mutually exclusive, the Daubert standard restricts the Frye standard and provides courts with considerations that may be used in determining whether expert witness testimony is admissible.

The Daubert Standard

The *Daubert* standard is based upon *Daubert v Merrell Dow Pharmaceuticals, Inc.*[47] where plaintiffs attempted to link birth defects in children to maternal ingestion of the sleep aid Bendectin. A thorough review of published studies showed no link between maternal Bendectin use and subsequent birth defects in their children, but multiple experts in their fields cited unpublished animal studies as evidence that Bendectin did cause birth defects in humans. Neither the trial court nor the appellate court allowed the plaintiffs to offer the unpublished studies as evidence, citing the Frye standard and stating that the evidence was inadmissible because it had not achieved general acceptance in the relevant scientific communities.

The US Supreme Court overruled the appellate court's opinion and instituted a new standard establishing trial court judges as gatekeepers, requiring them to perform inquiries to determine whether proffered testimony is "relevant and reliable." Among the recommended inquiries were whether the evidence had been tested, whether it was subject to peer review and publication, potential error rates, and existence of standards regarding the testimony—in addition to whether there was widespread acceptance of the evidence in question. The Daubert standard is used in most state courts and in all federal courts. Sixteen states still use the Frye standard to determine the admissibility of expert evidence in legal proceedings, including New York, Florida, California, and Illinois.[48]

Cross Examination of Experts

Once experts have finished providing "direct" testimony, opposing attorneys are permitted to cross examine the experts in order to expose any inconsistencies in that testimony. After cross-examination, redirect examination allows the party offering the witness to clarify any issues raised on cross-examination. For example, on direct examination, an expert may testify that the standard of care requires any patient experiencing an acute myocardial infarction to receive aspirin in the ED. On cross-examination, the expert might be forced to admit that patients who have aspirin allergies should not receive aspirin and that patients who have received aspirin in an ambulance do not need to receive an additional dose of aspirin in the ED. On redirect examination, the expert may note that in the current case, the patient had no allergies and did not receive aspirin in the ambulance.

Closing Arguments

Once all of the evidence in a case has been presented, attorneys for both parties have the opportunity to present their closing arguments. During closing arguments, attorneys summarize what they believe the evidence showed. In contrast to opening statements, during closing arguments, attorneys can interject arguments, innuendos, and hypothesis while trying to persuade a jury to believe their version of events. For example, a plaintiff attorney may use a defendant physician's poor recall of events, delay in obtaining repeat electrocardiograms, failure to give aspirin, and sloppily written notes to allege that the physician was "sloppy" in his practice of medicine and his sloppiness caused the patient's injuries.

A defense attorney may counter that the patient's failure to inform the physician of a history of tobacco use and a family history of heart attacks made the patient responsible for his own injuries and that a reasonable physician would not have suspected heart disease given the patient's complaints and physical findings.

Verdict

Once closing arguments are completed, the judge defines the law for the jury and instructs the jury on the burden of proof that the plaintiff has to meet in order to win the case. The jury then deliberates over the evidence provided and renders a verdict based upon the judge's instructions. Note that in 25 states, a jury's decision to find a physician liable for medical malpractice does not need to be unanimous but may be consensus of 9 or 10 out of 12 jurors for a finding of liability.[49]

THE ED LEADER'S INVOLVEMENT

An ED group leader naturally wants to assist a physician who is the subject of a malpractice claim. While it may be tempting to discuss the merits of a malpractice case with the physician being sued or with other providers, the ED leader should avoid doing so. Statements made about a case are often discoverable and must be disclosed if a plaintiff attorney formally inquires about them.

For example, statements a physician makes about what might have been done differently in managing a case with a bad outcome would likely be detrimental to the physician's defense, even if those options were not available when the physician was providing the allegedly negligent care. Statements made to one's attorney, one's insurance representative, and one's spouse are examples of privileged communications, which are usually not discoverable during litigation. Plaintiff attorneys may also seek to depose any person who has made statements about or who is aware of facts relevant to a malpractice case, including the ED manager.

An ED leader may even attempt to coach a defendant on how to respond to plaintiff attorney questioning. However, doing so may be similarly counterproductive. Inappropriate answers to plaintiff attorney questioning may inadvertently damage the theme of the case that the defense attorney is trying to establish or may even concede liability on issues where liability did not exist.

The best recommendation that an ED leader can give to a defendant in a medical malpractice case is to listen to the defense attorney's advice and to actively participate in the defense of the case. If the physician is uncomfortable with the defense attorney, believes that the defense attorney is not providing adequate preparation, or believes that a conflict of interest has arisen, the ED leader may suggest that the physician seek alternate counsel from the insurance company or recommend that the physician retain personal counsel to oversee the defense of the case.

CONCLUSION

Unfortunately, the effects of medical malpractice cases often do not end with the verdict. Malpractice fears affect a physician's clinical practice long after a case has been resolved. Physicians with higher risk aversion and malpractice fear tend to hospitalize more low-risk patients and order more low-yield testing.[50,51] Perception that one has committed a medical error is associated with significant elevations in physician burnout, depersonalization, and emotional exhaustion and a significant decrease in physician empathy.[52]

An ED leader who understands the adverse psychological and emotional effects on physicians involved in malpractice litigation may be able to help the emergency physician with the effects of a medical malpractice lawsuit. Reinforcing the ideas that malpractice lawsuits are not a reflection of the physician's competence and that the physician is a strong clinician who provides good medical care can help combat the negative thought processes that some malpractice defendants encounter.

Recognizing maladaptive behavior in a physician suffering from litigation stress and encouraging such physicians to seek psychological counseling can be career saving or even lifesaving (see Chapter 112). Many medical societies, including ACEP, also offer a peer support system.

In summary, medical malpractice lawsuits are stressful events that a majority of emergency physicians will experience in their careers. An ED manager who helps to familiarize physicians with the process of a malpractice lawsuit, who provides emotional support for physicians involved in litigation, and who is vigilant for maladaptive behaviors resulting from litigation stress will be a tremendous asset to the members of his department.

REFERENCES

1. National Practitioner Data Bank. Available at: https://www.npdb.hrsa.gov/analysistool/.

2. Singh H. National Practitioner Data Bank: adverse action and medical malpractice reports (1990-June 30, 2020). Generated using the Data Analysis Tool. 2020. Available at: https://www.npdb.hrsa.gov/analysistool. Accessed April 26, 2019.

3. Greve P. *HealthTrek: Medical Malpractice Claim Trends in 2017*. Willis Towers Watson Insurance Company; 2017.

4. Guardado JR. Medical professional liability insurance indemnity payments, expenses and claim disposition, 2006–2015. Policy Research Perspectives No. 2018-1. American Medical Association; 2018.

5. Rui P, Kang K. National hospital ambulatory medical care survey: 2015 emergency department summary tables. National Center for Health Statistics. Available at: https://www.cdc.gov/nchs/data/nhamcs/web_tables/2015_ed_web_tables.pdf

6. Jena AB, Seabury S, Lakdawalla D, Chandra A. Malpractice risk according to physician specialty. *N Engl J Med*. 2011;365(7):629–636.

7. 42 USC § 1395DD(a).

8. *Cogswell v Chapman*, 249 AD2d 865 (NY 1998).

9. *Bienz v Cent. Suffolk Hosp.*, 163 AD2d 269 (NY 1990).

10. *Hoover v Williamson*, 203 A.2d 861 (MD 1964).

11. *Millard v Corrado*, 14 S.W.3d 42 (MO 1999).

12. *Schrader v Kohout*, 522 S.E.2d 19 (GA 1999).

13. *McKinney v Schlatter*, 118 Ohio App. 3d 328 (1997).

14. *St. John v Pope*, 901 S.W.2d 420 (TX 1995).

15. *Tarasoff v Regents of University of California*, 551 P.2d 334 (1976).

16. *Tedrick v Community Resource Center, Inc.*, 920 N.E.2d 220 (2009).

17. O.C.G.A. § 51-1-29.5(c).

18. *Gliemmo v Cousineau*, 694 S.E.2d 75 (GA 2010).

19. American College of Emergency Physicians. Expert Witness Guidelines for the Specialty of Emergency Medicine. In: *College Manual*. American College of Emergency Physicians Web site. Available at: https://www.acep.org/patient-care/policy-statements/expert-witness-guidelines-for-the-specialty-of-emergency-medicine/. Accessed November 1, 2020.

20. *Thomas v Corso*, 288 A.2d 379 (MD 1972).

21. *Colbert v Georgetown University*, 623 A.2d 1244 (DC 1993).

22. *Robertson v LaCroix*, 534 P. 2d 17 (OK 1975).

23. 42 USC § 1395DD(d)(1)(B).

24. 45 CFR § 164.306.

25. *Walski v Tiesenga*, 381 NE 2d 279 (IL 1978).

26. *Lhotka v Larson*, 238 N.W.2d 870 (MN 1976).

27. *Ohligschlager v Proctor Comm. Hosp.*, 303 N.E.2d 392 (IL 1973).

28. *Sanzari v Rosenfeld*, 167 A. 2d 625 (NJ 1961).

29. *Seavers v Methodist Med. Cent. of Oak Ridge*, 9 S.W.3d 86 (TN 1999).

30. *Haddock v Arnspiger*, 793 S.W.2d 948 (TX Supreme Court 1990).

31. *Cangelosi v Our Lady of Lake Reg. Med. Ctr.*, 564 So. 2d 654 (LA 1989).

32. *National Practitioner Data Bank 2006 Annual Report*. US Department of Health and Human Services; 2006: 33.

33. *Schloendorff v Society of New York Hospital*, 105 N.E. 92 (NY 1914).

34. *Curtis v Jaskey*, 759 N.E.2d 962 (IL 2001).

35. *Watkins v Cleveland Clinic*, 719 N.E.2d 1052 (Ohio 1998).

36. *Estate of Leach v Shapiro*, 469 N.E.2d 1047 (Ohio 1984).

37. *Berrios v Our Lady of Mercy Medical Center*, 20 A.D.3d 361 (NY 2005).

38. *Sassali v DeFauw*, 696 NE 2d 1217 (IL 1998).

39. *Riffe v Armstrong*, 477 S.E.2d 535 (WV 1996).

40. 45 CFR §164.512(e).

41. 45 CFR §164.512 (e)(1)(ii)(A).

42. General Rules of Pleading, Affirmative Defenses. Fed. R. Civ. P. 8(c).

43. *Borrero, et al. v Lake Erie Women's Center, et al.*, No. 12060-2004 (Erie Co., PA [2004]).

44. Brown TW, McCarthy ML, Kelen GD, et al. An epidemiologic study of closed emergency department malpractice claims in a national database of physician malpractice insurers. *Acad Emerg Med*. 2010;17(5):553–560.

45. Golann D. Dropped medical malpractice claims: their surprising frequency, apparent causes, and potential remedies. *Health Aff*. 2011;30(7):1343–1350.

46. *Frye v United States*, 293 F. 1013 (D.C. 1923).

47. *Daubert v Merrell Dow Pharmaceuticals, Inc.*, 509 US 579 (1993).

48. Bernstein DE. Frye, Frye again: the past, present, and future of the general acceptance test. *SSRN Electronic J*. 2001.

49. Table 42: trial juries, size and verdict rules. In: Rottman DB, Strickland SM. *State Court Organization 2004*. NCJ 212351. US Department of Justice, Bureau of Justice Statistics. USGPO; August, 2006.

50. Katz DA, Williams GC, Brown RL, et al. Emergency physicians' fear of malpractice in evaluating patients with possible acute cardiac ischemia. *Ann Emerg Med*. 2005;46(6):525–533.

51. Wong AC, Kowalenko T, Roahen-Harrison S, et al. A survey of emergency physicians' fear of malpractice and its association with the decision to order computed tomography scans for children with minor head trauma. *Pediatr Emerg Care*. 2011;27(3):182–185.

52. West CP, Huschka MM, Novotny PJ, et al. Association of perceived medical errors with resident distress and empathy. *JAMA*. 2006;296(9):1071–1078.

ANATOMY OF A LAWSUIT

CHAPTER 114

Jennifer L'Hommedieu Stankus

Dr. Smith is an outstanding young emergency physician with several years of experience in a busy tertiary care center where you are the medical director. She is competent, energetic, positive, and thorough. You are working with her one evening and notice that she is being short with patients and staff and seems agitated. It is very out of character for her, so you pull her aside and ask if something is wrong. She burst into tears and says that she has been sued for missing an ovarian torsion.

Litigation is a part of medical practice for most emergency physicians and for all medical directors. More than 50% of emergency physicians will be sued at some point in their career, and over 30% will be sued multiple times.[1] As the leader of an emergency department (ED) or group, it is important to recognize the frequency of litigation, understand the effects these suits may have, and be prepared to support and protect your team.

On the other hand, being prepared, mitigating risk, and offering appropriate support can dramatically change the extent of the potentially negative impact a lawsuit can have on a department. To do this effectively, ED leaders must understand the different stages of litigation, malpractice insurance contracts and coverage, and the profound influence that being sued can and will have on clinicians.

STAGES OF LITIGATION

There are multiple stages of litigation, each with their own cadence and gravity. All stages require the thoughtful attention of those involved.

Notification

Being sued will cause 95% of clinicians to experience emotional distress during part or all of the litigation process.[2] This burden may impact health and well-being, personal and professional relationships, and clinician practice. The emotional stress can lead to an increase in diagnostic testing, strained physician–patient relationships, and decreased concentration, all of which can lead to cognitive errors. Many clinicians feel ashamed and incompetent when served with notice of a lawsuit. It is critical to let them know that they are not alone.

Dr. Smith was in the middle of a busy shift when a sheriff's deputy served her with official papers. Her stomach dropped and her heart raced as she opened the envelope. She was being accused of missing an ovarian torsion in a young patient who had to undergo emergency surgery two days later at another institution. The suit demanded an award of $5 million.

Dr. Smith felt that she had failed this patient, her group, and the hospital. She started worrying about losing her home, her job, and her friends. The rest of her shift was a blur, and she had a hard time providing patient care due to constant intrusive thoughts.

Dr. Smith has not told anyone about the lawsuit and has been unable to sleep or concentrate well. She also finds herself feeling antagonistic toward patients.

Notification of a lawsuit can be done in person or by mail. Not all notices from attorneys are actual lawsuits, but any official correspondence from an attorney related to patient care or medical records requires the involvement of the hospital, group risk manager, and/or the insurance carrier. Clinicians should never respond to an attorney's request for medical records. Such appeals should be directed to the medical records office, which can ensure proper disclosure and compliance with standards of the Health Insurance Portability and Accountability Act (HIPAA).

Action must be taken quickly to provide a response within the time frame defined in the notification (usually 20-30 days). Failure to properly respond to the complaint can result in a default judgment against the clinician. Default judgments can lead to an insurance company refusing to defend the clinician or pay for judgment. Failure to respond in a timely manner also makes the clinician appear guilty by failing to mount a defense.

Fortunately, Dr. Smith was served with notice of a lawsuit just last week, so there has not been a lengthy delay in her response. She relates that she has not told anyone because she is so embarrassed and ashamed. She feels depressed, inadequate, and is even wondering why she went into medicine in the first place. You meet with her after the shift and tell her that you and the group are there for her and will help her through this. You tell her that you want to talk about her feelings and to help her through this difficult time by providing technical advice about the legal process, but you also advise her not to discuss any facts or opinions about the case with anyone other than her attorney and spouse. You direct her to the appropriate agent with your malpractice insurance carrier and assure Dr. Smith that the defense team will spring into action on her behalf.

Once the insurance carrier receives notice of a lawsuit, a defense attorney is assigned. This is done without input from the defending clinician; however, the provider still has some power and influence in the process, and new counsel may be requested if there is good cause. A good working relationship with the defense counsel is crucial. Clinicians should get to know their counsel and become actively engaged in the defense process. The malpractice counsel is the clinician's advocate and must hear and understand all aspects of the case: "the good, the bad, and the ugly." The communication between the clinician and their counsel is privileged. This is an important distinction because communication with colleagues, friends, and family (other than a spouse) is not privileged and is therefore discoverable.

Dr. Smith explains that she was newly out of residency when this case occurred. You stop her and again remind her not to tell you any facts about the case or her decision-making process. You also tell her that it is important to express any concerns she may have with her defense attorney.

The lawyer will not judge the client but needs to know everything in order to provide the best defense. A lawyer's job is to vigorously advocate for their client, and part of the process is forming arguments and counterarguments against the opposing counsel. Preparation requires knowing what will be coming at them from the other side. The sooner they have all information, the better prepared the attorney will be to defend the case.

Many cases are voluntarily dismissed. The plaintiff may withdraw the complaint at any time. As an example, a voluntary withdrawal may occur when the plaintiff's attorney gets a case just as the statute of limitations is about to run out. In order to preserve the right to advance the case, the suit is filed. Then, additional time is spent to evaluate whether the case has merit. After a thorough review and expert evaluation of the records, the plaintiff's team will determine the strengths and weaknesses of the case. Because moving forward with a lawsuit is a gamble and the plaintiff's attorney pays out of pocket until there is a settlement or judgment, most will only proceed with "strong" cases.

While avoiding false reassurances, you explain to Dr. Smith that 65% of cases will close without a settlement; only 7% go to trial, and of those, the defense wins 85% of the time. So just based upon that, the odds are in her favor.[3] Dr. Smith admits this information does make her feel better, but she also says she wants to add something to the record that will strengthen her case.

The patient's medical records should not be altered.[4] Changes can always be detected through metadata analysis, and "after-the-fact" alterations of the medical record can make it appear as though the physician is lying or attempting to cover their tracks. In most cases, the clinician's credibility will be damaged, which may lead to a poor result. It may be possible to add a dated addendum only if approved by the defense counsel (rare), as these late additions to the chart usually hurt the defense of the case.

You advise Dr. Smith to wait until she is assigned counsel to discuss the possibility of adding an addendum. You explain that she will have ample opportunity to relate all information that she has to her attorney and, if deemed important, the information can be described during deposition or trial.

Occasionally, a plaintiff's attorneys will send inappropriate requests to other clinicians who are involved in or aware of the case. An example might be a request for a signature on an affidavit summarizing care or expressing an expert opinion about an injury that occurred to the client/patient. These requests should be denied. To properly obtain this information, the attorney can subpoena the provider to testify as a fact witness, in which case that provider would be compelled to do so. When testifying, the clinician should not stray beyond their direct observations and decisions. Communications with the patient are private, so unless the right of confidentiality has been waived, this information should not be divulged. **Box 114.1** summarizes "pearls and pitfalls" of the notification process.

BOX 114.1 ■ NOTIFICATION PEARLS AND PITFALLS

DO:
- Notify your insurance carrier, hospital risk management, and medical director.
- Actively engage in your defense from the beginning.
- Give all information to your attorney, both good and bad, about the case.
- Make copies of all legal documents for your own records.
- Discuss your feelings with your medical director and friends.

DON'T:
- Provide any medical records requested.
- Correspond with the attorney bringing suit.
- Express an opinion about the case or other providers.
- Delay or ignore a notice.
- Discuss any details or facts of the case with anyone other than your attorney and spouse.
- Sign any affidavits outlining care or opinions about injuries or illnesses.
- Change or add to the medical record.

Discovery

During discovery, the attorneys for the defense and the plaintiff build their cases. Expert witnesses are selected, medical records are reviewed, and depositions are taken. Defendants will begin receiving interrogatories (questions that must be answered) and requests for records. Note that peer-review documents are not typically discoverable in this process unless they have been voluntarily disclosed.

As a medical director, you review random charts of your providers and provide feedback on documentation and care. You explain that if something is not documented in the chart, there will be an assumption that it did not happen. Furthermore, in the event of a lawsuit, complaint, or peer review, the chart is the physician's lifeline, describing the clinical decision-making process and detailing the treatment that was provided.

A poorly documented chart looks sloppy, and assumptions will be made that patient care was similarly careless, undermining the clinician's credibility.[5,6] The most important part of the chart, particularly in a failure-to-diagnose claim, is medical decision-making. This information can sway an attorney to pursue or drop a case. It should outline differential diagnoses and justify the care provided.

Dr. Smith feels somewhat reassured that her charting is excellent. Her chart allowed her to see everything she did and revealed what she was thinking two years ago regarding a patient she would not otherwise remember.

The clinician should be actively involved when choosing the defense expert. In about half the states, the expert for the plaintiff must be of the same medical specialty as the defending clinician, but in the remaining states, other specialists are allowed to testify.

When discussing who should review the case as the defense expert, Dr. Smith suggests the chair of the ED where she trained. Her attorney reminds her that the expert cannot be someone she knows well personally or with whom she works, but assures her that there are many prominent emergency physicians who do expert witness work.

As her medical director, you provide names to her defense council upon request. You recognize that the more control the physician feels she has over the process and outcome, the more confident she will be. She also will be less likely to suffer the related ill effects.

After records are obtained and answers are submitted by both parties, depositions are scheduled. These include defense and plaintiff fact witnesses and expert witnesses. With counsel, the defending clinician should determine the plaintiff's strategy while preparing their defense. The plaintiff's approach will be evident in the official lawsuit complaint, where the case theory is outlined. Role-playing and mock testimony with defense counsel or a trial coach may help avoid pitfalls and prepare the defendant clinician.

It has been about eight months since Dr. Smith received notice of her lawsuit. She is anxious and frustrated that there has been so little activity. She then receives notice of her pending deposition and is fearful of the process and result. You (and her attorney) explain to her that this is a long process and that depositions constantly get rescheduled. Courts are full and often cannot schedule a case for up to a year. You encourage her to remain active in her defense. As the scheduled deposition nears, her attorney suggests that she practice her testimony to build her confidence and set her expectations.

Depositions are testimony taken under oath, usually at an attorney's office. These statements can be used in court to make specific points and are sometimes used to demonstrate inconsistencies and even discredit witnesses. The clinician should not be lulled into complacency by an apparently polite and reasonable plaintiff's attorney; that attorney's role is to win their case "against" the defendant clinician.

Dr. Smith has her deposition in the morning, and she is nervous. Her counsel gently explains that the plaintiff's attorney is not using this process to find the truth. Rather, he wants to evaluate how she will come across on the witness stand and possibly trick her into saying things that can impeach her subsequent testimony in trial. She sighs and says, "Yeah, I know. That's what you said when we were practicing for tomorrow. I just wish this would go away."

During the deposition, the plaintiff's attorney may ask the same question multiple times in different ways. The process can be prolonged and tiring. Remember that the plaintiff's attorney has multiple goals, including:

- Establishing inconsistencies in testimony
- Determining the clinician's qualifications, as well as strengths and weaknesses during testimony
- Developing a strategy for trial
- Uncovering previously undisclosed information

The plaintiff's attorney is gathering information that can be used in support of the plaintiff and against the defendant. In other words, they are "digging for pay dirt." Unprepared defendant clinicians may attempt to educate the plaintiff's attorney, thinking that the case will be dropped or dismissed. The clinician must go into the deposition rested and prepared with precise, carefully considered answers.

Defendants and their appointed attorneys should thoroughly review the deposition process and prepare for and role-play testimony. The clinician should spend as much time as needed to review the deposition process and likely lines of attack prior to the deposition. In particular, the defendant clinician should:

- Allow the attorneys to finish asking questions before answering.
- Pause and think before answering.
- Ask the attorney to rephrase any questions that are confusing or poorly worded.
    - It is common to be asked overly broad questions. Don't guess at the intent; ask for clarification. Defendants must avoid giving information that may subsequently be used against them. Remember, the plaintiff's attorney is not a friend.
    - If asked a complex question with multiple components, the clinician should ask the plaintiff's attorney to ask questions "one at a time."
    - Erratic questioning, friendliness, challenging answers, and so on, by the opposing counsel are often devices to throw the clinician "off guard."
    - The plaintiff's counsel may be silent after the clinician's answer, creating discomfort and hoping the defendant will continue to speak. This is another device that is often used to get more information. Be comfortable with silence, and don't speak unless asked a specific question.
- Give concise responses to questions. Avoid making the opposing counsel's job easier. Verbose answers may provide information that allows the attorney to open new doors that the clinician may regret. (When under oath, the answer to "Do you know the time?" is either "Yes" or "No," not "It's 3:46 p.m.")
- Never speculate or offer opinions. The defendant clinician is a fact witness, not an expert witness.
- Maintain composure, show humility, and be respectful. The opposing counsel may purposely attempt to agitate the clinician through intimidation and accusations

("Doctor, do you really expect us to believe . . . ?"). Demonstrating hostility may encourage the plaintiff's attorney to elicit the same response during trial.
- Use the record as reference. Be fully familiar with the case before the deposition. Never try to memorize the record; read from it in answer to specific questions.
- Read the deposition transcript carefully before signing it.

Attorneys typically argue and "object" during the deposition. These comments are really for the record because there is no judge to rule on them at the time. All discussion between attorneys should conclude before the clinician answers. Then, unless specifically instructed by defense council not to answer, the clinician should address the question.

The plaintiff's council will use the deposition to judge how the clinician will present in front of a jury and judge.[7,8] Many depositions are now video recorded. The clinician may find it helpful to participate in a mock video deposition with their attorney to observe comportment, such as eye contact, posture, tone, and expressions. A careful review may expose unintended and unflattering mannerisms.

During the preparation and deposition processes, the clinician should dress professionally, be polite, avoid arrogance, and always tell the truth. These qualities positively influence juries. Preparation is key to feeling comfortable and doing well. **Box 114.2** presents pearls and pitfalls of the discovery process.

> *As the medical director, you meet with Dr. Smith the next evening to talk about how the deposition went. She says it was mentally exhausting, but she felt very good about it because she was prepared, well rested, and felt like she had done everything she could. She also thanks you for the advice you gave her: Prioritize family and friends, and keep life in balance. Simply feeling like she was being supported and not judged by her colleagues has helped to keep her spirits up.*

Alternative Dispute Resolution

Alternative dispute resolution (ADR) may be required before a case can go to trial.[9,10] Typical forms of ADR include mediation and nonbinding arbitration. The court occasionally appoints the arbitrator and/or mediator, and sometimes the person chosen is agreed upon

---

BOX 114.2 ■ DISCOVERY PEARLS AND PITFALLS

DO:
- Prepare and practice.
- Actively participate in the defense.
- Understand that this is a long process.
- Be precise and succinct in answers.
- Dress for success.
- Be polite.
- Think before answering.

DON'T:
- Contact the patient or opposing council.
- Lie.
- Be arrogant or hostile.
- Speculate.
- Offer more than what was asked.

by both parties. If these processes fail to result in a settlement, the case will proceed to trial. If the malpractice contract includes a "consent to settlement" provision, the defendant clinician cannot be forced to settle.[11] In that situation, the malpractice insurer is required to seek the insured's approval prior to settlement.

When obtaining malpractice insurance, the group insisted on a "consent to settlement" provision, ensuring that the individual clinician has the right to determine whether or not to settle a case. Though she believes she provided the standard of care, Dr. Smith is worried that the malpractice insurance company will settle the case because of a bad outcome. You advise her, as does her defense counsel, that she has the final say (if indeed the policy language gives her that right). This information reassures her.

Trial

Insurance carriers typically pay defense costs, settlement or judgment costs, and sometimes compensation for time spent during trial. This insurance policy clause may significantly mitigate litigation stress if the clinician is an independent contractor and is required to take time away from their practice.

Your group is large enough to accommodate the three weeks away from work that Dr. Smith requires for trial. However, she is worried about loss of income because she works as an independent contractor in a relative value unit–based compensation model. You understand that the financial stress associated with the malpractice case could be an additional stressor and tell her that your insurance contract contains the important clause that compensates her for the lost income during trial.

Different jurisdictions have different standards for which a defendant can be held liable for medical malpractice. In most states, the standard is negligence. In some states, such as Texas, it is *gross* negligence. Knowing the standard can be reassuring. The opposing experts' testimonies should be monitored to ensure that they are testifying to the appropriate standard and meeting the ethical guidelines for expert testimony.[12] The defending clinician should remind their defense council to investigate any ethical infractions by the plaintiff's testifying expert.

In most jurisdictions, the trial will occur within a year after the lawsuit or complaint was filed, but sometimes the process can drag on for several years. A malpractice case is a marathon, not a sprint, so be prepared for the long haul. If the case has not been settled, dropped, or dismissed, each side will present their arguments to a judge or jury, who will then determine whether malpractice has occurred. This is the clinician's opportunity to truthfully explain their actions to the judge or jury. The advice of defense attorneys should be followed during trial; they are experienced professionals who understand how to effectively navigate the system.

Composure on the stand is important. The opposing attorney will try to unnerve the defendant in front of the jury. Because juries generally like doctors, whom the view as honest and humble, it is important that the clinician connect with the jurors. The clinician should look at the jury when answering questions and explain things in a way they can understand, just as if speaking to a patient or family member. The best outcomes occur when the jury members think, "This is the kind of doctor I would want if I were in the ED." Clinicians are in control of their testimony and should not allow an attorney to lead their answers. As in a criminal trial, the defendant clinician must be present during the medical malpractice

> **BOX 114.3 ■ TRIAL PEARLS AND PITFALLS**
>
> **DO:**
> - Come prepared and well rested.
> - Stay calm.
> - Dress professionally.
> - Ensure ethical expert testimony.
> - Know the liability standard in your state.
> - Check the record of the plaintiff's medical expert witnesses for any ethics violations.
> - Determine if your insurance contract has a clause that will compensate the physician during trial.
>
> **DON'T:**
> - Be arrogant.
> - Let opposing council lead you.
> - Get flustered by opposing council.

trial the entire time (typically one to three weeks). **Box 114.3** lists the pearls and pitfalls of malpractice trials.

To provide support, you attend Dr. Smith's trial during her testimony. She looks sharp and does an outstanding job of connecting with the jury and coming across as the compassionate, competent emergency physician that she is. You can see the relief on her face when she is done. Now the hard part will be waiting for the jury's decision; but it is coming, and the odds are in her favor.

Damages

If a jury reaches a verdict against the clinician, damages will then be awarded. The amount will depend in part on the jurisdiction where the trial is held, as some states have caps on damages. It will also depend on the makeup of a particular jury. Cases tried in federal court tend to be more predictable and are less likely to result in excessive awards.

The fear of damage awards that exceed the limits of the insurance policy is real. However, this rarely occurs. If the clinician asked to settle within the policy limit prior to judgment but the insurance company refused, there can be a bad faith action against the insurance carrier. Alternatively, if the insurance company requested settlement but the clinician refused, resulting in an excessive award, the insurance company might not be sympathetic. It is rare for clinicians to pay out of pocket for judgments.[4,13]

One of Dr. Smith's biggest fears as this process began was that she could lose her house and personal assets. It was a huge relief to her when you explained that it is extremely rare for this to happen, and there are caps on damages in your jurisdiction.

Settlement can take place at any point in the process, even once the trial has begun. Clinicians may wish to work with a malpractice insurer that does not settle claims without the consent of the defending clinician.

It has been almost three years since you discovered that Dr. Smith had been served with notice of a lawsuit. You meet with Dr. Smith and her husband at her favorite restaurant, where you are greeted with a glass of champagne. She informs you that her defense team won the case, and she thanks you for all of the support and guidance that not only helped her win but also allowed her to continue to give outstanding patient care.

Any settlement, regardless of dollar amount, will result in a report to the National Practitioner Data Bank (NPDB).[14] These records are maintained permanently in the NPDB files and will follow the defendant clinician indefinitely. Depending on the number and nature of these reports, they may have an impact on job availability, insurance coverage or rates, and credentialing.

Because Dr. Smith won her defense, she will not be reported to the NPDB. You all toast to her successful navigation through the difficult process of the malpractice system.

CONCLUSION

Lawsuits are an unfortunate part of doing business. In order to best support their team members, ED leaders must understand the malpractice process and how being sued might affect a clinician's ability to provide confident patient care. Determine if the malpractice insurance contract includes a consent-to-settle clause and provides compensation in case of a lengthy trial. Educate your team members on the importance of documentation, and caution them that after-the-fact changes to the medical record should never be made. Share what to do when being sued or given legal notice, and remind defendant clinicians to limit discussions about their case to only their attorney and spouse. Monitor the wellness of the provider who has been sued, and look for patient or staff complaints as a possible sign of distress. Encourage active engagement in the defense process. Urge the provider to prioritize family, friends, and work-life balance. Finally, reiterate that lawsuits are a predictable threat in the practice of emergency medicine.

REFERENCES

1. Guardado JR. Medical liability claim frequency among US physicians. American medical association. 2017. Available at: https://www.semanticscholar.org/paper/Policy-Research-Perspectives-Medical-Liability-U-.-Guardado/88a23279a327c110dc67e325c158ef7050098eea. Accessed October 1, 2020.
2. Charles SC. Coping with a medical malpractice suit. *West J Med.* 2001;174(1):55–58.
3. Brown TW, McCarthy ML, Kelen GD, et al. An epidemiologic study of closed emergency department malpractice claims in a national database of physician malpractice insurers. *Acad Emerg Med.* 2010;17(5):553–560.
4. Kern SI. Alter the records, bad idea. *Medical Economics.* May 18, 2007.
5. Medical charting errors can drive patient liability suits. *American Medical News.* March 25, 2013. Available at: https://amednews.com/article/20130325/profession/130329979/5/. Accessed December 31, 2019.
6. Butler M. Preventing healthcare's top four documentation disasters. *J AHIMA.* 2015;86(7):18–23.
7. Devine DJ, Caughlin DE. Do they matter? A meta-analytic investigation of individual characteristics and guilt judgments. *Psychol Public Policy Law.* 201;20(2):109–134.
8. Judice MW. The defendant physician at trial. 2011. Available at: https://www.judice-adley.com/Articles/Article1.html?id=2544. Accessed December 31, 2019.
9. Sohn DH, Bal BS. Medical malpractice reform: the role of alternative dispute resolution. *Clin Orthop Relat Res.* 2012;470(5):1370–1378.
10. Radic Z, Roncevic A, Yongqiang L. Alternative dispute resolution in medical malpractice disputes. In: *The Legal Challenges of Modern World, Book of Proceedings;* 2018:233–242. Available at: https://papers.ssrn.com/sol3/papers.cfm?abstract_id=3213596. Accessed January 2, 2020.
11. Armon B, Beidel JL. Consent to settle: who decides? *Legal Matters.* 2010. Available at: https://journal.practicelink.com/legal-matters/consent-to-settle-who-decides/2/. Accessed January 2, 2020.
12. American College of Emergency Physicians. Policy statement: expert witness guidelines for the specialty of emergency medicine. Available at: https://www.acep.org/patient-care/policy-statements/expert-witness-guidelines-for-the-specialty-of-emergency-medicine/. Accessed December 30, 2019. Revised June, 2015.
13. American College of Emergency Physicians. So you have been sued! An information paper. https://www.acep.org/globalassets/uploads/uploaded-files/acep/clinical-and-practice-management/resources/medical-legal/so-you-have-been-sued.pdf. Revised May 2019.
14. National Practitioner Data Bank. Available at: https://www.npdb.hrsa.gov/. Accessed January 2, 2020. Updated 2019.

CHAPTER 115

EXPERT WITNESS: TELLING THE STORY OF THE CASE

Thom A. Mayer

All sorrows can be borne if you can put them into a story or tell a story about them.

—Isak Dinesen (nee Baroness Karin von Blixen)[1]

Do any of you have any questions for my answers?

—Secretary of State Henry Kissinger, addressing reporters at a press conference[2]

The threat of a malpractice suit is one of the most intimidating aspects of the practice of emergency medicine and nursing, hanging like the sword of Damocles over the daily care of patients. Fortunately, while the literature is very clear that most emergency physicians and nurses will not be sued during their careers, a small percentage of providers are involved in an inordinate number of suits. Data from the National Practitioner Data Bank from 1992 to 2014 indicate that the malpractice claim rate decreased 56%, from 20 to nine claims per 1,000 physician years of practice.[3] Emergency department (ED) claims also decreased, although at a lesser rate of 47%, from 24 to 13 claims per 1,000 physician years. However, payments for successful claims in EDs increased 26%, from $249,000 to $314,000. Half of claims filed were for wrongful death and most alleged failure to adequately diagnose.[3]

With the number of claims falling and the average payments rising, the threat of a malpractice suits still looms large for EDs.

BASIC ELEMENTS OF MALPRACTICE

Professional liability suits involving EDs are typically referred to as "malpractice suits," which are a form of tort law, pitting claims alleged by an aggrieved party, the "plaintiff" for actions (or failure to act) on the part of those whose duty it was to provide the care (the "defendant").[4] While criminal law requires that allegations be proven "beyond a reasonable doubt," tort law typically states that liability generally must be proven as "more likely than not." Some states have statutes, like Georgia's, which has been tested by the Georgia Supreme Court, requiring patients who file a medical malpractice claim arising from ED care to provide "clear and convincing evidence" that the medical provider's actions "showed gross negligence." This statute is interpreted to mean that the provider failed to "exercise even a slight degree of care."[5] However, most states retain some version of the "more likely than not" standard.

While each state has their own vagaries governing professional liability cases, all states have four fundamental requirements for the plaintiff to prove in a malpractice case[6]: duty, breach of standard of care, causation, and damages.

Patients presenting to the ED generally are cared for by a team of physicians, nurses, ED staff, essential services (laboratory, imaging services, etc.), and, depending upon the condition, consultants who care for the patient. Malpractice suits generically name the physician, nurse, hospital, and consultant, based on the facts and nature of the suit. For many plaintiffs' attorneys, this process of casting a wide net is meant to, at best, name all possible plaintiffs while in the process of discovery and, at worst, seek to pit providers against each other in the process of evidence gathering and depositions. ("What I did was great, but what the nurse/doc/hospital/consultant did was the problem!")

Duty

In most cases, but not all, a *duty* to evaluate and appropriately treat the patient is present in ED cases. However, as will be discussed in more detail later, the story of the case is an important part of establishing duty in deposition or trial testimony:

Plaintiff's attorney: *"Doctor, isn't it true that you had a duty to treat Mrs. Jones?"*

Doctor: *"Sir, I treat all my patients with a commitment not only to my duty to treat any and all patients who present to the ED, regardless of the time of day or night and without any consideration of their ability to pay for their services, but also with the professionalism and courtesy they deserve, as I did with Mrs. Jones."*

In this case, the defense attorney and the doctor had answers well prepared, reflecting Kissinger's wisdom (noted above).

Breach of Duty

Breach of duty revolves around establishing that the provider failed to provide the "standard of care," which is generally defined as exercising the requisite skill, care, and knowledge that a reasonably well-qualified practitioner in the same specialty with the same resources in the same setting would apply in the same or similar circumstances. It is critical to note that the standard of care is *not:*

- Perfect care
- Ideal care
- Care that the author of the latest journal article recommends
- Care the chairman of the academic ED recommends to her residents
- Care that is delineated in the newest edition of an emergency medicine or nursing textbook
- Care that results in the best outcome
- Care that, on reflection, you wish you had provided

When named in a malpractice suit, the attorney will advise more specifically on the definition of "standard of care" as it applies in the state in which the case occurred, but it is important at the outset to have a fundamental understanding of the principles listed above.

Causation

If indeed there was a duty to provide care and assuming there was a breach of the standard of care (that a reasonable clinician would have provided in similar circumstances with similar resources), it must still be proved that the breach actually was responsible for *causing* any ensuing damages. Causation is usually referred to as "actual" or "proximate." Actual causation typically is referred to as the "but for" test, meaning that "but for" the alleged negligence, the injury would not have occurred. For example:

Assume a patient has fallen on his or her outstretched hand and presents with wrist pain, and the emergency physician fails to read the radiograph correctly as a displaced scaphoid fracture. Nonetheless, the physician refers the patient to the orthopedic surgeon for follow-up in 2 days, where the fracture is correctly diagnosed and surgery is performed.

In this case, there would not be actual causation in that the surgery would have had to be performed anyway, regardless of whether the diagnosis is made in the ED or several days later. However, given the same circumstances and a failure to refer to the orthopedic surgeon, if the patient presents 6 months later with osteonecrosis of the scaphoid that requires more extensive surgery, actual causation might be established.

Proximate causation establishes a direct temporal relationship between the alleged deviation from standard of care and the patient's injury.

Damages

If indeed there was a duty to provide care and assuming there was a breach of the standard of care, it must still be proved that the patient or the family suffered economic, noneconomic, or punitive damages *as a result of* (causation) the breach of the standard of care. Economic damages are the financial losses the patient or family incur and typically include medical bills, lost wages, or cost of future medical care. Noneconomic damages are typically "pain and suffering," words at which anyone who has been sued cringes but they are a part of legal practice and parlance. Punitive damages are typically reserved for only the most egregious of cases, in which the jury determines that there was a particularly gross case of negligence or wanton disregard for the patient's welfare.

DEFINING AN EXPERT WITNESS

Simply stated, an expert witness is someone permitted to testify at trial or in deposition because of special knowledge or proficiency in the area alleged to be the subject of malpractice. In ED malpractice cases, these "expert witnesses" might include those with expertise in emergency medicine, emergency nursing, ED operational issues, or consultants claiming to have expertise in these areas.

Once selected, an expert witness is expected to give her or his opinion, to a reasonable degree of medical certainty, regarding the care provided to the patient. They would typically explain: "What happened?" and "What should have happened?"

As will be discussed in more detail, the ability to tell the story of the case in a way the jurors can understand is as much a function of communication skills, trust, and believability as it is a function of the innate intelligence or knowledge of the expert witness.

Daubert Definitions and Challenges

The courts have increasingly determined the validity and admissibility of how an expert witness' testimony may be governed. The Daubert Challenge (1993) is a hearing conducted before the judge where the expert is required to demonstrate that his or her methodology, reasoning, and expertise are scientifically valid and can be applied to the facts of the case. There are five determinative factors:

- The method used can or has been tested.
- The method's known potential rate of error is acceptable.

- The method has been subjected to peer review.
- The method is controlled by generally accepted standards.
- The method has general acceptance within the relevant scientific community.

The term "Daubert Challenge" is eponymous and is derived from the 1993 US Supreme Court case *Daubert v Merrell Dow Pharmaceuticals, Inc. (509 US 579, 1993)* in which the five criteria were enumerated.[7] While a formal Daubert Challenge may not occur in a medical malpractice case, these are the five general criteria used. To be clear, in most cases, an experienced emergency physician involved in clinical practice will qualify as an expert witness in most jurisdictions.

THE THEORY OF THE CASE

One of the most important first steps in understanding what happened in a medical malpractice case is to develop a cogent "theory of the case." Both sides will try to develop a reasoned approach that is supported by the facts of the care provided and the time lines in which that care occurred. In other words, the set of facts, carefully considered and properly organized, highlights the four necessary elements of a malpractice case—duty, breach, causation, and damages—particularly breach of standard of care.

> *The theory of the case is a delineation of the factual details of the patient's presentation, the medical facts of the case, the time line in which they occurred, with the care and treatment overlaid against them.*

Both the plaintiff and the defense teams will each have their respective theory of the case, and they will share certain facts but will differ dramatically in the conclusions drawn from those facts. However, whether one is named in a malpractice suit or is acting as an expert witness, it is wise to develop not only one's own theory of the case but consider that of the opposing team as well, since this allows a better understanding of what to expect in deposition or at trial.

How the theory of the case and the story of the case relate is discussed below, but for now, think in these terms. The *theory* of the case includes factual details about the patient's presentation, medical data, diagnostic workup, and treatment within a time line. The *story* of the case uses those factual details to explain, "Here's what happened and why it happened and why this is good medical care."

To effectively develop a theory of the case supported by the known facts, it is necessary to follow these steps:

1. Make a detailed time line/spreadsheet of all the pertinent facts of the case. (This may be done using a roll of paper, because there are typically many details in even the simplest of cases.)
2. Define how those facts and the time line lead to a cogent theory of the case.
3. Correlate the theory of the case to duty, breach of standard of care, causation, and damages.
4. Consider what the opposing counsel and expert witness will allege as their theory of the case.

Creating a Detailed Time Line

Modern day medical records are long, often duplicative, separated into sections according to nursing, physician, pharmacy, laboratory, imaging, and so on. Further, in many cases, the electronic medical record makes it difficult to organize all the facts into a single cohesive flow of care in which the information can be viewed in context. For those and other reasons, it is necessary to make a detailed time line/spreadsheet in which all the pertinent facts of the case can be seen in one place and in context with all the other facts.

Use a roll of white paper laid out on a long table, upon which all these details from the myriad sources of the medical record (and information from depositions of witnesses, where available) can be captured. This method not only allows a visual representation of the facts but also helps place them in context within the time line. Others use a spreadsheet or pieces of paper. Regardless of the specific method, this is designed to capture all the pertinent factual details into a time line. For example:

> *An 8-year-old child was struck by an automobile and was resuscitated at a level III trauma center. During the care of this pediatric trauma patient, several sets of vital signs were obtained and recorded on the nursing flow sheet or the trauma flow sheet. The nursing and medical records showed that the child presented hypotensive (BP 80/40) and tachycardic (P 170). The emergency physician quickly obtained two intravenous lines and administered 20 mL/kg of isotonic fluid, after which several sets of vital signs showed the blood pressure rising to 105/60 and the pulse slowing to 100. Arrangements were made for transport to a level I pediatric trauma center for definitive care. After arrival, the patient became hypotensive and tachycardic and was taken to the operating room by the pediatric surgeon, where the right lobe of the liver was resected. The child did well, despite several weeks of hospitalization.*

A detailed review of the medical record revealed that just prior to transport, the emergency physician noted in his medical record that the child's heart rate rose to 135. (This information was not noted on the trauma flow sheet.) Instead of assuming this was due to anxiety, he gave a second bolus of 20 mL/kg of isotonic fluid, to be continued by the transport team, whose notes also reflected this.

The plaintiff's attorney and their expert witness (a pediatric emergency physician) alleged that the ED team—and the emergency physician specifically—deviated from the standard of care by *not* demanding that the local surgeon operate on the patient (despite the fact that the local surgeon had no training or experience in the care of pediatric trauma patients). They then concluded that this "misstep" resulted in a prolonged hospitalization, high costs, and complications. Their theory of the case is thus dramatically different from that of the defense team and their expert witness.

Far from breaching the standard of care, the emergency physician very astutely noted that while the child was not hypotensive after initial fluid resuscitation, the child did subsequently develop tachycardia and the emergency physician aggressively infused fluids, probably saving the child's life. However, the development of a clear time line showing this increase in heart rate extracted from the physician's notes, though not on the trauma flow sheet, supports the facts and the time line in which they occurred, as well as the entirely appropriate care provided by the referring emergency physician.

Defining a Cogent Theory of the Case

Once the facts and data are captured in one place, the records and depositions should be reviewed to ensure that all the pertinent components of the care provided have been captured. Overlay important information from the depositions on the time line. Then, the team should consider:

- What conclusions can be drawn regarding the theory of the case?
- What do the facts and the data indicate?
- What's missing? Are there pieces of data which should be there but aren't? If not, why not?

In reviewing the data, it will usually become clear what the theory of the case is likely to be. For example, one may think, "This is a patient presenting with atypical chest pain who was recognized and appropriately worked up for an acute coronary syndrome (ACS)." In that case:

- Are all the facts present and represented? If not, what's missing? Why?
- Did the ED have a policy or evidence-based guideline for the workup of ACS? If so, where is it, and how does it relate to the theory of the case?
- How do the depositions of the emergency physician and nurse relate to this theory of the case?"

Correlating the Theory of the Case

The total review of the facts and the depositions then need to be related to each of the four elements necessary to prove a malpractice case. In the pediatric trauma case above, the plaintiff's attorney argued that the standard of care was for a pediatric emergency physician, and she used one as her standard expert. However, the initial care of the child occurred in a general ED, so the standard of care was for a general emergency physician and the standard was, "what a reasonable general emergency physician would have done faced with similar circumstances and with similar resources." (And a general surgeon in a community hospital would likely not have agreed to operate on this child.)

Considering Opposing Viewpoints

Finally, it is wise to consider the facts and use them to anticipate what the opposing counsel and expert witness will allege at deposition and at trial. The filings on the malpractice suit typically outline the allegations in great detail. However, the facts and additional details should be reviewed with an open mind to determine which ones support or conflict with the theory of the case. Once the allegations are understood:

- What facts support their theory of the case?
- Which facts contradict their theory of the case?
- And how can these facts be used to tell "the story of the case"?

THE STORY OF THE CASE

In many ways, the theory of the case is what the facts are and the sequence in which those facts occurred. This information provides a frame in which to organize the picture. The story of the case is what it "means," the picture itself:

- What happened?
- Why did it happen that way?
- What does all the medical language mean (to a jury)?
- What do the facts imply with regard to standard of care, placed in context?

Far from simply saying, "The standard of care was met," telling the story of the case makes it meaningful to a jury of peers. Jurors often become confused, not just by the mind-numbing barrage of facts thrown at them but also by the fact they are being told two completely different versions of the case by the plaintiff's attorneys and by the defense.

Effective expert witnesses understand this dichotomy and have the capacity to use the facts (theory) to tell the jury the story of what actually happened and what it means. That requires *credibility* and *believability*, which is another way of saying it requires *skill* and *trust*. Juries understand statements like these:

> *There have been a lot of confusing facts thrown at you, but here's what really happened . . .*

> *Here's how to make sense of all these facts . . .*

> *It's my opinion, based upon a reasonable degree of medical certainty and based on the facts of the case, that Dr. Smith not only met but exceeded the standard of care by . . .*

Matt Hasselback was a Pro Bowl quarterback for 17 years in the NFL before building a highly successful career as a studio analyst for ESPN. When congratulated on how effective he was at making complex football issues understandable on air, he said:

> *Thanks, Doc. I just imagine I'm talking to my grandma and telling her the story of the game in a way she can understand*[8]

Effective expert witnesses are similarly successful precisely because of their ability to tell the story of the case. Another way of thinking of it is to consider the best teacher one ever had, how they taught, why they were loved, and why so much was learned from them. As an expert witness, it is necessary to become that best teacher when telling the story of the case. From the perspective of the emergency physicians and nurses, the expert witness creates a picture of what it was it like in the ED. In general, the story should not be based on the latest journal article but rather on the actual experience in the daily practice of emergency medicine or nursing when treating patients like the one in question. The picture should be about *people*—the patient first and foremost—and also the ED staff, who are dedicated to getting it right.

Perhaps the best way to illustrate the concept of the story of the case is through examples taken from real cases.

Case One: Chest Pain

The plaintiff's attorney and their expert witness had the following theory and story of the case.

> *A 65-year-old man was shoveling snow just prior to the Christmas holidays when he developed chest pain that radiated to the jaw. He went to the ED. Despite this history, an electrocardiogram (ECG) was not obtained, but instead cervical spine radiographs were ordered. He was discharged on opiate pain medication. The patient had a cardiac arrest in the hospital parking lot after leaving the ED and could not be resuscitated.*

The ED care might at first appear indefensible. The case was filed for statutory limits as well as punitive damages. In fact, no one would take the case as a defense expert, based on the plaintiff's attorney and expert's version of events.

However, a detailed review of the facts of the case, including reading the depositions of the emergency physician, nurses, and family members, led to a different theory and story of the case. The gentleman was in fact not shoveling snow but was working on a snowblower inside his heated garage, when he jerked hard on a wrench and developed radicular pain in his neck, not his jaw, which transiently went down his arm.

In the ED, he was extremely adamant that he had neck pain, not chest pain, and had had a full cardiac workup one month earlier, which was negative. The family admitted that he was a bit obstreperous and "set in his ways," but he maintained: "Doc, this isn't my chest. I know what that feels like." He refused an ECG and any further cardiac workup.

On completion of this further review, the theory and story of the case are completely different. While there were still potential problems with the defense of the case, the actual case and the way it transpired are completely different than the original story, which could only be known by taking a fresh look at the case, detailing the time line, and putting the facts into the correct context. The case settled out of court.

Case Two: Missed Aneurysm

The plaintiff's attorney and their expert witness had the following theory and story of the case:

> *A 28-year-old woman with a past history of complex congenital heart disease (double-outlet right ventricle with pulmonary stenosis requiring a Rastelli procedure as a child) presented to the ED with a chief complaint of chest pain "not like anything I have ever felt before." Vital signs, including heart rate, were all normal, including four separate readings. The patient underwent a detailed workup in the ED, including a computed tomography angiogram (CTA). The final report of the CTA showed a "new aneurysm at the base of the aortic root." Despite this finding, the patient was discharged from the ED with instructions to follow up with her cardiologist in 3 to 4 days. The patient died at home 2 days later.*

Again, the theory and story of this case seems to point to a serious lapse of care in which the emergency physician failed to provide appropriate care and clearly violated the standard of care. On initial review, "the story" appeared accurate. However, the story is illogical. Why would an emergency physician who had ordered a CTA showing a newly developed aneurysm fail to either admit the patient or at the least consult cardiovascular surgery?

This implausible discharge naturally leads to the question: "Did the emergency physician actually know the results of the CTA?" The physician and nurses' depositions made clear that they recalled the patient but did not recall the results of the CTA. The radiology records showed the "final read" of the CTA, but no record of a "wet read." The defense team asked several times for the "wet read," but it could not be found.

It was determined that there must have been a wet read, because there was a policy in place at that time and there was even a specific written form for wet reads at that hospital. An additional, in-depth search of the medical records *did* uncover a wet read that included, "No aneurysm noted." In retrospect, that wet read is the information upon which the emergency physician based his decision, even though he had no independent recollection of the wet read itself.

When the story does not make sense, it is necessary to dig deeper into the facts, including the communication processes. In this case, discovering what did and did not happen immediately changed the story of the case and made it clear that this was a radiology malpractice suit, not an ED malpractice case. In fact, the ED personnel were released from the case immediately, and it was settled by the radiologist who performed the wet read.

AN APPROACH TO PLAINTIFF'S EXPERTS

Plaintiff's expert witnesses typically do not have a positive reputation among emergency physicians and nurses who often feel such witnesses are unfairly criticizing their care. A disciplined approach should be taken to consideration of the plaintiff's expert's opinion.

Suspend Belief

It is important to recognize that "expert" witnesses do not always offer a professional opinion that is consistent with the standard of care. In fact, there is, in effect, an entire industry of plaintiff's experts willing to testify, seemingly to almost anything. While there are disingenuous "experts," there are also many principled, thoughtful experts whose honest opinion is that the standard of care in specific cases has been breached.

That said, it beggars the imagination to hear or read what some so-called expert witnesses have said to support their opinions. Here are a few expert witness testimonies:

Delay-in-care case: *"All ED patients should be seen within 5 minutes of arrival!"*

Failure-to-administer thrombolytic medication case: *"Yes, the thrombolytic window exceeded 3 hours, but the symptoms changed and the window 'reopened!'"*

Georgia ED case: *"Without question this is gross and willful negligence . . . the worst I have ever seen!"*

Plaintiff's experts may genuinely believe that standard of care has been breached. However, disreputable experts will say whatever is necessary to tailor their opinions and testimony to the case.

Start Calm, Stay Calm

While it varies by jurisdiction, in many cases, the defendant may choose to attend the plaintiff's witnesses' depositions. The defense attorney will advise on whether he or she feels this is a good idea or not, because it may be viewed as an attempt to intimidate or unduly influence the witness. The advantage of attending is that it can be highly effective at reducing excessive claims of deviation from standard of care or claims of gross and willful negligence. If advised to attend the deposition, stay calm and restrained, including your body language and other nonverbal communication. The plaintiff's attorney will be watching very closely for clues on how best to depose the defendant. The defense attorney will already have shared (with the defendant) the general line of questioning he or she will use in deposing the plaintiff's experts.

This will be one of the most difficult experiences of one's professional life. Prepare for it, stay calm in the storm, but expect to be upset or even depressed at times, as it is common to feel that one is being accused of being a "bad doctor."

American College of Emergency Physicians Resources

In recognition of the importance of expert witness testimony, the American College of Emergency Physicians (ACEP) Board of Directors has taken a strong and positive stance on the issue of appropriate testimony. Beginning in 1990 and every five years since, ACEP has published a policy statement that delineates criteria by which an expert witness should be judged, as well as an "Expert Witness Reaffirmation Statement."[10]

Expert Witness Guidelines for the Specialty of Emergency Medicine

In addition to board certification in emergency medicine, ACEP's "Expert Witness Guidelines for the Specialty of Emergency Medicine" require experts to have been in "active clinical practice of emergency medicine for at least 3 years (exclusive of training) immediately preceding the date of the occurrence giving rise to the case." This helps prevent physicians or professionals from other specialties opining as to standards of care in the ED.

The guidelines also are clear that emergency physicians should not engage in advertising that contains "false or deceptive representations about the physician's qualifications, experience, titles, or background."

Both the guidelines and ACEP's "Expert Witness Reaffirmation" statement (see Appendix 1 at the end of this chapter) indicate that expert witnesses should be willing to submit their testimony to peer review, which is a very powerful tool to help avoid capricious and misleading testimony. In fact, ACEP has censured several emergency physicians, including prominent and well-known "experts," due to their testimony.

Expert Witness Reaffirmation

ACEP's "Expert Witness Reaffirmation" statement provides an additional tool that has been helpful in defending malpractice cases.[10] Experts should be asked to sign this statement as a part of their deposition and/or testimony. While all of elements are important, item numbers 3 and 9 are critical. They state:

> 3. *I will provide evidence or testify only in matters in which I have sufficient clinical experience and knowledge in the areas of medicine that are the subject of the case or proceeding.*
>
> 9. *I will submit my testimony to peer review, if requested by a professional organization to which I belong.*

For example, a recent case involved care provided in the ED of a level I trauma center. In deposition, it was determined that the plaintiff's expert, who had signed the reaffirmation form, had never practiced in a trauma center of any kind since his residency training, 20 years earlier. His testimony was excluded.

Affirming that the testimony will be subject to peer review can have a powerful impact, effectively sending the message that one can say whatever they choose, but not with impunity.

Whether acting as a defense expert or as a defendant in a malpractice suit, it is wise to ensure that the defense attorney is aware of both ACEP's expert witness statements. For those offering testimony as an expert, it is important to make a point of signing the reaffirmation statement, which effectively challenges any all other experts to do so as well.

AN APPROACH TO DEFENSE EXPERTS

Just as there should be a disciplined approach to the testimony of plaintiff's experts, the same discipline should be applied to defense experts.

Just as it is hoped that the plaintiff's experts will not tailor their testimony to make the case against a defendant, neither should the defense expert be expected to agree 100% with everything that was done (or not done) in a given case. Instead, the defense experts' role is to render an opinion on the case, particularly about the standard of care. In most but not all cases, the defense expert will have had the opportunity to review the depositions of the defendants, the patient or family, and often the plaintiff's experts as well. This information gives him or her the chance to truly develop both the theory of the case (the facts and time line) and the story of the case (what happened, why, and what it means, in full context).

In selecting defense experts, credibility is key, as is the ability to tell the story to the jury in a clear and compelling fashion. That doesn't necessarily mean they are the person who has written the most on the subject, is the chair of an academic ED, or has the longest curriculum vitae. It does mean they are likely to be believable; someone others are likely to trust when clarifying the details of the often confusing elements of patient care.

One of the best ways to determine if an expert witness is likely to be believable and trusted is to speak with attorneys and physicians who have worked with the expert in the past. Don't expect to speak directly with the defense expert; that rarely happens and only in extremely limited circumstances. But do feel free to communicate your thoughts to your defense attorney, because that helps him or her defend your case in the most effective manner.

CONCLUSION

The four elements of a professional liability malpractice suit are duty to treat, breach of that duty (deviation from standard of care), damages, and causation (damage attributable to the breach). An expert witness is someone permitted to testify at trial or in deposition because of special knowledge or proficiency in the area alleged to be the subject of malpractice. The "theory of the case" is a delineation of the factual details of the patient's presentation, the medical facts of the case, the time line in which they occurred, with the care and treatment overlaid against them. "The story of the case" is not just the facts, but what those facts mean in the context in which the care was provided. It is a picture of what happened, why it happened that way, what all the complex medical care and language mean, and what it all means in relation to the standard of care. Far from simply saying, "The standard of care was met," telling the story of the case makes it meaningful to a jury of peers.

When confronted with testimony from the plaintiff's experts, be prepared to suspend belief (will the expert be honorable and rational?). Start calm and stay calm. Use the ACEP expert witness guidelines and the reaffirmation statement to limit the impact of the plaintiff's experts. In selecting defense experts, credibility is key, as is the ability to tell the story to the jury in a clear and compelling fashion. The defense expert needs to be able to combine the theory of the case (the facts) with the story of the case (what the facts mean).

APPENDIX 115.1: EXPERT WITNESS REAFFIRMATION

As a member of the medical profession and the ACEP, I hereby affirm my duty, when giving evidence or testifying as an expert witness, to do so solely in accordance with the merits of the case. Furthermore, I declare that I will uphold the following professional principles in providing expert evidence or expert witness testimony.

1. I will always be truthful, and I will abide by the Code of Ethics of the ACEP.
2. I will conduct a thorough, fair, and impartial review of the facts and the medical care provided, including any and all relevant information.
3. I will provide evidence or testify only in matters in which I have sufficient clinical experience and knowledge in the areas of medicine that are the subject of the case or proceeding.
4. I will evaluate the medical care provided in light of generally accepted clinical standards, neither condemning performance that falls within generally accepted practice standards nor condoning performance that falls below these standards.
5. I will evaluate the medical care provided in light of the generally accepted standards that prevailed at the time and the negligence standard of the jurisdiction of the occurrence giving rise to the case.
6. I will provide evidence or testimony that is complete, objective, scientifically based, and likely to assist in achieving a just resolution of the proceeding.
7. I will make a clear distinction in my testimony between a departure from accepted practice standards and an untoward outcome.
8. I will make every effort to determine and to specify whether I believe there is a causal relationship between any substandard practice and the medical outcome.
9. I will submit my testimony to peer review, if requested by a professional organization to which I belong.
10. I will not accept compensation that is contingent upon the outcome of the litigation.

Name _____

Signature _____

APPENDIX 115.2: PERSONAL REFLECTIONS ON BEING AN EFFECTIVE EXPERT WITNESS

It's been my privilege to have been a defense expert witness several times, defending the care of excellent emergency physicians and nurses, and working with very principled and talented defense attorneys. Very often, I receive cases that others have declined to defend, as indicated in some of the case examples. What follows here are the tips I give to physicians who want to diversify into expert witness work, but these tips also apply to those who find themselves as defendants and want to ensure they have the best expert witnesses for their case.

As I noted at the outset, I am not a lawyer, and I don't play one on TV. Being an expert witness has comprised less than 5% of my total work. But I did handle all risk management and defense expert selection for my group, BestPractices, for over 25 years. The following are my thoughts:

- If you've done one case, you've done one case. Each case is different and should be treated as such.
- Keep an open mind. Don't enter any case with preconceived ideas or opinions. If you do, you will only see what you thought you would see.
- Tell the story of the case, making it from both the patient's and the providers' perspectives.
- Make every attempt to distill the story into four to five short sentences.
- Be prepared to say, "I'm glad you asked that because this is so important to understanding what really happened . . ." (Remember Kissinger.)
- Never forget that bad outcomes do not equate to bad care.
- Look at the jury. Make eye contact.
- You "read" your patients all the time. Use those skills to "read" the jurors' reactions to your story.
- Be the best teacher you ever had. Teach, but don't lecture to them.
- Don't argue—ever. Lawyers argue; witnesses testify.
- Don't get angry, but there might be an opportunity to get even.
- Be calm, even when they aren't. Stay calm, especially when the opposing lawyer becomes obnoxious or argumentative. The judge and jury will see how composed you are.
- When an attorney asks if you are being paid for your testimony, tell them, "I'm not paid for my opinion. My opinion is not for sale. I'm paid for my time, just as you are."
- Don't try to memorize everything, just pertinent details, context, and the story of the case.
- Refer to the record when needed—no one expects you to have a photographic memory, plus it demonstrates that good doctors refer and defer to their documentation.
- Don't advertise your services as an expert witness.
- Don't discuss the specific details of a specific case with your colleagues. You will be asked if you have discussed the case with anyone when you are at deposition and trial.
- In making standard-of-care determinations, ask yourself: "Is that the way I would do it 100% of the time?" If the answer is yes, it's likely to be standard of care. If the answer is no, it probably isn't, even if it is excellent medical care.
- Take as much time as you need to understand the question.
- If the question is vague to you, it will be vague to the jury. Get clarity before answering.

- Think before answering, even if you think you know what they are going to ask before they ask it.
- Don't talk over the lawyers. Let them finish.
- Don't necessarily accept opposing counsel's statements, particularly when they ask you to "accept the following fact pattern." (I once answered a plaintiff's attorney by saying, "Just to be clear, you would like me to accept a fact pattern that has no bearing whatsoever on the facts of *this case*?")
- Use short declarative sentences in the active voice whenever possible.
- If you are handed a document, study it carefully before answering (especially if you think you know what the document is).
- Don't hesitate to correct mistakes if you have misspoken.
- Don't ever say, "To tell the truth..." or "To be honest..." It makes you sound like the rest of the time you might not have been telling the truth.
- If you don't know, say so. Don't apologize for what you don't know.

REFERENCES

1. Dinesen I. In an interview with Mohn B. *The New York Times Book Review*. November 3, 1957.
2. Kissinger H. *World Order*. New York, NY: Penguin; 2014.
3. Schaffer AC, Jena AB, Seabury SA, et al. Rates and characteristics of paid malpractice claims among US physicians by specialty, 1992–2014. *JAMA Intern Med*. 2017. Available at: http://dx.doi.org/10.1001/jamainternmed.2017.0311. Accessed September 29, 2020.
4. Brown TW, McCarthy MC, Kelen GD, et al. An epidemiologic study of closed emergency department claims in a national database of physician malpractice insurers. *Acad Emerg Med*. 2010 May; 17(5):553–560.
5. Georgia Code § 51-1-27.
6. Karcz A, Korn R, Burke MC, et al. Malpractice claims against emergency physicians in Massachusetts: 1975–1993. *Am J Emerg Med*. 1996;14(4):341–345.
7. Daubert v. Merrell Dow Pharmaceuticals, Inc. (509 US 579, 1993).
8. Hasselback M. Personal communication to the author, September 12, 2019.
9. American College of Emergency Physicians Policy Statement. Expert Witness Guidelines for the Specialty of Emergency Medicine. 2015. Available at: https://www.acep.org/globalassets/new-pdfs/policy-statements/expert-witness-guidelines-for-the-specialty-of-emergency-medicine.pdf. Accessed September 29, 2020.
10. American College of Emergency Physicians Reaffirmation Statement. 2015. Available at: https://www.acep.org/globalassets/uploads/uploaded-files/acep/clinical-and-practice-management/resources/medical-legal/expert-witness/board-approved---expert-witness-reaffirmation---6-15.pdf?_t_id=s_yGUswORhc9StQ823xZag==&_t_q=Approved&_t_tags=andquerymatch, language: en%7Clanguage:7D2DA0A9FC754533B091FA6886A51C0D, siteid:3f8e28e9-ff05-45b3-977a-68a85dcc834a%7Csiteid:84BFAF5C 52A349A0BC61A9FFB6983A66&_t_ip=&_t_hit.id=ACP_Website_Application_Models_Media_DocumentMedia/_460ebd9e-0515-46c6-a993-eb935ce764b1&_t_hit.pos=3. Accessed September 29, 2020.

CHAPTER 116

MEDICAL DEFENSE EXPERTS: A DEFENSE ATTORNEY'S PERSPECTIVE

Mark M. Jones

To be involved in a medical malpractice case is to experience a powerful life drama. In the aftermath of an unfortunate—and probably unexpected—patient outcome, a lawsuit may be used to challenge a defendant physician's skills, reputation, and possibly finances. The plaintiffs' attorneys may be aggressive and seemingly outraged at the defendant physician's conduct. Likewise, the defendant physician is faced with powerful feelings, including anger, worry, sadness, embarrassment, and guilt.

While plaintiffs are often tremendously sympathetic, the stories they tell are inherently incomplete. The primary role of the defense expert is to tell the *rest* of that story by illuminating the risk-laden medical issues that require the wise application of science and a commitment to doing the right thing for every patient. The defense attorney's job is to facilitate the expression of that story—a nearly impossible task without an expert witness who is fully engaged in the effort.

FIRST STEPS

When first contacted by a defense attorney, it is important for the expert to glean details about the expected timeline of litigation, including the following:

- Upcoming deadlines, such as when the *initial review* should be completed
- When a *written opinion* is needed (an element that is not always required or desired)
- When the deposition and trial dates are scheduled

To avoid potential conflicts, the medical expert should learn the identity of the parties and their counsel at the outset. Furthermore, the expert should review the *complaint* and the *answers to interrogatories* (written questions) to be prepared to address the plaintiff's claims. The attorney who retained the defense expert is likely to have only a limited knowledge of medical science; as such, the expert must provide a deeper and more contextual understanding of the facts.

Some medical experts mistakenly assume that simply offering an opinion is enough. However, the attorney who hires the defense experts usually expects them to stand by their opinions through sworn testimony and a trial appearance. Any expert who is unwilling to testify at trial should be clear about that during the first telephone call with the attorney.

Others' Opinions

Some experts may be tempted to seek input from their colleagues about the case, but it is necessary to refrain from doing so until such a consultation is specifically approved by the defense attorney. When deposed, defense experts will be asked to divulge the people to whom they have spoken about the case. Such revelations can put those potential witnesses in jeopardy of being deposed. If the expert admits relying on a colleague's opinions when formulating testimony, part or all of that testimony may be excluded from evidence because it is dependent on hearsay (an out-of-court statement offered for its truth but not subject to cross-examination).

Notes and Written Records

The medical defense expert should ask the defense attorney about the appropriateness of taking notes or creating any kind of written record. In some courts, these materials must be disclosed to the other side, so it is important to be thoughtful before putting anything in writing.

When reviewing the record, consider whether opinions from alternative medical specialties would be useful. There is a finite window in which to retain and disclose experts; the sooner the defense attorney is aware of additional experts, the more opportunity there will be to identify the best choices. Medical defense experts should ask the attorney what depositions have already been taken and thoroughly review the key witness testimony.

The Jury's Role

Most medical malpractice cases are tried before a jury. Despite popular lore, however, the jury is not comprised of the defendant's peers. The jurors are rarely physicians or even medically trained citizens; rather, they are qualified adults from the nearby geographic area. They may be moved to tears when a patient tells a story of suffering, but jurors may also be quite empathetic and receptive to the physician's attempts to make the best decision.

Jurors generally take their role very seriously and try their best to do the right thing by all parties. Jurors presume that a defendant physician is well trained and caring and tried their best to handle a complicated medical problem. Although the patient's attorney will strive to prove otherwise, the defendant physician and defense expert often prevail if they can be understood.

CRAFTING A SIMPLE STORY

Steve Jobs, who once said "simple can be harder than complex," was revered for his ability to make complicated technology accessible to everyday consumers. Similarly, the role of the expert witness is to express the complexities of medical science in plainspoken, relatable language that can be understood by lay jurors, who may have little to no knowledge of clinical terms.

Unfortunately, creating a simple, straightforward narrative can be quite complicated. In addition to years of medical training and experience, the task requires the expert to translate voluminous medical records and deposition transcripts into a simple, relatable story. Most importantly, experts must be effective teachers, using stories, analogies, and clear concepts that allow the jurors to assess the reasonableness of the defendant physician's medical decisions.

Establishing Credibility

While it is necessary to clearly state your conclusions, it is not nearly enough. Jurors (or, in a bench trial, the judge) must be fact finders who assess the credibility—the believability—of the plaintiff, defendant, and various witnesses. Once the case is turned over to a jury for deliberation, jurors must weigh the integrity of conflicting stories and opinions.

The jury's most critical job is not to understand what happened but to understand *why* it happened. The jurors must not only discern a timeline of events, they must also independently decide whether the defendant physician's medical choices were, in fact, reasonable. For example, they may ask:

- Why did the physician decide not to seek a surgical consultation?
- Why did the defendant believe that drug A was preferable to drug B?
- Why was a CT scan not ordered?

It is insufficient for an expert to assert that a particular choice is reasonable because "it is the way I and other good physicians do it." Such conclusions are unpersuasive and undermine the jury's mandate to determine *why* "good physicians" do something a certain way. Disagreements often arise during deliberations; to successfully express their points to the rest of the jury, each juror will need to call upon the stories, facts, and medical concepts they have been exposed to during the trial.

Presenting the Evidence

For the jury to understand those "whys," it is critical that experts consider the evidence from a real-time, contemporaneous perspective. No defendant can be fairly judged based on a bad outcome. When a patient tragedy is at the center of a case, that outcome can be hard to ignore, but it is essential to focus the jury on what was known at the time the medical decisions were made.

Unless the physician defendant was impaired during the event (e.g., by drug use, lack of sleep, mental health issues), the expert and defense attorney will generally maintain that every decision was medically sound at the time the care was provided. In some cases, new information may shed a negative light on the veracity of a physician's initial choices, but the expert's story must address a more specific timeline: what was the evidence available *at the time?*

Although the expert witness' in-depth understanding of the medical timeline is critical, medical lawsuits often boil down to a few essential questions. Mastering the intricacies of the case allows the defense expert to identify the most important issues, which may not be initially apparent to either the expert or the defense attorney. Finally, the expert must find the most effective ways to express the defense team's views of those central issues.

TESTIFYING AT TRIAL

Giving an expert opinion either in deposition or at trial constitutes *testifying*. Whether in a deposition during the discovery phase or at trial, the process requires hours of preparation and a comfortable knowledge of the facts of the case. Preparation is critical, particularly when testifying under the duress of the plaintiff's attorney's probing questions.

A testimony is not a test of memory; credibility sometimes demands a simple, truthful answer such as, "I don't know" or "I don't remember." The medical expert should not hesitate to say, "Let me consult the chart to be sure the facts are clear." Once again, it is far better to prepare your response to potential questions ahead of time than to scramble for answers in the courtroom, while a stenographer records every "uhm" and "uh."

Prepare, Prepare, Prepare

The medical defense expert should sit down with the defense attorney once or twice before the deposition and come prepared with the facts. The attorney should use the opportunity to present the practice questions and inquire about the expert's views. Although it is rare to put an expert through an entire mock deposition, a lot can be gained from wrestling with the most challenging questions.

Common legal phrases like, "whether, to a reasonable degree of medical probability, there was a breach of the standard of care" can cause confusion. The medical expert should understand how "standard of care" is defined in that jurisdiction. "Standard care" does not mean *ideal* care, but rather *reasonable* care. Almost invariably, the expert will be asked to relate their opinions to a reasonable degree of medical *probability*. This standard is not the same as medical *possibility*. A possibility can be lower than .001%, while a probability describes odds above 50%. When asked to state whether a treatment fell within the standard of care, the expert is expected to provide an answer under the "probability" standard.

Address Weaknesses

Every defense case has shortcomings. One of the most important tasks of the defendant, the defense attorney, and the expert is to confront, understand, and provide a reasonable explanation for the weaknesses in the defense's case. Defense witnesses who are unprepared to address these flaws will be caught by surprise at the worst possible time—in court, in front of a live jury.

Defense attorneys expect to deal with difficult facts, but it is devastating to be caught off guard by issues that were unanticipated before trial. The case's weaknesses should be discussed openly with the defense team during the investigative phase of the lawsuit. It is far better to prepare an explanation in the quiet of an office than in a high-pressure courtroom. Moreover, ignoring or brushing aside potential problems prior to or during the trial emboldens the plaintiff to establish the narrative of the case.

Listen Carefully and Attentively

While testifying, an adept medical expert listens carefully, avoids rushing, and answers only when the question is clear. No attorney wants to find out later that their expert responded without understanding what was being asked. In most cases, the medical expert is permitted to review the patient's record before answering; however, an attorney can ask the expert to address the question based on memory alone. Even if prevented from reviewing the record, the expert should consider making the request. Such an appeal makes it clear to the jury that the accuracy of an answer based purely on recollection will be limited.

The medical expert must be truthful and admit facts, even those that are uncomfortable. In a deposition, the opposing attorney is trying to assess the level of credibility that the medical expert will have with the jury. Not only is this credibility demonstrated by an expert's knowledge and memory of the events, it is also established by the expert's willingness to concede what is obvious.

Respect the Process

Jurors make substantial (sometimes involuntary) sacrifices to participate in these high-stakes cases, and they receive little in return. They expect every witness, including the experts, to be respectful of the process, patient with the tedium of trial, and honest in their answers. Every question, even those that seem repetitive or argumentative, is another opportunity to teach and tell the story.

No witness should get into a personal argument with the opposing counsel or be dismissive of the questions asked. Jurors might be inclined to punish experts who appear to be arrogant or close minded, who may remind them of an unsettling experience they had with a personal physician. If the attorneys are arguing with one another, or with the judge, the medical expert should just listen, wait, and avoid offering any thoughts until the legal concerns have been resolved.

For instance, the attorneys may argue about whether a question was previously "asked and answered," and experts may maintain that they have already answered the question. But it is not the expert's role to argue the point. In some cases, the attorney may simply have forgotten that the question was previously asked. In addition, an attorney who did not like a given answer may pose the question again, hoping the expert will answer differently. Regardless, the expert should just take it slow; be reflective; and calmly, clearly state or clarify the answer to the question. The jurors probably dislike the repetition more than the expert does, and remaining calm and respectful causes jurors to fault the attorney—not the expert—for the wasted time.

Be a Great Teacher

Some attorneys prefer to keep the answers to cross-examination questions as brief as possible. However, the defense expert is ultimately a teacher who must explain why the medical care provided was reasonable. Such explanations require more than simple yes-or-no answers. Every question asked by the defendant's or plaintiff's attorney should be viewed as an opportunity to clarify what may be confusing to the jury.

Nonetheless, it is generally best to answer in a sentence or two. Verbose answers sometimes seem like obfuscation or may demonstrate the witness's inability to explain something succinctly. Long answers can also convolute already complicated matters and inadvertently reveal unnecessary information, leading to multiple follow-up questions from the plaintiff's attorney.

If tasked with teaching "Grandmother" the facts of a case, most experts would try to minimize the medical jargon. There are countless abbreviations in medicine—many quite common—but it is best to presume that they're unfamiliar to a jury. If busy trying to remember what the "W" in "WBC" stands for, a juror is not listening to the expert's next two sentences. A better approach is to fully express the term (e.g., "white blood count"), so everyone can move forward in sync.

Sitting on a jury can be boring and exhausting, and it requires its jurors to process a heavy flow of auditory information. At any given time, one-third of the jurors may not even be listening to the testimony. Some may be thinking about a prior moment in the trial, while others are pondering what they need to get from the grocery store on the way home. While a portion of the plaintiff's medical record may be shown to the jury, it's important to remember that jurors seldom have access to the whole report. Jurors are only hearing the details in (sometimes nonchronological) pieces, which can prevent them from considering the full context of the case. In light of these challenges, experts should use clear language, an inflective voice, and an even pace to ensure their opinions are heard and retained.

In addition, an artfully used analogy can make the testimony more interesting, although this tool should be used carefully and sparingly. (Analogies usually use the word "like" or "as." For example, the expert might say that the fast and extreme blood loss from a burst aortic aneurysm is "like turning on a fire hose.") The defense attorney and expert should discuss how the most critical points should be presented. The positive aspects of the case are best described in finely sliced detail. If the blood values are crucial to the defense case, the expert can say, "All the blood values looked fine to me." Another approach is to isolate each component of significance, describe its role, and explain any relevant numerical values.

Once the jury understands the various components, the medical expert should explain why the data support his or her opinions. By breaking down the supporting facts piece by piece, experts can help the jury lock in on the most important parts of the case and better understand the physician's decisions.

A summary statement that all the blood values looked good asks the jury to trust the expert's judgment, although one essential role of the jury is to question the credibility of every witness. Jurors do not want experts to talk down to them; they want to be empowered to truly deliberate the merits of the case. A highly effective expert witness is confident, calm, good natured, comfortable with the facts, and eager for every opportunity to teach the jury through a clear, understandable narrative.

CONCLUSION

Being an expert witness requires the ability to tell the "the rest of the story," not only address the plaintiff's claims. The medical expert should start by consulting with the defense attorney, determining whether notes and a written opinion will be required, and establishing if other experts will be consulted about the case. It is equally important to understand the evidence and timeline of events, which can be woven into a simple, credible story for the jury.

The weaknesses of the case should be recognized and addressed by telling the story of why these shortcomings do not constitute breaches of the jurisdiction's standard of care. This responsibility requires an understanding of the terms "possibility" and "probability" in relation to the case. Before testifying, the physician expert should meet with the defense attorney to ascertain the questions that the plaintiff's team is likely to ask.

The expert is well served by listening carefully and attentively during the deposition and at trial. Good answers avoid medical jargon and aim to simplify complex issues. Patience and respect for the process are essential, as is respect for the jury's time. Experts must appreciate the jury's honest desire to understand what happened and—more importantly—why it happened.

The best experts are great teachers who are warm, engaging, personable, professional, and tell "the story" in a meaningful and comprehensible way.

HUMAN RESOURCES

SECTION 12

HUMAN RESOURCES MANAGEMENT: BASIC PRINCIPLES

CHAPTER 117

India J. Taylor Owens, Kevin M. Klauer

The concept and functions of human resources (HR) have changed significantly over the past 10 years. Hospital systems, which have rapidly become more complex, now require high-functioning employee management systems. As such, HR is now less of a department and more of a strategy for interacting with employees. As medical reform evolves, there is an increasing formation of corporations and integration of physician groups. The evolution of an advanced practice provider system, needed to bridge the gap left by too few primary care and emergency physicians, adds yet another layer of complexity.

Popular awards, including "100 Best Places to Work" and the surveys on which such awards are based, demonstrate the importance of a highly functioning workplace in today's consumer-driven medical culture. Effective HR management should create an environment that encourages fairness, productivity, and safety while ensuring individual rewards, recognition, and opportunities for growth. Personnel costs comprise the majority of a health-care organizations' operating budgets, and the need to deliver high-quality care to growing numbers of increasingly sicker patients establishes the critical importance of HR management skills in the emergency department (ED).

THE ROLE OF HUMAN RESOURCES

Department leaders must pay consistent and thoughtful attention to HR issues. Fully developed HR functions include employment, compensation and benefits, policy development, and employee relations and training. Aligning these functions to the corporate business and strategic objectives of the organization and the ED yields great value. In this sense, HR can take a proactive leadership role in helping organizations accomplish their objectives.[1]

A Brief History of HR

When HR was first invented as a separate entity, its role was one of record keeping and employee management. Then, between 1965 and 1975, HR departments reacted to increasing governmental mandates around equality and diversity, and their role expanded to managing conflict and protecting the organization from costly litigation. Collaborative and cooperative relationships between employees and their employers further evolved between 1975 and 1985. During that time, HR became increasingly proactive, and employees were perceived as the most important corporate resource. Since 1985, HR has become key to organizational survival. These indispensable departments are involved in policy development, defensive activities (e.g., background checks, labor dispute grievances), corporate communication, marketing strategies, and personnel asset management.

Current HR Roles

The evolution of HR has been contingent on the changing characteristics of work environments and labor laws. Today's work environment places a greater emphasis on cross training, collaborative practice, the pressure to substitute "cheaper" health-care workers for more expensive clinicians, and escalating pressures to provide continuing education—particularly leadership training. Current HR considerations include ethnic and cultural diversity, including gender identity and sexual orientation; gender equality in management roles; and schedule flexibility in the workforce. The increasing unionization of health-care workers and labor practices are another focus of today's HR team. Beyond these challenges, hospital HR departments contend with shortages of essential health-services professionals, such as pharmacists, physical therapists, nurses, and primary care physicians.[2]

As health-care organizations implement new leadership models, HR is evolving into a consultative service that is able to transfer the knowledge of HR principles to other leaders and staff. The pressures affecting health care require a continued focus on cost cutting while simultaneously aligning HR philosophies, functions, policies, and practices with the organization's strategic objectives. It is necessary in all of these functions to draw on the richness and value that diversity brings to the workplace.

Regulatory Mandates

External mandates that create a dynamic HR environment include federal oversight by organizations like the Occupational Safety and Health Administration (OSHA) and legislation, such as the Family Medical Leave Act, Uniformed Services Employment and Reemployment Rights Act, and the Americans With Disabilities Act (ADA). When an organization supports and ensures the deployment of HR functions and education that readily addresses corporate objectives, employee trust is enhanced. Conversely, frequent unexplained changes to benefits, compensation, or employee policies can reduce the credibility of management and lead to staff mistrust.[1]

LEGAL AND REGULATORY CONCERNS

The legal basis for most employer–employee relationships is known as *employment at will*. This concept defines the relationship as existing "at the pleasure" of either side. Fundamentally, this can be described as a noncontractual relationship, without specifying the duration of employment. There are limitations to the termination of at-will employees. For instance, despite the ability to fire an employee with or without cause, such terminations must be legal and may not be motivated by retaliation or discrimination. As a result, many organizations apply a system of documentation and progressive discipline, including an opportunity for grievance hearings.[1]

A number of federal laws apply to the employer–employee relationship, including those listed in **Box 117.1**. Although this chapter does not fully explore each of these statutory regulations, it is clear that the employment relationship is increasingly complex and, in many cases, externally mandated. The federal government is taking a greater role in advocating for employee (rather than employer) rights. These mandates apply to both job applicants and current employees.

These legislative mandates are generally intended to define and ensure both employee and employer rights. It is important to be aware of these laws and, when necessary, consult with HR professionals with respect to implementation and compliance.[1] The recent focus

> **BOX 117.1 ■ EMPLOYER-EMPLOYEE LAWS**
>
> - National Labor Relations Act
> - Fair Labor Standards Act
> - Occupational Safety and Health Act
> - Civil Rights Act of 1991
> - Americans With Disabilities Act
> - Equal Pay Act
> - Age Discrimination in Employment Act
> - Family and Medical Leave Act
> - Privacy Act
> - Immigration and Naturalization Service Policies and Procedures
> - Equal Employment Opportunity Act
> - Various state and local employment practice laws

on gender pay equality is one example of increasing regulation by the federal government. A best-practice employment climate can be established in anticipation of many federal mandates.[3]

Compensation and benefits practices are largely dictated by federal, state, or local statutes. One of the overriding external mandates is the Fair Labor Standards Act (FLSA) associated with state wage and hour laws. Additional legal issues related to compensation are addressed in the Equal Pay Act, which requires comparable pay for employees who perform the same or similar jobs, regardless of their gender. It is wise for organizations to have an equitable and consistently applied wage and salary system that includes objective methods for making hiring offers and internal wage adjustments (e.g., promotions).[1]

Gender Disparity

There is growing interest at the federal level in narrowing the gender pay gap. This applies not only to men and women as traditionally defined but also to transgender employees.[4] Men who were employed full time in professional, management, and related occupations in the fourth quarter of 2019 earned 19% more than women in the same fields.[5] Emergency medicine is not exempt from this phenomenon. Approximately 49.5% of men reported a salary (clinical hours only) between $240,000 and $400,000, while only 23.5% of women reported salaries in the same range. Approximately 76% of those reporting an annual clinical salary under $240,000 were female, while 51.5% were male. Controlling for appropriate variables, hour for hour, women earned less for the same work performed.[5]

Medical directors must be aware of this bias and work with HR to avoid pay disparities. Efforts to analyze the gender pay gap and pass laws to strengthen the Equal Pay Act are expected to continue. Salary systems that establish payment and rate adjustments based on employee experience and market data are increasingly being scrutinized by the Department of Labor. This is particularly true for organizations that are classified as federal contractors (i.e., those that accept federal Medicare and Medicaid monies).[1] Specifically, the market as a factor for determining hiring offers and salary adjustments is being reviewed more rigorously for its validity and effect on the gender gap.[6]

Job Categorization

Salary grids are a means to facilitate fair pay practices by considering each employee's experience, credentials, areas of responsibility, and decision-making authority. Those aspects can be placed into defined grids that are in line with internal and external market compensation structures. The large number of jobs and interdependent responsibilities in health care present unique challenges to the creation of appropriate job grades or groupings.

Job titles, responsibilities, and compensation packages must be created with careful attention to detail and a thorough understanding of the roles and responsibilities of the job itself. Positions must be categorized, and external market conditions must be reviewed on an ongoing (perhaps quarterly) basis.[1] Many organizations engage a professional health-care salary survey vendor that is well versed in the associated nuances of these organizations. As employees become skilled in salary negotiations, they may also engage salary survey organizations to gauge the economic trends for their positions.

Compensation Philosophy

In addition to ensuring a legal and internally equitable framework, organizations must strategically employ a compensation philosophy to help identify what they intend to accomplish. For instance, does the organization want to pay at the top of its market, at the middle, or toward the low end? Base-wage adjustments can be made by instituting merit pay, gain sharing, or bonuses.[1] These strategies can be used to achieve organizational objectives, including patient satisfaction goals, Centers for Medicare and Medicaid Services guidelines, and operational metrics (e.g., door-to-doctor time), overall length of stay for admitted or discharged patients, and even financial goals.

EMPLOYEE BENEFITS

The increasing cost of employee benefits has had a significant impact on employers, employees, and even consumers, as many of these costs are passed along to patients. Most organizations negotiate with insurance companies to obtain the best rate for their employees; however, despite these efforts, which put large organizations with expanded buying power at an advantage, costs have dramatically risen over a relatively short period. The frontline ED leader should understand the array of benefits available and be able to answer basic questions. The ability to refer the employee to a knowledgeable HR specialist will lead to the best results.

Rising Costs

Rising benefit costs have contributed to the desire of small organizations and even emergency physician practices to seek alliances with larger health-care delivery systems with enhanced buying power. To demonstrate that the cost of benefits should be considered part of the total compensation package, most organizations communicate this rising expense directly to their employees.

The rise of accountable care organizations, medical homes, and coordinated care delivery models has required many employees (who wish to maintain full benefits) to seek health care within the corporate environment. This is an attempt by hospitals to stem the loss of business generated when their own employees seek medical care "off campus." Mandating "local" care allows hospitals to recapture lost revenue. As a result, insurance plans provide coverage at a higher rate and with lower copays if consumers seek care in their own insitutions. To be effective, these rules require organizations to address questions about access to care, privacy, and the ability of the employer to take on an increased patient volume.

Health Incentives

Many organizations are also reimbursing a portion of benefit dollars or decreasing the cost of benefits for employees who demonstrate a more desirable health status (e.g., nonsmokers, significant exercise regimen) and those who comply with treatment plans for certain medical conditions. In addition, organizations are providing their employees with:

- Health surveys
- Access to nutrition and diet classes
- Nicotine testing
- Reduced or free smoking cessation aids
- Free stress management tools
- Testing for high cholesterol
- Testing for high blood pressure
- Body fat testing

COBRA

The Consolidated Omnibus Budget Reconciliation Act (COBRA) outlines an employer's responsibility to continue health insurance coverage for employees who are (voluntarily or involuntarily) terminated or had their hours reduced. However, there are some participant exclusions, such as loss of employment due to gross negligence. COBRA is applicable to private-sector employers with 20 or more employees, state and local governments, and employee organizations. Generally, minimal provisions of COBRA require that an employer provides, at group rates, a continuation of health insurance for a minimum of 18 months. There are programs and conditions that allow extensions. Former employees may find the expense daunting because they must pay the full insurance cost, including portions that both they and the employer previously paid.

The Affordable Care Act

The Affordable Care Act extended benefits to dependent children to age 26 (under their parents' workplace policies). As a cost-saving measure in response to this and other programs with increased premium costs, some employers began "gating" participation in their group health benefits. One mechanism excludes employees' spouses if the spouse is employed by an organization that provides insurance coverage, shifting the burden to the spouse's employer. This exclusion has resulted in increased out-of-pocket payments for married couples who are forced to purchase two plans. Additionally, some employers require validation, for example, proof of dependency for any children added to the plan.

A cafeteria-style benefit plan is often used, in which employees can pick and choose from specific components. In this way, employees can weigh the value of their benefits against the premiums. For instance, participation in a low-premium dental or vision plan may be worthwhile when compared to the risk of paying high out-of-pocket costs for associated medical services.

High-Deductible Health Plans

High-deductible health plans (HDHPs) are alternatives to the 80/20 insurance model that has been popular for decades. These plans offer lower premiums in exchange for the employee assuming more of the upfront (first payment) risk and are often combined with a health savings account (HSA). Employees choosing HDHPs pay out of pocket until they reach a preset deductible. Individuals may make pretax contributions to HSAs, from which out-of-pocket medical expenses can be paid. These plans have several advantages:

- Employees may be more apt to regulate unnecessary care.
- Employers get a break on premiums.
- The unspent savings accumulate year-to-year (unlike flexible savings accounts).
- Accumulated savings can be invested.

The disadvantage of these plans is that employees may be attracted to the low premiums but lack the financial shrewdness to budget for necessary care. It is critically important that employees understand the potential out-of-pocket costs and plan accordingly.

Other Benefits

Corporations can offer other types of benefits, including childcare at a reduced cost, early retirement options, matching contributions to the employees' retirement accounts, and fully funded retirement accounts without required employee contributions. An employer's status (i.e., for profit or not for profit) dictates the type of tax-deferred retirement program it can offer.

Benefits typically fall into the categories of health, disability, pension, life insurance, workers' compensation, unemployment insurance, leave time, and business and educational expenses. Additionally, mandated benefits accrue under social security.[1] Because of the complicated nature of benefits plans, technical and strategic expertise from HR professionals is more important than ever.

An additional benefit that has become a mainstay of most organizations is the employee assistance program (EAP), which provides personal counseling to deal with stress, financial difficulties, addiction-related disorders, and family and social concerns. Typically, these programs offer a basic service or set number of counseling encounters at no cost to employees and are offered as part of the standard benefits package. Referrals to the EAP can be voluntary but can also be provided as part of a disciplinary or remedial process, as a means of improving an employee's behavior and restoring their productivity.[1]

EMPLOYEE RELATIONS

Effective employee relations can be established by creating a strong legal framework, including HR policies and external requirements, and encouraging a positive employee-relations environment.[1] The desired outcome is satisfied employees who are loyal and equipped to meet patient needs, both of which result in improved retention.

Legal Framework

Many complex federal laws govern the relationship between the employee and employer. Regulatory agencies, including the Equal Employment Opportunity Commission, and laws such as the ADA and the FLSA, are intended to ensure that employees are treated with fair and consistent workplace policies, procedures, and practices. Department leaders should know that these legal mandates exist and know when to contact HR professionals if questions arise about their interpretations or applicability.[1]

Human resource policies should be consistent with the business objectives and strategic intent of the organization. For example, policies and procedures may address the promotion of internal candidates for open positions, as well as provide ways of recognizing and motivating current employees. It is essential for ED leaders to understand and ensure the consistent application of HR policies, particularly those that can infringe on an employee's employment status, basic working conditions, and ability to be promoted, demoted, or reassigned.[1]

Policies and procedures that relate to employee discipline are particularly important for creating supportive employer–employee relationships. A grievance or appellate process that allows an objective third party to consider both sides of a disciplinary case may be valuable. This process can either be open to any management action or be more restrictive in scope. It is important for the grievance process to include several steps in which a senior administrator or panel of employees reviews the grievance independently. However, the wise ED leader should have at least one third party present to verify the events and agreed-upon outcomes.

Grievance processes are not intended to shift accountability or authority for disciplinary actions; rather, they are designed to support managers in carrying forth their duties relative to employee discipline. Such processes should not be confused with arbitration for the purpose of resolving legal disputes, such as alleged wrongful termination. Grievance processes and structures that are set up with this approach typically result in an environment that can be endorsed and supported by both management and employees.[1] The basic tenet of employee relations and HR is consistency and fairness of action without surprises.

Strategic Employee Relations

Elements of a strategic approach include training supervisors and managers; focusing on communication practices and styles; and considering job scope, description, design, and organizational structure in general. Leaders can be thought of as designers of their organization or department, coaches, and stewards. In their role as designers, ED leaders must give careful consideration to the design of each job and its relationship to employee satisfaction, productivity, and the organization at large. In their role as coaches, leaders are tasked with identifying developmental needs, applying appropriate staff resources, and creating a real learning environment. In their role as organizational stewards, leaders must see themselves as servants, both to employees and patients.

Meaningful communication requires effective listening and a sincere understanding of employees' needs, ideas, and thoughts. Successful ED leaders are almost always good communicators who create a vision that allows the staff to align their goals with those of the institution. Communication is often taken for granted in terms of form and content, and yet it has great value in fostering job satisfaction.[1]

Involving employees in decisions that affect their jobs and informing them about the status of their work are key. For example, providing feedback on how effectively a staff member is meeting corporate quality goals, departmental expectations, patient satisfaction scores, or financial goals is essential to building a strong employer–employee relationship. Such feedback should be viewed as an opportunity for improved performance, as opposed to being punitive in nature. An old cartoon comes to mind, in which a pirate addresses his crew: "The beatings will continue until morale improves." Negative reinforcement is not a successful performance improvement strategy and may damage employer–employee relations. Attention to developing competencies and treating staff with respect are also necessary to establish trust and a foundation for retention.

Creating a balance between individual and corporate needs requires vision. A vision statement helps employees understand where the organization is going and how they might contribute. In addition, in periods of rapid change, a vision statement helps employees become more invested in the future.

Department leaders should frequently gather feedback to determine and understand the needs and expectations of their employees. This information should be obtained in a risk-free environment. In response to the feedback (e.g., surveys), action plans can be designed to address the gaps between the current and desired states. Responsive action plans demonstrate the value of employee feedback and help staff understand and validate future goals. Employee opinion surveys, focus groups, town hall meetings, and other methods effectively and symbolically reinforce the importance that an organization places on communication and feedback.

Training and Education

As with other HR functions, medical training and education have both internal and external components and mandates. For example, the Joint Commission requires providers to be trained on the age-related skills and criteria needed to manage specific patient populations. In addition, OSHA requires that employees be trained on infection control and potential workplace hazards.[1] Creating "centers of excellence" (e.g., stroke or trauma center designation) necessitates ongoing education for physicians and nurses to demonstrate continued competence. Educational issues that range from fire safety to specific licensing requirements are ubiquitous in health-care organizations.

Training is generally defined as the provision of job-related skills that can be directly applied to a given work situation. Education generally includes the development of skills and capacities that employees can use to perform their jobs. Effective ED leaders value the professional development of their employees and implement programs to address each component.

In addition to observation and feedback, such efforts require a formalized approach to pinpointing each employee's developmental requirements. It is often useful to have the employees identify these needs themselves (e.g., via an instrument or ranking system). The results can then be pooled to build consensus on training requirements and resources.[1]

It is most useful to identify training and education needs related to expected job outcomes and organizationally identified goals. This process ensures that these efforts are grounded in relevant activities that can be used immediately or in the near future. Training that is based solely on the needs of employees is less effective, as it does not incorporate the institution's goals and may be similar to an academic setting in which a variety of educational programs are offered in the hope that they will be useful to the organization. Although this kind of "employee perceived needs" approach to training can have a positive effect, it tends to be less efficient, consume more resources, and be off target.[1] True learning organizations create an environment that allows:

- Mistakes to be made
- Assumptions to be tested
- Openness to the ideas of others
- Dialogue and feedback
- Application of inquiry skills

The learning organization process requires a fundamental shift in the way most professionals think, feel, and act. It requires a willingness to take risks and make mistakes while recognizing that one's familiar approach may not be the best. This may be particularly difficult for highly trained professionals who have ascended the organizational hierarchy.[1]

Respect and Inclusion

The #MeTooMedicine movement has highlighted opportunities for cultural improvements in the medical field. It is important that ED leaders collaborate with their HR department to develop policies that address the needs of employees undergoing gender transformation; HR professionals must provide guidance for navigating these potentially novel waters. Policies must be implemented to address locker rooms and restroom facilities, dress code, benefits, and other relevant considerations. Creating guidelines for gender transition can be an essential step in communicating with those undergoing the process.[4]

Department leaders should look to HR for standardized and up-to-date education on gender terminology and ensure that a clear definition of sexual harassment is part of organizational policies, as this area is rapidly evolving. Importantly, they should be familiar with the process for handling any allegations of harassment. These situations must be approached with great sensitivity, as it is imperative to preserve the dignity of those involved by maintaining their privacy during the investigation. Tolerance and respect are the right of all employees. The expectation that employees can work with *all* individuals should be the norm.

CONCLUSION

Emergency clinicians tend to share a singular mindset grounded in the belief that the ED is unique and different from the rest of the hospital. While this is certainly true, independent thinking and action do not advance the goals of the organization or department. To be effective, ED leaders must interact and work across institutional barriers for the benefit of patients, staff, and the parent organization.

The link between health-care quality and HR is readily apparent. Employees have more opportunities to transfer jobs and locations than ever before, and they are more inclined to seek out employment that meets both their professional and personal needs and values. The function of HR is to identify and respond to these needs in an ongoing effort to recruit new talent and reward the existing staff. In conjunction with HR, ED leaders can create a progressive environment that is mutually safe and fulfilling for the staff while also protecting the interests of the group and hospital.

REFERENCES

1. Greene LE. General principles of human resource management. In: Salluzzo RF, Mayer TA, Strauss RW, et al, eds. *Emergency Department Management: Principles and Applications*. St. Louis, Mo: Mosby (Elsevier); 1997.
2. Leatt P, Shortell SM, Kimberly JR. Organizational design. In: SJ Williams, ed. *Healthcare Management: Organization Design and Behavior*. 4th ed. New York, NY: Delmar Thomson Learning; 2000:274–306.
3. O'Dell C. Building on received wisdom. *Health Forum J*. 1993;36(1):17–21.
4. Society for Human Resource Management HR Magazine, Milligan S. How HR can support transgender employees. 2015. Available at: https://www.shrm.org/hr-today/news/hr-magazine/pages/0915-transgender-employees.aspx. Accessed March 19, 2020.
5. *The Editor's Desk, Bureau of Labor Statistics. Median Weekly Earnings for Fourth Quarter 2019* (USDL 11-0062). Washington, DC: US Government Printing Office; 2020.
6. Wolfe J, Klauer K. Gender bias in the halls of medicine. *EP Monthly*. 2011;18(6). Available at: http://www.epmonthly.com/features/current-features/sexism-in-the-ed-how-pervasiveis-gender-bias/. Accessed July 5, 2013.

CHAPTER 118

PHYSICIAN RECRUITMENT, CREDENTIALING, AND ORIENTATION

Kevin M. Klauer

Physician staffing of an emergency department (ED) is a seemingly never-ending process. Although many view recruitment as merely a tool for filling available positions, this important undertaking has more significant implications. Particularly in emergency medicine, there is a constant ebb and flow of providers due to changing professional goals, personal priorities, family needs, illnesses, the rigors of shift work, physician burnout, and other, often unforeseen, circumstances. This unpredictability creates a dynamic seldom encountered in most other specialties: a comparative instability in physician staff. This relative instability creates opportunities to carefully consider the process of recruiting desirable candidates.

In a chronically understaffed department, opportunities to improve provider performance and accountability may be lost because of staffing pressures. In other words, when the priority is to fill the schedule, other objectives, such as quality of care, may inadvertently become secondary. Further, when the demand for physicians greatly outweighs an ED's supply, the existing providers find job security in their ability to simply ameliorate the staffing "crisis" and feel no pressure to improve their performance. However, in a fully staffed or slightly overstaffed department, it is not enough to simply fill shifts; every provider must perform to the institution's expectations. Continuous recruitment incentivizes the performance of existing providers while allowing ED leaders to seek out clinicians who are a better fit than those who cannot or will not improve.

Retention is a critical piece of recruitment. Stated simply, retention is putting forth effort to entice the current physicians to stay. Since these providers are already there, keeping them is usually far easier and less expensive than recruiting and orienting new physicians. One element of successful retention is a thorough and effective orientation process, which should create an easy transition to the facility and set the tone for the long-term success of the director–practitioner relationship.

RECRUITMENT

Hospital credentialing processes are complex and burdened by potential pitfalls. The skilled leader is adept at navigating this process and avoiding delays or the denial of hospital privileges.

The Relationship

Recruitment marks the beginning of the relationship between the director and provider. Many ED leaders believe the relationship exists only when a contract is signed or the provider begins clinical duties. This misconception results in a weakened foundation that may cause future problems. From the first contact (e.g., phone conversation or handshake), the practitioner and the director begin to form opinions of each other. All such communication—including discussions about scheduling, compensation, professional development, and departmental operations—form a basis for the psychological contract.

The Psychological Contract

A psychological contract, noted most frequently in the business world, is an unspoken agreement between the ED director and the ED provider. This agreement represents a mutual respect and trust on the part of both parties. Damage the psychological contract, and you damage the working relationship. Most provider agreements stay in the file cabinet until there's a problem; such issues usually indicate a violation of the psychological contract.

Potential violations often originate from miscommunication and lack of clarity in expectations or promised actions. Although less common, a substantially more concerning violation occurs when either party is intentionally misled by the other. Unfortunately, in the contract/relationship world, promises are sometimes made before the ability to execute them is confirmed; in other cases, promises are simply made to gain short-term negotiating advantages. This is a strategy for certain failure, as any intentionally misled party will be apt to sever the relationship abruptly. The most common psychological contract violations are listed in **Box 118.1**.

Financial Issues

Bonus structures are often discussed during recruitment; however, financial details may be intentionally omitted from the conversation. It is appropriate to advise candidates that a bonus is additional compensation based individual performance and is not guaranteed. Providing the candidate with a bonus history can help bridge the gap between true enticement and the implication of guarantee. The structure, eligibility requirements, and timelines and benefits of the partnership should be fully disclosed, defined contractually, and adhered to. Equitable scheduling and compensation are fundamental components of a sound psychological and financial contract. Nevertheless, unintentional inequity may arise due to certain circumstances, such as the hospital's group structure or compensation program. For instance:

> *If a group is structured to reduce the number of night shifts worked by older team members, the burden of additional night shifts must fall on the shoulders of younger physicians. Although well intentioned, such a plan would be deemed inequitable by many younger physicians, particularly in groups with a large percentage of older members.*

BOX 118.1 ■ COMMON PSYCHOLOGIC CONTRACT VIOLATIONS

- Failure to fulfill expectations, written or implied
- Bonuses not provided
- Partnership not offered
- Promotion timelines not adhered to
- Vesting schedules not understood or not followed
- Inequitable scheduling
- Inequitable compensation among providers
- Inadequate performance reviews and feedback
- Inadequate control
- Given less responsibility than promised

Incentive-based compensation programs may be a source of discontent for some physicians. Such programs should be structured to equalize the opportunity for all clinicians to earn available incentives. Unstructured compensation programs—in other words, inconsistently negotiated packages—are problematic and often result in inequity. For example:

> *If Physician A and Physician B are hired for the same position, but Physician B is a better negotiator than Physician A (e.g., securing an additional $10 dollars per hour and one less shift per month), Physician A will likely be incensed when this inequity is discovered (and rest assured, it will be discovered). If Physician B secures a signing bonus of $15,000 that existing group members didn't receive, should all of the group members be awarded the same bonus?*

To preserve everyone's psychological contract and the stability of the department, two logical options are available: 1) decline to provide a signing bonus to Physician B, the skillful negotiator, or 2) award the same bonus to everyone in the group. Emergency physicians should be compensated for seeing patients and fulfilling their various administrative responsibilities—not for their negotiating skills. "Special" deals for "special" people is a strategy that results in inequity, provider discontent, and retention issues.

Vision/Mission

Recruitment requires some degree of honest salesmanship. Although this may seem unprofessional to some, the reality is that candidates need to buy what is being sold: the "best opportunity" available. However, you can't sell what you can't define. Every department needs a vision and a mission, and every leader should work toward actualizing these elements and integrating them into their recruitment plan.

Recruitment Strategies

There are many strategies for recruiting physicians. However, recruitment efforts can and should be tailored to the needs of the individual ED and be flexible enough to address the particular needs of the candidate. For instance, an open position in the region's most sought-after location may attract applicants by nothing more than "word of mouth." However, most EDs aren't so lucky. As a framework for successful recruiting, the medical director may use a combination of the following techniques to close the deal.

Advertising and Promotion

Advertising is necessary to cast a wide net that generates the largest pool of candidates possible. Although beginning a recruitment campaign with a narrow focus may seem efficient and consistent with the thinking of an emergency physician (getting right to the point), too narrow a focus is unlikely to generate a sufficient candidate pool. It is wise to enlist the assistance of the institution's marketing staff, who are knowledgeable about and experienced with advertising.

Marketing can take many forms, but the goal is simple and universal. Although an advertisement won't fill an open position, it should prompt candidates to take the next step and explore the opportunity. Likely publications to showcase ED employment opportunities include:

- Emergency medicine magazines (e.g., *Emergency Physicians Monthly* and *EM News*)
- Specialty society publications (e.g., *ACEP Now*)
- Peer-reviewed journals (e.g., *Annals of Emergency Medicine* and *Academic Emergency Medicine*)
- Online versions of these publications

In addition to print and online media, advertising can be performed in real time at conferences and tradeshows. It is more labor intensive, depending on the size of the meeting; however, the number of solid leads generated at these events can be substantial. Because of the face-to-face interaction with potential candidates and the opportunity to address specific needs and issues, the quality of these generated leads is often better than those that result from print and online advertisements. Further, direct contact and a positive impression make a candidate much more likely to progress to the next step of the recruitment process. The tradeshows with the greatest yields are the high-attendance emergency medicine conferences and regional meetings.

Screening

Once the advertising campaign is underway and responses are received, candidates should be appropriately screened to make certain they meet the requirements of the position. For instance, if the facility will only hire residency-trained and board-certified emergency physicians, then only applicants with those qualifications should be considered.

Appropriate screening can be delegated to support personnel, such as an administrative assistant. Specific screening instructions and training should be provided to the staff who performs the screening function, including correspondence thanking the candidates for their interest. Names and contact information for candidates who meet the predetermined eligibility requirements should be forwarded to the medical director for a preinterview, which may be conducted via telephone, video call, or other means of communication. While support staff may assist with scheduling, the medical director should conduct the preinterview.

Preinterview

The preinterview is often the first conversation that ED leaders have with their new or prospective providers. The purpose of this process is to dig a little deeper than the position's baseline eligibility requirements. The fundamental qualifications are important, but they cannot distinguish one candidate from another. The preinterview should be structured to determine the personality behind the curriculum vitae. The screening process is objective, whereas the preinterview and interview processes are usually more subjective.

The qualities that are determined for a successful relationship should be sought in the preinterview. If work ethic is important, the candidate's employment history, conduct, and job commitment should be discussed. If the goal is to hire a full-time night physician, the candidate's interest in overnight shifts should be explored early. The preinterview should be conducted to determine if there seems to be a good fit between the ED group and practitioner. If that fit is found, the formal interview should be scheduled.

Interview

The interview is often the first face-to-face meeting between the ED leader and candidate. As an excellent rule of thumb, ED leaders should avoid interviewing candidates they do not intend to hire. Recruiting isn't the same as dating. Thus, the only desirable outcome is a long-term commitment. The time and money required to fly candidates and their spouses to a work location cannot be justified unless there is sincere interest in hiring that clinician.

Many medical directors misapply social rules to the interview process by avoiding difficult but important topics in order to evade conflict or awkwardness. However, the interview is an opportunity to identify the wants, needs, and "deal breakers" of both parties.

Doing a well-choreographed dance around the difficult subjects won't help anyone when those same topics inevitably come up after the new practitioner begins work. Uncomfortable subjects may include but are not limited to scheduling, benefits, compensation, and start dates. Direct discussion will strengthen the newly formed relationship and psychological contract. If potential issues cannot be amicably resolved for any reason, a successful match is unlikely.

Of note, behavioral-based interviewing techniques are an effective way to test the fit. Astute interviewers identify their key candidate attributes and ask questions that confirm whether applicants possess those qualities. For instance, if teamwork is a valued attribute, the interviewer might ask the following: "When was the last time you helped a colleague work through a difficult problem, and how did you assist them?" Less-revealing questions such as, "Where do you see yourself in five years?" should be replaced with those that more clearly demonstrate a candidate's behaviors and perceptions.

In addition to time spent between the candidate and the medical director, there are several other components of an interview that effectively cement the bond and result in a good psychological contract and hire. The applicant's significant other(s) (i.e., spouse, life partner, and at times, even parents) should be included, particularly at social events that are planned as part of the interview process. Interactions during a social event:

- Demonstrate a different, often more casual, perspective of the candidate
- Create an opportunity to observe the candidate with a group
- Provide an opportunity for others to meet the candidate, including the significant others of other physicians, nurses, and hospital administrators
- Remove barriers and offer an informal, relaxed setting to get to better know the candidate

Compliance

Although beyond the scope of this chapter, addressing compliance is necessary to the recruitment process. In particular, during the preinterview and interview processes, the interviewer must be careful to avoid any questions that could later be deemed civil rights violations. Questions regarding race, age, religion, and sexual orientation—and even gender-specific questions—may be inappropriate and should be avoided.

Closing the Deal

The ultimate goal of recruitment is to have the candidate "sign on the dotted line." It cannot be emphasized enough that appropriately screened candidates worth interviewing are usually worth hiring, assuming the fit is confirmed (**Figure 118.1**). Some medical directors have a contract on hand to offer the candidate at the conclusion of the interview. The contract can either be generic or personalized with the provider's name. Certainly, there should be no pressure to commit to the position on the spot; however, when appropriate, the candidate should leave with the understanding that the interview was successful and that the position is being offered.

Professional Recruiters

Although all of the recruiting and marketing strategies discussed can be handled directly by the medical director, assistance from experts and support personnel is almost always helpful. Emergency department leaders are experts in emergency medicine, and physician

FIGURE 118.1 ■ Finding the Right Fit

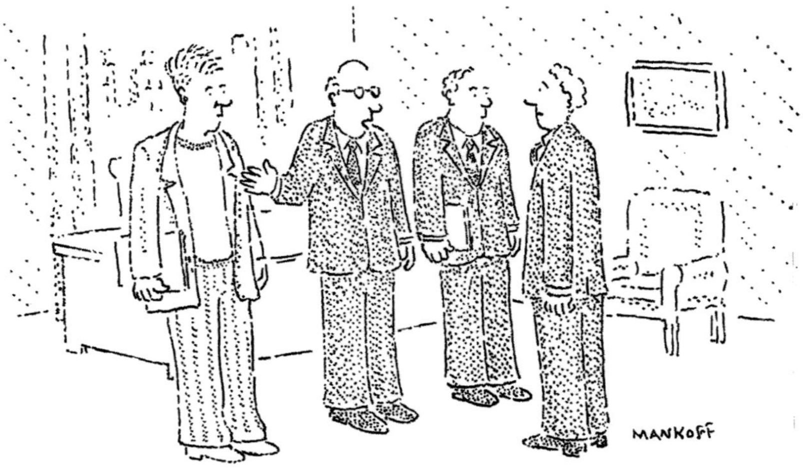

"And on my right is Mr. Darius, who'll fill you in on our corporate *counter*culture."

recruiters are experts at recruiting physicians. In general, there are three categories of assistance one might seek:

- *Hospital-based recruiters* are invaluable. Every hospital has a marketing department that typically supports physician recruiting efforts and integration strategies. These departments draft and place advertisements, may attend trade shows, and usually screen candidates. Human resources departments may also assist in this endeavor.
- *Group-based recruiters* are often career physician recruiters who are employed to recruit solely for that group. These recruiters are usually salaried and generally have incentives that are aligned with the success of the group.
- *Professional recruiting firms* can be excellent tools for getting candidates to sign a contract with the hiring organization. However, there are two caveats:
  - ☐ The recruiters work for the firm, not the hospital or the physician group. Thus, their primary loyalty resides with their firm.
  - ☐ Recruitment fees for successfully closing the deal with a qualified candidate may exceed $25,000. Although these services can be helpful, there may be more cost-effective ways to recruit.

The level and type of support needed will be determined by the medical director's desire and expertise as well as the degree of difficulty in recruiting for the practice. If positions are highly enticing and easily filled, limited resources may be needed. However, when recruitment challenges are noted, it may be necessary to bring in the professionals.

Retention

"Retention" is "recruitment" spelled differently. In other words, retention is the continual rerecruitment of current members of the group. Unfortunately, many leaders ignore this critical aspect of staffing. It takes much less effort to retain the current staff than recruit replacements for those who leave. In addition, current staff members are known entities. Ignoring retention creates the real risk of having to replace a valued provider with someone who is less desirable. Beyond the time, energy, and expense that go into recruiting, the additional efforts required to orient new staff members are substantial and better dedicated to other projects.

Retention requires managing relationships. If these relationships are left untended, practitioners will invariably feel ignored. It is key to constantly assess the pulse of the staff. Medical directors should ask whether their providers are fulfilled and happy in their professional and personal lives; both need to be frequently evaluated. The concerned director might even ask, "What can I do to help?"

From a professional perspective, regular formal performance evaluations should be provided; quarterly is reasonable. However, informal check-ins (monthly or even more frequently) to make certain providers' needs are met are valuable and easy to accomplish. All performance evaluations, formal or informal, should provide the equally important opportunity for clinicians to evaluate the ED and its operations, their career satisfaction and commitment to the practice, and the leader's performance.

It is important to schedule social events that include the providers and their significant others. These activities are fun and rewarding. It is also a necessary part of the successful ED leader's job responsibilities. Job commitment is a personal, emotional, and even visceral response—not necessarily an analytical decision. In short, people enjoy working with and care about those who care about them.

CREDENTIALING

Credentialing is the hospital's mechanism to ensure that expectations for patient safety and quality of care are fulfilled. Prior to 1965, hospitals focused on facility operations, while the medical staff was solely responsible for the quality of care. This structure dates back to the American College of Surgeons Hospital Standardization Program from the early 1900s. In the 1950s, the Joint Commission revised this program. The landmark medical malpractice case *Darling v. Charleston Community Hospital* assigned liability to the hospital for failure to properly credential a physician. In subsequent years, this liability has also been reassigned for inadequate recredentialing processes. Therefore, credentialing and recredentialing processes are responsibilities shared by the hospital and its medical staff.

Hospital Responsibility

The hospital bylaws govern all credentialing and recredentialing responsibilities and requirements, which include the delineation of provider privileges. Although every institution is governed by such bylaws, there is substantial variability in their content. Each hospital is afforded the necessary latitude to define its own mission and establish unique rules, regulations, and even limitations to medical staff membership. In other words, each hospital may restrict the number of physicians it will credential, the specialties they represent, and the qualifications each applicant must possess (i.e., residency training and board eligibility or certification). However, the hospital must apply those standards uniformly and consistently follow its defined processes. The inconsistent application of credentialing rules and regulations can result in liability (i.e., antitrust action).

Inherent Liability

If a hospital's credentialing process is deemed inadequate and a bad outcome results from care provided by an unqualified provider, the hospital might be deemed negligent. A detailed discussion of the liability between a hospital and its medical providers is beyond the scope of this chapter. However, it is important to note that, whether an employee of the hospital, an employee of an emergency group, or an independent contractor (IC), the emergency physician is generally assumed to be an "agent" of the hospital. As a result, the hospital is perceived to be responsible for the physician's negligence while performing in the ED. This legal relationship is called "agency."

Although they work independently of the hospital's influence or control, ICs are frequently regarded as hospital "agents." When a hospital, by its actions or policies, exerts control over the practitioner, an "agent–agency" relationship is more fully established. This relationship is termed "ostensible" or "apparent" agency. If ostensible agency is established, the hospital may be exposed to claims of negligence. This form of responsibility is distinct from the institutional liability that arises from negligent credentialing.

Medical Director Involvement

Credentialing may seem like a simple administrative task that can be delegated to the medical staff office, the physician group clerical staff, or both. When everything runs smoothly, this is probably true. However, credentialing is a complex and very detailed process, and things do not always run smoothly. Medical directors who fail to carefully shepherd the process often find out just days or hours before a shift that their providers will not be credentialed and are unable to work.

The wise medical director obtains a list of items required by the hospital's medical staff office and the expected dates of return. The medical staff office can be instructed to provide periodic reminders and updates. In addition to verifying receipt of the privileging application components, the medical director should follow up with the provider to ensure a timely response to requests made by the medical staff office.

Time Frame

New providers should begin the credentialing process immediately upon execution of the employment contract and complete it as soon as possible. Depending on the institution, the process may take as little as 30 days (the minority) or as long as 6 months. The majority of candidates with uncomplicated work histories are able to receive privileges within 90 days of application. Additional time will be necessary for providers without a current, unrestricted license to practice medicine in that particular state. However, the credentialing and licensure process may take place concurrently.

Process

The process usually consists of several steps, most of which are the responsibility of the applicant. Some institutions will initiate the process with a preapplication that is designed to quickly verify that the basic requirements for medical staff membership are met. If these are not met, then completing the formalized and more arduous medical staff application cannot be pursued, and the process ends there. Once the preapplication is successfully completed and basic requirements are confirmed, the full application should be sent to the provider.

Gathering data from the applicant and outside institutions or agencies is the most time-consuming portion of this process. Once completed with all of the components returned, the application formally enters the actual hospital medical staff credentialing process. The first stop is the hospital's credentials committee, which may recommend privileges be granted or request additional details, documents, or input before making its decision. Once satisfied that the applicant meets all requirements, the committee generally recommends appointment. Initial appointments are typically provisional and limited to the first year of membership. Barring any issues regarding quality of care or behavior, the renewal is granted with a change in status from "provisional" to "active." At each stage of membership, the committee's recommendations are forwarded to the hospital and medical staff leadership teams. If those individuals and/or bodies agree with the appointment recommendation, the application is forwarded to the hospital's board of trustees, which holds the ultimate authority to grant medical staff privileges.

Application Components

Several components of any medical staff privilege application are fairly constant from one institution to the next. These components are designed to:

- Assess the status of the applicant's license.
- Verify educational and previous work background.
- Confirm that any required certifications are up to date.
- Uncover any previous or current legal issues, state licensing actions, or medical staff sanctions taken at a former facility.
- Evaluate the applicant's risk management history through self-reported cases and the National Practitioner Data Bank (NPDB).

References

References, usually three, are requested by most hospitals when applying for medical staff privileges. Generally speaking, the goals of references are to verify employment history and identify any potential character flaws, behavioral issues, or clinical deficiencies the candidate may have. Although the practice of obtaining references is ubiquitous with respect to credentialing, their value can be questioned. It is rare to receive anything other than a positive reference, as most candidates choose people that they know will provide a glowing endorsement.

However, when a negative reference is received, the information is almost always of value and raises questions about the candidate's judgment and self-awareness. The candidate's former departmental chairperson will usually be sent a reference form. This additional requirement helps mitigate a candidate's attempts to avoid a potentially negative review or the disclosure of previous sanctions or disciplinary actions. Specific requests may be sent to individuals who can verify performance during key levels of training or education. Prior to soliciting references, the hospital may ask the applicant to sign a release, which allows those contacted to provide the requested information.

Reference forms will usually ask for dates of employment and information on the individual's clinical performance and personal attributes. As already noted, the references may be of limited value, as some colleagues may be hesitant to speak openly about a candidate's shortcomings. They may perceive potential liability for providing a negative reference if that individual ultimately isn't hired because of the information shared. To reduce this liability, some medical organizations will only provide nonevaluative references. Such references don't include value judgments about performance and only provide factual information about dates of employment and positions held.

This objective, nonevaluative approach, which has limited usefulness to the credentialing body or prospective employer, does offer protection to those providing the reference. Certainly, many hiring physicians contact colleagues directly to get more data; however, providing such information without the candidate's consent may confer a similar risk of liability.

Education and Training

Credentialing bodies always confirm a candidate's education and training. Copies of diplomas or certificates of completion are almost always required for credentialing.

Copies of state licenses as well as state and federal DEA numbers and certificates are also required. The credentialing body confirms that the applicant is in good standing with these organizations.

A final note regarding educational background: Many hospitals require "merit-badges," including course certifications for basic life support, advanced cardiac life support, pediatric advanced life support, and advanced trauma life support. Many emergency medicine experts feel that such requirements are redundant, onerous, and inappropriate. Depending on the physician's training and level of experience, these certifications provide no educational value. Particularly for physicians who are residency trained and board eligible and/or certified in emergency medicine, the training and board certification process far exceeds the requirements of these additional certifications. Any such requirement speaks to the lack of understanding of what an emergency physician does, what the training entails, and the skill set of those who practice in the ED. The medical director should approach the hospital leadership to have such requirements removed for emergency medicine applicants if possible.

Medicolegal History and Professional Liability Insurance

A candidate's risk-management history is important to the hospital. First, the hospital sees the physician's malpractice history as a marker of clinical acumen, and second—and perhaps a more accurate assumption—hospital leaders may fear that a history of multiple claims of significant severity (high dollar amounts) would subject the institution to greater financial risk. Thus, all candidates must disclose any case that has resulted in a claim or lawsuit. A limited time frame (e.g., in the past 10 years) may be specified, and the candidate should be given the opportunity to describe the case and its circumstances. Self-disclosure and/or annual queries of the NPDB are recommended, as claims from prior exposures may continue to be reported years after an employment transition. Thus, a single assessment may provide an incomplete picture of a clinician's professional liability experience.

In addition, a report from the NPDB is obtained on every candidate. In 1986, President Ronald Reagan signed the Health Care Quality Improvement Act into law. The underpinning of this legislation was that, given the increase in medical malpractice claims and lawsuits, mandating a more consistent and complete review of these cases would provide better information about a clinician's practice.

The NPDB was designed to function as a single repository of information regarding the competence and conduct of health-care providers. In addition to tracking medical malpractice judgments and settlements, the data bank also tracks adverse events related to licensure, credentialing, and privileges. In other words, if a physician is suspended (other than for medical record incompletions) or their clinical privileges are restricted, the event may be reportable to the data bank.

Verifying that the candidate has adequate professional liability insurance coverage is also accomplished during the credentialing process. Hospitals have certain minimum requirements that include policy limits, both individual and aggregate, as well as mandates regarding the quality of the insurance carrier. For instance, a hospital may require that the provider's insurer be AM Best rated as "A+" or better. This rating system reflects the financial strength of the insurance carrier. Having insurance with a company that cannot afford to pay all of its claims or goes bankrupt is of no help to the hospital or provider.

Although limits of coverage vary, most hospitals require a minimum of $1 million per occurrence and $3 million in aggregate per year. If the provider will be a hospital employee, then the insurance verification issue is nothing more than a formality, following underwriting of that provider's policy by the insurer. If a group that contracts with the hospital employs a provider, the hospital may require the group to carry certain minimal limits, as well.

ORIENTATION

The orientation process in emergency medicine has historically consisted of, "Here are the charts, and there are the patients." Not only does this minimalist approach lead to confusion and missteps, it also misses the opportunity to cement the psychological contract, further confirm the long-term fit, and ensure the provider's success by helping them get started on the right foot. An orientation program must be structured and yet flexible enough to meet the individual needs of the new hire.

An effective orientation program prepares new hires to function independently. The process should be clearly outlined, and the provider's understanding of key components (e.g., hospital policies) should be acknowledged in writing. In the unfortunate event that a new hire cannot successfully navigate the orientation, this failure should be well-documented. If the practitioner is terminated during this period, thorough documentation may be instrumental to avoid or defend against allegations of wrongful termination.

Group

Every new provider should be oriented to the physician group with a thorough explanation of the following:

- Description of the group structure
- Introduction to the group leader
- Description of benefits with completion of enrollment applications
- Reintroduction to group members and/or coworkers
- Managed care and/or third-party payer enrollments
- Advanced-practice provider supervisory agreements
- Applications
- Billing and coding requirements
- Credentialing processes
- Scheduling requirements
- Risk management education and responsibilities
- Compliance training

Much of this information can be compiled in an employee or orientation manual, including all of the necessary forms new hires are expected to review and complete on their own.

Hospital

The hospital orientation process is intended to provide introductions, build relationships, and familiarize the new medical staff member with policies and procedures. Each physician, prior to providing clinical care, should review the medical staff bylaws. It is better to understand these bylaws (e.g., disruptive physician policy) prior to confronting situations that they address. Avoiding a problem is much easier when the rules and expectations are clear. Just as in a court of law, ignorance is no defense. Particular areas of the bylaws to review include:

- Disciplinary processes and due process
- Credentialing and recredentialing requirements
- Medical malpractice coverage requirements
- Medical records completion policies
- Substance abuse and disruptive physician policies

Relationships

New physicians should be introduced to hospital leaders during the interview process. This level of involvement demonstrates and reinforces the existence of an authentic partnership between the hospital and the emergency medicine team and a mutually strong relationship between the ED medical director and the hospital CEO. The absence of such introductions during an interview day is conspicuous and may raise concerns for the candidate.

Medical Staff Office Personnel

The candidate should also be introduced to the personnel in the medical staff office. Although some physician leaders may consider these middle managers or administrative support staff as nonessential in the grand scheme of things, everyone recognizes their power and value when it comes time to get a new provider credentialed. Nothing gets past the medical staff office before it is ready to go. Once a credentialing file makes it to the CEO's desk or the credentials committee, it is likely to be approved. A personal relationship with the medical staff office personnel can help the candidate and medical director navigate the credentialing process more expeditiously, particularly when application issues arise. The value of this relationship cannot be overstated.

Key Medical Staff Leaders

It is essential for any new physician to meet key medical staff members and, in particular, the hospital's physician leadership (e.g., chief medical officer and the chief of staff). As most emergency physicians function as employees or agents of a third party (e.g., physician group), it is very easy for some staff to treat these "contracted physicians" as outsiders. Unfortunately, this dynamic often arises because some emergency physician groups do not recognize their responsibility as "good citizens" of the hospital. Physicians who haven't taken the time to become familiar with the medical staff and their habits should not be surprised if they are treated gruffly or even rudely. Put a face and a handshake with a name, and a now-familiar voice on the phone at 2 AM becomes a trusted colleague.

All new physicians should be celebrated with equal enthusiasm, whether they practice emergency medicine or cardiothoracic surgery. The same "red carpets" that roll out for nonhospital-based physicians should be rolled out for emergency physicians. The lack of such pomp and circumstance isn't benign; it devalues the clinicians who don't receive this treatment.

Other Key Introductions

- *Community*: The community, particularly if small, will notice the introduction of a new physician and generally regard it as an upgrade in services. A visit to influential community organizations may be worthwhile. At the very least, both internal (hospital newsletter) and external announcements (press release) are essential when welcoming a new physician.
- *Emergency medical services (EMS) personnel*: EMS drives many health-care decisions, probably more than they have been credited with in the past. Developing and nurturing these relationships is key to ensuring that when EMS members have discretion over facility choice, they choose the one with familiar and friendly faces. Introductions are necessary to make certain that EMS personnel feel that the ED is "their" department, too.
- *Hospital support services personnel (e.g., CT and ultrasound technologists)*: Support services are just that: services that support the ED. It is human nature for individuals to work harder for those they like and respect. Personalizing this relationship from the beginning may result in smoother operations and less interpersonal conflict.

Policy Review and Clinical Orientation

The ED clinical orientation is perhaps the most important orientation. Without developing an acceptable degree of comfort with the work environment, a practitioner shouldn't function independently. An ED "nonorientation" is unacceptable, for example:

> *Here are the charts, there are the patients, and those are the nurses. Call me if you have any questions.*

Without an appropriate orientation, a new provider is likely doomed to fail—or at least make multiple unnecessary missteps. A lack of departmental familiarity can result in reduced retention and job satisfaction. The ED orientation should cover all facets of clinical operations and may be divided into two primary components: a review of policies and procedures and a clinical orientation.

Every ED policy relevant to the new provider's practice should be reviewed. Such policies may include dress code, conduct, standard operating procedures, and disaster preparedness. Any operational or policy issue that may be encountered throughout the course of a shift should be addressed.

The most successful clinical orientation programs schedule new clinicians as additional (nonessential) providers, which affords them the opportunity to gain confidence with how the department works. New practitioners should not "fly solo" until the medical director has released them to do so. A provider who begins before understanding the system may prompt clinical staff dissatisfaction and even refusal to work with that individual. Negative first impressions are difficult to overcome and, in many circumstances, prevent new providers from integrating into their new department. An allegation of employer negligence may result from an inadequate clinical orientation. For example:

> *A new physician begins his first shift on a Monday morning at 7:00 AM. At 07:30 AM, a patient presents in severe respiratory distress. The new physician can't find the airway equipment and, while looking, the patient suffers a cardiopulmonary arrest. In this case, the physician's acts are deemed negligent, but so are the employer's. The employer failed to provide an adequate clinical orientation and is found liable for negligence.*

A clinical orientation should be customized to the individual's needs. As a provider progresses to the satisfaction of the medical director, more responsibility and autonomy can and should be allowed. However, if satisfactory progress is not made, the orientation should continue to address specific gaps. In practical terms, the clinical orientation should be provider-specific and should end only when the clinician is ready to function independently.

In some circumstances, the orientation will illuminate reasons why the provider may not be a good fit for the work environment or opportunity. When this happens, the orientation can provide the ED leader with ample information to suggest mutual separation or even termination. However, an individual who successfully passes the orientation should be given the green light.

Compensation During Orientation

Should the provider be compensated during the orientation process? This question addresses the fine balance between preserving the psychological contract (i.e., not requiring work without compensation) and economics. Most ED directors would agree that at least some portion of the orientation process should be paid. Some departments fully compensate new hires for the entire time spent during the orientation program, while others offer no compensation. A reasonable compromise is to provide compensation for the clinical portion of the orientation. Once a provider is generating revenue, even in restricted and supervised circumstances, pay is warranted.

Other Components of Orientation

Other ED orientation components include policies related to the formulary, charting, patient flow, essential provider scope, outside involvement, and clinical guidelines such as processes for referral, transfer, and radiology discrepancies. Department policies should be reviewed before any direct patient contact is allowed. After review, it is important to have the provider sign an attestation acknowledging that the policies have been read and are understood. A reasonable amount of time should be given for such review.

Formulary

Having the new provider review the ED formulary is a valuable exercise that may identify gaps in practice that can be addressed by adding or deleting certain medications. This will help ensure that new providers have access to all of the medications that they believe are necessary to deliver high-quality patient care. In addition, this process gives the medical director insight into the practice style of the new clinician. For instance, if a physician asks to add sublingual nifedipine to the formulary (proven to be harmful in the acute reduction of asymptomatic hypertension), this practice should result in a discussion about the rationale for the request.

Electronic Medical Record Documentation

Electronic health records (EHRs) are a fundamental component of ED workflow; however, some practitioners don't consider documentation an essential portion of their job. It is critical to stress the importance of adequate documentation as a core competency. Good "charting" improves the continuity of care, enhances risk management, and encourages effective coding and billing. Expectations in this regard should be made clear from the beginning. It is reasonable to expect that all patient records are completed on the same day of service and that any records that require additional information are completed at the provider's next available opportunity, either on site or online. This part of the orientation is an excellent time to review the medical record requirements outlined in the hospital's bylaws.

Patient Flow

New providers should be walked through the entire patient experience from registration to discharge. This will confirm that they understand the flow of the average patient. It is also important to ensure an understanding of the ED's processes for order documentation, EHR alerts, and patient tracking.

Essential Providers

Essential providers—such as transport personnel, patient care assistants, scribes, volunteers, flow techs, and even radiology techs—help support the function of the ED. Their roles, training, capabilities, and job responsibilities should be fully discussed. In addition, the role of outside providers must be considered. For instance:

- Are there any limitations placed on medical staff members evaluating patients in the ED?
- Are orthopedists allowed to sedate patients for procedures, or are those services provided exclusively by emergency physicians?
- Can patients be sent from the floor to the ED for procedures when the operating room staff isn't available?
- Are consulting residents allowed to order treatments and diagnostics without first discussing them with the ED attending?

These are all departmental- and institutional-specific components of the new provider's orientation. It is important to remember that any policies or issues related to legal and/or regulatory compliance must be covered. This part of the process should include policies related to the Emergency Medical Treatment and Labor Act, the Health Insurance Portability and Accounting Act, the Joint Commission, the Occupational Safety and Health Administration, and other such laws, agencies, and regulatory mandates.

CONCLUSION

As the US population ages and emerging infectious diseases become more prevalent, ED acuity will increase. Compensation pressures and a scarcity of clinician resources will continue to make timely hiring more difficult. The proficient leader must effectively recruit, orient, and retain a talented staff or be constantly overwhelmed by the need to fill shifts with competent providers. Successful hiring of the right clinicians, though expensive, should be a sustained process. Poor performance in this area is far costlier and may threaten a group's existence.

The savvy leader creates a vision by assembling a team of like-minded, high-performing, dedicated members, who trust their leaders and work within a culture that provides them with opportunities to grow. While there is art to the process, there is science as well. Success includes determining what motivates the candidate, screening effectively and thoroughly, interviewing to predict "fit," onboarding supportively, and creating a purposeful retention process.

CHAPTER 119

PHYSICIAN RETENTION AND PROFESSIONAL DEVELOPMENT

Randy Pilgrim, Ricardo Martinez

Building and maintaining high-performing teams requires a diligent approach to recruiting and retention. Effective physician recruiting requires a clear vision, an engaging mission, and a team environment in which a physician can envision success. Effective physician retention relies heavily on the same foundations. A successful retention plan engages physicians meaningfully in the practice, provides productive feedback, and generates individualized plans for professional development.

CHALLENGES AND OPPORTUNITIES

While most emergency medicine practices devote considerable proactive attention to recruiting qualified providers, relatively little focus is placed on retaining those same professionals. Surveys indicate that relatively few organizations have formal retention initiatives in place, and even when a plan exists, it may not meet the organization's needs adequately.[1,2] Loss of physicians can be very costly, involving recruiting and relocation expenses, orientation and onboarding costs, and losses from low initial productivity.[3-6] Physician turnover also affects the group's morale, team performance, and the reliable delivery of patient care. In addition, current staff must endure both the practicalities and the emotional toll of a new recruiting process. The reputation of the department (and even the stability of the contract) may suffer.

Physician retention is plagued by numerous challenges and sobering realities. Well-trained, experienced physicians usually have many options in the workplace. Increasing workforce shortages significantly increase competition for qualified emergency physicians and other providers.[7-9] The leadership and management skills required for successful retention programs may not be natural for (or viewed as important by) the physician group or its leaders. Some leaders may underestimate the need for a tailored approach to retention after professional training, including issues inherent in the transition from residency to full-time practice. Finally, certain practice environments may not be ideal, producing additional pressures on physician retention.

Changing the Paradigm

A successful retention program complements successful recruiting and supports sustainable excellence in patient care. In practical terms, a successful physician retention program equips new physicians for entry into a practice, while also addressing the needs of more tenured staff. Omitting key areas or missing simple steps can result in an otherwise avoidable departure. Optimal approaches involve basic "do's and don'ts" that produce a good work environment and promote engagement of each physician. Interestingly, the best retention plans result in the emergency department (ED) being "the place to be" and the "team to be on," while truly engaging high-performing, team-oriented physicians. Strong leadership is critical to success, especially when there is a strong mission-driven foundation supported with considerable focus on the quality of relationships with colleagues (**Box 119.1**).

Why Physicians Stay

Physicians remain with a practice when their career's foundational aspects are fulfilled, while at the same time personal, family, and professional needs are met. Fundamentally, physicians value five basic elements of a healthy practice environment: foundations, environment, leadership, personal factors, and professional factors:

- *Foundations*: Base pay, incentives, and benefits are fair and competitive and reasonably reflect effort and productivity. Employment arrangements and contracts are acceptable. Schedule and lifestyle are manageable and consistent with the desired work–life balance.
- *Environment*: The physician experiences an inspiring mission, a meaningful vision, an acceptable culture, and a common purpose. Issues are resolved fairly and promptly. The organization provides opportunities for meaningful input, demonstrates appropriate respect for individuality, and promotes appropriate diversity and inclusion.[10,11]
- *Leadership*: The medical director's role is paramount in maintaining high physician retention rates. One cannot pay providers enough to work in a bad environment, when other opportunities abound. Creating a culture that is collegial, collaborative, and team-oriented attracts and retains talented colleagues. The ability of the medical director to craft a vision, mold teamwork, coach and counsel providers, and lead the department's evolution improves physician performance, satisfaction, and ultimately, retention.
- *Personal factors*: Lifestyle, recreation, and time-away needs are met while social, family, and cultural issues are well addressed.
- *Professional factors*: Medical practice, teaching, research, and other career needs are consistent with the physician's requirements and aspirations.

BOX 119.1 ■ DRIVERS OF PHYSICIAN RETENTION

- Purposeful work
- Clear communication
- Effective feedback
- Feel part of a team
- Satisfying work
- Valued
- Respected
- Appreciated
- Fair, reasonable pay
- Acceptable contract
- Manageable lifestyle
- Meaningful contribution
- Pride of association with institution
- Continuous learning and development

How To: The Elements of an Effective Physician Retention Program

A successful approach to retention is a continuous process that requires careful planning, focus, and attention. A robust program effectively engages new physicians and concurrently addresses the ongoing needs of long-term staff (**Figure 119.1**).

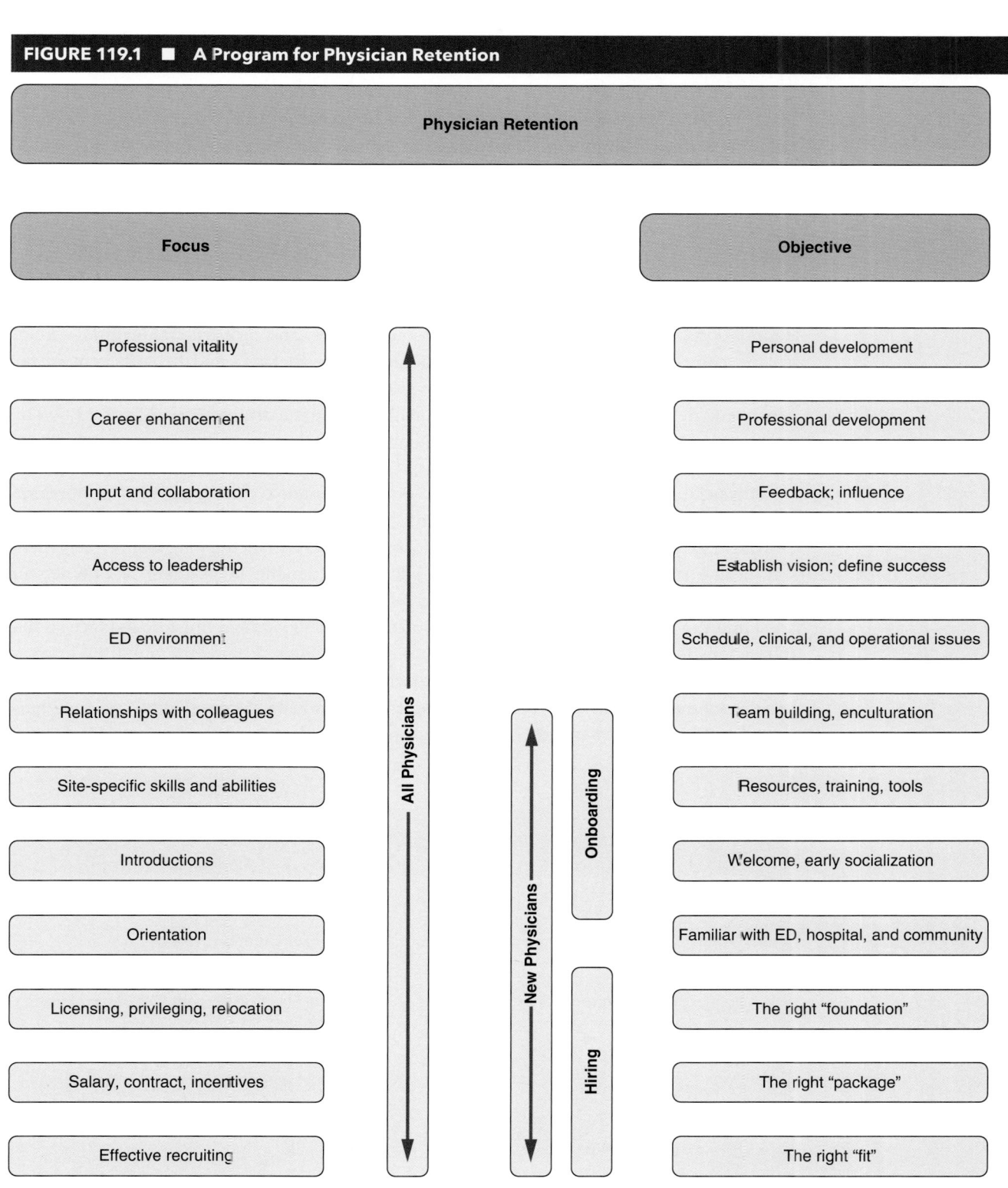

FIGURE 119.1 ■ A Program for Physician Retention

The New Physician: Orientation and Onboarding

The early stages of the relationship have the greatest impact on retention. Trust deepens and engagement is strengthened when a new physician perceives appropriate continuity with the recruitment process (contract, salary, benefits, privileges, relocation issues, etc.). For physicians new to a practice, it is especially important that the physician's expectations of the practice gained from the recruiting process are reaffirmed and remain consistent.[12,13] Thus, effective orientation and onboarding are important cornerstones of retention and require significant initial focus (**Box 119.2**). Early transitions are also supported with introductions, social activities, and involvement of family (including spouse or significant other, children, etc.).[14,15] Identifying a colleague who serves as a formal or informal mentor is a key element for onboarding. Mentorship also increases satisfaction, enhances performance, fosters engagement with the organization, and promotes higher rates of retention.[16,17]

Retention Strategies for Current Staff

Retention plans for current staff build on many elements involved in the "new physician" plan. Additionally, there should be more extensive, individualized strategies that cultivate long-term career satisfaction. The same five issues noted previously must be addressed (i.e., foundations, environment, leadership, personal factors, and professional factors). Annual salary, contract, and incentive reviews should ensure that pay and benefits remain fair and competitive. Physicians should be provided training on novel systems, such as a new electronic medical record, or updates on existing systems and processes in the ED. This training and retraining ensures that skills and competencies remain current, results are satisfactory, and frustrations are minimized.

Physicians value consistent feedback on performance, outcomes, and professional factors affecting their practice. Together with a robust annual evaluation, ongoing feedback is critical to building trust, supporting performance, and enhancing long-term engagement. Promoting physicians' access to ED and hospital leadership helps them feel ownership because they see their input considered and reflected in decision-making.[18,19]

Finally, a clear plan of personal and professional development must be in place so that physicians feel supported, allowing them to enhance their skills while pursuing areas of interest and adjusting to changes. Regularly discussing an individual's development plan encourages input and feedback along the way and helps physicians feel they have an advocate who is interested in more than just what they produce. Looking for "anchor

---

BOX 119.2 ■ ORIENTATION AND ONBOARDING

- Introductions
- Orient to ED, facility, community
- Department goals
    - Key performance indicators
    - Initiatives
    - Challenges
    - Desired outcomes
- Review sources of feedback
- Preview evaluation process
- Train on key competencies
    - Documentation system
    - Radiology system
    - Quality improvement (QI)/performance improvement (PI) processes
    - Clinical processes
- Opportunities for input and collaboration
- Family (spouse, children)

points" (things that resonate uniquely for the physician) assists in individualizing the plan, while emphasizing the quality and unique value of each physician in the practice. Further engagement and professional longevity are predictable results.[19-21]

Why Physicians Leave

Many factors may cause physicians to leave a practice, including professional issues, family and personal needs, changes in marital status, a more competitive offer, and an opportunity for professional advancement. However, factors often cited in avoidable departures include:

- Poor initial hiring decision
- Mismatch of the job with the physician's initial expectations
- Lack of feedback
- Other highly modifiable factors (**Box 119.3**)[22]

An effective retention process will address these common issues with a customized approach for each physician in the practice.[22,23]

The Bottom Line

An effective recruitment process identifies the necessary education, skills, knowledge, and experience for physician candidates while also ensuring an appropriate "fit" for the department. Even if that is well done, it is only half the battle. Effective physician retention involves both programmatic elements and individualized plans that effectively address foundational needs, the practice environment, relationships with leaders and colleagues, and a plan for personal and professional development. With a long-term view of a practice in mind, a focused approach to physician retention is one of the best investments an emergency medicine practice can make.

THE ROLE OF PHYSICIAN ENGAGEMENT

Health care can learn from other industries. Human resource departments have long recognized that people, as invaluable resources, need investment and development as much as any other part of an organization. Research into the productivity and effectiveness of workers sparked new insights about how people work and why they stay. The concept of engagement has direct application for physician groups and EDs.[24] Engagement is defined as the degree of an individual's positive or negative emotional attachment to their organization, their job, and their colleagues.[25] Engagement is a belief in one's work and unique value

BOX 119.3 ■ WHY PHYSICIANS REALLY LEAVE[22]

Analyzing data from close to 20,000 interviews conducted by the Saratoga Institute, Inc, Leigh Branham uncovered significant causes for employee turnover.

- Job or workplace not as expected
- Mismatch between job and person
- Too little coaching and feedback
- Too few growth and advancement opportunities
- Feeling devalued and unrecognized
- Stress from overwork and work-life imbalance
- Loss of trust and confidence in senior leaders

and also a belief in the organization itself with an understanding of the greater context in which work occurs. True engagement results in respect and helpfulness to colleagues, the willingness to "go the extra mile," and a desire for professional and personal development.

Engagement is not something one can mandate; it is purely related to effective leadership, management, and the environment's supportiveness and synergy with each person's needs and desires. Building high-performing teams requires a specific focus on developing actively engaged practitioners. As professionals, this group is not motivated solely by extrinsic rewards such as wages, benefits, titles, or bonuses. The actively engaged professional gains "intrinsic" value from internal characteristics, including:

- Sense of being part of something bigger than oneself
- Belief in the mission of the organization
- Opportunity to engage in meaningful work
- Relationship with one's manager
- Sense of teamwork and relationship with teammates (**Figure 119.2**)[26]

Why does engagement matter? Actively engaged practitioners are also highly committed, usually high-performing, and have high rates of retention. They believe that their actions make a difference, and they expend discretionary effort to further the organization's goals. Actively engaged providers also account for the majority of the positive influence on customer satisfaction, even though they may represent a minority of the group. Finally, highly engaged clinicians experience less professional burnout, which itself is a risk for nonretention.[27,28]

As a team leader, executive, or boss, one can craft job requirements in exquisite detail. The amount of work and effort to meet those requirements is the minimal effort required to maintain the job. On the other hand, the effort that goes beyond those minimal requirements is known as *discretionary effort*. Discretionary effort is just that—the effort exerted by the person at his or her discretion—and is a function of how much the person is engaged with the organization.

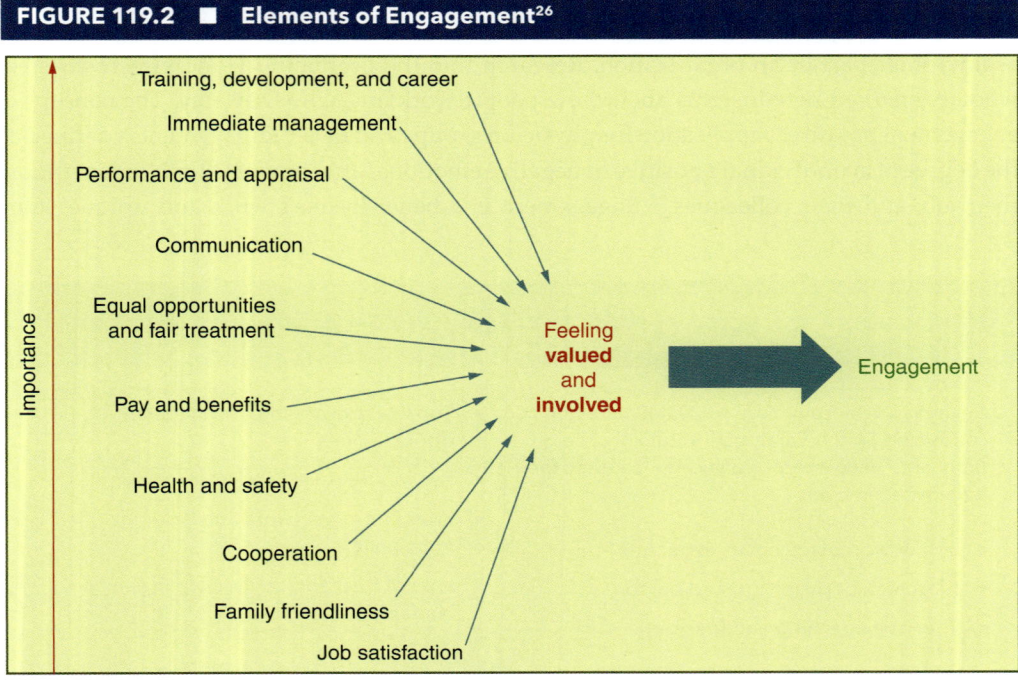

FIGURE 119.2 ■ Elements of Engagement[26]

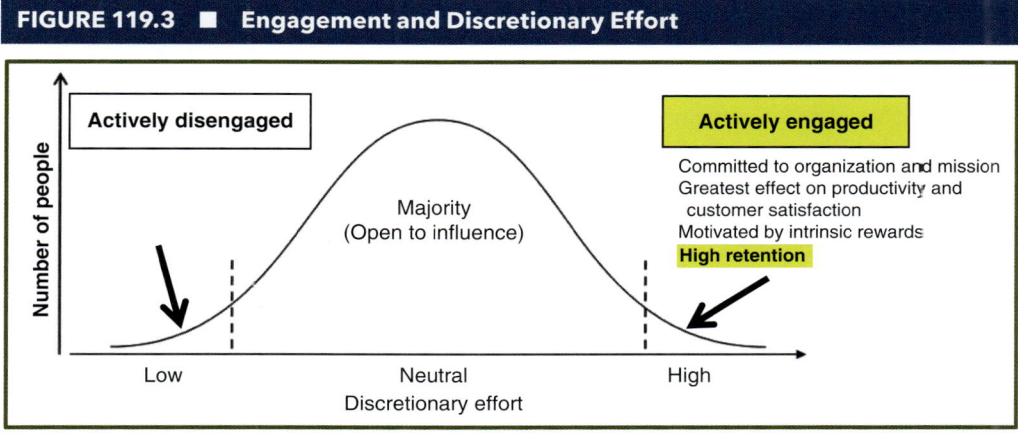

FIGURE 119.3 ■ **Engagement and Discretionary Effort**

Research has shown that there is a nearly bell-shaped "distribution curve" describing staff engagement that involves three basic categories (**Figure 119.3**):

- *Actively engaged:* Aligned with the mission and values of the company, staff feels that their work is important and that they can make a difference.
- *Not engaged:* Focused on accomplishing tasks required of the job and not on the overall outcome or performance of the organization, these staff members may believe that their contributions are not appreciated and do not feel connected to teammates or managers.
- *Actively disengaged:* This group does more than feel disconnected; they actually expend energy on negativity, undermining initiatives or goals.

Estimates of "employee" engagement vary, but recent literature suggests that approximately 20% to 30% of "employees" are actively engaged, while 10% to 20% are actively disengaged.

Most medical professionals appreciate engagement with their colleagues and their institutions. They also want to be a part of a mission-oriented team that provides feedback and coaching. All of these characteristics provide opportunities for medical leadership to invest in physicians and staff and to promote professional development while attracting and retaining high-quality staff (**Box 119.4**).[29]

BOX 119.4 ■ TOP 10 DRIVERS OF EMPLOYEE ENGAGEMENT[29]

1. Senior management sincerely interested in employee well-being
2. Ability to improve skills and capabilities
3. Organization's reputation for social responsibility
4. Employee's input into decision-making
5. Quick resolution of customer concerns
6. Setting high personal standards
7. Excellent career advancement opportunities
8. Challenging work assignments that broaden skills
9. Good relationships with supervisors
10. Organization encourages innovative thinking

PHYSICIAN FEEDBACK

Effective physician feedback supports good patient care, fosters teamwork, builds trust, and promotes physician engagement with the practice. To be meaningful, feedback must focus on results as well as *perceptions* of one's work, style, and results. Effective feedback mechanisms support successes, clarify roles and responsibilities, and identify and remediate performance issues early. Without appropriate feedback, physicians can become frustrated (or even fail) because they are unsure of what is truly valued in the practice, including how success is measured.

Focus groups reveal that physicians generally want more feedback than they are getting.[22] In fact, physicians would rather hear difficult feedback than no feedback at all. Physicians are concerned about important facts of their practice and perceptions about them that are often not communicated in a timely manner, if ever. Physicians often value periodic acknowledgment and appreciation more than formal incentives or rewards.

Frequently, however, feedback is ineffective, misapplied, or worse, entirely absent. The ED director or other leaders may not realize its criticality in creating a high-performing and engaging environment. Instead, the director may mistakenly rely solely on the physician's own self-reflection, experience, or professional judgment to create change. Leaders may lack training in how to deliver feedback, may feel uncomfortable addressing peers, or may never have experienced effective communication in a high-quality environment.

Feedback on What?

Feedback is most effective when it involves performance and results or teamwork and relationships. Feedback on performance and results should be grounded in the department's mission and vision and tied to its goals and objectives. For example, in a hospital whose mission involves good clinical care and a good *experience* of care, patient satisfaction and door-to-provider times in the ED are important measurements. Mechanisms for frequent feedback, both for individual rules and for the department, must be implemented accordingly (**Box 119.5**).

Although less quantitative in nature, feedback related to teamwork and relationships is also important. This feedback should also be grounded in a departmental vision, which often references quality care as a "team sport" and includes the need for dignified and respectful communication. As an example, because optimal patient safety requires effective communication and inclusion of others' observations, those who use workarounds instead of an established system for patient flow may need feedback about relevant concerns from the rest of the team in regard to avoidable frustrations, delays in care, risk and safety concerns, documentation issues, and so on.[30] Feedback, especially corrective messages, *without* a

---

BOX 119.5 ■ SOURCES OF FEEDBACK

- Medical director
- Departmental reports/data
- Compliments and complaints
- Quality improvement processes
- Committee/taskforce proceedings
- Colleagues and team members
- Hospital administration
- Risk management
- Annual evaluation
- Patients and families

shared vision and mutual objectives is often ineffective and may actually harm relationships. It can reduce feedback to a difference of opinion, rather than objective standards. Unhealthy power struggles and difficult emotions often result. However, in the context of a clear vision that yields goals and objectives for performance and teamwork, feedback has the requisite framework and serves as a critical tool for achieving those objectives.

Effective Feedback Is a Leadership Competency

Consistent, effective feedback is a core competency for leaders and a basic building block of high-performing teams. Whether scheduled or spontaneous, formal or informal, verbal or written, effective feedback mechanisms continually affirm key elements of quality emergency care. Positive feedback reinforces desired behavior and results, while corrective communications address marginal performance. Frequent "small doses" not only prevent serious remediation and interventions but also recognize exemplary efforts and consistent results. Communications that result in a two-way dialogue provide an invaluable opportunity for input and problem solving in the department. Effective feedback also supports personal and professional development plans, affirms aligned incentive programs, supports formal reward systems, and previews the formal performance appraisal.

Feedback: Principles, Pearls, and Pitfalls

Feedback is an opportunity to express a professional commitment to a colleague. It affords an opportunity for learning, development, and deeper engagement and is most useful when given regularly, honestly, and constructively, even when acknowledging suboptimal performance. Usually, a mentorship and coaching approach works best.

Physicians are trained to be logical, critical, and to prefer fact-based discussions. They often make quick judgments in the face of confusion or contradiction, value autonomy, and can become impatient with vague messages or nonactionable discussions. They may also believe that *what* gets done is always more important than *how* things are done and that outcomes or intentions may outweigh any difficulties for others on the team.

There are numerous models for communicating feedback effectively. Most approaches employ a few core principles supported by effective techniques. Although these models

---

BOX 119.6 ■ COMPONENTS OF EFFECTIVE FEEDBACK

- Timing
- Frequency
- Setting
- Preparation
- Opening
- Facts, behaviors, and results
- Context
- Manner
- Desired state
- Listening

- Forward-facing plan
- Individualizing the plan
- Assisting
- Closing
- Follow-up
- Providing constructive criticism
- Recognizing the positive
- Anchoring
- What really works

frequently focus on constructively critical (negative) feedback, the same principles apply to reinforcing (positive) feedback. A leader should use an individualized approach that affirms their native style, incorporating the following considerations (**Box 119.6**):

- *Timing*: Feedback is most effective when it is delivered as close to the event as possible, while the experience is fresh. For difficult conversations, however, promptly find a time when no other responsibilities interfere with it and, most importantly, have the discussion when you, as a leader, are prepared.
- *Frequency*: Deliver feedback consistently and regularly. Avoid acknowledging performance or results only once or twice a year and certainly not just when "negative" feedback is in order.
- *Setting*: Give feedback in person and in a private setting whenever possible. One-on-one is best and is required for most difficult conversations. Avoid giving feedback during a change of shift or meetings, unless public acknowledgment of success is the goal. Avoid feedback by phone unless it prevents an excessive delay. Almost never use e-mail, memos, or phone messages alone.
- *Preparation*: Especially for difficult conversations, take time to plan a thoughtful approach. This usually includes careful consideration of the delivery, possible reactions, and acceptable or unacceptable outcomes from the discussion. For most difficult discussions, it is helpful to prepare thoughts in writing and verbally practice at least the initial delivery. Simple and straightforward communication is best.
- *Opening*: Get to the point quickly and directly, which helps to clarify the concern and prevent defensiveness. For both positive and constructive (negative) feedback, identify the topic or issue in your first sentence.
- *Facts, behaviors, and results*: Specific feedback is more actionable. Communicate data, results, facts, objective observations, and behaviors. Avoid generalities, personal opinions, interpretations, and biases. Theoretical, professional, or philosophical discussions have their place, but not in early discussions. Focus on performance and results and/or teamwork and relationships.
- *Context*: Even the most self-assured physician inwardly wonders: "Why are we talking?" or "Where is this going?" Verbalizing a commitment to the mission and vision of the department *and* to the provider's success helps the physician digest the feedback in proper context and avoids over-personalization. Quality dialogue and better solutions will result.
- *Manner*: How you convey a message is more important than what you say. Be sincere, focused, concerned, and forward-looking.
- *Desired state*: With constructive (negative) feedback, identify specific behaviors or results that need to change. State clearly what you want to see and give examples. Reinforce expectations and a vision of success. The physician must understand why the feedback is important, where current performance stands, and the nature of your support for the clinician's success. A simple guide to verbalizing these issues succinctly is the "I statement" (**Box 119.7**).
- *Listening*: Listening promotes engagement and better solutions. Allow for additional insights to be shared by the physician without inappropriately diluting your perspective. How does the physician think things are going? What does he or she think success looks like? What are the physician's concerns? Allow time and space for a response. Be prepared for disagreement and further dialogue.
- *Forward-facing plan*: Rather than dwell on the issue itself, solicit a commitment to improve and move promptly to a plan. Agree on future goals. In positive feedback settings, discuss plans that support excellence and inspire others as well. Assist with advice as needed but allow the physician to "own" the plan.

- *Individualizing the plan*: People have unique skills, abilities, attitudes, strengths, and weaknesses, as well as different backgrounds and different perspectives. As a leader you should compare and contrast your communication and learning style with the other person's style and adjust the approach accordingly.
- *Assisting*: Ask how you can help. Offer techniques and tools, if needed. Affirm your support for a good outcome.
- *Closing*: Be sure the physician understands the issue, its impact, and what needs to change. Clarify possible consequences. Emphasize your support for an appropriate outcome. Address questions. Establish a time frame for follow-up and interval communications. Remind the physician of his or her strengths and what you value about them. Reiterate your willingness to support him or her in the process.
- *Follow-up*: Stay committed to the vision of success and support with additional feedback as needed. Follow the plan. Do not miss time lines. Report, trend, and document as appropriate.
- *Providing constructive criticism (negative feedback)*: Give feedback in private, rather than in a group. Do not apologize for addressing a performance deficit. Use a tone of concern and sincerity, rather than anger, frustration, or sarcasm, which dilutes the message. Talk about behavior and results rather than the person and his or her attitudes, opinions, character, or perceived motivations.
- *Recognizing the positives*: Recognize where your colleague has done well or improved. Stay focused on providing concrete examples, including the *impact* you see. This reinforces behaviors that are valued and sets a positive tone. Catch people at their best, using thank-you notes, rewards, and recognitions regularly.
- *Anchoring*: Tell the truth. Integrity speaks softly, but very convincingly. Refuse to personalize issues. Discuss issues, not people. Defuse resistance with respectful persistence. Every disagreement is an opportunity to improve a relationship.
- *What really works*: What really works is a meaningful mission, a clear vision, a winning culture, effective teamwork, personal integrity, proper skills, knowledge of risks and pitfalls, compassionate communication, and truth (**Box 119.8**).

Documentation

Documenting feedback serves several purposes. From a professional standpoint, shared documentation serves as a communication tool that affirms strengths and opportunities for improvement. It reflects agreed-upon plans for personal or professional development, while tracking progress and milestones. Documenting results informs the annual performance review and, ideally, is consistent with regular communication with the individual along the way.

From a legal or risk perspective, documentation can also demonstrate important communications in retrospect, including action plans and follow-up. Each practice should develop its own approach and standards for documentation, and consultation with hospital

---

BOX 119.7 ■ THE "I-STATEMENT"

"When I (see, hear) _____,

I become concerned about _____, or I feel _____."

"What I'd like instead is _____" so that _____."

> **BOX 119.8 ■ TOP 10 QUALITIES OF EFFECTIVE FEEDBACK**
>
> 1. Specific
> 2. Timely
> 3. Actionable
> 4. In person
> 5. Simple
> 6. Fair
> 7. Sincere
> 8. Respectful
> 9. Forward looking
> 10. Tied to mission and vision

or legal resources should advise contractual issues, discoverability concerns, labor law, and liability issues. In general, it is best to document feedback routinely, so that successes and excellent performance can be acknowledged, and when necessary, performance problems and action plans can be referenced accurately.

Difficult Issues

Feedback focuses on sharing *information*. Coaching suggests effective *actions* based on that information. A leader can coach the physician through an improvement process, requiring that specific results or behaviors must occur within a certain time frame. Difficult or repetitive situations require not only feedback and coaching but also counseling, remediation, or intervention. If these interventions prove unsuccessful, resignation or termination discussions may occur.

Most difficult or recurring issues are nonclinical in nature, involving communication, personality issues, and difficulties with teamwork. Certain issues require special skills and unique approaches, including sexual harassment, impairment, or significantly disruptive behavior (see Chapter 122). Some issues even have legal, regulatory, licensing, credentialing, or contractual implications.

Approaching significant issues that require extensive counseling, remediation, or intervention is outside the scope of this chapter. However, typical guidance includes the following[31-33]:

- Act promptly when addressing significant or repetitive problems.
- Be aware of laws, regulations, policies, and professional guidelines that may impact the approach.
- Engage assistance early (e.g., risk management, legal assistance, or intervention and recovery professionals).
- Document well.

PROFESSIONAL DEVELOPMENT

As noted previously, investing in physicians provides intrinsic rewards and leads to a greater level of engagement. Investment and engagement lead to enhanced performance for the individual, the team, and the organization. For physicians, a professional development program is important for individual growth, both as a person and as a member of the medical profession. Professional development also leads to greater rates of retention.

To address professional development, it is necessary to first define a profession: A profession is an occupation that has a covenant with society, and in return, the professional is given certain privileges by that society. The medical profession establishes the standards for training, certification, and privileges of physicians and is expected to set values, standards of practice, and competence and to self-police its members. This covenant is based on trust that the medical profession will place the needs of society above its own. Rather than an occupation alone, a profession may be considered a way of life.

The past few decades have seen an explosion of technology and information in medicine (see this book's Section 5, Informatics). This change has created a shift toward a more technical approach by many physicians and less emphasis on humanistic qualities.[34] As a result, the profession has failed to meet certain patient experience expectations, and there has been some loss of stature by the profession. In response, medical schools and professional societies are reengaging physicians and students on the behaviors and values associated with the medical profession.[35]

Despite many advances in modern health care, medicine remains essentially an apprenticeship learning model. Medical students transform into physicians through didactic training, experience-based learning, and tutelage by mentors and role models. This framework creates comprehension and context for learning and behaviors. Unfortunately, the environment for growth and development often disappears as one enters clinical practice, providing strong opportunity—and an imperative—for professional development programs.

The requirements for professional practice continuously evolve, but many of the core values of the covenant of medical professionalism remain the same (**Box 119.9**).[36] Literature shows that effective teamwork improves care and patient safety, and in most practice settings, teamwork is a core competency.[37-39]

An excellent professional development program, then, should focus on three main domains. The physician should develop as a:

- Clinician practitioner (medical skills and knowledge)
- Medical professional (behaviors and values of the profession)
- Team member (team skills)

Clinical Practitioner

Medical school starts physicians on a path of lifelong learning. Most organizations are familiar with a continuing medical education program for physicians, either required by the medical staff or licensing bodies. However, a more robust program that develops physicians and staff can improve clinical performance and raise the level of knowledge uniformly. More importantly, a well-published and formalized program of continuing education provides opportunity for individual training, personal growth, and feedback.

BOX 119.9 ■ PROFESSIONAL RESPONSIBILITIES[36]

- Commitment to professional competence
- Commitment to honesty with patients
- Commitment to maintaining appropriate relations with patients
- Commitment to improving quality of care
- Commitment to improving access to care
- Commitment to a just distribution of finite resources
- Commitment to scientific knowledge
- Commitment to maintaining trust by managing conflicts of interest
- Commitment professional responsibilities

For individuals to feel that they are active participants in this process, opportunities should be created for physicians to discuss or reflect on cases, provide short presentations on topics of interest (positioning each physician as a contributing expert), and generate ideas for further study.

The learning environment is also important. Knowledge transfer can occur at change of shifts, at monthly department meetings, and at breakfast or dinner meetings. Overall, this creates a learning culture where gaps in knowledge are proactively addressed and the physicians and staff are seen as constantly helping each other grow.

Medical Professional

As previously mentioned, technical mastery of medical knowledge is not enough; physicians are involved in issues that go beyond medical knowledge and involve ethics, values, and morals. They must become good medical professionals and team members. Physicians often discuss the sanctity of the doctor–patient relationship. However, that relationship is rooted in the physician's ability to demonstrate professional ethics and behaviors. In truth, the ability to act as a medical professional is key to influencing better patient care. Responsibilities within the profession require collaborative work to:

- Advance the quality of patient care
- Participate in medical staff governance
- Participate in self-regulation processes
- Engage in remediation and discipline of members who fail to meet professional standards.

Physicians also have professional obligations to both personal and group-provided care and should be open to outside review of their professional performance.[36] They also have duties to their patients, their medical community, and the community at large and should participate in committees, events, and initiatives that strengthen the role of the medical professional and fulfill its obligations to society.

While there is no generally agreed-upon definition of medical professionalism, there are some central tenets that are universally noted, including principles, values, virtues, and behaviors. A set of 10 virtues or character traits that are germane to the practice of emergency medicine have been proposed by the Society of Academic Emergency Medicine.[40] These include:

- Prudence
- Courage
- Temperance
- Justice
- Unconditional positive regard
- Charity
- Compassion
- Trustworthiness
- Vigilance
- Agility

In addition, the American College of Physicians and the American Board of Internal Medicine have issued a physician charter on medical professionalism. These provide a rich source of concepts upon which to shape a medical professional ideal (see **Box 119.9**).

Team Member

Characteristics of teamwork are different than individual actions (see Chapter 12). Team characteristics include:

- Shared goals and plans
- Coordination of actions
- Coaching
- Performance feedback
- Collaboration
- Enhanced communication (especially at handoffs)

The practice of medicine has moved from care by individuals to a "team sport," but most medical training does not optimally prepare physicians with the skills needed to be effective in a team. In fact, medical training often underscores and reinforces autonomy of decision-making, which can undermine teamwork.

However, physicians can be taught team skills within the proper learning environment. Research underscores that team skill training can lead to improved team performance, improved staff attitudes, and a reduction in errors.[37] Teamwork is a process with specified roles, responsibilities, and behaviors that ensure coordination and accomplishment of shared goals. Research suggests that educating even one or two members of a team can improve overall work of the team by introducing fundamental team processes into the team's work.[41] In 2011, the Association of American Medical Colleges called for greater training of team-based competencies for medical students and medical professionals.[42] In addition, physicians who feel that they are part of a dedicated, mutually respectful team are more likely to remain with that practice.[43]

Excellent resources on team skill training include the Emergency Team Coordination Course and TeamStepps.[37,38]

The Personal Development Plan

Creating a solid path for professional development requires a well-crafted personal development plan (PDP) for the individual. Each physician is different, with different strengths and weaknesses; a PDP becomes an internal roadmap for individual growth. The plan is generally a simple process that asks three questions: Where am I now? Where do I want to go? and How will I get there? While these questions seem simple, they are only effective if they are examined clearly and carefully and acted upon accordingly.

Where Am I Now?

For example, when asking "Where am I now?," physicians should develop a list of strengths and weaknesses based on feedback from others, identifying areas in which they generally have success and failure, common complaints and compliments, and areas in which they are comfortable or uncomfortable. This usually generates a fairly rounded view of one's current status.

External feedback is critical in this process. For example, research shows that surgeons grade their teamwork with nurses in the operating room as excellent, but operating room nurses rank it much lower.[44,45] In addition, physicians routinely overestimate their clinical competence against observed measures.[46] Honest evaluation is critical to understanding one's beginning point in a growth process. Appropriate candor and truthfulness in an environment of trust and support places the personal development process on a firm foundation.

Where Do I Want to Go?"

"Where do I want to go?" Visualizing oneself as having excellent clinical competence, great medical professionalism, a collaborative team member, or all three at a future point is important. A mentor should strive to understand what the physician wants to be and why, so that support and resources can be optimized. Progress toward that vision is important, and the process of growth can be its own intrinsic reward. Robust underpinnings for these ultimate goals give considerable meaning to the transition.

How Will I Get There?

The question, "How will I get there?" helps identify the knowledge, skills, behaviors, and experiences that one needs and provides specific milestones and objectives to attain both long-term and short-term goals. For example, if the physician wants to be a leader in the medical staff, the PDP might identify joining a committee as a short-term goal and chairing a committee as a longer term goal. However, success in these positions will likely require additional knowledge, skills, and mentorship. Appropriate learning resources should then be identified through the PDP with time frames for accomplishment. Fundamental to the PDP is routine feedback, objective assessments, personal reflection, and coaching and mentorship by a trusted colleague or leader. Physicians with a realistic PDP and good plans for professional development are more engaged, satisfied, and stay with their practice longer.

Creating the Culture for Continuous Growth

Individuals only grow in fertile ground. It is incumbent upon medical leadership to develop a culture that values the individual and team development and celebrates accomplishments. The three domains of professional development—clinical, professional, and team skills—must be reinforced through consistent communications within the group and the ED staff. It is incumbent upon medical and nursing leadership to embody the values and behaviors that they espouse. If leadership does not believe it, who will? Cultivate it, and it will grow.

Constant and consistent communications are important. Many people mistakenly believe that a memo suffices, but it is far more effective to continuously reinforce core messages in meetings, presentations, newsletters, and conversation. With consistent messages, people will begin to change behavior over time. Leaders should continue to coach their colleagues about the necessary behavior changes until those changes become habit, a process that usually takes longer than anticipated.

Professional character is formed over time and shaped by many factors, including values, attitudes, and behaviors espoused by role models. Most physicians can name a role model that influenced their personal growth and will recall an experience from which they learned. Role modeling, coaching, and mentorship are fundamental parts of learning and professional development for physicians.

Medical directors must understand that role modeling is both a blessing and a burden. By modeling desired professional behaviors in meetings, at the bedside, when resolving conflict and dealing with medical staff, during disciplinary actions, and within the community, the medical director has tremendous influence on the behavior and personal growth of other physicians. Learning and identity formation are strongly related, and role models contribute great influence to both aspects of growth. Observational learning is a powerful way to transmit values, attitudes, and patterns of behavior.[47] On the other hand, if the medical director's behavior stands in contrast to espoused beliefs, then credibility erodes and the behaviors of others decay accordingly.

Lastly, cultural values are transmitted and reinforced by[48]:

- The way leaders behave
- Recognizing individuals who demonstrate those values
- Celebrating the values within the organization and community
- Honoring those who exemplify the values that we hold dear

Building high-performing individuals, teams, and organizations requires that efforts are taken to instill, cultivate, and celebrate a set of core values that forms the foundation for professional growth.

CONCLUSION

Building and maintaining a high-performing ED requires effective recruiting, retention, and development of both individuals and teams. Each of these critical factors is positively influenced by crafting a clear vision and an engaging mission and by creating a team environment in which a physician can envision success. The most effective individuals are those who are truly engaged and see themselves as part of something bigger than themselves, with the personal reward of meaningful work and an opportunity for growth. More importantly, a team approach amplifies the efforts and enhances the delivery of quality patient care, improves patient safety, and builds a more collaborative workplace.

Leaders can develop individuals by supporting them as clinical practitioners, medical professionals, and team members. All of these domains require active feedback, opportunities for engagement, and an investment in personal growth. These combined efforts lead to greater provider engagement, improvements in individual and team performance, and long-term retention of key physician staff.

REFERENCES

1. NewsWise.com. Retention initiatives rise as physician turnover concerns increase. 2006. Available at: https://www.newswise.com/articles/retention-initiatives-rise-as-physician-turnover-concerns-increase. Accessed November 15, 2020.
2. Shah S. The real cost of emergency department physician turnover. 2016. Available at: https://www.studergroup.com/resources/articles-and-industry-updates/insights/january-2016/the-real-cost-of-emergency-department-physician-tu. Accessed November 15, 2020.
3. Waldman JD, Kelly F, Arora S, et al. The shocking cost of turnover in health care. Health Care Manage Rev. 2004;29(1):2–7.
4. Scott K. Physician retention plans help reduce costs and optimize revenues. Healthc Financ Manage. 1998;52(1):75–77.
5. Buchbinder SB, Wilson M, Melick CF, et al. Estimates of costs of primary care turnover. Am J Manage Care. 1999;5(11):1431–1438.
6. Berger JE, Boyle RL Jr. How to avoid the high costs of physician turnover. Med Group Manage J. 1992;39(6):80–91.
7. Ginde AA, Sullivan AF, Camargo CA Jr. National Study of the Emergency Physician Workforce, 2008. Ann Emerg Med. 2009;54(3):349–359.
8. Emergency Medicine: Physician Recruiting, Supply, and Staffing Considerations in Today's Healthcare System. White Paper Series. Merritt Hawkins, an AMN Healthcare Company; 2017.
9. Koski-Vacirca R, VanderVinne N, Burmeister B. Physician shortage and physician workforce challenge. In: Schlicher N, Haddock A, eds. Emergency Medicine Advocacy Handbook. 5th ed. Emergency Medicine Residents' Association (EMRA); 2019:103–110.
10. Shaw G. Building a diverse emergency medicine. Emerg Med News. 2020;42(3):20–21.
11. Choo EK, Kass D, Westergaard M, et al. The development of best practice recommendations to support the hiring, recruitment, and advancement of women physicians in emergency medicine. Acad Emerg Med. 2016;23(11):1203–1209.
12. Bretz RD, Judge TA. Realistic job previews: a test of the adverse self-selection hypothesis. J Appl Psychol. 1998;83(2):330–337.
13. Buckley RM, Fedor DB, Veres JG, et al. Investigating newcomer expectations and job-related outcomes. J Appl Psychol. 1998;83(3):452–461.
14. Bender C, DeVogel S, Blomberg R. The socialization of newly hired medical staff into a large health system. Health Care Manage Rev. 1999;24(1):95–108.
15. King H, Speckart C. Ten evidence-based practices for successful physician retention. Available at: https://docplayer.net/18332157-Ten-evidence-based-practices-for-successful-physician-retention-by-hannah-king-mph-carrie-speckart-ma.html. Updated 2020. Accessed November 16, 2020

16. Chao, GT, Walz PM, Gardner PD. Form and informal mentorships: a comparison on mentoring functions and contrast with nonmentored counterparts. *Personnel Psychology*. 1992;45(3):619–636.

17. Ragins BR, Cotton JL. Mentor functions and outcomes: a comparison of men and women in formal and informal mentoring relationships. *J Appl Psychol*. 1999;84(4):529–550.

18. Tallman K, Steinbruegge J. Successful practices in the physician work environment: we work together. *Perm J*. 2002;6(4):39–42. Available at: http://www.thepermanentejournal.org/issues/43-the-permanente-journal/original-research-and-contributions/6122-successful-practices-in-the-physician.html. Accessed November 16, 2020.

19. Rhoades L, Eisenberger R, Armeli S. Affective commitment to the organization: the contribution of perceived organizational support. *J Appl Psychol*. 2001;86(5):825–836.

20. TrissaConsulting.com. Personal Balanced Scoreboards: The Key to Organizational Alignment. 2011. Available at: http://www.trissaconsulting.com/articles/personal-balanced-scoreboards-the-key-to-organizational-alignment. Accessed November 16, 2020.

21. Amabile TM, Kramer SJ. Inner work life: understanding the subtext of business performance. *Harv Bus Rev*. 2007;85(5):72–83,144.

22. Branham L. The 7 hidden reasons employees leave. 2020. Available at: https://leadershipbeyondlimits.com/wp-content/uploads/2013/06/WhyPeopleLeave-Branham.pdf. Accessed November 16, 2020.

23. Ross JA. Dealing with the real reasons people leave. *Harvard Management Update*. 2008. Available at: https://hbr.org/2008/02/dealing-with-the-real-reasons. Accessed November 14, 2020.

24. James F, Gerrard F. Emergency medicine: what keeps me, what might lose me? A narrative study of consultant views in Wales. *Emerg Med J*. 2017;34(7):436–440.

25. Schaufeli W. *What is Engagement?* In: Truss C, Delbridge R, Shantz A, et al., eds. *Employee Egagement in Theory and Practice*. London: Routledge Company; 2013. Available at: https://www.wilmarschaufeli.nl/publications/Schaufeli/414.pdf. Accessed November 24, 2020.

26. Robinson D. Employee Engagement. 2003. Available at: https://www.employment-studies.co.uk/system/files/resources/files/op11.pdf. Accessed November 15, 2020.

27. Williamson K, Lank PM, Lovell EO. Emergency Medicine Education Research Alliance (EMERA). Development of an emergency medicine wellness curriculum. *AEM Educ Train*. 2017;2(1):20–25.

28. AMN Healthcare, Smith BE, Hawkins M. Room to grow: trends in hospital & health system physician leadership. *AMN Leadership Solutions*. 2019. Available at: https://www.merritthawkins.com/uploadedFiles/Physician_Leadership_Survey_Report.pdf. Accessed November 14, 2020.

29. Bijoor A. Employee engagement—A Towers Perrin Study. 2009. Available at: https://bijoor.me/2009/03/09/employee-engagement-drives-business-performance/. Accessed November 17, 2020.

30. Rosenstein AH. Nurse–physician relationships impact on nurse satisfaction and retention. *Am J Nurs*. 2002;102(6):26–34.

31. Brinkman R, Kirschner R. *Dealing With Difficult People: 24 Lessons for Bringing Out the Best in Everyone*. New York, NY: McGraw-Hill; 2006.

32. Patterson K, Grenny J, McMillan R, et al. *Crucial Conversations: Tools for Talking When Stakes are High*. New York, NY: McGraw Hill; 2002.

33. Patterson K, Grenny J, McMillan R, et al. *Crucial Confrontations: Tools for Resolving Broken Promises, Violated Expectations and Bad Behavior*. New York, NY: McGraw Hill; 2005.

34. Branch WT Jr, Weil AB, Gilligan MC, et al. How physicians draw satisfaction and overcome barriers in their practices: "it sustains me." *Patient Educ Couns*. 2017;100(12):2320–2330.

35. Swick HM. Toward a normative definition of medical professionalism. *Acad Med*. 2000;75(6):612–616.

36. American Board of Internal Medicine (ABIM) Foundation, ACP-ASIM Foundation, European Federation of Internal Medicine. Medical professionalism in the new millennium: a physician charter. *Ann Intern Med*. 2002;136(3):243–246.

37. Morey JC, Simon R, Jay GD, et al. Error reduction and performance improvement in the emergency department through formal teamwork training: evaluation results of the MedTeams project. *Health Serv Res*. 2002;37(6):1553–1581.

38. TeamSTEPPS. Homepage. Available at: https://www.ahrq.gov/teamstepps/index.html. Accessed July 11, 2013.

39. Barrett J, Gifford C, Morey J, et al. Enhancing patient safety through teamwork training. *Healthc Risk Manag*. 2001;21(4):57–65.

40. Larkin GL, Iserson K, Kassutto Z, et al. Virtue in emergency medicine. *Acad Emerg Med*. 2009;16(1):51–55.

41. Magrane D, Khan O, Pigeon Y, et al. Learning about teams by participating in teams. *Acad Med*. 2010;85(8):1303–1311.

42. Team-Based Competencies: Building a Shared Foundation for Education and Clinical Practice. *Proceedings of Interprofessional Educational Collaborative*. February 16-17, 2011. Accessed November 13, 2020. Available at: https://www.gih.org/files/IPE%20conference%20proceedings%20Report_5211.pdf.

43. Lemieux-Charles L, McGuire WL. What do we know about health care team effectiveness? A review of the literature. *Med Care Res Rev*. 2006;63(3):263–300.

44. Makary MA, Sexton JB, Freischlag JA, et al. Operating room teamwork among physicians and nurses: teamwork in the eye of the beholder. *J Am Coll Surg*. 2006;202(5):746–752.

45. Carney BT, West P, Neily J, et al. Differences in nurse and surgeon perceptions of teamwork: implications for use of a briefing checklist in the OR. *AORN J*. 2010;91(6):722–729.

46. Davis DA, Masmanian PE, Fordis M, et al. Accuracy of physician self-assessment compared with observed measures of competence: a systematic review. *JAMA*. 2006;296(9):1094–1102.

47. Kenney NP, Mann KV, MacLeod H. Role modeling and physicians' professional formation: reconsidering an essential but untapped educational strategy. *Acad Med*. 2003;78(12):1203–1210.

48. Cohen JJ. Viewpoint: linking professionalism to humanism: what it means, why it matters. *Acad Med*. 2007;82(11):1029–1032.

CHAPTER 120

NURSE RECRUITMENT, ORIENTATION, AND CREDENTIALING

Colleen Desai, Robert W. Strauss

> *Your days can be stressful and exhausting and sometimes thankless. But through long shifts and late nights—in the hectic scrum of the emergency room, or in those quiet acts of humanity—you are saving lives, you are offering solace, you're helping to make us a better nation.*
>
> —President Barack Obama

The emergency department (ED) is a dynamic, ever-changing environment that is often referenced as "the front door of the hospital." It is the portal of entry for about 70% of all hospital admissions.[1] With the advent of publicly reported data and the ease of electronic access by consumers, an ED's success is very much dependent on achieving or surpassing customer experience expectations. Consumers have choices and prefer to receive care where they feel like they are listened to, taken seriously, and kept informed about delays and treatment plans while receiving high-quality care.

Less than one half of all ED visits occur at the facility closest to where a patient lives.[2] This may suggest that patients are willing to travel for their care. To further emphasize the value of the patient experience, the Centers for Medicare & Medicaid services (CMS) has developed an Emergency Department Patient Experience of Care (EDPEC) survey that follows the model of the Consumer Assessment of Healthcare Providers and Systems (CAHPS) format. The survey was initially referred to as ED-CAHPS.[3] To incentivize ED leaders, CMS will likely tie results of EDPECs to reimbursements to the hospital and individual practitioners, similar to other pay-for-performance measures. Poor survey results are likely to result in less money.

Balancing the needs, desires, and requirements of consumers, regulatory agencies, and staff can be challenging for many ED leaders. A perfect staffing plan is impossible because it is difficult to predict the unpredictable, for example, daily patient census, times of arrival, patient acuity, and the overall hospital environment. Emergency departments across the world struggle to balance appropriate staffing and financial responsibilities; to consistently staff for the busiest and highest-acuity day would result in bankruptcy for many organizations. Alternatively, consistently staffing for the lightest census day would compromise the care of those in need.

For this reason, today's nurse leaders utilize data to drive informed decisions about their staffing plans. Once the plans are created, the next challenge becomes recruiting and retaining qualified staff to provide efficient, quality care. Nationwide nursing shortages require ED nurse leaders to develop creative staffing plans that also address the fact that seasoned nurses resign for a multitude of reasons.

Nurse leaders need to be innovative, adaptable, proactive, and informed to balance and/or navigate the external pressures of regulatory requirements, staffing, and the delivery of quality care successfully.

BRIEF HISTORY OF NURSING

The nursing profession and the health-care industry are experiencing dramatic changes in today's technological world. These shifts are compounded by significant nursing shortages. According to *The Future of the Nursing Workforce: National- and State-Level Projections, 2012–2025*, a report by the Health Resources and Services Administration, the national supply of registered nurses (RNs) and licensed practical nurses will not meet the projected demand. Additionally, distributional imbalances at various state levels are predicted, with some states in the west, south, and northeast having the greatest imbalance of RN supply.[4] Similar challenges are noted worldwide.

Historically, the field of ED nursing has been viewed as prestigious, competitive, and desirable.[5] Emergency nurses have continued to have valuable learning and professional growth opportunities, which have encouraged them to remain in their positions. The popularity of this career path has helped spare EDs from the negative effects of nursing shortages experienced by other specialties.

Staffing Shortages

Additional challenges, such as inpatients boarding in EDs—often because there are insufficient inpatient nurses to care for the patients—have complicated the current staffing shortages. While some RNs leave the ED for advancement experiences in other domains, others leave because of emotional exhaustion and burnout. Registered nurses also leave their jobs as a result of injuries or dissatisfaction with their department's leadership.[6] Generational values have also changed, and what previously motivated nurses to accept and remain in their positions may no longer be as appealing. As a result, nurse leaders are compelled to have a deep understanding of what motivates ED staff members to predict and plan for these workforce challenges.

Hospitals do not completely understand staff turnover, a complex issue with no single solution.[5] When ED nurse leaders anticipate turnover, they are better positioned to address it proactively. However, it is important that they do not accept these challenges as an unavoidable norm. When a staff member expresses a desire to leave, it is imperative to understand *why*. If the reason is a professional growth opportunity that cannot be met locally, then the RN leader can join in celebrating the employee's new path. If, however, the employee is leaving because of job dissatisfaction or unhappiness with the ED culture, the nurse leader should use this important clue to improve the situation. In EDs with high rates of employee turnover, the devastating effects on morale, compromised patient safety, poor community reputation, and the financial bottom line make it especially important to recognize and aggressively manage the problem.

Nursing shortages and vacancies can have multiple effects on an ED, pressuring the RN leader to perpetually "fill the gaps" by asking staff to work extra hours. The results of chronic understaffing are clinician burnout and poor morale. If these staffing gaps cannot be filled, patient care may be compromised. From a budget perspective, the resulting overtime or reliance on premium-paid agency staff can consume funds earmarked for other departmental needs.

It is important to note that the average cost to replace a single ED nurse is estimated to be anywhere between one to three times the annual salary of a typical RN in the United States.[7,8] This is all the more reason why nurse leaders must understand, articulate, advocate for, and implement proactive strategies for both recruiting and maintaining staff.

RECRUITMENT STRATEGIES

Successful recruitment is the action of enlisting new people to join an organization or support a cause.[9] In the ED, this translates into locating and hiring the most qualified and personable applicants. To accomplish this, nurse leaders should partner with their human resources (HR) colleagues for maximum impact. Human resources should have a clear understanding of the unit's culture, goals and objectives, market served, and candidate requirements. To facilitate this understanding, the ED nurse leader may choose to invite the HR liaison to routine department meetings and/or staff outings. This familiarity with the ED can provide the HR liaison with firsthand knowledge of the department's staff dynamics, culture, successes, and challenges.

When nursing shortages exist, marketing becomes an increasingly important strategy for recruitment. Organizational support, a unit with strong collaborative leadership, and a team that believes in the mission of the ED can easily promote a positive image in the community that will help attract the interest of potential candidates.

Anticipating staff turnover can be one of the more challenging concepts for a nurse leader; however, developing and maintaining a positive rapport with each employee and proactively facilitating periodic formal check-ins can limit turnover. For example, when meeting one-on-one with a staff member, the nurse leader should discuss professional goals with the employee. If an advanced practice RN has plans to obtain a position as a family nurse practitioner, the ED nurse leader can:

- Use this information to proactively post this nurse's position for replacement months before the nurse gives formal notice. Advanced posting allows proactive recruiting and training of a new hire, possibly even before or coinciding with the current nurse's actual departure.
- Support the nurse in their career goals by helping them find local opportunities in their specialty area. This enhances the nurse leader's reputation as someone who cares about the promotion of their staff.

Proactive recruitment combined with an effective retention program can help to maintain positive staff morale. If a nurse leader focuses only on recruiting and hiring and fails to address retention, the department may suffer from a revolving door, leading to poor staff morale and increasing the need to recruit new employees.

Community Relationships

Building community relationships is a valuable recruitment strategy. For example, contracting with a local nursing program at a college that provides student rotations promotes a nursing unit. These relationships also provide:

- Nurse leaders with an opportunity to assess the students' personality, work ethic, and potential for hire
- Students with an opportunity to meet potential colleagues, develop camaraderie, gain experience, and see what it is like to work at the facility

When working with local schools and universities, the nurse leader may participate in career days or mock interview days. By conducting mock interviews, the nurse leader provides a valuable service and can simultaneously scout for potential candidates. Additional community recruitment strategy ideas may include:

- Inviting students to attend planned educational sessions
- Conducting job fairs out in the community or on school campuses

- Attending community outreach events such as injury prevention events (i.e., Stop the Bleed) or wellness events (such as blood pressure or blood sugar screenings)

By encouraging participation in these events, nurse leaders can foster pride in the department. It further helps to demonstrate a true representation of the department to aid in recruiting new candidates.

Involvement of HR

Partnering with HR is critical to building an effective relationship with prospective candidates. The nurse recruiter often makes the first contact with applicants and conducts the initial screening interview. The nurse leader must provide the recruiter with a clear understanding of the desired candidate's required qualifications, personality, experience, motivation, and attitude, as well as an in-depth overview of the unit culture. After performing the initial screening, the nurse recruiter presents qualified candidates to the nurse leader. The presentation should include the nurse recruiter's assessment of the candidate.

Involvement of Departmental Staff

Involving the ED team in the recruitment process has a positive effect on staff morale and is beneficial to the prospective applicant. Current staff who are engaged in shared governance or unit-based councils can be instrumental in articulating the department's mission, goals, objectives, and culture to the candidate. These staff members are also in a prime position to assess the applicant's capacity to participate in the department's culture, goals, and initiatives.

Staff involvement is most effective when the nurse leader has collaborated with the team to develop and support a positive unit identity, including a collaborative culture, comprehensive performance improvement plan, and true employee engagement.

To successfully develop a comprehensive recruitment plan, the nurse leader should assess current team strengths and deficits and elicit input from department staff. That input should include a cultural assessment and frank feedback gathered via open forums or brainstorming sessions. While some nurse leaders may view such assessments as just one more thing on their to-do lists, investing the time up front will increase the odds of hiring quality candidates.

Recruitment Tools

It is important to keep in mind that recruitment is a two-way street. The organization is aiming to attract top-notch, qualified employees, but the candidates are also searching for positions that offer benefits, professional development opportunities, and a high-reliability culture. To maximize these opportunities, the recruitment team should use myriad tools to connect with applicants (**Box 120.1**). Regardless of the modality, any interaction with a candidate should include timely engagement and follow-up. This is especially true in times of nursing shortages, when qualified candidates become a particularly hot commodity. To ensure the timely tracking of applicants and follow-up, the ED nurse leader and HR recruiter should meet on a regular basis to review the status of job postings and incumbents.

Internet-Based Recruiting

Nurse leaders may also utilize internet-based recruiting to find qualified candidates. This process typically involves social media campaigns to announce open positions, online recruitment job sites, and virtual open houses.

> **BOX 120.1 ■ RECRUITMENT TOOLS**
>
> **Internet-based recruiting:**
> - Social media campaigns
> - Online job sites
> - Virtual open houses
>
> **Person-to-person recruitment:**
> - Employee referral programs
> - Word of mouth
>
> **On-site recruiting programs:**
> - Vendor tables at conferences/conventions
> - Open houses
> - Job fairs
> - Open interview days/walk-ins
>
> **Traditional media tools:**
> - Print advertising (journals, newspapers)
> - Direct mailings

Social Media Campaigns

Social media is an easy way to reach potential applicants. Messaging can be as simple as a text post or as sophisticated as a video or testimonial about the position or organization. Sites and apps like LinkedIn, Facebook, Instagram, Snapchat, YouTube, and Visual Supply Company are (at the time of this publication) reliable and popular forums for reaching a broad, diverse audience. However, with the advent of new technologies and the speed at which the social media vector advances, department leaders must stay abreast of this rapidly evolving market and employ the most effective sites.

Online Job Sites

Other online recruitment tools include job sites like Monster, Indeed, Glassdoor, and ZipRecruiter. Many applicants utilize these websites to search for potential jobs using filtered or individualized criteria, including geographical area. Additionally, some applicants will post resumes on these sites to broadly market themselves, allowing recruiting organizations to be more selective. Nurse leaders and their HR liaisons are well advised to regularly advertise on and peruse these forums.

Virtual Open Houses

Applicants may also value the opportunity to chat online with a nurse leader or nurse recruiter during a virtual open house or job fair. Interested applicants can register to participate in group or individual sessions, and employers can share information on benefits, location highlights, salary, position needs, and other important topics. Sophisticated virtual open houses may even offer video interviews. This modality of recruiting can give the hiring organization access to a broader range of candidates, who would otherwise have to travel for an in-person interview.

Person-to-Person Recruitment

Referrals from existing staff can be the most valuable and reliable source of new recruits. One report found that referrals are associated with a 2.6% to 6.6% greater chance of a candidate accepting a job, and approximately 30% of employee referrals lead to a new hire.[10] Organizations that are highly focused on employee referrals may successfully hire between 50% and 75% of all referred applicants.[11]

Since word of mouth can encourage or dissuade potential applicants from applying, the ED nurse leader should focus on internal recruiting and positive staff engagement. No matter how acute the need, department leaders must avoid making the situation worse by ignoring the current team. In fact, greater effort must be placed on retention. Employees who feel overwhelmed and unappreciated may leave and are unlikely to encourage new hires or participate in the employee referral campaign.

By virtue of their connection with an existing staff member, word-of-mouth applicants are typically well informed about the organizational culture and benefits prior to applying for a position. Simultaneously, the referring employee's direct knowledge of an applicant gives the nurse leader valuable information. Given the benefit of direct referrals, some organizations offer existing employees a monetary bonus for referred applicants who join the organization and stay for a certain amount of time.

On-Site Recruiting Programs

On-site recruiting programs are ideal opportunities to meet and vet potential job applicants. Hosting a table at a specialty nursing conference can provide valuable exposure for a hiring department or organization. This approach can be costly if it involves travel, lodging, and a fee for the booth or table; however, direct face time with a significant pool of qualified individuals may prove beneficial. Attending local or regional conferences or conventions may be a more affordable option.

Hosting periodic open houses can be another efficient way to coordinate multiple applicants and interviews in a consolidated period of time. If new graduates are considered, ED nurse leaders and HR can host biannual, large-scale open houses in advance of nursing school graduation. For EDs that do not hire new graduates, participation in hospital-wide events may still support new hires in other parts of the organization and will encourage new graduates to consider work in the ED in the future.

Job fairs are another relatively inexpensive way to attract an audience that might not otherwise express interest in the organization. A job fair also guarantees candidates face-to-face interactions that they may not get by blindly submitting an application. At the same time, the recruitment team will see potential applicants who may have previously been passed over based solely on a paper review. Additionally, these events can enable efficient workflow between the interviewing parties and HR colleagues who are responsible for making the offers. Ideally, a job fair can result in many positions getting filled in just one day.

Occasionally, departments encounter unannounced applicants who walk in to apply. Such visits can signal the applicant's confidence and be a clear indication of true interest in the organization. Given that the ED is a specialty area with occasional recruitment challenges, it may be prudent to remain open to the serendipitous opportunities provided by impromptu interviews.

Traditional Media Tools

Advertising in professional journals is generally an expensive way to target a direct audience, but it may be particularly useful for filling a high-profile position, such as a nurse director, manager, or educator. Newspaper advertising is also a viable option; however, given the cost and potentially limited audience, it is important for these ads to be catchy, relevant, and succinct. Printed direct mailings may be particularly valuable when promoting events like job fairs, signing bonuses, open houses, and so on. Zip code-specific mailing lists are usually available from various professional organizations.

While television and radio ads can reach large audiences, costs can vary widely depending on the desired number of airings, time of day, inclusion in certain broadcast segments, and so on. Costs can range from hundreds to tens of thousands of dollars, depending on the sophistication of the promotion. When considering a cost/benefit ratio, television and radio may only be a viable option for large organizations with broad recruitment needs.

Experiential Recruiting

Some hospitals have successfully implemented student nurse internships. These programs allow the student nurse to work as a nurse's aide, with some added responsibilities that are within the scope of practice of the Board of Registration of Nursing. This approach can provide an organization with access to graduating nurses early in their educational careers. While working in their internship roles, these nurses are simultaneously orienting to the organization. If they are subsequently hired, their onboarding time is expedited, and they will be rooted in the culture already.

The fact that few nursing schools offer clinical rotations in the ED creates an innovative opportunity to propose unique and exciting student experiences. The experience exposes nursing students to emergency nursing as a clinical discipline and career option. Marketing the profession of emergency nursing to students may encourage them to consider becoming an emergency nurse one day.

Internal Recruitment

Hiring employees from within the organization has several clear advantages:

- The staff member is already familiar with the organizational culture.
- The ED onboarding period is significantly shortened.
- Employees will likely feel satisfaction related to job advancement.
- The "new" employee will already know how to navigate the institution and its computer applications, rules and regulations, and so on.

There is a potential disadvantage in an institution that has "siloed" management. When these programs function independently and without consideration for other divisions, they tend to compete for limited nursing resources.

INTERVIEW STRATEGIES

Once a potential employee begins to fill the application pipeline, the wise ED nurse leader works to ensure the candidate is an excellent fit. In the long run, a strategy that ensures the applicant is talented, capable, dedicated, compassionate, and goal-oriented is more likely to decrease future recruiting needs. Just filling holes compromises team morale and increases staff turnover.

Behavioral Interviewing

One popular and effective approach that can provide deep insight into the candidate's actions is behavioral interviewing. This style poses specific open-ended scenarios, rather than simple yes-or-no questions, and assumes that the best predictor of a candidate's future performance is their past behavior.

For example, instead of saying, "Tell me about yourself," the nurse leader may ask, "Tell me about a time when you . . . and what was the result?" Or, "What did you do when . . . and what was the result?" Note that these questions are aimed at drawing specific examples from a candidate's past behavior and avoid hypothetical responses that might be elicited if a candidate were asked, "What would you do *if* . . . ?"[13]

Peer Interviews

Peer interviews can help leaders gain deeper insight into a candidate's personality, interactions, and core competencies. Should the ED nurse leader choose to use this modality of applicant screening, it important that the participating staff are identified as high performers and receive clear instructions on peer interviewing. Staff members should know the difference between legal and illegal questions, appreciate the value of open-ended questions, and understand the competencies that the department is seeking. Staff engagement in this arena is not only a benefit to the ED nurse leader, it is also a great way to empower the staff at the same time!

Credentialing and Certification

Credentialing and certification requirements are important to consider when recruiting for an existing or anticipated vacancy. The recruiting team must define both required and preferred candidate experience, certifications, prerequisites, licensure, and degree/education.

Licensure and Registration

An active state license is required for a nurse to practice. Nurses graduating from an accredited school of nursing are permitted to take the National Council Licensure Examination to obtain the right to apply for a state license. Each state has a board that defines the state's specific scope of practice and standards that nurses must maintain. For license maintenance and renewal, some states have specific educational requirements, including predefined topics that must be covered (**Table 120.1**).

Some states offer nurse licensure compact status, which allows a nurse to practice in another nurse compact licensure state without having to obtain additional licenses.[14] States that participate in the compact program agree to accept licensure from another state. Of course, even within the compact, the nurse's licensure status has to be verified by the hiring state, an expedited process within the compact agreement.

Nurses must maintain an updated license in good standing in their home state to ensure compliance with the compact agreement. "Good standing" entails meeting any and all continuing education and other mandated requirements necessary to renew the home state license, even if currently practicing in another state. Further, the compact requires nurses to meet the practice act standards for each state in which they work. Emergency departments that employ travel nurses should recognize the benefits of compact licensure, enabling quicker onboarding of potential candidates.

Certification

Certification recognizes expertise in a nursing domain or specialty. There are many certifications that an emergency nurse may achieve. Nurse leaders should hold applicants who have a certification in their field in high regard, as it demonstrates professionalism, pride, and a desire for success.

Certification in Emergency Nursing

Several emergency nursing certifications are offered by the Board of Certification for Emergency Nursing (BCEN), an American Board of Nursing Specialties-accredited agency. The BCEN cites board certification as, "a mark of *excellence* based on rigorous national standards that validate a nurse's specialty knowledge, skills, and clinical judgement."[15]

While it is unclear if nursing certification impacts patient outcomes, the BCEN attests that 90% of emergency nurses who have attained Certification in Emergency

TABLE 120.1 ■ License and Continuing Education by State (as of June 2018)

State	Compact Licensure	Continuing Education Requirement	State	Compact Licensure	Continuing Education Requirement
Alabama	Yes	24 hours/2 years	Montana	Yes	24 hours/2 years
Alaska		30 hours/renewal	Nebraska	Yes	20 hours/2 years
Arizona	Yes	None required	Nevada		30 hours/2 years
Arkansas	Yes	15 hours/2 years	New Hampshire	Yes	30 hours/2 years
California		30 hours/renewal	New Jersey		30 hours/2 years
Colorado	Yes	None required	New Mexico	Yes	30 hours/2 years
Connecticut		None required	New York		Content specific
Delaware	Yes	30 hours/2 years	North Carolina	Yes	30 hours/2 years
Florida	Yes	24 hours/renewal	North Dakota	Yes	12 hours/renewal
Georgia	Yes	20 hours/renewal	Ohio		24 hours/2 years
Hawaii		30 hours/renewal	Oklahoma	Yes	24 hours/2 years
Idaho	Yes	15 hours/2 years	Oregon		7 hours pain management; then none required
Illinois		20 hours/2 years	Pennsylvania		30 hours/2 years
Indiana	Yes	None required	Rhode Island		10 hours/2 years
Iowa	Yes	36 hours/3 years	South Carolina	Yes	30 hours/2 years
Kansas	Yes	30 hours/2 years	South Dakota	Yes	12 hours/renewal
Kentucky	Yes	14 hours/year	Tennessee	Yes	None required
Louisiana	Yes	5 hours/year	Texas	Yes	20 hours/2 years
Maine	Yes	None required	Utah	Yes	30 hours/2 years
Maryland	Yes	None required	Vermont		None required
Massachusetts		15 hours/2 years	Virginia	Yes	30 hours/renewal
Michigan		25 hours/2 years	Washington		45 hours/3 years
Minnesota		24 hours/2 years	West Virginia	Yes	12 hours/year
Mississippi	Yes	20 hours/2 years	Wisconsin	Yes	None required
Missouri	Yes	None required	Wyoming	Yes	20 hours/ 2 years

Nursing (CEN) feel pride in this accomplishment, and the overwhelming majority of nurse supervisors value certification.[16,17] Holding a current CEN is associated with the following:

- Earning more per year, on average
- Attaining a higher level in one's career
- Feeling confident of marketability
- Achieving higher satisfaction with career achievements

Furthermore, employers value achievement of the CEN among their staff. Specifically, supervisors rate nurses higher on emergency nursing expertise if the nurse has a CEN. Five job performance items, including technical skill and ethical behavior, are positively correlated with having a current CEN.[17]

Certification as a Flight RN

In addition to the CEN, emergency nurses may attain the Certified Flight Registered Nurse (CFRN), a distinction that was accredited by the Accreditation Board for Specialty Nursing Certification (ABSNC) in 2007. Currently, there are over 4,000 nurses who maintain CFRN certification, which is valid for four years.[17]

Certification as a Transport RN

In 2004, BCEN and the Air & Surface Transport Nursing Association collaborated to offer a four-year certification for ground transport nursing. The Certified Transport Registered Nurse certification program was introduced in 2006.[17]

Certification in Pediatric Emergency Nursing

The Certified Pediatric Emergency Nurse (CPEN) certification was developed through a collaboration between BCEN and the Pediatric Nursing Certification Board in 2009. The four-year certification was accredited by ABSNC in 2015. Those applying for this certification must demonstrate at least 1,000 hours of practice caring for pediatric patients. Approximately 5,000 nurses hold CPENs.[17]

Certification as a Trauma RN

The Trauma-Certified Registered Nurse certification was established in 2016, and over 3,600 nurses have attained the certification.[17]

Benefits of Certified Nurses

Most nurses recognize that certification demonstrates personal accomplishment, validates knowledge, provides personal satisfaction, indicates professional credibility, and offers a professional challenge.[18] Certification may lead to a more positive view of an applicant and result in a higher pay grade. Patients and families often assume that nurses with certifications are providing a higher level of care, which may create a marketing opportunity for the organization.

A nurse who has achieved certification demonstrates drive, professionalism, high achievement, and a solid dedication to the profession. Potential marketing opportunities have led some organizations to reimburse employees for the successful achievement of certification, further enhancing employee engagement, aspirations, and morale.

Some ED nurse leaders celebrate staff who have achieved certification by publishing their star employees' names and faces in a hospital newsletter, blog, community benefit publication, or local newspaper. An ED nurse leader can also post names on a plaque in a visible hallway or waiting area. Leaders who encourage excellence also motivate and reward nurses who strive to achieve certification. It should be made clear that all staff have an equal opportunity to achieve certification.

While some ED staff members may not achieve certification, effective leaders encourage all employees to seek additional skills and certificates of achievement to enhance their job function, increase their value, and build their sense of pride and engagement. Examples include courses on basic dysrhythmias, phlebotomy skill verification, advanced cardiac life support, nonviolent crisis intervention, and behavioral health first aid. To foster collaboration, certified nurses can teach these verification courses and encourage their teammates to take them.

Verifications and Other Credentials

Department leaders should conduct a needs assessment to determine which core competencies can be made available or even mandatory. Employees with other, nontraditional ED skills, such as out-of-hospital care, may be beneficial to an organization. Some states regulate the responsibilities of out-of-hospital physicians working in EDs. Although the National Registry of Emergency Technicians offers guidelines for EMTs and paramedics, they have not been adopted by all states, and individual state's rules supersede national protocols. As an example, when developing an ED technician role, the scope of practice and job description must align with the state's regulations to ensure that the employee provides the greatest value.

NURSING ORIENTATION

Nursing orientation is another critical component of a new hire's onboarding process. Once the pre-employment checklist is complete, the orientation may begin. Typically, new hires will attend a HR or general hospital orientation that covers generic, mandatory regulatory requirements, including blood-borne pathogen training, fire and emergency response training, and corporate compliance programs.

The department-specific clinical orientation usually begins once the general orientation is complete. The ED nurse leader should participate in the development and delivery of the employee's department-specific orientation and have a thorough command of the onboarding process.

Departmental Orientation

Departmental orientation may last weeks to months, depending on the skill and experience level of the newly hired staff member. A position statement by the Emergency Nurses Association asserts that a successful ED nurse orientation must rely upon a comprehensive, individualized, evidence-driven, competency-based approach, incorporating adult learning principles, active teaching and learning activities, and socialization strategies.[19]

A planned, structured orientation should be coordinated by the ED nurse leaders and include educators, preceptor(s), and the physician group. A clear set of objectives and goals should be available to the team and reviewed weekly or biweekly to track the employee's progress. This documentation serves as a communication between preceptors and leaders and demonstrates competence, a regulatory requirement.

Departmental Needs Assessment

The ED leadership should intermittently conduct a departmental needs assessment, particularly when developing an orientation training/competency checklist. This evaluation should include an assessment of high-risk/low-volume procedures to prepare employees to care for the community. Additionally, the nurse leader can gather input from other ED leaders, charge nurses, experienced staff, and new employees about their desired and necessary learning opportunities. Results of the needs assessment can then be used to enhance the orientation checklist.

As an example, a small community hospital may see very few critically ill children; patients who have experienced trauma, snake bites, or sexual assault; or human trafficking victims. Therefore, a directed orientation and training on these potential presentations ensures the employee learns the foundational concepts.

The needs assessment should also elicit feedback on specific education focused on the use of rarely used or complex equipment. The ED nurse leader, perhaps in conjunction with an educator, can often elicit the help of product representatives to aid in training and the creation of skills checklists.

Additionally, when conducting a needs assessment, policies and procedures should be reviewed to ensure they are up to date and relevant. Specific policies warrant dedicated orientation time, including the Emergency Medical Treatment and Labor Act, the Consolidated Omnibus Budget Reconciliation Act, procedural sedation, mandated reporting, standing/protocol orders, monitoring and assessment standards, suicide assessments, consent and refusal of care, ligature-free status, and restraints, for example. A new employee's completion of the orientation process, including the ED nurse leader's assessment, should be documented.

Precepted Orientation

Precepted orientation pairs new employees with a preceptor to guide and support them while they continue to grow professionally. New employees should attend a formal training session that may include topics such as:

- How to have a crucial conversation
- How to give constructive feedback
- The value of teamwork
- Adult teaching and learning styles
- Skill validation expectations
- Documentation requirements

It is important to choose the right preceptor–orientee fit. The nurse leader should consider personality styles, the needs and learning preferences of the new employee, and the natural teaching style of the preceptor, all with the goal of facilitating a successful pairing.

Becoming a preceptor requires special skills, including excellent interpersonal communication, leadership capability, patience, and teaching ability. Some organizations choose to compensate those who precept with a financial incentive, while others incorporate the demonstration of effective precepting into the clinical ladder program. Additional ways to recognize and honor preceptors may include an annual breakfast, letters of commendation, and a mention in the organization's newsletter.

During the orientation process, it is equally important to monitor the performance of the orientee and preceptor. The ED nurse leader (or the ED educator) should plan and conduct regular meetings at set intervals with both parties. The agenda for these meetings should include:

- What is going well
- A review of the past goals, setting of new goals
- Identification of any issues that need correction along with a detailed plan for correction and concrete due date by which compliance is expected

The orientee's skills checklist should also be reviewed, as it serves as a springboard for addressing these topics. Details of these meetings should be documented and tracked, with the documentation used as the basis for the next conversation. This documentation can also serve to support progressive discipline should an employee be unsuccessful in completing the orientation process.

Individualized Orientation

Using the orientation skills/competency checklist that was developed from the needs assessment, the ED nurse leader may find it valuable to have the new employee document a self-assessment of the topics listed in the orientation skills list. This exercise not only acknowledges the skills and experience that a new ED employee brings with them but also serves as a basis for determining the new employee's insight into their capacity.

Information obtained from the self-assessment can guide an individualized orientation plan by determining which topics simply require a quick validation versus those that need additional time for teaching, observing, practicing, and validating.

Resources

Many resources are available to address the needs of the unit identified by the needs assessment.

In-House Education

In large hospitals, ED leaders can collaborate with other units to address skills requiring validation. For example, focused experience in an ICU or with respiratory therapy can give a new employee targeted exposure to ventilators, expediting their skill, experience, and validation. Similarly, a new employee needing intravenous insertion exposure and validation could spend time in pre-op or endoscopy, or even as a member of an infusion team. An innovative approach to skill development might result in collaboration with other departments (and even vendors) to host a skills day, in which a round-robin teaching station format can facilitate skill learning and validation.

Commercially Available Education

Emergency department leaders may also recommend education through self-study or online programs. A variety of commercial programs designed to augment the assessment and orientation process are available for purchase.

One example is the Basic Knowledge Assessment Tool (BKAT), which offers tests that measure knowledge in critical care nursing. As of this publication, the most current ED critical care nursing test is the ED-BKAT3r.[20] If the exam results demonstrate a strong knowledge in particular aspects of nursing, that information may allow the nurse to "test out" of specific components of the orientation. Many ED nurse leaders find these tools valuable, as they can shorten a new employee's onboarding process while ensuring critical elements of performance are not overlooked.

Other commercially available tools include performance-based development system examinations, which can be purchased from several companies. These products test the following three domains of nursing:

- Critical thinking skills
- Technical skills
- Interpersonal skills

These tests can be modified to be ED-specific and, unlike the BKAT, may even be used in the application process to screen candidates based on their results. The test can also be used to develop and streamline orientation plans.

Documentation

It is important that the ED nurse leader ensures thorough record keeping of employees' orientations, competency validations, and ongoing competency assessments. Methods of documenting competence include skills checklists, post-tests, preceptor direct observations, and recorded completion of simulation exercises. In some facilities, electronic learning management systems can be used to complete and file documents. Regardless of the method used, it is essential to document the competence. **Figure 120.1** provides an example of a direct observation competency checklist.

FIGURE 120.1 ■ Example of Direct Observation Competency Checklist

[Organization Logo]

Name: _____ Employee# _____

PERFORMING AN ECG: COMPETENCY CHECKLIST

Performance Criteria	Yes	No	Comments
Verify practitioner's order.			
Gather and prepare the appropriate equipment.			
Perform hand hygiene, put on gloves as needed (to comply with standard precautions).			
Confirm the patient's identity using at least two patient identifiers.			
Provide privacy.			
Explain the procedure to the patient. Tell patient that the test records the heart's electrical activity and that it may be repeated at certain intervals.			
Raise the patient's bed to waist level when providing patient care to prevent caregiver back strain.			
Have the patient lie supine in the center of the bed with arms at the sides. Raise the head of the bed if the patient desires to promote comfort. Ensure that the patient's arms and legs remain relaxed to minimize muscle trembling, which can cause electrical interference.			
Expose the patient's arms, legs, and chest, and then cover appropriately with a bath blanket or sheet.			
Select the electrode sites. Select flat, fleshy areas on which to place the limb lead electrodes. Avoid muscular and bony areas. If the patient has an amputated limb, choose a site on the stump. (If the area is excessively hairy, clip the hair.)			
Apply a pregelled electrode at each electrode position on the patient's chest. If the patient is female, be sure to place the chest electrodes under the breast tissue. (Pediatric lead placement is the same as for adult.) To ensure accurate test results, position chest electrodes as follows: V_1: Fourth intercostal space at the right border of the sternum V_2: Fourth intercostal space at the left border of the sternum V_3: Halfway between V_2 and V_4 V_4: Fifth intercostal space at the midclavicular line V_5: In the horizontal plane of V_4 at the anterior axillary line (or halfway between V_4 and V_6 if the anterior axillary line is ambiguous) V_6: In the horizontal plane of V_4 at the midaxillary line			
Tell the patient to relax and to breathe normally. Tell patient to lie still and not to talk when you record the ECG to minimize artifact.			
Press the START button. Observe the tracing quality. The machine will record all 12 leads automatically, recording three consecutive leads simultaneously.			
After disconnecting the lead wires from the electrodes, you may leave the electrodes on the patient in case another ECG will be ordered.			
Return the bed to the lowest position to prevent falls and maintain patient safety. Clean, disinfect, and prepare the equipment for future use.			
Give the ECG to a physician for review and document the ECG in the computer in patient's record.			

Educator/Preceptor's Signature: _____ **Date:** _____

1. Measured in Learning Lab/Simulation Center ☐ **Measured During Direct Care**

CONCLUSION

Although emergency care is a basic need for the community, it is also a business that relies on consumerism to remain viable. Providing an exceptional patient experience as evidenced by positive publicly reported ratings has a strong effect on community perceptions and staff morale. The general population is living longer and is generally sicker with increasingly complex medical conditions. These facts, combined with the multiple stressors caused by nursing shortages, technology changes, and increasing regulatory mandates, have a profound impact on a hospital's ability to recruit and retain quality ED staff.

The successful ED nurse leader collaborates to recruit the most qualified and appropriate candidates for open positions. An in-depth, comprehensive orientation ensures a positive onboarding experience and confirms the employee is adequately prepared to provide safe, quality patient care. The ED nurse leader who develops and facilitates a deliberate, structured, and inclusive recruitment, credentialing, and orientation program will establish a team of professionals that meets the critical needs of the department, the staff, and the patients who rely on them.

REFERENCES

1. Augustine J. Latest data reveal the ED's role as hospital admission gatekeeper. 2019. Available at: https://www.acepnow.com/article/latest-data-reveal-the-eds-role-as-hospital-admission-gatekeeper/. Accessed June 6, 2020.
2. Brown AM, Decker SL, Selck FW. Emergency department visits and proximity to patients' residences. Published 2015. Available at: https://www.cdc.gov/nchs/products/databriefs/db192.htm, Centers for Disease Control and Prevention. Accessed May 22, 2019.
3. CMS.gov. Emergency Department Patient Experiences with Care (EDPEC) Survey. 2020. Available at: https://www.cms.gov/Research-Statistics-Data-and-Systems/Research/CAHPS/ED. Accessed June 4, 2020.
4. US Department of Health and Human Services, Health Resources and Services Administration, National Center for Health Workforce Analysis. The future of the Nursing Workforce: national-and state-level projections, 2012-2025. Rockville, Md; 2014. Available at: https://bhw.hrsa.gov/sites/default/files/bhw/nchwa/projections/nursingprojections.pdf. Accessed May 30, 2019.
5. Winters, N. Seeking status: the process of becoming and remaining an emergency nurse. *J Emerg Nurs*. 2016:42(5):412–419.
6. Brewere CS, Kovover CT, Greene W, et al. Predictors of actual turnover in a national sample of newly licensed registered nurses employed in hospitals. *J Adv Nurs*. 2011;68(3):521–538.
7. Jones CB. The costs of nurse turnover part 1: an economic perspective. *J Nurs Adm*. 2004;34(12):562–570.
8. Jones CB. The costs of nurse turnover part 2: application of the nursing turnover cost calculation methodology. *J Nurs Adm*. 2005;35(1):41–49.
9. Available at: www.webster-dictionary.net/definition/Recruiting. Accessed May 1, 2019.
10. Chamberlain A. Why interview source matter in hiring: exploring Glassdoor interviews Data. 2015. Available at: https://www.glassdoor.com/research/interview-sources/. Accessed June 1, 2019.
11. Sullivan J. Assessing employee referral programs: a checklist. 2005. Available at: https://www.ere.net/assessing-employee-referral-programs-a-checklist/. Accessed June 1, 2019.
12. American Express Global Customer Service Barometer—2017. 2020. Available at: https://business.americanexpress.com/sg/business-trends-insights/thought-leadership/american-express-global-customer-barometer-2017 Accessed June 1, 2020.
13. Studer Group. *The Nurse Leader Handbook*. Gulf Breeze, Fla; 2010.
14. NCSBN. Nurse Licensure Compact. Available at: https://www.ncsbn.org/nurse-licensure-compact.htm. Accessed June 1, 2019.
15. Available at: https://bcen.org/value-of-certification/. Accessed June 1, 2019.
16. ABNS Research Committee Subgroup. The relationship between nursing certification and patient outcomes: a review of the literature. 2014. Available at: http://www.nursingcertification.org/resources/documents/research/certification-and-patient-outcomes-research-article-synthesis.pdf. Accessed June 1, 2019.
17. Madsker G, Cogswell MS. Value of CEN® Certification Research Study: Results. 2017. Available at: https://bcen.org/wp-content/uploads/2018/09/2017-BCEN-Value-of-Certificaiton-Study-PPT.pdf. Accessed June 1, 2019.
18. Garrison E, Schulz C, Nelson C, et al. Specialty certification: nurses' perceived value and barriers. *Nurs Manage*. 2018;49(5):42–47.
19. ENA Position Statement: Emergency Nurse Orientation. 2019. Available at: https://www.ena.org/docs/default-source/resource-library/practice-resources/position-statements/emergencynurseorientation. Accessed June 1, 2020.
20. The Basic Knowledge Assessment Tool (BKAT) for the Emergency Department (ED-BKAT3r—Critical Care Nursing. 2020. Available at: http://www.bkat-toth.org/ED-BKAT3r.html. Accessed May 27, 2020.

CHAPTER 121

NURSE RETENTION

Michael D. Moon

According to the Agency for Health Care Research and Quality, emergency department (ED) visits have increased by 20% since 2006, a trend that shows no signs of slowing down.[1] The Centers for Disease Control and Prevention reports that there are 45.6 million ED visits in the United States every year, 8.7% of which result in hospital admission.[2] This increased patient volume and acuity require EDs to be well staffed with registered nurses (RNs).

Maintaining a strong and committed nursing staff is essential to consistently achieving positive patient outcomes. When large numbers of RNs intend to leave an ED, something within the organization must be addressed. The average turnover rate for emergency RNs is 19% to 20%, which is one of the highest turnover rates for any specialty area.[3] Registered nurses with 1 to 5 years of experience account for 48.3% of these turnovers.[3]

A high turnover rate within an ED is an expensive budgetary consideration. The Emergency Nurses Association (ENA) estimates that it costs an average of $82,000 to replace every RN that leaves an ED, and it takes on average 81.6 days to recruit and hire a replacement.[3] An increase or decrease of 1% in RN turnover can result in a $328,400 loss or gain for the hospital.[3] Therefore, maintaining a stable nursing staff can save the ED a significant amount of money while substantially improving patient outcomes.

There is no single solution to improving RN retention in an ED. Rather, it is important to understand the bigger picture and implement a multifaceted approach to this important issue (**Table 121.1**).

TABLE 121.1 ■ Factors Impacting Nurse Retention

Staffing and associated patient outcomes

Nursing shortage
- Shortage of new RNs entering the workforce
- Aging workforce and retiring RNs

Emergency department environment
- Complexity of patients
- Physical requirements
- Scheduling
- Workplace violence
  - Patient violence
  - Lateral violence and bullying

Interprofessional communication

Inadequate resilience/moral distress

Professional development needs

Work-life balance

Organizational structure

STAFFING CONSIDERATIONS

Staffing issues are a primary factor affecting RN retention.[4-9] An ED may be understaffed due to patient volume or heavily staffed with new, inexperienced or agency/temporary RNs. This can create an environment that interferes with the staff's ability to work effectively and can cause fatigue and/or burnout, which has a further negative impact on patient care. This is not to say that new RNs, agency/temporary RNs, licensed practical nurses/licensed vocational nurses, or unlicensed personnel should not be used in an ED, but rather that consideration should be given to balancing the staffing mix.

With appropriate staffing, RNs are better able to use their skills and clinical judgment to identify urgent issues that must be addressed to prevent the deterioration of patient conditions.[10] The staffing schedule should ensure that an appropriate skills mix is established so that staff have an appropriate level of competence to handle the ED's patient population. Furthermore, the schedule should include an adequate number of RNs who are confident and able to work unsupervised.[4,5,11] Adequate RN staffing has a significant positive impact on the delivery of safe, quality care and is essential to achieving positive clinical outcomes.[4,5,11] Appropriate staffing reduces medical errors, medication mistakes, lengths of stay, readmissions, patient mortality, and preventable events.[5,10]

A number of accrediting agencies have written standards regarding the ready availability of nurses in the ED.[12,13] Although these standards do not mandate particular staffing rules, they do require organizations to closely examine how RNs are used and integrated into the health-care system, including the ED. These accrediting agencies include the Joint Commission and the Centers for Medicare & Medicaid Services. Failure to comply with their standards can affect reimbursement rates and may result in fines and/or penalties depending on the nature of any violations. Other agencies like the Institute of Medicine (IOM) and the American Nurses' Credentialing Center also advocate for collaborative RN involvement in clinical decisions.

Department leaders must avoid the temptation to reduce the number of staff RNs as a cost-containment measure. Although nursing is one of the largest hospital budget items, accounting for an estimated 25% to 40% of annual operating expenses, decreasing RN staffing results in worse patient outcomes, particularly in the ED, where patients often present with multiple comorbidities.[14-16] Adequate RN staffing contributes to improved hospital economic performance and better value-based reimbursement.[5,15] More information regarding ED nursing staffing can be found in Chapter 22.

THE NURSING SHORTAGE

Health care has entered an unprecedented time, when shortages of key personnel threaten to affect the ability of EDs to provide safe, quality medical care. In the United States, it is predicted that there will be an estimated shortage of 41,000 to 105,000 physicians by the year 2030.[17] Alarmingly, the nursing shortage is expected to be at least four times greater, resulting in an estimated shortfall of 500,000 RNs worldwide by 2026.[18] The World Health Organization estimates that an additional 9 million RNs will be needed by 2030.[19] This international shortage will substantially limit the ability of hospitals to recruit RNs from other countries to fill vacancies in the United States—a strategy that has commonly been employed in the past. The resulting loss of human and intellectual capital will likely have a deleterious effect on patient outcomes. Therefore, it is imperative that hospitals develop strategies to maximize their ability to retain their valued team members.

Nursing Faculty Shortage

One of most significant factors affecting the supply of RNs entering the profession is an international shortage of nursing faculty. In 2018, the American Association of Colleges of Nursing reported 1,715 faculty vacancies in 872 schools with baccalaureate and graduate nursing programs.[21] Associate and diploma schools are also experiencing a shortage of nursing faculty. This lack of teaching faculty has resulted in more than 75,000 qualified applicants being turned away from baccalaureate and graduate nursing programs and 45% of qualified candidates being turned away from associate degree nursing programs.[21,22] An aging faculty and increasing rates of retirement compound the problem. The average age of nursing faculty ranges from 54 to 57 depending on the faculty member's level of education (**Table 121.2**).[21]

Furthermore, colleges and universities have been unable to compete in the salary market. Many graduate-prepared nurses decline to join a nursing faculty simply because higher compensation can be obtained in the clinical or private sectors.[21]

Shortage of New Graduates

The shortage of new RNs entering the workforce is directly related to the inability of nursing schools to keep up with the demand. The shortfall is indirectly related to the exodus of RNs from the workforce, which can be attributed to retirement and a stressful work environment (fatigue and burnout). The number of RNs leaving the workforce has steadily increased each year and is expected to double by 2020.[23]

Retiring RNs

The U.S. Census Bureau projects that by the year 2030, one in five Americans will be at retirement age.[24] This trend is also being felt within the nursing profession. The National Council of State Boards of Nursing and the Forum of State Nursing Workforce Centers reports that more than half of the RNs in the workforce are 50 years or older.[25] By 2030, more than 1 million nurses will have reached retirement age.[17,26,27] As these RNs leave the workforce, the pressures on recruiting and staffing will be substantial.

PROBLEMS AFFECTING THE ED ENVIRONMENT

The workplace plays a significant role in whether RNs will remain within an ED.[14,27,34–36] When comparing hospital environments classified as "poor" versus "better," researchers found that "better" workplaces experienced a 10% decrease in patient mortality when the RN workload was decreased by only one patient. Conversely, hospitals with "poor" environments experienced no change in mortality when the RN workload was decreased by one patient.[14]

Complexity of ED Setting

Large and unpredictable ED patient volumes are a significant challenge that is further compounded by having to board admitted patients who cannot be transferred to inpatient

TABLE 121.2 ■ Average Age of Nursing Faculty Based on Level of Education

Level of Education	Average Age
Doctoral degree	57 years
Master's degree	54 years

units yet. Regulatory agencies have stated that the level of care provided to these patients must be consistent with the care they would receive in any other hospital unit, regardless of the current holding location—a mandate that significantly increases the pressure on the ED staff.

Working in the ED is physically demanding. Clinicians are often on their feet for 12 to 13 hours, sometimes without a break. Nurses, in particular, also do a great deal of lifting, whether extricating a patient from the back seat of a car or transferring a patient to the CT table for a scan. Nurses must also push, pull, and lift various pieces of equipment, such as gurneys, oxygen tanks, monitors, and crash carts. These physical demands can be challenging for all ED staff, but they may present substantial obstacles for older or unfit RNs.

Scheduling

Many hospitals have adopted a staffing model that exclusively uses 12-hour shifts. However, clinical and administrative responsibilities that must be completed at the end of a shift may require RNs to stay much longer than their scheduled 12 hours. To further complicate matters, many hospitals mandate overtime to address their staffing issues. This practice is discouraged by most professional associations and some regulatory agencies.[4] Currently, 18 states have laws that restrict or heavily regulate mandatory overtime in health-care industries.[28] The need for adequate rest between shifts is paramount to ensure both patient and staff safety. While most RNs are satisfied with their schedules, there is mounting evidence that shifts longer than 10 hours increase the likelihood of errors.[29,30] This combined with an aging workforce may require hospitals to evaluate the benefits and disadvantages of prolonged shift work.

Workplace Violence and Bullying

Violence against medical professionals has been steadily climbing. Forty-six percent of all nonfatal assaults and violent acts in health care have been perpetrated against RNs—not to mention that 35% to 80% of hospital staff have reported being assaulted at least once during their careers.[31] In fact, one-third of emergency RNs have considered leaving the profession because of workplace violence.[32] Hospitals that downplay these types of violent acts, fail to report them to appropriate authorities, or discipline staff for reporting hostile behavior severely affect RNs' perceptions about the workplace. Lateral violence, horizontal violence, and bullying are all terms that typically encompass verbal threats, physical threats, and intimidation by other health-care personnel, including physicians, RNs, support staff, emergency services, and law enforcement personnel, against one another.

The most common types of violence are bullying and/or intimidation, which can include deliberate acts of aggression (e.g., verbal assaults, unjust disciplinary action, heavy patient assignments, and intimidation) or deliberate acts of exclusion (e.g., withholding information, assistance, support, or guidance).[33] This inappropriate behavior is not only perpetuated by the offender but also by witnesses who fail to take action. Violence of any kind is a symptom of a maladaptive culture, and immediate intervention is required to correct it. Department leaders must foster an environment in which staff at all levels feel safe when reporting such events, knowing that the complaint will be taken seriously and handled without retaliation.

Interdisciplinary Communication

When physician–RN relationships deteriorate, it directly affects the delivery of patient care and contributes to staff turnover.[7,9,36,37] Poor relationships occur when RNs perceive that physicians view them as assistants rather than independently licensed professionals. Team dynamics can further deteriorate when RNs disagree with the medical care plan or fail to inform physicians about significant changes in a patient's condition.

Inadequate Resilience/Moral Distress

Although there are numerous definitions associated with inadequate resilience/moral distress, it is defined here as a condition that develops when one is unable to cope with the demand to provide safe, effective care. This distress may arise when a clinician is overwhelmed and working in an environment of distrust. Only recently have there been studies examining this phenomenon within the context of the ED.[27,38,39]

Inadequate resilience/moral distress is a contributing factor to RN retention.[8,27,38,39] Inadequate resilience by ED staff is not necessarily based on a specific incident; rather, it is related to the overall work environment. A dysfunctional practice setting, feelings of being overwhelmed, and adaptive/maladaptive coping skills are significant contributors to moral distress in the ED.[38]

Professional Development

When hospitals fail to recognize and support the professional development of RNs, they are in effect limiting the RNs' ability to provide the most effective patient care. This creates what is known as the "silo" effect, in which professionals are only familiar with how care is provided within their own organization. When health-care professionals are isolated, they may not know if they are practicing according to current professional standards. Obstacles to professional development include:

- Limited financial support
- Failure of management to allow RNs' time off to participate in continuing educational activities
- Preferential treatment of some RNs while ignoring the needs of others

It is crucial to remember that all members of the nursing staff should have access to professional development. When these opportunities cannot be provided within the institution, other viable external or online opportunities should be sought. Lack of support for professional development is a contributing factor to RN turnover.[7,8,35,37]

Work-Life Balance/Integration

Work-life balance is essential to maintaining a positive attitude and both physical and psychological health. When work becomes all encompassing, it creates stress that affects the RN's work. Demands from employers for committee work, staffing, overtime, and mandatory competencies—coupled with demands for continuing professional development and certification—can exceed the time RNs have to commit to their job and limit the time needed to take care of themselves and their families. Employers must also consider the expectations of the newer generation of RNs. The willingness to work long hours commonly associated with baby boomers and Generation X is now shifting. Younger members of the workforce want a "real" life that allows time for family and friends.[40]

Organizational Structure

The willingness of RNs to commit long term has a lot to do with the structure and operations of an organization. Nurses are most likely to stay in an environment of shared governance that encourages them to:

- Have a voice in operations, particularly related to patient care.
- Become valued members of the organization.

- Advance within the organization.
- Practice to the full extent of their license.[4,7,8,35,37,41,42]

Organizations that take a top-down approach to leadership tend to alienate professional staff, including RNs. Clinicians are experts in their specialties and are often the most familiar with practice guidelines and standards of care. When leadership decisions are contrary to these established protocols or standards, leadership is no longer trusted. This disconnect between the business approach and clinical practice creates an environment in which RNs are more willing to leave an organization.[27] Such disparities are particularly noticeable when professional staff must report to leaders who do not have a clinical background. The trust gap escalates when shared governance is not incorporated.[4,43]

Charge nurses, nurse managers, medical directors, chief nursing officers, and other senior members of the ED team play a central role in staff perceptions. When these leaders demonstrate poor performance and are inaccessible and inflexible, RNs are more likely to leave the organization.[6-9,37,41] Changes to organizational policies, particularly regarding practice, require those in positions of authority to work collaboratively with frontline professionals. This approach ensures that clinical practice guidelines, standards of care, and any potential obstacles are considered.

Whether intentional or unintentional, organizations that do not empower RNs to advance or assume leadership roles increase staff attrition.[7,8,42] This stagnation can also occur when organizations hinder RNs from participating in their professional associations, limiting their ability to make a difference within emergency medicine as a whole. Failing to provide time away from work or financial support to participate in professional activities can create resentment toward the leadership and contribute to the "silo" effect. As a result, burnout and apathy may develop.

STRATEGIES TO IMPROVE RETENTION

Unfortunately, there is little department leaders can do to address the shortage of available RNs in health care. (Specific information regarding ED nursing staffing can be found in Chapter 22.) However, numerous strategies can be implemented to retain the RNs who are already working in the ED.

Leadership Approach

Increasing nurse retention starts with a leadership philosophy. The antiquated authoritative approach does not work in today's health-care environment. Many medical leaders learned how to manage through on-the-job training without any significant mentoring, often resulting in a trial-and-error approach. Modern leadership, however, requires the use of best practices and evidence-based strategies.

Leaders should consider embracing a transformational strategy, which encourages mutually respectful relationships that elevate each member of the organization. Implementing transformational leadership requires leaders to:[9,37]

- Engage others in a shared vision with shared goals.
- Empower team members and support them in their professional development.
- Encourage the sharing of ideas.
- Recognize individuals and teams for their accomplishments.
- Create trust between management and staff.

It is important to note that these relationships require constant work and encouragement to remain effective.

> **BOX 121.1 ■ IOM ESSENTIAL MANAGEMENT PRACTICES**
>
> 1. Use evidence-based practice and evidence-based management.
> 2. Create and sustain trust.
> 3. Actively manage the process of change.
> 4. Involve workers in work design and workflow decision-making.
> 5. Create a learning organization.

The IOM identified five essential management practices that should be integrated into any organization's leadership philosophy, regardless of which theoretical approach is used (**Box 121.1**).[44] A core tenet that must be woven throughout any management plan is the promotion of two-way communication and exchange of information/ideas between the interdisciplinary team and management. In addition to these management practices, common actions that will help leaders succeed include:

- Visibility within the ED
- Approachability at all times
- Active listening to team members
- Empowering staff to become leaders
- Encouraging new ideas with support for innovation
- Recognizing and rewarding excellence for both professional accomplishments and clinical outcomes

Leaders who stay behind closed doors lose credibility with staff and are perceived as out-of-touch with the realities of practice. The alienation is particularly acute if the only time staff see management is when they are scolding or disciplining staff. Occasionally assisting in the clinical area and providing accolades when something is well done help portray department leaders as supportive and approachable.[6] When leaders are seen as coaches and supporters rather than authoritarians, RNs are more willing to remain committed to the organization.[42] It is imperative that leaders actively listen when staff are talking and avoid reactionary, on-the-spot decisions as much as possible (see Chapter 8).

Evidence-Based Practice and Management

Managing an ED requires leaders and staff to ensure that their respective roles are based on the most current, evidence-based strategies (e.g., "best practices," validated research, new clinical practice guidelines).[45] Static ED leadership can be stagnating. The departmental culture should encourage leaders to articulate their rationales and the basis for their decisions.

A questioning approach fosters continuous quality improvement by examining how decisions are made, implemented, and evaluated from both a management and clinical perspective. This method addresses a concern identified by the IOM recommending a balance between efficiency, which stresses the need for cost-effective and timely services, with the need for reliability, which improves safety but may conflict with efficiency. Achieving the desired level of safety may involve strategies like cross training and redundancy.[44] Cross training requires time and money but helps fill the gaps when key personnel are unavailable. Using redundancy to "read-back" orders and implementing "time-outs" to ensure that all team members are focused on the same processes take time but create a culture of safety.

Creating and Sustaining Trust

A team is not a group of people who work together; it is a group of people who trust each other.[37,42] Developing standards of conduct that hold both leaders and staff accountable is necessary to build and sustain that trust. It is appropriate to have high expectations of the ED staff as long as everyone, including leadership, is held to the same standards. It is imperative that leaders are viewed as forthright and fair. The focus should always be on specific behaviors and actions, never on the individuals themselves. For example:

> *Consider an RN who is not well liked in the department and has been consistently showing up late for work. Leaders in the department place the nurse on notice, informing him that any further tardiness will result in immediate termination.*
>
> *Within the same unit, another nurse who is well liked by physicians and the staff has also been consistently showing up late for work. However, the only counseling that is issued to this second RN is a verbal reminder to try to be on time.*

A disparity like this creates an environment of mistrust. Both RNs should be counseled on the specific behavior that has occurred, the expectations for timeliness and attendance, and the consequences that will occur if those expectations are not met. The approach should be the same regardless of who is involved. This also applies when dealing with physicians and other staff within the department. If leaders hold the RN staff accountable but do not hold physicians, themselves, or other staff accountable, a similar level of distrust will emerge.

Inconsistent approaches most often occur in response to behavioral issues. Sometimes, leaders take actions against everyone for unacceptable behaviors that only occur among a few individuals. Rather than unfairly "cracking down" on everyone, counseling or disciplinary actions should be limited to the individuals who are failing to meet established expectations. Punitive action against the whole department should be avoided.

Besides being fair, leaders need to be reliable and keep their word. Unkept promises of any type build a pattern of disbelief and low morale. For example:

> *An ED leader promises to implement a differential for RNs who obtain certification in emergency nursing. The staff agrees that this is an excellent idea and are willing to participate in the initiative. As several RNs obtain their certification, the differentials are implemented. However, a number of nurses without the certification start to complain that the new plan is unfair. Compounding the matter is pressure from upper management to reduce operating expenses. The leader decides to eliminate the initiative, and an environment of mistrust results.*

The Process of Change

Change is inevitable in health care, and effective ED leaders create a plan for implementing it. However, multiple simultaneous changes create significant stress for physicians, RNs, and other staff. Too many modifications can cause confusion and decrease the likelihood that they can be appropriately sustained or evaluated for effectiveness. Changes in outcomes may not be attributable to one specific initiative.

Introducing change creates disruption as old behaviors are relinquished and new ones are solidified.[46] Because members of the ED staff will adopt and incorporate changes at different speeds, it is important to allow adequate time for implementation.[47,48] Additionally, adequate training may be required to maximize the success of the change process.

Leaders and staff will need to discuss, become familiar with, and agree on the change initiative ahead of time. A collaboratively developed process that includes the recognition

> **BOX 121.2 ■ Actively Managing the Process of Change**[45]
>
> - Ongoing communication
> - Training
> - Mechanisms for feedback, measurement, and redesign
> - Sustained attention
> - Worker involvement

of possible failure points and "in-process" feedback allows for an adequate evaluation of the initiative's effectiveness. Implementation should include ongoing and regular communication to ensure that any challenges are addressed. **Box 121.2** highlights the IOM's recommendations for actively managing the process of change.[44]

Shared Governance

Effective management requires leaders to have a good understanding of how the ED is functioning in real time. When solutions to departmental problems fail, the failure may be blamed on the staff charged with making the changes. However, these failures can also occur when leaders neglect to involve staff in formulating the plan of action. Frontline staff are expert innovators and frequently can find effective workarounds to obstacles in practice. These shortcuts may help improve patient care, particularly when the obstacles are interfering with the physician's or RN's ability to make practice decisions. On the other hand, some workarounds are designed to bypass safeguards in exchange for staff convenience or efficiency. Involving staff in this kind of analysis is key. When healthcare organizations approach management as a partnership between leaders and staff, all participants can contribute equally within the scope of their roles. These organizations are implementing the shared-governance model.[46] Mature shared-governance models provide RNs with autonomy and the power to participate in decisions that affect the entire ED staff.[4,7,8,41,43]

When delegating responsibilities to the staff, leaders must also provide the authority that goes with making decisions. Nothing will sabotage RN retention faster than a leader who delegates decisions only to micromanage or override them. Shared governance, which can become an essential structure to integrate core professional practice values and beliefs into the decision-making process, must be in place for a hospital to obtain magnet status.[43]

Creating a Learning Organization

To make sure the ED team is instituting best and evidence-based practices, department leaders should create a "learning organization." This entails active management of the learning process by allowing RNs and other staff the necessary time away from the clinical setting to grow professionally by attending professional conferences, obtaining certifications, conducting research, and carrying out quality-improvement projects.

Whenever possible, compensation or financial support should be considered. Examples include covering the cost of attending a conference, reimbursing tuition, and providing a differential for certification. An investment in professional development helps improve overall performance and increases RN satisfaction.[27,42]

When a failed process is discovered, the focus should be on improvement rather than on shifting blame. Effective leaders empower their staff to develop better ways of doing things and encourage them to learn from their own and others' mistakes.[6-8,27]

Developing Clinical Ladders

Clinical ladders are an excellent way to recognize the accomplishments of staff and encourage them to grow as leaders. Key components of a clinical ladder program usually consist of growth and active involvement in:

- Clinical experience
- Professional development and/or education
- Critical thinking and clinical reasoning
- Organizational leadership
- Unit- and/or hospital-based committees
- Professional associations
- Evidenced-based practice projects and/or research

Clinical ladder development should be in alignment with the organization's goals, and the criteria should explicitly describe how to achieve each promotional level.[47] Ideally, staff should be actively involved in the development of measurable clinical criteria. Without it, staff may view the ladder process as subjective, particularly when staff are unsuccessful in advancing to the next rank.[47] Failure to involve staff in the development process may also be seen as a means to limit the advancement of emergency RNs.

The value of creating a learning organization with clinical ladders will be determined by the resources that ED leaders devote to the process. If little recognition or compensation is provided to staff for their efforts, then the staff have little reason to value the learning process—a dynamic that can eventually cause an ED to become stagnant.

Environment

The workplace environment significantly contributes to RN retention. When staff feel supported, respected, and safe and can practice autonomously within their respective scopes of practice, job satisfaction increases.[6,8,35,41]

Safety

Patient and staff safety are top priorities in all EDs. As such, it is important for health-care organizations to develop a culture of zero tolerance for violence. This includes violence perpetrated by patients, family, staff, physicians, and even administrators. Numerous resources are available to help combat this epidemic, such as the ENA/American Organization of Nurse Executives toolkit for mitigating violence in the workplace. Nurse leaders should also encourage their RN staff to support state initiatives that help combat this issue. By collaborating with hospital administration and local law enforcement, policies can be developed that encourage the reporting and prosecution of violent offenders.

Policies about violence should also include and address horizontal/lateral violence and bullying.[33] Nurse leaders need to work collaboratively with medical directors to ensure that physicians, RNs, and other staff are aware that this type of violence is unacceptable; this includes the complacent behavior of witnesses who fail to report problematic behavior to the appropriate leaders.[33] This type of violence can be subtle, so leaders should be vigilant in investigating any reported incidents. Every attempt should be made to avoid a response intended to stifle the report.

Scheduling

Staff self-scheduling with specific guidelines helps increase satisfaction among RNs. It is important that the scheduling guidelines ensure fairness. As the RN workforce ages and approaches retirement, hospital systems might consider whether their employee guidelines could be made more flexible to accommodate various scheduling requests. For example, an older team member or an RN who wants part-time work may find that 12-hour shifts are not a viable option. Using strategically placed 4-, 6-, or 8-hour shifts might provide enough flexibility to allow these RNs to work while addressing critical staffing needs.

Interdisciplinary Team Dynamics

Dysfunctional teams create operational chaos, patient and staff dissatisfaction, disengagement, and staff exodus. Both physicians and RNs are independently licensed health-care workers who have been granted the right to practice autonomously within the scope of their training and are accountable to their respective regulatory boards. Mutual respect and effective communication between physicians and RNs are necessary to ensure that the best patient care is provided.[4] When physicians see nurses as subservient or approach them in an authoritarian manner, conflict will arise. Conversely, when RNs become dismissive about medical plans of care or fail to inform physicians about significant changes in a patient's condition, distrust will arise. Only when health-care workers recognize and honor the contributions that each discipline makes can the team work effectively.

Health of the Workforce

There is a growing body of evidence identifying the negative health effects of prolonged shift work. Department leaders and staff have multiple opportunities to develop strategies that will promote the wellness of the ED team, including:

- Ensuring appropriate immunizations for health-care workers
- Providing ergonomic equipment when possible
- Staffing and scheduling appropriately to allow breaks and meals and to address surges in the workflow
- Encouraging appropriate breaks when possible
- Collaborating with the health system or community to obtain discounts for wellness services, such as gym memberships
- Making healthy food choices available to all health-care workers on all shifts
- Safeguarding time away from work between shifts to allow for adequate periods of rest

Hiring and Orientation

Establishing an effective health-care team requires defining the competencies necessary for success. Department leaders should consider involving other physicians and RNs in the hiring process. A broader interview approach can help to evaluate the applicants' ability to use clinical reasoning, prioritize, and recognize when they need help. It also creates opportunities to evaluate how applicants interact with the rest of the team. Hiring RNs who fit well within the culture of the ED fosters retention and limits potential disruptions.

A comprehensive orientation will help new hires acclimate to the ED. It is a best practice to provide new staff with a personalized letter welcoming them to the unit and outlining the orientation process and schedule. The length and structure of the orientation will vary based on the experience and needs of the new hires. Inexperienced RNs will require a longer orientation that may include a residency training program. These in-depth programs generally include both didactic and clinical components focused on the delivery of safe, quality care that meets established professional standards.[45]

All new RNs should orient with a trained preceptor who can provide guidance and constructive feedback. These training programs increase staffing stability and retention while decreasing the costs associated with turnover.[45,9]

Peer Review

A peer-review process can improve care and encourage the reporting of inevitable errors. In peer review, practicing professional colleagues evaluate the quality and appropriateness of the care provided in order to:[49]

- Review the quality and quantity of care provided based on established practice standards
- Determine the strengths and deficiencies
- Provide evidence for change in practice protocols to improve care
- Identify practice patterns that indicate a need for more knowledge

The peer-review process is not meant to be punitive or anonymous; rather, it is a process by which one's peers can help improve an individual's practice. Rarely, an error may be significant enough to legally require a colleague to report the provider to an official regulatory board. Policies and procedures should clearly outline how the peer-review process will be implemented. Whenever possible, it is important that professional practice guidelines be used as the standard of care. When RNs feel that they are being treated fairly and held to objective standards, they are more likely to remain with an organization.

Professional Associations

Professional associations have been recognized as a key component of career growth as far back as 1928.[50] While these organizations originally served as gatekeeping/regulatory agencies, they now:

- Develop clinical practice guidelines
- Advocate for regulatory rules and laws to improve patient care and the well-being of practicing professionals
- Educate practicing professionals
- Validate the acquisition of knowledge
- Provide a network of practicing professionals who work within the same environment

Most staff and leaders participating in professional organizations find great value and describe multiple benefits (**Box 121.3**).[51] ENA serves as the primary professional association

---

BOX 121.3 ■ Professional Association Benefits[52]

- Allows health-care workers to connect with others outside of their own institution
- Promotes a broader perspective and avoids the silo effect
- Fosters networking
- Encourages sharing of advice and experience
- Supports health-care workers
- Encourages health-care workers to set the standards of practice
- Supports health-care workers in advocating for the profession
- Assists in keeping the profession current and safe
- Promotes professional development
- Improves and validates knowledge
- Fosters a sense of belonging
- Provides a voice for health-care workers for the specialty
- Encourages community involvement

for emergency RNs. Participation in a larger community allows RNs to see a broader picture beyond what is occurring within their own institutions. Engagement in a national organization can lead to the initiation of local innovations and improvements.

It is particularly important for ED leaders to participate in their professional associations as an example to the staff. Many organizations have included active participation in professional associations as a component of their clinical ladders. Engaged team members are more likely to advance within their institutions and are more likely to be satisfied with their role.

CONCLUSION

Nurse retention is a complex process that requires an understanding of many contributing factors. Successful RN retention programs often use a transformational leadership approach and incorporate IOM essential management protocols into their practice. Multiple lines of communication between leadership, staff, and members of the interdisciplinary team are essential for creating a culture that is focused on quality patient care and professional growth. Shared governance within the ED further allows RNs to integrate core professional values and beliefs into their clinical decisions.[43]

Ensuring the safety of ED staff is essential to creating a workplace environment that encourages RN retention. Staff safety requires leaders to foster effective communication between team members, including physicians. Civility creates a positive work environment that encourages staff to remain at an organization. Physically, psychologically, and spiritually healthy team members perform better and maintain a more positive approach to patient care. As members of the workforce age and begin to focus more heavily on work-life balance, ED leaders must consider how they can meet the evolving needs of their employees.

Encouraging clinician involvement in professional associations allows nurses to communicate with peers outside their respective organizations; encourages them to advocate for their patients; and helps them to pursue continuing education, develop a sense of professional identity, and become more engaged in the community. High RN retention rates improve the financial performance of the ED and significantly enhance patient outcomes. It is imperative that ED leaders consistently review other organizational environments to incorporate best practices that will help retain qualified emergency RNs.

REFERENCES

1. Sun R, Karaca Z, Wong HS. *Healthcare Cost and Utilization Project Statistical Brief #238: Trends in Hospital Emergency Department Visits by Age and Payer, 2006-2015.* Rockville, MD: Agency for Healthcare Research and Quality; 2018:1–11.

2. National Center for Health Statistics. FastStats: emergency department visits. Centers for Disease Control and Health Prevention. Available at: https://www.cdc.gov/nchs/fastats/emergency-department.htm. Updated Jan 19, 2017. Accessed May 22, 2019.

3. Hesse C. Executive synopsis: emergency nurse retention. Emergency Nurses Association. Available at: https://www.ena.org/docs/default-source/resource-library/practice-resources/other/emergency-nurse-retention-executive-synopsis.pdf?sfvrsn=b8b1a708_4. Accessed August 3, 2020.

4. American Nurses Association. *ANA's Principles for Nurse Staffing.* 2nd ed. Silver Spring, MD: American Nurses Association; 2012.

5. Avalere Health. *Optimal Nurse Staffing to Improve Quality of Care and Patient Outcomes.* Washington, DC: American Nurses Association; 2015.

6. Bakon S, Christensen M, Barker-Gregory N. Appropriate staffing in critical units: a review of the literature. *Singap Nurs J.* 2016; 43(2):16–24.

7. Khan N, Jackson D, Stayt L, Walthall, H. Factors influencing nurses' intentions to leave adult critical care settings. *Nurs Crit Care.* 2019;24(1):24–32.

8. Moloney W, Boxall P, Parsons M, et al. Factors predicting registered nurses' intentions to leave their organization and profession: a job demands-resources framework. *J Adv Nurs.* 2018;74(4):864–875.

9. Sandler M. Why are new graduate nurses leaving the profession in their first year of practice and how does this impact on ED nurse staffing? A rapid review of current literature and recommended reading. *Can J Emerg Nurs.* 2018;41(1):23–24.

10. Aiken LH, Clarke SP, Cheung RB, et al. Educational levels of hospital nurses and surgical patient mortality. *JAMA.* 2003;290(12):1617–1623.

11. Brennan CW, Daly BJ, Jones KR. State of the science: the relationship between nurse staffing and patient outcomes. *Western J Nurs Res.* 2013;35(6):760–794.

12. The Joint Commission. *2019 Comprehensive Accreditation Manuals.* Oak Brook, Ill: The Joint Commission; 2019.

13. Centers for Medicare and Medicaid. State Operations Manual Appendix A—Survey Protocol, Regulations and Interpretive Guidelines for Hospitals. Available at: https://www.cms.gov/Regulations-and-Guidance/Guidance/Manuals/downloads/som107ap_a_hospitals.pdf. Updated October 12, 2018. Accessed June 6, 2019.

14. Aiken LH, Cimiotti JP, Sloane, DM, et al. Effects of nurse staffing and nurse education on patient deaths in hospitals with different nurse work environments. *Med Care.* 2011;49(12):1047–1053.

15. American Nurses Association. Nurse staffing. American Nurses Association; Available at: http://www.nursingworld.org/practice-policy/work-environment/nurse-staffing. Accessed June 6, 2019.

16. Recio-Saucedo A, Pope C, Dall'Ora C, et al. Safe staffing for nursing in EDs: evidence review. *Emerg Med J.* 2015;32(11):888–894.

17. Buerhaus PI, Skinner LE, Auerbach DI, et all. Four challenges facing the nursing workforce in the United States. *J Nurs Regul.* 2017;8(2):40–46.

18. United States Department of Labor. U.S. Bureau of Labor Statics Registered Nurses. Available at: https://www.bls.gov/ooh/healthcare/registered-nurses.htm. Updated April 12, 2019. Retrieved May 10, 2019.

19. World Health Organization. Nursing and Midwifery. Available at: https://www.who.int/news-room/fact-sheets/detail/nursing-and-midwifery. Updated February 23, 2018. Retrieved June 6, 2019.

20. Covell CL, Sidani S. Nursing intellectual capital theory: implications for research and practice. *Online J Issues Nurs.* 2013;18(2):1–14.

21. American Association of Colleges of Nursing. Fact sheet: nursing faculty shortage. American Association of Colleges of Nursing. Available at: https://www.aacnnursing.org/News-Information/Fact-Sheets/Nursing-Faculty-Shortage. Updated April 1, 2019. Retrieved June 6, 2019.

22. National League for Nursing. NLN nurse educator shortage fact sheet. National League for Nursing. 2013. Available at: http://www.nln.org/docs/default-source/advocacy-public-policy/nurse-faculty-shortage-fact-sheet-pdf.pdf. Accessed June 6, 2019.

23. Auerbach DI, Buerhaus PI, Staiger DO. Will the RN workforce weather the retirement of the baby boomers? *Med Care.* 2015;53(10):850–856.

24. United States Census Bureau. Older people projected to outnumber children for first time in U.S. history. United States Census Bureau. 2018. Available at: https://www.census.gov/newsroom/press-releases/2018/cb18-41-population-projections.html. Accessed June 6, 2019.

25. National Council of State Boards of Nursing and The National Forum of State Nursing Workforce Centers. National Nursing Workforce Study. Available at: https://www.ncsbn.org/workforce.htm. Accessed June 6, 2019.

26. Health Resources and Services Administration. The registered nurse population. US Department of Health and Human Services. 2010. Available at: https://data.hrsa.gov/DataDownload/NSSRN/GeneralPUF08/rnsurveyfinal.pdf. Accessed June 6, 2019.

27. Gorman VL. Future emergency nursing workforce: what the evidence is telling us. *J Emerg Nurs.* 2019;45(2):132–136.

28. Wheatley C. Nursing overtime: should it be regulated? *Nurs Econ.* 2017;35(4):213–217.

29. Clendon J, Gibbons V. 12 h shifts and rates of error among nurses: a systematic review. *Int J Nurs Stud.* 2015;52(7):1231–1242.

30. Stimpfel AW, Aiken LH. Hospital staff nurses' shift length associated with safety and quality of care. *J Nurs Care Qual.* 2013;28(2):122–129.

31. Emergency Nurses Association. *ENA Toolkit: Workplace Violence.* Schaumburg, Ill: Emergency Nurses Association; 2010.

32. Emergency Nurses Association. Workplace violence in EDs. Emergency Nurses Association. Available at: https://www.ena.org/practice-resources/workplace-violence. Updated 2019. Accessed June 6, 2019.

33. Wolf LA, Perhats C, Clark PR, et al. Workplace bullying in emergency nursing: development of a grounded theory using situational analysis. *Int Emerg Nurs.* 2017;39(2018):33–39.

34. Aiken LH, Clarke SP, Sloane DM, et al. Effects of hospital care environment on patient mortality and nurse outcomes. *J Nurs Admin.* 2008;38(5):223–229.

35. Chang H, Shyu YL, Wong M, et al. Which aspect of professional commitment can effectively retain nurses in the nursing profession. *J Nurs Scholarsh.* 2015;47(5):468–476.

36. Djukic M, Kovner, CT, Brewer CS, et al. Work environment factors other than staffing associated with nurses' ratings of patient care quality. *Health Care Manage Rev.* 2013;38(2):105–114.

37. Shimp KM. Systematic review of turnover/retention and staff perception of staffing and resource adequacy related to staffing. *Nurs Econ.* 2017;35(5):239–266.

38. Wolf LA, Perhats C, Delao AM, et al. "It's a burden you carry": describing moral distress in emergency nursing. *J Emerg Nurs.* 2016;42(1):37–46.

39. Hopson M, Petri L, Kufera J. A new perspective on nursing retention: job embeddedness in acute care nurses. *J Nurses Prof Dev.* 2018;34(1):31–37.

40. Mokoka KE. Managing a multigenerational nursing workforce to strengthen staff retention. *Prof Nurs Today.* 2015;19(4):42–45.

41. Adams SL. *Influences of Turnover, Retention, and Job Embeddedness in Nursing Workforce Literature* [master's thesis]. Johnson City, Tenn: East Tennessee State University; 2016.

42. LaRock-McMahon C. *Factors Influencing Emergency Registered Nurse Satisfaction and Engagement* [master's thesis]. Minneapolis, Minn: Walden University; 2018.

43. Fisher CA, Jabara J, Poudrier L, et al. Shared governance: the way to staff satisfaction and retention. *Nurs Manag.* 2016;47(11):14–16.

44. Institute of Medicine. *Keeping Patients Safe: Transforming the Work Environments of Nurses.* Washington, DC: The National Academies Press; 2004.

45. Institute of Medicine. *The Future of Nursing: Leading Change, Advancing Health.* Washington, DC: The National Academies Press; 2011.

46. Guanci G, Medeiros M. *Shared Governance That Works.* Minneapolis, Minn: Creative Health Care Management; 2018.

47. Knoche EL, Meucci JH. Competencies within a professional clinical ladder: differences in understanding between nurse managers and staff nurses. *J Nurses Prof Dev.* 2015;31(2):91–99.

48. Batras D, Duff C, Smith BJ. Organizational change theory: implications for health promotion practice. *Health Promot Int.* 2014;31(1):231–241.

49. *Barbara Haag-Heitman and Vicki George; Peer Review in Nursing: Principles for Successful Practice.* Jones and Bartlett Publishers; 2011.

50. Carr-Saunders AM. *Professions: Their Organization and Place in Society.* Oxford, England: The Clarendon Press; 1928.

51. Moon MD. *Influences of the Emergency Nursing Professional Association on the Socialization of Emerging Emergency Nurses* [master's thesis]. San Marcos, Tex: Texas State University; 2013.

CHAPTER 122

MANAGING IMPAIRED PROFESSIONALS

Dennis C. Whitehead, Abbie G. Whitehead, Kirk R. Klemme

Few problems in emergency medicine management are as vexing as dealing with an impaired professional. Following the old saw "Judge not, lest ye be judged" is often harmful not only to patients but also to practitioners. Depending on the nature of the impairment, available treatment can usually resolve the problem or at least make it manageable. The worst thing that can be done is to ignore the issue or assume someone else will handle it. When lives are at stake, a conspiracy of silence, although often the easier and more tempting course, is not an acceptable option.

Impairment, defined here as a lessening of ability to perform professional duties, may be a result of several factors. In emergency medicine, most impairment is due to substance use disorder (SUD, previously called chemical dependence), which may be further subdivided into more specific categories such as opioid use disorder and alcohol use disorder. Other disorders, both behavioral and organic, also may appear in the differential diagnosis. Age itself may be a cause. All these factors need to be considered when evaluating the impaired professional.

CULTURE AND LEADERSHIP

Dealing with a complex problem like professional impairment takes planning and a carefully crafted mindset. Proactive planning is far more effective than *post hoc* reactionary measures. The goal is to create a work environment that encourages effective, nonblaming, and appropriate responses to potential and actual clinical impairment. Promoting a culture of safety in health care protects patients, clinicians, and institutional integrity (**Figure 122.1**).

FIGURE 122.1 ■ Culture of Safety

Medical Directors	Administrators	Clinicians
1. Lead by example.	1. Provide ongoing leadership coaching/training.	1. Collaborate and communicate.
2. Adopt open-door policies.	2. Define appropriate and inappropriate behavior.	2. Identify and report issues.
3. Adopt processes and provide resources to promote clinician well-being.	3. Estabilsh policies and procedures for predefined issues.	
4. Set expectations and intervene early.	4. Make process-improvement and wellness programs top priorities.	
5. Make difficult topics routine in team meetings.		
6. Form rapport with individual team members.		

The proactive strategy for provider impairment required for a safe culture in health care includes:

- Leadership recognition of the high-risk nature of health care and continuously working to improve the safety of the operations
- A "just culture" environment where individuals understand their role in speaking up about incidents, harmful processes, bottlenecks, and any other concerns without fearing administrative repercussions
- Collaboration and communication across all levels of health-care workers
- Organizational commitment to providing the necessary resources to improve safety and well-being of the health-care team[1]

Leaders play a crucial role in establishing a healthy team dynamic. High clinician stress levels often lead to burnout. A study by Medscape suggests that 42% of physicians are currently burnt out. Further, the study reveals that burnout occurs across all generations but is more prevalent during mid-career when, in addition to professional stressors, clinicians may be responsible for the care of multiple generations, including children and parents.[2] These stresses, compounded by any behavioral health factors, cause clinicians to be at high risk for impairment issues and burnout. It is imperative that leaders recognize and openly acknowledge the high risk for burnout and potential reliance on coping mechanisms that may include alcohol or illicit substances.[3,4]

Proactive Strategies

Clinical leadership should incorporate topics like burnout and impairment into routine discussions, both individually and as a group. Since a cardinal sign of impairment is denial, providers may be more apt to recognize and admit they have an issue when staff leaders recognize and empathize with the difficulties common to busy clinicians.

Clinicians typically believe they must live up to the public and their own view of a near-faultless performance.[3,5] Leaders may wish to provide statistics or share a recovered clinician's true story to gain credibility and acceptance of the issue. These statistics and stories decrease the stigma and may provide a sense of hope.

Just Culture

"Just culture" environments have preestablished responses to errors and issues.[1] Clinical leaders and their administrative human resource and legal partners should define what unsafe behavior and processes look like (e.g., provider impairment, disruptive or disrespectful confrontations to staff or patients) and implement policies to recognize and address these unsafe behaviors. Leaders are also responsible for establishing and communicating the procedures for individuals to report unsafe behavior in good faith. These policies and procedures may additionally be written into hospital bylaws.[5]

Testing

Administrators are expected to establish the necessary agreements with entities that can provide toxicologic testing, mental health assessments, cognitive functioning assessments, and diagnostic testing. When searching for partners, it is appropriate to consider nonaffiliated entities above internal entities. If an internal entity is used, it is necessary to ensure that both confidentiality and the chain of custody are maintained. Human resources should develop and distribute a process/form for staff to use when suspicious behavior occurs.

Additionally, disclosure forms must be developed for the impaired clinician to sign prior to any form of testing (**Box 122.1**). The form should list the individuals with whom the results will be shared and in what manner (i.e., lab value versus positive/negative). This process helps maintain confidentially of the impaired clinician. An impaired clinician should be offered the same privacy protections as that of any patient.[6]

Leadership Communication

Clinical leaders are responsible for communicating the established processes to their team members. Establishing open lines of communication allows leaders to both gather baseline information about individuals and more readily detect changes from normal behavior. Ideally, leaders regularly round on their team members, inquiring about each person's well-being and establishing a sense of normality around chatting with individuals.[3] Changes in behavior or lifestyle should result in inquiry about the individual's well-being through an in-person conversation. Much like a patient assessment, this direct process allows the clinical leader to visually assess for signs of impairment.

Leaders with open-door policies have the greatest potential to become aware of staff issues in the early stages. It is time consuming, as it requires being available; however, leaders build trust by following up diligently on these matters. It may be particularly difficult to identify early signs of provider impairment. Typically, clinicians mask their illnesses, and poor job performance is often a late sign of impairment.[7] By building a "just culture" environment centered around awareness, open communication, and accountability, clinicians may have a better understanding about the crucial role they play in appropriately reporting signs of their own or others' impairment early.

Clinician Reporting

When an impaired clinician reports their own impairment, the gesture is considered voluntary and is more likely to lead to advocacy as opposed to discipline.[5] When the clinician self-reports, effective leaders listen before responding and provide encouragement and show respect for the courage the clinician has displayed. It might be wise to pause and invite

---

BOX 122.1 ■ EXAMPLE DISCLOSURE FORM

Provider Permission to Disclose Results

I, _____, give permission to _____
  Print Clinician's Name   Name of Entity Performing Study/Diagnostics

to release the results of the study or assessment that are circled below. Results should be submitted directly to _____.
                        Administrator's Name

- Toxicology Screening
- Diagnostic Testing
- Alcohol Screening
- Mental Health Assessment
- Cognitive Testing
- Other _____

Results (positive/negative) will be shared unless specifically defined below.

_____

| Clinician's Signature | Date | Leader's Signature | Date |

a human resource representative to join the conversation, especially if impairment is caused by an SUD. Clinicians who self-report are still required to undergo toxicology screening and must report to the predetermined laboratory for testing immediately after the discussion.

If a clinician reports concerns about a colleague's potential impairment, the reporter's anonymity must be maintained. The reporting clinician should document the suspicious behavior and provide the documentation to the clinical leader. Reporting a colleague is a difficult decision that may require corroboration. The leader is obligated to take every concern seriously. A discussion with human resources is warranted to determine next steps. Ultimately, if the organization or impaired clinician fails to respond appropriately, reporting clinicians have an ethical responsibility to report the suspicious behavior to an appropriate supervisory agency.[7]

SUBSTANCE USE DISORDER

About 10% of all people become dependent on alcohol and/or other mood-altering substances. The incidence is higher in medical professionals than in the general population: About 15% of physicians will suffer SUD at some point in their careers.[8] Because physicians make decisions that impact the health of others, they are held to a higher standard. Thus, SUDs and other forms of impairment pose an even more consequential problem for health professionals than for most of the general population.

The physicians at greatest risk for addiction appear to be anesthesiologists, who have the easiest access to addictive substances.[9] Emergency physicians may well have the next highest risk.[10] Emergency medicine residents have been shown to be at higher risk for SUDs than those in other disciplines.[9] Emergency services personnel as a whole (doctors, physician assistants, nurse practitioners, nurses, EMTs, and paramedics) commonly have ready access to addictive drugs and the opportunity to use them. Furthermore, the demand for qualified emergency medicine practitioners makes professional mobility easy and hinders detection of the disease.

Since nearly all emergency physicians will need to deal with the difficult problem of a chemically dependent colleague or employee at some point in their careers, it is imperative to have as thorough an understanding of SUDs as other common life-threatening pathologies.

Disease Model

SUD, which includes alcoholism, has been recognized as a disease by the medical profession since 1953.[11] Like other disease processes, SUD has a characteristic symptom complex, clinical course, and treatment (**Box 122.2**).[12] Some aspects of the disorder that frustrate both those who have it and those who treat it are progression, denial, and a tendency to relapse.

In years past, chemical dependence was defined as "a cluster of cognitive, behavioral, and physiologic symptoms that indicate that the person has impaired control of psychoactive substance use and continues use of the substance despite adverse consequences. The symptoms of the dependence syndrome include, but are not limited to, the physiologic symptoms of tolerance and withdrawal."[13] Alcoholism, a specific form of chemical dependence, is a chronic, progressive, and potentially fatal disease characterized by tolerance and physical dependency.

SUD is a complex psychosocial disease with a genetic component. All races, professions, and socioeconomic classes are affected. Susceptible individuals become addicted through a combination of chemical/alcohol use and biogenetic tendency. The disorder does not appear

> **BOX 122.2 ■ DIAGNOSTIC AND STATISTICAL MANUAL OF MENTAL DISORDERS, 5TH EDITION (DSM-5) CRITERIA FOR SUBSTANCE USE DISORDER**
>
> A mild substance use disorder is diagnosed if three of the following criteria are met. People meeting four or five criteria are classified as having moderate substance use disorder, and severe substance use disorder is diagnosed in cases where six or more of the criteria are met.
>
> 1. Taking the substance in larger amounts or for longer than you meant to
> 2. Wanting to cut down or stop using the substance but not managing to
> 3. Spending a lot of time getting, using, or recovering from use of the substance
> 4. Cravings and urges to use the substance
> 5. Not managing to do what you should at work, home, or school because of substance use
> 6. Continuing to use, even when it causes problems in relationships
> 7. Giving up important social, occupational, or recreational activities because of substance use
> 8. Using the substance again and again, even when it puts you in danger
> 9. Continuing to use, even when you know you have a physical or psychological problem that could have been caused or made worse by the substance
> 10. Needing more of the substance to get the effect that you want (tolerance)
> 11. Development of withdrawal symptoms, which can be relieved by taking more of the substance

without exposure to mood-altering chemicals; thus, it will not be seen in those who never use such substances. The disorder cannot otherwise be predicted on an individual basis (**Box 122.3**).

Core Symptoms

Denial

Denial is the cardinal symptom of untreated SUD. Denial manifests itself as displaced blame, wherein problems related to the disease are perceived by the victim as stemming from anything except chemical use. Continued denials mystify those around the addict to whom the disease process is obvious. Recovering addicts say, "The disease tells you that you don't have a disease."

Compulsion

Compulsion is the obsessive drive to use the chemical despite real or potential adverse consequences. The addict eventually must recognize his or her complete inability to stop chemical use. The "spirit may be willing," but the disease is too strong. Thoughts of use

> **BOX 122.3 ■ SHORT DEFINITION OF ADDICTION**
>
> Addiction is a treatable, chronic medical disease involving complex interactions among brain circuits, genetics, the environment, and an individual's life experiences. People with addiction use substances or engage in behaviors that become compulsive and often continue despite harmful consequences. Prevention efforts and treatment approaches for addiction are generally as successful as those for other chronic diseases.
>
> *Adopted by the American Society of Addiction Medicine Board of Directors, September 2019.*

dominate waking hours and frequently intrude into dreams. This fits the commonly stated definition of insanity: "doing the same thing and expecting different results."

Progression

Progression leads to the inevitable deterioration of all aspects of life, spreading out from the addict like ripples in a pond. Social and family lives disintegrate first, with the job often the last thing to go. This is particularly true for professionals, whose only shred of self-respect as the world is collapsing around them is their work, which is also deteriorating. By looking at advanced cases retrospectively, one can see that chemical dependence has a clear pattern of progression (**Table 122.1**). It is difficult, however, to predict which drug users will progress to SUD and serious physical addiction. Early identification is important because of potential fatality. Experts now define impairment as an enduring condition that, if left untreated, is not amenable to remission and continued sobriety.

Relapse and Recovery

Relapse is common in individuals with SUDs. This powerful illness has a relentless tendency to resurface no matter how long the period of recovery. Psychosocial deterioration, often difficult to detect behaviorally, usually precedes actual use. Relapse is generally due to a resurfacing of denial, the cardinal symptom. Addicts who have survived relapse speak of a failure to respect the disease and treat it appropriately. If detected early, relapse may be a positive experience for the addict, reinforcing the seriousness of the disease. Recovery from SUD may begin at any point in the process before death.

Identifying Impaired Professionals

The most difficult aspect of helping an impaired professional is making the diagnosis. Denial is the cardinal symptom of the disease and may also be present in those closest to the subject (spouse, business partner) who have a vested interest in protecting the addict from

TABLE 122.1 ■ Typical SUD Progression	
Social use	• "Take it or leave it" • Does not preclude *infrequent* intoxication • Rare with intravenous drugs and smoked cocaine or heroin
Abuse	• Using interferes with life • Developing obsession with using • Frequent references to "getting loaded" noted • Increased solitary consumption • Absenteeism common
Addiction	• Life interferes with using • Obsessive/compulsive pattern well established • Waking state devoted to avoiding withdrawal • All other aspects of life (food, job) secondary • Institutionalization/insanity
Death	Either directly from toxicity or indirectly (accident, suicide)

> **BOX 122.4 ■ WORK-RELATED WARNING SIGNS OF SUD[16]**
>
> - Chronic tardiness
> - Missing shifts or frequent last-minute rearrangements
> - Sloppy charts
> - Incomplete or altered medical records
> - Inappropriate orders
> - Increasing complaints from patients and colleagues
> - Won't answer phone when on back-up call
> - Excessive irritability when contacted at home
> - Frequent use of strong cologne or breath mints
> - Solicits controlled drugs for self or family
> - Spends excessive time in bathroom
> - Frequent visits to car during shift
> - Erratic behavior with sudden, wide mood swings
> - Exaggerated exhilaration or negativism

scrutiny. Substance use disorder is notoriously difficult for professional colleagues to detect in the early stages, as troubles at home or in the community may not be generally known. Attitudes toward gender may play a role, as female physicians do not seem to be referred for treatment as frequently as male physicians.[14]

Suspicion and Warning Signs

Suspicions about chronic chemical dependence may arise when a professional presents for credentialing after a prolonged period between jobs, applies for a position for which they're clearly over qualified, or shows a willingness to work for low pay. The prospect may refuse to take a preemployment drug screen or may attempt to delay it by several days in hopes of producing a clean urine specimen. Most job applicants do not mind such testing, and those successfully recovering from SUDs welcome it. A period of probation with random drug testing may be appropriate for a new employee with a known history of SUD, especially if the period of recovery is less than 5 years.

It is the *pattern* of events, rather than a single precipitating incident, that aids in making the diagnosis of primary impairment. Physicians may benefit from education on the ethical and legal obligations of assisting impaired colleagues.[15] Emergency medicine administrators should be familiar with *work-related* warning signs of SUD (**Box 122.4**).[16]

The situation is less difficult to identify when there is an obvious alcohol or cannabis odor, slurred speech, ataxia, pinpoint pupils, or other observable signs. Substance use disorder is progressive, and work is almost always the last thing to deteriorate. Ample warning signs are usually evident to those who know the subject well before these signs occur on the job (**Figure 122.2**).

Medical Profession Denial

The medical profession has sometimes been accused of having a "code of silence" when it comes to dealing with its own, particularly those who have SUDs or behavioral problems. Although this view may be extreme, physicians are commonly reluctant to pass judgment on a colleague's behavior. Nonetheless, our role as patient advocates supersedes these concerns. Although colleagues should be given the benefit of the doubt, protection of the patient must always be the primary goal. It is useful in such cases to remember that SUD is a treatable disease and that the impaired professional is also a patient in need of care

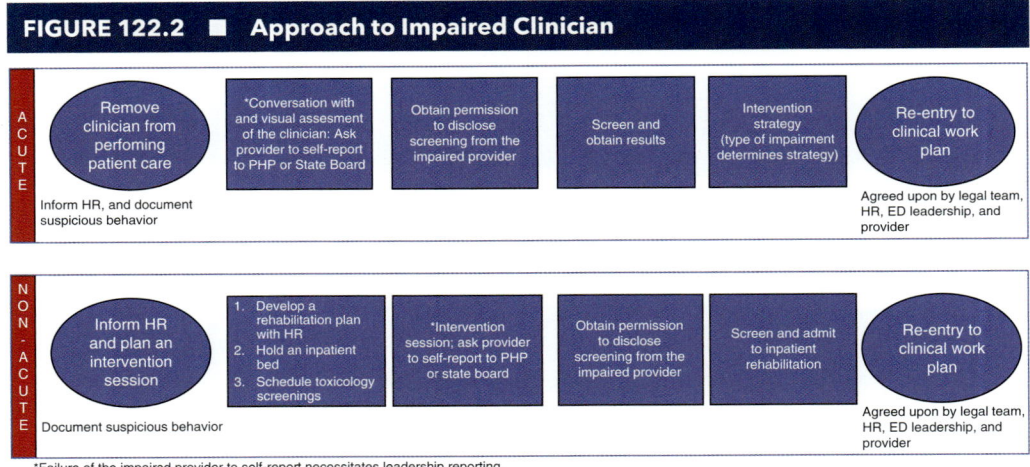

FIGURE 122.2 ■ Approach to Impaired Clinician

*Failure of the impaired provider to self-report necessitates leadership reporting.

and compassion. According to the Ethics Manual of the American College of Emergency Physicians (ACEP):

> The emergency physician may encounter colleagues or consulting physicians who are incompetent or impaired by drugs, alcohol, or psychiatric or medical conditions. The primary responsibility of the physician is to ensure patient safety. Having ensured patient safety, the emergency physician should attempt to help the impaired [professional].[17]

Special Considerations

Although emergency physicians have some access to addictive substances in the professional setting, emergency nurses have even more exposure as "gatekeepers" for psychoactive drugs dispensed in the emergency department (ED). Even computerized dispensing systems like Pyxis can be manipulated. While medically it may make sense to prescribe opiates as a PRN order with a range of doses (e.g., fentanyl 25-100 μg IVP q1-2h PRN), a nurse suffering from SUD would have little trouble diverting "excess" medication for personal use. Verbal orders may also be similarly abused, especially in busy EDs, where formal computer orders may not always be obtained in real time. Paramedics have the same opportunities as nurses in this regard. A good rule of thumb in such situations is:

> If you can think of it, an addict has, too.

While most addicts have a drug of choice, specific access to opiates, sedatives, and other addictive medicines may well determine what a professional with progressive SUD eventually becomes dependent on. A pediatrician would find it difficult to justify having great quantities of narcotics in the office, but stimulants prescribed for ADHD may be readily available. Anesthesiologists have wider availability to addictive substances. And alcohol is always an option, no matter what the professional situation.

Emergency professionals, who are in a unique position to assess other members of the medical staff, have been likened to the catcher on a baseball team. The catcher is the only player with the action right in front of him and the whole field in full view. Emergency professionals see consultants at their best and at their worst. A consultant with dependence issues may hide the problem adequately during regular office hours but not always so well when required to appear unexpectedly while on call. The ED staff may be the first to recognize such problems in a colleague.

INTERVENTION AND MANAGEMENT

Managing a case of SUD among ED staff requires early intervention and supervision at numerous steps along the way.

Acute Intervention

When immediate action is imperative, it is desirable to have medical staff or emergency protocols in place proactively to deal with an acute patient-safety problem. If a clinician is acutely impaired while managing patients, colleague clinicians are empowered and ethically required to intervene.[7] The intervening clinician should then immediately report the situation to the proper clinical leader. In most cases, however, the intervention can and should be planned beforehand. A prescribed approach is recommended (**Box 122.5**).[18] Because most properly performed interventions are successful in getting the subject to admit there is a problem, a treatment bed should be *immediately available*. If there is any delay, denial will quickly resurface and the window of opportunity may be lost.

A properly performed intervention can be lifesaving. The person suffering from SUD must be confronted by persons involved in all aspects of their life in such a way as to demolish the encircling wall of denial, which is the first step in recovery. A caveat: Since intervention is a potentially lifesaving process, planning should be as vigorous as for any difficult surgical or medical procedure. A professional facilitator should be involved.

Intervention is an emotionally taxing experience for all the participants, as the subject may initially claim those present are betraying him; preparation and rehearsal are imperative. The desired result is to get the subject into appropriate treatment immediately. As with all complex procedures, however, the participants should also be prepared for

---

BOX 122.5 ■ SUGGESTED INTERVENTION PROCEDURE

1. Preintervention planning with a professional facilitator is crucial. As this is a potentially lifesaving process, planning should be as vigorous as for any difficult surgical or medical procedure. Intervention is an emotionally taxing experience for all the participants as the subject may initially claim those present are betraying him, so preparation and rehearsal are imperative. The desired outcome will almost always be inpatient treatment, but participants also should be prepared for possible failure.

2. Include family, friends, professional colleagues, and successfully recovering persons the subject knows. It is especially important to include people the subject respects. Intervention should *never* be undertaken alone, as the subject is extraordinarily skilled at manipulating individuals to get out of jams.

3. The session should be nonjudgmental, focusing on indisputable facts (absenteeism, poor work performance, bizarre behavior) rather than on the cause of the problems. The inevitable negative consequences of the subject's behavior should be stressed (job loss, licensing problems, marital discord) after concern and friendship are expressed and facts as known to the intervenor are reviewed. Participants must be emotionally prepared to follow through on the consequences specified if the subject does not agree to be helped. An intervention is not a time for bluffing.

4. Intervenors speak first, each to completion of statement. Interruptions from the subject should not be permitted.

5. Subject speaks last.

6. Treatment or negative consequences should occur immediately as specified.

failure and should be resolute in seeing that the discussed consequences are effected if the subject is uncooperative or defiant.

Treatment of SUD

Most health-care professionals require initial intensive inpatient treatment, usually lasting 30 to 40 days. An intake assessment period of a few days may be necessary if the diagnosis is in doubt or if there are complicating psychiatric problems. Detoxification will proceed as indicated.

This initial treatment is customarily followed by some time in a recovery or halfway house. Additional rehab time is critical, as brain changes associated with longer-term SUDs may not fully heal for many months, or even years. This is an important consideration for professionals who make critical decisions every day. Additionally, health-care workers are used to being in control, frequently finding it difficult to adopt a matter-of-fact attitude toward their own disease the way many lay persons can.

Counselors and physicians at the treatment facility often involve family and employers/colleagues throughout the process. As described earlier, professional colleagues should be educated about SUD. When properly identified, treated, and monitored, the prognosis for physicians with SUDs is very good.[19] In fact, physicians in recovery do better than those in the general population.[20]

Relapse is a common feature of SUD, and relapse prevention and planning should be addressed before discharge home. A retrospective study from the Washington Physicians Health Program found that the risk of relapse was increased with major opioid use, a coexisting psychiatric disorder, and a family history of addiction.[21] Treatment of relapse must be individualized and may have positive features, as the subject may then become convinced of the pervasive power of the disease.

As with any patient, it is important to respect confidentiality, even though a health-care professional's problem will likely be well known. If asked, it is appropriate to say the person is on medical leave and is expected to recover.

Returning to Work

Victims of SUD who practice in health care are sometimes treated differently from the general population by their peers, as if medical training should somehow inoculate them from the disorder. Medical providers suffering from SUD may therefore be deemed more culpable for their plight and more deserving of punishment than laypeople.

The attitude toward the returning professional is important, but recovery must come from within. Agreements with the employer or medical staff should be formalized and

---

BOX 122.6 ■ ELEMENTS OF AN AFTERCARE PROGRAM

1. Individualized
2. Written agreement, including plan if relapse occurs
3. 12-step meetings
4. Drug screening, randomized
5. Practicing/prescribing monitoring
6. Continued contact with treating or other designated facility
7. Designated medical staff sponsor to ensure compliance
8. Advocacy for the professional enjoying successful recovery

specific, again focusing on the individual's welfare and recovery. There may be superseding licensing or legal requirements, which should be researched in advance to assist in compliance.

A structured aftercare program is extremely important for the recovering professional (**Box 122.6**). Not only is this of proven effectiveness for SUD recovery, it also ensures the protection of patients treated by the recovering professional. The goal of aftercare is not punishment; rather, its aim is to detect problems early when they are most amenable to correction. A brief relapse within the first year of recovery is not unusual for professionals and need not be greatly damaging if detected immediately. In one recovery program, monitored physicians achieved a 96% recovery rate, compared to 64% when physicians were not monitored.[21] Given that a prolonged time for the brain to heal from the ravages of SUD may be needed, it is reasonable to continue monitoring the individual for at least 3 years.

Because recovery rates for all health-care professionals are higher than for the general population (likely as a result of closer monitoring and a desire to avoid adverse consequences), a similar high success rate can be expected for all properly monitored personnel recovering from SUD.

State-Sponsored Programs

All 50 states and Washington, DC have developed professional monitoring programs for impaired professionals. Recognizing that many addicted and/or depressed practitioners are talented and skilled at their jobs, these programs stress the disease aspect of SUD and other behavioral health issues and strive to rehabilitate the subject rather than mete out punishment. The primary aim of these programs is always to ensure patient safety by helping the affected professional return to a monitored work environment in an appropriate fashion.

These state programs protect the patient by initially removing the impaired practitioner from unrestricted clinical practice. Except in egregious cases, compliance with the program generally protects the practitioner from legal proceedings and licensing suspension. After appropriate investigation by the state reveals an obvious impairment issue, most professionals choose cooperation with the program rather than prolonged (and generally unsuccessful) attempts to evade sanctions. Those who successfully complete such a program, which usually lasts 2 to 5 years depending on circumstances, can expect to have their records of participation expunged.

Most state and/or medical society programs provide skilled intervention specialists who are adept at getting recalcitrant professionals to admit their dilemma and comply with needed treatment. The threat of licensure action is a big stick that usually gets desired results when previous attempts have failed.

COGNITIVE DECLINE

We are an increasingly aging society, and as the number of practicing doctors over age 65 continues to increase, older practitioners are becoming more of a focus. In 2015, 23% of practicing physicians were 65 or older.[22] By 2050, the US population over age 65 will be greater than 88 million, more than a 50% increase from 2010.[23]

Aging Clinicians

Working beyond age 65 is becoming increasingly common for clinicians, and that trend will likely continue. Economic reasons are among the most likely drivers. The financial losses caused by the US economic recession of 2008 and the COVID-19 recession of 2020 have significantly contributed to the current economic uncertainty. Further, many practitioners look upon medicine as a calling that may be difficult to give up at any age. Some may describe their practice as a pure form of altruism. No matter what the reasons are for remaining in the workforce, it is critical to recognize the cognitive changes that occur with aging.[23] Cognitive decline is an important cause of physician impairment.

Other regulated professionals, including air transport pilots, air traffic controllers, FBI agents, and judges, are subject to periodic competency testing and/or mandatory retirement ages, but medical professionals generally are not. Increasingly, hospitals are instituting cognitive testing as a preventive measure, often with the encouragement of their insurers. This trend is likely to continue.

Cognitive changes can occur earlier than the "elder years."[24] Information processing, short-term memory, executive functioning, and visuospatial abilities/construction necessary for the practice of medicine all decline with age. Cognitive changes occur at different rates, given individual genetics, physical fitness, medical maladies, and psychological factors.[23]

Addressing Safety Concerns

Some organizations have implemented clinical programs and processes to decrease the risk of potential error and patient harm that may result from cognitive decline (**Box 122.7**). Because age discrimination is illegal in the United States, leaders should engage their organization's human resource and legal representatives to determine when cognitive testing is appropriate and then develop consistent policies.[23] In addition, designated workplace monitors may be employed to observe the continuing practice suitability of aging clinicians at risk for cognitive decline.[5]

As always, patient safety must come first. If a clinician is diagnosed with an illness known to cause more serious cognitive decline, such as Alzheimer's disease, there is a clear ethical responsibility to report the impairment issue. Because clinicians with disabilities are protected under the Americans with Disabilities Act, alternative solutions, likely nonclinical in nature, can be explored to allow the clinician to continue some sort of work.[25]

Since cognitive decline is notoriously insidious, the aging physician is frequently the last to recognize the problem. We suggest older practitioners consider using a "Fair Witness" (apologies to Robert A. Heinlein).[26] A Fair Witness should be a trusted coworker who knows the older practitioner well and is capable of recognizing incipient decline in skills that others might miss. The Fair Witness must be fiercely honest and completely trusted to act in the best interest of the practitioner and their mutual patients. The practitioner in question should agree beforehand to retire or switch to a nonclinical position if a loss of skill is observed. If the observed practitioner feels otherwise when so informed, formal cognitive testing by a neutral third party should be promptly accomplished per extant institutional protocols. Use of an appropriate Fair Witness may keep a competently practicing clinician on the job with reasonable assurance of patient safety.[27]

BOX 122.7 ■ PRACTICING SAFETY DURING MILD COGNITIVE DECLINE

- Fewer and shorter shifts
- Double coverage where feasible
- Lower-acuity patients
- Day shifts preferable
- Additional resources, such as scribe or resident coverage

OTHER CAUSES OF IMPAIRMENT

Substance use disorder and cognitive decline are certainly not the only reasons for professional impairment. Physical or psychological issues may be the cause of, or may complicate, other conditions. Health-care professionals have medical and behavioral problems like all human beings, so it is important to intervene with support, counseling, and professional treatment if needed. Psychiatric problems are perhaps more difficult to recognize. Trust the warning signs, remembering that intervention can always include a physical and psychological workup.

Organic Etiologies

Organic problems are usually straightforward. We see behavioral changes every day in our patients because of malignancies, thyroid dysfunction, diabetes, pharmaceutical side effects, electrolyte disturbances, strokes, and other causes. Some of the more challenging issues concern contagious diseases, such as hepatitis and HIV infections. State laws and hospital polices may offer guidance in these areas.

Stress and Burnout

The physical and mental costs exacted by chronic shift work have received attention in the academic emergency medicine literature since 1992.[28] More than any other medical specialty, emergency care professionals are at the greatest risk for recurrent short-term impairment from sleep deficit, disturbed sleep architecture, and circadian disharmony. Physician performance decrements have been documented during night shifts.[29] Aging worsens all aspects of shift work.

Physicians are being stressed by many factors in the workplace. Increasing numbers of patients, fewer resources (including staff), decreasing availability of consultants, and increasing expectations of mastery of an endless number of technical advances act in concert to create additional tension for emergency care workers. In addition to this, many aspects of life outside the hospital—including the demands of child rearing, aging parents, and marital conflict—can create the "perfect storm."

The COVID-19 pandemic is a good example of how unexpected serious developments can upset the lives of and place even more demands on emergency medicine practitioners. The coping mechanisms of even the most composed professionals can be insufficient. Some may turn to alcohol, as discussed earlier, while others may begin to argue with colleagues or be curt with patients. ACEP's Wellness Committee and Wellness Section are excellent resources for information and support on stress and burnout.

Disruptive Behavior

Any interaction that intimidates another individual can be a form of disruptive behavior; this can become even more concerning when patient safety and quality of care may be compromised.[30] Such behavior may be subtle at first, such as failing to return phone calls or showing up late for meetings. Other common forms include agitation, sarcasm, anger, blaming, harassment, and belittling behaviors. These behaviors lead to poor communication and hinder team trust and collaboration, all of which further jeopardize patient care and safety. Like other issues of professional impairment, disruptive behavior is important but often difficult to address. At best, the solution is finding resources to reduce life's stresses, while at worst, careers can be lost.

An individual peer coach, mental health professional, or anger management education may answer the needs of the troubled professional. The Joint Commission requires that hospitals have a code of conduct that defines unacceptable, disruptive, and inappropriate behaviors and a process for managing such behaviors. Recognizing the signs early and providing resources within the hospital can benefit struggling professionals.

Problems with sexually inappropriate behavior *per se* are beyond the scope of this chapter. Nonetheless, steps should be taken to ascertain that such behavior is not the result of primary impairment as discussed throughout this chapter.

SUMMARY

Key conclusions from this chapter include these:

- Impairment may be due to a variety of causes and may be multifactorial.
- SUD is a treatable disease with a high rate of recovery, particularly in programs that monitor the health-care professional.
- Successfully recovering professionals in monitored programs should be allowed to return to work when able.
- All forms of impairment (not just SUDs) must be considered and addressed.
- Cognitive decline should be addressed proactively, preferably on an individualized basis.
- A prospective approach establishing protocols and team discussions is the most successful approach.
- Early recognition and intervention are crucial to ensure patient safety.
- The impaired professional should be treated respectfully and nonjudgmentally, which improves the odds for a meaningful recovery.

REFERENCES

1. Agency for Healthcare Research and Quality. Patient Safety Network: culture of safety. 2019. Available at: https://psnet.ahrq.gov/primer/culture-safety. Accessed May 3, 2020.
2. Kane L. Medscape National Physician Burnout & Suicide Report 2020: The Generational Divide. 2020. Available at: https://www.medscape.com/slideshow/2020-lifestyle-burnout-6012460#8. Accessed May 3, 2020.
3. Frost M. Prevent, recognize impairment. ACP Internist. 2019. Available at: https://acpinternist.org/archives/2019/09/prevent-recognize-impairment.htm. Accessed May 3, 2020.
4. Cole A. Physician health programs and addiction among physicians. In: Earley PH. *ASAM Principles of Addiction Medicine*. 6th ed. Philadelphia, PA: Wolters Kluwer. Chapter 49.
5. Federation of State Medical Boards Policy on Physician Impairment. 2011. Available at: https://www.fsmb.org/siteassets/advocacy/policies/physician-impairment.pdf. Accessed May 3, 2020.
6. American College of Emergency Physicians. Physician impairment. 2020. Available at: https://www.acep.org/patient-care/policy-statements/physician-impairment/. Accessed May 3, 2020.
7. Ross S. Identifying an impaired physician. *AMA Journal of Ethics*. 2003. Available at: https://journalofethics.ama-assn.org/article/identifying-impaired-physician/2003-12. Accessed May 3, 2020.
8. Talbott GD, Gallegos KV, Wilson PO, et al. The Medical Association of Georgia's Impaired Physicians Program. *JAMA*. 1987;257:2927-2930.
9. Baldisseri MR. Impaired healthcare professional. *Crit Care Med*. 2007;2(35):S106-S116.
10. Booth JV, Grossman D, Moore J, et al. Substance abuse among physicians: a survey of academic anesthesiology programs. *Anesth Analg*. 2002;95(4):1024-1025.
11. Hughes PH, Baldwin CD, Sheehan DV et al: Resident physician substance use by specialty. *Am J Psychiatry* 1992;129:1348–1354.
12. Jellinek EM. *The Disease Model of Alcoholism*. Highland Park, NJ: Hellhouse Press; 1960.
13. American Medical Association Council on Mental Health. The sick physician: impairment by psychiatric disorders including alcoholism and drug dependence. *JAMA*. 1973;233:684-687.
14. Wunsch MJ, Knisely JS, Cropsey KL, et al. Women physicians and addiction. *J Addict Dis*. 2007;26:35.
15. Farber NJ, Gilibert SG, Aboff BM, et al. Physicians' willingness to report impaired colleagues. *Soc Sci Med*. 2005;61:1772.
16. Whitaker GR. Keeping the emergency physician healthy and effective. *NC EPIC*. 1990;1:2.
17. Sanders AB, Derse AR, Knopp RK, et al. *American College of Emergency Physicians Ethics Manual*. Dallas, Tex: American College of Emergency Physicians; 1991.
18. Collins GB, McAllister MS, Jensen M, et al. Chemical dependency treatment outcomes of residents in anesthesiology: results of a survey. *Anesth Analg*. 2005;101(5):1457.
19. Boisaubin EV, Levine RE. Identifying and assisting the impaired physician. *Am J Med Sci*. 2001;322(1):31.

20. Domino KB, Hornbein TF, Polissar NL, et al: Risk factors for relapse in health care professionals with substance use disorders. *JAMA*. 2005;293:1453.

21. Shore JH. The Oregon experience with impaired physicians on probation. *JAMA*. 1987;257:2931-2934.

22. Dellinger EP, Pellegrini CA. Gallagher TH. The aging physician and the medical profession. *JAMA*. 2017;152(10):967-997.

23. Harada CN, Natelson Love MC, et al. Normal cognitive aging. *Clin Geriatr Med*. 2013;29(4):737-752. Available at: https://doi.org/10.1016/j.cger.2013.07.002. Accessed May 3, 2020.

24. Centers for Disease Control and Prevention. The truth about aging and dementia. 2019. Available at: https://www.cdc.gov/aging/publications/features/dementia-not-normal-aging.html. Accessed May 3, 2020.

25. United States Department of Justice Civil Rights Division. The Americans with Disabilities Act of 1990 and Revised ADA Regulations Implementing Title II and Title III. 2017. Available at: https://www.ada.gov/. Accessed May 3, 2020.

26. Heinlein RA. *Stranger in a Strange Land*. Chapter XI. New York, NY: GP Putnam's Sons; 1961.

27. Whitehead DC. How to practice emergency medicine until you're 70. Paper presented at: ACEP BalancED Conference; Feb 2019; Ojai, Calif.

28. Whitehead DC, Thomas F Jr, Slapper D. A rational approach to shift work in emergency medicine. *Ann Emerg Med*. 1992;21:1250-1258.

29. Smith-Coggins R, Rosekind MR, Buccino KR, et al. Rotating shiftwork schedules: can we enhance physician adaptation to night shifts? *Acad Emerg Med*. 1997;4(10):951-961.

30. Lowen JT. Disruptive docs. *Minn Med*. 2011;94(1):16-18. [Ross S. Clinical pearl: identifying an impaired physician. In: Ross S, ed. *Ethics Journal of the American Medical Association*. Chicago: American Medical Association; 2003.

CHAPTER 123

GENERATIONAL DIFFERENCES IN EMERGENCY MEDICINE

Nicholas M. Mohr, Lisa Moreno-Walton, Rebecca Smith-Coggins, Angela M. Mills, Hollynn Larrabee, Pamela L. Dyne, Kathleen J. Clem, Marie-Laure Romney, Susan B. Promes

The magnitude of difference between the newer and older generations in the profession depends on how pronounced are the societal changes from one generation to the next.

—Richard Cruess, Sylvia Cruess, and Yvonne Steinert[1]

For the first time in history, four generations are working together—Traditionalists, Baby Boomers, Generation X, and Millennials (also referred to as Generation Y). Each generation carries a unique perspective of the world based on their shared experiences and common values. Every emergency department (ED) is an ecosystem of the people, processes, and systems comprising it. Wise leaders use an understanding of generational differences to improve this ecosystem across all boundaries.

Historically, generations have been classified based on changes in world values. These generational shifts have accelerated to meet the rapidly evolving new millennium. Each generational cohort includes members with similar childhood experiences and comparable world views, work traits, teaching and learning styles, communication preferences, and expectations that dictate how they interact with those around them.[2] Individuals born on the border between generational groups may engender attributes of more than one classically defined generation. These people, called "cuspers," historically play an important role in facilitating intergenerational understanding and harmony.[3-8]

OVERVIEW OF GENERATIONAL CHARACTERISTICS

Generational groups (**Figure 123.1**) tend to share major life experiences and societal events at similar stages of life development. This common history leads to mutual values, beliefs, attitudes, and behaviors. **Table 123.1** lists attributes of each of the four generations in the workplace today: the Traditionalists (born 1925-1945), the Baby Boomers (born 1945-1962), Generation X (born 1962-1980), the Millennials (born 1980-1999). It also includes the Post-Millennials (Generation Z, born 1999–2012) who will soon be entering the emergency medicine (EM) workforce.

Traditionalists (1925-1945)

The Traditionalists, also called the Silent Generation or the Veterans, are often described as dedicated, patriotic, conventional, respectful of order, and altruistic. The major life

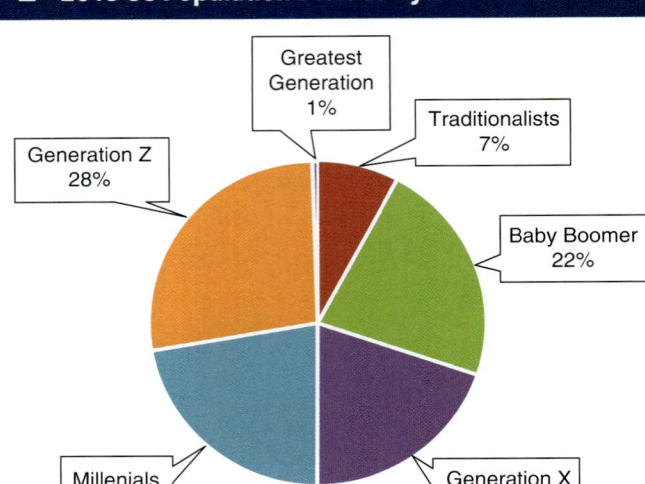

FIGURE 123.1 ■ 2018 US Population Divided by Generation of Birth

Source: Data Courtesy US Census 2018.

experiences members of this generation shared were the Great Depression and societal rebuilding after World War II. They lived in a world characterized by faith, patriotism, and justice.[9] Traditionalists abide by duty and honor and have a strong sense of community. They are committed to taking care of their world and the institutions they serve.[10,11] As they grew up in an era of limited resources, Traditionalists tend to be mindful of resources and waste.[12,13] They married young and lived in an era before divorce was common.

While most Traditionalists are now retired, they still comprise up to 10% of all active physicians, according to the 2016 census of physicians.[14,15] Many of these people are the founders of EM and have been the leaders of modern departments. Traditionalists value formality, hierarchy, and loyalty to their organizations, and they subscribe to conformity without challenging the systems in which they work. Members of this group work hard in their professions, expect rewards for their diligence, and value lifetime employment at a single institution.[16,17] Delayed gratification is an accepted norm. Many have an expectation that society will take care of them later (e.g., retirement benefits, pension plans) in return for their hard work. Traditionalists have made great sacrifices for their careers and value experience and seniority. The term "company man" was coined for members of this generation.

Dedicated to their careers, Traditionalists often remain in medical practice to teach and share their knowledge and skills with younger generations. They fulfill the role of a classic professor or chair emeritus and tend to focus more on the process of education rather than its outcomes.[18,19] They view medicine as a vocation rather than a day job.

Baby Boomers (1945-1962)

The Baby Boomers (also called Boomers or the Me Generation) were, until recently, the largest generation in the workforce.[15,20,21] They were born during the post–World War II years and are often described as optimistic, driven, and workaholics. The major life experiences Boomers shared were the Cold War, the Vietnam War, the civil rights movement, the space race, and the women's rights movement. They were born during great economic and educational prosperity. Their world was one of television, rock-and-roll or rhythm and blues music, and a traditional nuclear family characterized by a stay-at-home

TABLE 123.1 ■ Overview of Generational Characteristics[49]							
Generation (Birth Years)	Societal Events	Childhood/ Family Traits	Personal Traits	Work Traits	Education Traits	Communication Styles	Technology
Traditionalists (1925-1945)	Great Depression, rebuilding after WWII	Traditional family, married young, divorce uncommon	Loyal, reluctant to challenge status quo, dedicated, believe in honor and duty, patriotic	Value hierarchy, loyal "company man," job security	Process-oriented	Formal	Tend not to understand
Baby Boomers (1945-1962)	Civil Rights and Women's Rights movements, the Cold War, the Vietnam War, TV, economic and educational prosperity	Traditional nuclear family, many grew up with stay-at-home mother and hardworking father	Optimistic, desire personal gratification, highly competitive	Workaholics, competitive, consensus builders, mentors	Learners dependent on educators, lecture format, process-oriented	Diplomatic	Not particularly savvy
Generation X (1962-1980)	Limited economic prospects, fall of institutions, political scandals, divorce, AIDS, computers	Nontraditional families, single-parent homes, "latchkey kids," television as babysitter	Independent, self-directed, skeptical, resilient, more accepting of diversity, self-reliant	Value work-life balance, comfortable with change, question authority	Independent learners, problem solvers, desire to learn on the job, outcome-oriented	Blunt	Interested and facile
Millennials (1980-1999)	Economic globalization, terrorism, 9/11, multiculturalism, technology boom	Protective "helicopter parents," play dates, close family relationships	Optimistic, need for praise, collaborative, global outlook	Team-oriented, used to following rules and having structured time, career change/ mobility	Grew up in team-based educational environment, turn to internet, outcome-oriented	Polite	Very savvy, view technology as a necessity
Generation Z (1999-2012)	9/11, economic recession, global terrorism, income gap, mass violence, have never known the world without internet	Children of Generation X, economic stress, presence of social media, diverse family characteristics	Entrepreneurial, independent, cautious and practical, risk adverse, overwhelmed, lonely	Certainty and stability, creative and flexible, individualisitic, integrate multiple sources of content	Self-taught technology, job training emphasized vs well-rounded liberal arts, search for "truth"	Nonconfrontational	Digital natives

mother and a hardworking father. Boomers have always been a demographically powerful force in our society.[10] Per the 2016 physician census, Boomers account for 45% of active physicians and occupy the majority of leadership positions.[14]

Boomers are a driven cohort who equate work with self-worth, contribution, and personal fulfillment. Boomers are often early to arrive and late to leave their workplaces.[22,23] Many choose their professions, in part, for their desire to improve their world. Baby Boomers tend to be very competitive, aspiring to higher monetary compensation and professional titles, and they are willing to sacrifice their personal lives for professional success. Individuals in this group work hard out of loyalty, expect a long-term job, and view self-sacrifice as a necessary virtue.[9,24,25] Boomers were promised compensation for their loyalty, and they feel promotion should be earned over time. They value recognition, leadership, and management positions.[14] Members of this group value a strong chain of command and may be judgmental of differing views. Since computers were not a part of their upbringing and education, they adopted electronic technology somewhat later in life. Boomers tend to accept new medical knowledge and techniques because they are "tried and true," meaning they have undergone careful, often exhaustive peer review. The argument from authority or "eminence-based" medicine was a strong influence on their medical education, later evolving to evidence-based medicine.

Generation X (1962-1980)

Generation X (Gen X) is often described as independent, self-directed, pragmatic, and flexible, which contrasts sharply with some of the societal-based attributes of prior generations.[17,26] The major life experience this group shares was a childhood near the end of the Cold War in a nation with increasing national debt and limited economic prospects. Because the divorce rate had tripled by this time, some were raised in single-parent households, and many two-parent households had both parents working outside the home.[26,27] Some Gen Xers spent much of their childhood as latchkey kids, returning to an empty home after school where television served as a babysitter. As adults, Gen Xers seek a greater sense of family, tend to focus equally on personal life and work, and are less likely to place their jobs before family or friends. Gen Xers "work to live" rather than "live to work." Gen Xers account for 45% of active physicians and often hold mid- to upper-level leadership positions.[14]

This group tends to be loyal to themselves and their families rather than to institutions. Some watched their parents fall victim to downsizing and economic turmoil. As such, they are more likely to leave jobs with limited upward mobility for those with better prospects for advancement.[9] Gen Xers question authority and resent top-down management. They believe in being evaluated for their accomplishments rather than by the quantity of time they spend at work.[24]

Since computers were introduced while they were in school, Gen Xers are adept users of a wide range of technologies. They are voracious learners, assimilate changing information quickly, and engage in parallel thinking. They are problem-solvers who tend to learn better by participating in a cooperative experience.[28,29]

Millennials (1980-1999)

Millennials (also known as Generation Y, Generation Next, Echo Boomers, and the Net Generation) are often described as optimistic, collaborative, team oriented, and technology savvy.[30] The major life experiences this group share include economic globalization; the 9/11 attacks; school violence; multiculturalism; and widespread cell phone, email, and internet use. "Technology is so deeply embedded into everything [Millennials] do that they are truly the first native online population."[31] Millennials tend to be globally oriented, culturally diverse, and constantly connected worldwide. They expect instant results and access to information, which sometimes brands them as impatient. This generation is highly accomplished with rich and diverse curricula vitae, and many feel some commitment to global health and advocacy for the underserved in their work lives. They often have multiple interests in addition to medicine.[12] In 2020, Millennials accounted for approximately 50% of the workforce and are expected to exceed 75% of the US workforce by 2025.[20] Per the 2016 physician census, Millennials comprise 22% of physicians.

As children, many Millennials were doted on by protective parents concerned about their safety, education, and success. They have been described as the most rewarded, recognized, and praised generation. As such, Millennials expect frequent feedback and tend to have a need for praise. Members of this group cherish close family relationships and value being connected with others. They grew up with play dates and structured play, so they tend to be comfortable following rules that stress collaboration.[18] Conversely, they may be less spontaneous and introspective than prior generations.

Some refer to Millennials as Echo Boomers, and this is not a misnomer. Millennials are eager to contribute to positive social change with an ability to organize and mobilize. They expect flexibility with work–life balance, but they also want to connect deeply with colleagues. As their parents often solicited their opinions on family decisions, Millennials feel they should have input in decisions being made in their workplace.[18] They tend to be socially bold, and they are unafraid to express their opinions.[12]

Millennials have been exposed to technology their entire lives and often prefer internet resources to textbooks for learning. Instead of a "tried and true" approach, both Millenials and Gen Xers tend to trust new knowledge because it is socially appealing, pragmatic, and supported by YouTube as opposed to staid literature. Instead of eminence or evidence based, their knowledge acquisition is more "everyone based," as in, "Everyone I know and trust like this—so do I." Millennials are optimistic about their careers and are more trusting of authority than Gen Xers.[32-36]

TEACHING AND LEARNING

For centuries, traditional medical education has been based on the Socratic method. In contrast to lecture-based instruction, the teacher in the Socratic method questions one or two learners in the presence of a student group in order to prompt and guide students' thinking. It is a method well suited to the education of Traditionalists, who have a high regard for instruction, respect for hierarchy, and are willing to yield to authority almost without question.[10] It is also a method ideally suited to slower technological advancement—a condition virtually unfathomable today. The role of experience as a necessary requirement to attaining the requisite gestalt to distinguish normal from the subtly abnormal has also been an important concept in traditional medical education.

Traditionalists teach out of a sense of duty to their profession and its history.[29,36-40] They are comfortable teaching and learning in a large group lecture format, but they recognize that didactic instruction is incomplete learning without an experiential component. They are unlikely to have much respect for knowledge that learners glean from websites when this knowledge is not borne out by experience. Their bedside teaching is often characterized by anecdotes, and they see themselves as keepers of institutional memory.[3]

As the Baby Boomer generation entered US medical schools, their value of peer recognition and acknowledgment of hierarchy continued to lend support to traditional medical education.[14] Professional values were beginning to change to reflect those of the wider society, but Baby Boomers were still reliant on educators to teach them actively. The Socratic method, which is characterized by teaching through intimidation, appeared to demonstrate the ignorance of the student and the superiority of the teacher. For a generation that strongly valued equality, this approach was unacceptable, and mentorship became the norm.[33]

From the time that Gen Xers entered training in the 1980s, they were perceived by their Boomer supervisors as being unprofessional and reticent to embrace physician-hood. They were viewed as self-absorbed, cynical, and lacking a strong work ethic when compared to workaholic Boomers.[26]

The unique independence that Gen Xers experienced in their childhood facilitated their ability to assess quickly and manage complex and difficult situations, an essential skill to the successful practice of EM.[41] Growing up on *Sesame Street*, Gen Xers excel at cooperative and interactive learning, and they believe that education should be fun.[28] In the mentoring relationship, they appreciate immediate responses with frequent, face-to-face, and specific interactions.[3] They perceive themselves as entitled to mentorship and education in the workplace, and they critically evaluate their mentors and supervisors at the same time that they are being evaluated. They sometimes bypass traditional lines of authority in pursuit of what they view as pragmatic, timely solutions to pressing problems.

Millennials began their medical education in an era that included many rules, such as duty-hour limits and patient caps, which limited training and a created the perception of delayed independence. This, coupled with the stereotypical narcissism, self-confidence, and interest in "work–life balance," has earned this generation a self-entitled reputation. However, Millennials' attributes can be leveraged to become very effective teachers and leaders because of their generally egalitarian worldview and inclusivity, resulting in very effective multigenerational collaboration.

Emergency medicine as a specialty has changed dramatically in the past 30 years. With the advent of bedside ultrasound, regional anesthesia, the electronic medical record, digital radiography, and easy online access to medical knowledge, trainees today sometimes view their senior faculty as hopelessly out of touch and wonder how they could possibly be competent to instruct them on the current practice of medicine.[42] On the other hand, physicians in the 1970s and 1980s developed their skill set on the job, performing direct patient care, while younger physicians have engaged in simulation and technology-based study. The lack of appreciation for the skill sets possessed by colleagues of different generations can serve as a barrier to intergenerational learning.[1]

Since older physicians are staying in the workforce longer, they must learn new technology and adapt to other changes.[30,43] Simulation is one example, providing an opportunity to "rethink the way medical education is delivered across a continuum of professional lifetimes. If [simulation] is well executed, it may truly make medical education better, safer, and cheaper, and provide real benefits to patient care."[44,45] These are areas in which junior emergency physicians (EPs) can help instruct senior faculty. Traditionalists and Boomers, with their respect for the medical hierarchy, can be uncomfortable with the concept of learning from their residents and junior faculty, and there is often the conviction that learning styles are too different.[46] However, the true meaning of the Socratic tradition involves a learning environment which encompasses all lenses and all voices so everyone can learn.

TECHNOLOGY

One of the most profound defining characteristics of generational conflict is the use of technology. Although technology is recognized as a tool to enhance practice, its implementation in the ED has been one of the most rapidly evolving workplace transformations in the history of medicine.[47-50] Gen Xers and Millennials both had access to computer resources during their childhood, laying a critical foundation for use of these systems later in life.[51] Although Traditionalists and Baby Boomers have adopted systems they find useful, their lack of early experience may limit their enthusiasm about using computer-based tools in the workplace. In the ED, technology takes many different forms.

The Electronic Health Record

The electronic health record (EHR) is likely one of the most transformative workplace technology initiatives of the 20th and 21st centuries. The holy grail of the electronic health information movement is the implementation of computerized systems that allow for the creation of medical records, comprehensive review of medical records, computerized physician order entry, access to electronic data from other institutions, decision support, and direct patient communication.[52] Such an ideal has been unachievable by physicians who have thus far resisted complete adoption. Some have suggested that this resistance is a generational attribute.[53-58] Employees in nonmedical fields widely cite implementation of a new computer system as a barrier to productivity that affects senior employees more than those of Gen X and the Millennial generations.[54,55,59] Others suggest that shortcomings in the technology are the primary deterrents to widespread adoption.[60-63]

The adoption of new tools in the workplace is closely tied to their ultimate impact on physicians' personal productivity and success. The ultimate driver of change is its ability to make the job easier, tapping into intrinsic motivation. The EHR has not yet been proven to revolutionize physician capabilities.[64] For younger physicians who have more experience with computer information systems and are more comfortable with changing technology, imperfect systems are less of a barrier to functioning than for older physicians. With greater exposure to technological change, workers show an increased openness to change and an increase in job satisfaction, making it possible for all generational cohorts to be "very comfortable" with technology when given the right training.[43,65,66] As the systems used in the health-care workplace improve, their value to physicians is enhanced. With this improvement, resistance to adoption is likely to wane from members of all generational groups.[53]

Diagnostics

Bedside provider-performed ultrasound is one of the most sweeping diagnostic changes in the ED in the last two decades. It appears to be a model for an effective, novel diagnostic tool with varying degrees of acceptance and diffusion within the EM community.

The introduction of ultrasound opened a window into the way that practicing physicians educate themselves on new technology. Ultrasound applications have a learning curve, and the quality and utility of its use depend most on a combination of experience, education, and expert exposure.[67] Traditionalists and Baby Boomers were largely unexposed to ultrasound education during residency training.[68] Younger EM faculty members, in general, have had more formal training. Current trainees are looking for expertise in their clinical training, and they recognize ultrasound as one facet of the knowledge base they are looking to develop. Training faculty members alongside residents and medical students breaks down some of the traditional teacher–learner barriers, and this redistribution of knowledge can be very uncomfortable for faculty members.

Communication Technology

Generational differences are perhaps the most pronounced in communication advances. Office-based collaboration was once restricted to face-to-face meetings and travel to conferences. The telephone offered a degree of separation, but interactions were very individualized and very personal. The computer revolution has morphed into a communications revolution. More than half of US households have cell phone-only access, and greater than two-thirds of workers worldwide work remotely at least one day a week, with more than 50% reporting doing so for greater than half the week.[69,70]

The communication landscape has changed even more profoundly in the last decade. The ability to work from home computer connections means the expectation for availability has been expanded—one should be *selectively available*, able to access the digital world without necessarily being accessible to coworkers. However, Twitter, Facebook, and other social networking sites have become a staple for Millennials, who are often eager to integrate their work with their home lives.

Selective availability has also contributed to development of asynchronous communication forums. LISTSERVs, web forums, wiki sites, discussion pages, YouTube, and digital online collaboration systems have been used to collaborate and to innovate. Online social networking tools are becoming more popular among physicians, and the American College of Emergency Physicians and other EM organizations have adopted Twitter as a method of communicating with members.[71-73] All of these modalities allow individuals to optimize creativity on their own schedules—instead of being tied to an agenda. Asynchronous communication forums are becoming one of the preferred mechanisms national organizations use for collaborating. These solutions lead to the potential for the creation of gaps between the early adopters and those potentially intimidated by the technology.

The premise of selective availability is sometimes not completely understood by Traditionalists and Baby Boomers. Grown out of an intense loyalty to their organizations, Traditionalists and Boomer faculty members tend to be perennially available. Their younger colleagues are more wired but *less* available. Gen Xers and Millennials use technology as a means of keeping in touch with professional colleagues and personal friends, but they tend to closely guard their personal time.[74]

The Google Effect

The ease of accessing updated, relevant information at the click of a mouse has changed how Gen Xers and Millennials value knowledge, and correspondingly, the role that information resources play in EM.[72,73,75-80] Almost 80% of Americans have access to the internet in their everyday lives.[81,82] However, physicians are much less likely than the rest of the population to perform work-related tasks online. About one in three physicians use email to communicate with colleagues, and less than 50% use online journals or clinical decision support systems to support their daily practice. Unsurprisingly, younger physicians and those in academic medicine use technology much more.[47,83]

With computer technology playing such an important role in answering clinical questions, the value of information as a commodity has diminished. Expensive textbooks are not the only key to medical understanding. Quality resources are available at the point-of-care, usually for free. Instead of keeping a file with landmark clinical trials or review articles, Gen X and Millennial faculty members often rely on popular mainstream search engines and electronic library collections to retrieve information, and they use digital storage for the files that match their clinical interests. Such availability has had the unintended consequence of devaluing nondigital resources.[84]

Electronic knowledge resources further dichotomize academic faculty. More senior faculty retain ownership of their knowledge, using their resources for the benefit of their students and residents. They often study carefully and rely on the organization of their personal knowledge repository to apply new knowledge. Younger faculty members value medical resources as a commodity that should be made freely available for the benefit of all and one that does not necessarily need to be memorized in minute detail. They exchange citations and articles, and they maintain a "public library," using personally validated online information resources as justification for their practice.[85-87]

For more than a decade now, web-based medical education in the form of free open access medical education (FOAMed) content has fundamentally disrupted the way medical content is consumed. Learners from across the globe, both in developed and underdeveloped countries, have come to rely on these sites as reliable sources for up-to-date information.[85,88] Given the significant lag time between the discovery of novel care delivery methods and subsequent publication of peer-reviewed content, FOAMed websites have increasingly become the preferred source for education on current practice standards. Millennials, who are more comfortable with technology and prefer informal content delivery, have really embraced this modality.[2] Furthermore, this public accessibility has opened medical knowledge to patients through WebMD, eMedicine, UpToDate, and other online medical references.[89]

STRUCTURE AND FUNCTION OF DEPARTMENTS

As awareness of generational differences increases, questions arise about how these differences might impact the structure and function of EDs. Generational cohorts have different values regarding work–life balance and personal motivation, desire for control over their work experience, and effective productivity incentives.[90-94]

Junior physicians work to gain respect and opportunities, and the payoff is often a decreased clinical load. However, some experts predict that Gen Xers and Millennials will not adhere to this system.[29,95] Gen X is exemplified by self-interest and a need for work–life balance. For them, success in the professional arena is an expectation of fulfilling requirements rather than sacrificing their personal lives. It often may not include the desire to advance up the administrative ladder or to be in charge. Millennials, on the other hand, may be less independent and require more structure, guidance, and regular feedback.[40,96] They are interested in continuous development and expect rapid advancement as they master an area. Millennials also value social involvement and are drawn to roles that incorporate collaborative teams. Younger generations are willing to perform tedious tasks if they feel they meet their personal objectives, but they try to avoid stagnant environments. They have less loyalty to their organizations, and they thrive on change. To recruit effectively and retain these generations, leaders will need to plan actively for their mentorship and development, since conventional methods of distributing rewards based on Traditionalist- or Boomer-designed criteria may not be effective.

Historically, senior physicians were respected as mentors and revered as those who had set their departments' course. Time and hard work led to rewards of salary increases and retirement with benefits. Today, EPs are not retiring as early. An increased life expectancy and a global labor shortage mean that the Boomers will be in the workplace for some time to come.[97] The balance between desire of job complexity and time commitment and between workplace and personal success all are key to the discovery of best practices.

Gen Xers and the Millennials also have different expectations when it comes to quantity of hours worked. They value their product more than the time it required. Gen X especially is known for efficiency in the management of their work day, and this is a particular area of conflict for Boomers, who have put a great deal of time into their work and do not respect those who leave early. In addition, the ability to do administrative work or research remotely is attractive to Gen Xers.[98] Recent graduates, including Millennials and Gen Xers, are accustomed to more free time than resident physicians have ever had, potentially igniting a change for faculty members as they graduate.

The challenge for EM leadership is to understand how the culture in EM is viewed by each generation. A paradigm shift may be necessary to harness the energy and productivity of younger generations by considering flexible shifts, part-time options, and personal development plans.

ORGANIZATIONAL CULTURE CLASH

Generational differences often lead to a clash in the culture of the organization as they adapt to change over time, including several different areas.

Transparency

Traditionalists and Boomers feel that to ensure quality control and fairness, the promotion process must be confidential. Similarly, salaries and productivity should be a private matter to foster community in the minds of Traditionalists and Boomers.[99] Gen X and Millenial faculty members, on the other hand, seek openness and transparency to attain fairness and equity. Working in an environment based on the belief that secrecy ensures quality does not make sense to them. They feel that secrecy masks favoritism, cronyism, racism, and sexism.[99] Generally, they prefer that all reported performance data metrics be "unblinded" so comparisons can be made through transparency.

Loyalty

Baby Boomers are often concerned and frustrated by their younger colleagues' lack of loyalty to their employer and their appearance of lacking a work ethic, and this leads to intergenerational turmoil in the workplace. While Boomers have questioned authority as part of their collective generational history, they value organizational hierarchy and usually cite career as the major focus of their time and effort. Gen X is skeptical about organizations and the motivations that drive them, so they consider that time with their families and friends is equally important as time devoted to the development of a career.[100] Career change, unthinkable for a Traditionalist physician, is not considered an unusual option for Gen Xers or Millennials, and this mobility drives some EM administrators to be hesitant to invest heavily in new faculty members who may move to a new institution after only a few years.[3,27,101,102]

Given the extreme variability in both the sense and the focus of loyalty among the generations, it is no surprise that there is misunderstanding and sometimes even anger when commitment to the medical profession, dedication to the hospital, and willingness to sacrifice are considered. Boomers tend not to respect those whom they regard as practicing medicine as a hobby, leaving work early, and signing out patient care.[98] Gen Xers and Millennials focus on the quality of their product. If what they have done has been done efficiently and well, they are ready to go home at the end of the shift. Traditionalists, who emphasize loyalty to the patient and to the institution, often view younger physicians as lazy and lacking dedication. These divergent attitudes among the four generations can create tension in the already stressful environment of the ED.[103]

Priorities

Delayed gratification is the norm for Traditionalists and Boomers. They view medicine as a vocation rather than a day job. Time devoted to family means less time for career; they have created a distance between their professional lives and their home lives.[99] Younger physicians tend to value autonomy and work–life balance, feeling that quality of life is central to personal satisfaction. Because they feel that home life and work life need to blend constructively, Gen Xers and Millennials may be less willing to stay late or take on additional responsibilities. Intergenerational difficulty arises as the Gen X and Millennial colleagues tend to be viewed by Traditionalists and Boomers as less committed physicians with poor work ethics.[12,104,105] Their avocations are important to them, not just their vocation.

Workspace

Elements of the physical workspace can cause conflict. Older workers are dissatisfied with restless and noisy workrooms.[19,106,107] Emergency physicians from the Millennial and Gen X generations often prefer to work with music and lights up, which can be bothersome to older generations. There is evidence that music enhances quality of work and diminishes time on task.[108] The use of earphones while charting is a plausible solution to this generational issue.

Schedules

The physiologic ability to tolerate night shifts worsens with age. Although this is due to the aging process more than generational influences, it is important to consider in this context because it can be a source of friction between generations. A worsening ability to sleep is at the root of this attitudinal difference. Boomers and Traditionalists find that their sleep is more disturbed and shortened both at night and during day sleep between successive night shifts.[109-114] Unlike their younger associates, older physicians tend physiologically to shift toward "morningness, which suggests that senior physicians may have fewer problems with early morning shifts.[115,116] Departments may be choosing to accommodate their senior members by creating a shift differential, but how these decisions are made may be a source of intergenerational conflict as well. The Traditionalist and Boomer faculty members will likely view the expectation of fewer night shifts as a right that comes with seniority. Gen X and Millennials tend to be more egalitarian and thus may resent such expectations.

The impact of shift work on one's health is significant. Chronic disruptions in the sleep/wake cycle inherent in a career in EM may increase a variety of disease states, including heart disease, ulcers, cancer, and diabetes.[117,118] Although these health risks are not generational, it is known that advancing age increases the probability of disease.[106]

CHALLENGES AND OPPORTUNITIES

An understanding of generational differences should lead to a better understanding of both the challenges they present and the opportunities they offer. Each generation brings strength to the team's response to these challenges and opportunities.

Traditionalists

Traditionalists are battling fatigue and diminishing personal health. They are discredited by younger health-care workers because of their lack of familiarity with technological advancements. They are less able to accurately judge younger employees by using usual definitions of professionalism, and they may struggle to interact effectively with female physicians as greater numbers enter the workplace. They are extremely loyal to their institutions, which can be advantageous. They have deep personal commitments to others throughout the nation, and the networking that they do for their mentees carries weight. Traditionalists are very trustworthy individuals, and others can rely on their word. Given the right roles, these individuals can continue to flourish.

Baby Boomers

Baby Boomers face fatigue and personal health issues also, although less intensely than the Traditionalists. They often have trouble understanding the motivations of their younger colleagues, and they may interpret an interest in work–life balance as laziness or an inexcusable lack of commitment to their careers.[91,119] Boomers feel that their experience should be valued while younger members in their field place value more on merit. They struggle with rapidly advancing technology and have feelings of inferiority when faced with electronically savvy younger colleagues. They have difficulty accepting change and are not as prepared to move to new jobs or careers as their younger colleagues.[119] Their optimistic, diplomatic approach brings a wealth of benefit to EM. Their industrious, diligent nature can be harnessed to power forward progress. The sheer numbers of Boomers populating the workforce is advantageous. Creating roles for them as they continue to age will alleviate the potential strain created by "birth dearth."

Generation X

Gen Xers may have a distrustful approach that ruffles the feathers of their elders. They do not like being told what to do and prefer to work alone. They are unimpressed by authority and are quick to place limits on their roles in medicine. Their self-reliant nature can in fact be advantageous in the workplace. "Xers' weaknesses as employees are their strongest assets."[119] Since some Gen Xers may lack loyalty, some experts suggest giving them short-term assignments.[119] They rarely stay in one position for long, so rewarding them with benefits like time off and child care is better than compensating them with pension plans. Although they are considered by many to have short attention spans, they can process a great deal of information quickly and therefore benefit from being able to multitask superbly. This trait is a strength in the ED. They are voracious learners, master new software quickly, and can bring process efficiency and creativity to their roles in medicine.[120,121] They expect to be trained, no matter what the organizational cost. Gen Xers are looking for supervisors who are consistent in their handling of difficult conversations, who are direct and honest, and who admit and apologize when they are wrong.[29,74,122] Their positive influence on medicine can be considerable. Gen Xers feel strongly that work–life balance should be recognized, and not penalized, by department management. Their penchant for lifestyle can help set an example by which the Boomers can pace themselves and remain in the workforce longer.

Millennials

In their time in medicine, Millennials have been criticized for informal dress, manners, and speech. Each of these issues should be prospectively addressed during the recruitment, onboarding, and mentoring periods. These observations have been interpreted as a breach in professionalism which places a strain on their relationships with Traditionalists and Boomers in the workplace. Work and family time priorities are areas where this generation clashes with older generations. Generally, Millennials expect flexibility and prefer to work remotely if their task does not require physical presence.[98] A greater number of Millennials are moving back home with parents after college than other generations.[123] Recruiting Millennials means accommodating their busy lives and multiple interests.[12] They are hopeful, optimistic, ambitious, collaborative, polite, and civic-minded, which are all traits that serve them well in the multigenerational workplace.[12,74]

Shared goals and values allow senior and junior physicians to work well together through options like "reciprocal mentoring," in which Millennials teach Boomers about technology while Boomers teach professionalism, interpersonal skills, and medical knowledge.

BRIDGING THE GENERATIONAL GAP

Leaders in EM can consider a number of strategies as they try to mitigate generational tension and bridge gaps in their organizations.[124] An approach encompassing all lenses, all voices, and all learners is key.

Personal Communication

Emergency medicine leaders should make an effort to maintain an element of personalization in all professional communication. Email, electronic bulletin boards, LISTSERVs, and other collaborative systems should be used intentionally to *enhance* personal communication and build relationships, not to *replace* those interactions. Much of the life and personality of a department resides in the relationships that exist between its members, much more so than simply the efficiency or convenience of the workplace. Expectations around boundaries and response times for replies to emails and texts should be explicit.

Teaching and Learning

Recognition of the different learning styles that are part of the societal influence on the workplace is required in order to teach and learn maximally across generations.[40,125] Learning must be tailored to learners, whatever their ages or skill levels. Because Millennials are outcome-oriented and value doing more than knowing, it could be helpful for them to realize that Traditionalists and Boomers are capable, ready, and able to teach.[33] In the current age of exponential knowledge advancement, Traditionalists and Baby Boomers must accept "the premise that all teachers are learners first."[126]

Older learners prefer interaction, discussion, process, and relevance. When instructing Boomers in new technology or information, the younger "teacher" should recognize that this role reversal is uncomfortable to the older generation. To mitigate this, the younger teacher should focus on the relevance of the information and create an environment in which it is safe to ask questions and challenge the teacher. Gen Xers like a fast-paced, fun learning environment with clear ground rules and opportunity for individual participation.[23] Gen X tends to be cynical and challenge authority, and those who are engaged in teaching them should not feel threatened by this behavior. Millennials are often not as independent as their predecessor generations, requiring more structure, guidance, and regular feedback. They learn best by doing and discovering through collaborative work, prefer that information be individually tailored to them, and expect that technology is available to use.[96] Each generational cohort appreciates positive feedback and a safe environment with a supportive, understanding mentor who creates an atmosphere in which it is acceptable to admit that they need clarification or state that they disagree.[43]

Implementation of New Technology

Departments should resist the implementation of technology for the purpose of modernization. Technology is a tool designed to solve specific problems, and problems have optimal solutions. Inasmuch as technological innovation can be applied effectively to solve problems, it will be universally adopted as practice-changing by all generational cohorts. Intergenerational tension is only enhanced when suboptimum solutions are adopted because they are "modern technology."

Maintaining Nontechnical Work Systems

Much of the literature on technology implementation focuses on "training up" those senior employees for whom digital solutions are less intuitive. This strategy makes a sometimes invalid assumption that electronic technology and complex diagnostic systems are by their very nature *better*. Perhaps the most critical intervention with respect to innovations is to continue to recognize the value of nonelectronic technology and to continue to embrace these strategies among colleagues and learners alike. Ultrasound has not replaced the physical examination, the computerized EHR has not completely replaced the handwritten workarounds on which many EDs depend, and email has not replaced department meetings. These proven strategies are important for trainees to master, and senior faculty members are best prepared to teach them.

Retention

Emergency medicine must develop strategies for strengthening retention of outstanding physicians from all generations.[24,127]

Retention of Senior Physicians

Retention of senior physicians requires the creation of positions that capitalize on the strengths of Traditionalists and Boomers. Placing senior physicians in career development positions to influence Gen X and Millennial colleagues is one option. However, the job satisfaction and continued success of senior physicians require that they put effort into understanding the basic distinctions in the cultural characteristics, learning styles, and work–life balance expectations of younger colleagues. The experiential wisdom of the Traditionalists and Boomers, a priceless resource for hospital committees, is further enhanced when partnering them with others who embrace evidence-based medicine or web-based electronic programs. Developing guidelines for monitoring and coaching delinquent physicians, leadership training workshops, professionalism curricula, and institutional policies on retaining physicians and nurses are just a few suggestions. To enable senior physicians to devote time to important issues facing EM, a reduction in clinical time may be appropriate in some circumstances. These solutions will require institutions to provide more alternative models of success and increase flexible work options.[128]

Retention of Mid-Career Physicians

If one defines a mid-career physician as one who has been out of training for between 5 and 15 years, then the majority of mid-level faculty are members of Gen X. The major challenges for this group revolve around work–life balance. Some specific retention strategies might include flexibility in shift and meeting scheduling, shared departmental responsibilities, promotion roll-backs, and part-time work options. Gen Xers, who tend to view their careers as mobile, prize professional advancement over departmental loyalty, so overt succession planning of the departmental leadership and distribution of authority may improve retention. This group is ideal to lead teams and generate consensus among physicians at all levels.

Flexible Work Schedules

Older EPs may benefit from decreased night shifts or split shifts with other physicians. This allows physicians to remain in the workforce longer and have greater job satisfaction. Younger physicians also benefit from flexible time management, allowing for a solution to work–life conflicts.[24] One strategy might be to create and legitimize part-time opportunities. Part-time and flexible work schedules have been identified as attractive ways to achieve balance between career and family.[129]

TABLE 123.2 ■ Strategies for Workplace Intervention[49]		
Adjustments	**General Workplace**	**Emergency Medicine**
Physical work environment	Physical workload, rest/work schedule, and regulation of one's own work and breaks	Location of clinical work (urgent care/observation units vs ED), choices in shifts with adjustment in remuneration (e.g., no nights but less pay)
Psychosocial work environment	Flexible work schedules, teamwork, management skills based on generation for supervisors	Flexible work schedules, formal team-building, maintaining electronic distance for leadership (email, etc.), education on intergenerational differences and improvement of the work culture
Health and lifestyle promotion	Physical exercise, risk factor reduction, occupational health services	EM faculty health initiatives: stress reduction, weight reduction, and exercise promotion
Worker skills and competency building	Nonthreatening ongoing continuing education	Offer attending-only educational workshops for ultrasound and technology-based tools (EHRs, video clips in presentations, and asynchronous communication forums); faculty development, leadership skills programs, leadership coaches

Sleep and Performance

To preserve employment for our aging workforce, it is necessary to adopt solutions specific to the aging process. **Table 123.2** presents four strategies for intervention.[106] Awarding more reimbursement to the night shift in return for the physiologic burden and increased risk of disease is one possible solution. Encouraging "senior night shifts" that are shorter, fewer, or split among two individuals has also been successful. Improving the strategies used to mitigate the burden of shift work will benefit physicians at all stages of training and work.[113,116,130]

CONCLUSION

Generational issues have a significant impact on our daily lives, and EM is not immune to these generational influences. As clinicians, it is important to understand the unique characteristics of each of the four generations that are currently present in our workforce: the Traditionalists, Baby Boomers, Gen X, and Millennials. By appreciating our own generational characteristics, we have the opportunity to optimize our interactions with those of other generational cohorts. Additionally, it is important to recognize that the characteristics attributed to each of the generations are made with very broad strokes. Do not allow such distinctions to resemble discrimination or allow implicit bias to preclude effective multigenerational collaboration.

The authors would like to acknowledge Deb Roush for her assistance in preparing this manuscript for publication.

REFERENCES

1. Cruess RL, Cruess SR, Steinert Y, eds. *Teaching Medical Professionalism: Supporting the Development of a Professional Identity*. New York, NY: Cambridge University Press; 2009.
2. Howe N, Strauss W. *Millennials Rising: The Next Great Generation*. Vintage Books; 2000.
3. Lancaster LC, Stillman D. *When Generations Collide: Who They Are, Why They Clash, How to Solve the Generational Puzzle at Work*. HarperCollins; 2002.
4. Walsh DS. Mind the gap: generational differences in medicine. *Northeast Fla Med*. 2011;62:12–15.

5. Smit D. Do you have enough "Generational Glue" in your organisation? *HR Future.* 2017;12:22–23.

6. Codrington G. *Mind the Gap: Own Your Past, Know Your Generation, Choose Your Future.* Penguin Random House South Africa; 2012.

7. Keenan AC, Leffler TG, McKenna PH. Generational differences and resident selection. In: Kohler TSB, ed. *Surgeons as Educators.* Cham, Switzerland: Springer; 2018: 189–198.

8. Roodin P, Mendelson M. Multiple generations at work: current and future trends. *J Int Relationships.* 2013;11:213–222.

9. Sudheimer EE. Stories appreciating both sides of the generation gap: baby boomer and Generation X nurses working together. *Nurs Forum.* 2009;44:57–63.

10. Washburn ER. Are you ready for generation X? *Physician Exec.* 2000;26:51–57.

11. Lim A, Epperly T. Generation gap: effectively leading physicians of all ages. *Fam Pract Manag.* 2013;20:29–34.

12. Vanderveen K, Bold RJ. Effect of generational composition on the surgical workforce. *Arch Surg.* 2008;143:224–226.

13. Woods K: Organizational ambidexterity and the multi-generational workforce. *J Org Cul Comm Conflict.* 2016;20:95–111.

14. Shangraw RE, Whitten CW. Managing intergenerational differences in academic anesthesiology. *Curr Opin Anaesthesiol.* 2007;20:558–563.

15. Young A, Chaudhry HJ, Pei X, et al. A census of actively licensed physicians in the United States, 2016. *J Med Reg.* 2017;103:7–21.

16. Weingarten RM. Four generations, one workplace: a gen X-Y staff nurse's view of team building in the emergency department. *J Emerg Nurs.* 2009;35:27–30.

17. Shaw H. *Sticking Points: How to get 4 Generations Working Together in the 12 Places they Come Apart.* Tyndale Momentum; 2013.

18. Wieck KL. Motivating an intergenerational workforce: scenarios for success. *Orthoped Nurs.* 2007;26:366–371.

19. Smedley K, Whitten H. *Age Matters: Employing, Motivating and Managing Older Employees.* Routledge; 2017:360.

20. Fry R. Millennials are the largest generation in the U.S. Labor Force. Pew Research Center. 2018. Available at: https://www.pewresearch.org/fact-tank/2018/04/11/millennials-largest-generation-us-labor-force/.

21. Population distribution in the United States in 2018, by generation, 2019.

22. Cordeniz JA. Recruitment, retention, and management of generation X: a focus on nursing professionals. *J Healthc Manag.* 2002;47:237–249.

23. Martin TN, Ottemann R. Generational workforce demographic trends and total organizational rewards which might attract and retain different generational employees. *J Behav Appl Manag.* 2016;16:1160.

24. Bickel J, Brown AJ. Generation X: implications for faculty recruitment and development in academic health centers. *Acad Med.* 2005;80:205–210.

25. Steele MM, Fisman S, Davidson B. Mentoring and role models in recruitment and retention: a study of junior medical faculty perceptions. *Med Teach.* 2013;35:e1130–e1138.

26. Kupperschmidt BR. Understanding generation X employees. *J Nurs Adm.* 1998;28:36–43.

27. Stewart JS, Oliver EG, Cravens KS, et al. Managing millennials: embracing generational differences. *Bus Horiz.* 2017;60:45–54.

28. Rohrich RJ. Training the generation X plastic surgeon: dispelling the myths? *Plast Reconstr Surg.* 2001;108:1733–1734.

29. Toohey SL, Wray A, Wiechmann W, et al. Ten tips for engaging the Millennial learner and moving an emergency medicine residency curriculum into the 21st century. *West J Emerg.* 2016;17:337–343.

30. Williams VN, Medina J, Medina A, et al. Bridging the millennial generation expectation gap: perspectives and strategies for physician and interprofessional faculty. *Am J Med Sci.* 2017;353:109–115.

31. Data F. *Forrester's 2008 North American Technographics Benchmark Survey.* 2008.

32. Kupperschmidt BR. Understanding net generation employees. *J Nurs Adm.* 2001;31:570–574.

33. Mangold K. Educating a new generation: teaching baby boomer faculty about millennial students. *Nurs Educ.* 2007;32:21–23.

34. Generations X, Y, Z and the Others.

35. Keys Y. Looking ahead to our next generation of nurse leaders: generation X nurse managers. *J Nurs Manag.* 2014;22:97–123.

36. Jauregui J, Watsjold B, Welsh L, et al. Generational 'othering': the myth of the Millennial learner. *Med Educ.* 2020;54:60–65.

37. Busari JO. The discourse of generational segmentation and the implications for postgraduate medical education. *Perspect Med Educ.* 2013;2:340–348.

38. van Dam M, Noben C, Higgins M. Bridging generation gaps in medical education: a "light bulb moment" at the Association for Medical Education in Europe annual conference in Barcelona. *Med Teach.* 2017;39:1195–1196.

39. Boysen PG, Daste L, Northern T: Multigenerational challenges and the future of graduate medical education. *Ochsner J.* 16:101–107, 2016.

40. Northern T, Daste L, Boysen PG. An evaluation of the preferred learning styles of incoming faculty and housestaff: a multidisciplinary and multigenerational approach. *Anesth Analg.* 2015;120:S425.

41. Johnston S. See one, do one, teach one: developing professionalism across the generations. *Clin Orthop Relat Res.* 2006;449:186–192.

42. Meyer AA, Weiner TM. The generation gap: perspectives of a program director. *Arch Surg.* 2002;137:268–270.

43. Salopek JJ. The young and the rest of us. *Train Develop.* 2000;54:26–30.

44. Gorman PJ, Meier AH, Rawn C, et al. The future of medical education is no longer blood and guts, it is bits and bytes. *Am J Surg.* 2000;180:353–356.

45. Bullock A, Webb K. Technology in postgraduate medical education: a dynamic influence on learning? *Postgrad Med J.* 2015;91:646–650.

46. Goyal N, Tung A. "We're Not Like Them!" Intergenerational Perceptions of Teaching Skill and Role Models. New Orleans, LA: American Society of Anesthesiologists Annual Meeting; 2007.

47. Chisholm R, Finnell JT. Emergency department physician internet use during clinical encounters. *AMIA Annu Symp Proc.* 2012;1176–1183.

48. Dunmore D. *Has Technology Become a Need? A Qualitative Study Exploring Three Generational Cohorts' Perception of Technology in Regards to Maslow's Hierarchy of Needs.* Capella University; 2013.

49. Czaja S, Beach S, Charness N, et al. Older adults and the adoption of healthcare technology: opportunities and challenges. In Sixsmith AGG, ed. *Technologies for Active Aging.* Vol. 9, Boston, Mass: Springer; 2013: 27–46.

50. Menachemi N, Powers TL, Brooks RG. Physician and practice characteristics associated with longitudinal increases in electronic health records adoption. *J Healthc Manag.* 2011;56:183–198.

51. Gladwell M. *Outliers: The Story of Success.* New York, NY: Little, Brown and Co; 2008.

52. Tang PC. *Key Capabilities of an Electronic Health Record System: Letter Report.* Washington, DC: Institute of Medicine; 2003.

53. Dawidowski AR, Toselli L, Luna DR, et al. Changes in physicians' attitudes to computerized ambulatory medical record systems: a longitudinal qualitative study. *Gaceta Sanitaria.* 2007;21:384–389.

54. Berner ES, Detmer DE, Simborg D. Will the wave finally break? A brief view of the adoption of electronic medical records in the United States. *J Am Med Inform Assoc.* 2005;12:3–7.
55. English B. *Generational SharePoint: Understanding Generational Differences in Share-Point Adoption.* Share Point Mindsharp Blogs; 2009.
56. Abdekhoda M, Ahmadi M, Gohari M, et al. The effects of organizational contextual factors on physicians' attitude toward adoption of electronic medical records. *J Biomed Inform.* 2015;53:174–179.
57. Henry J, Pylypchuk Y, Searcy T, et al. Adoption of Electronic Health Record Systems among U.S. Non-Federal Acute Care Hospitals: 2008-2015. ONC Data Brief 35, The Office of the National Coordination for Health Information Technology; 2016.
58. Duke É, Montag C. Smartphone addiction, daily interruptions and self-reported productivity. *Addict Behav Rep.* 2017;6:90–95.
59. Sharpe A. *Solving the Productivity Paradox: The Mysterious Link Between Computers and Productivity.* Toronto, Ontario, Canada: National Post; 1997.
60. Zitner D. Physicians will happily adopt information technology. *CMAJ.* 2006;174:1583–1584.
61. Hebert MA. Impact of IT on health care professionals: changes in work and the productivity paradox. *Health Serv Manage Res.* 1998;11:69–79.
62. Garavand A, Mohseni M, Asadi H, et al. Factors influencing the adoption of health information technologies: a systematic review. *Electron Physician.* 2016;8:2713–2718.
63. Lee J, McCullough JS, Town RJ. The impact of health information technology on hospital productivity. *RAND J Econ.* 2013;44:545–568.
64. Viccellio P. Turnaround time and transaction costs. *Ann Emerg Med.* 2008;51:186–187.
65. Axtell C, Wall T, Stride C, et al. Familiarity breeds content: the impact of exposure to change on employee openness and well-being. *J Occup Organ Psychol.* 2002;75:217–231.
66. de Jong T, Wiezer N, de Weerd M, et al. The impact of restructuring on employee well-being: a systematic review of longitudinal studies. *Work and Stress.* 2016;30:91–114.
67. Costantino TG, Satz WA, Stahmer SA, et al. Predictors of success in emergency medicine ultrasound education. *Acad Emerg Med.* 2003;10:180–183.
68. Kendall JL, Hoffenberg SR, Smith RS. History of emergency and critical care ultrasound: the evolution of a new imaging paradigm. *Crit Care Med.* 2007;35:S126–S130.
69. Blumberg SJ, Luke JV. *Wireless Substitution: Early Release of Estimates From the National Health Interview Survey, January–June 2018.* National Center for Health Statistics; 2018.
70. International Workplace Group. The Annual IWG Global Workspace Survey. Welcome to Generation Flex—The Employee Power Shift; 2019.
71. Berger E. This sentence easily would fit on twitter: emergency physicians are learning to "tweet". *Ann Emerg Med.* 2009;54:23A–25A.
72. McGowan BS, Wasko M, Vartabedian BS, et al. Understanding the factors that influence the adoption and meaningful use of social media by physicians to share medical information. *J Med Internet Res.* 2012;14:e117.
73. Budd L. Physician tweet thyself: a guide for integrating social media into medical practice. *BCMJ.* 2013;55:38–40.
74. Larson DL. Bridging the generation X gap in plastic surgery training: part 1. Identifying the problem. *Plast Reconstr Surg.* 2003;112:1656–1661.
75. Gholami-Kordkheili F, Wild V, Strech D. The impact of social media on medical professionalism: a systematic qualitative review of challenges and opportunities. *J Med Internet Res.* 2013;15:e184.
76. Pearson D, Bond MC, Kegg J, et al. Evaluation of social media use by emergency medicine residents and faculty. *West J Emerg Med.* 2015;16:715–720.
77. Scott KR, Hsu CH, Johnson NJ, et al. Integration of social media in emergency medicine residency curriculum. *Ann Emerg Med.* 2014;64:396–404.
78. Kind T, Patel PD, Lie D, et al. Twelve tips for using social media as a medical educator. *Med Teach.* 2014;36:284–290.
79. Forgie SE, Duff JP, Ross S. Twelve tips for using Twitter as a learning tool in medical education. *Med Teach.* 2013;35:8–14.
80. Berger E. Web 2.0 in emergency medicine: specialty embracing the future of medical communication. *Ann Emerg Med.* 2012;59:A21–A23.
81. Taylor H. *Internet Provides Public with Health Care Information that They Value and Trust and Which Often Stimulates Discussion with Their Doctors.* Rochester, NY: Harris Interactive, Inc; 2009.
82. AlGhamdi KM, Moussa NA. Internet use by the public to search for health-related information. *Int J Med Inform.* 2012;81:363–373.
83. Grant RW, Campbell EG, Gruen RL, et al. Prevalence of basic information technology use by U.S. physicians. *J Gen Intern Med.* 2006;21:1150–1155.
84. Montgomery CH, King DW. Comparing library and user related costs of print and electronic journal collections. D-Lib Magazine: Corporation for National Research Initiatives. 8, 2002.
85. Cadogan M, Thoma B, Chan TM, et al. Free open access meducation (FOAM): the rise of emergency medicine and critical care blogs and podcasts (2002-2013). *Emerg Med J.* 2014;31:e76–e77.
86. Nickson CP, Cadogan MD. Free open access medical education (FOAM) for the emergency physician. *Emerg Med Australas.* 2014;26:76–83.
87. Mallin M, Schlein S, Doctor S, et al. A survey of the current utilization of asynchronous education among emergency medicine residents in the United States. *Acad Med.* 2014;89:598–601.
88. Otterness K. Incorporating FOAM into medical student and resident education. *Clin Exp Emerg Med.* 2017;4:119–120.
89. Fox S. *E-Patients With a Disability or Chronic Disease.* Washington, DC: Technology PRCI; 2007.
90. Kapur PA. The impact of new-generation physicians on the function of academic anesthesiology departments. *Curr Opin Anaesthesiol.* 2007;20:564–567.
91. Jobe LL. Generational differences in work ethic among 3 generations of registered nurses. *J Nurs Adm.* 2014;44:303–308.
92. Kaliannan M, Perumal K, Dorasamy M. Developing a work-life balance model towards improving job satisfaction among medical doctors across different generations. *J Develop Areas.* 2016;50:343–351.
93. Kupfer JM. The graying of US physicians: implications for quality and the future supply of physicians. *JAMA.* 2016;315:341–342.
94. Goldberg R, Thomas H, Penner L. Issues of concern to emergency physicians in pre-retirement years: a survey. *J Emerg Med.* 2011;40:706–713.
95. Alch ML. Get ready for the net generation. *Train Develop.* 2000;54:32–34.
96. Feiertag J, Berge ZL. Training Generation N: how educators should approach the net generation. *Educ Train.* 2008;50:457–464.
97. Costa G, Di Milia L. Aging and shift work: a complex problem to face. *Chronobiol Int.* 200825:165–181.
98. Hewlett SA, Sherbin L, Sumberg K. How Gen Y and Boomers will reshape your agenda. *Harv Bus Rev.* 2009;87:71–76, 153.
99. Trower CA. Making academic dentistry more attractive to new teacher-scholars. *J Dent Educ.* 2007;71:601–605.

100. Mackay B. Residents strive to raise public awareness of their role. *CMAJ.* 2003;168:1030.

101. Hagemann B, Stroope S. Developing the next generation of leaders. *Ind Commerc Train.* 2013;45:123–126.

102. Moore JM, Everly M, Bauer R. Multigenerational challenges: team-building for positive clinical workforce outcomes. *Online J Issues Nurs.* 2016;21:3.

103. Howell LP, Servis G, Bonham A. Multigenerational challenges in academic medicine: UCDavis's responses. *Acad Med.* 2005;80:527–532.

104. Haeger DL, Lingham T. A trend toward Work–Life Fusion: a multi-generational shift in technology use at work. *Technol Forecast Soc Change.* 2014;89:316–325.

105. Becton JB, Walker HJ, Jones-Farmer A. Generational differences in workplace behavior. *J Appl Soc Psychol.* 2014;44:175–189.

106. Silverstein M: Meeting the challenges of an aging workforce. *Am J Ind Med.* 2008;51:269–280.

107. Tuomi K, Ilmarinen J, Martikainen R, et al. Aging, work, life-style and work ability among Finnish municipal workers in 1981–1992. *Scand J Work Environ Health.* 1997;23(Suppl 1):58–65.

108. Lesiuk T. The effect of music listening on work performance. *Psychol Music.* 2005;33:173–191.

109. Marquie JC, Ansiau D, Tummino S, et al. Aging, shiftwork, and sleep disorders: results from the VISAT longitudinal study. Paper presented at: 18th International Symposium on Shiftwork and Working Time, Yeppoon, Queensland, Australia; 2007.

110. Folkard S. Shift work, safety, and aging. *Chronobiol Int.* 2008;25:183–198.

111. Drapeau C, Carrier J. Fluctuation of waking electroencephalogram and subjective alertness during a 25-hour sleep-deprivation episode in young and middle-aged subjects. *Sleep.* 2004;27:55–60.

112. Gaudreau H, Morettini J, Lavoie HB, et al. Effects of a 25-h sleep deprivation on daytime sleep in the middle-aged. *Neurobiol Aging.* 2001;22:461–468.

113. Smith-Coggins R, Broderick KB, Marco CA. Night shifts in emergency medicine: the American Board of Emergency Medicine Longitudinal Study of Emergency Physicians. *J Emerg Med.* 2014;47:372–378.

114. Almklov EL, Drummond SP, Orff H, et al. The effects of sleep deprivation on brain functioning in older adults. *Behav Sleep Med.* 2015;13:324–345.

115. Monk TH. Aging human circadian rhythms: conventional wisdom may not always be right. *J Biol Rhythms.* 2005;20:366–374.

116. Kecklund G, Axelsson J. Health consequences of shift work and insufficient sleep. *BMJ.* 2016;355:i5210.

117. Gibson EM, Williams WP, III, Kriegsfeld LJ. Aging in the circadian system: considerations for health, disease prevention and longevity. *Exp Gerontol.* 2009;44:51–56.

118. Viswanathan AN, Hankinson SE, Schernhammer ES. Night shift work and the risk of endometrial cancer. *Cancer Res.* 2007;67:10618–10622.

119. Corbo SA. The X-er files. They're young, techno-hip job-hoppers. And maybe the perfect health care workers. *Hosp Health Netw.* 1997;71:58–60.

120. Tulgan G. *The Manager's Guide to Generation X.* Amherst, Mass: HRD Press; 1997.

121. Smith TJ, Nichols T. Understanding the millennial generation. *J Bus Divers.* 2015;15:39–47.

122. Larson DL. Bridging the generation X gap in plastic surgery training: part 2. A proposed solution—identifying a "best practice" in a plastic surgery training program. *Plast Reconstr Surg.* 2003;112:1662–1665.

123. Vogt P. *Live With Your Parents After Graduation?* New York, NY: Monster.com; 2013.

124. Managing an Intergenerational Workforce: Strategies for Health Care Transformation. American Hospital Association Committee on Performance Improvement.

125. Hopkins L, Hampton BS, Abbott JF, et al. To the point: medical education, technology, and the millennial learner. *Am J Obstet Gynecol.* 2018;218:188–192.

126. Avegno J, DeBlieux PMC. Characteristics of great teachers. In: Rogers RLMA, Winters M, Martinez J, Mulligan T, eds. *Practical Teaching in Emergency Medicine.* Indianapolis, Ind: Wiley Blackwell; 2009:283–294.

127. Snadden D, Kunzli MA. Working hard but working differently: a qualitative study of the impact of generational change on rural health care. *CMAJ Open.* 2017;5:E710–E716.

128. Brown AJ, Swinyard W, Ogle J. Women in academic medicine: a report of focus groups and questionnaires, with conjoint analysis. *J Womens Health (Larchmt).* 2003;12:999–1008.

129. Caniano DA, Sonnino RE, Paolo AM. Keys to career satisfaction: insights from a survey of women pediatric surgeons. *J Pediatr Surg.* 2004;39:984–990.

130. Ginde AA, Sullivan AF, Camargo Jr., CA. Attrition from emergency medicine clinical practice in the United States. *Ann Emerg Med.* 2010;56:166–171.

CHAPTER 124

GENDER BALANCE

Jeannette Wolfe, Andrea Austin

> *Hiring and promoting talented women is the right thing to do for society—and it's an economic imperative...*
>
> —Carolos Ghosn, Chairman Renault-Nissan Alliance[1]

Although men, women, and gender nonbinary people may share the same job title, *how* they do that job and the challenges that they face are often quite different. The focus of this chapter is to better understand these differences and give both individuals and leaders better tools to enhance professional development and create more functional, inclusive, and high-performing teams.

Paying attention to gender-related issues facing emergency medicine (EM) should not be the result of an out-of-touch, compliance-oriented human resources (HR) directive. Rather it should spring from an effort to authentically recognize that creating diverse, gender-intelligent teams increases organizational value by elevating its creative capabilities, financial potential, institutional loyalty, and quality of medical care.[2-4] This rationale has been considered by many businesses:

> *More than hitting a number, this is about creating a more inclusive culture that values all dimensions of diversity—because a more diverse culture fosters a more innovative culture, and innovation moves our company forward.*[5]

THE GENDER PAY GAP

Over the past several decades, the medical workforce and its developing talent pool have dramatically changed. In 2019, 51% of first-year medical students were women. Within the specialty of EM, as of 2020, approximately 36% of current residents and 38% of full-time academic faculty were women.[6-8] Although studies confirm that women have the ability to lead as effectively as men, gender gaps in advancement opportunities and compensation remain. A recent study suggests that, even when career point and academic productivity are comparable, men are still far more likely to be at an associate or professor rank than women.[9] This aligns with 2019 American Association of Medical Colleges (AAMC) data that show only 19% of professors and 30% of associate professors in EM are female.[8] The AAMC data also show that, for all clinical academic faculty regardless of specialty, men, on average, still significantly outearn women: a 15% difference at the instructor level and a 21% difference at the chair level.[10] To better understand the root of these inequities and how to systemically address and mitigate them, it is necessary to review some basic definitions surrounding biological sex and gender.

Neurobiology

Biological sex is based on an individual's sex chromosomes, sex hormones, and anatomy. Generally, biological sex is regarded as binomial, with females having an XX pair of sex chromosomes and males an XY. In truth, this is an oversimplification. Some individuals are born intersex, having an unanticipated number of sex chromosomes or atypical hormonal function that precludes simple categorization.

Gender, on the other hand, is heavily influenced by social constructs and includes the experiences, opportunities, and expectations of an individual and is greatly influenced by the societal norms. Gender occurs on a spectrum in which the stereotypical behavior of men and women exists on opposite ends.

When noting an objective outcome difference between men and women, it can be helpful to determine if the main driver behind that difference is rooted in biological sex or gender. Although sometimes this is possible, often it can be rather difficult because an individual's biological sex can heavily influence their sociocultural experiences.[11] For example, boys (represented by Josh) are statistically more likely to play hockey and girls (represented by Annie) to play the flute. Hence, via the process of neuroplasticity, it is easy to imagine that Josh and Annie may have quite physically different functional connections in their brains if Josh spent 10 years playing club hockey with others while Annie spent the same amount of time practicing flute alone in her room.

This nature/nurture distinction gets even more complicated, however, after the consideration of epigenetics. It was once believed that sex chromosomes were simply important due to their programming of sex hormones, but now it is appreciated that sex chromosomes influence the functions of other chromosomes. Although males and females share about 98% of the same deoxyribonucleic acid (DNA), *which* genes get turned on or off after being exposed to the same experiences (or infections or toxins) may be quite different.[12] This suggests that even if Josh and Annie *both* played 5000 hours of high-level hockey, their brains would physically look quite different. Furthermore, if they both received a similar impact during a game that caused a head injury, their neurobiological responses could be quite different, leading to different clusters of symptoms and even recovery times.[13]

Gender Science and Behavior

Science relating to gender and behavior sets the groundwork that brains perceive, process, and react to situations based on both biology and gendered experiences. Objective examples include the vastly different vulnerabilities to certain neurological diseases that women and men face, including Alzheimer's, multiple sclerosis, post-traumatic stress disorder, autism, dyslexia, attention-deficit/hyperactivity disorder, and schizophrenia. A study by Ingalhalikar et al examined sex differences in our connectome (the map of neural connections or the *wiring diagram* of our brain). The study suggests that males are more likely to have increased intrahemispheric information transmission with strong connections between areas of visual input to motor processing, while females appear to have more interhemispheric crossing of information with increased connections between areas of the brain associated with intuitive and analytic thinking.[14]

Similarly, research on stress suggests that men and women have very different neural underpinnings in how they perceive anxiety. Men sense anxiety when they have less firing in certain areas of their executive cortices, while women sense it when those same areas are overstimulated.[15] Ultimately, data suggests that stressed men are at greater risk for impulsivity while women are more likely to experience excessive rumination. As researchers in one study explain, "Taken together, the observed differences in these regions suggest that men and women may differ in the extent to which they engage in verbal processing, visualization, self-referential thinking, and cognitive processing during the experience of stress and anxiety."[15]

In this view, it appears that the fundamental way in which men and women think is different and that the first step in creating diverse teams is recognizing and valuing the importance of this neurodiversity. To create better equity in EM, it is necessary to have a frank discussion about some of these differences.

WOMEN IN THE WORKPLACE

When learning about gender-based differences in the workplace, there is a risk that a barrage of statistics will overwhelm the reality that these differences impact the lives of real people. To better personalize the challenges that many women in medicine experience, this chapter presents five fictional characters who will repeatedly appear; they are:

- Tom, a department vice chair
- Sarah, a senior attending
- Josh and Annie who are both new junior attendings
- Maryanne, a charge nurse

For simplicity's sake, these characters are cisgender—their personal identities and genders correspond with their birth sex. This is not meant to downplay the very real challenges that nonbinary people experience in the workplace. Also, these characters represent biological sex and gender-based tendencies, which may or may not directly translate to the individual tendencies of a specific person. While the described challenges do not impact *all* women, the fact that they could highjack the careers of even *some* women (possibly including a woman or two in the reader's own department) is enough to merit thoughtful consideration if the specialty of EM wishes to optimize the productivity and contributions of all of its members.

The Playground

To better understand how and why men and women often behave differently at work, it is helpful to review evolutionary psychology. Darwin's theory of sexual selection demonstrates that organisms with reproductive advantages are more likely to transmit their DNA into the next generation's gene pool. From this lens, males and females are wired differently because characteristics that optimize their abilities to compete for the best mates and resources are different. Material resources and hierarchical status are important for males, and physical signs of fertility and social connections are important for women. For example, at a very basic level, a lactating female in a hunting/gathering community requires help with food access as foraging alone is unlikely to produce enough calories to support the metabolic needs of herself and her growing infant.

As mentioned previously, societal expectations also exert significant influence in interpersonal interactions. What follows is a liberally expanded example that is often used by Dr. Leonard Sax, one of the gurus of sex and gender-based differences and author of the excellent book *Why Gender Matters*.[16] It features an excellent anthropological observation area—an elementary school playground (**Box 124.1**).

Workplace Implications

In general, men are more comfortable with hierarchy, rotating alliances, competition, direct aggression, and challenging the rules. Men bond through teasing and sharing tasks, such as completing a project, watching football, playing music, and so on. Men are goal-oriented and often share a problem to seek a solution. They feel validated when they overcome a personal challenge or get a *win*. Finally, they are more comfortable with compartmentalizing and moving past interpersonal conflict.[16-18]

Women value loyalty and relationships. They often quickly pick up nonverbal cues, especially anger and fear, and can be wary of engaging in direct verbal challenges. They may seek empathy rather than solutions when sharing a problem. Connection often comes in the form of the exchange of personal information rather than working together to obtain a

> **BOX 124.1 ■ THE ELEMENTARY SCHOOL ALLEGORY**
>
> Tom and Sarah are elementary school students who are playing in the school yard during recess. Several kids are playing kickball. Children in the outfield taunt each new player stepping up to the plate. A child kicks the ball and runs to the base, and it is unclear if they are safe or out. Voices rise and a few kids start shoving each other. For a moment it looks like a fight might break out, but when one of the team captains reminds everyone that the game is tied and they only have 5 minutes left of recess, a truce is called, and the game is finished. An hour later in the classroom, the player who was shoved is laughing with the kid who did the shoving, and both are recounting just how mad the other kid looked during the game. Their conversation ends with loose plans to get together that weekend to watch a movie.
>
> If one had to guess whether Sarah or Tom was involved in the above scenario, chances are most would guess Tom.
>
> Where is Sarah? She is over on the swings in deep conversation with her best friend, Jenny. They are talking about an incident in history class in which a teacher called on a new boy who wasn't paying attention. Sarah listens intently to Jenny as she connects the story with other things that she has heard about the boy. Sarah pays close attention to Jenny's facial expression and body language and lets Jenny finish her sentence before she adds, "Well I don't really know him, but I wonder if maybe he's not that smart." When Jenny answers in agreement, Sarah more assertively adds additional comments about her own opinion of the new boy.
>
> Later in math class, students are asked to partner up for a math quiz game. Sarah picks Jenny to be her partner, even though she knows that Jenny struggles with math. Tom chooses Ben, a boy he knows is quite good at math, even though they are not close friends. When Tom's team wins, they start trash-talking the other teams while Sarah downplays her team's second-place finish (clearly carried by Sarah's own math skills) and states they were just "lucky."
>
> As school ends, Sarah and Jenny pass several girls who noticeably roll their eyes at them. Jenny whispers to Sarah that one of the girls was her best friend until they got into an argument at a party and have not talked since. Sarah empathizes, sharing her own story about an abruptly ended friendship and musing that although arguments with girls rarely cause bloody noses, they still seem to inflict real pain.

specific goal. Women are often process-oriented and able to identify confounding variables associated with goal attainment, as well as more tolerant of short-term sacrifices for long-term gains. They feel validated by inclusion and peer recognition. Finally, women may perceive conflict as a personal threat, and when direct verbal challenges occur, they may have more difficulty moving forward and repairing the relationship.[16-18]

The Gender Intelligence Group

Barbara Annis, chief executive officer (CEO) of Gender Intelligence Group, has written extensively about the differences between how men and women behave in the workplace.[19] Over the years, her company has done thousands of workshops in which she puts men and women in separate rooms and asks them to share the most difficult challenges that arise from working with the opposite sex.

Regardless of industry, the top answers in the breakout groups are universally the same. The primary challenge reported by men is that they are unsure of how to communicate with women in the workplace. Their concern stems from the fear that women they work with may become overly defensive or too emotional should they make a misstep in conversation. There is also concern that, if something goes wrong, it will never be forgotten and held against them. Among women, the greatest challenge is feeling dismissed and excluded by men at work. In the light of these differences, it is easier to understand how men and women get both confused and frustrated during some communications.

For example, in a meeting between the characters Josh and Annie, Annie might buffer her words when presenting a new idea. "I was thinking, maybe we should . . ." Josh may sense this as a sign of insecurity and indecision and repackage her words into a more declarative statement. While he might see it as *clarifying*, Annie might interpret this as *stealing*—especially if Josh is later given credit for the idea. Likewise, Josh and Tom may get quite frustrated in a meeting if they perceive that Sarah is going off agenda. Meanwhile, Sarah becomes annoyed because she believes she has identified a new issue that needs to be addressed if the group wants to accomplish their greater goal and that her input is being ignored.[17,19]

Implicit Bias

The real reasons that women are not moving up do not lie primarily with women. They are embedded in systems that have evolved over decades and reflect the values, motivations and views of a male majority. None of this is done intentionally or even consciously. It is simply the result of history and corporate evolutions. But so long as these issues remain unseen, they form an intractable barrier to a more inclusive work environment.

—Avivah Wittenberg-Cox[20]

It is necessary to discuss implicit bias to understand why women have been in the pipeline for the last two decades and yet not reached proportionate representation in leadership positions. As the words of Wittenberg-Cox suggest, implicit bias refers to the unconscious attitudes and stereotypes that affect individual decisions and behaviors. It is ubiquitous and affects everyone, regardless of gender, race, or background. Many examples may be manifest in the workplace; these include:

- *Affinity bias:* favoring someone because of perceived commonalities
- *Attribution bias:* judging an individual based on preconceived notions, rather than investigating specific circumstances
- *Gender bias:* preferentially hiring or advancing a male candidate based on assumptions about men and women
- *Confirmation bias:* seeking confirmation of an initial impression

Importantly, these behaviors are usually subconscious and may be in direct opposition to one's consciously held beliefs. Harvard's Implicit Association Test (IAT), available online, studies this phenomenon of subconscious conceptual linking.[21] Millions of people have taken the IAT that examines the participants' implicit biases in areas such as diversity, inclusion, and leadership. The timed responses of test-takers are measured when comparing pictures and names to attributes.

In the gender section of the IAT, pictures or names of men and women are projected and participants are asked to associate the names and pictures with career or family. The speed of association is measured. Tens of thousands of scored tests demonstrate that both men and women are slower to associate women to career and men to family, suggesting a bias that can lead to subtle gender discrimination.[22] The AAMC has an excellent slide set on the potential detrimental effects of unconscious bias.[23] **Tables 124.1** and **124.2** show how implicit bias can impact recruiting, hiring, promotion, and award recognition.

The Competence Hurdle

Along with an implicit sense that they are not meant to be traditional leaders, women often face setbacks because of how their leadership is viewed. Traditional leadership has been associated with traits that are stereotypically male, such as self-assertion and independence, while communal traits more common in women leaders have been viewed

TABLE 124.1 ■ Implicit Bias and Solutions for Fair Recommendations and Hiring Practices		
Scenario	**Unconscious Bias**	**Solution**
Search committee	• Committee made up of only men	• Ensure several women are on committee • Define desired objective qualifications of applicant
Letters of recommendation	• Men's tend to be longer, record-focused, and written with more professional respect • Women's tend to contain more "doubt" raisers, less "standout" adjectives, and include more information about temperament[58]	• Increase awareness • Encourage standardized letters of recommendation within your institution
CV	• In men and women with similar CVs, the man's may be judged to be stronger[59] • In addition, women who are mothers may be viewed as less capable as nonmothers[61]	• Increase awareness • Blinding name on CV • Objectively compare required qualifications with CV
Recruitment	• Word-of-mouth and certain advertising venues preferentially favor men • Recruiting ads written with male pronouns and stereotypical adjectives • Search firm may have own underlying bias	• Expand search efforts to seek out qualified women • Use gender neutral terminology • Require that search firm produces pool that includes at least 25% women[57] • Provide structured evaluation forms[65]
Interviews	• Same applicant behavior may be interpreted differently depending on the applicant's gender	• Unconscious bias training • Interview standardization • Legal and organizational interview best practices training

as weak. When women adopt traditional leadership styles, they are often penalized for being abrasive. To promote credibility, women must balance the right mix of socially expected communal behavior with charisma, aggression, and competition.[24]

Although literature suggests that men and women are equally competent at leading a resuscitation, women may face additional challenges.[25,26] This is illustrated in a survey of internal medicine residents who were asked to reflect on their codes.[27] Female residents voiced a need to show more masculine traits, such as speaking loudly and standing on a step to appear taller. Several also expressed a concern about potentially jeopardizing relationships with other team members if they were perceived as being too commanding or authoritarian. This sentiment illustrates the added mental energy women must expend to be viewed as both capable and approachable.

A more recent study conducted on EM residents in Boston, Massachusetts further highlighted the challenges that women, especially younger physicians, may face at work. This study suggested that residents are held to slightly different standards in gaining trust and respect among nursing staff, with the implication that women had to work much harder than men to prove their competence.[28]

Gendered Discordant Feedback

Two other recent studies underscore how implicit bias impacts women in EM. The first studied more than 33,000 milestone evaluations of EM residents in several different programs and found that, although there was no gender difference in how first-year EM residents were evaluated, by the third year, men were evaluated higher across all 23 core subcompetencies.[29]

TABLE 124.2 ■ Implicit Bias and Solutions for Fair Retention and Promotion

Scenario	Unconscious Bias	Solution
Advancement	• Men are more comfortable with self-promotion. • Women wait to be asked. • Women may be prematurely dismissed due to perception job would not "fit" their preferences (long hours or travel). • Men are often promoted for their "potential" to acquire new job skills; women are usually promoted after they have already "obtained" new skills.[15]	• Perform an annual structured review of employees' short- and long-term professional objectives. • Identify specific opportunities for employees to obtain skill sets, mentoring, and to network. • Post all positions with objective qualifications, encourage internal queries, and consider active solicitations. • Biannually remind managers of benefits of gender balance directive. • Hold managers accountable for tracking all of their employees' professional development. • If gender-based patterns emerge, analyze and address root causes.
Awards and recognition	• Subjective-based awards often favor men.	• Make award criteria as objective as possible. • Include award and recognition section on annual review. • Validate all award recipients privately and publicly.
Attrition	• Belief that attrition is due to personal conditions beyond the organization's control.	• Conduct structured exit interviews addressing root causes if patterns emerge.
Committees	• Committee is made up of only men, or men and one woman. • Committee's perspective is subtly male biased.	• Place at least 30% of women on a committee.[3]

To try and understand why this occurred, a qualitative follow-up study was done that examined 1,000 written-in comments.[30] This showed that senior male EM residents who were struggling were much more likely to receive consistent feedback, while female residents often received quite inconsistent feedback, especially surrounding the areas of autonomy and assertiveness.

The authors of these studies suggest that implicit bias likely plays a role in their findings in that, as residents progress through training, they are increasingly expected to run resuscitations and make independent critical decisions, which are traits more stereotypical of men. This may also contribute to why female faculty are evaluated less favorably than male faculty.[31] Hence, teams led by women are often caught in this razor-thin line between being viewed as not assertive enough or too assertive. As autonomy is integral to skill proficiency and career satisfaction, it should be consistently and intentionally taught in training programs to students of all genders.

Although strategies to address implicit bias are discussed later in the chapter, two main issues should be addressed here:

1. Implicit bias is real and can greatly influence professional advancement.
2. Meaningful change will not occur unless individuals and organizations recognize its impact and commit to improvement.

Stereotype Threat

Stereotype threat is closely related to implicit bias. To better understand, consider the sense of self as the sum total of many personal attributes: age, gender, ethnicity, social–economic class, and so on. Each person's behavior in any situation is influenced by several factors, including the external environment, implicit biases, and individual attributes relevant to the situation. Importantly, studies have shown that particular attributes can be subtly primed by certain cues. For example, mentioning sushi and egg rolls may provoke ethnicity considerations, while talking about boardrooms may trigger gender attributes. When an individual's specific personal attribute becomes primed and they find themselves in a situation in which there is an expected behavior associated with that attribute, if the association is perceived as a benefit, the individual's performance can improve; this is called stereotype boost. Conversely, if the primed attribute is associated with a negative bias, unchecked, their performance can actually decline; this is called stereotype threat.

Stereotype threat can impact performance because it can trigger psychological and physiological processes that increase arousal and anxiety and negatively impact working memory, test performance, and effort.[32] For example, triggering ethnic identity for Black and Latino test-takers decreases standard intelligence quotient scores.[33] Importantly, performance can be enhanced or impaired by priming different attributes within the same group. In a clever experiment involving Asian female college students taking math tests, scores could be improved by subtly triggering their Asian attribute and worsened when triggering their gender one.[34] In addition, stereotype threat can lead to disengagement of the threatened individual or group from areas that trigger the threat.

Fortunately, there are ways to avoid and decrease the impact of stereotype threat. As with implicit bias, the first step is to bring the threat to the conscious level and acknowledge its existence. The next step is to disconnect the task from the stereotype and to acknowledge that, at least in some situations, the task at hand may be challenging regardless of personal attributes. Recalling a personal experience in which a barrier was successfully overcome can help reframe the situation and facilitate self-efficacy. Similarly, seeking out others with shared attributes who have achieved a desired goal can also reinforce that success is obtainable.

ENHANCING COMMUNICATIONS AT WORK

The ability to effectively communicate with patients and team members is essential for both career advancement and patient safety. In an ideal world, we would all work in gender-intelligent organizations that prioritize cultures of safety and appreciate different communication styles.

Women Working With Men

Recognizing communication preferences among individuals in a workgroup can enhance communication. Many men prefer direct, concise communication, especially when in a meeting format. When speaking in a meeting, it may be helpful to clarify how the point being expressed is relevant to obtaining the desired goal, starting with the headline or main point, and then giving supportive data.

An area worth specific comment is the management of difficult conversations with male consultants. Due to the nature of EM, conflict is common, and having a framework to manage challenging interactions can be helpful. Start with the understanding that, although conflict may be inevitable, each participant has some control over how it is *managed*. A person can consider the conflict either as a challenge or as a threat. Choosing the former allows depersonalization of the situation. Another tip is the BRAVE pneumonic developed by Jeanette Wolfe, one of the authors of this chapter.

- *Breathe*: Take the time to exhale and help stimulate your parasympathetic nervous system.
- *Realign the conversation*: Fortunately most physicians want to deliver excellent medical care and act professionally. Acknowledging that the interaction has become challenging and that you want to reset it and refocus on shared goals can help. For example: "Wow, I think this has become a difficult conversation, as I know that we both want to do the right thing for this patient and to be professional. Do you think we could restart?"
- *Active listening*: Take the time to understand the other person's perspective. Sometimes they have new or different information that may shift decision-making.
- *Verbalize your own concerns*: Express them objectively and concisely.
- *Establish a next step*: It helps if this is time-specific to keep everyone on the same page.

Finally, because it can be challenging to find the right words in the middle of a heated disagreement, especially if there is any sense of intimidation, it can be helpful to have a few rehearsed statements on hand to increase self-efficacy, such as:

I need clarity. Please help me better understand why we are doing this.

I am concerned about your plan. Could you please clarify your thinking?

Of note, although occasional interdepartmental conflict is to be anticipated, patterns of recurrent disruptive behavior should not be tolerated as they are associated with medical error, decreased team performance, and decreased job satisfaction.[35] Repeat offenders should be appropriately reported to protect patients and other team members.

Women Working With Women

Ironically, little is written about professional conflict among women. The reasons are probably multifaceted. First, there is a misconception that women do not compete. Additionally, *indirect* aggression among women may be trivialized as it differs from traditional male direct aggression. Finally, some may also be concerned that studying conflict among women might produce data that could be misused to justify not hiring women into leadership positions.

However, how women interact with each other and their *expectations* of those interactions are different than similar content-based interactions that women have with men or men have with other men. One interesting study showed gender differences in workplace civility, with women reporting more microaggressions from other women than those reported from women/men and men/men dyads.[36] Importantly, these slight behavioral injustices were targeted more at women who acted in a traditionally more authoritarian or direct fashion.

Dr. Anne Litwin, an expert in human and organizational systems, did an international qualitative study examining women from different fields to better understand the obstacles and solutions that affect women working together. She published the results in

> **BOX 124.2 ■ EXAMPLES OF LITWIN'S "FRIENDSHIP RULES"**
>
> **Case One:** Sarah and Annie are the only two women on a hospital committee. Annie walks out of a meeting feeling blindsided because Sarah did not back her committee proposal. (Rule violation: loyalty.)
>
> To prevent the chance of being publicly blindsided, Annie could share her idea with Sarah before the meeting. Even if Sarah doesn't agree with the proposal, she could agree to professionally support Annie by ensuring that she got adequate time during the meeting to present the idea.
>
> **Case Two:** During a difficult resuscitation Annie gave clear directive orders to Maryann and corrected her when taking too long to restart CPR after a rhythm check, Annie she feels as though Maryann is giving her the cold shoulder. (Rule violation: acting hierarchical.)
>
> Annie could speak with Maryann privately and say, "I sense that code was challenging for us both. As I know that we both want to take excellent care of our patients, I'm hoping that we can talk about it so that we can work through it and continue to support each other."
>
> **Case Three:** Maryann and her friend Megan have worked together as nurses for years and are good friends. Maryann takes a new position as a charge nurse and abruptly fires a technician. Megan questions her about the details, and when Maryann says she can't tell her because it would violate employee confidentiality policies, Megan gets annoyed and thinks Maryann is taking her new position too seriously. (Rule violation: no longer sharing secrets or being professionally "equal.")
>
> Maryann could openly admit the difficult position that her new job creates and that she sincerely wants to continue her friendship with Megan but understands that there is now information that she can no longer share. Maryann might say, "This is really difficult because you are my friend, however right now I have to wear my 'professional hat' and simply cannot share specifics."

her book, *New Rules for Women*.[37] She states that, from a very early age (recall the playground example) girls develop "friendship rules" that direct the expected behavior of how they should interact with each other. These rules become problematic when women try to apply them to the workplace because the rules will predictably be broken. The rules consist of loyalty, equality, listening, sharing of secrets, and critically, the understanding that the rules shall implicitly be followed and thus are never explicitly discussed (**Box 124.2**).

Fortunately, Litwin provides concrete suggestions to help women address these professional disputes. She starts by having women normalize the realities of most workplaces, recognizing that competition, hierarchy, and difficult communications are usually inevitable. Next Litwin recommends that women commit to breaking the code of silence by directly communicating with each other and focusing on shared goals such as the desire to work in a supportive environment. These processes allow realignment after work-related conflict and further the opportunity to identify areas of shared alliance.

As the vast majority of health-care workers are women, most female physicians will be interacting with other women throughout their careers. Managing these relationships intentionally, like having a prerehearsed statement such as the following example, can help set the tone for a strong and supportive work environment:

> *When we come to work, I know that we both want to take excellent care of patients and that we both have slightly different roles within the team. Because our immediate responsibilities are different, there will be times in which our priorities will inevitably clash or be in conflict. I ask that when those situations occur that we try to commit to working through them in a direct and professional manner so that we can support each other and optimize the care of our patients.*

TABLE 124.3 ■ Tips for Women to Support Each Other in the Workplace	
General tips	• Anticipate that interpersonal conflict is inevitable. ○ Commit to addressing workplace conflicts with women directly and professionally. • Amplify another woman's good idea. • Redirect credit to a woman if her idea is being "re-presented" by a male colleague. • Support policies that increase flexibility and are family-friendly. • Encourage women to apply for high-profile committees and leadership opportunities. • Support the selection of consultants and presenters with diverse backgrounds.
Nurses/techs	• Appreciate that having different job descriptions can cause conflict due to occasional competing priorities. • Align goals such as excellent patient care and job satisfaction and commit to working together to achieve them. • Liberally use time-outs to ensure that everyone is on the same page and to open up the opportunity for all team members to voice concerns. • Sincerely recognize and validate team member efforts. • Celebrate professional wins together.
Junior faculty	• Formally welcome them. • Be flexible; women have different needs at different points in their professional careers and personal lives. • Encourage skill-based mentoring and connect them with colleagues possessing desired skills. • Invite them to accompany you to social events at outside meetings. • Publicly share their accomplishments.
Peers	• Acknowledge that competition is a reality in most workforces. • Align forces when able and be honest with each other when you can't. • Expand opportunities for skill acquisition, networking, and leadership development beyond your immediate department. • Invest in professional relationships with women outside your organization. ○ Helps foster perspective and resiliency.

Senior leadership	• Appreciate their position.
	   ○ They may be walking their own tightrope.
	• Target areas of potential collaboration.
	   ○ For example, asking for coaching on an important department presentation.
	• Identify "mutual" mentoring opportunities.
	   ○ For example, swapping technology tips for advice on grant writing.

See **Table 124.3** for more tips on how women can support other women in the workplace.

Women Working With Teams

As noted previously, running resuscitations is a challenging part of EM, and stepping into a team leadership position as a woman can be associated with additional considerations. One way to help meld a traditional masculine leadership style with a more collaborative one that many women may find more natural is the liberal use of time-outs. In this use of a time-out, the team leader briefly recaps and then outlines immediate critical actions to create a shared mental model of time-sensitive goals. Adding, "Does anyone have any questions or considerations we may have missed?" offers the opportunity for information exchange and

> **BOX 124.3 ■ THE SYRUP FEEDBACK ANALOGY**
>
> Imagine that maple syrup is feedback and that some recipients who accept the syrup like waffles and others like pancakes. The waffles accept and wall off the feedback, while the pancakes allow the syrup to spread widely. Each has its advantages and disadvantages.
>
> As the waffles see feedback as task-oriented and tied to expected behavior in expected situations, they may not generalize it to other areas in which it would also apply (e.g., being mindful of not raising one's voice when addressing a desk clerk may not generalize to similarly expected behavior involving other team members).
>
> The pancakes are much better at generalizing; however, they may be challenged by distinguishing between what they perceive to be content-based and character-based feedback (e.g., understanding the difference between not talking loudly to a patient versus being perceived as a bad person because they talked loudly to a patient). As pancakes, these feedback recipients can smear content and character together. The feedback syrup can spread far beyond its intended area to the point that it is internalized and perceived as a personal threat.

recognition that all team members are valued. Similarly, debriefings after a resuscitation can enhance effective team communication.

Giving and Receiving Feedback

Even without gender-associated dynamics, giving and receiving effective feedback can be challenging. Few clinicians have been trained in giving feedback effectively, often resulting in feedback either being given or received inappropriately, which may then cause reluctance or even avoidance of giving future feedback. Unfortunately, bringing in the added variable of gender amplifies these challenges.

Business research suggests that compared to men, women often receive more vague and less actionable feedback.[38] In addition, feedback to women who are working in more traditionally masculine roles can be heavily influenced by implicit bias. Various types of bias can lead to incongruent feedback. Some feedback to women may be further complicated because acting on it may violate a gender-expected norm. As constructive professional feedback is essential for career development, those who give and receive feedback should be given effective tools to manage the process. When contemplating feedback, it may be helpful to consider a syrup analogy (**Box 124.3**).

Feedback Example

Several excellent resources are available to improve feedback effectiveness, including the books *Thanks for the Feedback* by Stone and Heen, *Radical Candor* by Kim Scott, and an easy-to-use tool called "The Feedback Formula" developed by Lisa Stefanac (see **Box 124.4**).[38-42] Notably, all of these resources emphasize that effective feedback is closely tied into the

> **BOX 124.4 ■ FEEDBACK FORMULA[41]**
>
> - Ask permission.
> - State intention.
> - State behavior.
> - Describe impact.
> - Inquire about learner's experience.
> - Identify desire behavior.

TABLE 124.4 ■ Using Effective Feedback Tools

Concept	Language	Reasoning
Ask permission	"Hey, Josh. Do have a minute? I'd like to talk to you about something. Would now be a good time?"	People will not be receptive to feedback if it is given at an inappropriate time or inappropriate place.
State intention	"I know that you are new and have a lot going on with the transition. We are glad you are here and as we really want you to fit into our group, I'd like to give you some feedback."	Good feedback is geared toward helping an individual grow, and it is best received in situations in which they feel like they belong and that the person giving them feedback believes in their potential.
State behavior	"I noticed earlier this afternoon that you looked pretty upset and that your voice got loud when you were talking to Maryann about the urine sample."	Feedback is most effective if it is timely and based on observed, specific and objective behavior.
Describe impact	"You might not have noticed that there were other staff members and some patients who overheard your discussion with Maryann. Maryann was covering for another tech, and when you publicly criticized her, she looked upset and embarrassed. We have a hard job, but we are all a team here and it is important we support each other."	Projected impact is contextual and, depending on the scenario, may be associated with patient care, a missed deadline, etc.
Inquire about the other's experience	"Was there something that I missed?"	This allows the person receiving feedback the opportunity to share their perspectives/reflections.
Identify desired behavior	"Our techs have multiple responsibilities, if I really need a specific test quickly, I personally discuss it with them after I put in the order. On the rare occasions that there may be an unnecessary delay, I will ask to speak with the involved person privately. As our techs are often the first people who notice when a patient is getting worse, I work hard to have a good working relationship with them so that they are comfortable approaching me with issues."	Good feedback is actionable and associated with objective behaviors.

investment of relationship-building between both parties. Sarah is working with Josh and noticed that he publicly and inappropriately reprimanded a seasoned technician named Maryann for taking too long to collect a patient's urine. **Table 124.4** illustrates how Sarah might use the tools.[41]

When giving someone feedback, including a person whom you supervise, start by clarifying the intention and framing the discussion, "I'd like to give you some feedback." Anticipate that feedback sessions may become emotionally charged with participants becoming defensive, angry, or tearful. If this occurs, the person giving the feedback should consider taking a short break or scheduling a follow-up session. If no break is taken and the session continues, leaders should intentionally decide whether or not to pivot and directly address the emotional overlay as it can be extremely difficult to manage both the emotional component and the content-related substance of feedback simultaneously.

Receiving Feedback

There are tools that can help when receiving feedback (especially if one tends to receive feedback in the "pancake" category). For example, Annie recognizes that receiving feedback is extremely challenging for her. She can:

- Acknowledge that receiving feedback is difficult for a lot of people; she is not alone.
- Remind herself that feedback may provide an opportunity for significant professional growth.

- Find some way to embrace the feedback and take advantage of the opportunity.
- Appreciate that the person giving her the feedback requires a respectful response or that person might be reluctant to provide feedback in the future.
- Mentally rehearse receiving feedback and have a prepared plan or statement in case an emotional response is inadvertently triggered, for example, "I obviously have a powerful response to this information. Could we please take a 5-minute break and regroup?" or "Receiving feedback is sometimes difficult for me. However, I am committed to my own professional growth, so please continue."

Finally, when the feedback is valid and actionable, Stone and Heen, in their book *Thanks for the Feedback,* offer an excellent processing tool: the "Second Grade."[39] They suggest that receivers label the initial feedback from evaluators as the "First Grade." Although this grade can be disputed, in most situations, the perceptions of the person giving the feedback are relatively fixed, and the receiver does not have a lot of control in changing it. On the other hand, how the receiver uses the feedback for their own personal and professional growth is very much in their own power. This *effort* is the basis for this "Second Grade." Because this grade is fully dependent upon the receiver's response to the initial feedback, it can provide them with a greater sense of self-efficacy and control.

NEGOTIATION

Gender differences are particularly evident in the area of negotiation. Before discussing the differences in negotiation style, it is important to consider prequel negotiation factors that determine who engages in the negotiating process in the first place. Linda Babcock, a professor of economics at Carnegie Mellon University, has dedicated her career to researching this question and makes several observations.[43] First, women are traditionally more likely to have an *external* focus of control versus men, who have an internal (or innate) focus of control, a significant factor in self-promotion. When a person has the view that they control innate factors, such as hard work, but that promotion is controlled by an external force like a superior, the person is less likely to consider that negotiation is a viable option.

Reluctant Negotiators

Not only are women less likely to negotiate than men, they are also less likely to appreciate that a situation is actually negotiable. For example, most people know when they buy a new car that they are expected to bargain. Yet men are about four times more likely than women to consider other domains as being potentially negotiable, such as upgrading a hotel room, requesting a specific table at a restaurant, or asking for a new work computer.[43]

A study by Small et al has shown that women are much more likely to negotiate when they are given external cues that suggest that negotiation is possible and anticipated.[44] Figuring out what is truly negotiable may be difficult for women, especially if they are in predominantly male-dominated fields in which salary lines and perks may not be transparent. Men often get such information through informal networks that may be less accessible to women, leaving them at a disadvantage. **Table 124.5** suggests ways to determine when and what is negotiable.

A frequently quoted study by Babcock et al. reviewed the starting salaries of graduating business school students and found that men were going to make about $4,000 more than women.[45] Next, the graduates were asked if they had tried to negotiate their salaries. Fifty-seven percent of men versus seven percent of women said yes. Of note, this study was done in a generation of young adults who have grown up post Title IX and went to colleges

TABLE 124.5 ■ Negotiable Issues	
What is negotiable?	• Salary • Committee work • Nonclinical time • Office space/equipment • Conference fees • Administrative assistance
Sources for information	• Association of American Medical Colleges website • National salary surveys • Departmental peers • Recent hires at place that you are interviewing • Recruiters • Your current boss • Peers at national meetings • Academy of Women in Academic Emergency Medicine • American Association of Women Emergency Physicians • American College of Osteopathic Emergency Medicine • Committee for Women in Emergency Medicine • Feminem.org
Timing of negotiation	• Initial contract • Annual budget deadline • Administrative turnover • Year-end review • After an award • Around a life change

and graduate schools in which women were quite likely the majority. The underlying expectation was that they would be paid equally. It may not have occurred to them that grade point average or class standing may be less important than negotiation skills. Yet, good negotiation skills are even more relevant in a world where unions and tenure that have historically advocated for standardized benefits are slowly disappearing. Idiosyncratic deals or "I" deals describes a condition in which individual employees negotiate for conditions with their employer that are different from comparable peers.[46] "I" deals are becoming increasingly more common, and women must learn how to negotiate for them or risk greater gender benefit discrepancies. As more fellowship-trained EPs join the workforce, these types of deals will likely be more common.

Interestingly, simply using the word negotiation creates different responses from men and women. Considerable research in the area of priming has occurred in the last 20 years. Studies have shown that the word "negotiation" is subtly associated with competitiveness and maleness and consequently may subconsciously negatively prime vulnerable women and make them less likely to successfully, or even attempt to, negotiate. Simply reframing the process by substituting the literal word *negotiate* with *ask* can avert some of this negative priming. Small et al. showed in their series that simple word substitution increased a woman's likelihood to request additional money from 58% to 73%.[44] Most notably, it also erased the gender differences in the propensity to negotiate. This reframing tool, as well as using a positive priming cue, may be helpful when coaching women to negotiate.

Assertiveness, Competition, and Dominance

Unfortunately, even when women recognize what is negotiable and have the courage to assert themselves at the negotiation table, additional hurdles remain. Social theory psychology states that two of the most prescriptive stereotypes for men are competence and dominance. Traditional negotiation generally requires the negotiator to be assertive and competitive, characteristics that fall under the dominance domain. However, women who negotiate demonstrating these characteristics may be perceived more negatively than similarly qualified male negotiators. Bowles et al performed a series of experiments studying this point.[47] They gave participants written and video evaluations of job applicants, controlling for the applicant's gender and whether or not they attempted to negotiate for a better package. The study showed that male evaluators viewed women negotiators more critically than matched male negotiators. The male evaluators also perceived women who negotiated as more demanding and less likable. In other words, if Annie and Josh are equally qualified and they both use the same words in asking for the same raise, Annie risks being perceived more negatively than Josh because her behavior is violating gender rules.

Bridging the Negotiating Gap

So how do women overcome this dilemma? Linda Babcock described a series of workshops and classes at Heinz Graduate School that were aimed at giving women more tools surrounding negotiation. She reported that the percentage of graduating women who negotiated their first job offers went from 12.5% in 2002 to 68%, and their starting salaries increased by 14%.[43,45]

Ultimately, mitigating the negotiation gap between men and women requires engagement from both parties at the table. Organizations and administrators need to acknowledge that the process and risks for negotiation are gender- and situation-specific and that seemingly small salary gaps can lead to large inequities over time. Organizations that encourage "I" deals and expect negotiation as necessary for professional advancement should formalize this as a policy. Managers should be educated that negotiation should be encouraged and expected from both genders to help prevent unconscious backlash against female negotiators. In addition, managers should be accountable for the professional development and advancement of all of their department's members. When gender trends in promotion or salary emerge, the root causes of these differences should be sought out, explored, and rectified. Women in such organizations should be coached on negotiating.

An alternative approach to organizational negotiation is to minimize it by standardizing expectations. This model is more aligned with the traditional tenure "publish or perish" contract, in which transparent and objective criteria are used in conjunction with an expected time frame for advancement. At first glance, this model appears to be more gender-neutral, as it eliminates the expectation of formal negotiation. However, unconscious gender bias can still occur as women are less likely to self-promote their projects and may be less aware of or familiar with how to obtain resources to keep them on track with comparable male colleagues. Coaching women and managers about expectations and tracking allocations can help eliminate these differences.

Women may also be successful in negotiation if they focus on "expand the pie" negotiation techniques. In traditional win-lose or competitive negotiation scenarios, the negotiator is competing for a "slice of the pie," where what is negotiated is specific and limited to a particular domain or resource. For example, a negotiator may say, "I want you to pay me $100,000 or I'll take a different job." In an "expand the pie" or collaborative negotiation, a series of considerations, some clearly benefiting the negotiator, others the employer, are on the table. The final package is created by collaboration, which better aligns with most women's communication styles, and avoids the potential for subtle gender backlash.[48]

GENDER DIFFERENCES IN PHYSICIAN SALARY

> *If you take men and women physicians who have the same length of training, the same kind of training, have the same kind of CV publications, even have the same grants from the National Institute of Health, work in the same field, with the same exact time parameters—and you do a multivariate analysis with all things being equal, women are still being paid significantly less.*
>
> —Sareh Parangi, an endocrine surgeon at Massachusetts General Hospital[49]

The logistics of finance and physician reimbursement are quite heterogeneous in the field of medicine. Multiple factors besides specialty, benefits, hours worked, and number of patients seen influence salary structure. These include board certification, academic versus community practice, experience, practice type (independent contractor, hospital employee, or group member), partner or tenure status, Medicaid mix, location, and acuity.

Because so many variables influence a physician's annual salary, it can be difficult to figure out if and how gender plays a role. However, mounting evidence, such as that described by Parangi, demonstrates that even when the above variables are considered, a gender disparity remains in physician income and advancement. According to a Medscape analysis of pay gaps among men and women physicians, on average, male specialists and primary care physicians were paid $89,000 and $52,000 more per year, respectively.[50] A 2017 study looking at academic emergency physicians suggested that, even after adjusting for significant variables including years of practice, rank, experience, clinical hours, core faculty status, administrative roles, and fellowship training, the mean salary for women was almost $20,000 less than it was for men.[51]

In a 2008 Board of Trustees policy statement, the American Medical Association (AMA) systematically reviewed the research in this area and concluded that gender disparities remain and that the root causes are likely a combination of subtle micro-inequities and residual gender discrimination and bias. According to the AMA:

> *. . . examples include assigning women in disproportionate numbers to clinical positions that offer little hope of academic advancement; attitudes that categorize pregnancy as a disservice to the department, discouraging women from entering certain fields by questioning their stamina, or disparaging their professional commitment because of their family responsibilities.*[52]

In addition, Lo Sasso et al did a study of graduating New York state residents, and after controlling for such factors as specialty, practice setting, hours worked, and location, there was an unexplained starting salary difference greater than $16,000 between male and female physicians.[53]

How does EM fare in gender disparities? Direct comparison, even in a specialty with relatively straightforward shift work, remains difficult. Besides the above-mentioned variables, there is also the consideration of shift differentials for nights and weekends and how an organization accounts for nonclinical professional responsibilities. For example, it is difficult to directly compare a full-time Kaiser emergency physician (EP) in California to a full-time nocturnist independent contractor in Cape Cod, Massachusetts to an academic EP in Michigan who does research. Demonstrating this point, a 2010 study reviewed 15 different 2009 EP salary surveys and showed that the reported average salary ranged anywhere from $239,000 to $316,000, depending on the specific survey.[54]

Further complicating salary discrepancies are additional potential gender-specific factors. Clem and Wolfe noted that salary, in and by itself, may not be as important a factor for women EPs as men when narrowing down job options. Women may be more likely to consider things like collegiality, flexible scheduling, and the ability for long-term advancement when choosing a job.[55,56] With all these considerations, it may be tempting to conveniently discredit studies that display EP gender disparities. Unfortunately, this would be premature as it is increasingly clear that significant gender pay gaps exist in medicine, including EM. A 2019 study of emergency academic physicians by Wiler et al. demonstrated the persistence of a pay gap of $12,000 after controlling for a myriad of variables.[57] Importantly, over a career these slight differences can add up to significant amounts of money and impact retirement savings.[58]

It is important to note that even though some women may choose a job based on factors other than salary alone, their expectation is that in that job they will be paid equitably and be given appropriate professional advancement opportunities. Clem explains that both of these factors are directly related to long-term female EP career satisfaction.[55]

Self-Promotion

As with negotiation, some baseline gender differences appear to exist in the area of self-promotion. Men are often more attuned to rank and hierarchy and more comfortable with self-promoting for committee and promotion consideration. This is confounded by gender-influenced optimism in expected performance. Males may overestimate their perceived abilities, while females may underestimate their own skill set. This was shown nicely in a recent surgical laparoscopic simulation evaluation in which, although there was no difference in objective surgical skills noted in the test, men reported a higher anticipated performance than women.[59]

Women wait to be asked. They believe that if they do their jobs well, and concentrate 100% of their effort on that job, their work will be validated and rewarded by their superiors. In an interview by Dee Dee Myers for her book *Why Women Should Rule the World*, Judith McHale comments on some of her experiences as former CEO of Discovery Communications.[60] Discovery had a policy of posting new positions internally prior to an external search, and McHale was confused when no internal female candidates showed an interest in a prestigious programming position. She investigated and found a universal female thread: women assumed that if they were good enough for the job, they would have been invited to apply.

There also appears to be a gender difference related to how men and women accept and solicit credit for their work. Myers also interviewed Shirley Tilghman, president of Princeton University, who shared a story about two incoming freshmen, a man and a woman, who both had won Westinghouse Science Project Awards. When asked about their projects, Tilghman described the young man's response. He said, "Oh yeah, I had this great project, and it was really exciting and the judges loved it." The young woman, however, consciously downplayed her award, saying, "I was so surprised. I didn't think my project was that great." Similarly, Myers writes about a woman chief operating officer who had just presented at her first board meeting. After the meeting, she was advised by the CEO to substitute the "we's" in her presentation with "I's" at future meetings.

Ironically, many women's ability to redirect their limelight and work collaboratively with their colleagues may ultimately make them good transformational leaders. But, in the short run, it may slow their professional advancement. Women may erroneously assume that their directors are fully aware of their accomplishments, while their busy male director, used to self-promotion, may fail to appreciate this gender difference and mistakenly assume the woman physician is content with the status quo. This mismatch of expectations may lead to career stalling or turnover. Clem showed that validation and opportunity for professional advancement are considered two of the major job satisfiers for female EPs. If they do not receive validation and advancement at their current positions, they may look elsewhere.[55] Importantly, when women do leave, they often imply they are leaving for work–life choices, when in reality they are leaving due to an organizational culture in which they do not feel professionally accepted and validated.[61]

Women are also more likely to be promoted after they have *already acquired* the necessary skill set to succeed in a new position, whereas men are often promoted for their *potential to* rapidly acquire new skills on the job. According to research at Hewlett Packard, women did not apply for a job opening unless they had 100% of the requirements of the listing, while men often applied when they only had 60%.[62]

To quote another study, "On the same project, the men will demonstrate 100% ambition even if they only have 50% of the required skills, whereas the women will be concerned about only having 80% of the required skills."[63]

Recruiting

Issues in recruiting start with who is invited to interview. A search committee consisting of only men is likely to recruit the same. This is the implicit bias associated with perceived commonalities. Ensuring that a group has at least 30% women will change the group's dynamic and help avoid selection bias.[4]

Where and how an individual is recruited also affects the applicant pool. Word-of-mouth and certain recruiting venues may subtly favor men. In addition, the recruiting ad itself may include wording or pronouns that discourage women. When trying to recruit a qualified high-level executive, search committees who are interested in creating diversity and gender balance may need to expand beyond their typical search patterns by considering hiring a search firm or directly soliciting qualified women. In addition, if an applicant pool consists of at least 25% women, a woman is more likely to get hired.[64]

Curriculum Vitae and Letters of Recommendation

Trix and Psenka reviewed 300 letters of recommendations for hired faculty members at major US medical schools.[65] They found that letters written for men were more likely to be longer and to include more information about their objective accomplishments, including research and publications. Letters for women were less record-focused and more likely to comment on communication skills. In addition, men's letters were likely to include more standout adjectives and fewer doubt-raisers.

An individual's curriculum vitae (CV) may also be evaluated differently based on their gender. In the Steinpreis et al's[66] study, CVs were sent to randomly selected male and female psychologists. The psychologists were given identical CVs that bore either the name "Karen Miller" or "Brian Miller" and were asked about their qualifications. Psychologists, regardless of their gender, evaluated "Brian's" CV more positively. A similar 2012 study sent identical CVs to managers from either "John" or "Jennifer." Male applicants were viewed as more competent and hirable and more likely to be offered higher starting salaries and faculty mentoring.[67] In addition, Correll et al asked research participants to evaluate the hiring potential of two candidates who were equally matched, except one was a parent and the other one was not. They found that mothers, but not fathers, were rated as less competent candidates.[68]

The Interview

Unchecked, the perception of a candidate during an interview can be heavily influenced by implicit bias. In a classic study, Goldin and Rouse studied this phenomenon during orchestra auditions.[69] The audition is critical to obtaining a position and historically most positions were offered to men. In the 1980s, many large orchestras required blind auditions in which musicians played behind a partition. These blind auditions led to 50% more women getting past the first round and increased the overall percentage of hired women by 25%.[69]

Can inadvertent human bias during the interview process be minimized? Among the most promising suggestions are requirements for all members of the interview panel to undergo implicit bias training and interviewing best practices training.[70-72] In particular, interviewers should:

- be taught that unchecked gut feelings can be heavily influenced by implicit bias;
- use behavioral and situational questions (e.g., "What would you do if a patient became upset if you declined to prescribe them an opioid?"), which can increase reliability and validity of the evaluations;
- understand organizational policies and employment laws to ensure they are not inadvertently violating either of them by asking applicants about pregnancy, children, or marital status.[73]

Conversely, clearly messaging the organization's family-friendly policies can be an important recruiting tool for both women and men. Many of the practices suggested by the AAMC's Best Practices for Residency Interviews could be easily modified to help create standardized questions for EP interviews.[74]

Promotions

As stated earlier, women are less likely to self-promote and are more likely to be penalized by implicit bias, both of which can stall their professional careers. Wright et al surveyed medical school faculty about their attitudes, experiences, and goals.[75] They found no gender differences in leadership self-assessments or desire to take on time-consuming tasks. Women, however, were less likely to be asked to serve as section head or committee chair or participate in decisions over advancement and resource allocation.

Managers should be cognitive of the possible tendency to prematurely exclude a female candidate based on assumptions. For example, when looking for a new emergency medical services director, a candidate who had a baby a few months ago may be prematurely dismissed from consideration due to an assumption that she would not want to travel several times a month for regional meetings. This assumption may or may not be correct but can only be determined by directly asking.

Awards

Bias can exist when considering recognition awards, especially if the award criteria are subjectively based. Abbuhl et al studied all awards given at University of Pennsylvania by department, then compared the gender ratio of the departments to the gender ratio of the awards.[76] Their study found that when the award was based on objective criteria (publications, grants) that they roughly matched the department's gender ratio. However, when the awards were more loosely based, like "Best Clinician," men were far more likely to be recipients. This study emphasizes the importance of making qualifications for awards and selections as specific and as objective as possible.

DEVELOPING A GENDER-INTELLIGENT AND NEURODIVERSE INITIATIVE

To ensure gender equity progress, institutional solutions need to be developed that support inclusive and supportive environments along with opportunities for women to build their skills.

—Darrell G. Kirch, MD, President Emeritus of AAMC[77]

Organizations that invest in the creation of neurodiverse, gender-intelligent teams will become more competitive and better places to work. The first step in moving an organization in this direction is to appreciate that half-hearted efforts geared at satisfying quotas and photo opportunities will fail. A successful initiative is driven by the authentic belief that it will make an organization stronger. Fortunately, there are a growing number of resources, several specific to EM, that can be used as guides to help organizations move forward.[17,20,61,73,74,75,76,78-83]

To begin, it may be helpful to collect specific organizational data related to hiring, advancement, and transitions (**Box 124.7**). These data can clarify whether a promotion, salary increase, hour reduction, committee assignment, and so on, occurred because of a specific qualification or skill, or alternatively, it might provide a hint to hidden organizational bias. It is not uncommon for leaders to sincerely believe that they are making merit-based and gender-blind decisions only to have their own organization data reveal patterns of subtle but pervasive gender inequities. Some organizations have sought to address their initially misguided efforts:

> *We assumed that women were leaving to have children and stay home. If there was a problem at all, it was society's or the women's, not Deloitte's. In fact, most senior partners firmly believed we were doing everything possible to retain women. We prided ourselves on our open, collegial, performance-based work environment. How wrong we were, and how far we've come.*[84]

Thus, these baseline data are necessary to make an objective and convincing case that opportunities for organizational improvement exist. Reveal the opportunity for cost saving measures. For example, if it is noted that there is a particularly high attrition rate for female physicians, investing in a new initiative that fosters inclusivity may ultimately save the group hundreds of thousands of dollars by decreasing recruiting and onboarding costs.

The next step is to survey the current milieu of the organization to understand how much effort will be required to get buy-in. As both honesty and confidentiality are important, institutions may consider hiring outside consultants to assess the organization and its employees. Ideally, those sampled should include all of the executive branch, senior women, and a representative group of middle managers and new hires.

Wittenberg-Cox notes that the men in organizations will likely fall into three groups: progressive, neutral, or plodding.[20,78]

- Men in the *progressive* group have either worked in an environment that has successfully integrated women or have personal experiences that validate the unique and economically competitive role that women bring to an organization. These men will be champions of a successful initiation.
- Men in the *neutral* group generally support gender balance and may point to examples of where gender diversity is already visible and successful. Their belief is that the company is already headed in the right direction and that everyone just needs to be patient. This group will likely represent the swing vote in any initiative.

- The *plodders* are men who like the status quo (or even miss the old days.) They discard the benefits of gender balance and are suspicious that any initiative is just a well-disguised HR quota to help make the company look more politically correct. It is important to identify this group, as they will be most resistant to change and may try to sabotage the effort.

Women within the group may also have varying degrees of interest in participating in a new initiative, especially in the early stages of development. This is because many women have been involved in previous programs directed to "helping" women that have had limited success or worse, backfired and marginalized them. In addition, senior women may be particularly leery of anything that sniffs of tokenism, so messaging and marketing the initiative are important. Labeling the process as enhancing neurodiversity in leadership or as an initiative to create more competitive gender-intelligent teams may help facilitate greater organizational buy-in.

Once specific industry data and internal organizational qualitative and quantitative information are known, senior leadership, if not already involved, should be brought up to date. Leaders must be authentically convinced that investing in a long-term initiative is a fundamental business decision that will make the organization more innovative, competitive, and profitable or the project will have a greater likelihood of failure. Any program that doesn't have top-level support will fail. For example, a significant key to the success of Massachusetts's Institute of Technology's (MIT's) gender equity program in which they dramatically increased the number of tenured women in science was the early support of the dean of science and MIT's president. "I have always believed that contemporary gender discrimination within universities is part reality and part perception . . . but I now understand that reality is by far the greater part of the balance."[85]

Next, it is important to thoughtfully select the initiative's chair. At first glance, a diversity manager from HR or a respected senior woman may be obvious choices. Another alternative is to appoint a politically savvy man who may have greater influence in successfully recruiting additional men in the "swing votes" category to buy into the initiative.[20,78] This value of this choice is underscored by a recent study that suggests that women who advocate for leadership diversity are often looked upon as less competent that men who advocate for it.[86] **Box 124.5** provides a list of how men can support female colleagues.

BOX 124.5 ■ WAYS THAT MEN CAN HELP WOMEN ADVANCE

- Recognize that very real challenges still exist for many female colleagues.
- Take the Harvard IAT test on gender, and learn about implicit bias.
- Encourage data collection to access current gender-based departmental metrics.
- Increase gender diversity on committees.
- Support structured interviewing processes.
- Encourage development and funding of women's professional development groups.
- Increase gender diversity in outside speakers and consultants.
- Include diverse images of patients and providers in your own presentations.
- Develop formalized mentoring and sponsorship programs.
- Invite women to participate in your projects.
- Introduce women to individuals in your extended network at conferences.
- Support policies that provide flexible scheduling and meeting options.
- Push for pay transparency.
- Share your understanding of organizational negotiation.
- Encourage the development and use of family-friendly policies.
- Normalize and encourage the use of maternity and paternity leave.

The individual who leads this initiative must be supportive; the neurodiversity chair (NDC) must have broad support throughout the organization and be given leadership of an interdepartmental team that includes men, women, and nonbinary individuals. The team's primary responsibility is to consistently educate and engage employees concerning the economic and long-term value of investing in gender intelligent policies. Significant focus will be required for individuals in mid-managerial positions, as they are often the ones who make the decisions that are most influential to women during critical junctures in their early and mid-careers.

It is important that middle managers have the motivation and the tools to identify and prepare talented women for greater leadership roles by facilitating opportunities (committees, networks, and sponsors) that can lead to professional growth and organizational value. Ultimately, middle managers should be accountable for this facilitation in their own annual evaluations. The NDC will also be responsible for tracking data analyses, spotlighting successes, and working with resistant outliers. It is imperative that the NDC has ongoing access to the CEO and other powerful stakeholders to ensure the initiative remains a priority over the long haul to the organization. For a program to be successful, the initiative will require time and dedicated resources that include support for educational and training programs geared toward mitigating implicit bias and addressing gender-based differences in communication.

Professional Women's Groups

Historically, when organizations have tried to increase the number of women in leadership roles, they often encouraged the development of formal or informal women's groups. The oversimplified belief was that women would compete better in a male organization if they simply learned to act more like men. Now, as more organizations recognize the economic and innovative advantage that women, *as women*, can bring to an organization, the role of these groups has evolved. When appropriately developed and supported, professional women's groups (PWGs) offer great value to both individual women and their organizations. However, they must be viewed as just *one part* of a larger organizational initiative rather than the entirety of the initiative itself.

Professional women's groups offer a forum to learn new skills like negotiating or understanding larger operational issues, as well as offering unique opportunities for networking, support, and sharing of best practices and professional collaborations. (For guidance on how to start a PWG, see **Box 124.6**) Availability of PWG's is helpful throughout a woman's career from medical school through retirement, especially if they have programs dedicated to issues associated with those different career points. If organizational circumstances prohibit the development of a PWG in-house, women can still benefit from networking and mentoring at regional and national leadership seminars like Females Working in Emergency Medicine's Idea Exchange or by joining a national PWG like the Academy of Women in Academic Emergency Medicine or the American Association of Women Emergency Physicians.

Mentoring and Sponsorship

The concept of mentoring has evolved over the past two decades. Rather than seeking out a single individual to be an all-encompassing mentor, women are now encouraged to intentionally create mentoring teams. Women should define skills that they would like to develop, such as grant-writing or creating an effective lecture, and then approach individuals who have mastered these skills for mentorship. A good mentor shares their

> **BOX 124.6 ■ STARTING A PROFESSIONAL WOMEN'S GROUP**
>
> **Form a steering committee:**
> - Perform a assessment to identify unique organizational opportunities.
>
> **Develop mission statement that includes:**
> - Vision of group
> - Recognition and alignment of organizational goals
> - Trackable metrics
> - Identification of stakeholders and champions
>
> **Create infrastructure:**
> - Develop bylaws.
> - Establish core committees.
> - Secure funding.
> - Formalize organizational sponsorship.
>
> **Develop programming considering:**
> - Universal skills
>   - negotiation
>   - networking
>   - communication/conflict resolution
>   - CV development
>   - promotion requirements
>   - mentoring/sponsorship
> - Content specific to women at a particular rank or life stage
> - Traditional and nontraditional formats
> - Varied scheduling
> - The dissemination of content to members
>
> **Amplify:**
> - Publicly recognize accomplishments of members.
> - Nominate women for awards.
> - Highlight programming pearls.
>
> **Network:**
> - Connect with other professional women's organizations.
> - Share content and best practices.
> - Integrate programming.
> - Create speaking opportunities for members.
> - Partner for projects and research.
>
> **Formalize leadership succession:**
> - Create long-term sustainability.
> - Stimulate continued adaption and growth.

experience with a mentee. Although they overlap, sponsorship is slightly different from traditional mentorship in that a sponsor is an individual who has organizational *power and influence* which they ideally can utilize to advocate for their mentee. As professor and author Herminia Ibarra says, "While a mentor is someone who has knowledge and will share it with you, a sponsor is a person who has power and will use it for you."[87]

In a recent article for Harvard Business School, Ibarra suggests expanding the mentor/sponsor continuum to include several other potential advisors.[87] She includes a strategizer (someone with access to inside information and policies), a connector (someone with influential networks who is willing to make introductions), and an opportunity-giver (someone who has the ability to create a high profile experience). This approach may help women be more intentional in their professional development and to encourage them to seek out individuals who share different life experiences than themselves.

Finally, any long-term organizational initiative requires continued evaluation and honing. For example, 20 years ago when MIT invested in an initiative to address its significant gender inequities, one of the changes advocated for the inclusion of at least one woman to be on every committee. Ultimately, this led to some women having to sit on numerous committees which began putting a strain on the time they had available to do their own research. Being adaptive to these issues will help keep initiatives move forward. For real-life examples of successful implementation of these types of programs, see the Medtronic's initiative that won the 2020 Catalyst Award and MIT's Gender Equity Project (**Table 124.6**).[79,82,88]

TABLE 124.6 ■ MIT Gender Equity Project[72]

In 1999, MIT made public the findings and recommendations of a committee charged with studying gender equity issues in its School of Science:

- Percentage of female faculty in science had remained 8% for 20 years.
- Inequities were found in teaching assignments, salary distribution, university awards and distinctions, and committee representation.
- Women, especially senior women, felt marginalized and excluded from important committees and department and university leadership roles.
- Women felt challenged to meet work/family commitments.

Summary of committee recommendations:

- Resources
- Yearly review of salary lines and resource equity
    - Correct discovered inequities
- Access to power
    - Facilitate direct dialogue with women faculty and their heads/deans.
    - Hold individuals accountable for discriminatory practices.
- Conscious awareness
    - Promote awareness around gender equity.
    - Consciously voice that women with children are capable of achieving on par with men and childless women.
- Recruiting
    - Consciously remind departmental heads that effective recruitment of women requires a continuous conscious effort.
- Place women on search committee.
- Recognize and advance qualified internal women candidates.
    - *Female faculty applicants reviewed by dean's office*
    - *Education sessions about unconscious bias*
    - *Conscious techniques to increase pool of women applicants*

Professional development:

- Recognize and prevent the marginalization of senior women.
- Proactively involve junior female faculty with senior women and departmental heads to prevent isolation.
- Appoint qualified women to influential positions like heads and chairs of important thesis and grant committees.
    - *Educating departmental heads about the threat of marginalization*
    - *Pamphlet to standardize mentoring expectations*

Work/life issues:

- Develop and support uniform maternity leave and tenure programs.
- Address work-life issues within MIT to make it more competitive in attracting qualified women.
    - *Parental release of one term after birth/adoption*
    - *One-year tenure extension for birth of child*
    - *Emergency daycare*
    - *Help with work-related travel childcare expenses*
    - *Onsite daycare*

10-year update results:

- *Resources*: More gender-equitable distribution of resources
    - Effective mechanisms to discovered inequities
- *Awareness*: More acceptance of women in leadership
    - Recognition of the need to consciously recruit women

(Continued)

TABLE 124.6 ■ (Continued)

Recruiting:
- Women faculty in science increased from 8% to 20%
- Female MIT president
- Two female academic deans
- One female associate dean
- Two female department heads

Professional development:
- More uniform mentoring
- Assessable network to leadership

Work-life issues:
- Removed stigma associated with being a scientist and a parent

*Specific actions MIT took to advance initiative are italicized.

Part-Time and Flexible Scheduling

When promoting a neurodiverse or gender equitable initiative, it is important to message that work flexibility issues impact all employees:

> We have little or no trouble recruiting talented women. The challenge is providing them with a career that allows them to balance personal and professional ambitions. When we figure it out for women we will have created a better workplace for all employees, the men included. It's not about working less hard. It's about taking the shackles off and letting smart, ambitious people decide how best to work.[20]

Although it is likely that more women will utilize part-time options, having flexibility over one's schedule has become an increasing priority for most workers, and schedule flexibility is likely a main driver behind why many individuals chose EM in the first place.

Groups that recognize the importance of flexible scheduling and try to make reasonable schedule accommodations are likely to have a significant advantage in recruiting and retaining their workforce. For employees who desire to work full-time, often scheduling is the impeding factor. Returning to the idea of expanding the pie negotiation, there are some creative ways to meet a physician's individual needs while still fulfilling the department's scheduling demands such as by job-sharing or reducing clinical hours for nocturnal shifts.

A 2016 Boston Physician Foundation survey of over 17,000 physicians found that nearly 70% of respondents expressed a desire to change their employment status within three years by reducing their clinical hours, going part-time, working locum tenens, or finding an alternative employment situation.[89] Cejka Search recruiters noted that after women with young children, men nearing retirement were the largest growing sector of physicians looking for alternative scheduling.[90] These changes reflect the fact that many physicians desire to define themselves beyond their medical degree.

Achieving Work-Life Balance

Along with scheduling, groups should consider other innovative benefits that may promote career progression and work–life balance. For example, Stanford University's emergency department piloted a time-banking program. In this program, picking up a shift or teaching a class for a colleague provides credits. These credits can be used to pay for dry cleaning, grocery delivery, home cleaning, and even academic assistance, such as manuscript editing and grant writing.[91]

Many academic institutions allow a tenure track pause for 1 to 3 years following the birth of a child.[92] A tenure track pause should be available to all new parents, including men, adoptive parents, and gender-nonbinary parents. When tenure track pause is only available to women, it promotes the stereotype that childrearing is the sole responsibility of female parents. Expanding the reasons for a pause promotes overall wellness, retains talent, and may increase acceptance within institutions. Examples of other reasons for a tenure pause may include personal illness, family illness, or bereavement.

In many ways, EM is ideally set up for flexibility thanks to the nature of the work. Emergency physicians get to see the same proportion of acuity and mix of patients whether they work 15 shifts a month or 10. This is not the case in many other medical specialties. Surgery in particular has been resistant to the development of anything but full-time work scheduling. Many specialists who try to cut back their hours are often faced with subtle discrimination and resentment as they buck the traditional mentality embraced by many older partners. This can lead to the assignment of a less desirable patient and procedural load and the loss of networking and professional development opportunities. Ultimately the individual may grow resentful (ironically actually reinforcing the negative part-time stereotype) and may consider quitting medicine altogether.

Given the unique nature of EM, it is important to develop objective policies that clearly delineate scheduling and financial logistics. In addition, it is important for group leaders to set a tone of departmental acceptance and encouragement toward physicians who choose to use these policies. A 2011 *Emergency Physicians Monthly* readers' survey revealed that women who choose to go part-time may face subtle bias that their part-time male peers do not. Women EPs were more likely than men to report that cutting back their hours negatively affected their professional reputation (23% vs 15%) and limited their ability to achieve their long-term professional goals (20% vs 0%).[56] As validation and the ability to work toward professional aspirations are tied into women EPs' career satisfaction scores, it is important for directors to acknowledge the potential for marginalization of women who choose to work less than full-time. Engagement and validation will increase job satisfaction and loyalty.[55]

Ways to keep part-time employees involved and to visibly reinforce their value to the full-time employees include having part-timers serve on key committees, including them in recruiting (happy women recruit other happy women), promoting their own professional development goals even if they need to be time adjusted for reduced hours, and giving them equitable departmental resources to help accomplish them.

Finally, a few things are important to discuss with women who are thinking about cutting back their hours. The first is to encourage them to consciously develop and describe their long-term career goals. Many women choose to detour off the linear trajectory career path by sequencing their work with home commitments. It is important to remind them that a lot can be accomplished over the decades of a professional life with a little support and planning. Having long-term professional goals and access to mentors can help women stay on track.[93]

Parental Leave

As with flextime in general, taking the time to develop objective transparent parental leave policies is crucial to individual and group morale. If policies are haphazardly patched together or if they exist "only on paper," individuals who try and use them may find themselves ostracized. In addition, the wide variation in family leave policies, with many offering little or no time off for nonbirthing parents, creates potential bias and can even make an organization vulnerable to legal action.[94]

Policies that favor maternal time off may inadvertently send a message that child-rearing is the role of women. It is important that departmental directors set a tone of acceptance and encouragement during parental leaves. Realistically, parental leave represents only a very brief time in a provider's long professional career. Employers that support their providers during this critical time will likely be rewarded by that provider's increased productivity and wellness upon their return to work as well as their increased loyalty to the group.[95]

CONCLUSION

Emergency departments are positively impacted by diverse teams. Women are often more collaborative, process-oriented, and more tolerant of short-term sacrifices for long-term gains. These are important attributes when building health-care teams. Significant gender-based differences continue to adversely affect advancement opportunities and compensation for women in medicine. Women face implicit bias, the competency hurdle, suboptimal feedback, and the stereotype threat that impact their ability to succeed in the workplace. Emergency departments that want to grow and retain the best leaders will commit to comprehensive strategies to address these issues. Additionally, women benefit from tailored professional development programs designed to mitigate some of the pervasive gender bias still present in the workplace.

The gender pay gap is a persistent problem, including in EM. Best practices to address the pay gap include clear and transparent communication regarding compensation for all work (clinical, administrative, education, and research). Parental leave, flexible scheduling, and options to go part-time for *all* EPs are important strategies to neutralize the criticism that women receive more workplace benefits related to parenting, which also perpetuates gender stereotypes. These strategies are also necessary to increase retention and advancement of women EPs.

REFERENCES

1. Ghosn C. Closing the gender gap in Japan, the car industry and the world. World Economic Forum. 2015. Available at: https://www.weforum.org/agenda/2015/01/closing-the-gender-gap-in-japan-the-car-industry-and-the-world/. Accessed October 28, 2020.
2. Hoogendoorn S, Oosterbeek H, van Praag M. The impact of gender diversity on the performance of business teams: evidence from a field experiment. *Manag Sci*. 2013;59(7):1514–1528.
3. Gloor JL, Morf M, Paustian-Underdahl S, et al. Fix the game, not the dame: restoring equity in leadership evaluations. *J Bus Ethics*. 2020;161(3):497–511.
4. McKinsey and Company: Delivering on Diversity. 2018. Available at: https://www.mckinsey.com/~/media/mckinsey/business%20functions/organization/our%20insights/delivering%20through%20diversity/delivering-through-diversity_full-report.ashx Accessed May 24, 2020.
5. Ishrak O. Rooted in our mission. International Women's Day. Available at: https://www.internationalwomensday.com/Activity/14153/Rooted-in-our-mission. Updated 2020. Accessed October 28, 2020.
6. AAMC: 2019 Fall Applicant, Matriculant, and Enrollment Data Table. Available at: https://www.aamc.org/system/files/2019-12/2019%20AAMC%20Fall%20Applicant%2C%20Matriculant%2C%20and%20Enrollment%20Data%20Tables_0.pdf. Accessed May 25, 2020.
7. AAMC: Table B3: Number of Active Residents, by Type of Medical School, GME Specialty, and Sex (2017-2018). Available at: https://www.aamc.org/data-reports/students-residents/interactive-data/table-b3-number-active-residents-type-medical-school-gme-specialty-and-sex. Accessed May 25, 2020.
8. AAMC: U.S. Medical School Faculty by Sex, Rank, and Department. Available at: https://www.aamc.org/system/files/2020-01/2019 Table13.pdf. Accessed May 25, 2020.
9. Bennett C, Raja A, Kapoor N, et al. Gender differences in faculty rank among academic emergency physicians in the United States. *Acad Emerg Med*. 2019;26(3):281–285.
10. Boyle P. Faculty salaries rise 2.3%, and new data spotlight gender gap. 2020. Available at: https://www.aamc.org/news-insights/faculty-salaries-rise-23-and-new-data-spotlight-gender-gap. Accessed May 25, 2020.
11. Mackay R. Let's change the girls play flue boy's bash drums stereotype. The Conversation. 2019. Available at: https://phys.org/news/2019-08-girls-flute-boys-bash-stereotypes.html. Accessed June 9, 2020.
12. Violante C. Every Cell has a Sex and the Future of Health Care 2016 Yale School of Medicine blog. Available at: https://medicine.yale.edu/news-article/13321/. Accessed August 23, 2020.
13. Wolfe J, Snedaker K, Raukar N. Episode 7 Part 1: Concussions. Available at: https://www.sexandwhy.com/sex-why-episode-7-part-1-concussions/. Accessed August 23, 2020.
14. Ingalhalikar M, Smith A, Parker D, et al. Sex differences in the structural connectome of the human brain. *Proc Natl Acad Sci U S A*. 2014;111(2):823–828.

15. Seo D, Ahluwalia A, Potenza MN, et al. Gender differences in neural correlates of stress-induced anxiety. *J Neurosci Res.* 2017;125:115–125.
16. Sax L. *Why Gender Matters.* 2nd ed. Harmony; 2017.
17. Gurian M, Annis B. *Leadership and the Sexes: Using Gender Science to Create Success in Business.* San Francisco, Calif: Jossey-Bass Publishers; 2008.
18. Beneson J. *Warriors and Worriers: The Survival of the Sexes.* :Oxford University Press; 2014.
19. Annis B. *Same Words, Different Language: An Updated Guide for Improved Gender Intelligence at Work.* 2nd ed. Alpharetta, Ga: BookLogix; 2011.
20. Wittenberg-Cox A, Maitland A. *Why Women Mean Business.* Hoboken, NJ: Wiley; 2009:156.
21. Project Implicit®. Available at: https://implicit.harvard.edu/implicit/. Accessed May 25, 2020.
22. Gender Career Test. Gender-Career IAT, Harvard. Available at: implicit.harvard.edu/implicit/user/agg/blindspot/indexgc.htm. Accessed August 20.2020.
23. Lautenberger D. Understanding Unconscious Bias in the Health Professions and How to Mitigate It. AAMC. 2019. Available at: https://www.aamc.org/system/files/2020-01/profdev-affinity-groups-gip-understanding-unconscious-bias-webinar-013120.pdf. Accessed August 23, 2020.
24. Rhee K, Sigler T. Untangling the relationship between gender and leadership. *Gender Manag.* 2015;30(2):109–134
25. Abele A. The Dynamics of masculine-agentic and feminine-communal traits: findings from a prospective study. *J Pers Soc Psychol.* 2003;85(4):768–776.
26. Meier A, Yang J, Liu J, et al. Female physician leadership during cardiopulmonary resuscitation is associated with improved patient outcomes. *Crit Care Med.* 2019;47(1):e8–e13.
27. Kolehmainen C, Brennan M, Filut A, et al. Afraid of being "Witchy with a 'b'": a qualitative study of how gender influences residents' experiences leading cardiopulmonary resuscitation. *Acad Med.* 2014;89(9):1276–1281.
28. Linden JA, Breaud AH, Mathews J, et al. The intersection of gender and resuscitation leadership experience in emergency medicine residents. *AEM Educ Train.* 2018; 2(2):162–168.
29. Dayal A, O'Connor DM, Qadri U, et al. Comparison of male vs female resident milestone evaluations by faculty during emergency medicine residency training. *JAMA Intern Med.* 2017;177(5):651–657.
30. Mueller AS, Jenkins T, Osborne M, et al. Gender differences in attending physicians' feedback to residents. Qualitative analysis. *J Grad Med Educ.* 2017;9(5):577–585.
31. MacNell L, Driscoll A, Hunt A. What's in a name: exposing gender bias in student ratings of teaching. *Innovat High Educ.* 2015;40:291–303.
32. Nguyen H, Ryan H. Does stereotype threat affect test performance of minorities and women? A meta-analysis of experimental evidence. *J Appl Psychol.* 2008;93(6):1314–1334.
33. Burgess D, Warren Phelan S, Dovidio J, et al. Stereotype threat and health disparities: what medical educators and future physicians need to know. *J Gen Intern Med.* 2010;25 (Suppl 2):169–177.
34. Shih M, Pittinsky T, Ambady N. Stereotype susceptibility. Identity salience and shifts in quantitative performance. *Psychol Sci.* 1999;10(1):80–83.
35. Riskin A, Erez A, Foulk TA, et al. The impact of rudeness on medical team performance: a randomized trial. *Pediatrics.* 2015;136(3):487–495.
36. Gabriel A, Butts M, Yuan Z, et al. Further understanding incivility in the workplace: the effects of gender, agency and communion. *J Appl Psychol.* 2018;103(4):362–382.
37. Litwin A. *New Rules for Women.* Annapolis, MD: Third Bridge Press; 2014.
38. Kuhl J. Three Tips for Women to Close the Feedback Loop. Available at: https://www.forbes.com/sites/joankuhl/2018/12/27/three-tips-for-women-to-close-the-feedback-gap/#60f75d1e24d7. Accessed May 22, 2020.
39. Heen S, Stone D. *Thanks for the Feedback.* New York, NY: Penguin Books; 2014.
40. Scott K. *Radical Candor.* New York, NY: St. Martin's Press. 2019.
41. Gisondi M, Stefanac L. The Feedback Formula Part 1: Giving Feedback, International Clinician Educators. Available at: https://icenetblog.royalcollege.ca/2018/10/02/the-feedback-formula-part-1-giving-feedback/. Accessed May 22, 2020.
42. Gisondi M, Stefanac L. The Feedback Formula Part 2: Giving Feedback, International Clinician Educators. Available at: https://icenetblog.royalcollege.ca/2018/10/23/the-feedback-formula-part-2-receiving-feedback/. Accessed May 22, 2020.
43. Babock L, Laschever S. *Ask for It: How Women Can Use Negotiation to Get What They Really Want.* New York, NY: Bantam Books; 2008.
44. Small D, Gelfand M, Babcock L, et al. Who goes to the bargaining table? The influence of gender and framing on the initiation of negotiation. *J Pers Soc Psychol.* 2007;93(4):600–613.
45. Babcock L, Laschever S, Gelfand M, et al. Nice girls don't ask—women negotiate less than men—and everyone pays the price. *Harvard Business Review.* 2003;81:14. Available at: https://hbr.org/2003/10/nice-girls-dont-ask. Accessed August 23, 2020.
46. Rousseau DM, Ho V, Greenberg J. I-Deals: idiosyncratic terms in employment relationships. *Acad Manag Rev.* 2006;31(4):977–994.
47. Bowles H, Babcock L, Lai L. Social incentives for gender differences in the propensity to initiate negotiations: sometimes it does hurt to ask. *Organ Behav Human Decis Proc.* 2007;103(1):84–103.
48. Staff P. Expanding the pie: integrative versus distributive bargaining negotiation strategies. Harvard Law School Daily Blog. 2020. Available at: https://www.pon.harvard.edu/daily/negotiation-skills-daily/negotiation-skills-expanding-the-pie-integrative-bargaining-versus-distributive-bargaining/. Accessed May 26, 2020.
49. Ralph E. Which profession has the biggest gender pay gap? Politico. 2020. Available at: https://www.politico.com/newsletters/women-rule/2020/04/03/which-profession-has-the-biggest-gender-pay-gap-488800. Accessed May 26, 2020.
50. Medscape Physician Compensation Report 2020. Slides 12-13/33. Available at: https://www.medscape.com/slideshow/2020-compensation-overview-6012684#1. Accessed May 26, 2020.
51. Madsen TE, Linden JA, Rounds K, et al. Current status of gender and racial/ethnic disparities among academic emergency medicine physicians. *Acad Emerg Med.* 2017;24:1182–1192.
52. AMA Report of the Board of Trustees 19-A-08: Gender disparities in physician income and advancement. Available at: https://www.slideshare.net/patrick89/report-19-of-the-board-of-trustees-a08. Accessed May 26, 2020.
53. Lo Sasso AT, Richards MR, Chou C-F, et al. The $16,819 pay gap for newly trained physicians: the unexplained trend of men earning more than women health affairs. 2011;30(2):193–201.
54. Robeznieks A. Par for doc pay? Modern Health Care. 2011. Available at: https://www.modernhealthcare.com/article/20110718/MAGAZINE/110719992/par-for-doc-pay. Accessed August 23, 2020.
55. Clem KJ, Promes SB, Glickman SW, et al. Factors enhancing career satisfaction in among female emergency physicians. *Ann Emerg Med.* 2008;51:723–731.
56. Wolfe J, Klauer K. Sexism in the ED: How pervasive is gender bias? June EP Monthly 2011. Available at: http://www.epmonthly.com/features/current-features/sexism-in-the-ed-how-pervasive-is-gender-bias/. Accessed May 26, 2020.

57. Wiler J, Rounds K, McGowan B, et al. Continuation of gender disparities in pay among academic emergency physicians. *Acad Emerg Med*. 2019;26:286–292.

58. Frangou S. The butterfly effect in the economic gender gap in academia. *JAMA Netw Open*. 2018;1(8):e186053.

59. Flyckt RL, White EE, Goodman LR, et al. The use of laparoscopy simulation to explore gender differences in resident surgical confidence. *Obstet Gynecol Int*. 2017;2017:Article: ID 1945801:1-7.

60. Myers D. *Why Women Should Rule the World*. New York, NY: Harper Collins; 2008.

61. Annis B, Merron K. *Gender Intelligence. Breakthrough Strategies for Increasing Diversity and Improving Your Bottom Line*. New York, NY: HarperCollins; 2014.

62. Antoine C. General manager, country & business internet marketing services EMEA, speaking at the WIN Conference, Geneva. 2005.

63. McKinsey and Company Report Women Matter. 2007. Available at: www.mckinsey.com/locations/paris/home/womenmatter/pdfs/Women_matter_oct2007. Accessed November 20, 2020.

64. Heilman ME. The impact of situational factors on personnel decisions concerning women: varying the sex composition of the applicant pool. *Organ Behav Hum Perform*. 1980;26:386–395.

65. Trix F, Psenka C. Exploring the color of glass: letters of recommendation for female and male medical faculty. *Discourse Soc*. 2003;14(2):191–220.

66. Steinpreis RE, Anders KA, Ritzke D. The impact of gender on the review of the curricula vitae of job applicants and tenure candidates: a national empirical study. *Sex Roles*. 1999;41:509–528.

67. Moss-Racusin CA, Dovidio JF, Brescoll VL, et al. Faculty's subtle gender biases favor male students. *Proc Natl Acad Sci*. 2012;109(41):16474–16479.

68. Correll S, Benard S, Paik I. Getting a job: is there a motherhood penalty? *Am J Sociol*. 2007;112(5):1297–1339.

69. Goldin C, Rouse C. Orchestrating impartiality: the impact of "blind" auditions on female musicians. *Am Econ Rev*. 2000;90(4):715–741.

70. Choo EK, Kass D, Westergaard M, et al. The Development of best practice recommendations to support the hiring, recruitment, and advancement of women physicians in emergency medicine. *Acad Emerg Med*. 2016;23(11):1203–1209.

71. Girod S, Fassiotto M, Grewal D, et al. Reducing implicit gender leadership bias in academic medicine with an educational intervention. *Acad Med*. 2016;91(8):1143–1150.

72. Bauer CC, Baltes BB. Reducing the effects of gender stereotypes on performance evaluations. *Sex Roles*. 2002;47:465–476.

73. Prohibited employment policies/practices. US Equal Employment Opportunity Commission website. Available at: https://www.eeoc.gov/prohibited-employment-policiespractices. Accessed August 13, 2019.

74. AAMC Best Practices for Conducting Residency Program Interviews. Available at: https://www.aamc.org/system/files/2020-05/best practices for conducting residency program interviews.pdf. Accessed May 27, 2020.

75. Wright AL, Schwindt LA, Bassford TL, et al. Gender differences in academic advancement: patterns, causes, and potential solutions in one U.S. College of Medicine. *Acad Med*. 2003;78(5):500–508.

76. Abbuhl S, Bristol MN, Ashfaq H, et al. Examining faculty awards for gender equity and evolving values. *J Gen Intern Med*. 2010;25(1):57–60.

77. Kirch DG. Advancing women in academic medicine. AAMC. 2020. Available at: https://www.aamc.org/news-insights/advancing-women-academic-medicine. Accessed October 28, 2020.

78. Report of the Committees on the Status of Women Faculty Engineering at MIT. 2011. Available at: https://studylib.net/doc/14409498/a-report-on-the-status-of-women-faculty-engineering-at-mi. Accessed August 23, 2020.

79. Annis B, Merron K. Gender intelligence: breakthrough strategies for increasing diversity and improving your bottom line. *Harper Business*; 2014

80. Alwazzan L, Al-Angari SS. Women's Leadership in Academic Medicine: a systematic review of extent, condition and interventions. *BMJ Open*. 2020;10:e032232.

81. Agrawal P, Madsen T, Lall M, et al. Gender disparities in academic emergency medicine: strategies for the recruitment, retention, and promotion of women. *AEM Education and Training*. 2019.

82. AWAEM Toolkit. Society for Academic Emergency Medicine. 2020. Available at: https://issuu.com/saemonline/docs/saem_awaem_toolkit. Accessed May 27, 2020.

83. McCracken DM. Winning the talent war for women" sometimes it takes a revolution. *Harvard Business Review*. 2000. Available at: https://hbr.org/2000/11/winning-the-talent-war-for-women-sometimes-it-takes-a-revolution. Accessed October 28, 2020.

84. Goldberg C. M.I.T Admits Discrimination Against Female Professors. *New York Times*, Section A, Page 1, March 23, 1999. Available at: https://www.nytimes.com/1999/03/23/us/mit-admits-discrimination-against-female-professors.html. Accessed October 28, 2020.

85. Johnson SK, Hekman DR. Women and minorities are penalized for promoting diversity. *Harvard Business Review*. 2016. Available at: https://hbr.org/2016/03/women-and-minorities-are-penalized-for-promoting-diversity. Assessed May 24, 2020.

86. Ibarra H. A lack of sponsorship is keeping women from advancing into leadership. *Harvard Business Review*. 2019. Available at: https://hbr.org/2019/08/a-lack-of-sponsorship-is-keeping-women-from-advancing-into-leadership. Accessed May 24, 2020.

87. Metronics Igniting Women to Lead Initiative. Available at: https://www.medtronic.com/us-en/about/citizenship/supporting-a-global-workforce/inclusion-diversity/elevating-women-leaders.html. Accessed May 27, 2020.

88. The 2016 Physician's Foundation: Survey of America's Physician Practice Patterns & Perspectives. Available at: https://physiciansfoundation.org/wp-content/uploads/2017/12/Biennial_Physician_Survey_2016.pdf. Accessed May 27, 2020.

89. Staff Writer. More Doctors Work Part Time, Flexible Schedules. amednews.com. 2012. Available at: https://amednews.com/article/20120326/business/303269974/1/. Accessed August 23, 2020.

90. Berg S. Working overtime? At Stanford, physicians bank the time for later. AMA blog. Available at: https://www.ama-assn.org/practice-management/physician-health/working-overtime-stanford-physicians-bank-time-later. Accessed August 23, 2020.

91. Mitchell S. Parental leave policies for 50 of the top public universities. Available at: http://saramitchell.org/index.html. Accessed October 25, 2018.

92. Wolfe J. The Part time academic physician. ALIEM podcast. Available at: https://soundcloud.com/academic-life-in-em/the-part-time-academic-physician-dr-jeannette-wolfe. Accessed August 2020.

93. Rau H, Williams JC. A winning parental leave policy can be surprisingly simple. *Harvard Business Review*. 2017. Available at: https://hbr.org/2017/07/a-winning-parental-leave-policy-can-be-surprisingly-simple. Accessed October 25, 2018.

94. The Council of Economic Advisers. The Economics of Paid and Unpaid Leave. Executive Office of the President of the United States. Available at: https://obamawhitehouse.archives.gov/sites/default/files/docs/leave_report_final.pdf. Accessed May 27, 2020.

95. McKinsey and Co: Women Matter. Gender Diversity, a Corporate Performance Driver. 2007. Available at: https://www.mckinsey.com/~/media/McKinsey/Business%20Functions/Organization/Our%20Insights/Gender%20diversity%20a%20corporate%20performance%20driver/Gender%20diversity%20a%20corporate%20performance%20driver.pdf. Accessed August 23, 2020.

BURNOUT: DIAGNOSIS, TREATMENT, AND PREVENTION

CHAPTER 125

Thom A. Mayer

In the middle of the road of my life,

I awoke to find myself in a Dark Wood,

Where the True Way was wholly lost.

— Dante Alighieri, *The Inferno*[1]

Everything can be taken from a man but one thing–the last of the human freedoms–to choose one's own way in any given set of circumstances, to choose one's own way.

—Viktor Frankl, MD, *Man's Search for Meaning*[2]

What if half the emergency department (ED) physicians, nurses, and team members providing care to you and your family were burned out? How confident would you be that such a team could deliver optimal quality care? That unsatisfying prospect is today's unsettling reality. Burnout has reached epidemic proportions, affecting over half of ED nurses and physicians, with some studies quoting 70% burnout rates.[3-5] The work of providing emergency care is extracting a cost we can no longer afford. The consequences of physician and nurse burnout to the organization are well-documented and include:[6,7]

- Absenteeism
- Turnover
- Patient safety errors
- Medication errors
- Declining patient experience scores
- Declines in staff engagement

Far more importantly, the toll exacted on individual clinicians includes a broad range of mental and physical ailments, including depression, loss of energy, insomnia, hypertension, weight gain, stress, and so on.[8] Burnout is a mismatch between job stressors and the adaptive capacity or resiliency to deal with them. This cascade can result in three cardinal symptoms: emotional exhaustion, cynicism or depersonalization, and loss of meaning in work (**Figure 125.1**). Two additional insights drive the definition of burnout: Every member of the ED team is a leader and "athlete" who is engaged in a cycle of performance, recovery, and training. Emergency department leadership is ultimately an act of courage, a willingness to venture forward in uncertain times, as the 2020 coronavirus pandemic graphically demonstrated.[9,10]

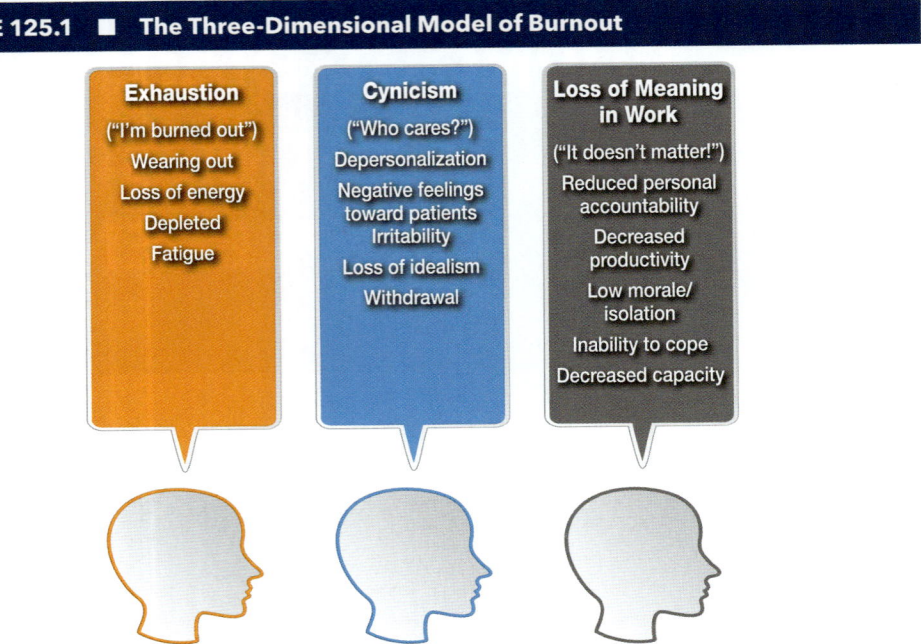

FIGURE 125.1 ■ The Three-Dimensional Model of Burnout

THE THREE-DIMENSIONAL MODEL OF BURNOUT

Exhaustion reflects the basic *strain dimension* on the individual experiencing burnout, with depleted mental, physical, psychological, and even spiritual resources needed to deal with the stressors. Cynicism represents the *interpersonal dimension*, reflecting a negative, callous, and fundamentally detached response to those being served. Finally, loss of meaning is the *self-evaluation dimension*, which is often excessively self-critical, reflected in feelings of incompetence, inadequacy, and lack of achievement.[11,12]

The term *burnout* was first used nearly simultaneously in the mid-1970s by Herbert Freudenberger, a New York psychiatrist working in an alternative medical clinic in the East Village, and Christina Maslach, a social psychologist at Berkeley studying human emotions in the workplace.[13,14] When the phenomenon of exhaustion, cynicism, and loss of effectiveness was described by Maslach to a poverty law professor working under stressful conditions, the attorney exclaimed, "Oh my God. We call that burnout!" Thus, like most syndromes, it was already present, waiting to be described and given its name.

Despite how wonderful and satisfying providing care to ED patients can be, there is a hidden danger in what we do. A disturbing paradox emerges precisely because the better you are, the more passionate you are, the more deeply you care for your patients, the greater the risk. Simply stated, A-Team members are at the highest risk for burnout. B-Team members, whose depth of passion and commitment can be questioned at times, seem to burnout at much lower and slower rates.[15]

Burnout is rarely discussed in EDs, as if admitting to it would weaken our relationship with the team. In that sense, it is a silent epidemic that robs us of the one resource we simply cannot do without—our passion. Burnout is a killer of joy, delight, and contentment in our work lives.[16] It creates a "passion disconnect," draining us of the fuel needed to do our jobs effectively.

This chapter provides a framework for effectively defining and diagnosing burnout and delineates ways to treat and prevent this insidious disease, which affects many emergency physicians and nurses. Pragmatic solutions are a major focus, as a review of the current literature indicates that more than 90% of what is written on burnout in health care focuses on diagnosing it; less than 10% is devoted to its prevention and treatment.[16]

IMPROVING BURNOUT

The framework for understanding burnout is made up of three elements:

- Instilling a culture of passion and professional fulfillment
- Hardwiring flow and fulfillment into systems and processes
- Reigniting passion and personal resilience

The cultures of our organizations and the systems and processes by which health care is provided revolve around organizational resilience, while reigniting passion is dependent on *personal* resilience. Far too much of the literature focuses on personal resilience, implying the fault lies with the team and neglecting the fact that fully two-thirds of the problems lie with the organization, whose culture and systems/processes have predictably produced burnout in the first place. When working with teams on burnout, it is common to hear the "C-suite" say, "We have a great culture here and incredible systems and processes." The only appropriate response is, "If your culture and systems are so great, why are half your people burned out?"

Changing Culture

Culture creates burnout when it espouses professional fulfillment, but the culture "in action" is different, as Harvard's Chris Argyris noted.[17] When the "words on the walls" aren't matched by the "happenings in the halls," burnout is inevitable (see Chapter 1). Culture is not just what people *do* in an organization, it's also what they *say* they do and how they *think*, particularly how they think about change, improvement, and innovation. Few things widen the gap further between job stressors and the resilience required to deal with them than leaders who espouse one culture but embody another.

Hardwiring Flow + Fulfillment

We are what we repeatedly do. Excellence is not a virtue, but a habit.

—Aristotle, Nichomachean Ethics[18]

If Aristotle is correct and we are what we repeatedly do, then *what we do* at work is guided by the systems and processes by which we do them. What we do in health care and how we do it create the types of warriors we will be. The majority of the work on burnout has focused on personal resilience to the relative exclusion of changing the nature of the work itself. Simply stated, hardwiring flow means doing "smart stuff"—the stuff that adds value, eliminates waste, and allows us to exercise our talents most effectively, leaving behind the "stupid stuff." Fixing the work requires changing the systems and processes by hardwiring flow + fulfillment. The "+" symbol that joins these two concepts is equally important precisely because flow and fulfillment are inextricable. Fulfillment cannot be attained or sustained unless systems and processes are hardwired for both flow *and* fulfillment. While it is common to measure flow exclusively by time, quality, and safety metrics and results, the impact of systems and processes on fulfillment must also be considered.

The Role of Stress

It is important to recognize the genesis of the concept of stress as *distress*, beginning with the work of Hans Selye.[19] While people commonly interpret stress in its negative connotation, Selye notes that there is good stress or *eustress*: positive, motivational stress that drives us to a higher performance. Working to get into medical or nursing school, improving our practices by updating our knowledge base, and keeping mentally and physically conditioned are all examples of eustress. As **Figure 125.2** indicates, performance improves as stress/eustress rises. Your stress response is a result of your experience and ability to adapt adequately to it in positive ways. As revered nurse educator Joan Keyes notes, it is only when the ability to deal with stress reaches the "stress tolerance level" (STL) near the top of the curve that stress plateaus and then tumbles down the far side of the curve, where performance declines as stress continues to rise.[20] (As discussed later in this chapter, developing the ability to recognize the signs and symptoms as we approach our respective STLs is an essential strategy to prevent and treat burnout.) Increasing or continuing stress past this point results in negative distress and declining performance.[20]

Burnout vs "Rustout"

When we experience burnout, we have a "passion disconnect," which leaves us without the necessary fuel to drive our engines. The Supreme Allied Commander in World War I was the French General Ferdinand Foch, who famously declared: "The greatest force on Earth is the human soul on fire!"[21] Passion is the fire that burns within us in EDs, helping us through the stresses we face.

Some emergency physicians and nurses are perhaps less likely to burnout than they are to "rustout." Rustout is an appropriate metaphor for those whose passion has gradually atrophied such that the skills of adaptive capacity have gradually "frozen" over the course of time, much like the Tin Man in *The Wizard of Oz*. To get them moving again, the "joints"

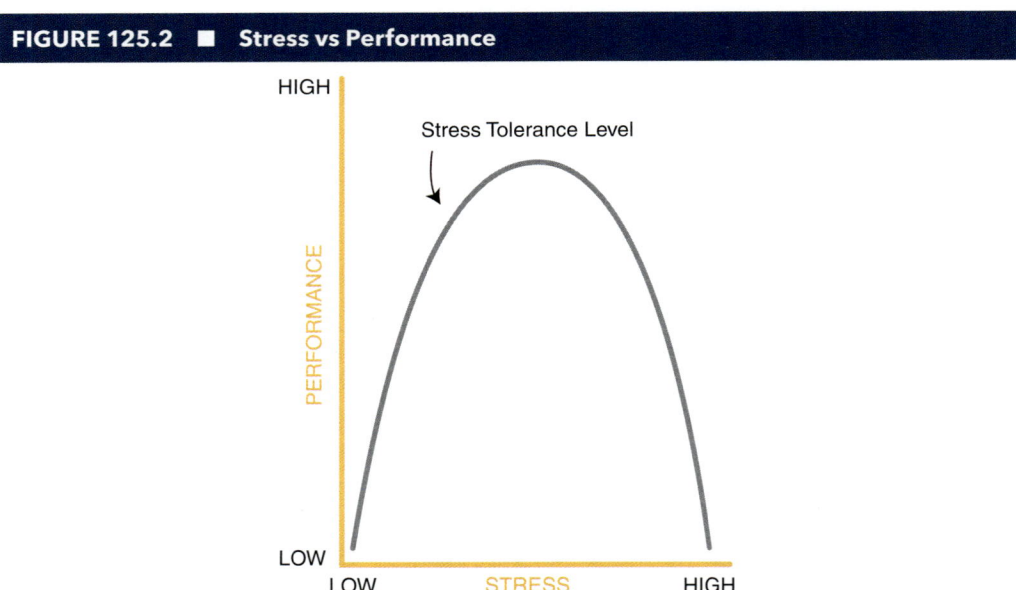

FIGURE 125.2 ■ Stress vs Performance

The Selye model of stress shows that on the left side of the curve, stress is positive because it results in improved performance. On the right side of the curve, increases in stress cause a steady decline in performance. As the top of the curve is reached, the individual reaches their "STL," where further increases in stress will produce poorer performance.

of these team members simply need the right "oil": a combination of organizational and personal resiliency strategies.

Engagement and Resiliency

The solution to burnout is restoring passion, not just attaining engagement. *Passionate engagement*, as opposed to engagement alone, is a helpful construct in which to consider health-care burnout. *Resiliency* is defined as the adaptive capacity required to thrive in the face of adversity. Simply stated, resiliency is a measure of adaptive stress-coping ability, particularly in the midst of change. The scale most commonly used to measure resiliency is the Connor-Davidson Resilience Scale, which began as a 25-element, four-point Likert scale but has since been shortened to 10- and two-element tools.[22]

Are There Gender Differences in Burnout?

Do women and men experience burnout at the same rates and in the same way? The answers, if available, could help develop prevention and treatment strategies. While there is surprisingly little written on this important topic, a Dutch study of 212 general practitioners gives some valuable insight.[23] Researchers found that men experienced burnout first in cynicism/depersonalization followed by emotional exhaustion; however, the male cohort experienced no significant progression to the dimension of loss of efficacy/effectiveness. (Almost as if the male physicians ignored the consequences of cynicism and exhaustion and failed to recognize the possibility of loss of efficacy—and just kept working.) Female physicians in the study experienced exhaustion as the first and most dramatic dimension, followed by cynicism and finally loss of efficacy.

While this study has not been replicated in emergency physicians and nurses, if accurate in those populations, it implies that recognition patterns and treatment alternatives may be different in men versus women. Research into gender differences in emergency medicine is a priority to understand these issues.

LEADERSHIP SKILLS TO BATTLE BURNOUT

Burnout cannot be battled successfully without effective leadership at all levels of every health-care organization. *Without question, the failure of leadership at all levels is what created the burnout crisis.* While this may seem a harsh judgment, the logic that increased job stressors were allowed to make their way into the fabric of the organization is at the heart of understanding burnout. All of us who were charged with making changes—or allowing those changes to make their way into our systems—simply did not fully realize the impact they would have on our teams. That is not meant as an indictment of leadership; rather, it acknowledges how we arrived at a place where half of our team members are burned out.

Is there evidence that improved leadership results in lower levels of burnout and increased fulfillment? While the number of studies supporting this idea is currently small, the data are nonetheless compelling. A study of 2,800 physicians practicing at the Mayo Clinic used a 60-point scale to assess physicians' ratings of their leaders and compared it to burnout rates using a modification of the Maslach Burnout Inventory (MBI).[24] Each one-point increase in physicians' ratings was associated with a 3.3% decrease in the likelihood of burnout. There was also a 9% increase in satisfaction for individual physicians (correcting for age, sex, and specialty). Further, 11% of the variation in burnout and 47% of the variation in satisfaction were tied to the aggregate leadership score.

Other studies—and considerable practical experience—have shown remarkably similar results, so it can be confidently said: *Leadership is essential to battling burnout.* Leadership is essential in all three areas in which we have framed burnout: culture of passion, hardwiring flow + fulfillment (systems and processes), and reigniting passion and personal fulfillment. Leaders cannot shield their teams from all the increasing job stressors on the horizon, but they should at least anticipate them and consider ways to blunt their impact. As Harvard Professor John Kotter explains:

> *The fundamental purpose of management is to keep the current system functioning. The fundamental purpose of leadership is to produce change, particularly non-incremental change. Most companies are over-managed and under-led.*[25]

Leaders Think, Act, and Innovate

Managers are maintainers, and leaders are innovators. To be successful in producing results while minimizing burnout, leaders must think, act, and innovate (**Figure 125.3**). The first step is to help the team think about burnout in a radically different way and get engaged on the takeoff. Second, leaders must challenge their teams to act quickly, usually within the week a solution is considered, to show progress and generate hope. (Generally, if new ideas aren't acted upon in some way within a week, they aren't acted upon at all.) Finally, leaders must be catalysts for innovative cultures, systems, processes, and behaviors to combat burnout and enhance both personal and professional resiliency/adaptive capacity.

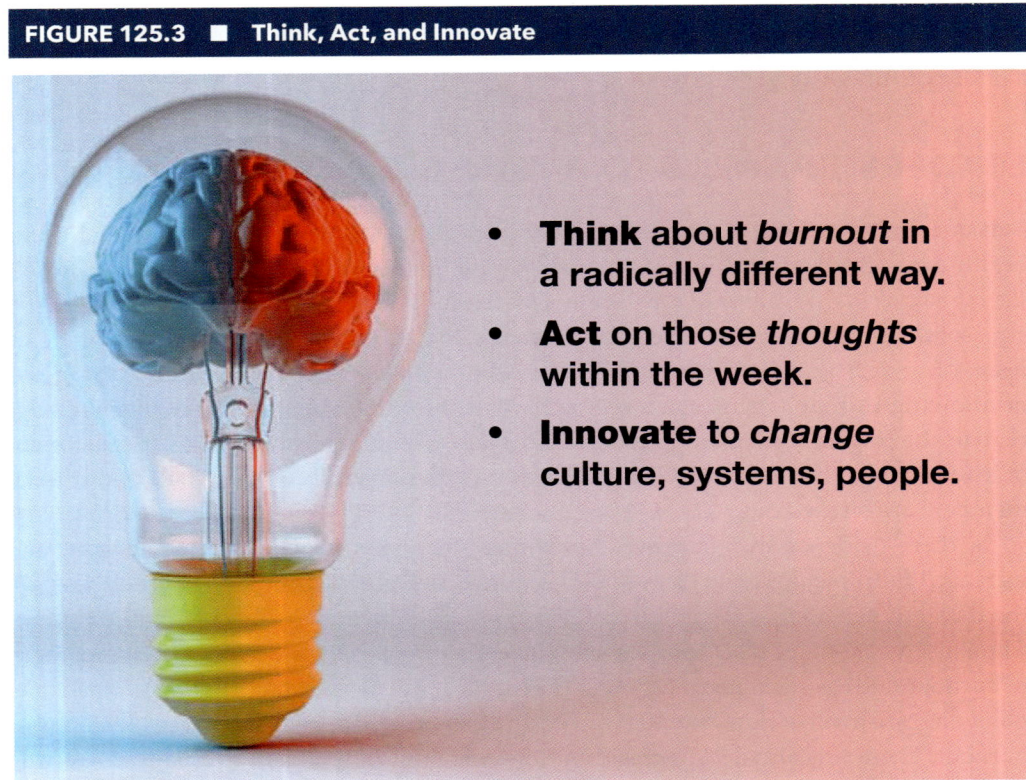

FIGURE 125.3 ■ Think, Act, and Innovate

- **Think** about *burnout* in a radically different way.
- **Act** on those *thoughts* within the week.
- **Innovate** to *change* culture, systems, people.

"Learning to love the job you have" focuses on individuals' roles in promoting change within themselves and their organizations. This entails a combination of personal and professional resilience strategies. "Creating the job you love" addresses solutions to change the culture and the systems and processes of health care, or *organizational resilience/adaptive capacity*. All of this speaks to the importance of leaders as innovators. Innovation requires a working understanding of "what is," a respectful appreciation for "what has been," and the audacity to create "what hasn't yet been dreamed."[26]

MEANINGFULLY MEASURING BURNOUT

Maslach Burnout Inventory

While there are numerous scales used to measure burnout, the most widely recognized and well-validated "gold standard" for quantifying the problem is the MBI, a 22-question survey that integrates questions on emotional exhaustion, cynicism/depersonalization, and loss of efficacy or personal accomplishment (**Table 125.1**).[27] Two other scales seek to measure burnout and professional fulfillment—the Well-Being Index and the Stanford Professional Fulfillment Index (PFI).[28,29]

TABLE 125.1 ■ Maslach Burnout Inventory (Abbreviated)

How often?	Never	A few times a year	Once a month or less	A few times a month	Once a week	A few times a week	Every day
	0	1	2	3	4	5	6
1. I deal very effectively with the problems of my patients.							
2. I feel I treat some patients as if they were impersonal objects.							
3. I feel emotionally drained from my work.							
4. I feel fatigued when I get up in the morning and have to face another day on the job.							
5. I've become more callous towards people since I took this job.							
6. I feel I'm positively influencing other people's lives through my work.							
7. Working with people all day is really a strain for me.							
8. I don't really care what happens to some patients.							
9. I feel exhilarated after working closely with my patients.							

Burnout should be viewed as a continuous rather than a dichotomous variable, ranging from low to moderate to high:

- *High burnout*: High scores on the "emotional exhaustion" and "cynicism/depersonalization" subscales and low scores in the "personal accomplishment" subscale
- *Average burnout*: Average scores across all three subscales
- *Low burnout*: Low scores in the "emotional exhaustion" and "cynicism" subscales and high scores on the "personal accomplishment" subscale

Each of the three elements should be considered, as well as their connection to the integrated model using the "domains of burnout" discussed in detail later.

Free-Form Questions

The use of free-form questions and interviews is critical to capturing the fundamentally human cost of burnout. Leading teams through the fires of burnout requires a granular understanding of its sources and consequences. That requires "the voice of the patient"—in this case, the voice of the team members. Marry the metrics from survey analysis, regardless of the survey used, with the results from free-form questions and interviews. Free-form questions include:

- What are the biggest sources of burnout for you?
- What strategies have you used to battle burnout?
- What is the biggest single thing that would reduce your burnout?
- How exhausted do you feel and why?
- Tell me if you feel more cynical about work and how we could work together to improve that?
- Do you feel a sense of meaning and purpose at work?
- What is your "deep joy" and have you been able to sustain that?
- What have been your biggest frustrations at work?
- What are your biggest job stressors?
- What could we do together to decrease those stressors?
- Do you feel you have enough adaptive capacity to deal with your stressors?
- What could the team work on to help?
- What could you work on to help?

Here are some free-form interview responses that give insight into the problem:

- "I'm burned out! I feel like I don't have the energy to get up and go to work."
- "I'm beyond burnout."
- "Exhaustion doesn't begin to express how I feel."
- "My compassion tank is running on empty."
- "I have compassion fatigue."
- "On days I'm scheduled to work, I can barely drag myself out of bed."
- "I've come to believe that what I do no longer makes a difference. The sad thing is, I'm not sure it ever did."
- "When I come home at night, I look back at the day and wonder if all that effort was worth it."
- "I used to feel like a great nurse. Now I feel like a glorified robot."
- "A monkey could do what I do. Actually, that's probably an insult to monkeys."
- "To me, my job has become fundamentally sad. It's a ton of effort for an ounce of making any real difference."
- "I think about my work, and I just sigh and think: Really? Why am I doing this?"

- "Honestly, it's just a job to me these days."
- "Does anyone really care what we do?"
- "It just doesn't matter anymore."
- "My patients don't seem to care about themselves. Why should I?"
- "You don't really buy this 'engagement' nonsense, do you?"

To assess the impact of exhaustion, cynicism, and loss of efficacy on burnout, consider both the results of the MBI and the nuanced narrative of the free-form staff interviews to decipher the complex mosaic of the effects on the team.

Maslach Two-Question Survey

Due to the time required to conduct and analyze the full 22-item MBI-HSS survey, West and colleagues culled two questions from that survey with the highest loading factor on the emotional exhaustion and depersonalization/cynicism subscales: "I feel burned out from my work" and "I have become more callous toward people since I took this job." The two-item survey has been shown to have high correlation with the full MBI on the emotional exhaustion and depersonalization scales and has been used in some health-care systems to reduce responder burden. Others have used the full MBI initially, followed by the two-item scale for follow-up.

Stanford PFI

The Stanford PFI measures burnout and professional fulfillment in physicians with the intent of extending it to other health-care professionals.[29] The 16-item, five-point Likert scale survey was designed by the Stanford WellMD program. The responses range from "not at all true" to "completely true" for professional fulfillment and "not at all" to "extremely" for work exhaustion and interpersonal disengagement items. The items fall into the following categories:

- Professional fulfillment items
- Work exhaustion items
- Interpersonal disengagement items

It may be used at no cost by nonprofit organizations for research or program evaluation. Cost of for-profit use may be obtained by emailing wellness.surveyteam@TheRiskAuthority.com. The PFI is currently in use by the Stanford Wellness Consortium, which comprises over 20 not-for-profit health-care systems across the United States.[30]

THE SIX DOMAINS OF BURNOUT

Maslach and Leiter developed the "six domains of burnout" in an effort to more specifically describe the problem and guide specific solutions to address its causes (**Figure 125.4**).[31]

Mismatch of Workload Demands and Capacity

Mismatches in workload occur when too many demands relative to the capacity to deal with them exhaust an individual's energy (and that of the team) to the extent that recovery is difficult, if not impossible. Thus, it's not the workload itself necessarily, but rather the capacity and ability to deal with the workload that creates exhaustion. This is innately understandable to members of the ED team, where considerations of demand–capacity mismatches are a part of understanding departmental flow.

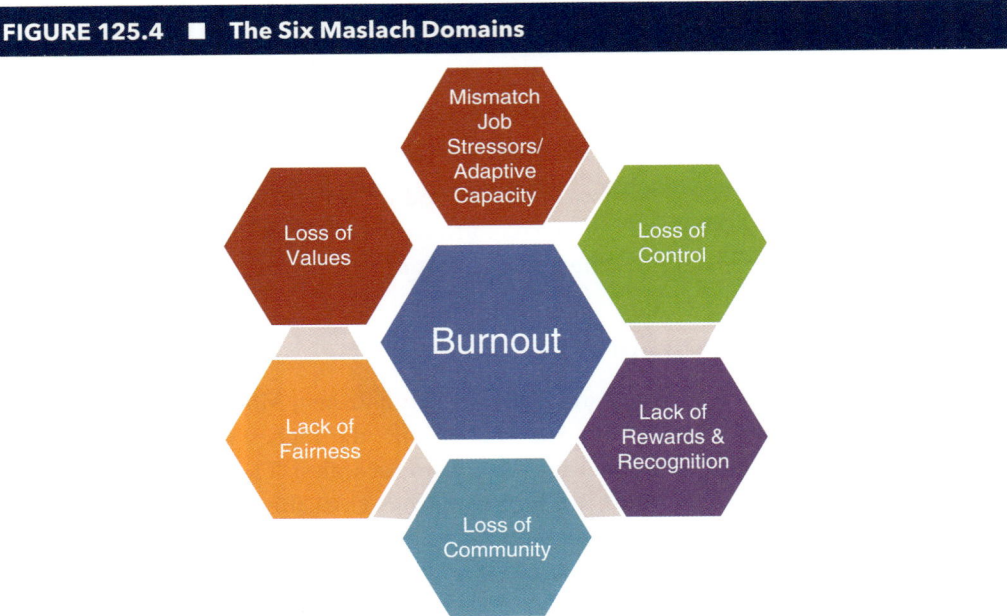

FIGURE 125.4 ■ The Six Maslach Domains

Loss of Control

Emergency department teams often have insufficient control over the resources needed to do their work and have inadequate authority to obtain the necessary tools. In working with medical and nursing directors at ACEP's Emergency Department Directors Academy, this question is posed to the participants: "How many of you feel you are held accountable for a system over which you have no control?"[32] Without exception, every hand is raised (enthusiastically!), indicating that this is an issue in every ED, where people feel their responsibility exceeds their authority. As Leiter and Maslach note, "Control problems occur when workers have insufficient authority over their work or are unable to shape the work environment to be consistent with their values."[12] Unsurprisingly, when people have more control over their work, their actions are more freely chosen, which leads to higher engagement.

Lack of Rewards and Recognition

The cemeteries of the world are full of indispensable men.

—Charles De Gaulle[33]

The third type of mismatch involves a lack of appropriate rewards and recognition for the work people do. In the vast majority of cases, the lack of rewards is not primarily financial in nature but rather refers to a fundamental devaluation of the work and talents requisite to care for ED patients and their families. The lack of intrinsic rewards, such as a deep pride in doing something of importance extremely well, is often a part of this mismatch. Lack of rewards and recognition is closely associated with the loss of efficacy/effectiveness portion of the MBI. Problems arise when the lack of rewards and recognition creates situations in which the ED team is considered fungible. And the journey from "indispensable" to "fungible" is a sure pathway to burnout.

Loss of a Sense of Community

The fourth area of mismatch occurs when people lose their sense of a positive, proactive participation in the team or community in which they work. (Chapter 12 discusses teams in more detail.) People innately thrive in common communities where praise, happiness, comfort, and even the trials of the job are shared. Sebastian Junger captures this well in his book *Tribe*.[34] As cynicism and exhaustion rise, the seams of the community are threatened, and people feel isolated.

Essential Fairness

Fairness is a fundamental human need, but it is also one that is felt even more acutely in professionals. Fairness communicates mutual respect, confirms self-worth, and creates a level playing field. Conversely, environments in which inequity rules are toxic by nature and dismissive of those required to work in them. A lack of fairness creates burnout because it is exhausting and creates deep cynicism about the workplace and its leaders.

In EDs, one of the most common areas of perceived unfairness is when there are high demands for performance metrics, but the means to attain those metrics are lacking, which may be referred to as "metrics mania without means."[35] This exposes a patently unfair mismatch between what is demanded of emergency physicians and nurses, the resources to attain the metrics, and even the assigned metrics themselves. Substantial experience shows that the first element to mark the descent to burnout in high-performing teams is a sense of unfairness.

Strong Values

The sixth area of mismatch is a conflict of values or confronting realities in which the stated mission, vision, and values are not matched by the resources necessary to attain them. Worse, in some cases, the values espoused by the leadership team conflict with the stated values of the organization. For example, a hospital and the ED say they value high-quality service and patient experience, but their mantra is "Move 'em, move 'em, move the meat!" That conflict of values risks creating deep cynicism among the staff. Leadership teams who communicate, directly or indirectly, "Get it done. I don't care how you do it" are at deep risk of subjugating values for results. Most importantly, an increasing amount of research shows that values play a central role in multiple areas of the organization.[36,37] This is important in both the diagnostic phase, where a discordance in values is a clear harbinger of burnout, and also in the treatment phase, where clear steps to realign processes with values help move the team to a place where other burnout treatment strategies can be used effectively.

SOLUTIONS FOR BATTLING BURNOUT

There are many evidence-based solutions to preventing and treating burnout. This discussion focuses on crosswalking the three elements of the burnout framework (culture, hardwiring flow + fulfillment into systems and processes, and reigniting passion and personal resilience) with the six Maslach domains.

Workload Demands vs Adaptive Capacity

Several highly specific strategies help diminish workload demands while increasing the adaptive capacity to meet them.

Culture of Passion and Resilience Solutions

Leaders everywhere at every level: Every ED team member at every level is a leader. "Lead yourself, lead your team" should be a guiding principle.

Leadership development and training skills: Invest in your teams by giving them effective leadership training, regardless whether they have a formal title. Communication skills, the ability to coach/mentor, empowerment, values, and fairness consistently rank as desired characteristics among effective ED leaders. Institutions that are committed to decreasing burnout and increasing engagement should ensure that hiring, training, and mentoring of ED leaders is a priority.

Culture continuity: Ensure that the espoused leadership attributes are reflected in action. Ensure that "the words on the walls match the happenings in the halls." Support those who point out discrepancies when they occur.

Stop doing stupid stuff, start doing smart stuff: While this aspect applies more specifically to hardwiring flow, a culture that allows systems and processes to burnout the staff is ultimately and inexorably a culture that cannot be sustained. Change to one that seeks out and eliminates stupid stuff.

Taking on the EHR: While this topic is discussed in more detail below, very few things negatively reflect the culture of an ED more than hearing "That's just the EHR. Get used to it!" Have the courage to make the machines work for the team, not the opposite.

Hardwiring Flow + Fulfillment Solutions

Stop doing stupid stuff and send a signal of hope: Hardwiring flow + fulfillment involves doing "smart stuff," the evidence-based best practice systems and processes that produce superior flow metrics and allow the team to feel fulfilled. One of the hardest things for leaders at all levels to accept is that a lot of what we do in health care simply doesn't make sense to patients or the people who take care of them.[15] (*Certainly, some folks would use a different, more scatological word after stupid, but I won't go there.*) "Stop doing stupid stuff" is a way of harvesting "low-hanging fruit," which everyone can see but no one has had the courage to address. Most importantly, stopping stupid stuff creates hope that leaders are paying attention and are serious about creating a common-sense culture. There are countless examples of stupid stuff, including these:

- In the morning hours in the ED, patients often wait in line to be triaged when there are rooms, doctors, nurses, and essential services staff in the back waiting to see them. They wait in a line when there should be no line.
- Nursing units operate with fewer nurses than scheduled but are expected to produce top-decile metrics. They use the same systems and processes when "working short" that they use when fully staffed. And we are somehow surprised when they think, "Seriously? You know we need this level of staffing, but nothing gets done."
- Patients "board" in ED hallways for hours (sometimes days) and are taken care of by ED nurses, who are thus unavailable to care for incoming patients. Once a bed is identified in the hospital, it takes hours to have it cleaned and almost as long until the inpatient team is ready to take the patient.
- An orthopedic surgeon is on-call over a busy holiday weekend, when there are a highly predictable number of ED patients with orthopedic problems who will require follow-up the next week. Instead of ensuring that there are enough designated appointments for these patients, the surgeon's schedule is completely filled, meaning those patients from the ED won't be seen in a timely fashion and some will return for follow-up care.

Each problem can be fixed with relatively simple actions that change the systems and processes by which patients are cared for. Leadership at all levels must seek out and resolve stupid stuff whenever and wherever it is identified. Fortunately, fixing stupid stuff sends a jolt of hope to the team, who think: "Well, I'll be darned. Maybe they are finally serious about correcting things around here."[38]

The five demand–capacity questions: One of the key tools of hardwiring flow is the use of demand–capacity tools, including the following five questions, which can also help us understand patient demands, the expectations that accompany them, and the capacity to deal with them:

- Who is coming? (What are the demands?)
- When are they coming? (What's the timing of the demands?)
- What will they need? (What is the specific nature of the demands?)
- Will we have what they need? (Capacity)
- What will we do if we don't? (Adaptive capacity)

Within each shift, these tools should be used to maximize adaptive capacity and mitigate the stressors the workload entails.

Around-the-clock care: Emergency clinicians, by nature, work 24 hours a day, 7 days a week, 365 days a year, which produces a workload that is predictable yet unrelenting. We can and should use the demand–capacity tools to inform us of who is coming and what they will need. Yet even with that, it should be recognized that many of the resources needed to care for ED patients are only available 12 to 18 hours a day, 5 days a week, 250 days per year.[30] Magnetic resonance imaging (MRI), consultative services, physical therapy, behavioral health services, and many others are only available certain times of the day (12–18 hours, typically) and on limited days of the week (5 days).

The better the ED understands this demand–capacity mismatch and is prepared to deal with it by developing proactive strategies, the more the ED adaptive capacity increases. The migration of ultrasound skills from radiology to the bedside of the ED is an excellent example.

Variation That Adds Value

What's true in the morning is a lie by the afternoon.

—Carl Jung[39]

The concepts of hardwiring flow often stress reducing variations whenever possible, but the more penetrating insight is to recognize when variation adds value. For example, at 10 am on a weekday, the ED may use a process of "direct bedding" or "triage bypass," in which patients are taken directly back to an ED bed instead of getting delayed at triage. But once the beds are full, that process no longer works and a different set of processes must be put in place, including advanced triage orders for certain patients or, if beds will not be available for extended periods of time, a physician or provider at triage. All of these are examples of ED teams prospectively understanding that, in some cases, variation adds value because the flow circumstances vary. This concept increases capacity and smooths workload.

Reigniting Passion and Personal Resilience

Most clinical care has been focused on a disease paradigm in which questions are focused on the patient's presentation and how it can be treated. "What's the matter *with you*?" is the primary question. That is appropriate when a clearly delineated pathology can be identified and a mandated treatment is available. However, even when the diagnosis and treatment are clear, the "patient experience diagnosis" begs the question, "What matters *to you*?"—a question with fundamentally different implications for successful treatment.

What you love, hate, and tolerate: One of the most powerful tools to maximize adaptive capacity is a thought exercise, which asks these three questions about the work done: *What do I love? What do I hate?* and *What do I tolerate?* It's important to be specific when answering

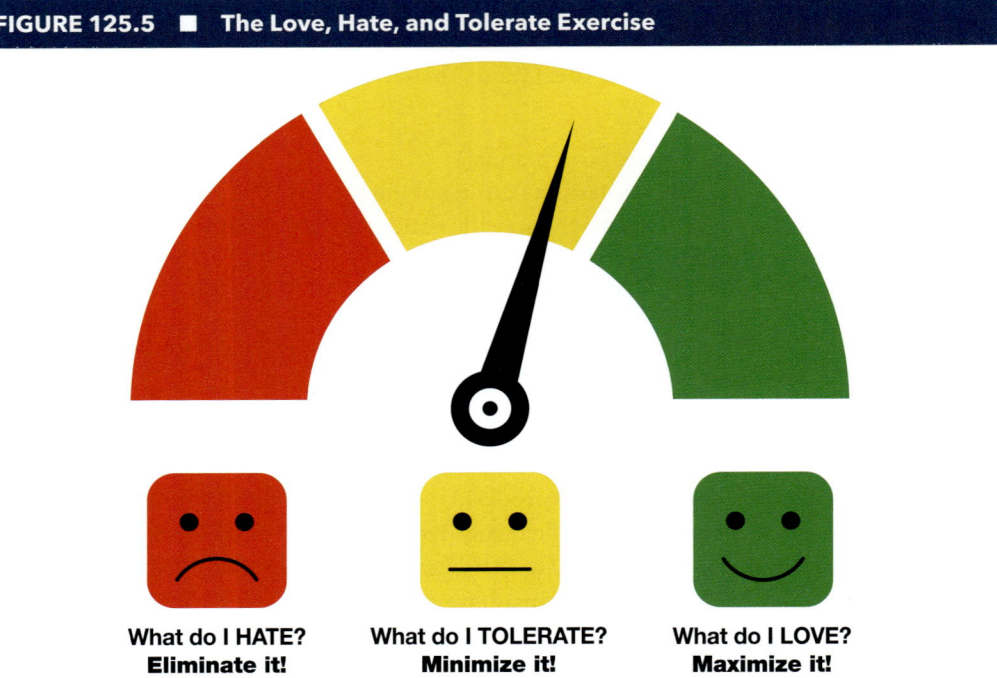

FIGURE 125.5 ■ The Love, Hate, and Tolerate Exercise

each question. Once that list is complete, move to the next step of accentuating what is loved, eliminating what is hated, and minimizing what is tolerated (**Figure 125.5**).

For example, emergency physicians and nurses might identify the demands of chronic pain patients as something they "hate." While eliminating this population from the ED is highly unlikely, the problem can be mitigated by developing evidence-based strategies to deal with these patients. The things we "tolerate" might include the vagaries of dealing with the EHR, difficulty in obtaining timely consults, and the lack of a functioning behavioral health system. Minimizing these interactions might entail developing specific order sets or the use of scribes, defining responsibilities and time frames for consultants to return calls, and creating task forces to develop better behavioral and mental health resources.

Creative energy: Just as exhaustion is an element of burnout, energy is the bellwether of passion and engagement. Joan Kyes, RN, developed a wonderful concept she called "creative energy," an approach that allows people to creatively invest energy by completing tasks in a timely manner; thus, the energy returns so it can be used for other projects. Everyone has had the experience of being around people who seem to have an inexhaustible energy reservoir; they are always ready to take on the next challenge. Others, who are burned out, always seem to have "nothing left in the tank."

Kyes makes the point that all humans have basically the same energy reserves in their reservoir; when we take on a project, we take an "energy packet" out of the tank. The size of the packet varies according to the magnitude and complexity of the requisite work needed to complete it. However, the energy expended on the task does not return to the energy reservoir until the project is fully completed. Develop the skill of having evidence-based plans to deal with tasks to decrease the amount of energy spent on thinking about what to do instead of knowing in advance, from experience, how to proceed.

Using the discipline of patient experience-survival skills: Balancing workload with adaptive capacity requires a proactive approach to the core aspect of patient experience, which is an increasingly demanding part of ED practice. Chapters 11 and 73 to 75 cover this topic in detail, but several points deserve emphasis here. First, understand the "why" of patient experience. The number one reason to get patient experience right is *it makes your job easier!*[15] Because all meaningful and lasting change is intrinsically not extrinsically motivated, the work of creating an excellent patient experience needs to be understood as a set of disciplines, all of which are designed to reduce job stressors.

Have a pain flight plan: Patients with chronic pain are among the most challenging for ED staff. Without preparation and a widely known approach to managing these patients, they make the workload seem much more onerous than it needs to be. Discuss among the emergency physicians and nurses an evidence-based approach to alternatives to opioids (ALTO) as a routine way to practice. Being proactive and consistent in this area expands adaptive capacity while making the workload far more manageable. Because treating chronic pain is so stressful, an evidence-based, structured approach to ALTO in the ED shows great promise as a tool to prevent and treat burnout.[40]

Regaining/Seizing Control

Empowerment solutions: Very few health-care systems can be successful without a culture of empowerment, which means never making a decision at a higher level that can better be made at a lower level, where the work gets done. At a major academic medical center, a question was posed to an audience of over 500 team members: "Are you empowered?" Frankly, the silence was a bit uncomfortable, until a small voice from the back of the room said, "They *tell us* we are." Empower your staff to make decisions and change the culture. One such tool is the "point-of-impact intervention" tool (**Figure 125.6**).[15]

Leading for passion, wellness, and fulfillment: If your ED claims to be committed to making change to deal with burnout and creating leaders at levels, shouldn't there be both a nursing and physician advocate for wellness with compensated protected times and budgets to deliver? Of course there should be. At the hospital or health-care system level, is there a chief wellness officer or chief human experience officer? Do they answer directly to the chief executive officer or to the chief operating officer? If not, how will they ever make the needed changes?

Hardwiring Flow + Fulfillment Solutions

Scribes as personal performance assistants: Using scribes as personal performance assistants has many advantages, which are discussed below, but these adjunct team members also help hardwire flow and increase fulfillment by improving systems and processes.

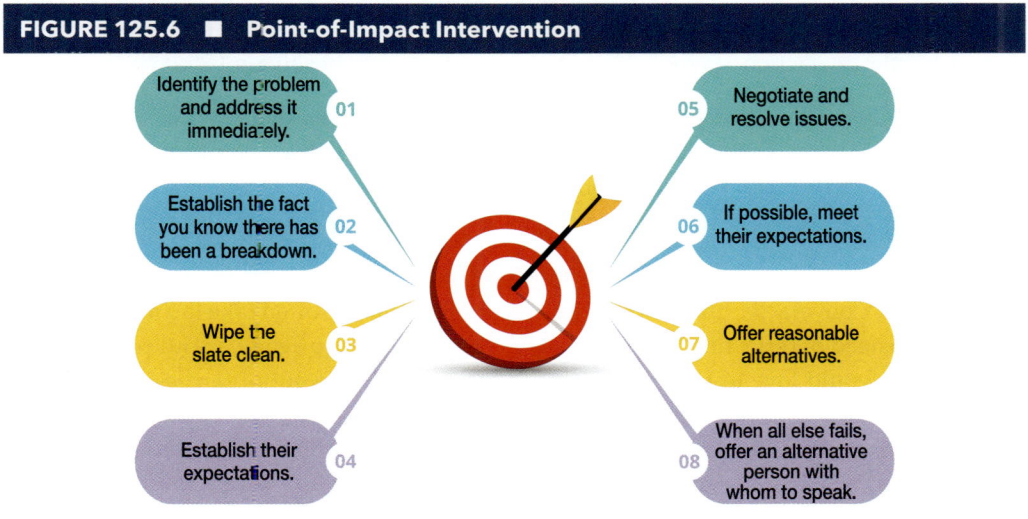

FIGURE 125.6 ■ Point-of-Impact Intervention

Practicing at the top of your license: Allow teams to practice at the top of their licenses by ensuring that "doctors do doctor stuff" and "nurses do nurse stuff." Non-value-added procedures and duties should be delegated to the essential service staff, thereby helping them regain control of their day.

Multitasking strategies: Multitasking strategies (discussed below) each have an important impact on hardwiring flow into the system and reducing of unnecessary interruptions.

Constant redesign: Regaining control partially comes from understanding that all systems and processes are undergoing constant, iterative redesigns with the input of the team members.

Reigniting Passion and Personal Resilience Solutions

Chief storyteller: Patients come to the ED because their day was disrupted by pain, injury, and many other symptoms, which they don't fully understand. Nurses and physicians have the role of the chief storyteller, whose job it is to make sense of things that otherwise don't make sense. Emergency doctors and nurses explain patients' symptoms and tell them the story of how the team will use diagnostic tools and studies to determine the etiology of their complaint and the most effective treatment.

What could be more of a position of control than "guiding the journey" of patients and explaining what will happen to them through their ED peregrinations? Control should be embraced and respected; we make a difference in people's lives, in part by appropriately exercising control on behalf of our patients.

Scribes as personal performance assistants: One of the most consistent aggravations for physicians and nurses in EDs is the necessity of dealing with the EHR. Clinicians feel that this pulls them away from the patient, often for extended periods of time and seemingly unnecessarily. One solution to this is the use of scribes or "personal performance assistants" who are specifically trained and tasked with ensuring that the EHR needs are met but that the physician or nurse interaction with the system is confined to value-added situations. This fundamentally changes the workload to help regain control of the environment.

The power of yes and the power of no: Rob Strauss emphasizes "the power of yes," which recognizes that acknowledging a person's thoughts and feelings is not the same as agreeing with them or with the solutions proposed.[41] It builds strength and trust without acquiescence. For example, if a patient requests an MRI scan of their knee at 3 am for chronic pain, a typical response might be, "No, we don't do that study in the ED at 3 am." Not only is the patient's request denied, but the interaction is handled in a negative way. A more positive approach is to say:

> *Yes, I can understand that you would like to get the scan done immediately. However, for problems like yours, we've found that getting your primary care physician's approval and coordinating with insurance actually ensures you aren't responsible for any unnecessary costs.*

The "power of yes" helps the workload by proactively using effective language to manage expectations. Conversely, "the power of no" recognizes that we often take too much work on ourselves instead of reflecting how the task fits with the others already on our plate. Saying, "Normally I would love to help, but I have to say no this time out of fairness to the other commitments I've already made." Too often, emergency professionals try to be superheros by taking on whatever they are asked to do without thoughtfully reflecting on their energy packets and ability to manage the task.[20]

Disconnect hot buttons: Everyone has "hot buttons." Not everyone knows what they are. If you don't know, ask the people you work with. "Hot buttons" are situations or types of patients who get an involuntary, seemingly uncontrollable response from us—invariably negative. Those responses increase our workload unnecessarily and should be avoided.

Once you have identified hot buttons, disconnect them. Mentally place yourself in an encounter where your hot buttons would be pushed. Imagine your typical response—the negative, nonproductive ways you have been handling them in the past. Now push the "rewind button" and take the scenario back to the start. Visualize yourself handling this in a calm, considered, and professional fashion, as the situation unfolds with equanimity. This allows for a different and more positive response, which consumes less energy and reduces the workload. Now do it for all your hot buttons.

Don't be surprised: Workload and adaptive capacity to deal with that workload are dependent on what we were prepared for as we approach our work. The good news is that, with some exceptions, most experienced emergency physicians and nurses have an innately informed sense of what they will see during a typical shift. Don't let work be a surprise. On the way to work, reflect upon the number and types of patients likely to be seen, what their likely expectations will be, and how best to most positively and proactively care for them.

Do the things we tell patients to do: Health-care professionals frequently provide advice to patients. It would be wise for them to follow their own recommendations, a partial list of which includes:

- Eat healthy meals regularly.
- Don't skip breakfast.
- Get 7 to 9 hours of sleep each night.
- Get aerobic exercise for 50 minutes or more four to five times per week.
- Leave work at work.
- Pursue mindfulness (for those so inspired).
- Reflect positively and regularly on the contribution you are making.
- Stop smoking.
- Drink alcohol in moderation.
- Take the time to reflect.
- Take care of yourself. You are the CEO of ME, Inc.[42]
- Make "electronic-free zones" or times when smart phones and computers are off-limits.
- Enjoy your family.

Have a multitasking strategy: While multitasking seems like an unavoidable occupational hazard in the ED, the literature is quite clear that multitasking *makes you stupid!*[43-45] The rate of errors, miscommunication, patient safety incidents, and even malpractice claims rise commensurate with the number of interruptions to which clinicians are subjected. Having a strategy for multitasking is critical for each person, but it also is important for the team to have a healthy discussion among all members of the team to distinguish between value-added and non-value-added interruptions.

Use evidence-based, mutually agreed-upon language to communicate: "I apologize. I am entering a critical medication order. Please let me finish to avoid any chance of error." Strategies to deal effectively with the multitasking burden decrease burnout by increasing control.

Giving and Getting Rewards and Recognition

Servant leadership: Leaders must seek to serve first, then to lead, which creates a powerful servant culture. Perhaps no area in health care is more fertile for servant leadership than the

ED. (The concept of "servant leadership" as developed by Robert Greenleaf is discussed in detail in Chapter 1.)

Reward yourself, the power of one: The first step in ensuring rewards and recognition is rewarding and recognizing ourselves. Many people aren't ever sure if they make a difference. That's not true for the ED team. One doctor, one nurse, one team, taking care of one patient: we *will* make a difference, and what will the difference be? Rewarding ourselves by recognizing the control we have over our clinical encounters is a powerful way to prevent and combat burnout.[36]

Say "thank you" 50 times a day: Since rewards and recognition are contagious, one of the most obvious solutions is to ensure that routinely thanking others is a part of work life, preferably in a disciplined, thoughtful way. Consider this:

- Most emergency physicians see at least 20 patients a day.
- Most emergency nurses see at least 10 patients a day.
- The nurses spend more time with the patient and the family.
- If each emergency physician thanks the patient when he or she first sees the patient and again when the patient leaves, and thanks the nurse for his or her care, that's at least 60 times a day.
- If the nurse thanks the patient and the family when they arrive and leave and thanks the doctor and the ED tech, that is at least 60 times as well.
- And of course, the more "thank you" is said, the easier and more natural it becomes.

Thank the "least important" team members: During a visit to the Denver Broncos, I noticed that every door out of the training room had a sign above it with the Broncos' logo and these words: "You can easily judge the character of a man by how he treats those who can do nothing for him." When I asked about it, the head athletic trainer told me the head coach insisted on the signs being placed. When I asked him who the quote was from, he shrugged, "The coach, I guess." In fact, as you may recognize, that quote is from Goethe![46] Goethe in the NFL? Hospital staff lounges would be wise to have such a sign above their doors.

The *entire team* should receive thanks and praise, including the techs, registrars, and environmental services (EVS) folks. Making sure to offer gratitude every chance you get is a sound investment in preventing and treating burnout. After a difficult trauma resuscitation, it's not uncommon for the nurses and doctors to thank each other for handling the patient well. But thanking the EVS folks who clean up the mess made during the resuscitation is also a discipline that should be developed. Well-deserved recognition is always noticed.

Catch people doing things right: In a profession built on a disease model, we often find ourselves focusing on what went wrong instead of proactively focusing on what went right and should be celebrated. Unexpected rewards and recognition arise from "catching" people doing things right and publicly complimenting them on their work. No one is immune to the power of praise.

Reconnecting passion: There is nothing abstract about a great work environment: It is great people with great leaders doing great work in service to their patients. The more this principle is articulated in what is said and done, the more the team will reconnect their passion and feel appreciated. "You did a great job on that case. Well done!" is a powerful reward and recognition. Writing a letter or email commending the team and copying the C-Suite is also effective.

Returning Community to the Workplace

Culture of teamwork: "Community" in health care refers to the team members with whom we work each day. Don't just *say* team but instead ensure that everyone can *play* team in their actions. (Detailed discussion is offered in Chapter 12.)

Gratitude creates community: Increasing the team's commitment to rewards and recognition also increases the sense of community, tying the members together in a bond of mutual appreciation. Developing the habit of ending each clinical shift with these words is a discipline worth developing: "Thanks for your help—you made a difference today." and "What could I have done to make your job easier?"

Rerecruit yourself and the A-Team: A great deal of time, effort, and energy goes into recruiting, training, and orienting physicians, nurses, and other members of the ED team. On the other hand, far too little time, effort, and energy go into "rerecruitment," which is the process of continuously reminding the members of the team or community how valued their contributions are. In addition to changing the character of performance evaluations to consider how the work itself can be improved, letting the A-Team members know how much their efforts mean to their colleagues and patients is an important part of daily rerecruitment.

Use clinical huddles to reinforce community: Huddles develop shared mental models that regularly reinforce a sense of community while delineating specific contributions that team members are making for the good of patients (see Chapter 12). Huddles also encourage the entire team to interact and prevent people from working in relative isolation through the course of the day.

Rounding on next: Rounding is an important tactic within the ED, which ensures sharing information across boundaries and enriching communication. It owes its origins to the concept of "MBWA" or "management by walking around," originally described by Tom Peters in *In Search of Excellence* and reaccentuated in *The Excellence Dividend*.[47,48] The rounding concept should be extended to "rounding on next," which refers to rounding on patients admitted from the ED to the hospital.[15] Keeping a log of patients each physician and nurse admits and having them visit the patient on the inpatient unit have incredible value in helping them understand their important role in the health-care community. It is also deeply appreciated by the patient and family, increasing gratification and preventing burnout.

Follow-up phone calls to discharged patients are another way to round on next. While this process has clear value in reestablishing a sense of community, it is less effective than face-to-face interactions.

Preventing withdrawal: Once the symptoms of burnout and cynicism develop and the individual starts to withdraw, it is critical that they be encouraged to reconnect to the team and their patients before burnout progresses further. That is the time to accentuate the elements of community discussed here. As the burned-out team members begin to retreat into themselves, systems that force them to focus outward on the team can be very effective.

Reestablishing Fairness in an Unfair Environment

Leadership candor: Fairness is also reflected in leaders at all levels who have the candor and transparency to notice when "the words on the walls don't match the happenings in the halls."[49] That is a sure sign of unfairness and needs to be eliminated to change the culture.

Mutual accountability: Eliminating functional silos and ensuring there is mutual accountability across boundaries is a clear way of ensuring fairness. Part of mutual accountability involves eliminating statements such as, "Well, the physicians' patient experience scores are great. It's the nurses' scores that are pulling us down." Instead, a focus on a fairness approach uses language like, "We are all in this together. Let's see what worked to raise the physician scores and apply it in other areas." Accountability across boundaries is essential to creating transparent fairness. The language we use also reinforces both community and fairness.

Deny metrics mania without means: "Metrics mania" refers to hospitals, health-care systems, or leadership teams that focus nearly manically on attaining metric targets without regard for the means required to meet those goals. It is one of the most common sources of creating a sense of unfairness among ED teams, resulting in a milieu of nascent burnout.[9,16] While metrics (particularly flow and patient experience metrics) are a part of modern EDs, leadership teams should discuss with the C-Suite the requisite resources to meet such targets. Making progress in this area goes a long way in preventing and treating burnout arising from unfairness.

Bounty hunt for unfairness; treasure hunt for fairness: Fairness does not return automatically. It must be cultivated and advocated for aggressively. The ED team must organize a "bounty hunt" to search for unfairness and quickly correct it. Perhaps the most obvious example of this is a hospital administration that holds the department accountable for flow and patient experience metrics while tolerating sustained boarding. That is a patently unfair double standard that should be called out and confronted. Otherwise, we not only tolerate unfairness, we condone it. As discussed above, matching metrics mania with the appropriate means to attain those metrics is also a powerful strategy to "right size" fairness. So will having a "treasure hunt" for fairness, acknowledging and praising it whenever and wherever it is found.

Druckenbrod's queries: Glenn Druckenbrod, the medical director at Virginia's Inova Fairfax Medical Campus's Department of Emergency Medicine, stresses the importance of the discipline of using three questions during the "landing" portion of the ED visit: "Have we met your expectations? "What questions do you have that I can answer?" and "How did we do?" These questions reflect a deep awareness of the fairness we commit to our practice.

The elevator speech: A medical director and her nursing director partner are waiting for an elevator as they go to round on inpatients admitted from the ED. The elevator door opens to reveal the following people: the CEO, CMO, CNO, COO, CFO, and the board chair, who are making their own rounds. Inevitably, they will ask, "How is it going today in the ED?"

The physician and nurse should have already prepared their elevator speech and discussed it with each other, as both will serve as chief storytellers when explaining the complex adaptive system of the ED. The story should always begin and end with the patient, not the staff, since that is their main focus—and power. Committing the time and effort to coordinate an elevator speech focusing on the patient also helps create a sense of fairness in those who hear it.

Become the "problem" doctor and nurse: This advice seems counterintuitive; however, it is wise to develop a reputation for being proficient at solving problems. Because the ED is a complex adaptive system, problems are a part of the nature of its operations. Emergency nurses and physicians solve problems seemingly all day, every day, so it is a skill set that is very familiar to them. Being known as a problem-solver of the highest skill is an effective pathway toward building community, both within the ED and throughout the hospital.

Reinfusing Values Into Your Practice

Leave a legacy: Values should be clear and clearly communicated among all the team members. If people feel strongly enough to state their values, they must also feel strongly enough to exemplify them in their actions. And as will be discussed below, the culture must be one of leaving a legacy through daily actions with each patient.

Every action = values: While ED personnel typically feel they have a set of values to which they hold themselves accountable, it is far less common for people to formally express what those values are. If we cannot clearly and succinctly express our values, how will we or others know them?

Some go as far as to write their own personal vision statement a personal vision statement is completed, compare those values with the stated values of the hospital and the ED. Are the two sets of principles consistent? If not, how do they differ? Are those differences fundamental enough to raise concern if people will be happy in their work? Does the experience at work lead them to believe that the actual values of the workplace are different than those proclaimed? Reflect on how they or the practice could change to better reflect the values to which the individual and their colleagues aspire. Until values are understood and articulated, it is difficult to embody them in action.

Reconnecting passion to purpose: Doesn't everyone who works in an ED deserve a life of passion connected to a great purpose? If not, who does? If someone has become a victim of "passion disconnect" and are feeling the symptoms of burnout, take steps to reconnect that passion. When my sons were still young, I always said the same thing to them when I dropped them off at school each day: "One more step in the journey of discovering where your deep joy intersects the world's deep needs."[15]

The point is that the proper starting place is one's own "deep joy," the passion that drives the person and not the relative abstraction of what the world needs. Sometimes, especially when the threat of burnout is looming, reconnect passion to the work.

Keep a patient journal: It's a natural human tendency, perhaps accentuated in professionals, to focus on the negative in hopes of finding ways to become better. But emergency physicians and nurses aren't always great at recalling and reflecting on the good things they do during a normal day. Those good things are not just the saving of lives or making a complicated diagnosis; they are also the simple kindnesses we express to our patients and each other. One way to ensure that these critically important moments aren't forgotten is to write them down. Keep a journal, preferably at the end of each shift, but no less than weekly, where a brief note is written, recalling a patient and their family, or a nurse who made a great pickup, or a doc who was especially kind to others, or an ED tech who was mentored.

Don't be hesitant to praise yourself in thoughts and journal entries. Give yourself credit for what you do well. You deserve it! And don't be surprised that keeping this journal will help you adopt even more habits of kindness and gratitude.

Be like Praveen: Everyone has heroes in their work, heroes whose values inspire us to do better, care more, and care more often. One of mine is Dr. Praveen Kache, with whom I worked at Sentara Northern Virginia Medical Center. Praveen is one of the kindest people I know, but this story is about much more than kindness. He was working an overnight shift when an 85-year-old lady was brought in from Brightview, the nearby nursing home/assisted-living facility. She was mentally sharp and had a French accent, having lived in Normandy during the Nazi Occupation in World War II. Using his patient experience skills, Praveen asked her, "What's the most important thing I can do for you to make this a great ED visit?" She replied, "Just get me well enough to go back to Brightview."

Praveen took great care of her, hydrating her, and getting appropriate diagnostic tests. He also took the time to sit and talk with her, letting her tell her story. True to his word, he got her back to the nursing home, as she wanted. But 1 week later, I received a note from the lady (with beautifully flowing penmanship, which is no longer taught) expressing her delight with "Dr. Kache Praveen" (she reversed his name) who "couldn't have been kinder and got me back to the nursing home, as I asked." Enclosed was a check for $10,000 made out to the ED.

We recognized Praveen at the annual medical staff meeting as a complete physician and commented on his taking the time to sit and talk with an old lady. He said, "Oh, it was my privilege! I treat these folks like they are 'time machines.' When I talk with them, I get to go back in time and experience what they lived through." Be like Praveen!

Taking on the EHR

Section 5, Informatics, is an excellent compendium of solutions to make the EHR work for the team. As physician and essayist Atul Gawande wisely notes, "I've come to feel that a system (the EHR) that promised to increase my mastery over my work has, instead, increased my work's mastery over me."[50] Here are some ideas that help us show courage by taking on the EHR on behalf of the team:

- Improving coaching and mentoring for the EHR
- Using physician and nurse champions on each unit to coach as "super users"
- Shadow shifting with EHR A-Team members
- Increasing leadership efforts through EHR optimization teams
- Meeting quarterly with system optimization teams
- Making progress transparent
- Mitigating "type, point, and click" with other solutions
- Natural language processing and speech recognition technology
- Using personal performance assistants/scribes and virtual scribes
- Using virtual assistants like Siri or Alexa to "show me"
- Using multiple screens in patient care areas to decrease screen switching
- Unroofing the abscess of the "inbox"
- Adopting "doing = documenting = decision" concepts
- Address work–life balance issues in the process
- Using AI and application program interfaces to liberate the teams
- Improving clinical decision support to smooth flow
- Exploring the use of mobile phones to simplify access to the EHR

Hope is on the horizon if leaders empower their teams to "take on the EHRs."

Redesigning Performance Assessments

In far too many hospitals and health-care institutions (including EDs), the performance-assessment process reeks far too much of hierarchical, authoritarian interactions and far too little of a chance to compare the demands of the job with the resources needed to complete the tasks. As experts in the field of leadership have noted, such sessions often have an almost neocolonial feel in which professionals believe they are fundamentally being told:[48,51,52]

- "Here are your deficiencies."
- "Here are the data supporting your deficiencies (which you had no voice in generating)."
- "Here's the time line for reassessing your deficient performance."
- "Fix it!"
- "Oh, by the way, I basically own you."

A far more productive approach is to use these assessments as a means of coaching and mentoring team members, including where they stand on burnout (both objectively and subjectively). This would include ways individuals can augment their capacity to deal with job stressors, but also ways in which the job itself can be changed to make it more manageable. (What a revolutionary concept—a performance assessment that takes into consideration both how the person is performing but also *how the job is performing for the person!*)

Other Voices

Regarding both diagnosis and treatment, there are several other constructs that attempt to define alternate means of identifying and treating burnout, the most prominent of which are the AMA STEPS Forward program, "Being Well in Emergency Medicine: ACEP's Guide to Investing in Yourself," the Emergency Nurses Association's "Compassion Fatigue," the white paper "IHI Framework for Improving Joy in Work," and the National Academy of Medicine's recent work *Taking Action Against Clinician Burnout*.[53-57]

THE FUTURE OF BURNOUT

As rich as the existing literature on burnout is, there are, in many respects, as many questions as answers on this intriguing topic. Important questions regarding this evolving topic are:

- Why do some clinicians burnout and others don't?
- Does emotional intelligence effect an individual's ability to deal with burnout? If so, what, specifically, are those factors?
- If we think that "only the strong survive," are we asserting that those who don't burn out are better than those who do? If so, why and how are they better?
- Are there those who are in "a state of uninformed bliss, awkward contentment, naïve happiness" who do not experience burnout?
- If so, what are those characteristics, and how are they best communicated to the staff and ingrained in others?
- Are there differences between males/females, docs/nurses, length of career and millennials in symptoms, prevention, and treatment?
- Can education and training in medical schools, nursing schools, and residency training programs circumvent the cycle of burnout by providing tools early?

These and many other rich factors will need to be explored to fully understand how to foster a healthy work environment that succeeds in eliminating burnout. No lesser goal can be tolerated.

CONCLUSION

Burnout is extremely common in EDs, affecting 70% of emergency physicians and up to 50% of nurses. Burnout in health care represents a failure of adaptive capacity to balance job stress with the resources required to deal with it, resulting in three highly negative yet completely predictable responses: overwhelming emotional exhaustion, cynicism born of detachment and depersonalization, and loss of effectiveness and personal accomplishment. The framework for organizational and personal resiliency is:

- Culture of passion and fulfillment
- Hardwiring flow + fulfillment into systems and processes
- Reigniting passion and personal resilience

Burnout manifests itself across six core domains:

- Mismatch in workload demands and capacity
- Loss of control
- Lack of rewards and recognition
- Lack of community
- Fairness
- Values

Diagnosing burnout is best done with a combination of the MBI, the PFI, and interviews with team members across the three-dimensional model and six domains. There also are effective means of preventing and treating burnout by focusing on specific strategies across the six domains. The literature on improving work environments and decreasing burnout is increasing, providing hope that the passion reconnect necessary can be attained.

REFERENCES

1. Alighieri D. *Inferno.* Ciardi J, trans. New American Library; 1954.
2. Frankl VE. *Man's Search for Meaning.* Beacon Press; 1992.
3. Arora M, Asha S, Chinnappa J, Diwan AD. Review article: burnout in emergency medicine physicians. *Emerg Med Australas.* 2013;25(6):491–495.
4. Shanafelt TD, Hasan O, Dyrbye LN, et al. Changes in burnout and satisfaction with work-life balance in physicians and the general US working population between 2011 and 2014. *Mayo Clin Proc.* 2015;90(12):1600–1613.
5. Adriaenssens J, De Gught V, Maes S. Determinants and prevalence of burnout in emergency nurses: a systematic review of 25 years of research. *Int J Nurs Stud.* November 11, 2014. Accessed June 1, 2020.
6. Sinsky CA, Dyrbye LN, West CP, et al. Professional satisfaction and career plans of US physicians. *Mayo Clin Proc.* 2017;92(11):15–16.
7. Toker S, Melamed S, Berliner E, et al. Burnout and risk of coronary heart disease: a prospective study of 8838 employees. *Psychosom Med.* 2012;74(8):840–847.
8. Shanafelt TD, Balch CM, Dyrbye LN, et al. Special report: suicidal ideation among American surgeons. *Arch Surg.* 2011;146(1):54–62.
9. Dzau VJ, Kirch D, Nasca T. Preventing a parallel pandemic—a national strategy to protect clinicians' well-being. *N Engl J Med.* May, 2020. Accessed June 1, 2020.
10. Hartzband P, Groopman J. Physician burnout, interrupted. *N Engl J Med.* May 1, 2020. Accessed June 1, 2020. doi:10.1056/NEJMp2003149
11. Maslach C, Leiter MP. Understanding the burnout experience: recent research and its implications for psychiatry. *World Psychiatry.* 2016;15(2):103–111.
12. Maslach C, Leiter MP. *The Truth About Burnout: How Organizations Cause Personal Stress and What to Do About It.* Jossey-Bass; 1997.
13. Freudenberger HJ, Richelson G. *Burnout: The High Cost of High Achievement.* Anchor Press; 1980.
14. Maslach C, Jackson SE. The measurement of experienced burnout. *J Organ Behav.* 1981;2(2):99–113.
15. Mayer T, Cates RJ. *Leadership for Great Customer Service: Satisfied Employees, Satisfied Patients.* 2nd ed. Health Administration Press; 2014.
16. Mayer T. Getting back to the job you love. *Healthcare Executive 2020.* March-April, 2020: 40–43.
17. Argyris C. *Knowledge for Action: A Guide for Overcoming Barriers to Organizational Change.* Jossey-Bass; 1993.
18. Aristotle. *Nichomachean Ethics.* University Michigan Press; 1990.
19. Selye H. *The Stress of Life.* McGraw-Hill; 1956.
20. Mayer T. *Leadership in Times of Crisis – Lessons from the NFL.* Invited keynote lecture presented to the Huron/Studer What's Right in Healthcare conference, August 28, 2020.
21. Foch F. *The Principles of War.* Henry Holt and Company; 1920.
22. Connor KM, Davidson JRT. Development of a new resilience scale: the Connor-Davidson Resilience Scale (CD-RISC). *Depress Anxiety.* 2003;18(2):76–82.
23. Prins JT, Hoekstra-Weelers JE, van de Weil HB, et al. Burnout among Dutch medical residents. *Int J Behav Med.* 2007;14:119–125.
24. Shanafelt TD, Noseworthy JH. Executive leadership and physician well-being: nine organizational strategies to promote engagement and reduce burnout. *Mayo Clin Proc.* 2017;92(1):129–146.
25. Kotter J. *What Leaders Really Do.* Free Press; 1999.
26. Mayer T, Jensen K. The patient flow advantage: how hardwiring hospital-wide flow drives competitive advantage. Lecture presented at: American College of Healthcare Executives Congress, 2017; Chicago, Ill.
27. Maslach C, Jackson SE, Leiter MP. *Maslach Burnout Inventory Manual.* Available at: https://www.mindgarden.com/117-maslach-burnout-inventory-mbi, 1997. Accessed June 2, 2020.
28. Dyrbye LN, Satele D, Shanafelt T. Ability of a 9-item well-being index to identify distress and stratify quality of life in US workers. *J Occup Environl Med.* 2016;58(8):810–817.
29. Trockel M, Bohman BD, Lesure E, et al. A brief instrument to assess both burnout and professional fulfillment in physicians: reliability and validity, including correlation with self-reported medical errors, in a sample of resident and practicing physicians. *Acad Psychiatry.* 2018;42:11–24.
30. Swensen SJ, Shanafelt TG. *Mayo Clinic Strategies to Reduce Burnout: 12 Actions to Create the Ideal Workplace.* Oxford University Press; 2020.
31. Maslach C, Schaufeli WB, Leiter MP. Job burnout. *Annu Rev of Psychol.* 2001;52:397–422.
32. Mayer T. Developing leadership and communication skills. Lecture presented at: American College of Emergency Physicians (ACEP)

Emergency Department Directors Academy (EDDA), March 2, 2020; Dallas, Tex.

33. de Gaulle C. *The Complete War Memoirs of Charles de Gaulle*. Simon and Schuster; 1955.

34. Junger S. *Tribe: On Homecoming and Belonging*. Hachette Book Group; 2016.

35. Mayer T. Leadership, management, and motivation. In: Strauss R, Mayer T, eds. *Strauss and Mayer's Emergency Department Management*. 2nd ed. American College of Emergency Physicians Press; 2020.

36. Collins JC, Porras JI. Building your company's vision. *Harvard Business Rev*. 1996:74:65–72.

37. Collins JC, Porras J. *Built to Last: Successful Habits of Visionary Companies*. Harper Collins; 1994.

38. Mayer T, Jensen K. Hardwiring hospital-wide flow to drive sustainable competitive performance. *Management in Healthcare*. 2018;2(4):373–387.

39. Jung C. *Man and His Symbols*. Random House; 1964.

40. LaPietra AM, Motov S. A country in crisis: opioid sparing solutions for acute pain management. *Missouri Med*. 2019:116(2):140–145.

41. Strauss R, Garmel G. Conflict management. In: Strauss R, Mayer T, eds. *Strauss and Mayer's Emergency Department Management*. 2nd ed. American College of Emergency Physicians Press; 2020.

42. Peters T. *Re-Imagine! Business Excellence in a Disruptive Age*. DK Press; 1993.

43. Skaugset LM, Farrell S, Carney M, et al. Can you multitask? Evidence and limitations of task switching in emergency medicine. *Ann Emerg Med*. 2016;68(2):189–195.

44. Westbrook JI, Woods A, Rob MI, et al. Association of interruptions with an increase risk and severity of medication administration errors. *Ann Intern Med*. 2010;170(8):683–690.

45. Mayer T. Rewarding the champions, corralling the stragglers. Lecture presented at: American College of Emergency Physicians (ACEP) Emergency Department Directors Academy (EDDA), February 4, 2020; Dallas, Tex.

46. Goethe W. *Poetry and Truth*. Princeton Press; 1987.

47. Peters TJ, Waterman RH. *In Search of Excellence: Lessons from America's Best-Runs Companies*. Harper Essentials; 2012.

48. Peters TJ. *The Excellence Dividend: Meeting the Tech Tide with Work that Wows and Jobs that Last*. Vintage Books; 2018.

49. Mayer T. Teams and teamwork. Lecture presented at: American College of Emergency Physicians (ACEP) Emergency Department Directors Academy (EDDA), February 4, 2020; Dallas, Tex.

50. Gawande A. Why doctors hate their computers. *The New Yorker*. November 12, 2018. Available at: https://www.newyorker.com/magazine/2018/11/12/why-doctors-hate-their-computers. Accessed June 2, 2020.

51. Block P. *Stewardship: Choosing Service Over Self-Interest*. Berrett-Koehler; 1994.

52. Drucker P. *Managing in the Next Society*. St. Martins Griffin; 2002.

53. StepsForward. American Medical Association. Available at: https://edhub.ama-assn.org/steps-forward. Accessed June 2, 2020.

54. American College of Emergency Physicians. Manfredi RA, Huber JM, eds. Being well in emergency medicine: ACEP's guide to investing in yourself. Available at: https://www.acep.org/globalassets/uploads/uploaded-files/acep/membership/sections-of-membership/wellness/ww_bwem_wellnessguide_0384_1116-.pdf.

55. Emergency Nurses Association. Compassion fatigue. Available at: https://www.ena.org/shcp/catalog/education/practice-resources/compassion-fatigue/c-23/c-104/p-315. Accessed June 2, 2020.

56. Perlo J, Balik B, Swensen S, et al. *IHI framework for improving joy in work*. IHI White Paper. Institute for Healthcare Improvement; 2017. Available at: http://www.ihi.org/resources/Pages/IHIWhitePapers/Framework-Improving-Joy-in-Work.aspx. Accessed June 2, 2020.

57. National Academy of Medicine. *Taking Action Against Clinician Burnout: A Systems Approach to Professional Well-Being*. National Academies Press; 2020.

CHAPTER 126
COMPASSION FATIGUE RESILIENCY

Kathleen Flarity, J. Eric Gentry, Jeffrey "Jim" Dietz, Vikhyat S. Bebarta

If I get to a point where I can't cry, I don't want to do it anymore.
—Bruce Janiak, MD, The First Emergency Medicine Resident

Compassion fatigue (CF) is an issue faced by emergency department (ED) clinicians, including registered nurses, physicians, residents, advanced practice providers, ED technicians, pharmacists, respiratory therapists, and others. These providers perform some of the most valuable and challenging mental and emotional work in our society. CF is not something abnormal to be ashamed of or to keep buried within until the pain is too great to bear. Those suffering from it are not alone nor defective, and this problem is not a permanent struggle with no escape. Healing, satisfaction, and resilience are possible and within reach of any clinician.

While researchers have spent much time defining and measuring burnout and CF, little effort has gone into exploring what resiliency resolution looks like, and, more importantly, how to attain it, leading to the following questions:

- Are resiliency and quality of life achievable in the chaotic demands of the ED?
- Can medical professionals and leaders hope to sustain caregiving amid the toxicity of the ED environment?

The answer is a resounding yes! Empirical evidence validates that ED clinicians are at high risk for CF (**Table 126.1**). The effects of cumulative exposure to others' distress and suffering (secondary trauma) may lead to a myriad of symptoms, including an altered world view, emotional withdrawal, depersonalization, anxiety, fatigue, and empathy blunting.[1-3] Compassion fatigue affects not only providers' job satisfaction and emotional and physical health but also the patients and department by decreasing productivity, increasing errors, and sparking turnover.[3] It is vital that individuals and organizations take measures to increase resiliency and mitigate the risk and negative effects of CF.

TABLE 126.1 ■ Professional Challenges Contributing to Compassion Fatigue
Caring for the critically ill/injured
Witnessing the pain and suffering of others
Caregivers' personal health and safety
Shift times (weekend, overnights)
Electronic health record issues
High patient acuity, overcrowding, unrealistic patient expectations, violence, trauma, and death
Rapidly responding to constantly changing time-sensitive situations[1,4,5]

Compassion fatigue may result from secondary traumatic stress (STS) in the ED, leading to burnout.[1,4,6] (See Chapter 125 for a more in-depth discussion.) Because of the debilitating nature of CF symptoms, many ED professionals need training and support to build resiliency and manage the negative effects of their work.[2,7,8] Resiliency helps individuals reduce the effects of stress, anxiety, and depression, leading to a more satisfying life.[9] Some small studies have shown that resiliency training has mitigated the negative effects of the challenging work, and it is postulated that ED staff can receive protective benefits from resiliency training.[1,7,8,10]

CASE STUDY

Ed has recently been appointed as the medical director of a Level 1 trauma center with approximately 110,000 annual patient visits. He was promoted by his peers and is well-liked and respected by all. Upon assuming the position, he was excited and had some great ideas on potential wins for the ED and the organization.

However, for the past several months, Ed has experienced both personal and professional uneasiness. He is fatigued, is having difficulty sleeping, and has been feeling moody and impatient around his coworkers and family. He initially blamed these problems on sleep deprivation, but he continues to feel increasingly unwell—emotionally and physically. His performance as a physician and medical director has been diminished.

Ed recently caught himself just as he was about to administer the wrong medication to a patient. He has also stopped doing some of the things that he usually enjoys, such as flying and spending time with his kids. In spite of his many past successes, he is starting to question whether he is capable of being a good physician and department leader.

Ed has not discussed his discomfort with anyone, fearing he would be perceived as weak and concerned that others' confidence in him might erode. Drinking more Scotch than usual, eating unhealthy food, watching television, and spending time alone are the only things that provide him with any respite. He has begun avoiding family activities and has become increasingly estranged from his wife and children. He occasionally considers discussing these difficulties with his wife, but he always stops himself, assuming that she wouldn't understand and might worry about their future.

Ed is secretly concerned that something is seriously wrong with him and suspects that he is in over his head with this new position. He is afraid that all his difficulties stem from his own weaknesses and inadequacies. When he looks at other physicians and medical directors in the hospital, they do not seem to share his struggles. They all seem to have acquired some secret formula for successfully navigating the demands of medical practice that are slowly killing him. Although he is unsure where to go from here, he vows to soldier on.

OVERVIEW OF COMPASSION FATIGUE

Compassion fatigue may result from the repeated exposure to pain and suffering that accompanies the provision of sustained, empathic care. The inability to provide short- or long-term resolutions can be a causative factor in caregiver burnout.[6,11] Compassion fatigue leads to emotional-, physical-, and work-related symptoms that negatively impact patient care and personal and professional relationships.[2,12,13] It may limit the ability of ED providers to endure in the profession.[1,6,7,12,14-16]

It is theorized that resiliency interventions might offer protective factors to mitigate the negative effects of CF.[2,6,12,16,17] Compassion fatigue is cumulative. It is not the result of caring for one memorable patient in the most extreme circumstances; instead, it is the result of providing empathetic care to hundreds if not thousands of patients over time. The collective effects of witnessing pain and suffering (secondary trauma) and working in a challenging practice environment may cause physiologic symptoms (e.g., sleep disturbances, headaches, gastrointestinal issues), emotional withdrawal, or empathy blunting.[1,7,10,19]

Compassion fatigue can mirror post-traumatic stress disorder (PTSD) but is typically more insidious in presentation. In many cases, caregivers are unaware they have CF, but family members, friends, and colleagues are often the first to notice changes in mood, behavior, and engagement.[2,20] Symptoms and distress are often related to intrusions, avoidance, traumatic memories, rumination, hyperarousal, and exhaustion.[1,10,19,21] Many clinicians ruminate over all the things they could have done better—the losses and failures. Negative health effects from CF may be in the short term or long term with significant comorbidities such as hypertension, excess weight, and chronic sleep loss but also have a negative effect on overall mortality. Exposure to chronic stress may provoke sustained physiological-perceived stress arousal and is associated with shortened telomeres (caps at the end of each strand of DNA that protect the chromosomes) and may also affect premature aging and quality of life.[22,23]

Although there is strong recognition of the prevalence and risk of CF in ED nurses, a paucity of published studies exist regarding the implementation and effectiveness of CF resiliency interventions for ED providers and none in health-care leaders.[24] In 2013, Flarity et al published a study to examine the effectiveness of an education program on CF in ED nurses.[1] The Passion in Practice program resulted in a statistically significant increase in compassion satisfaction (CS; $P = .004$) and a decrease in burnout ($P < .001$) and STS ($P = .001$) symptoms. The same intervention was evaluated in forensic nurses and nurse residents with similar results, but there are no similar studies in ED providers, so more research is needed.[7,10,24]

Operational Definitions

Compassion satisfaction is described as the fulfillment, joy, and passion arising from doing a job well and contributing to the well-being of others.[2,7,10,12,25] It is the powerful experience of emotional engagement and compassionate caring of others, despite the challenges of providing care in the ED. Compassion satisfaction also enjoys significant convergent validity with resilience.[25]

Resiliency is an individual's external and internal resources and strengths that provide the capability to endure, recover, and thrive despite life stressors and challenging demands.[2,9] Resiliency has also been referred to colloquially as *bounce*, highlighting that resilience is the individual's ability to recover after a stressful event and "regain their shape."[27] Resiliency can also be considered *adaptive capacity to deal with job stressors*.

Compassion fatigue consists of two components: burnout and STS.[2,6,12,18,28,29] Secondary traumatic stress refers to the caregiver negative effects from witnessing the pain and suffering of others. Secondary traumatic stress can be prompted by caring for trauma patients, ill or injured children, abuse, fear, or feelings of professional inadequacy.[1,2,6,7] Mayer describes a multidimensional model of burnout, which includes depersonalization, emotional exhaustion, and diminished personal accomplishment in those in the helping profession, all of which result from an excess of job stressors compared to the resiliency/adaptive capacity needed to deal with those stressors. Burnout has further evolved in health care and is linked with occupational stressors such as staffing, high patient acuity, work overload, organizational dysfunction, lack of control, unrealistic patient expectations, and lack of organizational and/or leadership support. Burnout may include feeling hopelessness, exhaustion, depression, frustration, and resentment, causing some ED providers to feel that their work does not matter.[30,31]

Risks and Protective Resiliency Factors

Reported rates of CF/burnout/STS among health-care professionals vary, with some studies showing as high as 100 or as low as 13%.[7,32] Most of the studies have considered organizational factors (caseload, acuity, training, and leadership) and demographic variables (younger, more novice caregivers are at higher risk). Fewer studies have assessed interpersonal protective factors like empathy, mindfulness, or self-regulation. These factors may influence providers' capacity to sustain an engaged healing relationship without experiencing the negative effects of witnessing the pain and suffering of others.[33,34] Risks of CF and protective factors are influenced by the amount, duration, and type of exposure to traumatized patients, supervisory support, social support, and personal resiliency practices such as self-regulation.[2,25]

While age has been shown to be a significant predictor of risk in burnout, research regarding the effect of gender has shown mixed results.[31] Occupational variables traditionally assumed to be important (such as type of caseload and supervision) were significant predictors for burnout in Siebert's (2006) research. Siebert also contends that certain personal variables should be examined as well. These include feeling overly responsible for clients and having difficulty asking for help, which her study also showed to be significant predictors of burnout.[35] Sprang and colleagues found that specialized knowledge and training are associated with higher CS and lower CF and burnout among practitioners.[32] While empathy is commonly considered a primary path of vulnerability for the development of secondary stress disorders, little empirical research has examined this relationship.[6,20,33-36]

It is postulated that clinicians can develop practices or abilities that may have protective factors on their work-related stressors, including caring for the victims of trauma. Ideally, health-care workers remain empathically engaged with patients and families and resilient, without succumbing to the negative effects of their work. Increasing the longevity of work satisfaction is discussed later in this chapter.[33]

Biological Basis for Empathy

Those who are drawn to health care may be more empathetic than the general population. An increased empathy for others may improve their caregiving but may also place the caregivers at greater risk for experiencing CF. According to the prevailing theory, empathy for the victim of trauma may be associated with some degree of experiencing it as our own (co-living the traumatic experience). Empathy is an innate human characteristic with research offering evidence for the neurobiological foundation of empathy. Mirror neurons create empathic responses when observing the actions of others and, in some cases, contribute to the negative effects of CF.[20,37]

For example, in a resiliency seminar by the lead author, participants are shown a slide with smiling happy babies, and the joy in the room is observable. Then the participants are shown a slide with pictures of children suffering, and the discomfort of the participants is also observable. In contrast to a classroom picture, the reality of actively caring for a pediatric trauma patient has a significantly more profound effect on the caregiver.

Mirror neurons are active in these situations by stimulating both the brain's empathetic centers and autonomic arousal. In nursing and physician training programs, students learn stoicism and objectivity, suppressing, repressing, and dissociating from distressing feelings. This process is learned and becomes involuntary and unconscious. However, over the long term, avoidance is an ineffective strategy for developing and maintaining resilient caregiving. The research in CF—especially the STS associated with an ED practice—demonstrates that painful experiences can resurface later in a variety of negative ways.[42] The very thing that can make caregivers good at their jobs (empathy) can contribute to unrecognized or delayed suffering.

Conversely, connection and support are primary factors of resilience among human beings. An empathetic connection with another human being interrupts the threat response (i.e., stress) and restores more optimal functioning.[42] Chronic lack of empathetic connection can exacerbate CF and the toxicity of the medical environment. Restoring and utilizing empathetic and supportive relationships can decrease the symptoms of and enhance immunity to the toxicity of the environment.

TOOLS AND INTERVENTIONS FOR RESILIENCY

The most joyful, productive, engaged staff feel physically and psychologically safe, experience purpose and meaning from their work, have some choice and control over their work environment, and experience camaraderie with others at work. There are proven methods for creating a positive work environment that create these conditions and ensure the commitment to deliver high-quality care to patients, even in chaotic times.[1]

The goal of CF research is to develop healthy caregivers who, after exposure to highly demanding and traumatic experiences, are able to master the practice of real-time resiliency and return quickly to high-functioning behaviors. Experiencing secondary trauma is an inherent risk for ED clinicians. Therefore, interventions that promote individual resilience and effective strategies in response to these adverse job exposures are likely to have significant health and economic benefits. These strategies reduce not only STS, burnout, and CF but also the risk of anxiety and depression, with their well-documented consequences on the quality of life and productivity.[43]

In an effort to mitigate support for their caregivers, many organizations have implemented resiliency or wellness programs. The 2015 Commission on Collegiate Nursing Education (CCNE) Entry-to-Practice Nurse Residency Program Standards require that residency programs include approaches to prevent CF during their education experiences.[10] Leaders in graduate medical education at the Accreditation Council for Graduate Medical Education (ACGME) and directors of individual programs and institutions acknowledge these important issues and have taken steps to address them. The ACGME outlines an expectation that institutions consider wellness initiatives to educate residents about burnout and train them in resiliency skills.[37]

Department leadership must develop a proactive approach. It is not sufficient to identify that the ED team is suffering. Leaders should also work to mitigate and resolve CF within their health-care systems. Although more research is needed, there are resiliency interventions that decrease the negative effects of CF and burnout. Tools, interventions, and programs aimed at improving resiliency in the individual and workplace are described in the next section.

Passion in Practice

Passion in Practice is a 4-hour interactive seminar adapted with permission from Dr. J. Eric Gentry's *Compassion Fatigue Prevention & Resiliency, Fitness for the Frontline* course.[44] It has shown efficacy in small limited studies among ED nurses, forensic nurses, and nurse residents.[1,7,10,25] Efficacy for the intervention was supported in a systematic review by Cocker on interventions to prevent or manage CF among emergency workers.[45] Cocker's systematic review, reported "[Flarity et al's. work was], the one study to achieve reduction in burnout and STS and an increase in CS."[45] The program is described in more detail in **Appendix 1**.

Joy in Work

The Institute for Healthcare Improvement (IHI) identifies the restoration of joy in the work environment as an important solution to burnout.[46] This positive focus avoids concentrating only on burnout and poor staff engagement. The IHI developed steps for leaders to improve joy in work to create a joyful, engaged workforce. To accomplish these steps, health-care leaders should identify the factors that diminish joy in work, take care of their workforce, and address issues that decrease joy in work.[46] A military adage that applies is: "Take care of your people, and the mission takes care of itself."

These IHI methods can help:

- Decrease medical errors
- Improve quality of care
- Increase patient satisfaction
- Improve staff health
- Reduce staff turnover

The concept of finding joy in work stresses the importance of communicating the top contributors to burnout, including chaotic work environment, work not valued by others, insufficient documentation time, and inefficient teamwork.[1] The *IHI Framework for Improving Joy in Work* white paper describes the:

- Importance of joy in work (*why*)
- Four steps leaders can take to improve joy in work (*how*)
- Nine critical components of a system for ensuring a joyful, engaged workforce (*what*)
- Key change ideas for improving joy in work, along with examples from organizations that helped test them
- Measurement and assessment tools for gauging efforts to improve joy in work

HeartMath

Some health-care organizations have implemented HeartMath as resiliency support for their employees. Although not evaluated for CF resiliency, the program provides a set of techniques aimed at lowering stress and boosting resilience, while at the same time engaging the power of positive emotions to promote well-being and self-care. In this workshop series, participants learn to build and sustain resiliency. These techniques may be shared with patients and families to lower anxiety, facilitate self-healing, and improve mood and positive outlook. In some small studies, HeartMath as a workplace intervention has shown positive personal and organizational impacts as an educational intervention on the stress of health team members.[47] In 2011, Pipe conducted a study of oncology staff (n = 29) exploring the impact of the HeartMath on Personal and Organizational Quality Assessment–Revised (POQA-R) scores at baseline and 7 months. In this small study, personal and organizational indicators of stress decreased during the time interval. (See **Appendix 2** for a more in-depth program description.)

Mindfulness-Based Stress Reduction

Mindfulness-based stress reduction (MBSR) is an evidence-based skills approach, drawing heavily from Buddhist practices. Mindfulness-based stress reduction was originally developed by Dr. Jon Kabat-Zinn at the University of Massachusetts Medical Center in the early 1970s, and it was used as an adjunctive or primary treatment for patients with chronic pain, anxiety, and/or depression. It applies the simple skills of attentional focus and relaxation to assist individuals with lessening distress and enhancing functioning.

Kabat-Zinn integrated the Buddhist practice of mindfulness meditation, also called walking meditation, to assist his patients in pain management. He discovered that when patients suffering from chronic pain could detach and divert their attention to an *observational* perspective, instead of engaging with the pain, the distress and pain level was significantly diminished. Over the next two decades, Dr. Kabat-Zinn and others began applying mindfulness to address psychiatric symptoms of anxiety and depression with great success.[48] To date, there have been over 100 randomized controlled trials demonstrating MBSR's effectiveness to a myriad of symptoms. In the 21st century, mindfulness has become an accepted and much-utilized component of medicine and psychotherapy. (For more details on MBSR and mindfulness meditation, see **Appendix 3**.)

Meditation

Meditation has been an effective method for treating stress and distress for over 5,000 years, with the first writings appearing in 1500 BC. Herbert Benson, assisted by the Dalai Lama, was one of the first 20th century physicians to develop and advocate the practice of mind–body medicine. Benson discovered the relaxation response using meditation with his patients at Harvard in the mid-1960s and found that his patients, when coached to develop these skills, improved in both physical and emotional functioning.[49]

Many mindfulness apps have been developed as meditation aids. Other apps are geared toward helping one stay more present throughout the day, using a periodic bell or reminder. Numerous apps are available, such as Headspace, Calm, and Waking Up, and numerous others have been shown to be an effective modality for encouraging meditation, improving mindfulness, and promoting self-compassion.[50]

Meditation has long been advocated for those suffering from stress. Research has demonstrated that Transcendental Meditation (TM) is a powerful adjunct for the treatment of pain, stress, depression, and anxiety.[51,52] In 2007, Maria Ospina reviewed 813 studies to determine the effectiveness of meditation on health. In her review, she subdivided the studies on meditation into five separate categories (see **Table 126.2**).[53]

In her meta-analysis, Ospina evaluated both randomized control trials (RCTs) and non-RCTs for three conditions most represented in the literature.[53] These were hypertension (27 trials), other cardiovascular diseases (21 trials), and substance abuse disorders (17 trials). Her results were the failure of any of these methods of meditation to produce robust effectiveness in lessening symptoms to the level of efficacy for any of the three conditions when compared with control groups. Her conclusions pointed out that the better designed the study, the smaller the effect size for the meditation practice(s) being investigated. However, she did not paint a completely bleak picture for the use of meditation practices in health. She found that TM, RR, and MBSR all demonstrated moderate effectiveness with the symptoms of cardiovascular disease—especially the stress-related symptoms.[53]

TABLE 126.2 ■ Types of Meditation Studies

- Mantra meditation
  - Transcendental meditation (TM)
  - Relaxation response (RR)
  - Clinically standard meditation (CSM)

- Mindfulness meditation
  - Vipassana (2500-year-old Indian meditation practice that helps practitioners see things as they really are and utilized to treat all ills in India)
  - Zen Buddhist meditation (i.e., sitting meditation)
  - Mindfulness-based stress reduction (MBSR)
  - Mindfulness-based cognitive therapy (MBCT)

- Yoga

- Tai chi

- Qigong

Several studies have identified TM as effective in lessening the symptoms of burnout and other work-related stress; however, there is yet to be well-designed RCTs that demonstrate that this practice is significantly effective when compared to control groups employing less demanding methods such as education groups or self-care activities.

Yoga

Over the past several years, yoga has emerged as a powerful adjunct to medical and psychiatric treatment.[52,54] For some conditions, such as PTSD, yoga has demonstrated powerful effects as a primary treatment.[55,56] As the research demonstrates, yoga is being increasingly used as both an adjunctive and primary treatment for physical and mental illness.

Understanding that CF shares many symptoms with PTSD, interventions that are effective for lessening the symptoms of one disorder may also be effective for managing the other.[19,57] Although several journal articles advocate the use of yoga as an ameliorative and preventive measure, no existing studies detail the effectiveness of this method in ED clinicians. However, among nurses and mental health professionals, studies exploring the use of yoga to treat and prevent burnout symptoms have demonstrated good to excellent results.[55,58] A recent meta-analysis demonstrated yoga as a useful complementary, and likely primary, method for lessening and preventing stress and burnout among health-care workers.[54]

Moving meditation methods (yoga, tai chi, qigong) will both lessen and prevent the effects of work-related stress. These effects may be due to two primary factors: developing mastery in interception (i.e., felt-sense, real-time awareness of one's physiological process) and relaxation skills. Adoption of any discipline that develops these skills is likely to have lasting positive effects in both treating and preventing the effects of work-related stress.

As was outlined by Ospina (2007) and others, the state of the research investigating the effectiveness of meditation practices is still in its adolescence.[53] Most published studies on the use of meditation, especially in the area of work place stress, have focused on simple effectiveness studies. While limited studies suggest that meditation practices are helpful, MBSR has emerged as an efficacious and recommended approach for the treatment of symptoms associated with workplace stress, burnout, and CF. As the research evolves and matures, there is reason to believe that yoga will also emerge as an effective treatment and prevention practice for these symptoms. More studies are needed.

ACEP Physician Wellness and Resiliency

The American College of Emergency Physicians (ACEP) has focused on improving the well-being of emergency physicians and residents, including developing and implementing the Well-Being Committee. The Well-Being Committee has developed educational resources on the elements of a healthy workplace environment and implemented an annual Wellness Week among a plethora of other resources on wellness.[59] The ACEP Well-Being Committee has created the *Wellness Guide Book: Being Well in Emergency Medicine: ACEP's Guide to Investing in Yourself* written by wellness champions Rita A. Manfredi and Julia M. Huber. The guide is an excellent resource that presents the emotional, physical, financial, spiritual, social, and intellectual well-being spokes of life in emergency medicine.[59] Additionally, the Well-Being Committee has compiled many resources to help emergency physicians stay healthy that are available on the ACEP website to both members and nonmembers.[59]

Institute of Healthcare Improvement Quadruple Aim

In a recent effort to improve medical care and optimize health-system performance, the IHI introduced its landmark Triple Aim approach in 2008. IHI mapped out the following three goals believed to be necessary in new designs of health care[60]:

1. Improving the patient's experience of care (including satisfaction and quality)
2. Improving the health of populations
3. Reducing the per capita cost of health care

A 2014 commentary in the *Annals of Family Medicine* by Bodenheimer and Sinsky examines how this widely accepted initiative for enhancing health systems is missing a vital ingredient for success: a framework to improve the work life of clinicians and health-care staff. Burnout is associated with lower patient satisfaction, reduced outcomes of healing, and higher overall cost, which means that its exclusion from the Triple Aim's goals for improvement imperils the whole approach.[60] The article recommended that the Triple Aim be broadened to a Quadruple Aim, one that includes the fourth objective of facilitating provider wellness.[61] Although the IHI has yet to expand their Triple Aim concept to include this fourth goal, it has begun promoting the IHI framework for improving joy in work, which incorporates nine components (among them being physical and psychology safety, autonomy, purpose, and teamwork) meant to better enable the health-care workforce to be joyful and engaged.[46,48]

Additionally, recognition of these impactful effects on productivity and patient safety has led many large health-care institutions and medical schools to add programs focused on physician wellness to their programs and curricula, with many institutions creating a chief wellness officer role to join their senior leadership team. The development of these initiatives is promising for the prevention and treatment of CF, but until more locations develop similar programs and work to refine their workplace efficacy, the caregiving field will continue to lose competent, highly qualified professionals.

Self-Assessment

Studies indicate that more than 60% of caregivers experience some elements of CF. A commonly used tool is the Professional Quality of Life Measure self-assessment (www.ProQOL.org). The reliability and validity of the tool has been previously established and is the most commonly used tool to measure the two components of CF: STS and burnout as well as CS (**Appendix 4**).

ED Debriefing Tool

In an ED survey at the University of Colorado Hospital, 78% of the respondents indicated they would like to see more debriefings after traumatic events. To support staff, Julia Lehman BSN, RN, and Barbara Blok, MD, created a debriefing tool aimed at not only education and quality improvement but also emotional processing for staff. The Permission to Pause tool is intended to be brief (less than 10 minutes) following a traumatic event. Any ED staff member can call for a debrief, which is typically led by a senior nurse or emergency physician. Emotional support is a key component as research has indicated that providers who share their experiences help to process and mitigate CF. After the debrief, staff are encouraged to return the form with the patient's medical record number. A member of the ED vitality committee then follows up with staff who were present at the debrief, offering emotional support to the ED team, resources, and referral to the department's case review committee.

Forward-Facing Professional Resilience

Forward-Facing Professional Resilience (FFPR) is a one-day training session focused on prevention and resilience components. The program has shown significant statistical and clinical effectiveness in both reducing CF symptoms and enhancing professional quality of life and resilience. With over 20 years of research and development, this resilience and *training-as-treatment* program has identified the following five core professional resiliency skills whose practice contributes to professional maturation:

- Self-regulation
- Intentionality
- Perceptual maturation
- Connection and support
- Self-care and revitalization

The FFPR process teaches providers that stress results from perceived threat where little or no danger exists.[62,63] Humans respond to perceived threat by activating the threat response and engaging systems that innervate the entire body. Health-care providers are taught self-regulation skills by engaging interoception (real-time body awareness) paired with acute relaxation to 1) reestablish comfort (reduce stress), 2) restore maximal motor and cognitive skills, and 3) maintain intentional behavior instead of aggressive or reactive conduct. (See **Appendix 5** for a more in-depth program description.)

ED LEADERSHIP RESPONSIBILITES

Imagine a workplace where all ED team members are self-regulated, connected, and supportive. *Where does the responsibility lie to reduce clinician suffering and ensure professional fulfillment?* Does it belong to leadership/organizations, or with each individual? The answer to this fundamental question is a resounding *both*. All ED clinicians will experience some negative effects from being a professional care provider. It is important that leaders see that as *normal*, not abnormal, and is a function of the way in which providers perceive and respond to their environments. Health-care providers cannot refer back to training nor the currently established paradigm and expect different results—that much is abundantly clear based on the rampant amount of discomfort, pain, and burnout afflicting many areas of modern-day professional caregiving.

Much in the work environment is in the circle of control of leaders who can help identify, mitigate, and resolve to support to ED teams. Institutional approaches that mitigate the impact of burnout in health care include assessing provider needs and returning some autonomy and control over workload to the provider.[35] It is important for leaders to regularly check in with staff rather than waiting for them to approach them. Leaders need to lead by example and implement their own self-care programs that renew, reenergize, and re-passion them. Strive to stay self-regulated and support staff who are suffering from CF or other stress-related issues.

Our vision is that when leadership and ED providers understand this dynamic and are able to each interrupt their own threat responses, there is the possibility of true collaboration. As each stakeholder is able to dial down their sympathetic nervous system (SNS) response, this restores the creative, empathetic, problem-solving, and communicative parts of their brains. With a comfortable body and a fully active neocortex, individuals are empowered to come together and work with each other to create the strategies, programs, and procedures that evolve the workplace environment away from toxicity toward health, engage providers to provide effective and satisfying care to patients, and maximize the profitability of our services.

This vision represents a revolutionary change in the fields of professional health care. Providers working comfortably at the top of their scope of practice; administrators working with providers and ED staff to make the workplace less chaotic and more supportive of the work being performed; patients receiving better care from providers who are in control of their own bodies and minds. Win. Win. Win.

CONCLUSION

Compassion fatigue is an important issue faced by ED clinicians who are providing some of society's most challenging work. Work in the ED is difficult and requires self-regulation and resiliency both personally and professionally to mitigate the negative effects of caregiving. Those suffering from CF are not alone, and it is not an inevitable result of the work; there are evidence-based resiliency solutions. Healing, satisfaction, and resilience are possible and within reach of any ED provider. This chapter discussed how individual and organizational health-care leadership can embrace and initiate methods to create a more efficient, empathetic, and effective system for future generations of caregivers, administrators, and patients.

The effects of work-related stress and burnout—CF—are real, significant, and devastating. The costs of unmitigated CF are immense due to many factors resulting from its effects, including staff attrition, sick time taken, medical errors, low morale, patient dissatisfaction, and work place violence. It is emergent and incumbent upon health-care leaders to address the issues stemming from work-related stress conditions. From a cost perspective, prevention dedicated to training staff to become more resilient can save millions of dollars resulting from the negative effects of CF both professionally (medical errors, patient dissatisfaction, staff turnover, etc.) and personally (health issues, relationship issues, fatigue, sleep disturbances, etc.).[57]

This chapter outlined some ways in which ED team members and leaders can pursue the lessening of their work-related symptoms and prevent future ones. Programs offering MBSR training are likely to be highly effective and are enthusiastically recommended. Yoga, tai chi, and qigong are also likely to be effective adjunct to any program. The FFPR workshop and Passion in Practice have brought elements of all the effective components together in one training activity and has good research on its effectiveness.[56]

There are methods that can help professionals navigate the toxic environment of health care without succumbing to its negative effects. Studies support that CF interventions can be beneficial for caregivers. More research is needed to examine the optimal timing, content, and delivery of CF prevention interventions. The need for additional research is underscored by the fact that CCNE and ACGME recently included CF and stress reduction education in their standards for accreditation.

APPENDIX 126.1: PASSION IN PRACTICE

Passion in practice is an intensive, two-level intervention.

First level: A 4-hour, interactive group seminar with multimedia resources focusing on:

- Origins of CF
- Physiological effects
- Signs and symptoms of CF and burnout
- Factors associated with working in health care that may lead to CF and burnout
- Information about how to prevent and treat CF using the following five elements identified by Gentry et al.[44,57]
    - Self-regulation
    - Intentionality

□ Perceptual maturation/self-validated caregiving
□ Social connectedness
□ Self-care

Second level: Participants are provided multimedia resources such as printed seminar handouts, a guided imagery CD, access to a website with CF, CS, and resiliency educational resources and publications.[45]

The Passion in Practice seminar includes an interactive lecture with slides, videos, group discussions, and individual and group exercises. The individual and group activities provide the participants an opportunity to apply the various intervention techniques. The participants do the following:

- Learn about the effects of chronic sympathetic stimulation on behavioral and cognitive function, laying the foundation for conceptualizing the importance of CF resiliency.
- Engage in several individual and group exercises to apply each strategy tool, including self-regulation, deep breathing, progressive relaxation, meditation, and guided imagery.
- Learn parasympathetic dominance as a technique to reduce the negative impact of stressors through demonstration and return demonstration of self-regulation skills.
- Utilize actionable relaxation techniques to apply while in highly stressful situations, such as caring for critically ill or injured patients or in emotionally charged situations. These techniques help clinicians to reduce the impact of the SNS. The SNS is responsible for the fight-or-flight response (release of catecholamine, neurotransmitters, and cortisol).
- Practice methods of perceptual maturation, self-regulation, and social connection. These exercises were designed to build critical skills of self-regulation to maintain a calm focus, foster critical thinking, and achieve peak performance during high-stress situations, stabilizing the wide biochemical swings produced by acutely stressful events.
- In addition to maintaining mental and physical fitness, early evidence suggests that practice with these tools can provide extra protection against the later development of CF.[1,2,17] This is due to the way the tools train the body to settle its biochemistry back down after intense, stressful, or chaotic events. These exercises teach simple but powerful relaxation skills, including self-regulation through conscious breathing, word and phrase repetition, and progressive body relaxation.
- Experienced, guided imaging for deep relaxation. The intervention included training on living with intentionality and application, as well as the importance and methods of social connectedness and sharing of personal trauma narratives for mitigating professional stress. The participants explore self-care actions necessary for reenergizing, renewing, and recharging, which included strategies related to healthy diet, exercise, optimal sleep, and stress mitigation.

Cocker further expands in the systematic review, "Unlike the other twelve interventions evaluated, this intervention focuses on teaching participants: i) about CF; ii) how to recognize, and actively prevent and treat CF in themselves and their colleagues; and iii) provides them with tools and resources to consolidate these learnings which is likely to increase the probability of these positive outcomes remaining long term."[45]

APPENDIX 126.2: HEARTMATH

HeartMath, used primarily in non-medical settings, is taught by certified trainers and consists of two, three-hour training workshops scheduled two weeks apart. It is a structured educational program designed to teach individuals to recognize their stress symptoms and to apply learned skills to counteract the negative effects of stress.[64,65] Several techniques are taught in a workshop format. The techniques are based on behavioral interventions that focus on improving self-regulation of physiological responses through various approaches that may be used in the moment and during the day. The program also offers participants the opportunity to use heart rate variability feedback, which is designed to help individuals learn self-regulation for a healthier physiological state.[64-66]

APPENDIX 126.3: MINDFULNESS MEDITATION

Mindfulness can be cultivated through a variety of meditation practices. It functions as an intentional (instead of autopilot) perspective through which personal stories are contemplated, reorganized, and refined. Formal meditation and relaxation practices are combined in MBSR to enhance the participant's awareness of the steam of thoughts, flow of feelings, and presence of sensations that often go unnoticed, yet inform action and behavior from moment to moment (**Table 126.3**).

Mindfulness-based stress reduction is a training program designed to teach these skills with participants to foster relaxation and nonjudgmental awareness. Since its inception in 1979, there have been more than 1,000 certified MBSR trainers who have completed this training in the United States and 30 countries abroad. The program is an eight-week training process that builds mastery of the skills listed in Table 126.3 with participants. As they begin to develop a skills mastery sufficient to implement relaxed awareness during the courses, participants are then coached to bring the mindfulness skills to all areas of their lives to lessen distress and improve functioning.[67]

Over the past few decades, MBSR has begun to be applied toward to treatment of burnout in medicine and in all caregiving industries with significant success. In a 2018 article published in an open-access journal, Dutch and United Kingdom researchers explored the effectiveness of MBSR for work-related symptoms in a quasi-meta-analytic review of previously published studies.[67] In the study, the authors reviewed 24 outcome studies that tested the effectiveness of MBSR on employee health. They found strong evidence that MBSR provided significant relief from of emotional exhaustion (a dimension of burnout), stress, psychological distress, depression, anxiety, and occupational stress. Some improvement was found for personal accomplishment (a dimension of burnout), (occupational) self-compassion, sleep quality, and relaxation. The conclusion they reached after reviewing the 24 studies of MBSR applied toward the treatment of work-related symptoms was: "The results of this systematic review suggest that MBSR may help to improve psychological functioning in employees."[67]

At least five studies have explored the effectiveness of MBSR with health-care professionals. The first study by Rosenweig et al found that MBSR was significantly effective for relieving mood disorder symptoms among 140 medical students.[48] In 2005, Shapiro et al found that MBSR was effective for burnout symptoms and significantly effective in lessening perceived stress among 10 health-care professionals. In a study looking at burnout symptoms among 29 health-care professionals (physicians, advanced practice providers, and nurses), Martin-Asuero et al found that MBSR was a statistically and clinically significant intervention for the reduction of work-related stress symptoms.[68] Goodman and Schorling found MBSR had a significantly ameliorative effect upon all three burnout symptoms as well as enhancing physical and mental well-being among 93 health professionals.[69] Finally, in 2016, several Irish researchers found that MBSR was very effective with medical students.[70]

TABLE 126.3 ■ Mindfulness Meditation Practices	
Body scan	A guided exercise to promote awareness of each part of the body. With this awareness comes the ability to effect immediate relaxation, therefore lessening anxiety and distress associated with the situation.
Mindful movement	Also called mindful yoga, in which participants are guided through a series of gentle movements, postures, and stretching exercises in the training programs to be able to self-engage these skills to lessen anxiety and to stimulate relaxed movement.
Sitting meditation	Quiet sitting to develop the skill of simply noticing—without intention—breath, thoughts, feelings, and sensations. Cultivating these skills diminishes arousal, provides clearer thinking, and lessens automaticity.
Walking meditation	Slow or fast walking with relaxed awareness of self and the environment without judgment and constantly turning away from intrusive thoughts to simply focus upon the present sensory stimuli.

Reviewing the evidence, it seems that MBSR is a useful, effective, easy-to-learn, and cost-effective method for helping care professional lessen the effects of work-related stress in their professional lives. It is interesting that MBSR, in addition to symptom reduction, also produces a significant enhancing of a sense of well-being among those who regularly practice its skills.

APPENDIX 126.4: THE QUALITY-OF-LIFE SCALE

When you help people you have direct contact with their lives. As you may have found, your compassion for those you help can affect you in positive and negative ways. Below are some questions about your experiences, both positive and negative, as a helper. Consider each of the following questions about you and your current work situation. Select the number that honestly reflects how frequently you experienced these things in the *last 30 days*.[25]

Scoring

Based on your responses, place your personal scores below. If you have any concerns, you should discuss them with a physical or mental health-care professional.

Compassion Satisfaction

Compassion satisfaction is about the pleasure you derive from being able to do your work well. For example. you may feel like it is a pleasure to help others through your work. You may feel positively about your colleagues or your ability to contribute to the work setting or even the greater good of society. Higher scores on this scale represent a greater satisfaction related to your ability to be an effective caregiver in your job.

The average score is 50 (SD: 10; alpha scale reliability: .88). About 25% of people score higher than 57 and about 25% of people score below 43. If you are in the higher range, you probably derive a good deal of professional satisfaction from your position. If your scores are below 40, you may either find problems with your job, or there may be some other reason—for example, you might derive your satisfaction from activities other than your job.

Burnout

Most people have an intuitive idea of what burnout is. From the research perspective, burnout is one of the elements of CF. It is associated with feelings of hopelessness and difficulties

TABLE 126.4 ■ Professional Quality-of-Life Scale (PROQOL)

		1 = Never	2 = Rarely	3 = Sometimes	4 = Often	5 = Very Often
1.	I am happy.					
2.	I am preoccupied with more than one person I [help].					
3.	I get satisfaction from being able to [help] people.					
4.	I feel connected to others.					
5.	I jump or am startled by unexpected sounds.					
6.	I feel invigorated after working with those I [help].					
7.	I find it difficult to separate my personal life from my life as a [helped].					
8.	I am not as productive at work because I am losing sleep over traumatic experiences of a person I [help].					
9.	I think that I might have been affected by the traumatic stress of those I [help].					
10.	I feel trapped by my job as a [helper].					
11.	Because of my [helping], I have felt "on edge" about various things.					
12.	I like my work as a [helper].					
13.	I feel depressed because of the traumatic experiences of the people I [help].					
14.	I feel as though I am experiencing the trauma of someone I have [helped].					
15.	I have beliefs that sustain me.					
16.	I am pleased with how I am able to keep up with [helping] techniques and protocols.					
17.	I am the person I always wanted to be.					
18.	My work makes me feel satisfied.					
19.	I feel worn out because of my work as a [helper].					
20.	I have happy thoughts and feelings about those I [help] and how I could help them.					
21.	I feel overwhelmed because my case [work] load seems endless.					
22.	I believe I can make a difference through my work.					
23.	I avoid certain activities or situations because they remind me of frightening experiences of the people I [help].					
24.	I am proud of what I can do to [help].					
25.	As a result of my [helping], I have intrusive, frightening thoughts.					
26.	I feel "bogged down" by the system.					
27.	I have thoughts that I am a "success" as a [helper].					
28.	I can't recall important parts of my work with trauma victims.					
29.	I am a very caring person.					
30.	I am happy that I chose to do this work.					

in dealing with work or in doing your job effectively. These negative feelings usually have a gradual onset. They can reflect the feeling that your efforts make no difference, or they can be associated with a very high workload or a nonsupportive work environment. Higher scores on this scale mean that you are at higher risk for burnout.

The average score on the burnout scale is 50 (SD: 10; alpha scale reliability: .75). About 25% of people score above 57 and about 25% of people score below 43. If your score is below 43, this probably reflects positive feelings about your ability to be effective in your work. If you score above 57, you may wish to think about what at work makes you feel like you are not effective in your position. Your score may reflect your mood; perhaps you were having a "bad day" or are in need of some time off. If the high score persists or is reflective of other worries, it may be a cause for concern.

Secondary Traumatic Stress

The second component of CF is STS. It is about your work related, secondary exposure to extremely or traumatically stressful events. Developing problems due to exposure to other's trauma is somewhat rare but does happen to many people who care for those who have experienced extremely or traumatically stressful events. For example, you may repeatedly hear stories about the traumatic things that happen to other people, commonly called *vicarious traumatization*. If your work puts you directly in the path of danger, for example, field work in a war or area of civil violence, this is not secondary exposure; your exposure is primary. However, if you are exposed to others' traumatic events as a result of your work, for example, as a therapist or an emergency worker, this is secondary exposure. The symptoms of STS are usually rapid in onset and associated with a particular event. They may include being afraid, having difficulty sleeping, having images of the upsetting event pop into your mind, or avoiding things that remind you of the event.

The average score on this scale is 50 (SD: 10; alpha scale reliability: .81). About 25% of people score below 43 and about 25% of people score above 57. If your score is above 57, you may want to take some time to think about what at work may be frightening to you or if there is some other reason for the elevated score. While higher scores do not mean that you do have a problem, they are an indication that you may want to examine how you feel about your work and your work environment. You may wish to discuss this with your supervisor, a colleague, or a health-care professional.

APPENDIX 126.5: FORWARD-FACING RESILIENCE

Forward-Facing Professional Resilience (FFPR) is a single-day, evidence-informed treatment program demonstrating significant statistical and clinical effectiveness in reducing CF symptoms and in enhancing professional quality of life and resilience.[19,71] Keys to FFPR include self-regulation and an internal locus of control. Environmental factors (physical demands, politics, etc.) are responsible for the deleterious effects associated with providing patient care; therefore, the provider tacitly believes this must change in order to realize a professional quality of life. FFPR teaches that stress results from perceived threat where little or no danger exists. Brief stress response activation is innocuous, but extended periods may lead to symptoms mimicking anxiety or depressive disorders.[72,73] Self-regulation through interoception paired with acute relaxation executed within a defined temporal window:

- Reduces stress
- Restores maximal motor and cognitive skills
- Supports intentional behavior

Over 20 years of research and development on this *training-as-treatment* program has identified five core professional resiliency skills.

Skill 1: Self-regulation is the central resilience skill, and FFPR focuses on modulating the autonomic nervous systems to combat CF genesis. Emergency clinicians discover how chronic activation of the threat response system generates deleterious stress (including secondary and posttraumatic stress), and they learn stress management strategies like reciprocal inhibition (exposure + relaxation). Self-regulation is distinct from relaxation (i.e., meditation), which require extended periods of dissociation from life activities (work, family, play). Self-regulation interrupts the threat response while the professional is fully engaged in life activities, relying on neuroception and interoception. Neuroception is the ability to discern safety in one's environment. This skill empowers providers to cognitively interrupt their physiological threat response. Interoception is a tangible, real-time awareness of physiological processes. This skill develops the ability to mentally locate and then actively calm physical tension to recover optimal neocortex function. Mastering these foundational skills requires diligent practice, but the benefits are permanent and life-changing.

Skill 2: Intentionality requires a focus on deliberate behavior throughout the workday to distance environmental stimuli from provider reactions. This separation is critical to reducing stress which may trigger self-defense behaviors and potential integrity violations. Behavior code breaches (sarcasm, avoidance) result from an unmitigated threat response. Realizing integrity violations are temporary hyperstimulation events is a relief to the provider affected by these lapses. Intentionality requires self-control over emotional stress responses threatening to siphon energy to the brain's emergency centers (thalamus, amygdala).[72] It also requires mission focus, which gives work purpose, meaning, and accomplishment.

Skill 3: Perceptual maturation focuses on how the professional's *perception* of the workplace causes physical distress. This insight reveals the pathway to burnout prevention and resolution: relax the body and change your perception. Shifting perceptions profoundly diminishes workplace toxicity. A physician may *perceive* a threat when 50+ patients are awaiting care, but shifting her perception quiets the physiological threat response, allowing her to perform her duties. FFPR also champions an internal locus of control, giving the provider power over their fate and providing vision and direction for professional career management.

Skill 4: Connection and support, especially relationships and attachment, are crucial to resilience, well-being, and quality of life.[74,75] Empathetic attachment relieves stress in humans and other mammals.[73,76–78] Stress elicits an instinctual desire to isolate and avoid relationship demands, which ultimately exacerbates symptoms; social support robustly mitigates work-related stress and burnout.[79] Developing and *utilizing* social support networks lessens STS by sharing difficult experiences with an empathetic peer accountability partner, and this social engagement enhances well-being.[57]

Skill 5: Self-care and revitalization in FFPR is about creating the buoyancy and energy to sustain work intensity. Sustaining medical practice and leadership skills requires active, ongoing, and intentional *re-fueling* through self-care. Many CF programs focus on self-care as the primary intervention for the effects of work-related stress, but FFPR enhances self-care in multiple needs areas: physical, psychological, emotional, spiritual, and professional.

REFERENCES

1. Flarity K, Gentry JE, Mesnikoff N. The effectiveness of an educational program on preventing and treating compassion fatigue in emergency nurses. *Adv Emerg Nurs J*. 2013;35(3):1–12.
2. Gentry JE. *Forward-Facing Trauma Therapy: Healing the Moral Wound*. Sarasota, Fla: Compassion Unlimited; 2016.
3. Lombardo B, Eyre C. Compassion fatigue: a nurse's primer. *Online J Issues Nurs*. 2011;16(1):3
4. Dominguez-Gomez E, Rutledge DN. Prevalence of secondary traumatic stress among emergency nurses. *JEN*. 2009;35(3): 199–204.

5. Zavotsky KE, Chan GK. Exploring the relationship among moral distress, coping, and the practice environment in ED nurses. *Adv Emerg Nurs J.* 2016;38(2):133–146.

6. Figley CR, Kleber RJ. Beyond the "victim". In: Figley CR, Kleber RJ, eds. *Beyond Trauma.* Boston, Mass: Springer; 1995:75–98.

7. Flarity K, Nash K, Jones J, Steinbruner D. Intervening to improve compassion fatigue resiliency in forensic nurses. *Adv Emerg Nurs J.* 2016;38(2):1–10.

9. American Psychological Association. 2015 Stress in America. http://www.apa.org/news/press/releases/stress/2015/snapshot.aspx. Accessed January 5, 2021.

10. Flarity K, Jones W, Reckard P. Intervening to improve compassion fatigue resiliency in nurse residents. *J Nurs Educ Pract.* 2016;6(12):1–6.

11. Vahey DC, Aiken LH, Sloane DM, Clarke SP, Vargas D. Nurse burnout and patient satisfaction. *Med Care.* 2004; 42(2 suppl):1157–1166.

12. Gentry JE, Baranowsky AB, Dunning K. ARP: The Accelerated Recovery Program (ARP) for compassion fatigue. In: Figley CR, ed. *Treating Compassion Fatigue.* New York, NY: Brunner/Mazel; 2002:123–137.

13. Hunsaker S, Chen H-C, Maughan D, Heaston S. Factors that influence the development of compassion fatigue, burnout, and compassion satisfaction in emergency department nurses. *J Nurs Scholarsh.* 2015;47(2):186–194.

14. Huggard P. Compassion fatigue: how much can I give? *Med Educ.* 2003;37(2):163–164. PMID: 12558888.

15. Laposa JM, Alden LE, Fullerton LM. Work stress and posttraumatic stress disorder in ED nurses/personnel. *J Emerg Nurs.* 2003;29(1):23–28.

16. Gillespie GL, Gates DM, Succop P. Psychometrics of the healthcare productivity survey. *Adv Emerg Nurs J.* 2010;32(3):258–271.

17. Naparstek B. Guided meditation guided imagery and visualization-health journeys. 2016. Available at: http://www.healthjourneys.com/. Accessed January 5, 2021.

18. Radey M, Figley CR. The social psychology of compassion. *Clin Soc Work J.* 2007;35(3):207–214.

19. Gentry JE. Compassion fatigue: a crucible of transformation. *J Trauma Pract.* 2002;1(3–4):37–61.

20. Iacoboni M. Imitation, empathy, and mirror neurons. *Ann Rev Psych.* 2009;60:653–670.

21. El-bar N, Levy A, Wald HS, Biderman A. Compassion fatigue, burnout and compassion satisfaction among family physicians in the Negev area—a cross-sectional study. *Isr J Health Policy Res.* 2013;2(1):31.

22. Mathur MB, Epel E, Kind S, et al. Perceived stress and telomere length: a systematic review, meta-analysis, and methodologic considerations for advancing the field. *Brain Behav Immun.* 2016;54:158–169.

23. Thimmapuram J, Pargament R, Sibliss K, Grim R, Risques R, Toorens E. Effect of heartfulness meditation on burnout, emotional wellness, and telomere length in health care professionals. *J Community Hosp Intern Med Perspect.* 2017;7(1):21–27. PMID: 28634520.

24. Sorenson C, Bolick B, Wright K, Hamilton R. Understanding compassion fatigue in healthcare providers: a review of current literature. *J Nurs Scholarsh.* 2016;48(5):456–465.

25. Flarity K, Moorer A, Jones-Rhodes WC. Longitudinal study of an intervention to improve compassion fatigue resiliency in nurse residents. *J Nur Ed Pract.* 2018;8(9):61–67.23.

26. Greene RR, Galambos C, Lee Y. Resilience theory. *J Hum Behav Soc Env.* 2004;8(4):75–91. doi:10.1300/J137v08n04_05

27. Smith BW, Tooley EM, Christopher PJ, Kay VS. Resilience as the ability to bounce back from stress: a neglected personal resource. *J Pos Psych.* 2010;5(3):166–176.

28. Stamm BH. The ProQOL (Professional Quality of Life Scale: Compassion satisfaction and compassion fatigue). Pocatello, Idaho: ProQOL.org; 2010. Available at: www.proqol.org. Accessed January 5, 2021.

29. Sabo BM. Compassion fatigue and nursing work: can we accurately capture the consequences of caring work? *Int J Nurs Pract.* 2006;12(3):136–42. PMID: 16674780.

30. Maslach C, Jackson SE, Leiter MP. *Maslach Burnout Inventory.* 3rd ed. 1997. Available at: https://www.researchgate.net/profile/Christina_Maslach/publication/277816643_The_Maslach_Burnout_Inventory_Manual/links/5574dbd708aeb6d8c01946d7.pdf. Accessed January 5, 2021.

31. Maslach C, Schaufeli WB, Leiter MP. Job burnout. *Ann R Psych.* 2001;52(1):397–422.

32. Sprang G, Clark J, Whitt-Woosley A. Compassion fatigue, compassion satisfaction, and burnout: factors impacting a professional's quality of life. *J Loss Trauma.* 2007;12:259–280.

33. Thomas JT. Does personal distress mediate the effect of mindfulness on professional quality of life? *Adv Soc Work.* 2012;13(3):561–585.

34. Thomas JT, Otis MD. Intrapsychic predictors of professional quality of life: mindfulness, empathy, and emotional separation. *J Soc Work Res.* 2010;1(2):83–98.

35. Babineau T, Thomas A, Wu V. Physician burnout and compassion fatigue: individual and institutional response to an emerging crisis. *Curr Treat Options Pediatr.* 2019;5(1):1–10.

36. Decety J, Lamm C. Human empathy through the lens of social neuroscience. *Sci World J.* 2006;6:1146–1163.

37. Jennings ML, Slavin SJ. Resident wellness matters: optimizing resident education and wellness through the learning environment. *Acad Med.* 2015;90:1246–1250.

42. Crumpei I, Dafinoiu I. The relation of clinical empathy to secondary traumatic stress. *Procedia Soc Behav Sci.* 2012;33:438–442.

43. Carter CS, Harris J, Porges SW. 13 Neural and evolutionary perspectives on empathy. *Soc Neurosci Empathy.* 2011;169.

44. Gentry J. Compassion fatigue prevention & resiliency, fitness for the frontline course [handout]. Unpublished—participant handout and personal conversation with author. 2012.

45. Cocker F, Joss N. Compassion fatigue among healthcare, emergency and community service workers: a systematic review. *Int J Environ Res Public Health.* 2016;13:618.

46. Perlo J, Balik B, Swensen S, Kabcenell A, Landsman J, Feeley D. *IHI Framework for Improving Joy in Work.* IHI White Paper. Cambridge, Mass: Institute for Healthcare Improvement; 2017. Available at: http://www.ihi.org/Topics/Joy-In-Work/Pages/default.aspx. Accessed January 5, 2021.

48. Rosenzweig S, Reibel DK, Greeson JM, Brainard GC, Hojat M. Mindfulness-based stress reduction lowers psychological distress in medical students. *Teach Learn Med.* 2003;15(2):88–92

49. Weggelaar-Jansen AM, van Wijngaarden J. Transferring skills in quality collaboratives focused on improving patient logistics. *BMC Health Serv Res.* 2018;18(1):224.

50. Huberty J, Green J, Glissmann C, Larkey L, Puzia M, Lee C. Efficacy of the mindfulness meditation mobile app "Calm" to reduce stress among college students: randomized controlled trial. *JMIR Mhealth Uhealth.* 2019;7(6):e14273. doi:10.2196/14273

51. Cabral P, Meyer HB, Ames D. Effectiveness of yoga therapy as a complementary treatment for major psychiatric disorders: a meta-analysis. *Prim Care Companion CNS Disorder.* 2011;13(4).

52. Cramer H, Lauche R, Langhorst J, Dobos G. Yoga for depression: a systematic review and meta-analysis. *Depress Anxiety.* 2013;30(11):1068–1083.

53. Ospina M. *Meditation Practices for Health State of the Research.* Darby, PA: DIANE Publishing; 2007.

54. Hagins M, Selfe T, Innes K. Effectiveness of yoga for hypertension: systematic review and meta-analysis. *Evid Based Complement Alternat Med*. 2013;2013:649836.
55. Mitchell KS, Dick AM, DiMartino DM, et al. A pilot study of a randomized controlled trial of yoga as an intervention for PTSD symptoms in women. *J Trauma Stress*. 2014;27(2):121–128.
56. Van der Kolk BA, Stone L, West J et al. Yoga as an adjunctive treatment for posttraumatic stress disorder: a randomized controlled trial. *J Clin Psychiatry*. 2014;75(6):e559–565.
57. Gentry E, Dietz J. A forward-facing® professional resilience: preventing & resolving burnout, toxic stress and compassion fatigue. 2019.
58. Alexander GK, Rollins K, Walker D, Wong L, Pennings J. Yoga for self-care and burnout prevention among nurses. *Workplace Health Saf*. 2015;63(10):462–470.
59. Manfredi RA, Huber JM. Being well in emergency medicine: ACEP's Guide to Investing in Yourself. 2017. Available at: https://www.acep.org/globalassets/sites/acep/media/wellness/acepwellnessguide.pdf. Accessed March 5, 2019.
60. Institute for Healthcare Improvement. IHI Triple Aim Initiative: Better Care for Individuals, Better Health for Populations, and Lower per Capita Costs. Available at: http://www.ihi.org/Engage/Initiatives/TripleAim/Pages/default.aspx. Accessed February 5, 2019.
61. Bodenheimer T, Sinsky C. From triple to quadruple aim: care of the patient requires care of the provider. *Ann Fam Med*. 2014;12(6):573–576.
64. Childre D, Rozman D. *Transforming Stress*. Oakland, Calif: New Harbinger Publications; 2005.
65. Pipe TB, Buchda VL, Launder S, et al. Building personal and professional resources of resilience and agility in the healthcare workplace. *Stress Health*. 2012 28:11–22.
66. Institute of HeartMath, IHM®. Available at: https://www.heartmath.org. Accessed January 5, 2021.
67. Shapiro SL, Astin JA, Bishop SR, Cordova M. Mindfulness-based stress reduction for health care professionals: results from a randomized trial. *Int J Stress Manage*. 2005;12(2):164.
68. Martín-Asuero A, García-Banda G. The Mindfulness-Based Stress Reduction Program (MBSR) reduces stress-related psychological distress in healthcare professionals. *Span J Psychol*. 2010;13(2):897–905.
69. Goodman MJ, Schorling JB. A mindfulness course decreases burnout and improves well-being among healthcare providers. *Int J Psych Med*. 2012;43(2):119–128.
70. Aherne C, Moran AP, Lonsdale C. The effect of mindfulness training on athletes' flow: an initial investigation. *Sport Psychol*. 2011;25(2):177–189.
71. Gentry E, Baranowsky AB, Dunning T. Compassion fatigue: Accelerated recovery program (ARP) for helping professionals. In meeting of the International Society for Traumatic Stress Studies on Linking Trauma Studies to the Universe of Science and Practice, Montreal, Quebec, Canada, September 1997.
72. Brosschot JF, Verkuil B, Thayer JF. The default response to uncertainty and the importance of perceived safety in anxiety and stress: an evolution-theoretical perspective. *J Anxiety Dis*. 2016;41:22–34.
73. Porges SW, Center BB. *The Polyvagal Theory: A Primer. Clinical Applications of the Polyvagal Theory: The Emergence of Polyvagal-Informed Therapies*. New York, NY: WW Norton and Company; 2018.
74. Porges SW. The polyvagal perspective. *Biol Psychol*. 2007;74(2):116–143.
75. Perry BD, Szalavitz M. *The Boy Who Was Raised as a Dog: And Other Stories from a Child Psychiatrist's Notebook--What Traumatized Children Can Teach Us About Loss, Love, and Healing*. New York, NY: Basic Books; 2017.
76. LeDoux JE. *Anxious: Using the Brain to Understand and Treat Fear and Anxiety*. Penguin; 2015.
77. Porges SW. Neuroception: a subconscious system for detecting threats and safety. *Zero to Three (J)*. 2004;24(5):19–24.
78. Porges SW. *The Polyvagal Theory: Neurophysiological Foundations of Emotions, Attachment, Communication, and Self-Regulation (Norton Series on Interpersonal Neurobiology)*. New York, NY: WW Norton & Company; 2011.
79. Schore AN. *Affect Regulation and the Origin of the Self: The Neurobiology of Emotional Development*. Abingdon: Routledge; 2015.

LATE CAREER TOOLKIT

Robert M. Bramante, Kathleen J. Clem

Physicians at varying stages of their careers must prepare for career change, transition, and retirement. As a relatively young field, emergency medicine still has many active late career physicians who were pioneers in the field and had no mentors for guidance. This chapter is intended for those clinicians who are thinking forward and considering options for the later parts of their careers. Physical health and personal burnout level must be taken into account when considering options for late career. The goal is to formulate a plan and walk through steps to get to those individual goals. Decisions about retirement, financial planning, and career change must be thoroughly explored and effectively navigated. Decisions for full or partial retirement or a second encore career include careful examination and optimally a network of trusted advisors.

CLASSIC GENERATIONAL EXPECTATIONS

Classic descriptions of the generations include the Silent Generation or Traditionalists, Baby Boomers, Generation X, and Millennials (see Chapter 123). While there is much debate about other generational descriptors and divisions, stereotypical members of these four generational groups are distinct and require characterization.[1] Late career physicians at the time of this writing are primarily from the Baby Boomer generation. Emergency medicine physicians of the Silent Generation were born between 1928 and 1945. Few members of this group can be found in the emergency department (ED), and having faced their own late career challenges may make superb mentors.

Silent Generation (1925–1945): Experienced the Great Depression and World War II, maintained traditional nuclear family values, and value set structure and hierarchy.

Baby Boomers (1945–1962): Experienced economic prosperity, the space race, the civil rights movement, the Vietnam War, and the COVID-19 pandemic. They also maintain traditional nuclear family values and have optimistic and competitive characteristics.

Generation X (1962–1980): Experienced political scandal, the AIDs epidemic, COVID-19 pandemic, increasing divorce, and the computer age. Change in the traditional household to single parents or dual parent employed households; are often more independent, accepting of diversity, and less structured.

Millennials (1980–1999): Experienced globalization, terrorism, COVID-19 pandemic, and rapidly advancing digital technology. Raised in child-centric households. Expect technology use, collaboration, and praise.[2]

While the Baby Boomers are currently the primary group looking at late career issues, Generation X and Millennials members can benefit from the universal lessons lived and learned by preceding generations. Despite the adjustments late career physicians have to make over time, burnout and satisfaction are experienced differently at different career stages. In a study (not specific to emergency physicians), physicians early in their careers report the lowest career choice satisfaction, and late career physicians were more likely to experience career satisfaction. Additionally, late career physicians were more likely to experience work–life balance than middle career physicians.[3,4]

While these positive attributes may be due to a self-selection bias among those who remained in their physician careers to become late stage, it is also important to consider generational influences. Expectations about wellness, work–life balance, and feedback can differ due to generational influences. A 2002 publication reported the desire for and frequency of feedback were lowest among the Traditionalists and steadily increased in subsequent generations. Additionally, an increased desire to balance career and nonwork activities noted in the younger generations.[5] While it is important to recognize and consider generational influences, it is important to recognize that these associations are broad generational characterizations and should not be attributed to individual physicians.

TECHNOLOGY

Over the past decade, the electronic health record (EHR) has become universal. Physicians under 50 years old have a higher EHR adoption rate than those aged 50 or older.[6] Overall physician satisfaction with EHRs and computerized physician order entry is low and considered a contributor to professional burnout.[7] At its inception, the EHR was the factor that drove late career decisions for some individuals. Nonadopters were essentially forced out of emergency medicine clinical practice. At least one academic center demonstrated a peak in provider attrition in the month prior EHR implementation.[8] Currently, EHR is central to, and a requirement of, practice, and while EHRs are negatively perceived, those physicians still in clinical practice have already overcome, or at least adjusted to, the burden of learning and adopting this technology.

Exponential Growth of Medical Knowledge

As medicine advances, those early in their careers have been exposed and trained in the newest techniques and practices. Late career physicians have had to seek continuing education or other training to learn and incorporate new skills and techniques, a daunting task late in one's career. This phenomenon is particularly true as the pace of change in medical practice is accelerating. Discoveries in medical science and evidence-based medicine have increased exponentially. Whereas in 1950 the doubling time for medical knowledge was thought to be 50 years, it is now as little as 73 days![9]

In emergency medicine, exponential growth has been most evident in point-of-care ultrasound. While the technology has existed for years, its proliferation, required residency education, and wide acceptance occurred after many late career physicians completed their residencies. Limited training availability is cited as one of the greatest barriers to its use.[10] As with any advancement, there are early adopters and late adopters. Typically, young clinicians are more open to change compared to late career clinicians whose patterns of practice may be more defined and less adaptable to new technologies.[11]

Expanded Educational Opportunities

Late career physicians should be encouraged to seek education and training in newer technologies in order to practice and provide up-to-date patient care. It is also crucial to recognize the difference between traditional self-education with fewer sources of information and newer guided learning with numerous new ways to obtain advanced education. Some may need direction to utilize modern apps, online evidence-based clinical decision support programs, and free open access medical education resources like podcasts, webinars, smartphone apps, and blogs. While the sheer volume of information available may be overwhelming, many learners find they can obtain information on more topics by utilizing these cultivated sessions of education.

Communication and Social Media

Communication methodologies can lead to friction for late career physicians both due to technology and generational norms. As home internet and mobile communication expanded, the concept of availability became dominant. This is another area of potential conflict as the earlier generations were accustomed to personalized and individualized communications often in the form of in-person communication, meetings, and phone calls, whereas newer generations demonstrate more broadcasted and asynchronous communication in the form of posts, text messaging, and social media.[12] Additionally, the collaborative rather than hierarchal view of the workplace by younger generations can lead to frequent less formal communications that late career physicians potentially view as not following established processes and less respectful.[3,12]

Social media (e.g., Facebook, Instagram, Twitter, online forums, etc.) presents both a benefit in terms of communication and a potential liability due to the public nature of communication. For instance, if the HIPAA privacy rules are violated, social media presence of personal posts and communications can lead to professional liability, ethical questions, and legal action by the patient and employer. It is generally in online users' best interests to remember that acceptable online behavior and commentary from physicians is no different than in an in-person communication. It is advisable to consider the axiom—once posted, always posted—since even deleted social media postings may remain forever.[13]

LATE CAREER OPTIONS

Prior to retirement, physicians should consider numerous considerations. Will retirement be a traditional full retirement or some combination of partial retirement with clinical work or an encore career? A full range of options, including clinical, nonclinical, and nonmedical, are available. The first planning step is evaluating an individual's goals, financial situation, and needs. General considerations for late career options include:

- Full-time clinical work
- Part-time clinical work (with or without other professional activities)
- Alternative professional activities (without clinical work)
- Professional retirement

Financial Planning

Some of the early financial planning questions to consider are:

- What financial requirements must be addressed?
- How much money will be needed beyond that which has been saved and invested?
  - If "retired," will continued paid professional activity (i.e., part-time work) be required?

It is a rule of thumb that a retiree can withdraw 4% of his or her portfolio each year without depleting the principle or incurring a substantial risk of running out of money. Using this rule, for every $100,000 you have, you would withdraw $4,000 a year. This rule has been based on solid academic research.[14] This formula provides 80% to 90% assurance that savings will last about 30 years. However, if the underlying assumptions no longer hold true, that is, consistent moderate interest rates will fall well below historical averages, then mathematical assumptions based on historical calculations will be incorrect.[15] Finding a trusted financial advisor is a good idea (see Chapter 90). It is best to start planning for retirement as early as possible.

Retirement affects an individual's mental health, family relationships, social network, and work-related friendships in anticipated ways.[16] Having a solid financial footing helps these other parts of retirement or career changes.

Late Career Physicians in the ED

Physicians late in their careers working in the ED both have unique challenges and bring valuable benefits. Wise department leaders find ways to capitalize on the benefits of late career physicians while making appropriate allowances for their unique needs.

Challenges include the toll shift work takes on biorhythms. With aging, the ability to tolerate night shifts decreases. However, the ability to be an early riser may benefit staffing as newer and midcareer physicians may prefer evening or even night shifts. Some late career physicians decrease their clinical time (without adding other professional responsibilities) prior to retirement if their finances allow this transition.

Recognizing the previous contributions and looking for ways to prolong the ongoing participation of late career physicians, some departments have adopted programs that allow physicians past a certain age to forgo night shifts.[3,17] One example program recommends "half-nights" at age 55 and "no-nights" at age 60. Medically, working night shifts is a known cardiac risk factor.[18] Continually changing the circadian rhythms decreases longevity, increases burnout, and has serious effects on family life, compounded by the fact that ED shift hours are not experienced or understood by the general public.

Career changing may also differ by gender. Women are more likely to modify (or even exit) clinical medicine to deal with family responsibilities. They may work part-time or not at all while their children are young. When their children are older, they may rethink their careers and choose a job outside of clinical practice. A study by the American Medical Group Association found that 44% of female physicians were working part-time in 2011, twice the level of male physicians.[19]

Cutting back on the number of clinical shifts can breathe new life into a career and for some improve attitude and enthusiasm. It provides opportunity to focus on physical fitness and allows pursuit of other life interests. Those late career physicians who decrease their shifts can serve as mentors and collaborators and bring unique viewpoints to problem-solving based on years of experience.[3]

Additional Roles Associated With the ED/Hospital

Many options exist for clinical late career clinicians. They include continuing to practice in a different capacity, such as a free-standing ED or new practice location, locums work, urgent care or primary care, and telemedicine. Administrative ED roles can lead to decreased clinical time and include creating and overseeing the schedule and paid opportunities for teaching and mentoring.

Clinical and nonclinical opportunities outside of the ED may allow clinicians to continue to support patients, colleagues, the hospital, and its leadership. A clinical example of working closely and collaboratively with the ED is working in observation medicine. This practice can be an effective alternative to the intensive emergency medicine practice, as in some locations, it allows more time for decision-making and information processing.

Typically, career path changes are preceded by earlier demonstration of interest including previous involvement, and ideally leadership, in related hospital committees or programs. Lacking experience, those appointed to new roles will be expected to address business issues with which they have had little or no experience.

Those clinicians thinking about, or accepting, physician advisor roles should consider joining professional organizations that specifically focus on the skills and development of physician leaders. One such organization is the American Association for Physician Leadership, whose goal it is to provide physicians the knowledge and skills require to become better leaders.[20]

Another form of networking and professional growth education with like-minded clinicians may be found in specialty specific groups. For instance, the American College of Emergency Physicians has sections, groups of clinicians, who "Network with other experts in the diverse areas of emergency medicine..."[21] **Box 127.1** lists several of the many section examples that might inform and professionally advance a late career physician.

Hospital Administration

Emergency physicians can and do serve in hospital administration. Although chief medical officer is the traditional role of physicians, more key hospital administration positions are opening. The opportunities are expanding as hospitals try to align more closely with physicians. For a practicing physician who wishes to decrease or discontinue patient care, these activities represent an opportunity to make a valuable difference across an entire institution and its staff and still earn a good living.

Some hospitals require continuing clinical involvement in addition to the administrative responsibilities. A physician may consider pursuing these options when they are matched by personal passion and aptitude. Networking with physicians who serve in these positions may provide insight into a career move that includes leadership in nontraditional roles.

The advantages of working in hospital administration are its financial rewards and an opportunity to stay clinically involved while using skills already gained. Administration is perceived by many as a great way to give back, and emergency physicians can and do well

---

BOX 127.1 ■ ACEP SECTIONS THAT MIGHT INTEREST LATE CAREER PHYSICIANS

- Careers in Emergency Medicine
- Emergency Medicine Informatics
- Event Medicine
- Freestanding Emergency Centers
- Pain Management and Addiction Medicine
- Quality Improvement and Patient Safety
- Rural Emergency Medicine
- Social Emergency Medicine
- Undersea and Hyperbaric Medicine

- Cruise Ship Medicine
- Emergency Telehealth
- Forensic Medicine
- Medical Humanities
- Observation Medicine
- Palliative Medicine
- Sports Medicine
- Wellness

in these roles.[3,22] The minuses of a hospital administration position include the possibility that assuming a new nonclinical role may cause a lack of credibility with former colleagues. It can also be difficult to find the right open positions, and the learning curve can be steep.

Telehealth

Physicians can play an active role in developing a variety of new software applications, ranging from at-home patient monitoring to telehealth. Telehealth is a rapidly expanding field as evidenced by the COVID-19 rapid deployment of this modality.[23]

The pluses of a role in telehealth are the variety of career paths are available to those who are computer-savvy. Learning to provide telehealth is simple and allows clinicians to continue to practice medicine, be reimbursed for rendered services, and provide value for both patients and hospitals. Further, many telehealth programs allow practice from home. Its drawbacks include that some learning is required and reimbursement for these services vary by state and payor.

Physician Advisor

A physician advisor works closely with doctors and other clinicians to improve a variety of quality, safety, well-being, and operational processes. A physician advisor can also interface with or be employed by multiple external organizations, such as Medicare's recovery audit contractors, The Joint Commission, and other regulators.

Physician advisors working at a hospital are usually chosen from within the hospital medical staff and generally are selected because they have earned their colleagues' respect and understand the particular nuances of practice at the facility. This role is best suited for a physician who is comfortable with evidence-based medicine, able to handle conflict, and effectively deals with different personality types.[24]

A key part of this job frequently involves monitoring admissions and educating colleagues with documentation, as well as offering feedback to reduce denials and improve care. A positive benefit of this role is challenging work for those interested in evidence-based medicine. It provides a valuable opportunity to improve patient quality and care and the well-being and satisfaction of colleagues. Minuses include the fact that physician advisors have to deal with pushback, and sometimes anger, from physicians. There may be goal misalignment among physicians, hospitals, and regulators, making this role complicated and frustrating.

Utilization Review

Another example of hospital-related activities that keep a late career physician intimately involved in quality is utilization review. Added benefits include the possibility of working from home and, if working full time, it may be possible to replace the clinical salary. Pluses include that reviewing claims pays relatively well, and in many cases, you can work part time from your home, while a minus is that the work is becoming more and more regimented.

Education

Physicians can serve as in-person or online educators. If already working in an academic medical center, options may exist to decrease or eliminate clinical practice time while increasing education time. In a community ED, opportunities to develop and provide staff education on specific topics such as infectious disease management or patient safety, for example, may exist.

Certain educators leave the institution entirely to work as freelance writers or even volunteer at local high schools, middle schools, and elementary schools. Many doctors dream of becoming teachers, and for some, it is a good fit. Physicians know how to talk to people about complicated medical concepts in simple terms, and they have had to speak in front of small groups. College teaching can be another excellent teaching opportunity.

Pluses of a role in education are the fact that teaching represents an opportunity to share experience and mentor others, while realizing personal satisfaction. This may be a good fit for physicians raising families or entering retirement. A minus is that education does not provide high reimbursement. The time invested in preparation for teaching is generally not reimbursed. A late career clinician should ensure teaching is a passion or potentially create an experience that is low paying and feels like drudgery.

What to Do in Retirement

Successful retirement generally involves significant forethought. It is wise to consider passions, hobbies, and even list enjoyable activities that are opportunities for expanded involvement. Ideally, increasing these experiences prior to retirement will provide a sense of the satisfaction that may occur after retirement.

Global Health

Some physicians combine their love of travel with opportunities in global health work. It is crucial to work with experts in this field to ensure the achievement of maximum benefit and to minimize potential harms. An example of the latter occurs when the programs are developed for the wrong reasons, including meeting the volunteers' needs rather than those being served, or the programs is poorly prepared to address the needs of the intended beneficiaries.[25]

Pluses are that it is gratifying work and provides opportunities for travel, new experiences, and intellectual challenges. Minuses of global health work are that it is often a voluntary rather than career path, concerns about medical *tourism*, and the potential for pathogen exposure.

Practice Management Consultancy

Thousands of physicians have begun or joined practice management consultancy firms, based on skills they learned while running a medical practice, including coding, claims processing, or practice efficiency. The transition can be an expensive, long-term process. Some physicians who start consulting firms generally continue to practice medicine to maintain credibility.

A plus is that the work can build on basic skills learned in clinical care. Minuses include the fact that it may take many years to establish the business, and many independent consultants are not successful, particularly if lacking experience or clients prior to changing careers.

Hobbies

It is a valuable exercise to determine if a beloved hobby or passionate interest has the potential to create personal financial gain, an encore career. Exploring these options before retirement can make the transition easier. Some examples might include painting, photography, or working outdoors.

Pluses include a chance to pursue a personal passion while heading into retirement, both following a passion and an existing skill. However, one minus is that it is important that the hobby is fulfilling as income from these jobs is generally low. The market may be saturated, and it can be a challenge to become established.

Career Coach

Physicians who enjoy mentoring and coaching may also consider professional coaching as an encore career. Professional training would be required to establish a coaching career, but for some clinicians who are effective listeners and counselors, this transition would be a joy and well worth the effort to develop the nuanced skills required. Once a clinician has attained the credentials, she or he could provide great value counseling others on career change, as well as helping physicians to develop their current careers, enhance their management skills, and develop new sources of income for their practices.[26]

Pluses include the high demand for coaching. Success would be rewarding both personally and financially, once trained, credentialed, and established. A minus is that it can be a challenge to develop expertise and build a client base.

COGNITIVE FUNCTION

Most adults face declining cognition in their later years (see Chapter 122). This issue is of particular concern in the fast-paced ED environment where patient safety is paramount, and the fluid intelligence which is utilized in processing new information and problem solving has been shown to decline with age.[11] Clinically, this decline may be somewhat balanced by the experience and knowledge gained with practice and time.

Unfortunately, it has been shown that physicians are often unaware of their own cognitive declines.[27] Physicians should seek out the opinions of trusted family and colleagues due to this difficulty with self-assessment. Department leaders must be aware of this issue and recognize early symptoms of cognitive decline to allow for early intervention. Clinical issues and personality changes can be subtle and develop over time. Physicians tend to have good cognitive reserves, making detection even more difficult.[28]

On the positive side, physicians can become involved in several of the described late career volunteer or paid activities without requiring the intellectual finesse required to practice emergency medicine. However, if there is some concern about cognitive decline, it should not be ignored. In cases where concern is identified, support should be provided to evaluate and understand alternate career paths, retirement options, and medical care for the identified concerns.

CONCLUSION

Regardless of the path to or type of retirement, it is critical to start planning early. Seek advice from respected authorities. Carefully evaluate your desires, financial situation, and life goals. Throughout your career, explore pathways that interest you with consideration of further development. Performing a self-evaluation and seeking and accepting feedback from colleagues may be crucial to creating a planned retirement when desired rather than required. Finally, remember the hard work, extensive training, good memories, hard times, and the many lives you have helped and forever changed.

REFERENCES

1. Walters E, Reibling E, Leung N, et al. Working with generations in emergency medicine toolkit. *Am Coll Emerg Phys*. 2017. Available at: https://lluh.org/sites/medical-center.lomalindahealth.org/files/docs/gme/EM-Workingin4s-GenerationsToolkit.pdf?rsource=medical-center.lomalindahealth.org/sites/medical-center.lomalindahealth.org/files/docs/gme/EM-Workingin4s-GenerationsToolkit.pdf. Accessed May 14, 2020.
2. Lieber LD. How HR can assist in managing the four generations in today's workplace. *Employ Relat Today*. 2010;26:85–91.

3. Mohr NM, Smith-Coggins R, Larrabee H, et al. Generational influences in academic emergency medicine: structure, function, and culture (part II). *Acad Emerg Med.* 2011;18(2):200–207.
4. Dyrbye LN, Varkey P, Boone SL, et al. Physician satisfaction and burnout at different career stages. *Mayo Clin Proc.* 2013;88(12):1358–1367.
5. Lancaster LC, Stillman D. *When Generations Collide: Who They Are, Why They Clash, How to Solve the Generational Puzzle at Work.* New York, NY: HarperCollins; 2002.
6. Jamoom E, Beatty P, Bercovitz A, et al. Physician adoption of electronic health record systems: United States, 2011. *NCHS Data Brief.* 2012;98. Available at: https://www.cdc.gov/nchs/data/databriefs/db98.pdf.
7. Shanafelt TD, Byrbye LN, Sinsky C, et al. Relationship between clerical burden and characteristics of the electronic environment with physician burnout and professional satisfaction. *Mayo Clin Proc.* 2016;91(7):836–848.
8. Crowson MG, Cail C, Eapen RJ Influence of electronic medical record implementation on provider retirement at a major academic medical centre. *J Eval Clin Pract.* 2015;22(2):222–226.
9. Densen P. Challenges and opportunities facing medical education. *Trans Am Clin Climatol Assoc.* 2011;122:48–58.
10. Sander JL, Noble VE, Raja AS, et al. Access to and use of point-of-care ultrasound in theemergency department. *West J Emeg Med.* 2015;16(5):747–752.
11. Lee L, Weston W. The aging physician. *Can Family Phys.* 2012;58(1):17–18.
12. Mohr NM, Moreno-Walton L, Mills AM, et al. Generational influences in academic emergency medicine: teaching and learning, mentoring, and technology (Part 1). *Acad Emerg Med.* 2011;18(2):190–199.
13. Ventola CL. Social media and health care professionals: benefits, risks, and best practices. *PT.* 2014;39(7):491–499, 520.
14. Anspach D. Don't cheat yourself with the 4% rule. *MarketWatch.* August 12, 2019. Available at: https://www.marketwatch.com/story/dont-cheat-yourself-with-the-4-rule-2018-05-04.
15. Kagan J. Four Percent Rule. Investopedia. May 1, 2020. Available at: https://www.investopedia.com/terms/f/four-percent-rule.asp. Accessed May 16, 2020.
16. McGurk WS. Retirement: making a successful transition. *Am Psychol Assoc.* 2005. Available at: https://www.apaservices.org/practice/ce/self-care/retirement.
17. Longevity, finances, and retirement in emergency medicine. *The Student Doctor Network.* 2015. Available at: https://forums.studentdoctor.net/threads/longevity-finances-and-retirement-in-emergency-medicine.1164727/.
18. Here's why working nights could be killing you. *World Economic Forum.* February 12, 2018. Available at: https://www.weforum.org/agenda/2018/02/working-nights-is-far-worse-for-your-health-than-you-probably-thought/.
19. More doctors work part time flexible schedules. *American Medical News.* March 26, 2012. Available at: https://amednews.com/article/20120326/business/303269974/1/.
20. American Association of Physician Leadership. 2020. Available at: https://www.physicianleaders.org/. Accessed May 16, 2020.
21. American College of Emergency Physicians. Sections of Membership. 2020. Available at: https://www.acep.org/how-we-serve/sections/. Accessed May 15, 2020.
22. Falcone RE, Satiani B. Physician as hospital chief executive officer. *Vasc Endovascular Surg.* 2008;42(1):38–94.
23. Smith AC, Thomas E, Snoswell CL, et al. Telehealth for global emergencies: implication for coronavirus disease 2019 (COVID-19). *J Telemed Telecare.* 2020;26(5):309–313.
24. Huff GL, Fee JP, Clesi W, et al. Selecting the ideal CDI physician advisor. *J AHIMA.* 2014;85(7):30–33.
25. Bauer I. More harm than good? The questionable ethics of medical volunteering and international student placements. *Trop Dis Travel Med Vaccines.* 2017;3:5.
26. Sabo K, Duff M, Purdy B. Building leadership capacity through peer career coaching: a case study. *Nursing Leadership.* 2007;21;27–35.
27. Davis DA, Mazmanian PE, Fordis M. Accuracy of physician self-assessment compared with observed measures of competence. *JAMA.* 2006;296(9):1094–1102.
28. LoboPrabhu SM, Molinari VA, Hmilton JD, et al. The aging physician with cognitive impairment: approaches to oversight, prevention, and remediation. *Am J Geri Psych.* 2009;17(6):445–454.

HEALTH-CARE POLICY

SECTION 13

INCLUSION, EQUITY, AND DIVERSITY

CHAPTER 128

Bernard L. Lopez, Andrea Green, Ugo Ezenkwele, Ava Pierce, Jeffrey Druck

Those who have the privilege to know have the duty to act.

—Albert Einstein

Diversity, inclusion, and equity are essential to excellence in health care. *Diversity* refers to the richness of human differences in race, ethnicity, socioeconomic status, language, nationality, sexual orientation, gender identity, religion, geography, abilities, age, personality, learning styles, and life experience.[1,2] Diversity incorporates all of the elements that make individuals unique. A diverse workplace employs a team of people that is reflective of the society in which the organization exists and operates.[3] Diversity is a pillar of good governance and leadership. And a diverse leadership team in health care has lasting effects on care delivery.[4] *Inclusion* is the active, intentional, and ongoing engagement with diversity.[2] Inclusion is achieved by creating a climate and culture within an institution or a society that fosters belonging, respect, and value for all.[2,5] Creating an inclusive environment is essential for the success of diversity efforts. *Equity* is the absence of avoidable or remediable differences among groups of people, whether those groups are defined socially, economically, demographically, or geographically. Conversely, health inequities involve inequality with respect to health determinants and access to the resources needed to improve and maintain health or health outcomes; they entail a failure to avoid or overcome inequalities that infringe on fairness and human rights norms.[6]

HISTORICAL IMPORTANCE OF HEALTH QUALITY AND EQUITY

The Institute of Medicine's (IOM) reports, "To Err is Human: Building a Safer Health System" (2000) and "Crossing the Quality Chasm: A New Health System for the 21st Century" (2001), brought attention to the inconsistent quality in the United States health system.[7,8] These reports documented the existence of differential access to quality care based on race and socioeconomic status and concluded that "bias, prejudice, and stereotyping on the part of health-care providers may contribute to differences in care." The reports highlighted that our health system cannot claim to deliver quality care to all patients while health disparities exist and included equity of care as one of the six pillars of quality health care.[2,8] The 2003 IOM report, "Unequal Treatment: Confronting Racial and Ethnic Disparities in Health Care," concluded that racial and ethnic minorities tend to receive a lower quality of health care than nonminorities, even when access-related factors, such as patients' insurance status and incomes, were controlled.[6]

Before June 26, 2003, the Association of American Medical Colleges (AAMC) used the term *underrepresented minority* (URM), which consisted of Blacks, Mexican Americans, Native

Americans (that is, American Indians, Alaska Natives, and Native Hawaiians), and mainland Puerto Ricans. The AAMC adopted URM on June 26, 2003, to shift the focus from a fixed aggregation of four racial and ethnic groups (Blacks, Mexican Americans, Native Americans [American Indians, Alaska Natives, and Native Hawaiians], and mainland Puerto Ricans) to accommodate the inclusion and removal of underrepresented groups on the basis of changing demographics of society and the profession. Underrepresented minority as defined by the AAMC identifies those racial and ethnic populations that are underrepresented in the medical profession relative to their numbers in the general population.[9] The AAMC workforce data for 2018 document that among active physicians, 56.2% identified as White, 17.1% identified as Asian, 5.8% identified as Hispanic, and 5.0% identified as Black or African American.[10] The number of minorities in the United States is continually increasing, but the number of URM physicians has remained relatively unchanged. The need to diversify the health-care workforce to help address health disparities is of paramount importance. The development of the chief diversity officer role in health-care organizations is one step in improving diversity.[2]

Benefits of Diversity, Equity, and Inclusion

The US Equal Employment Opportunity Commission enforces laws to protect individual employees in the workplace who commonly face discrimination based on specified social categories. These social categories typically include nondiscrimination on the basis of race/color, religion, sex (including pregnancy and gender identity), national origin, political affiliation, sexual orientation, marital status, disability, genetic information, age, membership in an employee organization, retaliation, parental status, and military service. There are certainly more visible and invisible elements that make individuals diverse from one another than those defined by these statements.[11] While these elements clearly do not define diversity alone, these categories can help identify gaps in diversity and provide measurable metrics for organizations to set goals to improve diversity in the workplace.

Benefits of a diverse health workforce include the ability to deliver quality, patient-centered care to more people through:

- *Improved access to care*: URM physicians are more likely to practice in underserved communities, including rural areas and minority communities[12,13]
- *Improved physician–patient concordance*: Patients with demographic concordance with their provider have increased trust of their physician
- *Higher patient satisfaction and improved treatment adherence*: Patient adherence generally leads to better outcomes[2,14]
- *Increased cultural competence*: Providers who work with people from different backgrounds may recognize cultural differences more easily[2,15]
- *Greater recognition of inequities in care*: A more diverse workforce may recognize inequitable care more readily[2,16]
- *Improved learning environments in medical education*: When diverse groups learn together, they become more comfortable learning about different backgrounds and are better able to pull from those experiences when treating patients.[17-22]

Political scientist Scott E. Page, author of *The Difference: How the Power of Diversity Creates Better Groups, Firms, Schools, and Societies*, states that diversity, more than ability alone, leads to improved performance and innovation, and therefore, diversity is a driver of excellence. His research documents that groups of people with different backgrounds, heuristics, experiences, and attributes can solve complex problems more quickly and completely than a homogeneous group.[2,23] Increasing diversity expands our potential to find creative solutions to our health-care challenges, mitigate against health disparities, and improve overall care and health outcomes for all patients.[2]

Despite decades of calls demanding increased representation of women and URMs in the health-care workforce, the numbers remain woefully suboptimal. Increasing efforts are required to achieve equity in representation in practice, academia, and in leadership positions for women and URMs. Focusing solely on increasing diversity in composition is not sufficient. To effectively enact change and leverage the benefits of diversity, leaders must focus their efforts on developing inclusive, equity-minded environments.[24-26] Health-care leaders must create teams with a shared desire for change and then provide those teams with the resources needed to ensure that change. With the appropriate mission and vision, a diverse health-care workforce can create innovative solutions that improve the institution's capacity for diversity, equity, and inclusion and improve the ability to deliver excellent quality care to all patients.[2,26]

THE CASE FOR DIVERSITY AND INCLUSION

Two schools of thought continue to emerge in discussions concerning the need for diversity, inclusion, and equity in hospitals and emergency departments (EDs). One consideration involves the business case for diversity and the other the moral case for diversity. As Darrin L. Williams, CEO of Southern Bancorp, Inc. states, "The business case for diversity will do more than the moral case."[27] Indeed, as this section shows, current research and industry publications have made a compelling argument concerning the business case for diversity, inclusion, and equity in EDs.

The Business Case

The racial and ethnic diversity of the United States has evolved significantly over the past 20 years and continues to increase. Extrapolations from census bureau reports show that the current racial majority will be the minority by 2050, changing the face of this nation. Hospitals and EDs must reflect the heterogenous communities that they serve to continue to be relevant and thrive in the marketplace. The conversation is no longer whether diversity, inclusion, and equity are good or bad. The conversation is about diversity as the reality and how do hospitals manage diversity and equity for successful outcomes of creating talented workforces, increasing profitability, influencing community dynamics, and decreasing cost.

Research has demonstrated that racial and gender diversity are related to business outcomes.[28,29] The heterogenicity of a company brings about increased creativity due to consideration of broader perspectives, ideas, and approaches, leading to superior problem-solving. A few studies have shown that there is higher cognitive flexibility among women and racial or ethnic minorities.[30] As EDs address metrics and risk management issues that impact hospital performance and revenues, a diversified team inclusive of gender, racial, cultural, and disability should be involved in facility policy and procedure decision-making. Staff members from diverse cultural backgrounds can serve as "cultural informants" to their peers, explaining differences in cultural norms firsthand, which can then, in turn, facilitate interactions with patients from diverse backgrounds.[31,32]

Clearly, diversity impacts the bottom line for hospitals and EDs. Organizations in the top quartile in racial and ethnic diversity are 35% more likely to have financial performance above medians, and the top quartile for gender diversity is 15% more likely to have financial performance above medians.[28] Among net results, innovation in diverse companies accounts for 19% higher revenues.[33] This translates into increased revenues, increased customers, more significant market share, and greater relative profits.[34] Research shows that a 1% increase in racial diversity increased revenues by approximately 9%, and a 1% increase in gender diversity increased revenue by approximately 3% and had a combined effect of approximately 16.5%.[34]

Most hospitals, as in other sectors of business, must generate revenues and profit. The inherent nature of EDs can create a considerable strain on the revenues and finances of a hospital due to losses from the uninsured and underinsured. Data show that in hospital EDs, most of the revenue is generated from the insured customers.[35] In a study examining ED profit margin for hospitals in 2009, patients having private insurance were the only group producing a profit margin at 39.6%. The estimated revenues would be higher with shifts in the marketplace that provide opportunities for the uninsured to obtain private insurance.[35]

Since revenues generated from the insured customers are necessary to cover the financial losses from the uninsured, it becomes imperative to increase the customer base and market share, particularly of the insured population. These customers have more choices for selecting where to get their health care. Hospitals and EDs must recognize and respond to the demographic diversity taking shape in communities and make themselves more attractive to these customers. Institutional diversity and cultural competence are crucial to developing a competitive edge and maintaining a viable market share. Racial diversity is the most critical predictor of relative market share.[34]

The Moral Case

In hospitals and EDs, community dynamics significantly influence the utilization of local services. There is no doubt that the image of the hospital and ED within a community impacts its customer base and satisfaction. A diverse workforce, as well as the quality of services provided to the community, are essential factors in customers' decision-making. Employing a diverse workforce appeals to a customer base as demonstrating to the community respect for fairness, tolerance, and human rights.

The benefits of diversity extend beyond team and workplace functioning and influence consumers' perceptions and purchasing practices.[35,36] A study evaluating the relationship between gender diversity on corporate boards and company reputation concluded that diversity positively affected the company's social responsibility ratings, which in turn positively influenced the company's reputation and attracted more customers.[31,37] Groups understand that companies like hospitals can drive positive changes within their communities. In doing so, hospitals protect their business and build customer loyalty. Building a strong culture creates conditions for hospitals and their ED to thrive and survive. This moral case is sobering, but the business case is proven and impactful.

Customer satisfaction is a critical part of ED metrics. It also plays an essential role in hospital image within the community, specialty referral patterns, evaluation by private insurers for contracting, and Centers for Medical and Medicare Services reimbursement. Patients' perceptions of personal similarity to their physicians can be a strong predictor of patients' satisfaction with care, trust in the physician, and intent to adhere to recommendations.[38] A 2001 study by the Commonwealth Fund uncovered disparities, by race and ethnicity, with patient satisfaction with their care:

> *African Americans, Asians Americans, and Hispanics are more likely than Whites to experience difficulty communicating with their physicians, feel that they are treated with disrespect when receiving health-care services, and to experience barriers to care, including lack of insurance or a regular doctor.*[39]

Cultural competence, which can be achieved by demographic diversity and inclusion, plays a significant role in ED customer satisfaction. In summary, there is a clear link between demographic diversity and the bottom line in the ED. Research and literature have shown the significance of demographic diversity in building more robust and more resilient organizations, improving profitability and financial outcomes, creating superior institutional problem solving and decision-making, building community relations, and helping to mitigate losses. Undoubtedly, demographic diversity, inclusion, and equity are increasingly a prerequisite for successful and profitable EDs.

HEALTH-CARE DISPARITIES

Much of the work that is done in creating an inclusive and diverse clinical environment is aimed at providing the most equitable health care to those served. When the environment is not inclusive and diverse, disparities ensue. In the United States, although the term disparities is often interpreted to mean racial or ethnic disparities, many dimensions of disparity exist, particularly in health care. A health disparity is:

> ... a particular type of health difference closely linked with social, economic, and/or environmental disadvantage. If a health outcome is seen to a greater or lesser extent between populations, there is disparity. Health disparities adversely affect groups of people who have systematically experienced greater obstacles to health based on their racial or ethnic group; religion; socioeconomic status; gender; age; mental health; cognitive, sensory, or physical disability; sexual orientation or gender identity; geographic location; or other characteristics historically linked to discrimination or exclusion.[40]

Disease risk factors, abject health status, and limited access to health care are often interrelated. It is essential to recognize the impact that social determinants have on the health outcomes of specific populations.

The conditions and social context in which people live can explain, in part, why specific populations in the United States are healthier than others and why some are not as healthy as they could be. According to the World Health Organization, "the social determinants of health are mostly responsible for health inequities—the unfair and avoidable differences in health status seen within and between countries."[41]

The World Health Organization defines the social determinants of health as "the conditions in which people are born, grow, live, work, and age," including the health-care system.[41] Health-care disparities refer to differences between groups in quality of care, access to and use of care, and health insurance coverage. Health disparities refer to differences that are not explained by variations in health needs, patient preferences, access-related factors, appropriateness of interventions, or treatment recommendations. They are closely linked with economic, social, and/or environmental disadvantage. The terms health inequality and inequity also are used to refer to disparities.[42,43]

Addressing health disparities is increasingly crucial as the population becomes more diverse. Since, by 2050, people of color will account for over half (52%) of the populace,[44] disparities in health and health care not only affect the groups facing inequity but also limit overall gains in quality of care and health for the broader population. These disparities will result in unnecessary direct and indirect costs. Experts estimate that disparities amount to approximately $93 billion in excess medical care costs and $42 billion in lost productivity per year and economic losses due to premature deaths.[45] So, what has been done to address these disparities?

The Result of Disparate Care

These disparities in care are evident in the acute emergency care system, an essential part of the US health-care safety net.[46] About 20% of the US population visits an ED each year, making it a relatively common site of care, and it has been suggested that care delivered in the ED provides a window into the state of health care in the United States.[47] Although the emergency care network can claim many successes, overall, the system is in trouble. A seminal report by the IOM in 2007 concluded that emergency care in the United States is underfunded, overburdened, and highly fragmented.[48] Furthermore, as the use of EDs continues to grow, the number of these facilities is declining, increasing the pressure on already-strained EDs.[49]

Upon arrival to the ED, minority populations, when compared to White patients, have also been found to receive disparate treatment for many common presentations, including:

- Chest pain and acute coronary events[50-54]
- Trauma[55-57]
- Stroke symptoms and brain injuries[58,59]
- Pain management for bone fractures, migraines, and back pain[60-62]

Even during their care, Black patients compared to White patients with similar presentations received lower emergency severity index scores in triage, were less likely to have tests ordered in the ED, were less likely to be admitted to the hospital and intensive care unit, and had a higher death rate in the ED and hospital.[63] Disturbingly these trends were true for children as well. Black, Hispanic, and Asian children were significantly less likely than White children to receive blood tests, x-rays, and computerized tomography scans in the ED and were subjected to substantially longer wait times and overall length of stays during their visits.[64] Such disparities are concerning given the strong association between emergency care quality and mortality risk, particularly given the heightened threat of racial biases affecting providers' decision-making in the fast-paced, information-poor ED.[65]

Efforts to Address Health-Care Disparities

The first significant legislation that focused on reducing disparities, the Minority Health and Health Disparities Research and Education Act of 2000, created the National Institute on Minority Health and Health Disparities and authorized the Agency for Healthcare Research and Quality (AHRQ).[66] The purpose of the AHRQ is to measure progress on systematic reduction of disparities. In 2003, the IOM released the seminal report "Unequal Treatment: Confronting Racial and Ethnic Disparities in Health Care," emphasizing the importance of health-care disparities.[67] The 2012 National Healthcare Disparities Report and the 2012 National Healthcare Quality Report found that almost none of the disparities in access to care were improving. Furthermore, the quality of care varied across the types of medical care and parts of the country.[68,69]

At the federal level, the Department of Health and Human Services (HHS) engaged in various initiatives focused on addressing disparities. Over the last decade and building on the Healthy People 2020 goals to achieve health equity and eliminate disparities, HHS has developed the "HHS Action Plan to Reduce Racial and Ethnic Health Disparities."[70-72] Since the report's release, HHS has undertaken various efforts to implement the plan, including coordinating programmatic and policy measures to advance health equity, expand access and quality of coverage and care, and strengthen health-care infrastructure and workforce. Unfortunately, despite overall improvements in population health over time, many disparities have persisted and, in some cases, worsened.

The Affordable Care Act (ACA) included provisions that advanced efforts to reduce disparities.[73] However, although the ACA did lead to gains in health-care coverage, some groups continue to lack access to care, be uninsured, and experience worse health outcomes. For instance, as of 2018, Hispanics were more likely than Whites to be uninsured (19.0% vs

7.5%) by over a two-fold margin. Individuals with incomes below poverty were four times as likely to be uninsured compared to those with incomes at 400% of the federal poverty level or above (17.3% vs 4.3%).[74]

Key initiatives to reduce disparities have been promulgated at the federal, state, and city levels and include the promotion of:

- Workforce diversity and cultural competence
- Increased funding for health-care professionals, cultural competence training, and education materials
- Data collection and research efforts

Unfortunately, actions within individual EDs remain variable and fragmented. No nationally coordinated effort among EDs exists to address disparities and the health inequities that invariably follow. Fortunately, professional organizations within the specialty recognize this issue. The American College of Emergency Physicians's (ACEP) Diversity, Inclusion and Health Equity Section, the Society of Academic Emergency Medicine's Academy of Diversity in Emergency Medicine, and the National Medical Association's (NMA) Section of Emergency Medicine are advocating for increased awareness and improvements.

UNCONSCIOUS BIAS

The previous section outlined disparities in certain groups and examples abound. Black patients with acute myocardial infarction (MI) receive percutaneous coronary intervention (PCI) at a lower rate than White patients. They also wait longer to receive care in the ED for their chest pain. A transgender patient gets asked questions about their sexual orientation that have nothing to do with their clinical condition. A Latino woman does not get adequate pain medication because she is being "dramatic." Women have a higher rate of missed MI. Male physicians receive higher pay and achieve leadership positions more often than female physicians. All of these scenarios are commonly cited in the literature and are examples of disparities that exist in health care.[75-77]

Generally, these disparities are not intentional—most health-care providers are committed to giving the best care possible to help people get and stay healthy. While the causes for these disparities are multifactorial and systems-related, unconscious bias plays a major role.

Unconscious bias, also known as implicit bias, refers to attitudes or stereotypes that are outside our awareness and affect our understanding, our interactions, and our decisions without our conscious knowledge. Evolutionarily, unconscious biases allow humans to act instinctively and protect one from harm. These same biases allow us to act quickly and efficiently in our daily actions. We all harbor automatic associations—both positive and negative—about other people based on a wide variety of characteristics such as race, ethnicity, gender, gender identity, sexual orientation, religion, age, ability/disability, social class, and appearance. These unconscious associations may influence our feelings and attitudes and have the potential to result in unconscious discriminatory practices. Given the ubiquitous and unconscious nature of these biases, they affect us in all aspects of our individual and organizational lives.

The effect of unconscious bias is greater in high-stress, demanding situations and environments and can thus have potentially life-altering consequences.[78-80] The 2003 IOM report "Unequal Treatment: Confronting Racial and Ethnic Disparities in Health Care" suggests that "bias, stereotyping, prejudice, and clinical uncertainty on the part of health-care providers may contribute to racial and ethnic disparities in health care."[8]

The Effect of Bias on Patient Care

Unconscious biases play a role in how important clues in the history and physical exam of a patient are interpreted. An unconscious bias may result in the over- or underemphasis of certain aspects, which then has the potential to negatively affect patient care, resulting in actions such as misdiagnosis, reduced analgesic treatment, and longer wait times. Unconscious bias also affects interpersonal interactions in the workplace such as the physician–nurse and director–employee and may create a certain patient care environment that may or may not be conducive to optimum care.

Consider this scenario. A 52-year-old African-American female presents to a tertiary care, academic ED with several hours of intermittent chest pain. The White male emergency medicine physician (whose peers consider him to be one of the most compassionate and knowledgeable physicians around) performs a history and physical examination and elicits a history of waxing and waning anterior chest pain, nonradiating and slightly worsened with exertion. Her pain at the time was 4 on a scale of 1 to 10. He orders the typical workup for chest pain. The electrocardiogram shows 1-mm ST-segment elevation across the precordial leads. The patient ends up being diagnosed with an acute MI and is admitted for medical therapy. No PCI is performed. In a day and age where PCI is considered the gold standard for the care of acute coronary syndrome (ACS), how does this happen? While treatment decisions are complex and are affected by many factors, studies have demonstrated that women and Black patients often do not receive the same care that men and White patients receive.

In 1998, Anthony Greenwald[81] and two colleagues created the Implicit Association Test (IAT). This online tool measures the strength of automatic associations between concepts (e.g., Black people, gay people) and evaluations (e.g., good, bad).[82] It is the most recognized and commonly used test to measure unconscious bias. The IAT score is based on how long it takes a person, on average, to associate certain evaluative words with the concept being tested. Thus, if one quickly associates "good" words with "white" and "bad" words with "black," there may be a preference of White over Black (a more detailed description can be found at https://implicit.harvard.edu/implicit/takeatest.html).

A study by Green et al in 2007[83] used the IAT to test whether physicians show implicit race bias and whether the magnitude of such bias predicts thrombolysis recommendations for Black and White patients with ACS. They presented vignettes of a patient presenting to the ED with ACS followed by a questionnaire and three IATs. A total of 287 internal medicine and emergency medicine physicians at four academic medical centers in Atlanta and Boston completed the study. Among the participants, there was explicit preference for White over Black patients on perceived cooperativeness. However, the IATs demonstrated implicit preference for White Americans and implicit stereotypes of Black Americans as less cooperative with medical procedures and in general. As the physician's pro-White implicit bias increased, so did their likelihood of treating White patients and not Black patients with thrombolysis. The authors conclude that unconscious bias may contribute to racial/ethnic disparities in the use of medical procedures, such as thrombolysis for MI. While the study is a bit dated (many physicians use PCI over thrombolytics for MI), it is the one study linking IAT results to treatment choices. A number of other studies have demonstrated the existence of implicit bias in physicians in regard to race,[78] obesity, gender, and age.[79,80]

Consider another scenario. A middle-aged Black male presents to the ED with a nondisplaced distal fibula fracture. The treating physician, who is White, administers acetaminophen for pain, discharges the patient, and tells him to continue with acetaminophen and to take ibuprofen if this does not work. Later that day, a middle-aged White male presents with a similar fibular fracture, and the same White physician administers intravenous morphine and discharges the patient with a prescription for oxycodone in case acetaminophen and ibuprofen are not effective in analgesia. How does this happen? Is it possible that the initial treating physician (again, considered to be a fine caretaker) interpreted pain and pain tolerance differently based on race?

Research has shown that racial and ethnic minorities are undertreated for pain as compared with White patients, and that it is likely related to unconscious attitudes.[84-88] In a 2016 study from the University of Virginia, researchers surveyed over 400 medical students and residents. Over half of the respondents endorsed false statements such as Blacks' nerve endings are less sensitive to pain than Whites' nerve endings; Blacks' skin is thicker than Whites' skin; Whites have a more efficient respiratory systems than Blacks; and Black people's blood coagulates more quickly than White people's blood.[89] While scientific evidence does not support these statements, the study demonstrates the existence of attitudes that would affect clinical decision-making with the potential for a poorer outcome.

It is not only the health-care provider who has bias; patients and their families also harbor biases. Thus, a patient's bias against the physician will negatively affect care. In his book *Black Man in a White Coat: A Doctor's Reflections on Race and Medicine*, Dr. Damon Tweedy describes a scenario in which a White patient for whom he has cared was initially resistant to care based purely on the fact that Dr. Tweedy was Black.[90] This scenario occurs commonly. Think of the unconscious biases that the patient may have had, such as "He's Black; they must have let him into medical school to fill a quota so he can't be as good" or "He won't really give me good care because I am White," and how these biases will affect the patient's ability to accept care. And consider this—Black patients may also harbor similar unconscious biases, seeking the "more educated and better" White physician. A minority patient may not follow the recommendations from a White physician because of their subconscious views that are based on their past experiences.

Strategies to Mitigate Bias

Research suggests that awareness coupled with a desire to overcome unconscious bias can change attitudes and lead to strategies to mitigate the effect of bias.[91,92] The American Association of Medical Colleges, in its publication "Proceedings of the Diversity and Inclusion Innovations Forum: Unconscious Bias in Academic Medicine," highlights mitigation strategies such as bias education and training and systematic identification of bias in all aspects of health care, including hiring practices and diagnosis and treatment delivery.[93] In his groundbreaking book *Everyday Bias: Identifying and Navigating Unconscious Judgments in Our Daily Lives*,[94] Howard J. Ross makes the following recommendations:

- Recognize and accept the ubiquity of unconscious bias and that these biases affect our interpersonal interactions and our decision-making
- Develop the capacity for introspection and self-examination—active assessment of one's biases
- Practice constructive uncertainty—are our first reactions to a person or situation unconscious biases at work?
- Explore awkwardness and discomfort—recognition of our biases can be unpleasant at times and it requires further exploration.
- Engage with those considered to be *others*, especially with exemplars from that group
- Seek feedback on your thoughts and actions from trusted individuals

Unconscious bias—the attitudes or stereotypes outside of awareness—affect understanding, interactions, and decision-making and is universal in humans. These biases serve as shortcuts to simplify the world and to help individuals understand their surroundings more quickly. Individual experiences shape these shortcuts and are continually changing in an ongoing dynamic process. Evidence abounds showing that unconscious bias in medicine can have life-altering consequences. Recognition that these biases exist is the first step in bringing them into our consciousness. This realization enables us to challenge our biases and ultimately creates the proper environment in which to work and learn that will allow us to provide optimal, culturally competent patient care.

MICROAGGRESSIONS

The harmful effects of unconscious bias are often seen in the form of *microaggressions*, defined as "a statement, action, or incident regarded as an instance of indirect, subtle, or unintentional discrimination against members of a marginalized group such as a racial or ethnic minority."[95] Underrepresented groups, such as racial/ethnic minorities and LGBTQ+, are treated differently within the workplace; one component of this variable treatment is related to microaggressions. These microaggressions are not limited to marginalized groups and commonly occur in the hospital; examples include a(n):

- Consultant's haughty attitude toward an EM physician
- Emergency physician's dismissive attitude about a nurse's observations
- Patient assuming that a female physician is a nurse

As ED leadership will have to contend with the impact of such events, it is crucial that leaders understand the elements of microaggressions and their effects on minority populations to avoid them as well develop appropriate responses when they occur.[96]

Types of Microaggressions

Microaggressions are subdivided into three groups:

- Microassault
- Microinsult
- Microinvalidation[97]

A microassault is most easily characterized by explicit derogatory remarks about a group, for example, referring to a Black person as *colored* or a gay person as a *homo*. Microassaults are usually cloaked in the background of history, with perpetrators thinking terms are not offensive.

Microinsults occur when someone demeans a group through comments to an individual. An example is "You are very well spoken for a Black person," implying Black people are not well spoken. Commonly referred to as backhanded compliments, perpetrators may not realize the implications of their words and instead only see the compliment of the statement. Another example that occurs frequently is the assumption that females are nurses and males are physicians.

Microinvalidations are statements or actions that exclude or minimize the thoughts, feelings, or experiential reality of a minority group. For example, attributing work done by one person to another person is a microinvalidation; similarly, telling someone to not be offended by a racial, ethnic, or gender identity-based slur is a microinvalidation. A common microinvalidation is the statement "we are all one race, the human race," implying that all people have the same experiences and that the experience of a minority group is no different.

Addressing Microaggressions in the Workplace

Commonly, perpetrators of microaggressions do not realize the effect of their words and actions and often do not realize that they have done anything offensive. As a result, it is incumbent upon leaders to ensure that the employees (physicians, nurses, support staff, and administrators) have all been educated on the types and effects of microaggressions.

These trainings can be uncomfortable but are essential as the first step to avoid microaggressions.

Good relationships among employees allow victims of microaggressions to discuss the occurrence of microaggressions when they happen. Efforts to improve relationships within a department can focus on creating a safe environment to allow immediate, real-time feedback. There are guidelines for victims of microaggressions on how and when to respond,[98] but little has been written about appropriate administrative methods of intervention to prevent or to respond to microaggressions.

A third crucial element to address microaggressions requires a culture of reporting. Only if employees feel comfortable with their leaders will they be willing to report on issues they have in their work environment. It is common for employees to feel uncomfortable confronting others about wrongs they have experienced.[99] As a result, having alternative conflict resolution methods, which include approaching leaders about microaggressions, is important to empower employees who otherwise may not feel like they have the authority or standing to confront a perpetrator directly.

In association with reports, a mechanism to discuss issues with perpetrators and for feedback to victims that something was done must be in place. During these conversations, additional educational material should be provided, as well as a discussion of the ramifications of repeated behaviors. Feedback to victims should include that a discussion with the perpetrator occurred and that any future issues should be reported for an escalated response.

In summary, administrative responses to microaggressions should start with preemptive education, overall good relationships among team members, a reporting mechanism, and a method of addressing the perpetrator with a feedback response. Knowing the prevalence of microaggressions, preparation to deal with microaggressions is critical for successful management of the ED.

CONCLUSION

An ED that is diverse (with people from a variety of backgrounds and ways of thought) and inclusive (in which each person is valued for their whole identity) is ideal for providing the optimal environment to provide outstanding medical care to all. The more diverse and inclusive the organization, the more successful it is from a patient care and a business perspective. This kind of success is even more crucial given that the ED is the safety net for those who lack access to medical care and who encounter the most disparities in health and health care. Thus, along with diversity and inclusion, understanding health disparities is paramount in providing optimum and equitable care to all that emergency medicine serves.

REFERENCES

1. Group on Diversity and Inclusion. Definitions. Association of American Medical Colleges website. Available at: https://www.aamc.org/members/gdi/about/. Accessed November 13, 2014.
2. Martin ML, Heron S, Moreno-Walton L, et al. eds. *Diversity and Inclusion in Quality Patient Care*. New York, NY: Springer International; 2016.
3. Builtin.com. 2020. Diversity & Inclusion: Definition, Benefits & Stats | Built In. [online]. Available at: https://builtin.com/diversity-inclusion. Accessed November 20, 2020.
4. Beckershospitalreview.com. 2020. The New Look of Diversity in Healthcare: Where We Are and Where We're Headed. Available at: https://www.beckershospitalreview.com/hospital-management-administration/the-new-look-of-diversity-in-healthcare-where-we-are-and-where-we-re-headed.html. Accessed September 16, 2020.
5. Group on Diversity and Inclusion. Definitions. Association of American Medical Colleges website. Available at: https://www.aamc.org/members/gdi/about/. Accessed November 13, 2014.
6. Smedley BD, Stith AY, Nelson AR, eds. *Unequal Treatment: Confronting Ethnic and Racial Disparities in Health Care*. Washington, DC: National Academies Press; 2003:780.
7. Institute of Medicine. *To Err Is Human: Building a Safer Health System*. Washington, DC: The National Academies Press; 2000.

8. Institute of Medicine. *Crossing the Quality Chasm: A New Health System for the 21st Century*. Washington, DC: The National Academies Press; 2001.
9. AAMC. Underrepresented in Medicine Definition. 2020. Available at: https://www.aamc.org/what-we-do/mission-areas/diversity-inclusion/underrepresented-in-medicine. Accessed November 20, 2020.
10. AAMC. Figure 18. Percentage of All Active Physicians by Race/Ethnicity, 2018. 2020. Available at: https://www.aamc.org/data-reports/workforce/interactive-data/figure-18-percentage-all-active-physicians-race/ethnicity-2018. Accessed November 20, 2020.
11. Builtin.com. Diversity & Inclusion: Definition, Benefits & Stats | Built In. 2020. Available at: https://builtin.com/diversity-inclusion. Accessed November 20, 2020.
12. Association of American Medical Colleges. Analyzing physician workforce racial and ethnic composition associations: geographic distribution (Part II). *Anal Brief*. 2014;14(9).
13. Komaromy M, Grumbach K, Drake M, et al. The role of black and Hispanic physicians in providing health care for underserved populations. *N Engl J Med*. 1996;334(20):1305–1310.
14. Street RL, O'Malley KJ, Cooper LA, et al. Understanding concordance in patient physician relationships: personal and ethnic dimensions of shared identity. *Ann Fam Med*. 2008;6:198–2005.
15. Saha S, Guiton G, Wimmers PF, et al. Student body racial and ethnic composition and diversity-related outcomes in US medical schools. *JAMA*. 2008;300(10):1135–1145.
16. Cohen JJ, Gabriel BA, Terrell C. The case for diversity in the health care workforce. *Health Affairs*. 2002;21(5):90–102.
17. Milem JF, Chang MJ, Antonio AL. *Making Diversity Work on Campus: A Research-Based Perspective*. Washington, DC: Association of American Colleges and Universities. 2005. https://www.aacu.org/sites/default/files/files/mei/MakingDiversityWork.pdf. Accessed November 20, 2020.
18. Racial and ethnic diversity in academic emergency medicine: how far have we come? next steps for the future. *AEM Educ Training*. 2018;(2) S1.
19. Komaromy M, Grumbach K, Drake M, et al. The role of black and Hispanic physicians in providing health care for underserved populations. *N Engl J Med*. 1996;334:1305–1310.
20. Keith SN, Bell RM, Swanson AG, et al. Effects of affirmative action in medical schools. A study of the class of 1975. *N Engl J Med*. 1985;313:1519–1525.
21. Marrast LM, Zallman L, Woolhandler S, et al. Minority physicians' role in the care of underserved patients: diversifying the physician workforce may be key in addressing health disparities. *JAMA Intern Med*. 2014;174:289–291.
22. Whitla DK, Orfield G, Silen W, et al. Educational benefits of diversity in medical school: a survey of students. *Acad Med*. 2003;78:460–466.
23. Page SE. *The Difference: How the Power of Diversity Creates Better Groups, Firms, Schools, and Societies*. Princeton, NJ: Princeton University Press; 2008.
24. Acosta D, Ackerman-Barger K. Breaking the silence: time to talk about race and racism. *Acad Med*. 2017; 92(3): 285–288.
25. Page SE. *The Diversity Bonus: How Great Teams Pay Off in the Knowledge Economy*. Princeton, NJ: Princeton University Press; 2017
26. AAMC. Fostering diversity and inclusion. Available at: https://www.aamc.org/data-reports/workforce/interactive-data/fostering-diversity-and-inclusion. Accessed November 20, 2020.
27. Moritz G. The business case for diversity. *Arkansas Business*. July 29, 2019:18. Business Insights: Global. Web. August 27, 2020.
28. Hunt V, Layton D, Prince S. Why diversity matters. 2015. Available at: https://www.mckinsey.com/business-functions/organization/our-insights/why-diversity-matters. Accessed November 20, 2020.
29. Reynolds A, Lewis D. Teams solve problems faster where they're more cognitively diverse. *Harvard Business Review*. 2017. Available at: https://www.hbr.org/2017/03/teams-solve-problems-faster-when-they're-more-cognitively-diverse. Accessed November 20, 2020.
30. Kochan T, Bezrukova K, Ely R, et al. The Effects of diversity on business performance: report of the diversity research network. *Human Resource Management*. 2003;42(1):3–21.
31. Norbash A, Nadja K. The business case for diversity and inclusion. *J Am Coll Radiol*. 2020;17:676–680.
32. Costantini SD. Leveraging diversity to improve patient care. Hospitals and Health Networks. 2017. Available at: https://www.hhnmag.com/articles/8416-levaraging-diversity-to-improve-patient-care. Accessed November 20, 2020.
33. Powers A. A study finds that diverse companies produce 19% more revenue. 2018. Available at: https://www.forbes.com/sites/annapowers/2018/06/27/a-study-finds-that-diverse-companies-produce-19-more-revenue/207785d0506f. Accessed November 20, 2020.
34. Herring C. Does diversity pay? Race, gender, and the business case for diversity. *Am Sociol Rev*. 2009;(74):208–224.
35. Wilson M, Cutler D. Emergency department profits are likely to continue as the Affordable Care Act expands coverage. *Health Affairs*. 2014;33(5):792–799.
36. Sen SC, Bhattacharya B. Does doing good always lead to doing better? Consumer reactions to corporate social responsibility. *J Market Res*. 2001;38:225–243.
37. Bear S, Rhaman N, Post C. The impact of board diversity and gender composition on corporate social responsibility and firm reputation. *J Business Ethics*. 2010;97:201–221.
38. Street RL, O'Malley KJ, Cooper LA, et al. Understanding concordance in patient-physician relationships: personal and ethnic dimensions of shared identity. *Ann Fam Med*. 2008;6.
39. Dreachslin JL. Diversity management and cultural competence: research, practice and the business case. *J Healthcare Manage*. 2007;52(2):79–86.
40. US Department of Health and Human Services. The Secretary's Advisory Committee on National Health Promotion and Disease Prevention Objectives for 2020. Phase I report: Recommendations for the framework and format of Healthy People 2020 [Internet]. Section IV: Advisory Committee findings and recommendations.
41. World Health Organization. Social Determinants of Health. Available at: http://www.who.int/social_determinants/sdh_definition/en/index.html. Accessed November 20, 2020.
42. Carter-Pokras O, Baquet C. What is a health disparity? *Public Health Rep*. 2002;117(5):426–434.
43. "NCHHSTP Social Determinants of Health: Frequently Asked Questions." Centers for Disease Control and Prevention. Available at: https://www.cdc.gov/nchhstp/socialdeterminants/faq.html. Accessed November 20, 2020.
44. US Census Bureau. 2017 National Population Projections, Race by Hispanic Origin, 2017–2060. Available at: http://www.census.gov/data/tables/2017/demo/popproj/2017-summary-tables.html. Accessed November 20, 2020.
45. Ani Turner. *The Business Case for Racial Equity, A Strategy for Growth*. Available at: https://altarum.org/publications/the-business-case-for-racial-equity-a-strategy-for-growth. Accessed November 20, 2020.
46. Owens PL, Barrett ML, Gibson TB, et al. Emergency department care in the United States: a profile of national data sources. *Ann Emerg Med*. 2010;56(2):150–165.
47. Institute of Medicine. *How Far Have We Come in Reducing Health Disparities? Progress Since 2000: Workshop Summary*. Washington, DC: National Academies Press (US). Available at: https://www.ncbi.nlm.nih.gov/books/NBK114236/. Accessed November 20, 2020.

48. Institute of Medicine. *Hospital-Based Emergency Care: At the Breaking Point*. Washington, DC: National Academies Press; 2007.
49. Hsia RY, Kellermann AL, Shen YC. Factors associated with closures of emergency departments in the United States. *JAMA*. 2011;305(19):1978-1985.
50. Bradley EH, Herrin J, Wang Y, et al. Racial and ethnic differences in time to acute reperfusion therapy for patients hospitalized with myocardial infarction. *JAMA*. 2004; 292:1563-1572.
51. Chen J, Rathore SS, Radford MJ, et al. Racial differences in the use of cardiac catheterization after acute myocardial infarction. *N Engl J Med*. 2001;344:1443-1449.
52. Maynard C, Fisher LD, Passamani ER, et al. Black patients in the Coronary Artery Surgery Study (CASS): race and clinical decision making. *Am J Public Health*. 1986;76:1446-1448.
53. Venkat A, Hoekstra J, Lindsell C, et al. The impact of race on the acute management of chest pain. *Acad Emerg Med*. 2003;10:1199-1208.
54. Syed M, Khaja F, Wulbrecht N, et al. Effect of delay on racial differences in thrombolysis for acute myocardial infarction. *Am Heart J*. 2000;140:643-650.
55. Marcin JP, Pretzlaff RK, Whittaker HL, et al. Evaluation of race and ethnicity on alcohol and drug testing of adolescents admitted with trauma. *Acad Emerg Med*. 2003;10:1253-1259.
56. O'Connor RE, Haley L. Disparities in emergency department health care: systems and administration. *Acad Emerg Med*. 2003;10:1193-1198.
57. Selassie AW, McCarthy ML, Pickelsimer EE. The influence of insurance, race, and gender on emergency department disposition. *Acad Emerg Med*. 2003;10:1260-1270.
58. Johnston SC, Fung LH, Gillum LA, et al. Utilization of intravenous tissue-type plasminogen activator for ischemic stroke at academic medical centers: the influence of ethnicity. *Stroke*. 2001;32:1061-1068.
59. Bazarian JJ, Pope C, McClung J, et al. Ethnic and racial disparities in emergency department care for mild traumatic brain injury. *Acad Emerg Med*. 2003;10:1209-1217.
60. Todd KH, Samaroo N, Hoffman JR. Ethnicity as a risk factor for inadequate emergency department analgesia. *JAMA*. 1993;269:1537-1539.
61. Todd KH, Deaton C, D'Adamo AP, et al. Ethnicity and analgesic practice. *Ann Emerg Med*. 2000;35:11-16.
62. Tamayo-Sarver JH, Hinze SW, Cydulka RK, et al. Racial and ethnic disparities in emergency department analgesic prescription. *Am J Public Health*. 2003;93:2067-2073.
63. Zhang X, Carabello M, Hill T, et al. Trends of racial/ethnic differences in emergency department care outcomes among adults in the United States From 2005 to 2016. *Front Med (Lausanne)*. 2020;7:300.
64. Zhang X, Carabello M, Hill T, et al. Racial and ethnic disparities in emergency department care and health outcomes among children in the United States. *Frontiers Pediatr*. 2019;7:525.
65. Richardson LD, Babcock Irvin C, Tamayo-Sarver JH. Racial and ethnic disparities in the clinical practice of emergency medicine. *Acad Emerg Med*. 2003;10:1184-1188.
66. Public Law 106-525, Nov 22, 2000, 114 Stat. 2495.
67. Smedley B, Stith A, Nelson A. *Unequal Treatment: Confronting Racial and Ethnic Disparities in Healthcare*. Washington, DC: The National Academies Press; 2003.
68. US Department of Health and Human Services. National healthcare disparities report, 2012. AHRQ Publication No. 12-0006, Rockville, MD; 2012. Available at: http://www.ahrq.gov/research/findings/nhqrdr/nhdr11/key.html. Accessed November 20, 2020.
69. US Department of Health and Human Services. National healthcare quality report, 2012. AHRQ Publication No. 13-0003. Rockville, MD; 2013. Available at: https://www.ahrq.gov/research/findings/nhqrdr/index.html. Accessed November 20, 2020.
70. "About Healthy People," Office of Disease Prevention and Health Promotion. Available at: https://www.healthypeople.gov/2020/About-Healthy-People. Accessed January 21, 2020.
71. US Department of Health and Human Services. *HHS Action Plan to Reduce Racial and Ethnic Health Disparities*. Washington, DC; 2011. Available at: https://www.minorityhealth.hhs.gov/npa/files/Plans/HHS/HHS_Plan_complete.pdf. Accessed November 4, 2020.
72. US Department of Health and Human Services. *HHS Action Plan to Reduce Racial and Ethnic Disparities: Implementation Progress Report 2011-2014*. Washington, DC: US Department of Health and Human Services; 2015. Available at: https://minorityhealth.hhs.gov/assets/pdf/FINAL_HHS_Action_Plan_Progress_Report_11_2_2015.pdf. Accessed November 20, 2020.
73. Andrulis DP, Siddiqui NJ, Purtle JP, et al. *Patient Protection and Affordable Care Act of 2010: Advancing Health Equity for Racially and Ethnically Diverse Populations*. Washington, DC: Joint Center for Political and Economic Studies; 2010. Available at: https://nashp.org/wp-content/uploads/sites/default/files/files/webinars/joint.center.ppaca_.health.equity.report.pdf}. Accessed November 20, 2020.
74. Artiga S, Orgera K, Pham O. Disparities in Health and Health Care: Five Key Questions and Answers, KFF Disparities Policy. 2020. https://www.kff.org/disparities-policy/issue-brief/disparities-in-health-and-health-care-five-key-questions-and-answers/view/footnotes/.
75. Alrwisan A, Eworuke E. Are discrepancies in waiting time for chest pain at emergency departments between African Americans and Whites improving over time? *J Emerg Med*. 2016;50(2):349-355.
76. Griffith D, Hamilton K, Norrie J, et al. Early and late mortality after myocardial infarction in men and women: prospective observational study. *Heart*. 2005;91(3):305-307.
77. Mosey JM. Defining racial and ethnic disparities in pain management. *Clin Orthop Relat Res*. 2011;469(7):1859-1870.
78. Cooper LA, Roter DL, Carson KA, et al. The associations of clinicians' implicit bias attitudes about race with medical visit communication and patient ratings of interpersonal care. *Am J Public Health*. 2012; 102(5): 979-987.
79. Schwartz MB, Chambliss HO, Brownell KD, et al. Weight bias among health professionals specializing in obesity. *Obes Res*. 2003;11(9):1033-1039.
80. Uncapher H, Arean PA. Physicians are less willing to treat suicidal ideation in older patients. *J Am Geriatr Soc*. 2000;48(2):188-192.
81. Greenwald AG, McGhee DE, Schwartz JLK. Measuring individual differences in implicit cognition: the Implicit Association Test. *J Pers Soc Psychol*. 1998;74:1464-1480.
82. About the IAT: Project Implicit. 2011. Available at: https://implicit.harvard.edu/implicit/iatdetails.html. Accessed September 25, 2020.
83. Green AR, Carney DR, Palin DJ, et al. Implicit bias among physicians and its prediction of thrombolysis decisions for black and white patients. *J Gen Intern Med* 2007;22(9):1231-1238.
84. Burgess DJ, Van Ryn N, Crowley-Matoka M, et al. Understanding the provider contribution to race/ethnicity disparities in pain treatment: insights from dual process models of stereotyping. *Pain Med*. 2006;7(2):119-134.
85. Elliot AM, Alexander SC, Mescher CA, et al. Differences in physicians' verbal and nonverbal communication with black and white patients at end of life. *J Pain Symptoms Manag*. 2016;1(51):1-8.
86. Epps CD, Ware LJ, Packard A. Ethnic wait time difference in analgesic administration in the emergency department. *Pain Manag Nurs*. 2008;9(1):26-32.
87. Heins A, Homel P, Safdar B, et al. Physicians race/ethnicity predicts successful emergency department analgesia. *J Pain*. 2010;11(7):692-697.

88. Telfer P, Bahal N, Lo A, et al. Management of acute painful sickle cell crisis in sickle cell disease—a re-evaluation of the use of opioids in adult patients. *Br J Haematol*. 2014;166(2):157-162.

89. Hoffman KM, Trawalter S, Axt JR, et al. Racial bias in pain assessment and treatment recommendations, and false beliefs about biologic differences between blacks and whites. *Proc Natl Acad Sci USA*. 2016;113(16):4296-4301.

90. Tweedy D. *Black Man in a White Coat—A Doctor's Reflections on Race and Medicine*. New York, NY: Picador; 2015:302.

91. Schaa KL, Roter DL, Biesecker BB, et al. Genetic counselors' racial attitudes and their relationship to communications. *Health Psychol*. 2015;34(2):111-119.

92. Teal CR, Gill AC, Green AR, et al. Helping medical learners recognise and manage unconscious bias towards certain patient groups. *Med Educ*. 2012;46(1):80-88.

93. Lewis D, Paulsen E, eds. *Proceedings of the Diversity and Inclusion Innovations Forum: Unconscious Bias in Academic Medicine*. Washington, DC: American Association of Medical Colleges; 2017:105.

94. Ross HJ. *Everyday Bias*. Lanham, MD: Rowman and Littlefield; 2014:204.

95. Dictinary.com. Microaggression. Available at: https://www.dictionary.com/browse/microaggression? s=t. Accessed September 13, 2020.

96. Byrd CM. Microaggressions self-defense: a role-playing workshop for responding to microaggressions. *Soc Sci MDPI Open Access J*. 2018;7(6):1-11.

97. Sue DW, Capodilupo CM, Torino GC, et al. Racial microaggressions in everyday life: implications for clinical practice. *Am Psychologist*. 2007:62(4):271.

98. Thurber A, DiAngelo R. Microaggressions: intervening in three acts. *J Ethn Cult Divers Soc Work*. 2018;27(1):17-27.

99. Pinder CC, Harlos KP. Employee silence: quiescence and acquiescence as responses to perceived injustice. *Res Pers Hum Resour Manag*. 2001;20:331-370.

CHAPTER 129

HEALTH POLICY AND ADVOCACY

Fred Neis, Nathaniel R. Schlicher, Steven J. Stack

Do what you can, with what you have, where you are.

—Theodore Roosevelt[1]

Though speaking more than a century ago, long before emergency medicine had been conceived, President Theodore Roosevelt could not have more succinctly described the world of the emergency department (ED) and role of the ED leader. As any emergency clinician is keenly aware, we are called upon daily to make lemonade out of lemons, get by with less than we need, and improvise novel solutions to difficult problems while remaining accountable for providing high-quality, compassionate medical care. Roosevelt's words address these realities of our specialty; they also lead us into this chapter for reasons more closely related to his role as a politician.

Teddy Roosevelt was a president the establishment never wanted. While serving as governor of New York, the Republican Party thrust him into the White House as President William McKinley's vice president in the election of 1900. Eager to be rid of Roosevelt, they considered the vice president's office a good way to render him ineffectual by parking him in a position about which John Adams, our nation's first vice president, once commented, "My country has in its wisdom contrived for me the most insignificant office that ever the invention of man contrived or his imagination conceived." Roosevelt himself commented on the job, "I would a great deal rather be anything, say professor of history, than vice president." And yet, when President McKinley unexpectedly died from complications following an assassination attempt, Roosevelt went on to be one of the more colorful and impactful presidents in our nation's history.

Emergency departments leaders can no doubt relate to President Roosevelt's plight, as they and their teams are frequently entangled in confusing and uncertain political battles, adored by some and despised by others, and often given impossible assignments with inadequate resources. The most effective emergency leaders, however, can also relate to Roosevelt's skillful navigation of the political process through their own advocacy efforts to influence health-care policy. With undeniable frustrations and sometimes-undesirable results, politics and policymaking have deep and far-reaching implications for health care.

WHY ADVOCACY IS IMPORTANT

Health care may be the most heavily regulated industry in the United States, possibly second only to nuclear waste disposal. Putting health care in the same regulatory category as nuclear waste underscores both the importance and challenge of delivering such care in a complex, highly regulated, and intensely scrutinized environment. Added to its innate complexity, the ED serves as the front door to both the hospital and, in many cases, the health-care system at large.

With its high-profile role amid the tangle of laws and regulations, the ED is at the epicenter of health care. Therefore, by extension, educated and effective ED managers are essential to leading policy and practice discussions that impact both the care provided in the ED and the broader social and health issues that drive patients to our front doors. Our laws, regulations, and policies dictate much of how, when, where, and why care is delivered. In the 114th Congress (2015-2017) alone, more than 1,400 health-related bills were introduced, only 20 of which made their way to the president's desk for his signature and enactment into law.[2] Despite this low completion rate, a reported $3.1 billion was spent on lobbying activities for health-related bills in 2016.[3]

With health-care laws and policies having so many moving pieces and such a large impact on emergency care, it is imperative that ED leaders get involved to advocate on behalf of our specialty and the patients who rely upon us. If we do not, others will do it for us, with profound implications for both clinicians and patients. Fortunately, we begin from a strong position of influence since physicians, nurses, and other clinicians are among the most respected professionals in society. In fact, in all but one year since 2000, nurses have been judged by the public to be the most trusted professionals in the United States. When clinicians advocate to improve the health of our fellow Americans, we are a force to be reckoned with.[4]

The Impact of Health Policy

There is no shortage of examples of how policy directly influences emergency care and alters the final outcomes and cost for consumers. A prime example, many might suggest, is the bedrock of laws affecting the ED: the Emergency Medical Treatment and Active Labor Act (EMTALA). Since its inception in 1986, the law has had a profound impact on the delivery of emergency care. Though advocates have argued both for and against this law, it remains largely intact more than 30 years after its adoption.

While EMTALA applies specifically to emergency care, many other laws have also had far-reaching consequences for emergency medicine. To name just a few, the Health Insurance Portability and Accountability Act (HIPAA), the Emergency Medical Services for Children (EMSC) program, the Children's Health Insurance Program (CHIP), and the Patient Protection and Affordable Care Act (PPACA) have all had an enormous impact on patients, and every one of these laws has needed advocacy from experts in the field to guide lawmakers in its design and package.

Adding to the complexity, government is not the only source of policies that directly impact emergency care. Just one prominent example: As high medical costs now feature prominently in the public conversation, emergency providers have felt increasing pressure from the insurance industry through attempts to deny coverage to patients when the insurer retrospectively determines that the treatment and final diagnosis were nonemergent.

The government and insurance companies, however, are only two of many forces pushing the ED to evolve. The health-care delivery system also faces pressure from patients, medical suppliers, employers, media outlets, advocacy groups, and even clinicians themselves. Lately, these groups are pressing the whole system to shift its focus from volume to value as a measure of success. This shift to value-based care is disrupting the traditional delivery system, changing the ways success is measured, and compelling advocates to speak with even stronger voices. With so much at stake, it is imperative that ED leaders design a better system, ensure appropriate funding, and advocate for both patients and clinicians.

ADVOCACY IN EMERGENCY MEDICINE

Advocacy is defined by Merriam-Webster as "the act or process of supporting a cause or proposal."[5] For ED leaders, this process can take several forms and requires an understanding of the topic and a willingness to publicly take a side. In the usual course of business, ED leaders encounter numerous opportunities to advocate in their departments, hospitals, states, and even nationally by sharing their input and opinions on a wide array of topics.

Successful advocacy requires the presentation of data-driven, topic-specific information in a way that can be understood by the general public. For the ED leader, this requires knowledge of the issue and its potential impact and a clear position on the topic. And, to be most effective, ED leaders should make their points using real-world stories about the impacts, both good and bad, of health-care policies on patients and their families.

With so many moving pieces on so many different levels, effective leaders recognize the value of pooling resources, sharing expertise, and collaborating with larger groups to amplify their voices. In this regard, professional associations are invaluable assets in the ED leader's armamentarium. Professional organizations—such as the American College of Emergency Physicians (ACEP), the American Academy of Emergency Nurse Practitioners (AAENP), and the Society of Emergency Medicine Physician Attendants (SEMPA)—can provide educational opportunities, bring leaders together to create policies, and often communicate these policy positions on a plethora of topics. Effective ED leaders should be familiar with these opportunities and actively engage in them to set the vision and take steps to positively impact emergency care.

Active advocacy for emergency care can also take other forms, ranging from the simple to the more time consuming. Direct engagement with policymakers can be as simple as writing a letter, sending an email, or calling their offices to influence decision-making. Personal contact back home in the district, either in the community or their legislative office, can be an even more effective means of engaging elected leaders. Engaging the media or providing legislative testimony will reach both policymakers and a wider public audience (**Figure 129.1**).[6]

Advocacy can be more than just policy work. Politicians and policy leaders must be elected or appointed to public office. Engagement in the political process through campaigning, doorbelling, and fundraising is important to ensure that leaders who understand the challenges of patients and the ED are well represented in government positions. Beyond direct individual support, working with larger organizations and their political action committees can help clinicians expand their influence.[7,8] Before engaging in partisan political activities, however, it is important for ED leaders to carefully consider any associated limitations of and ramifications on their employment.

What an ED Leader Should Know

The view from our vantage point as ED leaders is unique and powerful. We share experiences as patients, family members, clinical experts, and through data. In addition, we engage with other stakeholders, both within and outside the industry, who regularly take actions that

FIGURE 129.1 ■ Joint Position Statement from ACEP

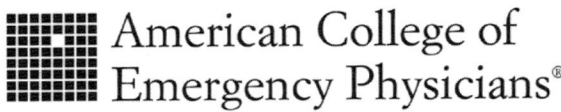

POLICY STATEMENT

Approved April 2017

Optimizing the Treatment of Acute Pain in the Emergency Department

Approved by the American Academy of Emergency Nurse Practitioners, the Emergency Nurses Association, and the Society of Emergency Medicine Physician Assistants August 2017

Approved April 2017

Replaces 2009 policy titled "Optimizing the Treatment of Pain in Patients with Acute Presentations" rescinded April 2017

A joint policy statement of the American College of Emergency Physicians, the American Academy of Emergency Nurse Practitioners, the Emergency Nurses Association, and the Society of Emergency Medicine Physician Assistants

The American College of Emergency Physicians seeks to improve acute pain management for patients in the emergency department (ED) and recognizes the need for prompt, safe, and effective pain management. <u>Although a very important topic, treatment of patients with chronic pain, especially those receiving hospice, palliative or end-of-life care, is beyond the scope of this document.</u>

Optimal acute pain management is patient-specific and pain syndrome-targeted when feasible, using a multimodal approach that includes pharmacological and non-pharmacological interventions. Base the assessment of pain and need for therapy on an overall accounting of patient status, including functional assessment, rather than solely on patient reported pain scores.

Acute Pain Management in the ED

Pharmacologic Treatments:

- Pharmacologic treatment of many acutely painful conditions should optimally begin with a non-opioid agent.

- Choose non-steroidal anti-inflammatory drugs (NSAIDs) based on their analgesic ceiling dose (which is lower than the anti-inflammatory maximal doses) and prescribe at the lowest effective dose for the shortest expected duration to avoid complications. Use NSAIDs with added caution in those with pre-existing renal insufficiency, heart failure, a predisposition to gastrointestinal hemorrhage, and in elderly patients.

- Oral (or rectal) acetaminophen is a good initial analgesic for mild-moderate pain. Intravenous acetaminophen (APAP) has similar effects as

Copyright © 2017 American College of Emergency Physicians. All rights reserved.

American College of Emergency Physicians • PO Box 619911 • Dallas, TX 75261-9911 • 972-550-0911 • 800-798-1822

influence and even dictate aspects of the emergency-care environment. From prevention, to treatment, to access, to quality, to funding, and more, there are innumerable opportunities for leaders to influence public and private policies (**Figure 129.2**).

As ED leaders mastering the craft of delivering emergency care, managing the business, and aligning it with the larger medical infrastructure, we should further expand our personal development to shape the future of emergency care. To advocate effectively, however, we

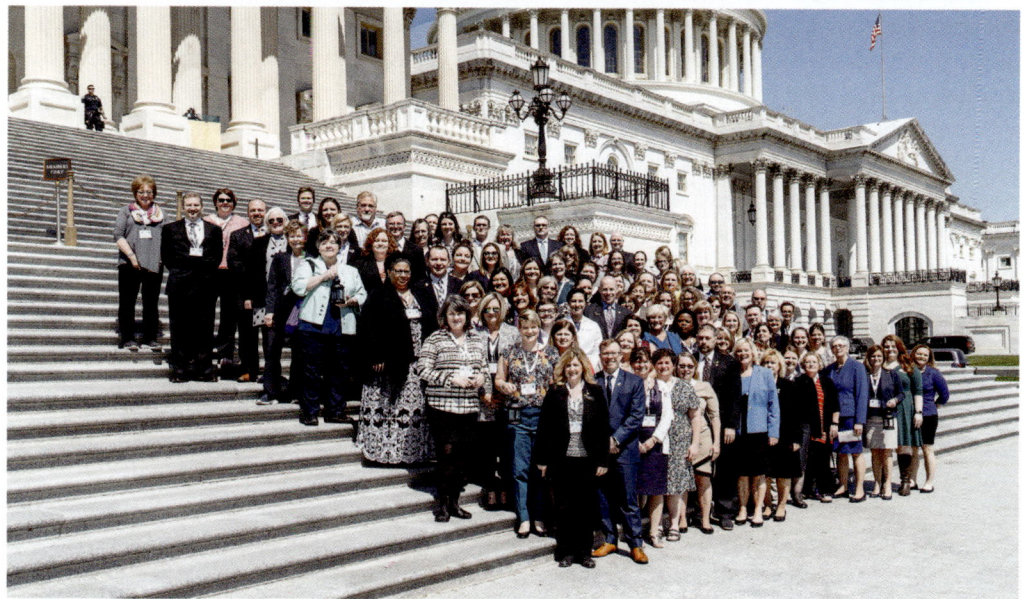

FIGURE 129.2 ■ Emergency Nurses Association's Day on the Hill, 2018

Photo credit: Brian McCarthy, www.corporatecloseups.com

must have at least a basic understanding of the structure and function of the federal and state government as they relate to health-care policy—in particular, emergency care.

CONCLUSION

Advocacy is at the core of shaping how patients receive safe, high-quality, and cost-conscious emergency care. While this section will not make ED leaders advocacy or policy experts, we hope it will support them in recognizing the need to advocate for the specialty and inspire them to engage as architects and meaningful contributors to the future of emergency care.

REFERENCES

1. Brainyquote website. Available at: https://www.brainyquote.com/quotes/theodore_roosevelt_100965. Accessed July 3, 2018.
2. Govtrack website. Available at: https://www.govtrack.us/congress/bills/subjects/health/6130#congress=114. Accessed July 4, 2018.
3. Rappleye E. Top 25 lobbyists by spending: who spent on healthcare issues in 2016. *Becker's* website. 2017. Available at: https://www.beckershospitalreview.com/finance/top-25-lobbyists-by-spending-who-spent-on-healthcare-issues-in-2016.html. Accessed July 8, 2018.
4. Brenan M. Nurses keep healthy lead as most honest, ethical profession. 2017. Available at: https://news.gallup.com/poll/224639/nurses-keep-healthy-lead-honest-ethical-profession.aspx. Accessed July 8, 2018.
5. Merriam-Webster website. Available at: https://www.merriam-webster.com/dictionary/advocacy. Accessed July 7, 2018.
6. ACEP, AAENP, ENA, SEMPA Policy Statement. Optimizing the treatment of acute pain in the ED. 2017. Available at: https://www.acep.org/globalassets/new-pdfs/policy-statements/optimizing-the-treatment-of-acute-pain-in-the-ed.pdf. Accessed November 7, 2018.
7. Longley R. About PACs - political action committees. ThoughtCo website. Available at: https://www.thoughtco.com/about-pacs-political-action-committees-3322051. Updated August 2, 2019. Accessed August 3, 2020.
8. FEC website. Available at: https://www.fec.gov/help-candidates-and-committees/taking-receipts-pac/contribution-limits-nonconnected-pacs/. Accessed October 5, 2018.

MECHANICS OF ADVOCACY

L. Anthony Cirillo, John Proctor

CHAPTER 130

Never doubt that a small group of thoughtful, committed, citizens can change the world; indeed, it is the only thing that ever has.

—Margaret Mead[1]

The Constitution of the United States and the Bill of Rights articulate the respective roles of the federal and state governments (**Figure 130.1**). The 10th amendment to the US Constitution reserves for the states and the people all powers not granted to the federal government. These powers are managed by state and local governments.

LEGISLATURES

Legislatures in the states are the primary mechanism by which laws are passed, which are then typically signed into law by the executive branch or governors and are subject to interpretation by the judicial branch, through state Supreme Courts. All 50 states sustain a state legislature with elected representatives to the legislature's upper house, or Senate, and lower house, or House of Representatives. Some states refer to a state legislature as the General Assembly or House of Delegates. Only one state, Nebraska, operates its legislative branch as a single chamber rather than a bicameral one.

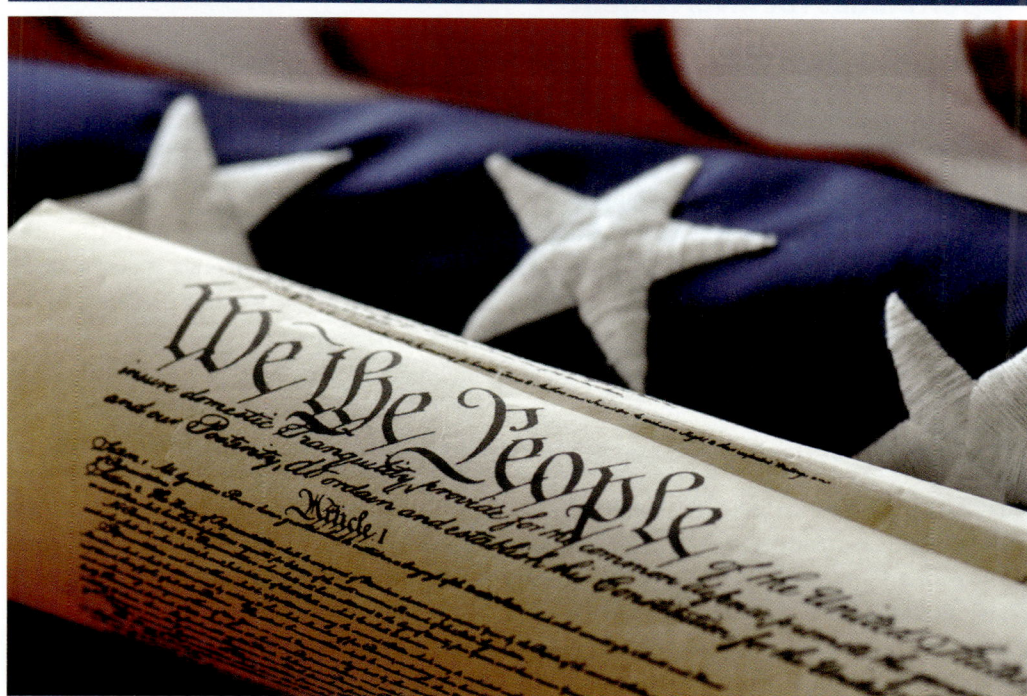

FIGURE 130.1 ■ US Bill of Rights

State senators typically serve four-year terms; state representatives typically serve two-year terms. These legislators are elected by and serve the populace of legislative districts. Hence, each citizen of a state is represented in its state legislature by an elected senator and house member. US senators serve six-year terms, and US representatives serve two-year terms. Elected officials maintain a high awareness of issues of importance to their constituents. Additionally, those who provide medical care and health-care leadership in a congressperson's district can be sought-after advisors to congressional representatives and their staff on matters related to health, wellness, and safety.

Legislative bodies deliberate matters brought forth by their members, state governors, or the president of the United States. Typically, an issue of interest is addressed in a draft bill or a draft amendment to existing law. The legislative leaders assign draft bills to committees, each of which is led by a chairperson. It is in these committees (and sometimes subcommittees appointed by the committee chair) that the details of draft bills are deliberated, modified, combined with other related bills, and ultimately supported or not supported. It is through committee support—generally through a majority vote of its members—that a draft bill moves to the full House of Representatives or Senate floor for consideration. If parallel bills are considered by both the House and Senate, legislative leaders sometimes appoint a conference committee comprised of both House and Senate members to work out differences between the two versions. Ultimately, in order for a bill to be sent to the governor or president for signature into law, it must pass both House and Senate by majority vote. Some issues, such as constitutional bylaws or amendments, require a two-thirds vote for passage.

Upon receipt of a bill successfully passed by the Senate and House of Representatives, the governor or president may sign the bill into law, veto it (essentially sending it back to the legislative branch for reconsideration or modification), or in the case of state bills, allow the bill to pass into law unsigned by the governor. This latter action may occur if the governor disagrees in principle with a bill but does not wish to veto it. In some states, the governor also retains the option of a line-item veto, allowing the governor to remove certain items from a bill prior to signing it into law.

Opportunities for Involvement

It is through participation in the drafting and deliberation of a bill that emergency clinicians, emergency department (ED) leaders, hospital leaders, and other constituents in the health-care space may impact state legislation related to the care of patients and other matters vital to medical delivery. Legislators and their staff members typically look to organized medical organizations for advice and collaboration on health-care matters. These organizations include national and state levels of the American College of Emergency Physicians (ACEP), the Emergency Nurses Association (ENA), and many other professional societies. State medical, nursing, and hospital associations often maintain significant expertise and presence in the legislative arena and can be important legislative partners to the generally smaller professional organizations representing particular medical specialties, such as emergency medicine.

Connecting With Representatives and Senators

Elected officials and their staffs often identify key contacts for legislative and public issues, such as health care, safety, and population health and wellness. Health-care professionals and leaders can serve as vital sources of information and advice on legislative considerations. Emergency physicians, advance practice providers (APPs), nurses, and hospital administrators are uniquely positioned to provide insight on a variety of concerns, including emergency care access, quality, risk, and operations. EDs provide care to the entire spectrum of socioeconomic and geographic populations, positioning its professionals as opinion leaders on community issues and challenges. Hence, state representatives and senators characteristically value the opinions of emergency medicine administrative and clinical leaders.

In political matters, there is strength in numbers. While presenting views to a legislator may be useful, the position of an organization or a coalition of organizations on an issue commands greater attention than an individual constituent. State chapters or affiliates of the ACEP, ENA, American Medical Association (AMA), American Nurses Association (ANA), American Hospital Association (AHA), and other key organizations often can agree in principle on a legislative initiative, thereby creating a unified and influential voice for legislative decision makers.

In addition to maintaining an office in the state legislative plaza or capital, state senators and representatives typically have an office locally in their district. One may connect or arrange a meeting with a legislator or legislative staff member by e-mailing or calling the congressional or district office, describing one's individual role (individual, district constituent, organization leader or representative, or coalition spokesperson) and the issue that will be discussed. Congressional members and staffers tend to appreciate knowing the advocate's general position on an issue in advance. Some congressional members may prefer to meet in a more casual atmosphere, such as a coffee shop or restaurant. There are significant restrictions and reporting requirements for congressional members relative to the acceptance of gifts, including meals, so be aware of these in advance of the meeting. It is always best to defer the meeting location to the congressional representative or staff member. Once a meeting is scheduled, plan for it by employing a focused process (**Box 130.1**).

Elected leaders often are barraged with disparate and passionate opinions on high-visibility and controversial legislative matters. Hence, congressional representatives appreciate presentations that communicate an understanding of various opinions on an issue while acknowledging and maintaining diplomacy toward alternate positions. Therefore, verbal communication and the written single-page summary should create a rational and compelling case on the issue.

Provide contact information for follow-up. Offer to serve as an ongoing resource on the issue at hand and other pertinent issues going forward. This offer provides a springboard

---

BOX 130.1 ■ A PLAN FOR MEETING WITH A LEGISLATOR[5]

- Perform due diligence.
- Be familiar with all sides of the issues to be discussed, including opposing views.
- Prepare a one-page position and rationale summary to give to the congressperson at the initiation or conclusion of the discussion.
- Attend the meeting dressed professionally, although formal business attire may be unnecessary, depending on the setting.
- Arrive promptly or early for the meeting with cell phone or smart device in silent mode.
- Address the representative as "Senator," "Representative," or gender appropriate "Congressman" or "Congresswoman," as applicable.
- Allow the representative to control the initial dialogue and be prepared to succinctly tell him or her about yourself and the organization or coalition that you represent, if applicable.
- If you reside and vote in the congressperson's district, it is important to note this connection.
- If multiple members of your organization are in attendance, plan the assignment and order of prepared comments in advance of the meeting.
- Do not overwhelm the congressperson with attendees; a limit of three or four in your party is judicious.

> **BOX 130.2 ■ BALANCE BILLING MEDIATION[2]**
>
> The Texas College of Emergency Physicians (TCEP) has a long and successful record of advocacy. In 2017, TCEP leaders partnered with the Texas Medical Association and multiple Texas physician specialty societies to lead legislative change on the thorny issue of "balance billing." Briefly, when payors and providers cannot agree on fair reimbursement for provider medical services to a payor's covered population, balance billing can occur, leading to the unexpected receipt by a patient of a bill from the provider for the medical expense not covered by his or her health insurer.
>
> TCEP successfully led a collaborative effort to pass legislation, which the Texas governor subsequently signed into law. That law establishes a Texas Department of Insurance mediation system for consumers caught in a balance billing nightmare. The law allows mediation for emergency care balance bills over $500 generated from an out-of-network provider at any health-care facility, including freestanding EDs.

for ongoing communication and collaboration on important issues for years to come. A brief handwritten note in follow-up to the meeting adds a personal and professional touch.

Drafting and Collaborating on Bills of Interest

State-level legislative actions directly affect ED patients and the providers and institutions that provide care to them. Consequently, it is essential that constituencies and institutions with a direct interest in the provision of quality emergency care engage in the legislative process. Such engagement must include participation in the submission, deliberation, and passage of legislation (**Box 130.2**).[2] The passage of new legislation, or the modification of existing legislation, begins with the submission of a bill. A proposed, or draft, bill originates from a state's governor or from a legislator. A legislator may, with the assistance of their legislative staff, draft a bill for submission to the legislature or may partner with an outside entity—such as a professional organization or lobbyist representing an organization—to draft a bill. An organization seeking to act legislatively on behalf of its patients or other interests may approach a senator or representative to seek their sponsorship of a draft bill. Senators and representatives who submit a bill to the legislative assembly for consideration function as the bill sponsor. In most circumstances, a House bill has an associated, or companion, bill in the Senate and vice versa. This requires at least one House sponsor and one Senate sponsor to take the lead on the draft bill and the issue therein.

A variety of issues impact ED patient care and those who provide it: quality, safety, medical liability, reimbursement, insurance company and governmental payor practices, and others. Clinician and hospital professional organizations often engage actively in the legislative process in order to impact these issues in a manner that positively affects ED patients and their providers. Active engagement includes identifying potential legislative sponsors for draft bills that the organization and its lobbyists, if applicable, compose or produce in collaboration with the legislator or staff. Such a draft bill subsequently is submitted by the respective Senate and/or House bill sponsors. The draft bill then is assigned by legislative leaders to the appropriate committees for deliberation and potential passage out of committee for a full floor vote.

Collaboration with multiple constituent organizations (including, whenever feasible, with organizations that are potentially adversarial to the draft bill) can strengthen the chance for ultimate passage of a draft bill into law. ACEP provides an online resource regarding coalition building.

Partnering With Lobbyists

Health-care professionals, medical societies, hospitals, and health insurance companies have much to gain through government advocacy on behalf of their patients, providers of care, and compensation for that care. However, these constituents cannot devote all or even a majority to their time to advocacy efforts. Professional lobbyists bridge this gap by devoting their professional lives to the promotion of their clients' interests. Professional lobbyists can provide significant value to organizations and legislators by gaining intrinsic knowledge of particular issues and then serving as a readily available resource to legislators and other government officials. Additionally, lobbyists spend significant time at the legislative plaza or capital during legislative sessions monitoring the progress of committee deliberations and communicating vital information to clients. Lobbyists are often positioned to arrange meetings with legislators and to facilitate the presentation by their clients of expert testimony to legislative committees.

Many medical societies and hospital associations contract with lobbyists to assist with the organization and execution of legislative efforts. When an organization decides to draft a bill or to collaborate with a legislator in the drafting of a bill, a lobbyist often assists with draft language and the coordination of efforts between the organization and the legislators. A skilled lobbyist may also take the lead in the development of coalitions with other constituent organizations that share an interest in a particular issue or draft bill. ACEP— and possibly other professional associations—provides an online guide to working with a lobbyist.[3] Before getting started, however, employed health-care providers should confirm that contractual or organizational restrictions do not prohibit certain lobbying activities.

Political Action Committees

By aggregating individual contributions of members, political action committees (PACs) provide financial support to legislators and candidates in an effort to positively influence the interests of patients and providers.

A national or state PAC is a stand-alone business entity, separate and distinct from a professional society, medical association, or hospital association. Although there are variations, a state PAC typically must form a domestic nonprofit organization with its department of state, create and maintain a constitution and bylaws, establish a federal employer identification number with the US Internal Revenue Service, and appoint a board of directors. ACEP provides a guide to state-level PACs.[4]

Through the financial support of certain legislator and candidate–legislator campaign funds, PACs can acknowledge a representative's particular interest in the welfare of patients and the challenges faced by medical providers. To maximize the opportunity for impact, it is important that ED leaders and clinicians contribute to their PACs to ensure they have sufficient resources to support candidates receptive to their concerns and inclined to take positive action in support of emergency patients and providers.

Technical Advisory Committees

Governors and legislative bodies occasionally appoint technical advisory committees (TACs) or technical advisory groups to study and provide structured direction and advice on a particular issue. This predominately occurs for complex issues with multiple interested constituents. Issues like health-care reimbursement and medical liability concerns are examples. Subject matter experts are often appointed to such TACs, along with governmental representatives and legislators. Emergency physicians, emergency nurses, APPs, and hospital leaders are well positioned to obtain appointment to TACs that deal with complex emergency medicine issues. Such appointment typically requires that the individual has a track record of sustained involvement in the pertinent issue. Additionally, a history of involvement by the subject matter expert in legislative and regulatory matters can heighten visibility and lead to appointment to a TAC. The final report of a TAC to the pertinent legislative committees or legislative assembly can significantly influence the outcome of a particular issue or draft bill.

REGULATORY BODIES

Both federal and state governments maintain a state department of health and human services (HHS) to oversee the delivery of certain health and social services to the citizens within their borders.

Departments of Health and Human Services

The HHS organizations play a major role in the execution of health-care bills that pass into law through a process known as "rule making." Once a bill is signed into law, rules must be developed to newly implement or amend implementation of previously existing law. A rule essentially interprets the law and develops a practice and procedure for the law's enactment. Rules, once adopted, hold the force of law. Hence, it is vital that constituents impacted by a particular law participate in the rule-making process.

There are generally two opportunities for health-care leaders to impact the final language of a rule:

- *During the initial drafting of a proposed rule*. Typically, this process is internal to the agency, HHS in this case. However, on occasion, the HHS appoints an advisory committee, or TAC, to advise and assist in drafting a proposed rule. Emergency clinicians, ED leaders, hospital leaders, and others with specific expertise applicable to a law can lobby for inclusion on such an advisory committee.
- *During the comment period*. The HHS announces a public comment period, inclusive of a start and end date, for each proposed rule. Frequently, the HHS also announces a date for a public hearing to receive commentary directly from the public pursuant to a particular proposed rule. During the comment period and public hearings, interested constituents may submit written and verbal concerns and recommend changes to the language of a proposed rule.

Typically, the HHS organization has a keen interest in the successful implementation of new laws and the adopted rules associated with them. Hence, written and verbal input from credible and expert individuals, organizations, or coalitions can substantially influence the final language of an adopted rule.

In collaboration with their federal counterpart, state HHS organizations oversee the operations of the Medicaid program in each state. Many states secure federal waivers for Medicaid participation that allow states to test new and innovative approaches to health-care delivery for the Medicaid-eligible population of the state. This includes access to ED care and payment model innovations that can dramatically affect ED patient care and compensation to those who provide it. Emergency physician, APP, nursing, and facility leaders should actively engage with their state Medicaid administrative organizations in order to collaborate and partner on the delivery of care to Medicaid-eligible patients.

Other Regulatory and Executive Branch Agencies

Multiple regulatory agencies touch the health-care space. Changes in law or regulation often impact the work of these agencies, making them key collaborators in many advocacy efforts. Examples within the federal government include:

- Agency for Healthcare Research and Quality, which supports health-care quality, cost reduction, and patient safety.
- Centers for Disease Control and Prevention, which promotes and supports disease and injury control and prevention.
- Centers for Medicare and Medicaid Services, which oversees and administers the Medicare, Medicaid, and the Children's Health Insurance Program.
- Other key executive branch organizations include the Federal Trade Commission, the Department of Justice, and the National Highway Transportation and Safety Administration.

State Medical and Nursing Boards

Unique to the state level of government, state medical and nursing boards issue licenses to practice within the state, conduct disciplinary procedures for practitioners who fall below the standard of care, and in some cases define the scope of practice based upon a practitioner's credentials. While there is limited opportunity for advocacy relative to their work, these organizations make important decisions impacting licensure and practice. Maintaining a professional relationship with one or more board members may create an opportunity to opine on matters related to a particular specialty or clinical practice.

MEDICAL ASSOCIATIONS

National umbrella organizations and their state counterparts, such as the AMA, ANA, AHA, and the ACEP, often maintain significant influence on legislative and regulatory considerations at the federal and state levels. Many of these organizations partner with lobbyists to sustain a presence in the legislative arena.

There are multiple opportunities for active participation by clinicians, ED leaders, and hospital administrators in these organizations. Each typically maintains a legislative committee that creates an annual legislative agenda and list of priorities. Interaction with or membership on such a legislative committee offers the opportunity to directly influence the legislative priorities of these organizations. State medical, nursing, and hospital associations also appoint or elect delegates to participate in national assemblies of the parent organizations where vital practice and health-care environment issues are deliberated. Election to the board of directors of one of these organizations is a particularly high-impact avenue to help drive the priorities of the organization as a whole and to add the valuable insights of an ED professional.

State Professional Society Chapters

State chapters of national medical societies provide a ready prospect for provider and health-care executive participation in advocacy. Examples of such organizations include

> **BOX 130.3 ■ PROFESSIONAL LIABILITY SAFEGUARDS[5]**
>
> Approximately 33 states adhere to some form of statutorily imposed damages cap when calculating the amount of damages a jury may award a successful plaintiff. State ACEP chapters often participate in the passage of medical liability noneconomic damage caps in their respective states. Noneconomic damages include compensation for nonmonetary losses such as pain and suffering or the loss of enjoyment of life caused by medical malpractice.
>
> In 2011, the North Carolina College of Emergency Physicians (NCCEP) was instrumental in the passage of a law limiting noneconomic damages in medical malpractice cases to $500,000. Beginning in 2014, this amount is adjusted upward for inflation each year. NCCEP leadership maintained an active presence in the North Carolina State Legislative Building during the deliberation of this bill, advocating for a fair and equitable solution to the issue of runaway jury awards and the consequent practice of defensive medicine by many physicians and other providers of health-care services. The NCCEP collaborated with multiple professional organizations throughout this successful legislative effort.

the American College of Healthcare Executives (ACHE), ACEP, ENA, and AHA. These organizations can provide valuable expertise to advocacy efforts (**Box 130.3**).[5]

Chapter Meetings

State ACEP and ENA chapters typically conduct regular meetings on a monthly, quarterly, or annual basis. These meetings offer networking opportunities and the chance to directly interact with chapter leaders. State chapters often solicit members who wish to get involved with legislative and other advocacy initiatives. Elections and appointments of chapter officers and national meeting delegates often occur in the course of annual membership meetings.

Committee and Board of Directors Membership

State ACEP and ENA chapters often appoint members to committees that focus on legislation, education, and other areas of priority. Volunteering for committee participation can lead to a leadership role in the organization. This may include election to the chapter's board of directors and other officer designations. These positions and their titles lend influence and reputation when seeking an audience with state legislators, executive branch officials, and regulatory authorities.

ACEP Council and ENA General Assembly

State ACEP and ENA chapters elect councilors (ACEP) and delegates (ENA) for attendance and participation in their respective national ACEP councils and ENA general assemblies. These national representatives deliberate and reach consensus on a wide variety of issues vital to the practice of emergency medicine and emergency nursing. Participation as a counselor or delegate provides the opportunity to fully engage in the most contemporary challenges facing the practice of emergency medicine and emergency nursing, better preparing the individual emergency physician and emergency nurse for advocacy on behalf of ED patients and those who provide care to them.

LOCAL GOVERNANCE

County, city, and municipal government bodies comprise a final and influential layer of governance. County and city commissions act as the legislative body of their communities, through approval of municipality budgets and spending, hiring of employees, and enforcement of local ordinances. This most local level of government oversees key public health and safety services, such as public health clinics and emergency medical services.

BEING AN EFFECTIVE ADVOCATE

Throughout our personal lives and professional careers in health-care leadership, challenging situations are regularly encountered that require change in order to generate improvement. Change management is personally rewarding, yet its greatest challenge is not devising solutions and policies. The fundamental challenge of change leadership is convincing *others* to embrace change and to help drive it. Dr. Martin Luther King once proclaimed:

> *There comes a time when one must take a position that is neither safe nor politic nor popular, but he must take it because his conscience tells him it is right.*[6]

Perhaps a prototypical advocate, Dr. King fully committed to convincing others of what he believed was the right path and to creating real change in American culture.

According to Webster, advocacy is "the act or process of supporting a cause or proposal."[7] There are a number of guiding principles and specific actions one can deploy to maximize the ability to convince individuals critical to the success of the change process to contribute to success. Some team members become early converts to the change process. It is the "nonbelievers," those with certain personal, political, or financial agendas, who are reluctant to contribute to the solution process or are obstructionists to change.

Effective advocacy includes the creation of a vision for change, communicating this vision to all parties, including supporters, neutrals, and opponents, and then driving all team members to achieve the vision. Effective advocacy is mostly about people, not just the issue—and people are complicated. The reader likely knows well that managing processes is easy, but managing people is hard. In the next sections of this chapter that follow, the guiding principles and specific advocacy actions are discussed. Although the primary purpose will be to apply certain concepts and actions to the state and federal levels of government, the same concepts and actions can apply more broadly to one's personal and professional life.

Guiding Principles of Effective Advocacy

Successfully advocating for a cause can be incredibly rewarding, but successful advocacy can also be hard work. Given the myriad of issues that may need to be fixed in personal or professional lives, how does one prioritize which to address first? Using a two-by-two analysis matrix can be helpful when categorizing issues into "easy" versus "hard" and "big impact" versus "little impact" (**Figure 130.2**). Once completed, this exercise leads to the most important question: "What issue do I care about the most?" On a more instinctive level, the question is: "What issue bothers me the most?" Bearing in mind that successful advocacy on an issue may require days, weeks, months, or years. One can then create an advocacy project chart to map planned advocacy efforts.

Be a People Person

As described previously, the ultimate success or failure of an advocacy project comes down to the ability to convince others to take an action that is different from their current behavior. Depending upon the size and scope of the issue and solution, this may involve just one individual (e.g., a partner in a two-person medical practice) or multiple levels of people (e.g., convincing all the surgeons, anesthesiologists, nurses, and techs performing duties in a

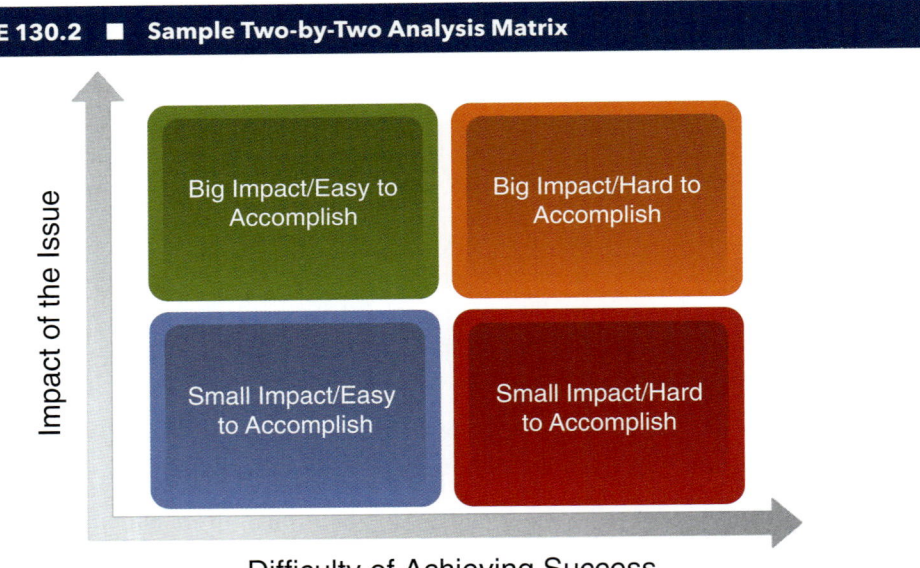

FIGURE 130.2 ■ Sample Two-by-Two Analysis Matrix

surgical suite to improve the surgical patient experience). Building a successful relationship, whether personal or professional, takes time and requires persistent investment in the relationship. This is no less true in the advocacy arena.

Turn One Voice Into Many

While one individual can sometimes change the world, it certainly is generally more effective to create change through engagement of multiple interested parties or constituents. When defining the issue, consider the impact on other individuals, groups, and organizations with which a common goal is shared. Reaching consensus with others may garner their support. Advocacy includes conveying to policymakers the scope of the issue's impact and involvement of multiple constituent groups. Offering concise statistics or evidence in support of a position is compelling and can emphasize the impact on multiple individuals and groups. For example, a strategy to improve acute stroke care may involve collaboration with the ACEP, American Heart Association, American Stroke Association, and the American Academy of Neurology.

Be Persistent

Simply stated, the advocacy process can take time and lots of it. This is particularly true when advocating for legislation. It is not uncommon for successful passage of legislation to require 3 years at the state level and 5 years at the federal level. And these time frames come with no guarantees, because election cycles can alter the blend of supporters and opponents and because the political priorities of a legislative body evolve. Successful advocacy requires being present on a regular basis. A persistent message or request to policymakers creates a greater chance of success when the political opportunity arises. Also, frequent presence by the advocate helps policymakers to know the constituency group will hold them accountable for action or inaction on the issue of importance.

Be Ready to Give

In the advocacy arena, there is no more precious commodity than time. In order to be successful, advocates must give of themselves and their time. Those who choose to advocate for one paramount issue generally find the time committed rewarding, despite the personal costs required. Giving time involves compromise and sacrifice. Fighting for an issue also means less time spent on other personal and professional matters. For these reasons, effective time management is critical. Although the issue may be very important to those affected by it, it is still important for the advocate to maintain a healthy life balance.

While time is a key asset in advocacy, it is not the only one. Money is often a critical factor in the success or failure of an advocacy effort. Money is not mandatory for every advocacy initiative, especially smaller scale efforts, but for engagement in a large-scale effort that impacts multiple interests, substantial financial resources are often essential. Many aspects of an advocacy program such as media exposure, printed materials, and consultants or lobbyists require financial investment. When advocacy involves elected officials, it may be appropriate to consider creating a budget to provide campaign contributions to those legislators and candidates for elected office who support the issue. While many people are unhappy with the current system of campaign finance in this country, it is a current political reality. Contributing to an elected official or candidate does not guarantee their favorable position on an issue, and it remains incumbent on an advocate to develop a legislative solution that an elected official can support. Campaign contributions do, however, augment the opportunity to interact with elected officials privately or during political gatherings. Practically speaking, contributing to the campaigns of supportive elected officials drives support within the legislative body when it comes time for voting.

Those who are interested in advocating for an issue that affects their own workplace should first discuss strategies with institutional leadership. Offering to take the lead on an issue that affects the workplace may be welcomed by senior leadership, but not if it conflicts with their priorities and perspectives. Public advocacy efforts must be undertaken within the authority of an individual's position and with approval of senior leadership if an individual's actions could impact the institution as an enterprise.

Be the Expert on Your Issue

While there are some aspects of an advocacy project that may be out of a person's control, all potential advocates can certainly control their own knowledge of the issue. The saying "knowledge is power" is definitely true in the advocacy arena. Demonstrating a commitment to an issue by being the most knowledgeable on the topic creates immediate credibility with policymakers. Depending on the community within which an advocate is working, the other stakeholders may be experts on the subject or completely naive. Using expertise to educate other stakeholders and policymakers can therefore be very powerful. This is especially true when working with legislators at the state and federal level, given the broad scope of issues they are responsible for understanding and voting on.

Being the expert on a topic includes mastering the data, particularly the financials when requesting additional resources. Understanding the total cost of a proposed solution is mandatory; however, one must also develop an understanding of potential revenue sources and how current resources are deployed. Understanding trends in the demographics of those affected by the issue may also provide an opportunity to request additional funds if a specific demographic is increasing in size.

Follow the Plan

Like successful project management, a successful advocacy campaign requires a plan. After selecting the issue, the next step is to craft a solution to which the other stakeholders can agree. Developing a list of "must haves" that are non-negotiable is important. Likewise, creating a list of issues that could involve acceptable compromise can help advance a solution with which all stakeholders can live. Identify the best strategies for the campaign and create a time line for implementation of these strategies. Implement the process and, following each step of implementation, reevaluate the progress and adjust tactics. A successful advocate must be prepared to adapt a plan because the people and political environment may change during the campaign. Like a seasoned sailor, advocates must know their destination but adjust to the changing tides and winds during the journey.

Using the Tools in Your Toolbox

Bearing in mind the aforementioned guiding principles, some common tactics deployed in successful advocacy are considered in the following text. As an advocacy campaign plan is being developed, consider which of these applies most effectively in the ultimate quest to make a positive change by convincing other stakeholders to support the proposed solution.

Be Visible and Vocal

As an advocate it is important to clearly share the critical issue and requested change with others. Wear the pin, ribbon, or wrist bracelet that shows the world the issue. Don't be shy, and talk to "everyone" about the issue. It's the only way to know who shares the concern.

Join a Professional Organization

Professional societies are created to represent those with a common background (e.g., AMA, ANA, ACEP, ACHE, etc.). These organizations provide a network of others who share common experiences and may also harbor an interest in "the" issue. Tapping into the personal and organizational strengths of a professional society can provide significant educational, financial, and people resources.

Join or Form an Issue-Based Organization

Issue-based organizations by definition are focused. Take advantage of the work that has already been done by others. Avoid reinventing the wheel if possible, but do not hesitate to create an organization around the critical issue if one does not exist. Having an "official" organization provides the campaign a more established and professional appearance. Create a logo, slogan, and image, and apply them consistently.

Attend a Rally

Participation in a rally with others who share passion about an issue is invigorating and can serve to recharge the participants' advocacy batteries. Signs, banners, and chants can be powerful tools to communicate advocacy messages. Using a "day on the hill" event can produce a highly visible show of support to legislators. Provide the media with an official notice of the event to gain maximal coverage.

Testify on a Bill

Take expertise to where the policymakers are. Testifying on a bill at a legislative or regulatory committee hearing proposes solutions directly to the policymakers. The testimony should be tailored to the allotted presentation time. Similarly, it is essential to be cognizant of the rules of testimony to ensure that there is adequate opportunity to speak. When reading prepared testimony, it should be written in a large font with spacing that permits sufficient opportunity to maintain some eye contact with the committee members. Another copy of the testimony should be prepared in standard font and format for submission to the official record of the hearing.

Use the Media

Successful advocacy requires a strategy of effective communication with stakeholders and those who are potential supporters. Develop a comprehensive communication plan that considers all forms of media—print, radio, television, mail, and social. While each of these media forms may contribute to the success of advocacy work, targeting the appropriate audience determines which is most effective.

Attend and Host a Fundraiser

Participating in a fundraiser event (which includes contributing to the elected official or candidate) not only connects the advocate with the office holder but also with those who support him or her in the race. These people are also potential supporters of the critical issue, and fundraisers are a great opportunity to network and "build a contact list." Hosting a fundraiser or serving on the host committee of an event demonstrates an "above and beyond" level of commitment to the elected official.

Directly Lobby Elected Officials (and Staff)

Ultimately, an advocacy campaign may require a specific action by a policymaker with authority over an issue. While building coalitions and support from the "community" affected can be helpful, having a direct conversation with a policymaker is a powerful opportunity to convey perspective on both the issue and the proposed solutions. Meeting with a policymaker is also an opportunity to listen and understand what he or she feels are hurdles to the successful outcome of the issue being proposed.

Never underestimate the importance of meeting with and building a relationship with staff members who work for policymakers. Staff members are often the subject matter experts for policymakers. Staff also provide issue analysis and recommendations for action to the policymaker or elected official.

HOW TO RUN FOR OFFICE... AND WIN

How wonderful it is that nobody need wait a single moment before starting to improve the world.[8]

—Anne Frank

Most medical professionals want all citizens to have ready access to quality, cost-effective health care. This goal sounds simple, but health-care delivery is very complicated. Each of the aspects of access, quality, and cost are interwoven. Changing one facet of this three-legged stool affects the other two. Change any one of the three and it ultimately affects the delivery of care to individual patients.

For those involved in leading health care—some at the bedside and some in the C-suite—it is clear that there are policymakers outside of the health-care delivery system who affect the system's daily operations. At the federal, state, county, and local levels, policymakers exist in the legislative, regulatory, and judicial arenas. Legislators are charged with enacting laws that authorize health-care programs and are responsible for appropriating funds to finance those programs. Regulators then operationalize the enacted programs and retain authority to oversee the people and organizations that deliver health care to the population. Lastly, the courts can play a major role in interpreting the statutes and regulations that have been enacted and promulgated and may render decisions that dramatically change the accepted standard of care.

There is likely significant agreement among the various constituents on the main tenets of an ideal health-care system. Yet such agreement has not been achieved. This failure is largely due to a lack of consensus about "what" to fix, with pervasive disagreements regarding the "how." While each potential solution may be valid, gaining consensus around any individual solution is challenging both inside and outside of the legislative and regulatory seats of power. At some juncture, some advocates decide that it's time to become a policymaker on the inside by running for an office that directly effects change within the system on a large scale.

Define Key Positions

Before deciding to run, it is necessary to develop a focused purpose for serving. Running for and serving in office, whether in the public sector or professional organizations, requires commitment and sacrifice. Without a driving policy passion, it is challenging to be a great candidate or public servant. So, each person considering candidacy should consider:

What is the one problem you would fix if you were queen or king for a day?

Though knowledge of multiple issues is necessary, passion should direct the candidate who is seeking office. For instance, those who want a single-payer medical system in the United States may wish to run for the House of Representatives or the Senate. For those who wish to change the standards of ethical testimony within a profession, running for the national board of the professional association or society may be the right choice.

Identifying the "why" should dictate what office is chosen. Bear in mind, just being passionate about running does not guarantee a win. Typically, multiple people will compete for the position. However, in 2016, the president of the United States was elected despite having never held public office before, so anything is possible!

Still Want to Run? Hold on There . . .

After considering running for elective office, it is wise to take time to consider several important points. Running for office entails sacrifice of personal time and probably commitment of personal financial resources. Consider carefully how the time to campaign and serve in office might affect personal and professional income and what possible conflicts of interest exist.

The commitment to serve in elected office deeply affects family and friends. Be certain to hold an open and honest discussion with family members about the challenges of office and its potential effect on their lives. Running for office, especially public office, will open candidates and their families to scrutiny from others, including the press and media. It is essential to honestly identify any personal or professional issues that might emerge during a campaign and, if present, consider the potential if compelled to address those issues publicly. Be mindful, as well, that information available on the Internet generally remains discoverable in perpetuity. So, clean up social media accounts now!

Regardless of the office sought, many elected officials spend countless hours preparing for meetings and being visible and accessible to the voting community. What are the terms of office? Are there term limits? What is the filing deadline? Must signatures from registered voters be gathered to earn a position on the ballot? Is there a nomination process within the party?

A personal passion to fix an issue does not ensure that voters share that passion or have interest to engage on the issue. It is important to assess the community and key leaders in order to identify the most pivotal issues in their view. Keep in mind that merely identifying problems facing the community is not enough. People will want to hear articulate solutions.

And yes, it is necessary to perform a self-assessment. A policy expert might be a terrible public speaker. It's easy to focus on one's strengths, but it may be more important to focus on those aspects of being a candidate that may be weaknesses.

Unless running unopposed, there will be at least one and potentially many other candidates. Study the dynamics of the competitors in the race. Is there an incumbent? If so, how long has he or she been in office? What were their previous margins of victory? Is the election partisan, meaning are candidates sorted by party affiliation? Deciding to run as a democrat against a democratic incumbent is often viewed as a noncollaborative move, especially among the party faithful. What about other new competing candidates? What are their similarities and differences that can be demonstrated when campaigning?

Ready, Set, Run!

Once the considerations described above are assessed, it is time to operationalize the campaign. A successful campaign requires people, planning, and persistence.

Every Campaign Needs a Team

No matter how strong candidates are, they cannot win an election on their own. An inner circle of people who commit their time to the candidate's success is necessary. Depending upon the office sought, it may take no more than a few good people or it may take a full professional campaign team. Prospective candidates should reach out to those who have run for similar office to research the particulars of the size and scope of their campaign and its effectiveness.

At a minimum, it is necessary to work with a campaign manager who can manage the day-to-day campaign operations. When selecting the campaign manager, confidence in their capability and dedication is essential, because a candidate cannot micromanage all aspects of a campaign. Agreement on what functions will be managed by the campaign manager in advance fosters an effective professional relationship, especially as the campaign heats up.

Another key position to consider is the fundraising/finance director who is responsible for helping develop a budget and fundraising strategy. The finance director may also serve in the role of treasurer of the official campaign committee. The finance director must command a thorough knowledge of the statutes and rules governing campaign contributions and reporting requirements in the jurisdiction.

Strong consideration should also be given to identifying a communications director who manages both internal campaign team and external, public-facing communications. Developing and maintaining a database of supporters and contact information enables the candidate to stay in touch with the base.

Party People

For elections in the public sector, races may be designated as *partisan* or *nonpartisan*. For partisan races, one must be engaged with the leadership of the party to be represented on the ballot. Within political parties, there often is an expectation that prospective candidates "pay their dues" prior to running for office. While this does not mandate active party involvement ahead of seeking elected office, one must respect the influence of the party faithful. It is these party members who show up to help with events and conduct the unglamorous work of walking neighborhoods to distribute door flyers and standing on busy intersection corners holding campaign signs. Without the party's support, a candidate faces a significant uphill battle in identifying volunteers and donors who will support and contribute their efforts to the campaign in general.

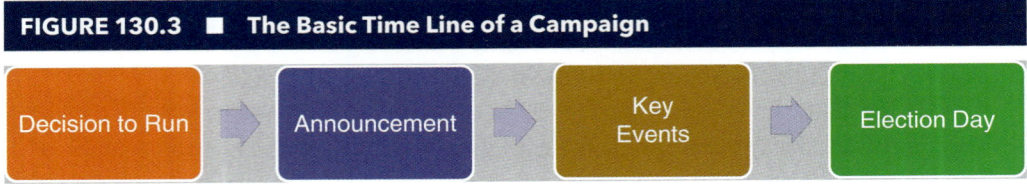

FIGURE 130.3 ■ The Basic Time Line of a Campaign

The Plan

Every successful campaign has a thoughtful strategy and time line, which begins with the date a candidate first considers running, followed by the date of the official regulatory filing as a candidate for public office (**Figure 130.3**). Other important time line entries are the date of the candidate's official public announcement and election night itself. It is appropriate to plan the campaign strategy backward from Election Day, identifying critical events, public appearances, campaign material production and acquisition, and participation in public debates.

The Message

Once the campaign is designed and plotted, develop campaign themes, key messages, and the branding that must be developed. This process directly correlates with the reasons chosen to run for office and the identified needs of the community. The campaign staff and trusted friends and advisors can help hone and refine the messaging, which defines who the candidate is to voters who may not know the candidate personally. It is appropriate to focus on three key campaign issues that help to demonstrate differences from competitors. For each of the three issues, develop three bullet points that clearly elucidate solutions to the problems or challenges those issues present to the voting community. Be certain to do the necessary homework ahead of time to become an expert on the key issues. Candidates lose credibility quickly if they fail to demonstrate comprehensive knowledge of their issues, particularly if they propose solutions that were previously proposed or attempted.

It's a Marathon, Not a Sprint

Campaigns for office, when well planned and well executed, require a paced and measured persistence of effort (**Figure 130.4**). Many people will be excited and energized following the decision to run and the official kickoff of the campaign. It is difficult, though, to maintain this initial level of intensity throughout an entire campaign. Identify times within the campaign cycle to "recharge batteries" (for the campaign team as well). Develop timed strategies to maintain a presence within the community in order to preserve a high profile with the voters. Plan for a ramp up of activities, including traditional media, social media, and other visual reminders such as lawn signs (in compliance with local ordinances regarding sign placement).

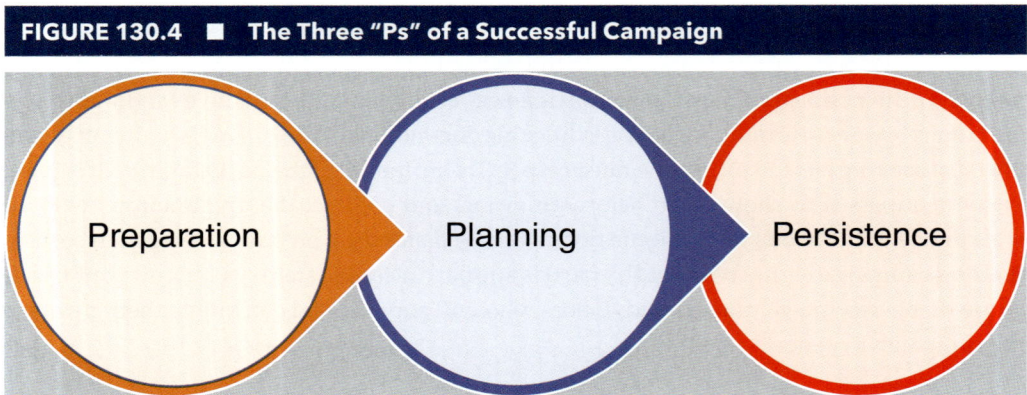

FIGURE 130.4 ■ The Three "Ps" of a Successful Campaign

The Election

Eventually, Election Day will come and go. To win, it is necessary but not sufficient to work hard, be surrounded by good people, and run an effective campaign, because each of the other candidates is trying to accomplish the same goal. Successful campaigns require hard work, dedication, and often a little luck, too. The harsh reality of running for office is that not everyone wins, and there are no consolation prizes or participation trophies for coming in second. However, even in defeat, the unsuccessful candidate achieves name recognition and, with good comportment, respect from the community.

Those who do not win should immediately consider how to build upon the experience to increase the chances of winning future races. It is wise to find ways to demonstrate continued commitment to the community. This can be done by serving on a committee or a task force that ideally focuses on the previous campaign's key issues.

Lastly, it is important to remember that service to the public or an organization is about making things better for the public and solving community problems. Especially in health care, this approach ultimately benefits the patients.

CONCLUSION

Change in the health-care system is inevitable, and the pace of change continues to accelerate. It is critical for medical professionals to guide and direct this change because they command a deep understanding of how policy affects the care of patients. Identifying critical issues within the health-care system and effectively influencing policymakers in the public and private sector can result in significant improvements in the wellness of individuals and the broader health of a population. Effective advocacy requires a passion to improve the health-care system, knowledge of an issue, and the skill set to positively influence legislative or administrative policymakers who can affect change. Every medical professional who possesses these three qualities has the potential to drive positive change.

REFERENCES

1. Mead M. Christian Science Monitor. June 1, 1989.
2. Tran TQ. Elections Matter. 2019. Texas College of Emergency Physicians. Available at: https://www.texacep.org/empact. Accessed November 17, 2020.
3. American College of Emergency Physicians. Working with a professional lobbyist. 2020. Available at: https://www.acep.org/globalassets/sites/acep/media/advocacy/state-advocacy/tools/physiciansguidesec07.pdf Accessed November 17, 2020.
4. American College of Emergency Physicians. State advocacy overview. 2020. Available at: https://www.acep.org/state-advocacy/state-advocacy-overview/. Accessed November 17, 2020.
5. North Carolina College of Emergency Physicians. Limits on non-economic damages. Available at: https://www.acep.org/globalassets/uploads/uploaded-files/acep/advocacy/state-issues/liability-reform/pursuing-special-liability-protection-for-emergency-care/samptest/bobbittermantestimonyandreferencedexamplesnchousemptaskforcejan2004.pdf. Accessed November 17, 2020.
6. King ML. A proper sense of priorities. Speech in Washington, DC. 1968. Available at: https://pnhp.org/news/martin-luther-king-jr-a-proper-sense-of-priorities/. Accessed November 17, 2020.
7. Merriam-Webster. Definition of "advocacy." Available at: https://www.merriam-webster.com/dictionary/advocacy#:~:text=%3A%20the%20act%20or%20process%20of, his%20advocacy%20of%20gay%20rights. Accessed November 17, 2020.
8. Frank A. *The Diary of Anne Frank*. New York, NY: Knopf; 1991.

CHAPTER 131

FEDERAL ADVOCACY

Taylor DesRosiers, Aaron George, Steven Stack

We must always take sides. Neutrality helps the oppressor, never the victim. Silence encourages the tormentor, never the tormented.

—Elie Wiesel (1928-2016), Nobel Prize Speech
The Night Trilogy: Night, Dawn, the Accident

The term *advocacy* is often perceived as overwhelming, something someone else should be doing, and incompatible with our daily clinical or administrative duties. This sentiment is exacerbated by the lack of formal guidance within medical training. This chapter provides a framework for the composition of the US Federal Government and its role in advocacy as well as offering practical tools for success in advocacy at the national level. Readers from other countries may find this chapter interesting, as it may help to explain how the process works in the United States, especially given that US policies may positively or negatively influence policies in other countries.

THE PLAYERS

Before diving into the details of the importance of federal advocacy, it is essential to understand the players in the arena. The federal government is composed of three branches: executive, legislative, and judicial. The primary focus of this chapter will be on the legislative branch, as this is traditionally where physicians, nurses, emergency department (ED) leaders, and health-care advocacy groups have interacted. However, a general understanding of the interplay of all three branches is essential.

The Executive Branch is overseen by the president and vice president. Fifteen additional cabinets and departments act as advisory bodies to the president. Most relevant to health care are the Department of Health and Human Services (HHS) and the Department of Veterans Affairs. Collectively, the cabinet departments and federal offices are often referred to as the "fourth branch" of government, the administrative or regulatory branch.

The Judicial Branch includes the Supreme Court, the highest federal court. Comprised of nine justices, the Supreme Court can make decisions that can have a large impact on the practice of medicine.

The Legislative Branch, the main focus of this chapter, consists of 435 voting members serving two-year terms in the House of Representatives and 100 voting members serving six-year terms in the Senate. The Senate and the House of Representatives collectively form Congress which has the authority both to enact legislation and to declare war. While many of the roles of the House and Senate are parallel in terms of creating and voting on legislation, they differ slightly. Legislative bills for raising revenue originate from the House of Representatives, while the Senate has the additional responsibility of providing its counsel and consent to presidential appointments to selected executive branch offices.

House Leadership

Leadership in the House of Representatives includes the following roles:

- *Speaker of the House*: Presiding officer of the House of Representatives who serves as both political and parliamentary leader. As administrative head, the speaker does not regularly participate in floor debates or vote. The speaker is also second in presidential line of succession, after the vice president.
- *Majority and minority leaders*: The majority leader is responsible for direct management and coordination of the House committees as well as scheduling the legislative calendar. Majority and minority leaders serve as the de-facto influential leaders of their respective party, guiding campaign assistance and promoting the party's agenda.
- *Majority and minority whip*: Manage the legislative actions and function of the party on the House floor, where they are considered to be the *floor* leaders. Serve to monitor legislation, assess and tally vote counts, and ensure that members are present for voting.

A significant amount of the work of the federal government is accomplished at the committee and subcommittee levels. Committees help to inform legislative language, funding, and governmental oversight, which serves to direct voting and actions of the Senate and House. **Tables 131.1** and **131.2** briefly outline the roles of those committees that have the most influence on health care. Each of these committees holds regular meetings to consider new legislation as well as to oversee agencies, programs, and activities within their jurisdictions. Each also has the prerogative to hold special hearings or inquiries as issues arise, such as hearings on opioids within the Senate Committee on Health, Education, Labor, and Pensions (HELP) and the Congressional Subcommittee on Health within the Energy and Commerce Committee. These hearings invite experts to report on issues, thus providing a public forum that informs and guides both the law-making process and budgeting.

Given the overwhelming number of national and international issues, it is impossible for any representative to be an expert on all matters that come before Congress. The committee structure allows members to focus on unique areas of expertise. Committees act as a vetting mechanism for legislation and provide oversight to their respective bodies of government. From a federal advocacy standpoint, this means that those members serving on important committees, as identified in Tables 131.1 and 131.2, have a more prominent impact on

TABLE 131.1 ■ House of Representatives Committees Relevant to Health Care

Committee	Role
Appropriations	Responsible for overseeing expenditures of money and thus controls spending of the Federal Government. Has jurisdiction over the budget for Health and Human Services (HHS).
Budget	Responsible for drafting the annual budget plan and for monitoring the budget of the Federal Government.
Energy and Commerce	Maintains jurisdiction over Medicaid, the Food and Drug Administration (FDA), and public health. The subcommittee on Health has oversight of private health insurance, medical malpractice, HHS, National Institutes of Health (NIH), and the Centers for Disease Control and Prevention (CDC).
Ways and Means	Responsible for originating all revenue-raising measures, with additional oversight of Medicare.
Veterans Affairs	Responsible for monitoring and evaluating the operations of the Veterans Affairs Administration (VA).

TABLE 131.2 ■ Senate Committees Relevant to Health Care

Committee	Role
Appropriations	Maintains jurisdiction over all discretionary spending in the Senate. Reviews supplemental spending bills for emergency expenses.
Budget	Responsible for drafting annual budget plan and for monitoring the budget of the Federal Government.
Finance	Responsible for oversight of health programs created under the Social Security Act, including Medicare, Medicaid, and Children's Health Insurance Program (CHIP). Responsible for general issues of taxation and revenue collection. Functions in a similar role to the House Committee on Ways and Means.
Health, Education, Labor and Pensions (HELP)	Responsible for oversight of HHS, FDA, CDC, NIH Agency for Healthcare Research and Quality (AHRQ), public health and health insurance, biomedical research and development, Occupational Safety and Health Administration (OSHA), and student loans. Additionally holds a subcommittee on Primary Health and Retirement Security.
Veterans Affairs	Responsible for legislative jurisdiction of veterans' compensation, rehabilitation, medical care, etc.

decisions relevant to health care. Thus, understanding which members sit on relevant committees improves messaging and advocacy efforts.

Additionally, professional staff serve as valuable resources to extend the knowledge and expertise of both individual representatives and committees; successful advocacy often requires extensive interaction with these topic area experts upon whom representatives rely for input and guidance on a broad array of issues.

Department of Health and Human Services

The US HHS serves as an executive-level agency with a primary goal of improving the health of all Americans. Working alongside local, state, and national projects, HHS provides more grant funding than all other federal agencies combined. Therefore, this office has a tremendous impact on the delivery of emergency medicine. **Table 131.3** briefly outlines those offices that have the most influence on health care as well as their fundamental roles. While an advanced knowledge of each of these offices is not necessary for engagement in advocacy, a basic understanding of the structure and relative function is useful.

HOW A BILL BECOMES LAW

While the legislative process may seem complex, it can be distilled to a few key steps. First, an issue is brought to the attention of Congress, where a member of the House or Senate can write and introduce a bill to address it. This is where individuals, ED leaders, organized medical societies, special interest groups, and lobbying groups can have the greatest impact, as they are often the most involved in raising the attention of issues that require legislative action. Bills introduced in the House are given the designation H.R. and in the Senate S., after which a number is assigned to each. For example, H.R. 3590 ultimately transitioned into the Patient Protection and Affordable Care Act, often referred to as the ACA.

Bills are typically introduced by a single or small group of representatives. To garner further support, additional representatives can sign on as cosponsors. This provides a

TABLE 131.3 ■ Offices Within HHS Relevant to Health Care

Office	Role
Centers for Disease Control and Prevention (CDC)	Serves as the national public health institute with a primary goal to protect and advance public health and safety. Focused on disease control, prevention, and improvement of the health of US citizens through research, education, and health promotion.
Agency for Healthcare Research and Quality (AHRQ)	Serves as the federal agency tasked with improving the safety and quality of the US medical system. Focused on research of health-care delivery with education for health systems as well as policymakers.
Food and Drug Administration (FDA)	Serves to oversee the safety and quality of pharmaceuticals, vaccines, and medical devices. Additionally responsible for regulating tobacco products as well as supervising cosmetics and dietary supplements.
National Institutes of Health (NIH)	Serves as the primary source for biomedical research and funding for discovery and advancement of knowledge in medical and associated sciences.
Health Resources and Services Administration (HRSA)	Serves as the primary federal agency for improving access to health-care services, such as those who are isolated, uninsured, or in vulnerable populations.
Office of the Assistant Secretary for Preparedness and Response (ASPR)	Created following Hurricane Katrina, this office focuses on federal emergency operational capabilities, disaster preparedness, and planning in medical catastrophes.
Office of Emergency Management (OEM)	Provides expertise and leadership for worldwide disaster response.
Office of the National Coordinator for Health Information Technology (ONC)	Serves to promote, support, and develop electronic exchange of health information.
Centers for Medicare and Medicaid Services (CMS)	Responsible for administration of the Medicare program as well as for working with states for the administration of Medicaid and CHIP.

second opportunity for ED leaders to contact their representatives and urge them to sign on for cosponsorship.

Newly introduced bills are first discussed in subcommittees and committees wherein public hearings are held to discern more about the issue, devise legislative language, and generate public and expert input. Once a bill is approved by a committee, it is eligible for open debate on the respective Senate or House floor. This is a third crucial period for political advocacy, as individuals and groups can make representatives aware of concerns before voting. Bills can be passed, defeated, or amended.

It is often the case that both the House and Senate will pass slightly different versions of the same bill. When this occurs, several members of each chamber will form a *conference committee* to attempt to generate compromise language. Once both the House and Senate have successfully voted and passed a bill, it is forwarded to the President's desk for signature or veto.

If Congress fails to pass a bill within a given two-year period, or term, the bill must be reintroduced and assigned a new number, and the process begins again for that Congressional period.

Federal Directives

The actions of the federal government go beyond just the passage of individual bills. While the legislative actions outlined in the preceding section are some of the most important for advocacy efforts, other actions of federal government directly impact health care—notably regulations and executive action.

Regulations

Once a bill is passed, agencies have the responsibility for carrying out the intent of that law. However, many details are not addressed directly within the law, new circumstances arise, and legislative language can often be vague. Therefore, federal agencies are granted the authority to issue regulations as a mechanism for interpreting and conveying the intent of the law. When an issue that is not explicitly defined by law arises, an agency is responsible for publishing a public statement in the *Federal Register*. Over the course of the subsequent 30 to 180 days, comments from the public and special interest groups are accepted and public discussion is encouraged. Any refinement to the regulation is published as a final rule in the *Federal Register* and an announcement is made of the date of implementation.

Executive Action

The President of the United States has the authority to take executive action on any issue, and this serves as an immediate directive and has the same force as law. Such orders are subject to judicial review and must not conflict with the Constitution. Famously, President Lincoln's Emancipation Proclamation was an executive action, and Franklin Delano Roosevelt issued over 3,500 of them during his presidency. One example that impacted health care was the first executive order by President Trump, "Executive Order Minimizing the Economic Burden of the Patient Protection and Affordable Care Act," on January 20, 2017, that called for providing relief from the ACA. This order allowed the Secretary of Health and Human Services, as well as the heads of other departments and agencies, to waive or delay the implementation of any ACA provisions that would impose a financial burden on states or any financial or regulatory on individuals.

Case Study One

The Emergency Medical Treatment and Labor Act (EMTALA) demonstrates how the various levels of government and private sector have contributed to the effective reality experienced by physicians, nurses, and ED leaders today.

Relevance to Emergency Medicine

Originally only four pages in length and barely noticed at the time of its creation, EMTALA has become a central paradigm in the practice of emergency medicine and is now considered "one of the most comprehensive laws guaranteeing nondiscriminatory access to emergency medical care and thus to the health-care system."[1]

Where It Started

In 1985, CBS aired a *60 Minutes* broadcast entitled "The Billfold Biopsy" that detailed the dumping of indigent patients from other medical facilities to Parkland Hospital in Dallas, Texas.[2] Specifically, concern existed that certain hospitals, "based only on a patient's financial inadequacy, failed to provide a medical screening that would have been provided a paying patient, or transferred or discharged a patient without taking steps that would have been taken for a paying patient."[3]

Who Was Involved

- *States*: As the topic gained popularity as a public safety issue, Texas adopted state legislation requiring all counties to provide health care for indigent residents, and an additional 20 states soon passed similar legislation. Funding was often lacking, however, in these otherwise well-intended bills.
- *Private sector*: At approximately the same time, two articles appeared from Cook County Hospital in Chicago detailing a similar practice of patient dumping, stating that the lack of insurance was the driving cause in 87% of cases, and only 6% of patients had given informed consent for transfer.[1]
- *Organizations*: Policy safeguards against this practice via The Joint Commission, the American College of Emergency Physicians (ACEP), and the Hill–Burton Act of 1946 already existed, but lacked enforcement.[1]
- *Congress*: Congressional concerns existed over a 1983 law outlining the practice of bundled payments to hospitals for Medicare patients. Worry existed that these Medicare patients would receive fewer services under a bundled model. These concerns were reinforced and echoed by Medicare Diagnostic-Related Groups guiding payment and policy at the time and a legislative fix was needed to financially protect Medicare patients from this outcome.[2]

This combination of lay press articles, professional reports, and the impotence of preexisting laws led to the creation of EMTALA to ensure nondiscriminatory access to emergency medical care. The legislation was enacted by Congress in 1986 as part of the Consolidated Omnibus Budget Reconciliation Act of 1985.[4]

Process, Influences, and Outcomes

The statute's original four pages of language lacked punitive measures for noncompliance which was a major reason this legislation itself did not drive actual behavioral change. However, with the addition of interpretive guidelines via the Health Care Financing Administration (now Centers for Medicare and Medicaid Services) as well as multiple federal court cases on the subject, patient dumping behavior in the United States changed drastically. The legislative steps that were required to take a transformative idea and turn it into a policy that effectively changed hospital behavior are detailed next.

Rules on enforcement of the EMTALA were not published in the *Code of Federal Regulations* until 1994 (8 years after its initial passage).[5] This code, however, was incomplete and created more confusion than actual change. In June 1996, a task force was created to further delineate and clarify the regulations, and interpretive guidelines were published in 1998.[5] It was not until 2003 that CMS published a final rule codifying interim guidance. This is also the time that a general guideline was drawn stating EMTALA guidelines ended upon the admission of a patient to a hospital service.[5] While the original language included only Medicare facilities, 98% of US hospitals were affected and the law became ubiquitous.[1]

Approximately 50 to 400 EMTALA violations have been investigated each year since 1994.[1,2] Additionally, the hospital now bears the burden to prove it did not break the statute after a complaint is made. Investigations of the violations are the responsibility of CMS. Enforcements of penalties fall under the Office of the Inspector General of the HHS, who has full enforcement authority, including prosecution. Over time, a complex set of changes and regulatory stipulations have been produced, thereby altering the impact of the law from the original four pages of published language.

Discussion

The EMTALA was minimally enforced in its first decade of life until the regulatory body of CMS enacted rules for enforcement. This process was guided by multiple iterations of the language and with the help of many levels of the federal government. This is a good example of where a law by itself is only as strong as the regulatory body that enforces it.

This case is also an example of the first time Congress used the Medicare statute to create policy applying to all people receiving health care, thereby becoming a national standard of care for emergency services. This highlights a unique lever of EMTALA through its standing as a federal statute, thereby requiring cases to be heard in federal courts, including and up to the US Supreme Court. The federal legislation supersedes all state and local laws, including tort reform limitations, statutes of limitation, and other aspects of lower courts.[5] Civil, state, and federal courts also have free access to all information gathered in EMTALA cases and can use this to bolster malpractice claims that often come bundled with EMTALA complaints.

The law remains controversial, as many consider it to be an unfunded government mandate. In an article about the statue, one author discusses, "It's a double-edged sword. The good side is that patients with emergency conditions are being taken care of; they must have an evaluation exam and they have to be stabilized. The negative side is that EMTALA is the largest unfunded mandate [on providers] that the government has ever instituted."[2] Congress has partially addressed this concern by including EMTALA in the Medicare Conditions of Participation by requiring that hospitals must comply with EMTALA to receive Medicare payments. In practice, this regulation has lifted the burden from local and state bodies to provide charity or unfunded care and placed it instead on hospitals and systems themselves. As a result, many *free* clinics have been closed and EDs have become a safety net for all-comers.[5]

Despite multiple iterations of this statute, questions still exist over its applicability to certain situations encountered in the ED daily. For example, what constitutes an appropriate transfer or discharge? How should providers handle a homeless patient or undocumented immigrant who has limited ability to follow up if the patient is considered stable? Also controversial has been a CMS proposition that EMTALA be expanded to the entire hospital stay—a proposal against which ACEP, the American Hospital Association (AHA), and the National Association of Public Hospitals stand in united opposition.[2]

This legislation now extends beyond emergency care providers. As on-call specialty physicians can be a necessary part of a medical screening exam (MSE), there have been friction and misunderstanding in specialties concerning their EMTALA-related obligations. It has been well established, though, that hospital on-call medical staff consulted through the ED as part of the MSE are obligated to evaluate the patient. This was not the case before 1989, however, and only became part of the legislative language through a subsequent congressional add-on. While traditionally each department had been in charge of its own on-call list, EMTALA legislation made hospitals responsible for these lists.[1] Specialist behavior has changed due to this language. Some specialists now avoid taking call or being placed on these lists, as they must accept additional obligations and potential liability when taking calls under EMTALA. Systems have also changed with the advent of *specialty* hospitals that provide practice settings with less EMTALA exposure.[5]

In addition, the implications of ever-growing ED wait times and record numbers of patients utilizing the ED are not yet fully understood are. Ongoing questions include the disposition of chronically ill patients without access to care elsewhere, as well as what to do with visits for socioeconomic or other needs that do not require medical treatment. Some argue that this legislation has enabled safety net hospitals to establish protocolized behavior standardizing the transfer of patients, theoretically preventing disability and saving money in certain cases.[2] Even so, others insist that patient dumping remains a serious problem.[6] And, ambiguity and uncertainty persists as to what determines failure to complete the MSE. Despite Congress having expanded the scope of EMTALA five times as of the publication of this chapter, many questions remain, leaving room for inconsistent application and interpretation of the law.[5]

Overall, debate, advocacy, and discussion continue on this complex piece of federal legislation, highlighting the need for ED leaders to have knowledge about the law-making process and its subsequent downstream effects.

OTHER PLAYERS IN FEDERAL ADVOCACY

Numerous organizations influence federal legislation, too many in health care alone to individually name or outline. There are, however, larger umbrella organizations that are particularly important to the practice of emergency medicine, some of which will be outlined here.

The American Medical Association (AMA), founded in 1845, represents the voice of physicians as a whole and includes representation from nearly all specialties, all states, various training levels (i.e., medical students, residents, fellows), and numerous other demographics. Currently, the organization maintains a substantial office in Washington, DC, where advocacy efforts occur year-round. AMA runs a yearly legislative conference at which timely topics for all physicians are discussed and advocated. Additionally, AMA holds a biannual meeting, the House of Delegates, where elected representatives from the aforementioned specialties, states, practice stages, and so on, gather. During these publicized and widely attended meetings, national health-care policy is debated, created, and implemented. AMA also has its own political action committee (AMPAC) that serves to support and communicate with representatives supportive of physician concerns.

Founded in 1968, ACEP was initially created with the goal of ". . . getting practitioners together to determine the best ways to run and maintain a viable emergency department."[7] Now the largest national medical specialty organization representing emergency medicine, ACEP is the leading advocacy and continuing education association for emergency physicians. The organization runs a public affairs department in Washington, DC, and provides up-to-date reporting of specialty-specific legislative actions relevant to emergency medicine practice. ACEP also runs a yearly Leadership and Advocacy Conference with rotating topics of interest.[8] Notably, it is ACEP that sends emergency medicine delegates to each AMA House of Delegates meeting.

The Society for Academic Emergency Medicine (SAEM), formed in 1989 from the amalgamation of the University Association for Emergency Medicine and the Society of Teachers of Emergency Medicine, has a slightly different focus than ACEP. SAEM dedicates itself to the improvement of care predominantly through research and education but also influences health policy through "forums, publications, interorganizational collaboration, policy development, and consultation services for physicians, teachers, researchers, and students."[9] While this organization has a smaller role in advocating for the practice of EM at the federal level when compared to ACEP, it contributes substantially to advancing the specialty from an education and research perspective.

The American Academy of Emergency Medicine (AAEM) was formed in 1993. It is dedicated to the protection of physician rights. The AAEM promotes "fair and equitable practice environments" so that "emergency physicians can deliver the highest quality of patient care," with each physician afforded an "equitable ownership stake in the practice."[10] As such, AAEM has advocated for physician autonomy, physician ownership of practices, and due process. It opposes restrictive covenants and the nonreciprocal right of termination without cause. It also believes in board certification for all physicians providing emergency care. The AAEM supports the "establishment and recognition of EM internationally as an independent specialty."[10] It also provides an annual educational forum and an advocacy day.

The Emergency Nurses Association describes itself as "the global emergency nursing resource and advocate for Safe Practice and Safe Care."[11] This organization produces specific resources for emergency nurses and additionally maintains a broad policy platform committed to the advancement of emergency nursing and patient care at a federal level. A government relations team heads federal, state, and grassroots advocacy efforts.

The American Nurses Association (ANA) is the nursing counterpart to the AMA, acting as an umbrella organization for all nurses regardless of specialty. ANA additionally has its own Political Action Committee, with complementary goals of supporting and influencing representatives.[12]

The American College of Healthcare Executives is an international professional society of more than 40,000 executives who lead hospitals, health-care systems, and other medical organizations. The American Association for Physician Leadership is another related organization that has promoted the development of physician leadership skills for more than four decades.[13]

Founded in 1898, the AHA is a national organization that represents approximately 5,000 hospitals, health-care networks, and other providers of care as well as 43,000 individual members. The organization's goal is to address "national health policy development, legislative and regulatory debates, and judicial matters." AHA's advocacy efforts include the legislative and executive branches as well as legislative and regulatory arenas.[14] The American Organization of Nurse Executives, founded in 1967, is a subsidiary of AHA and focuses on nursing leadership.

Case Study Two

H.R. 3590, commonly known as The Patient Protection and ACA, was signed into law in 2010, and its passage has been met with both praise and contention. While this bill has had a tremendous impact on health care and insurance, a study of the pathway to passage provides insight into the legislative process and players. This case study highlights how the aforementioned organizations interacted with the various levers of government, each with their own voice and unique pattern of influence.

Relevance to Emergency Medicine

The ACA has had a broad and far-reaching impact on health-care reform, payment, insurance, and practice. Access to private health insurance, frequently with federal subsidies, and expansion of Medicaid for persons up to 135% of the federal poverty level markedly reduced the national uninsured rate by 2016. Additionally, health systems and hospitals have redirected systemic focus as a result of ACA-created initiatives, such as accountable care organizations and hospital readmission reduction programs that have influenced ED and hospital-wide delivery efforts as well as associated payments.

Where It Started

For much of the 20th century, attempts were made to increase insurance coverage and improve regulation of the health-care industry. Most of these efforts were met with incomplete success or outright failure in the 50 years that followed the introduction of Medicare and Medicaid in 1965. Continuing along this path into the 21st century, unsustainable growth in medical costs, including spiraling ED expenditures, again made health-care reform and cost control a continuing major legislative and presidential focus.

Who Was Involved

The national discussion on health-care reform throughout 2009 saw input from essentially every corner of American society. In particular, the American public was quite vocal, and estimates indicate that various industries spent nearly $400 million in lobbying efforts.[15]

- *Presidential politics*: The Presidential election of 2008 highlighted health-care reform as candidates positioned themselves with their goals for reforming the health-care system. This emphasis stemmed from findings, such as a 2007 Kaiser poll, that found health care to be the top domestic issue among voters. It appeared very likely that the next elected President would have the opportunity to champion and ultimately sign or veto comprehensive health-care reform legislation, and the presidential debates therefore highlighted these issues.[16]
- *Insurers*: The major insurers were of diverging opinions, as were many others, on the specifics of the legislation. Initially, the insurance industry was skeptical and generally negative toward the ACA. Their primary concern was that the ACA would mandate insurers to expand services without adequate compensation and would lead to increased regulation of the industry. For example, leading up to the vote on the ACA, Anthem Blue Cross of California projected that passage of the bill would lead to a 39% increase in premium costs. The prospect of mandated health care driving more covered lives and reducing some of the restrictive language in the final version did ultimately bring most insurers to a supportive stance.[17]
- *The American people*: One poll in mid-2009 found that Americans were split on their opinion of the bill, with 46% in support and 48% opposed. While many demanded increased coverage, others were worried about the possible expansion of government.[18] When representatives returned to their home districts for congressional recess in the fall of 2009, they were met by constituents, some expressing mob-like anger, others offering unwavering support, at town hall meetings across the country.
- *AARP*: Sensing the opportunity to expand coverage and increase services for senior citizens, AARP offered general support for the ACA. Representing more than 30 million Americans over the age of 50, this nonpartisan, nonprofit organization maintains tremendous political clout across the country. Further, as their members have a large stake in the US health-care system, their general support was paramount to the success of the passage of the bill.[19]
- *AMA*: Initially having some concerns about the bill, the AMA House of Delegates ultimately voted to support it. Recognizing that this would have a profound impact on medicine, the group released the statement that the ACA is . . ." not a perfect representation of our views, but is close enough to warrant this group's support and keep the reform process moving forward."[20]
- *AHA*: The AHA desired to maintain as much revenue as possible to its member hospitals, particularly through the Medicare and Medicaid programs. As such, the group was willing to compromise with a proposed $155 billion overall cut in reimbursements to prevent even more substantial cuts to funding. Additionally, the AHA hoped that many uninsured Americans gaining access to health insurance would markedly reduce their burden of uncompensated care and thereby offset some of these payment reductions.[21]
- *The pharmaceutical industry*: The Pharmaceutical Research and Manufacturers of America (PhRMA) invested heavily in lobbying to avoid increased regulations of drug manufacturing and delivery. The group was particularly concerned about the risks of direct federal negotiations over prices as well as the potential approval for importation of drugs from Canada and Europe.[22]
- *Labor industry*: The Service Employees International Union (SEIU) represents labor unions from more than 100 different industries, and the group saw health-care legislation as an opportunity to initiate or expand coverage for workers. The group was quick to join in support of the ACA.[19]

Process and Influences

- *January 18, 2007*: The Healthy Americans Act (HAA) is introduced in the Senate. Often viewed as an immediate precursor to the ACA, the HAA included regulation of insurance markets and an individual mandate to purchase health insurance. The bill stalled and died in the Senate Finance Committee.
- *January 20, 2009*: President Barack Obama is sworn in as the 44th President of the United States.
- *February 24, 2009*: President Obama announces in his first joint session of Congress his intention to work toward a health-care reform bill.
- *March 4, 2009*: President Obama convenes a health summit of lawmakers, doctors, health-system leaders, insurers, consumer advocate groups, and pharmaceutical company leadership. This includes over 50 members of Congress and more than 80 interest group representatives.
- *May 15, 2009*: A joint statement of support is released by AMA, AHA, PhRMA, America's Health Insurance Plans, the Advanced Medical Technology Association, and SEIU.
- *June 17, 2009*: Senate HELP committee begins markup on the bill.
- *July 14, 2009*: The House introduces its own bill.
- *November 7, 2009*: House approves its bill in a 220-215 vote along party lines.
- *December 24, 2009*: Senate approves its bill 60-39.
- *December 2009 to January 2010*: House and Senate conference committee derails when Democrats lose 60-seat supermajority in Senate with the election of Senator Scott Brown (R-MA).
- *March 21, 2010*: House adopts Senate-amended version of the bill.
- *March 23, 2010*: President Barack Obama signs the ACA into law.
- *June 10, 2010*: First provisions of the ACA are implemented with the initiation of high-risk insurance pools.

Outcome

Though the ultimate impact of the ACA is still evolving, the passage of the bill has undeniably left an enormous imprint, unparalleled since the creation of Medicare and Medicaid, on the American health system.

Discussion

The time line and passage of the ACA provide insight into the legislative process of how a bill moves through Congress. More importantly, it demonstrates the spectrum of players and interest groups involved and how vocal advocacy can influence legislation. Nationwide, an intense overarching health-care debate ensued, and congressional and senate offices received an overwhelming barrage of constituent contact during the legislative process. Interest groups and professional medical societies played an influential role in much of the final bill's language, as well as in generating support and momentum for its eventual passage.

The passage of this bill was unique in that during the first few weeks of 2010, the balance between democrats and republicans in the Senate shifted with the special election of Republican Scott Brown in Massachusetts. When the Democrats lost their 60-vote supermajority in the Senate, they no longer fully controlled the legislative process and the opportunity to resolve differences in House and Senate bills through a conference committee was derailed. This change of events empowered Republicans and, as a result, the Democrats employed a less common process called reconciliation to make limited changes to the Senate bill. Ultimately, the House Democrats voted to support the Senate bill even though some of their concerns were not resolved. This unanticipated legislative curveball resulted in a final law that differed in certain key elements from what many legislators and advocacy groups had envisioned.

This case study of the ACA highlights some of the many opportunities for emergency physicians and ED leaders to influence the federal political process. Using their individual voices, physicians were afforded substantial opportunity through direct contact with representative offices as well as at town hall meetings. E-mails, letters, and phone calls from constituents were all counted and tallied throughout Capitol Hill. In addition, through membership and/or participation in professional medical societies, or even hospital or trade groups, physicians amplified their voices and leveraged their combined voices to express both support and opposition to elements of the legislation. The lesson is that in watching a bill move through Congress, there are many touchpoints for advocacy, numerous opportunities to effect change, and frequently dramatic and unanticipated twists and turns along the way.

WHY INVOLVEMENT MATTERS

The involvement of ED leadership in federal advocacy efforts is essential. If the above case studies have failed to provide enough evidence as to why our voice matters, consider the case study below. (**Box 131.1**).

Case Study Three

The Balanced Budget Act of 1997 (BBA) was an omnibus legislative package enacted by Congress with the goal of balancing the federal budget by 2002 via the budget-reconciliation process. This case study is an example of how large and complex federal legislation seemingly unrelated to health care has had a profound effect on how physicians train and practice.

Relevance to EM

This bill aimed to balance the entire federal budget, and health-care spending was the main lever utilized to do so. Medicare cuts totaled 73% of the projected savings, reducing payments for hospitals, physicians, and other providers.[23] The BBA also formed the basis of the current graduate medical education (GME, e.g., residency and fellowship training) environment by placing caps or limitations on the number of Medicare-funded residency training spots.

Where It Started

Cost-saving goals driven by a republican-led Congress during the Clinton presidency formed the basis of this legislation. When completed, the congressional and executive branches reached compromise by coming together on a bill that was the largest structural adjustment to Medicare since 1981.[24] Prior legislation dictated Medicare payments to hospitals training residents,

---

BOX 131.1 ■ FEDERAL BUDGETING

The federal budget is divided into two categories, discretionary and mandatory spending. In a fiscal year, which is the period between October 1st and September 30th of the following year, a federal budget is passed that sets spending ceilings that serve as a guide for both the House and Senate to make appropriations and tax decisions. An appropriations bill assigns money for specific federal government departments, agencies, and programs to provide funding for operations, personnel, equipment, and activities.

indirectly forming the base of residents' salaries. Due to the potentially unlimited nature of this funding stream, there was concern that "there were too many physicians in general and too many specialists in particular," and that Medicare support for GME would balloon out of control.[25]

Legislative Process and Influence

A static number of funded residency positions was set for hospitals already training residents. This could not be adjusted for population growth increases, changes in ratios of specialty, or the creation of new specialties. The legislation essentially froze the number of funded GME training spots in 1996.[24] The intent of the freeze was to provide a cushion for Medicare patients and to create an incentive for outside entities to initiate funding for GME training positions in addition to the cap.[25,26] There was consideration to recalculate this cap on a three-year basis, but that has not occurred.

The Balanced Budget Refinement Act of 1999 increased this GME limit for rural training hospitals to 130% of the previously defined resident cap.[27] Section 5503 of the ACA and Section 422 of the Medicare Modernization Act created a mechanism to reduce funding to programs with below-cap residency counts and redistribute them to hospitals hoping to expand their caps.[28] **Table 131.4** lists the parties involved.

Outcome and Discussion

Studies analyzing the distribution of residents and the impact of this bill show fascinating and conflicting outcomes. One paper reported an increase in the absolute number of

TABLE 131.4 ■ Who Was Involved in the Balanced Budget Act of 1997	
Association of American Medical Colleges (AAMC)	Called to increase medical school class size by 30% after an analysis of the physician workforce in the 90s (which has now been met as of 2018), but could not increase residency training positions as well, exacerbating the bottleneck between medical school and residency. There was an unsuccessful attempt on the organization's behalf to increase funding by 15,000 residency positions during the negotiation of the ACA, and efforts to maintain GME funding continue.[24]
American Hospital Association (AHA)/Hospitals	Initial concerns centered around the projected decreased payments to specifically larger academic medical centers, leading to the unintended consequence of limiting the scope of specialty services.[25] The argument was based on the idea that residents are expensive to train and would require additional money, more so than what was being provided.
American Medical Association (AMA)	Worked alongside AAMC to advocate for GME funds. Continues to have both joint and independent advocacy efforts to maintain funding.
Council on Graduate Medical Education (COGME)	Authorized by Congress in 1986 to provide ongoing assessment of physician workforce trends; it reports to the HHS as well as Senate and House committees. Gave recommendations towards the creation of the bill and placed in charge of determining outcomes of this legislation.
Private sector	Multiple unique inputs. As an example, Georgetown University's analysis suggested the "all-payer" model as early as 1997 to replace government funding towards training doctors.[23]
States	Multiple unique inputs. Florida and Texas each created new medical schools over the last decade, but did not increase GME slots accordingly. Governor Rick Scott proposed state support at $80 million, only a fraction of what Medicaid would cover. Texas gave $8.76 million toward GME, and California has had success as well.[24]

trainees in Accreditation Council for Graduate Medical Education-accredited locations by 20.6% in the decade preceding the legislation and only 8% from 1997 to 2007. More interestingly, a large part of the latter growth was attributed to the lengthening of training time instead of increasing the number of training slots, as well as adding international medical graduates into specialties less sought out by US medical graduates.[29] This implies at least a temporary slowing of the growth of training positions after the implementation of this bill.

There was an even greater impact on the specialty of family medicine. In the years prior to implementation of the BBA, this specialty had seen growth by an annual rate of 11% to 12%. But in the year after passage, this number was reversed and growth declined. Additionally, this specialty was disproportionately affected as one-third of residents worked in ambulatory, not hospital, settings at the time of implementation and therefore were not considered when determining the cap.[30] While parallel data in EM are not readily available, EM was likely disproportionately affected as a new and growing specialty during this integral funding period.

This legislation provides an example of how a large bill, seemingly unrelated (a budgetary act) directly to health care, can have small elements that massively impact our profession and the practice of emergency medicine. This highlights the importance of the continued advocacy efforts required to influence profound changes to the medical practice environment and compellingly demonstrates the importance of having a "seat at the table" when decisions are made. While it is debatable whether the government should be the primary funding stream for the training of physicians, there is a compelling need for a stable training pathway for providers in this uncertain time of health-care delivery. With health care consuming an ever-larger part of the federal budget at a time of escalating deficits, the likelihood of future cost savings and reductions coming from medicine is significant.

This case study also highlights the importance of feedback from constituents. For example, patient advocacy groups have called for increasing access to care. At the time of publication of this chapter, waiting times to see providers has increased 30% since 2014, with an average waiting time of 24 days to receive an appointment.[31]

Part of decreasing wait times is increasing the number of available providers, which has been exceedingly difficult with the cap on training positions. Some of the need has been met by introducing advanced practice providers, a change welcomed by many. Even so, the inflexibility of this law makes it impossible to have a dynamic training pool where deficiencies of certain providers, such as primary care doctors, can be immediately addressed. Lawmakers benefit from hearing how this policy plays out in the real world. Whether that is done through your professional societies or as an individual, your input and that of your patients is paramount. Your voice matters!

Opportunities for Success

Advocacy efforts at the federal level start with having a basic awareness of issues, monitoring bills, and keeping track of health care-related activities. The good news is that the digital age provides easy access to a wealth of up-to-date resources. The use of mobile apps or enrollment in daily or weekly health policy e-mails can be a good place to start.

Even a minimal understanding of the issues at hand provides the opportunity to get involved and be an active voice for emergency medicine. Emergency physicians, nurses, and other ED leaders are experts on issues relevant to their patients, practice, and business. The next step is to voice *your* concerns and share *your* story. On a daily basis, this can be as simple as speaking with others about shared barriers or concerns. At the federal level, this involves communicating these concerns and barriers to your representatives.

Every US citizen has one congressperson and two senators who represent them in Washington, DC. Each congressional member is elected to serve a distinct congressional voting district, allocated based upon population. To determine who represents you, go to:

- https://www.house.gov/representatives/find-your-representative
- https://www.govtrack.us/congress/members

Representatives have both local offices, typically situated in the higher-density population areas of their districts, and DC-based offices. Though a constituent can reach out to either office at any time, meeting the team at the local office is often easier and more direct. Establishing relationships with representative offices is a critical component of advocating at the federal level. The representative should strive to understand, vocalize, and fight for the concerns and well-being of their constituents. That is their job!

The first call, letter, or visit to a representative's office may go to a member of their staff. Since office roles can be confusing, **Table 131.5** serves as a list of the different office members whom you may encounter. Visiting a representative's office may not lead to an audience with the representative. Keep in mind that many staff members have substantial influence on voting decisions and some, such as the health legislative assistant, often understand specialized issues better than the representative.

While the sheer number of bills moving through Capitol Hill at any one time can be overwhelming, it is a much less daunting task to monitor those bills that are directly relevant to emergency medicine. Many organized medical societies can help to identify bills worth following or advocating for.

TABLE 131.5 ■ Congressional Staff and Roles

Role	Description
Chief of Staff	Oversees each congressional office, supervising staff, and often serving as a Member's top political advisor. May divide time between the DC and local office.
Deputy Chief of Staff	Not all offices have a deputy, but this staff member will often be second in command or assistant to the chief.
Legislative Director	Oversees the office planning for legislative initiatives and coordinates strategy.
Legislative Assistant	Serves as a specialist for a given issue, such as health care. Responsible for monitoring bills, running committee meetings and preparing office statements on these specialized issues. Will often meet or communicate with constituents on these areas as well.
Communications Director	Serves as press secretary and primary spokesperson for the representative. Will often coordinate with the media, but also responsible for communicating priorities and actions to constituents.
Legislative Correspondent	Responsible for sorting and responding to constituent communication, effectively monitoring for trends in constituent concerns.
District Director	Serves as the head of the home state office, and thus often works as a liaison to the community directly.
Staff Assistant	Entry-level permanent staff and the most numerous position on the Hill.
Intern	Non-permanent staff who are often unpaid, or receive a small stipend. Interns may be the first person greeting you at the front doors or answering your phone call. Serve various administrative tasks as needed.

Becoming Involved

Involvement in advocacy at any level as a tiered approach, with many different steps and levels of investment.

Step 1: Awareness

- The first step is to be aware of the major issues impacting health care. At times this may feel overwhelming, but there are many resources available through your specialty, state, or professional society, as well as online and on various apps to help guide and breakdown content. The act of reading just a few moments each day or week can go a long way to understanding the scope of federal politics and policy.

Step 2: Discussion

- Once you are aware of important issues, discussing them with those in your immediate ED, health system, and community is essential. This allows the dissemination of important information as well as the opportunity to engage others in addressing the issues at hand.
- Invite others to become politically active as well.

Step 3: Individual Action

- The most fundamental element is the simple act of voting regularly. By voting, and encouraging others to do so, you improve the likelihood of electing representatives that align with the goals of your ED and protecting patient care.
- Contact your representative's office and vocalize your concerns and viewpoints, as outlined above.
- Attend your respective advocacy organization's policy meetings, both to create internal policy in that organization and to attend in-person visits to Congress through organized efforts.

Step 4: Mobilizing Your ED

- As a leader in your ED, you can influence others to impact federal advocacy efforts. Place agenda items to be discussed at department meetings, create a political advocacy committee or task force, and send representatives to organized medical society meetings.
- Most importantly, if you recognize any specific issue or concern in the business or practice of medicine, you can raise this issue to your hospital, hospital system, state, or advocacy organization to be addressed at the national level.

Step 5: Further Investment in the Process

- Consider both direct financial support of candidates and joining national political action committees. It is costly and demanding to run for elected office and your support of candidates receptive to your concerns is an integral part of our representative democracy.
- Get to know your local representative; if you are able to form a relationship with them, offer to host or support fundraising events. A recent Congressional Management Foundation publication quotes, "Constituents who make the effort to personally communicate with their Senators and Representatives—except via fax—are more influential than lobbyists and news editors."[32]

Risks and Barriers to Involvement

Congress continues to reflect intense national partisan division resulting in increased difficulties passing legislation. Even so, the voices of American citizens have never been more important, and this highly politicized era creates an opportunity for ED leadership to lead our nation in improving health-care policy for all.

Emergency department leaders' schedules are busy. Most professional societies lower the barriers to involvement by having resources for your use, outlined previously, and also in both the additional readings and the appendix of this chapter. For instance, template e-mails, Twitter statements, and fill-ins are available online through organized medical, nursing, and administrative societies.

These societies also lead in-person meetings on Capitol Hill where you can visit your representative's offices yourself. Unfortunately, for many clinicians, these are difficult to attend as there is an associated cost as well as the loss of income while away from clinical work. Styles of advocacy are changing, though, and traditional influence through these in-person visits and phone calls are more frequently being supplemented or replaced by social media. At the time of publication, Twitter and likes on social media sites are starting to receive similar weight to in-person visits. A recent publication by the Congressional Management Foundation suggests that, "Most staffers (87%) thought email and the Internet have made it easier for constituents to become involved in public policy. Almost all (97%) felt electronic communications have increased the number of constituents who communicate with their offices. A majority of staff (57%) felt email and the Internet have made Senators and Representatives more accountable to their constituents."[30]

CONCLUSION

This chapter outlines the structure of the federal government, the interplay of EM in federal advocacy through case studies, and how you and your ED can get involved. In summary, take these steps today to be a leader in advocating for your ED at the national level:

- Discuss these topics in department meetings
- Support time away from the ED for members to engage in federal advocacy efforts
- Promote understanding about the mechanisms of your local, state, and federal governments
- Encourage protected and respectful discussion of policies relevant to the practice of EM and health care in general

Federal advocacy is not an all-or-nothing activity, and getting involved is easy when using the available resources. Even a small amount of personal investment can have a major impact on your department, how you care for patients, your department's bottom line, and the direction of policy and health care as a whole.

REFERENCES

1. Zibulewsky J. The Emergency Medical Treatment and Active Labor Act (EMTALA): what it is and what it means for physicians. *Proc (Bayl Univ Med Cent)*. 2001;14(4):339–346.
2. The history of EMTALA. Available at: https://www.emtala.com/history.htm. Accessed August 18, 2018.
3. Friedman E. The law that changed everything—and it isn't the one you think. 2011. Available at: https://www.hhnmag.com/articles/5010-the-law-that-changed-everything-and-it-isn-t-the-one-you-think. Accessed August 18, 2018.
4. ACEP EMTALA Fact Sheet. Available at: https://www.acep.org/life-as-a-physician/ethics--legal/emtala/emtala-fact-sheet/#sm.001tn088l1azpdizynw1hw3aowc7l. Accessed August 18, 2018.
5. Taylor TB. *EMTALA: Advanced Cases. Emergency Department Directors Academy – Phase II.* American College of Emergency Physicians; 2011.

6. Stricker TL Jr. Emergency Medical Treatment & Active Labor Act: denial of emergency medical care because of improper economic motives. *Notre Dame Law Review.* 2014;67(4):1120–1159.
7. ACEP 50 years making every moment count. Available at: https://www.acep.org/50Years/#sm.001tn088l1azpdizynw1hw3aowc7l. Accessed August 18, 2018.
8. ACEP Federal Advocacy Overview. Available at: https://www.acep.org/advocacy/ Accessed August 18, 2018.
9. SAEM Website. Available at: http://www.saem.org/utilitymenu/about. Accessed August 18, 2018.
10. AAEM Website. Available at: https://www.aaem.org. Updated 2020. Accessed November 4, 2020.
11. ENA Website. Available at: https://www.ena.org/about#mission. Accessed August 18, 2018.
12. American Nursing Association Leadership and Governance. Available at: https://www.nursingworld.org/ana/leadership-and-governance. Accessed August, 18, 2018.
13. American Association of Physician Leaders Website. Available at: https://www.physicianleaders.org. Accessed November 4, 2020.
14. American Hospital Association. About the AHA. Available at: https://www.aha.org/about. Accessed August 18, 2018.
15. Steinbrook R. Lobbying, campaign contributions, and health care reform. *N Engl J Med.* 2009;361:e52.
16. Kaiser Family Foundation Health Tracking Poll: Election 2008. 2007. Available at: https://kaiserfamilyfoundation.files.wordpress.com/2007/12/7728_election-tracking-findings_final.pdf. Accessed August 18, 2018.
17. Helfand D. Anthem blue cross dramatically raising rates for Californians with individual health policies. *Los Angeles Times.* February 4, 2010.
18. Cohen J, Balz D. Opposition to Obama's health-reform plan is high, but easing. *Washington Post.* September 14, 2009.
19. Starr P. *Remedy and Reaction: The Peculiar American Struggle Over Health Care Reform.* New Haven, CT: Yale University Press; 2011.
20. Bush D, Desjardins L, Walsh D. AMA, AARP back house health care bill. 2009. Available at: http://www.cnn.com/2009/POLITICS/11/05/health.care/. Accessed August 18, 2018.
21. Associated Press. Will safety new hospitals survive health reform? 2009. Available at: http://www.nbcnews.com/id/32672409/ns/health-health_care/t/will-safety-net-hospitals-survive-health-reform/#.W3gZiehKiUl. Accessed August 18, 2018.
22. Norman B, Karlin-Smith S. The one that got away: Obamacare and the drug industry. 2016. Available at: https://www.politico.com/story/2016/07/obamacare-prescription-drugs-pharma-225444. Accessed August 18, 2018.
23. Moon M. An examination of key Medicare provisions in the Balanced Budget Act of 1997. The Commonwealth Fund. 1997. Available at: https://www.commonwealthfund.org/publications/fund-reports/1997/sep/examination-key-medicare-provisions-balanced-budget-act-1997?redirect_source=/publications/fund-reports/1997/sep/an-examination-of-key-medicare-provisions-in-the-balanced-budget-act-of-1997. Accessed August 18, 2018.
24. Schneider A. Overview of Medicaid provisions in the Balanced Budget Act of 1997, P.L. 105-33. Center on Budget and Policy Priorities. 1997. Available at: https://www.cbpp.org/archives/908mcaid.htm. Accessed August 18, 2018.
25. Reuter JA. *The Balanced Budget Act of 1997: Implications for Graduate Medical Education. Institute for Health Care Research and Policy.* Georgetown University; 1997.
26. Iglehart JK. The Residency mismatch. *N Engl J Med.* 2013;369;4.
27. Davis PH. The Effects of the Balanced Budget Act of 1997 on Graduate Medical Education. A COGME Review. Council on Graduate Medical Education Resource Paper. 2000.
28. Medicare Resident Limits ("Caps"). AAMC Website. Available at: https://www.aamc.org/advocacy/gme/71178/gme_gme0012.html. Accessed August 18, 2018.
29. Resident Caps. AAMC Website. Available at: https://www.aamc.org/advocacy/gme/276130/residentcaps.html. Accessed August 18, 2018.
30. Salsberg E, Rockey PH, Rivers KL, et al. US residency training before and after the 1997 Balanced Budget Act. *JAMA.* 2008;300(10):1174–1180.
31. Terry K. Wait times for new-patient appointments rise 30%. *Medscape Medical News.* March 22, 2017. Available at: https://www.medscape.com/viewarticle/877616. Accessed August 18, 2018.
32. Communicating with Congress. Perceptions of Citizen Advocacy on Capitol Hill. Congressional Management Foundation. 2011. Available at: http://www.congressfoundation.org/storage/documents/CMF_Pubs/cwc-perceptions-of-citizen-advocacy.pdf. Accessed August 18, 2018.

ADDITIONAL READINGS

- https://wire.ama-assn.org/ama-news/what-physicians-need-know-about-how-reach-lawmakers?utm_source=BulletinHealthCare&utm_medium=email&utm_term=021018&utm_content=physicians&utm_campaign=article_alert-morning_rounds_weekend
- A quick guide to effective grassroots advocacy for scientists: https://www.ncbi.nlm.nih.gov/pmc/articles/PMC5531731/

CHAPTER 132

STATE ADVOCACY

Alison Haddock, Brad Uren

In politics, nothing happens by accident. If it happens, you can bet it was planned that way.

—Franklin D. Roosevelt
Speech at The Citadel University, October 23, 1935

Policymaking at the state level can be a highly rewarding experience that provides opportunities to make a meaningful impact without the encumbrances often encountered at the federal level, where agreement across 50 diverse states is necessary and difficult to achieve. Similarly, some issues can be approached legislatively, while others require a more administrative and regulatory approach.

On the federal level, a total of 329 laws were passed in the two years that made up the 114th Congress.[1] A large number of those laws consisted of the renaming of federal buildings and post offices, leaving little room to address issues specific to a particular care setting, such as the emergency department (ED). In contrast, numerous states will pass that many laws in a single year, even with a much shorter partial-year legislative calendar. As a result, many advocates find state-level work to be more immediately rewarding because it is more common to see rapid action on important issues.

Many health-care issues are legislated and regulated almost entirely at the state level. While some insurance regulation occurs at the federal level due to ERISA (Employee Retirement Income Security Act of 1974), every state individually regulates health insurance. Each state also individually regulates licensing for physicians, nurses, and other health-care providers. Medicaid and CHIP (Children's Health Insurance Program) are state–federal partnership programs that take on a huge importance at the state level because the cost of providing Medicaid within the state can consume more than 20% of a state's budget.[2] Another source of state spending on health care is expenditures on health insurance for state employees, such as teachers. Because of the costs associated with those programs, state legislators are often concerned with containing the costs of health care within their state.

With all of the state-level health policy decisions to be made, there are countless opportunities for leaders in emergency medicine to help shape the care of their patients. Moreover, the individual ED leader can have a constructive and personal relationship with his or her legislator in a way that is not always possible for national health policy. Understanding how state government is organized, how to engage in the process, and the various ways issues can be tackled will arm the ED leader with the tools for success.

STRUCTURE AND MECHANICS OF STATE GOVERNMENT

State governments are similar but not identical to the federal system. Their systems vary from state to state. As such, it is impossible to describe each state's individual structure in this chapter, so it remains incumbent upon advocating leaders to investigate their particular state's system of government and to understand their own local variation and nuances.

Legislative Branch

With the exception of Nebraska, every state has a bicameral legislature made up of two branches, similar to the federal government. In all of these states, the upper branch, or chamber, is called the Senate, which is made up of a small number of members, each representing a large number of citizens. The name of the lower chamber varies by state. The majority use "House of Representatives," as the federal government does, but some states call it the "Assembly" or "House of Delegates." This larger house varies greatly in size from state to state, with 40 members in Alaska and 400 members in New Hampshire. As of October, 2020, a total of 7,383 Americans currently serve as state legislators.[3]

In order to enact a state law, legislation must be shepherded through and passed by both chambers before being signed into law by the governor. Intrinsic to this process, there is often a diversity of opinion that can vary from party to party, chamber to chamber, and geographically within a given state. Before advancing any particular initiative, therefore, it is important that it is structured to survive such a process. It is also important to consider the makeup of current leadership in both the legislative and executive branches of the state government. When dealing with controversial issues, the odds of successfully passing legislation may change significantly when the majority leadership of one of the state houses changes, thereby requiring the advocate to alter the legislative approach to find success.

After being introduced into one of the legislative chambers, a bill must be assigned to a committee. While a variety of committees impact the health-care realm, most states have a committee specifically devoted to these issues, such as the Texas Senate Committee on Health and Human Services[4] or the California Assembly Committee on Health.[5] Additional committees of potential importance include those that are responsible for overseeing insurance, medical licensing, administration of benefits for state employees, and funding for graduate medical education.

State legislatures uniquely operate on a partial-year calendar with a limited duration session in many states. These shorter sessions allow legislators to return to their communities and work in their daily jobs because the role is seen as a part-time position, unlike the full-time federal equivalent. With this truncated time line, many states also implement specific deadlines known as cutoff days for policies to move through various stages of the process (committee, rules, floor action, and other chamber adoption).

Compared to advocacy at the federal level, the differences inherent in passing legislation at the state level—especially the accelerated time line—impact the advocate's approach.

Executive Branch

The state executive branch of government includes the office of the governor, the state's chief executive, and the individual departments responsible for the implementation and enforcement of laws created by the legislature or directed by the state constitution. The executive branch is therefore responsible for a great deal of rulemaking through the development of regulations necessary to supplement the laws passed by the legislature.

Administrative rulemaking involves working with policymakers in the state departments responsible for health care, insurance, or other relevant area over which they have oversight responsibility. Since there is substantial variation across the nation, it is imperative to understand the specific structure and processes of one's individual state government. In some cases, it may be easier to affect a legislative solution than an administrative solution. In others, it may be more expedient to pursue a rule change through the executive branch rather than pursuing change through the legislative process.

Many executive branches also create statewide taskforces, advisory committees, and other technical work groups to advise the executive and administrative process. These entities rely on local citizens with content matter expertise to help guide state policy. Examples include a state trauma committee, Medicaid technical advisory group, or opioid response taskforce, all of which benefit from physician and nursing leadership engagement. Some of these executive agencies and groups will also serve a role as advocates on issues important to their jurisdictions, making them well-connected allies or opponents in creating legislation.

Judicial Branch

As part of the balance of powers, states have a judicial branch, as seen on the federal level. Typical state structure includes a lower level district court or circuit court, with a court of appeals for matters not resolved, followed by a supreme court as the final court of appeal for state judicial matters. Note that these naming conventions are not the same in every state and can be very confusing when a state's supreme court is the lowest appellate level instead of the highest, so it is necessary to research the court hierarchy in advance.

Advocacy can sometimes involve a lawsuit at the state level in order to resolve a disagreement. An example of this is the 2018 joint American College of Emergency Physicians (ACEP)/Georgia Medical Association lawsuit against Anthem for its policies violating the prudent layperson standard.[6] In other instances, court decisions can be used to influence legislative policymaking; thus, it is important to understand where a case is in the legal process. Legislatures will work to change what they perceive as bad law, but rarely while a case is being actively litigated.

Relationship to Federal Government

State governments are responsible for the implementation and enforcement of laws within the state itself. The individual states, however, are also responsible for implementing some programs that have a substantial federal funding component, such as transportation, public assistance programs, and health-care programs such as Medicaid. Though there are significant limitations to the discretion that state governments have in the local implementation of federal–state partnerships, states do have opportunities to shape these programs.

For example, states have had discretion to make adjustments in the Medicaid reimbursement rates paid to physicians and hospitals. This regional determination has generated wide discrepancies across the country for emergency physician reimbursement for Medicaid patients despite Medicaid being a single federal program. States have also had the ability to apply for waivers from the federal government to make substantive changes to the state's Medicaid program, such as expanding coverage, changing benefits, or adding copays and cost sharing. It is therefore imperative that physicians understand the state-level decision-making that may affect the implementation of such programs because effective engagement in a perceived federal issue may in fact be needed at the local capitol.

ENGAGING IN THE LEGISLATIVE PROCESS

When legislation has an impact on emergency medicine patients or the practice of emergency medicine, ED leaders may find themselves engaged in the legislative process either proactively (by bringing forth legislation) or reactively (by responding to legislation put forth by others). If legislation has already been introduced, mounting a rapid and

> **BOX 132.1 ■ KEY POINT**
>
> An effective relationship with your legislator will create a long-lasting opportunity to influence health policy in your community and state.

effective reaction to the proposed legislation is critical. Because in many states the legislature is in session only a portion of the year, the need for swift engagement is more critical than in the year-round federal legislative process. Ideally, however, identifying legislative opportunities proactively and engaging the legislature to pursue passage of legislation to benefit emergency care is the preferred mode of action (**Box 132.1**).

Team Building

A team approach will usually be the most successful. Ideally, a state-based emergency care organization interested in working with legislators will have a standing legislative committee. This committee will typically take direction from the board of directors when deciding legislative objectives for the organization in any given legislative session. This committee should be chaired by individuals who have experience working with the legislature in crafting legislation, the election process, and/or the implementation of health policy. It is also helpful to have a cochair or vice-chair identified to ensure a clear line of succession as well as "bench strength" for the organization and committee.

Most state chapter organizations are smaller and frequently have limited budgets compared to their national partners. As a result, economic realities may lead to volunteer members serving as key legislative contacts. When resources allow, it can be effective to have professional staff engaged in the legislative process who can maintain routine contact with members of the legislature. A more economical solution is employing a part-time contract lobbyist from a multiclient firm to engage on behalf of the organization. These individuals already have relationships with legislators that can be leveraged to create organizational benefit. Regardless of the presence of a lobbyist, the individual providers' personal relationships with their legislators can help immensely to influence legislation.

Whatever form of lobbying is chosen, it is critical that an individual responsible for contact with the legislature is identified, effectively represents the organization, and is regularly available for questions or feedback regarding proposed legislation. This individual must also monitor bills as they are introduced in the capitol. Some monitoring can occur electronically with web services performing keyword searches and alerting the appropriate individual when potentially relevant legislation is introduced. Even so, this approach is no substitute for having a representative who has established and constructive relationships with relevant stakeholders in the capitol. The best time to learn about legislation is before it is introduced, so meetings can be set up and legislators influenced to introduce language that protects emergency patients and the practice of emergency medicine. Given the breadth and scope of the practice of emergency medicine, reviewing these bills can be a very time-consuming process in states actively engaged in shaping health care in their state.

Local Community Advocate Members

In addition to legislative committee leaders and professional lobbyists, it is imperative to have a team of people who actively work in EDs and are available to interact with legislators and the media. In contrast to national issues that have shared reporting, local news outlets often want a story angle that involves their community and is told by local voices. Likewise, state legislators are often more connected to their local communities and thus want to hear from their constituents directly. A ready team of local community leaders and advocates that is prepared to quickly respond to these requests can substantially magnify advocacy efforts. These individuals must be familiar with the issues and ready to help lead messaging and engage with the requesting entities. They should also be geographically located throughout the state to cover as many legislative districts and media markets as possible. It is also important to have some members with easy access to the capitol. After legislation is introduced, there may be little time to prepare before a committee hearing is convened and experts are needed to provide testimony. As such, it is critical to understand the state's rules and have an advocate ready on short notice to ensure that emergency medicine is represented in the press, at conversations with legislators, and during hearings.

Personal Legislative Relationships

State-based advocacy is often a more personal event than national advocacy due to smaller districts, legislators who often live and work in their communities, and a need for numerous content experts drawn from a smaller pool of individuals at the state level. Even when not actively pursuing legislation, it is essential to have members interacting with legislators whether at fundraisers, town halls, "coffee hours," or other constituent meetings to ensure a constant engagement with the legislature (**Box 132.2**). Legislators often have their own kitchen cabinet of experts on topics such as health care, which creates opportunities for leaders to be a resource and ally on difficult issues and, by so doing, build a personal relationship.

Tours of the ED, with proper preapproval from the hospital administration, can often be a good opportunity to engage with lawmakers and a big source of enjoyment and positive public relations for elected leaders. In addition to legislative relationships, it is equally useful to maintain similar contact with members of the media. Remaining engaged with and serving as a resource for the media will keep the organization and issues front of mind and makes it more likely that media will seek out and be responsive to members when urgent legislative issues arise.

The Legislative Plan

It is appropriate to develop an action plan to address difficult issues in emergency medicine. The first consideration is whether a legislative or a regulatory plan is needed. After an issue has been identified for legislative action, potential key components of the legislation should be reviewed with the appropriate stakeholders. In some cases, the bill to be introduced may have already been written by a national organization as model legislation and may not require or not be easily amenable to editing. Even if that is the case, it is important to ensure that all stakeholders are familiar with and supportive of the proposed language prior to it being brought to the legislature to minimize disagreements and fracturing of the coalition.

BOX 132.2 ■ BUILD YOUR ADVOCACY TEAM

- Members of your legislative committee
- Lobbyists
- Local community leaders
- Media
- Patient advocates
- Members of allied medical groups

Though it may involve bringing in additional professional help at considerable cost, it is advisable to have an attorney skilled in state-specific legislative language review any proposed legislation prior to it being introduced. The review is intended to ensure that the language accomplishes the coalition's objectives. Most states will also have professional legislative staff that a legislator can utilize to write or revise a bill if he or she is interested in an issue, but these professionals are not directly available to members of the lay public.

Bill Sponsors

In some cases, members of the legislature may approach a coalition about a bill they plan to introduce. In other cases, the coalition may need to seek out a legislative sponsor to champion the legislation. If legislators have not been involved during the building of the coalition, it is important to identify a member of the legislature who would be willing to support the legislative goals of the coalition early in the process. Ideally, members of the coalition will already have existing relationships with several members of the legislature and can engage in discussions to seek out an appropriate sponsor.

The ideal sponsors are likely to be those who have a personal passion or connection to the issue, serve on key committees to which the bill will be assigned, or hold leadership posts in the caucus. It is also important to consider which party is in power and who will be the prime sponsor. This choice may impact the likelihood of passage (e.g., if the minority party is the prime sponsor). Unlike at the federal level because state legislatures are smaller in most jurisdictions, a natural division of labor often occurs, and individual legislators may act as the content experts on an issue by one or both parties. These individuals become even more important allies or opponents in the legislative process.

When deciding how many sponsors to seek, it may be helpful to approach members in both chambers of the legislature to introduce the bill simultaneously in both houses. In most states, it provides an opportunity for the legislation to be simultaneously considered in both chambers and for the coalition to take advantage of a more rapid two-chamber approach, rather than the slower approach of one chamber, followed by the other.

It also may be easier late in a legislative session to work out disagreements on a bill that has already passed both chambers independently with minor differences. Compared to the continuous national congressional process that may address an issue for an indefinite period of time, the condensed time line for legislative activities in most states makes the advocate's timing decisions much more important.

In many cases, having more than one sponsor is encouraged because it demonstrates broad support from parties and members from across the state. Additionally, members with their name on the bill may be more likely to push for its advancement. Legislators with a background in health care may be especially valuable. Some legislators may have personal or family experience with a particular health problem being addressed by the legislation. Still others will have heard from constituents affected by a certain health-care issue and may be particularly motivated to assist in such an effort. Developing long-standing relationships well in advance will help the coalition identify those most inclined to assist.

Bill Introduction

Bill introduction can be as subtle as dropping it at the code reviser's office. Alternatively, rolling out controversial or exciting bills may entail grand public affairs. Because legislators are typically interested in the concerns of constituents, it is helpful to engage the public by sharing the message of the legislation and, broadly, what it would accomplish. State legislators often compete against the coverage of larger national issues in their local and state media, so helping to make a bill introduction a big event can build momentum.

A professional public relations firm can be especially helpful to organize the media messaging around the legislation. Stories about survivors can be collated into press releases. Op-ed pieces can be placed in influential newspapers within the state. Even if unable to work with a professional firm, every member of the coalition has a local newspaper. Members of the coalition can write letters to the editor or volunteer to write guest op-eds that may be published in the newspaper to help build public support. These efforts should be timed to coincide with the introduction of the legislation or other key moments in the process, such as cutoff dates for committee passage, movement out of a chamber, or final passage.

When the bill is introduced, the sponsor may wish to hold a press conference. This will provide an opportunity for the legislator to speak directly to the media and the public about the benefit of the legislation he or she is proposing. It is important for the coalition to work closely with the sponsor to assist with this media opportunity and promote the event. It may be helpful to have physicians, nurses, hospital leaders, impacted patients, and even educators present at such a press conference to discuss the importance of the legislation from a variety of perspectives. Having white coats in photographs is also something that many legislators appreciate and is a resource you can offer when you join a press event.

Legislative Testimony

The coalition should identify early those members who will be involved in testifying about the legislation (**Figure 132.1**). The bill sponsor may wish to speak first regarding the legislation and then be followed by supportive organizations and individuals. Members of the coalition representing other constituent groups may also wish to speak. Testimony should be coordinated by the coalition, ideally in cooperation with professional government

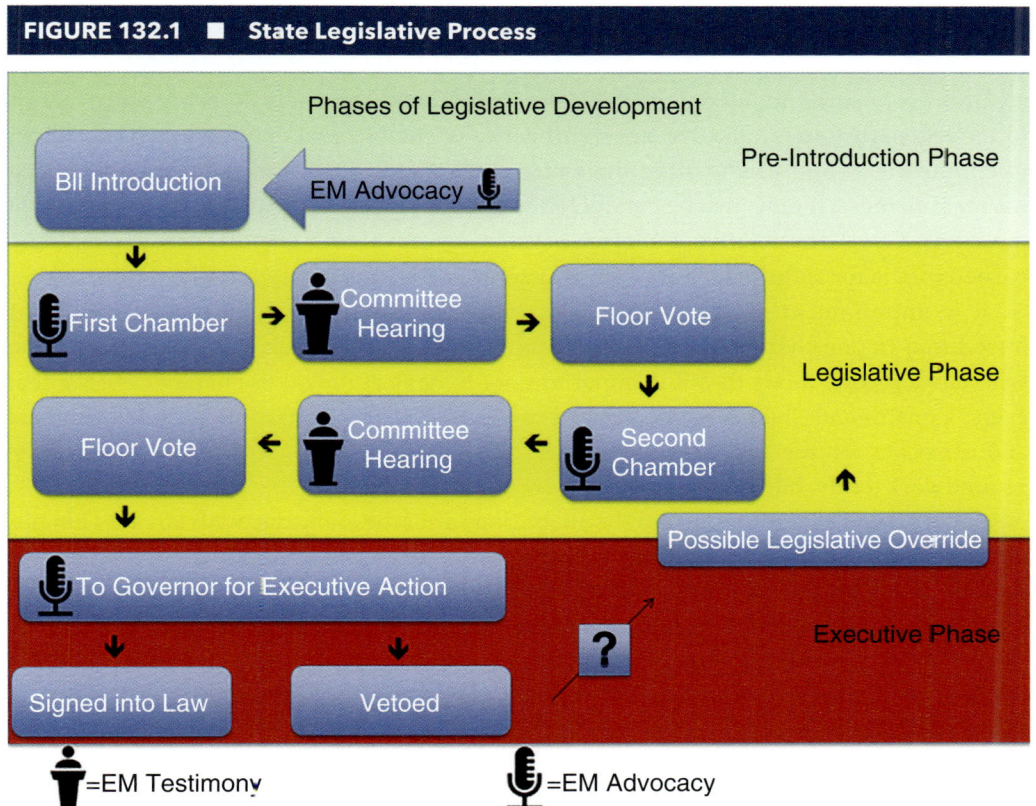

FIGURE 132.1 ■ State Legislative Process

> **BOX 132.3 ■ KEY POINT**
>
> Whenever legislation is introduced, the emergency medicine coalition should be sure to bring both solid data and personal patient stories.

relations staff, to ensure minimal overlap and cohesive messaging. Most committees also limit the duration of time allotted for testimony on a topic. If this limitation impacts the presentation of the bill, it may be important to consider who speaks and in what order to ensure key talking points are heard in committee. Many state legislators will have committee days or work sessions that are more informal, allow for a deeper dive on a topic, and that can create opportunities to educate members on the issue.

Though different states have different rules, customs, and traditions regarding testimony, it is universally important to balance the potential human impact of the legislation with the factual and science-based impact. Patient stories can bring an important humanity to the testimony. This should never be underestimated. However, it is important for medical professionals to clearly lay out the evidence-based considerations behind the legislation to ensure that the emotional appeal is supported by strong science (**Box 132.3**).

Excessive medical or administrative jargon should be avoided in both storytelling and data presentation. Also addressing financial or administrative burdens proactively can help the bill when controversy arises. In the end, it is essential to comprehensively address the many facets of the bill because it will enhance the likelihood of passage as it moves through the legislative process.

Bill Advancement

Passing a bill into law can be an arduous process that may seem far too complicated for even the simplest issue. To help overcome this barrier, it may be helpful to have a coalition-sponsored lobby day at the state capitol. It is important to bring constituents to the legislature to emphasize the significance of the bill and explicitly ask legislators to support it. While this is often most effectively held within the state capitol during normal business, it may also be conducted within the district during regular constituent meetings. Given the relatively shorter distance of travel and importance of garnering earned media for state legislators, may be useful to have the coalition rally at the capitol.

It is important to recall that in a bicameral legislature the legislation may only be introduced in one chamber at the time of the lobby day. Because it may be impractical to schedule a second lobby day, it is important not to neglect the other chamber during that event. Constituents should be encouraged to meet with their legislators in both chambers and advocate for the bill currently under consideration. This can help to prepare the groundwork for the bill after passage in the original chamber.

Follow-through is essential and should be done after the lobby day with targeted emails, phone calls, and in-person meetings to members of the legislature asking them to support the bill. There are many Internet-based services that can assist organizations in creating e-mails to be sent to members of the legislature based upon a constituent's address. These can be quickly sent out to members of the coalition who can then send e-mails in a matter of minutes to individual legislators asking them to support the legislation.

Bill Passage

When a coalition has delivered a successful legislative solution to the governor's desk for signature, it is important not to take for granted the role of the chief executive of the state. Ensuring that his or her signature will be on the bill by way of ongoing advocacy and engagement is critical. Some states still have line-item veto authority that allows portions of bills to be struck before signing the overall package. Being mindful of this risk is important when constructing the bill and advocating for final passage.

Once the bill has been confirmed to receive the governor's signature, a signing ceremony is often held. In most states, the governor will invite the supporting coalitions to the event. This is an excellent opportunity to do a final wrap on the coalition's activities and celebrate in a unique way that is often harder to do with federal legislation. A photograph with the governor means a lot to individual leaders and can serve as a simple gesture of thanks for all their hard work.

VARIATIONS IN STATE LEGISLATIVE ISSUES

Issues addressed at state-level advocacy can come in varying formats, from single local jurisdictional issues to large national concerns with local implications. While it is impossible to discuss all variations, there are three large categories that can be explored: single state issues, coordinated multistate concerns, and state implementation of national laws.

Single State Issues

With 50 states and countless local municipalities, there are abundant opportunities for local advocacy and engagement on health policy by emergency medicine leaders. Single state issues often have to do with nonhealth laws that impact the delivery of health care. For instance, zoning laws that ban certain types of businesses might be a barrier to establishing a medication-assisted treatment clinic to combat the opioid epidemic and require emergency leader advocacy to "put a face" on the victims of the disease. Some states have seen mental health interest groups lobby for and achieve success in creating special taxing authority to fund expanded treatment. Motorcycle and bicycle helmet laws are public health issues addressed on the state level in the transportation committees. Some of these local efforts will then spark a national response that further expands the impact of the issue (**Box 132.4**).

Case Study One: Out-of-Network Billing

Out-of-network billing is one of the most problematic issues facing EDs, since insured patients understandably feel that they should not be billed for anything beyond their copay.

BOX 132.4 ■ KEY POINT

The possibility for advocacy on health-care delivery and public health topics is endless.

Background

Issues surrounding billing and payment of physicians have historically been locally regulated by states when disputes over insurance company network coverage exist. Insurance commissioners and regulators are state-level entities that develop rules and regulations governing the administration of all insurance products, including health insurance. As a result, advocacy on the issue of balance billing has customarily been done through local approaches on a state-by-state basis given the unique nature of each state's regulation and governing entities.

Out-of-network billing has been an increasingly hot topic in emergency medicine. As insurance companies seek new strategies to cut costs, they increasingly rely on narrowing their networks, thereby leaving more patients without in-network to emergency care. ED leaders support the patient's right to seek care wherever is closest in the event of a medical emergency. However, patients may end up at a hospital that is (or is not) in-network with their insurance company but that has hospital-based physicians (emergency physicians, as well as radiologists, anesthesiologists, pathologists, hospitalists, and other specialists) who are not in their insurance network. Emergency physicians seeking in-network status with insurance companies are not always able to find common ground with insurers to arrive at reasonable compensation rates. Insurance companies know that emergency physicians are obligated by federal law (the Emergency Medical Treatment and Active Labor Act, or EMTALA) to provide care to all patients, which may create a disincentive for reasonable compromise. Insurance companies may pay unreasonably low rates for out-of-network patients, leading some physician groups to "balance bill" the patient.

In contrast, private practice clinicians can refuse to provide service to patients of the insurers with whom they do not contract. Because the private clinician is unencumbered by EMTALA, they have greater leverage to negotiate a reasonable rate with the insurer.

Policymaker Response

Policymakers have been increasingly attentive to the burden of balance billing on "insured" patients. Insurance companies have also drawn attention to this issue as they seek to lower their costs. The potential solutions for emergency physicians are complex, and resolution must involve large multistate insurers, medical groups, and other advocacy groups.

State responses to this issue usually originate in the legislature. One state passed legislation that required physician payment to be limited to the "usual and customary" charge. However, determination of a usual and customary charge was deferred to the regulatory process. As a result, advocacy work must continue beyond the legislative arena to the regulatory environment even if legislation is successful.

The development of a coalition to address the balance billing concern has been unique in each state. Some have been unable to find common ground across specialties, creating an additional source of conflict. Others have been coordinated in their efforts and fought for a single solution for medicine. Generally, the EMTALA-mandated specialties have worked together, given their desire for adequate compensation for their services. This is particularly relevant when a contractual prohibition disallows balance billing of patients. Historically, the response has occurred at the state level. More recently, hospital-based groups have joined to form national advocacy groups.

National Coalitions

Support from national organizations can provide assistance and resources to individual state coalitions, as each confronts its own unique challenges. National emergency medicine and anesthesiology specialty societies have convened leaders from several specialties. The coalition developed a consensus document to address state-based legislation that impacts insurance coverage for out-of-network physicians.[7] The American Medical Association (AMA) House of Delegates, highly regarded by state legislators, has also adopted a similar set of principles.[8]

National advocacy coalitions can provide resources for public relations, education, and legislative advocacy. Physicians for Fair Coverage (PFC) was created to help bring together physician professional specialty associations with large group practices. Physicians for Fair Coverage has created public relations campaigns that support state-level advocacy efforts to educate the public and state legislators. Physicians for Fair Coverage has also financially supported hiring lobbyists to engage at the local level. Physicians for Fair Coverage is an example of a unifying organization that can access the groups most heavily impacted by reimbursement changes. Similarly, the Emergency Department Practice Management Association (EDPMA) supports emergency medicine groups.

Moving Forward

State legislation has emphasized strong network adequacy standards appropriately reinforced by better patient education, insurer transparency that describes patient financial responsibilities, and reasonable minimum benefit standards and "allowables" for out-of-network care. Some states have developed separate solutions for out-of-network emergency care and out-of-network scheduled care. It is important to work closely with the other hospital-based specialties because legislators respond poorly when physician groups take opposing approaches. Further, a disjointed physician strategy makes solutions advocated by insurance companies more likely to succeed.

The development and promotion of model legislation can be a reasonable starting point for negotiations with coalition members and potential sponsors. Legal counsel should be sought to tailor the legislation to current state laws. An appeal to a national standard that seeks uniformity can help to address these complex issues. When large coalitions like PFC, the AMA, and EDPMA provide education and support a unified approach, legislators are supported when they take a stance on complex and contentious issues such as balance billing and fair coverage. When educating legislators, patient stories and data-driven examples should demonstrate that advocated solutions are patient centered.

The out-of-network billing debate has sometimes been driven by misleading press coverage. For instance, extraordinary bills for out-of-network air ambulance services have been used to show why new legislation on hospital billing practices is needed. In some situations, fair-billing coalition opponents have been unable to demonstrate unreasonable hospital-based physician medical bills that the proposed legislation would supposedly address. Further, some patients receive large bills related to their high-deductible plans but inaccurately believe they are receiving them because they are out-of-network.

Introduction of the Bill

After the bill is introduced by a sponsor, media coverage can substantially impact your bill's success or failure. Obtaining media support on reimbursement issues can be particularly challenging due to the complexity of the topic. Once a bill is introduced, it is critical to interact with the media to discuss the legislation from the perspective of patient and health systems advocacy. Potential avenues for media communication include:

- Press releases and letters to the editor
- Availability of coalitions members as resources
- ED visits by journalists and state legislators

> **BOX 132.5 ■ SUPPORTING BILL ADVANCEMENT**
>
> - Press releases
> - Letters to the editor
> - ED visits by journalists and legislators
> - Coordinated legislative testimony
> - Public relations campaigns

During discussion of the bill, testimony should be coordinated among various members of the coalition. This is particularly important when the legislation will have an impact on patient access and the delivery of care. Actively involved state medical societies can help coordinate testimony. State medical societies are often larger than state specialty societies and are more likely to have lobbyists present in the capitol. Long-term relationships between medical society advocates and state legislators and their staffers can lead to ready access and even the outreach to "go-to" organizations to get the "physician" view of legislation. Ensuring state medical society support can ensure thorough consideration of an issue.

Case Conclusion

States legislatures have adopted widely varying solutions to out-of-network billing legislation. Some have passed legislation ensuring patients have fair coverage and physicians receive fair payment for their services. In others, the deep pockets of the insurance companies and the public and media confusion have led to laws that are unfavorable to emergency patients and their care providers. A coordinated approach to legislative process remains strong (**Box 132.5**). It can lead to passage of bills that ensure access to emergency care and EDs that are financially sustainable.

Multistate Advocacy

When the same challenge is presenting itself simultaneously across the country, there can be a great advantage when physicians partner together on the national level to share strategies. Strategies that are highly successful in one state can then be spread to additional states to improve the likelihood of successful bill passage. Failed strategies can be abandoned to avoid investing resources in a program less likely to be successful. However, careful attention must be paid to the differences between states.

Case Study Two: CPR in Schools

The "CPR in Schools" program is a successful, multistate-based policy initiative that emergency medicine leaders have supported and helped to implement in a majority of states. The program has been advanced by the American Heart Association and supported by ACEP. Some states have enacted "CPR in Schools" legislation, requiring school systems to teach cardiopulmonary resuscitation (CPR) to their students prior to high school graduation. This legislation is referred to as "white hat" because it represents a noncontroversial position and is in the best interest of public health.

Background

In cases of cardiac arrest, immediate bystander CPR is associated with higher rates of survival.[9] The "CPR in Schools" initiative seeks to require CPR training in all states to increase the number of trained responders in the community. Most commonly, CPR-mandated

TABLE 132.1 ■ Natural Alliances for CPR Training Legislation

Specialty-Specific Organizations	Nonspecialty Societies
American College of Emergency Physicians	American Heart Association
American Cardiology Association	American Hospital Association
American Academy of Pediatrics	State medical societies
Urgent Care Association	US First-responder associations
Emergency Nurses Association	State nursing societies
Society of Emergency Medicine Physician Assistants	

training has occurred through state legislative initiatives. This route ensures that teaching CPR prior to graduation is carried out by individual school districts. While regulatory changes to required curriculum may occur, a legislative change is not subject to removal, even by budget changes or competing priorities. As such, a legislative mandate is considered the preferred way to make a permanent change.

Developing a Coalition

Building a strong coalition for an initiative such as the CPR education initiative can be critical to its success. Prior to introducing a bill, proponents should find and enlist other interested stakeholders within the state. For instance, natural allies to support CPR training might include those listed in **Table 132.1**. Additionally, lay advocates should be sought. In the case of CPR training, survivors of cardiac arrest and the families of those who have suffered cardiac arrest can share compelling stories of how their lives were impacted.

When developing a strategy for white hat issues, those impacted by the result should be advised and recruited to the coalition. If they are against the approach, they should be informed to minimize their opposition because failure to plan for potential adversaries can derail the legislation. School districts and teachers themselves might be adversaries to mandated CPR, if the mandate is perceived to interfere with the curriculum or if it is an unfunded mandate in an underfunded curriculum.

Developing this initiative at the national level as a multistate effort confers multiple benefits, including advanced preparation educational materials, standardized legislation, and a public relations campaign, which are already available when a state coalition decides to take up the cause. Talking points for media interviews and identification of survivors of sudden cardiac arrest saved with CPR all help the messaging. National coalition leaders can provide additional support by testifying on behalf of the initiative and may help propel initiatives like "CPR in Schools." This process has been utilized in many states, resulting in the successful passage of "CPR in Schools" legislation in the majority of states, thereby improving outcomes in emergency medicine for patients with cardiac arrest.

Federal Programs With Local Implications

State-level legislation and regulation may be created in response to federal legislation and programming that requires active local engagement. The administration of Medicaid is an example of one of the most complex state and federal policy intersections. Since the passage of the Affordable Care Act (ACA) and the subsequent litigation that went to the Supreme

Court, the variability among states on Medicaid implementation has continued to increase. While many states have expanded Medicaid, many others have not. Adding even more complexity, some states have used Medicaid waivers to create programs to expand coverage, but in a manner completely unique to their particular situation. In the end, while Medicaid is a federal program, it is state administered and partially state funded.

Hybrid state and federal programs exist both in the health-care delivery system and for public health issues. Some programs are developed to avoid issues with the Commerce Clause of the United States Constitution. The clause limits the federal government's power to influence issues that infringe upon state rights. To accomplish the program intent, issues like a national drinking age of 21 were not directly passed by the federal government but instead incentivized by linking it to federal highway funding to motivate states to pass a universal drinking age.[10] ED leaders should engage in these issues to ensure that the local implementation protects the patients they care for in their departments.

Case Study Three: Prudent Layperson

Medicaid is a federal–state jointly administered program that has been the target of significant state-level advocacy efforts. Since the passage of the ACA, an increasing number of ED visits have involved Medicaid as a payor.[11] The large numbers of patients with Medicaid as a payor in the ED can create administrative and reimbursement challenges.

Background

The state-based administration of Medicaid can provide opportunities for state medical leaders to engage with the leaders of their state Medicaid program. Medicaid administrators face a difficult challenge as rising health-care costs of the Medicaid budget can consume more than one-fifth of the entire budget for the state. As a result, Medicaid administrators are under significant pressure to cut costs, which may directly impact the ED, which is frequently blamed for the high cost of medical care. The administrators may also have difficulty addressing the underlying issues of primary care access, specialty contracting, and network adequacy given the complex challenges of these issues. Thus, the cost of care in the ED is often an easy target for perceived cost savings while numerous other unresolved contributing factors are overlooked.

In 2011, Washington State Medicaid administrators introduced a plan that would have limited Medicaid patients to three "nonemergency visits" each year. A list of conditions was created that would retroactively deem the visit to be nonemergent. This list was a violation of the prudent layperson standard, which states that if a prudent layperson believes they are having a medical emergency, those symptoms are enough to require the insurance company to cover the visit, regardless of the final diagnosis.

A Coalition of Stakeholders

Rather than attempting to argue about each of the more than 700 items on the diagnosis list, the leaders in Washington State built a coalition to find a new approach to this issue. Leaders from the state specialty society for emergency physicians, state hospital association, and state medical association worked together with the Washington State Health Care Authority to create the "Seven Best Practices" to address the challenges of ED high utilizers (**Table 132.2**).[12] Their best practices included improved health information exchange technology, care plans for frequent ED utilizers, opiate use guidelines, and patient education.

Together, these changes were implemented across the state and resulted in a reduction in ED visits by patients with Medicaid, with particularly large differences seen in the high-utilizer and low-acuity diagnosis population.[12] The state benefited by a reduction in costs,

TABLE 132.2 ■ Washington State's "Seven Best Practices"	
May 2011	Medicaid administrators first propose program limiting Medicaid visits for "nonemergent diagnoses"
July 2011	The workgroup consisting of the Washington State Chapter of the American College of Emergency Physicians (WA-ACEP), Washington State Medical Association (WSMA), and the Washington State Hospital Association (WSHA) convenes to meet with administrators regarding the list.
August 2011	Medicaid administrators reject collaborative list and create expanded list of 700 diagnoses.
October 2011	Medicaid implements program with limit of three "nonemergent visits."
October 2011	WA-ACEP takes legal action.
November 2011	Thurston County Superior court imposes stay on program.
January/February 2012	Collaborative workgroup generates alternative program.
March 2012	State budget passes with "Seven Best Practices" codified.
April 2012	Governor suspends any further implementation of a "nonemergent visits" program.

and emergency physicians and hospitals benefited by preventing the implementation of a program that would have endangered patients and their access to care.

The Outcome of the Coalition's Efforts

Getting to this successful outcome was not assured, given the starting point proposed by the Medicaid authorities to just not pay the bill. The coalition initially attempted to negotiate a compromise list supported by evidence-based medicine. Unfortunately, the regulators did not support this and attempted to implement their policy over the coalition's objections. National contact was made directly with the Center for Medicare and Medicaid Services to inquire about the legality of the regulators' approach. This conflict resulted in litigation over the legality of nonpayment for services provided. The Thurston County Superior Court eventually ruled in favor of the coalitions and halted the program's implementation.[13]

As most state legislatures are part time, legislative solutions could not be initiated until the legislature reconvened. During the delay, the coalition was able to bring forward their "Seven Best Practices" to the legislature for adoption. To achieve success, they leveraged personal relationships with legislators, engaged lobbyists from across the medical specialties on the issue, and even reached out to congressional members who were strong proponents of the prudent layperson standard to send supportive letters to the state legislature. Patient advocacy groups were engaged where possible to meet with legislators and to testify on the issue. As a result, the "Seven Best Practices" were enacted as part of the budget bill and became law after more than a year of advocacy and engagement in the legislative process.

The coalition then worked to implement the program again, with additional guidance from the federal entities that supported the prudent layperson standard in addition to the state legislature's endorsement of the "Seven Best Practices." The program resulted in $33 million in savings in the first year and and a 10% reduction in ED visits by high-utilizer patients.[13] Emergency medicine leaders must monitor state-level efforts on federal programs and engage in advocacy when the care of their patients is threatened.

CONCLUSION

State legislative and regulatory issues have many similarities to national issues, but the process takes place on a more local and personal scale. This local advocacy offers more opportunities for relationship building with state legislators, state executive branch leaders, state and local regulators, and journalists because they tend to be more easily available to their local constituents than are their national counterparts. Building these relationships as an ED leader will lead to access when issues arise that impact local practice. In the current era of national legislative gridlock, coalition-led state bills are more likely to pass, benefiting patients and emergency providers across the state.

REFERENCES

1. Public laws: 114th Congress (2015–2016). Congress.gov. Available at: https://www.congress.gov/public-laws/114th-congress. Accessed December 12, 2018.

2. Medicaid's share of state budgets. MACPAC (Medicaid and CHIP Payment Access Commission). Available at: https://www.macpac.gov/subtopic/medicaids-share-of-state-budgets/. Accessed December 12, 2018.

3. List of United States state legislatures. Wikipedia: The Free Encyclopedia. 2020. Available at: https://en.wikipedia.org/wiki/List_of_United_States_state_legislatures. Accessed October 17, 2020.

4. Senate Committee on Health and Human Services. The Texas Senate. Available at: https://senate.texas.gov/cmte.php? c=610. Accessed December 12, 2018.

5. Welcome to the Committee on Health. California State Assembly Committee on Health. Available at: https://ahea.assembly.ca.gov/. Accessed December 12, 2018.

6. Livingston S. Anthem ED policy draws lawsuit from docs. *Modern Healthcare*. Available at: https://www.modernhealthcare.com/article/20180717/NEWS/180719919. Accessed December 12, 2018.

7. Physicians for Fair Coverage. End the Surprise Insurance Gap. Available at: https://www.physiciansforfaircoverage.org/impacts/physicians. Accessed December 1, 2020.

8. Issue brief: balance billing. AMA (America Medical Association) Advocacy Resource Center. 2016. Available at: https://www.ama-assn.org/sites/default/files/media-browser/balance-billing-issue-brief-final.pdf. Accessed December 12, 2018.

9. Hasselqvist-Ax I, Riva G, Herlitz J, et al. Early cardiopulmonary resuscitation in out-of-hospital cardiac arrest. *N Engl J Med*. 2015;372:2307–2315.

10. *South Dakota v Doe,* 483 US 203 (1987).

11. Pines JM, Zocchi M, Moghtaderi A, et al. Medicaid expansion in 2014 did not increase emergency department use but did change insurance payer mix. *Health Affairs*. 2016;35(8):1480–1486.

12. Pines J, Schlicher N, Presser E, et al. Washington State Medicaid: implementation and impact of "ER is for Emergencies" program. The Brookings Institution. 2015. Available at: https://www.brookings.edu/wp-content/uploads/2016/07/050415EmerMedCaseStudyWash.pdf. Accessed December 12, 2018.

13. Report to the Legislature. Emergency department utilization: update on assumed savings from best practices implementation. Washington State Health Care Authority. 2014. Available at: https://app.leg.wa.gov/ReportsToTheLegislature/Home/GetPDF?fileName=HCAReport_3ESHB2127_EmergencyDeptUtilization_ae99b680-c5be-4788-a9a3-91537bdc555d.pdf. Accessed December 12, 2018.

CHAPTER 133

PRIVATE SECTOR ENGAGEMENT

Ashley Booth Norse

I think whenever there's something that affects the public good, then there does need to be some form of public oversight.

—Elon Musk, American Inventor[1]

As medical spending in the United States approaches 18% of the gross domestic product (GDP), the private sector is increasing its engagement in the health-care system with significant implications for emergency medicine.[2] Emergency medicine leaders must participate in these private-sector activities to ensure that those delivering and receiving care are involved in the decision-making process. With their increasing scope and scale, these private stakeholders will be increasingly important advocates for myriad issues that affect emergency department (ED) patients, including clinical safety, medical costs, and access to care.

Frequent players in the private sector that drive the medical industry include large health systems, direct employer purchasers of health insurance, and large nonprofit organizations like the Joint Commission (TJC). Over the last decade, corporations and individual consumers have also emerged as powerful new drivers in the medical market. Large corporations, the largest nongovernmental purchasers of health insurance in the United States, are directly engaging medical entities in an attempt to decrease cost and improve health outcomes for their employees. Likewise, consumers are now paying more for their health care, and as a result, they are demanding more price transparency. These forces are causing significant market disruptions that may compel changes to the current delivery and payment systems.[3,4] Leaders in emergency medicine must be aware of these payment pressures to adequately represent the needs of their patients and providers.

HOSPITAL-BASED ADVOCACY

In order to stay competitive, hospitals have begun employing physicians and purchasing physician practices at a rate that has not been seen previously. In addition, hospitals are selling and merging with other hospital systems at a rapid pace to form larger and more integrated health systems. The result has been the commoditization of health care reminiscent of the 1990s, which ushered in the large-scale push for health maintenance organizations. With this increasing consolidation of the market, many decisions that directly impact patient care and quality will occur inside the organization instead of externally through public discourse.

The effects of health policy changes, positive or negative, are usually experienced by the ED first. For example, following the implementation of the Affordable Care Act (ACA), the expansion of coverage without increased primary care provider access resulted in increased ED utilization. Emergency visits increased 14.8% from 2006 to 2014 compared to only a 6.9%

increase in the US population over the same period.[6] Anything that affects a hospital—from policy changes regarding quality, patient safety, or delivery of care to issues surrounding reimbursement—affects the ED and emergency medicine providers. Emergency physicians and nurses must work closely with their hospital to implement change when mandated and advocate for change when needed.

Case Study One: Addressing ED Overcrowding

ED overcrowding continues to be a major quality, safety, and throughput issue for the delivery of emergency care. Overcrowding occurs when the influx of ED patients needing admission exceeds hospital capacity. This has become a national epidemic as hospitals now continuously operate at near or full capacity. Due to the requirements of the Emergency Medical Treatment and Active Labor Act (EMTALA), EDs cannot turn patients away and are obligated to provide stabilizing services, including admission when medically indicated. Because EDs have no ability to control the influx of patients and limited capacity to control outflow, emergency providers are left to deal with the challenges resulting from this squeeze, including full waiting rooms, long wait times, inpatient boarding in the ED, and adverse events related to prolonged inpatient care in the ED. Full waiting rooms and long wait times additionally result in increased numbers of patients who leave without being seen by an emergency provider.

Where It Started

The practice of boarding admitted patients in the ED has been a topic of debate in the media and the academic literature since the 1980s and was the feature of a 1990 *Time Magazine* article titled "Do You Want to Die? The Crisis in Emergency Care Is Taking a Toll on Doctors, Nurses, and Patients."[7] Hospitals are now operating at much smaller profit margin, driving them to keep their beds full and to downsize staffing, leaving no room for surges in patient volumes.

The common misconception is that crowding is an ED issue caused by poor departmental leadership and misuse by patients with nonemergent complaints. In reality, ED crowding is a complex problem stemming largely from inpatient hospital throughput challenges and, in some instances, the local or regional health-care system. Systems issues that contribute to overcrowding include but are not limited to:

- Primary care access issues
- Surgery scheduling
- Turnaround times and throughput delays
- Decreased inpatient capacity[8,9]

In addition, broader health system issues with access to care, such as increased volumes of mental health and substance abuse complaints presenting to the ED, have contributed to the crowding epidemic.[6] All of these issues trickle down to the ED, which bears the brunt of the impact but controls few of the levers that cause the problem.

Discussion

Emergency visits have consistently increased over the past decade with approximately 150 million ED visits in 2018.[5] However, there has been a corresponding decrease in the number of hospital-based EDs.[2] Additionally, though the inappropriate use of the ED for nonemergent complaints by both insured and uninsured patients has often been cited as the cause of ED crowding, this is a misconception that has been disproven.[8,9]

What, then, are the factors contributing to ED crowding? The first is the aging of the US population. Emergency department visits have increased due to more patients in the older age bracket seeking care for true emergent complaints. Another is injury comprising 30% of the ED patient volume, with the highest injury rates in patients over 75 years of age. Increased ED volume has corresponded with older, more complex and higher acuity patients seeking care. Increased ED utilization along with decreasing inpatient bed availability have contributed to the problem of ED crowding.[6,9]

Other factors contributing to ED crowding include systems issues like access to care. Often primary care clinics are not open after regular business hours or may not have the ability to schedule visits for emergent complaints. Therefore, patients have no choice but to go to the ED for acute care. In addition, complex patients are often sent to the ED by their primary doctor who is unable to have testing completed expeditiously due to multiple system constraints such as insurance prior authorization requirements, limited resources and availability of advanced testing, and patient expectations. Even the Centers for Medicare and Medicaid (CMS) data have shown that as many as two-thirds of ED visits occur after business hours or on weekends and holidays when primary care offices are closed.[2,9]

Hospital operational factors that impact overcrowding include systems issues like surgery scheduling and hospital bed management (**Figure 133.1**). Operating rooms often have standard Monday through Friday business hours with declining admission and case complexity throughout the week. This causes the stacking of admissions in the hospital early in the week, which leads to increased crowding since patients coming out of the operating room compete with ED patients for inpatient beds. If the hospital's operating room hours coincide with peak ED admission times, the result is a throughput bottleneck. In many institutions, surgical patients will have priority for inpatient beds and potentially even have beds held for them for the day of their surgery. This constricts the number of available inpatient beds, which can cause ED patients to remain in the department until all the postoperative patients with priority have beds assigned, directly leading to ED boarding.

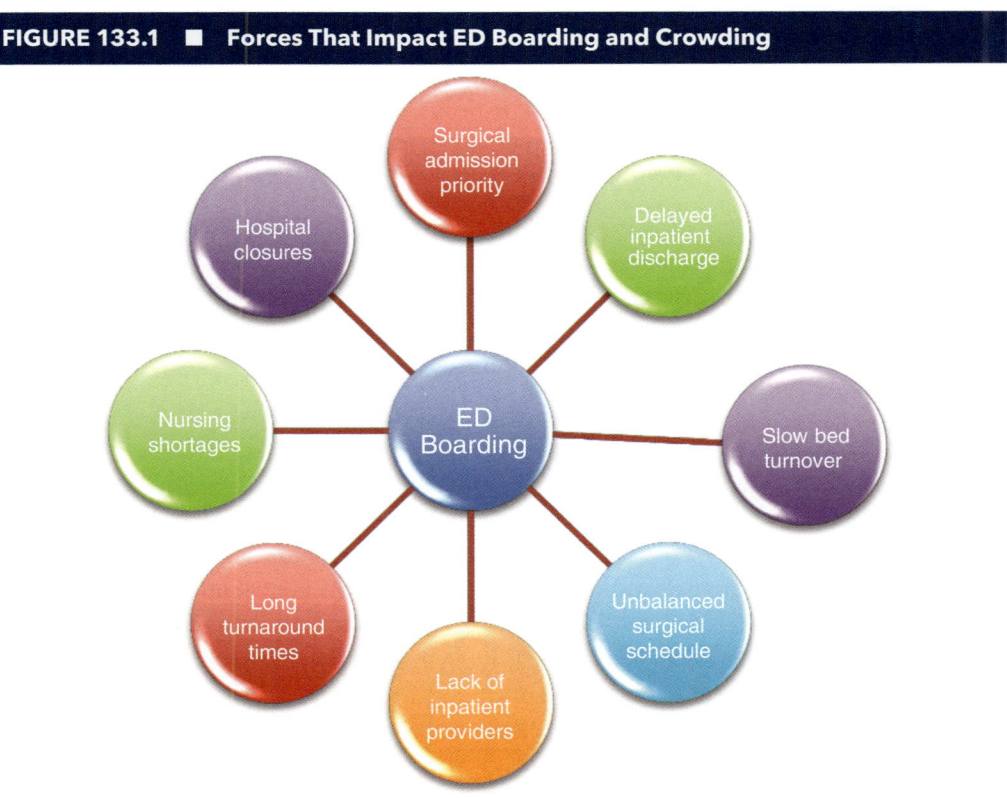

FIGURE 133.1 ■ Forces That Impact ED Boarding and Crowding

There are multiple other systemic hospital issues that impact patient throughput (see Chapters 33 and 34). Seemingly simple items such as the time of day that inpatients are discharged, morning versus afternoon, can keep beds occupied into the evening, which is peak admission time for the ED. Late discharge delays cleaning and turnover of rooms by environmental services, which can further compound the problem. Inefficient turnaround times for inpatient discharges once orders are written and slow turnaround time for essential services (such as lab, radiology, and transportation) are other examples of complex systems issues that negatively affect throughput. The systems issues that contribute to ED crowding and boarding are multifactorial and require a multidisciplinary and a multidepartmental team approach to find solutions.

The consequences of ED crowding are far reaching and include delays in patient care, increased complication rates, increased hospital length of stay, and increased mortality rates.[10] It stands to reason that if all the beds in an ED are full of admitted patients waiting on inpatient beds, then there is no place for newly arriving emergency patients to receive treatment. This includes patients who are critically ill and those with time-sensitive disease processes, such as trauma, stroke, heart attack, and sepsis.

Delays in these patient populations can lead to worse outcomes. In addition, overcrowding and boarding are associated with a higher rate of patients leaving without being seen (LWBS) visits. Those who LWBS are not always lower-acuity patients; many ultimately require hospitalization. The delays in care associated with the LWBS population often result in patients presenting later and with more serious disease. Studies show that patient's length of stay in the hospital is at least a day longer for patients who board in the ED. Similarly, the mortality rate is higher for patients who board more than 12 hours, with intensive care unit patients being at an even higher risk.[11-17]

Boarding and overcrowding is the result of overall health system challenges that directly impact patient outcomes and thus begs for leadership and advocacy. Without the voice and concerns of ED leaders pushing for change in their institutions, few will see the problems and even fewer will seek solutions for what they perceive to be other people's problems.

Solutions

In an effort to force hospitals to address crowding, CMS has tied ED throughput measures to reimbursement as part of the hospital quality reporting measures. Hospitals must report these data to CMS as part of their participation in Medicare and Medicaid. These measures include the median times of ED:

- Arrival to medical screening exam
- Arrival to departure for discharged patients
- Arrival to ED departure for admitted patients
- Admit decision to ED departure for admitted patients

These measures are tied to reimbursement by way of the hospital quality incentive program.[18,19] The metrics help identify the problem and provide monetary incentives for change, but the work of process improvement requires active local advocacy. Often simple solutions like adding nursing and physician coverage during peak hours via schedule alignment to patient flow, increasing the number of transportation staff, or streamlining lab or radiology processes can help. More commonly, though, the contributing factors are more complex. One solution to boarding that has been cited is the practice of moving admitted patients to inpatient hallways as opposed to leaving them in the ED to wait for a bed.[11] Despite numerous examples of solutions, each hospital faces unique constraints and challenges that require local problem solving to move admitted patients out of the ED as rapidly as possible in order to optimize operations.

All emergency providers must be engaged in the internal politics of the hospital to address the system factors that impact throughput and crowding. Clinicians must provide feedback and data to their directors on issues as they arise, as well as recommendations on solutions to bring about positive change. Emergency nurses and physicians should consider becoming involved in hospital throughput committees to target processes changes that can positively impact ED boarding and overcrowding. While CMS and others may examine the issue of overcrowding and boarding, effective solutions will only come from leaders engaging in their local health system to solve their own throughput challenges.

Hospital-Based Advocacy

One thing is certain: Hospitals face many challenges and must constantly change and adapt in the current health-care environment. Payment reform, drug shortages, and the lack of mental health resources are just a few of the many daunting issues they face that require tough local decisions in which emergency medicine leaders must be involved.

According to the Agency for Healthcare Research and Quality, the rate of mental health- and substance abuse-related ED visits increased 44% from 2006 to 2014, with ED visits associated with suicidal ideation increasing more than visits for any other condition. Hospital admission for mental health and substance abuse visits had a corresponding increase of 32% during the same time period.[6] The lack of inpatient beds for mental health admissions, along with the increasing rate of mental health-and substance abuse-related visits are forcing emergency providers to work with their hospital to look for local, city, and state-wide solutions to these crises.

Local efforts to advocate within a health system might include pushing for medication-assisted treatment programs for substance dependency in your institution or from your ED, working with local government entities to secure funding for new psychiatric services, or advocating for a treatment center in a high-risk neighborhood. The solutions to mental health problems will not be derived within the four walls of the ED but instead come from our active engagement in the community.

Payment reform is driving significant change in hospitals as the overall health system converts from the traditional fee-for-service model to bundled payments with reimbursement based on quality measures. These changes are placing added pressure on health systems that trickles down to the EDs as they work to avoid readmission penalties, keep patients in their organization, and achieve other metrics that impact overall system payments. To control the expenditures as reimbursement becomes capitated, some hospitals are hiring physicians and buying practices in order to form large integrated health systems or even their own accountable care organizations (ACOs) to adapt and be competitive in the new reimbursement models. Hospitals are also merging and forming partnerships to increase their buying power to combat the issues associated with other cost drivers such as drug shortages. These new practice arrangements can have implications for call coverage, expectations for payment of duties, and other human resource issues that will have indirect but substantial impact on the care of emergent patients.

Emergency providers are an integral voice as health systems adapt to new payment models and are playing a bigger role in the coordination of care across the spectrum of disease, from reducing avoidable admissions and readmissions to coordinating patient placement in the outpatient environment. As health-care dollars are divided up, emergency providers must speak up to make sure that hospitals and health systems understand the essential role they play in providing safe, efficient patient care. Emergency medicine leaders must engage in advocacy within their hospital system as they would any governmental entity.

REGULATORS AND THEIR IMPLICATIONS

The role of regulators in the health-care system has been steadily increasing in quantity and impact. Large governmental agencies and the nongovernment private sector organizations with whom they contract can place enormous burdens on the emergency health system and potentially cause harm if not done with the input of those providing care. Some state Medicaid programs, for example, have enacted programs that seek to limit emergency care by denying reimbursement, use contracted managed care insurers to mandate prior authorizations for hospital admissions, or place hurdles in the way of care with additional burdensome rules and regulations.

Not all regulatory actions are adverse, however. An example of a more positive impact has been recent efforts to address substance dependency and misuse through support for Medication-assisted treatment with agency grants and case management services for those who have complex medical disease. Regardless of the direction of the impact, it is important that emergency medicine leaders are actively engaged in helping to shape these policies proactively instead of dealing reactively with the consequences of bad policy making.

Centers for Medicare and Medicaid Services

The CMS is a federal agency within the US Department of Health and Human Services (HHS) that administers the Medicare program and works in partnership with state governments to administer Medicaid. Medicare is a national health insurance program that began in 1966 under the Social Security Administration to provide health insurance to Americans, 65 and older, who have paid into the Medicare system. It also provides health insurance to people with certain disabilities or chronic medical conditions, such as end-stage renal disease. In 2015, Medicare provided health insurance to more than 55 million people.[19]

The future of Medicare has been the topic of debate for the last decade focused around the issues of the rising cost for care and increasing Medicare enrollment numbers. As the baby boomer generation retires and becomes Medicare eligible, the number of workers per Medicare enrollee continues to decline. What does this mean for taxpayers? There will continue to be a decrease in the number of US citizens funding Medicare through payroll taxes, but there will be an increase in the number of citizens enrolled and consuming Medicare services. In addition, Americans are now living longer and with more chronic medical conditions, which adds to increasing health-care costs. In 2016, Medicare spending exceeded $672 billion (roughly 20% of total national health expenditures).[2,20]

Unlike Medicare, Medicaid is a combined federal and state insurance program "for people of any age whose income and resources are insufficient to pay for health care."[21] Medicaid is jointly funded by federal and state governments with states funding as much as 50% of the cost of Medicaid. Within broad federal parameters, states primarily manage Medicaid, independently determine eligibility requirements, and have broad latitude in implementation of the program within their boundaries.[22] Medicaid is the largest source of funding for medical and health-related services for people with low income in the United States. In 2017, it provided health insurance to 74 million low-income and disabled people.[23] Medicaid spending exceeded $565 billion in 2016 (roughly 17% of total national health expenditures).[2]

Quality Reporting

Given the sheer size and scope of Medicare and Medicaid, CMS is a driver of change across the entire health-care system, exercising a great deal of power to set delivery and payment policies. One example of CMS driving change was the development of the Hospital Inpatient Quality Reporting Program.[18] In collaboration with the Hospital Quality Alliance, CMS began collecting data on quality in 2002. The original intent of the Hospital Quality Alliance was to make it easier for consumers to make informed decisions based on hospital quality metrics. Congress expanded the program, however, and in 2003, the Medicare Prescription Drug, Improvement, and Modernization Act authorized CMS to pay hospitals a higher annual update to their payment rates when they successfully report designated quality measures.

In 2005, the first set of 10 "core" process-of-care measures related to heart attack, heart failure, pneumonia, and surgical care were released. As a result of this program's evolution, hospital quality reporting measures became directly linked with CMS reimbursement through incentives for high performers and penalties for low performers. Over the past 10 years, private insurers have followed CMS's lead with their own quality metrics and increased linkage of reimbursement to these metrics through incentive payments or alternative payment models. Notwithstanding its modest beginnings, CMS now administers more than 270 quality measures for 2018.[18,24]

The CMS drives health policy not just for hospitals but for physicians as well. Quality reporting initially began as a hospital initiative but quickly expanded to physicians. The Physician Quality Reporting System (PQRS), formerly known as the Physician Quality Reporting Initiative, began in 2006 as a quality improvement incentive program that rewarded providers financially for reporting health-care quality data to CMS.[25] The program was initially voluntary, but after the passage of the ACA, physicians were required to report in order to prevent a decrease in Medicare reimbursement.[26,27] Then, through subsequent legislation, the Medicare Access and CHIP Reauthorization Act of 2015 ended the sustainable growth rate formula as the determinant for physician reimbursement by CMS and required CMS to instead implement the Quality Payment Program (QPP).[28] As a result, PQRS ended in 2016 and transitioned to the Merit-Based Incentive Payment System under the QPP. Private insurance companies have followed CMS's direction and have started implementing quality incentives for physicians through various models.[28]

Payment Policies and Alternative Payment Models

Though CMS conceptually only controls policy for Medicare and Medicaid beneficiaries, CMS's actions have widespread impact on the overall health system compensation model and quality reporting for health care. The benefits and reimbursement rates set by CMS for Medicare, for example, are often used as a benchmark by many private insurers when setting their own benefits and rates. The CMS also collects extensive data on utilization and cost, which is publicly reported and utilized by private entities for rating, payment, and reporting. Private insurance companies often enact similar policies to Medicare and will try to contract for reimbursement rates that are based on percentages of Medicare rates, increasing the effective role of CMS regulatory decisions in health policy advocacy. Thus, engagement as ED leaders in the regulatory space is critical, given the downstream impacts on all of health care.

Another recent example of CMS driving change is the development of ACOs. The ACA gave CMS the mandate to promote cost containment throughout the health-care system by promoting the creation of ACOs and replacing fee-for-service payments with bundled payments.[29] Once Medicare started developing rules for the development of ACOs, private insurance companies began to do the same. Private insurers also started negotiating contracts with hospitals and physician groups that would allow reimbursement incentives for quality care and cost-effective care through shared savings models.

Insurance companies have also attempted to enact policies established by state Medicaid authorities In some states, Medicaid will not cover visits to the ED if the diagnosis is retrospectively not deemed serious enough to warrant emergency care. Following Medicaid's lead, commercial insurance plans are now developing diagnoses lists and other retrospective review tools to deny or reduce payments for emergency services. Many feel these policies violate federal and state prudent layperson standards in failing to evaluate each case based upon the patient's presentation but instead retrospectively denies care based on final diagnosis.

Under the prudent layperson standard, the patient's presenting chief complaint, not final diagnosis, is intended to determine the necessity for an emergency medical evaluation. The perverse consequence of these retrospective denials is to compel patients to self-diagnose their medical condition or risk retrospective insurance company second-guessing and denial of their insurance benefits. This is dangerous for patients and unfair to emergency physicians who are required by federal law—EMTALA—to treat patients who come to the ED for care. It applies unsafe and unfair 20-20 hindsight. Thus, engagement in the regulatory space and work with private insurers to impact these types of payment policies can have significant implications for the delivery of care.

The Public-Private Interface

Regulations by governmental agencies such as CMS often initiate dramatic and sweeping changes in the health-care system that are implemented by private sector partners and enhanced by other health system agents, including commercial insurers. It is not possible for every ED leader to engage in federal regulatory advocacy, but it is critical that their voices are heard.

NONGOVERNMENTAL ORGANIZATIONS

Nongovernmental organizations (NGOs) serve important roles in the health-care industry. While not government agencies, organizations such as TJC often work closely with regulators and governmental entities and have substantial impact on the delivery of health care.[30] Other organizations, such as The Leapfrog Group, have become arbiters of hospital quality with whom health-care entities are *de facto* obligated to engage for public perception and marketing.[31] The list of NGOs that evaluate and influence the medical delivery system is constantly expanding to include patient advocacy groups, commercial insurer groups, large business purchasers, and others, all engaging the health system in an attempt to control cost, improve quality, or advance other causes. The impact of these NGOs is substantial and requires the ED leader to ensure that proper recommendations are created and implemented safely.

The Joint Commission

The Joint Commission, originally called the Joint Commission on Accreditation of Hospitals (JCAH), is an independent nonprofit organization created in 1950 by the American College of Surgeons, the American College of Physicians, the American Hospital Association, the American Medical Association, and the American Dental Association for the primary purpose of voluntary accreditation of hospitals. The role of TJC has evolved over the last decade, but its primary purpose remains the accreditation of hospitals and other health-care entities.[30]

While TJC is an independent organization, it has close ties to governmental entities that fund health care. In 1965, Congress passed the Social Security Act Amendments, which included a provision that hospitals accredited by TJC (then called the Joint Commission on Accreditation of Hospitals, or JCAH) were "deemed" to be compliant with most of the Medicare conditions of participation for hospitals and thus were allowed to participate in the Medicare and Medicaid programs. In 1971, the Social Security Act was amended to require that the Secretary of the HHS validate JCAH findings. Since the 1960s and 1970s, the ability to participate in Medicare and Medicare programs has been closely linked with

TJC accreditation. Over the years, as its scope broadened beyond hospitals, JCAH changed its name to the Joint Commission on Accreditation of Healthcare Organizations in 1987 and then, more succinctly, to TJC in 2007.[30]

Today, TJC accredits many types of health-care organizations, including hospitals, doctor's offices, nursing homes, office-based surgery centers, behavioral health treatment facilities, providers of home care services, and hospice providers. While TJC's primary role is accreditation, it has become a powerful private sector advocate for patient care and patient safety. The Joint Commission does not have direct governmental authority over hospitals; however, hospitals that participate in TJC accreditation must pass an on-site survey every 3 years in order to participate in Medicare and Medicaid programs. If TJC "deems" something as a requirement in their standards, then hospitals must comply in order to pass their TJC survey and thus become a Medicare participating hospital. **Table 133.1** lists a sampling of the actions TJC has taken over the years.[30]

The Joint Commission's "standards," as they are formally titled, focus on patient safety and quality of care. There are currently more than 250 standards that address issues such as patient rights, infection control, medication management, prevention of medical errors, credentialing of medical staff, and emergency preparedness. These standards are updated regularly to reflect changes or advancements in health-care delivery.

Pain Management: Good Intentions, Unintended Consequences

One of TJC's more controversial standards was the 2001 pain assessment and management standard.[32] During the late 1990s, many pain societies and organizations began a campaign to address the widespread problem of underassessment and undertreatment of pain. In response, TJC created standards addressing pain management within its accredited health-care organizations. One of the more controversial aspects of the standard was that pain should be assessed in all patients. Another controversial element was the utilization of a 10-point pain scale. During the same time frame, the Food and Drug Administration approved the use of oral sustained-release opioid medications. After initial accolades in 2002, reports began to emerge about the adverse effects of aggressive pain treatment. Physicians saw these standards as an intrusion into their practice. Many raised concerns

TABLE 133.1	■ Actions of the Joint Commission
Date	**Action**
1996	Established the sentinel event policy
2001	Established new pain assessment and management standards for hospitals and organizations providing ambulatory care, assisted living, behavioral health care, and long-term care
2002	Established its first annual national patient safety goals
2002	Launched *Speak Up* in partnership with the Centers for Medicare and Medicaid Services (CMS)
2003	Developed a primary stroke care certification program with the American Stroke Association, providing the first nationwide certification program to evaluate stroke care provided by hospitals
2004	Announced a universal protocol for preventing wrong site, wrong procedure, wrong person surgery
2012	Created a certification program for comprehensive stroke centers
2016	Released new behavioral health-care standards

> **BOX 133.1 ■ TJC PAIN-MANAGEMENT STANDARDS**
>
> - Hospitals must have a process to address pain assessment when necessary.
> - Hospitals must have a process for the clinical determination to either treat patient's pain or refer patients for pain treatment, which may include nonpharmacologic or pharmacologic approaches.
> - Hospitals must have a process for the clinician to reassess and respond to a patient's pain based on reassessment criteria.

that the standards could lead to inappropriate use of opioids. In response to the criticism and concern for unintended consequences, the standards were quickly modified, but the standard that pain "should" be assessed in all patients remained.[32,33]

In 2016, in response to the national opioid crisis, TJC began to revise its pain assessment and management standards and develop new standards for the safe and judicious prescribing of opioids.[33] The new standards were published in July 2017 for implementation on January 1, 2018. They require hospitals to establish policies and procedures that address comprehensive clinical assessment, treatment, and reassessment of pain[32,33] (see **Box 133.1**).

Regardless of TJC's decision to amend the pain standards, many clinicians and patient advocates see the initially well-intentioned mandates by a nongovernmental entity as a major driver in the current national opioid crisis. Emergency providers were some of the first to witness the devastation of the epidemic as overdoses increased, and they have had a vocal voice in advocacy efforts to roll back the perceived overreach on pain management.

Suicide Risk Screening: Good Intentions, Substantial Implications

More recently, TJC has released new standards for suicide risk screening of ED patients.[34] The Joint Commission standards state that universal suicide screening is required for all behavioral health chief complaints, although many EDs are now screening all patients in response to these standards. In addition, TJC issued a statement on inpatient suicides. The Joint Commission suggests that ED patients with suicidal ideation be placed in a "safe room" that has been assessed for ligature risk and had these risks mitigated. In the event that the ED does not have a safe room, the standard states that patients need to have one-to-one monitoring because most in-hospital suicides are a result of hanging.[34] These accreditation standards can have significant physical plant and staffing implications and represent an important opportunity for clinical leaders to engage with TJC, their hospital system, and other NGOs in standard creation and implementation.

Nongovernmental Organization Engagement

The Joint Commission is just one of the many NGOs that have substantial direct and indirect impacts on health-care delivery. Engagement with these NGOs is extremely important to increase the likelihood that their actions improve health-care delivery and, whenever possible, minimize risk of unintended consequences. These interactions can be done directly by ED leaders or through large emergency medicine organizations, such as the American College of Emergency Physicians, Emergency Medicine Residents Association, Emergency Nurses Association, and so on. Participation in an individual hospital's response plan to accreditation surveys or quality rating reviews can be another method for participation. Regardless of how emergency leaders engage, their participation is critical because ignoring NGOs is unlikely to prevent them from impacting the delivery system.

NEW PRIVATE SECTOR DRIVERS OF HEALTH CARE

In recent decades, the health-care industry has been the target of increased attention from nontraditional sectors of the economy looking to cause significant disruption in health-care delivery and its associated cost in the United States. Technology companies are working to market direct-to-consumer health solutions to bypass the more traditional health system delivery models. Employers and large corporations have emerged in the market wanting increasing voice in the delivery of care to employees. Consumers are purchasing more health care with after-tax dollars and demanding price transparency unlike ever before. The impact of these new private sector agents is disrupting the legacy health-care system in both intended and unintended ways that directly impact emergency care.

Technology-Empowered Patients

Technology companies such as Apple, Google, Microsoft, and Amazon are increasingly disrupting the health-care market by stepping into the technology side of the health-care arena with software and devices to improve consumer access. Wearable health-care devices are a booming market with heart rate monitors embedded in wrist watches, apps for tracking sleep cycles, at-home electrocardiogram devices, and many more that will facilitate direct patient access to health information not previously available without engaging legacy clinicians. These devices, while helping patients become more active owners of their own health care, can have unintended consequences when patients are presented with data that they are unable to process. This dynamic leads some to seek care in the traditional medical system.[20,21,35-37]

Employers Driving Change to Contain Cost

Employers and large corporations have emerged on the health-care scene as a major driver of change. Employer-sponsored health insurance provided coverage to 155 million Americans in 2017, well in excess of the 55 million Americans covered by Medicare.[19,20] In an effort to control rising cost, Amazon partnered with Berkshire Hathaway and JP Morgan in 2018 to create their own health-care company for their employees. They aim to cut out the "middle man" and use technology to provide cheaper care. Walmart is also driving innovation on the health-care delivery side by setting up their own ACO. Other large corporations are trying to bypass traditional insurance by directly contracting with a narrow provider network and providing incentives for controlling cost while improving health outcomes for their employees.[3,4,38] As employers see rising health-care costs as one of the largest drivers of their overhead and cost of goods delivered, their active and aggressive engagement in the health-care delivery system is only likely to increase.

Patients as Consumers

Patients, as newly empowered consumers, are also driving change. With patients now paying a larger share of their health-care costs, they are becoming more engaged consumers and demanding more price transparency in the market. Consumers have started questioning the disparity in charges at hospital-based facilities versus outpatient facilities. Consumers are also being challenged with better understanding of in-network versus out-of-network coverage and are forcing change at the state and federal levels around cost of care and network adequacy. Consumers are also using additional after-tax dollars to pay for health care that is squeezing out their ability to afford the overall cost of living. With the average American having less in liquid savings than the health insurance deductible, the voice of consumers in cost containment is likely to grow louder.

Case Study Two: High-Deductible Health Insurance Plans

High-deductible health insurance plans have shifted more of the cost of health care away from insurance companies and onto the patient for first-dollar coverage. According to the Kaiser Family Foundation's 19th annual employer health benefits survey that looks at the insurance coverage of more than 155 million people provided by more than 2,100 companies, in addition to paying their monthly health insurance premiums, workers now pay an average of $1,318 in out-of-pocket expense before health insurance coverage begins to cover part of their bills, up from $584 a decade ago.[37,38] According to CMS, out-of-pocket spending grew over 5% in 2016 and was 11% of total national health expenditures.[2]

Emergency care is often the first point of contact with the health system for many patients and triggers their requirement to pay unaffordable out-of-pocket expenses. Patients with high-deductible insurance plans that have not met their yearly deductible at the time they seek emergency care can often be responsible for all or a large portion of their ED bill. In reimbursement language, these patients effectively become "self-pay," even though they have insurance. Reimbursement data show that a very small percentage of self-pay patients ultimately pay their bill. As a result, emergency physicians commonly provide substantially more uncompensated care than other physicians.[19] As more health insurance transitions to high-deductible health plans, the amount of bad debt involved in emergency care has the potential to increase significantly, thereby putting revenue pressures on hospitals and clinicians with substantial adverse impacts on service availability.

Where It Started

The rise in high-deductible insurance plans began in the early 2000s but has escalated since the passage of the ACA in 2010.[26] The ACA defined a set of essential benefits that all insurance products must include. This protects patients but also increases cost. In addition, the legislation included a future provision that employer-paid health plans that include benefits sufficiently in excess of the "essential benefits" would be taxed. The tax was to be levied on the employer paying for the health insurance and became known as the "Cadillac tax." These provisions of the ACA, along with increasing cost of health insurance, compelled many employers to look for more cost-effective insurance options. What emerged was an increase in high-deductible health insurance plans because insurers could no longer reduce covered benefits to save costs and control premiums. For the year 2021, deductibles in some plans are set at a maximum of $7,000 for individuals and $14,000 for families.[39]

High-deductible insurance plans have been on the insurance market for many years but prior to the passage of the ACA in 2010 had a fairly low penetrance. Over the past 5 years, however, enrollment in preferred provider organization insurance plans has fallen and been increasingly replaced by enrollment in high-deductible plans, either with or without a concomitant health savings account (HSA). A decade ago, only 55% of plans even had a deductible, but that number is now over 80%. Approximately 51% of workers in 2017 are in plans with an out-of-pocket expense that exceeds $1,000 for individuals. This is a significant increase from 34% in 2012.[38]

Discussion

Overall, health-care costs continue to increase. The causes are multifactorial but are due in part to increased utilization of medical services, higher prices for services, new technologies, and an aging population. In addition, the per-capita cost of private health insurance has grown faster than the per-capita cost of Medicare since 1970. Over the next decade, projections continue to show a higher rate of increase for those privately insured. Most experts and policymakers agree that containing health-care costs is essential to the nation's fiscal stability.[40-42]

Corporations remain the largest purchaser of health insurance in the United States and continue to be significantly impacted by the rising cost of insurance.[38] Employer-sponsored health-care spending rose to its highest point in 2018, even though health-care service provided to patients remained about the same.[43] As a result, premiums for employer-sponsored family and individual coverage have also increased and the cost of insurance is growing at a rate that is faster than both inflation and the average employee's wages. The average family premium, including the amount contributed by both the employer and the employee, was $18,764 in 2017.[38] The increasing cost of health insurance premiums is a real threat to many employers, especially small businesses.

Some companies have used HSAs to offset the cost of the high deductibles. An HSA is an account that can be established either by an employer or the employee. It allows for money to be deposited from the employee's wages prior to being taxed into the HSA, with the provision that the money can only be used to pay for health-care cost. The Internal Revenue Service sets the limits for HSAs. The limits established for 2021 were $7,200 for family coverage under high-deductible health plans and $3,600 for those with individual plans.[44] Health savings accounts have allowed companies to purchase more affordable health insurance while keeping their employers' out-of-pocket cost neutral.[45]

For emergency medicine providers and patients, the rise in high-deductible health-care plans has caused a shift in the payer mix of patients who are seen in EDs. Previously, patients with employer-provided commercial insurance would typically be responsible for their copay, plus or minus a small deductible. Health insurance companies would be billed for the emergency services after care was rendered. Now, patients with employer-provided commercial insurance may be responsible for their entire ED bill if they have not met their deductible for the year. Due to EMTALA requirements, insurance coverage, deductible responsibility, and the patient's out-of-pocket cost cannot be taken into consideration before services are provided in the ED. As a result, high-deductible health plans have resulted in a pronounced increase in the out-of-pocket cost to patients for emergency services. As increasing costs are borne by patients, they are changing their location of engagement with the health-care system.

The cost associated with high-deductible health insurance plans should not be confused with the issue of out-of-network balance billing. Balance billing refers to the practice of billing patients for services that their health insurance does not cover as a result of physician or hospital being out of network. If an emergency medicine provider is not in an insurance company's provider network, some insurance companies deny coverage or reduce payments for emergency care. This trend has led to practice of "balance billing." Balance billing is often confused with high-deductible insurance plans. Many consumers do not know what is covered or what their deductible responsibility is under their insurance plan. In addition, many consumers have no idea which hospitals and physicians are in their insurance company's provider network. This leads to confusion between high-deductible payments and out-of-network insurance coverage and coinsurance responsibility.[46]

As a result of both balance-billing and high-deductible insurance plans, patients are becoming more informed about the cost of health care and pressing for more transparency in cost within the health-care system. An example of this cost transparency is the recent push for hospitals to publicly post a list of their charges. Patients have driven this change in the outpatient setting, especially in the outpatient lab and radiology venues. The change has not yet been widely adopted.

Solution

High-deductible health-care plans are not going away. The drivers that have led to the emergence of these plans are complex. High-deductible insurance plans combined with mandatory HSAs can mitigate out-of-pocket cost to the patient. However, the real solutions lie in solving the issues surrounding the increasing cost of health care both in the insured and uninsured populations. Since EDs remain the first point of contact for many patients with high deductibles, this issue will have an increasing impact in these settings and result in additional scrutiny of both the care provided and costs incurred. As such, emergency medicine leaders must engage on the issues of deductible coverage, importance of emergency care, and addressing the cost of emergency care where possible.

CONCLUSION

Health care is evolving with new private sector actors entering the field to disrupt and innovate the traditional health delivery system. Emergency physicians, nurses, and other staff are uniquely positioned to take an active role in advocacy on behalf of patients. While advocacy varies among providers, emergency physicians and nurses are now becoming chief medical officers, chief nursing officers, chief quality officers, and even chief executive officers of hospitals and health systems. Emergency providers work at the interface of the outpatient and inpatient environments, possess a unique understanding of both landscapes, and play an active role in the coordination of care and stewardship of health care resources. The ED is in many ways the epicenter for health care policy. Nearly anything that affects patients—from changes in CMS reimbursement or documentation requirements to new Joint commission standards on the care of the suicidal patient—affects the ED either directly or indirectly. This makes ED leaders excellent advocates for patients and the profession of emergency care.

Emergency physicians, nurses, and other providers of emergency care have to work with our health-care partners—hospitals, policymakers, NGOs, as well as patients and employers—to ensure that our EDs continue to provide quality patient care that is cost-effective and available to all. Advocacy is not someone else's job. It is everyone's job. It is critical that we as emergency medicine leaders advocate for our patients and our profession. A small investment in time can have a big impact!

REFERENCES

1. Musk E. in an interview with Gayle King, March 11, 2018. Available at: https://www.viacomcbspressexpress.com/cbs-news/shows/cbs-this-morning/releases/view?id=49941. Accessed December 7, 2020.
2. Centers for Medicare and Medicaid Data. National Health Expenditure Data, NHE Fact Sheet. 2016. Available at: https://www.cms.gov/Research-Statistics-Data-and-Systems/Statistics-Trends-and-Reports/NationalHealthExpendData/NationalHealthAccountsHistorical. Updated December 17, 2019. Accessed October 31, 2020.
3. D'Urbino L. Apple and Amazon's moves in health signal a coming transformation. *The Economist*. February 3, 2018.
4. Tracer Z. Amazon isn't the only retail giant trying to remake health care. *Modern Healthcare*. 2018.
5. Augustine JJ. Latest data reveal the ED's role as hospital admission gatekeeper. *ACEP Now*. 2019;38(12). Available at: https://www.acepnow.com/article/latest-data-reveal-the-eds-role-as-hospital-admission-gatekeeper/. Accessed November 20, 2020.
6. Moore BJ, Stocks C, Owens PL. Trends in emergency department visits, 2006–2014. HCUP (Healthcare Cost and Utilization Project) Statistical Brief #227. Agency for Healthcare Research and Quality; September, 2017.
7. Gibbs N. Do you want to die? The crisis in emergency care is taking a toll on doctors, nurses—and patients. *Time*. 1990;135(22):58–65.
8. Sommers AS, Boukus ER, Carrier E. Dispelling myths about emergency department use: majority of Medicaid visits are for urgent or more serious symptoms. HSC Research Brief No. 23. Center for Studying Health System Change; 2012.
9. Roberts DC, McKay MP, Shaffer A. Increasing rate of emergency department visits for elderly patients in the United States, 1993 to 2003. *Ann Emerg Med*. 2008:51(6):769–774.
10. Morley C, Unwin M, Peterson GM, et al. Emergency department crowding: a systemic review of causes, consequences, and solutions. *PLoS One*. 2018:13(8).
11. ACEP Task Force on Boarding. *Emergency Department Crowding: High Impact Solutions*. American College of Emergency Physicians (ACEP); 2008.
12. Richardson DB, Bryant M. Confirmation of association between overcrowding and adverse events in patients who do not wait to be seen. *Acad Emerg Med*. 2004:11(5):462.
13. Cowan RM, Trzeciak S. Clinical review: emergency department overcrowding and the potential impact on the critically ill. *Crit Care*. 2005:9(3):291–295.
14. Liu SW, Thomas SH, Gordon JA, et al. A pilot study examining undesirable events among emergency department-boarded patients awaiting inpatient beds. *Ann Emerg Med*. 2009:54(3):381–385.

15. Singer AJ, Thode HC, Viccellio P, et al. The association between length of emergency department boarding and mortality. *Acad Emerg Med.* 2011:18(12):1324–1329.

16. Chalfin DB, Trzeciak S, Likourezos A, et al. Impact of delayed transfer of critically ill patients from the emergency department to the intensive care unit. *Crit Care Med.* 2007:35(6):1477–1483.

17. Hong KJ, Shin SD, Song KJ, et al. Association between ED crowding and delay in resuscitation effort. *Am J Emerg Med.* 2013;31(3):509–515.

18. Hospital inpatient quality reporting program. CMS.gov. Available at: https://www.cms.gov/Medicare/Quality-Initiatives-Patient-Assessment-Instruments/HospitalQualityInits/HospitalRHQDAPU. Updated September 19, 2017. Accessed June 15, 2018.

19. Centers for Medicare and Medicaid Services. 2016 Annual Report of the Boards of Trustees of the Federal Hospital Insurance and Federal Supplementary Medical Insurance Trust Funds. 2016. CMS.gov. Available at: https://www.cms.gov/Research-Statistics-Data-and-Systems/Statistics-Trends-and-eports/reportstrustfunds/downloads/tr2016.pdf. Accessed November 20, 2020.

20. Potez L, Cubanski J, Neuman T. Medicare spending and financing: a primer. Report #7731-03. The Henry J. Kaiser Family Foundation; 2011. Available at: https://www.kff.org/wp-content/uploads/2013/01/7731-03.pdf. Accessed June 13, 2018.

21. America Health Insurance Plans. Introduction to Medicare-Medicaid Dual Eligibles and Service Models. 2018. Available at: https://www.ahip.org/introduction-to-medicare-medicaid-dual-eligibles-and-service-delivery-models/. Accessed December 7, 2020.

22. Medicare program—general information. *CMS.gov*. Available at: https://www.cms.gov/Medicare/Medicare-General-Information/MedicareGenInfo/index.html. Accessed June 10, 2018.

23. Gottlieb JD, Shepard M. Evidence on the value of Medicaid. *Econofact.* 2017. Available at: https://econofact.org/evidence-on-the-value-of-medicaid. Accessed December 7, 2020.

24. Hospital compare. Available at: https://www.cms.gov/Medicare/Quality-Initiatives-Patient-Assessment-Instruments/HospitalQualityInits/HospitalCompare#:~:text=Hospital%20Compare%20is%20a%20consumer, to%20go%20for%20health%20care.&text=General%20information, Survey%20of%20patients'%20experiences. Accessed December 7, 2020.

25. Physician Quality Reporting System (PQRS) Overview. Available at: https://www.cms.gov/Medicare/Quality-Initiatives-Patient-Assessment-Instruments/PQRS/Downloads/PQRS_OverviewFactSheet_2013_08_06.pdf. Accessed December 7, 2020.

26. About the Affordable Care Act. HHS.gov. Available at: https://www.hhs.gov/healthcare/about-the-aca/index.html. Updated October 23, 2019. Accessed November 1, 2020.

27. Compilation of Patient Protection and Affordable Care Act. HHS.gov. 2010. Available at: https://www.hhs.gov/sites/default/files/ppacacon.pdf. Accessed November 1, 2020.

28. Quality Payment Program. CMS.gov. Available at: https://www.cms.gov/Medicare/Quality-Payment-Program/Quality-Payment-Program.html. Last Modified March 23, 2020. Accessed July 20, 2018.

29. Accountable Care Organizations. CMS.gov. Available at: *https://www.cms.gov/Medicare/Medicare-Fee-for-Service-Payment/ACO*. Last Modified February 11, 2020. Accessed November 1, 2020.

30. The Joint Commission: over a century of quality and safety. The Joint Commission. 2020. Available at: https://www.jointcommission.org/-/media/tjc/documents/about-us/tjc-history-timeline-through-2019-pdf.pdf. Accessed December 7, 2018.

31. The Leapfrog Group. Available at: https://www.leapfroggroup.org/. Updated October 30, 2020. Accessed November 1, 2020.

32. Baker DW. The Joint Commission's pain standards: origins and evolution. The Joint Commission. 2017. Available at: https://www.jointcommission.org/assets/1/6/Pain_Std_History_Web_Version_05122017.pdf. Accessed June 5, 2018.

33. The Joint Commission. Standards for Accredited Organizations. Available at: https://www.jointcommission.org/resources/patient-safety-topics/pain-management-standards-for-accredited-organizations/. Accessed December 7, 2020.

34. Special report: suicide prevention in health care settings. TJC Perspectives. 2017;37(11). Available at: https://www.jointcommission.org/-/media/tjc/documents/resources/patient-safety-topics/suicide-prevention/november_perspectives_suicide_risk_reduction.pdf.

35. Kacik A, Livingston S. Disrupted: American healthcare has reached its tipping point. *Modern Healthcare.* 2018. Available at: http://www.modernhealthcare.com/article/20180203/NEWS/180209961. Accessed November 20, 2020.

36. Arndt RZ. Google, Amazon, Microsoft, and others have a long road ahead in healthcare. *Modern Healthcare.* 2018. Available at: http://www.modernhealthcare.com/article/20180827/TRANSFORMATION02/180829916/google-amazon-microsoft-and-others-have-a-long road-ahead-in-healthcare. Accessed November 20, 2020.

37. Claxton G, Rae M, Long M, et al. *Employer Health Benefits—2015 Survey.* Henry J. Kaiser Family Foundation; 2015:118. Available at: http://files.kff.org/attachment/report-2015-employer-health-benefits-survey. Accessed November 1, 2020.

38. 2017 Employer Health Benefits Survey. The Kaiser Family Foundation and Health Research & Educational Trust. 2017. Available at: https://www.kff.org/report-section/ehbs-2017-summary-of-findings/. Accessed June 15, 2018.

39. What are HDHPs and HSAs? HealthCare.gov. Available at: https://www.healthcare.gov/high-deductible-health-plan/hdhp-hsa-information/. Accessed November 1, 2020.

40. Tikkanen R, Abrams MK. US health care from a global perspective, 2019: higher spending, worse outcomes? The Commonwealth Fund. 2020. Available at: https://www.commonwealthfund.org/publications/issue-briefs/2020/jan/us-health-care-global-perspective-2019. Accessed November 1, 2020.

41. Gondi S, Chokshi DA. Financial stability as a goal of payment reform—a lesson from COVID-19. *JAMA Health Forum.* 2020. doi:10.1001/jamahealthforum.2020.1012. Accessed November 1, 2020.

42. Mathews AW. Why America's doctors are struggling to make ends meet. *The Wall Street Journal.* March 16, 2012. Available at: https://www.wsj.com/articles/SB10001424052970204603004577271340816194320. Accessed November 1, 2020.

43. Health care cost and utilization report (HCCUR). Health Care Cost Institute. Available at: https://healthcostinstitute.org/health-care-cost-and-utilization-report/annual-reports. Accessed November 1, 2020.

44. Miller S. IRS announces 2021 limits for HSAs and high-deductible health plans. SHRM. 2020. Available at: https://www.shrm.org/resourcesandtools/hr-topics/benefits/pages/irs-2021-hsa-contribution-limits.aspx. Accessed November 1, 2020.

45. Where can I learn more about Health Savings Accounts (HSA) and Health Reimbursement Arrangements (HRA)? Available at: https://www.irs.gov/government-entities/federal-state-local-governments/where-can-i-learn-more-about-health-savings-accounts-hsa-and-health-reimbursement-arrangements-hra. Updated June 17, 2020. Accessed November 1, 2020.

46. Berger E. Finding a balance on balance-billing. *Ann Emerg Med.* 2017;70(2):A15-A18.